CLINICAL
LABORATORY
MEDICINE

CLINICAL
LABORATORY
MEDICINE

Edited by

Richard C. Tilton, Ph.D.
President and Chief Scientific Officer
North American Laboratory Group
New Britain, Connecticut

Albert Balows, Ph.D.
Department of Clinical Pathology and Laboratory Medicine
Emory University School of Medicine;
Director Emeritus
Center for Infectious Diseases
Centers for Disease Control
Atlanta, Georgia

David C. Hohnadel, Ph.D.
Director
Genesee Hospital
Rochester, New York

Robert F. Reiss, M.D.
Professor of Clinical Pathology and Clinical Medicine
College of Physicians and Surgeons
Columbia University;
Director, Transfusion Service
Columbia–Presbyterian Medical Center
New York, New York

with 587 illustrations and 65 color plates

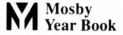
Mosby
Year Book

St. Louis   Baltimore   Boston   Chicago   London   Philadelphia   Sydney   Toronto

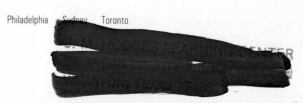

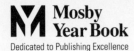

Mosby
Year Book
Dedicated to Publishing Excellence

Editor: Stephanie Manning

Developmental editor: Maureen Slaten

Assistant editor: Anne Gunter

Project supervisor: Barbara Bowes Merritt

Book design: Susan Lane

Editing and production: The Wheetley Company

Printed in the United States of America

Mosby–Year Book, Inc.
11830 Westline Industrial Drive
St. Louis, Missouri 63146

Library of Congress Cataloging-in-Publication Data

Clinical laboratory medicine / edited by Richard C. Tilton . . . [et al.].
    p. cm.
    Includes bibliographical references and index.
    ISBN 0-8016-5873-X
    1. Diagnosis, Laboratory. I. Tilton, Richard C.
    [DNLM: 1. Diagnosis, Laboratory. I. Tilton, Richard C.
  RB37.C583 1992
  616.07'54—dc20
  DNLM/DLC
  for Library of Congress   92-8370
                                   CIP

92 93 94 95 96   GW/MV   9 8 7 6 5 4 3 2 1

Contributors

Nancy L. Anderson, M.M.Sc., M.T. (ASCP)
Associate
Department of Pathology and Laboratory Medicine
Emory University School of Medicine
Atlanta, Georgia

Albert Balows, Ph.D.
Department of Clinical Pathology and Laboratory Medicine
Emory University School of Medicine;
Director Emeritus
Centers for Disease Control
Atlanta, Georgia

Peter A. Benn, Ph.D.
Associate Professor
Director of Laboratory Services
Division of Human Genetics
Department of Pediatrics
University of Connecticut Health Center
Farmington, Connecticut

Mary Kay Boehmer, M.T. (ASCP)
Assistant Administrative Director, Laboratory
Overlook Hospital
Summit, New Jersey

Lawrence W. Bond, Ph.D.
Clinical Chemist and Toxicologist
Department of Pathology
St. Vincent Medical Center
Toledo, Ohio

Marge Brewster, Ph.D.
Professor
Pathology and Pediatrics
University of Arkansas for Medical Sciences;
Clinical Biochemist
Arkansas Children's Hospital
Little Rock, Arkansas

Malcolm L. Brigden, M.D.
Director of Hematology and Microscopy
Island Medical Laboratories
Victoria, British Columbia

Edward R. Burns, M.D.
Associate Professor
Laboratory Medicine and Medicine
Albert Einstein College of Medicine;
Director, Laboratory Hematology
Weiler Hospital of the Albert Einstein College of Medicine
Bronx, New York

Donald J. Cannon, Ph.D.
Associate Professor
Department of Pathology
University of Cincinnati
College of Medicine;
Director of Toxicology
Department of Pathology
Bethesda Hospitals
Cincinnati, Ohio

I-Wen Chen, Ph.D.
Professor
Department of Pathology and Laboratory Medicine, and Radiology
University of Cincinnati
Cincinnati, Ohio

David Ciavarella, M.D.
Associate Professor
Clinical Pathology
New York Medical College;
Director, Hudson Valley Blood Services
Vice-President, New York Blood Center
Valhalla, New York

Norman B. Coffman, Ph.D.
Clinical Chemist
Department of Pathology
Abington Memorial Hospital
Abington, Pennsylvania

John K. Critser, Ph.D.
Director of Andrology Center for Reproduction and
    Transplantation Immunology
Methodist Hospital of Indiana, Inc.;
Assistant Professor
Department of Physiology and Biophysics and
    Department of Obstetrics and Gynecology
Indiana University Medical School
Indianapolis, Indiana

Mario R. Escobar, Ph.D.
Professor of Pathology
Medical College of Virginia
Richmond, Virginia

William Daniel Follas, M.S.
President
Follas Laboratories, Inc.
Indianapolis, Indiana

Lynne S. Garcia M.S., C.L.S., M.T.

Manager
Clinical Laboratories/Microbiology
Department of Pathology and Laboratory Medicine
University of California at Los Angeles
Los Angeles, California

Petrina V. Genco, Ph.D.

Department of Laboratory Medicine
Medical University of South Carolina
Charleston, South Carolina

Michael A. Gerber, M.D.

Associate Professor
Department of Pediatrics
University of Connecticut School of Medicine
Farmington, Connecticut

Arlene S. Gingras, M.T. (ASCP), SBB

Transfusion Service
Columbia-Presbyterian Medical Center
New York, New York

Joanne M. Griffith, M.A., M.T. (ASCP)

Laboratory Manager
Department of Laboratory Medicine
The Christ Hospital
Cincinnati, Ohio

R. Ian Hardy, M.D., Ph.D.

Department of Obstetrics, Gynecology, and Reproductive Biology
Brigham and Women's Hospital
Harvard Medical School
Boston, Massachusetts

Michael Hassan

Assistant Director
Department of Pathology and Laboratory Medicine
University of Cincinnati School of Medicine
Cincinnati, Ohio

Janet A. Hindler

Senior Specialist
Clinical Microbiology
Department of Pathology and Laboratory Medicine
    Clinical Microbiology Section
University of California at Los Angeles
Los Angeles, California

Gordon N. Hoag, M.D., Ph.D.

Director of Clinical Chemistry
Island Medical Laboratories
Victoria, British Columbia

David C. Hohnadel, Ph.D.

Director
Genesee Hospital
Rochester, New York

Gayle B. Jackson, M.S.

Director
Hematology/Immunology
Department of Laboratory Medicine
The Christ Hospital
Cincinnati, Ohio

Sarah H. Jenkins, Ph.D.

Associate Director
Chemistry
Department of Pathology and Laboratory Medicine
University of Cincinnati
Cincinnati, Ohio

Stephen G. Jenkins, Ph.D.

Clinical Assistant Professor of Medicine
University of Florida Medical School;
Director of Clinical Microbiology
Baptist Medical Center
Jacksonville, Florida

Robert C. Jerris, Ph.D.

Director
Clinical Laboratory Sciences Program
Department of Pathology
Emory University School of Medicine
Atlanta, Georgia;
Director, Clinical Microbiology
DeKalb Medical Center
Decatur, Georgia

Carol L. Johnson, M.T. (ASCP) SBB

Coordinator, Technical Education
The New York Blood Center
New York, New York

Harold S. Kaplan, M.D.

Professor and Director, Transfusion Medicine
Department of Pathology
University of Texas
Southwestern Medical Center
Dallas, Texas

Lawrence A. Kaplan, Ph.D.

Associate Professor
Department of Pathology
New York University Medical Center;
Director, Clinical Chemistry and Toxicology Laboratories
Bellevue Hospital
New York, New York

Michael P. Kiley, Ph.D.

Director of Research and Development
Salk Institute
Swiftwater, Pennsylvania

Richard Kowalczyk, Ph.D.

Director of Manufacturing
Boston Biomedica, Inc.
West Bridgewater, Massachusetts

Sandra Larsen, Ph.D.

Chief, Treponemal Pathogenesis and Immunobiology Branch
Division Sexually Transmitted Diseases Laboratory Research
Centers for Disease Control
Atlanta, Georgia

Bonnie Lupo, M.S, (ASCP) SBB

Clinical Instructor
Department of Medical Technology
State University of New York
Stony Brook, New York

Linda M. Mann, Ph.D.

Postdoctoral Fellow
Department of Pathology and Laboratory Medicine
Clinical Microbiology Section
University of California at Los Angeles
Los Angeles, California

Stanford Marenberg, Ph.D.

Clinical Chemist/Scientific Director Chemistry
Department of Pathology and Nuclear Medicine
Kettering Medical Center
Kettering, Ohio

Melissa Martincich, B.S., M.B.A.

Chief Executive Officer
North American Laboratory Group
New Britain, Connecticut

Charles G. Massion, M.D.

Cincinnati, Ohio

Michael D.D. McNeely, M.D.

President
Island Medical Laboratories
Victoria, British Columbia

J. Michael Miller, Ph.D.

Chief, Clinical Bacteriology Laboratories
Centers for Disease Control
Atlanta, Georgia

Victor Mondy, M.B.A., M.T. (ASCP)

Assistant Supervisor, Chemistry
Department of Laboratory Medicine
The Christ Hospital
Cincinnati, Ohio

Mark A. Neumann, Ph.D.

Co-Director
Clinical Microbiology, Immunology, and Virology
Department of Pathology and Laboratory Medicine
Diagnostic Services, Inc.
Naples, Florida

David H. Persing, M.D., Ph.D.

Director
Bacteriology Referral Laboratory
Section of Clinical Microbiology
Department of Laboratory Medicine and Pathology
Mayo Clinic
Rochester, Minnesota

Amadeo J. Pesce, Ph.D.

Professor
Pathology and Laboratory Medicine
University of Cincinnati Medical Center
Cincinnati, Ohio

Marie Pezzlo, M.A., F(AAM)

Senior Supervisor
Medical Microbiology Division
Department of Pathology
University of California Irvine Medical Center
Orange, California

Robert F. Reiss, M.D.

Professor of Clinical Pathology and Clinical Medicine
College of Physicians and Surgeons
Columbia University;
Director, Transfusion Service
Columbia-Presbyterian Medical Center
New York, New York

Willie Ruff, Ph.D.

Associate Director
Clinical Laboratories
Howard University Hospital
Washington, DC

Paul T. Russell, Ph.D.

Division of Reproduction and Fertility
The Christ Hospital
Cincinnati, Ohio

Michael A. Saubolle, Ph.D.

Director, Microbiology/Serology Sections
Department of Clinical Pathology
Good Samaritan Regional Medical Center
Phoenix, Arizona

Ron B. Schifman, M.D.

Director, Clinical Pathology
Tucson Veterans Affairs Medical Center;
Associate Professor of Pathology
University of Arizona
Tucson, Arizona

David L. Sewell, Ph.D.

Associate Professor of Pathology
Oregon Health Sciences University;
Chief, Microbiology Division
Laboratory Service
Veterans Administration Medical Center
Portland, Oregon

John E. Sherwin, Ph.D.

Director of Chemistry
Valley Children's Hospital
Fresno, California;
Clinical Assistant Professor of Laboratory Medicine
University of California, San Francisco Medical School
San Francisco, California

Howard Smith, M.D.

Albany Medical Center Hospital
Albany, New York

Juan R. Sobenes, M.D.

Director of Clinical Pathology
Valley Medical Center
Fresno, California;
Clinical Assistant Professor of Laboratory Medicine
University of California, San Francisco
Medical School
San Francisco, California

Louis H. Steinert, Ph.D.

Technical Director
Doctors Clinical Laboratory
Cincinnati, Ohio

Richard C. Tilton, Ph.D.

President and Chief Scientific Officer
North American Laboratory Group
New Britain, Connecticut

Thomas J. Tinghitella, Ph.D.

Assistant Clinical Professor
Department of Laboratory Medicine
Yale School of Medicine
New Haven, Connecticut;
Department of Pathology
Bridgeport Hospital
Bridgeport, Connecticut

Joan Uehlinger, M.D.

Assistant Professor
Department of Medicine
Albert Einstein College of Medicine
Bronx, New York;
Director, Blood Bank and Transfusion Service
Assistant Attending in Medicine
Montefiore Medical Center
Bronx, New York

Jay E. Valinsky, Ph.D.

Associate Director
Special Diagnostics
The New York Blood Center
New York, New York

Kathy V. Waller, Ph.D.

Assistant Professor
School of Allied Medical Professions
The Ohio State University
Columbus, Ohio

Kory M. Ward, Ph.D.

Assistant Professor
School of Allied Medical Professions
The Ohio State University
Columbus, Ohio

Ann Warner, Ph.D.

Associate Professor
Department of Pathology and Laboratory Medicine;
Associate Director
Division of Toxicology
University of Cincinnati
Cincinnati, Ohio

Melvin P. Weinstein, M.D.

Professor of Medicine and Pathology
University of Medicine and Dentistry of New Jersey
Robert Wood Johnson Medical School;
Director, Microbiology Laboratory
Robert Wood Johnson University Hospital
New Brunswick, New Jersey

Barry Wenz, M.D.

Professor of Laboratory Medicine
Albert Einstein College of Medicine
Bronx, New York;
Director of Clinical Pathology and Immunohematology
Albert Einstein College of Medicine
Bronx, New York

Donald A. Wiebe, Ph.D.

Associate Professor
Department of Pathology and Laboratory Medicine
University of Wisconsin
Madison, Wisconsin

Marie Zureick, M.T. (ASCP)

The Christ Hospital
Cincinnati, Ohio

Preface

Continued growth and increasing complexity are words frequently used to describe many scientific disciplines. Laboratory medicine, a multifaceted discipline with seemingly unabated growth and complexity, definitely falls under this rubric.

Technological advances, coupled with a growing battery of diagnostic skills, have led to the development of many innovative and far-reaching approaches to the laboratory diagnosis of disease. Some of these new approaches include rapid screening tests that provide prompt and useful general information, whereas other analyses are highly automated, sensitive, and specific, which not only yield results in support of a diagnosis, but other levels of information as well. Laboratory medicine provides data that help formulate therapy, promote the patient's recovery, and help establish the need for dietary, environmental, and physiological changes that contribute to the maintenance of good health.

Laboratory medicine specialists not only determine the methodology of the tests offered and control technical quality, but also consult with the medical staff to interpret test results and give advice on the role of the laboratory to resolve diagnostic dilemmas.

Other facets of laboratory medicine include the provision of laboratory support for public health activities and epidemiological investigations, evaluation of persons for drug abuse, and medicolegal investigations. The staff of the clinical laboratory also frames and implements institutional guidelines and procedures to control nosocomial infections, monitors sterilization and disinfection procedures, and con-

sults for the proper disposal of medical waste. The laboratory staff must also be familiar with the growing number and variety of rules, regulations, and recommendations that come from local, state, and federal government and professional organizations.

At times it may appear that these constraints place added emphasis on the test results and diminished emphasis on the knowledge and skill of laboratory personnel. Regardless of such appearances, and regardless of the size, location, or scope of services offered by a clinical laboratory, the one requirement that transcends all others is the need for a staff of individuals who are knowledgeable and technically proficient.

This textbook attempts to bring together the method selection and decision-making processes that ensure quality laboratory testing and to correlate the laboratory data obtained with current understanding of disease pathophysiology and clinical management of patients. The editors and authors have labored diligently to produce a book that will be a companion to students, a resource to the laboratory medicine specialist, and a reference to the clinician who wishes to optimally utilize the clinical laboratory.

Richard C. Tilton
Albert Balows
David C. Hohnadel
Robert F. Reiss

Contents

PART ONE

INTRODUCTION TO LABORATORY MEDICINE

1 Laboratory organization and management

Richard C. Tilton
Melissa Martincich

This chapter briefly presents some guidelines for the organization and management of a clinical laboratory. The presentation is neither exhaustive nor comprehensive. Rather, it is designed to stimulate questions regarding laboratory management, to provide an outline of necessary administrative functions, and to introduce fundamental information to laboratorians whose primary tasks may be analytical rather than administrative.

LABORATORY STRUCTURE

Traditional laboratory administrative structure has developed from an organization plan that was originally designed to implement laboratory testing in the most efficient manner. Figure 1-1 depicts this simple structure.

The laboratory was usually administered by a pathologist whose chief role in the hospital was in anatomic pathology. Supervisors in each of the laboratory sections reported to the chief technologist. There was little administrative distinction between the clinical laboratory and pathology department. The laboratory, being a high profit center, underwrote losses incurred by other non-revenue generating hospital functions. The last decade, however, has seen significant change, not only in how the laboratory relates to the hospital in a fiscal sense, but how the laboratory interacts in an increasingly complex and highly regulated health care environment. Figure 1-2 more typically portrays the laboratory of the 1990s. This table of organization is more characteristic of a commercial laboratory, but as hospital clinical laboratories develop outreach programs or spin-off for profit facilities, the distinctions become less apparent.

Whereas tables of organization may differ markedly from institution to institution, the point to be made is the growing complexity of laboratory medicine as a discipline, now separate and distinct from pathology services. Doctoral scientists and pathologists may not be hospital employees, but may be partners in a group practice that lease laboratory space from the hospital.

New health care financing plans (DRGs, Medicare, HMO's) have seriously limited profitability of the laboratory. Consequently, as a result of regulatory constraint, a new focus on laboratory management has emerged. Lines of authority once traditionally controlled by the laboratory are now managed by hospital administration. No value judgment should be placed on these changes, only the recognition that hospital ancillary services management has become an enigma; that is, how to administer a technologically burgeoning organization in an environment of severe fiscal constraint, regulation, and oversight.

THE INTERFACE OF LABORATORY SCIENCE AND BUSINESS

Laboratory services annually constitute a multibillion dollar health care expenditure. Yet, in many respects, the laboratory has not caught up with the changing face of medical practice. The clinical laboratory must provide service in a complex environment of:

- Decreased hospital inpatient census
- Expanded outpatient medicine, i.e., surgery centers, and so on
- Shortened inpatient stays
- Inpatients requiring major therapeutic intervention and intensive support systems, i.e., critically ill inpatients
- Demand for rapid turnaround time for laboratory tests
- Point-of-use testing
- Long-term (non-hospital) care facilities with an increasing role in acute care
- Large group practices with increased need for a wide variety of tests
- Increased patient expectations of quality and cost containment

Laboratories have struggled to meet these needs and changes in a variety of ways, including the following:

- Active marketing of laboratory services within the community to maximize profit.
- Satellite laboratories specializing in point-of-use testing, particularly to support single day medical intervention clinics, operating rooms, intensive care units.
- Electronic communication and information transfer to reduce turnaround time.
- Mechanization and automation of laboratory procedures to minimize use of a shrinking work force.
- Increased use of private reference laboratories for non-profitable testing.

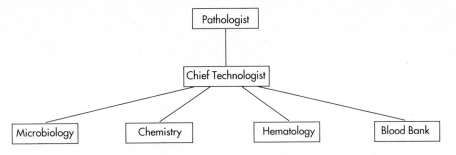

Fig. 1-1 A traditional table of organization for a small clinical laboratory.

Laboratory Organizational Chart

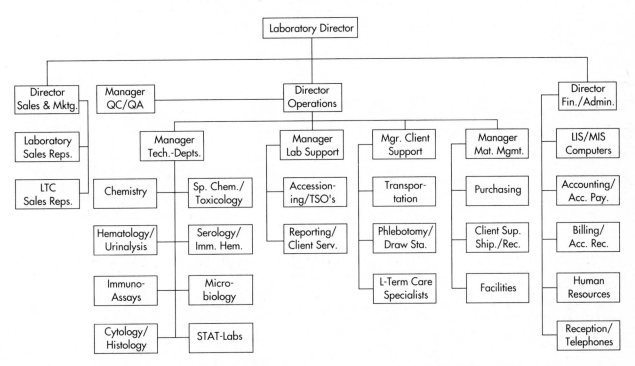

Fig. 1-2 A typical laboratory table of organization. (Modified from Mattice and Associates, Vancouver: 1991.)

• Trends toward centralization of laboratories within communities or specialty allocation (hospital A does endocrinology, hospital B does immunology).

There has also been a blurring of intralaboratory turf because of changing technology and manpower utilization. For example, hepatitis and human immunodeficiency virus (HIV) serology may be done through the blood bank, automated testing for infectious disease through the chemistry laboratory, and urinalysis through the microbiology laboratory. Almost all primary care physicians in the United States have access to an office laboratory. There is active marketing and sales of small, cost-effective analyzers that can perform chemistry profiles and enzyme-linked immunosorbent assays (ELISAs), as well as single use rapid tests for group A streptococcus, *Chlamydia,* and several other infectious disease agents. Such changes may radically alter the balance of testing between the hospital laboratory and

the physician office laboratory (POL). Existing and emerging restrictions on POLs regarding personnel qualifications and quality control, promulgated in 1992 as a result of the Clinical Laboratory Improvement Act of 1988 (CLIA 1988), may again affect this delicate balance.

The increase in self-testing cannot be ignored and is best illustrated by home pregnancy and ovulation kits, as well as home monitoring of blood glucose by diabetics.

LABORATORY FINANCIAL PLANNING

The contemporary laboratory is financially complex as well as technically sophisticated. Annual budget development time is not the favorite time of year for most laboratories. However, because of the changing nature of laboratory services, all must recognize that the operating budget and the financial plan are the critical interfaces between medicine and business. In fact, most organizations now rely on accounting professionals to organize and prepare their periodic financial status reports. However, it is critical for laboratory staff to appreciate the variety of management tasks and reports required to ensure the success of what is often a multimillion dollar business. For even a small laboratory, some elements of financial planning include:

- Income from laboratory tests (prediction of increases or decreases in test volume by laboratory section)
- Numbers of personnel required to satisfy sales forecasts
- Assessment of personnel productivity (e.g., College of American Pathologists [CAP] Workload Recording Plan)
- Anticipated needs in reagents, supplies, disposables
- Anticipated union contracts or budgeted pay increases
- Cost of continuing education
- Debt service (if any)
- Capital equipment (new and replacement)
- Quality assurance costs (external proficiency testing, etc.)
- Plan for monitoring variable costs
- Plan to control costs once budget is accepted
- Analysis of individual test fees; determination of margin for each test performed in laboratory
- Estimate of laboratory overhead (utilities, etc.)

PERSONNEL

Regardless of the layers of federal, state, and private regulations of the clinical laboratory, innumerable quality assurance (QA) probes, and internal and external test quality control, the best assurance that a laboratory reports accurate, reproducible results is the quality of personnel who perform the tests. Several personnel issues are critically important and are outlined here.

Educational background

There has been a tendency for federal agencies to attempt to lower personnel standards by minimizing the need for formal education in the clinical laboratory sciences. Increasingly complex instruments, molecular diagnosis, and demands for increased quality and rapid turnaround time clearly indicate that all laboratory personnel must be better educated and trained. For example, that a baccalaureate degree should be the minimum requirement for a technologist, and an associate degree the minimum requirement for a technician.

Certification

Certification of scientific and clinical competency by examination is a necessary prerequisite for a quality work force. There are a number of certifying agencies, such as the American Society for Clinical Pathology (ASCP), the American Academy of Microbiology, and the American Association of Clinical Chemistry. Personnel must be encouraged to become certified and their successful efforts rewarded with salary increases.

Continuing education

Continuing education is becoming increasingly expensive. However, continuing education is essential (mandatory if the laboratory is CAP accredited) to guarantee that workers who are judged competent by possession of a degree and certification continue to remain knowledgeable of the many changes in laboratory medicine. Some of the best continuing education classes are sponsored by local and regional groups such as the American Society for Medical Technologists (ASMT) and the laboratory specialty associations. Similarly, local programs exist for all specialty areas of the laboratory.

Once the laboratory has set in place a system for judging initial quality of applicants and increasing their competency through education, then other personnel issues become critically important to both the professional and the technical staff.

These issues include:

- Laboratory safety and health
- Career development and advancement (career ladders)
- Pleasant working environment
- Schedules of time off, vacations, etc., that are fair and consistent with the need to provide adequate clinical laboratory support

MANAGEMENT PHILOSOPHY AND STYLE

Volumes have been written about, degrees have been given for, and courses have been designed around the philosophy of management and how best to select a style that maximizes the talent of the employees and the strength of the management team. Some caveats that may prove useful include:

- Manage By Objectives (MBO): Set reasonable, attainable goals and provide tools for the work force to achieve those goals. An example of a goal might be to achieve 100% success in the parasitology proficiency testing program or in an area in which the laboratory has been weak.
- Manage By Example (MBE): Don't expect high performance of others if you cannot or are unwilling to measure up to the same standards of performance.
- Manage By Consensus (MBC): Seek advice of staff before making a management decision, recognizing that some decisions cannot be made by consensus and may not be popular.
- Avoid or discourage destructive conflict: In any group of interacting individuals, conflict management may be the skill that is most difficult to learn and the hardest to practice.
- Praise in public, admonish in private: Publicize the efforts of exemplary employees, but do not publicly chastise an employee or hold him or her up to criticism in the presence of fellow workers.

Whereas MBO is still the favorite management style in most laboratories, a combination of MBO, MBE, and MBC may be preferable in certain instances.

QUALITY CONTROL/QUALITY ASSURANCE

The scope of most clinical laboratories is now so broad and the interactions between laboratory technical operations, professional consultation, marketing, and finance so complex that the laboratory management is better served by the professional manager. Thus, the medical or scientific director of the laboratory should be relieved of much of the responsibility of the day-to-day management functions. However, the advent of professional laboratory managers has not diminished the role of the pathologist or clinical laboratory scientist; it has allowed them to play a much more proactive role in what is clearly the most important and also the most difficult part of the laboratory operation—quality assurance. The dilemma faced by all laboratorians is how to maintain the balance between financial constraints and high quality output. The clinical laboratory exists to provide data that assist clinicians in making medical decisions. Laboratory medicine uses successful outcome to measure quality. That is, quality is result-oriented. One has only to look at new stringent proficiency testing requirements in CLIA 1988 in contrast to a growing egalitarianism in personnel standards to understand the trend. Throughout this book, the chapters that follow discuss and review quality control guidelines. The laboratorian is advised to pay close attention to avoid some very unpleasant sanctions by one or more regulatory agencies.

REGULATION

Laboratories are regulated by local, state, private, and federal agencies. A single laboratory may be inspected and/or proficiency tested by the state in which it resides, the city in which it intends to do business, the College of American Pathology (CAP), the American Association of Blood Banks, the American Board of Bioanalysts, the Joint Commission on the Accreditation of Hospitals (JCAOH), HCFA, and other agencies of the Department of Health and Human Services. Regulations are in dynamic flux to the extent that guidelines presented today may be changed tomorrow. It is impossible to even summarize all of the regulations pertaining to the operation of a clinical laboratory. However, some of the more pertinent ones are presented with the understanding that they are subject to change and may vary as some state regulations take precedence.

The basis for federal regulation of laboratories, in particular those involved in interstate testing, has been the Clinical Laboratory Improvement Act (CLIA) of 1967. An outline of the evolution of CLIA from 1967 to 1991 follows.

Clinical laboratory improvement act of 1967

- Regulates interstate testing for independent laboratories
- Adopts Medicare standards for technical personnel
- Exempts hospital laboratories
- Requires proficiency testing
- Is administered by the Centers for Disease Control (CDC) in Atlanta

Initially, a laboratory designated as being able to receive fees for service for tests performed on Medicare and Medicaid patients had to operate under somewhat different regulations than a laboratory (even the same laboratory) operating under CLIA-67. In 1988, new legislation under CLIA-88 brought all laboratories under a single set of rules for payments and regulations for patients, personnel qualifications and provision of certain laboratory tests. Final rules were published in 1990 and were effective September 10, 1990. Proficiency testing under these new rules was effective January 1, 1991. It should be noted that many of these revisions were incorporated into CLIA 1988.

There are some exceptions to CLIA 1967 (revised). Rules *do not apply* to physician office laboratories who only test their own patients, health maintenance organizations (HMOs) and rural health clinic laboratories, insurance testing laboratories, and specimen collection and mailing facilities who do not perform tests.

Under the CLIA 1967 (revised) and CLIA 1988, laboratories must comply with all federal, state, and local laws regarding health and safety of patients, laboratory licensure, staff licensure, fire safety, and handling, storage, and disposal of hazardous materials.

One of the most important aspects of the CLIAs is proficiency testing. Proficiency testing specimens must be tested using the laboratory's routine procedures. There may be no discussion of proficiency testing results among laboratories. Unsuccessful participation is defined as two consecutive or two out of three unsatisfactory testing events, or two out of three failing scores for the same analyte. The number of samples has been increased to five per event. A satisfactory score is at least 80% (100% for immunohematology). Before Medicare or CLIA certification can be issued, a laboratory must receive a satisfactory score in one proficiency testing event.

The most radical changes brought about by CLIA 1967 (revised) and CLIA 1988 are evident in cytology. Changes include the following:
- Workload limit of 120 slides in 24-hour period
- Maximum number of 120 slides must be examined in no less than 6 hours
- Limit of 80 unevaluated slides per day, the remaining 40 slides can be examined for quality control purposes only
- More stringent requirements for record keeping, quality control, and quality assurance

Cytology proficiency testing is summarized as follows:
- One proficiency test performed annually at designated testing site
- One proficiency test performed annually that was unannounced on-site
- Each cytotechnologist must take part in two proficiency test events per year
- A score of at least 80% must be attained
- If a score of less than 80% is achieved, the last 500 slides examined by that individual must be reexamined by a cytotechnologist who passed

For all sections of the laboratory, there are new requirements for patient test management:
- Written specimen labeling instructions for clients
- Test requisition to include age, sex, date of birth, and clinical information
- Preliminary laboratory results must be kept for 2 years
- Pathology reports must be kept for 10 years
- "Panic" (results that require immediate attention) value reporting procedure must be in place

Quality assurance/quality control measures for all laboratory sections include the establishment of policies and procedures to: (1) monitor and evaluate quality; (2) identify and correct problems; (3) assure prompt, accurate, and reliable result reporting; and (4) assure that the laboratory is adequately and competently staffed.

More specifically, the following measures should be taken:
- Facility ventilation must be adequate for testing and reporting.
- Temperature and humidity must be monitored.

- There can be no mixing of kit components of different lots.
- A procedure manual including instructions for slide preparations and calculations must be maintained.
- Daily equipment function checks must be performed before patient testing.
- Adherance to equipment manufacturers' quality control recommendations.
- Quality control procedures for equipment are to be performed at least each day of use.
- More stringent calibration and verification requirements are necessary.
- Control samples should be tested in the same manner as patient's samples.
- Immunohematology records should be kept for 5 years.

For hospital-based laboratories, the laboratory director must be either a pathologist (MD/DO) with laboratory training and experience, or have a PhD in the life sciences with laboratory training and experience, or be a director qualified under state law.

Technical supervisors are required if the laboratory performs testing in the following areas:
- Histocompatibility
- Histopathology
- Blood banking
- Cytology
- Clinical cytogenetics
- Dermatopathology
- Transfusion services
- Oral pathology

Other personnel standards have been proposed under CLIA 1988 based on the complexity of laboratory testing. However, it is not anticipated that personnel requirements for hospital laboratories will change. The Clinical Laboratory Improvement Act of 1988, to be administered by the Health Care Financing Administration (HCFA), was prompted by the "Pap Smear Scandal" and the fact that relatively few states (14) have laboratory licensure laws. The process of rule making has been tortuous and final rules, after much debate, are to be published by January of 1992. Some additional features of CLIA 1988 include:
- Varying standards based on test complexity: "simple testing, moderately complex, highly complex" testing
- The requirement that all laboratories, except Department of Veteran Affairs (VA) laboratories, research laboratories, and insurance testing laboratories must have either a waiver or a certificate
- User fees to finance the program
- Proficiency test standards, further tightened over CLIA 1967 (revised), to come into effect in January of 1994
- Provision for publishing a list of problem laboratories

Under the present proposed rules, a waiver will be granted to laboratories performing only the following tests (these laboratories will, in most instances, be physician office-based):
- Urine dipstick or tablet urinalysis
- Ovulation tests
- Urine pregnancy tests
- Fecal occult blood
- Hemoglobin (copper sulfate)
- Erythrocyte sedimentation rate

The majority of these tests are available to patients in over-the-counter test kits. There are no personnel requirements for a laboratory performing only waived tests. Personnel requirements have been published, however, for a moderately complex laboratory. They include requirements for laboratory director, technical consultant, clinical consultant, and testing personnel. For a highly complex laboratory, all of the above are included along with technical supervisor, general supervisor, and testing personnel assistant.

There are enforcement procedures that will interconnect state, federal, and private accrediting agencies. It will be impossible to be sanctioned by one agency and continue to operate under another agency. Sanctions include suspension, revocation, or limitation of license, denial of Medicare payment, and civil penalties including fines and jail terms.

Not all sanctions can be appealed. For example, if it is determined not to reinstate a CLIA certificate, this action cannot be appealed. In addition to CLIA 1967 (revised) and CLIA 1988, there are a number of other laws that have been introduced or passed. They include:
- The Stark Amendment: This deals with physician test referral to laboratories in which physicians have an interest
- Safe Harbors: delineates fraud and abuse practices relevant to clinical laboratories
- Medicare/Medicaid Anti-Kickback Act of 1977
- Rural Laboratory Personnel Shortage Act
- A variety of health care reform bills

INTERACTION WITH REFERENCE LABORATORIES

Very few, if any, clinical laboratories performs all of their requested testing in-house. Therefore, the use and selection of a reference laboratory is virtually universal. Choosing a reference laboratory should be based on quality, service, turnaround time, and accessibility of experts for consultation. Fiscal restraint often dictates that the decision may be made based on the lowest bid for laboratory services. Such low bid situations are not always satisfactory. The laboratory is usually left to make a most important decision, whether or not to send out the test or perform it in-house. Certain elements outlined in Box 1-1 should be considered when making such a decision.

It is recommended that laboratories designate one person to coordinate reference laboratory testing and develop a workflow for the referral process. Box 1-2 outlines some typical tasks of a "send out" section.

There are many problems that can arise when using reference laboratories. Most can be avoided by developing a working relationship with a responsible and knowledgeable person at the reference laboratory. This is most often the client services coordinator. Problems such as STAT pickups, unreliable courier service, inaccessibility of technical people, lost specimens, or misunderstood or missing interpretation of data must be reconciled before a professional partnership between the client and the reference laboratory is a reality. The most common problem encountered is too long a turnaround time, which results in physicians calling to find out test results. Many reference laboratories provide a list of expected turnaround times, but they produce a test schedule less often. With both lists, the referring laboratory

---

Box 1-1   Aspects of a make-or-buy decision

Personnel:	Is your staff skilled enough to do the test you have in mind, or must you train or hire skilled personnel?
Equipment:	Will you have to acquire new instrumentation?
Reagents:	Will reagents be readily available?
Service:	Will you be able to run the test often enough to permit acceptable turnaround time?
Economics:	Will the new test make money? If not, can your laboratory afford to perform it?
Longevity:	Is the new test a fad?
Setting up:	Will the end result compensate for the difficulties of establishing the new test?
Time frame:	How much time will it take to develop a workable assay?
Projections:	In planning equipment purchases, have you devoted sufficient time and effort to envisioning the future?

(*Medical Laboratory Observer* 6:30, 1991).

Box 1-2   Workflow in the laboratory's send-out section

SENDING SPECIMENS

1. Receive specimen on hospital requisition slip
2. Enter patient's name and other pertinent data in log book or computer
3. Fill out reference laboratory test request slip:
   a. Copies 1 and 2 accompany specimen
   b. Copy 3 is stapled to hospital requisition form, which is placed in work-in-progress file
4. Label transport tube as instructed by referral laboratory
5. Prepare specimen as instructed by referral laboratory
6. Place specimen in plastic bag; store for courier or mail pickup

RECEIVING REPORTS

1. Report arrives by mail, courier, or fax
2. Match patient identification number with number on hospital requisition form in work-in-progress file
3. Enter results in log book or computer
4. Distribute report forms:
   a. Attach original to patient's chart
   b. Place one copy in general laboratory files
   c. Place one copy in daily envelope, alphabetize by patient name, write date on envelope, file in send-out laboratory
   d. Make additional copies for attending physician, if requested
   e. Make additional copies for all appropriate physicians if patient has been discharged from hospital
5. Send billing information to hospital billing department

(*Medical Laboratory Observer* 6:62, 1991).

---

is much better able to determine when a test result should be available. Figure 1-3 depicts typical turnaround times and test schedules for a few tests.

INFORMATION SYSTEMS

In today's competitive environment, it is difficult to imagine a laboratory operating effectively without a well-designed laboratory information system (LIS). When computers were first introduced into the laboratory environment, their applications were limited largely to statistical analysis in conjunction with the reporting of assay results. Today's LIS impacts all levels of a laboratory's operations. A good LIS allows the laboratorian to monitor and control operations much like any other business, thereby improving performance and turn-around-time. As more laboratories are expected to perform as profit centers, timely information on clients or clinicians, productivity, quality, and costs are critical. The well-designed LIS should decrease turnaround time, increase productivity of both administrative and technical personnel, improve responsiveness to clients and clinicians, and enhance access to information that is essential to the laboratorian making operational and competitive decisions. In fact, what was once a laboratory information system is now perhaps better described as a management information system (MIS), as its applications, in most cases, extend far beyond the confines of the laboratory.

Overview

Depending upon the size and complexity of the laboratory, the MIS can range in complexity from a simple program that runs on one personal computer (PC) to a highly sophisticated and complicated system that requires the power of a mainframe computer. In essence, however, all MISs are simply data management systems that are set up as a series of data bases. A computerized data base is a list of individual pieces of similar information that can be quickly accessed and arranged according to whatever criteria are deemed important. The four primary data bases in a laboratory MIS are the *patient* data base, that contains all relevant information with regard to the patient; the *specimen* data base, that contains information on a particular test request; the *test* data base, that contains information on each of the tests performed in the laboratory, including normal ranges, pricing, and interpretation of results; and the *client* data base, that contains information on clients who utilize the laboratory, including billing and reporting information, and special pricing. Depending upon the laboratory, the contents of each of these data bases may vary considerably, but in general, all laboratory MISs maintain data bases that parallel those described. Figure 1-4 illustrates a typical laboratory data management system, its functions, and the interaction of each of the data bases just described.

Practical application

Laboratory MISs are divided into the following:
   1. Order entry: Order entry takes place when a specimen is received with a test request. Order entry is the entry of all information regarding the test request into the specimen databank, including patient information, specimen information, client identification data, tests requested, and billing information. Figure 1-5 depicts a typical order entry screen. At order entry, the spec-

TEST SCHEDULE

| PROCEDURE | SET-UP DAYS | | | | | TEST TIME | TAT | |
	M	T	W	Th	F		MIN	MAX
AFB Stain	x	x	x	x	x	1 day	1	4
AFB Culture	x	x	x	x	x	6 weeks*	6 weeks	
Amikacin	x	x	x	x	x	4 hours	SD	
Antibiotic MBC	x	x	x	x	x	2 days	2	5
Antibiotic MIC	x	x	x	x	x	2 days	2	5
ASO			x			1 day	1	7
Bacterial Ag Detection	x	x	x	x	x	1 day	SD	
Bacterial Isolate ID	x	x	x	x	x	1-7 days[2]	1	10
Blood Culture	x	x	x	x	x	5 days*	5	8
Chlamydia Culture	x	x	x	x	x	3 days	3	6
C. difficile toxin	x	x	x	x	x	3 days	3	6
CMV Culture	x	x	x	x	x	3 weeks	3 weeks	
CMV Culture Early Ag	x	x	x	x	x	2 days	2	5
CMV IgG/IgM		x				1 day	1	8
Cold Agglutination			x			2 days	1	8
Cryptococcal Antigen	x	x	x	x	x	1 day	SD	
EBV	x		x			1 day	1	6
Fungus Culture	x	x	x	x	x	4 weeks*	4 weeks	5 weeks
HBsAg	x		x		x	1 day[1]	1	4
Hepatitis markers - Other		x		x		1 day	1	6

Fig. 1-3 Typical turnaround times and test schedules.

imen is assigned an accession number, a unique code that identifies each specimen and allows each order to be traced through the system. The accession number is usually assigned by the computer, which will then generate a label for the specimen that contains all the information a technologist will need to process the sample. A label can either be a text label that must be read by the technologist, or a bar code label that is read using a bar code wand. The bar code system is a much more efficient system for tracking the progress of a specimen through the laboratory, as the bar code can be read and the accession number entered into the MIS at each stage of processing. Bar coding also speeds up data entry by eliminating manual entry of accession numbers at each stage of specimen processing, and gets specimens into the laboratory more quickly. These benefits must be weighed, however, against the capital investment necessary for installation of the system, which can run as high as $50,000. In general, bar coding can usually be jus-

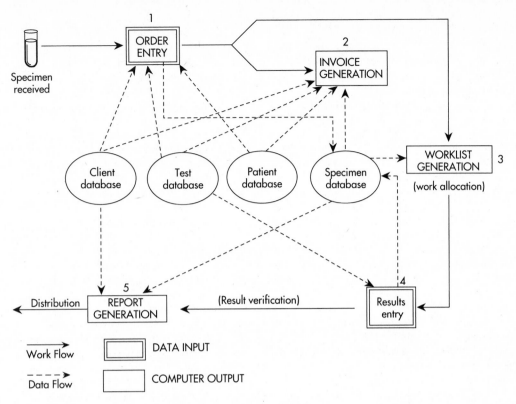

Fig. 1-4 Data management system.

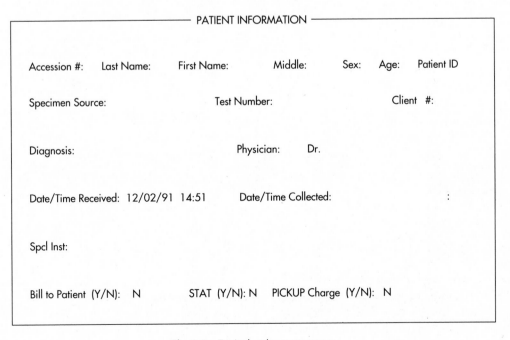

Fig. 1-5 Typical order entry screen.

tified in laboratories processing 400 or more samples a day.

2. Worklist processing: Once a test request is entered into the specimen data base, the specimen is available to the technologist for testing. In worklist processing, each test requested is automatically assigned to a worklist, which is used by technologists to build their workload. The printed worklist is also often used to record test results during the testing procedure, if necessary.

3. Results entry: Once a specimen has been processed and results are available, these results must be entered into the specimen data base. Results may be entered manually by the technologist by using preprogrammed results that are stored in a separate data base, or results may be automatically entered via an instrument interface. During result entry, an LIS should be able to perform a delta check, that is comparing entered results with reference values and flagging abnormal entries. It should also perform "nonsense" checks to ensure that preprogrammed comments coded for a result are appropriate for the test performed, or that the values entered for a result fall within certain defined limits. For example, a hemoglobin of 1120 g/dl would be flagged a nonsense result. Figure 1-6 shows a typical results entry screen.

4. Reporting: Once results have been entered and verified, a report is generated for each requisiton. Generally, reports are printed in the laboratory and forwarded to the client. More sophisticated MISs can send reports to remote printers that may be installed in a client's office or laboratory. In this way, reports are printed directly on-site and there is no transportation delay. Reports may be cumulative or single event reports. The advantage of a cumulative report is that the patient's laboratory history can be readily observed. The disadvantage is that the report can be very complicated, and most recently reported results may be difficult to locate unless flagged. A sample report form (Figure 1-7) incorporates data required for most clinical laboratory test reporting functions.

5. Inquiry: A fifth important function of the MIS is inquiry. Inquiry allows the laboratory to quickly acertain the status of a test or test results. Inquiries can be based on patient name or accession number. Depending upon the extent of terminal distribution, inquiry may be initiated at a remote site such as the patient floor.

6. Billing: A sixth important function of many laboratory MISs is billing. Although not all laboratory MISs have a built-in billing function, to do so improves billing efficiency and thereby cash flow. Laboratory billing systems in general can generate invoices immediately upon order entry if desired. The billing function will use the specimen data base to determine which tests are available for billing, the test data base to determine the price of a test to be billed, and the client data base to determine to whom invoices need to be sent. In addition, a well-designed MIS should allow for special pricing for each client. This information will be captured by the billing function directly from the client data base.

In addition to the basic operational function, an MIS must perform a management reporting function. This function produces reports for use by laboratory management. These reports may include information on the numbers of specimens processed and laboratory productivity (workload reporting), client activity, sales, types and numbers of tests

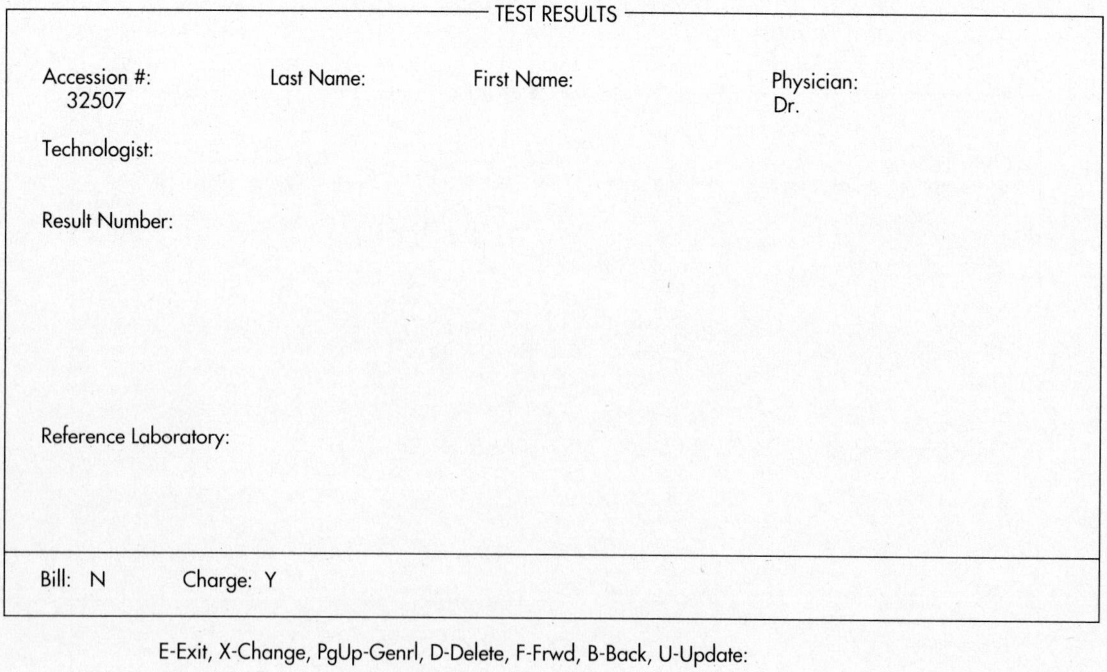

```
┌──────────────────────── TEST RESULTS ─────────────────────────┐
│                                                                │
│   Accession #:      Last Name:      First Name:       Physician:│
│     32507                                             Dr.      │
│                                                                │
│   Technologist:                                                │
│                                                                │
│   Result Number:                                               │
│                                                                │
│                                                                │
│                                                                │
│                                                                │
│                                                                │
│                                                                │
│   Reference Laboratory:                                        │
│                                                                │
│                                                                │
│                                                                │
├────────────────────────────────────────────────────────────────┤
│   Bill:  N      Charge:  Y                                      │
└────────────────────────────────────────────────────────────────┘
```

E-Exit, X-Change, PgUp-Genrl, D-Delete, F-Frwd, B-Back, U-Update:

Fig. 1-6   Typical results entry screen.

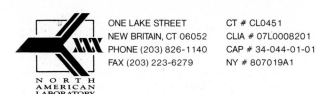

ONE LAKE STREET   CT # CL0451
NEW BRITAIN, CT 06052   CLIA # 07L0008201
PHONE (203) 826-1140   CAP # 34-044-01-01
FAX (203) 223-6279   NY # 807019A1

NORTH
AMERICAN
LABORATORY
GROUP

REPORT DATE

M I C R O B I O L O G Y - S E R O L O G Y R E P O R T

TEST REQUESTED BY	CLIENT ACCESSION	NALG ACCESSION

| | PATIENT |

ORDERING PHYSICIAN	AGE	SEX	SPECIMEN SOURCE	COLLECTION DATE	DATE RECEIVED

TEST REQUESTED	CPT CODES

RESULTS

X

SPECIAL INSTRUCTIONS

FAX RESULTS TO: PHONE SIGNIFICANT RESULTS TO:
ATTN: ATTN:
RESULTS FAXED BY: DATE: RESULTS CALLED BY: DATE:

Fig. 1-7   A sample report form.

performed, quality control results, and epidemiology reports. Ideally, an MIS should be flexible enough to allow managers to design their own reports, although more often than not, this is not the case.

Hardware

An MIS can be designed to operate on any number of hardware platforms. A small laboratory can manage its information on nothing more than a PC if the operating system is well designed. Larger laboratories need to upgrade to networked systems, which provide access to the main data bases from multiple locations or to mainframes.

As PC networks become more powerful and sophisticated, their use is becoming more prevalent in the industry. Personal computer networks provide flexibility, are easily expandable, are low cost, and are relatively easy to administer. Networks can be composed of computers from any number of vendors including IBM, NCR, Digital, Hewlett Packard, and Texas Instruments.

The most common software for setting up PC networks is Novell Netware Ethernet or Tokenring. The type of network set up will depend on the MIS vendor and the size of the laboratory. Most packaged LIS systems are designed to work with specific hardware and within a specified operating environment.

Operating software

The two most common operating systems in use for laboratory MISs are UNIX and MUMPS, although DOS is also commonly used in a network environment. UNIX and MUMPS are probably more flexible and powerful as operating systems, but they are also more complex and less familiar to the average user. Furthermore, the numbers and types of software that can be run on DOS makes available many other tools to assist in laboratory management. In most cases, the operating system is transparent when using the MIS, so the choice of operating systems will often be a function of the type of MIS package that is preferred. Only the systems administrator need actually be familiar with the operating system.

The first choice a laboratorian must make when installing a new MIS is whether or not to design and develop a customized system or to buy a turnkey laboratory MIS. A number of excellent laboratory software packages exist on the market. Some of the better known are Antrim, Sunquest, and SCC (Software Computer Consultants), although a large number of other packages exist and thorough research should be conducted before deciding on a system. If a software package is chosen, it may be important to specify that the source code of the program be made available so that the laboratory can program custom modifications if necessary. Laboratory information systems are relatively expensive when purchased from a vendor. Costs will run anywhere from a minimum of $70,000 to over $1,000,000, depending on the numbers of workstations required, the type of hardware specified, and the numbers of software features supplied or the amount of custom changes to the package required. An alternative is to hire a programmer to design a custom system that performs all of the specific functions required by your laboratory. Depending upon the operating system chosen, a custom-designed system can cost significantly less than a turnkey system but will probably have fewer features. A custom-designed DOS-based network system could cost as little at $40,000.

Regulatory issues

In addition to the impact on laboratory operations, today's regulatory environment directly affects the design of the laboratory MIS. Both state and federal regulations require clinical laboratories to keep records for a designated minimum amount of time and these records must be easily accessible. Therefore, the laboratory MIS must have a system for both downloading and storing historical files and uploading them for access as needed. In addition, in order to maintain patient confidentiality, several levels of security must be built into the laboratory MIS, especially in regard to accessing patient information. Finally, most regulatory agencies require that the laboratory MIS be well documented. A complete computer manual must be available to the user at all times to guide them in correct use of the system. A lack of any of the aforementioned features will lead to deficiencies according to a number of regulatory bodies.

In the highly sophisticated, technologically complex, and highly regulated laboratory environment of the 1990s, virtually no clinical laboratory should be without an information system. An LIS, no matter how small, cheap, or unsophisticated, has the capability of making a reality the recommendations for budget, personnel, quality assurance, and regulatory compliance as outlined in this chapter.

2 Clinical laboratory safety, biohazard surveillance, and infection control

Michael P. Kiley

Absolute safety in the clinical laboratory should be the aim of every laboratory worker and laboratory manager. Although this lofty goal may not be realistically attainable, we do possess the means to reduce laboratory accidents to a minimal level. In his 1979 historical review of laboratory-acquired infections, Pike concluded "the knowledge, the techniques and the equipment to prevent most laboratory infections are available." It is now up to laboratory technical personnel and laboratory managers to take advantage of current knowledge and techniques to reduce the number of laboratory-acquired infections and laboratory accidents to the lowest possible level. In recent years the concept of management's responsiblity to provide a safe working environment, including proper training opportunities, has become an operational reality. This chapter will describe the typical components of a prudent clinical laboratory safety program. Topics to be discussed include facilities, containment, work practices, biohazard surveillance, infection control, chemical hazard control, chemical hygiene, waste management, training, and record keeping.

Much has been published on the topics of laboratory safety and biosafety, and there are several good sources that are considered to be essential in the field of laboratory biosafety; these are highlighted in the Suggested Reading at the end of the chapter.

HISTORICAL PERSPECTIVE

Clinical and research laboratory workers are in work areas where the risk of infection is higher than in the general population, although the risk of exposure of laboratory workers to infectious agents is somewhat less than in other groups of health-care workers.

To determine the proper components of a laboratory safety program, it was first necessary to determine, to the extent possible, the risk of infection associated with working in a clinical laboratory. Pike compiled the best collection of data to date dealing with accidental infections of laboratory workers with pathogenic microorganisms. Pike analyzed and reported on the global experience with laboratory-acquired infections since the beginning of the current century. Although much of the data cover the period before the age of antibiotic chemotherapy and laminar flow biosafety cabinets, the review still presents some idea of the

potential risks to those working in laboratories. The weaknesses of the studies relative to clinical laboratories are that most of the reported infections occurred in research rather than in clinical laboratories, and the denominator, or the populations at risk, were unknown, so that attack rates could not be calculated. Additionally, the data do not take into account the changing pattern of laboratory techniques or relative importance of different groups of infectious agents through the years (Table 2-1).

It is obvious from examining the data that a major shift away from bacteria and rickettsia as the chief causes of laboratory-acquired infections has occurred. The majority of laboratory-acquired infections reported in the recent past have been of viral origin. In general, this has followed the trend of a decrease in aerosol infections with an increase in blood-borne diseases.

The decrease in aerosol infections in the laboratory is most likely due to the development of the laminar flow biosafety cabinet, an increased awareness of routes of infection, and a greater awareness of the need for safety in the laboratory. The discovery of antibiotics, as well as the increase in the number of available vaccines, has also played a role in the decrease in illness due to laboratory infections. In spite of the general trends, there are still laboratory-acquired infections that occur on a regular basis; because of the lack of a reporting system and the lack of adequate medical surveillance, the true extent of laboratory-acquired infections may never be known. This is illustrated by a recent report of a laboratory-acquired *Brucella* infection by a microbiologist in a reference laboratory who had worked

Table 2-1 Changing trends in cause of laboratory-acquired infections

Microbe	Time periods		
	1925-1934 (%)	1945-1954 (%)	1965-1974 (%)
Bacteria	67	40	13
Viruses	15	22	59
Rickettsia	6	22	3
Fungi	2	8	20
Other	10	8	6

From Pike RM: Ann Rev Microbiol 33:41, 1979.

with the agent for at least 20 years without a laboratory-related infection. This is merely one example that points to the need for a strong, continuing, and vigorous biosafety program in every clinical laboratory.

COMPONENTS OF A BIOSAFETY PROGRAM

Rules and regulations covering the use, management, and disposal of hazardous and carcinogenic chemicals in the laboratory have been in place for some time. The National Fire Protection Agency NFPA codes, as well as Occupational and Safety Health Administration (OSHA) regulations are the usual source of the regulations. Prior to 1989, criteria for working safely with biological materials consisted of a series of guidelines and recommendations emanating from the Centers for Disease Control (CDC), the National Institute of Health (NIH), or certain professional groups such as the ASM. A great concern for the safety and protection of laboratory and health-care workers was generated by the sudden appearance of the human immunodeficiency virus (HIV) as the agent responsible for acquired immune deficiency syndrome (AIDS). Also, because of the continuing problem of hepatitis B infections among all health-care workers, a regulation to reduce occupational exposure to blood-borne pathogens, specifically HIV and hepatitis B has been promulgated. These regulations have taken the form of a proposed OSHA rule dealing with occupational exposure to blood-borne pathogens published in the Federal Register of May 30, 1989. The proposed rules essentially codify most of the information present in previously published guidelines and recommendations. The emphasis in the proposed rules is on employee training and education, use of safety equipment, and the responsibility of employers to provide a worksite that is maintained in a "clean and sanitary condition." In fact, the new OSHA rules spell out, in a performance-oriented regulatory approach, the legal obligations of an employer to provide a safe worksite. Although the new regulation covers many areas relating to laboratory safety, it should only be considered as the starting point for a comprehensive laboratory safety program. A laboratory safety program should consist of:

1. The commitment by top management to develop and support a strong laboratory safety program.
2. The establishment of a safe workplace, including the provision of the proper safety equipment and personnel protective equipment where needed.
3. The recognition of the collective responsibilities of management, front-line supervisors, and laboratory workers to support the program.
4. The establishment of appropriate on-the-job training and training courses so that laboratory workers understand proper safety practices and the components of the infection control program at the institution for employees and patients.
5. The development and implementation of an effective and comprehensive infection control program.

CONSIDERATIONS IN DEVELOPING A LABORATORY SAFETY PROGRAM

Each laboratory safety program, while having general objectives, will vary depending upon the nature of the institution involved. Factors to be considered include the scope of laboratory work being done, the level of technical expertise of the laboratory staff, and the availability of equipment designed to ensure a safe work environment. Of equal importance is engineering support to ensure proper installations of biosafety cabinets, fume hoods, eye washes, and the proper air balance.

INFECTION CONTROL/EPIDEMIOLOGY PROGRAM

The goal for all clinical laboratories is to provide the safest possible working conditions for all employees. In order to accomplish this it is necessary to understand the possible risks involved in working with clinical specimens such as microbial cultures or chemical reagents and the procedures required to prevent laboratory infections or exposure to a chemical hazard. It is also necessary for top-level management of the laboratory to be aware of the levels of risk to their employees.

The exact incidence of occupational infections among laboratory workers is unknown. Although there are a number of published reports detailing individual or small group outbreaks of laboratory-acquired infections, there is no report that has successfully determined the population at risk for any of these incidents. These reports have dealt largely with single cases or outbreaks, retrospective studies, and passively acquired anecdotal information. The overall mortality for reported cases is approximately 4%, but this number is most likely very high considering the unknown denominator and the great number of unreported nonfatal laboratory illnesses.

It is important when establishing an infection control/medical surveillance program that institutional authorities understand the relative risks that their employees face in their own institutions. This requires information regarding infectious agents and other potential sources of employee risk that are likely to be found at their workplace and the laboratory as a whole. A hospital in the rural midwest is less likely to have HIV-positive serum or blood samples in its laboratory than one located in a major metropolitan area. On the other hand, the likelihood of *Brucella* being present in a specimen may be many times more likely in a laboratory located in a rural area. State public health laboratories and large commercial diagnostic and reference laboratories should be especially alert because of the large number and wide variety of specimens they process.

Knowledge of infectious disease processes is necessary because the cornerstone of an infection control program is the need to identify employees whose duties include routine and anticipated tasks involving, or potentially involving, exposure to infectious material. Particular duties must be evaluated for their infectious potential. It is the job that is rated and not the individual, although some individuals, because they are highly susceptible to infection, should be excluded from duties that are not risky to the normal population. Especially vulnerable are those people whose immune system has been compromised, regardless of the reason. The infectious potential of any job is usually arrived at by asking a series of questions about the job. Questions that might be asked include: does the individual routinely come in contact with blood or blood products, or does the individual routinely handle incoming shipments of biological material? Other information required for a determination may include the type of laboratory equipment that is used and the nature of the clinical samples received.

By evaluating the duties of the position and determining that a worker is at risk, a written infection control plan for that position must be developed. This plan should contain an exposure determination (the criteria used to evaluate the position), a schedule and method for meeting any applicable safety standards (including those of OSHA), and the contents of a worker training program. A good training program, including a record of all training received, is especially important to an overall effective laboratory safety program. Training should include familiarization with the nature of laboratory pathogens and safe and proper use of laboratory equipment. A laboratory safety manual must be available for all employees that includes approved protocols for all laboratory procedures, as well as a list of duties and responsibilities. One of the responsibilities of any laboratory worker should be to report to the supervisor any incident that occurred and has the potential for an occupational exposure to an infectious agent.

An infection control program should also contain a medical surveillance component. This component should include a medical evaluation, including an occupational/medical history and a physical examination covering conditions that a physician feels may interfere with a worker's ability to use protective clothing or laboratory safety equipment. It is also essential to ensure that all workers are adequately immunized. This should include immunization with all of the vaccines usually required for entry into primary school, as well as access to hepatitis B virus (HBV) vaccination. With the development of the recombinant HBV vaccine, there is no reason for all laboratory workers not to be vaccinated against hepatitis B virus.

A major goal of a good medical surveillance program is to educate workers of the need, and indeed the institutional requirement, to report any occupational exposure. Employees should also have the right to a confidential medical evaluation and follow-up after reporting such an incident. Elements of such a follow-up would include documentation of the events surrounding the exposure, the source patient (if known), and the documentation of the route of exposure. For a laboratory incident with possible HIV exposure, a medical consultation and decision as to whether or not to begin AZT (zidovudine) treatment may be necessary. For this reason it is prudent to have a pre-established policy covering this situation (*Morbidity and Mortality Weekly Report*, vol 39, 1990). Continued follow-up, including counseling and illness reporting, should also be part of the program.

It is evident that a good institutional infection control/medical surveillance program requires well-designed and clearly written procedures and protocols, as well as good definitions for terms used in the document. It is also essential that the program be made known to all employees and that any information derived from any in-house investigations be used for educational purposes. Laboratory workers should understand and support the program; not fear it.

FACILITIES AND WORK PRACTICES

Working with potentially infectious microorganisms in the clinical microbiology laboratory requires an appreciation of the facilities and work practices needed to make such laboratories a safe environment in which to work. Guidelines on the safe handling of pathogens have evolved over the last decade and have reached the point where there is general agreement on the basic principles of biosafety in the laboratory. Four biosafety levels (BL) have been described (BL1 through BL4) that consist of combinations of laboratory practices and procedures, safety equipment, and laboratory facilities appropriate for the operations performed and the hazards posed by the infectious agents, and for the laboratory function or activity (Richardson and Barkley, 1988). The levels are almost identical to the "P" levels (P1 through P4) described for studies employing recombinant DNA molecules (United States Public Health Service recombinant DNA guidelines). Essentially, the numerical designation of a safety level increases with an increase in the risks and a corresponding increase in precautionary and safety procedures involved in working with an agent (Table 2-2).

Biosafety level 1

Biosafety level 1 practices, safety equipment, and facilities are appropriate for work with organisms that present no danger to humans. Examples of laboratories that may be operated at this level include undergraduate and secondary educational training and teaching laboratories. In these laboratories, work is done with well-characterized agents that do not produce disease in normal healthy adult humans. Examples of some microorganisms that meet the criteria for BL1 are bacteriophages, *Bacillus subtilis*, and most animal viruses that do not infect humans, such as infectious canine hepatitis virus. Use of BL1 biocontainment conditions for these and similar agents is routine, but there are microbes that are usually benign in the human host but may present problems for certain groups of people. Many agents not normally able to produce disease in healthy individuals may produce severe illness in the aged, the immunodeficient or immunosuppressed, and even in children. Also, vaccine strains, because they are attenuated in virulence, may not produce disease in healthy individuals, but may produce severe disease in others. The latter two categories of organisms should be manipulated under BL2 conditions.

Biosafety level 2

Conditions described for BL2 are usually applicable to clinical, diagnostic, research, and teaching laboratories in which work is done with a wide variety of microorganisms that are present in the community at large and are associated with human disease of varying severity. When applying good microbiological techniques and reducing aerosol production to a minimum, most of the samples that may contain the organisms assigned to this level may be worked with at the open bench. Hepatitis B virus, human immunodeficiency viruses, salmonellae, and *Toxoplasma* spp. are among those that can be manipulated at the BL2 level. Generally, the agents that are assigned to this level cause blood-borne diseases and do not have a history of infection through the respiratory route. It is not surprising, then, that the usual

Table 2-2 Brief description of the four biosafety levels

Biosafety level (containment)	Work practices and procedures (use)	Engineering considerations
1 (Basic)	Standard microbiological practices; work can be done on an open bench (undergraduate teaching laboratory)	No special engineering requirements; containment achieved by adherence to standard laboratory practices
2 (Basic)	Standard laboratory practices, plus lab coats, infectious waste decontamination, proper waste disposal including sharps, limited access, use of gloves, and proper biohazard signage (clinical/diagnostic laboratory, routine microbiological research laboratories)	Procedures that produce potentially infectious aerosols performed in a biological safety cabinet; barriers used to reduce droplet dispersal
3 (Containment)	Standard and special practices listed above plus special lab clothing (long sleeve wrap-around gown and mask); controlled access. (TB laboratories and research labs working with a variety of aerosol-spread organisms)	Inward air flow and two sets of doors between outside and laboratory; one pass air, BSC's air can be recirculated if fillers are monitored.
4 (Maximum containment)	Change to special lab clothes prior to entering lab; personnel shower on exiting lab; all wastes autoclaved before leaving facility	HEPA filtered supply and exhaust air work done in class 3 cabinet or in BSC using an air-supplied positive pressure suit in an airtight lab

routes of laboratory-acquired infections with agents in this group are through autoinoculation, ingestion, and mucous membrane exposure to the infective agent. Procedures that have a high probability of aerosol production should be conducted in primary containment equipment or devices. Additional information on equipment and work practices used in BL2 is discussed shortly. Biosafety level 2 is the safety level commonly employed in clinical laboratories. The main features of a prototypical BL2 laboratory are presented in Figure 2-1 and a picture taken in a modern BL2 research laboratory is shown in Figure 2-2.

Biosafety level 3

The work practices, safety equipment, and facilities described for BL3 are applicable to work with indigenous or exotic agents where aerosol infection, through either the respiratory or droplet route, is a real possibility and the disease may have serious, or even fatal consequences. Familiar agents for which BL3 safeguards are routinely recommended include *Mycobacterium tuberculosis*, St. Louis encephalitis virus, and *Coxiella burnetii*, the rickettsial agent that causes Q fever. One of the more exotic agents that requires BL3 containment is Rift Valley fever virus, a hemorrhagic fever virus from Africa that can be handled at this level by adequately immunized workers.

Whereas autoinoculation, ingestion, and mucous membrane contamination are a hazard with these agents, the major concern is with aerosol infection. Because of this, the requirements for BL3 are more stringent than those for BL2 and are aimed at controlling aerosol production and

spread through this route. Access to the BL3 laboratory is restricted and there must be two sets of doors between general access areas and the laboratory. These laboratories must also contain a ducted exhaust system so that air is not recirculated within the laboratory or to other areas, and so that the system can be made to assure that air is always flowing into the laboratory (i.e., the laboratory is under negative pressure). Figure 2-3 is a schematic of an example of a BL3 laboratory design. Work with infectious material is done within laminar flow biosafety cabinets by workers wearing full frontal gowns, gloves, and surgical masks. Full-face respirators are not required because the aerosols produced by routine laboratory manipulations are larger than 5 µm and will be stopped by the surgical mask. Laboratory wastes are decontaminated prior to disposal. If they must be removed from the laboratory for decontamination, they are transported in leakproof containers to an approved decontamination site. Other microbiological practices employed at this containment level are also used at BL2 and will be described in more detail.

Biosafety level 4

This containment level is to be used when working with exotic viruses that have a high mortality rate and for which there is no vaccine or reliable treatment. A variety of agents causing viral hemorrhagic fever, including Lassa, Marburg, Ebola, and related viruses, are those most commonly studied at BL4. It is extremely rare for a patient with viral hemorrhagic fever to be admitted to a U.S. hospital, but if such a patient is to be admitted, the Centers for Disease Control

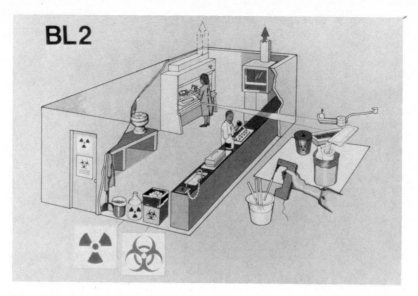

Fig. 2-1 Schematic diagram presenting the main features of a typical BL2 laboratory. Not all of the laboratories will have all of the features indicated.

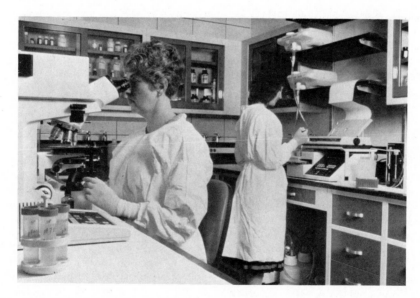

Fig. 2-2 Photograph of one of the new BL2 laboratories in the Viral and Rickettsial Diseases Laboratory at the Centers for Disease Control. Courtesy of CDC.

does have a mobile laboratory especially designed to be moved to a hospital in order to provide the necessary laboratory support for such patients.

THE CLINICAL LABORATORY

As mentioned earlier, clinical microbiology laboratories operate under BL2 conditions. Facilities design, recommended personnel protective equipment, and work practices suggested for work at BL2 have been defined. Clinical/diagnostic laboratory personnel should also be aware that certain conditions may exist in a laboratory for a given period of time that may call for more stringent work practices. Laboratorians should also be aware that certain laboratory equipment, particularly automated analytical devices, may

present an increased risk of exposure to pathogens present in clinical specimens. This may occur either because of an increased risk of aerosol (droplet) production or an increased risk of parenteral exposure.

Laboratory facilities

Laboratories should be designed so that the floors, walls, windows, and are easily cleanable. This should include having as few as possible nooks and crannies where dust and dirt are likely to collect. Bench tops should be of a material that is impervious to water and resistant to acids, alkalis, organic solvents, germicides, and moderate heat. Laboratory furniture should be of similar resistant materials and should not interfere with the proper circulation of workers

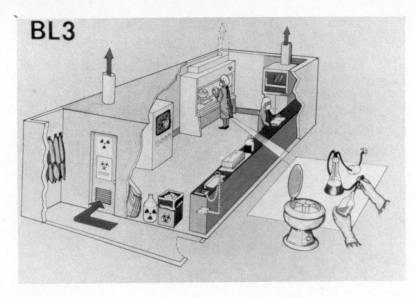

Fig. 2-3 Schematic drawing of a typical BL3 laboratory design. Note the presence of an anteroom and the indication of inward airflow, the two cardinal features of BL3 construction.

while performing their duties. Equipment should be placed in a location where it is easily accessible for cleaning and where, if it is likely to produce an aerosol, it is in the safest possible location. Attention should be paid to door swings since a door opening in the wrong direction has the potential to knock items from peoples' hands. Equipment must not be placed near thermostats since this can create a situation in which temperature control is erratic and work conditions may not be ideal. Floors should be non-skid so as to reduce the likelihood of slipping.

Each laboratory should contain a wash basin, preferably near the door, so that laboratory workers can wash their hands before leaving the laboratory. If the laboratory contains windows that open, they must be fitted with fly screens. An autoclave, for decontaminating laboratory waste, must be available. Although the autoclave does not have to be directly in the laboratory, this is the preferred location. If potentially infectious material must be transported out of the laboratory for decontamination, it must be done in containers that preclude aerosolization and/or leakage of the contents. Each laboratory should also have at least one, preferably two, eye wash stations, either fixed or transportable, for emergency use. Face shields and glasses or goggles should be available when personnel are handling corrosive, caustic or explosive chemicals. Caps, gowns, face masks, and respirators should also be available in the laboratory ready for use as needed.

Containment equipment

Clinical laboratories in which laboratory personnel anticipate working with potentially infectious material should contain a biosafety cabinet, preferably a class II laminar flow biosafety cabinet (Figure 2-4). Procedures with the potential for creating infectious aerosols should be done inside the hood. These procedures may include centrifugation, grinding, blending, vigorous shaking or mixing, sonic disruption, and opening containers of infectious materials or centrifuge tubes. Intranasal inoculation of animals and harvesting in-

fectious tissues from animals or eggs should also be done in a biosafety cabinet. If it is not possible for the laboratory to obtain a biosafety cabinet, at least some means to prevent droplet contamination should be employed. This may be as simple as a plastic shield or possibly a transparent plastic box that may be placed over the work during any manipulations. This is important since most laboratory infections with blood-borne agents, other than those produced by parenteral inoculation, are probably due to droplet contamination of broken skin or mucous membranes.

Any work with high concentrations of infectious agents should be done in a containment cabinet. Reduction of aerosols is also a consideration when working with many of the analytical instruments found in a modern diagnostic laboratory. Special precautions should be taken when operating instruments such as cell sorters or when loading analytical instruments where the sample may be under pressure and at an increased risk for aerosol production. In many cases a splash guard may suffice.

Work practices

Previous investigations of laboratory accidents indicate that it is often a break in good laboratory practice that is the direct cause of an accident. Information derived from the investigation of laboratory accidents, experience obtained from working in clinical laboratories, and the application of common sense have contributed to the development of a list of good work practices. The practices and procedures listed here are considered to be de rigueur for most clinical laboratories conducting work at the BL2 level. There are instances (work with *Mycobacterium tuberculosis*) in which more stringent precautions should be taken and these will be indicated. Situations also arise, especially in smaller laboratories, in which the specific item of equipment called for may not be available; where possible, optional or substitute procedures will be suggested, but short cuts are to be avoided. The work practices described are applicable throughout the clinical laboratory. Improper handling or

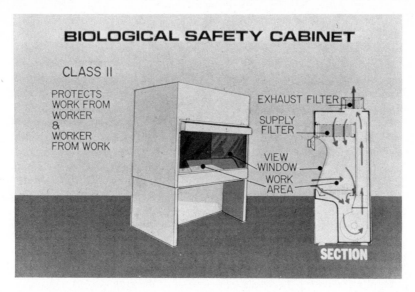

Fig. 2-4   Schematic drawing (including cross-section) of a Class II, Type A laminar flow biological safety cabinet. Air from this cabinet can be either recirculated within the laboratory or exhausted to the outside.

unsafe exposure to chemicals in the laboratory may pose hazards that are as great, or greater, than exposure to infectious agents. The same may also be said for exposures to radioactive materials.

1. Access to the laboratory is controlled; free access or through traffic is not allowed. The laboratory door should remain closed and a sign should be *prominently displayed* on the door, indicating that the room is a clinical laboratory where potentially infectious material and hazardous chemicals may be present. It is impossible to list the actual etiologic agents or chemicals present, but a sign will serve as a warning that a variety of infectious agents or chemicals may be present at any time. This warning is especially useful as an aid to traffic control throughout the laboratory.

2. The laboratory director should be the individual responsible for granting or limiting access to the laboratory. In general, people with immunological deficiencies who are at increased risk of infection or for whom infection may be particularly dangerous, should not be allowed in the laboratory. Other situations, such as pregnancy, should be decided on an individual basis. Children under the age of 16 should not be allowed in the laboratory. Animals not involved in laboratory procedures should never be allowed in the laboratory.

3. Work surfaces should be decontaminated at least once a day and immediately following any spill involving potentially infectious material. In most cases, surfaces can be decontaminated with 70% alcohol, 10% bleach solution, or any other effective disinfectant. The general procedure for handling spills of potentially infectious material is to first absorb any liquid with sorbent paper towels or similar material and then add an appropriate disinfectant, such as sodium hypochlorite solution. When possible, first put on disposable surgical gloves; if not

readily available, all exposed skin should be thoroughly washed with soap and water. The rationale for this procedure is to minimize the potentially infectious aerosol or splatter that may be produced while pouring one liquid directly onto another liquid. Spills should always be reported to the laboratory supervisor and a written report of the incident should be generated as soon as is practical.

4. Mouth pipetting should *never* be permitted. There are mechanical pipetting devices for every laboratory situation and this requirement deals with applying common sense.

5. Eating, drinking, smoking, and applying cosmetics should be strictly prohibited. Food may be stored in cabinets or refrigerators located outside of the work area; these cabinets or refrigerators should not be used for storage of any microbial cultures or microbiological or chemical reagents and supplies.

6. The creation of aerosols should be minimized to the greatest extent possible. This usually requires the development of standard operating procedures (SOP) for all laboratory procedures likely to produce aerosols and the timely review of these SOPs to ensure that personnel are abreast of current technology and take advantage of the latest innovations in safety.

7. Procedures that may produce an infectious or chemical aerosol should be done within a laminar flow biosafety cabinet. It is important that all people who operate such cabinets understand the principles of operation. If a biosafety cabinet is not available in the laboratory, the principles of containment may be achieved by other means. The major concerns in the laboratory are usually of bloodborne and respiratory diseases; protection of open skin and mucous membranes is why aerosols are minimized in the laboratory. What we refer to as an aerosol might better be defined as "splatter" and the aerosols in this case usually consist of particles larger than 5 μm and not

the smaller particles that are small enough to penetrate the deeper reaches of the respiratory system. If a biosafety cabinet is not available, the work should be done in a manner that reduces the risk of droplets coming in contact with skin or mucous membranes. One approach is to perform the work behind a Plexiglas shield or in a Plexiglas box with armholes in either side. Gloves, mask, eye protection, and a laboratory gown with full-length sleeves should be worn if the work must be done at the open bench.

8. Special care should always be taken to avoid contact between broken skin or mucous membranes and potentially infectious material. This usually means wearing gloves for most laboratory work, including drawing blood. Gloves used in the laboratory are usually made of latex or of a vinyl compound, usually polyvinylchloride (PVC). There seems to be no difference in barrier effectiveness between good quality gloves made of either material. One consideration in choosing gloves is the toxic products, such as vinyl chloride and hydrochloric acid, produced when PVC gloves are incinerated.

One area of debate that has arisen regarding the use of gloves by phlebotomists is whether or not they are required to be worn under all conditions in which blood is drawn. Under the concept of "universal precautions," all blood is considered to be potentially infectious, and the current feeling is that gloves should be worn during all phlebotomies. However, some institutions have relaxed these requirements for skilled and experienced phlebotomists in settings where the prevalence of blood-borne pathogens is known to be very low. The argument presented by experienced phlebotomists is that their sense of touch is more acute when not wearing gloves, and therefore, risk of an accidental needlestick is lower. This may be true, especially since gloves do not really act as an effective barrier against needlesticks. With these arguments in mind, the CDC has recommended that institutions that have a "relaxed" glove policy periodically reevaluate that policy. In addition, the CDC has promulgated the following guidelines:

a. Gloves should be worn for phlebotomy whenever the phlebotomist has cuts, scratches, or other skin breaks.

b. Gloves should be worn in situations in which the phlebotomist judges that hand contamination with blood may occur, for example, when drawing blood from an uncooperative patient.

c. Gloves should be used when performing finger and/or heelsticks on infants and children.

d. Gloves should always be used by trainees in phlebotomy.

In addition to these recommendations, several other comments on glove use are in order. Surgical or examination gloves should never be washed or disinfected for re-use. Washing with detergents or surfactants may cause "wicking," the enhanced penetration of liquids through undetected holes in the glove. Also, disinfectants can cause deterioration of the glove material.

9. Hypodermic needles, syringes and needles, and scalpels, collectively referred to as "sharps" are the major source of accidents and infections in health-care workers, including laboratory technologists and phlebotomists. For this reason, it is especially important that laboratory workers, as well as others, use extreme caution in the use and disposal of these items. Needles and syringes should only be used when necessary, for example, as parenteral injection and aspiration of fluids from patients or diaphragm-stoppered bottles. Only needle-locking syringes or disposable syringe-needle units should be used. Needles should not be recapped or removed by hand. Attempts to perform recapping or separating syringes and needles by hand are major causes of needlesticks. Whenever a person's free hand is in the proximity of a syringe, with a needle in the other hand, the potential for an accident is very high. The proper handling of sharps in the hospital and laboratory setting requires common sense, prudence, and knowledge. Needlesticks have occurred when used syringes, capped or uncapped, are placed in the pocket of a laboratory coat, and either the individual wearing the coat or a colleague was subsequently stuck. Using syringes and needles to replace pipettes is not good procedure. Although the syringe, in this case, is clean and the risk of infection is minimal, these syringes often are discarded in the general trash, and their presence is a potential source of injury to the housekeeping staff.

Any soiled sharp, except nondisposable items, should be placed in a sharps disposal container. Needles should be placed in such a container, uncapped, along with used scalpels and other sharps. The sharps container itself must be of rigid construction and leakproof. The top opening should be large enough so that the used sharps can be dropped in the container without the need to force the material into the container. These containers should be placed at convenient locations throughout the laboratory and should have a top that closes easily and tightly when the container is full. When full, the containers should be decontaminated by autoclaving and then the container and its contents should be incinerated. If direct access to an incinerator is impossible, then the container can be sealed and incinerated directly.

Sharps that are to be reused should be discarded into a clean pan, preferably stainless steel, containing a mild detergent and autoclaved promptly after use. These items can then be carefully cleaned, dried, and repackaged for resterilization. It should be noted that too much time in the detergent may dull or cause rust to form on the instruments.

10. All workers must wash their hands immediately after handling any infectious materials, chemicals or animals, and upon leaving the laboratory. Sinks, preferably with foot or elbow controls and located near the exit door, should be available in each laboratory. Because of the number of times hands are washed,

it is probably best to use a mild soap with a lanolin base. Although these soaps are not disinfectants, their use usually removes most of the surface microbes from the skin.

11. Laboratory coats, gowns, smocks, or uniforms should be worn in the laboratory and removed before leaving. Although a regular laboratory coat is sufficient for most clinical laboratory situations, a rear-closing, solid front gown is required when practicing BL3 procedures, such as those used when working with *Mycobacterium tuberculosis*. As a general rule, no special treatment is required for laboratory clothing prior to laundering.

12. In the modern clinical laboratory, sophisticated as well as fairly simple instruments are a potential source of laboratory accidents that may lead to an infection with a biological agent or harmful contact with a chemical or physical agent. Centrifuges are examples of a potential source of aerosols. Centrifuge tubes containing infectious or harmful material should be loaded and unloaded in a biosafety cabinet. It is also prudent to use sealed tubes or safety heads when centrifuging these potentially harmful materials. Automated analyzers are another potential source of danger in the laboratory. Blood or serum samples are often introduced into the instrument under pressure. The potential for splatter is increased if tubing were to come loose or some related malfunction were to occur. Loading samples with a needle and syringe may also increase the potential for aerosolization. It is best to equip such machines with a shield that will protect the worker from splatter while loading the machine. If such shields are not available, the operator should wear eye protection as well as a laboratory coat and gloves while loading the machine. Also, if living cells are used in a cell sorter, a shield should be present, proper personal protective equipment should be worn, and the apparatus should be placed in a separate room that is under negative pressure. Even Vacutainer tubes present some risk from the splatter that may occur when the cork is "popped." There are available blood collection tubes that have screw-on caps that may reduce the likelihood of splatter.

13. The ubiquity of chemicals throughout the clinical laboratory (and the entire institution) is often taken for granted and the potential hazards associated with chemical substances are often ignored. The clinical laboratory must have as part of its overall laboratory safety program a segment that recognizes and deals with the control, prevention, and management of incidents arising from chemical agents. Consequently, all chemical agents, those we work with and those in our day-to-day environment (e.g. toilet bowl cleaners, lead in crystal ware, and ultrafine particles of asbestos in building material), when exposed to or used excessively or indiscriminantly, may result in a reaction ranging from slight discomfort to sudden, acute illness and death. It is an OSHA mandate that laboratories have in place a Chemical Hygiene Plan that includes material safety data sheets (MSDS) on each chemical substance in the laboratory and a continuing education program on chemical safety. The laboratory must have on hand and available for all to read a list of all chemicals stocked and used in the laboratory and the potential hazard category to which each chemical belongs. The hazard categories should be clear and understood by all employees. Some commonly used hazard categories are: toxic substance, corrosive agent, carcinogen, mutagen or teratogen, inflammable agent, explosive agent, and cytotoxic or sensitizing agent. The director of the clinical laboratory is responsible for developing the overall chemical safety guidelines as part of the safety program for the entire laboratory. These guidelines should address risk assessment of chemical agents, protective measures, health hazards, and emergency measures following exposure. The guildines should ensure that chemicals are stored and used properly and that all containers of chemicals have clear, readable labels with appropriate color code approved by the NFPA. (Samples of these color coded labels and their interpretation can be obtained form the National Fire Protection Association, Batterymarch Park, Quincy, MA 02269. Ask for "704 Diamond Identification System.") Additionally each laboratory department should have at least one copy in each major laboratory room of The National Institute for Occupational Safety & Health (NIOSH) "Pocket Guide to Chemical Hazards." These can be obtained from NIOSH, Publications Office, 4676 Columbia Parkway, Cincinnati, OH 45226. This pocket book is an invaluable aid in establishing the required written chemical safety and hygiene program and the MSDS for the clinical laboratory.

14. A rodent and pest control program should be in place for the laboratory as well as all other locations in a health-care setting.

In addition to the above described general work practices that are applicable throughout the clinical laboratory, all laboratory personnel should be mindful of the increasing number of federal, state, and local laws, regulations, guidelines, and standards that are periodically promulgated and apply to activities or procedures conducted in clinical laboratories. To illustrate: On December 6, 1991, OSHA, an agency of the U.S. Department of Labor, published in the Federal Register "The OSHA Bloodborne Pathogens Final Standard." This standard lists a series of key provisions designed to limit exposure of *all* employees who could be reasonably anticipated to come into contact with blood or other potentially infectious materials (all body fluids, excreta, exudates, transudates) as a result of performing their duties. Employers are required to have a written exposure control plan that spells out in some detail the tasks and procedures and job classifications of those laboratory personnel where occupational exposure to blood and other body fluids may occur. The bloodborne pathogens include, but are not limited to, Hepatitis B virus (HBV) and Human immunodeficiency virus (HIV). The standard also mandates work practices such as universal precautions, use of protective equipment, decontamination of work site, handling sharps, wastes, and specimens, use of appropriate warning labels and biohazard symbols on containers, refrigerators, etc., record keeping on all employees and an ongoing periodic training program for all employees on how to comply with all aspects of the standard. Every laboratory should obtain a copy of the OSHA Bloodborne Standard (and other OSHA directives) and review it frequently to ensure compliance with all of the requirements. It can be obtained from OSHA Technical Data Center, 200 Constitution Ave. NW, Washington, D.C. 20402.

MEDICAL WASTE

Considerable interest has been generated on the topic of medical waste, especially following the washup of debris that included some medical waste on East Coast beaches. It was felt that some of this waste may have been generated by hospitals and related health-care facilities. The culmination of this interest in medical waste has been the passage of a federal law, the Medical Waste Tracking Act of 1988 (MWTA). Under the act, in certain coastal states, the United States Environmental Protection Agency (EPA) has established demonstration projects designed to track medical waste from "cradle to grave." The purpose of the demonstration projects is to assess whether or not such tracking systems are necessary at the national level. The act also requires the EPA to determine: the types, number, and size of generators of medical waste (including small-quantity generators) in the United States; the types and amounts of medical waste generated; and the on-site and off-site methods currently used to handle, store, transport, treat, and dispose of the medical waste, including the extent to which such waste is disposed of in sewer systems. The EPA is also examining the present or potential threat to human health and the environment posed by medical waste and its incineration, and will assess other available and potentially available methods for tracking medical waste.

The act also mandates the Agency for Toxic Substance and Disease Registry (ATSDR) to prepare for Congress a report on the health effects of medical waste. This report will include a description of the potential for infection or injury from the segregation, handling, storage, treatment, or disposal of medical waste. The report will also include estimates of the number of people injured or infected annually by sharps and an estimate of the number of people infected by other means related to waste segregation, handling, storage, treatment, or disposal and the nature and seriousness of those infections, if any. Finally, ATSDR has been asked to report diseases possibly spread by medical waste, including acquired immune deficiency syndrome and hepatitis B, and an estimate of what percentage of the total number of cases nationally may be traceable to medical wastes.

Regardless of what may happen in the future, for the time being, most medical waste regulations, except in those states participating in the EPA demonstration program, emanate from the individual states and are variable but have general themes. The definition of medical waste found in the MWTA is "any solid waste which is generated in the diagnosis, treatment, or immunization of human beings or animals, in research pertaining thereto, or in the production and testing of biologicals." There may be several other definitions of medical waste, but they are all quite similar. Of the estimated 160 million tons of solid waste generated each year in the United States, 3.2 million tons is thought to be medical waste from hospitals. This waste includes administrative papers and records, wrappers from medical devices, containers such as intravenous bags and used vials, syringes, and needles, and other disposable items such as tongue depressors and thermometer covers. The Environmental Protection Agency estimates that 10% to 15% of medical waste is potentially infectious.

Until a national policy for the handling of medical waste is developed, each institution must develop a rational medical waste program based on good infection control practice and local waste regulations. To begin with, there is no evidence that presently accepted waste disposal methods are contributing to human or environmental health hazards. Moreover, there is no documented epidemiologic evidence that current health-care related waste disposal practices have ever caused disease in a community. There is also no epidemiological evidence to suggest that most waste generated by hospitals, other health-care facilities, or clinical/diagnostic/research laboratories is any more infectious than residential waste. Nonetheless, there are four classes of medical waste that are generally considered to be potentially infectious. These are: microbiology laboratory waste, pathology laboratory waste, blood specimens or blood products, and the general category of sharps. Every health-care institution should establish an infectious waste disposal plan. Such a plan should consist of three basic elements: identification of potentially infectious material; proper handling, transportation, and storage of such material; and appropriate processing and disposal of this waste.

It is important to identify potentially infectious waste so that it can be segregated from the main waste stream and treated properly to comply with local regulations. It is also important to segregate potentially infectious waste, because if all waste is treated as potentially infectious, the cost of waste management can become prohibitive. Proper handling usually involves the assurance that waste is placed in designated containers and decontaminated in a timely manner using proper technology. Containers should be leakproof and of construction rigid enough to preclude leakage or puncture during transportation. Waste should only be handled by those who have been trained in the proper handling procedures. If contaminated waste must remain for any length of time before proper disposal, it should be placed in a secured area accessible only to those who are responsible for waste disposal.

The EPA estimates that about 70% of hospital waste is incinerated on-site, which is the method of choice. The alternate method is to decontaminate the waste in an autoclave followed by removal to a landfill. This is a well-documented means of decontamination and is another method of choice. Some local laws require that any infectious waste not only be decontaminated, but that it be rendered unrecognizable as medical waste. All animals and human body parts must be incinerated. If infectious waste is to be transported off-site for treatment, it must be packed in a sealed container and transported via a certified carrier who will ensure that the waste arrives at the proper location and that it is disposed of properly.

Other waste disposal technologies are currently being developed and must be evaluated regarding effectiveness and applicability. New technology includes chemical inactivation of waste, oxidation of waste materials, and thermal disinfection.

PACKING AND SHIPPING OF DIAGNOSTIC SPECIMENS, BIOLOGICAL PRODUCTS, AND ETIOLOGICAL AGENTS

Operation of a clinical laboratory usually requires receiving or shipping diagnostic materials or etiologic agents to or from the laboratory. Because these shipments may contain infectious agents, their transportation is regulated by three U.S. government agencies, each of which has issued guidelines or regulations. The Department of Transportation (DOT) is responsible for the safe transportation of hazardous materials between states and to foreign countries. The DOT governs all means of transportation except shipping by mail, which is covered by the U.S. Postal Service (USPS). The DOT regulations are found in the Code of Federal Regulations (CFR), Title 49, Parts 100-199 and the USPS regulations are found in 39CFR, Part 123. The Postal Service regulations have recently been updated (Federal Register, vol 54, no. 156, August 15, 1989). The USPS requirements applicable to the mailing of "diseased tissue, blood, serum, and cultures of pathogenic microorganisms" are listed in the *Postal Service Manual.*

The U.S. Public Health Service's (PHS) authority to govern the shipment of etiologic agents was delegated to the Centers For Disease Control (CDC) in 1971. The current regulation, entitled "Interstate Shipment of Etiologic Agents" (42CFR, Part 72), was last revised in 1980 and is currently undergoing another revision (see Federal Register, vol 55, no. 42, March 2, 1990). The regulation defines the terms "diagnostic specimen," "biological product," and "etiologic agent" and gives minimum packaging requirements and volume limits for each.

The regulation defines a diagnostic specimen as "any human or animal material including, but not limited to, excreta, secreta, blood and its components, tissue, and tissue fluids shipped for the purposes of diagnosis." With regard to packaging, the rule states that no person may knowingly transport or cause to be transported, in interstate traffic, directly or indirectly, any material including, but not limited to, diagnostic specimens and biological products that such person reasonably believes may contain an etiologic agent unless such material is packaged to withstand leakage of contents, shocks, pressure changes, and other conditions incident to ordinary handling in transportation. The major decision to be made then, when determining the transport requirements for any sample, is whether or not it contains an etiologic agent. It is prudent to be conservative in this matter and assume that each specimen may contain an agent unless you are certain that it does not. The current USPS regulations do not require an outside package label for diagnostic samples. The revised regulation will require a sticker on the mailing container and may also require upgraded, performance-oriented, packaging requirements.

The current requirements for mailing etiologic agents are somewhat more strict. For the regulation, an etiologic agent means "a viable microorganism or its toxin which causes, or may cause, human disease." The packaging of etiologic agents requires triple packaging that includes a securely closed, watertight, primary container that is enclosed in a second durable watertight container. Several primary containers may be placed in a single secondary container as long as the total volume does not exceed 50 ml. The space between each single or multiple primary container and the secondary container must contain enough absorbent material to absorb all of the contents of the primary container in case of leakage (Figure 2-5). Each set of primary and secondary containers is then enclosed in an outer shipping container constructed of fiberboard, cardboard, wood, or other material of equivalent strength. An etiologic agent/biomedical

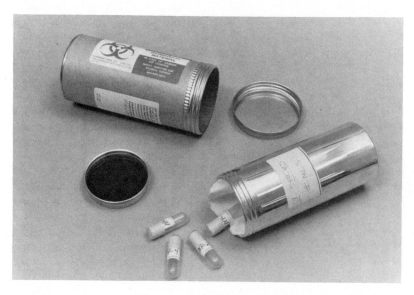

Fig. 2-5 Photograph demonstrating a proper way to package etiologic agents for shipment. Shown are the sealed primary containers, a secondary container with absorbent material, and a properly labeled shipping container.

material adhesive label is required for the outer mailing package.

A benchmark of all good, reliable clinical laboratories is the ability to produce accurate analyses on clinical specimens in a timely manner in a safe and pleasant work environment. Laboratory safety does not just happen; it is the end result of everyone who works in the laboratory. Laboratory safety must be part of an ongoing, in-house continuing education program with the laboratory's safety manuals the focus for discussion, improvement, and necessary implementation. With a positive approach to safety and good health for the entire staff, the clinical laboratory can become the model for safety and health in the work place for the entire institution.

SUGGESTED READING

Centers for Disease Control: Recommendations for prevention of HIV transmission in health-care settings, Morbidity and Mortality Weekly Report 36(2S):1987.

Centers for Disease Control: Update: human immunodeficiency virus infections in health-care workers exposed to blood of infected patients, Morbidity and Mortality Weekly Report 36:285, 1987.

Centers for Disease Control: Agent summary statement for human immunodeficiency viruses (HIVs) including HTLV-III, LAV, HIV-1 and HIV-2, Morbidity and Mortality Weekly Report 37(S-4):1, 1988.

Centers for Disease Control: Update: universal precautions for prevention of transmission of human immunodeficiency virus, hepatitis B virus, and other bloodborne pathogens in health-care settings, Morbidity and Mortality Weekly Report 37(24):377, 1988.

Centers for Disease Control: Public Health Service Statement on management of occupational exposure to human immunodeficiency virus, including considerations regarding zidovudine postexposure use, Morbidity and Mortality Weekly Report 39(RR-1):1990.

*Committee on Hazardous Biological Substances in the Laboratory, Board on Chemical Sciences and Technology, Commission on Physical Sciences, Mathematics, and Resources National Research Council: Biosafety in the laboratory: prudent practices for the handling and disposal of infectious materials, National Academy Press, 1989.

Department of Labor: Occupational safety and health administration. 29 CFR Part 1910. Occupational exposures to hazardous chemicals in laboratories. Agency: Occupational Safety and Health Administration (OSHA), Labor. Action: final rule, 1990.

*Miller BM and others (editors): Laboratory safety: principles and practices, Washington, DC: American Society for Microbiology, 1986.

*National Committee for Clinical Laboratory Standards (NCCLS): Protection of laboratory workers from infectious disease transmitted by blood and tissue. Proposed guidelines 7(9):325. NCCLS Document M29-P, Villanova, Pa: NCCLS, 1987.

Pike RM: Laboratory-associated infections: incidence, fatalities, causes, and prevention, Ann Rev Microbiol 33:41, 1979.

*Richardson JH and Barkley WE (editors): Biosafety in microbiological and biomedical laboratories. U.S. Public Health Service. Centers for Disease Control and National Institutes of Health. HHS publication no. (CDC) 84-8395, Washington, DC: U.S. Government Printing Office, 1988.

Rayburn SR: The foundations of laboratory safety: a guide for the biomedical laboratory, New York, 1990, Springer-Verlag.

Richardson JH and others (editors): Proceedings of the 1985 institute on critical issues in health laboratory practice: safety management in the public health laboratory, Wilmington, Del: E.I. du Pont de Nemours and Company, 1986.

U.S. Department of Health and Human Services: Laboratory safety monograph: a supplement to the NIH guidelines for recombinant DNA research. Bethesda, Md: U.S. Public Health Service, National Institutes of Health, 1979.

U.S. Department of Health and Human Services: Code of Federal Regulations Title 42, Part 72, Interstate shipment of etiologic agents, Washington, DC: U.S. Government Printing Office, 1980. (Proposed revision of 42 CFR, part 72, published in the Federal Register, vol 55, no. 42, March 2, 1990).

U.S. Department of Health and Human Services, National Institutes of Health: Guidelines for research involving recombinant DNA molecules: notice. Federal Register, vol 51, no. 88, May 7, 1986.

*U.S. Department of Health and Human Services, Department of Labor: Occupational safety and health administration occupational exposure to bloodborne pathogens (proposed rule), Federal Register, vol 54, no. 102, p. 231-34.

U.S. Department of Transportation: U.S. Code of Federal Regulations, Title 49, Parts 100-199, Washington, DC: U.S. Government Printing Office.

3

Sample collection and processing

Joanne M. Griffith

The quality and reliability of laboratory results depend on the proper and timely collection and processing of specimens. The most expensive and technologically advanced equipment; the most highly skilled, dedicated laboratory scientists; the most modern, well-designed facility will produce erroneous laboratory data if the specimen is drawn from the wrong patient, transported too late to be useful, or processed improperly.

TEST ORDERING
Patient preparation and sample collection manual

In order to provide information to the medical and nursing staff, laboratory personnel must publish a manual that outlines the laboratory's important characteristics and describes the services it provides. This manual should state the location of the laboratory and its operating hours, list key staff members, and provide other useful demographic information. It should list the following for each test:

Laboratory test name (with synonyms)
Assay schedule and turnaround time
Patient preparation instructions
Specimen type and amount
Collection container and instructions
Requisition or computer code used to order the test

Requisition forms and computer order entry

An order for laboratory work is initiated by the patient's physician. This order is transferred to the laboratory, usually by a nursing clerk, by either filling out a paper requisition or mark-sense card, or by entering the order into a computer terminal. The information that should be included as a part of the test order is listed in Box 3-1.

BLOOD COLLECTION EQUIPMENT

Blood, a suspension of cells in a protein- and salt-rich liquid, is the sample most frequently used for laboratory analysis. It is used in one of three forms:

1. Whole blood prevented from clotting by exposing it to an anticoagulant during collection
2. Serum, the liquid, noncellular portion of clotted blood
3. Plasma, the liquid, noncellular portion of anticoagulated blood

The phlebotomist is a person who obtains a blood sample; the term is from the Greek word for "vein" (phlebos) and "to cut" (tome), literally meaning "one who cuts a vein." The phlebotomist may collect a venous (venipuncture), or capillary (heel, finger, or earlobe puncture), or arterial blood specimen.

The phlebotomy tray and blood collection equipment

The equipment used to obtain a blood specimen is ordinarily organized and transported on a tray or cart. Supplies commonly used in phlebotomy are listed in Box 3-2.

Venipuncture equipment
Needles

Needles are made in many lengths and diameters. The diameter of a needle is referred to as gauge; the larger the diameter, the lower the gauge number. Needles used for collecting blood samples for laboratory tests are usually 20, 21, or 22 gauge. A needle should be selected based on the patient's physical characteristics and the amount of blood to be drawn. Patients with poor or small veins should be punctured using a smaller needle, such as 22 gauge, or 23 gauge winged infusion sets.

Box 3-1 Information required on a laboratory requisition

Patient name	Person placing the order
Identification number	Collection date/time or
Date of birth	expected time
Sex	Collection and testing
Location	priorities
Admitting physician	Specimen (for non-blood
Requesting physician	specimens)
Ordering date/time	Test(s) to be performed

Optional

Diagnosis
Infectious diagnosis
Antibiotic therapy

Box 3-2 Supplies carried on a phlebotomy tray or cart

Evacuated collection sets needles, adapter, tubes
Syringes and syringe needles
Butterfly sets (multiple sample luer adapter)
Tourniquets
Lancets
Microcollection containers and caps or sealing clay
Infant heel warmers (sodium thiosulfate packs)
Microscope slides
70% isopropyl alcohol preps

Iodine
Green soap swabs
Gauze pads
Adhesive bandages or sterile gauze with tape
Bleeding time templates
Filter paper
Needle removal and disposal container
Personal protective equipment (gloves, masks, goggles)
Marking pen

Table 3-1 Color coding of evacuated tubes

Color	Additive	Yields	Use
Red	None	Serum	Chemistry, serology, blood bank
Lavender	Na or K EDTA	Whole blood	Hematology
Blue	Sodium citrate	Plasma	Coagulation
Green	Na or Li heparin	Plasma	Chemistry
Gray	K oxalate (inhibits glycolysis)	Plasma	Glucose testing
Royal	None or heparin	Serum or plasma	Trace elements

The length of the needle varies between ½ to 1 ½ inch; the size chosen depends on the depth of the vein and the preference of the phlebotomist. Some phlebotomists feel they have better control with a shorter needle.

The sharp tip of the needle is known as the bevel, the shaft gives it its length, and the hub is the part that attaches to the holder or syringe. The lumen is the inside diameter of the needle and determines the rate of flow of the blood through a needle. A smaller lumen may contribute to hemolysis because of the more rapid flow and greater shearing action.

Evacuated collection system

An evacuated collection system consists of a needle, a tube-needle holder (or "adapter"), and collection tube(s). The needle used in an evacuated collection system is pointed on both ends; the longer end penetrates the vein, the shorter end extends into the barrel and penetrates the rubber stopper of the vacuum tube. When the stopper of the tube is punctured by the recessed end of the needle, the vacuum inside the tube draws the blood into the tube. This needle may also have a rubber sleeve to prevent blood from leaking into the adapter when multiple tubes are collected.

The adapter is the device that holds the needle and tube together during collection. It is made of a see-through plastic so that blood flow can be observed. Each manufacturer of blood-collecting supplies has engineered its adapter to precisely fit its own needle, so an adapter should not be used with another brand of needle.

Evacuated collection tubes are manufactured to draw a measured volume of blood, which is determined by the size of the tube and its vacuum. A variety of fill volumes are available, from as small as 2 ml up to 20 ml. The most commonly used sizes are 5, 7, and 10 ml, although, because of the smaller volume of blood used by most of today's

analyzers, many laboratories are using tubes that draw a smaller volume of blood.

The interior of all collection tubes should be sterile so that bacteria are not introduced into the bloodstream if a backflow of blood from the tube to the vein occurs. Trace metal analysis (e.g., analysis for lead, mercury, arsenic, aluminum) requires tubes that are certified to be metal-free.

Silicon prevents a blood clot from dragging or adhering to the wall of a tube. There is less chance of hemolysis when silicon-coated tubes are used.

A variety of collection tubes are available that contain additives or anticoagulants used to prepare specimens for different testing needs. Tubes may contain a gel and/or clot enhancer. The color of the stopper of a collection tube is coded to indicate what, if anything, has been added to the tube. A list of the most commonly used evacuated tubes is presented in Table 3-1. While there is some uniformity in the color coding of stoppers, variability of color codings exists among different manufacturers.

Syringes

Most syringes in use today are made of plastic, although glass ones are occasionally used for special procedures. They are available in many sizes (e.g., 5, 12, 20, 35, and 60 ml).

Syringes have two primary parts, the barrel and the plunger, which fit tightly together. When the plunger is drawn back, the vacuum created draws blood into the barrel. The blood is then dispensed into test tubes, usually the same tubes used in evacuated collection systems.

Winged infusion set

A winged infusion ("butterfly") set is a stainless steel beveled needle that is connected by a length of tubing to a blood delivery device. A syringe is attached to this device when drawing blood from fragile veins like those in the hand. The winged infusion set may alternately be fitted with a luer adapter, which has a needle, possibly with a multisample sheath, to directly fill evacuated tubes.

The winged infusion set is held by gripping together the plastic winglike (hence the term "butterfly set") tabs on either side of the needle. The beveled needle (usually 23 gauge, ¾ inch long) is inserted into the vein; when vacuum is supplied at the other end, by a syringe or an evacuated tube, blood flows through the tubing into the evacuated tube or syringe barrel.

The use of this type of collection device is indicated in patients with small or fragile veins because it gives the phlebotomist much finer control of the needle. When performing a foot puncture, the phlebotomist can get a better angle on the vein without being hindered by the adapter or syringe.

Tourniquets

Tourniquets are usually strips or tubing made of latex or rubber, ¾- to 1-inch wide and 14- to 18-inches long. The tourniquet is tightly wrapped around the patient's arm 2 to 3 inches above the venipuncture site. The ends may be tucked under or tied, or some are fastened with Velcro pieces at either end.

Skin puncture equipment
Lancets

Lancets are small plastic devices with sharp metal tips used to puncture the skin and cause blood to flow from the capillaries. The depth of the puncture is controlled by a protective flange surrounding the tip. Lancets are sterile when packaged and should be used only once, then discarded.

Spring-loaded devices can be used with lancets to deliver an automatic and quick puncture. These are often used by diabetic patients who must draw their own capillary samples for glucose monitoring.

Microsample containers

There are many types of microsample collection containers available (Box 3-3). Skin puncture specimens may be collected drop by drop through the collector top of a microcollection device or by capillary action into small or large bore capillary tubes.

Microsample tubes are available with or without additives; they should be chosen based on the type of test(s) to be performed. Heparin is the most commonly found additive for plasma samples. Hematology specimens should be collected into tubes containing ethylenediamine tetraacetic acid (EDTA) because this additive is least likely to distort blood cell morphology.

Heel warmer

A heel warmer is a packet of chemicals (sodium thiosulfate and glycerin) that reacts to create an exothermic chemical reaction. It provides a controlled temperature (40° C) heat source, which is helpful when trying to increase blood flow to skin puncture sites.

The chemicals should be activated by wrapping the packet with a towel or cloth, holding it away from the

---

> **Box 3-3** Microsample collection containers
>
> Plastic microsample tubes (e.g., Microtainer, Becton Dickinson and Company)
> Small-bore capillary pipettes (e.g., microhematocrit tubes)
> Large-bore capillary pipettes (e.g., Caraway/Natelson pipettes)
> Micropipette and dilution systems (e.g., Unopette, Becton Dickinson and Company)
> Test tubes

---

face, and squeezing the packet. It should then be gently kneaded to mix the chemicals, and the cloth-covered packet should be applied to the skin puncture site for 3 to 5 minutes.

Miscellaneous blood collection equipment
Skin cleaning supplies

Isopropyl alcohol (70%) is the antiseptic most commonly used to cleanse the puncture site of skin flora bacteria. It should not be used, however, when collecting blood for ethanol determinations (especially in legal cases) since not all methods of assay are specific for ethyl alcohol. An iodine-containing antiseptic must be used, however, when blood cultures are drawn, so that the skin is made as sterile as possible. Iodine should not be used when collecting skin puncture samples for chemical testing. Green soap swabs or a second vigorous alcohol scrub can be used if the patient is allergic to iodine.

Gauze pads or cotton balls may be used with the disinfectant when cleansing the puncture site. Gauze is also used when removing the needle to apply pressure to the wound. Adhesive bandages or tape can be used to help control bleeding from the site of a venipuncture.

Needle removal/disposal containers

Needles, lancets, razor or scalpel blades, broken glass, or any other similarly sharp item that might cause a cut or puncture, must be disposed in a specially designed "sharps" container. Most of these containers have needle removal devices to safely remove the needle from an evacuated collection holder. Needles must never be recapped using two hands.

Each of these devices works in a slightly different manner and a description of each follows.

The Vacutainer Brand sharps container (Becton Dickinson Vacutainer Systems, Becton Dickinson and Company, Rutherford, NJ) consists of a yellow box with a red lid; it has slots to place a needle cap to assist recapping after the venipuncture.

- When ready to begin the venipuncture, remove the sheath of the needle and place it in the small opening in the lid of the needle box.
- After drawing the blood specimen, insert the contaminated needle down into the sheath, securing tightly.
- Pull out the entire device and unscrew the capped needle from the adapter or syringe.
- Discard the dirty needle into the large opening of this box.

The Sharps-A-Gator sharps container (Sharps-A-Gator sharps collection system, Devon Industries, Inc., Chatsworth, CA) consists of a large red box; it has slots to place a needle cap to assist recapping after the venipuncture. It is used in the same way as the Vacutainer system, but because of its size, it is better suited for use at a stationary site.

A simple block of wood that has holes drilled to hold needle caps can be used to recap a vacuum-tube type needle without risking a needlestick injury. This is an easy, portable device to carry to the bedside.

- When ready to begin the venipuncture, remove the sheath of the needle and place it in the opening of the wooden block.
- After drawing the blood, insert the contaminated needle down into the sheath, securing it tightly.
- Pull out the entire device and unscrew the capped needle from the adapter or syringe.
- Discard the dirty needle in an approved sharps container.

Marking pens

Marking pens with indelible ink are used to write identification information on the specimen label. Microscope slides should be carried in the event that direct peripheral or malarial blood smears have been requested.

Protective equipment

A laboratory coat that is impervious to blood should be worn when performing venipunctures and capillary punctures.

Gloves should be made available to all phlebotomists for use at their discretion. However, gloves must be worn (1) if the phlebotomist has cuts, scratches, or other breaks in the skin; (2) when performing a phlebotomy on an uncooperative patient; (3) when performing finger or heel sticks; and (4) by all persons receiving phlebotomy training. If gloves are worn, they should be put on immediately before applying the tourniquet. If it is difficult to palpate the vein, this may be done bare-fingered and the gloves should be donned immediately preceding the puncture. Gloves should be removed right before leaving the room, after contact with each patient.

Because of the potential for blood to spray, facial protection is recommended during an arterial puncture.

METHODS OF BLOOD COLLECTION
Blood collection by venipuncture
The venipuncture procedure

Good venipuncture technique assiduously follows a step-by-step protocol without exception. These steps are summarized in Box 3-4.

Step 1: Prepare accession order. Orders for tests to be collected by laboratory personnel are assembled and sorted in the laboratory according to patient and collection time. The paper requisitions or computer-printed labels must be organized and allocated to the phlebotomist or the phlebotomy team in a time-efficient manner. Usually, specimen accession numbers are assigned at this time.

Step 2: Interview the patient. The patient will form opinions about the competence of the phlebotomist, and

---

Box 3-4   Venipuncture procedure

1. Prepare accession order
2. Interview the patient
   a. Introduction and informed consent
   b. Identification
   c. Determining patient readiness
   d. Reassuring the patient
3. Assemble supplies
4. Verify paperwork and tubes
5. Position the patient
   a. Seated patient
   b. Patient lying down
6. Apply tourniquet
7. Select vein site
   a. Preferred veins
   b. Procedure for vein selection
   c. Factors to consider in site selection
8. Cleanse venipuncture site
9. Perform the venipuncture
10. Bandage patient's arm
11. Fill the tubes (if collection is by syringe)
12. Dispose of puncturing unit
13. Chill or warm specimen (if indicated)
14. Identify specimen
15. Eliminate diet restrictions
16. Record collection time

---

secondarily of the laboratory, within seconds after the phlebotomist enters the room, based on the manner and appearance of the phlebotomist. The ability to project a professional appearance and manner comes from the confidence of being well trained and prepared; it reassures the patient that he or she is dealing with a competent member of the health care team.

When greeting a patient, the phlebotomist should introduce himself or herself and state that he or she is from the laboratory and is going to draw a blood sample for a test ordered by the patient's physician. As a part of the principle of informed consent, the patient must understand what is to be done and have the opportunity to refuse this procedure.

The most important step (and the easiest one to take for granted) in the venipuncture procedure is to properly identify the patient. Drawing blood from the wrong patient can have serious repercussions—from being transfused with an incompatible blood type to having a physician make an incorrect diagnosis or give the wrong treatment based on erroneous results.

The patient should be asked to state his or her name; ill or elderly patients might not hear or understand and incorrectly agree to the question, "Are you Mrs. Price?"

A hospitalized patient should be wearing an identification bracelet displaying his or her name and identification number. This information should be compared to that on the paper requisitions or computer-printed labels. If the patient is not wearing an identification bracelet, the nurse should be asked to identify and place the correct identification bracelet on the patient.

In an outpatient setting it might be appropriate to ask the patient to state his or her full name and some additional information listed on the requisition, such as date of birth, address, or doctor's name.

If the test to be done requires a special state of readiness such as fasting, the phlebotomist should verify that the patient is properly prepared. Common procedures that are affected by eating are glucose (increased), inorganic phosphorus (decreased), and triglycerides (increased).

Reassuring the patient. The phlebotomist must gain the confidence of the patient and reassure him or her that, while the procedure won't be painless, it will be only of a short duration. At each step the patient should be told exactly what is going to happen. If, during the venipuncture, the patient becomes alarmed by the amount of blood being taken, reassure him or her that the quantity (usually 5 to 50 ml) is really quite small. Compare it to his or her total blood volume (5 L) or to the amount safely taken when a unit of blood is donated (450 ml).

Step 3: Assemble supplies. The phlebotomist should assemble all of the equipment needed to properly perform the venipuncture. In most cases an evacuated collection system will be used; a syringe or winged infusion set will be used, however, if the phlebotomist determines that the patient has fragile or rolling veins.

The appropriate size needle should be selected based on the patient's physical characteristics and amount of blood to be drawn. All collection tubes should be assembled for the tests ordered; prechilled or prewarmed tubes should be prepared, if necessary. The phlebotomist should also choose the antiseptic and gather the necessary tourniquet, gauze pads, and bandages.

If an evacuated system is used, the phlebotomist should assemble the system by screwing the needle into the plastic adapter until it is secure. The first collection tube to be drawn should be inserted into the holder, onto the recessed needle tip, up to the guideline on the holder.

If a syringe is indicated, a syringe needle should be twisted onto the hub of the syringe. The collection tubes needed should be left on the tray so that they can be filled while standing in a rack and on a stable surface.

Step 4: Verify paperwork and tubes. This step must be done to check that the equipment and tubes selected are appropriate for the tests ordered on the requisition.

Step 5: Position the patient. The patient should be placed in a comfortable and safe position, either seated or lying down. Avoid startling the patient, such as by sudden awakening, and be sure there is nothing such as food, gum, or a thermometer in the patient's mouth.

Seated patient. If seated, the patient's arm should be extended across the arm of a phlebotomy chair or firmly positioned on a table or bed. The arm should be straight from shoulder to wrist. A roll of towels or a pillow may be used to help comfortably position and secure the arm.

Patient lying down. If lying down, the patient should be asked to lie on his or her back with an arm extended so that it is straight from shoulder to wrist.

Step 6: Apply tourniquet. A tourniquet is used to help visualize and gain access to the vein by slowing the return of venous blood from the arm. It should be applied 2 to 3 inches above the vein to be punctured.

If using a vein in the antecubital fossa, the tourniquet should be placed around the patient's arm between the elbow and shoulder. The patient should be asked to make a fist, but should avoid vigorous "pumping." This pumping action might cause hemoconcentration, an increased concentration of formed elements and other large molecules in the blood sample.

The tourniquet should be applied tight enough to restrict venous flow, but not tight enough to occlude arterial flow. Because restricted blood flow disrupts the normal balance of blood cells and fluids, and consequently affects test results, the tourniquet should never be left on the arm for more than 1 minute. If the venipuncture is delayed, the tourniquet should be loosened and reapplied immediately before the puncture, or hemoconcentration might result.

Step 7: Select vein site

Preferred veins. For most adult patients, the preferred sites for the puncture are the three veins located in the center of the arm at the bend of the elbow—the antecubital fossa. The median cubital vein, the center of the three veins, is the first choice because it is usually large, easily accessible, and less painful to the patient.

The second choices would be either the cephalic or basilic veins located to the right and left of the median cubital vein. However, these veins tend to roll and are also more easily bruised. Also, blood will flow more slowly from the cephalic vein.

Hand and wrist veins should only be used after checking both arms. They are much more fragile and painful to draw from. Avoid the 2-inch area on the volar surface of the wrist; this area is concentrated with many nerves. Small-bore butterfly needles should be considered when drawing from these sites.

Venipuncture from the lower extremities is not recommended because frequent complications arise from their use for venipuncture. It is often best to call in another phlebotomist before using leg, ankle, or foot veins.

Procedure for vein selection. The phlebotomist should always palpate the vein and trace its path with the index finger; the vein should feel soft and spongy. A pulsating vessel is an artery and should not be punctured. Anything that feels hard or nonpliable should be avoided; it may be a tendon, muscle, or scarred vein.

If a suitable vein is not apparent, the phlebotomist can tap the site with the index and second finger a few times, massage the arm from wrist to elbow, or apply a warm (40° C) cloth to the site. If there is still no vein apparent, the opposite arm should be checked.

Factors to consider in site selection. Other factors that will affect which site is selected for venipuncture are described.

Intravenous therapy. The most frequent problem to deal with in vein selection is the presence of an intravenous IV device in a patient's arm. Specimens should be collected from the arm without the IV device, if possible. If it is necessary to draw blood from an arm with an IV device, never draw from above the IV needle. Satisfactory samples may be obtained by drawing below the IV needle by having it turned off for at least 2 minutes before the venipuncture. Select a vein other than the one with the IV device; draw a 5-ml discard sample before drawing the specimen for analysis.

Scarring. Avoid healed burn areas or sites that are scarred because of repeated venipunctures, surgery, or trauma.

Mastectomy. Because of lymphostasis, specimens taken from the side on which a mastectomy was performed may not be representative samples. The arm may also be very sensitive and subject to swelling.

Hematoma. Specimens collected near a hematoma may be affected by the bruise. If the site must be used, make the puncture distal (in a line away from the heart) to the hematoma.

Lines, catheters, heparin locks. These are all indwelling devices used to maintain vascular access. Specimens should only be drawn by specially trained personnel; ordinarily, phlebotomists do not draw from these devices.

Because heparin is frequently used to flush these lines, a specimen at least three times the volume of the line should be removed and discarded before the specimen is collected.

Fistula. A fistula is a surgical fusion of an artery and vein to facilitate vascular access for dialysis. An arm bearing an arteriovenous fistula should not be used for venipuncture unless the physician authorizes it.

Step 8: Cleanse venipuncture site. The venipuncture site should be cleansed with an antiseptic such as 70% alcohol. Vigorously rub the site with the antiseptic-soaked pad in concentric circles, working from the inside out. The antiseptic should be allowed to dry because it may interfere with the test, and it will also cause stinging when the skin is punctured. If the site is touched again, it must be cleansed again.

An antiseptic other than alcohol should be used if a legal blood alcohol test is to be performed on the sample.

If blood cultures are to be drawn, a special decontamination procedure is needed to obtain a sterile site. Refer to Chapter 39 for a complete description of this procedure.

Step 9: Perform the venipuncture. Before performing the venipuncture, inspect the needle (and syringe, if used). When ready to begin the puncture, remove the cap from the needle by pulling in an even outward motion that avoids nicking the tip. The sterile needle should not be contaminated by touching anything. Check the needle for burrs on the tip and for obstructions in the opening. If a syringe is to be used, the plunger within the barrel should be aspirated by pulling back and forth to assure its free movement. (This motion, however, should be avoided when drawing blood for culture to maintain an anaerobic state.)

Next, the phlebotomist should anchor the vein by placing his or her thumb 1 or 2 inches below the venipuncture site and drawing the skin taut by stretching it toward the patient's hand. The phlebotomist's other four fingers should be used to grasp the back of the patient's arm. In this position, the vein will be held stationary; the patient's pain will also be lessened.

To align and insert the needle, the syringe or adapter should be held in the dominant hand with the thumb on top, fingers underneath. The needle should be aligned in the direction of the vein. With the bevel up, the needle should be inserted at a 15° angle to the skin. There will initially be some resistance, but the phlebotomist will feel a release when the needle has penetrated the wall of the vein. The patient's arm should be kept in a downward position to prevent backflow of blood from the collection tube.

Grasp the adapter and push the tube onto it. With one hand holding the adapter, the phlebotomist should grasp the flange of the adapter with fingers of the other hand. The tube is pushed forward with the thumb while gripping the adapter with the fingers and thumb of the other hand (to minimize movement of the needle) until the cap is pierced by the inside needle.

The vacuum of the tube will draw the blood into it; the tube should be filled until the vacuum is exhausted and the flow stops. The assembly should be held downward so that the blood does not contact the stopper. When full, the tube should be gently removed from the adapter. Tubes containing additives should be immediately mixed by gentle inversion.

If a syringe is used instead of an evacuated collection set, the phlebotomist should pull gently on the plunger when the needle is located in the vein. If the plunger is pulled back too quickly, the strong vacuum created may cause the vein to collapse, especially if the vein is small.

The inability to draw a specimen can be caused by several factors. Blood may not flow into the evacuated tube or the syringe because the needle may not have been inserted into the vein deeply enough, or it may have gone all the way through the vein. The phlebotomist may be holding the bevel of the needle against the vein wall, or may have laterally missed entering the vein at all.

When this happens, the phlebotomist should feel the point of the needle under the skin with the forefinger of the free hand. The following procedure should be used to redirect the needle:
- If the needle is touching the wall of the vein, pull the needle back slightly and redirect the needle into the vein, then apply vacuum (syringe or evacuated tube).
- If the needle is not inserted all the way into the vein, move the needle deeper using minute movements and apply vacuum.
- If the needle has gone through the vein, pull the needle back using minute movements until it is in the lumen of the vein. It is quite likely in this case that a hematoma is forming; unless the venipuncture can be quickly completed, withdraw completely and try again at a new site.

Blood may sometimes fail to flow because the tube has lost its vacuum, either during manufacturing or by puncture. It is wise to keep a spare set of tubes within arm's reach to be ready for this circumstance.

If the vein is small, the strong vacuum force of the evacuated tube may have caused the vein to collapse; a syringe usually works better in this case because the phlebotomist can better control the vacuum generated.

If the phlebotomist is unable to obtain the blood needed, he or she should withdraw and look again for a better site. No more than two venipunctures should be attempted by the same person, however.

Once the blood flow is established (or optionally, after the blood is drawn, but before the needle is withdrawn), the tourniquet should be released and the patient instructed to open his or her hand. To obtain valid results, it is important that the tourniquet not be fastened for longer than 1 minute.

If multiple collection tubes are to be drawn, the next tube should be pushed into the holder. (A multiple sample needle has a rubber sheath, which recovers the tip of the inner needle to prevent blood leakage during tube changes.)

The order of drawing multiple tubes is important to minimize tissue fluid and additive contamination of the specimen. The National Committee for Clinical Laboratory Standards (NCCLS) recommends the following order for drawing multiple tubes:

First: Blood culture tube (to maintain sterility)
Second: Nonadditive tubes (e.g., red stopper)
Third: Coagulation tubes (e.g., blue stopper)
Fourth: Heparin tubes (e.g., green stopper)
Fifth: EDTA-K3 (ethylenediamine tetraacetic acid-K3) tubes (e.g., lavender stopper)
Sixth: Oxalate/fluoride tubes (e.g., gray stopper)

If a blue-stoppered tube for coagulation testing is the only tube to be drawn, a 5-ml discard tube should be filled first.

Once all tubes have been drawn, remove the last tube and lightly place a gauze pad above the venipuncture site.

Apply slight pressure to the pad and remove the needle gently. Immediately apply pressure to the wound and keep the arm straight. Apply pressure and elevate the arm for 3 minutes; the patient may assist, if he or she is able.

Bandage patient's arm. Gently tap around the site with the fingers to assure all bleeding has stopped (i.e., no visible "beading"). Apply an adhesive or gauze bandage that the patient should leave in place for 15 minutes. If the patient continues to bleed, hold a pressure patch on the site and call for nursing assistance.

Fill the tubes (if collection is by syringe). If the blood was collected by syringe, transfer the blood to evacuated tubes. Place the tubes to be filled in a rack, and using one hand to avoid a needlestick injury, puncture the stopper of the tube and allow the vacuum to correctly fill the tubes. Fill the tubes in the reverse order of draw used for collecting evacuated tubes. To avoid hemolysis, do not force the blood into the tube. Promptly mix tubes containing additives.

Step 12: Dispose of puncturing unit. Needlesticks are one of the most serious causes of work-related injuries in health care workers. Proper use and disposal of all sharp instruments in rigid containers will prevent the phlebotomist, as well as other workers such as housekeepers and incinerator operators, from dangerous exposure to blood. Should a needlestick injury or mucous membrane exposure occur, the phlebotomist must report this incident to the employee health department.

Needles should never be clipped. Syringes should be disposed with the needle attached. If a nondisposable adapter has been used, the needle should be resheathed and removed using one of the devices that allows this procedure to be done using only one hand. The needle should then be carefully removed from the reusable adapter by grasping the adapter in one hand and the needle cap in the other. While placing hands side by side, twist the needle off the adapter and discard it.

Needles should never be reused even when making a second attempt on a failed venipuncture.

Step 13: Chill or warm specimen (if indicated). Some analytes require that the blood specimens be collected into tubes that have been prechilled for 3 to 5 minutes and/or should be chilled immediately following venipuncture so that the metabolic processes that alter blood specimens are retarded. Common tests that require chilling of the blood

specimen are tests for activated partial thromboplastin time, renin activity, ammonia, lactic acid, serum gastrin, fibrinogen, acid phosphatase, and catecholamines.

When drawing a specimen for cryoglobulin or cryofibrinogen, tubes should be prewarmed and maintained at 37° C throughout transportation and processing.

Step 14: Identify specimen. Each specimen should be properly labeled with certain essential information:
Patient's name
Patient's identification number
Collection date and time
Phlebotomist's initials
Optional information the institution may require includes:
Accessioning number
Doctor's name
Patient's location
Comments related to how collection was done

In laboratories that use manual requisitions, some of this non-identification information may be recorded on the requisition instead of the label. Computer-generated labels usually contain most of the aforementioned data elements. Only the exact collection time and phlebotomist's initials need be handwritten on these labels.

Collection tubes should only be labeled after the blood specimen has been collected. There is too great a possibility of mixing up blood and tubes when prelabeling is done.

Step 15: Eliminate diet restrictions. If the patient fasted before the blood test, diet restrictions should now be removed.

Step 16: Record collection time. The exact time of specimen collection should be recorded. In a laboratory that uses manual requisitions, a time stamp should be used to record the time the specimens arrive in the laboratory.

The laboratory's information system (LIS) may require that a collection verify program be run. This program usually records the collection and receipt date and time, as well as the phlebotomist's identification.

Sources of error in venipuncture

The most common and possibly the most harmful error made when performing a venipuncture is to misidentify the patient or the sample. Box 3-5 lists some of the more common errors that are made when performing a venipuncture.

Age limitations for venipuncture

If a venipuncture is to be done on a child under 2 years of age, NCCLS recommends using a 21- to 33-gauge butterfly set attached to either a tuberculin or 3-ml syringe, or to a vacuum tube holder.

The child's arm should be secured by another person if possible; the phlebotomist should be prepared for sudden movements. Only superficial veins should be used, and every attempt should be made to minimize the volume of blood withdrawn.

In children under 6 years of age it is usually better to obtain the blood specimen, if feasible, by skin puncture.

Blood collection by skin puncture
The skin puncture procedure

A skin puncture might be necessary to obtain a blood specimen on adults whose veins are fragile or small, or are inaccessible due to obesity, intravenous therapy or scarring.

Box 3-5 Sources of error in venipunctures

Improper patient identification
Patient not properly prepared for testing (e.g., not fasting)
Inadequate fill of tube with an anticoagulant
Tourniquet left on too long (causing hemoconcentration)
Venipuncture done in unacceptable area (volar surface of the wrist, scarred areas, in hematoma, above an IV device, from arm with fistula, lower extremities)
Wrong collection tube used
Improper order of drawing multiple tubes
Failure to mix sample and anticoagulant (causing clotted sample)
Vigorous mixing of tubes (causing hemolysis)
Excess force used on syringe barrel when filling tubes (causing hemolysis)
Improper disposal of sharps (causing needlestick injury)
Improper sample identification
Failure to keep samples at proper temperature
Failure to transport specimens within required time limit

Box 3-6 Skin puncture procedure

1. Interview the patient
2. Assemble supplies
3. Verify paperwork
4. Select skin puncture site
5. Warm skin puncture site
6. Cleanse skin puncture site
7. Perform the skin puncture
   a. Discard the first blood drop
   b. Collect blood
   c. Close (and mix) the collection container
8. Apply pressure
9. Dispose of puncturing unit
10. Identify specimen
11. Chill or warm specimen (if indicated)
12. Eliminate diet restrictions
13. Record collection time

Box 3-7 Skin puncture supplies

Lancet
Microsample containers
Alcohol and gauze pads
Heel warmer (optional)

In most cases skin puncture is preferable to a venipuncture on newborns to both minimize the amount of blood loss and to avoid the trauma that venipuncture might cause in this small a patient. The steps followed in a skin puncture procedure are listed in Box 3-6.

Step 1: Interview the patient. The initial steps in which the phlebotomist introduces himself or herself and the patient is interviewed, identified, and assessed for testing readiness are the same as described for the venipuncture procedure.

Step 2: Assemble supplies. The phlebotomist should then gather the supplies needed for the skin puncture, as listed in Box 3-7.

Step 3: Verify paperwork. This step is the same as described in the venipuncture procedure.

Step 4: Select skin puncture site. In newborns and infants who have not yet begun to walk, the medial or lateral sections of the bottom surface of the heel should be used. Imaginary lines can be drawn from the middle of the great toe to the heel and from the fourth toe to the heel; the areas outside these lines are least hazardous. The posterior curvature of the heel should not be punctured because there is a possibility of hitting the bone at this point. In infants 6 to 18 months, the great toe may be used.

With adults and children over 18 months old, the preferred skin puncture site is the fleshy palmar surface of the distal portion of the middle finger. The other fingers may be used; the thumb, the great toe (except as noted), and the earlobe are rarely used. The puncture should not be made in an edematous area or through a previous puncture site.

Step 5: Warm skin puncture site. The puncture site can be warmed to facilitate blood flow. This can be done by heating a washcloth with warm (40° C) water and wrapping it around the site for 3 to 5 minutes. Alternately, a chemical heat pack can be applied to the puncture site for 3 to 5 minutes to warm it.

Step 6: Cleanse skin puncture site. This step is the same as described in the venipuncture procedure. It is especially important, however, that the antiseptic be allowed to thoroughly dry before puncturing the skin to avoid hemolysis and specimen contamination. A dry, sterile gauze pad may be used to dry the site.

Step 7: Perform the skin puncture. If performing a heel puncture, lie the baby on his or her stomach; firmly grip the newborn's heel, placing the forefinger at the arch of the foot and the thumb below the heel away from the puncture site, at the ankle. The leg should be extended from the hip as straight as possible; a bent leg may obstruct blood flow at the hip joint. In a heel puncture, the depth should be between 1.6 and 2.4 mm and be 2- 2.5-mm wide.

If performing a finger stick, hold the finger firmly between the thumb and the forefinger. The puncture should be done in a deliberate, continuous motion perpendicular to the print lines of the skin. The depth of a finger puncture should be between 2 to 3 mm.

Discard the first blood drop. The first drop of blood should be wiped away with a gauze pad because it contains excess tissue fluid from the puncture.

Collect blood. The blood should be collected into the selected microsample container (see Box 3-3). The phlebotomist can enhance the flow of blood by holding the puncture site downward and gently applying pressure to the surrounding tissue. Squeezing or milking the site should not be done as it will contaminate the blood specimen with tissue fluid and may cause hemolysis. Do not scoop the blood; it causes platelet clumping. Collect additive tubes first to avoid clotting of the specimen.

Close (and mix) the collection container. If capillary pipettes have been used, they should be sealed with clay or closed with commercially made covers. Lids should be placed on plastic, round-bottomed collection tubes.

If an additive-containing plastic collection tube has been used, the sample should be mixed by inversion. For capillary tubes, 2 to 3 small metal stirring wires should be inserted into the tube before sealing and the sample should be mixed by rubbing a magnet along the length of the tube.

Step 8: Apply pressure. Pressure should be applied to the puncture site using a small gauze pad; elevate the site above the patient's heart. Bandaging is not recommended.

Step 9: Dispose of puncturing unit. The lancet should be discarded into a puncture-proof container.

Step 10: Identify specimen. The specimen should be appropriately labeled with the same information described in the venipuncture procedure. If an identification label is placed on the collection tube, the label can be wrapped around the collection tube like a flag. However, because of the small size of these sample containers, they are most easily labeled by placing them into a larger test tube and writing the identifying information on that outer container.

Step 11: Chill or warm specimen (if indicated). Specimens requiring special temperature handling should be properly chilled (by placing them in water containing ice chips) or kept warm (by placing them in a warming block).

Step 12: Eliminate diet restrictions.

Step 13: Use time stamp to record collection time. These steps are the same as described in the venipuncture procedure.

Analyte concentrations in skin-punctured blood

Capillary specimens are chemically very similar to venous blood except for a few known variances. The concentration of glucose is higher in serum from a capillary sample than from a venous sample. The levels of potassium, total protein, and calcium are higher in venous serum than capillary serum.

Sources of error in skin punctures

Collecting an acceptable blood specimen by skin puncture is a difficult procedure. Some of the errors commonly made performing this procedure are listed in Box 3-8.

Special blood collection procedures

Arterial punctures

Blood samples are collected by arterial puncture for blood gas analysis and when samples cannot be collected by skin or venipuncture.

The radial artery, accessed at the wrist, is the most commonly used site for arterial punctures. Other sites used are the brachial, femoral, temporal (especially in infants), and the dorsalis pedis arteries.

Allen's test should be performed to assure that the patient has good collateral circulation through the ulnar artery before puncturing the radial artery. The patient should make a fist; the phlebotomist should then apply pressure to both the radial and the ulnar arteries to fully obstruct blood flow. The patient should open and close his or her hand until it has blanched. The phlebotomist should then release the ulnar pressure and observe the hand. It should become flushed within 15 seconds with blood supplied by the ulnar artery. If it does not turn pink again, the ulnar artery does not adequately supply blood to the hand. The radial artery

---

Box 3-8 Sources of error in skin puncture

Improper patient identification
Patient not properly prepared for testing (e.g., not fasting)
Puncture site not dried after cleansing
Skin puncture done in unacceptable area (puncturing fingers or wrong area of heel on infants, puncturing fifth or wrong area of finger on adults)
Failure to wipe away first drop of blood
Squeezing or milking puncture site
Collecting air bubbles in blood gas sample
Wrong collection tube used
Inadequately sealing/capping tubes
Failure to mix with anticoagulant (causing clotted sample)
Vigorous mixing of tubes (causing hemolysis, introducing air)
Improper disposal of sharps (causing needlestick injury)
Improper sample identification
Failure to keep samples at proper temperature
Failure to transport specimens within required time limit

---

should not be used for puncture in this case because damage to it might result in total loss of circulation to, and possibly loss of, the hand.

Bleeding times

A phlebotomist may be assigned to perform a bleeding time on a patient. This test assesses platelet and capillary performance in the control of bleeding. It is used as a preoperative screening test as well as to help diagnose problems with hemostasis.

It is performed by making a measured incision (5 × 1 mm) in the forearm (Ivy's or template method), or by puncturing the earlobe (Duke's method). Filter paper is used to blot the site every 30 seconds, and the time interval until bleeding stops is measured.

Blood alcohol levels

When cleansing the venipuncture site before drawing a blood alcohol level, it is important that alcohol not be used as the disinfectant. Either soap and water or an iodine preparation should be used to cleanse the site. See Chapter 28 for a discussion of how to collect a specimen for legal purposes.

Blood cultures

When collecting a blood specimen for culture, sterile technique must be used to avoid introducing skin and environmental bacteria into the specimen. The site must also be swabbed with an iodophor and alcohol scrub. See Chapters 39 and 49 for a complete discussion of blood culture techniques.

Blood gas analysis

Heparinized whole blood samples for blood gas analysis may be collected by skin or by arterial puncture. If a skin puncture is done, the site must be warmed so that the sample is more similar to arterial blood. The sample must be collected without introducing air bubbles, which would distort the pO_2 level, into the capillary tube or syringe.

If the sample is not going to be tested immediately, it should be placed in ice water. In any case, the sample should be delivered to the laboratory within 15 minutes of collection.

Positive identification for crossmatch samples

Because of the potentially fatal complication of a hemolytic transfusion reaction, patient samples collected to prepare blood for transfusion must be thoroughly identified.

The American Association of Blood Banks requires that the patient and the patient's blood specimen be labeled with name, date of collection, and an identification number at the time the sample is collected. Many institutions accomplish this by having the phlebotomist apply a separate identification band that bears a unique transfusion number. This number is applied to the specimen and the unit to be transfused. At the time of transfusion, the number on the unit is compared to the number on the patient's special identification bracelet. The numbers must exactly match before the unit can be given to the patient.

Timed collections

Some tests, such as cortisol, serum iron, or glucose, must be drawn at specific time intervals because of biologic variations of certain compounds in the body. Also, the measurement of therapeutic drugs (or their actions) in the body require that blood be drawn at defined times.

It is important that the phlebotomist obtains the specimen at the required collection time, and notes the exact collection time on the sample and the requisition and enters this information in the computer system.

Phlebotomy complications

There are several complications commonly associated with collecting blood samples. The phlebotomist must understand and be prepared to deal appropriately with these situations.

Fainting

Fainting is a common side effect during phlebotomy. The phlebotomist should be observant of the patient's condition throughout the sample collection procedure. If a seated patient feels faint, the phlebotomy should be stopped and the patient's head lowered between the legs. (Patients having their blood drawn while lying down will rarely feel faint.) When possible, a patient who is feeling faint should be assisted to a lying position.

Hematomas

A hematoma is a swelling around a puncture site caused by the leaking of blood from a vessel into the surrounding tissues. When a needle goes completely through a vein, the needle opening is partially in the vein, or when inadequate pressure is applied to a puncture site, a hematoma can form. If this happens during the venipuncture, the phlebotomist should remove the tourniquet and needle immediately and apply pressure to the site.

Petechiae

Petechiae are small, red dots that appear on the skin when the tourniquet is applied. They are caused by small amounts of blood entering the epithelium and may indicate a bleeding disorder. The phlebotomist should be especially alert for excessive bleeding from the puncture site.

Allergic reactions

Some patients may be allergic to the agents used to cleanse the puncture site, especially the iodine-containing agents. Others might be allergic to adhesive tape or bandages. These patients are often aware of this sensitivity; the phlebotomist should use an alternative method when alerted to this situation.

URINE COLLECTION

It has been said that the composition of blood is determined less by what the body produces than by what the kidneys keep. In a normal healthy person, over 1 L of urine is produced per day. This body fluid is used in the laboratory to help diagnose and treat urinary tract disorders as well as many metabolic and systemic diseases.

Tests on urine may be performed on a single specimen or on the entire urinary output during a defined time period, most frequently 24 hours.

Single-specimen collection

Routine urinalysis is one of the most frequently requested laboratory procedures. This test usually includes chemical tests for glucose, protein, blood, bilirubin, ketones, urobilinogen, and others, as well as pH and specific gravity measurements. A microscopic analysis of the urine for the presence of red and white blood cells, bacteria, crystals, casts, and other formed elements might also be included.

Some other tests that can be performed on "random" urine specimens are urine pregnancy test, hemosiderin, iodide, myoglobin, and porphyrin. Random urine is also the specimen of choice when screening for illegal drugs, although a chain of custody procedure, as described in Chapter 28, should be used if a legally defensible result will be required.

The preferred "random" or single urine specimen is the first voided urine of the morning, when urine is the most concentrated. A clean, plastic cup with a tight-fitting lid should be used for collection. The container should hold a volume of 50 ml.

Another very commonly performed single specimen urine test is the urine culture. This specimen must be collected in a sterile container as aseptically as possible. The patient should not have voided in the 3 hours prior to collection. Instructions must be given to the patient to cleanse the genital area thoroughly before specimen collection. Caution should be used if cleansing with disinfectants. Soap and water are satisfactory. A midstream collection will cleanse the urethral canal of contaminant bacteria. The specimen should be cultured within 1 hour of collection. If it cannot be immediately brought to the laboratory, the specimen should be kept refrigerated to prevent an overgrowth of contaminant bacteria. Refer to Chapters 39 and 48 for additional information.

Timed collection

Many of the tests performed on urine require a collection of all the urine produced over a 24-hour (or other timed) period. Some analytes exhibit a diurnal variation in urinary excretion, and the variable hydration of a patient throughout the day may effect the quantitation of chemical analytes in urine. The sample collected over a 24-hour period yields an average concentration of the analyte.

Collection containers

Collection containers for 24-hour urine specimens should hold 3 to 4 L, be clean, and have tight-fitting lids. They should be labeled with:

Patient's name
Patient's identification number
Starting collection date and time
Ending collection date and time
Name of the test
Preservative
Storage requirements during collection

Optional information the institution may require includes:

Accessioning number
Doctor's name
Patient's location
Tare weight of bottle (if volume is measured by weight)
Warning to patient if preservative is harmful when spilled.

Preservatives

Many analytes require preservatives to maintain their viability during the collection period by minimizing oxidation and bacterial growth. Some analytes require an acidic pH for stability, while others are most stable in an alkaline pH. Some of the commonly used preservatives are described here:

- Acetic acid, to maintain acidity, is the preferred preservative for aminolevulinic acid, catecholamines, chloride, cortisol, deoxycorticosteroids, metanephrines, porphobilinogen, and vanillylmandelic acid.
- 6 N Hydrochloric acid is added to containers for timed collection to measure calcium, oxalate, and serotonin.
- Boric acid, another agent to maintain a low pH, is the preservative of choice for aldosterone dehydroepiandrosterone (DHEA), estriol, estrogen, 5-hydroxy indoleacetic acid (5-HIAA), homogentisic acid, homovanillic acid, 17-hydroxycorticosteroids, iron, pregnanediol, pregnanetriol, 17-ketosteroids, and testosterone.
- Toluene inhibits oxidation and is used as a preservative for creatine, glucose, hydroxyproline, urea, and uric acid.
- Sodium carbonate is used to maintain alkalinity in coproporphyrin, porphobilinogen, and porphyrins.
- Some analytes are best preserved by refrigeration or by keeping on ice. These include ammonia, amylase, creatinine, cortisol, follicle-stimulating hormone (FSH), glucose, heavy metals, hemosiderin, iron, luteinizing hormone (LH), melanin, methymalonic acid, phosphorus, potassium, protein, sodium, and sulfate.
- Analytes that must be protected from light by either wrapping the container with foil or using a dark container are porphobilinogen, porphyrins, and urobilinogen.

Storage during collection

If at all possible, all timed urine samples should be refrigerated during collection.

Procedure for collection

The collection of a timed urine sample requires much cooperation on the part of the patient and/or the nursing staff. The following procedure should be used:

- At the time selected to begin the collection (often the first thing in the morning), the patient should empty his bladder.
- This specimen should be discarded, and the exact time of this void should be noted.
- If a urine preservative has been used, advise the patient in advance of any problem that might arise from inadvertent spillage.
- Patients should be warned, prior to the use of bed pans, to urinate before having a bowel movement. Else, they might forget and urinate into the pan while having a bowel movement, losing a part of the urine collection.
- Collect all urine passed after the initially discarded specimen in a clean container and transfer it to the timed urine collection container.
- Have the patient try to void the last specimen just when the timed period is ended. Include this in the total specimen collected. Record the exact time this last specimen was obtained.

Measuring total volume

When performing a timed urine (e.g., 24 hour, 12 hour) quantitation, the measured concentration units are multiplied by the total volume of urine excreted during that period. The final result is reported as quantity excreted per timed (e.g., 24 hour) period. Therefore, it is necessary that the total urine volume collected during the time interval be measured.

One way to perform this measurement is to weigh the container with the sample and subtract the tare weight of the empty container, which was previously recorded. The weight of the urine is equated to its volume at 1 g = 1 ml. Alternately, volume can be determined directly by measuring the urine in a graduated cylinder.

Aliquoting

After the total volume is measured and recorded, an aliquot of urine should be made for each test to be performed (plus an extra aliquot for the stored sample file). The remainder of the urine may be discarded.

Sources of error in timed urine collections

Box 3-9 lists some of the more common errors that are made in the collection of timed urine specimens.

COLLECTION OF OTHER SPECIMENS
Cerebrospinal fluids

Cerebrospinal fluid (CSF) is usually collected in three or four sterile containers numbered in the order in which they are filled. The first (and sometimes second) tube is often contaminated with blood and should not be used for analysis. The second (or third) tube should contain enough CSF for

---

Box 3-9   Sources of error in timed urine collections

Inadequate preservative used
Loss of voided specimens
Inclusion of two morning specimens
Measuring volume and/or aliquoting from only one of several containers
Incorrectly measuring and/or recording total volume

---

all tests requested. The last tube is reserved for bacteriologic examination.

Tests commonly performed on CSF might include:
Albumin
Cell count (and differential)
Chloride
Cryptococcal antigen
Culture
Glucose
Gram's stain
IgG
IgG/Albumin ratio
Immunoelectrophoresis
Oligoclonal bands
Protein electrophoresis
Total protein
VDRL (Venereal Disease Research Laboratories)

Fecal specimens

Most tests on feces require that the sample be collected in a clean cardboard container with a lid. The stool sample should not be contaminated with water or urine. If an enema must be given, Epsom salts or Fleet enemas should be used; do not use mineral oil, castor oil, or liquid petrolatum enemas.

For a culture, 0.3 to 2 g of stool is sufficient; portions of the stool that contain mucus or blood should be chosen because they usually harbor larger numbers of organisms. (Refer to Chapter 39 for additional information on collecting fecal specimens.)

Tests performed on feces might include:
Bilirubin
Clostridium difficile toxin assay
Culture or Leukocyte Stain
Fat, qualitative or quantitative
Occult blood
Ova and parasite exam
Potassium
Sodium
Trypsin
Urobilinogen (wrap in foil)

Other body fluids

Laboratory personnel are called on to perform tests on a variety of other body fluids and drainages. It is important to avoid contamination of fluid with blood or other body fluids. Usually, these specimens are collected into evacuated containers with the same additives used for the same tests done on blood specimens.

SAMPLE TRANSPORTATION
Transport time

Once specimens are collected, they should be promptly transported to the laboratory. Because the blood cells continue to live in the collection tube, they continue to metabolize some of the substances in the blood. The glycolytic action of erythrocytes may alter the true values of many analytes (glucose, phosphorus, blood pH) or material may leak from the cells (enzymes).

Erythrocytes are also potassium-rich cells that may falsely elevate the measurement of potassium if the plasma is subjected to prolonged or traumatic erythrocytic exposure. Consequently, blood specimens should be delivered to the laboratory for processing within 30 to 45 minutes, depending on the test. Stat specimens should be drawn and delivered immediately. It is equally important that other specimens be transported to the laboratory within a short time after their collection.

Urine specimens should be brought to the laboratory within 1 hour of collection. Formed elements (cells, crystals, and casts) that might be observed on microscopic analysis will quickly disintegrate unless preserved by refrigeration. Bacterial contaminants will overgrow and mask the presence of pathogens in specimens for culture.

Methods of transport

There are several methods that can be used to transport specimens to the laboratory. They should be properly used to ensure that specimens are delivered soon after collection, in a manner that preserves the integrity of the sample, and in a biologically safe manner.

Hand delivery

Hand delivery of specimens can either be accomplished by the phlebotomy team, by a centralized transport department, or by the nurse or physician who has collected the sample.

Pneumatic tube systems

Many institutions use pneumatic tubes for the transport of specimens to the laboratory. Such systems must be evaluated for their suitability. Factors to be considered are mechanical reliability and the conditions of transport that might cause hemolysis of the specimen.

Plasma hemoglobin, potassium, and lactate dehydrogenase (LDH) values are particularly susceptible to false elevations due to the destruction of blood cells during transport. This destruction can be minimized if the pneumatic tube system operates at a low velocity, has no low radius bends, and uses slow deceleration.

Specimens should always be transported in carriers with shock-absorbent liners that pad and protect the tubes from breakage. They should be placed in closed plastic bags to minimize contamination in case there is breakage.

Dumbwaiters

Dumbwaiters are in use in some hospitals to transport specimens from those areas located vertically above or below the laboratory. There need be no special considerations taken for this mode of transport except that the system must be mechanically reliable.

Mechanized vehicles

There are a variety of other transport systems in use, from robots to electronic track vehicles. The same criteria for evaluating these systems should be used for pneumatic tube systems.

External transport

Transport of specimens to reference laboratories or other outside agencies requires that special considerations be made regarding packaging and labeling.

According to the Rules and Regulations of the United States Department of Transportation as published in the Code of Federal Regulations, "Etiologic agent preparations, clinical specimens and biological products are nonmailable except when . . . it is determined that such items are properly prepared for mailing to withstand shocks, pressure changes, and other conditions incidental to ordinary handling in transit."

Etiologic agent preparations

According to the U.S. Postal Service, "Etiologic agent preparations are cultures or suspensions of microbiological agents or their toxins that may cause human or animal disease."

Packaging

- The primary container should be labeled with the patient's name, laboratory number, date, and specimen source.
- The screw cap of the primary container should be tight and secured with tape.
- Bacterial specimens should be shipped on agar slants whenever possible. If it is necessary to send a liquid specimen, sufficient space for liquid expansion must be provided so that the primary container will not be liquid-full at 130° F. The total liquid volume must not exceed 50 ml per outer container. The primary container and a liquid absorber should be placed into a locking plastic bag before proceeding with the next step.
- The primary tube should be wrapped with a thick layer of cotton and placed inside a durable, watertight, secondary container. A layer of cotton should be put on the bottom of the container and on the top after the primary tube is inserted. Tightly secure and tape the lid of the secondary container.
- The requisition form should be wrapped around the secondary container and placed in the outer shipping container. The lid of the outer container should be secured.
- The outer container should be labeled with an "Etiologic Agents/Biomedical Material" sticker as well as the usual address information. (See Chapter 2).

Mailing. If shipping via U.S. Mail, the parcel must be sent by First-Class Mail, Priority Mail, or Express Mail.

Clinical specimens

According to the U.S. Postal Service, "Clinical specimen means any human or animal material including but not limited to, excreta, secreta, blood and its components, tissue, and tissue fluids."

Packaging

- The primary container should be labeled with the patient's name, laboratory number, and any specific information required by the reference laboratory.
- The lid of the primary container should be securely fastened, the container placed in a locking plastic bag with a liquid absorber packet, and the bag rolled up and sealed.
- The bag(s) containing the primary container(s) should be placed in a secondary Styrofoam container.
- The Styrofoam secondary container should be placed in an outer cardboard sleeve, which should be labeled as "Clinical Specimens" and should display address information.

Additional requirements for shipping packages containing dry ice by air transport

- Packages containing more than 5 pounds of dry ice must have a shipper's declaration for dangerous goods attached in triplicate.
- Packages containing less than 5 pounds of dry ice should be marked with the weight of the dry ice and "Dry Ice" or "Carbon Dioxide Solid." They must also be constructed to permit the release of carbon dioxide gas to prevent a buildup of pressure that could rupture the packaging.

SAMPLE ACCESSIONING AND PROCESSING

Once the specimens have been collected and transported to the laboratory, accessioning and pretest processing must take place. This may occur in the individual laboratories or in a centralized processing area. Centralized processing has become commonplace in large and in computerized laboratories.

Wherever the specimens are processed, there should be either a processing procedure manual or a card file (Rolodex) defining all processing instructions. It should contain an alphabetized list of all tests, with synonyms, and all information about the specimen needed to process it:

Type and amount of specimen
Container type
Special collection and processing instructions
Storage instructions
Test availability
Laboratory performing test

Accessioning and sorting specimens

As specimens are received in the laboratory, they should be "accessioned," which is to make a record in order of acquisition and assign a specimen number. In computerized laboratories it additionally means to log the specimen into the computer, a function that makes the specimen available to the technologist's workpool and records the time it is received in the laboratory.

Also, in this process the technologist or technician must match the patient's name, identification number, and computer specimen number on the labels with the information in the computer or on the requisitions. One must also check that the specimens received are appropriate for the tests ordered.

Specimens not needing any further processing, such as hematology or blood bank specimens, can be immediately distributed to the laboratory.

Centrifugation

Serum samples, that is, blood with no anticoagulants, should be allowed to clot for 30 minutes before centrifugation, unless the blood has been drawn in a tube with a special clot activator. Plasma samples can be centrifuged immediately upon receipt. Samples being tested for an unstable analyte should be kept cold during centrifugation by using a refrigerated centrifuge.

Stoppered tubes (to minimize the creation of aerosols) should be placed in the centrifuge so that all tubes are balanced—tubes of the same size and weight should be placed in opposite buckets. Blood samples should generally be centrifuged for 10 minutes at 1000 x G, although the manufacturer's instructions for the centrifuge and the evacuated tube should be consulted first.

Serum and plasma separation techniques

Gel separation tubes have been a great help in safe and efficient processing of serum and plasma specimens; this closed system also prevents evaporation and creates a barrier between the liquid and the cells.

Other separation devices include beads or crystals added prior to centrifugation that similarly form a barrier between the serum or plasma and the cells, although this barrier is not as effective as the gel barrier.

Serum skimmers are the third separation technique commonly used. The skimmer is a small plastic tube with a rubber squeegee at the bottom. It is inserted into the tube after centrifugation to a point above the layer of cells. The serum or plasma is forced through a filter in the squeegee into the plastic tube, away from the cells. An aliquot can then be poured without spilling cells into the sample. Skimmers are less convenient to use than gel tubes and the primary tube cannot be easily re-stoppered. They also should not be used in tubes requiring that sterility be maintained; sterile pipettes should be used instead.

Aliquoting of specimens

While the tubes are in the centrifuge the technologist should prepare any needed aliquot tubes. The labels for these tubes should contain the patient's name, identification number, accession number, and test name. Aliquot tubes can be glass, although plastic tubes are preferred if specimens are to be frozen or sent out for testing.

When centrifugation is complete, the serum or plasma should be transferred to the labeled aliquot tube, taking care to correctly match the labels of both tubes.

Determining specimen acceptability

Laboratories should have written criteria to determine when to reject a specimen as unacceptable for testing. Some common criteria for rejecting a sample are listed in Box 3-10.

Hemolysis will falsely elevate measurements of potassium, LDH, aspartate aminotransferase (AST), and plasma hemoglobin because of high amounts of these substances in the erythrocytes. Additionally, the hemoglobin released by hemolysis may cause a methodological interference in the assay. Similarly, samples might be unsuitable for use in some assays due to interference of bilirubin (icteric) or chylomicrons (lipemic).

Distribution of specimens

When distributing specimens to the individual laboratories, some sorting into racks by urgency or by test might be

---

Box 3-10 Criteria for sample rejection

Inadequate or improper sample identification
Improper collection tube used
Insufficient quantity of sample
Sample hemolyzed, lipemic, or icteric
Anticoagulated blood clotted
Sample improperly transported (e.g., not on ice, when required)
Anticoagulated tube insufficiently filled

Box 3-11 Sources of error in processing

Aliquot misidentified
Specimen misplaced
Specimen tube broken in centrifuge
Specimen centrifuged at wrong temperature (e.g., at room temperature instead of refrigerated)
Specimen repeatedly frozen and thawed
Serum/plasma contaminated with red blood cells
Specimen stored at wrong temperature (e.g., refrigerated instead of frozen)

---

required. In a laboratory with centralized processing, samples for tests, which are not continuously run but are run in batches, might be gathered in racks or buckets in a central refrigerator or freezer.

Sample storage
Storage before analysis

In general, specimens should be tested within 1 hour of collection. If this is not possible because of test performance schedules, the sample may need refrigeration, freezing, or deep freezing, depending on the compound to be tested. Some blood and urine analytes may need acid or alkaline stabilization before testing or storage.

Stored sample file

After testing, the remainder of the sample should be refiled with a portion of the "master" sample. Samples must be capped and should be filed by day of week and accession number. These samples can then be easily retrieved for retesting or for use in additional tests ordered by the patient's physician. When an "add-on" request is received, the sample is pulled from storage. The technologist checks if the test ordered can be performed on a stored sample (depending on the period of stability and the effect of temperature on the analyte). This program often can save the patient from additional venipunctures.

Sources of error in processing

Box 3-11 lists some of the more common errors that are made in specimen processing.

SUGGESTED READING
Garza D and Becan-McBride K: Phlebotomy handbook, Norwalk, Conn, 1989, Appleton & Lange.

Lotspeich CA: Specimen collection and processing. In Bishop M, Duben-Von Laufen JL, and Fody EP, editors: Clinical chemistry: principles, procedures, correlations, Philadelphia, 1985, JB Lippincott.

National Committee for Clinical Laboratory Standards: Collection and preservation of timed urine specimens; proposed guidelines, Villanova, Pa, 1987, NCCLS.

National Committee for Clinical Laboratory Standards: Collection and transportation of single-collection urine specimens; Proposed guideline, Villanova, Pa, 1985, NCCLS.

National Committee for Clinical Laboratory Standards: Procedures for the collection of diagnostic blood specimens by skin puncture—ed 2, Approved standard, Villanova, Pa, 1986, NCCLS.

National Committee for Clinical Laboratory Standards: Procedures for the collection of diagnostic blood specimens by venipuncture—ed 2, Approved standards, Villanova, Pa, 1984, NCCLS.

National Committee for Clinical Laboratory Standards: Procedures for the handling and processing of blood specimens; Tentative standard, Villanova, Pa, 1984, NCCLS.

Rapp Marji and others: Introduction to phlebotomy, Denver, 1986, Colorado Association for Continuing Medical Laboratory Education.

Slockblower JM and Blumenfeld TA: Collection and handling of laboratory specimens, Philadelphia, 1983, JB Lippincott.

US Postal Service (39 CFR Part III): Mailability of etiologic agents, Federal Register, August 15, 1989, 54(156):33523-33525.

4

Weights, measures, and principles of instrumentation

Marie Zureick

The primary function of the clinical laboratory is to quantify or qualify analysis of analytes in body fluids and tissues. Normally, body fluid analyte composition fluctuates within defined limits. This chapter presents some of the basic analytical concepts of the measurement process and includes weights and measures, and basic principles of simple instrumentation.

WEIGHTS AND MEASURES

Quantities can be expressed as basic or derived properties. A basic property is one that is defined only in terms of itself; a derived property is one defined in terms of combinations of other basic properties. Quantitative analytical results are usually expressed as the quantity of the measured component per unit volume or weight of sample. A unit of measure is defined as an amount of some quantitative property. A system is a group of units of measure used together.

In laboratory medicine two systems of measurement are commonly used; these are the metric system and the SI (the Systéme International d'Unités). Both systems have been attempts by international groups of scientists represented at the Conference Generale des Poids et Measures (CGPM) to standardize weights and measures on the international level.

Metric system

The metric system employs the gram, meter, liter, and second as the standard units of measurement for weight, length, volume, and time, respectively. The advantage of the metric system is that larger or smaller units of the system are derived by multiplying the standard unit by some power of 10.

Identical prefixes are used with all the basic units to denote larger or smaller size. Thus, 1 milligram refers to one thousandth of a gram (10^{-3} g), 1 milliliter refers to one thousandth of a liter (10^{-3} L). Table 4-1 summarizes the relationship of the prefix to the multiple of the basic unit. The metric unit, while convenient, legitimately allows for variation in the expressions of measurement. For example, the concentration of blood constituents can be expressed in

Table 4-1 Relationship of the metric system prefix to the multiple of the basic unit

Prefix	Multiple name	Power of 10	Symbol
Giga-	Billion	10^9	G
Mega-	Million	10^6	M
Kilo-	Thousand	10^3	k
Hecto-	Hundred	10^2	h
Deca-	Ten	10^1	da
No prefix	Standard unit	10^0	—
Deci-	One tenth	10^{-1}	d
Centi-	One hundreth	10^{-2}	c
Milli-	One thousandth	10^{-3}	m
Micro-	One millionth	10^{-6}	µ
Nano-	One billionth	10^{-9}	n
Pico-	One trillionth	10^{-12}	p

either mg/dL or g/L and this sometimes can lead to confusion as both sets of units are considered correct.

Systéme International d'Unités

To stem the confusion generated by variation in units in the metric system, CGPM, in 1960, adopted a more coherent system that uses nine basic properties from which all other properties are derived. This is the Systéme International d'Unités, which is abbreviated SI in all languages. Table 4-2 shows the nine basic properties and their associated units and symbols. Many of the units used in the laboratory, for reasons of convenience and tradition, are not consistent with the SI system; that is, they are not derivable from one of the nine basic SI units. The liter is an example of an inconsistent volume unit. Strictly defined, the SI unit for volume is the cubic meter, which, because of its large size, is inconvenient for laboratory use. The liter is 0.001 cubic meter or cubic decimeter and is the volume term in common use. In 1964 the CGPM approved the use of the liter as a special name for the cubic decimeter. Commonly used prefixes of the liter are milli-, micro-, and nano-.

Table 4-2 Basic SI properties

Basic property	Property symbol	Basic unit	Unit symbol
Length	l	Meter	m
Mass	m	Kilogram	kg
Time	t	Second	s
Electric current	I	Ampere	A
Thermodynamic temperature	T	Degree Kelvin	°K
Luminous intensity	l^v	Candela	cd
Amount of substance	n	Mole	mol
Plane angle	α, β, γ, θ, or φ	Radian	rad
Solid angle	ω or Ω	Steradian	sr

The CGPM recommends that whenever the molecular weight of an analyte is known, its concentration should be expressed in molecular terms (moles/L) instead of mass terms (mg/L).

VOLUMETRIC MEASUREMENTS

Correct, meaningful laboratory measurements involve the preparation of reagents, standards, controls, and transfer of samples. All of these efforts require the use of volumetric equipment. The accuracy and precision of volumetric devices can vary widely, depending on the material the device is made from and the tolerance to which it is made.

Ideally, laboratories should purchase class A volumetric glassware whenever it is available. Class A glassware conforms to the specifications listed in the National Bureau of Standards (NBS) circular C-602 and is the highest standard available commercially. Volumetric glassware that is not class A must be calibrated and checked for precision and accuracy to avoid analytical error.

Manual pipettes

The laboratory employs two basic types of pipettes: To Deliver (TD) and To Contain (TC). To Deliver pipettes are marked "TD" at the upper edge of the tube and are designed to deliver the stated volume when allowed to drain for a specified time at room temperature. Many sizes of these pipettes are available manufactured to class A specifications. The To Contain or "rinse out" pipettes hold a certain volume that must be completely transferred. They must be refilled or rinsed out with the diluting mixture after the initial solution is transferred. To Contain pipettes do not meet class A specifications. Table 4-3 lists some of the pipettes found in the laboratory, classified according to their degree of accuracy.

Volumetric or transfer pipettes are TD pipettes and are used when greatest accuracy is required. The pipette is an open-ended tube, tapered at the delivery tip, with a bulb near the middle of the tube. This type of pipette delivers one fixed volume, indicated on the pipette, within a specified drainage time. The accuracy of the volumetric pipette varies with the volume. For example, the accuracy of a 1-mL class A pipette is stated to be accurate within 0.6% of 1 mL, and a 25-ml pipette is said to be accurate within 0.12% of 25 ml. A specialized version of the volumetric pipette is the Oswald-Folin pipette. Because it is designed to accurately transfer fluids more viscous than water, it has a shorter tube

Table 4-3 Accuracies of the different types of manual pipettes (in mL)

Type of pipette	1.0 mL	5.0 mL	10.0 mL	25.0 mL
NBS standard	—	0.01	0.02	0.025
Class A volumetric	0.006	0.01	0.02	0.03
Mohr	0.01	0.02	0.03	0.10
Mohr long tip	0.02	0.04	0.06	—
Serological	0.01	0.02	0.03	0.10
Serological large opening	0.05	0.10	0.10	0.20
Serological long tip	0.02	0.04	0.06	—

From Steiner P and Byrne EA: Basic laboratory principles and calculations. In Kaplan LA and Pesce AJ, editors: Clinical chemistry: theory, analysis, and correlation, ed 2, St Louis, 1989, Mosby–Year Book, Inc.

with the bulb located nearer the delivery tip. The residual volume left after drainage must be blown out. Any pipette requiring that the residual volume be blown out is readily identified by the presence of two frosted bands near its mouthpiece.

Mohr or measuring pipettes are a kind of TD pipette that consists of a long straight tube tapered near the delivery tip with calibration intervals marked between two points on the straight portion of the tube. Solution must be delivered between the two points because the tapered tip is not calibrated.

Serological pipettes are similar to the Mohr pipettes but are calibrated to the tip. If the full volume of the pipette is to be delivered, the residual volume must be blown out. These pipettes are calibrated at intervals and so are used for point-to-point measurements in the straight part of the tube but not in the tapered tip. Serological pipettes are also available with large opening tips (for faster draining) and with long tips. Stated accuracies for the Mohr and serological pipettes are for the full volume. Accuracy decreases as the size of the aliquot pipetted decreases. Figure 4-1 shows several types of manual pipettes.

Pipetting technique

Correct use of pipettes ensures that accuracy requirements are met. A list of correct pipetting technique follows:

1. Always use a bulb or mechanical device to aspirate fluid into the pipette.
2. Pipette must be clean and the delivery tip intact. Only a clean bore will support a uniform film of fluid and

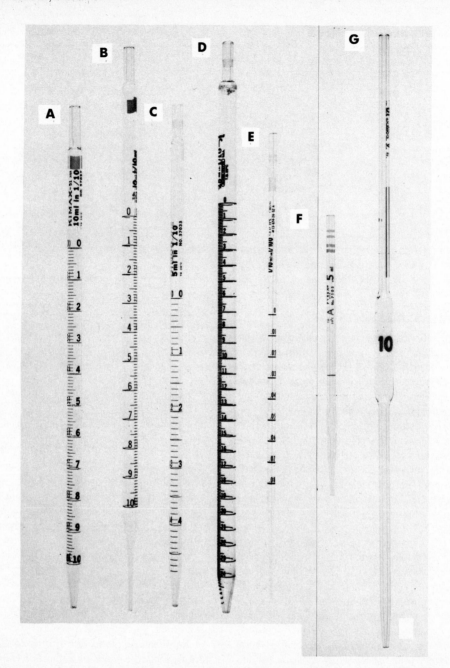

Fig. 4-1 Examples of transfer to deliver (TD) pipettes. **A,** Mohr. **B,** Mohr long tip. **C,** Serological. **D,** Serological large opening. **E,** Serological long tip. **F,** Oswald-Folin. **G,** Class A volumetric. *From Steiner P and Byrne EA: Laboratory techniques. In Kaplan LA and Pesce AJ: Clinical chemistry: theory, analysis, and correlation, ed 2, St Louis, 1989, Mosby-Year Book, Inc.*

conform to the calibration marks. Dirt or traces of dried material in the bore are indicated by the presence of residual droplets in the bore after the drainage is complete.

3. With the pipette held in the vertical position, aspirate fluid to just above the top calibration ring. Drain the fluid to the upper desired ring and wipe the pipette tip with a lintless tissue.

4. Transfer the pipette to the receiving vessel and allow the fluid to drain with the pipette held with its tip against the side of the vessel.

When setting the liquid level at any time during the pipetting procedure, the lowest part of the meniscus should be level with the calibration mark when viewed at eye level. If not viewed at eye level, parallax can introduce significant error.

Semiautomatic pipettes

The need to conserve patient sample for the large number of tests ordered, the use of expensive immunological reagents, and the prevalence of automated analyzers in the laboratory contributed to the development of automated micropipettes. These pipettes are designed to deliver 2 to 500 µl of sample or reagent and operate on one of two principles: air displacement or positive displacement. Both types are To Deliver (TD), piston-operated devices with disposable or semidisposable tips. Plastic or glass tips are fitted onto the pipette barrel. The volume of solution pipetted is dependent on the piston stroke length and bore size. When the piston is depressed, the tip is placed into the fluid and as the piston is allowed to return to its resting position, fluid fills the tip. The outside of the tip is wiped and another depression of the plunger dispenses the fluid. With the positive displacement pipette, the Teflon-tipped plunger wipes the pipette wall free of sample. Tips are not usually changed between samples. Some carryover does exist, making it necessary to evaluate the use of these pipettes in assays for analytes that can be present in widely varying concentration. Two examples of this type of problem analyte are glucose with a range of 400 to 6000 mg/L and beta-human chorionic gonadotropin (hCG), with an even larger range of less than 4 to greater than 100,000 mIU/mL. Pipettes utilizing air displacement usually require that the tips be changed between all patient samples, removing all chance of carryover.

Micropipettes are available in single volume, multiple set volumes, and adjustable volume models. As with manual pipettes, accuracy decreases with decreasing volume. Manufacturers typically claim accuracies with an error of less than 0.5% and precisions of less than 0.2% with water at 20° for full volume use of pipettes between 50 and 1000 µl. Accuracy and precision of pipettes between 10 and 25 µl are somewhat less, with errors in accuracy ranging from less than 1.2% to less than 0.6% and precision less than 0.4% to less than 0.3%. Calibration should be verified by an independent spectrophotometric, gravimetric, or radioisotopic method.

Good precision and accuracy with micropipettes requires adherence to manufacturers' directions for consistent and smooth operation and regular maintenance. Maintenance varies according to pipette type. Air displacement devices require intact, well-lubricated seals and unobstructed airways. Positive displacement pipettes require smoothly functioning springs, intact plunger tips, capillary retainers, and capillaries.

CALCULATIONS
Solution concentration

The concentration of a solution can be expressed in a variety of terms: percent solution, molarity, and normality.

Percent solution

Concentrations given as percent solutions are expressed as parts of solute present in 100 parts of total solution and are noted in one of three ways: weight per volume (W/V), volume per volume (V/V), or weight per weight (W/W). The most common of the three expressions is weight per volume, written as grams % (g%) or g/dL. Less commonly, it indicates mg/dl (mg%) or µg/dL (µg%). When the term *percent solution* is used without specification, that is W/V, V/V, or W/W; it is assumed to designate g/dL. Although the convention of the percent solution to describe concentration was commonly used, laboratory organizations such as the American Association for Clinical Chemistry (AACC)

or College of American Pathologists (CAP) discourage this use because of the inability to always explicitly understand the units. In addition, while it is possible to add more than 100 g/dL of some materials, it makes no sense to refer to more than 100 parts per 100 parts of solution. With the SI units, these solutions would be expressed as weight or moles/L, weight or moles/mL, or weight or moles/µL.

EXAMPLE: (weight/volume) Prepare 200 mL of 10% NaOH (W/V). By definition, a 10% (W/V) solution contains 10 g of NaOH per 100 mL solution. To calculate the grams required for any other than a volume of 100 mL, use a ratio proportion method and solve for *x*.

$$\frac{10 \text{ g NaOH}}{100 \text{ mL}} = \frac{x \text{ g NaOH}}{200 \text{ mL}}$$

$$x \text{ g NaOH} = \frac{10 \text{ g NaOH} \times 200 \text{ mL}}{100 \text{ mL}}$$

$$x = 20 \text{ g}$$

Add 20 g of NaOH to a 200-mL volumetric flask and dilute to volume with water.

EXAMPLE: (volume/volume) Prepare 100 mL of 5% H_2SO_4 (V/V). This solution contains 5 mL of concentrated H_2SO_4 (V/V) per 100 mL. Since acid must always be added to water, add about 50 mL of water to a 100-mL volumetric flask then slowly add the 5 mL of H_2SO_4 to the flask. After this solution cools to room temperature, fill to volume with water. NOTE: With this type of solution, the fact that concentrated acids contain varying percentages of the acid is ignored.

Molarity

The molarity of a solution expresses concentration as the number of moles of substance per liter of solution (mol/L), millimoles per milliliter (mmol/mL), or nanomoles per nanoliter (nmol/nL). A mole of a substance is the number of grams equal to the atomic or molecular weight of a substance. A millimolar (1mM) solution contains one millimole per liter. When atomic or molecular weight is expressed in milligrams, it refers to a millimole. This weight is the actual mass of the chemical particles, either atom or molecule, relative to the mass of carbon and for an atom or element is found in the periodic table. The molecular weight of a compound is the sum of the molecular weights of the atoms comprising the molecule. One mole of any chemical contains Avagadro's number (6.02×10^{23}) of particles. Designations for mole include gram molecular weight (gmw) and molecular weight (MW). The mathematical formula for molarity (M) from which all calculations involved in the preparation of molar solutions derive is:

$$\text{Molarity} = \frac{\text{mol}}{\text{L}} = \frac{\text{g/L}}{\text{gram molecular weight (gmw)}}$$

Other factors are added to this basic formula to account for variation in concentration units or volumes other than 1 L.

EXAMPLE: Prepare 1 L of a 2.5-molar solution of NaOH.

1. By definition: Molarity $= \dfrac{\text{g/L}}{\text{gmw}}$
2. Determine the molecular weight of NaOH:

ELEMENT	ATOMIC WEIGHT
Na	23 g
O	16 g
H	1 g
	40 g

The molecular weight of NaOH is 40 g.

3. Using the basic equation:

$$2.5 = \frac{x \text{ g/L NaOH}}{40 \text{ g}}$$

Solve for x g/L NaOH
x g/L NaOH = 2.5 × 40 g
x g/L NaOH = 100 g/L

To prepare the solution, add 100 g of NaOH to a 1-L volumetric flask half filled with water. When the solution returns to ambient temperature, fill to volume with water.

The classic and safest method to solve these problems is the unit cancellation method. With this method, the basic mathematical relationship is combined with factors to convert any concentration units and volumes into the desired units. The equation is designed so that all units except those desired cancel out. When solving a problem with this method, first determine the given and desired units, then set up the equation to cancel all units except the desired units.

EXAMPLE: (See last example) Given units are mol/L; desired units are g/L.

$$\frac{2.5 \text{ mol}}{L} \times \frac{40 \text{ g NaOH}}{1 \text{ mol}} = \frac{100 \text{ g NaOH}}{L}$$

After canceling out the like units, the desired units of g/L are obtained.

EXAMPLE: What is the molarity of a solution containing 49 g H_2SO_4 in 500 mL of solution?

1. Determine the molecular weight of H_2SO_4.

ELEMENT	ATOMIC WEIGHT
H_2	2
S	32
O_4	64
	98 g H_2SO_4

The molecular weight of H_2SO_4 is 98 g.
2. Given units are g/mL.
   Desired units are mol/L.
3. Arrange the equation as follows:

$$\frac{49 \text{ g } H_2SO_4}{500 \text{ mL}} \times \frac{1 \text{ mol } H_2SO_4}{98 \text{ g } H_2SO_4} \times \frac{1000 \text{ mL}}{L} = \frac{x \text{ mol } H_2SO_4}{L}$$

$$\frac{49}{500} \times \frac{1 \text{ mol}}{98} \times \frac{1000}{L} = \frac{1 \text{ mol}}{L}$$

Therefore this is a 1-molar solution. A 1-millimolar solution of H_2SO_4 would contain 98 mg of H_2SO_4 per liter of solution.

Normality

Once the concept of molarity is understood, that of normality follows. *Normality* is defined as the number of gram equivalents per liter (gEq/L). It is closely related to gram molecular weight because the gram equivalent weight (gEq) of a substance is its gram molecular weight divided by its total positive valence. By definition, *gram equivalent weight* of an element or compound is the mass that will replace or combine with 1 mole of hydrogen. Equivalent weight represents the combining weight of an element or compound, and the equivalent weights of all substances are equal in terms of combining power. In other words, normality indicates the ability of ions to combine with other ions and is useful in acid-base calculations, such as those required for acid-base titrations. The equation describing normality is:

$$\text{Normality (Eq/L)} = \frac{\text{g/L}}{\text{gEq}}$$

EXAMPLES:
A. Calculate the gram equivalent weights for each chemical listed.
   1. HCl gmw = 36 g, valence (V) = 1 since 1 mole of H or Cl^- reacts for every mole of HCl.
      36 g/1 = 36 g per equivalent weight.
   2. H_2SO_4 gmw = 98 g, valence = 2
      98 g/2 = 49 g per equivalent weight.
   3. $CaSO_4$ gmw = 136, valence = 2, since 2 mole volume electrons are available for reaction with either Ca^{++} or SO_4.
      136/2 = 68 g per equivalent weight.
B. A 2000-mL solution contains 14.8 g $Ca(OH)_2$. What is its normality?
   The units desired are Eq/L (this is the definition of normality).
   The units given are g/mL.
   To solve this problem, determine the equivalent weight of $Ca(OH)_2$, then set up the equation to cancel out all but the desired units of Eq/L.
   1. Equivalent weight of $Ca(OH)_2$ = gmw/V = 74 g/2 = 37 g.

ELEMENT	ATOMIC WEIGHT
Ca	40 (the valence of a $Ca(OH)_2$ is 2)
O_2	32
H_2	2
	74

   2. $$\frac{14.8 \text{ g}}{2000 \text{ mL}} \times \frac{1 \text{ gEq}}{37 \text{ g}} \times \frac{1000 \text{ mL}}{1 \text{ L}} = 0.2 \text{ gEq/L}$$

By definition, a solution containing 0.2 gEq/L of $Ca(OH)_2$ is a 0.2-N solution.
Normality and molarity are related to one another by the following equation: Molarity(M) × Valence (V) = Normality. From this equation it follows that the normality of a *given* solution is always equal to or greater than its molarity. For example, if the molarity of a divalent solution such as $Ca(OH)_2$ is 5, then its normality is: 5M × 2 = 10 N.

Conversions

Conversion operations are used to solve several types of laboratory problems, for example, to express the quantity of one substance as an equivalent quantity of another, to account for differences in procedural quantities, or to change units of concentration.

EXAMPLE: A physician received calcium results in mg/dL units. He requests the result in mEq/L. What is the conversion factor?

A. Use the unit cancellation method.
   Units desired are mEq/L.
   Units given are mg/dL.
   Equivalent weight of calcium = 40 g/2 = 20 g.

$$\frac{x \; \cancel{mg}}{100 \; \cancel{mL}} \times \frac{1 \; \cancel{g}}{1000 \; \cancel{mg}} \times \frac{1 \; \cancel{Eq}}{20 \; \cancel{g}} \times \frac{1000 \; mEq}{1 \; \cancel{Eq}} \times \frac{1000 \; \cancel{mL}}{1 \; L} = \frac{mEq}{L}$$

   The calculated conversion factor is 0.5. The factor of 0.5 is used to convert any calcium result in mg/dL units to mEq/L. For example, a calcium result of 12 mg/dL equals 6 mEq/L.
B. The conversion factor can also be determined in a two-step procedure that converts mg/dL to mEq/dL and then adjusts for the change in volume from dL to L.
   1. To convert mg/dL to mEq/dL:

$$\frac{\dfrac{mg}{dL}}{mg/mEq} = mEq/dL$$

   For calcium, the mg/mEq is its millimolecular weight of 40 mg divided by its valence of 2 = 20 mg.
   2. To account for the tenfold change in volume:

$$\frac{mEq}{\cancel{dL}} \times \frac{10 \; \cancel{dL}}{1 \; L} = \frac{mEq}{L}$$

   Combining the two equations:

$$\frac{\cancel{mg/dL}}{\cancel{mg}/mEq} \times \frac{10 \; \cancel{dL}}{1 \; L} = mEq/L$$

   For calcium, this translates to:

$$\frac{mg/dL}{20 \; mg/mEq} \times \frac{10 \; dL}{L} = \frac{mEq}{L}$$

   Therefore the conversion factor is 10/20 or 0.5.

EXAMPLE: An assay requires a 500 mg/100 mL solution of bromide. Sodium bromide must be used to prepare the solution. Find the milligrams of NaBr required.

A conversion factor using the gram molecular weights of bromide and sodium bromide as the basis of comparison is used to solve this problem.

1. Molecular weight of Br = 80 g.
   Molecular weight of NaBr = 103 g.
2. Conversion factor = $\dfrac{103 \; (NaBr)}{80 \; (Br)}$ = 1.29.
3. Weight of NaBr that is equivalent to 500 mg Br is 1.29 × 500 mg = 644 mg.

To prepare the solution, add 644 mg NaBr to a 500-mL volumetric flask and fill to volume with water.

Water of hydration

Some chemicals are available in both anhydrous and hydrated forms. The state of hydration (number of water mol-

ecules per compound) is listed on the reagent bottle. When a chemical specified for reagent preparation is unavailable but one of its other hydrated or anhydrous forms is available, then a calculation can be performed to adjust for the chemical on hand. This is accomplished by using molecular weights as the basis of comparison in a ratio proportion equation.

EXAMPLE: A procedure calls for 100 mL of a 10% $CaCl_2$ (W/V) solution. Only $CaCl_2 \cdot 10 \; H_2O$ is on hand. How is the solution prepared?

1. A 10% (W/V) solution contains 10 g $CaCl_2$/100 mL.
2. Use gram molecular weight as the basis of comparison between the specified and available chemicals.

$$Mol \; wt \; CaCl_2 = 110 \; g.$$
$$Mol \; wt \; CaCl_2 \cdot 10 \; H_2O = 290 \; g.$$

3. Set up a ratio proportion equation and solve for x.

$$\frac{290 \; (mol \; wt \; CaCl_2 \cdot 10 \; H_2O)}{110 \; (mol \; wt \; CaCl_2)} = \frac{x \; g/100 \; mL \; CaCl_2 \cdot 10 \; H_2O}{10 \; g/100 \; mL \; CaCl_2}$$

$$x \; g/100 \; mL \; CaCL_2 \cdot 10 \; H_2O = \frac{290 \times 10 \; g/100 \; mL \; CaCl_2}{110}$$

$$x = 26.4 \; g$$

Transfer 26.4 g $CaCl_2 \cdot 10 \; H_2O$ to a 100-ml volumetric flask and fill to volume with water.

Dilutions
Simple dilutions

The most frequent use of dilutions in the clinical laboratory is to bring the concentration of some body fluid component into the linear range of an assay. Dilutions can also be an economical and efficient method of preparing reagents and standard solutions. By definition, dilution is the addition of some substance (the diluent) to another substance (the solute) to reduce the concentration of the solute. Dilution usually means that so many parts of the solute are diluted in the total parts of the final solution. As such, dilution indicates the relative amount of the solute in the dilute solution, that is, it is an indicator of concentration not volume. To illustrate, a 1 to 10 dilution can be prepared in any of the following ways:

1 mL serum + 9 mL saline
10 mL serum + 90 mL saline
0.1 mL serum + 0.9 mL saline

Dilution statements are written in various ways. The following terms all designate a 1-to-10 dilution:
   1 to 10
   1:10
   1/10

The dilution factor that is used to calculate concentration before dilution is the inverse of the dilution statement—for a 1-to-10 dilution, the dilution factor is 10. A less common meaning of dilution is that so many parts of diluent are added to so many parts of solute. The correct term for such a procedure is ratio so that a dilution prepared as a 1 to 10 ratio results in a dilution statement of 1 to 11 and a dilution factor of 11.

EXAMPLE: Three milliliters of concentrated standard solution are available to prepare a 1:50 dilution of the standard with saline. What is the maximum amount of dilute standard that can be prepared?

Method 1. Set up a ratio proportion using the dilution of statement as the known relationship:

$$\frac{1}{50} = \frac{3 \text{ mL}}{x \text{ mL}} \text{ ; solve for x mL}$$

$$x \text{ mL} = 50 \text{ x } 3 \text{ mL}$$

$$x = 150 \text{ mL}$$

Method 2. Use the equation $V_1 \times C_1 = V_2 \times C_2$ where:

V_1 = volume of the concentrated solution
C_1 = concentration of concentrated solution
V_2 = volume of dilute solution
C_2 = concentration of dilute solution

$$3 \text{ mL} \times 1 = x \text{ mL} \times 1/50; \text{ solve for x mL:}$$

$$x \text{ mL} = \frac{3 \text{ mL} \times 1}{1/50}$$

$$x = 150 \text{ mL}$$

Note that what is actually expressed on each side of the $V_1 \times C_1 = V_2 \times C_2$ equation is the amount of solute. Use of this equation requires that all volume and concentration units be the same or equivalent. It can be used for any type of units: percent solution, molarity, or normality.

EXAMPLE: Prepare 100 mL of 0.25 N NaOH from 1.0 N NaOH. Use the $V_1 \times C_1 = V_2 \times C_2$ equation to determine the volume of 1.0 N NaOH required
where:

V_1 = x mL of 1 N NaOH
C_1 = 1.0 N
V_2 = 100 mL
C_2 = 0.25 N

$$x \text{ mL} \times 1.0 \text{ N} = 100 \text{ mL} \times 0.25 \text{ N}$$

$$x \text{ mL} = \frac{100 \text{ mL} \times 0.25 \text{ N}}{1.0 \text{ N}}$$

$$x = 25 \text{ mL}$$

This is a 1 to 4 dilution of 1.0 N NaOH. The dilution statement is:

$$\frac{25 \text{ mL (solute)}}{100 \text{ mL (total solution)}} = \frac{1}{4}$$

To prepare the solution, transfer 25 mL of 1.0 N NaOH to a 100-mL volumetric flask and fill to volume with water.

EXAMPLE: One millileter of spinal fluid is diluted with 5 mL of saline. The protein result obtained on the dilute sample is 52 mg/dL. What is the original concentration?

This is a 1 to 6 dilution:

$$\frac{\begin{array}{l}1 \text{ mL spinal fluid}\\5 \text{ mL saline}\end{array}}{6 \text{ mL total solution}}$$

Therefore the dilution factor is 6. Original spinal fluid protein concentration is $\frac{6 \times 52 \text{ mg}}{\text{dL}} = 312$ mg/dL.

Serial dilutions

Serial dilutions are a special type of dilution series in which all dilutions except the first are prepared from the previous dilution and all dilutions made after the initial dilution are the same. With this type of series, samples containing widely varying concentrations of a component are easily prepared with a minimum of solute and solvent. Because of this property, serial dilutions are used to prepare samples for analyses of components that can exist over a wide concentration range, for example, antibody titers and beta-hCG concentrations. Serial dilutions are also used to prepare sets of standard solutions. These should always be compared with standards made individually as errors can be compounded with the serial technique. As with all dilutions, the procedure can be designed to yield the most desirable concentrations.

EXAMPLE: A serum sample is diluted 1:2 with buffer and then a five-tube series of 1:10 dilutions with buffer are prepared. What is the dilution and dilution factor for each of the five tubes?

TUBE:	INITIAL	1	2	3	4	5
Dilution:	1:2	1:20	1:200	1:2000	1:20000	1:200000
Dilution factor:	2	20	200	2000	20000	200000

1. Initial tube contains 1 mL serum and 1 mL buffer.
2. Tubes 1 through 5 contain 9 mL buffer.
3. One milliliter of the initial dilution (1:2) is added to tube 1.
4. One milliliter of the solution in tube 1 is added to tube 2.
5. Continue for all tubes in sequence.

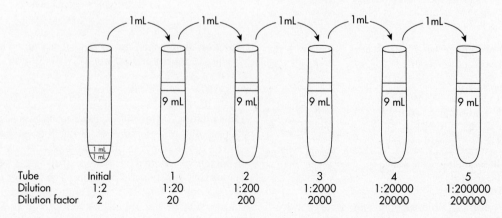

Tube	Initial	1	2	3	4	5
Dilution	1:2	1:20	1:200	1:2000	1:20000	1:200000
Dilution factor	2	20	200	2000	20000	200000

The dilution of any tube in the series is the product of all dilutions made up to that point. The final dilution is 1:200000 and the dilution factor is 200000. Note that if one were to prepare each dilution separately, more serum and large quantities of buffer would be required.

Clearance

Creatinine clearance calculations are used as a simple measure of kidney function since they express the volume of blood "cleared" of a substance (creatinine) in milliliters per minute. The formula for calculating the creatinine clearance (CL) is as follows (see also Chapter 6):

$$CL \text{ (mL/min)} = \frac{U}{P} \times Vol \times \frac{1}{T \times 60 \text{ min/hr}}$$

where:
U = Urinary creatinine concentration (mg/dl)
P = Plasma creatinine concentration (mg/dl)
Vol = Volume of urine in milliliters collected
T = Time (collection period) in hours

EXAMPLE: What is the creatinine clearance for a patient whose urinary creatinine concentration is 87 mg/dl, plasma creatinine concentration is 0.8 mg/dl, and volume of urine collected is 1300 ml for 24 hours?

$$CL \text{ (mL/min)} = \frac{87}{0.8} \times 1300 \times \frac{1}{1440}$$
$$CL = 98 \text{ mL/min}$$

The clearance formula may also be corrected for body surface area to give a clearance adjusted to the body surface area of a "standard person."

$$CL \text{ (mL/min)} = \frac{U}{P} \times Vol \times \frac{1}{T \times 60 \text{ min/hr}} \times \frac{1.73}{A}$$

The definitions for CL, U, P, Vol, and T are the same and A represents the surface area in square meters. The 1.73 factor is the surface area of a standard (average) person.

EXAMPLE: What is the creatinine clearance for a patient whose urinary creatinine concentration is 65 mg/dL, plasma creatinine concentration is 1.1 mg/dL, and volume of urine collected is 1500 ml in 24 hours? Correct the clearance for surface area; the patient weighs 100 pounds and is 4 feet, 10 inches tall, so the surface area is 1.36 m².

$$CL \text{ (mL/min)} = \frac{65}{1.1} \times 1500 \times \frac{1}{24 \times 60} \times \frac{1.73}{1.36}$$
$$CL \text{ (mL/min)} = 59.1 \times 1.042 \times 1.27$$
$$CL = 78 \text{ mL/min}$$

Buffers

Solutions that resist changes in pH are called buffers. Often these solutions are made from combinations of weak acids and their salts, or weak bases and their salts. The expression relating the solution pH to the concentrations of the weak acid and salt of the weak acid is called the Henderson-Hasselbalch equation. A similar form can be used for weak bases.

$$pH = pKa + \log \frac{\text{(concentration of salt)}}{\text{(concentration of acid)}}$$

where *pKa* is the negative logarithm of the association constant for the weak acid.

EXAMPLE: Calculate the pH of an acetate buffer composed of 0.2 M sodium acetate and 0.1 M acetic acid. The pKa for acetic acid is 4.76. Solve using the Henderson-Hasselbalch equation.

$$pH = 4.76 + \log \frac{(0.2 \text{ M})}{(0.1 \text{ M})}$$
$$pH = 4.76 + \log 2$$
$$pH = 4.76 + 0.3$$
$$pH = 5.1$$

EXAMPLE: How would you make 1 L of a 0.1 M acetic acid buffer with a pH of 4.90? The gmw of acetic acid = 60, the gmw of sodium acetate = 82.

First, express salt and acid concentration in terms of one unknown variable. Since buffer = 0.1 M = salt + acid, let x = acid. Therefore, salt = 0.1 − x. Then use the Henderson-Hasselbalch equation:

$$pH = pKa + \log \frac{\text{(salt)}}{\text{(acid)}}$$
$$4.90 = 4.76 + \log \frac{(0.1 - x)}{(x)}$$
$$0.14 = \log \frac{(0.1 - x)}{(x)}$$

Taking the anti log of both sides of the equation:

$$1.38 = \frac{0.1 - x}{x}$$
$$1.38 x = 0.1 - x$$
$$\underline{+ x \qquad + x}$$
$$2.38 x = 0.1$$
$$x = 0.042 \text{ M} = acid$$

Salt = 0.1 − 0.042 = 0.058 M
Therefore: 0.042 M acetic acid × 60 g/mol = 2.52 g acetic acid
0.058 M Na acetate × 82 g/mol = 4.75 g Na acetate

EXAMPLE: What is the pH of a buffer made up of 10 mL of 0.1 M $NaHCO_3$ and 5 mL of 0.14 M H_2CO_3? The pKa for bicarbonate is 6.1.

First, determine how many moles of salt and acid are in the buffer.

$$0.1 \text{ M } NaHCO_3 \times 10 \text{ mL} \times \frac{1 \text{ L}}{1000 \text{ mL}} = 0.001 \text{ moles of salt}$$

$$0.14 \text{ M } H_2CO_3 \times 5 \text{ mL} \times \frac{1 \text{ L}}{1000 \text{ mL}} = 0.0007 \text{ moles of acid}$$

Then use the Henderson-Hasselbalch equation:

$$pH = pKa + \log \frac{\text{(salt)}}{\text{(acid)}}$$
$$pH = 6.1 + \log \frac{(0.001)}{(0.0007)}$$

$$pH = 6.1 + \log \frac{(1)}{(0.7)}$$

$$pH = 6.1 + \log 1.4286$$

$$pH = 6.1 + 0.155$$

$$pH = 6.255$$

CENTRIFUGES

Centrifuges are pieces of laboratory equipment that are required for most other laboratory work. They are used to separate components of a mixture on the basis of particle size or density. The most common application is the separation of blood into cells and a serum or plasma supernatant. Other uses are the separation of chylomicrons from serum or plasma and the fractionation of lipoproteins. Each application requires a specific centrifugal force and a defined time period.

All centrifuges contain three basic parts: the motor, drive shaft, and rotor. They are available with either horizontal or fixed angle rotor heads in floor or tabletop models. General operation centrifuges attain speeds up to 6000 revolutions per minute (rpm), producing relative centrifugal force (RCF) of 7300 times the force of gravity (G). Ultracentrifuges produce much greater RCF and are required for the separation of lipoproteins from other components. Although it is common to see centrifugation instructions specify the rpm to be used, the only time this is valid is if the centrifuge and its rotor head radius are also listed. The more valid parameter is the RCF required. Relative centrifugal force and rpm are related to each other by this formula:

EQ. 4-1

$$RCF = 1.12r \frac{(rpm)^2}{(1000)}$$

where r = radius in millimeters measured from the center of rotation (center of the centrifuge head) to the bottom of the rotor cavity. Figure 4-2 shows a nomogram relating revo-

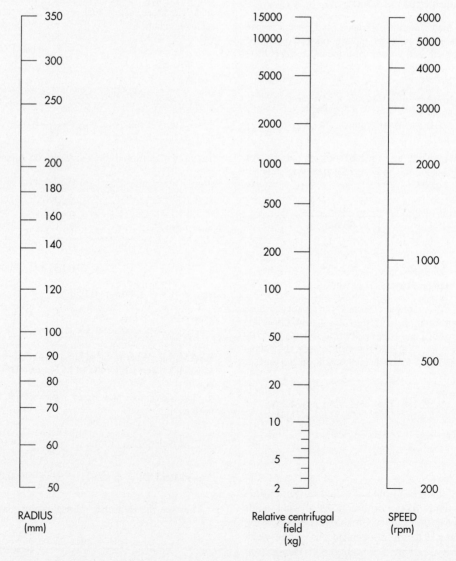

Fig. 4-2 Nomogram for centrifuge speed selection. Centrifugal force is a function of radius and speed. The speed required to obtain the desired force is obtained by aligning a straight edge through the radius and required centrifugal force. The required speed is then read from where the straight edge intersects the speed column.

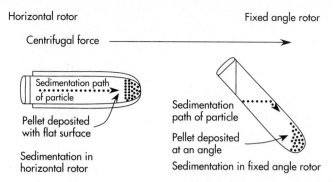

Fig. 4-3 Pellet formation in horizontal rotor and fixed angle rotors. *From A centrifuge primer, Palo Alto, CA, 1980, Spinco Division of Beckman Instruments.*

lutions per minute and radius to relative centrifugal force. Relative centrifugal force is measured in multiples of the earth's gravitational field and is designated G. Separation of cells from serum or plasma requires an RCF of 1000 × G for a minimum of 10 minutes. Serum or plasma separator tubes contain a material of density intermediate between that of cells and the liquid component of blood. These tubes require a specific RCF and time for proper positioning of the separating material. Follow manufacturer's guidelines when using these tubes. Certain laboratory procedures require strict adherence to centrifugation conditions because some components can be damaged or lost by either excessive RCF or time.

Fixed angle rotors are capable of higher speed than horizontal angle rotors and are desirable when quick separation of small particles is required. Horizontal rotors form a more compact pellet because only the tube bottom and not the sides are aligned with the direction of the centrifugal force. Figure 4-3 shows the quality of pellet formation obtained with both rotor types.

Verification of centrifuge calibration

The correlation of RPM with the meter speed indicator should be checked with a tachometer every 3 months and any corrections to the calibration dial posted near the speed indicator.

Maintenance and operation

Limits for speed and load weight must be observed to avoid rotor failure. All loads must be balanced and all buckets must be in place even if empty. Opposing loads must be equal within the tolerance limits specified by the manufacturer. If opposing buckets are spun with partial loads, the tubes must be arranged symmetrically.

Centrifuges must be cleaned and lubricated regularly. Brushes must be replaced at intervals dictated by usage and the manufacturer's recommendations. Any broken glass must be removed immediately to avoid damage to the rotor. Accumulation of fine gray dust is evidence that glass fragments are bombarding the inside of the rotor chamber of the rotor. Liquids spilled in the centrifuge, particularly hazardous chemicals or biological specimens, must be removed before the centrifuge is operated again because the centrifuge forms a stable aerosol of the fluid and can disperse it into the surroundings. Tubes containing biological hazards

should be centrifuged with stoppers in place to reduce the danger of exposing operators to this material.

BALANCES
Mass vs. weight

Underlying every good analysis is an accurate measurement of mass or volume. Mass is a constant measure of the quantity of matter as opposed to weight, which is the force of attraction between that matter and the earth. Mass and weight are related to one another by the equation:

EQ. 4-2

$$W = M \times G$$

where W = weight, M = Mass, G = acceleration caused by gravity. This equation demonstrates that weight is dependent on gravitational force, which varies with distance from the earth's gravitational center. Mass is independent of this variable.

In the laboratory the analytical balance is used to determine mass by comparison with objects of known mass. Commonly, this process is called "weighing" and the objects of known mass are called "weights."

Balance types

There are two types of analytical balances in common use; the equal arm balance and the single pan balance. In both types the beam pivots on a prism-shaped knife-edge that rests on a flat surface. The knife-edge of an equal arm balance is positioned at the center of the beam and both pans are supported by knife-edges. In the single pan balance, the main knife-edge is positioned asymmetrically on the beam and the pan requires only one additional knife-edge. Balances are equipped with dampers that reduce the time required for the beam to return to rest when the weights are in equilibrium. Single pan balances usually utilize an air damper; magnetic dampers are common in equal arm balances.

With the equal arm balance shown in Figure 4-4, *A*, the weight is obtained by adjusting the position of the counterbalancing weights on the extension of the beam called the balance arm bridge.

The single pan balance shown in Figure 4-4, *B*, has three balance arm bridges supporting the counterbalancing weights. Both of these balances are useful for quick weighing operations that require no more than a 0.1 g sensitivity. Typical maximum capacities for these types of balances are about 200 g.

Single pan balances have several advantages over the equal arm balances; they have two knife-edges instead of three, reducing frictional interference and wear and tear over time. In addition, the sensitivity is independent of the weight of the object being weighed because the beam is subjected to constant loading.

Since 1960 the analytical balance offering the greatest precision and accuracy is the substitution balance—a modified single pan balance with a set of weights suspended above the pan. These weights are counterbalanced by one weight located at the opposite end of the beam, which also serves as the moving portion of the air damper (Figure 4-5). When an object is placed on the pan unequal loading results. The beam is restored to within 100 mg or less of

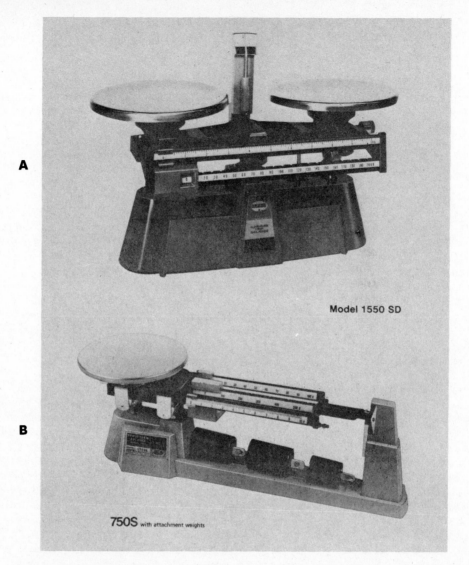

Model 1550 SD

750S with attachment weights

Fig. 4-4 **A,** Double beam trip balance (type of equal arm balance). **B,** Single pan trip balance. *From Alexander RL and Bauer JD: Basic laboratory principles. In Kaplan LA and Pesce AJ: Clinical chemistry: theory, analysis, and correlation, St Louis, 1984, Mosby-Year Book, Inc.*

the object's weight by the addition of the weights above the pan. The operator does this by turning dials to adjust the internal weights. The final 100 mg is determined by the deflection of a light beam from its original position to a position that is proportional to the difference between the weight of the object and the final weight added. This difference is translated by an optical system to mass units that display the fractional weight on a frosted glass surface. The substitution balance eliminates errors caused by unequal arms because the weighed objects and weights are compared on the same arm and the weights are manipulated mechanically so they are not damaged by the operator.

Top-loading balances are modified substitution balances. They are quick and more rugged than the analytical balance but are less sensitive and precise.

Electronic balances are available with precision and accuracy as good or better than that offered by mechanical balances. They are single pan balances that use electromagnetism to counterbalance the load. When an object is

placed on the pan, current to the coil supporting the pan is increased until the pan returns to its original position. The current required is proportional to the object's mass and is converted to a digital display of mass.

Care of balances

Balances should be placed on a weighing table or on a heavy slab of material in an area away from air currents. The balance should be located far from instruments or machines that cause vibration (elevators and centrifuges) and away from corrosive chemicals that can erode the weights. Materials to be weighed should be placed on weighing paper, or in weighing boats or bottles. Before use, ensure that the balance is level by centering the bubble in the spirit level with the foot screws and adjusting the optical zero with the zero control knob. If the capacity of the zero adjustment knob is exceeded, follow the manufacturer's instructions to adjust the zero counterweight located near the main knife-edge. Protect the knife-edge and bearing surfaces by en-

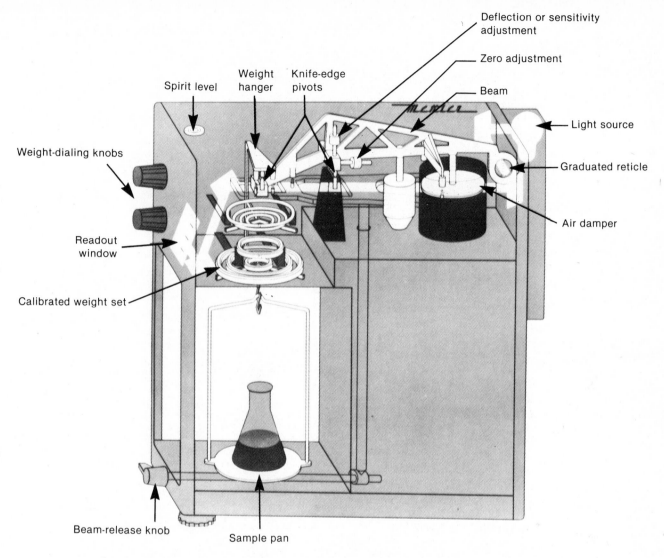

Fig. 4-5 Single pan substitution balance showing internal designs. *From Steiner P and Byrne EA: Laboratory techniques. In Kaplan LA and Pesce AJ: Clinical chemistry: theory, analysis, and correlation, ed 2, St Louis, 1989, Mosby-Year Book, Inc.*

gaging the beam support when changing the pan load or weights.

Verification of calibration

Most analytical balances are equipped with internal weights that meet the class S weight tolerance limits as defined in the National Bureau of Standards (NBS) circular 547, section I (1962). The internal weights should be checked at regular intervals with an external set of class S weights. Table 4-4 lists the class S weights with their NBS maintenance tolerance limits. If the tolerance limits are exceeded, service is required.

pH METER

The pH meter is a highly sensitive potentiometer used to measure the hydrogen ion concentration, or more accurately, the hydrogen ion activity of solutions. The activity of an ion is an expression of its ability to react in or influence chemical reactions.

Table 4-4 Individual National Bureau of Standards tolerances for class S weights

Nominal mass	Individual tolerance (mg)	Maintenance tolerance (mg)
1, 2, 3, 5, 10, 20, 30, 50 mg	±0.014	±0.014
100, 200, 300, 500 mg	±0.025	±0.05
1, 2, 3, 5 g	±0.054	±0.11
10, 20, 30 g	±0.074	±0.148
50 g	±0.12	±0.22
100 g	±0.25	±0.5

From Steiner P and Byrne EA: Laboratory techniques. In Kaplan LA and Pesce AJ, editors: Clinical chemistry: theory, analysis, and correlation, ed 2, St. Louis, 1989, Mosby-Year Book, Inc.

Concentration vs. activity

Activity and concentration are related by an activity coefficient:

EQ. 4-3

$$a = \gamma c$$

where a = activity; γ = activity coefficient, always less than 1.0; and c = concentration. For most clinical laboratory purposes, the distinction between activity and concentration is ignored since in the dilute solutions often used by the laboratory the concentration approaches the activity.

For the sake of convenience, hydrogen ion concentration is expressed in pH units. pH is defined as the negative logarithm to the base 10 of the hydrogen ion concentration, pH = $-\log [H^+]$. For example, the hydrogen ion concentration of pure water is 10^{-7} mol/L and the pH = 7. The pH scale ranges from 0 to 14, corresponding to concentrations of 1 mol/L to 1×10^{-14} mol/L of hydrogen ions. Each increase of 1 pH unit from 0 indicates a tenfold decrease in the concentration of hydrogen ions.

In the clinical laboratory the pH meter is used in the preparation and quality control of reagents. pH is a most important consideration because the rate, extent, and type of chemical reaction is often pH-dependent. A specialized version of the pH meter, miniaturized and thermostated, is an integral part of the blood gas analyzers used to monitor the acid-base status of acutely ill patients.

Basis of pH measurement

The basic principle of pH analysis, is that a voltage difference develops across a thin, conducting glass membrane used to separate two solutions of different pH. This difference in voltage is detected by two reference electrodes of known, constant voltage that are placed in the solution on either side of the membrane (Figure 4-6).

With this arrangement, the voltage across the reference electrodes varies in relation to the ratio of the hydrogen ion activities in the two solutions (a1 and a2). The voltage obtained is derived from the Nernst equation:

EQ. 4-4

$$E \text{ measured} = E_o + 2.303 \frac{RT}{nF} \log \frac{a1}{a2}$$

where:
E = measured voltage
E_o = difference in standard half-cell potentials
R = gas constant
T = absolute temperature
n = electrons transferred
F = Faraday's constant (96,500 C)
a1, a2 = activities of the ions being measured

In all cases the electrode voltage of a half-cell is measured with respect to the standard hydrogen electrode, which is 0 volts.

For any pair of half-cell reactions, the measured voltage is the difference between the measuring electrode half-cell and the reference electrode half-cell corrected for the concentration of the active species. At 25°C for one electron transfer this becomes:

EQ. 4-4a

$$E_{\text{measured voltage}} = k_1 + 0.059 \log \frac{a1}{a2}$$

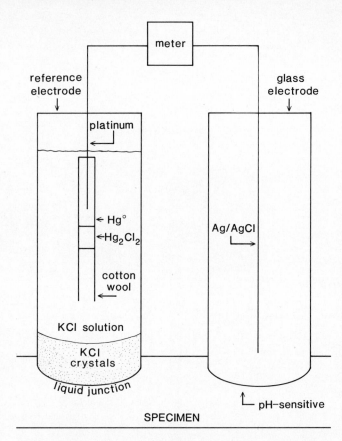

Fig. 4-6   Scheme of contact sequence of specimen, glass electrode, and reference electrode. The potential of interest occurs as a result of the difference between the hydrogen activity of the specimen *(a1)* and the hydrogen activity inside the glass electrode *(a2)* when the two solutions are separated by pH-sensitive glass. Since a2 is constant, potential is a function of a1. *From Bruegger BB and Sherwin JE: Blood gas analysis and oxygen saturation. In Pesce AJ and Kaplan LA: Methods in clinical chemistry, St Louis, 1987, Mosby-Year Book, Inc.*

where k_1 is a constant. With the use of a pH meter, the pH of the solution inside of the indicator electrode (a2) is constant, and since the voltage of the two reference electrodes are constant, any change in measured potential is a function of the pH of the test solution and is described by the formula, where k_2 includes the log of the constant activity (a2).

EQ. 4-4b

$$E_{\text{measured voltage}} = k_2 + .059 \log a1$$

or using the definition of pH.

EQ. 4-4c

$$E_{\text{measured voltage}} = k_2 - .059 \text{ pH}$$

The value of k_2 is obtained by measuring E for a solution of known hydrogen ion concentration, namely, a standard acid.

Instrumentation

The first commercial pH meter was introduced by Arnold O. Beckman in 1935. Its use for the selective measurement of hydrogen ion concentration was made possible by the development of the "glass electrode." The three basic components of the pH meter are the indicator or glass electrode, the reference electrode, and the voltmeter.

Indicator electrode

The indicator electrode is constructed with a tip made of a special glass sensitive to the conductance of hydrogen ions, hence its name "glass electrode." It is across this glass membrane that the potential difference indicative of hydrogen ion concentration of the test solution develops. Investigation into the sensitivity and selectivity of different compositions of glass membranes to protons and other cations has led to the development of several commercial glass electrodes. In general, they all contain varying amounts of Na_2O, CaO, and SiO_2.

The glass electrode is filled with a reference solution of known pH that is resistant to changes in pH. Suspended in this solution is the internal reference electrode, usually a Ag-$AgCl_2$ half-cell. Since the pH of the electrode interior is constant, any voltage changes detected are caused by hydrogen ion concentrations of the exterior test solution. The glass membrane does not actually permit electron transfer through the membrane, but establishes an ion exchange equilibrium between the hydrogen ions in the test solution and the positive ions in the glass membrane.

Reference electrode

The reference electrode consists of an internal element or reference electrode, a filling solution, and a liquid junction through which the filling solution can slowly flow. It serves two basic functions: it provides a constant reference voltage against which the indicator electrode voltage is measured, and, through the liquid junction, it completes the electrical circuit between the pH meter and the test solution. The internal element of the reference electrode is usually a Hg-$HgCl_2$ half-cell, also called a calomel electrode. The filling solution is usually saturated KCl so that the difference in ionic strength and composition of the test solution does not greatly affect the potential of the reference electrode.

Voltmeter

When the indicator and reference electrodes are immersed into a test solution, a small voltage difference, which is proportional to the hydrogen ion concentration of the test solution, develops at the glass membrane surface. The voltmeter supplies an equal and opposing voltage. This voltage is amplified and converted to a digital or meter display of pH.

Combination electrodes

Electrodes that combine the indicator and reference electrodes in one glass probe are called combination electrodes. These make the pH measuring system more compact. They are especially useful for measuring the pH of small volumes of solution.

Errors affecting pH measurement

The glass calomel electrode system is a powerful tool for the accurate determination of pH. However, the electrode is subject to several limitations that must be taken into account so that pH data can be obtained with little error.

Alkaline error

The conventional glass membrane shows excellent selectivity to other cations for hydrogen ions up to a pH of 9; at higher pH values the membrane becomes sensitive to sodium and other alkali metals as well as the hydrogen ion concentration. This sensitivity to other cations causes a negative pH error. New electrode compositions have been developed to reduce the alkaline errors to an insignificant level, but both types of electrodes are commercially available.

Acid error

In strongly acidic solutions when pH values would be less than zero, values obtained with the glass electrode are inappropriately high. The cause of acid error is uncertain but occurs because hydrogen ion activities on either side of the glass membrane are no longer related to hydrogen ion concentration in the test solution.

Junction potentials

Ideally, the only voltage measured should be the boundary voltage at the glass membrane surface. However, because of the additional junction voltages that arise at the surface between the reference electrode and the analytical solution in the glass electrode system, a composite voltage is measured. This voltage includes the unknown sample voltage plus the additional contributions of the reference junction voltages. Errors in junction voltage cannot be entirely compensated for by standardization because of matrix differences between standards and test solutions. For dilute solutions, these errors are usually small. In blood gas pH, pCO_2, and pO_2 measurements, a larger error of this type exists because the sample measurements are made in whole blood. This complex sample of liquid and cellular material has a matrix that does not correspond to the aqueous buffer and gas standards used to calibrate the instrument.

Dehydration errors

The glass membrane must be hydrated for some time prior to being used. A dry electrode that is used immediately will drift excessively and may have accuracy problems. If an electrode must be used before hydration is complete, restandardization must be completed frequently during the measurement process.

Standard solutions

Standard buffer solutions that have been contaminated by bacteria or fungi, have evaporated, or have beeen prepared incorrectly will cause deviations from stated standard values and introduce serious analytical error. Sometimes these problems are not immediately apparent. This problem is prevented when pH determinations are performed on control samples with known pH values.

pH meter controls

The meter has three basic controls: the standardizing control, the slope control, and the temperature control. Standardizing with buffers of known pH must be done frequently to correlate meter response with pH by adjusting for changes in electrode response. The slope control adjusts the millivolts per pH unit to accommodate changes in electrode performance. Temperature control is necessary because the voltage to activity conversion factor is temperature-dependent. Some pH electrodes make this unnecessary as they are temperature-compensated.

pH standards

Standardization is done with standard buffer solutions. The primary buffers recommended by NBS have been chosen to minimize the effects of temperature, air exposure, and other contaminants. Three of the common buffers that can be used for this purpose with their pH at 25° C are:

BUFFER	pH
Phthalate	4.01
Phosphate	6.06
Borax	9.15

Ideally, standardization should be done using the standard with a pH closest to the pH of the solution to be measured. This standard should also be similar in ionic strength. A second standard buffer is used to set the slope control in the direction it is anticipated most measurements will be from the first standard.

Use and care of the pH meter

Successful use of the pH meter requires adherence to a few simple guidelines.
1. Adjust the meter for temperature by carefully measuring the temperature of a standard buffer with a thermometer and setting the dial to the indicated temperature.
2. Standardize using the buffer with a pH close to the pH of the test solution.
3. Adjust the slope with a second buffer. For example, if standardization is done with a buffer of pH = 7 and it is expected that the unknowns will be between pH 5 and pH 7, then adjust the slope with a buffer of pH = 4.
4. Ensure that all samples are thoroughly mixed. If the solution is to be mixed during the measuring process, make sure that the stirrer is well removed from the electrode surfaces and the solution is insulated from any heat produced by the mixer. Stop mixing just before measuring, if possible, since the electrodes can be affected by magnetic and electric fields.
5. Avoid carryover between buffers and test solutions by rinsing the electrode with distilled water and gently blotting the tip with lintless tissue before transfer of the electrode to each successive solution. Do not wipe the tip as a static charge may result and can affect the measurement.
6. Maintain the reference electrode filling solution to above the internal element. Replace the filling solution at intervals recommended by the manufacturer.
7. Proper electrode function depends on hydration of the glass membrane; therefore, store electrodes in the solution recommended by the manufacturer (water or buffer). Not all electrodes are stored wet. Some specific ion measuring electrodes are stored dry.

Rejuvenating electrodes

Electrodes that exhibit erratic performance or long measuring times may have their measuring surface partially coated with contaminating material or the reference electrode junc-

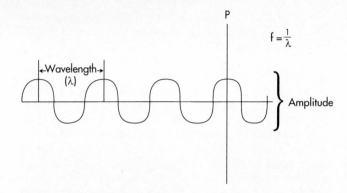

Fig. 4-7   Electromagnetic radiation as wave motion. Wavelength is the distance between wave peaks in nanometers (nm) and amplitude as the height of each wave. The number of waves passing a fixed point (P) per unit time is the frequency. Given constant velocity, frequency and energy are inversely proportional to wavelength.

tion may be partially clogged. These problems can often be corrected by the following procedures:
1. To strip organic buildup on the glass membrane of the indicating electrode:
   a. Immerse the tip in 0.1 M NaOH for 1 minute.
   b. Immerse the tip in 0.1 M HCL for 1 minute.
   c. Repeat the process and rinse thoroughly with distilled or deionized water.
2. To unclog the reference electrode junction:
   a. Replace the filling solution.
   b. Soak electrode for 1 hour in saturated KCl.
   c. Apply gentle pressure to the filling hole to dislodge material blocking the junction.

SPECTROPHOTOMETER

The spectrophotometer is a laboratory instrument used to measure the intensity of light. The photometer is also used to measure light of known wavelengths. Chemical substances can be characterized by their pattern of absorbance or transmittance when placed in the path of a light beam. In the ultraviolet (UV) and visible (VIS) ranges of the light spectrum, this pattern of light transmission is the result of changes in the energy levels of certain chemical groups due to their light-absorption properties. Many of the assays done in the clinical laboratory isolate some component of interest by a chemical reaction that convert it to a colored product. The amount of color produced is proportional to the concentration of the component being studied.

Properties of light

Light is a form of electromagnetic or radiant energy whose movement must be described in two ways, as an oscillating wave and as a linear particle movement. Both descriptions are useful for basic understanding of the spectrophotometer and the microscope. Most pertinent to absorption spectrophotometry is the wave theory. Because light travels in oscillating waves, it possesses properties of wavelength, amplitude, and frequency. Wavelength, symbolized by the Greek lambda, λ, is defined as the length in nanometers or micrometers between two wavepeaks; amplitude is the height of each wave; and frequency is the number of waves passing a fixed point per second (Figure 4-7).

Wavelength and frequency are related as follows:

EQ. 4-5

$$V = \lambda F$$

where V = velocity, λ = wavelength, and F = frequency. In air or in a vacuum, the velocity of light is 3×10^8m/sec. Given constant velocity, wavelength and frequency are inversely related so that an increase in wavelength is associated with a decrease in frequency. Commonly, wavelength is thought to determine color when velocity is constant. For example, blue light is of wavelength 400 nm, red light of 700 nm. However, when velocity changes, such as when light travels from air to glass, neither color nor frequency change, rather the wavelength is shortened. Therefore, color is actually a function of frequency.

The electromagnetic spectrum includes a wide range of wavelengths (≤ 0.1 nm for gamma radiation to $> 25 \times 10^7$ for radio waves). In the laboratory the portions of the spectrum employed for absorption spectroscopy are the visible range (390 to 780 nm) and the ultraviolet or UV range (180 to 390 nm).

When light is conceived as a linear particle movement, it travels through a homogenous (isotropic) medium as a straight beam until it passes into another medium. If the medium is a lens, it will be refracted or bent. If it is a solid substance, it will be either reflected or absorbed. In most spectroscopy specimens, a portion of the light is absorbed.

Light from the sun or a tungsten filament lamp used in absorption spectrophotometry is a mixture of visible light of all wavelengths and appears "white." Table 4-5 shows a breakdown of white light into its components with associated absorbed and transmitted colors. The color of a solution is its transmitted color. For example, a solution that absorbs violet light at 400 nm reflects or transmits all other light and appears yellow-blue. If one were to picture the absorbance of the colored solution vs. wavelength, the resulting graph is known as an absorption spectrum. Spectrophotom-

Table 4-5 The visible spectrum*

Approximate wavelength (nm)	Color of light absorbed	Color of light reflected (transmitted)
400-435	Violet	Green-yellow
435-500	Blue	Yellow
500-570	Green	Red
570-600	Yellow	Blue
600-630	Orange	Green-blue
630-700	Red	Green

*The wavelengths are an approximation because in reality there is no clear demarcation between colors—the colors of the absorbed and reflected light change gradually with wavelengths. Observed color of a solid object is the sum of the wavelength reflected; for a solution, the observed color is the sum of the wavelengths transmitted by the solution.

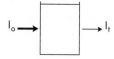

Fig. 4-8 Transmittance of light through a cuvette. I_o is the incident light; I_t is the transmitted light.

etry takes advantage of the ability of colored solution to absorb light of a specific wavelength; the amount of absorbance is directly related to the amount of color. For example, to measure the concentration of a blue solution, light of about 600 nm is passed through the solution and the amount of light *absorbed* is proportional to the concentration of the blue-colored substance in the solution.

Beer's law

Beer's law describes the relationship of absorbance to concentration. Absorbance is not a directly measurable quantity but is computed from transmission data. When light of a particular wavelength passes through a cuvette that contains a colored solution, some of the light is absorbed; the rest of the light is transmitted through the sample (Figure 4-8). The portion of light transmitted when expressed as a percent is known as the percent transmission (%T) and is represented by the equation:

EQ. 4-6

$$\frac{I_t}{I_o} \times 100\% = \%T$$

where I_o is the intensity of the light beam striking the sample and I_t is the intensity of the transmitted light.

As the concentration of the colored substance in solution in the cuvette increases, absorbance increases and the amount of light transmitted decreases. The percent transmission varies inversely and logarithmically with concentration as shown in Figure 4-9, *A*, but if the negative logarithm of the %T is plotted against concentration, a straight line is obtained (Figure 4-9, *B*); absorbance increases linearly with concentration and is defined as:

EQ. 4-7

$$A = 2 - \log \%T.$$

The linear relationship between absorption and concentration is expressed in the equation known as the Beer-Lambert law:

EQ. 4-8

$$A = abc$$

where A = absorbance, a = absorptivity coefficient (a constant for each molecular species having units that are

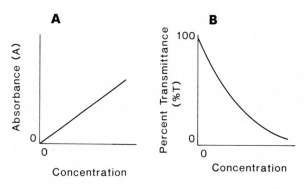

Fig. 4-9 Relationships of absorbance, **A,** and percent transmittance, **B,** to concentration. *From Frings CS and Gauldie J: Spectral techniques. In Kaplan LA and Pesce AJ: Clinical chemistry: theory, analysis, and correlation, ed 2, St Louis, 1989, Mosby-Year Book, Inc.*

reciprocal to those for b and c), b = length of the light path in centimeters, and c = concentration of the substance of interest (mol/L).

Once a chromogen is known to follow Beer's law at a certain wavelength, then the concentration of an unknown solution is derived by comparison with a standard solution:

EQ. 4-9

$$\frac{A_u}{A_s} = \frac{C_u}{C_s}$$

or more conveniently:

EQ. 4-9a

$$C_u = \frac{A_u}{A_s} \times C_s$$

where A_u and A_s are the absorbances of the unknown and the standard, respectively; C_u and C_s are the concentrations of the unknown and standard, respectively.

A standard curve in which standard concentrations are plotted against absorbance of the standards can be made and concentrations of test samples determined from the graph by comparison of their absorbance values.

Limitations of Beer's law

Beer's law is an ideal mathematical relationship that applies to a limited concentration range, which must be determined for each assay. In any assay, there is a point when the reactants or products limit the reaction and therefore color formation is no longer linearly related to concentration.

Several other factors cause deviation from Beer's law and are summarized as follows:
1. The incident light (striking the cuvette) is not monochromatic and therefore not specific for the measured substance.
2. Sample matrix other than the substance of interest interferes with absorbance.
3. Stray light enters the system and is detected.
4. Cuvette surfaces are not uniform or parallel.

Instrumentation

A spectrophotometer separates light into its component wavelengths, passes a portion of this light through a sample, and measures the light transmitted at each wavelength to produce an absorption spectrum. The pattern of absorption can be used to identify a substance. The amount of absorption is related to concentration.

A single-beam spectrophotometer is constructed of five basic components: (1) a stable light source comprised of a power supply and a lamp; (2) a wavelength selector; (3) a sample holder or cuvette; (4) a photodetector, which responds to light by the production of current; and (5) a meter or other measuring device.

If the wavelength selector is a colored filter that isolates a certain wavelength, the instrument is called a "photometer." If the wavelength selector is a monochromator (prism or grating) that provides monochromatic light over a continuous range of wavelengths, the instrument is a "spectrophotometer."

In the double-beam spectrophotometer, two light beams pass through the sample compartment—one beam passes through the sample cuvette and the second beam passes through a reference cuvette. The detector measures both transmitted beams. The reference cuvette transmittance is electronically subtracted from the transmittance of the sample cuvette; the difference is proportional to the transmission of the material in the sample cuvette. The use of the double-beam configuration compensates for variations in reference absorption as a function of wavelength, thereby making the use of a blank cuvette at each wavelength unnecessary. It also automatically compensates for variations in the intensity of the light source and in detector sensitivity and response. Components of the single-beam and double-beam spectrophotometer are shown in Figure 4-10.

Light source

The lamps used in UV and VIS spectrophotometry are usually a tungsten bulb for work in the visible range (390 to 700 nm) and a deuterium discharge or hydrogen lamp for the ultraviolet range (200 to 390 nm). Mercury vapor lamps emit a discontinuous or line spectrum and because of the very specific wavelengths emitted, are useful for checking wavelength calibration. Since light sources vary in the amount and wavelength of light emitted, their suitability for a specific analysis should be verified by checking with a standard curve before use in the analysis.

Wavelength selectors

In a photometer, wavelength is selected by use of colored filters. Early photometers employed glass or Wratten filters, composed of layers of colored gelatin between clear glass plates. In general, these filters transmitted a wide segment of the spectrum, 50 nm or more, centered about their specific wavelength.

A more recent development is the interference filter, composed of a thin layer of magnesium fluoride crystal with a semitransparent silver coating on each side. Because these filters transmit only light for which a multiple of the wavelength is equal to the thickness of the crystal, they have much smaller bandpasses (5 to 8 nm) than glass or Wratten

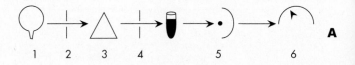

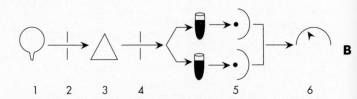

Fig. 4-10 Spectrophotometer configuration. Configuration for **A,** single beam and **B,** double beam spectrophotometer. Individual components are *1,* light source; *2,* entrance slit; *3,* monochromator; *4,* exit slit; *5,* detector; *6,* readout device (meter).

filters. The bandpass describes the width of the spectrum transmitted by the filter.

Monochromator

The monochromator is a device that can isolate wavelengths over the entire spectrum emitted by the source lamp. It consists of: (1) an entrance slit, (2) a series of focusing lenses, (3) a prism or diffraction grating, and (4) an exit slit.

Both the entrance and exit slits in a filter photometer serve the same purpose: to make the light beams parallel and to reduce stray radiation. In the spectrophotometer the two types of slits perform separate functions. The entrance slit focuses light onto the prism or grating. When light enters a prism, the shorter wavelengths are refracted more than the longer wavelengths. Prisms provide higher optical efficiency than gratings because all of the incident radiant energy is distributed; however, the dispersion is nonlinear above wavelengths of 550 nm. Because of this nonlinearity, wavelength validation for an instrument containing a prism must be done at least three wavelengths.

Diffraction gratings consist of a large number of parallel grooves (10,000 to 50,000) cut into a surface of polished metal, glass, or quartz. Dispersion of the incident light into a continuous spectrum is linear so that only two wavelengths must be checked to verify wavelength accuracy.

Exit slits control the width of the light beam entering the sample cuvette. The narrower the slit, the smaller the instrument bandpass. Although it seems that the exit slit could be used to obtain the desirable narrow bandpass, the fact that a narrow slit reduces the light energy passing through the system imposes a practical limit on slit size. If the slit is too narrow, the light energy could be insufficient for measurement.

Variable wavelength instruments are equipped with a manually adjustable slit width. Large slit widths can be used only when measuring compounds that have broad absorption peaks. Some instruments are equipped with exit slit widths that vary automatically with wavelength. Their purpose is to compensate for variation in: (1) intensity of different wavelengths and (2) photometer sensitivty to different wavelengths. In these instruments sensitivity remains constant over the entire spectrum.

Bandpass or bandwidth

Bandpass or bandwidth describes the degree of monochromicity or spectral purity attainable with a spectrophotometer. It is defined in terms of the range of wavelengths that pass through the exit slit of the monochromator at some nominal wavelength, for example, 340 ± 2 nm. The nominal wavelength of a range of wavelengths is the one at which peak intensity occurs. The nominal wavelength of a filter is noted on the filter; for a monochromator, it is the number corresponding to the instrument wavelength setting.

More specifically, the bandpass of a filter is noted by its half-band width, which is the width, in nanometers, of the spectral transmittance curve at a point equal to 50% of the transmittance (Figure 4-11). For monochromators, spectral purity corresponds to the width, in nanometers, of the wavelengths centered about the peak wavelength that transmit 75% of the radiant energy.

Cuvettes

Samples for spectrophotometric analysis are transferred to cuvettes or cells. Square or rectangular cuvettes with parallel flat optical surfaces are most desirable, but round cuvettes matched to within 1% tolerance in light transmission have been used in some cases because the analytical errors are often larger than this variation. Figure 4-12 shows the transmission characteristics of several types of cuvettes.

Glass cuvettes can be used for the 320 to 950 nm range; quartz cuvettes must be used for testing in the range below 320 nm.

Most cuvettes have inside dimension (pathlength) of 1 cm and a 3 to 4 ml capacity. For smaller sample volumes, about 1 ml, cuvettes with thicker side walls are available. The optical pathlength in these cuvettes remains 1 cm.

Photodetectors

Several types of photodetectors, varying in sensitivity, amplification, and cost are available. The basic component

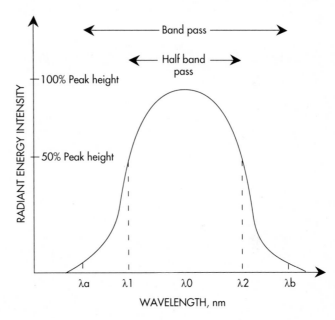

Fig. 4-11 Bandpass of a filter. The curved line represents the intensity of light of various wavelengths transmitted by a filter when the nominal wavelength is λ_0 . The wavelengths at which the intensity of light is one half of that at peak height (λ_0) are λ_1, and λ_2. These two wavelengths encompass the half bandpass of the filter ($\lambda_2 - \lambda_1$, in nm).

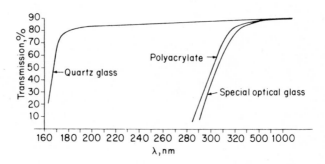

Fig. 4-12 Transmission characteristics of several types of optical materials used for cuvettes. *From Keller H: In Richterich R and Colombo JP (editors): Clinical chemistry, New York, 1981, John Wiley & Sons.*

in all detectors is a light-sensitive surface that responds proportionally to the light striking it by the release of electrons.

Photocell detector (barrier layer cell; selenide cell). These detectors consist of a bottom layer of copper or iron, a semiconducting layer of selenium or cadmium, and a light-transmitting layer of metal that acts as a collector electrode.

When light strikes the transparent electrode, it induces electron flow in the semiconductor, which is measured by an ampmeter. The current generated is a direct function of the quantity of light striking the photocell.

Photocells are rugged, relatively inexpensive, and useful in the UV to 1000-nm range. Generally, they are insensitive detectors and not readily amplified so they are not useful for measuring low light levels or small changes in intensity. Because they exhibit a "fatigue" effect (gradual return to the ground state after illumination), a resting interval of 30 seconds is required between readings. This further limits uses to relatively slow measuring systems.

Photomultiplier tube detectors (PMT). The PMT is sensitive and capable of fast response. It consists of a light-sensitive cathode and an anode separated by several dynodes (Figure 4-13). Light striking the cathode causes emission of electrons that are attracted to the first dynode. Every electron hitting this first dynode causes the release of several electrons, which are attracted to the more positive charge on the second dynode. This process is repeated at as many as 15 dynode surfaces, resulting in significant amplification of the original signal. Because of their sensitivity and fast response time. photomultiplier tubes are used in spectrophotometers with narrow bandwidths and in scanning electrophotometers.

Phototransistor and photodiode detectors. These detectors are constructed of two semiconductors joined together so that there is resistance to the flow of current between them. When light strikes the junction, this resistance is overcome and current flows between them. These conductors are comparatively inexpensive, sturdy, and capable of amplification.

Display devices

Display devices respond to the current from the detector and convert it to a meter display, digital display, or printed answer. Information can be presented as %T, absorbance, or concentration.

Selection of optimum conditions

The wavelength at which particular chromogen should be measured is determined from an absorbance spectrum (plot of absorbance vs. wavelength) of that chromogen. Selection of wavelength and bandpass must strike a balance between the conditions offering the peak of greatest absorbance and width. This will produce the greatest sensitivity and be least subject to slight errors in wavelength setting. In addition, the absorption peaks should be chosen that best isolate the chromogen of interest from absorption peaks in the spectrum of any potentially interfering materials.

Quality control of spectrophotometers

Four instrument parameters must be checked to verify adequate performance: (1) wavelength accuracy, (2) detector linearity, (3) photometric accuracy, and (4) stray light.

Wavelength accuracy

When wavelength calibration drifts (the wavelength of the incident light is not the wavelength selected), absorbance measurement is subject to significant error because it is being taken from the slope of the peak and not the maximum.

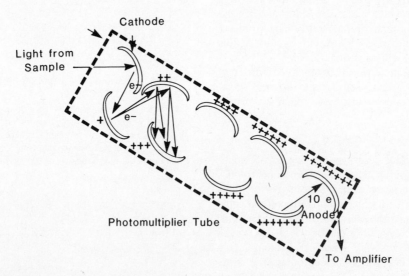

Fig. 4-13 Schematic of photomultiplier tube. Each dynode (electrode used to generate secondary emissions of electrons) is represented by a crescent. Light impinges on cathode and frees an electron. Electron is drawn toward first dynode (stage) by applied voltage. Secondary electrons are released and pass on to successive dynodes, which are at increasingly higher voltages, as depicted by the + symbols. Increasing numbers of secondary electrons are generated at each stage. In this diagram a tenfold amplification of the initial signal is produced at the anode. A photomultiplier tube may increase signal several thousandfold. *From Simonson MG: In Kaplan LA and Pesce AJ (editors): Nonisotopic alternatives to radioimmunoassay, New York, 1981, Marcel Dekker.*

Several methods, all employing some means of producing very specific absorbance or transmission peaks, are available to ensure wavelength accuracy.

1. Holmium oxide, a rare-earth metal can be purchased as a stable glass filter mounted in a special holder. It has strong absorbance peaks at 241, 279, 287, 333, 361, 418, 453, 536, and 636 nm, and is easily used as a daily check for wavelength accuracy.
2. Spectrophotometers containing hydrogen or deuterium source lamps have a built-in source for checking wavelength accuracy. Both lamps exhibit strong emission lines at specific wavelengths. For example, the deuterium lamp shows emission lines at 486 and 656 nm (Figure 4-14).
3. Solutions of stable chromogens can be used as secondary wavelength calibrators. They should not be used in place of primary wavelength calibration standards because they usually have broad absorbance peaks and are subject to spectral shifts caused by contaminants, aging, and preparation errors.

Detector linearity

Linearity is checked with a series of stable solutions of increasing concentration of analyte known to follow Beer's law. Absorbances of the solutions are plotted against concentration. Deviation from linearity, assuming correct preparation of the solutions, indicates instrument failure. Some solutions in common use for linearity checks with their respective wavelengths are: cobalt ammonium sulfate (512 nm), copper sulfate (650 nm), and p-nitrophenol (405 nm).

Factors other than nonlinear detector response can also cause deviations. These include a too large slit width and unintentional measurement of stray light.

Photometric accuracy

A photometric analysis is accurate when a solution of known concentration gives a particular absorbance value. Consideration of Beer's law shows that the absorbance value is dependent on the molar absorptivity of a substance, its concentration, and the pathlength of the measurement. Therefore, absorbance of a standard solution is ideally independent of spectrophotometric variation.

A check of photometric accuracy is particularly important when the spectrophotometer is used to perform assays in which the standard is different, or treated differently, than the unknown solutions; or for assays for which there is no available standard. Two sets of absorbance accuracy standards, SRM 930 and 931, developed through the joint efforts of CAP, NBS, and the AACC, are available. SRM 930 is a set of three neutral density filters with known absorbance values at four wavelengths. The cost of these standards is offset by their stability and ease of use.

Stray light

Stray light is light that reaches the detector of any wavelength other than the set wavelength. Stray light is caused by many factors. Causes inside a spectrophotometer are created by unwanted reflections from mirrors, prisms, and gratings, or by optical misalignment or dirt and corrosion on the optical surfaces. External causes of stray light are due to light leakage into the sample compartment or detection housing from the outside.

During analysis, stray light manifests itself as gradual, negative deviation from Beer's law at the high end of the known linear range (Figure 4-15). If this is observed, a stray light check at a wavelength close to the wavelength used in the assay should be done. Regular stray light checks are done with solutions that have very high absorbances at the test wavelength so that any unmeasured transmission is due to stray light.

Test materials for stray light checks are commercial absorbing filters or potassium dichromate (K_2CrO_4) and copper sulfate ($CuSO_4$) solutions. Transmission caused by stray light should be less than 1%.

If excessive stray light is observed, the operator should follow corrective procedures outlined in the instrument manual. The problem is often solved by changing the lamp or aligning the light beam. Further actions to clean optical surfaces or align the monochromator are best left to instru-

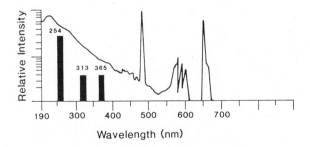

Fig. 4-14 Intensity of radiant energy vs. wavelength for a deuterium lamp. *From Frings CS and Gauldie J: Spectral techniques. In Kaplan LA and Pesce AJ (editors): Clinical chemistry: theory, analysis, and correlation, ed 2, St Louis, 1989, Mosby-Year Book.*

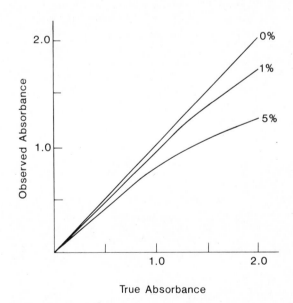

Fig. 4-15 Effect of stray radiation on true absorbance. The straight line *(0%)* represents true absorbance. As stray light increases, measured absorbance decreases as represented by the two curved lines labeled *1%* and *5%. From Frings CS and Broussard LA: Clin chem 25:1013, 1979.*

ment manufacturer service representatives as these surfaces are easily damaged and difficult to align.

MICROSCOPY

Brightfield microscopy employs several properties of light to produce a magnified and resolved image of an object. Classically, the pinhole camera is used to demonstrate how magnification occurs. Light emitted from each point on an object's surface travels through the small aperture to the back plane of the camera (Figure 4-16), forming a magnified virtual image of the object, that is, upside down and laterally reversed. As the size of the aperture increases, the image blurs or becomes less resolved because light from each object point starts to overlap. If a suitable lens is inserted into the enlarged aperture, it refocuses the light from each point to form a distinct image point.

Properties of light

The aspects of light pertinent to brightfield microscopy include: (1) reflection, (2) refraction, (3) dispersion, and (4) diffraction.

Reflection

When a ray of light strikes a surface at an angle measured from a line extended perpendicularly from a planar surface or the arc of a curved surface, and it bounces back at an angle of equal size (angle of reflection), it is said to be reflected (Figure 4-17). Reflection occurs not only when light passes through air and strikes an object, but also when it strikes the interface between glass and air. Stray reflections inside a microscope interfere with the optical path and degrade the sharply defined image.

Refraction

Refraction produces a magnified image of an object. It is simply the bending of a light ray from the "normal" angle when it passes into a different optical medium. A normal line is the line perpendicular to a planar (flat) surface or to the tangent of a curved surface. Optical mediums include glass (lenses, filters, slides, and coverslips), air, immersion substances, and mounting media (Figure 4-18).

Refraction is caused by changes in the speed of light as it passes through different media. When light enters a more dense field, it bends toward the normal line; when entering a less dense medium, light bends away from the normal line. Refractive index is the measure of refraction expressed as:

EQ. 4-10a

$$n \text{ (refractive index)} = \frac{\text{velocity in a vacuum (Km/sec)}}{\text{velocity in medium (Km/sec)}}$$

It is proportional to the density of the medium. Refractive index can also be defined as the relationship between the sine of the incident angle[a] to the sine of the refracted angle[b] (Figure 4-18):

EQ. 4-10b

$$n = \frac{\text{sine}^a}{\text{sine}^b}$$

Dispersion

Dispersion occurs because light of different frequencies is refracted to different degrees; the greater the frequency, the greater the angle of refraction. It is the phenomenon observed when a prism is used to separate white light into its separate components. Dispersion causes chromatic ab-

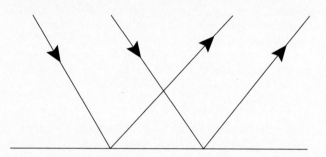

Fig. 4-17   When light rays encounter surfaces such as those between air and glass, secondary rays are sent out in all directions. Those that bounce back at the same angle as the incident ray are the reflected rays.

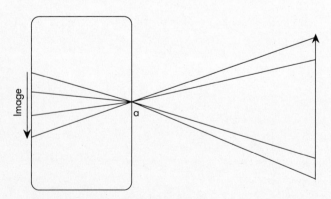

Fig. 4-16   The pinhole camera. Light from each object point travels in a straight line through the aperture *(a)* to the back plane, forming an image upside down and laterally reversed. If the back plane is moved forward or backward, the image changes sizes. *From Wilson MB: The science and art of basic microscopy, Bellaire, Tex, 1976, American Society of Medical Techology.*

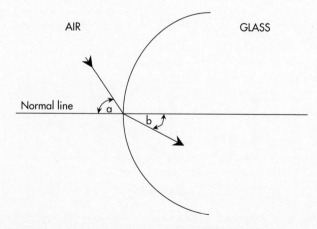

Fig. 4-18   A ray of light bends (is refracted) as it crosses the surface between air and glass because of a change in the speed of light. The refractive index *(n)* is the sine a/sine b.

erration and is a major obstacle to correct image formation in the microscope.

Diffraction

Formation of a magnified image is mainly due to the practical application of refraction. Just as important as magnification is the quality or sharpness of that image, which decreases as magnification increases. This sharpness or resolution of an image is dependent on diffraction.

As light waves pass through a nonhomogenous object such as a tissue specimen, each detail of the specimen acts as if it were an exit slit for the light ray, causing new light rays to appear. The size and direction of the new waves depends upon the size of the slit (Figure 4-19). The smaller the slit (or the greater the morphological detail), the greater the angle of diffraction and the more difficult for the rays to be directed into the optical path of the microscope.

Diffraction, like refraction, is also dependent upon wavelength—the longer the wavelength, the greater the diffraction. Another important factor is the medium through which the rays travel. A thinner medium, such as air, allows more diffraction than oil because the wavelength is shortened in the denser medium.

The resolving power of the microscope depends on how well the optical system collects the diffracted rays. This ability is referred to in terms of "orders of diffraction." The direct ray is called the zero order, the first diffracted rays to the left and right of the zero order ray are the first order, the second diffracted rays to the left and right are the second order, and so on. In order to resolve a point, the microscope must collect at least two orders of diffracted rays.

Lenses

In an optical system the lens collects light rays from an object and redirects them to form a sharp, magnified image of the object in what is termed the image plane. The magnification produced by a lens is defined as the distance between the lens and the image plane (b) divided by the distance between the object and the lens (a); magnification = b/a.

Lens descriptions and limitations

There are two basic types of lenses used in microscopy: converging or positive lenses and diverging or negative lens. The converging lens is convex and directs light to a point; the diverging lens is concave so that it bends light outward. Since lenses are two-sided, several combinations of the two basic types are possible. The type commonly referred to when describing microscopy is the double convex lenses. With this lens, light rays entering the top portion of the lens are refracted downward; those entering the bottom portion are refracted upward (Figure 4-20).

The plane in which the refracted rays converge is termed the focal plane and the distance from lens to focal plane is termed the focal length. The relationship between object to lens distance (a), lens to image distance (b), and focal length is defined as follows:

EQ. 4-11

$$\frac{1}{a} + \frac{1}{b} = \frac{1}{f}$$

When a fat biconvex lens with a short focal length is brought very close to a specimen, then $1/a$ approaches $1/f$. This means that $1/b$ is small or that b is very large. Since magnification is defined as b/a, this lens configuration and small object-to-lens distance results in a large order of magnification (Figure 4-21).

The standard used to define magnification is based upon the visual angle encompassed (subtended) when viewing an object 250 mm from the eye, this being magnification X1. As an object is brought closer to the eye, the angle encompassed becomes larger and increases its "apparent" size. From the standard point of 250 mm, magnification is defined

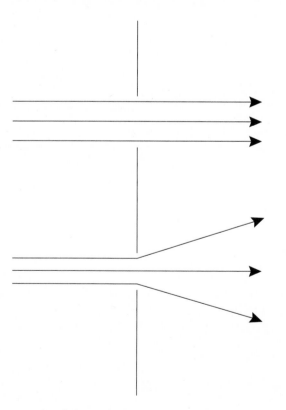

Fig. 4-19 When light passes through a slit, the central rays, termed direct rays, pass through unaffected. The waves emanating from the slit edges are termed diffracted. The smaller the slit, the greater the angle of diffraction (angle between the direct rays and diffracted rays).

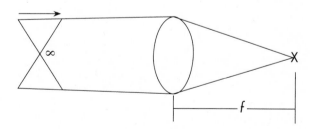

Fig. 4-20 With the double convex (biconvex) lens, light striking the upper portion of the lens is reflected downward, light striking the lower part of the lens is reflected upward. The light rays converge at the focal point. The focal length (f) is the distance from the focal point to the lens. *From Wilson MB: The science and art of basic microscopy, Bellaire, Tex, 1976, American Society of Medical Technology.*

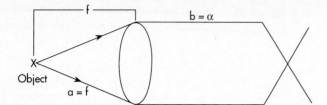

Fig. 4-21 When a lens with a short focal length is brought close to an object so that *a* (the lens to object distance) equals *f* (focal length), then *b* (lens to image distance) approaches infinity and magnification (*b*/*a*) is very large.

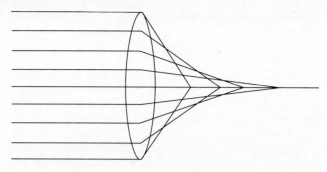

Fig. 4-22 Spherical aberration is caused by differences in angles of refraction in various sections of the lens. These differences result in the formation of multiple focal planes and therefore a blurred image. *From Wilson MB: The science and art of basic microscopy, Bellaire, Tex, 1976, American Society of Medical Technology.*

as the ratio of the tangents of the encompassed angle at various distances, so that an object at 250 mm is X1, at 125 mm is X2, and at 50 mm is X5. In other words, magnification is the reciprocal of the ratio between the standard 250-mm distance and the actual distance.

The lens system of the microscope increases the subtended visual angle, thereby enabling the formation of a sharp magnified image on the retina of the eye. While lenses provide the desirable aspect of magnification, they also have limitations caused by the behavior of light. In microscopy, these limitations arise from two basic causes: (1) the shape of the lens and (2) the presence of light of different wavelengths. These limitations are corrected by compounding lenses of varying refractive indices and dispersing abilities to one compound lens.

Spherical aberration. A lens system is composed of spherical surfaces and by definition cannot produce a perfect image. Because of the curvature of the lens, light strikes its surface at a unique angle in each section of the lens and is refracted differently. For example, light striking the center of the lens at 90° to the tangent travels through with no refraction. Light striking the top of the lens is refracted more than light striking halfway between the center and the top of the lens (Figure 4-22). The result of the differences in the angle of refraction is the formation of an indistinct image plane (curvature of field). Spherical aberration increases with the thickness of the biconvex lens and is compensated for by compounding the positive biconvex lens with a negative biconcave lens that brings the image plane into focus (flat field).

Chromatic aberration. Chromatic aberration is caused by the differential refraction of light inside a lens, the surface of which acts as a prism. When white light passes through a prism, light within a shorter wavelength is refracted more strongly than that with a longer wavelength. Thus, the light of one color is projected at a greater magnification than another. Chromatic aberration in the modern microscope is controlled by a proper combination of lenses. Achromatic lenses are corrected for one color; apochromatic lenses are corrected for three colors.

Astigmatism. Several other types of distortion can affect the image. Astigmatism occurs when a point image is cut into separate lines at multiple angles and so cannot be focused as a sharp point. It results from a defect in the objective lens and is not correctable by the microscopist.

Coma. Coma is an aberration in which different concentric zones of the lens surface cause different magnifications. It is due to a combination of spherical aberration and astigmatism. If a coma occurs in the center of the field, it usually indicates damage to the objective lens.

Pincussion distortion. Pincussion distortion renders a square object as an image with curved sides and is generally not a problem with the modern microscope.

Compound microscope

A compound microscope (Figure 4-23) contains at least two lens systems with magnifying power equal to the product of the magnifying power of each system. The two lens systems are mounted on either end of a tube; the lens nearest the object is called the objective lens, whereas the one nearest the eye is the ocular lens or eyepiece. Most good quality microscopes incorporate a third system of lenses that make up the condenser, which concentrates and focuses light from the light source directly through the specimen. An iris diaphragm on the condenser is used to control the diameter of the light beam. Positioning screws on the condenser allow precise alignment of the beam for each objective lens.

The eyepiece limits the viewing field and magnifies the real intermediate image formed in the tube body so that it appears as a virtual image 10 inches from the eye. Some eyepieces contain compensating lenses to correct for aberrations in the objective lens system; these eyepieces are marked with a "COMP" or "C," and have magnifying powers of X4 to X30.

Objective lenses

The objective lens system is the component most responsible for the magnification and resolution of detail in a specimen. The set of lenses in the objective lens system collects the light from every detail in the specimen and forms a magnified image in the eyepiece focal plane. Degree of magnification is dependent upon the focal length of the objective lens and tube length.

Apochromatic objectives correct for three colors; red, blue, and green, and contain at least four lenses. If the objective also corrects for flatness of field, it is called planochromatic and contains seven or more lenses.

The resolution of detail is defined as the numerical aperture (NA) of the objective lens and it is usually noted on each objective lens. This figure indicates the orders of dif-

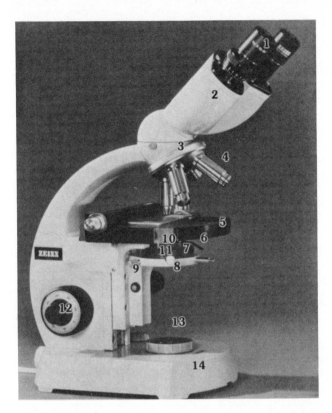

Fig. 4-23 The compound microscope and its components: eyepiece *(1)*, body tube *(2)*, nosepiece *(3)*, objective *(4)*, stage *(5)*, condenser iris diaphragm *(6)*, condenser *(7)*, condenser front lens lever *(8)*, knobs for centering condenser *(9)*, filter holder *(10)*, auxiliary lens holder *(11)*, fine and coarse adjustment knobs *(12)*, field iris diaphragm *(13)*, and base with built-in, low-voltage illuminator *(14)*. *From Wilson MB: The science and art of basic microscopy, Bellaire, Tex, 1976, American Society of Medical Technology.*

fracted rays that the objective can collect—the greater the NA, the better the resolving power of the microscope. Mathematically, NA = n sin θ, where θ = the angle between the central direct ray and the most diffracted ray collected by the objective and *n* = the refractive index of the medium.

Since the refractive index of air is 1 and the greatest possible angle of diffraction is 90° (sine 90° = 1), a dry objective can never have a NA greater than 1. This relationship also explains why the use of oil between a coverslip and a special oil immersion lens increases the resolving power of a microscope—it is because the refraction index of glass (slide and coverslip) and oil are both about 1.51. These oil immersion objective lenses are marked as OIL or OEL.

Oil does not improve the resolving power of a dry objective because dry objectives are designed to take refractive index and dispersion by the coverslip and air into account. The quality and thickness of a coverslip is important—its refraction index should be equal to glass (~1.51) and it should be 0.17 mm in thickness. Plastic coverslips are not ideal because their low refractive index and varying thicknesses cause aberration.

Most microscopes have multiple objective lenses mounted on a nosepiece turret, centered on an axis, so that they are all in focus when rotated into position. Such arrangement is termed parfocalized.

The tube length (distance from the mounting shoulder of the objective to the upper rim of the tube) is usually 160 mm. This length, along with the focal length of the lens, can be used to calculate magnification, where magnification is defined as: M = b/a; *b* is 160 mm (image to objective distance) and the focal length of the lens = *a* (in mm). This figure, multiplied by the magnification power of the eyepiece, gives the total magnification. For example, an objective with a focal length of 8 mm used with a X5 eyepiece will give a total magnification of:

EQ. 4-12

$$M = \frac{160 \text{ mm}}{8 \text{ mm}} \times 5 = X100$$

Illumination systems: Brightfield

Ideal illumination of an object viewed under the microscope requires even light distribution and that the objective's aperture be entirely filled with light from the condenser. To fulfill these requirements, the illumination system contains several elements: the source, the collector, the field iris diaphragm, and the condenser iris diaphragm.

Ernst Abbe, in the later nineteenth century, introduced the first condenser, a system of lenses to improve and control the illumination source. Prior to that time, the illumination source was used directly without imposition of optical devices to distribute and focus the light. Even though more complex systems have been developed, the two-lens Abbe condenser is adequate for most brightfield applications.

The most common type of illumination in use today is Köhler illumination, developed by Dr. August Köhler. With this type of illumination, the source is imaged by the collector lens onto the back focal plane of the condenser. From here, the source light is projected in a cone-shaped beam, the angle of which is controlled by the aperture diaphragm so that it fills the objective's aperture (Figure 4-24).

The ability of the condenser to capture, enhance, and focus light from the source is rated in terms of numerical aperture. For maximum performance, the numerical aperture of the objective and condenser lenses should match. Therefore, condensers of NA >1.0 are to be used with oil between the top lens of the condenser and the specimen slide.

In the modern microscope most illumination sources are either tungsten or tungsten-halogen bulbs. The intensity of the source is usually adjustable via a transformer. Because these sources emit light that is excessive in yellow color, a blue filter is placed over the condenser to produce a more white source.

Use of the compound microscope

Two basic adjustments are necessary to attain the best resolution with each objective lens: focusing the specimen with the chosen objective lens and optimization of the illumination system. The second of these adjustments is often overlooked, resulting in significant loss of resolution.

The stage holding the specimen has two knobs to control horizontal movement. Some stages have scales to measure their position and these can be used to pinpoint a location

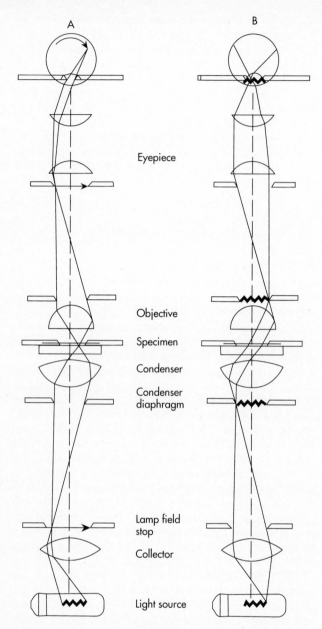

Fig. 4-24 Image formation light path *(A)* and illumination light path *(B)* in Koehler illumination. *From Wilson MB: The science and art of basic microscopy, Bellaire, Tex, 1976, American Society of Medical Technology.*

on the slide for future reference. Once the intensity of the source has been adjusted with the field iris diaphragm to adjust for the different field diameters of the objective, the specimen is brought into focus.

Focusing is done with a coarse and fine control knob to move the stage up and down. Its position is dependent on the objective used. High-powered objective lenses of short focal length must be brought closer to the specimen than objectives of lower power. Slowly move the stage up close to the objective lens (most objective lenses are spring-mounted for specimen protection). Then, while looking through the microscope, use the coarse control knob to drop

the stage until the specimen comes into focus. Exact focus is accomplished with the fine control knob.

Adjustment of the illumination system is of critical importance for proper resolution. To attain Köhler illumination so that the entire field viewed by the objective is evenly lit and properly resolved, the following general procedure can be used:

1. With the low-powered objective lens, focus on a specimen.
2. Move the condenser to its highest position, and close down the field iris diaphragm. Move the condenser down until a shape image of the field iris diaphragm appears.
3. With the condenser centering screws, center the circle of light.
4. Open the field iris diaphragm just to the point when the circle of light fills the entire field.
5. Remove an eyepiece and adjust the condenser iris diaphragm until it covers 75% of the illuminated circle, which represents the objective lens aperture. Replace the eyepiece.

Ideally, the illumination and condenser should be adjusted for each objective. In practice, such as when viewing urine sediment that must be observed with both low- and high-power objective lenses, this is impractical. Often times in this situation, the technologist racks down the condenser to effect more contrast with the low-power objective. Although this does increase contrast, important resolution is lost. A preferable approach to adjust for different objectives is to set the condenser iris diaphragm for the highest objective while setting the field iris diaphragm for the lowest objective. If this is done, the condenser iris diaphragm can be slightly adjusted to compensate for the field diameter of the different objectives. When using the low-power objective, stopping down the condenser iris diaphram will increase contrast with minimum loss of resolution.

Special microscopy

In addition to brightfield microscopy in which the condenser illuminates the objective lens aperture evenly, other forms of microscopy are useful for the visualization of objects exhibiting low contrast with surrounding media. Some types of microscopy require only modification of the usual light microscope, whereas other types require use of a special microscope.

Darkfield microscopy

Some objects such as spirochetes, protozoa, unstained tissue, and cells do not contrast sufficiently with their background to be viewed with conventional microscopes. If staining to effect contrast causes undesirable changes in the specimen, darkfield microscopy can often be used to view these specimens.

With the darkfield technique, a hollow cone of light enters the specimen at an angle too large to be received by the objective lens so that the intense rays that usually enter the objective lens pass by it. This creates the dark background and allows only those rays diffracted by the specimen to enter the objective lens, thus rendering the specimen visible. Darkfield condensers produce the hollow cone of light by the placement of a stop or darkspot in the center of the condenser (Figure 4-25). The numerical aperture of the objective lens must be less than that of the condenser.

Immersion oil must be used between the condenser and the bottom surface of the slide for some darkfield apparatus so that light from the condenser passes directly to the object with no change in direction.

Extreme cleanliness of all the components used in darkfield microscopy is of critical importance. These include slides, coverglasses, and immersion substances. Dirt and air bubbles are refractile and so interfere with darkfield applications. Chemically cleaned quartz glass slides and coverslips are preferred for critical darkfield work.

Polarized light microscopy

A polarizing filter allows passage only of light oriented in a single plane. Therefore, when two polarized filters are rotated at 90° with respect to one another, no light passes through. Birefrigent or anisotropic substances rotate light 90°. If such a substance is placed between two polaroid filters that are rotated at 90°, it will rotate light and allow passage of light through the filter. Many substances important in the clinical laboratory—crystals, fat, barium—are birefringent.

Because there is a phase difference between refractive indexes of a crystal, some wavelengths will be enhanced and others canceled, producing a pattern of colors specific to the thickness and birefringence of the crystal. These specific patterns allow for identification of crystals.

Ordinary microscopes can be used with polarizing filters: one filter is placed beneath the specimen, usually in the condenser and the other above the specimen, often in the ocular lens.

Phase-contrast microscopy

In brightfield microscopy, contrast between objects and their surrounds results from differences in color and absorption. Many of the components of biological specimens are not capable of producing sufficient contrast, but do cause phase changes in the light that strikes them. Unfortunately, the eye does not detect these phase changes, but phase-contrast apparatus converts these phase changes into amplitude changes, which are visible to the eye as differences in intensity.

In 1935 Zernike produced the first phase-contrast microscope. A phase-annular aperture diaphragm is placed in the front focal plane of the condenser, producing a hollow cone of light. Fine structures in the specimen produce diffraction spectra, which are imaged in the rear focal plane of the objective lens. A phase-shifting element (or phase ring) is placed in the plane, in which it acts as a neutral density filter to reduce the intensity of all nondiffracted wavefronts. The end result is improved contrast as a function of the diffraction. Because phase-contrast microscopy depends on wavefronts, it performs optimally only within a certain wavelength range. A green filter is used to isolate this range. Phase-contrast microscopy is particularly useful for the study of cellular detail in unstained, living material and for the detection of casts in urine sediment.

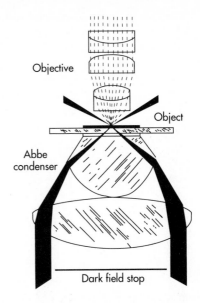

Fig. 4-25 Darkfield illumination.

Care of the microscope

A few simple guidelines ensure that a good quality microscope will perform optimally for many years:

1. Place the microscope in a clean, vibration-free area away from windows and other bright lights.
2. Dust the microscope daily with a brush or lint-free cloth. Keep covered when not in use.
3. Clean the ocular lenses with lens paper moistened with water. If grease or oil persist, clean with a cotton swab moistened with denatured ethanol.
4. Periodically remove the objective lenses one at a time from the turret. Clean the lower lens surface with a cotton swab moistened with denatured alcohol.
5. Never soak any lens system in any organic solvent (including alchohol).
6. A microscope field engineer should clean and align the microscope on a yearly basis.

SUGGESTED READING

A Centrifuge primer, Palo Alto, Calif., 1980, Spinco Division of Beckman Instruments.

Alexander LR and Barnhart ER: Photometric quality assurance instrument check procedures, Atlanta, 1980, U.S. Department of Health and Human Services, Centers for Disease Control, Bureau of Laboratories.

Campbell JB: Laboratory mathematics, medical and biological applications, ed 2, St Louis, 1980, Mosby–Year Book, Inc.

Kaplan LA and Pesce AJ: Clinical chemistry, theory, analysis, and correlation, ed 2, St Louis, 1989, Mosby–Year Book, Inc.

The National Committee for Clinical Laboratory Standards: Quantities and units (SI), Clin Chem 25:657–658, 1979 (position paper).

Pesce AJ and Kaplan LA: Methods in clinical chemistry, St Louis, 1987, Mosby–Year Book, Inc.

Wilson MB: The science and art of basic microscopy, Bellaire, Tex., 1976, American Society of Medical Technology.

5

Laboratory statistics, reference ranges, and quality control

Mary Kay Boehmer

STATISTICS

There is certainly no limit to the numerical data that are generated within a clinical laboratory and statistics is the area of mathematics that deals with the collection, computation, and interpretation of these data. Statistical tests provide a useful means by which one can make decisions about the data that have been collected. These decisions might be concerned with changing methods, from an expensive assay to a more economical one, or deciding if a shift in a month's quality control data is actually significant. The first step in this decision-making process involves the application of the null hypothesis, which states that there is no difference between two values or two groups of data being compared. This hypothesis holds true unless calculated probabilities show that a significant difference does exist.

This chapter will review statistical terminology and some basic and frequently used equations that will be helpful in dealing with tests of significance. The main reason for learning and applying these statistical tools in the laboratory setting is so that one can apply them to the concepts of method comparison and evaluation, the establishment of reference ranges, and the surveillance of quality control.

A single result generated by a chemical measurement is not enough insurance that a particular analysis is acceptable. It is only by comparing that result to each and every other result that one can determine if the result is acceptable and if the analysis as a whole is satisfactory.

Terminology and equations
Central tendency

The most common and easily used statistical tests are those that determine the central tendency of populations. The mean, median, and mode describe the values about which these populations are centered. The arithmetic mean, designated as $\bar{x}$ (x bar), is the average of two or more values. It is calculated by the formula:

EQ. 5-1

$$\text{Mean} = \frac{\sum x_i}{n}$$

The average value equals the summation of each and every individual value x_i divided by n, which equals the number of values measured.

The median is the value that falls in the middle of a group of numbers when the values are listed from smallest to largest. In the sample group of numbers, 57, 58, 60, 61, 62, 62, 63, the median equals 61 because this group contains an odd number of values. If the group contained one more number, a 64 for example, there would be an even number of values and the median would be the average of the two middle numbers, 61 and 62, or 61.5. In designating the median it can be said that 50% of the values will fall below it and 50% will lie above it. It is also known as the 50th percentile.

The mode is the value in a population that occurs the most frequently. In the group of numbers, 101, 99, 100, 101, 102, 101, and 98, the mode is 101 because it occurs three times, more often than any other number. A population of numbers can have more than one mode if there is more than one number that occurs more frequently.

Distribution

The distribution of data refers to the way a group of numbers are spread around a central point. For a symmetric, continuous distribution, these three terms, mean, median, and mode, will equal the same value. Symmetric distributions are those that have mirror-image shapes from the mean to the highest value and from the mean to the lowest value. Continuous distributions are those in which a data point can occur at any value. A glucose result on an individual, for example, can occur at any point in the biological range between approximately 20 mg/dL and 2000 mg/dL. The result may occur at 70 mg/dL, 85.2 mg/dL, or 101.02 mg/dL and is not limited to a discrete value that occurs at any defined interval. A special case with a specific relationship of the mean and standard deviation to the total distribution is known as a normal distribution or a Gaussian distribution (Fig. 5-1).

A distribution that is skewed to one side or the other is considered an asymmetric distribution. If it is positively skewed, the distribution tails to the right and the mean value is greater than the value of the median. On the other hand,

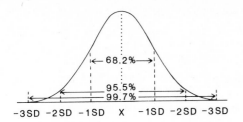

Fig. 5-1 Gaussian distribution curve. *From Garber CC and Carey RN: Laboratory statistics. In Kaplan LA and Pesce AJ (editors): Clinical chemistry: theory, analysis, and correlation, ed 2, St Louis, 1989, Mosby-Year Book, Inc.*

if it is negatively skewed, the distribution tails to the left and the value of the mean is less than that of the median. If a distribution is not symmetrical, the arithmetic mean will not describe the center of the distribution. When there is a difference between the mean, median, and mode of a population of numbers, then the distribution of that population can be assumed to be asymmetric.

On occasion, a population of numbers can have two distinct peaks in its distribution. This is referred to as a bimodal distribution. It will be encountered again when referring to reference groups. A distribution of this type might lead one to separate the group into two separate and distinct subpopulations.

Variance

Variance is the general term used to describe the differences in values that are obtained when multiple determinations are taken on a single sample. When a large number of measurements are taken, the dispersion about the mean of the results can be measured by the calculation of the variance:

EQ. 5-2

$$\text{Variance} = \frac{\Sigma \, |\overline{X} - X_i|^2}{n - 1}$$

In this equation, the difference of each value from the mean is squared and summed and then divided by $n-1$, where n equals the number of values used in the analysis. In the equation, $n-1$ is used rather than n because one degree of freedom (df) has been lost. Degrees of freedom designate the number of values that carry new information from one calculation to another and the value of n has already been used in the calculation of the mean.

The term *range* indicates the spread of data from the smallest value to the largest value. The range does not give any indication as to the shape of the distribution. This is especially true if the spread of data points is large.

In the laboratory a statistical term more commonly used than variance is standard deviation. It is designated as s or SD. It is simply the square root of the variance:

EQ. 5-3

$$\text{Standard deviation (SD)} = \sqrt{\frac{\Sigma \, |\overline{X} - X_i|^2}{n - 1}}$$

A problem encountered when attempting to compare data using either variance or standard deviation is that units are

attached to their values. A demonstration of why this can be misleading is given in the following example. A set of multiple glucose determinations are performed on a sample and the mean is determined to be 100 mg/dL with a standard deviation of 5 mg/dL. A second sample is analyzed the same number of times and its mean is determined to be 200 mg/dL with a standard deviation of 10 mg/dL. A comparison of the deviations seems to indicate less precision with the second sample than the first sample since 10 mg/dL is twice as large as 5 mg/dL. If the coefficient of variation (CV) is determined instead, relating the standard deviation to the mean as a percentage, then one finds the variation for both samples to be exactly 5%. This proves that there is no difference in variation after all. The coefficient of variation also known as the relative standard deviation, is calculated using the following formula:

EQ. 5-4

$$\text{Coefficient of variation (CV)} = \frac{\text{SD}}{\overline{\text{x}}} \times 100\%$$

When gathering data for a method comparison or a reference range interval, it is impossible to test the entire human population. Since this is the case, it is usually assumed that the sample data collected will be a reasonable representation of the overall population. Theoretically, the larger the sample size measured, the closer the sample mean will be to the true mean of the population. If several small groups of data are analyzed from a sample population, the means of each of these groups will scatter around the actual mean of this sample population. The standard error of the mean (SEM) is an estimation of that scatter. It can be calculated by dividing the standard deviation of the means of the groups by the square root of the number of groups used:

EQ. 5-5

$$\text{Standard error of the mean (SEM)} = \frac{\text{SD}}{\sqrt{\text{n}}}$$

If the data from the sample population are normally distributed, it can be assumed that the calculated standard deviation of the group will determine the confidence intervals for this particular population. In other words, it will follow the probability distribution of a Gaussian curve (Fig. 5-1), where 68.2% of all future observations will fall within ± 1.0 SD of the mean, 95.5% will fall within ± 2.0 SD of the mean, and 99.7% will fall within ± 3.0 SD of the mean. There is only a 0.3% chance that a value will occur outside of ± 3.0 SD due to random error.

Comparison of errors

The main objective of a clinical laboratory is to deliver accurate results. If a result is not accurate, it is of little use to the physician. Unfortunately, an incorrect result may be detrimental to a patient if a physician orders treatment based on the inaccurate information.

There are two main types of errors a good laboratory has to be acutely aware of: random error and systematic error. These errors may be inherent in the test methodology or instrumentation that a laboratory uses, or they can be introduced by the technologist performing the analysis. Both errors cause a result to be different from its true value. Each error is caused by a different reason and each is independent of the other. Both types of errors must prove to be minimal before a test methodology is used. If the test is replacing an assay already in use, the new method should be just as accurate and precise as the one it is replacing.

Random errors are a reflection of precision. Precision is defined as how closely a measurement repeats itself. Precision can be determined by calculating the standard deviation between multiple measurements. Systematic errors reflect the accuracy of a method. Accuracy is how close a measured result matches the expected result. Accuracy is determined by the mean. If an assay is inaccurate, it does not matter if it is precise.

When measurements are plotted on a graph, random error, namely, imprecision, is revealed as a scatter of points around a line drawn to fit the expected or theoretical values (Fig. 5-2). Different types of systematic errors, or bias, can also be demonstrated by means of graphical presentations. Two primary systematic errors are constant error and proportional error. If a constant error is present, the comparison line will not go through the origin of the graph. Constant error (Fig. 5-3) causes the line to shift proportionally in one direction or the other while the slope remains unaffected. Results containing a proportional error, on the other hand, may or may not go through the origin of the graph. With proportional error, the slope of the line is different than the expected or theoretical slope of the line. In statistical terms the difference between two values at any given point along the actual or theoretical lines is not the same as the difference between any other two points on the same lines.

There is another type of systematic error known as random bias. Bias refers to the accuracy of the measurement and random means that it cannot be predicted. This is an effect that can vary from sample to sample and might be due to individual specimen interferences, such as the presence of lipemia, hemolysis, or bilirubin.

Method comparison

While graphs are visual pictures of analytical errors, there are also statistical equations that can be used to evaluate

these same errors in comparison data. The F test is a standard equation used to compare differences in precision. It determines if the standard deviations between two methods are statistically different. It is calculated by dividing the larger of the two standard deviations squared by the smaller of the standard deviations squared:

EQ. 5-6

$$F = \frac{(SD_1)^2}{(SD_2)^2}$$

The calculated F value is compared to a critical F value that can be found in widely available F-distribution tables. As an example, an abbreviated F-distribution table is shown in Table 5-1. To determine the critical F value from the table, the degrees of freedom *(df)* for both the numerator and denominator are necessary. The *df* for each is equal to n-1, *n* being equal to the number of samples analyzed by each test method. To find the critical F value, one must go down the left-hand vertical column stopping at the *df* corresponding to the denominator and across the table to the column corresponding to the *df* of the numerator. If the calculated F value does not exceed the critical F value determined from the table, then no statistical difference exists between the standard deviations of the two test methods. On the other hand, if the F value does exceed the critical F value, then one can assume that there exists a statistical difference between the two standard deviations and that the precision of one method varies significantly from the other. The confidence level at which these values are determined depends upon the F-distribution table used. For most laboratories, the use of $p = 0.05$ or 95% confidence is the most widely accepted value. It should be noted that the F test can be used for a statistical comparison of two methods but it does not determine if the precision of the method in question is acceptable for laboratory use.

To study the statistical significance between two means, it is appropriate to use the Student's *t*-test. This calculation determines if the mean of one method is significantly different than the mean of another. In the first form of the

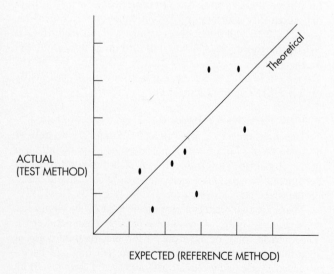

Fig. 5-2　Graph of random error (precision).

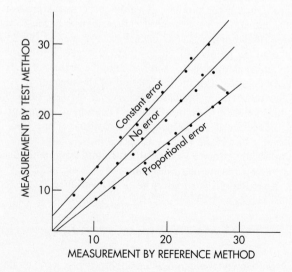

Fig. 5-3　Graph of systematic error (accuracy). *From Tietz N: Fundamentals of clinical chemistry, ed 3, Philadelphia, 1987, WB Saunders.*

calculation, the unpaired t-test, the difference between the means of two separate population groups is compared. This form of the test compares two different groups of samples tested by two different test procedures. The equation for this form of the calculation is:

EQ. 5-7

$$t = \frac{|X_1 - X_2|}{SD_d}$$

where t equals the absolute value of the difference between the means, divided by the standard error for that difference. The standard error is calculated as follows:

EQ. 5-8

$$SD_d = \sqrt{\left(\frac{n_1 + n_2}{n_1 n_2}\right)\left(\frac{(n_1 - 1)SD_1^2 + (n_2 - 1)SD_2^2}{n_1 + n_2 - 2}\right)}$$

where:

n_1 = the number of observations in the first group,
n_2 = the number of observations in the second group,
SD_1 = the standard deviation of the first group, and
SD_2 = the standard deviation of the second group.

In another form of this test, the paired t-test, the comparison of means is between two methods using the same sample population. This test determines if a significant statistical difference exists between values determined by a test method and values obtained by a reference method. The t-value is calculated by the following equation:

EQ. 5-9

$$t = \frac{|bias|\sqrt{n}}{SD_d} = \frac{|\overline{Y} - \overline{X}|\sqrt{n}}{SD_d}$$

In equation 5-9, the square root of n (n equals the number of samples analyzed) is multiplied by the bias. The bias is the absolute value of $\bar{y} - \bar{x}$ ($\bar{y}$ being the test method mean and $\bar{x}$ being either an assigned value or the mean obtained from a reference method. This product is then divided by SD_d, which equals the standard deviation of the results obtained from the two methods. SD_d is calculated as follows:

EQ. 5-10

$$SD_d = \sqrt{\frac{\Sigma[(y_i - x_i) - (\overline{Y} - \overline{X})]^2}{n - 1}}$$

In this equation, y_i are the results obtained from the test method and x_i are the results obtained by the reference method. The bias, or the difference between the average of the test values and the average of the reference values, is represented as $\overline{Y} - \overline{X}$. By using a table for critical T values for selected probabilities (p) and degrees of freedom (df), a critical T value can be determined and compared with the t-test value. An abbreviated T table can be found in Table 5-2. If the t-test value calculated is larger than the critical T value obtained from the table, then the difference between the means of the methods is significant. If the critical T value is smaller than the t-test value, then a significant statistical difference does not exist. Again, the t-test does not determine if the difference between the means is clinically significant.

Just knowing if the mean and standard deviation are statistically different than the reference method is not sufficient information to make a decision concerning the adoption or rejection of a new method. It is also useful to know how well all the data points correlate and if a straight line can be obtained through a graph of the data. This can be determined by a linear regression, also known as a least square analysis.

The equation for a straight line is:

EQ. 5-11

$$y = a + bx$$

where x is the reference value, y is the test value, a is the y-axis intercept, and b is the slope of the line. The slope of the line is calculated using the following equation:

EQ. 5-12

$$b = \frac{n\Sigma xy - \Sigma x \Sigma y}{n\Sigma x^2 - (\Sigma x)^2}$$

The y-intercept (a) is calculated by the equation:

Table 5-1   Critical values of F for $p = 0.05$ and selected degrees of freedom (df)

	Degrees of freedom for numerator						
df for denominator	**5**	**10**	**15**	**20**	**30**	**60**	**∞**
1	230.00	242.00	246.00	248.00	250.00	252.00	254.00
2	19.30	19.40	19.40	19.40	19.50	19.50	19.50
3	9.01	8.79	8.70	8.66	8.62	8.57	8.53
4	6.26	5.96	5.86	5.80	5.75	5.69	5.63
5	5.05	4.74	4.62	4.56	4.50	4.43	4.36
6	4.39	4.06	3.94	3.87	3.81	3.74	3.67
7	3.97	3.64	3.51	3.44	3.38	3.30	3.23
8	3.69	3.35	3.22	3.15	3.08	3.01	2.93
9	3.48	3.14	3.01	2.94	2.86	2.79	2.71
10	3.33	2.98	2.85	2.77	2.70	2.62	2.54
15	2.90	2.54	2.40	2.33	2.25	2.16	2.07
20	2.71	2.35	2.20	2.12	2.04	1.95	1.84
30	2.53	2.16	2.01	1.93	1.84	1.74	1.62
60	2.37	1.99	1.84	1.75	1.65	1.53	1.39
∞	2.21	1.83	1.67	1.57	1.46	1.32	1.00

Modified from Barnett RN: Clinical laboratory statistics, ed 2, Boston, 1979, Little, Brown.

Table 5-2   Probability points of the student's t-distribution with v degrees of freedom; α is the upper tail probability

v \ α	0.40	0.25	0.10	0.05	0.025	0.01	0.005	0.0005
1	0.325	1.000	3.078	6.314	12.706	31.821	63.657	636.619
2	0.289	0.816	1.886	2.920	4.303	6.965	9.925	31.598
3	0.277	0.765	1.638	2.353	3.182	4.541	5.841	12.941
4	0.271	0.741	1.533	2.132	2.776	3.747	4.604	8.610
5	0.267	0.727	1.476	2.015	2.571	3.365	4.032	6.859
6	0.265	0.718	1.440	1.943	2.447	3.143	3.707	5.959
7	0.263	0.711	1.415	1.895	2.365	2.998	3.499	5.405
8	0.262	0.706	1.397	1.860	2.306	2.896	3.355	5.041
9	0.261	0.703	1.383	1.833	2.262	2.821	3.250	4.781
10	0.260	0.700	1.372	1.812	2.228	2.764	3.169	4.587
11	0.260	0.697	1.363	1.796	2.201	2.718	3.106	4.437
12	0.259	0.695	1.356	1.782	2.179	2.681	3.055	4.318
13	0.259	0.694	1.350	1.771	2.160	2.650	3.012	4.221
14	0.258	0.692	1.345	1.761	2.145	2.624	2.977	4.140
15	0.258	0.691	1.341	1.753	2.131	2.602	2.947	4.073
16	0.258	0.690	1.337	1.746	2.120	2.583	2.921	4.015
17	0.257	0.689	1.333	1.740	2.110	2.567	2.898	3.965
18	0.257	0.688	1.330	1.734	2.101	2.552	2.878	3.922
19	0.257	0.688	1.328	1.729	2.093	2.539	2.861	3.883
20	0.257	0.687	1.325	1.725	2.086	2.528	2.845	3.850
21	0.257	0.686	1.323	1.721	2.080	2.518	2.831	3.819
22	0.256	0.686	1.321	1.717	2.074	2.508	2.819	3.792
23	0.256	0.685	1.319	1.714	2.069	2.500	2.807	3.767
24	0.256	0.685	1.318	1.711	2.064	2.492	2.797	3.745
25	0.256	0.684	1.316	1.708	2.060	2.485	2.787	3.725
26	0.256	0.684	1.315	1.706	2.056	2.479	2.779	3.707
27	0.256	0.684	1.314	1.703	2.052	2.473	2.771	3.690
28	0.256	0.683	1.313	1.701	2.048	2.467	2.763	3.674
29	0.256	0.683	1.311	1.699	2.045	2.462	2.756	3.659
30	0.256	0.683	1.310	1.697	2.042	2.457	2.750	3.646
40	0.255	0.681	1.303	1.684	2.021	2.423	2.704	3.551
60	0.254	0.679	1.296	1.671	2.000	2.390	2.660	3.460
120	0.254	0.677	1.289	1.658	1.980	2.358	2.617	3.373
∞	0.253	0.674	1.282	1.645	1.960	2.326	2.576	3.291

From Tietz N: Fundamentals of clinical chemistry, ed 3, Philadelphia, 1987, WB Saunders.

EQ. 5-13

$$a = b\bar{x} - \bar{y}$$

where b is the slope obtained from equation 5-12, $\bar{x}$ is the average of all the reference values, and $\bar{y}$ is the average of all the test values.

Of course not all the data points will fall directly on the regression line. The scatter of the points about the line can be determined by measuring the standard deviation about the regression line. This standard deviation is measured by $s_{y/x}$ and is calculated as follows:

EQ. 5-14

$$s_{y/x} = \sqrt{\frac{\sum (y_i - Y_i)^2}{n - 2}}$$

where y_i are the measured values for each data point and Y_i are the values calculated from the regression equation.

A perfect or ideal line will have a slope (b) of 1.0, a y-intercept (a) of 0.0, and a standard deviation ($s_{y/x}$) of 0.0. As mentioned before, various errors can cause a skewed line. Slope changes will occur due to proportional errors, shifts in the y-intercept will occur due to constant errors, and random errors will cause an increase in the standard deviation about the regression line.

The correlation coefficient (r), (Fig. 5-4), is another common statistical calculation that is performed when comparing methods. It determines whether the test data correlated positively or negatively to the reference data. It is calculated using the equation:

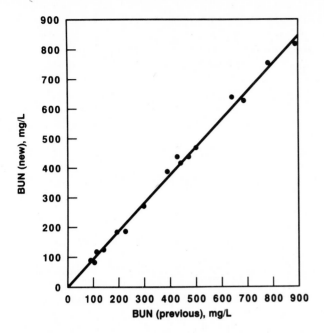

Fig. 5-4   Graph of Correlation Coefficient. *From Garber CC and Carey RN: Laboratory statistics. In Kaplan LA and Pesce AJ: Clinical chemistry: theory, analysis, and correlation, ed 2, St Louis, 1989, Mosby-Year Book, Inc.*

EQ. 5-15

$$r = \frac{n\sum xy - \sum x \sum y}{\sqrt{[n\sum x^2 - (\sum x)];[n\sum y^2 - (\sum y)^2]}}$$

When the two methods correlate exactly, r will equal either $+1.00$ or -1.00. Random errors are the cause of a result that does not equal 1.00. A result of zero indicates no correlation between the methods. Systematic errors do not affect r and therefore r might be close to ideal even though a method is inaccurate.

As stated earlier, it is laboratory personnel's top priority to report the most accurate results possible at all times. However, errors can never be totally eliminated. Both accuracy and precision are dependent upon methodology and technique. Whereas the precision of a method might be improved by automation, accuracy can be improved by evaluating standardization and calibration procedures and materials. Constant error, on the other hand, may be corrected by better specificity of the assay.

REFERENCE RANGES
Definition of normal results

Once laboratory data reaches the physician, the question becomes one of whether the patient's results are normal or abnormal. There is not always a clear answer to that question, for what is normal for one person may not be normal for another. This can be true even when the result is the same. The situation then requires the interpretation of the concept of "normal."

In the statistical sense, normal refers to a distribution that follows a Gaussian probability distribution. This distribution is a bell-shaped curve and the value that occurs the most frequently is the mean. The rest of the values will

fall evenly to either side of this central value. Although this is the case when multiple measurements are made on a single sample, for example, quality control serum tested for glucose, it is rarely true when single measurements are made on many individual samples, for example, all glucose determinations performed on every patient during a given day.

In another setting, normal might be equated with the terms common, typical, or usual. However, just because a result is referred to as typical or usual, it does not necessarily imply a state of good health. This can be demonstrated by the fact that it is common to find an average American cholesterol value that is greater than 200 mg/dL. Elevated levels of cholesterol have been shown to be associated with an increased risk of coronary artery disease. However, not all people with cholesterol levels greater than 200 mg/dL show symptoms of heart disease. There are also many cases in which people suffering from atherosclerosis have cholesterol values less than 200 mg/dL.

Normal has also been used to describe a patient known to be free of a particular disease. At the same time, one can define the presence of that disease by obtaining a measurable difference from this normal result. It is uncommon, especially during the process of chronic illness, to be able to distinguish exactly when a patient changes from a state of good health to a state of pathological illness. Most of the time it is a very gradual process.

Selection of reference ranges

It has been recommended that the use of the term *reference ranges* be substituted for the more traditional one, *normal values*. This recommendation comes from the International Federation of Clinical Chemistry (IFCC). These reference ranges should be determined by performing multiple analyses on a population of individuals who are selected to fit the population of people to which they will be compared.

When beginning a reference range study, it is best to begin with a population that is as random as possible, but at the same time is a sampling of subjects who are free of disease. It is typical in a hospital setting for the laboratory staff to be used as the sample population. This is due to the ready availability of volunteers and the fact that an invasive procedure is used to obtain the blood samples. However, the use of this population has certain limitations. Most laboratory populations tend to be of a younger average age than the general population and they tend to be in better health and physical condition. Therefore, they may not be representative of the general population and may not always provide the best reference range.

The number of participants in the study is highly important. Theoretically, the greater the number of participants in the study, the closer the mean of the study will be to the overall population. A large number of participants in the study will also help lower the range of variability between measurements. If the test data are likely to follow a Gaussian distribution, it is recommended that there be a minimum of 40 participants in the study. Even though this number can give a good representation of a limited geographical area, there are bound to be a few samples with results that are considered to be outliers and which will eventually be excluded from the rest of the test data. Therefore, it would be preferable to start with a slightly larger test population so that if a few results are excluded, the sample statistics would not be compromised. On the other hand, studies of 200 or more subjects will more than likely expose subgroups within the general population. When the test data seem to support the fact that more than one population exists, statistical tests such as the F test and the *t*-test can be performed to determine if significant statistical differences between the various subpopulations really exist. It should also be determined if the group variation is larger or smaller than individual variations. If individual variations are larger than a group's variation, the group's variation would be considered clinically insignificant.

The two most common major subgroups encountered during reference range determinations are age and sex. These can be a major concern when measuring and referencing certain analytes. The enzyme alanine aminotransferase (ALT) can be used as an example of an analyte with an age dependency. The values found in normal adults usually run between 0 and 55 IU/L when analyzed at 37°C. Newborns, on the other hand, have a reference range up to twice that of adults (0 to 110 IU/L). γ-Glutamyltransferase (GGT) has a reference range that is dependent on the sex of the individual. When analyzed at 37°C, males typically measure less than 50 IU/L, whereas females usually measure less than 30 IU/L.

The stage a woman is in during her menstrual cycle can have a profound influence on the results obtained for certain hormonal studies. For example, luteinizing hormone (LH) concentrations are fairly low early in the menstrual cycle (up to 15 mIU/mL). Later in the menstrual cycle, increasing concentrations of follicle stimulating hormone (FSH) stimulate follicular growth and the release of estrogens. The rising estrogen concentrations cause the LH values to increase. The rise in LH at midcycle (up to 50 mIU/mL) then leads to the maturation and release of the ovum approximately 24 hours after the LH concentrations reach their peak. When progesterone is released by the corpus luteum, LH production is again inhibited and falls sharply back down to early cycle values.

Other health-related factors that can influence data distribution are:

1. Exercise. If it is vigorous, tests may show an elevation of muscle enzymes, especially creatine kinase.
2. Diet. Both the type and quality of food eaten will have an impact on food metabolites. Diets high in protein will elevate blood urea, ammonia, and urate levels, whereas foods such as bananas and avocados will increase urinary excretion of 5-HIAA (5-hydroxyindoleacetic acid).
3. Smoking. If it is moderate to heavy and done over extended periods of time, smoking may affect blood gas values, carbon monoxide concentrations, and possibly induce elevated levels of carcinoembryonic antigen (CEA).

These subpopulations may be included in the overall calculations of the reference ranges as long as these factors do not cause a skew in the data range.

Data summary

There are also preanalytical and analytical considerations that must be taken into account when obtaining samples and analyzing the test data. Some of the preanalytical criteria are concerned with the posture of the person when obtaining the blood sample, the time of day the sample is collected, and also the person's state of fasting. Many times the results obtained on an ambulatory person will differ from that of a hospitalized person who is more prone to bed rest. This is noticeable with analytes such as albumin, which tends to be lower in recumbent patients. Cortisol, which shows a diurnal variation, is an analyte whose reference range is dependent upon the time of day it is collected. This means cortisol levels should be higher in the morning before rising and lower in the evening. Glucose levels, which vary according to food intake, are a good example to use when comparing states of fasting.

Analytically, a laboratory should be concerned with the instrumentation used for the analyses. Sensitive instrumentation needs to be properly maintained by routine preventive maintenance and servicing. Temperatures at which samples are analyzed must be documented and maintained within narrow limits (usually ±0.2°C). This is especially important in the case of enzyme results, which are very temperature-dependent. The age of the reagents and how the material is reconstituted can also affect results. Calibrations or standardizations should always be performed according to manufacturer recommendations. Quality control samples should also be included with the analysis of unknown samples to ensure that the instruments are performing properly.

An easy way to overview the accumulated reference data is to display data in the form of a histogram (Fig. 5-5). This technique identifies the frequency of the data points compared to the analyte concentration. Not only does a histogram provide an idea about the shape of the data distribution, but it also makes it easier to pinpoint any outliers. An outlier is a value that appears to be different from the majority of the measurements. Any value suggestive of being an outlier should first be checked by reviewing the analytical records, correcting any transcription errors, and possibly rerunning the sample. A statistical test is performed on a value to determine if it is a true outlier. First, the apparent outlier is subtracted from the mean of all the values. The absolute value of this difference is then divided by the standard deviation of all the values:

EQ. 5-16

$$y = \frac{|\bar{x} - \text{outlier}|}{\text{SD}}$$

The value of *y* is then compared to the table of critical values for rejection of a single outlier (Table 5-3). If *y* is larger than the critical value for *n*, *n* equaling the number of measurements that determined the mean, then the value is a true outlier and should be discarded. Once discarded, the mean and standard deviation of the group must be recalculated.

After identifying and removing any outliers, the reference range can then be determined. Either parametric or nonparametric statistical techniques can be implemented. Usually, the nonparametric methods are the easiest to use. Calculation of percentiles is the most commonly used technique. A percentile is a value on a scale of 1 to 100 that describes the percentage of the reference distribution that is equal to or lower than itself. The usual reference range is

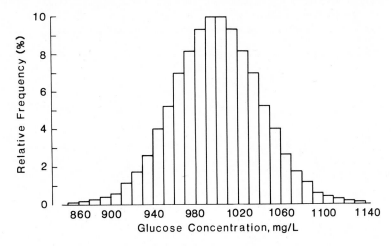

Fig. 5-5   Histogram. *From Garber CC and Carey RN: Laboratory statistics. In Kaplan LA and Pesce AJ: Clinical chemistry: theory, analysis, and correlation, ed 2, St Louis, 1989, Mosby-Year Book, Inc.*

Table 5-3   Critical values for rejection of a single outlier

No. of observations	Reject suspect value if ratio $(X_s - \bar{X})/SD$ or $(\bar{X} - X_s)/SD$ greater than:
8	2.126*
9	2.215
10	2.290
11	2.355
12	2.412
13	2.462
14	2.507
15	2.549
16	2.585
17	2.620
18	2.651
19	2.681
20	2.709
21	2.733
22	2.758
23	2.781
24	2.802
25	2.822
26	2.841
27	2.859
28	2.876
29	2.893
30	2.908

From Standard practice for dealing with outlying observations, Designation: E 178–80. In Annual book of ASTM standards, sec 14; General methods and instrumentation, 1989.
*At 2.5% level of significance considering one side only; at 5% level of significance considering outliers occurring on either side.

described as the central 95% of a distribution curve bounded on either side by the 2.5th and 97.5th percentiles. This means that 2.5% of the upper and 2.5% of lower values are cut off and are not included in the reference range. To determine the interpercentile intervals using a nonparametric technique, the system of sort and rank can be employed.

The first step is to sort all the data points and rank them in numerical order from the lowest result to the highest result. Each result is then assigned a rank number, the lowest value being assigned the number 1. Results of equal values are given consecutive rank numbers. Rank numbers for the 2.5th and 97.5th percentiles are calculated using the following equations, *n* equaling the number of data measurements:

EQ. 5-16a

$$0.025 (n + 1)$$
Calculation of 2.5th percentile

EQ. 5-16b

$$0.975 (n + 1)$$
Calculation of 97.5th percentile

After calculating the rank numbers for the 2.5th and 97.5th percentiles, the corresponding reference values to these rank numbers are determined and are considered to be the cutoff values for the reference range.

The parametric methods for calculating interpercentile estimations include the use of the mean and standard deviation. Parametric methods, of course, assume that the distribution is Gaussian or that the data can be mathematically manipulated to fit a Gaussian distribution. Testing the assumption that the reference data fit a normal distribution can be done visually by means of a graph (such as a histogram) or mathematically by means of equations.

The Chi-square (χ^2) goodness-of-fit test compares the frequency of an occurring number to that which would be expected for an assumed distribution, in this case, a Gaussian distribution. Chi-squared is calculated as follows:

EQ. 5-17

$$\chi^2 = \sum_{i=1}^{n} \frac{(O_i - E_i)^2}{E_i}$$

where *n* equals the total number of data points being compared, O_i refers to the observed frequency of each number, and E_i corresponds to the expected frequency of those numbers. The differences between the expected and observed values are squared and then divided by E_i. All of the values

Table 5-4   Critical values of the χ^2 distribution; the table gives values of the number t_o such that $PR(\chi_k^2 \geq t_o) = p$

Degrees of freedom (k)	Probability level, p						
	0.25	0.10	0.05	0.025	0.01	0.005	0.001
1	1.323	2.706	3.841	5.024	6.635	7.879	10.83
2	2.773	4.605	5.991	7.378	9.210	10.60	13.82
3	4.108	6.251	7.815	9.348	11.34	12.84	16.27
4	5.385	7.779	9.488	11.14	13.28	14.86	18.47
5	6.626	9.236	11.07	12.83	15.09	16.75	20.52
6	7.841	10.64	12.59	14.45	16.81	18.55	22.46
7	9.037	12.02	14.07	16.01	18.48	20.28	24.32
8	10.22	13.36	15.51	17.53	20.09	21.96	26.13
9	11.39	14.68	16.92	19.02	21.67	23.59	27.88
10	12.55	15.99	18.31	20.48	23.21	25.19	29.59
11	13.70	17.28	19.68	21.92	24.72	26.76	31.26
12	14.85	18.55	21.03	23.34	26.22	28.30	32.91
13	15.98	19.81	22.36	24.74	27.69	29.82	34.53
14	17.12	21.06	23.68	26.12	29.14	31.32	36.12
15	18.25	22.31	25.00	27.49	30.58	32.80	37.70
16	19.37	23.54	26.30	28.85	32.00	34.27	39.25
17	20.49	24.77	27.59	30.19	33.41	35.72	40.79
18	21.60	25.99	28.87	31.53	34.81	37.16	42.31
19	22.72	27.20	30.14	32.85	36.19	38.58	43.82
20	23.83	28.41	31.41	34.17	37.57	40.00	45.32
21	24.93	29.62	32.67	35.48	38.93	41.40	46.80
22	26.04	30.81	33.92	36.78	40.29	42.80	48.27
23	27.14	32.01	35.17	38.08	41.64	44.18	49.73
24	28.24	33.20	36.42	39.36	42.98	45.56	51.18
25	29.34	34.38	37.65	40.65	44.31	46.93	52.62
26	30.43	35.56	38.89	41.92	45.64	48.29	54.05
27	31.53	36.74	40.11	43.19	46.96	69.64	55.48
28	32.62	37.92	41.34	44.46	48.28	50.99	56.89
29	33.71	39.09	42.56	45.72	49.59	52.34	58.30
30	34.80	40.26	43.77	46.98	50.89	53.67	59.70

Abridged from Pearson ES and Hartley HO: Biometrika tables for statisticians, vol 1, ed 3, London, 1966, Biometrika Trustees, Cambridge University Press. It appears here with the kind permission of the publishers.

are then summed up. If the observed frequencies are larger or smaller than expected, then chi-squared will be a large number. If the calculated value of χ^2 is greater than the critical value of χ^2 (Table 5-4), then it can be assumed that a significant statistical difference exists between the observed and expected distributions. This would mean that the observed distribution is not Gaussian.

Before plotting a distribution graph, a table of the data points vs. frequency and cumulative frequency should be constructed. This can be done by sorting the data points from lowest to highest (as in the ranking procedure) and listing them in a columnar form as shown in Table 5-5. In the second column, the frequency (number of times the data point occurs) is listed. The third column lists the frequency of each data point added to all the previous data point frequencies. This is considered the cumulative frequency. A fourth column, F_x, or cumulative percent, designates the ratio of each cumulative frequency to the total number of frequencies. The last data point on the list will have the highest cumulative frequency and F_x will equal 1.000. Once the cumulative frequency for each concentration value is

determined, the data can be plotted on normal probability paper as concentration vs. cumulative percent (Fig. 5-6). If the plot is a straight line, the distribution is assumed to be Gaussian. In the example shown in Fig. 5-6, the line is not straight.

If the distribution is basically Gaussian but is positively skewed, the same data can be plotted on log-normal probability paper as shown in Fig. 5-7. In this case, a straight line will indicate that a log-normal association exists.

It is highly unlikely that a physician will order only one test on a patient. Since this is often the case, and because of the automated equipment that is available, it is often more economical to offer a variety of tests in what is commonly termed a profile. Profiles can encompass a large spectrum of assays for a general overall picture of health, or a profile might concentrate on a particular tissue (renal panel) or on an area of special interest, such as a variety of hormone tests to determine fertility.

Even if a patient is healthy and free of disease, the more tests that are performed, the greater the statistical chance of finding an abnormal result on that patient. Assuming the

Table 5-5   Parathyroid hormone data

x (pg/mL)	Frequency	Cumulative frequency	F(x)
≤160	6	6	0.100
180	1	7	0.117
190	1	8	0.133
200	1	9	0.150
230	4	13	0.217
240	1	14	0.233
290	1	15	0.250
320	1	16	0.267
330	3	19	0.317
350	1	20	0.333
360	2	22	0.367
380	5	27	0.450
400	2	29	0.483
410	2	31	0.517
430	1	32	0.533
450	1	33	0.550
470	4	37	0.617
500	1	38	0.633
520	1	39	0.650
530	2	41	0.683
560	1	42	0.700
570	2	44	0.733
580	2	46	0.767
600	1	47	0.783
650	2	49	0.817
670	1	50	0.833
730	3	53	0.883
800	1	54	0.900
920	1	55	0.916
1150	1	56	0.933
1280	1	57	0.950
1370	2	59	0.983
1520	1	60	1.000

From Buncher CR and Weiner D: Reference values. In Kaplan LA and Pesce AJ editors: Clinical chemistry: theory, analysis, and correlation, ed 2, St Louis, 1989, Mosby-Year Book, Inc.

usual 95% prediction interval and the fact that each constituent is measured independently of the others, the percentage of constituents that can be expected to fall outside reference range limits can be calculated as follows:

EQ. 5-18

$$100 [1 - (.95)^n]$$

where *n* equals the number of constituents measured. As the number of constituents measured increases, the higher the percentage of values that will fall outside the reference range. The physician might choose to have an abnormal result repeated and it may be normal. Alternatively, if it can be determined that the abnormal result is not due to a disease process, then it may be assumed that the result is normal for that patient.

Sensitivity and specificity. The sensitivity of a test defines the test's ability to give a true positive (TP) result when a certain disease is present. If a test is 100% sensitive, then it will give a positive result every time a patient suffers from that disease. Specificity, on the other hand, defines the ability of a test to obtain a true negative (TN) result in a patient free of that specific disease. If a test is 100%

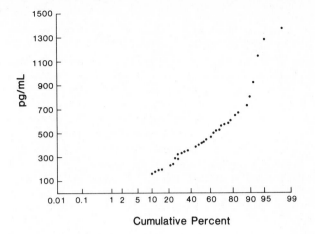

Fig. 5-6   Concentration vs. cumulative percent—normal. *From Buncher CR and Weiner D: Reference values. In Kaplan LA and Pesce AJ: Clinical chemistry: theory, analysis, and correlation, ed 2, St Louis, 1989, Mosby-Year Book, Inc.*

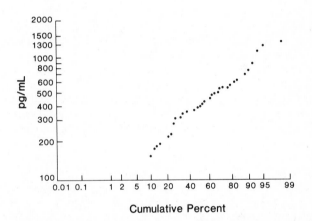

Fig. 5-7   Concentration vs. cumulative percent—log normal. *From Buncher CR and Weiner D: Reference values. In Kaplan LA and Pesce AJ: Clinical chemistry: theory, analysis, and correlation, ed 2, St Louis, 1989, Mosby-Year Book, Inc.*

specific, it will be negative all of the time when performed on patients who do not suffer from that given disease. The predictive value of a positive result is the percentage of true positives obtained when a test is performed on a combined group of healthy and diseased people. Equations that are variations on Bayes' theorem and that more easily define these concepts are shown:

EQ. 5-19

$$\text{Sensitivity} = \frac{TP}{TP + FN} \times 100$$

EQ. 5-20

$$\text{Specificity} = \frac{TN}{TN + FP} \times 100$$

EQ. 5-21

$$\text{Predictive value of a positive} = \frac{TP}{TP + FP} \times 100$$

where

TP = true positive, TN = true negative, FP = false positive, and FN = false negative.

Clinically, it is not possible to achieve 100% sensitivity and 100% specificity at the same time. If the cutoff level of the assay is adjusted to a lower concentration to pick up all the patients with a certain disease, there will be some healthy people who will be considered positive for the disease. These results are called false positives (FP). If the cutoff of the assay is raised to prevent all healthy patients from giving a positive result, a few diseased patients with a value lower than the cutoff will be missed. These results are called false negatives (FN). It would, of course, be optimal if both high sensitivity and high specificity could be achieved at the same time. The decision of which to choose, however, depends upon the nature of the disease and how many false positives and/or false negatives are acceptable. If a screening test is relatively expensive, then fewer false negatives would be desirable. On the other hand, if the screening test is inexpensive and the confirmation testing on a positive result is not expensive or difficult to perform, then more false positives could be accepted. In other words, high sensitivity is desired when disease prevalence is low in a population and high specificity should be achieved when disease prevalence is high.

Previous results. Instead of comparing a patient's test results to a previously determined reference range group, it might be more feasible to compare the results of the patient's own personal history. With the mass health screenings that are becoming so popular and the acceptance of preventive medicine by health insurance carriers, it is becoming more common to find previous results taken at a time of good health. With the advent of better computerization, it will be easier to track patient data and to have it readily accessible for previous result comparisons. If what is normal for one person is not necessarily normal for another, then at least a change from the previous result will indicate a change in the individual.

QUALITY CONTROL

Internal quality control in the clinical laboratory is absolutely necessary to ensure that the highest level of job performance is enforced by all. Quality control should set limits and direction for those involved in test performance. It should encompass all procedures from sample collection, processing, and analysis, to the timely transfer of the test results to the physician. Hopefully, these procedures will lead to less result variation due to individual subjective interpretation of test data.

Patient identification and preparation

The most important aspect of sample collection is patient identification. It is absolutely necessary that the patient be positively identified before a sample is taken. This is most commonly done by verifying the patient's name and identification number from his or her identification band usually found on one of the wrists. If this band is missing, it is best to have the nurse in charge of the patient give a positive identification. It is never proper to identify the patient by room and bed number.

Next, it is important to make sure that the patient was properly prepared. For example, the phlebotomist should make sure the patient was fasting, if necessary. This is important for such tests as fasting glucose or triglycerides. If a therapeutic drug level is being monitored, it should be noted when the last dose of the medication was given. Since some things are very difficult for a laboratory to monitor, it is important that the laboratory provide an easy-to-use procedure manual to which all nursing staff can refer. It should contain all information regarding each test, from how to request a test to any instructions that should be followed before and while a sample is being collected. In the case of a xylose tolerance test, the patient will first need to be fasting. A urine sample should be collected before the dose of D-xylose is ingested by the patient since the assay for xylose can be affected by high values of glucose that might be in the patient's urine. The nursing unit will need to notify the laboratory staff of the time the dose was given so that a blood sample can be collected exactly 2 hours later. The nursing unit will also need to inform the patient that all urine voided for the next 5 hours will need to be saved for analysis. If all of these steps are not properly followed, the information the physician receives from the results could be incomplete and/or compromised.

Specimen acquisition and transportation

The procedures for the collection of samples should follow the specific guidelines established by the National Committee for Clinical Laboratory Standards (NCCLS). The type of collection tubes used will be determined by the tests that are ordered. Many times it will be necessary to collect more than one sample tube per patient because more than one type of anticoagulant will be required. Each tube should be labeled with the patient's entire name, his or her hospital identification number, the patient's room number, the date and time of sample collection, and the initials of the phlebotomist collecting the sample.

It is important that the samples collected be transported to the laboratory in a timely manner. Sometimes it will also be necessary to have them delivered either in a preheated block or on ice. As an example, ice is extremely important to reduce metabolic processes when transporting a sample to be tested for an ammonia value. Ammonia concentrations in whole blood begin to rise immediately after venipuncture because of the deamination of the amino acids present in the sample. Ice slows down this process. A specimen collected for an ammonia determination should also be centrifuged at 0 to 4°C within 20 minutes of collection; the plasma should be removed from the cells immediately thereafter and analyzed as soon as possible.

Sample log-in and processing

When a sample arrives in the laboratory, it should be logged in so that the appropriate personnel know that it is available for testing. This can be done by means of manual written logs or, as is more common these days, via a computerized laboratory log. This is the beginning of the paper trail that will follow each step of the specimen's journey throughout the laboratory.

If the sample will not be analyzed immediately after processing, the proper storage recommendations must be followed. Some samples, such as serum for lactate dehydrogenase (LDH) isoenzymes, will need to be stored at room temperature as the LDH-4 and LDH-5 fractions are unstable at cold temperatures. Most other samples will require either refrigeration at 0 to 8°C or freezing at −20°C. Not only is temperature important, but the effect of light in some cases can dramatically affect the results of certain analytes. This is especially true for bilirubin, which is very photosensitive, decomposing when exposed to light of certain wavelengths.

After the sample is properly logged in, processed, and distributed for testing, analytical system checks are implemented to ensure that the results are accurate. Before the actual analysis is performed, it is necessary to go through a complete checklist of items to make sure all laboratory systems are monitored and in control. Water quality is an item of extreme importance in the preparation and reconstitution of analytical reagents and in sample dilutions. In general, type I water, fitting the specification of NCCLS, should be used whenever possible. This reagent grade water will give the minimum amount of interference.

Analytical checks

Balances and mechanical pipettes need to be kept clean and properly maintained. They should be periodically checked for accuracy and precision. Balances should be checked with weights from the National Bureau of Standards (NBS). Glassware should also be cleaned properly and discarded when it becomes chipped or cracked. Glassware checks for residual detergent should be done weekly. As a rule, only class A glassware should be used for precision work. Volumetric glassware must be used when accuracy is important.

All temperature-dependent equipment should be checked and the temperature should be recorded daily or just prior to use. This includes waterbaths, dry heating blocks, refrigerators and freezers, incubators, and ovens. All should have an established acceptable temperature range listed on the laboratory daily maintenance log.

To ensure that all instruments are performing up to expected standards, all scheduled maintenance should be performed on a timely basis. This should include all preventive maintenance checks done by the manufacturer. A scheduled maintenance sheet for each instrument should be available for the regular checkup of operating characteristics. Any function tests should be recorded and checked against specified tolerance limits. This way, any trends or malfunctions can be detected as soon as possible. Any major or minor troubleshooting repairs should be recorded on an instrument problem and maintenance report form. This should be filed near each instrument for easy reference.

Procedure manuals with essential information are needed for each test method. They must be available at the workstation. Step-by-step instructions should include procedure name, clinical significance of the test, principle of the method, all acceptable specimen types, any reagents and/or equipment necessary for testing, detailed procedure steps, reference values for healthy individuals, any notes important to the assay, and any references upon which any of the procedure is based. A good procedure manual should help maintain consistency between different technologists performing the analyses.

Standards and calibrations

Definitive test methods are the most accurate way to measure a compound. These methods are usually not economical for hospital laboratories as they require the most sophisticated instrumentation available and the purest standards attainable. Reference methods have been compared to a definitive method and have been found to give results within ±1% to 2% of the true value. Derived methods have been compared to reference methods and fall within an acceptable range stated by the Food and Drug Administration (FDA). Either reference or derived methodologies are usually found in clinical laboratories.

The dependability of a method to give reliable results depends upon the quality of the standards used for the calibration or standardization of that method. Definitive methods, in addition to validating reference methods, are used to verify values of primary reference materials. These certified reference materials (CRM) are then used to develop and verify reference methods, as well as to calibrate these definitive and reference methods. Secondary reference materials, or calibration and test materials (CTM), are developed from primary reference materials and are used as working standards for the derived or field methods. Control materials are analyzed solely as unknown samples to monitor the calibration of methods and instrumentation. They are never used as calibrators or standards.

Internal quality control
Choice of material

Control material needs to be stable over a long period of time and have little vial-to-vial variability. This material should also consist of the same matrix as the constituent being measured, that is, serum, whole blood, urine, or spinal fluid. It is important that at least two different concentration ranges be monitored. One of those should be the reference range and the other an abnormal or critical range.

Control materials can be prepared in the laboratory from leftover patient sera, but this is very time consuming and the safety of such pools is questionable. Commercial pools come either as lyophilized material, which is then reconstituted with type I water or with a purchased diluent, or as a frozen/refrigerated liquid. Although liquid pools will have lower bottle-to-bottle variation than lyophilized controls, the cost of liquid controls is usually much higher. All commercial control pools are required by the FDA to test free of the human immunodeficiency virus (HIV) and the hepatitis B virus. In the future, control pools will also be tested for hepatitis C virus. It is in the best interest of the laboratory staff to purchase a large enough supply to last approximately 1 to 2 years. If storage facilities are insufficient, many companies that distribute commercial control supplies will sequester large amounts of controls for an institution and will deliver it in predetermined shipments.

The next decision to make is whether to purchase assayed or unassayed material. Unassayed controls are usually much less expensive than assayed controls, but are accompanied only by a list of target values. On the other hand, assayed controls are more expensive than unassayed controls, but include expected values as well as a list of ranges for various analytical methods. This might be preferable when a control is only used in small quantities and a control range analysis would cost more than the money saved by buying an unassayed control. They are also handy when there is not sufficient time to do a control range determination before use. Although assayed controls have assigned values, it is a good idea for the laboratory to check new lots of controls before use against the existing control lot number. An adjustment in the listed standard deviation might also be needed.

Limits determination

Unassayed control material requires a range limit determination to be performed before use. New lot numbers of controls should be run in parallel with the existing lot number for a minimum of 2 weeks or for a minimum of 20 measurements. The initial mean and standard deviation calculated from these values can be used until more data have been accumulated. Once the mean and standard deviation are determined, the control limits can be set at the mean ± 2 SD. These values are then applied to a control chart. Daily control values are then plotted on the control charts. This way, quality control can be quickly and easily reviewed on a daily basis. Deciding whether the control data is "in range" or "out of range" depends upon the decision criteria or control rules established within the laboratory.

Chart development

Shewhart/Levey-Jennings chart

Probably the most commonly used chart in the chemistry laboratory is the Shewhart/Levey-Jennings chart (Fig. 5-8) developed in 1952. A Shewhart/Levey-Jennings chart allows the technologist to view data on a day-to-day basis and scan the chart for overall patterns. After a minimum of 5 to 7 days, trends and shifts become noticeable. A slow deviation from the mean value in either direction is considered a trend, whereas a sudden jump from the established mean to a new mean is considered a shift. The precision of an instrument or method can also be determined by the scatter of points plotted above and below the mean. To construct a Shewhart/Levey-Jennings chart, the vertical axis is labeled with the control values and the horizontal axis is labeled with the run number or date. Horizontal lines are drawn off the vertical axis and represent the mean and upper and lower limits set either at ± 2.0 or ± 3.0 SD. Each control result is plotted as a point intersecting the control concentration and the day or run number. A run is considered "in control" and results can be reported when both control values fall within their predetermined ranges. If the limits are set at ± 3.0 SD, then the false rejection rate will be low, namely, 0.3%, but its error detection will also be low.

If the limits are set at ± 2.0 SD, then the false rejection rate will be higher, namely, 5%, but error detection will also be higher.

To help sort through all of the confusion to decide which is better, a low false rejection rate or a high error detection rate, many control procedures using various decision criteria have been developed. These control procedures vary from laboratory to laboratory. Some laboratories use the ± 2.0 SD range as a warning rule and ± 3.0 SD range as an error limit. Simply, if a two-control system is used and one control was within its ± 2.0 SD range and the other control was between the ± 2.0 to 3.0 SD range, the run would be accepted but a warning would be issued for the next analysis. If instead, one control was within ± 2.0 SD and the other control was outside of ± 3.0 SD, then an error condition would exist and the run would be rejected.

Westgard and associates (1981) have developed a valuable flowchart for making decisions concerning control data. False rejection is kept low with rules whose probabilities for false rejection are low and the probability of error detection is kept high by choosing rules that are sensitive to random and systematic errors. These rules can be applied to charts adapted to the Levey-Jennings format with limits set at the mean, ± 1.0 SD, ± 2.0 SD, and ± 3.0 SD.

A list of abbreviated rules are listed here. They follow the logic diagram shown in Fig. 5-9.

1. 1_{2S}: This is a warning rule. One control observation exceeds the mean ± 2.0 SD. Test other control data with the following rules.
2. 1_{3S}: This is a rejection rule. One control observation exceeds the mean ± 3.0 SD. This rule is sensitive to *random* error.
3. 2_{2S}: This is a rejection rule. It can be applied to either two consecutive control observations on the same control sample exceeding the same ± 2.0 SD limit or it can be applied to control observations on two different controls exceeding their respective ± 2.0 SD limits. This rule is sensitive to *systematic* error.
4. R_{4S}: This is a rejection rule. The difference between two control observations within one run exceeds ± 4.0 SD. This means that one control value exceeds the mean $+2.0$ SD and the other control exceeds the mean by -2.0 SD. This rule is sensitive to *random* error.

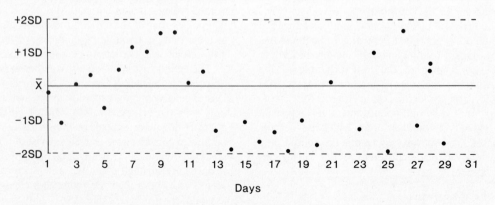

Fig. 5-8   Shewhart/Levey-Jennings chart. *From Copeland BE: Quality control. In Kaplan LA and Pesce AJ: Clinical chemistry: theory, analysis, and correlation, ed 2, St Louis, 1989, Mosby-Year Book, Inc.*

5. 4_{1S}: This is a rejection rule. Four consecutive control observations exceed the same 1.0 SD limit. This rule can also be applied across two control materials, which would require checking the controls for both the present run and the previous run. This rule is sensitive to *systematic* error.

6. $10_{\bar{x}}$: This is a rejection rule. Ten consecutive control observations occur on the same side of the mean. This can also be applied across two control materials. This would require checking the controls for the present run and the four previous runs. This rule is sensitive to *systematic* error.

If neither control exceeds the ±2.0 SD limit, the run is considered "in control" and the results can be reported. If one control exceeds ±2.0 SD, the 1_{2S} rule is implemented and a warning is imposed. The other control result is then tested by the 1_{3S}, 2_{2S}, R_{4S}, 4_{1S}, and $10_{\bar{x}}$ rules. If no further rules are violated, the run is considered "in control" and the results can be reported. If the other control does violate one of the rejection rules, the run is considered "out of control" and results must be held until the error is rectified.

It can be helpful when interpreting analytical errors to review the rule(s) violated. When the 2_{2S}, 4_{1S}, or $10_{\bar{x}}$ control rules are violated, a systematic error usually exists. If the 1_{3S} or R_{4S} rule is violated, random error is usually the problem. The 1_{3S} rule, however, can also be sensitive to a large systematic error. Once the type of error has been determined, possible causes can be investigated. When a systematic error exists, the most probable causes are problems with standards, calibration of an instrument, or reagent blanking. These errors affect results all in the same direction. Violation of the random error rules points to reagent instability, unstable instrument conditions, or too much variability between individual techniques in timing or pipetting. Once

the error condition has been corrected, quality control data obtained during the period of instability should not be used in future calculations.

Probability of rejection is the chance that a rejection rule will occur. The probability will lie between 0 (no chance of occurring) and 1 (100% chance of occurring). Power function graphs are plots that show the probability of rejecting a run when various control rules are violated. Probability of rejection (p) is plotted on the y-axis, whereas the size of the error (random or systematic) is plotted on the x-axis. The point at which the curve intersects the y-axis is the probability of false rejection. That is, the point at which no analytical error exists except the inherent imprecision of the method. Any point along the curve designates the probability of error detection when an error exists that corresponds to the size shown on the x-axis. In both the case of random error (Fig. 5-10) and systematic error (Fig. 5-11), the size of the error is measured in multiples of the standard deviation of the method. That means a value of 2.0 is equivalent to twice the test standard deviation. The number of controls or observations is designated by N. As N increases, error detection also increases. These charts are used only when deciding the acceptability of individual runs. They are not used when reviewing monthly quality control charts.

Cusum

A not so commonly used control system is the cumulative sum (cusum) control procedure. The cusum analysis is based on the theory of random scatter. The control values that lie above the mean will be canceled out by the control values that lie below the mean. The eventual outcome will be a cumulative sum that nears zero when a system is in control. Control limits are set at the mean ±2.0 to ±3.0 SD. If five to six consecutive values fall on the same side of the

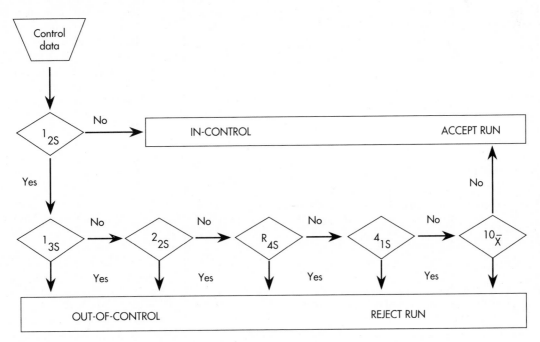

Fig. 5-9 Logic diagram for applying a series of decision criteria (control rules) in the multi-rule Shewhart procedure. *From Westgard J and others: A multi-rule Shewhart chart for quality control in clinical chemistry, Clin Chem 27(3):495, 1981.*

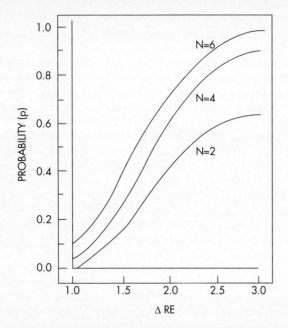

Fig. 5-10   Power graph of the $1_{3S}/2_{2S}/R_{4S}/4_{1S}/10_{\bar{x}}$ multi-rule Shewhart procedure for detecting random error. *From Westgard J and others: A multi-rule Shewhart chart for quality control in clinical chemistry, Clin Chem 27(3):498, 1981.*

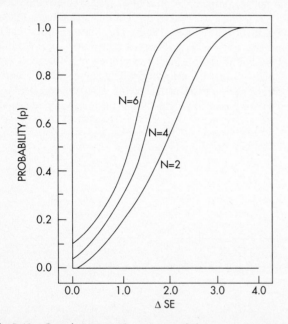

Fig. 5-12   Cumulative sum (Cusum) control chart. *From Tietz N: Fundamentals of clinical chemistry, ed 3, Philadelphia, 1987, WB Saunders.*

mean, there is a high probability that an out-of-control situation exists. Shifts and trends add up, or down, rapidly.

To set up a cusum control chart (Fig. 5-12), the days or observation numbers are recorded on the x-axis. Zero is located at the midpoint of the y-axis and represents the mean, or a cusum of zero. Values corresponding to approximately ±10.0 SD are marked on either side of zero.

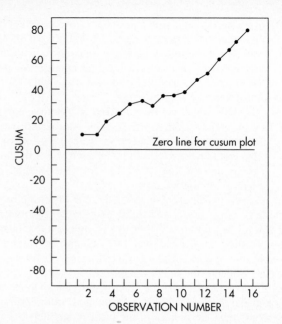

Fig. 5-11   Power graph of the $1_{3S}/2_{2S}/R_{4S}/4_{1S}/10_{\bar{x}}$ multi-rule Shewhart procedure for detecting systematic error. *From Westgard J and others: A multi-rule Shewhart chart for quality control in clinical chemistry, Clin Chem 27(3):498, 1981.*

A table is constructed to include the run number, the control value, the difference of the control value from its mean, and the cumulative sum of the differences (Table 5-6). On day number one, the control value obtained from the test run is recorded on the chart. The mean value is subtracted from the control value. This difference is recorded on the chart and plotted as a point on the cusum chart. When the next control value is obtained, the difference of the value from the mean is added or subtracted to or from the point that was plotted previously. A line is drawn connecting the new point to the one before. Each step is repeated for each successive quality control result. When inspecting the chart, a line that wanders back and forth across the zero line indicates an in-control situation. A steep angle up or down is strongly suggestive of systematic error. Because all previous data are compounded with each point plotted, this control system is very sensitive to systematic error. Unfortunately, this type of system is weak at detecting random error and therefore should be used in conjunction with a system that is sensitive to random error.

Youden plot

This chart is also known as a two-way convergence plot. It blends two quality control pools into one chart (Fig. 5-13). One pool is plotted on the horizontal axis and the other is plotted on the vertical axis. The means of each control pool intersect at the center of the grid. Intersecting points from each of the control's ±1.0 SD and ±2.0 SD create lines to form an inner box (1.0 SD) and an outer box (2.0 SD). Both control values from an analytical run are plotted simultaneously. If the resulting point lies outside the 2.0 SD box, the system is out of control. Trends and shifts are apparent early in the chart's development. As long as successive plotted points lie within the 2.0 SD box, the system is in control.

Table 5-6 Example of cusum calculations (for control material with $\bar{x} = 100$, $s = 5.0$)

Control observation number	Control value	Difference from $\bar{x}$, d_1	Cumulative sum of differences, CS_1
1	110	+10	+10
2	100	0	+10
3	108	+8	+18
4	105	+5	+23
5	105	+5	+28
6	101	+1	+29
7	96	−4	+25
8	105	+5	+30
9	101	+1	+31
10	101	+1	+32
11	111	+11	+43
12	102	+2	+45
13	110	+10	+55
14	107	+7	+62
15	107	+7	+69
16	107	+7	+76

From Tietz N: Fundamentals of clinical chemistry, ed 3, Philadelphia, 1987, WB Saunders.

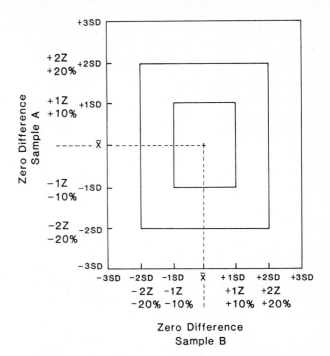

Fig. 5-13 Youden control plot. *From Copeland BE: Quality control. In Kaplan LA and Pesce AJ: Clinical chemistry: theory, analysis, and correlation, St Louis, 1984, Mosby-Year Book, Inc.*

Use of patient results

The monitoring of patient results is another type of quality control that does not incur any additional expense by the laboratory. Although it would be tedious and time consuming for a laboratory to correlate all test results with a patient's clinical symptoms, it is practical to overview an analytical run to determine if the results, as a whole, lie within the expected reference range of the assay. If an analytical run produces results that lean heavily to either the low or high side of normal, then it would be a good idea to repeat the run, regardless of the quality control results.

Testing samples in duplicate is a very good way to detect random errors. Since this technique is more expensive, it is usually reserved for procedures that are long and tedious, or ones that involve extractions.

With the advent of computerization, it is much easier to compare results with previously reported values. This is not only a good idea for checking the feasibility of current results, but it can be a good way to catch sample collection and identification errors.

When building a computer data base, it is common to include certain safety checks, such as limit checks and delta checks. Limit checks include reference ranges, critical (panic) and technical limits, and therapeutic values. Since the reference ranges of many analytes are age- and sex-dependent, computer flags are extremely helpful in alerting technologists to situations in which many combinations for error are possible.

It is a good policy to recheck critical values before reporting them. When the person in charge receives a value that has already been rechecked, he or she can be more assured that the value is correct and can proceed with patient treatment more rapidly. Since the clinicians are the people who will ultimately rely on the integrity of test results, they should be included as part of the quality control program.

They should be encouraged to report questionable or unreasonable results in a timely manner so that any problems can be thoroughly investigated as soon as possible.

External quality control

Internal quality control involves the day-to-day monitoring of laboratory activities. It helps ensure that systematic and random error are caught before patient data are released. External quality control, on the other hand, is a way by which laboratories can compare their performance to other laboratories that perform the same analyses. These types of quality control are also known as proficiency surveys. The material that is used for surveys is produced in large quantities by various sources. Some are professional organizations, such as AACC and CAP, while others are product manufacturers. Survey material is distributed at various time intervals throughout the year. For example, the AACC distributes their therapeutic drug monitoring and ligand surveys monthly, while the CAP distributes all their surveys quarterly. All laboratories that participate in a survey program receive aliquots of the survey material and analyze it according to their established methods. These methods are noted on the survey form along with the survey results.

After laboratory data are submitted and analyzed, each participating laboratory receives a personal survey evaluation. Data from each laboratory are compared to the expected results or those determined by a few reference laboratories. Each laboratory's data are also compared to the average data of the group as well as compared to those laboratories that use only the same methods for analyte determination as themselves.

Survey results are presented in several different ways. The AACC, for example, displays assay results in the form of histograms. Each laboratory is represented by a symbol on the graph. Statistical tests may include the *t*-test or the SDI (standard deviation interval/index). The SDI is a calculation of the number of standard deviations a laboratory's value is from the group's mean. It is calculated by the following formula:

EQ. 5-22

$$SDI = \frac{\text{Lab result } - \text{ group mean}}{\text{Group standard deviation}}$$

A result greater than or less than 2.0 indicates that the laboratory's result varies more than 2.0 SD from the rest of the group. This usually means that a systematic error occurred at the time of testing.

When a laboratory receives a survey report that indicates a SDI greater than or less than 2.0 for any test value, a review of the situation is necessary, followed by an action to correct the situation. The laboratory must try its best to determine what caused the erroneous result so that the same circumstances will not affect patient results.

SUGGESTED READING

American National Standards Institute/ASTM E 178-80. National Committee for Clinical Laboratory Standards: Nomenclature and definitions for use in the national reference system in clinical chemistry, NCLLS document PSC-13, Villanova, Pa, 1979.

Galen R and Gambino S: Beyond normality, New York, 1975, John Wiley & Sons.

Kaplan L and Pesce A, editors: Clinical chemistry: theory, analysis, and correlation, ed 1, St Louis, 1984, Mosby–Year Book, Inc.

Kaplan L and Pesce A, editors: Clinical chemistry: theory, analysis, and correlation, ed 2, St Louis, 1989, Mosby–Year Book, Inc.

Matthews D and Farewell V: Using and understanding medical statistics, Basel, 1985, S Karger AG.

Tietz N, editor: Fundamentals of clinical chemistry, ed 3, Philadelphia, 1987, WB Saunders.

Westgard J and Hunt M: Use and interpretation of common statistical tests in method-comparison studies, Clin Chem 19(1):49–57, 1973.

Westgard J, and others: A multi-rule Shewhart chart for quality control in clinical chemistry, Clin Chem 27(3):493–501, 1981.

PART TWO

MEDICAL CHEMISTRY AND CHEMICAL ANALYSIS

6 Renal physiology and water and electrolyte balance

Lawrence A. Kaplan

STRUCTURE OF THE KIDNEY

The kidney plays a central role in the body's metabolic processes, especially those regulatory processes designed to maintain homeostasis. The body contains two kidneys placed symmetrically on either side of the spinal cord in the lower abdomen. Each kidney can be divided into two major parts, the outer part, called the *cortex* and the inner part, called the *medulla* (Figure 6-1).

The primary functional unit of the kidney is the *nephron* (Figure 6-2). Each of the approximately 1 million nephrons begins with a *glomerulus,* which is a net of capillaries formed between the incoming (afferent) arterial and the outgoing (efferent) arterial. Surrounding the glomerulus is the open end of the renal tubule, called the *Bowman's capsule.*

The renal tubule has three sections, each with a discrete function (Figure 6-2). The first section is the *proximal convoluted tubule* located primarily in the cortical region of the kidney. As the proximal tubule enters the medulla, it forms the descending limb of the *loop of Henle.* This portion of the renal tubule descends through the medulla and then

reverses back up through the medulla as the ascending limb of the loop of Henle. As the ascending limb emerges into the cortex, it forms the *distal convoluted tubule.* As two or more of the distal tubules emerge from the cortex, they form the beginning of the *collecting duct.* The collecting ducts continue to merge within the medulla to form larger ducts in the papilla portion of the kidney (Figure 6-1). These large ducts merge in the renal pelvis to form the *ureter,* which empties into the *bladder.* The bladder empties into the *urethra* which forms the channel to the outside of the body.

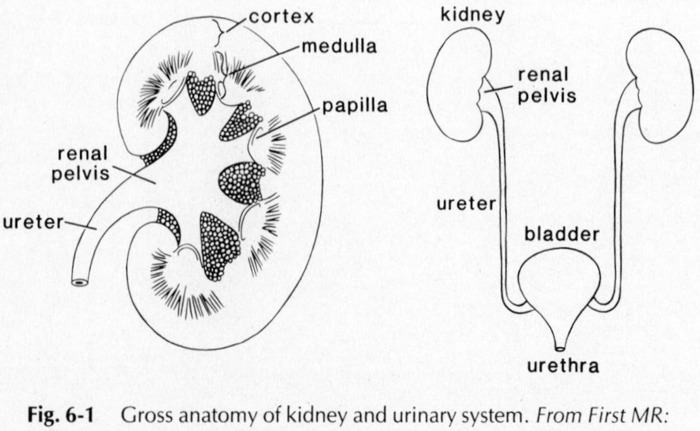

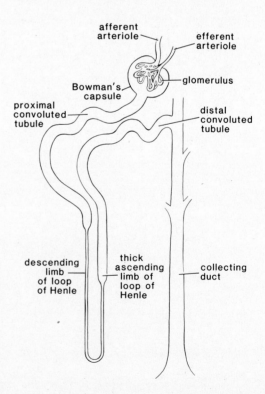

Fig. 6-2 Components of nephron. *From First MR: Renal function. In Kaplan LA and Pesce AJ: Clinical chemistry: theory, analysis, and correlation, ed 2, St Louis, 1989, Mosby-Year Book, Inc.*

Fig. 6-1 Gross anatomy of kidney and urinary system. *From First MR: Renal function. In Kaplan LA and Pesce AJ: Clinical chemistry: theory, analysis, and correlation, ed 2, St Louis, 1989, Mosby-Year Book, Inc.*

84

RENAL PHYSIOLOGY AND BIOCHEMISTRY

The importance of the kidney is demonstrated by the fact that 25% of the total blood output of the heart is pumped through the kidneys. There are five primary functions of the kidney:

1. Removal of waste products (nitrogenous wastes, acids, etc.)
2. Retention of nutrients (electrolytes, protein, water, glucose)
3. Acid-base balance
4. Water and electrolyte balance
5. Hormone synthesis (erythropoietin, renin, and vitamin D)

Renal functions

Removal of waste products

The removal of body wastes is important since most of these substances are toxic to the body at elevated levels. The wastes removed from the body by the kidney include acids derived from the body's general metabolic processes and nitrogenous wastes. The nitrogenous wastes include:

1. *Urea*—which is the end-product of the catabolism (breakdown) of amino acids and proteins. Urea is formed by the *urea cycle* in the liver (see Chapter 13).
2. *Creatinine*—which is formed by the spontaneous hydrolysis and cyclization of muscle creatine. Creatine serves as the primary energy reservoir of muscle cells by forming creatine-phosphate (see Chapter 13).
3. *Uric acid*—which is the end-product metabolite of the nitrogenous purine bases, adenine and guanine, used for DNA and RNA synthesis

Other biochemicals eliminated by the kidney include organic acids, conjugated bilirubin, and exogenous drugs and toxins. The metabolic wastes are eliminated by the kidney in an aqueous solution. The final solution that contains the body's waste products is called *urine*.

Nutrient conservation

Just as it is important for the body to rid itself of the waste products of metabolism, it must also conserve important body nutrients and other important substances. These nutrients, which are important because they help maintain body functions, include:

1. Protein and amino acids
2. Glucose

3. Electrolytes, especially sodium, calcium, chloride, and bicarbonate
4. Water

Table 6-1 summarizes the typical excretory and conservatory roles of the kidney for these analytes.

Acid-base, water, and electrolyte balance

Intimately linked with its excretion and conservation functions, is the kidney's role in maintaining the pH of the body's fluids. The kidney achieves this by eliminating mineral (fixed) acids and conserving alkali (as bicarbonate) as needed. Similarly, the excretion and retention of salts and water is the basis of the kidney's role in maintaining overall water and electrolyte balance.

Hormone synthesis

The kidney also serves as the site of synthesis of three endocrine hormones: erythropoietin, renin, and vitamin D. These compounds are synthesized in the parenchymal cells of the non-nephron portion of the kidney.

Erythropoietin is an approximately 55,000 dalton glycoprotein whose gene is located on chromosome 7. Its function is to stimulate the bone marrow and spleen to produce red blood cells by inducing stem cell differentiation. Although most of the erythropoietin found in plasma (mean concentration, 25 mU/mL) is probably synthesized in peritubular cells of the kidney, 10% to 15% of the erythropoietin can be produced in the liver (the primary site for synthesis in the fetus). Erythropoietin in patients with no kidneys (anephric) is totally derived from hepatic synthesis. The major stimuli for the conduction of erythropoietin are tissue hypoxia and anemia. Anemia is a common clinical finding in renal disease as a result of decreased erythropoietin synthesis by the diseased kidney.

The metabolism of *vitamin D* is complex, involving the liver as well as the kidney (see Chapter 10). However, the step producing the most biologically potent vitamin D metabolite occurs in the kidney as follows:

7-dehydrocholesterol $\xrightarrow[\text{light}]{\text{UV}}$ cholecalciferol — skin

cholecalciferol $\xrightarrow{\text{25-hydroxylation}}$ 25-(OH)-cholecalciferol — liver

$$
25\text{-(OH)-cholecalciferol} \begin{cases} 1,25\text{-(OH)}_2\text{-cholecalciferol} \\ \text{(active vitamin D}_3\text{)} \\[4pt] 24,25\text{-(OH)}_2\text{-cholecalciferol} \\ \text{(inactive)} \end{cases} \text{ — kidney}
$$

Table 6-1   Filtration, reabsorption, and excretion by kidney

Component	Amount filtered per day	Amount excreted per day	Percentage reabsorbed
Water	180 L	1.5 L	99.2
Sodium	24,000 mEq	100 mEq	99.6
Chloride	20,000 mEq	100 mEq	99.5
Bicarbonate	5000 mEq	2 mEq	99.9
Potassium	700 mEq	50 mEq	92.9
Glucose	180 g	0	100
Albumin	360 mg	18 mg	95.0

From Kaplan LA and Pesce AJ: Clinical chemistry: Theory, analysis, and correlation, ed 2, St. Louis, 1989, Mosby-Year Book, Inc.

The third renal hormone, *renin*, is a protein produced in the juxtaglomerula cells situated between the afferent and efferent arterioles of the glomerulus. In response to decreased blood pressure or to increased concentrations of plasma sodium, these cells produce and release renin. Renin is a protease that acts in the renin-angiotensin-aldosterone cascade shown in Figure 6-3. Renin degrades the liver protein angiotensinogen to angiotensin I. This in turn is degraded to angiotensin II by the protease, *angiotensin converting enzyme (ACE)* which is produced primarily in the lung. Angiotensin II is a powerful vasoconstrictor that causes small blood vessels to narrow, increasing blood pressure. Angiotensin II also acts on the adrenal cortex to produce aldosterone and stimulates the brain to induce thirst and to release antidiuretic hormone (ADH). Aldosterone, in turn, acts on the distal convoluted tubule to increase the renal retention of sodium and water. The net result of the actions of angiotensin II and aldosterone is to increase blood volume, blood pressure, and plasma sodium levels. This in turn inhibits synthesis and release of renin to close the homeostatic loop. The renin-angiotensin-aldosterone system maintains blood pressure within a fairly narrow range under a variety of conditions.

The nephron—formation of urine

In order to understand how the kidney accomplishes its regulatory functions, the path of the nephron and each step of the formation of urine will be followed.

Glomerulus

The thin walls of the glomerular basement membrane covering the capillaries act essentially as molecular filters, allowing compounds whose molecular weight is less than approximately 69,000 daltons to filter out of the capillaries and into the Bowman's capsule. Blood cells and larger molecular weight compounds are retained in the vascular compartment so that the glomerular filtrate is essentially free of protein. Because the glomerular filtrate contains most of the low molecular weight solutes of plasma, it has approximately the same osmolality of plasma, that is, it is *isoosmolar* with plasma (282-300 mOsm/L).

The rate at which plasma is filtered by the glomerulus is called the *glomerular filtration rate* (GFR). This value, which decreases with age, varies with the method of measurement. When the glomerular filtration rate is measured by the clearance of inulin, it is estimated to be approximately 130 mL of plasma filtered per minute. Diseases of the kidney affecting the glomeruli can be diagnosed and monitored by measuring decreases in GFR, usually by estimating the creatinine clearance.

Proximal tubule

Approximately 80% of the fluid and electrolytes filtered by the glomerulus is reabsorbed in the proximal tubule. Thus, quantitatively and qualitatively, most of the conservation function of the kidney occurs here. It is important to note that the retention of nutrients by the proximal tubule

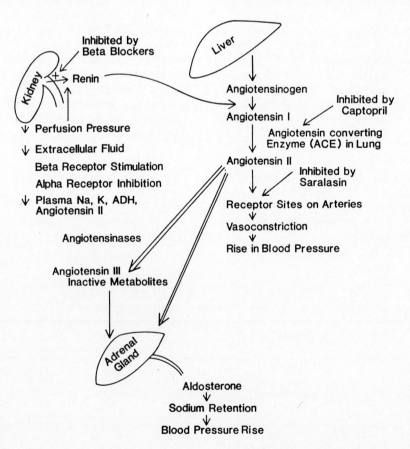

Fig. 6-3 Renin-angiotensin system. *From Bremner WF: Cardiac disease and hypertension. In Kaplan LA and Pesce AJ: Clinical chemistry: theory, analysis, and correlation, ed 1, St Louis, 1984, Mosby-Year Book, Inc.*

is obligatory at this stage; that is, it is not controlled by regulatory processes.

The proximal tubule has a limited capacity to reabsorb analytes (tubular maximal reabsorption, Tm) and this capacity varies with each analyte. The reabsorptive capacity of the nephron is defined by a plasma concentration of the analyte, the *renal plasma threshold*. Below the renal threshold value, essentially all of the filtered analyte is reabsorbed by the nephron. Above this threshold, the tubule's reabsorptive capacity is exceeded and the analyte begins to appear in urine. Renal plasma thresholds have been determined for glucose, bicarbonate, and phosphate. The renal plasma threshold for glucose is approximately 180 mg/dL. Thus, diabetics will have glucose in their urine only when their blood glucose levels exceed 180 mg/dL. The actual renal threshold for an analyte usually decreases with age, leading to increased renal losses of these substances in older individuals.

Analytes are reabsorbed from the glomerular filtrate by two mechanisms. In the first, *active reabsorption,* an expenditure of energy is required for the analyte to be reabsorbed, usually against a concentration gradient. That is, the analyte is moved from a region of lower concentration to one of higher concentration. The second mechanism for reabsorption is called *passive reabsorption,* in which an analyte moves passively down a concentration gradient, that is, from a region of higher concentration to a region of lower concentration. Alternatively, an analyte can move passively along with another analyte that may be actively reabsorbed. For example, the chloride and bicarbonate anions move passively with the sodium cations, which are actively reabsorbed. This maintains electrical neutrality. Water is also passively reabsorbed as the solvent which hydrates the solutes being reabsorbed. No energy is consumed during passive reabsorption of an analyte.

Some of the important analytes that are reabsorbed in the proximal tubule are listed below:

ACTIVE	PASSIVE
Sodium (some passive)	Chloride (some active)
Glucose	Bicarbonate
Protein (albumin)	Water

ACTIVE—cont'd	PASSIVE—cont'd
Amino acids	Potassium
Uric acid	Urea
Calcium	
Potassium	
Magnesium	
Phosphate	

Active secretion of body wastes also occurs in the proximal tubule. This includes the secretion of hydrogen ions, phosphate, organic acids, and certain drugs, such as penicillin. The secretion of hydrogen (H^+) is related to the kidney's role in maintaining acid-base balance, that is, the excretion of excess acids and the conservation (reabsorption) of base, as bicarbonate ions.

The renal excretion of H^+ and the reabsorption of bicarbonate is depicted in Figure 6-4. Central to this mechanism is the enzyme *carbonic anhydrase (CA),* found in renal proximal and distal tubule cells and in red blood cells. CA rapidly hydrates dissolved CO_2 to form H_2CO_3, which dissociates to form H^+ and HCO_3^-. The H^+ is secreted in exchange for a sodium ion (Na^+), and Na^+ and bicarbonate together are taken up into plasma. The excreted H^+ can react non-enzymatically with bicarbonate in the glomerular filtrate (now modified and termed the presumptive urine) to form CO_2, which can enter the tubular cell and form more bicarbonate by the carbonic anhydrase reaction.

The net result of the processes in the proximal convoluted tubule is the absorption of 80% of the glomerular filtrate. Because solutes and water are reabsorbed in equal proportions, there is no concentration of the tubular fluid at this point and it is still iso-osmolar with plasma.

Loop of Henle

The function of the descending and ascending segments of the loop of Henle is to reduce the volume of the presumptive urine in the tubule and to continue to recover additional sodium and chloride. As the descending, or concentrating, segments pass into the medulla, the interstitial fluid outside the tubules becomes increasingly hypertonic as a result of increased concentrations of sodium, chloride, and urea. The descending segment is freely permeable to

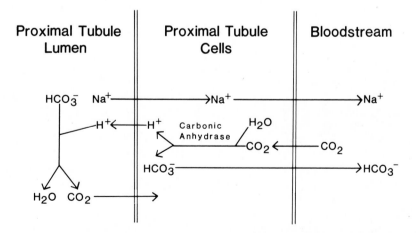

Fig. 6-4 Kidney reabsorption of bicarbonate with excretion of H^-. *From Sherwin JE and Bruegger BB: Acid-base control and acid-base disorders. In Kaplan LA and Pesce AJ: Clinical chemistry: theory, analysis, and correlation, ed 2, St Louis, 1989, Mosby-Year Book, Inc.*

Table 6-2 Composition of body compartments

	Plasma (mEq/L)	Plasma water (mEq/L)	Interstitial fluid (mEq/L H₂O)	Intracellular water (mEq/L H₂O)
Cations	153	164.6	153	195
Na$^+$	142	152.7	145	10
K$^+$	4	4.3	4	156
Ca^{++}	5	5.4	(2-3)	3.2
Mg^{++}	2	2.2	(1-2)	26
Anions	153	164.6	153	195
Cl$^-$	103	110.8	116	2
HCO$_3^-$	28	30.1	31	8
Protein	17	18.3	—	55
Others (HPO$_4^{-2}$, HSO$_4^-$)	5	5.4	(6)	130
Osmolarity (mOsm/L)		296	294.6	294.6
Theoretical osmotic pressure (mm Hg)		5712.8	5685.8	5685.8

From Kaplan LA and Pesce AJ: Clinical chemistry: Theory, analysis, and correlation, ed 2, St. Louis, 1989, Mosby-Year Book, Inc.

water but not to solutes. As the segment passes farther into the medulla, water increasingly and passively moves from the loop into the interstitium, concentrating the presumptive urine remaining in the tubule. The water released into the interstitium does not remain there, but is absorbed by the blood vessels passing from the medulla back into the cortex, in a counter or reverse direction to that of the descending limb. Thus, this mechanism for concentrating the urine is called the *counter-current mechanism*.

The lower, thick portion of the ascending, or diluting, segment of the loop of Henle has the ability to actively secrete sodium and chloride, but prevent water loss. Thus, the concentrated presumptive urine steadily loses sodium and chloride as it passes through the ascending portion of the loop of Henle, becoming progressively more dilute until, by the time it enters the distal convoluted tubule, it is either hypertonic or isotonic compared to plasma.

Distal convoluted tubule

This segment of the nephron has two major functions. Sodium is reabsorbed, for the last time, thus maintaining water and electrolyte balance, and excess body acid is removed.

Sodium is actively reabsorbed along with some bicarbonate in this portion of the tubule. The primary mechanism for sodium reabsorption, however, is by the sodium/potassium pump. This pump is under the hormonal control of *aldosterone*. Aldosterone is released from the adrenal medulla in response to angiotensin II, which is one of the products of the renin response to hypotension or low plasma sodium. Aldosterone stimulates the sodium/potassium pump to *actively* absorb sodium from the presumptive urine in exchange for potassium excreted by tubular cells. The net result is an increase in plasma sodium and water with a decrease in body potassium levels. The increase in the plasma concentration of sodium and water results in an expanded plasma volume and increased blood pressure. Aldosterone also acts on the collecting ducts, sweat glands, and the large intestines to conserve body sodium and water.

An interesting, potentially life-threatening side-effect of the sodium/potassium exchange can occur when a patient is receiving certain diuretic medications for hypertension. The goal of many diuretic medications is to decrease blood pressure by reducing blood volume. This, in turn, can be achieved by increasing the elimination of sodium and accompanying water. In fact, this is the opposite of the effect of the renin-aldosterone axis. There are two types of diuretics commonly used; the "loop-acting" and the distal tubule acting diuretics. The loop diuretics act by inhibiting sodium excretion in the ascending segment, while the distal tubule diuretics, for example, spiralactone, inhibit the action of aldosterone. When a loop diuretic is used alone to prevent sodium reabsorption, a larger than normal amount of sodium enters the distal tubule resulting in increased action by the sodium/potassium pump. Although excess sodium is still excreted in the urine, an unwanted side effect is often a severe reduction in body potassium levels. To prevent life-threatening hypokalemia, that is, low blood potassium levels, patients receiving a loop diuretic also take potassium supplements or a spiralactone-type drug to inhibit the sodium/potassium pump in the distal tubule.

If the nephron is to excrete hydrogen ions, there must be salts available to neutralize the ions and buffer the urine. The primary buffer of urine is phosphate, the most prevalant extracellular inorganic ion (see Table 6-2). The lowest pH attainable by phosphate salts in urine is approximately pH 4.5. Below this pH harmful free acid is excreted. A mechanism does exist to excrete additional acid during a prolonged period of harsh acidosis. In these cases, the distal tubular cells convert glutamine into glutamic acid with a net release of ammonia (NH₃) into the presumptive urine:

in tubular cells: glutamine $\xrightarrow{\text{glutaminase}}$ glutamic acid + NH$_3$

in urine: NH$_3$ + H$_2$PO$_4^{-1}$ $\longrightarrow$ NH$_4^+$ + HPO$_4^{-2}$

The excreted NH₃ reacts with dihydrogen phosphate (H$_2$PO$_4^-$) to form NH$_4^+$, thus allowing the monohydrogen phosphate (HPO$_4^{-2}$) that is formed to buffer additional hydrogen ions excreted from the tubular cell. The net result is the excretion of the acid cation NH$_4^+$. The distal tubule also actively excretes uric acid and small amounts of creatinine.

Collecting ducts

The isotonic fluid leaving the distal tubule enters the collecting ducts. The collecting ducts, like the descending segment of the loop of Henle, pass through the renal cortex down through the increasingly hypertonic layers of the medulla. Although the collecting ducts are also permeable to water, their permeability is not passive, as in the descending loop of Henle, but under the control of the antidiuretic hormone (ADH, or vasopressin). This hormone, produced by the pituitary gland in response to increased plasma osmolality, increases the water permeability of the collecting duct and the distal tubule and prevents an excretion, or diuresis, of excess water. In the absence of ADH, a diuresis occurs and the kidney produces a more dilute urine. In the presence of ADH, water is retained by the body and a more concentrated urine is produced. Thus, the final concentration of urine occurs in the collecting ducts.

The fluid leaving the collecting ducts and entering the ureter is now called urine. The urine is stored in the bladder before being excreted from the body during micturation, or urination.

ELECTROLYTE AND WATER BALANCE
Body electrolyte composition

Figure 6-5 describes the body water compartments while Table 6-2 lists the major cations and anions found in these three major compartments. Sodium and chloride are, respectively, the primary cation and anion of extracellular fluids, while potassium and phosphate are, respectively, the primary intracellular cation and anion. The extracellular compartment accounts for approximately 20% of an adult's body weight, but it is approximately 45% of a newborn's body weight. Plasma, the only body fluid easily sampled

and analyzed, represents only 5% of the body's weight and only about one-quarter of the extracellular water compartment. *Interstitial* fluid is essentially a protein-free filtrate of plasma and is the fluid that directly bathes all tissue cells.

The sum of the concentrations of all cations must equal the concentration of all anions in serum in order to maintain electrical neutrality. However, most laboratories routinely analyze only sodium, potassium, chloride, and bicarbonate. The difference between the measured cations, sodium plus potassium, and the measured anions, chloride plus bicarbonate, does not equal zero but averages between 10 and 20 mmol/L in serum or plasma. This difference is called the *anion gap* and is equal to the concentration of the anions not measured. Although the anion gap is only a calculated result and not a measured analyte, it can be a useful indication of clinical or laboratory problems. Increased anion gaps are usually associated with metabolic acidoses such as diabetic ketoacidosis (see Chapter 7), while decreased anion gaps are most often the result of errors in analysis (usually chloride). Less frequently, decreased anion gaps may be seen in cases of hypoalbuminemia and hypergammaglobulinemia.

Regulation of body fluid volume and osmolality

Body water homeostasis is maintained by balancing the loss of body water with sufficient water intake. Table 6-3 demonstrates the primary routes of water losses and sources of body water. Note that while most of the routes of water

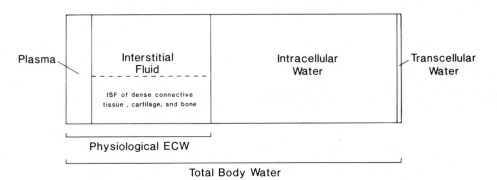

Fig. 6-5 Body water compartments. Note that anatomical extracellular water *(ECW)* includes physiological extracellular water and transcellular water. *ISF,* Interstitial fluid. Numbers in parenthesis indicate approximate percentage of total body weight for each compartment. *From Kleinman LI and Lorenz JM: Physiology and pathophysiology of body water and electrolytes. In Kaplan LA and Pesce AJ: Clinical chemistry: theory, analysis, and correlation, ed 2, St Louis, 1989, Mosby-Year Book, Inc.*

Table 6-3 Water balance in average adult under various conditions

	Intake (ml/day)				Output (ml/day)		
	Normal	Hot environment	Strenuous work		Normal	Hot environment	Strenuous work
Drinking water	1200	2200	3400	Urine	1400	1200	500
Water from food	1000	1000	1150	Insensible water			
Water of oxidation	300	300	450	Skin	400	400	400
				Lungs	400	300	600
				Sweat	100	1400	3300
				Stool	200	200	200
Total	2500	3500	5000	Total	2500	3500	5000

From Kaplan LA and Pesce AJ: Clinical chemistry: Theory, analysis, and correlation, ed 2, St. Louis, 1989, Mosby-Year Book, Inc.

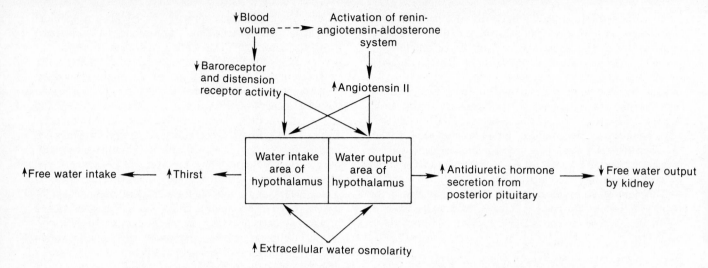

Fig. 6-6 Hypothalamic regulation of water balance. *From Kleinman LI and Lorenz JM: Physiology and pathophysiology of body water and electrolytes. In Kaplan LA and Pesce AJ: Clinical chemistry: theory, analysis, and correlation, ed 2, St Louis, 1989, Mosby-Year Book, Inc.*

input and output are relatively constant, the kidney can change its concentrating ability by approximately three-fold in response to losses of water by other routes. The kidney plays a central role in the maintenance of the electrolyte concentration of the body by its ability to retain or excrete electrolytes and water. Water balance and extracellular osmolality is controlled by regulating water intake (thirst response) and renal excretion of water.

The hypothalamus plays a key role in controlling both water intake and water loss. The hypothalamic water input center contains specialized neurons that are sensitive to extracellular osmolality. As the extracellular osmolality increases, these hypothalamic nerves respond by producing a conscious feeling of thirst, which stimulates body water intake. Baro- (pressure) receptors in the atria of the heart and other areas of the body also sense changes in blood volume and blood pressure and stimulate the water output center of the hypothalamus, which results in the release of ADH from the posterior pituitary. ADH acts to increase retention of water by the kidney. Thus, control of the hypothalamic water input and output areas can cause an increase in body water content by increasing water input and decreasing water output. This restores extracellular osmolality and plasma blood pressure to normal. A decrease in extracellular osmolality or an increase in blood volume or pressure causes the opposite changes to occur in order to reduce the body's water load and restore these parameters to normal.

The other mechanism for regulating body fluids is the renin-angiotensin-aldosterone system described previously. Whereas the hypothalamic-ADH mechanism controls renal water conservation, the renin system controls renal sodium conservation in order to maintain a constant extracellular water volume. Both of these control mechanisms maintain the body's fluid and electrolytes within reasonably narrow limits when the body is subject to stress such as extreme heat, strenuous exercise, or excessive or insufficient salt or water intake that can cause increased losses of water and electrolytes. Figure 6-6 shows the interrelationships between the kidney and the hypothalamic thirst-control center in maintaining electrolyte and water balance.

RENAL DISEASES AND ELECTROLYTE DISORDERS

Renal disease can result from a dysfunction of the glomerulus, the proximal and distal tubules, the collecting duct and ureter, or the entire organ including the parenchymal cells. Many of these diseases can occur either singularly or in combination with other diseases.

Disorders of the kidney
Glomerular dysfunction

There are two basic types of disease entities resulting from glomerular dysfunction: *glomerular nephritis* and the *nephrotic syndrome*. Glomerular nephritis is caused by an acute inflammatory attack on the glomerular basement membrane. This inflammation can be secondary to deposits of immunoglobulin complexes or hypertension. The filtering ability of the glomerulus is compromised as a result of the nephritis and there is decreased glomerular filtration rate and decreased urine formation, or *oliguria,* or no urine formation, *anuria.* The decreased renal function results in an increase in blood concentrations of waste products such as urea, creatinine, and hydrogen ions. As a result of the inflammatory attack on the glomerulus, there is also increased leakage of red blood cells (hematuria) and protein (proteinuria) into the urine. The presence of red blood cell casts is an important finding associated with glomerular nephritis.

The nephrotic syndrome can result from a variety of causes including infectious agents, toxins and allergens, and immunological destruction of glomerulii secondary to other diseases (e.g., cancer, diabetes). The nephrotic syndrome is defined clinically by a massive protein loss into urine (greater than 5 Gm/d) with edema, that is, the transfer of water from intracellular to extracellular spaces; hypoalbuminemia, hyperlipidemia, and lipiduria. Most of these clinical signs are the result of the increased glomerular permeability, resulting in the loss of lipoprotein and serum albumin in the urine.

Tubular disease

Defects in tubular function result in a reduced ability of the tubules to excrete or reabsorb specific biochemicals. This, in turn, can lead to an inability to produce concentrated or dilute urine and affect electrolyte and acid-base balance. Renal *tubular proteinuria* is the result of an inability of the proximal tubule to reabsorb small amounts of low molecular weight proteins normally filtered through the glomerulus. This can result from genetic abnormalities or tubular damage.

Renal tubular acidosis can be caused by defects in either the proximal or distal tubules. *Proximal tubular acidosis* is caused by an inability of these tubules to reabsorb bicarbonate. Instead of absorbing bicarbonate, chloride is reabsorbed leading to a hyperchloremic acidosis. A tubular acidosis is associated with *Fanconi's syndrome* in which defects in proximal tubular absorption of analytes lead to losses of glucose, amino acids, phosphate, and protein along with a metabolic acidosis. The inability of the proximal tubules to reabsorb filtered protein can result in a tubular proteinuria of approximately 2 Gm/d.

Distal tubular acidosis is often associated with an inability of the distal tubules to excrete hydrogen ions, potassium or uric acid leading to hyperkalemia and hyperuricemia. The unabsorbed HCO_3^- is excreted, leading to an alkaline urine (pH > 7.0) even though a metabolic acidosis is often present.

Urinary tract infection

Urinary tract infections can occur in the bladder or the kidney. When the infection occurs in the kidney, this is termed *pyelonephritis*. A urinary tract infection is noted by an increase in white blood cells in the urine and by an increase in leukocyte esterase activity in the urine.

Renal vascular disease

Renal vascular disease can result in loss of renal function. Certainly the microvascular changes associated with diabetes and long-standing hypertension can result in damage to the glomerulus and tubules, leading to progressive renal failure. Approximately 25% to 30% of end-stage renal patients are diabetics, usually insulin-dependent, and renal failure is a leading cause of deaths among insulin-dependent diabetics. Occlusive disease of the small blood vessels of the kidney can result in an increase in plasma renin concentration, which is a cause of secondary hypertension. Occlusion of larger veins in the kidney can lead to renal failure.

Acute and chronic renal failure

Acute renal failure (ARF) occurs when there is an abrupt cessation of renal function. Acute renal failure can be caused by:
1. Prerenal causes: cardiovascular failure, hypovolemia
2. Renal causes: acute tubular necrosis from toxins, glomerular nephritis, vascular obstruction
3. Postrenal causes: rupture of bladder, obstruction of lower urinary tract

Chronic renal failure (CRF) is the result of long-standing, gradually progressing renal disease seen often in people with hypertension; diabetes; chronic inflammatory diseases; chronic exposure to poisons (e.g., cadmium); chronic obstructive disease; and inflammatory diseases of the kidney. In early CRF, when the GFR is still >25 ml/min (~25% of normal), most patients show few symptoms and have few biochemical abnormalities. As chronic renal failure progresses to a GFR below 25 ml/min, many of the regulatory processes become affected, resulting in electrolyte and acid-base disturbances and other biochemical abnormalities. In addition, the kidney loses its hormonal functions. Decreased production of erythropoietin results in an anemia, while decreased vitamin D synthesis can result in secondary hyperparathyroidism, loss of bone calcium, and eventually renal rickets. Chronic renal failure is associated with increased morbidity and mortality. If the blood levels of toxic wastes, that is, acids and other materials like phosphate and urea, become too great, the patient must be *dialyzed* to remove these waste products. Long-term treatment of patients with chronic renal failure with aluminum-containing phosphate binders can result in aluminum toxicity. The only permanent treatment for irreversible chronic renal failure is a renal transplant and life-long treatment with an immunosuppressive reagent such as cyclosporine.

Change of analyte with disease

The relationship between various clinical signs and symptoms, urine analyte concentrations, and plasma analyte changes and the various types of pathological conditions affecting the kidney are summarized in Table 6-4. Many of the biochemical changes and clinical symptoms become readily apparent when the GFR decreases below 25 ml/min. Important analyte changes are discussed as follows:

Nitrogenous compounds. In general, one does not see significant changes in serum BUN or creatinine concentrations until approximately half the glomerular function is lost. However, there is a correlation between the increase in serum concentrations of urea (BUN), creatinine, and uric acid and the loss of renal function. The ratio of serum BUN to creatinine concentrations can be used to predict the nature of acute renal failure. With most renal diseases, the ratio is similar to that normally seen, approximately 10:1 to 20:1. If the cause of renal failure has an extra-renal origin (e.g., cardiac insufficiency, hypovolemia resulting from bleeding, or excessive protein intake with borderline renal function), the ratio is often greater than 20:1. Borderline elevated BUN concentrations can be seen in individuals who consume large amounts of protein. Low concentrations of serum urea can be seen in severe liver disease and with low dietary protein intake. Because changes of the serum creatinine levels are not dependent on diet, as are changes in BUN levels, serum creatinine is a more specific indicator of renal dysfunction. However, serum urea concentrations change faster than plasma creatinine concentrations with renal disease, and thus changes in serum urea concentration can indicate renal dysfunction earlier than changes in serum creatinine levels.

Table 6-4 Association of pathological conditions affecting the kidney and clinical and biochemical abnormalities*

	AGN	NS	TD	UTI	HT	RVT	DM	UTO	RC	ARF	CRF
Hypertension	++	+	0	0	++	±	±	0	0	+	+
Edema	+	++	0	0	0	+	+	0	0	+	+
Oliguria or anuria	+	±	0	0	0	±	0	+	0	+	+
Polyuria	0	0	+	0	0	0	+	0	0	0	0
Nocturia	0	±	+	±	0	0	+	±	0	0	+
Frequency	0	0	0	+	0	0	0	±	±	0	0
Loin pain	0	0	0	+	0	+	0	+	+	0	0
Anemia	+	0	0	0	0	0	0	0	0	0	++
↑ Blood urea nitrogen	+	0	0	0	±	±	±	±	0	+	+
↑ Serum creatinine	+	–	–	–	±	±	±	±	0	+	+
↓ GFR	+	0	0	0	±	±	±	±	0	+	+
↑ Serum potassium	±	±	0	0	0	0	0	0	0	+	+
↑ Serum phosphorus	±	0	0	0	0	0	0	0	0	+	+
↓ Serum calcium	0	+	0	0	0	0	0	0	0	+	+
↑ Serum uric acid	0	0	+	0	±	0	±	0	±	+	+
Acidosis	0	0	+	0	0	0	0	0	0	+	+
Proteinuria	+	++++	+	±	±	++	+	0	0	±	±
Hematuria	++	+	±	+	0	+	0	0	++	+	±
RBC casts	+	0	0	0	0	0	0	0	0	±	0
Pyuria	±	0	0	++	0	0	0	±	±	0	0
WBC casts	0	0	0	+	0	0	0	+	0	0	0
Glucosuria	0	0	+	0	0	0	++	0	0	0	0

From Kaplan LA and Pesce AJ: Clinical chemistry: Theory, analysis, and correlation, ed 2, St. Louis, 1989, Mosby-Year Book, Inc.
*AGN, Acute glomerulonephritis; ARF, acute renal failure; CRF, chronic renal failure; DM, diabetes mellitus; HT, hypertension; NS, nephrotic syndrome; RC, renal calculi; RVT, renal vein thrombosis; TD, tubular disease; UTI, urinary tract infection; UTO, urinary tract obstruction. 0 = absent; ± = variable; + = present. RBC, red blood cell; WBC, white blood cell.

Uric acid levels do not become abnormally elevated until the GFR drops below 20 ml/min, about one-fifth of normal. Thus, uric acid levels are not very sensitive to changes in GFR.

Protein. Renal protein losses into urine can be the result of either *glomerular proteinuria* or *tubular proteinuria*. In glomerular proteinuria, large as well as small protein molecules are lost in urine because of increased glomerular permeability. Such losses can range from >2 Gm/d to the >5 Gm/d seen in the *nephrotic syndrome*. Tubular proteinuria, caused by an inability of the proximal tubule to reabsorb the normally small amounts of filtered protein, can result in losses in urine of no more than 1 to 3 Gm/d of low molecular weight proteins.

Small, but abnormal levels of proteinuria may, in some clinical situations, be predictive of impending chronic renal disease. For example, approximately one-third of insulin-dependent diabetics are at an increased risk for developing end-stage renal failure. Measurement of low levels of proteinuria has been advocated to detect loss of renal function earlier in these patients. Usually albumin or beta$_2$-microglobulin are the proteins measured. The very low levels of albumin that might be indicative of early glomerular proteinuria (*microalbuminuria*, 30-300 mg/dL) require sensitive immunoassays.

Tubular proteinuria is often detected by measuring low molecular weight proteins, such as beta$_2$-microglobulin, acid alpha$_1$-glycoprotein, or retinol-binding protein, in urine. Beta$_2$-microglobulin is an 11,000 dalton protein, normally present in urine at less than 300 ug/L. Sensitive immunoassays are employed for these assays.

Losses of protein in urine will not affect serum total protein concentrations unless there are massive losses of protein, as seen in the nephrotic syndrome. Then, a hypoalbuminemia can occur which results in loss of plasma oncotic pressure and a shift of water from the plasma compartment to the interstitial fluid compartment resulting in edema. As an attempt to correct the hypoproteinemia, the liver produces excess lipoprotein, resulting in a hyperlipoproteinemia with increases in VLDL and LDL lipoproteins.

Hemoglobin and hematocrit. In advanced chronic renal failure, a decreased hemoglobin and hematocrit is commonly observed, probably as a result of the decreased renal synthesis of erythropoietin. This is usually seen when the GFR falls below 25 ml/min and the BUN increases to 60 to 80 mg/dL. The hematocrit can fall to approximately 18 to 20%. The resulting normochronic, normocytic anemia rarely requires transfusions and usually responds to chronic hemodialysis treatment. Chronic anemia of renal failure can now also be treated with preparation of a properly glycosylated human erythropoietin produced by recombinant DNA techniques.

Calcium and phosphate. Advanced chronic renal failure results in a hyperphosphatemia and a decreased formation of 1,25 dihydroxy vitamin D$_3$. Decreased vitamin D$_3$ synthesis in turn causes a decrease in absorption of calcium from the intestines, resulting in hypocalcemia. The hypocalcemia results in a secondary hyperparathyroidism as the body attempts to raise the plasma calcium levels. The hyperphosphatemia is usually treated with phosphate binders, usually aluminum hydroxide antacids that bind phosphate in the gastrointestinal tract.

Acid-base changes associated with renal failure. Acute renal failure is associated with a metabolic acidosis because of a general inability to excrete fixed acids. As outlined previously, proximal tubular disease can result in a tubular acidosis. The changes in concentration of several blood analytes in the acidosis of severe renal failure are typical of most metabolic acidoses: low pH, low bicarbonate, low PCO_2 as part of a respiratory compensation, and an increased anion gap. Chronic renal failure is usually associated with a mild acidosis and the blood pH is rarely below 7.35. However, with progressive loss of renal function, there is usually a reduced ability to excrete ammonia. Because renal failure may affect the ability of the distal tubules to excrete potassium, and because an acidosis may cause displacement of potassium in cells by H^+, an acidosis associated with renal failure is usually accompanied by hyperkalcemia.

Water and electrolyte changes associated with renal failure. An adequate glomerular filtration rate (GFR) allows the kidney to concentrate urine to a level that is three to four times greater than that of serum, that is, approximately an osmolality of 1,200 mOsm/kg (specific gravity, 1.032). One of the first losses of a progressively diseased kidney is its ability to form a concentrated urine. The urine becomes more dilute, finally falling to a level of < 100 mOsm/kg (specific gravity, 1.005). In order to excrete the same amount of solids, a larger urine volume must be produced. This is usually manifested clinically by nocturia (increased frequency of urination during sleeping hours) and polyuria (increased urine volume). A very dilute urine is also produced in *diabetes insipidus,* a disease resulting from an inadequate production of ADH or from cells that have become unresponsive to normal levels of ADH. In these cases, the cells of the proximal tubule and collecting ducts become impervious to water, and large amounts of urine are produced. The urine that forms in these conditions can have an osmolality below 50 mOsm/kg and a specific gravity < 1.005.

The kidney's ability to produce a dilute urine when faced with a water load is another function that is lost in a diseased kidney. An inability to produce a urine with an osmolality < 100 mOsm/kg in the presence of a water load can be indicative of renal disease.

As renal disease progresses and the glomerular filtration rate decreases, the kidney also loses its ability to excrete the excess water needed to excrete solute. The urine volume becomes reduced until finally no urine is produced. A hyponatremic, hypo-osmolar state can result from the excess of retained water.

Disorders of water and electrolyte balance
Dehydration

Although the simplest definition of "dehydration" is lack of water, physiologically dehydration can be caused by a deficit of water, a deficit of sodium, or a combination of the two deficits. *Simple dehydration* caused by insufficient replacement of obligatory water losses (see Table 6-3), is a deficit of water relative to a normal amount of body sodium. Simple dehydration, associated with *hypernatremia* and hyperosmolality, can be caused by food and water deprivation, excessive sweating, and diuretic therapy.

If water losses equal the loss of sodium from the body, then the osmolality of body fluids remains normal as does the serum sodium concentration. This is known as *normonatremic* or *iso-osmolar dehydration.* However, the total

body sodium and water contents are decreased and the plasma volume is also decreased. Normonatremic dehydration can be seen with excessive vomiting or diarrhea and when lost fluids are replaced with liquids low in sodium.

If sodium losses exceed water losses from the body, then the extracellular osmolality decreases resulting in a *hyponatremic, hypoosmolar dehydration.* In this type of dehydration, water shifts from extracellular fluid (plasma) into cells, resulting in edema. Hyponatremia dehydration may be associated with diuretic therapy, excessive sweating, and adrenocortical insufficiency. Table 6-5 summarizes the water and sodium changes seen in various types of dehydration. In all cases of dehydration a sensation of thirst is associated with dry mucus membranes, decreased urine output, increased hematocrit, increased BUN, and, if the dehydration is the result of kidney failure, an inability to conserve water and a decreased urine osmolality. Depending on the severity of the dehydration, there may also be an accompanying weakness, hypotension, renal failure, and shock.

Overhydration

Whereas dehydration is defined as a water deficit, overhydration can occur when there is an excess of body water content. The retained body water is usually associated with an increase in total body sodium. However, if the retained water exceeds the retained sodium, the extracellular water compartment's osmolality decreases and hyponatremia results. This is called *dilutional hyponatremia* or *water intoxication.* The excess water in the extracellular compartment moves into cells resulting in edema. If the serum sodium concentration falls below 125 mEq/L, nausea, vomiting, seizures, and coma may also occur. Causes of water intoxication include psychiatric disorders, injury to the anterior hypothalamus, ectopic secretion of ADH from a cancer, and hypothyroidism.

Water and sodium may be equally retained in congestive heart failure, oliguric renal failure, nephrotic syndrome, cirrhosis, and primary hyperaldosteronism. The excess body water may be associated with normal or lower body sodium concentration resulting in a normonatremic or hyponatremic condition.

Change of analyte with disease

Hypo- and hypernatremia can be caused by a number of clinical conditions such as renal disease, liver disease, heart failure, diabetes, inappropriate (iatrogenic) treatment with fluids and electrolytes, gastrointestinal diseases, burns, and adrenal insufficiency (Table 6-5). Note that clinical conditions of hypo- or hypernatremia may be associated with either increased or decreased body levels of sodium.

Hypokalemia (low serum potassium levels) can have a renal origin in patients treated with diuretics without sufficient supplementation with potassium. Prolonged treatment with corticosteroids may also result in a hypokalemia. Hyperkalemia may result from acute or chronic renal failure. As in the case of sodium, clinical conditions associated with hypo- or hyperkalemia may be associated with increased or decreased levels of total body potassium. Clinical conditions associated with hyperkalemia include acidosis, crush injuries, hypoxia, renal failure, while hypokalemia may be associated with alkalosis, diuretic therapy, and increased potassium loss from renal or gastrointestinal diseases.

RENAL FUNCTION TESTS AND ANALYTE MEASUREMENTS
Urine analysis

Microscopic and chemical determinations of urine constituents can provide extremely important information about renal function and the presence of disease states. If renal disease is suspected, bright-field microscopic examination of urine for cells, casts, crystals, bacteria, or parasitic organisms is a critical procedure. The microscopic examination should accompany a chemical examination of urine constituents. Semi-quantitative measurements of urine glucose, ketones, red blood cells, hemoglobin, white blood cells, nitrate, pH and specific gravity can be reproducibly performed by means of "dipsticks." Dipsticks are strips of plastic with individual pads containing reagent for the measurement of each of the above.

The presence of red cells in urine is indicative of glomerular nephritis while white blood cells in urine are indicative of pyelonephritis (See Tables 6-5 and 6-6.). The etiology of renal disease can be determined in part by finding abnormal results for glucose and ketones (diabetes) and protein.

A chemical dipstick analysis is commonly used as a screening test to identify urine samples that require microscopic analysis. If a dipstick screen is positive for protein, nitrate (bacteria), leukocyte esterase activity (bacteria), or red blood cells (hemoglobin), there is a greater probability that the urine will also have significant findings by microscopic analysis. On the other hand, a totally negative dipstick screen is usually associated with a negative microscopic analysis. Microscopic urinalysis is rarely needed in the absence of a suspicion of renal disease. Both chemical and microscopic analyses can be performed on randomly collected urines or on a 24-hour urine collection. The best sample for a random urine analysis is one obtained early in the morning when the urine constituents are most concentrated.

Creatinine clearance

Glomerular dysfunction can occur in many renal disorders. Thus, it is important to be able to assess glomerular function when diagnosing or monitoring renal disease. This can be accomplished by measuring the rate of *clearance* of a substance from plasma into urine. A clearance can be defined as the volume of plasma from which a measured amount of a substance is eliminated into a volume of urine per unit time. Since the clearance of many substances is also affected by tubular uptake and excretion rates, an accurate measure of glomerular filtration can only be determined if the clearance can be calculated for a substance which is not absorbed or excreted by the renal tubules to any appreciable extent. The substance routinely used to estimate the glomerular filtration rate is creatinine. Although there is some renal absorption and secretion of creatinine, creatinine clearance is routinely measured because of its close approximation to the true glomerular filtration rate, because of the relative ease of creatinine analysis, and because plasma levels of creatinine are essentially independent of diet. Thus, the amount of creatinine found in urine depends primarily on the functioning of the kidney, that is, glomerular filtration.

Signs and symptoms of renal disease are usually not apparent until approximately two-thirds of the glomerular filtration rate is lost. In addition, a slightly abnormal level of plasma creatinine may not reflect a true *increase* in the

Table 6-5   Changes in total body water volume and distribution, total body sodium content, and plasma sodium concentration with dehydration and overhydration

	Total body water	Extracellular water	Intracellular water	Total body sodium	Plasma sodium concentration
Dehydration					
Hypernatremic	↓	sl ↓	↓	nl or sl ↓	↑
Normonatremic	↓	↓	nl	↓	nl
Hyponatremia	↓	↓ ↓	↑	↓ ↓	↓
Overhydration					
Water intoxication	↑	↑	↑	nl	↓
Extracellular water volume expansion					
Normonatremic	↑	↑	nl	↑	nl
Hyponatremic	↑	↑	↑	sl ↑	↓

From Kaplan LA and Pesce AJ: Clinical chemistry: Theory, analysis, and correlation, ed 2, St. Louis, 1989, Mosby-Year Book, Inc.
nl, Normal; *sl,* slightly.

Table 6-6   Characteristic urine microscopic findings in renal disease

Condition	Protein	Red blood cells (per high-power field)	White blood cells (per high-power field)	Bacteria	Casts (per low-power field)
Normal	0-Trace	0-3	0-5	0	Hyaline, occasionally
Glomerulonephritis	1-2+	>20	0-10	0	Granular red blood cells
Nephrotic syndrome	4+	0-10	0-5	0	Oval fat bodies; hyaline
Pyelonephritis	0-1+	0-10	<30	+ +	Granular white blood cells

From Kaplan LA and Pesce AJ: Clinical chemistry: Theory, analysis, and correlation, ed 2, St. Louis, 1989, Mosby-Year Book, Inc.

plasma creatinine level as a result of renal disease. Thus, securing an accurate assessment of the glomerular filtration rate by measuring creatinine clearance can be important in the diagnosis of renal disease.

The most appropriate sample for creatinine clearance measurement is an accurately timed 24-hour urine sample. The patient is usually requested to empty the bladder at the beginning of the time period, discarding the urine, and then collecting all of the subsequent urine for the next 24 hours. A serum or plasma sample is usually drawn at the end of the 24-hour collection period.

The formula for calculating the creatinine clearance (CL) is as follows:

EQUATION 1A (GENERAL EQUATION):

$$CL(ml/min) = \frac{U}{P} \times Vu \times \frac{1}{T \times 60 \, min/hrs}$$

EQUATION 1B (EQUATION FOR 24-HOUR COLLECTION):

$$CL(ml/min) = \frac{U}{P} \times \frac{Vu}{1440 \, min}$$

where U and P, respectively, are the creatinine concentrations in urine and plasma samples expressed as mg/dL respectively, Vu is the volume in ml of the urine and T is the time of collection in hours. For a 24-hour collection, this reduces to equation 1B where 1,440 minutes is the number of minutes in a 24-hour time period. Because plasma creatinine levels are related to an individual's muscle mass, creatinine clearance reference ranges are gender dependent. Males have creatinine clearances from 97 to 137 ml/min, while females have creatinine clearances ranging from 88 to 128 ml/min. The 24-hour creatinine clearance can be normalized to a body surface area of 1.73 m^2 as shown in equation 1C, where A is the surface area in square meters. The reference range for normalized creatinine clearance is 90 to 120 ml/min. Nomograms connecting a patient's height and weight to body surface are available for both adults and children.

EQUATION 1C:

$$CL(ml/min) = \frac{U}{P} \times \frac{Vu}{1440} \times \frac{1.73}{A} \, m^2$$

Concentration and dilution studies

To assess the kidney's ability to produce a concentrated urine, a patient is deprived of any fluid intake for 15 hours. Dehydration will normally stimulate the production of ADH to produce a concentrated urine. Urine is then collected hourly for the next three hours. If the kidney's concentrating power is normal, the urine's osmolality should be at least three times that of plasma or approximately greater than 850 mOsmol/L. The specific gravity of the urine should be greater than 1.025. Significantly lower values are indicative of renal disease.

To test the urinary diluting capacity of the kidney, the following procedure is used. The patient empties the bladder and is given 1000 to 1200 ml of water. Urine specimens are then collected every hour for the next four hours. Under these circumstances, the urinary specific gravity should fall to 1.005 or less or have an osmolality of less than 100

mOsm/kg. In patients with chronic renal disease who are unable to dilute the urine, there may be a danger of fluid overload with this test and proper precautions should be taken.

Measurement of analytes (see Table 6-7)
Electrolytes (Na, K, Cl)

Sodium and *potassium* can be accurately and precisely measured by ion-selective electrodes (ISE). Automated ISE analysis can be accomplished by direct analysis of whole blood, serum, or plasma or following an approximately 35-fold dilution of the sample with buffer.

Dilutional ISE measurements yield results for sodium and potassium that are slightly lower than those obtained for non-dilutional ISE analysis since ISE's measure the amount of electrolyte present in the water portion of the sample only. Plasma or serum is approximately 93.5% water, 5.4% protein, 0.6% lipid, and 0.9% other molecules. Sodium and potassium ions are present in the water fraction. However, when the sample is diluted, the final concentration of analyte in the sample is calculated based on the analysis of the diluted sample and the calculation may not take into account the fact that the analyte was not present in the entire sample volume. Thus, sodium and potassium concentrations of serum or plasma may be 7% lower when measured by dilutional ISE's than when measured by direct, non-dilutional ISE measurements. The directly measured ISE analyses are probably closer to the true physiological levels of sodium and potassium.

Many instrument manufacturers adjust the calibration of non-dilutional ISE instruments so that the analyses of most samples yield results that match the lower results of dilutional ISE's. However, any pathological processes that change the fraction of water in samples can affect the measurement of sodium and potassium when measured by dilutional ISE but not when measured by direct, non-dilutional ISE's. This can be seen in cases of significant increases in serum protein or lipid levels. In these cases water is displaced by protein and lipid causing the fraction of water per volume of sample to be decreased. As a result, the sodium levels appear to be greatly decreased when measured by dilutional ISE's. This is called *pseudo-hyponatremia*. The term "pseudo" is used since the low sodium that is measured is not a real value but is an artifactual result. A very low serum sodium level (< 120 mmol/L) should alert a technologist to the possibility of pseudo-hypernatremia. The sample should then be checked for interferences. This can be achieved by simply looking at the specimen and checking for the abnormal turbidity of a hyperlipemic sample, or by measuring the sample's protein level.

Changes in the volume fraction of water can affect the measurement of other analytes measured in diluted samples, but the effect is not as striking as that seen in the case of sodium. Other analytes usually have much wider reference ranges than sodium. For example, sodium has a reference range of approximately 135 to 145 mmol/L, representing a 7% change in concentration while the reference range for potassium shows an approximately 33% change in concentration (3.6 to 5.0 mmol/L). A 10% decrease in the apparent sodium concentration because of water displacement will result in a sodium level of 135 mmol/L being measured as

Table 6-7 Methods of analysis

Analyte	Most frequently used methods	Advantages	Disadvantages
Sodium	Ion-selective electrode:		
	Dilutional —	Smaller sample volume	Negative error with decreasing water fraction in sample
	Non-dilutional —	Can perform measurement on whole blood	Larger sample volume
Potassium	Ion selective electrode:		
	Dilutional —	Smaller sample volume	Small neg. error with decreasing water fraction in sample
	Non-dilutional —	Can perform measurement on whole blood	Larger sample volume
Chloride	Ion selective electrode:		
	Dilutional —	Smaller sample volume	Small neg. error with decreasing water fraction in sample
	Non-dilutional —	Can perform measurement on whole body	Larger sample volume
			Largest positive interference by Br and I for both types
	Mercuric thiocynate	Easily automated	Negative interference by lipemia, positive interference by Br and I
	Coulometric	Can measure Cl in other body fluids, larger range of linearity, minimal interference from Br and I	Not automated, slow
Creatinine	Alkaline picrate, end-point	Readily automated	Interferences by hemoglobin, bilirubin, and ketones
	Alkaline picrate, kinetic	Readily automated	Negative interference by bilirubin and hemoglobin; positive interference by ketones and cephalosporins
	Enzymatic	Might be most specific method	
Urea	Urease/GLDH	Readily automated to add most instruments	Fl^- inhibits urease
	Urease/Conductivity	Readily automated	Fl^- inhibits urease
	Urease/Dye	Readily automated	Fl^- inhibits urease
Osmolality	Freezing point depression	Relatively rugged, precise instruments	Relatively large sample volume
	Vapor point depression	Smallest sample volume	Relatively imprecise, delicate instruments

The advantages and disadvantages listed in this table may not apply to every instrument and reagent combination, but are general concerns for the listed method.

121 mmol/L, while a potassium level of 3.5 mmol/L would only decrease to 3.1 mmol/L. The sodium value of 121 mmol/L is much more significantly abnormal than is the potassium value of 3.1 mmol/L.

Analysis of sodium and potassium by ISE has few chemical interferences. The selectivity of the sodium electrode is 1000 times greater for sodium than for potassium, while the selectivity ratio of potassium to sodium for the potassium ion selective electrode is approximately 10^5. If ammonium heparin is used as an anticoagulant, the ammonium ions will result in a positive interference in potassium measurements.

Serum *chloride* is most frequently measured by ion selective electrodes. The chloride ISE's are usually very accurate, although their reliability may not be as great as the ISE's for sodium and potassium. The next most frequently used automated method for serum chloride analysis is the mercuric thiocyanate method. In this procedure, chloride reacts with mercuric thiocyanate to form mercuric chloride and thiocyanate (SCN^-). The free thiocyanate ions react with ferric ions to form ferric thiocyanate. The intensity of the red-color at 525 nm of the ferric thiocyanate is proportional to the chloride concentration.

$$2Cl^- + Hg(SCN)_2 \longrightarrow HgCl_2 + 2SCN^-$$
$$Fe^{+3} + 3SCN^- \longrightarrow Fe(SCN)_3$$
$$\text{red}(A_{525})$$

Chloride in other fluids, especially urine, can be measured by the coulometric titration method. In this procedure, the sample is diluted into an acidic solution. A silver generating electrode produces free silver ions that immediately react with chloride ions to produce insoluble silver chloride. When all the chloride ions are consumed, excess silver ions appear in the reaction mixture. These are quickly detected by a silver ion-sensing electrode. Since the silver ions are generated at a constant rate, the time required to titrate all the chloride ions is directly proportional to the chloride concentration.

All three methods for chloride analysis have positive interferences from bromide and iodide ions. However,

Table 6-8 Reference ranges of analytes used to assess renal function and electrolyte status

Analyte	Sample	Method	Reference range
Blood gases (See Chapter 7.)			
Carbon dioxide, Total	S	Enzymatic	24-32 mmol/L
Chloride	S	Mercuric thiocynate	101-111 mmol/L
	U		110-150 mmol/24 hrs
Creatinine			
	S	Alkaline picrate	0.64-1.04 mg/dL (Male)
			0.57-0.92 mg/dL (Female)
	U		1.0-2.0 g/24 hrs (Male)
			0.8-1.8 g/24 hrs (Female)
		Creatinine clearance—adjusted for surface area	97-137 ml/min (Male)
			88-128 ml/min (Female)
Osmolality	S	Freezing point depression	282-300 mOsm/kg
	U		50-1200 mOsm/kg
Potassium	S	Dilutional ISE	3.6-5.0 mmol/L
	U		2.5-125 mmol/24 hrs
Protein, total	S	Biuret	6.6-6.8 g/dL
	U	TCA, turbidimetric	<150 mg/24 hrs
Sodium	S	Dilutional ISE	135-145 mmol/L
	U		40-220 mmol/24 hrs
Urea	S	Urease-glutamate dehydrogenase	5−.17 mg urea nitrogen/dL
	U		7-16 g urea nitrogen/24 hr

S = Serum; U = Urine; TCA = Trichloroacetic acid; ISE = Ion selective electrode

bromide and chloride do not react equivalently on all analytical systems. Bromide ions show a reactivity equivalent to 2.3 chloride ions with some ion selective electrodes but an equivalency to 1.6 chloride ions with the mercuric thiocyanate method, and an equivalency of 1:1 with the coulometric titration method. The thiocyanate method also has a positive interference from lipemia (triglycerides > 600 mg/dL).

Creatinine

Creatinine is usually quantitated by measuring the red complex (absorbance between 510 and 520 nm) formed between creatinine and picric acid in a highly alkaline solution. The alkaline picrate procedure has significant interferences from hemoglobin (positive or negative), bilirubin (negative), ketones (positive), and cephalosporin (positive, if measured within about two hours of receiving a dose of cephalosporin).

Some of the interferences can be minimized if the alkaline picrate reaction is monitored as a kinetic rather than as an endpoint procedure.

Enzymatic methods for creatinine analysis are also available. The most widely used enzymatic procedure employs the following set of reactions:

$$\text{Creatinine} + H_2O \xrightarrow[\text{amidohydrolase}]{\text{creatinine}} \text{creatine}$$

$$\text{Creatine} + H_2O \xrightarrow[\text{amidohydrolase}]{\text{creatine}} \text{Sarcosine} + \text{Urea}$$

$$\text{Sarcosine} + O_2 \xrightarrow[\text{Oxidase}]{\text{Sarcosine}} \text{Glycine} + \text{Formaldehyde} + H_2O_2$$

$$H_2O_2 + \text{Dye} \xrightarrow{\text{Peroxidase}} \text{colored dye} + H_2O$$

This method has few reported interferences.

Urea

Urea is most frequently measured in most body fluids by the urease/glutamate dehydrogenase (GLDH) method involving the following reactions:

$$NH_2 - \overset{\overset{\displaystyle O}{\|}}{C} - NH_2 + 2H_2O \xrightarrow{\text{Urease}} 2NH_4^+ + CO_3^{-2}$$

$$NH_4^+ + NADH + \alpha\text{-Ketoglutaric acid} \xrightarrow[\text{ADP}+H^+]{\text{GLDH}} NAD^+ + \text{Glutamic acid}$$

The decrease in absorbance at 340 nm is directly proportional to the urea concentration in the sample. Automated methods which monitor only the urease reactions are widely available. This can be accomplished by measuring the change in conductivity resulting from the production of the ions NH_4^+ and CO_3^{-2} or by measuring the absorbance change of a dye when the dye comes into contact with the NH_4^+. All urease methods are very accurate and precise with very few reported interferences.

Osmolality

Osmolality measurements or serum in urine can be accomplished by either freezing point depression or vapor pressure methods. The former method is more widely used because of its greater reliability and precision. The major advantage of the vapor pressure osmometer is its very small sample volume requirement (8 uL).

Reference ranges for the analytes discussed in this section are listed in Table 6-8.

7 PH and blood gases

Sarah H. Jenkins

ACID BASE CONTROL
Acids and bases
Acid

The Bronsted-Lowry definition of an acid is any substance that donates or releases hydrogen ions or protons (H^+) in solution and a base is any substance that accepts hydrogen ions. The dissociation of a hypothetical acid (HA) can be represented by the equilibrium:

EQ. 7-1

$$HA \leftrightharpoons H^+ + A^-$$

The above reaction is reversible so that A^- can act as a base by accepting a proton and is referred to as the conjugate base of the acid, HA.

Qualitatively, the strength of an acid can be thought of in terms of how well it dissociates or how far to the right the equilibrium in Equation 7-1 lies. If HA were a strong acid like HCl the equilibrium would lie very far to the right and the acid would be virtually completely dissociated. Weak acids, on the other hand, only partially dissociate so that significant amounts of both HA and A^- exist at equilibrium.

Quantitatively, the relative strength of an acid can be expressed in terms of its K_a or its dissociation constant which is expressed as:

EQ. 7-2

$$K_a = \frac{[H^+][A^-]}{[HA]}$$

Since the dissociated form of the acid is represented in the numerator, then the stronger the acid the larger the K_a.

pH

The activity of the hydrogen ions in a solution is a measure of the acidity of the solution. The hydrogen ion activity is related to the hydrogen ion concentration as follows:

EQ. 7-3

$$\alpha H^+ = \gamma H^+ [H^+]$$

where γH^+ is the activity coefficient of the hydrogen ions. The activity coefficient varies inversely with ionic strength and directly with temperature. In concentrated solutions,

the electrostatic interactions substantially reduce the hydrogen ion activity so that the activity coefficient would be less than 1.0. For more dilute solutions, such as biological fluids, the γH^+ can be assumed to be unity. Since the temperature and physiological concentrations of many analytes in biological fluids are closely maintained, the activity coefficients have very little variance.

The common unit of measurement of acidity is the pH unit. The pH of a solution is defined as the negative logarithm of the hydrogen ion concentration when it is expressed in moles/liter:

EQ. 7-4

$$pH = -\log_{10}[H^+]$$

The greater the hydrogen ion concentration or the more acidic the solution, the lower the pH. Since hydrogen ion concentrations usually encountered are between 1 and 10^{-14} mol/L, the pH of 1 to 14 provides a simple way to express these concentrations without using powers of ten. The normal hydrogen ion concentration in blood is 4.0×10^{-8} mol/L which is a pH of 7.4.

Sources

Physiologically, there are two classifications of acids that are important, fixed acids and volatile acids. Fixed acids are those nongaseous acids such as: the inorganic acids, phosphate (HPO_4^-) and sulfate (HSO_4^-) and the organic acids, lactic acid, acetoacetic acid and beta-hydroxybutyric acid. Carbonic acid (H_2CO_3) is the physiologically important volatile acid and is classified due to its ability to form from or dissociate into carbon dioxide and water:

EQ. 7-5

$$CO_{2(gas)} \Leftrightarrow CO_{2(dissolved)} + H_2O \Leftrightarrow H_2CO_3 \Leftrightarrow H^+ + HCO_3^-$$

The major physiological source of acids is metabolism. Carbohydrates are metabolized to pyruvic and lactic acids under anaerobic conditions such as respiratory distress or strenuous exercise. Triglycerides are metabolized to ketone bodies, acetoacetic acid, and beta-hydroxybutyric acid under anaerobic conditions. All of these acids are further oxidized to carbon dioxide under aerobic conditions. Proteins are hydrolyzed to amino acids which are then metabolized, in part, to carbon dioxide. Sulfur-containing amino acids are oxidized to the salt of sulfuric acid.

Buffers

A buffer is simply a solution that resists changes in pH. It consists of a weak acid and its conjugate base or a weak base and its conjugate acid. The solution resists changes in pH due to the presence of a reservoir of both the acid (proton donating) and base (proton accepting) components of the conjugate pair. For example, if a small amount of acid (H^+) were added to a HA/A^- buffer (Equation 7-1) one might expect the pH of the solution to drop, but the A^- present in solution would accept the added H^+, resulting in a shift of the equilibrium to the left leaving the pH of the solution virtually unchanged. On the other hand, if a small amount of base (A^-) were added to the HA/A^- buffer, one might expect the pH to rise. However, the reservoir of HA present in the solution would dissociate and shift the equilibrium to the right, restoring the H^+ concentration, and leaving the pH again virtually unchanged.

The pH of a buffer will be a function of the pK_a and the relative concentrations of the two components of the solution. Using the equilibrium expression of Equation 7-2 and rearranging as follows:

EQ. 7-6

$$[H^+] = \frac{K_a\,[HA]}{[A^-]}$$

and then taking the negative logarithm of both sides of the equation and rearranging to obtain the general form of the Henderson-Hasselbalch equation:

EQ. 7-7

$$pH = pK_a + \log \frac{[A^-]}{[HA]}$$

Thus, the resulting pH of a buffer is dependent upon the pK_a of the weak acid and on the ratio of the base to the acid component. When the concentration of A^- is equal to the concentration of HA, the pH is equal to the pK_a and the solution is at its maximum buffering capacity. Adding acid or base changes the $[A^-]/[HA]$ ratio. However, the log function causes little change in pH until quantities of added strong acids or bases are large enough to substantially change the ratio. The major physiological buffers are listed in Table 7-1, with their pK_a and concentrations.

Bicarbonate buffer

The bicarbonate buffer system, though not the major blood buffer, is extremely important. In addition to containing the physiologically important volatile acid, carbonic

Table 7-1 Physiologically important buffers

Buffer	pK_a	Concentration (mmol/L)
Bicarbonate	6.33	25
Hemoglobin	7.2	53
Phosphate	6.8	1.2

acid, the bicarbonate buffer system neutralizes fixed acids that enter the blood. Carbonic acid is formed when carbon dioxide combines with water as shown below:

EQ. 7-8

$$CO_{2(gas)} \leftrightarrows CO_{2(dissolved)} + H_2O \Leftrightarrow H_2CO_3$$

Although the reaction of dissolved carbon dioxide with water occurs spontaneously, the reaction rate is very slow. This is overcome in vivo by the enzyme carbonic anhydrase which greatly enhances the reaction rate.

Carbonic acid is a weak acid that dissociates into bicarbonate ion and a proton:

EQ. 7-9

$$H_2CO_3 \Leftrightarrow H^+ + HCO_3^-$$

The pH of this carbonic acid/bicarbonate buffer equilibrium can be represented by the Henderson-Hasselbalch equation:

EQ. 7-10

$$pH = pK_a + \log \frac{[HCO_3^-]}{[H_2CO_3]}$$

The pH can be measured easily, but there are no direct analytical methods for determining bicarbonate and carbonic acid. Equation 7-8 shows that the concentration of carbonic acid is directly proportional to the concentration of dissolved carbon dioxide. It can also be shown that the concentration of a gas dissolved in a liquid is directly proportional to the pressure exerted by the gas above the solution, or its partial pressure. Therefore, the $[H_2CO_3]$ term of Equation 7-10 can be replaced by αP_{CO_2} where α is the solubility coefficient for CO_2 in plasma at 37°C and P_{CO_2} is the partial pressure of CO_2. Substitution into Equation 7-10 yields:

EQ. 7-11

$$pH = pK' + \log \frac{[HCO_3^-]}{[\alpha P_{CO_2}]}$$

This effectively combines Equation 7-8, the hydration of CO_2 and Equation 7-9, the dissociation of carbonic acid, thus creating a new equilibrium expression with a new equilibrium constant. Therefore, the equilibrium constant in Equation 7-11 is now denoted by K'. The new Equation 7-11 still contains a quantity that cannot be measured directly, the bicarbonate concentration. A related quantity that can be measured is the total CO_2 concentration. The total carbon dioxide content of plasma is made up of dissolved carbon dioxide, carbonic acid, and bicarbonate ion:

EQ. 7-12

$$T_{CO_2} = CO_{2(dissolved)} + H_2CO_3 + HCO_3^-$$

The concentration of carbonic acid is very small relative to the other two components and can be disregarded. The dissolved carbon dioxide, as has already been shown in Equation 7-8, can be replaced by αP_{CO2}. The bicarbonate ion can now be expressed by measurable quantities so that Equation 7-12 becomes:

EQ. 7-13

$$HCO_3^- = T_{CO_2} - \alpha P_{CO_2}$$

Substituting for the bicarbonate ion in Equation 7-1, the pH of the bicarbonate buffer system is now represented by:

EQ. 7-14

$$pH = pK' + \log \frac{T_{CO_2} - \alpha P_{CO_2}}{\alpha P_{CO_2}}$$

The solubility coefficient, α, for CO_2 in plasma at 37°C is 0.031 mmol $\cdot$ L^{-1} $\cdot$ mmHg^{-1} and pK' is 6.1 mol/L.

In the bicarbonate buffer system, the concentration of the base component, HCO_3^-, exceeds the concentration of the acid component, H_2CO_3, by a factor of 20. The primary products of the body's metabolism are acids (excess H^+) which create the need for the large excess of the base component of the bicarbonate buffer system. The 20:1 ratio is maintained primarily by the lungs, which expel the CO_2 produced by the body's metabolism.

Hemoglobin

Hemoglobin is the major physiological buffer and is localized within the red blood cells. Hemoglobin is responsible for the buffering of the volatile acid, CO_2. The actual buffer activity of hemoglobin, at physiological pH, is due to the imidiazole group of the histidine amino acids, particularly the C-terminal histidines of the β chains, as shown in Figure 7-1. The imidiazole residues have a pKa of 7.3 which, in addition to the relatively high concentration of hemoglobin, accounts for the dominant role of this protein in buffering the blood.

As oxygenated hemoglobin delivers O_2 to the tissues, the resulting deoxygenated hemoglobin, a weaker acid than oxygenated hemoglobin, will bind a proton. This causes a slight increase in pH which in turn causes the ionization of H_2CO_3. This decrease in H_2CO_3 allows the passage of more CO_2 into the blood from the tissues. The various equilibria involved are shown in Equation 7-15. The overall process of deoxygenation results in an increase in the total CO_2 content of blood.

EQ. 7-15

$$CO_2 + H_2O \leftrightharpoons H_2CO_3$$
$$H_2CO_3 \leftrightharpoons HCO_3^- + H^+$$
$$H^+ + HbO_2 \leftrightharpoons HHb^+ + O_2$$
Net: $$CO_2 + H_2O + HbO_2 \leftrightharpoons HCO_3^- + HHb^+ + O_2$$

Dominant in the lungs $\leftrightharpoons$ Dominant in the tissues

In the lungs, the reverse reaction occurs; hemoglobin is oxygenated and the proton is released because oxygenated hemoglobin is a stronger acid than deoxygenated hemoglobin. The proton combines with HCO_3^- to form H_2CO_3 which is then dehydrated. The resulting CO_2 is then expelled by the lungs. The overall process of oxygenation drives CO_2 out of the lungs and lowers the CO_2 content of the blood.

Protein and phosphate

Compared to the bicarbonate or hemoglobin buffer systems, protein and phosphate constitute a minor class of blood buffers. The proteins have prosthetic groups and amino acids such as histidine, lysine, arginine, glutamate, and aspartate that function to bind or release H^+. Albumin accounts for much of the buffer capacity of plasma proteins. This is

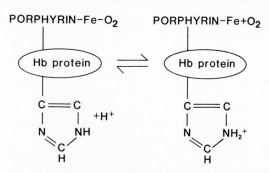

Fig. 7-1 The immidazole ring of histidine responsible for the buffering capacity of hemoglobin at physiological pH. *From Sherwin JE and Bruegger BB: Acid-base control and acid-base disorders. In Kaplan LA and Pesce AJ: Clinical chemistry: theory, analysis, and correlation, ed 2, St. Louis, 1989, Mosby-Year Book, Inc.*

largely due to the 16 histidine residues per molecule of albumin and the large albumin concentration in plasma.

Both inorganic and organic phosphate compounds function as buffers in body fluids. Although there are three equilibria associated with the ionization of inorganic phosphate, only one (shown in Equation 7-16) has a pKa that would allow it to function to an appreciable degree at physiological pH of 7.4.

EQ. 7-16

$$H_2PO_4^- \Leftrightarrow H^+ + HPO_4^{-2} \text{ pKa} = 6.8$$

In plasma, the normal phosphate concentration is approximately 1 mmol/L. Thus, the inorganic phosphate buffer system contributes little to blood buffering compared to hemoglobin (53 mmol/L) and bicarbonate (25 mmol/L). On the other hand, inorganic phosphate plays an important role in urine buffering because it tends to absorb the H^+ excreted.

Significant concentrations of organic phosphates such as 2,3 diphosphoglycerate (2,3-DPG), glucose-1-phosphate, and various nucleotide phosphates are present in intracellular fluids. The phosphate in these compounds functions as a buffer just as inorganic phosphate does, yet the individual organic portions of these compounds influence the hydrogen ion affinity. The pKa values for these compounds therefore range from 6.0 to 7.5.

Gases

Partial pressure

The partial pressure of a gas is defined as the pressure any one gas exerts, whether it is alone or in a mixture of gases. Partial pressure is denoted by a P followed by the chemical symbol for the particular gas. For example, P_{O_2} refers to the partial pressure of O_2. The partial pressure of a gas depends on the number of moles of gas in a specified volume and on the temperature, but is independent of the presence of other gases. The partial pressure of gas A can be written as:

EQ. 7-17

$$P_{gas\ A} = \frac{(n_{gas\ A}\ R\ T)}{V}$$

where n is the number of moles of gas occupying volume, V, at absolute temperature, T, and R is the ideal gas constant.

The total pressure exerted by a mixture of gases is simply the sum of the partial pressures of the individual gaseous components:

$$P_{total} = P_{gas\ A} + P_{gas\ B} + P_{gas\ C}$$

EQ. 7-18

or

$$P_{total} = \frac{(n_{gas\ A} + n_{gas\ B} + n_{gas\ C})\ R\ T}{V}$$

EQ. 7-19

If Equation 7-17 is divided by Equation 7-19, it can be shown that the ratio of the partial pressure of gas A to the total pressure is equal to the ratio of the moles of gas A to the moles of gas present, as shown below:

EQ. 7-20

$$\frac{P_{gas\ A}}{P_{total}} = \frac{n_{gas\ A}}{n_{total}}$$

where $n_{total} = n_{gas\ A} + n_{gas\ B} + n_{gas\ C}$. Equation 7-20 can also be written as:

EQ. 7-21

$$P_{gas\ A} = (P_{total})(F_A)$$

which states that the partial pressure of gas A in a mixture is equal to the product of the total pressure exerted by all the gases and the fraction of the total moles of gas that is gas A (F_A).

Equation 7-21 becomes important when the composition of a gas mixture and the total pressure are known so that the partial pressures of the individual gases can be calculated. For the blood gas analysis, the total pressure is equal to barometric pressure, the composition of the gas components are measured and the partial pressures of the gases of concern, P_{CO_2} and P_{O_2}, are calculated.

Composition of alveolar air

Inspired air, or inhaled air, mixes with air already present in the lungs. Some of this mixture then fills the alveoli where contact between the alveolar air and lung capillaries is made. Alveolar air not only contains the three major components of inspired air, O_2, CO_2, and N_2, but is also saturated with water vapor from the evaporation of water from the trachea and lung tissue surface.

The total pressure in the alveoli is the same as the barometric pressure. The pressure exerted by the water vapor, because the air is saturated, is constant at 47 mm Hg at normal body temperature of 37°C. The pressure exerted by the dry gases is equal to the barometric pressure minus 47 mm Hg.

Under normal conditions, the composition of alveolar air remains relatively constant. In a normal patient at rest the P_{CO_2} is about 40 mm Hg. If this same patient were to begin strenuous exercise, the rate of CO_2 production would increase from approximately 250 cc per minute to 2500 cc per minute, but the alveolar ventilation also rises proportionately so that the P_{CO_2} remains nearly constant at 40 mm Hg. Disturbances in this P_{CO_2} arise when the alveolar ventilation increases or decreases without a proportional change in CO_2 production.

Gas exchange

Venous blood arriving in the lungs normally has a lower P_{O_2} and a higher P_{CO_2} than alveolar air. This creates a diffusion gradient that results in the diffusion of gases from a region of higher partial pressure to the region of lower partial pressure. Oxygen therefore diffuses from the alveoli to the blood and carbon dioxide diffuses in the opposite direction, from the blood to the alveoli. This movement of the gases converts the venous blood to arterial blood.

Arterial blood then passes through the tissues where the P_{O_2} is lower and the P_{CO_2} is higher than that of the arterial blood. Oxygen will diffuse from the arterial blood to the tissues and carbon dioxide diffuses from the tissues to the blood. This process results in the conversion of arterial to venous blood.

Gas transport
Carbon dioxide transport

The majority of carbon dioxide diffusing from the tissues to the blood enters into the erythrocytes. A significant amount of the carbon dioxide remaining in the plasma reacts nonenzymatically with accessible amino groups of plasma proteins to form carbamino groups:

EQ. 7-22

$$CO_2 + H_2N\text{—Protein} \rightleftharpoons {}^-O_2C\text{—NH—Protein} + H^+$$

The remainder of the plasma carbon dioxide is dissolved in solution. A small amount of the CO_2 is hydrated to form H_2CO_3 (Equation 7-8) but the equilibrium lies far to the left. As the CO_2 increases in venous blood, the equilibrium is forced to the right so that a slightly larger amount of H_2CO_3 is formed.

The CO_2 that enters the erythrocytes is distributed among three forms. Some CO_2 remains dissolved within the erythrocyte and some reacts with hemoglobin to form the carbamino compound. The largest fraction of CO_2 entering the erythrocyte is hydrated. This reaction is normally slow, but carbonic anhydrase present in the erythrocytes greatly enhances the reaction rate. The resulting carbonic acid ionizes to form H^+ and HCO_3^-. This reaction proceeds because the reaction products are removed as they are formed. The deoxygenated hemoglobin, being a weaker acid than oxygenated hemoglobin, binds the protons formed and the HCO_3^- formed diffuses into the plasma. This process of removing the reaction products results in a shift of the carbonic acid dissociation equilibrium to the right so that more CO_2 can be removed from the tissues.

The law of electroneutrality requires an equal number of positive and negative charges in the erythrocyte. When carbonic acid ionizes, it forms an equal number of H^+ and HCO_3^- ions. The H^+ binds with hemoglobin and HCO_3^- is then balanced electrically against sodium or potassium cations and electroneutrality is maintained.

As mentioned earlier, the HCO_3^- formed in the erythrocytes diffuses into the plasma. The electroneutrality is unbalanced as the negatively charged HCO_3^- leaves. To correct this, cations must also diffuse out or other anions must diffuse into the erythrocytes. Because the membrane is relatively impermeable to cations it is the chloride anion (Cl^-) that diffuses into the erythrocyte to maintain electroneutrality. This exchange of HCO_3^- for Cl^- within the eryth-

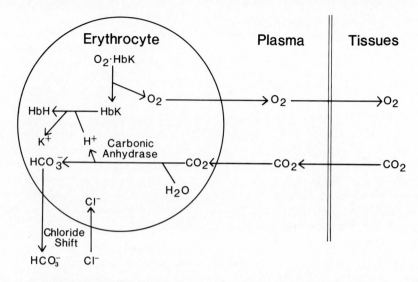

Fig. 7-2 Hemoglobin buffering action in the tissues. *From Sherwin JE and Bruegger BB: Acid-base control and acid-base disorders. In Kaplan LA and Pesce AJ: Clinical chemistry: theory, analysis, and correlation, ed 2, St. Louis, 1989, Mosby—Year Book, Inc.*

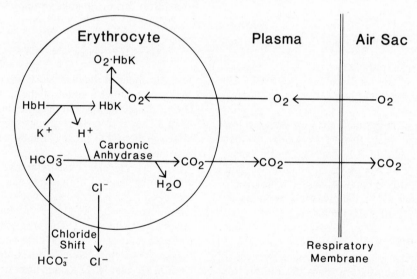

Fig. 7-3 Hemoglobin buffering action in the lungs. *From Sherwin JE and Bruegger BB: Acid-base control and acid-base disorders. In Kaplan LA and Pesce AJ: Clinical chemistry: theory, analysis, and correlation, ed 2, St. Louis, 1989, Mosby—Year Book, Inc.*

rocyte is termed the "chloride shift." These processes are summarized in Figure 7-2.

The formation of HCO_3^- and the subsequent diffusion of Cl^- into the erythrocytes as HCO_3^- diffuses out may disrupt the osmotic equilibrium between plasma and the erythrocyte. Osmotic equilibrium means that a specific volume of water in the plasma outside the red blood cell must contain the same number of osmotically active molecules as the same volume of water inside the erythrocyte. Osmotically active molecules are small ions such as Na^+, Cl^-, HCO_3^-, and K^+. Large molecules such as plasma proteins and hemoglobin only have a slight osmotic activity. When hemoglobin binds protons, the net negative charge of hemoglobin is reduced. This loss of negative charge is balanced by the addition of the osmotically active anions, HCO_3 and Cl^-. The result is an increase in osmotic pressure within

the erythrocyte. In order to reattain osmotic equilibrium, water diffuses from the plasma into the erythrocyte. Consequently, the red blood cells of venous blood are slightly larger than those of arterial blood.

The opposite reactions occur in the lungs. The dissolved CO_2 diffuses from the erythrocyte to the plasma and then into the alveoli. The drop in HCO_3^- within the erythrocyte results in the diffusion of more HCO_3^- into the red blood cell. Simultaneously, O_2 diffusing from the alveoli into the erythrocytes binds to hemoglobin causing the release of a proton. The proton combines with the incoming HCO_3^- forming $H_2CO_3^-$. The carbonic acid is then dehydrated by carbonic anhydrase to form water and dissolved carbon dioxide to be given off through the lungs. To maintain electroneutrality, the chloride diffuses out into the plasma. The overall process is summarized in Figure 7-3.

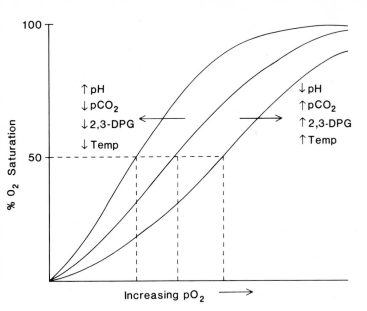

% O_2 Saturation

Increasing pO_2 ⟶

↑ pH
↓ pCO_2
↓ 2,3-DPG
↓ Temp

↓ pH
↑ pCO_2
↑ 2,3-DPG
↑ Temp

Fig. 7-4 Hemoglobin-oxygen dissociation curves and factors that shift the curve right and left. *From Sherwin JE and Bruegger BB: Acid-base control and acid-base disorders. In Kaplan LA and Pesce AJ: Clinical chemistry: theory, analysis, and correlation, ed 2, St. Louis, 1989, Mosby-Year Book, Inc.*

Oxygen transport

Oxygen transported in the blood is primarily dissolved in solution or chemically bound to hemoglobin. The amount dissolved is relatively small and is a function of the solubility of oxygen in blood at physiological temperature and on the P_{O_2}. Each of the four subunits of hemoglobin contains a heme group whose iron can reversibly bind one oxygen molecule. The heme iron has six valence bonds; four of these positions are occupied by the pyrrole rings of heme, one attaches the heme to the protein (globin) portion, and the sixth valence bond is available for the reversible binding of oxygen or other ligands. The binding of oxygen by hemoglobin is dependent on the temperature, pH, P_{O_2}, and on the presence of other ligands that bind to hemoglobin, such as CO_2 and 2,3-DPG. Approximately 1.34 cc of oxygen can be bound by one gram of hemoglobin.

The oxygen dissociation curve of hemoglobin at a plasma pH of 7.4 and temperature of 37° C is shown in Figure 7-4. The percent saturation of hemoglobin is defined as the fraction of oxygenated hemoglobin (HbO_2) to total hemoglobin (HbO_2 + Hb) multiplied by 100:

EQ. 7-23

$$\% \text{ Saturation} = \frac{HbO_2 \times 100}{(Hb + HbO_2)}$$

As shown by the curve, an increase in the P_{CO_2} causes the dissociation curve to shift downward and to the right. This causes a decrease in the hemoglobin saturation for any given P_{O_2}. This occurs because CO_2 reacts with the α-amino groups of the N-terminal valine residues on the four polypeptide chains of hemoglobin. The binding of CO_2 causes a conformational change in the hemoglobin molecule that results in the dissociation of O_2. An increase in CO_2 is accompanied by a decrease in pH. Therefore, a decrease in

pH also causes a shift downward and to the right. This dependence of oxygen dissociation from hemoglobin upon pH and CO_2 is called the Bohr Effect.

Organic phosphates also combine with hemoglobin as 2,3-diphosphoglycerate (2,3-DPG) is produced by a side reaction outside the main glycolytic pathway and is the major organic phosphate in the erythrocyte. The concentration of 2,3-DPG rises during anaerobic metabolism (hypoxia). DPG binds to hemoglobin in the same fashion as CO_2 except that the DPG binds only to the amino acid valine of the β-chains. Nevertheless, the effect is the same as when CO_2 binds to valine in both the α- and β-chains; an increase in 2,3-DPG causes hemoglobin to bind less oxygen.

Acid-base balance

The control of physiological pH is crucial to the functioning of enzymes, maintaining conformation of structural proteins, and for the uptake and release of oxygen. Two systems, the respiratory and renal systems, also play important roles in acid-base balance through the regulation of the bicarbonate:carbonic acid ratio.

Respiratory control

The bicarbonate buffer system is responsible for neutralizing fixed acids entering the blood as shown below:

EQ. 7-24

$$HA + HCO_3^- \rightleftharpoons H_2CO_3 + A^- \rightleftharpoons H_2O + CO_2 + A^-$$

The respiratory system can quickly remove or add the volatile acid, CO_2, to adjust the $HCO_3^-/\alpha P_{CO_2}$ ratio and hence, the pH. A decrease in the respiratory ventilation causes less CO_2 to be removed resulting in an increase in HCO_3^-. The increase in P_{CO_2} is greater than the increase in HCO_3^-. Therefore, both the ratio and pH decrease. Conversely, if the ventilation were to increase, too much CO_2 is given off, and the bicarbonate:carbonic acid ratio and pH both increase. The respiratory system therefore represents a rapid adjustment of acid base balance through the addition or removal of the volatile acid, CO_2.

Renal control

The renal system, on the other hand, represents a slower, more long-term control through the regulation of H^+ excretion and HCO_3^- uptake. The first function of the renal system is the excretion of acid with the concurrent generation of bicarbonate. This process occurs in the renal tubule cells. Carbonic anhydrase present in the renal tubular cells catalyzes the hydration of carbon dioxide (Equation 7-8). The carbonic acid ionizes to HCO_3^- and H^+. The hydrogen ions are excreted by the renal cells in exchange for sodium ions, which are retained, and the excreted protons buffered in the urine by HPO_4^{-2} and ammonia. The bicarbonate ion is transported with the sodium ion into venous blood. The excretion of acid functions, therefore, to add HCO_3^- (base) to the blood and to facilitate the reabsorption of sodium ions. The second function of the renal system is to prevent bicarbonate loss into the urine by reabsorption from the glomerular filtrate. This process occurs in the lumen. The bicarbonate present in the glomerular filtrate is associated with sodium ions. When the filtered sodium and bicarbonate ions reach the region of the tubules where acid is secreted,

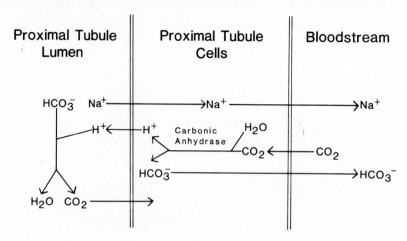

Fig. 7-5 Kidney reabsorption of bicarbonate with excretion of H^+. *From Sherwin JE and Bruegger BB: Acid-base control and acid-base disorders. In Kaplan LA and Pesce AJ: Clinical chemistry: theory, analysis, and correlation, ed 2, St. Louis, 1989, Mosby–Year Book, Inc.*

the sodium is reabsorbed in exchange for the hydrogen ion and the secreted hydrogen ion combines with the bicarbonate to form carbonic acid. The carbonic acid is dehydrated to give water and carbon dioxide. The carbon dioxide then diffuses into the renal tubular cells and into the blood. The overall process is shown in Figure 7-5.

ACID-BASE DISORDERS

The isohydric principle (constant pH) is based on the fact that minor physiological buffers, such as proteins and phosphate, are in equilibrium with the carbonic acid/bicarbonate buffer system. This creates the need only for the accurate description of the carbonic acid/bicarbonate buffer system in order to assess the pH status of the body. Since the plasma pH is a function of the ratio of Pco_2 (a respiratory component) to the HCO_3^- (a metabolic component), then any change in plasma pH results only from changes in this ratio and therefore all acid-base disorders result from changes in either of these two variables. Disorders initiated by a change in Pco_2 are classified as respiratory disorders while those stemming from changes in the bicarbonate concentration are metabolic disorders. Respiratory acidosis is created by increased Pco_2 while respiratory alkalosis is caused by a decreased Pco_2. Metabolic acidosis results from a decreased bicarbonate concentration while an increased bicarbonate concentration causes metabolic alkalosis.

Respiratory and metabolic acid-base disturbances not only result in physiological pH changes but also initiate secondary responses that adjust the member of the bicarbonate/carbonic acid pair not affected by the initial disturbance. Therefore, metabolic disturbances will be compensated by a secondary ventilatory response that will change the Pco_2. Similarly, respiratory disturbances trigger a secondary response that alters the bicarbonate concentration.

Acidosis
Metabolic acidosis

Causes. Metabolic acidosis is characterized by a lowered physiological pH due to a decrease in the bicarbonate concentration and can be a result of three factors. An increase in organic acids other than carbonic acid will result in an excess acid load. Hydroxybutyric and acetoacetic acids can

accumulate in uncontrolled diabetes. Strenuous exercise or systemic infection result in an increase in lactic acid. Ingested compounds that are themselves acids or are metabolized to acids (salicylate) can induce an acidosis. Ingestion of carbonic anhydrase inhibitors such as acetazolamide or sulfonamides, disrupt the normal formation of bicarbonate in the erythrocytes and renal tubule cells and lead to a metabolic acidosis. In these cases, the excess acids enter the plasma and react with bicarbonate to form carbonic acid that is immediately converted to CO_2 and expelled. The overall effect is a decrease in bicarbonate, no change in Pco_2, and a lowered pH.

A metabolic acidosis can not only be caused by an excess of acid but also by a loss of base. Diarrhea results in the rapid loss of intestinal fluid which contains high concentrations of bicarbonate.

The decrease in the kidney's ability to excrete acid by exchanging H^+ for Na^+ results in renal tubule acidosis. Acute renal failure is an extreme example of acid excretion ceasing, thus causing a progressive decrease in plasma bicarbonate concentration.

Secondary response. The immediate response to a metabolic acidosis is hyperventilation. Hyperventilation lowers the Pco_2 and to a smaller extent lowers the bicarbonate concentration. But the overall effect is an increase in the bicarbonate/carbonic acid ratio and the return of plasma pH toward normal. This process is referred to as compensatory respiratory alkalosis.

If the metabolic acidosis does not involve kidney impairment, the kidney will excrete acid and exchange H^+ for Na^+ in the distal tubule, resulting in a more acidic urine. The renal tubule cells also respond by increased excretion of ammonia into the urine allowing for even more H^+ excretion. The renal involvement is more long term and will only occur when the primary cause of the acidosis is removed but will eventually correct the plasma pH and bicarbonate concentration.

Respiratory acidosis

Causes. A respiratory acidosis results from a decrease in the bicarbonate/carbonic acid ratio due to an increase in carbonic acid. The increased carbonic acid also causes a slight increase in the bicarbonate ion concentration due to buffering but the increase in bicarbonate is less than the increase in carbonic acid.

A respiratory acidosis results when the respiratory system is depressed so that CO_2 is not removed efficiently or is not removed at the same rate it is produced. Respiratory disorders that interfere with normal CO_2 expulsion include pneumonia, emphysema, bradycardia, and bronchoconstriction. Drugs that depress the respiratory system such as morphine and barbituates can, in excessive amounts, cause respiratory acidosis.

Premature infants commonly suffer from respiratory distress syndrome (RDS) because they lack sufficient amounts of surfactants in their lungs. As a result, the alveoli are unable to expand properly and the smaller-than-normal surface area impairs normal gas exchange. Respiratory acidosis results.

Secondary Response. The secondary response is increased renal excretion of acids with the retention of sodium and bicarbonate. This renal response is termed *compensatory metabolic alkalosis.*

Alkalosis
Metabolic alkalosis

Causes. Metabolic alkalosis results from an increase in plasma bicarbonate concentration coupled with little or no change in carbonic acid. This can occur through excessive ingestion of bicarbonate of soda for gastrointestinal distress, which raises the blood bicarbonate and hence, the plasma of pH. Prolonged vomiting can cause a metabolic alkalosis due to the loss of gastric hydrochloric acid. This condition is known as hypochloremic alkalosis and is caused by the increased renal retention of bicarbonate to counter the sodium reabsorption due to the lowered chloride concentration. The increased retention of bicarbonate then causes the increase in plasma pH.

Secondary response. The compensation for a metabolic alkalosis is respiratory. The respiratory system slows, decreasing the expulsion of CO_2, while only slightly increasing the bicarbonate concentration, thereby decreasing the plasma pH.

Respiratory alkalosis

Causes. Respiratory alkalosis is caused by a lowered P_{CO_2} due to increased ventilation or hyperventilation. Conditions that lead to this include hysteria, asthma, fever, pulmonary embolism, and excessive use of a mechanical respirator.

Table 7-2 Changes in blood gas parameters associated with disorders of acid-base balance

| | Disorder | | | | | |
| | Acidosis | | Alkalosis | | | |
Analyte	Met	Resp	Met	Resp	RDS	Renal failure
pH	↓	↓	↑	↑	↓	↓
P_{CO_2}	N*, ↓	↑	N*, ↑	↓	↑	N*
pO_2	N	↓	N	↑	↓	N
HCO_3^-	↓	N*, ↑	↑	N*, ↓	N	↓
Base Excess	↓	N*, ↑	↑	N*, ↓	N	↓

N* = normal initially

Secondary response. The secondary response for respiratory alkalosis is the increased excretion of bicarbonate by the kidneys caused by the decreased reabsorption of bicarbonate in the proximal tubules. This lowers the plasma bicarbonate concentrations so that in the presence of the lowered P_{CO_2}, the plasma pH returns toward normal. Table 7-2 shows the changes in blood gas parameters for the conditions discussed in this section.

BLOOD GAS MEASUREMENT
Measured parameters

pH. The blood pH is measured with a pH electrode consisting of a glass membrane selective for hydrogen ions. A voltage change caused by the H^+ association with the membrane is a measure of the hydrogen ion activity.

P_{CO_2}. This electrode is covered with a membrane that is permeable to CO_2 which diffuses through the membrane and into a weak bicarbonate buffer solution inside the electrode. The CO_2 entering the weak buffer compartment changes the pH of the internal solution which is detected by a pH electrode. The change in pH is a measure of the concentration of CO_2.

P_{O_2}. Oxygen is also measured electrochemically. The Clark oxygen electrode is covered with a membrane permeable to oxygen. The oxygen diffuses through the membrane and undergoes electrochemical reduction at an internal platinum electrode. The current generated as oxygen is reduced is a measure of the partial pressure of oxygen in the sample. This electrode is diagrammed in Figure 7-6.

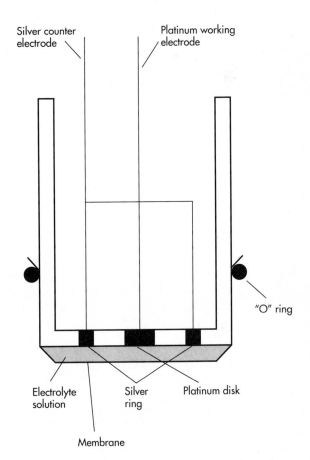

Fig. 7-6 Schematic diagram of the oxygen electrode.

Calculated parameters

Bicarbonate ion. Bicarbonate ion concentration is calculated using the measured pH, P_{CO_2}, and the rearranged Henderson-Hasselbalch equation:

EQ. 7-25

$$HCO_3^- = (\alpha P_{CO_2}) \text{ antilog } (pH - pK'_a)$$

A nomogram, such as the one shown in Figure 7-7, can also be used to determine the bicarbonate concentration using the pH and P_{CO_2}.

Total CO₂. Total CO_2 can also be calculated from the pH and P_{CO_2} using Equation 7-12. The concentration of carbonic acid is insignificant and is ignored in this calculation. The nomogram shown in Figure 7-7 can also be used

SIGGAARD-ANDERSEN ALIGNMENT NOMOGRAM

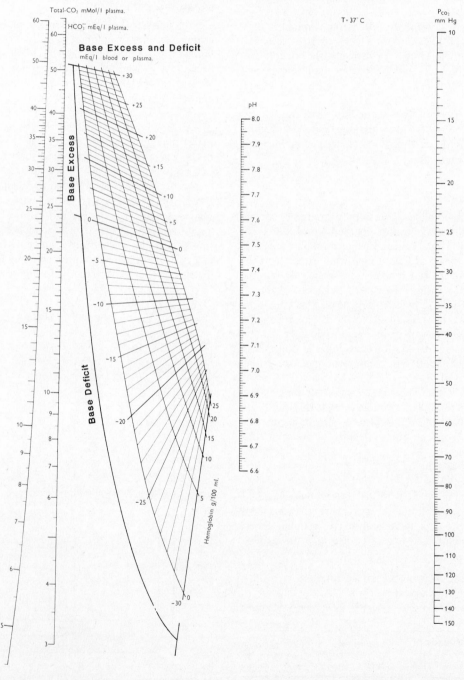

Fig. 7-7 Nomogram of the relationship between P_{CO_2}, pH, base excess, hemoglobin, bicarbonate, and total CO_2. A straight line through a pH and P_{CO_2} value will intercept the corresponding calculated concentrations for bicarbonate and total CO_2. The base excess can be derived from that straight line if the hemoglobin concentration is known. *From Sherwin JE and Bruegger BB: Acid-base control and acid-base disorders. In Kaplan LA and Pesce AJ: Clinical chemistry: theory, analysis, and correlation, ed 2, St. Louis, 1989, Mosby–Year Book, Inc.*

to determine the total CO_2 from the pH and Pco_2.

Base excess. Base excess is a calculated parameter used to assess acid-base status. A positive base excess indicates an excess of bicarbonate while a negative base excess indicates a deficit of bicarbonate. The base excess of a normal patient with a blood pH of 7.4, Pco_2 of 40 mm Hg, hemoglobin of 15 mg/dL, and a temperature of 37°C is zero. The base excess can be calculated using Equation 7-26, the measured pH and Pco_2, and either a measured or assumed hemoglobin concentration.

EQ. 7-26

$$\text{Base excess} = (1.0 - 0.0143\ \text{Hb})(\text{HCO}_3^-) - \\ (9.5 + 1.63\ \text{Hb})(7.4\ \text{pH}) - 24$$

The hemoglobin concentration must be included in the calculation due to its crucial role in the buffering of blood. The base excess can also be calculated from the nomogram in Figure 7-7.

Oxygen saturation. Oxygen saturation is calculated from the measured values of pH and P_{O_2}, and is used to assess the effectiveness of oxygen therapy. The oxygen saturation can be calculated using Equation 7-23 or using the nomogram in Figure 7-8.

Reference ranges

Reference ranges for the important blood gas parameters can be found in Table 7-3.

Sample handling

Blood consists of living cells and will continue to consume oxygen and produce carbon dioxide during transport to the laboratory. This process is minimized if the sample syringe is placed in an ice slush immediately after drawing. This rapidly lowers the temperature of the sample to 4°C so that changes in blood gas parameters are insignificant over several minutes. Samples that are acceptable are those that have been properly iced and transported to the laboratory within 15 minutes of drawing.

Noninvasive methods

Noninvasive methods of analysis are becoming increasingly important in all areas of clinical chemistry. For blood gas analysis, transcutaneous methods are important for continuous monitoring of neonates with respiratory distress syndrome and are significantly less traumatic for the patient than a static arterial puncture.

P_{O_2}. The transcutaneous measurement of P_{O_2} takes advantage of the small amount of diffusion of gases from the capillary bed in the skin toward the surface of the skin. The P_{O_2} of the surface correlates well with arterial P_{O_2} if the temperature of the skin is raised to 42°C to achieve maximal blood flow. The transcutaneous P_{O_2} (tcP_{O_2}) operates under the same principle as the Clark oxygen electrode except that the electrode apparatus includes a heating device and a sealing ring placed around the outer edge of the electrode to prevent atmospheric oxygen from interfering. Because the electrode is placed directly on the skin, the heating device

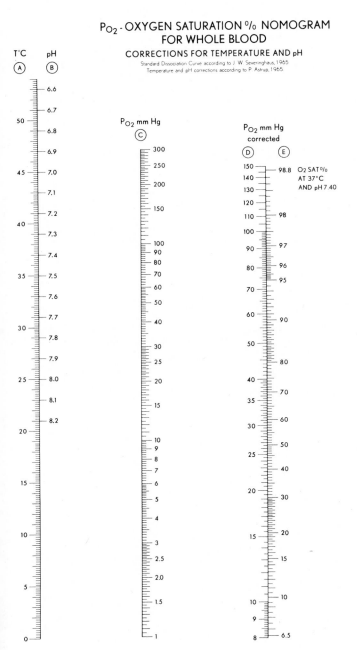

Fig. 7-8 Nomogram of the relationship between pH, P_{O_2}, and O_2 saturation. A straight line through pH and P_{O_2} values will intercept the corresponding calculated O_2 saturation at 37° C. *From Sherwin JE and Bruegger BB: Acid-base control and acid-base disorders. In Kaplan LA and Pesce AJ: Clinical chemistry: theory, analysis, and correlation, ed 2, St. Louis, 1989, Mosby–Year Book, Inc.*

Table 7-3 Reference values for adult blood gas parameters in arterial and venous blood

Parameters	Arterial	Venous
pH	7.35-7.45	7.33-7.43
Pco_2	35-45 mm Hg	38-50 mm Hg
Po_2	80-100 mm Hg	30-50 mm Hg
HCO_3^-	22-26 mmol/L	23-27 mmol/L
Total CO_2	23-27 mmol/L	24-28 mmol/L
O_2 saturation	94-100%	60-85%
Venous anion gap	5-14 mmol/L	
Base excess	-2-$+2$ mEq/L	

must be capable of precise temperature control to minimize the risk of burns.

P_{CO_2}. The transcutaneous P_{CO_2} (tcP_{CO_2}) electrode operates as the standard P_{CO_2} electrode found in blood gas instruments. It is also similar to the tcP_{O_2} electrode in that it too contains a heating device and must be sealed from atmospheric interference.

Oxygen saturation. The pulse oximeter measures O_2 saturation and relies on the differential absorption of red and infrared light of oxyhemoglobin and deoxyhemoglobin. The light passes from the pulse oximeter through pulsating tissue and the absorbance at each wavelength is measured by the instrument. By comparing the measurements obtained between pulses (baseline) to those obtained during the pulse of arterial blood, the saturation of hemoglobin is determined. Using this data the pulse oximeter calculates the relative amount of oxyhemoglobin and deoxyhemoglobin in blood, expressing the results in terms of oxygen saturation or sPO_2.

Pulse oximeters can have some interferences. Since the pulse oximeter makes measurements timed with the pulsing of blood, patient motion can sometimes cause the instrument to make a false reading. The pulse oximeter must be shielded from bright light sources that will interfere with the absorbance determination. Also the calculations performed by the pulse oximeter include only oxyhemoglobin and deoxyhemoglobin. The instrument is blind to abnormal forms of hemoglobin unless the spectral absorption characteristics are similar to normal adult hemoglobin.

SUGGESTED READING

Davenport HW: The ABC of acid-base chemistry, ed 6, Chicago, 1974, The University of Chicago Press.

Kaplan LA and Pesce AJ: Clinical chemistry: theory, analysis, and correlation, ed 2, St. Louis, 1989, Mosby-Year Book, Inc.

Shapiro BA, Harrison RA, and Watson JR: Clinical application of blood gases, ed 3, Chicago, 1982, Year Book Medical Publishers, Inc.

8 Carbohydrates

Juan R. Sobenes
John E. Sherwin

STRUCTURE AND CLASSIFICATION OF CARBOHYDRATES

Carbohydrates are organic molecules that contain carbon, hydrogen, and oxygen. They were once thought to be hydrates of carbon—thus the name carbohydrate. Many carbohydrates do have the ratio of two hydrogen atoms to one oxygen atom (as in H_2O) for every carbon atom. Carbohydrates are either aldehyde or ketone derivatives and also contain hydroxyl groups. Thus they can be defined as polyhydroxyl aldehydes, polyhydroxyl ketones, or substances that produce these compounds—upon hydrolysis—and their derivatives.

Carbohydrates are classified according to the size of their molecules and in some cases the number of carbon atoms. The largest carbohydrates are polymers called polysaccharides, which contain many simple sugars linked together. The simplest carbohydrates are called monosaccharides. Polysaccharides can be hydrolyzed (broken down in a reaction with water) to produce monosaccharides. The monosaccharides cannot be changed to simpler molecules. Carbohydrates composed of a few monosaccharides are called oligosaccharides. They contain generally two to 10 monosaccharide units bonded together. The most important oligosaccharides are the disaccharides, which consist of two monosaccharide molecules joined by a chemical bond.

The term "sugar" generally applies only to those monosaccharides and oligosaccharides that are soluble in water and taste sweet.

Monosaccharides

Monosaccharides are classified, according to their functional group, into aldoses (compounds containing an aldehyde group) and ketoses (compounds containing a ketone group). "ose" is characteristic of simple carbohydrates.

A triose, a three-carbon sugar, is the smallest possible carbohydrate. Glyceraldehyde, the simplest of all the monosaccharides, is an aldotriose and is formed from the breakdown of hexoses in muscle tissue.

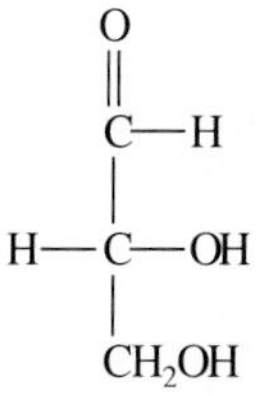

Glyceraldehyde

Tetroses, or four-carbon monosaccharides, are not of major importance biologically.

The pentoses, carbohydrates with five carbon atoms, are biologically very important. Two aldopentoses, five-carbon monosaccharides, make up part of the complex nucleic acids, which are most important in gene structure. They are ribose and deoxyribose, building blocks of RNA and DNA, respectively.

The prefix "deoxy" means that the molecule contains one less oxygen atom, at carbon 2, as shown by its structural formula.

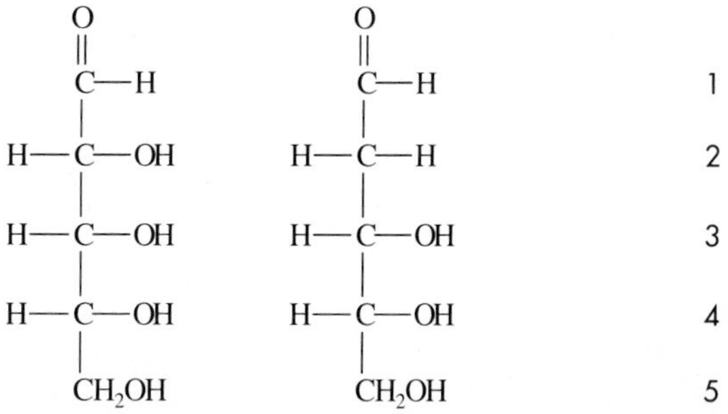

Ribose   2-deoxyribose   Number of carbon atoms

Hexoses

Hexoses, carbohydrates containing six carbon atoms, are the most important group of monosaccharides. Of these, only glucose, also called dextrose or blood sugar, plays a major role in metabolism. This molecule, which has the formula $C_6H_{12}O_6$, follows:

109

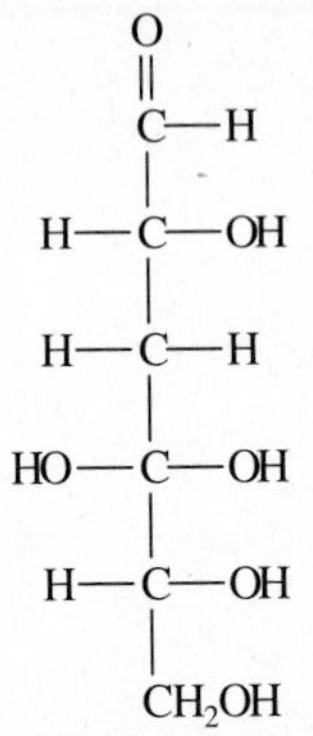

D-glucose

All monosaccharides found in nature are stereoisomers. Steroisomerism is defined by the ability of a molecule to rotate the plane of incident polarized light. This occurs when a molecule contains at least one asymmetric carbon atom. That is, a carbon with four different groups attached to it. The other physical and chemical properties of isomers are the same. The aldohexoses exist as eight isomers because C2, C3, C4, C5 are symmetric and two isomers are possible for each carbon atom. Except for their different action on polarized light, they are exactly the same.

All the monosaccharides in human biochemistry are of the dextroisomeric (D) form. Some examples are given in Figure 8-1.

The pentose and hexose monosaccharides have the ability to form ring structures. The six-membered ring forms of the sugars are called pyranoses, the five-membered rings are called furanoses. The aldohexoses, such as D-glucose, form six-membered rings; the aldopentoses, such as D-xylose, form five-membered rings.

Glucose can form two types of six-membered rings depending on the position of the hydroxyl group at carbon number 1 with respect to the plane of the ring. When the hydroxyl group is on the same side of the molecule as oxygen at C6, the isomer is known as beta-D-glucose. If the OH group is on the opposite side of the ring it is called alpha-D-glucose.

Another aldohexose, galactose, is an isomer of glucose. The structural formulas of the open form and the beta-ring form are as follows:

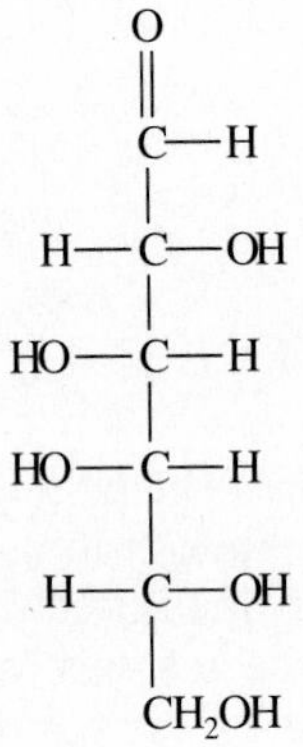

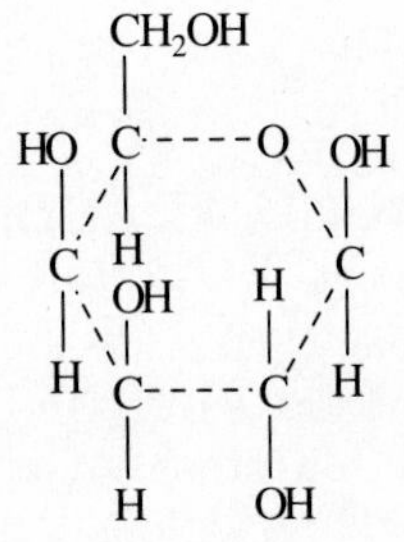

Beta-D-galactose

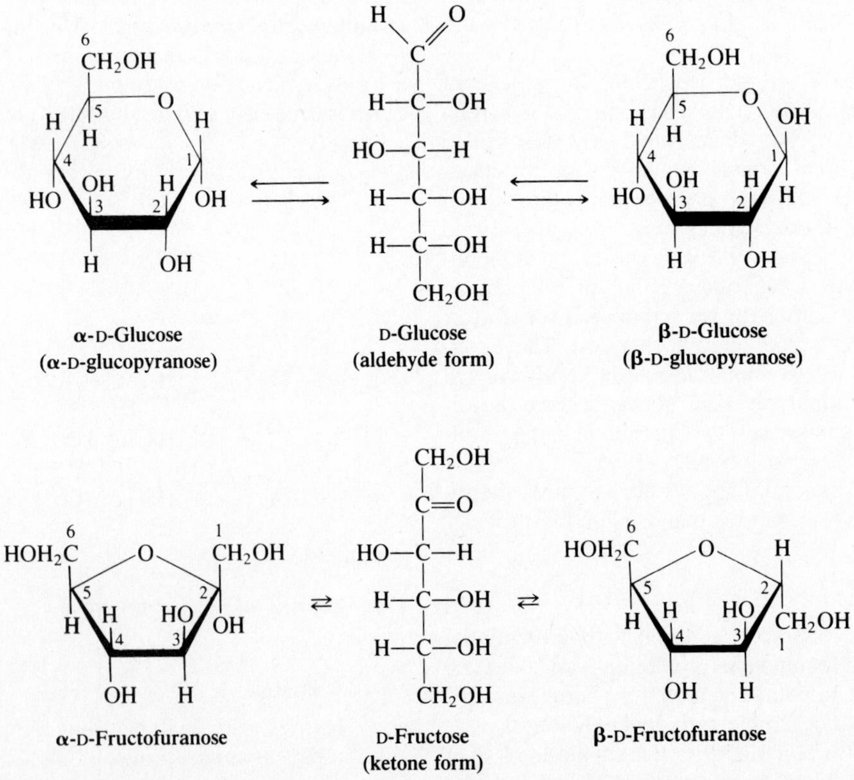

α-D-Glucose
(α-D-glucopyranose)

D-Glucose
(aldehyde form)

β-D-Glucose
(β-D-glucopyranose)

α-D-Fructofuranose

D-Fructose
(ketone form)

β-D-Fructofuranose

Fig. 8-1 Interrelationships between straight-chain and ring forms of D-glucose and D-fructose, which form pyranose and furanose rings. *From Orten, JM, and Neuhaus, OW: Human biochemistry, ed 10, St. Louis, 1982, Mosby–Year Book.*

Galactose and glucose are called epimers because they differ only in the arrangement of groups at a single C4 carbon atom.

A few six-carbon sugars, aldoketoses, form five-membered rings. The most important of these is D-fructose, a six-carbon aldoketose. It also has both alpha- and beta-forms (see Figure 8-1).

Derived monosaccharides

These compounds are formed by reduction or oxidation of carbonyl groups. When derived monosaccharides are the products of reduction, they are called polyols, polyalcohols, such as D-sorbitol or D-mannitol. The products of oxidation are acids such as D-glucuronic acid, formed from D-glucose. Acid forms of monosaccharides are important constituents of more complex carbohydrates like mucopolysaccharides. Acid forms are also used metabolically by the body to increase the solubility of some xenobiotic compounds, which aid the excretion of acids into the urine.

Sialic acid, an important derivative of N-acetyl neuraminic acid, which is often found covalently linked to proteins, is a monosaccharide derivative formed by replacement of a hydroxyl group by an amino group.

Disaccharides

Disaccharides consist of two monosaccharides joined together by an oxygen atom, with the removal of a molecule of water.

Maltose

Maltose is formed by combining two glucose units, marked A and B in the figure that follows. Carbon 1, the anomeric carbon atom of glucose A, in the alpha form, is connected by an oxygen "bridge" to carbon 4 of glucose B. This is the beta form due to the C1 of glucose B. Maltose, or malt sugar, does not occur abundantly in nature, although it is found in sprouting grain. Maltose is the main product of the hydrolysis of starch and is used commercially in baby formulas and other beverages.

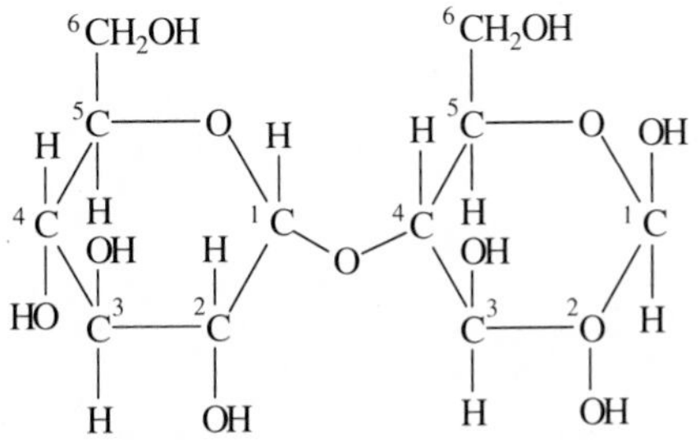

Glucose (A)　　　　Glucose (B)

Maltose (beta form)

Lactose

Another disaccharide is lactose, or milk sugar. It consists of glucose combined wtih galactose. Lactose is found almost exclusively in milk; human milk contains about twice as much lactose as milk from cows.

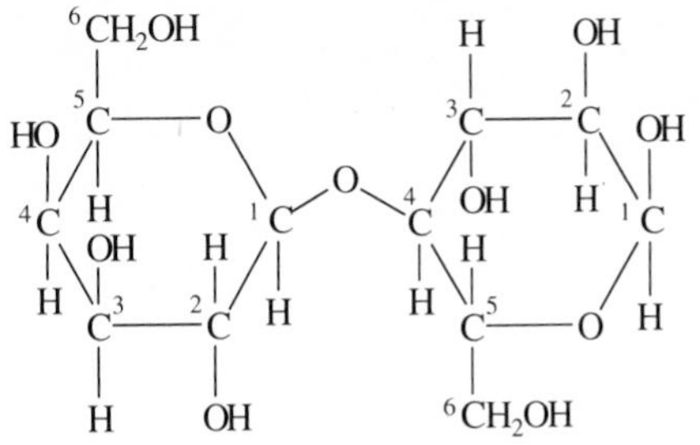

Galacose　　　　Glucose

Lactose (alpha form)

Sucrose

The most common disaccharide is sucrose, formed by the linkage of glucose and fructose. Unlike other diasaccharides, the anomeric carbons of both the monosaccharides are "tied up" in a new bond. As a result, sucrose does not have alpha and beta forms and is not a reducing sugar.

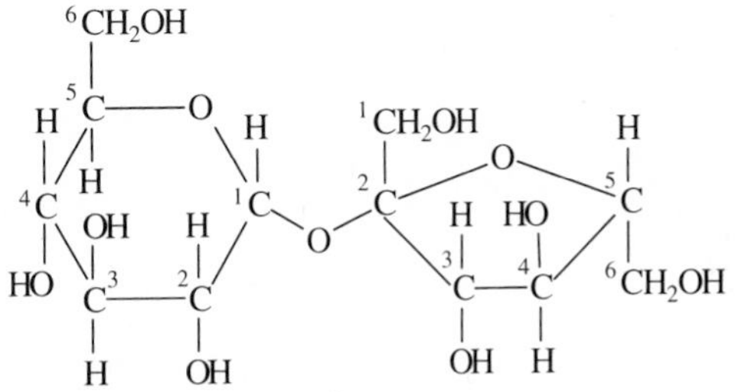

Glucose　　　　Fructose

Sucrose

Sucrose is found primarily in sugar cane, sugar beets, and fruits and vegetables. It is the table sugar used as a sweetener at home.

Polysaccharides

Polysaccharides are polymers, generally containing hundreds of monosaccharide molecules, joined together through bridging oxygen atoms. Molecular weights vary from a few thousand to several million daltons. The most abundant polysaccharides in nature are glucosans, so called because they are formed from repeating glucose units.

Starches

Starch is formed by a mixture of two types of polysaccharides—a straight chain glucose polymer (20% to 30%) called amylose and a highly branched polymer (70% to 80%) called amylopectin (see Figure 8-2).

Amylose consists of 250 to 500 glucose units linked together in the alpha form with a bond of C1 of one unit to C4 of its neighbor. Amylopectin contains about 1000 glucose units with large numbers of branches with C1-6 linkages, each consisting of about 25 monosaccharide units.

Starch is the most important carbohydrate as a soure of metabolic energy and can be considered the basis of the human diet, since more carbohydrates are ingested than any other type of food. When broken down by hydrolysis, starch produces smaller pieces called dextrans. Further hydrolysis results in maltose and finally glucose molecules.

Glycogen is similar in structure to the branched amylopectin, although it is larger, about 5000 monosaccharides,

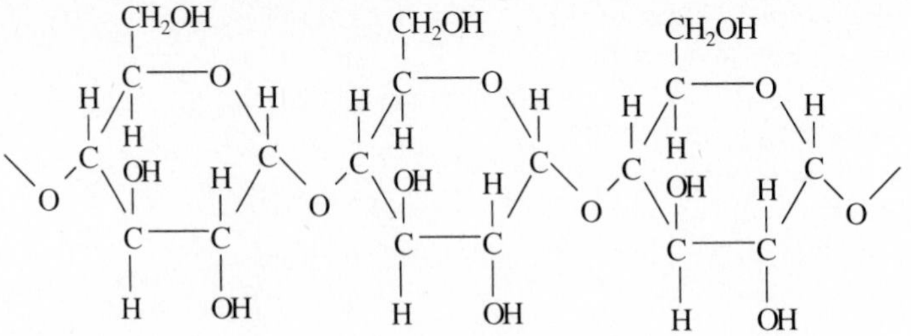

Amylose

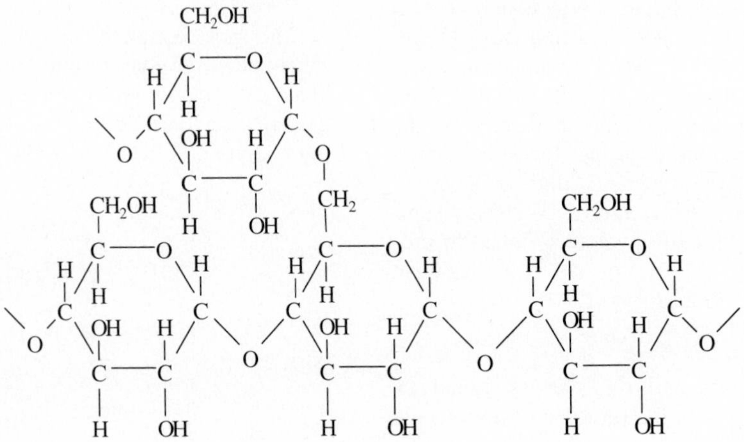

Amylopectin

Fig. 8-2 Starch is a mixture of 20% to 30% amylose and 70% to 80% amylopectin. As shown, amylose is a straight-chain polymer and amylopectin contains branches.

and has shorter chains, averaging 12 glucose units. This polysaccharide is the storage form of carbohydrate in the body. It is found primarily in the liver and muscle tissues and is drawn upon when needed as a source of energy. After eating, part of the glucose produced by digestion is converted to glucogen by a process called glycogenesis. Later, when the concentration of glucose in the blood falls, glycogen is hydrolyzed back to glucose through glycogenolysis. Glycogen is well suited for storage because its large size prevents it from diffusing through the cell membranes.

Cellulose

Cellulose is the most abundant organic substance in nature. Unlike starch and glycogen, cellulose consists of beta-glucose units in a straight chain, 900 to 6000 units per molecule. Because the glucose molecules are joined in their beta forms, cellulose cannot be digested. Humans lack the enzyme capability for hydrolyzing beta glucose linkages. Only certain species like cows and termites can digest cellulose-containing materials because they harbor microorganisms with the necessary enzymes. Since cellulose is not digested, it forms part of the diet's roughage and aids in the formation of normal stools.

Metamucil is a trademarked preparation of a psyllium hydrophilic mucilloid, a powdered preparation of the mu-cilagenous portion of bland psyllium (*Plantago ovata*) seeds. It is used in the treatment of simple constipation resulting from lack of bulk.

CARBOHYDRATE METABOLISM

Dietary carbohydrates are usually complex carbohydrates such as starch. Disaccharides (sucrose, lactose, and mannose) and simple carbohydrates (glucose, galactose, and fructose) are also available.

Glucose is the major hexose derivative used as a source of metabolic energy. Enzymatic activity in the gastrointestinal system reduces starch to its hexose components and disaccharides to monosaccharides.

Biochemical pathways

Starch and glycogen ingested as foods undergo partial digestion under the enzymatic action of salivary amylase with the production of intermediate forms of dextrans and maltose. In the small intestine, the amylase of the pancreas completes the digestion of starch and glycogen to maltose. Maltose and other disaccharides are split by disaccharidases including maltase, lactase, and sucrase from the intestinal mucosa to form the monosaccharides glucose, galactose, and fructose, which can then be absorbed.

The rate of absorption of glucose, being an active process, is greater than similar molecules absorbed by passive

Stage 1
Collection of simple sugars
and conversion
to the common
product glyceraldehyde
3-phosphate

Stage 2
Conversion of
glyceraldehyde
3-phosphate
to lactate and
coupled formation
of ATP

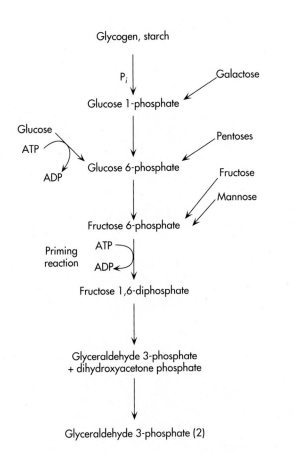
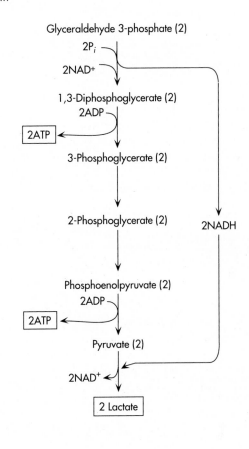

Fig. 8-3   Stages of glycolysis.

diffusion (e.g., xylose). Fructose is absorbed more slowly than glucose, and galactose is absorbed by a carrier-mediated process independent of the glucose and galactose transport mechanisms.

The intestinal absorption of glucose routes these hexoses into the liver via the portal vein. Depending on the physiologic needs of the body, glucose can follow one of several paths, which include:

1. Conversion to and storage as liver glycogen (glycogenesis)
2. Metabolism to carbon dioxide and water to provide immediate energy.
3. Conversion to keto acids or amino acids
4. Conversion to fatty acids
5. Anaerobic glycolysis to pyruvate and lactate
6. Release from the cell to maintain blood glucose for other peripheral cells

Glucose metabolism

Metabolism of glucose inside cells requires phosphory-

lation to glucose-6-phosphate, which uses ATP. This compound is further phosphorylated to fructose, 1,6-diphosphate and broken down by the Embden-Meyerhof pathway yielding two molecules of pyruvate and two molecules of ATP per mole of glucose (Figure 8-3).

Anaerobic glycolysis

The catabolism of glucose to pyruvate and lactate is anaerobic metabolism. The net reaction in the transformation of glucose into pyruvate is:

$$\text{Glucose} + 2\ \text{Pi} + 2\text{ADP} + 2\text{NAD}^+ \longrightarrow$$
$$2\ \text{pyruvate} + 2\text{ATP} + 2\text{NADH} + 2\text{H}^+ + 2\text{H}_2\text{O}$$

Two molecules of ATP are generated in the conversion of glucose to pyruvate.

Pyruvate can be converted to lactate when the amount of oxygen is limited, as in muscle tissue during intense exercise. The reduction of pyruvate by NADH to form lactate is catalized by the enzyme lactic dehydrogenase.

The chemical equation showing conversion of Pyruvate to L-Lactate:

Pyruvate + NADH + H$^+$ $\xrightarrow{\text{Lactate dehydrogenase}}$ L-Lactate + NAD$^+$

Hypoxia is a determining factor in the blood concentration of lactate. A large increase in blood lactate is an ominous sign when a patient is in shock—it indicates the development of an irreversible stage in this condition.

Severe exercise may increase the lactate concentration to values of 16 mEq per liter or higher. Such accumulation of anions in the plasma represents considerable acidosis with marked lowering of the bicarbonate concentration. Fortunately the rise is fleeting; it subsides when the oxygen debt is overcome and even more rapidly if renal excretion of lactate is maximal.

Aerobic glycolysis

Aerobic glycolysis is a more energy-efficient process. Glucose is converted to pyruvate as in anaerobic metabolism. The pyruvate is then converted to two molecules of acetyl CoA with production of 14 mol of ATP per moles of glucose. Acetyl CoA is then degraded in the citric acid cycle with the production of an additional 24 moles of ATP. Thus aerobic glycolysis produces a net balance of 38 moles of ATP per mol of glucose or nineteen times the energy of anaerobic glycolysis (Figure 8-4).

Hormonal control

Many hormones are involved in the control of carbohydrate metabolism. Their effects are aimed at producing glucose in exactly the right amount for the metabolic needs of various organs. This balance is necessary to maintain the concentration of blood glucose between relatively narrow limits.

The two main hormones that control glucose concentrations in the blood and have apparent antagonistic effects are

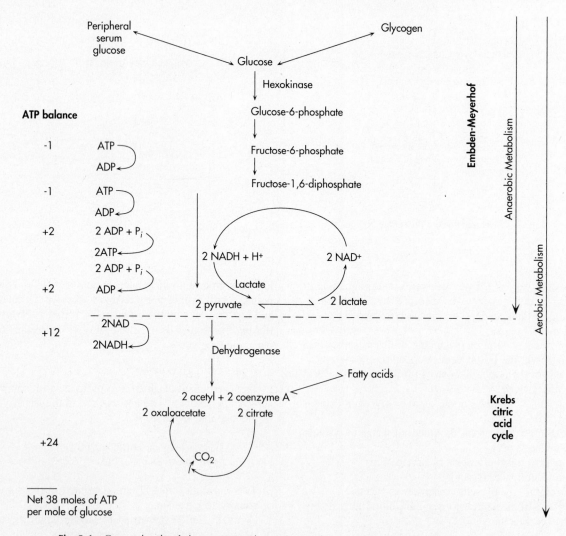

Fig. 8-4   One molecule of glucose (a 6-carbon compound) is converted to two molecules of pyruvate (a 3-carbon compound), which in aerobic glycolysis is further converted to two molecules of acetyl coenzyme A with production of 14 moles of ATP per mole of glucose. Acetyl CoA is then degraded in citric acid cycle with production of a further 24 moles of ATP. Thus aerobic glycosysis produces a net balance of 38 moles of ATP per mole of glucose.

glucagon and insulin. Glucagon produces increases in blood glucose; insulin reduces blood glucose.

Glucagon

Glucagon produces increases in glucose values by hydrolyzing stored glycogen. Glycogenolysis occurs by activating hepatic phosphorylase under the influence of cyclic AMP. A second hyperglycemic mechanism occurs with the hypophysis through the actions of growth hormone and ACTH. This gluconeogenesis mechanism acts to produce glucose from aminoacids, glycerol, and triglycerides. At the same time, the metabolism of fatty acids provides the necessary energy for this process. These are the so-called stress hormones. Other factors can influence test results when evaluated under non-resting conditions.

Insulin

Insulin plays an essential and continuous role in the utilization of glucose derived from the reactions described previously. Insulin is secreted by the beta cells of the islets of Langerhans in the pancreas. The hormone is primarily synthesized as a larger inactive precursor composed of a single polypeptide chain called proinsulin. This polypeptide is cleaved at several points by peptidases, which break the polypeptide into an N-terminal fraction and a central protein called C-peptide. The amount of C-peptide released into blood is equivalent to the amount of insulin produced.

Glycogen synthesis

Glucose values are also reduced by stimulating the formation of glycogen. The rate of glycogen formation is controlled by the enzyme glycogen synthetase (GS). Increases in the concentration of glucose stimulate this enzyme and the production of glycogen.

Glucose-1-phosphate is activated to UDP-glucose and then glycogen synthetase transfers UDP-glucose to the C-4 terminus of glycogen to form a 1,4 glycosidic linkage and UDP.

$$\text{UDP-glucose} + \text{glycogen} \xrightarrow{\text{GS}} \text{glycogen} + \text{UDP}$$
$$\text{(n residues)} \qquad \text{(n+1 residues)}$$

Synthetic pathways employ branching enzymes that create large numbers of non-reducing terminal residues, thus increasing the rate of glycogen synthesis. The result of increased glycogen formation is a reduction in glucose.

DISORDERS OF CARBOHYDRATE METABOLISM
Hyperglycemic syndromes

Hyperglycemic syndromes can be the result of conditions that reduce the pancreas' capacity to secrete insulin. These conditions include pancreatitis, carcinoma of the pancreas, hemochromatosis, and pancreatectomy. Hyperproduction of insulin antagonistic hormones, growth hormone, cortisol, epinephrine, or glucagon can cause the same result. Acromegaly, hypercortisolism, pheochromocytoma, and glucagonoma will therefore be the cause of these hyperglycemic syndromes. Also, hyperglycemia can be an iatrogenic condition as a result of corticotherapy or the use of progestational steroids or certain drugs that can sometimes elicit a latent anomaly to glucose tolerance.

Diabetes mellitus

The most important hyperglycemia syndrome is diabetes mellitus. The etiologic considerations of diabetes suggest an underlying hereditary role. There are two primary forms of diabetes mellitus:
1. Insulin-dependent diabetes mellitus (IDDM)
2. Noninsulin-dependent diabetes mellitus (NIDDM)

Usually IDDM is seen in young idividuals with infantile or juvenile diabetes; occasionally it is seen in older people. IDDM appears to be related to diverse causes, but particularly to viral infections of the beta cells of the islets of Langerhans that exhibit an exaggerated immunologic reaction and a genetic background characterized by the predominance of certain human leukocyte antigenic (HLA) groups (DW3, DW4, B8, Bw15).

NIDDM, type II, or maturity onset diabetes mellitus, is far more common (80% of cases) and is usually accompanied by obesity. NIDDM is manifested as a peripheral resistance to insulin associated with a reduction of insulin secretion, which is responsible for glucose intolerance.

The presence of insulin results in the passage of glucose into peripheral cells. Reduced insulin values give rise to elevated blood sugar and decreased intracellular glucose values.

The end result of diabetes, regardless of its type, is related to diffuse tissue damage involving chiefly the vascular basal membranes caused by chronically elevated blood glucose values. The deposition of glucose by covalent linkage to proteins is responsible for the microangiopathy in the retina and glomeruli and involvement of the nervous system. Diabetes and glucose intolerance are factors in the risk of atheroma formation.

The concept of reversal of dysfunctional angiopathy with normalization of glycemia reinforces the need to control diabetes mellitus as closely as possible. It has been postulated that the tissue damage is due to the fact that glycosylated hemoglobin binds oxygen with greater affinity and probably deprives the endothelium of adequate oxygenation.

These disorders affect more than 6 million Americans and significantly contribute to medical-care costs. Screening for disease is only justified when early treatment in asymptomatic patients is more effective than treatment begun after symptoms have appeared. Presently, early treatment is available only for gestational diabetes.

Gestational diabetes mellitus (GDM)

Gestational diabetes is glucose intolerance that appears for the first time during pregnancy. It occurs in approximately 3% of pregnancies and is considered by some physicians a third type or diabetes type III. Untreated gestational diabetes mellitus can cause macrosomia of the fetus, increased risk of birth trauma, hyperbilirubinemia, hypercalcemia, hypoglycemia, or respiratory distress syndrome (RDS).

Plasma glucose in the mother usually can be controlled by diet alone, though insulin treatment is required in 10% to 15% of patients with GDM. Oral hypoglycemic agents are contraindicated in GDM because of possible teratogenesis. Desirable values are fasting blood glucose of less than 100 mg/dL and a post prandial plasma glucose of less than 120 to 140 mg/dL. After delivery, patients with GDM usually revert to a normal glucose tolerance, but there is increased risk (30% to 40%) of developing NIDDM later.

Complications of diabetes mellitus

The main complications of diabetes mellitus are retinopathy, neuropathy, angiopathy, nephropathy, increased susceptibility to infection, hyperlipidemia, ketoacidosis, and hyperglycemic hyperosmolar nonketotic coma (HHNC).

Diabetic ketoacidosis

One consequence of the altered glucose metabolism is ketosis with the possibility of keto-acidosis. In comatose patients, the condition is related to the acute deficiency of insulin and to the absence of glycolysis with lowered amounts of oxalacetic acid.

Acetyl CoA is a compound at the metabolic junction of glucose, protein, and lipid metabolism and is produced in excess during this condition. Acetyl CoA can be carboxylated to acetone (in the lungs) and combined with a second acetyl CoA to produce acetoacetate or reduced enzymatically to beta-hydroxybutarate. Acetoacetate and beta-hydroxybutarate are commonly called "ketoacids." Ketoacids are excreted in the urine with sodium and potassium ions, which results in the retention of hydrogen ions. If a significant amount of ketoacids are produced, acidosis will be the result.

In nondiabetics, ketoacid formation is a minor pathway. In Type I diabetics, muscle and fat cells are deprived of glucose due to the lack of insulin, which facilitates the passage of glucose through the plasma membrane. The cellular response to this type of starvation is the mobilization of fatty acids from triglycerides. Fatty acid catabolism produces excessive quantities of acetyl CoA, which is only partly metabolized to produce energy via the tricarboxylic acid cycle. Increased amounts of ketoacids elevate the hydrogen ion concentration in the blood and lowers the pH, producing acidosis.

Diagnosis of ketoacidosis

A low pH with normal pCO_2 or a large anion gap with low bicarbonate and high glucose suggest ketoacidosis. The abnormal anion gap is caused by accumulation of ketoacids, i.e., acetoacetic acid, beta-hydroxybutrate, and acetone. The acetoacetic acid can be demonstrated with the nitroprusside test commonly known as Acetest, which can evaluate blood or urine. Nitroprusside does not react with beta-hydroxybutyrate (HBA) and reacts only weakly (20%) with acetone.

In the early stages of diabetic ketoacidosis, acetoacetate values are often normal or only mildly elevated (AcAc: HBA—1:3). However, sometimes beta-hydroxybutyrate values can be highly elevated (AcAc:HBA—1:30). Under these conditions the nitroprusside test, which does not react with HBA, can underestimate the severity of the ketoacidosis. As ketoacidosis becomes controlled, the beta-hydroxybutyrate is metabolized to acetoacetic acid and the nitroprusside test can become strongly positive. The screening test for ketoacids thus may appear negative when it should be positive and positive when it should be negative. The failure of the screening test to measure the principal

ketoacid constituent may suggest a lab error to an unsuspecting clinician.

Hypoglycemic syndromes

Evaluating a patient with suspected hypoglycemia requires consideration of both the presence of symptoms associated with this condition and the concentration of glucose in the circulation. Patients with glucose values less than 50 mg/dL in males and less than 40 mg/dL in females are prone to produce symptoms.

The increased output of hormones that would tend to reduce hypoglycemia (i.e., glucagon, glucocorticoids, growth hormone, and catecholamines) may be responsible for the clinical manifestations of diaphoresis, tachycardia, tremulousness, and weakness, which are especially prominent when blood glucose values fall rapidly. If blood glucose concentrations fall to values inadequate to support normal metabolism in the CNS, then manifestations of headache, changes in vision, altered mental status, focal neurological deficits, seizures, and ultimately coma and death may ensue. The potential diagnosis of hypoglycemia is supported if the symptoms decrease as blood glucose values return to normal.

Reactive hypoglycemia

The classification of specific disorders as reactive, (occurring between one and five hours after food ingestion) or fasting (occurring more than five hours after the last meal) is important. This distinction gives insight into the pathophysiology of the process. The most common cause of reactive hypoglycemia in adults is a poorly defined syndrome designated as idiopathic, functional, or simply reactive hypoglycemia. Patients develop hypoglycemic symptoms generally two to four hours after a meal. Alimentary hypoglycemia, also known as the dumping syndrome, develops one to three hours after food ingestion. This condition, which results from the rapid entry of gastric contents into the upper intestinal tract, occurs in 5% to 10% of patients who have undergone surgery in the pyloric region. A third form of reaction hypoglycemia occurs early in the course of adult onset diabetes. Most patients are asymptomatic but a few develop characteristic adrenergic symptoms that correlate with the fall in glucose concentration.

Insulinomas/Neoplasia

Fasting hypoglycemias can be caused by insulinomas functioning benign (90%) or malignant (10%) tumors of the beta cells of the islets of Langerhans or rarely by diffusely hyperplastic beta cells. Extra pancreatic non-islet cell neoplasia also occasionally causes hypoglycemia. This has been attributed to ectopic insulin synthesis in a few cases. Hypoglycemia most often occurs through insulin-independent mechanisms, which include consumption of glucose at an excessive rate by large tumors like sarcomas, or production of insulin-like growth factors, somatomedins. In addition, hypoglycemia may be due to the possible elaboration of yet unidentified factors that inhibit hepatic gluconeogenesis and glycogenolysis.

Endocrine disorders

Hypoglycemia can also occur with endocrine deficiencies. Decreased concentrations of the hormones raise blood glucose in the fasting state, including glucocorticoids, primary and secondary adrenal insufficiency and forms of the adrenogenital syndrome, growth hormone, and possibly glucagon. Catecholamine deficiency is not believed to cause hypoglycemia. Other causes include severe liver failure, renal failure, and several uncommon immunologic syndromes. Patients with large amounts of insulin antibodies that arise spontaneously or in response to insulin administration can develop fasting or reactive hypoglycemia that appears to result from sequestration and intermittent release of large amounts of insulin from circulating immune complexes.

Insulin overdose (reaction) in diabetics represents the most common exogenous cause of hypoglycemia, but this is usually not a diagnostic problem. Hypoglycemia from other pharmacologic or toxic agents, however, can be difficult to diagnose and may threaten life. Agents to consider include insulin (administered surreptitiously), oral hypoglycemia agents, ethanol, beta-adrenergic blocking agents, and many other drugs including aspirin and pentamidine.

Inborn errors of carbohydrate metabolism

Disorders of galactose metabolism

There are several disorders of galactose metabolism. The most common is classic galactosemia, in which patients are unable to metabolize galactose. If untreated, the condition is severe enough to cause death. Several less severe conditions are also found to be enzyme defects in the metabolic pathways of galactose metabolism.

Galactosemia is inherited as an autosomal-recessive trait and is caused by a deficiency of the enzyme galactose-1-phosphate uridyl transferase. Patients with this disease appear normal at birth. After a few days of breast feeding, or feeding with milk containing formula, symptoms of diarrhea, vomiting, and dehydration develop. Subsequently, jaundice, hepatomegaly, and abnormal liver function ensue. Eye examination with a slit lamp reveals the development of cataracts within a few days to a few weeks. E. coli or Klebsiella infections may complicate the course of the deficiency.

Some patients present a less dramatic course with hepatomegaly, failure to thrive, progressive cataracts, and developmental delay. These children have milk intolerance due to the disaccharide lactose, which is metabolized to glucose and galactose. Consequently, a reduced galactose and lactose intake is desired to reduce the symptoms.

The diagnosis of galactosemia can be established by measuring galactose-1-phosphate values and uridyl transferase activity. Finding a positive reducing substance in the urine using clinitest—with the copper sulfate reaction—that is not positive in a glucose oxidase dipstick test may be used as a screening procedure.

Elimination of galactose from the diet, by using a lactose-free formula, reverses growth failure and hepatic and renal dysfunction. Cataracts regress and most patients have no impairment of eyesight. Mental retardation is preventable when therapy begins very early, even just after birth. With early detection and treatment the prognosis in galactosemia is excellent. Successful treatment is one of the incentives for neonatal screening for the disease. Neonatal screening is mandatory in many states. The incidence of this disorder is approximately 1 in 60,000.

Galactokinase deficiency

The constellation of symptoms and organs involved in classic galactosemia are not present. Cataract formation is usually the only manifestation of this autosomal recessive trait. The affected infant is otherwise asymptomatic. It presents increased concentration of blood galactose with normal transferase activity in erythrocytes. The treatment of galactokinase deficiency is effective and consists of dietary control of galactose intake. Sources of galactose or lactose are removed from the diet.

Uridine diphosphate galactose-4-epimerase deficiency

This disorder is usually an incidental finding in neonatal screening programs. The defect is limited to leukocytes and erythrocytes, the course is usually benign, and affected persons do not present cataracts, failure to thrive, or other symptoms.

Disorders of pentose metabolism

Pentosuria is an asymptomatic, harmless autosomal recessive metabolic derangement characterized by the excretion of L-xylulose in the urine, due to the absence of the enzyme L-xylulose dehydrogenase. It occurs almost exclusively in people of Jewish ancestry, with an incidence of 1 in 2500 in American Jews. As in fructosuria, pentosuria's only clinical importance is that the presence of this sugar may lead to an erroneous diagnosis of diabetes mellitus. With current specific testing for glucose in urine by glucose oxidase methodology, instead of reducing substance testing, this differentiation should not represent a problem. Treatment is not required in pentosuria.

Disorders of fructose metabolism

These are inherited as autosomal recessive traits. Three types are known.

Essential fructosuria (fructokinase deficiency)

An asymptomatic metabolic anomaly caused by a deficiency of fructokinase activity in the liver, kidney, and intestine. Affected persons are usually discovered when urine is tested for reducing substances. The identification of fructose by thin layer, paper, or gas-liquid chromatography confirms the diagnosis.

Hereditary fructose intolerance (fructose-1-phosphate aldolase deficiency)

The lack of fructose-1-phosphate aldolase in the liver, kidney, and intestine causes the accumulation of fructose-1-phosphate and initiates severe symptoms. Normally the fructose-1-phosphate is hydrolyzed to triose-1-phosphate and glyceraldehyde. Patients with fructose intolerance are healthy and asymptomatic until fructose is ingested either with fruit, fruit juice, or sweetened cereal. When given fructose, the infant becomes acutely ill with vomiting, abdominal pain, sweating, lethergy, and even convulsions. Repeated exposure to fructose leads to hepatosplenomegaly and failure to thrive. The symptoms are accompanied by hypoglycemia, hypophosphatemia, hyperuricemia, hyperfructosemia, fructosuria, elevation of transaminases, and proximal tubular renal dysfunction. Reducing substances in urine are increased during an attack. The diagnosis is supported by an intravenous fructose tolerance test, which causes a rapid fall of serum phosphate followed by a lowering of blood glucose value and a rise in uric acid and magnesium. Definitive diagnosis requires assessment of fructaldolase activity in the liver.

Management of the patient consists of complete elimination of sources of sucrose and fructose from the diet. As the patient matures, symptoms become milder, even after fructose ingestion. The long-term prognosis is good. Liver and kidney dysfunction are reversible and catch-up growth is common. There is no mental retardation.

Fructose 1-6-diphosphate deficiency

This disorder is characterized by life-threatening episodes of lactic acidosis and ketotic hypoglycemia with hyperventilation or apnea. Episodes are triggered in infants when oral food intake is decreased. In this type of fructosuria there is no renal nor liver dysfunction. Treatment consists of avoiding fasting and eliminating fructose and sucrose from the diet. Patients surviving into childhood seem to develop normally.

Disorders of glycogen metabolism

Glycogen storage disease. These are inherited disorders where glycogen is abnormal either in quality or quantity. Virtually all enzymes involved in the degradation or synthesis of glycogen and glucose have been discovered to be causes of glycogen storage disease. (See Figure 8-5.)

Traditionally, glycogen storage diseases have been assigned numerical types in accord with chronologic order of identified enzymatic defects. For simplicity, glucogenoses are grouped as disorders primarily of the liver, muscle, or both. Incidence of glycogenoses is low (less than 1 in 200,000 live births).

Symptoms and signs in glycogen storage diseases are due to accumulation of glycogen or other intermediate metabolites or to the hypoglycemia resulting from the lack of glycogen breakdown. Glycogen can be detected non-invasively by nuclear magnetic resonance. The definitive diagnosis is made by demonstrating the absence of the specific enzyme in a biopsy of the affected tissue.

Liver glycogenoses. Liver glycogenoses present with hepatomegaly and hypoglycemia.

Type Ia (von Gierke disease, glucose-6-phosphatase deficiency). Patients with this disorder convert glycogen to glucose-6-phosphate but cannot produce glucose due to the lack of glucose-6-phosphatase. Patients may demonstrate hypoglycemia in the neonatal period, but more commonly it occurs somewhat later with an enlarged liver and/or hypoglycemic seizures, often at three or four months of age, when nighttime feedings are discontinued or when febrile illness causes a decreased oral food intake. These children usually have protuberant abdomens due to hepatomegaly. They also present with a short stature and thin lower extremities.

A rare form (Type Ib) is due to a defect in the transport of glucose-6-phosphate across the microsomal membrane,

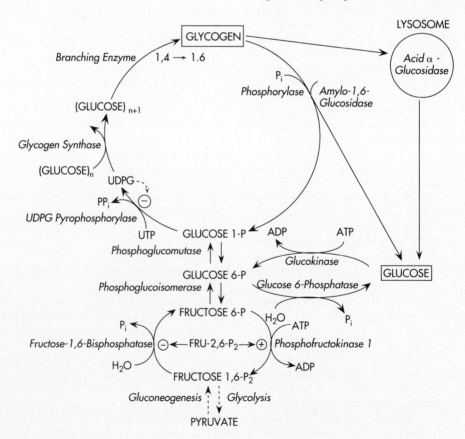

Fig. 8-5 Glycogen and related metabolism in the liver. *From Scriver, CR, et al (eds): The metabolic basis of inherited diseases, ed. 6, vol I, New York, 1989, McGraw-Hill Information Services Co.*

a translocase deficiency. The lack of glucose-6-phosphatase activity or the translocase in the liver leads to a rapid onset of hypoglycemia with fasting because of inadequate production of glucose from glucose-6-phosphate through normal glycogenolysis and gluconeogenesis.

The kidneys are enlarged, but the spleen is of normal size. Xanthoma and diarrhea may be present and nose bleeds (epistaxis) are a frequent problem. As the child grows older, disturbed kidney function is a serious complication. In addition, Type Ib may demonstrate neutropenia and in some cases regional enteritis.

Hypoglycemia, hyperlipidemia, hyperuricemia, and hyperlactenemia are characteristic findings. Hypoglycemia and lactic acidemia occur after a short fast. The administration of glucagon or epinephrine, which are glycogenolysis-promoting compounds, reveals little or no rise in blood glucose.

Treatment of this disorder is aimed at maintaining a normal glucose concentration. For infants less than two years, nocturnal nasogastric infusion of a glucose containing solution, plus frequent diurnal feedings, are part of the treatment. As the child grows older and the amount of amylase increases, uncooked cornstarch every six hours is a good therapy. Allopurinol, a xanthine oxidase inhibitor, is given to control hyperuricemia.

Type VI (liver phosphorylase deficiency, Hers' disease) and Type IX (liver phosphorylase kinase deficiency). Both are benign forms of glycogenoses. The clinical manifestations resemble Type I but are much milder. Growth retardation and hepatomegaly are usually seen in childhood. Hypoglycemia occurs only after a longer fast and is not as severe as in other types. Treatment is symptomatic with high complex carbohydrate diet and frequent feedings to maintain normal blood glucose values. Patients attain adulthood with normal stature and minimal hepatomegaly. Family studies suggest an X-linked inheritance in many cases of liver phospharylase kinase deficiency.

Muscle glycogenoses

Type V (muscle phosphorylase deficiency, McArdle disease). This is usually manifested in adolescence or early adult life by cramps or exercise with no rise in lactic acid values. Muscle wasting is not a prominent feature but may occur in older patients. There is no cardiac involvement. Myoglobinuria due to injury to skeletal muscle may occur after severe exercise.

A congenital myopathy and a fatal infantile form of this disease has been described. Most patients with the disease are men, although it is an autosomal recessive disorder. It is not clear whether this is due to men being likely to engage in strenuous physical activity or some other, unknown factor.

The diagnosis is supported by an abnormal ischemic exercise test during which patients have characterisitic forearm "contraction" and no rise in lactate concentration. Definitive diagnosis requires a muscle biopsy and enzyme assay to demonstrate a reduced phosphorylase value. There has been no consistently effective treatment.

Generalized glycogenoses. Glycogen is stored in most tissues, and the clinical expression in some forms of the disorder is more widespread, involving many organ systems.

Type II (alpha-1,4-glucosidase deficiency, Pompe's disease). Infantile, juvenile, and adult forms have been de-

scribed. In the infantile form, infants appear normal at birth but soon develop generalized muscle weakness, poor feeding, hepatomegaly, macroglosia, and congestive heart failure. In severely affected infants, enzyme activity is generally undetectable. Light microscopy demonstrates a vacuolar myopathy with storage of glycogen; with electron microscopy the glycogen accumulation is seen within the membranous sac and in the sarcoplasm. Patients with juvenile and adult forms usually present with a myopathy but the heart is rarely affected.

Laboratory findings include elevation of blood creatine kinase and lactic dehydrogenase. Electromyography reveals myopathic features with excessive electric irritability of muscle fibers and pseudomyotonic discharges. No effective treatment is available. Death from cardiorespiratory failure or aspiration pneumonia usually occurs before the age of two in the infantile form. Patients with the adult form who have reduced diaphragmatic function may need nocturnal ventilatory support.

Type III (Debrancher deficiency, limit dextrinosis, Forbes' disease). In this form of glycogenoses, a saccharide resembling the structure of limit dextran accumulates. This saccharide is a glycogen with short outer branch chains. Patients with this disease may present as adults with chronic myopathy. Most patients have both muscle and liver involvement. They show hypoglycemia, hepatomegaly, muscle weakness, and growth retardation. Progressive muscle weakness and cardiomyopathy may also occur.

In childhood, hypoglycemia, hyperlipidemia, and elevation of transaminases may be present. Heptomegaly and hypoglycemia diminish with age, and by puberty patients may have normal liver size and normal stature. Progressive myopathy, however, is a major concern in some older patients.

Treatment in children is symptomatic and aimed at maintaining normal glucose values with a high carbohydrate diet and cornstarch supplement.

Type IV (Branching enzyme deficiency, amylopectinosis, or Andersen's disease). Abnormally structured glycogen with unbranched long outer chains accumulates in various tissues. Progressive cirrhosis with splenomegaly occurs, usually leading to death before five years of age. The disease may also present with neuromuscular symptoms consisting of hypotomia, decreased or absent deep tendon reflexes, muscle atrophy, and cardiomyopathy. There is no specific treatment.

A summary of the main characteristics of the glycogenoses and the enzyme systems affected are listed in Table 8-1.

Muscle glycogenoses associated with hemolytic anemia. These include generalized deficiencies of glucose phosphate isomerase and triose phosphate isomerase. Deficiencies of muscle isoenzymes of phosphofructokinase, phosphoglycerate kinase, phosphoglyceromutase, and lactate dehydrogenase are found in some forms of the disorder. All are associated with non-spherocytic hemolytic anemia.

Analyte measurement and function testing

Glucose measurement. Both blood and urine have been traditionally used as specimens for the diagnosis of diabetes. Due to the presence of sugar in urine, it was observed by Hindu physicians of early times that urine from patients

Table 8-1 Characteristics of the glycogenoses

Type	Enzyme system affected	Organs involved	Clinical symptoms	Eponym
O	UDPG-glycogen transferase	Liver, muscle	Large fatty liver, fasting hypoglycemia	—
Ia	Glucose-6-phosphatase	Liver, kidney	Large liver & kidney; growth retardation; severe hypoglycemia; acidosis; hyperlipemia; hyperuricemia	von Gierke
Ib	Glucose-6-phosphatase	Liver, leukocytes	As above but less severe; neutropenia, recurrent GI infections	—
II	Lysosomal glucosidase (various types)	All organs	Large liver & heart; no abnormal blood chemistry	Pompe
III	Debrancher enzyme system	Liver, muscle, heart, leukocytes	Enlarged liver, fasting hypoglycemia, variable muscle involvement	Forbes'
IV	Brancher enzyme system	Liver, muscle, & most tissues	Progressive cirrhosis in juvenile type; myopathy & heart failure in late-onset type	Andersen
V	Muscle phosphorylase	Skeletal muscle	Cramps on exercise with no rise in blood lactate	McArdle
VI	Liver phosphorylase	Liver	Enlarged liver, fasting hypoglycemia but often no symptoms at all	Hers'
VII	Phosphofructokinase	Skeletal muscle erythrocytes	Cramps on exercise but no rise in blood lactate, hemolysis	Tarui

VIII, IX, X: Rare disorders involving various components of the liver phosphorylase activating-deactivating cascade

with a tendency to "boils" attracted ants when disposed outdoors. This probably represents the first urinalysis for "sugar." More scientific methods start with the idea of taking advantage of the reducing properties of some sugars to include glucose and its ability to transform cupric ions (Cu^{+2}) to monovalent cuprous (Cu^{+}). In the presence of heat, the reduced cuprous ions can produce cuprous oxide (Cu_2O), which can be detected in a variety of ways. One of the most popular methods in the past, the Folin-Wu method, utilized a phosphomolybdate containing reagent. Several other methods, like the Somogyi-Nelson and Neocuproine methods, were successfully used, but they lack specificity since several sugars and other non-carbohydrate reducing substances can produce positive results. These procedures are no longer used to detect glucose, and they are mentioned only for their historical interest. Benedicts modification of the copper-reducing methods is still marketed by the Ames Division of Miles Laboratories (Elkhart, Ind.) as Clinitest. This procedure, sensitive to reducing substances in urine, yields red Cu_2O and yellow CuOH precipitates. The greater the concentration of sugar, the redder the color. Currently Clinitest is used in combination with a more specific enzymatic assay (glucose oxidase). When dealing with a pediatric patient, a Benedict reaction is useful in screening for genetic disorders of carbohydrate metabolism, like galactosemia. A negative glucose oxidase color reaction in urine, coupled with a positive Clinitest, is indicative of the presence of other reducing sugars, predominantly galactose, which can be confirmed by thin layer chromatography or other enzymatic methods.

The most common procedures for glucose analysis use enzymatic reaction to increase analytical specificity. (Table 8-2). One of the most frequently used assays is the glucose oxidase method, which uses two coupled enzyme reactions. In this combination, the initial enzymatic reaction is specific, and the indicator reaction is nonspecific.

$$\text{Glucose} + O_2 \xrightarrow{\text{GO}} \text{Glucuronic acid} + H_2O_2$$

The hydrogen peroxide formed by the glucose oxidase reaction is consumed by a peroxide-dye indicator reaction in which the oxidized dye is colored and as such can be measured quantitatively in a spectrophotometer. The enzyme involved in this second portion of the assay sequence on glucose analysis is catalyzed by horseradish peroxidase (HPO) and is not specific, allowing for a variety of indicators to be used, among them 4-amino phenazone, 3-methyl-2-benzothiazolin hydrazone/N, N-dimethylaniline (MBTA/DMA) and o-dianisidine.

The coupled glucose oxidase procedure has been adapted to many automated instruments and to urine dipsticks. The Ames strip employs the oxidation of iodine to monitor the peroxidase reaction:

$$\text{Glucose} + O_2 \longrightarrow \text{glucuronic acid} + H_2O_2$$
$$H_2O_2 + 2KI \longrightarrow I_2 \text{ (brown)} + 2KOH$$

These strips can be read visually or by reflectance photometry for a semiquantitive analysis.

Other ways to detect the coupled glucose oxidase reaction use chromophore to attenuate the fluorescence of fluorescein. However, these techniques are somewhat costly and not yet widely used.

Tolerance function testing
Glucose challenge

Early treatment of gestational diabetes mellitus (GDM) has been proven to reduce neonatal risk. Consequently, early detection is desirable and since GDM is asymptomatic, a systematic screening program for its detection is justifiable. Glucose intolerance is more prevalent in the second and third trimesters of pregnancy, so screening should be done at 24 to 28 weeks gestation. The recommended procedure,

Table 8-2 Clinically useful methods of glucose analysis*

Methods	Type of analysis	Principle	Usage	Comments
1. Benedict's	Qualitative, semi-quantitative	$Cu^{+2} + Glucose \xrightarrow[OH^-]{Heat}$ $Cu_2O \downarrow + CuOH \downarrow$ $(red) \quad (yellow)$	Basis of semiquantitative tests for total reducing sugars in *urine*	Used in combination with more specific glucose oxidase/peroxidase urine screen to differentiate glucosuria from other sugars in urine, especially in neonates
2. Alkaline ferricyanide	Quantitative, EP	$Fe(CN)_6^{-3} \xrightarrow[Glucose]{Heat, OH^-} Fe(CN)_6^{-4}$ (ferricyanide) (ferrocyanide) (yellow) (colorless) Decreased absorbance at 420 nm because of consumption of ferricyanide	Rarely used, sometimes seen in Technicon systems; of historical interest	1 mg of creatinine = 1 mg of glucose; 0.5 mg of uric acid = 1 mg of glucose; very poor specificity
3. *o*-Toluidine	Quantitative, EP	Increased absorbance at 630 nm	Serum or urine; rarely used in automated analysis	*o*-Toluidine is a suspected carcinogen; other sugars, especially mannose and galactose, give positive interferences; turbidity can cause a positive bias

O-Toluidine + B-D-Glucose ⟶ Glycosamine (colored)

Enzymatic

Methods	Type of analysis	Principle	Usage	Comments
4. Hexokinase (HK)	Quantitative, spectrophotometric, EP	$Glucose + ATP \xrightarrow{HK}$ $Glucose\text{-}6\text{-}phosphate + ADP$ $Glucose\text{-}6\text{-}phosphate + NADP^+$ $\xrightleftharpoons{G6PD}$ $6\text{-}Phosphogluconate +$ $NADPH + H^+$ Increased absorbance at 340 nm related to glucose concentration	Serum, CSF, urine; automated; most commonly used method	Has been proposed as basis of reference method; very good accuracy and precision
5a. Glucose oxidase coupled reaction ("Trinder")	Quantitative, using various types of dyes as final O₂ acceptor; K or EP	$Glucose + O_2 \xrightarrow{Glucose\ oxidase}$ $Gluconic\ acid + H_2O_2$ $H_2O_2 + Reduced\ dye \xrightleftharpoons[peroxidase]{Horseradish}$ (colorless) $Oxidized\ dye + H_2O$ (colored) Peroxidase indicator reaction Increased absorbance related to glucose concentration	Serum, urine, CSF; easily and usually adapted to automated analysis	Second indicator reaction susceptible to false-positive interferences from a variety of compounds; good accuracy and precision
	Quantitative or semiquantitative in dipstick screen, visual or reflectance photometry		Used in all dipstick screens; serum, urine	
5b. Glucose oxidase (GO) oxygen consumption	Quantitative, polarographic measurement using O₂ electrode, K	$Glucose + O_2 \xrightarrow{Glucose\ oxidase}$ $Gluconic\ acid + H_2O_2$ H_2O_2 consumed in side reactions O₂ consumption measured polarographically by oxygen electrode	Serum, CSF; semiautomated and fully automated systems	Correlates best with proposed reference method; very good accuracy and precision
6. Radiation energy attenuation	Quantitative, EP	Reaction described in method 5a is used; chromogen absorbs light used to excite fluor or absorbs fluorescent light itself; glucose concentration related to attenuation of fluorescence	Rare, serum	Used only on TDx automated assay
7. Glucose dehydrogenase	Quantitative, EP, K	$Glucose + NAD^+ \xrightarrow{GDH}$ $\text{D-}Gluconolactone +$ $NADH + H^+$ Increased absorbance at 340 nm related to glucose concentration	Rare, serum, CSF	Can be adapted to automated instruments

From Kaplan LA and Pesce AJ: Clinical chemistry: theory, analysis, and correlation, ed 2, St. Louis, 1989, Mosby-Year Book, Inc.
*EP = End-point analysis mode; K = kinetic analysis mode; CSF = cerebrospinal fluid; GDH = glucose dehydrogenase; GGPD glucose-6-phosphate dehydrogenase.

sometimes called a "glucose challenge" or the O'Sullivan test, is to give the patient a 50 gm glucose load and measure plasma glucose one hour after ingestion. The test can be given any time of day without regard to previous meals. A positive result is a plasma glucose of greater than 150 mg/dL (83% sensitivity and 87% specificity). A positive screening test should be followed by an oral glucose tolerance test (OGTT) to confirm the diagnosis.

Oral glucose tolerance test (OGTT). The OGTT, although still used by clinicians, is not as frequently requested now as in the past. The National Diabetes Data Group has proposed a standard set of criteria for use in the diagnosis of diabetes mellitus. According to these criteria, no OGTT would be necessary if fasting blood glucose is greater than 140 mg/dL or if the two hour post prandial is 200 mg/dL or greater.

An oral glucose tolerance test is indicated in the following situations:

1. Diagnosis of gestational diabetes
2. Further evaluation of borderline elevations of fasting or post prandial blood sugar
3. Risk counseling in an individual with previously abnormal glucose tolerance test
4. Evaluations of patients with unexplained retinopathy, nephropathy, or neuropathy, which are usually seen in diabetes
5. The evaluation of post-prandial hypoglycemia (usually extended to five to six hours in this case)

When a glucose-tolerance test is ordered, the following conditions should be met:

1. It should be performed in the morning, after three days of unrestricted diet containing at least 100 gm of carbohydrates and normal activity.
2. The patient should fast for at least 10 hours (10 to 16 hours).
3. Plasma glucose should be measured during fasting and every 30 minutes for 2 hours after a glucose load of 75 gm (for adults) and 1.75 gm/kg for children, up to 75 gm total. In pregnancy, if used to confirm GDM, a 100 gm glucose load is used.

Several factors affect the glucose-tolerance test, including carbohydrate intake, length of fasting, prior GI surgery and malabsorption conditions, age, inactivity, weight, and stress. Some medications are also known to affect glucose tolerance, such as thiazides, estrogens, dilantin, propanolol, and cortisol.

The test is considered positive when the sum of the fasting one hour, two hour, and three hour plasma glucose is greater than or equal to 600 mg/dL.

Intravenous glucose tolerance test (IVGTT)

Patients unable to tolerate an oral glucose load because of vomiting, gastric surgery, or other causes may require an IV glucose tolerance test.

The dose of glucose should be 0.5 gm/kg of body weight and should be given as a 25 gm/dL solution administered intravenously within a three-minute period. Blood is drawn for glucose before infusion and at one, three, five, 10, 20, 40, 60, and 120 minutes. Glucose disappearance constants (K values) are calculated from a plot of the log of the glucose concentration in relationship to time. A K value of 1.2 is considered diagnostic of diabetes mellitus. This test is not as reliable as the oral GTT information 40% of the time. Because of this and lack of standardization, IVGTT is not a commonly used diagnostic tool.

Time averaged testing

Glycosylated hemoglobin. Determining stable, glucose ketoamine complexes of hemoglobin provides an assessment of the timed-averaged control of the plasma glucose concentration for the preceeding eight to 12 weeks.

In normal adults, hemoglobin typically consists of HbA (97%) of total HbA_2 (2.5%) and HbF (0.5%). Chromatography of HbA shows that a number of fast-migrating hemoglobins can be identified as HbA_{1a}, HbA_{1b}, and HbA_{1c}. Collectively, they are referred as HbA_1, "fast hemoglobins," glycosylated hemoglobins, glycated hemoglobins, or simple glycohemoglobins.

Hemoglobin A_{1c} is formed by the condensation between glucose and N-terminal valine amino acid of each beta chain to form an unstable Schiff base (aldimine), which then undergoes an Amadori rearrangement to form a stable ketoamine (Figure 8-6).

The formation of glycohemoglobin is a nonenzymatic process and occurs over the 120-day life span of the erythrocyte. The amount of glycosylation is determined by the glucose concentration present over the two or three months before obtaining the plasma sample. It provides the clinician with a means for judging control of diabetes in a new patient or when urine glucose recoveries are inadequate. It covers a longer span of assessment of the blood glucose as compared to specific blood glucose analysis on the day of ex-

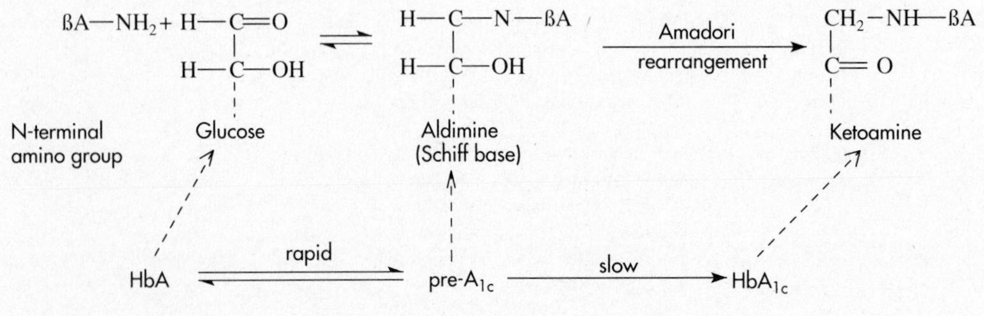

Fig. 8-6 Formation of Hb A_{1c}. Hb A_{1c}. Hb A_{1c} is the major fraction of the "fast hemoglobins." *From Tietz N: Textbook of clinical chemistry, Philadelphia, 1986, WB Saunders Co.*

amination, which can be manipulated by a noncompliant patient.

Non-enzymatic attachment of sugars to amino acid groups in proteins other than hemoglobin also occurs. In the case of albumin, the half-life of this glycation is about 19 days and monitoring of glycosylated albumin would provide a more recent time averaging of the blood glucose (Table 8-3).

Fructosamine

The monitoring of other glycated serum protein fractions, fructosamines, has been suggested as a way to monitor glucose control in diabetic patients. The HbA$_{1c}$ monitors control over a two- to three-month period and the fructosamine levels provide a measure of short-term control for a period of one to three weeks.

The analytical method takes advantage of the ability of fructosamines to reduce nitrotetrazolium blue (NTB) at an alkaline pH. The normal reference range for nondiabetic patients is 2.14 to 2.75 mmol/L (mean 2.4 mmol/L). Diabetic patients have values approximately 50% higher.

Related protein measurements

Insulin. Insulin was the first protein hormone to have its amino acid sequence completely determined. It was the first substance to be measured by radioimmunoassay, and the first compound produced artificially by recombinate DNA techiques. Insulin release is stimulated by glucose, amino acids, other pancreatic and gastrointestinal hormones, and some medications (e.g., sulfonylureas and beta-adrenergic stimulators such as isoproterenol. Insulin release is inhibited by hypoglycemia, somatostatin produced in the pancreatic delta cells, and a variety of drugs that are beta-adrenergic stimulators. Insulin is degraded by the liver and the kidney. The half-life of insulin in the circulation is between five and 10 minutes. Insulin is produced as a prohormone. Proinsulin is stored in secretory granules in the Golgi complex, where proteolytic cleavage to insulin and C-peptide occurs.

RIA has become the technique of choice for measuring insulin in biologic fluids. Various RIA methods and commercial kits are available.

The antibody is produced against porcine insulin in guinea pigs, since porcine and human insulin react identically. Samples and dilutions of an insulin standard are incubated with antiserum and ^{125}I-insulin. Antibody-bound insulin is then separated, and the radioactivity of this fraction

is determined. The amount of insulin in the sample is calculated by comparing the percent of bound radioactivity in the sample with the standard curve.

C-peptide. Proinsulin is enzymatically cleaved to insulin by removing a 32-amino acid connecting peptide between the A and B peptide chains of insulin called C-peptide. C-peptide does not have a role in carbohydrate metabolism. C-peptide and insulin are secreted in equimolecular amounts. Because of the longer half-life (by about 20 minutes) of C-peptide, the concentration of C-peptide is greater than that of insulin in circulating blood.

C-peptide determinations in blood or urine are useful in assessing beta cell function in the presence of exogenous insulin or circulating antibodies to insulin. Exogenous insulin as a synthetic product contains no C-peptide, and insulin elevations without corresponding C-peptide increase would indicate external sources of insulin.

The primary diagnostic use of C-peptide measurement is in patients with fasting hypoglycemia and suspected insulin-producing, beta-cell tumor in which both the insulin and the C-peptide are elevated. In surreptitious hypoglycemia cases due to exogenous administration of insulin, the C-peptide will remain low. The reference interval for C-peptide as measured by RIA is 0.5 to 2.0 mg/mL.

Glucagon. Glucagon increases blood glucose by stimulating glycogenolysis in the liver. It has no effect on muscle glycogen. Glucagon is produced by the alpha cells of the pancreatic islets of Langerhans. Glucagon is elevated in cases of tumors of the alpha cells of the islets of Langerhans which tend to be malignant and prone to metastasize.

The diagnosis of glucagonoma is established by the appearance of symptoms and a plasma glucagon level exceeding 500 pg/mL. The clinical symptoms include migratory necrolytic erythema in the face and extremities and in areas associated with friction, such as groin and buttocks; substantial weight loss; and a mild, easily controlled hyperglycemia.

Somatostatin. This is a tetradecapeptide initially isolated from hypothalamic tissue and later also found in the gastrointestinal tract. In addition, somatostatin can be localized in endocrine-like and paracrine-like cells in the pancreatic islets and in the mucosa of stomach and intestine. Somatostatin inhibits acid and pepsin secretion by the stomach while stimulating gastric mucus secretion. Somatostatin inhibits gastrin release from the G cells in the gastric antrum. Somatostatin also inhibits the release of other gastrointestinal

Table 8-3 Comparison of methods for glycohemoglobin analysis

Method	Coefficient of variation (%)	Temperature dependence of separation	pH dependence of separation	Assay time of one sample	Interferences
HPLC (ion exchange)	3	Significant	Significant	10-20 min*	Hb F
Minicolumn ion exchange	2-16	Significant	Significant	20-40 min†	Hb F
Minicolumn affinity	1-3	Negligible	Minor	15-30 min†	None
Electrophoresis	4-10	Negligible	Minor	20-45 min†	Hb F
Colorimetric	4-18	‡	‡	hours†	None

From Pesce AJ and Kaplan LA: Methods in clinical chemistry, St. Louis, 1987, Mosby-Year Book, Inc.
*Samples cannot be batched.
†Samples can be batched.
‡No hemoglobin separation step.

peptides including secretin, cholecystokinin (CCK), gastric inhibitory peptide (GIP), motilin, enteroglucagon, pancreatic polypeptide (PP), insulin, and glucagon.

A few years after the discovery of somatostatin, pancreatic tumors containing somatostatin-like material were found in association with high-circulating concentrations of this hormone in the blood. Somatostatin may also be secreted ectopically by a variety of neoplasms including medullary carcinoma of the thyroid, oat cell carcinoma of the lung, and bronchial carcinoids. The pancreatic tumor may also secrete adenocorticotropic hormone and calcitonin.

The symptomatology of somatostatinoma are related to inhibition of insulin and glucogen secretion, and a mild hyperglycemia is usually present. Delayed gastric emptying and inhibition of gastric secretion produce dyspensia and achlorhydria. Gallbladder contraction is also inhibited, which, together with inhibition of pancreatic juice secretion, can lead to diarrhea and steatorrhea.

The diagnosis of somatostatinoma requires a very high suspicion index and familiarity with the symptomatology of this process. Unfortunately, most cases are diagnosed when evidence of metastasis to liver, skin, or bone are the presenting signs, and only palliative chemotherapy is the management of choice.

SUGGESTED READING

Bouriotis V, Stolt J, Galloway A, et al: Measurement of glycosylated hemoglobins using affinity chromatography, Diabetologia 21:579-580, 1981.

Charles MA, Hofeldt F, Shakelford A, et al: Comparison of oral glucose tolerance tests and mixed meals in patients with apparent idiopathic postabsorptive hypoglycemia. Absence of hypoglycemia after meals. Diabetes 30:465-470, 1981.

Dolhofer R, and Wieland OH: Increased glycosylation of serum albumin in diabetes mellitus, Diabetes 29:417-422, 1980.

Fajans SS and Floyd JC Jr: Fasting hypoglycemia in adults, N Eng J Med 294:766-772, 1976.

Gordon P, Hendricks CM, Kahn CR, et al: Hypoglycemia associated with non-islet-cell tumor and insulin-like growth factors, N Eng J Med 305:1452-1455, 1981.

Horwits DL, Kuzuya H, and Rubenstein AH: Circulating serum C peptide: a brief review of diagnostic implications, N Eng J Med 295:207-209, 1976.

James TM, Davis JE, McDonald JM, et al: Comparison of hemoglobin A_{1c} and hemoglobin A1 in diabetic patients, Clinical Biochem 14:25-27, 1981.

Johnson DD, Dorr KE, Swenson SM, et al: Reactive hypoglycemia, JAMA 243:1151-1155, 1980.

Kaplan LA and Pesce AJ, Clinical chemistry: theory analysis and correlation, ed 2, St. Louis, 1989, Mosby-Year Book, Inc.

National Diabetes Data Group: Classification and diagnosis of diabetes mellitus and other categories of glucose intolerance, Diabetes 28:1039, 1979.

Olefsky JM: Insulin resistence and insulin action, Diabetes 30:148-162, 1981.

Pryor TW, Chapman JF, and Bankson DD: Sensitivity of serum fructosamine in short term glycemic control, Ann Clin Lab Sci 19:107, 1989.

Tietz NW, ed: Textbook of clinical chemistry, Philadelphia, 1986, WB Saunders Co.

9 Lipids

Donald Wiebe

There are a wide variety of natural chemicals produced by living organisms. Most of these chemicals are soluble in water, such as peptides, enzymes, and carbohydrate metabolites. However, lipids are natural products that are *not* soluble in water (aqueous media) but are readily soluble in organic solvents such as alcohol, chloroform, hexane, and diethyl ether. Lipids include a variety of compounds that have different metabolic or physiologic functions but share the characteristic of limited solubility in water.

Lipid compounds are commonly referred to as fat and generally fat is thought of as something to avoid. "Fat" is a term that generates negative thoughts, especially relative to physical appearance and certain disease states. However, fats and lipid compounds are necessary for life. Cells could not function properly without the presence of lipids.

This chapter is organized first to introduce specific lipid compounds that have significant metabolic roles and have become routine analytes in clinical laboratories for diagnostic purposes. Next, lipoproteins are discussed and both exogenous and endogenous metabolic pathways show the role of lipoproteins. Finally, apolipoproteins are introduced and discussed as proteins that control the fate of individual lipoproteins or lipid molecules. In addition, analytical methods available to clinical laboratories for the measurement of lipids, lipoproteins, and apolipoproteins are presented.

LIPID CLASSES

The importance of lipids was recognized in medicine long before laboratory analyses were available for measuring individual lipid compounds. Total lipid content of serum or other biological specimens were determined by extracting lipids from serum or plasma with organic solvents, such as chloroform/methanol, and reporting the weight of the extractable material versus the volume of fluid extracted. Sterols (cholesterol), triglycerides, phospholipids, and fatty acids are the four major classes of lipids. Laboratory methods are generally available to analyze these compounds.

Cholesterol

Cholest-5-en-3β-ol (cholesterol) belongs to a group of 3β hydroxy sterols that share the same basic steroid structure. Mixtures of 3β hydroxy sterols can be isolated from plant tissue and fish but cholesterol is the principal sterol in higher forms of life. In man, cholesterol is present in all body tissues and most cells can synthesize cholesterol. (Erythrocytes, red cells, are an exception.) Cholesterol can be isolated from biological specimens in two forms: the free hydroxyl form and as cholestryl esters. Cholesterol esters have long-chain fatty acids attached to cholesterol through the hydroxyl group by an ester linkage. Serum and biological specimens contain a higher percentage of cholesterol esters (75%-85%) than free cholesterol (15%-25%).

The physiologic role of cholesterol can be divided into two components: a cellular membrane structure and a metabolic precursor for other biological steroids. Cholesterol is one of the major constituents of cellular membranes. It is easy to understand the importance of cholesterol and other lipids in cellular membranes because of their limited solubility in water. Cellular membranes must control the flow of water soluble product in and out of cells and lipids help to serve this need. Thus, small molecules or ions like sodium, potassium, and chloride that are present in different concentrations within and outside the cells can be maintained. Yet larger molecules, such as glucose, are also capable of passing through the cellular membranes to be metabolized. The other major function of cholesterol is as a metabolic precursor for other biological steroids which meet the physiologic requirements to generate small quantities of female and male sex steroids (estrogens and androgens), adrenal steroids (aldosterone and corticosterone), and bile acids. Specific cells in the ovaries, testes, adrenal, and liver that function to synthesize these steroids utilize cholesterol as the primary precursor.

Triglycerides

"Triacylglycerols" is a more descriptive term for these compounds that are derived from mixtures of long-chain fatty acids esterified to glycerol. Triglyceride is the major component of glycerides (mono-, di-, and triglycerides) in circulating blood and tissues with only minor amounts of di- and monoglycerides.

Human bodies store energy very efficiently and triglycerides are the primary constituents used for long-term energy storage. A gram of triglyceride oxidized to CO_2 and H_2O produces 9 kcal of energy as compared to 4 kcal from a gram of glycogen. Adipose tissue can intercellularly store triglycerides as concentrated fat droplets. Some tissues, such as heart muscle, rely on long-chain fatty acid oxidation as their main source of energy. Therefore, triglyceride metabolism is a key component of man's ability to store and derive energy for many of the body's functions. The primary source of triglycerides is from the diet. Diets high in fat and carbohydrates will usually present weight problems. However, since the ability to process triglycerides for storage is so efficient, the short-term effect of diet may not be reflected in a fasting serum triglyceride concentration.

Phospholipids

Structurally, phospholipids (phosphoglycerides) are similar to triglycerides. Both compounds utilize glycerol and long-chain fatty acids within their basic structure. Phosphatidic acid, a 1,2 diacylglycerol with a phosphate group attached to the free, nonesterified hydroxyl group, is the key structural variation from triglycerides. Other alcohol-functional compounds are esterified through the phosphate group to form a family of phospholipids. Alcohol-functional compounds associated with phospholipids include ethanolamine, choline, serine, and inositol. As a result of this association, phospholipids usually are charged, polar compounds with both hydrophobic and hydrophilic characteristics. Therefore, phospholipids provide an ideal interface between nonpolar lipids and highly polar water molecules.

Phospholipids are one of the principal components of cellular membranes. Having both hydrophobic and hydrophilic properties makes phospholipids ideal for the task. Scientific studies have been performed to determine the impact on the fluidity of cellular membranes with specific phospholipids. Such studies have included changing the fatty acids from saturated to polyunsaturated within the phospholipids and analyzing the alterations in membrane properties.

Fatty acids

Nonesterified free fatty acids are a minor constituent in circulating plasma lipids or tissue stores. However, fatty acids are an integral part of most lipids through ester bonds. The length of natural fatty acids ranges from 14 to 22 carbon atoms (including the carboxylic acid carbon) and only fatty acids with an even number of carbon atoms occur naturally in mammals. Fatty acids are grouped according to the absence or presence of double bonds in the chain. Saturated fatty acids have no double bonds and are the primary fatty acid in animal tissues. Monounsaturated fatty acids contain one double bond, whereas polyunsaturated fatty acids have two or more double bonds. Plants are an excellent source of polyunsaturated fatty acids. Polyunsaturated fatty acids, essential for mammals, are required dietary components since man cannot synthesize these fatty acids.

The primary physiologic function of long-chain fatty acids is to provide energy to cells and muscle tissue by an oxidative process referred to as β-oxidation. Fatty acids are oxidized sequentially, generating one acetyl-CoA for each cycle. The starting fatty acid is reduced by a two-carbon fragment from the carboxyl terminal end, or the beta position along the fatty acid. For example, the complete oxidation of palmitic acid, which has a chain length of 16 carbon atoms, will generate eight acetyl-CoA molecules. Acetyl-

Table 9-1 Lipoprotein terminology

Electrophoretic mobility	Ultracentrifuge fractions
Chylomicron	Chylomicron
Pre-beta	Very Low Density Lipoprotein
Beta	Low Density Lipoprotein
Alpha	High Density Lipoprotein

CoA will enter the tricarboxylic acid cycle and ultimately be further oxidized to CO_2 and H_2O. Considerable energy is generated by β-oxidation of fatty acids and half the energy released can be used by the cells to perform their functions. The remainder of energy released is in the form of heat. Essential fatty acids are necessary precursors for prostaglandins that play an important role in clot formation and several other physiologic functions.

LIPOPROTEIN CLASSES

Lipid compounds must be capable of movement from cell-to-cell or tissue-to-tissue to meet their physiologic function. In order to transport lipid material in the aqueous environment, the lipid must be bound to specific proteins to form lipoproteins. Lipoproteins are composites of lipid and protein that provide solubility characteristics in aqueous media that enable the occurrence of lipid movement and metabolism. Lipoproteins have a spherical shape with neutral lipid (triglycerides and cholesterol esters) at the center surrounded by free cholesterol, phospholipids, and proteins on the surface. Specific proteins (apolipoproteins) are associated with lipoproteins that have both hydrophilic and hydrophobic characteristics, such that part of the apolipoprotein prefers an aqueous environment while the other portion wants to interact with lipid material. In general, the primary function of the lipoproteins is to provide a mechanism for intracellular transport.

Nomenclature for lipoproteins has been operationally based on the methods used to isolate the lipoproteins. Therefore, if electrophoresis is used for separation, the individual lipoprotein families are classified by their electrophoretic mobility relative to serum protein mobility. Chylomicrons, triglyceride-rich lipoproteins, do not migrate from the point of sample application and therefore are not classified by mobility. Ultracentrifugation separates lipoproteins on the basis of density. Table 9-1 compares the nomenclature based on electrophoretic mobility with ultracentrifugation terminology for the various lipoprotein classes.

Lipoprotein families usually are referred to by the initials from ultracentrifugation—VLDL, LDL and HDL. Chylomicrons are the exception. This family of lipoproteins has a density less than that of serum (<1.006 g/mL). The nomenclature based on the method of separation may seem difficult to remember as opposed to names that relate to function. The system becomes further complicated because each lipoprotein family represents a mixture of lipoprotein complexes that have similar characteristics. For example, HDL may be further subdivided into HDL-2 and HDL-3 fractions. Similarly, investigators are beginning to explore the heterogeniety of LDL by size and composition. The composition of lipoprotein classes is presented in Table 9-2.

Table 9-2   Lipoprotein composition

Lipoprotein	Density*	Chol (%)	TG (%)	PL (%)	Prot (%)
Chylomicron	0.95	4	85	9	2
VLDL	0.97-1.006	19	50	18	10
IDL	1.006-1.019	?	?	?	?
LDL	1.019-1.063	45	10	20	23
HDL	1.063-1.120	17	4	24	55

*Ultracentrifugation density (g/mL)
Chol = cholesterol, TG = triglycerides, PL = phospholipids, Prot = proteins

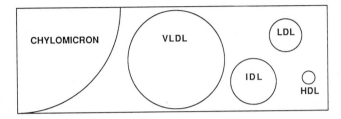

Fig. 9-1   Relative sizes of lipoproteins.

Density is related to both triglyceride and protein content of the lipoprotein class. Lower densities are associated with increased content of triglycerides and decreased amounts of protein. Size is also useful in distinguishing lipoprotein classes (see Figure 9-1).

Lipoprotein metabolism

A discussion of lipoprotein metabolism must be divided into two separate but related topics. The first focuses on exogenous metabolism and deals with lipids and lipoproteins derived from outside sources—food and nutrients. The second topic concerns endogenous metabolism which involves lipid and lipoproteins derived from the normal biological process of living cells using acetyl-CoA to synthesize complex lipid compounds in the liver and other tissues.

Exogenous metabolism

In the typical American diet, fat accounts for about 40% of calories, with protein and carbohydrate contributing the remainder. As the food passes into the stomach, pancreatic digestive enzymes (amylase, peptidases, and lipases) are released and activated to reduce complex molecules to metabolites that are readily absorbed. Fats (triglycerides) are hydrolyzed by lipases to free fatty acids and monoglycerides that can be absorbed through the intestinal cell lining (intestinal mucosal cells). Once inside these cells, the free fatty acids and monoglycerides are used to synthesize triglycerides and phospholipids. These newly formed lipids are packaged into large triglyceride-rich lipoprotein complexes, chylomicrons, that are passed into the lymph as an interstitial fluid. Chylomicron containing lymph enters the circulating blood through the thoracic duct. Absorption of dietary triglycerides occurs rapidly following a meal and peak serum triglyceride concentrations can be observed in serum within 30 to 90 minutes. After the triglyceride-rich chylomicrons enter circulation, they interact with lipoprotein lipase, an enzyme bound to the capillary surface of the blood vessel walls. The function of lipoprotein lipase is to hydrolyze the triglyceride to fatty acids and glycerides. These metabolites are readily absorbed by the cells to which the enzyme is bound. Once inside the cell, the hydrolyzed products are resynthesized to triglyceride for energy storage. Repeated lypolytic action upon the chylomicron reduces the triglyceride content of the lipoprotein, leaving a chylomicron remnant that is rapidly cleared from the blood stream by the liver.

Endogenous metabolism

The liver is considered the principal organ for lipid metabolism and the primary site of synthesis for lipoproteins. Triglyceride and cholesterol in the hepatic cells are packaged and secreted into circulation as triglyceride-rich VLDL. Lipoprotein lipase interacts with VLDL in the same manner that the enzyme interacts with chylomicrons—hydrolyzing triglyceride. In the case of VLDL, loss of triglyceride results in intermediate density lipoproteins (IDL) of increasing cholesterol content. IDL is rapidly processed to LDL or cleared by hepatocytes and thus, IDL normally is not found in fasting specimens. LDL is the final product from extensive lipolysis of VLDL.

LDL is the principal material used to transport cholesterol to peripheral tissues. LDL binds to cell receptors located on the cell surface and is incorporated into the cell. The cholesterol content of the LDL complex is added to the intercellular pool and provides a negative feedback mechanism for regulation of cholesterol synthesis. As the cholesterol pool increases, the rate of synthesis is reduced, and as the intercellular cholesterol pool decreases, the cell increases its ability to synthesize cholesterol.

HDL is derived from liver and intestinal sources and is released into circulation as a nascent form that does not resemble typical spherical lipoproteins. However, nascent HDL acts like a sponge and can absorb lipid from other lipoproteins or peripheral tissue and take on a spherical shape. HDL is thought to function as the reverse cholesterol transport system, such that HDL can regulate the movement of cholesterol from peripheral tissue back to the liver. Free cholesterol from the cells is esterified within HDL by an enzyme, lecithin-cholesterol acyl transferase (LCAT). HDL can exchange cholesterol esters with triglycerides from the VLDL but requires a cholesterol ester transport protein to facilitate this interchange. The ability to exchange cholesterol and triglyceride between HDL and VLDL probably explains, in part, why individuals with increased triglycerides generally have lower HDL cholesterol (HDL-C).

Thus, VLDL, LDL, and HDL interact to maintain the necessary intracellular lipid needs. Transporting lipid to peripheral tissue provides necessary substrate for the cells' requirements to function properly. Lipoproteins transport lipids from sites of synthesis to areas for metabolic needs, storage, or catabolism. An example is the transport to the adrenal cortex where cholesterol is required to synthesize cortisol and aldosterone, hormonal steroids that are involved with different but vital physiologic functions.

APOLIPOPROTEINS

Apolipoproteins control the variety of manipulations and transformations that lipid and lipoproteins undergo. Some of the important functions of apolipoproteins are listed in Box 9-1. Apolipoproteins are specialized proteins capable of binding lipid material and interacting with aqueous media. Portions of apolipoproteins have hydrophobic properties that associate with lipid material while other sections of the protein exhibit hydrophilic characteristics that interact with the aqueous phase. Apolipoproteins function as the interface between lipid and water and allow lipid to function in the adverse aqueous media. In addition to the transport needs of lipid, apolipoproteins mediate enzyme activities, such as lipoprotein lipase, or provide the recognition of receptor sites for lipoprotein metabolism.

The unique ability of apolipoproteins to associate with lipid have had a significant impact on methods used to analyze and quantitate apolipoproteins in biological specimens. The usual analytical procedures and techniques used for proteins cannot be directly applied to apolipoproteins. First, the lipid material must be removed from lipoproteins by tedious extraction techniques to isolate apolipoproteins. Antisera (antibodies) to apolipoproteins can be produced by the methods applied to proteins.

Measurement of apolipoprotein content of lipoproteins must first include a delipidation step to free the apolipoprotein from lipid and expose all the antigenic binding sites of the protein for the antisera. A variety of delipidation procedures exist and the analytical result depends on the procedure selected. The problems associated with delipidation have caused considerable disagreement over methods developed for apolipoprotein analysis. The protein structure of apolipoproteins often is altered when lipids are removed and they may aggregate and self-associate when concentrated for use as calibration material. In addition, some purified apolipoproteins have limited solubility in aqueous media, especially apolipoprotein B. These difficulties have had a negative impact on calibration and standardization of the various apolipoprotein assays and limited the application of these methods for routine clinical work (Table 9-3).

Apolipoprotein AI (apoAI)

ApoAI is the major protein constituent of HDL with lesser amounts found in chylomicrons and trace quantities found in VLDL. The reverse cholesterol transport system may be the primary role of apoAI, especially as it associates with HDL. LCAT, the enzyme that esterifies cholesterol in the reverse cholesterol transport system, requires apoAI for activation. ApoAI is synthesized in both the liver and intestine. It is released into circulation associated with either nascent HDL or chylomicrons.

Apolipoprotein AII (apoAII)

HDL is the principal lipoprotein containing apoAII. As with apoAI, it is found to a lesser extent in chylomicrons and trace amounts are associated with VLDL. ApoAII and apoAI are associated with the same lipoproteins and apparently act as antagonists, such that apoAII inhibits LCAT activity. ApoAII, like apoAI, is synthesized in both the liver and intestine.

Apolipoprotein B (apoB)

ApoB is the largest of the apolipoproteins—its molecular weight is approximately 500,000—and has been difficult to study because delipidated apoB is insoluble in aqueous media. The majority of apoB in serum is associated with LDL, but lesser amounts are found in both chylomicrons and VLDL. Recently, apoB has been shown to exist in two forms, apoB-100 and apoB-48. ApoB-100 is synthesized in the liver and is the primary constituent of LDL and VLDL. ApoB-48 is derived from the intestine and is associated with chylomicrons. Therefore, apoB-100 is the principal transport protein for endogenous cholesterol and apoB-48 serves to transport exogenous lipid. ApoB-100 has affinity for the LDL receptor located on cell surfaces in peripheral tissue and is involved with cellular deposition of cholesterol. ApoB-48, half the size of apoB-100, lacks the affinity for the LDL receptor.

Apolipoprotein C (apoC)

There are three distinct C apolipoproteins, CI, CII, and CIII, that vary in both size and amino acid composition. The C apolipoproteins are low in molecular weight and can be easily separated on polyacylamide electrophoresis. The apoC's nomenclature is derived from their electrophoretic mobilities; apoCI is the slowest and apoCIII the fastest. Liver is the likely source of the C apolipoproteins in circulation and they are functionally involved with metabolism of triglyceride-rich lipoproteins. ApoCII has been shown to be an activator for lipoprotein lipase activity, the enzyme required to hydrolyze triglyceride from chylomicrons and VLDL. It is likely that apoCI and apoCIII are also involved

---

Box 9-1   General apolipoprotein functions

1. Transport and bind lipophilic compounds
2. Regulate lipoprotein metabolism
3. Express lipoprotein immunogenicity
4. Recognize tissue receptors
5. Provide lipoprotein structure

Table 9-3   Apolipoproteins

Abbreviation	Quantity (mg/dL)	Lipoprotein association
A-I	70-180	Chylo, HDL
A-II	20-50	HDL
A-IV	10-15	Chylo, HDL
B-48	—	Chylo
B-100	50-160	VLDL, LDL
C-I-III	20-100	Chylo, VLDL, HDL
E	10-60	Chylo, VLDL, HDL

Chylo = chylomicron

in this process as either activating or inactivating agents for lipolytic enzymes. All three readily transfer from HDL to VLDL of chylomicrons. The C apolipoproteins may also function in the reverse cholesterol transport system by activation of LCAT. Thus, there is much to learn about these apolipoproteins and their role in lipid metabolism.

Apolipoprotein E (apoE)

ApoE is a single polypeptide synthesized in the liver and primarily found in VLDL and to a lesser extent in HDL. Plasma concentrations of apoE range from 2 to 6 mg/dL, lowest of the apolipoproteins. Functionally, however, apoE is quite active in the metabolic process with chylomicrons, VLDL, and HDL. ApoE has a specific receptor on hepatocytes that binds remnants of chylomicrons and VLDL for removal from circulation. Similarly, HDL may have a selective receptor in the liver, mediated through apoE, which closes the feedback loop for the reverse cholesterol transport system. Thus, even though apoE is not the most abundant of the apolipoproteins, its role in lipid metabolism is of major importance. Individuals with apoE abnormalities present with increased serum triglyceride and cholesterol concentrations and increased amounts of IDL (intermediate density lipoproteins) that are intermediate byproducts between VLDL and LDL. Also, apoE has such a strong affinity for the apoB receptor site of LDL on adipose tissue that HDL with apoE will readily displace LDL.

Isoelectrophoresis separates proteins based on their isoelectric points and isoelectrophoresis of apoE reveals four isoforms EI, EII, EIII, and EIV. An isoelectric point is the pH at which the protein has an apparent neutral charge. Three isoforms, EII, EIII, and EIV, are alleles from a single gene and are present in the general population as three possible homozygote (EII/II, EIII/III, and EIV/IV) or three heterozygote (EII/III, EII/IV, and EIII/IV) states. The isoforms are different in molecular structure in that EII has two additional cysteines, EIII one cysteine and one arginine, and EIV two arginines. As a result of the different amino acid composition, EIII and EIV have significantly greater affinity and recognition for the liver receptor and they are cleared faster from circulation. Patients with EI and EII

homozygote phenotypes will often present with increased IDL. This is likely due to the decrease in apoE receptor recognition on the hepatocytes.

Apolipoprotein a (apo[a])

Apo(a) is a single polypeptide with a molecular weight of about 500,000 daltons that has gained considerable attention in most lipid specialty laboratories. Apo(a) binds through a disulfide linkage with LDL to apoB to give rise to the lipoprotein complex Lp(a). Lp(a) may be the most atherogenic of all lipoproteins. Atherogenicity refers to the ability of a lipoprotein to cause or increase vascular lesions that can lead to advanced atherosclerotic disease. Researchers have demonstrated that apo(a) is structurally similar to plasminogen. Homology with plasminogen could account for the atherogenicity of apo(a) and Lp(a). There may be two key interactions of Lp(a) that result in increased risk of CHD: 1) competitive inhibition to activate plasminogen to lyse clots and 2) interaction with platelets at the site of vascular injury resulting in an increased lipid content (Figure 9-2). In addition, research studies have suggested that Lp(a) interacts directly with foam cells in the endothelium, thus adding to the development of fatty lesions. Individuals with increased concentrations of Lp(a) apparently have significantly higher risk of coronary heart disease. As a result, Lp(a) has taken a prominent position in laboratories that investigate lipid and lipoprotein abnormalities.

METHODS

Lipid methods have been through a major transition since the 1970s. The traditional tedious extraction procedures and the use of caustic reagents have given way to the enzymatic approaches that are commercially available. Enzymatic lipid assays offer several advantages when compared to traditional procedures. The obvious advantage is the ability to perform the analysis directly on the serum specimen without a pretreatment step to isolate the lipid. The second and equally important aspect of enzymatic assays is the ability to automate the procedures. Automation for traditional methods was quite limited but enzymatic procedures could be simply added to existing automated equipment. Table 9-4 lists some of the advantages and disadvantages of traditional and enzymatic methods.

Cholesterol

As the first lipid method to have enzymatic reagents readily available, cholesterol led the way for other lipid procedures to develop similar approaches. Enzymatic methods are the principal methods used in clinical laboratories to measure cholesterol in biological fluids. Historically, cholesterol was assayed using cumbersome extraction techniques to remove

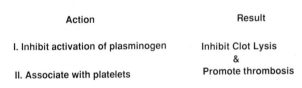

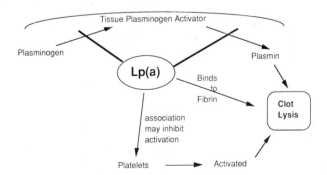

Fig. 9-2   Possible Lp(a) impact on coagulation.

Table 9-4   Traditional vs. enzymatic methods

Method	Advantages	Disadvantages
Sulfuric acid	1. Primary standards 2. Reference method	1. Large sample 2. Not automated 3. Extraction required
Enzymatic	1. Micro sample 2. Automated	1. Secondary standards 2. Matrix effects 3. Direct analysis

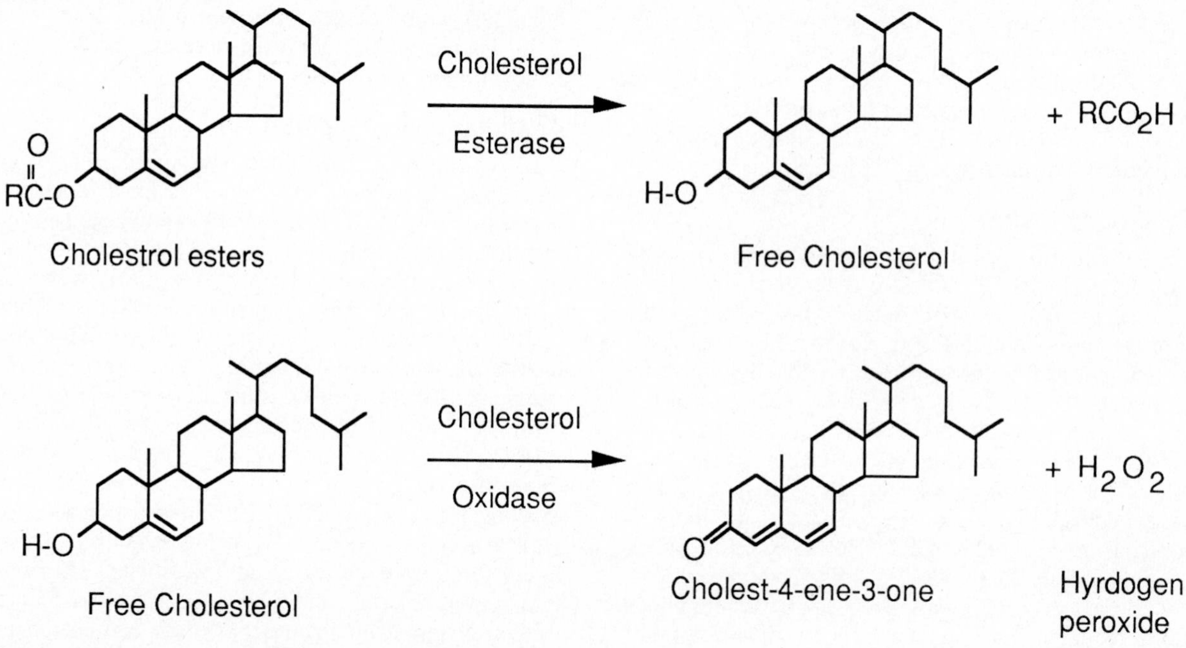

Fig. 9-3 Key enzymatic cholesterol reactions.

cholesterol from the biological protein matrix. Caustic reagents were used to detect and quantitate the amount of cholesterol present. Enzymatic procedures were readily accepted by clinical laboratories as they became commercially available during the 1970s. Cholesterol esterase and cholesterol oxidase are common ingredients for all commercial procedures. Cholesterol esterase catalyzes the hydrolysis of esterified cholesterol to cholesterol and free fatty acids (see Figure 9-3). Cholesterol oxidase catalyzes the oxidation of cholesterol in the presence of oxygen to form cholest-4-ene-3-one and hydrogen peroxide (H_2O_2).

Schemes for cholesterol quantitation with enzymes have used both the consumption of oxygen and formation of hydrogen peroxide as indicators. The majority of commercial procedures couple a peroxidase system that is driven by hydrogen peroxide, such as the Trinder reaction. In this reaction, peroxidase catalyzes the oxidative coupling of 4-aminoantipyrene and phenol by H_2O_2 to form a quinoneimine dye and water. This quinoneimine dye absorbs maximally at 500 nm and may be readily quantitated spectrophotometrically.

Various derivatives of phenol or a substituted aniline have been reported to increase the absorptivity of the quinoneimine dye and thus the sensitivity of the assay. The general Trinder reaction is presented in Figure 9-4.

Enzymatic cholesterol methods typically are designed to use the patient's specimen directly and, therefore, the presence of hemolysis, elevated bilirubin, and turbidity may result in significant spectral interference by direct absorption. Interestingly, bilirubin contributes additional positive interference to enzymatic procedures as bilirubin competes with the intended chromogen system for peroxide.

Patients usually are asked to observe a 12-hour fast before blood collection. The fast is not an absolute requirement for cholesterol or HDL-C since fasting will not influence these tests. However, other lipid tests (e.g., triglycerides) must be assayed on fasting samples to obtain clinically useful information.

Triglycerides

Several enzymatic approaches have been used to measure triglycerides in patient specimens. Some methods have included extracting triglycerides with organic solvents and subsequent hydrolysis with alcoholic alkali prior to enzymatic analysis of the free glycerol. The methods presented here are complete enzymatic assays that incorporate enzymes into the hydrolysis of the triglycerides and subsequent analysis of byproducts to estimate the triglyceride present. Typically, triglyceride assays rely on mixtures of lipase and esterase to cleave the fatty acids and generate glycerol. Glycerol kinase is another common reaction to most enzymatic assays. Glycerol kinase coupled with ATP phosphorylates glycerol at the 3-position to form glycerol-3-phosphate and ADP (see Figure 9-5). Glycerol and ultimately triglyceride concentrations are monitored by the production of ADP. ADP is coupled with pyruvate kinase and phosphoenolpyruvate to generate ATP and pyruvate. Pyruvate, in turn, reacts with lactate dehydrogenase in the presence of NADH and a source of protons to yield lactate and NAD^+. The process can be followed spectrophoto-

$$H_2O_2 + \text{4-aminoantipyrene} + \text{Phenol} \xrightarrow{\text{Peroxidase}} \text{Quinoneimine dye}$$

Fig. 9-4 Trinder reaction.

$$\text{Triglycerides} \xrightarrow{\quad\text{Lipase/Esterase}\quad} \longrightarrow \longrightarrow \text{Glycerol} + \text{Free fatty acids}$$

$$\text{Glycerol} + \text{ATP} \xrightarrow{\frac{\text{Glycerol}}{\text{Kinase}}} \text{Glycerol-3-phosphate} + \text{ADP}$$

$$\text{ADP} + \text{Phosphoenolpyruvate} \xrightarrow{\frac{\text{Pyruvate}}{\text{Kinase}}} \text{ATP} + \text{Pyruvate}$$

$$\text{Pyruvate} + \text{NADH} + \text{H}^+ \xrightarrow{\text{LDH}} \text{Lactate} + \text{NAD}^+$$

Fig. 9-5 Glycerol kinase reaction assay.

metrically at 340 nm from the disappearance of NADH. This analytical approach is not very sensitive at low triglyceride concentrations.

Glycerol-3-phosphate dehydrogenase has been used as an alternate approach for measuring triglycerides. This assay also uses glycerol kinase to generate the phosphorylated derivative. The dehydrogenase enzyme is coupled with glycerol-3-phosphate in the presence of NAD^+ to form dihydroxyacetone phosphate and NADH (see Figure 9-6). Monitoring the increase in NADH at 340 nm provides a direct relationship with the amount of triglyceride present and this approach offers increased sensitivity at lower concentrations.

The use of glycerol-3-phosphate oxidase to measure triglycerides has permitted the approach that has been successful with cholesterol to be applied to triglycerides. Glycerol-3-phosphate oxidase in the presence of oxygen will oxidize the substrate to dihydroxyacetone phosphate and generate hydrogen peroxide.

The use of an alpha-glycerolphosphate oxidase coupled system for the determination of serum triglyceride levels was the next advancement for enzymatic triglyceride assays. The state-of-the-art oxidase coupled reaction sequence was initially applicable only to the dry-film technology of the Kodak Ektachem equipment.

Coincidental to the commercial availability of the alpha-glycerolphosphate oxidase, new lipases with higher activities and broader specificities became available. These two enzymes have facilitated the production of reagents that produce complete hydrolysis, with more specific, more sensitive, and broader dynamic ranges than provided by previous reagent systems.

The obvious advantages of these enzymatic assays are that automated analytical methods could be developed that utilize the serum/plasma specimen directly. Several variations of these procedures are available to clinical laboratories and selection should be made on the basis of specific application requirements, such as availability of spectrophotometric instrumentation for the procedure. Occasionally, the manufacturer supplies the triglyceride reagents in single or multiple vials that the user must reconstitute. Single vial reagent systems are often easier to handle and may be most desirable. However, the multiple vial reagent systems offer laboratories the additional capability of "blanking" their triglyceride systems to account for free glycerol. In general, the serum/plasma specimen is mixed with the triglyceride reagent minus lipase, and free glycerol in the specimen reacts with the reagent as if it came from triglyceride. An initial spectrophotometric reading is taken and next lipase is added to the reaction mixture. After appropriate time to allow the reaction to proceed, a second absorbance measurement is taken and the difference represents the triglyceride concentration minus the free glycerol contribution. Free glycerol based corrections are important in several clinical situations. For example, diabetes, in which patients have two to three times the normal amount of free glycerol (0-15 mg/dL). In another case, specimens from a liver-transplant patient presented with over 2000 mg/dL triglyceride using a nonblanked procedure and less than 200 mg/dL with a blanked method.

High-density lipoprotein cholesterol (HDL-C)

Clinical laboratories universally utilize solutions of polyanions with divalent cations to alter the solubility of specific lipoproteins, which results in precipitation of the lipoproteins affected. The reagents listed in Box 9-2 have been extensively used to precipitate VLDL and LDL as methods to isolate HDL supernates from serum.

$$\text{Glycerol} + \text{ATP} \xrightarrow{\frac{\text{Glycerol}}{\text{Kinase}}} \text{Glycerol-3-phosphate} + \text{ADP}$$

$$\text{Glycerol-3-phosphate} + \text{NAD}^+ \xrightarrow{\frac{\text{GP}}{\text{Dehydrogenase}}} \text{Dihydroxyacetone} + \text{NADH} + \text{H}^+$$

Fig. 9-6 Glycerol-3-phosphate dehydrogenase assay.

Box 9-2   Common HDL-C reagents

Heparin and $MnCl_2$
Heparin and $CaCl_2$
Dextran Sulfate and $MgCl_2$
Phosphotungstate and $MgCl_2$
Polyethylene Glycol

There are several variations of each method, including the use of different molecular weights of the polyanions, such as 50,000 or 500,000 daltons for dextran sulfate procedures. Concentration of the divalent cation is critical to achieve complete precipitation of both VLDL and LDL. The apparent cation concentration can be altered if EDTA plasma is used as the sample and EDTA chelates the Mn^{2+} or Mg^{2+}. When heparin/$MnCl_2$ is used for HDL analysis with EDTA plasma, the 2.0 M/L $MnCl_2$ should be used. Typically, 1.0 M/L $MnCl_2$ is required with serum specimens. Thus, there is not a common method used in clinical laboratories that could simplify standardization of HDL methods. Currently, laboratories must ensure their method is optimized for the cholesterol method to provide appropriate reproducibility. Comparison of the HDL method with results from other laboratories and survey sample data is important to have confidence in the answers being reported.

There are several reasons for the generally wide acceptance of these precipitation techniques by clinical laboratories (Box 9-3).

HDL-C is more easily quantitated by the relatively simple and inexpensive selective precipitation techniques compared to either ultracentrifugation or electrophoresis methods. Currently, the majority of clinical laboratories use either dextran sulfate or sodium phosphotungstate procedures for HDL-C analysis. Future approaches may include more direct and selective isolation of lipoprotein fractions using immune complexes (antigen-antibody reactions) to permit analysis of HDL-C, LDL-C, or even VLDL-C, independently.

Apolipoproteins

There are several options available to both research and clinical laboratories for apolipoprotein assays. Box 9-4 lists some of the analytical approaches that are available on a commercial basis.

Selection of the proper method for a given laboratory depends on several factors, such as: 1) instruments required or available; 2) cost factors (e.g., reagent, instrument, labor); and 3) performance requirements (accuracy, precision, and turn-around time). Each issue needs to be considered

---

Box 9-3   Popularity of routine HDL-C analysis

1. Routine quantitation of HDL-C as a CHD risk factor
2. Inexpensive equipment required
3. Analysis performed directly on supernate
4. Easily automated for high-volume laboratories

Box 9-4   Immunoassay procedures

Radioimmunoassay (RIA)
Electroimmunoassay (EIA)
Radial immunodiffusion (RID)
Enzyme-linked immunoassays (ELISA)
Nephelometric immunoassay (NIA)
Turbidometric immunoassay (TIA)

Box 9-5   Method evaluation studies

1. Precision studies to optimize the method
2. Interference studies: hemolysis, bilirubin, and lipemia
3. Sample comparison with other laboratories or reference materials (CDC)

---

before selecting a method. In many clinical laboratories, instruments are already available and the primary need is to select a reagent system compatible with those instruments. For example, a turbidometric immunoassay can be performed on a variety of spectrophotometric systems. Many of these instrument systems have automated sample/reagent processing programs and the user needs only to determine appropriate sample and reagent volumes, wavelength, incubation times, and temperature to perform the assay. Once a laboratory selects a procedure, the method evaluations must be performed (Box 9-5).

The purpose of these studies is to ensure that the apolipoprotein method will meet the clinical needs. The precision of the apoprotein method should have a coefficient of variation (CV) of less than 5%. The sample comparison and reference materials can be used to establish the relative accuracy of the method.

NATIONAL CHOLESTEROL EDUCATION PROGRAM

Laboratory analysis of the various lipid, lipoprotein, and apolipoproteins have become routine requests for most clinical laboratories. The National Cholesterol Education Program (NCEP) was established in 1988 by the National Heart, Lung, and Blood Institute of NIH in response to medical research data indicating the direct involvement of lipids and lipoproteins in coronary heart disease (CHD). As a result, NCEP was formed with three specific goals (Box 9-6).

NCEP has been a successful program. Both physicians and the public have been deluged with information about cholesterol. The Adult Treatment Panel established a set of

---

Box 9-6   NCEP goals

1. Inform both the public and clinicians about the concerns of CHD risk and increased cholesterol
2. Develop uniform treatment recommendations for individuals with increased cholesterol
3. Improve accuracy and precision of cholesterol assays in clinical laboratories

Table 9-4 CHD risk assessment

Two or more risk factors	Definitive disease
Male	Previous MI
Family CHD history	Angina
Hypertension	
Cigarette smoking (>10/day)	
Low HDL (<35 mg/dL)	
Diabetes mellitus	
Vascular disease	
Obesity (30% overweight)	

recommendations for providing an approach to treating hypercholesterolemia. In addition, the Laboratory Standardization Panel set performance criteria that laboratories are expected to achieve when measuring cholesterol. These are unprecedented moves that have an immediate impact on cholesterol management and testing but will also carry over to other medical and laboratory disciplines.

The Adult Treatment Panel used the scheme illustrated in Table 9-4 to assess an individual's risk for CHD.

Physicians manage patients based on specific risk factors. For example, hypertension, diabetes, cigarette smoking, and obesity are potential cardiovascular heart disease risk factors that can be managed through proper therapy, diet, or behavior modification. Other risk factors are beyond the control of the physician or patient, such as age, sex, and family history of cardiovascular disease. As patients are

evaluated for increased cholesterol values, the physician must rule out possible secondary causes for hypercholesterolemia (Box 9-7).

To further establish a patient's risk for CHD, cholesterol testing must be performed and possible follow up with additional lipoprotein analyses (Table 9-5 and Figure 9-7).

Cholesterol analysis is only the first step the physician uses to assess an individual's potential hyperlipidemia. Since cholesterol can be performed on nonfasting specimens, this assessment serves as a good screening test. Actual follow up and treatment guidelines for adults with increased cholesterol are based on the individual's CHD risk factors and LDL-cholesterol value (Table 9-6 and Figure 9-8).

Cholesterol analysis must be performed on more than a single specimen and the time between specimens must be

Box 9-7 Hypercholesterolemia secondary causes

Medications
  β-blockers, diuretics, esterogens
Diabetes mellitus
Hypothyroidism
Nephrotic syndrome
Liver disease
  Obstructive liver disease

Table 9-5 Cholesterol CHD risk assessment

Cholesterol (mg/dL)	CHD risk
<200	Desirable
200-239	Borderline high
≥240	High

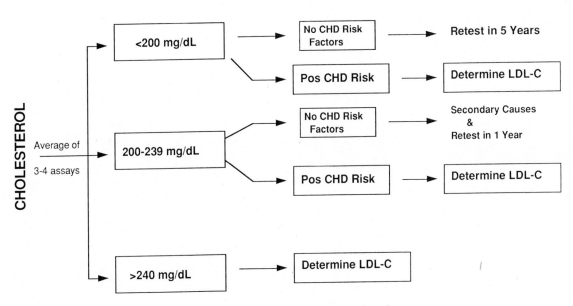

Fig. 9-7 Assessment of initial cholesterol results.

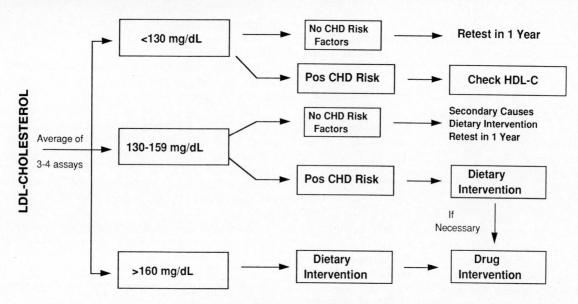

Fig. 9-8 Assessment of LDL cholesterol results.

two or more weeks. To account for biological variability in an individual, the cholesterol analysis may require three, four, five, or more samples to accurately assess typical cholesterol concentration. Factors that determine the number of specimens required include changes in lifestyle, recent illness, and laboratory variability. Table 9-7 lists accuracy and performance standards recommended by the Laboratory Standardization Panel.

Standard laboratory practice requires all laboratories to maintain a methods manual that contains written descriptions of all analyses performed. The methods manual must describe the instruments, source of reagents, method of calibration, validation studies, interference studies, reference-range studies, and linearity studies performed. Also, the methods manual must specify quality-control procedures

used to ensure the proper performance of the method over time.

The NCEP has played a key role in leading the clinical laboratories to improving methods and materials used for cholesterol analysis. Establishing performance goals for laboratories is only part of the overall need. Developing reference materials readily available to all laboratories will transfer accuracy for all methods. National reference laboratories, through which both general laboratories and manufacturers have ready access to reference cholesterol analysis, have been established by NCEP and CDC. As a result, the capability of determining the performance of any cholesterol method or material is a reality. Now the focus for improving laboratory performance must be aimed at other lipid parameters and NCEP will provide support.

Table 9-6 LDL-Cholesterol CHD risk assessment

LDL-Cholesterol (mg/dL)	CHD risk
<130	Desirable
130-159	Borderline high
≥160	High

Table 9-7 Cholesterol performance standards

Year	Accuracy	Precision (%CV)
1988	≤5%	≤5%
1990	≤4%	≤4%
1992	≤3%	≤3%

10 Bone and mineral metabolism and parathyroid hormones

Willie Ruff

NORMAL PHYSIOLOGY AND METABOLISM OF BONE
Anatomy and physiology

Bone is an extremely hard, highly specialized form of connective tissue. The hardness is the result of the presence of a complex mineral substance which contains mostly calcium, phosphate, and carbonate. The intercellular matrix of bone consists of both organic matter and inorganic salts. The organic matter includes blood vessels, nerves, bone cells, and collagen. The primary substance of the organic matter is collagen fibers embedded in an amorphous ground substance. The inorganic material contains calcium phosphate salts and small amounts of calcium fluoride and calcium carbonate.

There are four types of bone cells—osteogenic cells, osteoblasts, osteocytes, and osteoclasts. Osteogenic cells are precursor cells which differentiate further into osteoblasts. Osteogenic cells are active during normal bone growth and participate during the healing of fractures and in the continual replacement of worn-out bone tissue by producing osteoblasts. Osteoblasts are bone-building cells responsible for bone-matrix formation often occurring in areas of active bone metabolism (i.e., trabecular bone). Osteocytes are mature osteoblasts responsible for maintaining the bony matrix; they synthesize small amounts of matrix and can resorb bone. Osteoclasts remove the organic matrix and the bone mineral as part of the normal turnover of bone material.

Composition

Bone matrix is approximately 90% collagen fibers, which have a high content of the amino acids proline and hydroxyproline. A homogeneous medium called *ground substance* constitutes the remaining 10%. Although the collagen fibers extend in all directions, they are most prominent along the lines of tensional force. Bone gains its powerful tensile strength from these fibers. The ground substance, or noncollagenous components, include chondroitin sulfate, bone sialoprotein, albumin, osteocalcin (Gla protein) lipids, and small peptides.

Bone mineral is composed principally of calcium phosphate and calcium carbonate, with smaller quantities of other divalent metal salts including magnesium. The minerals are present as a mixture of hydroxyapatite crystals [Ca_{10} $(PO_4)_6(OH)_3$], amorphous calcium phosphate, and other materials. Divalent cations other than calcium can replace this ion in the crystal lattice to which it is bound by a hydration shell. Ions are transferred through the hydration shell to and from the crystal surfaces. Hydroxyapatite crystals have three zones—crystal interior, crystal surface, and an outer hydration shell. The exchange of ions in the hydration shell or the crystal surface is relatively fast compared to the ion exchange to the crystal interior. In addition to calcium and phosphate, other ions, including the following, are found in the hydroxyapatite crystal lattice: potassium, sodium, magnesium, strontium, radium, zinc, chloride, citrate, carbonate, and fluoride.

Amorphous calcium phosphate does not have a rigidly defined chemical composition. Molar ratios of Ca to PO_4 vary from 1 to 44 to about 1 to 55, which is lower than the ratio found in hydroxyapatite. Amorphous calcium phosphate is the source of ions that control production of apatite crystals.

Structure and function

Cancellous (spongy) bone, found in the interior of bones, is made up of trabeculae—a network of fine interlacing partitions with cavities that contain either fatty or red marrow and osteoblasts. The red marrow is the source of stem cells, which proliferate and differentiate into monocytes, neutrophils, platelets, and erythrocytes. The majority of flat bones and the ends of long bones are made of cancellous bone. The large surface and blood supply permit a rapid response to changes in plasma mineral concentrations.

Hard compact cortical bone, with its densely packed calcified intercellular matrix, is more rigid than spongy bone. Compact cortical bone is found largely in the shafts of the long bones that surround the marrow cavities. Hard bone provides structural support for the skeleton and protects the material in the marrow.

Biochemistry and homeostasis

In bone formation, osteoblasts produce bone matrix, or osteoid, material. Collagen and some carbohydrate-protein complexes found in osteoid are synthesized by these cells. Calcification of bone involves depositing calcium salts—crystalline and amorphous hydroxyapatite—in the osteoid.

135

Osteoblasts probably control the availability of calcium and phosphate to and from bony storage. Osteoblasts secrete alkaline phosphatase, an enzyme, which is found in excess in areas of calcification. It is believed that the enzyme hydrolyzes stored phosphate esters, producing excess-free inorganic phosphate ions. The calcium-phosphate ion product is increased above the solubility point and precipitation occurs.

Osteoclasts, under the influence of parathyroid hormone and calcitonin, function to increase bone dynamics. Parathyroid hormone increases the resorptive function and the number of osteoclasts. Calcitonin has the opposite effect, increasing bone deposition.

During resorption of bone, both the mineral content and the organic matrix are removed. Osteoclasts are thought to secrete acid, which liberates calcium from the osteoid and exposes the collagen fibers to digestion by mononuclear cells or other osteoclasts. However, the exact mechanism of bone resorption remains obscure.

Bone serves as a reservoir for calcium, the most plentiful cation in the body. Only a small portion of bone calcium is exchangeable. Some of the exchangeable calcium is found in other tissues such as the liver and the gastrointestinal tract. However, most of the pool of exchangeable calcium is in bone, specifically, the parts of the bone that are undergoing active bone resorption and deposition. There is an equilibrium between the exchangeable calcium in bone and calcium in the extracellular fluid.

Total calcium exists in equilibrium with ionized calcium (46%), calcium bound to albumin (32%), calcium bound to globulins (8%), and 14% as soluble calcium salts ($CaCO_3$, $CaPO_4$). Ionized calcium is biologically active. The protein-bound calcium and dissolved calcium salts serve as a small active reserve pool of calcium. Changes in the equilibrium by a rise or fall in the ionized calcium concentration results in compensatory hormonal action.

Magnesium is stored principally in bone, about 60%, with the remaining 40% divided between muscle and other soft tissue. Magnesium is the primary intracellular cation, with only about 1% present in the plasma. That means most of the laboratory measures of this ion are not a good estimate of the changes that occur in bone, muscle, or soft tissues where most of this ion is stored.

For acute changes in magnesium concentration, magnesium is absorbed by the intestine and conserved by the kidney in a feedback mechanism with PTH similar to that observed in calcium metabolism. Magnesium is deposited in and removed from the bone like calcium but to a lesser extent.

Chronic changes in magnesium concentrations seem to disconnect from this PTH feedback. Perhaps this is due to an overriding importance for the organism to maintain normal calcium feedback cycles with the bone, in spite of abnormal magnesium concentrations. In addition, there is a reserve intracellular magnesium pool available for magnesium homeostasis.

Three hormones are involved in regulating the concentration of calcium and, to a lesser extent, magnesium and phosphate found in plasma—parathyroid hormone, 1,25-dihydroxycholecalciferol (calcitriol), and calcitonin. Para-

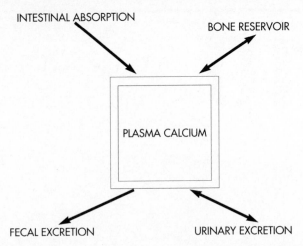

Fig. 10-1 Principal factors in the maintenance of plasma calcium concentrations.

thyroid hormone (PTH) and calcitriol act by increasing and decreasing the calcium concentration, and calcitonin acts independently and less directly by decreasing the concentration of calcium.

Normally the plasma calcium concentration represents an equilibrium between the sites of absorption and storage and the sites of mobilization and excretion. Figure 10-1 illustrates, in simplified form, the dynamics of these interrelationships. Intestinal absorption of dietary calcium and calcium mobilization from the bone reservoir both serve to increase the plasma calcium concentration. But mobilization from bone is quicker and quantitatively more important. The bone is the site of storage and mobilization for the body's reservoir of calcium. Calcium concentration is lowered through excretion by both the fecal and urinary routes. Because of the central role of calcium in muscle contractility and the need to carefully control the concentration, processes that increase the plasma calcium concentration are subject to hormonal regulation (see Figure 10-2). The parathyroid glands secrete parathyroid hormone (parathormone) when the plasma calcium concentration is low. Parathormone rapidly stimulates bone resorption of calcium, phosphorus, and magnesium, and the hydroxylation of calcidiol to calcitriol. Parathormone also rapidly stimulates renal tubular reabsorption of calcium and urinary phosphate excretion. Less rapidly, calcitriol promotes the absorption of dietary calcium and phosphorus in the intestines. The quantitative effect of PTH in response to low calcium is to gain a large increase in plasma calcium (and some phosphate and magnesium) from bone and from the kidney to retain calcium and discard a large amount of phosphorus. The net effect in the plasma is to increase plasma calcium and decrease phosphate. A high plasma calcium produces the reverse effect, a reduction in the amount of PTH secreted, thus increasing bone deposition of calcium and phosphate and a reduction in the amount of calcitriol produced, with subsequent lowering of calcium and phosphate absorbed in the GI tract.

Calcitonin, not depicted in Figure 10-2, is a hormone secreted by the C-cells of the thyroid gland which, when

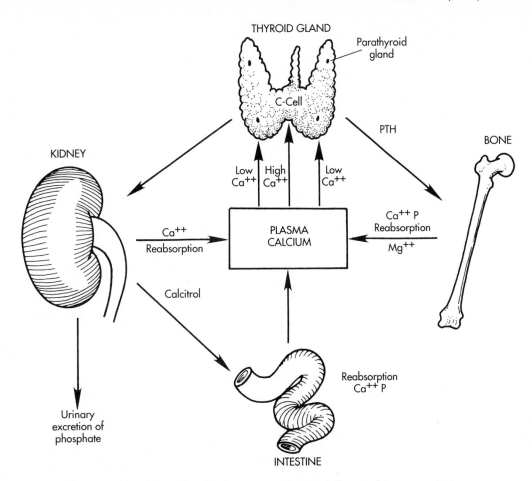

Fig. 10-2 Interrelationships of various organ systems and plasma calcium concentrations.

elevated, promotes the lowering of calcium concentration. It does not seem to direct or reverse PTH action but acts by a separate mechanism.

Calcitonin acts on both kidney and bone. In the kidney, elevated calcitonin causes a decrease in reabsorption of calcium, phosphorus, magnesium, potassium, and sodium, and decreases in hydroxyproline excretion in urine. In bone, calcitonin inhibits osteoclastic bone resorption. Neither excess nor deficiency of the hormone is clearly associated with bone disease or alterations in plasma calcium homeostasis, perhaps because the separate PTH response may overwhelm the calcitonin effect. In the parathyroid glands, PTH is synthesized as a 115 amino acid precursor, preproparathyroid hormone. Proteolytic cleavage of amino acids from this hormone results in the loss of 25 amino acids, thus yielding proparathyroid hormone. Further proteolysis from the same point to remove a six amino acid piece produces an 84 amino acid peptide, parathormone, which is then secreted. In the peripheral circulation, PTH is cleaved into an amino terminal fragment and a carboxy terminal fragment. The half-lives of the amino terminal and carboxy terminal fragments are a few minutes and about an hour, respectively. Biological activity resides in the first 34 amino acids of the amino terminal end of the hormone.

Calcitonin, a peptide hormone secreted in precursor form, is produced primarily by the C-cells of the thyroid gland. However, some hormone is produced by the pituitary gland, the liver, and the gastrointestinal tract. The precursor hormone undergoes proteolytic cleavage in the peripheral circulation to the active hormone. The half-life of calcitonin, approximately 10 minutes, is relatively short. Hormonal secretion is stimulated by hypercalcemia and inhibited by hypocalcemia. The concentration of calcitonin is affected to a lesser extent by estrogens and gastrointestinal hormones (e.g., cholecystokinin and gastrin).

Vitamin D plays an important role in helping to regulate the plasma calcium concentration. Vitamin D is a generic name that refers to two compounds—ergocalciferol and cholecalciferol. Although the compounds differ by the presence of a double bond, they have identical biological activities. Figure 10-3 depicts the sources and pathways for conversion of Vitamin D to active metabolites. There are two sources of Vitamin D—intestinal absorption and skin photoconversion of 7-dehydrocholesterol; of the two, photoconversion is the most important. In the liver there is an enzymatic 25-hydroxylation of the cholecalciferol that is absorbed or produced, which gives rise to calcidiol. This compound undergoes further hydroxylation in the kidney by one of two pathways. Renal enzymatic hydroxylation of calcidiol at the one position yields 1,25-dihydroxycholecalciferol (calcitriol), the most potent vitamin D metabolite. Alternatively, hydroxylation at the 24 position yields 24,

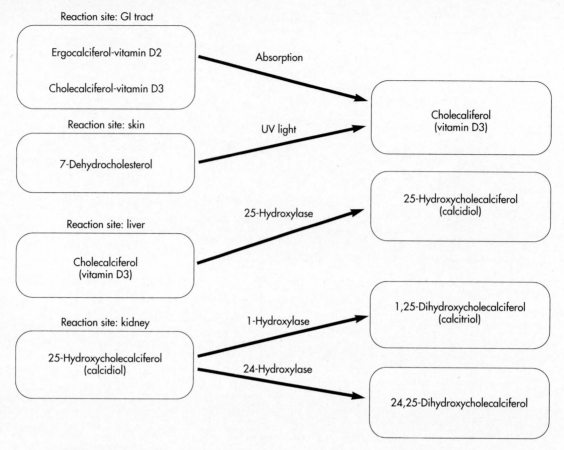

Fig. 10-3   Reactions and reaction sites of the metabolic conversions of Vitamin D_3 to calcidiol and calcitriol.

25 dihydroxycholecalciferol, an inactive compound. The formation of calcitriol is favored during a deficiency of cholecalciferol, calcium, or phosphate. Upon replenishment, calcidiol is hydroxylated in the kidney at the C-24 position to form 24,25-dihydroxycholecalciferol.

In the intestines calcitriol promotes calcium and phosphorus absorption. Calcitriol has a similar effect on the kidney. Together with parathormone, calcitriol increases bone resorption by increasing osteoclastic activity.

When the concentration of ionized calcium falls, the parathyroid gland secretes PTH. PTH acts in an acute fashion to raise the plasma calcium concentration by osteoclastic bone resorption. Low levels of plasma calcium stimulate production of calcitriol, which acts within hours to promote intestinal absorption of calcium.

When the ionized calcium concentration rises above normal, calcitonin is secreted by the C cells of the parathyroid gland. Calcitonin decreases the tubular reabsorption of calcium and phosphorus allowing more to be lost in the urine. The hormone also decreases the resorption of calcium and phosphorus from bone by inhibiting the action of osteoclasts (and probably osteocytes) and the concentration of plasma calcium returns to normal.

Metabolic changes in disease

A number of similar biochemical abnormalities can occur as a result of certain types of parathyroid disease and bone disease. The biochemical changes in parathyroid disease for calcium, phosphorus, PTH, magnesium, and urine calcium are given in Table 10-1. Similarly, a basic summary of the changes found in bone disease for calcium, phosphorus, PTH, calcidiol, and calcitriol is given in Table 10-2.

Parathyroid disease

Primary hyperparathyroidism results in the increased secretion of PTH. The high PTH excessively stimulates osteoclastic bone activity and renal 1-hydroxylase activity, both of which cause elevations of calcium concentration. In this disorder, the major defect is in the parathyroid gland. Two types of problems are found—adenomas and glandular hyperplasia. Adenomas are lesions found in single glands. Hyperplasia generally involves stimulation of multiple glands. Some malignant diseases, such as those that lead to osteolytic and skeletal metastases, cause bone destruction and concomitant release of calcium. Hypervitaminosis D producing toxicity also causes hypercalcemia.

Patients with primary hyperparathyroidism, when symptomatic, present with renal stones or bone disease. Pain and hematuria or obstruction may be associated with renal stones. Occasionally the renal stones may cause renal failure. Bone changes include osteoporosis and subperiosteal resorption. Some patients may present with nonspecific symptoms such as gallstones, hypertension, mild lethargy,

Table 10-1 Biochemical abnormalities associated with parathyroid disease

	Ca^{+2}	PO$_4^{-2}$	PTH	Mg^{+2}	Urine Ca^{+2}
Primary hyperparathyroidism	H	N/L	N/H	H	H
Secondary hyperparathyroidism (osteomalacia)	L	L	H	L/N	L
Primary hypoparathyroidism	L	H	L	L	L
Pseudo hypoparathyroidism					
I	L	H	N/H	L	—
II	L	H	N/H	L	—
Sarcoidosis	H	N/L	L	H	H

N = normal; L = decreased; H = increased

Table 10-2 Biochemical abnormalities associated with bone disease

	Ca^{+2}	PO$_4^{-2}$	PTH	Calcidiol	Calcitriol
Osteoporosis	N	N	N	N	L
Osteomalacia Vitamin D deficiency	L	L	H	L	L/N
Vitamin D dependency					
I	L	L	H	H	L
II	L	L	H	H	H
Vitamin D resistant	N	L	N	N	N/L
Phosphorus deficiency	N	L	N	L	H
Osteitis fibrosa	H/N	L/H	H	N	H/L
Paget's disease	N	N	N	N	N

N = Normal; L = decreased; H = increased

vague neuromuscular symptoms, pancreatitis, and nonspecific abdominal pain.

Secondary hyperparathyroidism is associated with chronic hypocalcemia, which results in stimulation of the parathyroid gland. The chronic hypocalcemia is caused by either a deficiency of cholecalciferol or a high-phosphate load. The cholecalciferol deficiency decreases the intestinal calcium absorption. Plasma calcium and phosphorus concentrations tend to rise and fall in the opposite directions. Hence, a high phosphorus load (caused by either the infusion or ingestion of fluids that are high in phosphorus or excess renal phosphorus retention) will result in a secondary decrease in plasma calcium concentration.

In pseudohypoparathyroidism, the plasma calcium concentration is low. The hypocalcemia results from decreased renal responsiveness to PTH and not from a decrease in PTH synthesis. Patients with this disorder present with short stature, short metacarpals or metatarsals, a round face, and mental retardation in addition to signs and symptoms of hypocalcemia.

Sarcoidosis is a chronic, progressive disease that affects multiple tissues including the small bones of the hands and feet. Some patients with the disease present with hypercalcemia resulting from increased conversion of calcidiol to calcitriol. In sarcoidosis plasma PTH is either normal or decreased. Elevated plasma PTH suggests a coexisting hyperparathyroidism.

Hypoparathyroidism and pseudohypoparathyroidism are diseases of the parathyroid gland that result in low plasma calcium concentrations (hypocalcemia). In hypoparathyroidism low or undetectable levels of PTH are secreted. As a result, PTH-stimulated osteoclastic bone resorption with subsequent release of calcium does not occur. Moreover, the renal reabsorption of calcium and phosphorus is hindered because of decreased calcitriol production and increased urinary calcium. In pseudohypoparathyroidism, the PTH concentration is normal or high but the end organs (bone and kidney) are unresponsive. Despite the presence of PTH, there is no tubular reabsorption of calcium or mobilization of bony calcium.

Patients with hypoparathyroidism and pseudohypoparathyroidism present with symptoms of hypocalcemia. A prominent feature of hypocalcemia is directly referable to enhanced neuromuscular excitability—tetany or muscle spasm. This may be demonstrated by tapping the facial nerve in front of the ear and observing muscle contractions around the eye and nose.

Vitamin D deficiency, renal failure, and malabsorption syndromes also may lead to hypocalcemia. A vitamin D deficiency (osteomalacia) results in insufficient amounts of hormone available for conversion to the active metabolite, calcitriol. Renal failure prevents the hydroxylation of calcidiol to calcitriol. The malabsorption syndrome is characterized by the inability to transport calcium from the intestinal lumen to the blood stream.

Bone disease
Osteoporosis

Osteoporosis is a metabolic bone disease in which osteoblasts fail to lay down bone matrix. In this disease the rate of bone formation is usually normal or may actually be decreased. However, bone resorption occurs at a greater rate than the rate of bone formation. When examined histologically, the bone cortex is decreased in thickness, and the number and size of trabeculae of the coarse cancellous bone are decreased.

Generally, the skeletal mass begins to decrease after the fourth decade of life at a faster rate in women than in men. The cause for this age-related decrease in bone mass is unknown. Parathyroid hormone, calcium, and calcitonin are normal in osteoporotic patients. However, calcitriol may be decreased.

In the United States osteoporosis is the most common metabolic bone disease. Bone fractures secondary to osteoporosis tend to occur by age 65. These fractures usually occur in the hip, pelvis, lower forearm, spine, and proximal humerus.

Clinically, there are two phenotypes of osteoporosis after age 50. Osteoporosis Type I occurs in a small subset of women age 51 to 65. These patients have vertebral or wrist fractures that involve mostly trabeculae bone. Osteoporosis

Type II is found in both women and men over 75 who sustain fractures of the tibia, hips, or humerus.

The diagnosis of osteoporosis is made primarily on radiological findings of thin and hollow bone cortices and the loss of coarse cancellous bone.

Osteomalacia

Osteomalacia refers to a group of diseases in which calcium phosphate deposition in the organic matrix of bone is abnormal (defective mineralization). Histologically, there is increased thickness of osteoid and an increased area of bone surface covered by osteoid. In adolescents osteomalacia is known as rickets.

The most common cause of osteomalacia is Vitamin D deficiency secondary to inadequate dietary intake and photoconversion in the skin of 7-dehydrocholesterol.

Clinically, patients usually have nonspecific complaints: diffuse aches and pains and muscle weakness. Patients with mild forms of the disease, characterized by slow progressive bone changes, may be totally asymptomatic for years. When the disease is advanced, tenderness or poorly localized bone pain is common, especially in the pelvis, spine, and proximal parts of the extremities.

Some common causes of osteomalacia are Vitamin D deficiency, Vitamin D dependent Types I and II, Vitamin D resistance and phosphorus deficiency. Generally, a deficiency of Vitamin D results in a deficiency of calcidiol and calcitriol. Insufficient calcitriol decreases the intestinal absorption of calcium, producing hypocalcemia. Parathyroid hormone secretion is stimulated in response to hypocalcemia, causing calcium mobilization from the bone reservoir and phosphaturia. A plasma hypophosphatemia occurs because of the increased phosphaturia.

In Vitamin D-dependent osteomalacia Type I, the biochemical abnormalities mirror those found in the Vitamin D deficiency state, except plasma calcidiol is normal and calcitriol is low. Patients with this disease heal when they are prescribed physiological doses of calcitriol. The biochemical defect in this disorder presumably is a deficiency of the renal 1-hydroxylase enzyme. Vitamin D-dependent osteomalacia Type II patients have similar biochemical abnormalities to Type I patients, except calcitriol is normal. These patients are resistant to physiological doses of calcitriol suggesting end-organ resistance.

Vitamin D-resistant osteomalacia patients present with biochemical markers different from patients who have other variants of the underlying disease. Both parathyroid hormone and plasma calcium concentrations are normal. However, there is a severe hypophosphatemia secondary to a renal tubular defect which interferes with phosphate reabsorption. The hypophosphatemia would be expected to be a major stimulus for calcitriol biosynthesis. In fact, measured plasma calcitriol concentrations are normal or below normal. The low plasma calcitriol suggests an enzyme defect that affects the renal 1-hydroxylase enzyme.

Osteomalacia may also result from phosphorus deficiency. Hypophosphatemia stimulates calcitriol synthesis which increases intestinal calcium absorption and urinary phosphorus reabsorption. Plasma PTH and calcium are normal in this disorder.

Osteitis fibrosa

Osteitis fibrosa is a disorder usually caused by either primary hyperparathyroidism or chronic renal failure, in which bone destruction exceeds bone formation. On histologic examination, numerous osteoclasts are seen resorbing bone, and adjacent marrow fat is replaced by fibrous tissue.

Osteitis fibrosa caused by chronic renal failure is termed renal osteodystrophy. In renal osteodystrophy, glomerular damage yields phosphate retention causing a hyperphosphatemia. Renal tubular damage causes a reduction in calcitriol. This results in decreased intestinal calcium absorption leading to a profound hypocalcemia. Parathyroid hormone is secreted in response to the hypocalcemia. The severity of the hypocalcemia provokes a marked increase in PTH, which does not effectively promote either intestinal calcium absorption or renal tubular calcium reabsorption. With the hyperphosphatemia and the absence of Vitamin D, the principle action of PTH is bone resorption of calcium.

Paget's disease

Paget's disease is characterized by excessive bone resorption and apposition. The disease shows no sex preference and generally affects people in the sixth decade of life. Although the exact etiology of the disease is unknown, it is believed to be of viral origin. Some evidence suggests that viral stimulation of osteoclastic activity produces excessive bone resorption.

Histologically, the disease is triphasic. In the first phase, which occurs early in the disease, osteoclastic resorption predominates. Bone formation predominates in the second phase. The rate of bone resorption declines in the third phase, yet continued bone formation produces hard, dense bone.

In Paget's disease plasma calcium and phosphorus are usually normal.

Analytes changes in disease
Calcium

The body of the average adult contains between 20 to 25 g of calcium per kg of fat-free tissue for a total of 1.0 to 1.5 kg. Approximately 99% of body calcium is in the skeleton. The remaining 1%, found in blood and other tissues, serves important functions unrelated to bone. When needed, the skeleton is the major reservoir for calcium. However, calcium is liberated from the skeleton only by bone resorption.

Plasma calcium is exquisitely regulated. Irritability, contractile, and conductive abnormalities of smooth and skeletal muscle and convulsions result when plasma calcium is low.

Phosphorus

Phosphorus is a ubiquitous cellular substance. The plasma concentration represents the equilibrium between dietary intake, compartmental distribution within the body, renal tubular reabsorption, and excretion by the kidneys. Disturbance of this equilibrium may produce either hypophosphatemia or hyperphosphatemia.

The diagnosis of hypophosphatemia and its cause can be made after plasma phosphorus assay and interpretation in the context of the clinical findings. In primary hyperparathyroidism, a decreased plasma phosphorus concentration is a typical finding. About 50% of patients with primary hyperparathyroidism present with hypophosphatemia. The hypophosphatemia results from the urinary excretion of phosphate to maintain the proper solubility product of calcium and phosphate ions for precipitation. Skeletal mineralization occurs when the solubility product of calcium and ions is great enough to cause precipitation on the bone matrix. Hypophosphatemia of hyperparathyroidism is associated with skeletal demineralization secondary to PTH stimulation of osteoclasts and osteocytes. Decreased serum concentration of phosphorus is often associated with osteomalacia (bone softening) muscle and neurological abnormalities.

Hyperphosphatemia does not produce direct clinical symptoms. Abnormalities of phosphorus occur secondary to changes in calcium homeostasis. Decreased bone resorption is found in hyperphosphatemia due to the movement of phosphorus and calcium into bone. Hyperphosphatemia favors skeletal mineralization. Severe hyperphosphatemia can cause metastatic calcification in soft tissues. The most common cause of hyperphosphatemia is renal insufficiency.

Magnesium

Magnesium is a constituent of bone salts and tends to move with calcium in and out of bone. The concentration of magnesium is higher in cells than in extracellular fluids. Hence, it tends to enter and leave cells under the same conditions as phosphorus. Magnesium is an essential cofactor of enzymatic reactions such as phosphorylation reactions catalyzed by kinases. Protein synthesis and oxidative phosphorylation also require magnesium. Moreover, magnesium is a modifier of the parathormone-calcium interaction.

Normally there is an equilibrium between magnesium in cells and magnesium in extracellular fluid. Disturbances lead to a redistribution of magnesium in an effort to restore that equilibrium. Hypomagnesemia is more common than hypermagnesemia.

Causes of depression of the plasma concentration of magnesium include decreased intake from dietary sources, internal redistribution, and increased loss from the body. Gastrointestinal disorders such as malabsorption syndrome and steatorrhea contribute to magnesium deficiency.

Defective renal tubular reabsorption of magnesium also can cause hypomagnesemia. Acute lowering of serum magnesium promotes an increase in the secretion of parathormone. However, chronic hypomagnesemia has the opposite effect. Magnesium deficiency causes a decrease in tissue response to PTH.

Hypomagnesemia may be found in a number of conditions including hypoparathyroidism, cirrhosis, chronic diarrhea, and hemodialysis. Patients with hypomagnesemia present with symptoms similar to patients with hypocalcemia. Specifically, they have severe neuromuscular irritability with tetany, hyperreflexia, and electrocardiographic changes.

Hypermagnesemia is rarely found in the absence of other abnormalities such as hypercalcemia or renal failure. Increased medicinal intake of magnesium may cause the plasma concentration of magnesium to increase. The wide-spread availability of patent medicine preparations containing magnesium is a contributing factor to the incidence of hypermagnesemia. In association with calcium, magnesium is released from the bone reservoir under the influence of PTH. It appears that magnesium also plays a role in the feedback regulation of PTH secretion. Hence, acute hypermagnesemia may decrease the secretion of PTH.

Depressed neuromuscular and cardiac activity are common symptoms of hypermagnesemia. Patients with this abnormality may have nausea, hypotension, drowsiness, and respiratory depression. Cardiac arrest may accompany hypermagnesemia.

Vitamin D

Vitamin D exists in two forms, calcidiol and calcitriol. However, Vitamin D has little or no activity until it is metabolized to compounds that mediate its activity. The regulation of vitamin D activity is influenced by several hormones: PTH, prolactin, and calcitonin. PTH and prolactin stimulate calcitriol production by the kidney. Calcitonin inhibits calcitriol synthesis. Changes in the concentration of phosphate and calcium exert an effect on calcitriol and 24,25-dihydroxycholecalciferol production. Hypocalcemia and hypophosphatemia result in increased calcitriol production. Hypercalcemia and hyperphosphatemia have the opposite effect.

PTH

Parathyroid hormone (PTH) is the name given to the secretory product of the parathyroid gland. First, a 115 amino acid pre-proparathyroid hormone is synthesized. This peptide undergoes successive proteolytic cleavage to a 90 and then 84 amino acid product, parathyroid hormone. Secretion of parathyroid hormone into the systemic circulation results in further proteolytic degradation to PTH fragments. To be biologically active, a PTH fragment must contain the 30 to 34 amino acid residues proximal to the amino terminus. The majority of carboxyterminal fragments are biologically inactive. PTH is a generic name for freely circulating fragments and intact molecules.

Changes in ionized calcium directly affect PTH secretion. In response to hypocalcemia, PTH is secreted and stimulates bone resorption of calcium, phosphorus, and magnesium, and the renal hydroxylation of calcidiol to calcitriol. Hypercalcemia suppresses PTH secretion.

Calcitonin

Calcitonin exerts a direct action on bone resorption. It appears to inhibit bone resorption, perhaps by a reduction in the number of osteoclasts. Chronic administration of calcitonin to patients with Paget's disease yields relief from pain and induces histological, biochemical, and radiological improvement. In medullary thyroid carcinoma, calcitonin values are elevated. It is interesting that in medullary thyroid carcinoma, plasma calcium and phosphorus levels are usually normal.

LABORATORY MEASUREMENT OF ANALYTES
Calcium

Approximately 40% of calcium is protein bound, mostly to albumin. The remainder of the calcium is free (46%) and

Table 10-3   Methods of calcium analysis

Method	Principle	Notes
1. Total Calcium		
A. Atomic absorption spectro-photometry	$Ca^{+2} \xrightarrow{+2e-} Ca^0$ $Ca^0 + light \rightarrow Ca^*$	Excellent precision, sensitivity and accuracy
B. Spectrophotrometric	$Ca^{+2} + $ 0-cresolphthalein $\rightarrow$ complex (A_{578nm})	Subject to interference by bilirubin and some drugs
C. Flurometric complexometry	$Ca^{+2} + $ calcein $\rightarrow$ Ca-calcein (flourescent) Ca-calcein + EGTA $\rightarrow$ Ca-EGTA + Calcein (diminished flourescence)	Highly sensitive subject to fluorescense quenching
2. Ionized Calcium ion-selective Electrode	$E_1 = E_0 + 2.3 \left\{ \dfrac{RT}{nF} \right\} \log (Ca^{+2})$ $E_1 = Ca^{+2}$ electrode potential $E_0 = $ standard potential of the reference half cell $R = $ Universal gas constant (8.3143 J X K^{-1} X mol^{-1}) $T = $ temperature in degrees Kelvin $F = $ Faraday's constant (96,487 coulombs $\times$ mol^{-1}) $n = $ charge of the measured ion	Subject to a variety of influences (See text.)

A = absorbance

complexed as organic and inorganic salts (14%). Table 10-3 lists some of the methods available for determination of both total and ionized calcium.

Total calcium

Atomic absorption spectrophotometry is a reference method widely used because of its excellent sensitivity, accuracy, and precision. Atomic absorption is used for the analysis of total calcium in both serum and urine.

There are two analytical approaches to atomic absorption spectrophotometry: flame and flameless. In flame atomic absorption spectrophotometry, a sample containing calcium is burned in an air-acetylene flame. The burning causes the calcium atoms to dissociate while remaining in the ground state. These atoms absorb incident light from a calcium hollow cathode lamp which is passed through the flame. The degree of light absorption is concentration dependent. Flameless atomic absorption spectrophotometry in principle is the same as the flame technique except a heating element such as a graphite furnace is used in lieu of the flame.

Before analysis by atomic absorption spectrophotometry, several types of interferences must be removed or compensated. Most importantly, calcium must be dissociated from protein or ionic and molecular phosphate complexes. Protein-bound calcium is dissociated by acid; and lanthanum ions or strontium ions are used to break calcium phosphate complexes. Calcium and magnesium phosphate complexes do not dissociate in the flame. Since lanthanum and strontium bind preferentially to phosphate, calcium and magnesium are released for analysis. Magnesium interference is removed by the use of a narrow band pass spectrophotometer for the specific isolation of the calcium absorption line at 422.7 nm. Sodium ions are added to the calcium standards to eliminate sodium interference in the analysis. The disadvantage of atomic absorption is that the method is relatively slow and does not lend itself to applications such as mass screening. A potential pitfall is that samples containing chelators, unknown to the analyst, may produce anomalous results. Serum and heparinized plasma are the samples of choice. Oxylated and EDTA anticoagulated blood are unacceptable for analysis because of their propensity for chelating calcium.

Calcium can also readily be measured when complexed with a chromophore that absorbs light in the visible region of the spectrum. A commonly used chromophore is o-cresolphthalein. In alkaline solution o-cresolphthalein forms a colored complex with calcium, which is measured spectrophotometrically at 578 nm. The addition of potassium cyanide stabilizes the calcium complex and eliminates interference by heavy metals. To minimize interference by other cations, particularly magnesium, 8-hydroxyquinoline is added to the solution. Protein interference is removed by dialysis against an acidified solution or by dilution. Acidification releases the bound calcium from the protein; and dialysis allows the free flow of the ionized calcium. This method is subject to interference by bilirubin and some drugs.

An alternative to the spectrophotometric method uses a fluorometric chromophore. The fluorometric procedure offers enhanced sensitivity, but is subject to problems of quenching. Hence, the analyst must assay blanks and controls to assess the effects of quenching on the result.

The reference range for total calcium is 2.10 to 2.55 mmol/L for adults and 2.2 to 2.7 mmol/L for children.

Ionized calcium

Ionized calcium is measured with an ion-selective electrode. Both a reference electrode and a calcium-selective electrode are used to measure the potential of an unknown solution. A calcium-selective membrane separates the electrode from the sample. The presence of calcium ions in the membrane yields a voltage across the membrane surface producing a change in potential, which is recorded and converted to concentration.

The measurement of ionized calcium is influenced by several factors: temperature, pH, ionic strength, protein,

Table 10-4 Methods of phosphorus analysis

Method	Principle	Notes
1. Phosphomolybdate Reduction	$PO_4^{-3} + MoO_4^{-2} \xrightarrow{H^+} Mo\text{-}PO_4$ (Complex 1) $MoPO_4$ (Complex 1) + reducing agent $\rightarrow$ Complex 2	
Reducing Agents		
A. p-methylaminophenol sulfate (PMAPS) and NaHSO3	(A_{max}, 340 nm)	Subject to lipemic and hemoglobin interference
B. semidine·HCL N-Phenyl-p-phenylenediamine (semidine)	(A_{max}, 740 nm)	Good sensitivity and Color stability
2. Enzymatic	1. HPO_4^{-2} + Inosine $\xrightarrow{PNP}$ R-1-P + H	Easily automated accurate and sensitive
	2. Hypoxanthine + $2H_2O$ + $2O_2 \xrightarrow{XOD} UA + 2H_2O_2$	
	3. $2H_2O_2$ + chromogen $\xrightarrow{P}$ purplish complex (A_{max}, 555 nm)	

DNP = purine nucleoside phosphorylase; R-1-P = ribose-1-phosphate; XOD-Xanthine oxidase; P = peroxidase; H = hypoxanthine; UA = uric acid; A = absorbance

and anticoagulants. Temperature affects the equilibrium between calcium bound to protein and other anions. To avoid this problem, assays are performed under conditions of controlled temperature. To compensate for differences in ionic strength, electrodes are calibrated with standards containing salts at normal serum concentrations. Anticoagulants such as EDTA bind calcium. Therefore, heparin is the anticoagulant of choice. An increase in pH lowers the concentration of ionized calcium. This problem can be eliminated by collecting and handling the sample anaerobically.

The reference range for ionized calcium is 1.14 to 1.29 mmol/L.

Phosphorus

Table 10-4 lists two major approaches to the determination of phosphorus. The first is the classical formation of phosphomolybdate and its subsequent reduction. In an acid medium, molybdate reacts with inorganic orthophosphate to form a phosphomolybdate complex. A variety of reducing agents have been used to reduce the colorless phosphomolybdate complex to a chromogenic product. Two reducing agents commonly used are p-methylaminophenol sulfate (PMAPS) and n-phenyl-p-phenylenediamine, hydrochloride (semidine·HCL). When PMAPS is used the complex is determined spectrophotometrically at 340 nm. Reduction with semidine·HCL yields a complex read at 740 nm. PMAPS reagent, when properly constituted with a solubilizing agent such as sodium dodecyl sulfate (SDS) and sodium hypochlorite, eliminates interferences due to protein and bilirubin. However, hemoglobin and lipemia interference is still a problem with this method.

In the enzymatic approach inorganic phosphate is coupled to inosine, in the presence of purine nucleoside phosphorylase to yield ribose-1-phosphate. Through a coupled reaction a reddish-purple complex is formed and is read at 555 nm. Enzymatic methods are relatively new and, unlike chemical reduction methods, add stability of the organic phosphate compounds under the assay conditions. Furthermore enzymatic methods eliminate the need for the use and handling of caustic and corrosive chemicals. A disadvantage of this procedure is the relatively high cost of the reagents.

Either heparinized plasma or serum is suitable for analysis. Some anticoagulants such as EDTA, citrate, and oxalate interfere with the formation of the phosphomolybdate complex. Hence these anticoagulants should not be used. Grossly lipemic samples cause falsely elevated results. Hemolyzed samples give results with a negative bias due to interference with color formation. Ideally, patients should be fasting because serum values are lower after meals.

The reference range for phosphorus is 1.45 to 2.76 meq/L.

Magnesium

The methods of choice for the determination of magnesium, listed in Table 10-5, include atomic absorption, nonenzymatic and enzymatic spectrophotometry, and fluorometry.

Atomic absorption is the reference method because of its accuracy, precision, and sensitivity. Unlike calcium measurements, lanthanum solution does not have to be used to eliminate interferences from divalent cations.

Nonenzymatic spectrophotometric methods such as the one using Calmagite are very common because of the good correlation between reference methods and the dye-binding results. The chromogenic product which absorbs at 532 nm is subject to interference by lipemia. However, the reagent formulation includes 9-ethylene-oxide adduct of p-nonylphenol (Bion NE9) and polyvinylpyrrolidine (Bion PVP) to remove protein interference with dye-complex formation. Cyanide and EGTA are added to prevent heavy metal and calcium interferences, respectively. Methylthymol blue is another substance that forms a chromogenic product when reacted under appropriate conditions with divalent magnesium. This procedure also requires the use of calcium chelators.

Enzymatic methods for the measurement of magnesium are being used with increasing frequency. They offer the advantage of easy automation, accuracy, and precision of analysis. Like previous enzymatic methods, the main disadvantage is that they are expensive.

Fluorometric methods of magnesium determination have enhanced sensitivity. However they are subject to quenching.

The reference range for magnesium is 0.6 to 1.1 mmol/L.

Table 10-5 Methods of magnesium anaylsis

Method	Principle	Notes
1. Atomic absorption	$Mg^{+2} \xrightarrow{+2e-} Mg^0$ $Mg^0 + light \rightarrow Mg^*$	Accurate, sensitive, and precise

2. Spectrophotometric
  A. Non-enzymatic
    1) Calmagite
	$Mg^{+2} + dye \xrightarrow{PVP} Complex (A_{532nm})$	Lipemia interference widely used

2) Methylthymol blue	$Mg^{+2} + methylthylmol\ blue \rightarrow Complex$ (A_{510nm})	Must be used with calcium chelatives
B. Enzymatic	$Mg{\cdot}ATP + D\text{-}glucose \xrightarrow{HK} D\text{-}G6P + MG{\cdot}ADP$ $NADP^+ + D\text{-}G6P \rightarrow NADPH + H^+ + DGl\text{-}6\text{-}P$ (A_{340nm})	Easily automated, accurate, sensitive
3. Fluorometric	$Mg^{+2} + calcein \rightarrow Mg{\cdot}calcein\ complex$ (420 nm, excitation 530 nm, emission)	Very sensitive, subject to fluorescense quenching

HK = hexokinase; D-G6P = D-glucose-6-phosphate; 6-PG = 6-Phosphogluconate; PVP = Polyvinylpyrrolidone; A = absorbance; D-Gl-6-P = D-gluconolactone-6-phosphate

Parathyroid hormone and calcitonin

Parathyroid hormone and calcitonin are determined by radioimmunoassay. In this procedure, labelled and unlabelled hormones are allowed to compete for a limited number of binding sites on an antibody. Separation of bound and unbound hormone is effected by a second antibody or adsorption on charcoal. Radioactively labelled hormone is counted in a gamma scintillation counter. A standard curve is used to calculate the concentration of hormone in the patient sample. For standard curve preparation, plot the percent of bound isotope against the concentration of the standards.

The reference range of PTH is 0 to 96 pg/mL; calcitonin's reference range is less than 40 pg/mL.

Vitamin D

As discussed previously, Vitamin D exists in two forms. Calcidiol and calcitriol are the two principal biologically active forms of Vitamin D. The regulation of Vitamin D activity is influenced by several hormones: PTH, prolactin,

and calcitonin. PTH and prolactin stimulate calcitriol production by the kidney. Calcitonin inhibits calcitriol synthesis. Changes in the concentration of phosphate and calcium exert an effect on calcitrin and 24,25-dihydroxycholecalciferol production. Hypocalcemia and hypophosphatemia result in increased calcitriol production. Hypercalcemia and hyperphosphatemia have the opposite effect.

The reference range of Vitamin D is 20 to 76 pg/mL.

SUGGESTED READING

Blick K and Liles SM: Principles of clinical chemistry, New York, 1985, John Wiley.

Kanis JA, Peterson AD, and Russell RGG: Disorders of calcium and skeletal metabolism. In Williams DL and Marks V, eds: Biochemistry, New York, 1985, Elsevier.

Kaplan LA and Pesce AJ: Clinical chemistry: theory analysis and correlation, ed 2, St. Louis, 1989, Mosby–Year Book, Inc.

Porth CM: Pathophysiology: concepts of altered health states, ed 2, Philadelphia, 1986, JB Lippincott.

Vaughn J: The physiology of bone, ed 3, Oxford, 1981, Clarendon Press.

11

Hemoglobin and iron

Gayle Jackson

HEMOGLOBIN
Structure and assembly of hemoglobins

Hemoglobin is the red pigmented protein (molecular weight of 68,000 daltons) in the red blood cells of vertebrates. It is made up of four protein chains, each containing an iron-porphyrin complex. These chains are folded into a macro-molecular complex whose principle function is to transport oxygen from the lungs to the peripheral tissues.

Human hemoglobin is composed of two pairs of poly-peptide chains. Variations in the primary amino acid sequences are responsible for the different types of globin chains. The polypeptide chains are designated by the following Greek letters: α, β, γ, δ, ϵ, ζ. The alpha chain consists of a sequence of 141 amino acids. The beta, gamma, delta, and epsilon chains consist of 146 amino acids with a different amino acid sequence for each chain. There are two types of gamma chains differing by one amino acid at position 136. G-gamma contains glycine, whereas A-gamma has alanine at this position. Both gamma chains normally appear as a mixture in fetal blood.

The principal hemoglobin in humans, hemoglobin A, consists of two alpha protein chains and two beta protein chains. Each polypeptide globin chain is conjugated to one

heme moiety, a ferroprotoporphyrin IX, in which one iron atom is complexed in the center of a porphyrin ring (Figures 11-1 and 11-2).

Hemoglobin A normally represents approximately 97% of normal adult hemoglobin. Hemoglobin A_2 represents 3.5% of adult human hemoglobin and is composed of two alpha and two delta globin chains. Fetal hemoglobin, which makes up 80% of the hemoglobin in newborns but less than 1% of the hemoglobin in normal adults, is composed of two alpha and two gamma chains.

Hemoglobin F and three embryonic hemoglobins, Gower I, Gower II, and hemoglobin Portland are found during fetal development. Gower I is composed of two zeta and two epsilon chains. Gower II is composed of two alpha chains and two epsilon chains. The Gower hemoglobins are not detectable after the first few months of gestation. The third embryonic hemoglobin, Portland, is composed of two zeta and two gamma chains and may persist in small amounts into fetal life. Hemoglobin F predominates from about the third gestational month until about 3 months after birth.

Normally, monomers of alpha and beta chains are released from the ribosomes into the cytoplasm of developing red blood cells. Both alpha and beta chains are synthesized

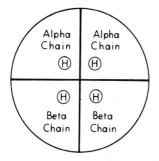

Fig. 11-1 Diagram of structure of Hb A molecule. Four heme groups are attached to one globin molecule, which consists of four polypeptide chains, two of which have an identical amino acid sequence of one type (α chain) and the other two an identical amino acid sequence of another type (β chain). Each polypeptide chain is conjugated to one heme moiety. *H,* Heme. *From Bauer JD: Clinical laboratory methods, ed 9, St Louis, 1982, Mosby-Year Book, Inc.*

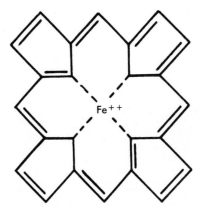

Fig. 11-2 Diagram of structure of heme. One iron atom is related to four pyrrole rings, which are joined to each other through methylene bridges. *From Bauer JD: Clinical laboratory methods, ed 9, St Louis, Mosby-Year Book, Inc.*

in equal amounts. Each monomer immediately incorporates a heme moiety. Two single peptide chains of the same type combine to form dimers and the dimers of different hemoglobin types then combine to form tetramers, which completes the molecule.

Six structural genes control the synthesis of the six different globin chains (α, β, γ, δ, ϵ, and ζ). The α and ζ genes are on chromosome 16 and γ, β, δ, and ϵ genes are linked on chromosome 11. The usual protein synthetic pathway is followed in translating the genetic code into the final globin polypeptide chains (Figure 11-3).

The primary function of hemoglobin is to serve as an oxygen-transport protein. It is the major constituent of the red cell cytoplasm, accounting for about 90% of the dry weight of the mature cell. Therefore, hemoglobin is found primarily as oxyhemoglobin or deoxyhemoglobin; however, other chemically modified forms exist.

Chemically modified forms

Carboxyhemoglobin is a toxic compound that forms when carbon monoxide (CO) rather than oxygen binds with the ferrous ion of hemoglobin. Although carbon monoxide binds to heme in a similar manner to oxygen, the union is much firmer because carbon monoxide has an affinity for hemoglobin that is 218 times greater than oxygen. A carbon monoxide concentration of 0.1% in the inhaled air combines with more than 50% of the available hemoglobin, making this hemoglobin unavailable for oxygen transport. The release of CO is 10,000 times slower than the release of O_2 from hemoglobin. Therefore, hemoglobin with bound carbon monoxide is effectively removed from the oxygen-carrying system.

A small amount of carboxyhemoglobin (CO-Hb) is produced endogenously during the degradation of heme to bilirubin (1 mole of CO produces 1 mole of carboxyhemoglobin). However, the amount of CO-Hb produced endogenously is harmless unless exhaled air is concentrated in an ill-ventilated small space. The exogenous CO from the exhaust of automobiles, smoking, and industrial pollutants such as the burning of coal and charcoal contribute to health hazards. Under the most favorable conditions, CO-Hb concentration in blood is 0.2% to 0.8%. The concentration in smokers varies between 4% and 20%. Long exposure to low CO concentrations can lead to toxic accumulations. Headaches and slight dyspnea occur at values of 10% to 15% with the addition of fatigue and impaired vision and judgment at values of 20% to 30%. Coma and convulsions accompany 50% saturation with death occuring at 60%. Chronic exposure to CO may lead to a relative polycythemia.

Methemoglobin is oxidized hemoglobin in which the ferrous (Fe^{2+}) ion has been oxidized to the ferric (Fe^{3+}) state. It cannot act as an oxygen carrier because the O_2 dissociation curve of methemoglobin is flat over the physiologic pO_2 levels. Normally, methemoglobin that has formed within erythrocytes by the spontaneous oxidation of hemoglobin constitutes less than 1% of total hemoglobin. Various drugs and chemicals (nitrites, nitrates, aniline dyes, sulfonamides, and phenacetin) may oxidize hemoglobin at such a rate that the reductive capacity of the red cell is overwhelmed.

Hereditary methemoglobinemia may result from the presence of hemoglobin M, a variant hemoglobin that stabilizes methemoglobin and renders it resistant to reduction. A second form of hereditary methemoglobinemia is caused by deficiency of the enzyme NADH-methemoglobin reductase, resulting in a decrease of the methemoglobin-reducing ability of the red cells. In methemoglobinemia, the methemoglobin may be present at over 30% of the total hemoglobin, thus resulting in hypoxia and cyanosis. If the oxidation of methemoglobin continues, greenish ferric compounds called hemochromes are formed. Hemochromes precipitate to form Heinz bodies, which are seen as inclusions in red blood cells.

Sulfhemoglobin forms when sulfur rather than oxygen is linked to hemoglobin. Exposure to sulfonamides, phenacetin, acetanilide, and trinitrotoluene may lead to sulfhemoglobinemia as well as methemoglobinemia. The symptoms include anoxia and cyanosis, which are clinically indistinguishable from methemoglobinemia. Sulfhemoglobin is a stable compound. Its formation is irreversible and remains with the red cell throughout its life cycle.

Hemoglobin function

The primary function of hemoglobin is to carry oxygen to the peripheral tissues. Each of the four heme ions can reversibly bind one oxygen molecule, thus resulting in oxy-

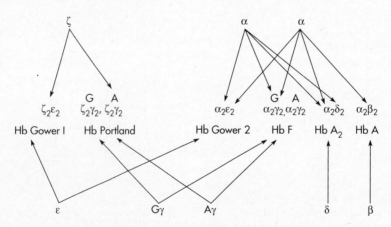

Fig. 11-3   Formation of normal human hemoglobins. *From D Harmening Pittiglio: Clinical hematology and fundamentals of hemostasis, Philadelphia, 1987, FA Davis.*

genation, not oxidation of hemoglobin. The heme iron does not change its oxidation state, it remains ferrous iron whether or not hemoglobin is picking up or discharging oxygen.

Hemoglobin can release oxygen under the relatively high oxygen tension that can exist in peripheral tissues. An examination of the oxygen dissociation curve of hemoglobin in Figure 11-4, which plots the oxygen content (% oxygen saturation) against the partial pressure of oxygen (pO_2), shows a sigmoid curve. Oxygen is released at relatively high partial pressures between 20 to 80 mmHg. In contrast, the oxygen dissociation curve of myoglobin results in a hyperbolic curve showing appreciable oxygen release at very low pressures of only 1 to 20 mmHg. Conventionally, the oxygen dissociation curve is indexed by the P_{50} value, which is the 50% O_2 saturation point. Normally, 50% O_2 occurs at 27 mm Hg for hemoglobin A. Thus, a decreased P_{50} value represents an increased oxygen affinity of hemoglobin and an impaired release of oxygen to the tissues.

Several other factors, including pO_2, temperature, pH (the Bohr effect), and the 2,3-diphoglycerate (DPG) concentration affect O_2 affinity and oxygen transport. The tissues accumulate carbon dioxide and acid metabolites, thus decreasing the pH. When the pH is decreased, the affinity of hemoglobin for oxygen decreases and the oxygen dis-

sociation curve shifts to the right. The fact that oxygen affinity varies with pH is known as the Bohr effect. Deoxyhemoglobin binds H^+ more actively than oxyhemoglobin, which is a stronger acid. In addition to the Bohr effect, the cellular concentration of 2,3-diphosphoglycerate affects oxygen affinity. The compound 2,3-DPG is an intermediate in the glycolytic pathway from glucose to pyruvate. The concentration of 2,3-DPG is equimolar with that of deoxyhemoglobin.

When the pH drops, as in acidosis, the 2,3-DPG concentration increases and the dissociation curve moves to the right. At a decreased pH, O_2 release increases and oxyhemoglobin is converted to deoxyhemoglobin. Deoxyhemoglobin binds H^+ ions and combines with 2,3-DPG. The 2,3-DPG binds to the beta chains bordering the central cavity of deoxyhemoglobin, thus stabilizing deoxyhemoglobin. Increased deoxyhemoglobin concentration raises the pH, correcting the shift to the right of the dissociation curve by an equal change to the left. The rate of glycolysis is the common denominator of the DPG-Bohr effect. Glycolysis is stimulated by alkalosis (thus increasing the concentration of 2,3-DPG) and suppressed by acidosis (decreasing the concentration of 2,3-DPG).

Laboratory testing

The photometric determination of hemiglobincyanide (cyanmethemoglobin) is the reference method for the determination of hemoglobin concentration in human blood. All forms of hemoglobin likely to occur in blood, with the exception of sulfhemoglobin, are quantitated with this method. The International Committee for the Standardization in Haemotology (ICSH) recommended in 1967, and revised in 1978, that any other method (i.e., photometric determination of oxyhemoglobin, iron determination, or gas analytic methods) should be adjusted to obtain compatibility with the cyanmethemoglobin method.

The test principal for the cyanmethemoglobin method is described shortly. The ferrous ions (Fe^{2+}) of the hemoglobins are oxidized to the ferric state (Fe^{3+}) by potassium ferricyanide, $K_3Fe(CN)_6$, to form hemiglobin. Hemiglobin reacts with the cyanide ions (CN^-) provided by potassium cyanide, KCN, to form hemiglobincyanide, HiCN. Either the transmission (%T) or the absorbance (A) of the unknown sample is determined spectrophotometrically at a wavelength of 540 nm. The hemoglobin concentration is determined by use of a standard curve. The absorbance of HiCN at $\lambda = 540$ nm is proportional to its concentration according to the Beer-Lambert law.

A suitable reagent can be prepared as follows: Dissolve 200 mg of $K_3Fe(CN)_6$, 50 mg of KCN, 140 mg of KH_2PO_4 (analytic grade chemicals), and 0.5 to 1.0 ml of nonionic detergent in type I reagent grade water. Dilute to 1L. The pH should be between 7.0 to 7.4 and the solution can be stored in brown borosilicate glass for several months.

The reaction with the aforementioned solution (National Committee for Clinical Laboratory Standards (NCCLS) February 1984) should be carried out at temperatures between 18° C to 25° C. Full color development occurs in 3 minutes. The original Drabkin's reagent contained $NaHCO_3$ rather than KH_2PO_4, resulting in an incubation time of 15 minutes or more. Drabkin's reagent did not contain a nonionic de-

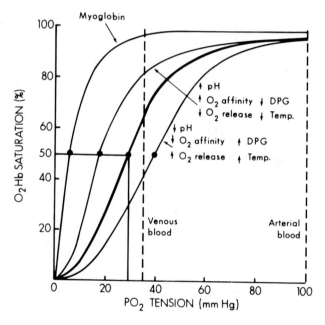

Fig. 11-4 Oxygen-dissociation curves of normal human hemoglobin. Heavy middle line, Dissociation curve of normal adult blood (temperature 37 C, pH 7.4, PCO2 35 mm Hg). Dots, P50 values, partial pressure of oxygen (27 mm Hg) at which hemoglobin solution is 50% oxyhemoglobin and 50% deoxyhemoglobin. If temperature increases, pH decreases, or carbon dioxide tension (PCO2) increases, the curve shifts to right. This shift increases release of oxygen from hemoglobin at given oxygen tension by decreasing its oxygen affinity. If temperature decreases, pH rises, or carbon dioxide tension decreases, oxygen-dissociation curve moves to the left. This shift increases oxygen-binding capacity of hemoglobin at given oxygen tension; thus there is a decrease in oxygen release. *From Bauer JD: Clinical laboratory methods, ed 9, St Louis, 1982, Mosby-Year Book, Inc.*

tergent to enhance erythrocyte lysis and minimize turbidity resulting from lipoprotein precipitation.

The preferred specimen is venous blood, anticoagulated with 1.5 to 1.8 mg Na_2EDTA. Ideally, the blood should be analyzed on the day of collection, but storing blood for 1 week at room temperature does not affect the hemoglobin value. After the sample and reagent are mixed, the resulting HiCN solution is stable. For storage periods exceeding 6 hours, the HiCN should be stored at 4° C to 10° C in the dark. Lipemia or the presence of large amounts of lipoproteins may falsely elevate the hemoglobin value because of turbidity.

In the United States the primary hemoglobin standard, the International Haemiglobincyanide Reference Preparation, is available to manufacturers and distributors of secondary HiCN calibration standards through the Standards Laboratory of the College of American Pathologists, or, on a limited scale, from the Hematology Laboratory, Centers for Disease Control, Atlanta, Georgia. Secondary calibrators are available from commercial sources for clinical laboratories. The manufacturers of secondary HiCN calibration standards can have their products certified as meeting ICSH specifications by the Standards Laboratory of the College of American Pathologists.

The most common procedures for measuring chemically modified forms of hemoglobin are spectrophotometric methods. The preferred method for carboxyhemoglobin is to mix hemoglobin in blood with sodium hydrosulfate ($Na_2S_2O_4$) to convert oxyhemoglobin and methemoglobin to reduced hemoglobin. After converting a multicomponent system to a two-component system (carboxyhemoglobin and reduced hemoglobin), absorbance measurements are made at 420 and 432 nm. A narrow bandpass spectrophotometer is used, which, if properly calibrated, allows the application of literature values for molar absorbance of Hb and HbCO. The following equation can be used:

$$\% X = \frac{(1 - [AR][F_1]) * 100\%}{AR(F_2 - F_1) - F_3 + 1}$$

Calculate $AR = A_{420}/A_{432}$ for each unknown.

$$F_1 = aHb_{432}/aHb_{420}$$
$$F_2 = aHbCO_{432}/aHb_{420}$$
$$F_3 = aHbCO_{420}/aHb_{420}$$
$$\% X = \text{percentage of HbCO}$$

The following literature constants can be substituted:

$$F_1 = 1.3330, F_2 = 0.4787, F_3 = 1.9939.$$

The literature constants must be confirmed for use in each laboratory and reverified as often as the spectrophotometer is subjected to source lamp changes or electronic repair.

A spectrophotometric method can be used to screen for methemoglobin or sulfhemoglobin. A characteristic peak can be observed between 620 and 640 nm in the presence of methemoglobin or sulfhemoglobin. One drop of 5% potassium cyanide solution should be added to the sample. The mixture should be mixed and scanned again. CAUTION: Cyanides are among the most deadly poisons known. For safety, amyl nitrate capsules should be present before per-

forming the procedure, to be used as an antidote. After scanning, no change in the absorption spectrum indicates the presence of sulfhemoglobin and rules out the presence of methemoglobin. Disappearance of the peak indicates the presence of methemoglobin and rules out sulfhemoglobin. Only methemoglobin is converted to cyanmethemoglobin by the addition of cyanide. A quantitative method for methemoglobin involves a measurement of total hemoglobin at 630 nm after the addition of $K_3Fe(CN)_6$. Potassium cyanide (KCN) is then added to the tubes and a second absorbance reading is made. The decrease in absorbance between the first and second readings is proportional to the methemoglobin concentration. It can be used to determine the percentage of methemoglobin in the total heme pigment.

IRON METABOLISM
Normal distribution and intake

Iron is biologically indispensable because it is needed to bind reversibly with oxygen and functions in electron transfer reactions. Most of the iron in humans is contained within cells in the porphyrin ring of heme and in proteins such as myoglobin, peroxidases, catalase, and cytochromes. Of all body iron, 25% to 30% is contained in the iron storage pool (Table 11-1).

Daily iron requirements vary depending on age, sex, and physiological status. Approximately 1 mg of iron is lost per day through the normal shedding of intestinal mucosa cells, skin epithelial cells, and the loss of erythrocytes in urine and feces. Thus, men and postmenopausal women require 1 mg per day of iron intake. Women in their reproductive years require 1.5 to 2 mg of iron per day since 20 to 40 mg of iron are lost with each menstrual cycle. Pregnant and lactating women, because of their greater needs, require 3 mg per day. The average North American diet contains 10 to 20 mg of iron per day.

Absorption and turnover

Iron absorption is rather inefficient and only 5% to 10% of dietary iron (1 to 2 mg) is absorbed through the duodenum and upper small intestine. Dietary iron is usually in the oxidized ferric (Fe^{+3}) state and must be reduced to the ferrous (Fe^{+2}) state by gastric secretions and hydrochloric acid for efficient absorption. In addition, iron forms insol-

Table 11-1 Iron distribution and function in a normal adult

Compound	Function	Iron (mg)
Hemoglobin	O_2 transport, blood	2500
Myoglobin	O_2 storage, muscle	
Enzymes		
Catalase	H_2O_2 decomposition	300
Peroxidases	Oxidation	
Cytochromes	Electron transfer	
Iron-sulfur*	Electron transfer	
Transferrin*	Iron transport	4
Ferritin* and	Iron storage	1000 (men)
hemosiderin*		100-400 (women)

Modified from Schreiber WE: Medical aspects of biochemistry, Boston, 1984, Little, Brown.
*Nonheme iron compounds.

uble complexes with many foods such as with phosphates in dairy products and oxalates and phytates in vegetables, which makes absorption difficult. Heme iron from meat and fish is absorbed more readily than the complexes of nonheme iron, even though these other dietary iron sources are smaller in molecular size.

In addition to dietary iron, the body recovers iron (10 to 25 mg/day) from the destruction of old erythrocytes. Phagocytic cells engulf the red blood cells (RBCs), then break open the porphyrin ring and release iron. The iron is transported in the plasma by transferrin to the bone marrow for hemoglobin synthesis. A small amount of this iron is conserved in other tissues and in the storage pool of the liver, spleen, and bone marrow.

Iron loss is largely unregulated, so iron absorption controls the body's iron supply. Within the intestinal cells, iron is absorbed and transported by a carrier protein to mitochondria for heme synthesis, stored as ferritin, or transferred directly into plasma to join the circulating iron pool.

The mechanisms for controlling iron by the intestinal cells is poorly understood. However, iron deficiency leads to increased uptake and transfer of iron from the intestinal cells to plasma and mitochondria and decreased transfer to ferritin storage forms. Conversely, iron load leads to normal uptake with decreased transfer to plasma and increased deposition to intracellular ferritin as a storage form.

Normally, the iron in mitochondria and ferritin is lost with the shedding of intestinal mucosa cells into the stool. New intestinal cells are grown and iron stores build up as cellular replacement occurs.

Transport and storage

Iron is transported in the blood by transferrin, a transport protein consisting of a single chain polypeptide with a molecular weight of 79,500 daltons. Each transferrin molecule has two binding sites for ferric iron and these sites are normally 20% to 50% saturated. Free iron is highly toxic and relatively insoluble, so all plasma iron is protein-bound. Iron is delivered to cells with transferrin-specific surface receptors.

Body iron is stored in the liver (one third), bone marrow (one third), and the remainder is stored in the spleen and other tissues. Storage is in the form of ferritin and hemosiderin. Since free iron is highly toxic, it is surrounded by a protein coat that isolates it from the cellular contents until needed. Ferritin has a multisubunit protein shell (apoferritin), which surrounds an iron core composed of hydrated, ferric oxide-phosphate complex. Iron in the ferrous form (Fe^{2+}) is taken up by ferritin and oxidized to the ferric (Fe^{3+}) form, where it is stored in the iron core. When iron is released from ferritin, it is reduced back to the ferrous form. Ferritin is found in nearly all cells, especially hepatocytes.

Hemosiderin is an insoluble complex derived from ferritin. The ferritin loses some of its surface protein, increasing the relative amount of iron to protein, and becomes more aggregated and dense. Although hemosiderin has a higher concentration of iron than ferritin, it releases the iron more slowly into circulation. Hemosiderin granules of 1 to 2 μm in diameter can be readily observed in mononuclear phagocytes of the bone marrow, spleen, and liver when stained with Prussian blue and viewed by light microscopy.

Changes of analyte in disease
Iron deficiency

As might be expected, iron deficiency leads to anemia. Iron deficiency anemia is found in about 2% of men in the United States and in about 20% of women of childbearing age. The most common cause is blood loss. The loss of blood through the menstrual cycle is a common cause of iron deficiency in women, whereas bleeding from the gastrointestinal tract (peptic ulcer, malignancy) is found in both men and women. Iron-poor diets containing large amounts of cereal and junk foods may lead to iron deficiency in young children and adolescents, whose growth demands increased supplies of iron. Pregnant women have an increased iron requirement as well. Weakness, fatigue, dizziness, pallor, and tachycardia are common symptoms of iron-deficiency anemia. However, in addition to the symptoms of anemia, iron deficiency has a wide ranging biological impact. A myriad of iron-containing enzymes, which include oxidases, catalases, reductases, peroxidases, and dehydrogenases, require iron for proper function. Iron deficiency in neonates and young children can lead to irreversible defects in cognitive ability. Iron deficiency during pregnancy increases maternal mortality as well as prenatal and perinatal infant death. Iron deficiency may result in lowered resistance to infection and to a lower resistance to cold exposure.

The complete blood count will reveal a reduced red cell count, hemoglobin, and hematocrit. The mean cell volume (MCV) will be low as will be the mean corpuscular hemoglobin (MCH) and mean corpuscular hemoglobin concentration (MCHC). The smear will show microcytic (smaller), hypochromic (less colored) red cells. These hematologic features may not be observed in the early stages of iron depletion. Iron loss will not be apparent in a bone marrow smear.

Serum iron levels will be decreased and the total iron-binding capacity (TIBC) will be increased. Transferrin saturation will be below normal. The single most reliable indicator of iron deficiency is a decrease in serum ferritin, which is a reflection of reduced iron storage in the tissues. Free erythrocyte protoporphyrin may be used as a screening test, but it is not specific for iron deficiency.

Iron overload

Iron overload may be either a congenital or acquired disorder. Hereditary hemochromatosis is characterized by an increase in body iron stores, leading to deposition of iron in the major organs. Inheritance is autosomal recessive, although only a fraction of hemozygote individuals actually develop the disease. Symptoms usually occur after 40 years of age. Iron deposition in the liver, pancreas, heart, and other organs leads to tissue injury and ultimately to organ failure.

Acquired hemochromatosis may be a complication of chronic anemias such as thalassemia and sideroblastic anemia. In addition to increased iron absorption in these patients, the iron load of the body may be increased by frequent blood transfusions used to treat the anemia.

The most definitive test is a liver biopsy with the direct measurement of hepatic iron and a microscopic evaluation of tissue damage and iron stores. However, because of the cost and risk to the patient, other procedures are often used. The serum iron is increased and the TIBC decreased in hemochromatosis, and serum ferritin is also increased. These procedures are more commonly used to evaluate iron excess because they are relatively inexpensive and do not place the patient at risk.

Laboratory testing
Hematology

The hematologic parameters simply define the presence or absence of anemia and its morphological character. Anemia is defined by the World Health Organization as a hemoglobin concentration below 130 g/L for men, below 120 g/L for menstruating women, and below 100 g/L for pregnant women. Since the anemia associated with iron deficiency is microcytic and hypochromic, the MCV, MCH, and MCHC are decreased. The blood smear shows variation of size in the erthrocytes with many smaller than normal and pale RBCs. Because microcytic anemias are seen with thalassemias, and sometimes with sideroblastic anemia and the anemia of chronic disease, this procedure is not specific enough to define iron deficiency anemia. The blood smear in thalassemia may show basophilic stippling, whereas these inclusions will be absent in pure iron deficiency. Nevertheless, once the presence of a hypochromic, microcytic anemia has been established, other tests are necessary to determine the cause.

Serum iron, total iron-binding capacity, and transferrin saturation

Colorimetric procedures are the most commonly used methods for measuring serum iron. The first step is a reduction of ferric iron (Fe^{3+}) to a ferrous state (Fe^{2+}) by a strong reducing agent. The second step is the binding of the ferrous iron to an iron-complexing agent and a colorimetric measurement of the resulting color. The general reaction is as follows:

1. Transferrin $(Fe^{3+})_2$ $\xrightarrow[\text{reducing agent}]{\text{buffer}}$ Transferrin + $2Fe^{2+}$
2. Fe^{2+} + complexing chromogenic agent → Colored complex
   (magneta, red)
   measured at 530
   to 560 nm

The most common chromogenic agents are bathophenanthrolene and Ferrozine, which form highly colored complexes with ferrous iron.

The measurement of serum iron is usually accompanied by the measurement of the total iron binding capacity (TIBC). Normally, only a portion of the transferrin molecule is saturated with iron. The unsaturated iron-binding capacity (UIBC) of transferrin measures the available iron-binding sites of serum. The amount of iron that serum transferrin can bind when completely saturated is the total iron-binding capacity. The TIBC is measured by first saturating the transferrin with excess ferric iron. The remaining unbound iron is removed by a chelator. The total amount of iron saturating the transferrin is measured by the aforementioned colorimetric method for serum iron. The reference interval for serum iron for men is 500 to 1600 μg/L and is 400 to 1500 μg/L for women. The range for TIBC, which is an indirect measurement of transferrin levels, is 2500 to 4000 μg/L and transferrin saturation is normally 20% to 55%. See Table 11-2 for the correlation of iron measurements to disease.

Serum ferritin

Ferritin circulating in plasma is normally in equilibrium with tissue iron stores. Serum ferritin can be measured by radioimmunoassay (RIA), enzyme immunoassay (EIA), or immunoradiometric assay (IRMA). The reference interval is generally between 20 and 200 ng/mL. A serum ferritin level below 10 ng/mL almost always indicates iron deficiency anemia. Significant tissue destruction or rapid cellular turnover such as with inflammation, liver disease, or malignancies, will result in a serum ferritin level that is disproportionately high when compared to bone marrow iron.

Free erythrocyte protoporphyrin

In the final steps of heme synthesis, the erythrocyte enzyme, ferrochetalase, inserts the ferrous iron into the protoporphyrin. Protoporphyrin without the iron is not incorporated into hemoglobin. The ferrochetalase reaction is a rate-limiting step in the heme synthetic pathway and the insertion of iron into protoporphyrin facilitates a negative feedback. Thus, in the absence of iron, there is no negative

Table 11-2 Laboratory measurements of iron status*

Disease	Serum iron (μg/L)	TIBC (μg/L)	Transferrin saturation (%)	Serum ferritin (μg/L)	Free erythrocyte protoporphyrin (μg/L cells)	Tissue iron stores
Normal	500-1600	2500-4000	20-55	15-200	170-770	N
Storage iron depletion, no anemia	N	N	N	↓	N	↓
Iron-deficiency anemia	↓	↑	↓	↓	↑	↓
Anemia of chronic disease	↓	↓	↓	N or ↑	↑	N or ↑
Thalassemia	↑	↓	↑	↑	N	↑
Sideroblastic anemia	↑	N	↑	↑	N or ↑	↑
Hemochromatosis	↑	↓	↑	↑	N	↑

From Schreiber WE: Iron, porphyrin, and bilirubin metabolism. In Kaplan LA and Pesce AJ: Clinical chemistry: theory, analysis, and correlation, ed 2, St Louis, 1989, Mosby—Year Book, Inc.
*N, Normal; ↓, decreased; ↑, increased.

feedback for protoporphyrin production and free erythrocyte protoporphyrin (FEP) increases several-fold.

Actually, the excess protoporphyrin is not really free, but is bound primarily to zinc in the absence of iron. Red cell protoporphyrin assays involve an acid extraction that removes the zinc and increases the metal-free compound left behind. After extraction, FEP is measured by fluorescence or by direct assessment with a hemofluorometer.

The reference range for FEP depends on the laboratory, but is generally between 15 to 80 μg/dL of RBCs. In the presence of iron deficiency and chronic disease states, FEP can increase fivefold. Free erythrocyte protoporphyrin remains with the RBC for its entire life span so that iron deficiency can be diagnosed even after iron therapy. Free erythrocyte protoporphyrin is a useful method for distinguishing thalassemia (normal FEP) from iron deficiency (elevated FEP). Nevertheless, FEP is only a screening test. It can be elevated in iron deficiency, sideroblastic anemia, the anemia of chronic disease, and lead poisoning. Thus, an elevated FEP when testing for iron deficiency should be followed by specific tests for iron status.

HEME SYNTHESIS AND THE PORPHYRIAS
Structure and function

The structure of heme is an organometallic complex of protoporphyrin IX and ferrous iron (Figure 11-5). The porphyrin ring contains alternating single and double bonds that absorb light, thus imparting the red color to hemoglobin. Porphyrin rings also fluoresce a reddish-pink color when illuminated with an ultraviolet light. This property can be used to detect porphyrins in body fluids. The four nitrogen atoms at the center of the ring enable the chelation of metal atoms. The most important of these is the iron in heme.

All cells synthesize heme, but the bone marrow producing red cell precursors and liver cells are the primary sites of heme synthesis. Heme synthesis can be divided into the following two steps: (1) the formation of the porphyrin ring by the condensation of precursors and (2) modification of the side chains and insertion of iron. Figure 11-6 summarizes the porphyrin pathway and shows the localization of the synthetic pathway between the mitochondria and cytosol. The first step of the pathway, the condensation of succinyl CoA and glycine to form δ aminolevulinic acid (ALA), is catalyzed by the enzyme ALA synthase and is the rate-limiting step in heme synthesis. Excess heme inhibits the enzyme activity and a deficit of heme stimulates the enzyme. There are three major classes of porphyrins in humans: (1) uroporphyrin (URO), (2) coproporphyrin (COPRO), and (3) protoporphyrin (PROTO). They differ by the type and position of the side chains located at the corners of the pyrrole rings; each class has several principle isomers. The route of a specific type of porphyrin excretion is a function of its solubility. Uroporphyrin is the most water-soluble and is excreted in urine. Protoporphyrin, the least water-soluble,

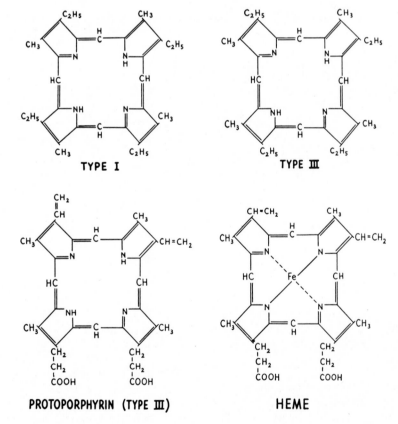

Fig. 11-5   Structure of porphyrin compound: types I and III isomers, protoporphyrin (type III), and heme.
From Miale JB: Laboratory medical hemotology, ed 5, St Louis, 1982, Mosby–Year Book, Inc.

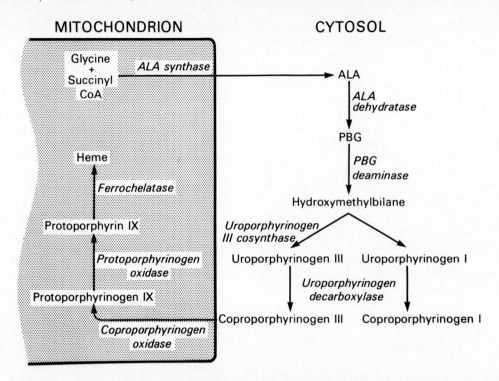

Fig. 11-6 Distribution of the porphyrin pathway between mitochondria and cytosol. *From Kaplan LA, Pesce AJ: Clinical Chemistry: theory, analysis, and correlation, ed 2, St. Louis, 1989, Mosby-Year Book, Inc.*

Table 11-3 Biochemical and clinical features of the porphyrias

	Acute intermittent porphyria	Variegate porphyria	Coproporphyria	Congenital erythropoietic porphyria	Protoporphyria	Porphyria cutanea tarda
Enzyme defect	Porphobilinogen deaminase	Protoporphyrinogen oxidase	Coproporphyrinogen oxidase	Uroporphyrinogen III cosynthase	Ferrochelatase	Uroporphyrinogen decarboxylase
Inheritance	Autosomal dominant	Autosomal dominant	Autosomal dominant	Autosomal recessive	Autosomal dominant	Autosomal dominant
Signs and symptoms						
Abdominal pain and neurological symptoms	Yes	Yes	Yes	No	No	No
Photosensitivity and cutaneous lesions	No	Yes	Yes	Yes	Yes	Yes
Metabolic expression	Liver	Liver	Liver	Erythroid cells	Erythroid cells and liver	Liver

From Schreiber WE: Iron, porphyrin, and bilirubin metabolism. In Kaplan LA and Pesce AJ: Clinical chemistry: theory, analysis, and correlation, ed 2, St Louis, 1989, Mosby-Year Book, Inc.

is excreted exclusively in feces. Coproporphyrin is found in both urine and feces. The porphyrin precursors ALA and porphobilinogen (PBG) are excreted in urine.

Porphyria disorders

The porphyrias are generally classified by signs and symptoms into neurological porphyria or cutaneous porphyria. The neurological porphyrias can be divided into three disorders: (1) acute intermittent porphyria, (2) variegate porphyria, and (3) coproporphyria. All three disorders are char-

acterized by abdominal pain, constipation, neuromuscular signs and symptoms, and psychotic behavior. In each case, the disorder occurs because of a deficiency of a specific enzyme in the biosynthetic pathway (Table 11-3). The enzyme defects are inherited as autosomal dominant traits. However, their biochemical basis is not completely understood because a number of people have the enzymatic defects, but do not develop acute attacks. These individuals are said to have *latent porphyria*. The attacks may occur spontaneously or may be precipitated by exposure to alcohol, toxins like lead, hormones like estrogens, and a wide variety of drugs. The signs and symptoms of porphyria are usually absent between attacks.

The enzyme defect in acute intermittent porphyria is a partial deficiency of porphobilinogen deaminase. As a result, the porphyrin precursors ALA and PBG accumulate in the body. Thus, the major diagnostic finding is an increase in urine ALA and PBG during attacks. Between attacks the values or urinary ALA and PBG return to normal and it is unclear whether or not enzyme concentrations are higher at this time. The patients suffer abdominal pain and neurological symptoms. Fecal porphyrins are normal.

Variegate porphyria differs clinically from acute intermittent porphyria in that in addition to abdominal pain and neurological symptoms, these patients also suffer from sensitivity of the skin to sunlight and mechanical trauma. The photosensitivity is caused by the accumulation of protoporphyrin and coproporphyrin in the body. The enzyme defect is a partial deficiency of protoporphyrinogen oxidase. δ-Aminoleulinic acid and PBG are increased in the urine during acute attacks. However, in addition, there is an increased excretion of protoporphyrin, as well as some coproporphyrin, in feces. King George III of England is thought to have had variegate porphyria.

The clinical symptoms of coproporphyria are similar to those of variegate porphyria except that only one third of the patients suffer from photosensitivity. The biochemical defect is a partial deficiency of coproporphyrinogen. Urinary ALA and PBG values are increased during acute attacks. Coproporphyrin accumulates and is excreted in feces and urine.

Patients with cutaneous porphyria have an excess of porphyrins in the body tissues. These molecules absorb light at about 400 nm. The energy from the light absorption may be transferred to molecular oxygen, creating an excited oxygen species capable of attacking cellular components. These events translate into photosensitivity and the production of skin lesions. The cutaneous porphyrias differ from the neurological porphyrias in that ALA and PBG are not excreted in excess and no neurological signs and symptoms are present.

Congenital erythropoietic porphyria is the most severe of the porphyrias. The disease manifests itself in early childhood. Extreme photosensitivity leads to extensive scarring and mutilation of body areas exposed to light such as the fingers, nose, and ears.

Erythrodontia, a unique reddish-brown staining of teeth, is caused by porphyrin deposition. The excessive amounts of uroporphyrins and coproporphyrins cause pink or red urine. Uroporphyrins and coproporphyrins also cause the red cells to fluoresce. Fecal porphyrins are increased. Hemolytic anemia and hypersplenism also occur. The disease is caused by a deficiency of uroporphinogen III cosynthase. Type III isomer is limited in production and type I isomer is produced in its place. The type I isomers are oxidized to form uroporphyrin I and coproporphyrin I. Fortunately, erythrodontia is inherited as an autosomal recessive trait and is relatively rare.

Protoporphyria is caused by a partial deficiency of ferrochelatase, the last enzyme in the pathway for heme synthesis. Photosensitivity caused by the accumulation of protoporphyrin begins in early childhood. Burning and itching, followed by swelling and redness, occurs in sun-exposed areas of the skin. Scarring is rare. A few patients develop liver disease because the liver is involved in the excretion of large amounts of protoporphyrin. Urine porphyrins, ALA, and PBG are normal. Fecal protoporphyrin is increased. Free erythrocyte protoporphyrin is increased.

The most common of all porphyrias is porphyria cutanea tarda. Patients afflicted with this disease suffer from photosensitivity, hyperpigmentation or hypopigmentation, mechanical fragility of skin, and blister formation. Onset is in adulthood and the disease remains dormant until some form of liver dysfunction develops, such as overload of hepatic iron stores or alcoholic liver disease. A partial deficiency of uroporphyrinogen decarboxylase leads to high levels of uroporphyrin and especially the 7-carboxyl porphyrin in urine. Fecal porphyrins are usually normal. The presence of an unusual porphyrin, isocoproporphyrin, is distinctive.

Secondary disorders of porphyrin metabolism may occur with lead poisoning, iron deficiency, and coproporphyrinuria. In lead poisoning, urinary ALA (but not PBG), the erythrocyte concentration of zinc protoporphyrin, and urinary coproporphyrin are increased. Lead inhibits ALA dehydrase and ferrochelatase, enzymes in the porphyrin pathway. However, a diagnosis of lead poisoning is made by the measurement of lead concentrations in whole blood. Conditions such as iron deficiency, malignancies, and infections lead to a decrease in available iron. As a result, zinc protoporphyrin accumulates to above normal concentrations in red cells and free erythrocyte protoporphyrin will be increased. A small, isolated increase in urinary coproporphyrin is a nonspecific finding in liver disease, acute illness, or exposure to toxic compounds.

Laboratory testing

The laboratory work-up for a prophyrin disorder might begin with screening tests on random urine and stool specimens (about 1 g of stool). Qualitative tests should be positive on both urine and feces for all forms of porphyria. Qualitative testing may also be performed on whole blood samples (any commonly used anticoagulant), but this test is less useful as an initial screen because blood porphyrins are elevated in the cutaneous porphyrias but not in the neurological porphyrias (Table 11-3). The qualitative screen for total porphyrins is based on the extraction of the porphyrins into an organic solvent (ethyl acetate) containing glacial acetic acid. The pH of this solution is close to the isoelectric point of the porphyrins, thus rendering them less soluble in water and more soluble in the organic solvent. The porphyrins are back-extracted into 3 M HCL to leave behind interfering materials such as drugs or abnormal metabolites that also fluoresce. The aqueous layer is removed and examined under long-wave ultraviolet light. Moderate elevations of porphyrin give a lavender fluorescence and greatly elevated porphyrin concentrations appear pink or even red.

Normal urine and feces should show no color after the back extraction. Normal blood may show a trace of porphyrin fluorescence. A porphyrin concentration in blood of two to three times normal will give a distinct reddish pink fluorescence. Because erythrocytes contain almost all of the porphyrins in whole blood, this screen really detects erythrocyte porphyrins. The screening tests show a trace of fluorescence at the following concentrations:

urine: 200 μg of porphyrin per liter of urine

stool: 60 mg of porphyrin per gram of dry weight of stool

blood: 500 to 600 μg of porphyrin per liter of whole blood.

When the urine screening test by extraction is positive or difficult to interpret, it may be helpful to identify the porphyrin (uroporphyrin or coproporphyrin) by thin-layer chromatography.

Ten microliters of the organic layer containing the porphyrins can be spotted onto a silica gel G-coated slide, approximately 10 mm from the bottom of the slide. The slide is placed in a covered staining jar containing 3 ml of chromatographic solvent, such as chloroform:methanol:ammonium hydroxide:water (12:12:3:2, V/V), and allowed to develop until the solvent has moved about half way up the slide (5 to 10 minutes). The coprophorphyrin (COPRO) spot should be clearly separated from the origin. The slide is observed under ultraviolet light. With normal urine, a COPRO spot shows about two thirds of the distance from the origin to the solvent front (R_f = 0.60 to 0.65), with little or no fluorescence remaining at the origin (URO). A noticeable increase in the intensity of the COPRO spot or a clearly visible URO spot indicates a higher than normal concentration for that porphyrin.

When the aforementioned screening tests are positive, then quantitative tests should be performed. The most widely used method is a solvent extraction technique. Coproporphyrin is extracted by adjusting urine to pH 4.5 and then shaking with an organic solvent (ethyl acetate). The urine is then adjusted to a pH of 3.1 and shaken with n-butanol to extract uroporphyrin. The organic layers are both back-extracted into 3 M HCl. The concentrations of coproporphyrin and uroporphyrin are measured spectrophotometrically (A_{max} = 401 to 406 nm). This extraction method only provides two fractions, coproporphyrin and uroporphyrin. These extracts may contain significant amounts of

porphyrins with intermediate numbers of carboxyl groups. The original method attempted to correct for nonspecific absorbance. However, the assumption of a linear background absorbance may not always be valid, thus lessening the desirability of the correction.

The most specific and sensitive method for quantitating porphyrins is high-performance liquid chromatography (HPLC). Porphyrins adsorb strongly to silica, so reversed-phase chromatography (C_{18} column) is used to isolate the porphyrins. Gradient elution with either a continuous or step gradient gives the best results. The porphyrin solutions are then separated by high-performance liquid chromatography. The porphyrins are identified by comparison of retention times to an external standard of known concentration. The concentration of each porphyrin is determined by fluorescence detection. The HPLC method detects less than 1 μg/L of urinary porphyrins as compared to the qualitative screening test sensitivity of 200 μg/L.

In addition to testing for the presence of porphyrins and identification and quantitation of porphyrins when present, quantitation of urinary δ-aminolevulinic acid (ALA) and porphobilinogen (PBG) may also be useful. The concentrations of these substances are increased with acute intermittent porphyria, variegate porphyria, and coproporphyria. Urinary ALA and PBG are normal in congenital erythropoietic porphyria, protoporphyria, and porphyria cutanea tarda (Table 11-4).

The modified Watson-Schwartz technique with butanol extraction is the best qualitative screening test for porphobilinogen (PBG). The urine specimen should be collected during or immediately after an attack of acute abdominal pain. The assay should be conducted within several hours to prevent the degeneration of porphobilinogen or the formation of an inhibitor to Ehrlich's reagent.

The qualitative test mixes modified Ehrlich's aldehyde reagent (p-dimethylaminobenzaldehyde, 134 mmol/L; HCl, 2.92 mol/L; acetic acid, 13.2 mol/L) combined with concentrated HCl and a urine specimen. Sodium acetate solution, 100 g/L, is added to adjust the pH to 4.0 to 5.0. A red color is observed in the supernatant when PBG is pres-

Table 11-4 Laboratory diagnosis of the porphyrias*

Porphyria	Urine ALA and PBG†	Urine porphyrins	Fecal prophyrins	Blood porphyrins
Neurological				
Acute intermittent porphyria	↑ ↑	URO ↑	N	N
Variegate porphyria	↑ ↑	COPRO ↑	PROTO ↑ ↑ COPRO ↑	N
Coproporphyria	↑ ↑	COPRO ↑	COPRO ↑ ↑ PROTO ↑	N
Cutaneous				
Congenital erythropoietic porphyria	N	URO ↑ ↑ COPRO ↑ ↑	COPRO ↑ PROTO ↑	URO ↑ ↑ COPRO ↑ ↑
Protoporphyria	N	N	PROTO ↑	PROTO ↑ ↑
Porphyria cutanea tarda	N	URO ↑ ↑ COPRO ↑	N	N

From Schreiber WE: Iron, porphyrin, and bilirubin metabolism. In Kaplan LA and Pesce AJ: Clinical chemistry: theory, analysis and correlation, ed 2, St Louis, 1989, Mosby-Year Book, Inc.
*N, normal; ↑, increased; ↑ ↑, greatly increased.
†May be increased only during acute attack.

ent. However, the color production at this phase is not specific for PBG. Urobilinogen, indole, and indicane also cause a red color. A chloroform extraction brings urobilinogen and other red pigments into the chloroform layer. Color remaining in the supernatant aqueous phase is generally caused by porphobilinogen.

The quantitative test for PBG employs an Ehrlich-HCl reagent to partially purify the PBG. Since the color fades slowly when a second molecule of porphobilinogen reacts with the colored product to form colorless dipyrryl phenylmethane, all measurements should be made at a consistent time after the addition of Ehrlich's reagent. Porphobilinogen is then separated from interfering compounds by column chromatography or by batch ion-exchange chromatography. Whereas the column chromatography technique is the standard method, the batch ion-exchange chromatography is probably more suitable for the clinical laboratory. With the batch technique, the PBG is bound to a resin (Dowex 2-X8 resin in the acetate form) and then eluted with acetic acid. The purified porphobilinogen solution is reacted again with Ehrlich's reagent and the colored solution is measured for absorbance spectrophotometrically at 525 and 555 nm. The reference interval is less than 2 mg/L of urine.

In addition to porphobilinogen, the second urinary substance that is positive with neurological porphyrias and negative with cutaneous porphyrias is ALA. Since ALA is also elevated in lead poisoning, the test is less specific for porphyria than PBG.

The most widely used screening method for ALA is performed by spectrophotometry. In some modifications, a urine specimen is passed through two chromatographic columns. The first column removes endogenous pyrrole species and the second column removes ALA. δ-Aminolevulinic acid is then eluted from the column and reacted with acetylacetone to yield ALA pyrrole. Ehrlich's reagent is reacted with the ALA pyrrole to form a colored complex that is quantitated colorimetrically at an absorbance of 553 nm. The spectrophotometric methods lack sensitivity below 0.5 μg/ml.

The best quantitative method for δ-aminolevulinic acid employs gas chromatography with the use of an internal standard. Both urine and plasma can be used for analysis. This method appears specific as no interferences for the analysis of ALA in human specimens have been reported. The reference intervals are 4 to 17 ng/mL for plasma and 25 to 100 μg/hour for urine. However, this method requires special instrumentation and is, therefore, out of reach for many clinical laboratories.

Porphobilinogen deaminase is the only red cell enzyme that is routinely measured in patients with porphyria. It is decreased by 50% of normal in all patients with acute intermittent porphyria.

BILIRUBIN
Production, transport, and excretion

Bilirubin is a breakdown product of heme-containing proteins. Most bilirubin (80% to 85%) is derived from aged erythrocytes. The destruction of red cell precursors in the bone marrow (ineffective erythropoiesis) and the turnover of hemoproteins in nonerythroid tissues account for the remaining 15% to 20% of bilirubin. Heme degradation occurs

in cells of the reticuloendothelial system. The protoporphyrin ring is opened by heme oxygenase (assisted by NADPH and O_2), releasing iron, carbon monoxide, and biliverdin, a yellow-orange pigment (Figure 11-7). Biliverdin is reduced by the enzyme biliverdin reductase to bilirubin. Bilirubin is bound to albumin for transport through the plasma to the liver.

In the hepatocytes, bilirubin is conjugated with glucuronic acid to reduce its toxicity. The conjugation of bilirubin increases its water solubility and aids in its excretion into bile. Conjugated bilirubin passes through the hepatic and common bile ducts and into the intestinal lumen. In the intestine, conjugated bilirubin is reduced to urobilinogen. Urobilinogen may be reabsorbed and returned to the liver. Urobilinogens are excreted in both urine and feces.

Total bilirubin values measure the unconjugated and conjugated bilirubin. Unconjugated bilirubin is the form that is bound to albumin en route to the liver from the reticuloendothelial system, where it is formed. It is nonpolar and not very soluble in water. Conjugated bilirubin is bilirubin that is combined in the liver with glucuronic acid. It is polar and water-soluble.

Van den Bergh first demonstrated bilirubin in serum by reacting serum with Ehrlich's diazo reagent (diazotized sulfanilic acid) and alcohol. Some bilirubin pigment in bile reacted with the diazo reagent without the alcohol addition, indicating that a change had occurred to the bilirubin in the liver. The bile pigment was called direct bilirubin since it reacted directly and did not require the alcohol addition. The terms have been replaced by total bilirubin and conjugated bilirubin. Directly reacting bilirubin is conjugated bilirubin. Unconjugated bilirubin is the indirect bilirubin that is calculated as the difference between the total and direct reacting fractions of bilirubin. Measurements of the total and direct bilirubin can help to determine the type of clinical problem and whether or not the liver is functioning normally.

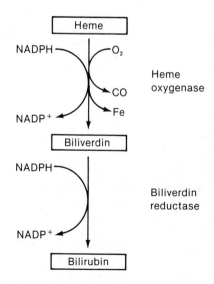

Fig. 11-7   Formation of bilirubin from heme. *From Kaplan LA, Pesce AJ: Clinical chemistry: theory, analysis, and correlation, ed 2, St Louis, 1989, Mosby-Year Book, Inc.*

Table 11-5 Concentrations and changes in concentrations of bilirubin and its metabolites in normal persons and those with jaundice

Condition	Serum		Urine		Feces pigment
	Total bilirubin	Conjugated bilirubin	Bilirubin	Urobilinogen	
Normal	2-10 mg/L	0-2 mg/L	Negative	0.5-3.4 mg/day	Brown
Prehepatic jaundice	Increased	Normal	Negative	Increased	Normal
Hepatic jaundice					
Hepatocellular disease	Increased	Increased	Positive	Decreased (normal)	Light brown
Gilbert's disease	Increased	Normal	Negative	Decreased (normal)	Normal
Crigler-Najjar syndrome	Increased	Decreased	Negative	Decreased	Light brown
Dubin-Johnson syndrome	Increased	Increased	Positive	Decreased (normal)	Light brown
Posthepatic obstructive jaundice	Increased	Increased	Positive	Decreased	Light brown

Form Sherwin JE: Liver function. In Kaplan LA and Pesce AJ: Clinical chemistry: theory, analysis, and correlation, ed 2, St Louis, 1989, Mosby-Year Book, Inc.

HYPERBILIRUBINEMIA

When the serum concentration of bilirubin reaches about 25 mg/L, jaundice (a yellowish discoloration of the skin and sclera) occurs. In neonates and premature infants, the threat of hyperbilirubinemia is significant. The liver in these patients is immature and takes days to a week or more to mature to the extent that bilirubin can be conjugated normally and excreted. With an immature liver, bilirubin values rise and unconjugated bilirubin is deposited in the brain and central nervous system. The deposition produces a condition known as kernicterus, which leads to mental retardation and death. When serum values are greater than 160 to 200 mg/L, these infants are treated by irradiation with ultraviolet lights, which causes photodecomposition of the excess bilirubin, while waiting for the liver to mature. Extreme cases are treated with exchange transfusions to lower the blood bilirubin values.

The clinical significance of hyperbilirubinemia is as an indicator or abnormal bilirubin production and metabolism, or of hepatic dysfunction. Excess bilirubin is easily bound to albumin and thus detoxified, not producing a health threat.

The five processes that lead to hyperbilirubinemia are as follows:

- Overproduction of bilirubin
- Impaired uptake by liver cells
- Defects in the conjugation reaction
- Reduced excretion into the bile
- Obstruction to the flow of bile

Overproduction is usually the result of accelerated red cell breakdown. This usually occurs in chronic hemolytic states such as sickle-cell disease or hereditary spherocytosis, or with ineffective erythropoiesis, as in thalassemia or pernicious anemia.

With hemolytic jaundice, the amount of unconjugated bilirubin in the blood exceeds the conjugating capacity of the liver. As a result, the hyperbilirubinemia is largely due to unconjugated bilirubin. Fecal urobilinogen is increased as a result of the increased bilirubin production, a characteristic finding of hemolytic jaundice. The urine content of urobilinogen also may be increased.

The Gilbert syndrome is a mild condition that results from a genetic defect of impaired uptake of bilirubin by the liver cells. The result is a large increase in the blood of unconjugated bilirubin. Urine and fecal urobilinogen are normal because bilirubin must be conjugated before the formation of these products.

Another congenital deficiency, the Crigler-Najjar syndrome, results in physiological jaundice because the intracellular microsomal conjugating system is not functional. The result is a large increase in blood concentrations of unconjugated bilirubin. Urine and fecal urobilinogen are normal.

Reduced excretion of bilirubin into the bile is found in Dubin-Johnson syndrome. In this syndrome, a biochemical defect prevents secretion of conjugated bilirubin, resulting in a backflow in the blood. Thus, the hyperbilirubinemia is caused by large increases in conjugated bilirubin.

Obstruction to the flow of bile is referred to as posthepatic jaundice. This type of jaundice is caused by biliary obstructive disease, resulting from spasms or strictures of the biliary tract, ductal occlusion by stones, or compression by neoplastic disease. The hepatic functions of transport and conjugation of bilirubin are normal. Therefore, conjugated bilirubin increases in the serum and urine. A summary of changes for serum bilirubin in several disease states is given in Table 11-5.

SUGGESTED READING

Franco RS: Ferritin. In Pesce AJ and Kaplan LA: Methods in clinical chemistry, St Louis, 1987, Mosby–Year Book, Inc.

McNeely MD: Porphobilinogen. In Pesce AJ and Kaplan LA: Methods in clinical chemistry, St Louis, 1987, Mosby-Year Book, Inc.

Nipper HC: Carboxyhemoglobin (carbon monoxide). In Pesce AJ and Kaplan LA: Methods in clinical chemistry, St Louis, 1987, Mosby–Year Book, Inc.

Perrotta G: Iron and iron-binding capacity. In Pesce AJ and Kaplan LA: Methods in clinical chemistry, St Louis, 1987, Mosby–Year Book, Inc.

Schreiber WE: Iron, porphyrin, and bilirubin metabolism. In Kaplan LA and Pesce AJ: Clinical chemistry, (ed 2), St Louis, 1989, Mosby–Year Book, Inc.

Schreiber WE: Porphyrin fractionation. In Kaplan LA and Pesce AJ: Methods in clinical chemistry, St Louis, 1987, Mosby–Year Book, Inc.

Scrimshaw NS: Iron deficiency, Scientific American, October, 1991.

Tabor MW: Delta-aminolevulinic acid. In Pesce AJ and Kaplan LA: Methods in clinical chemistry, St Louis, 1987, Mosby–Year Book, Inc.

Tietz NW: Determination of methemoglobin and sulfhemoglobin. In Fundamentals of clinical chemistry, Philadelphia, 1987, WB Saunders.

12 Proteins

Kory M. Ward
Kathy V. Waller

STRUCTURE, CLASSIFICATION, SYNTHESIS, METABOLISM, AND BIOLOGICAL FUNCTION
Structure

Proteins are found in all the cells and fluids of the body. They are synthesized within the cells of the body and released into the interstitial fluid of the tissues, and then into the plasma. The number and kind of amino acids, as well as their sequence in the polypeptide chain, give each plasma protein its characteristic shape and influence its biological function. There are several designations given to the protein structure that relate to its shape or conformation. The sequence of the amino acids in the polypeptide chain is known as the *primary structure*. This specific sequence is determined by the DNA code, which subsequently determines its biologic properties. The *secondary structure* is the winding of the polypeptide chain and the formation of hydrogen bonds, resulting in amino acid residues in close proximity to one another. This secondary structure can form alpha helices, beta pleated sheets, or random coils. The *tertiary structure* refers to the way the chain folds over on itself to form the three-dimensional structure. This folding is caused by the formation of covalent bonds (i.e., disulfide bonds, S-S), electrostatic bonds, hydrogen bonds, and hydrophobic bonds that occur from the bonding of amino acid residues that are far apart in the linear sequence. Consequently, the tertiary structure confers the specific biologic properties. The *quaternary structure* is the arrangement of two or more polypeptide chains to form a complex protein. Albumin, for example, is a protein composed of only one polypeptide chain and thus has no quaternary structure. Conversely, an enzyme, such as creatinine kinase, made of two polypeptide chains, has three major isoenzyme forms that result in various quaternary structures of this protein.

Classification, properties, and functions
Classification

Because of the great structural and functional diversity of proteins, it is difficult to arrange them in a simple classification scheme. Proteins have been traditionally classified by their physicochemical properties, for example, their solubilities: globular proteins are water soluble and fibrous proteins are not water soluble. Proteins can be further classified into simple and conjugated.

Conjugated proteins are those that have a nonprotein group attached to them. The conjugated protein consists of two components—the protein, referred to as the apoprotein and the nonprotein prosthetic group. The particular prosthetic group may be a metal ion, a carbohydrate moiety, a lipid, a nucleic acid, or a phosphate. These specific prosthetic groups impart certain functional characteristics to the protein (Figure 12-1). The names assigned to these conjugated proteins are self-descriptive. Nucleoproteins contain nucleic acids; an example of this type of protein is a histone. Several terms are used to describe those proteins that contain carbohydrates. Glycoprotein is the term applied to a protein containing 10% to 15% carbohydrate. A conjugated protein containing greater than 15% carbohydrate is referred to as a mucoprotein or proteoglycan. Tamm-Horsfall protein, for example, is a mucoprotein synthesized by the epithelial cells in the distal tubules of the kidney. Other examples of mucoproteins include chondroitin sulfate found in bone tissue and keratin found in hair and nails. Hemoglobin is a type of metalloprotein. Lipoproteins consist of lipids such as cholesterol, triglycerides, and phospholipids combined together inside a protein coat. Examples of lipoproteins include low-density lipoprotein, high-density lipoproteins, very low density lipoproteins, and chylomicrons. Many of the phosphoproteins in the body include enzymes that become phosphorylated and subsequently, become physiologically active (or inactive) depending upon the specific metabolic pathway.

Physicochemical properties

The general physicochemical properties of proteins are often utilized as a basis for identification, separation, and quantitation of the numerous proteins found in body fluids. These properties of proteins are used as the principles of analysis. Proteins can be physically separated based on size. Since proteins are typically macromolecules of high molecular weight, they can be easily separated from other, smaller molecules by techniques based on size, such as dialysis or gel filtration. The density of most proteins is

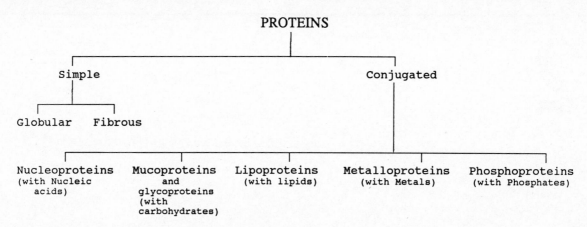

Fig. 12-1   General classification scheme of proteins.

approximately 1.33, with the exception of lipoproteins, which are between 1.006 and 1.21 and which can be separated by density-gradient ultracentrifugation.

Another property of proteins, solubility, is associated with the ability of proteins to denature and, thus, precipitate out of solution. Loss of solubility is the loss of affinity of the solute (e.g., the protein) for its solvent. Physicochemical properties of the solvent such as pH, ionic strength, dielectric constant, and temperature will influence the affinity of the protein for the solvent. Proteins can denature, and thus precipitate out of solution by exposure to high temperatures; they can also undergo hydrolysis by strong acids or alkalis, enzymatic action, or exposure to urea, detergents, or ultraviolet light.

One of the earliest methods employed to purposely remove proteins from solution were salting-out procedures. Decreasing the dielectric character of the solvent, typically by adding salts or organic solvents to the solution, will promote aggregation of the protein. Raising the temperature of a solution will promote breaking of the intramolecular secondary and tertiary bonds of the protein, subsequently exposing the less polar interior of the protein. As a result, the protein becomes less soluble (denatures), aggregates, and precipitates out of solution. By using a range of salt solutions or organic solvents with a range of dielectric constants, a wide variety of proteins can be separated from solution. This separation technique has been used in analysis of protein-containing body fluids.

Depending upon the pH of the surrounding medium, proteins can exist with an overall positive, neutral, or negative charge. The ability of the protein to exist in three ionic forms is referred to as amphoterism. The reactive acidic or basic groups on the protein, not involved in the peptide linkage, can be manipulated by altering the pH, which will change the surface charge on the protein. At physiologic pH (i.e., 7.4), both the alpha amino group and the carboxylic group of an amino acid will be in the ionized form. Compounds such as amino acids on a polypeptide chain with two opposite charges present at the same time are called zwitterions. In a body fluid, which contains a mixture of many proteins, proteins can also be separated by their rate of travel in an electrophoretic field. Electrophoresis is a

biochemical technique that is based on this physicochemical property of proteins. Isoelectric focusing, a highly specific method of separation in an electromagnetic field, takes advantage of the phenomenon of proteins precipitating out at their isoelectric point (i.e., when the net charge on a specific protein is zero).

Alteration of the pH of the suspending medium is a technique that is also applied in ion-exchange chromatography. A mixture of proteins can be separated by manipulating the electrostatic charge on the protein through the alteration of the pH so an opposing charge on a column will attract it. Both electrophoresis and ion-exchange chromatography are two frequently employed methods for protein separation in the clinical laboratory.

Another frequently utilized method of separating proteins is based on the principle of adsorption of proteins on inert, hydrophobic, nonpolar materials such as charcoal. Adsorption of proteins can also occur with polar substances such as silica or alumina, owing to hydrogen bonding or ionic interactions. Separation of proteins in a mixture is then accomplished by eluting the absorbed material with various buffers.

Protein immunogenicity is a property of proteins, which is the basis for the newer immunochemical methods utilized in the clinical laboratory. Proteins will recognize and subsequently bind to a complementary compound with a high degree of specificity. The ability of a protein to bind to its specific antibody is the property that has become the principle for radio-fluorometric, nephelometric, and enzymatic immunoassays.

A final property of proteins is that the peptide bond of proteins is capable of absorbing light in the ultraviolet region of the spectrum, especially near 280 nm. The binding of proteins to a specific dye such as Coomassie brilliant blue will shift the wavelength of absorption so that it can be detected by a spectrophotometer. Measurement of total protein in body fluids is usually determined based on this property of proteins.

Biological functions

Plasma proteins serve a number of biological functions in the body. Each protein performs specific functions within

Table 12-1 General biological functions of selected plasma proteins

Biological function	Protein	Specific function
Transport	Albumin	General transport
	Alpha-lipoprotein	Transports lipids
	Transferrin	Transports iron
	Ceruloplasmin	Transports copper
	Haptoglobin	Binds hemoglobin
	Hemoplexin	Binds heme
	Beta-lipoprotein	Transports lipids
	Thyroxine-binding globulins	Transports thyroxine
	Prebeta-lipoproteins	Transports lipids
	Alpha-macroglobulin	Transports hormones
	Transcobalamin	Transports cobalt
Nutrition	Albumin	General transport of nutritive substances
	Prealbumin	Indicator of nutritional status
	Retinol-binding protein	Transports vitamin A
Osmotic pressure regulation	Most plasma proteins	Regulate distribution of water in body fluid
Coagulation	Fibrinogen	A coagulation factor
Immunity/defense	Alpha globulins (IgG, IgA, IgM, IgD, IgE)	Antibody formation
	Complement proteins (C_4, C_2, C_{1q})	Immune response
	Alpha-fetoprotein	Believed to protect the fetus from immunologic reaction from the mother
	Alpha$_1$-antitrypsin	Acute phase reactant
	Alpha$_1$ acid glycoprotein	Acute phase reactant
	C-reactive protein	Acute phase reactant

these broad categories. Table 12-1 outlines the functions of selected plasma proteins. Although the exact biological functions of some plasma proteins have not been elucidated, several proteins have become useful biochemical markers of disease. Beta$_2$-microglobulin, for example, is a plasma protein that becomes elevated in renal failure, inflammation, and certain neoplasms. The most common purpose of the beta$_2$-microglobulin assay is to monitor renal tubular function. Many proteins have specific binding properties and appear to serve as carriers. The binding of metals, vitamins, hormones, or drugs to proteins serves to transport the bound substance to a location where it can be utilized (e.g., thyroxine with thyroxine-binding globulin), maintain the bound substance in the soluble state (e.g., lipids with apolipoproteins), provide a site for removal of excess of a substance (e.g., hemoglobin with hemoplexin), and prevent loss of substances (e.g., iron with transferrin) through the kidneys.

Synthesis, metabolism, and catabolism of proteins

Most plasma proteins, with the exception of some immunoglobulins and protein hormones, are synthesized in the liver. Albumin, alpha-globulins, beta-globulins, and some gamma-globulins are secreted by the hepatocytes and enter the general circulation via central veins of the liver. Most immunoglobulins originate from plasma cells in the bone marrow. Synthesis of proteins occurs as a result of covalent linking of amino acids. The amino acid sequence is predetermined by the genetic code within the cell. Deoxyribonucleic acid is transcribed into messenger RNA, which becomes translated in the cytoplasm of the protein-synthesizing cells. Protein synthesis then occurs at a rate of approximately 2 to 6 peptide bonds per second. Synthesis of intracellular proteins is not only controlled by the genetic code, but is also influenced by certain anabolic hormones (e.g., thyroxine, insulin, growth hormone, somatomedin-C, and testosterone).

Plasma proteins circulate both in the intravascular and extravascular fluid compartments. Movement of plasma proteins between these fluid compartments occurs by passive diffusion and active transport. Because of differences in molecular size of some plasma proteins, the proportions of individual proteins may vary within the different body fluids. Certain disease states may alter the amount and proportion of plasma protein within the body fluids in characteristic ways.

Catabolism of plasma proteins occurs in the liver. Following hydrolysis of the protein, removal of the amino group from the amino acids occurs within the hepatocytes. Subsequently, ammonia and keto acids are formed. Ammonia is detoxified by conversion to urea and is excreted in the urine. The keto acids enter the Krebs cycle and are recycled to amino acids or become converted to glucose or fat to be utilized for fuel. Catabolism of proteins is promoted by the presence of glucagon and cortisol.

In a healthy, nondiseased individual, a balance exists between protein anabolism and catabolism. Nitrogen balance, the difference between intake and excretion of nitrogen, is one of the most widely used indicators of assessing relative protein change. In healthy individuals, anabolic and catabolic rates are in equilibrium and the nitrogen balance is zero. During periods of growth and pregnancy, anabolism exceeds catabolism of proteins, thus a positive nitrogen balance occurs. Conversely, if protein catabolism exceeds anabolism, a negative nitrogen balance occurs. Starvation or malnourishment typically results in a negative nitrogen balance.

Table 12-2   Selected plasma proteins: molecular weights, reference ranges, and interpretative comments

Protein	Molecular weight (D)	Reference range (g/L)	Interpretative comments
Prealbumin	54,400	0.20-0.40 Values vary with age	Serves as a transport protein for thyroxine and triiodothyronine Rarely seen as a distinct band on electrophoresis Migrates ahead of albumin Increased in some cases of nephrotic syndrome Decreased in liver damage, burns, salicylate poisoning, malnutrition, and inflammation
Albumin	66,000	29-55 (0-1 yr) 35-50 (1-31 yrs) Values begin to decline after age 40	Serves as transport protein for fatty acids, bilirubin, etc., and maintains oncotic pressure Migrates the fastest on cellulose acetate electrophoresis Generally used on a marker of nutritional status Measured in urine to follow proteinuria Found in highest concentration in plasma Increased values occur in dehydration Decreased values occur in malnutrition, starvation, malabsorption, and protein losing disorders (i.e., nephrotic syndrome) Retinol binding protein
ALPHA-GLOBULINS			
Alpha$_1$-antitrypsin	55,000	0.78-2.0 Neonates have values much lower than adults	Comprises 90% of the protein that migrates immediately behind albumin A protease inhibitor A deficiency is associated with severe, degenerative, emphysema-like pulmonary disease Increases are seen in inflammatory reactions, pregnancy, and with oral contraceptive therapy
Alpha$_1$-acid glycoprotein	44,000	0.55-1.4	Associated with steroid binding Found in platelets Increased concentrations are associated with inflammation Increases also occur in pregnancy, cancer, pneumonia, rheumatoid arthritis, and other conditions associated with cell proliferation
Alpha$_1$-fetoprotein	76,000	$<1 \times 10^{-5}$	Proposed function: protects fetus from immunologic attack by its mother Measured in maternal serum and amniotic serum to determine fetal disorders, or neural tube defects, spina bifida, etc., prior to term of baby Used to monitor antineoplastic drugs Used to aid in diagnosis of hepatocellular carcinoma (hepatoma) or germinal neoplasms
Alpha-lipoprotein (high-density lipoprotein)	200,000	2.5-3.9	Alpha-lipoprotein is composed of cholesterol, phospholipids, and apolipoprotein AI and AII, predominantly There is an inverse relationship between the serum concentration of alpha-lipoprotein and risk of coronary artery disease Hyper-alpha-lipoprotein is associated with longevity syndrome
Haptoglobin	100,000-400,000	0.4-1.8	Associated with free hemoglobin binding An acute phase reactant protein Elevations occur in inflammatory disorders (e.g., neoplasma, infections) Decreased values occur in hemolytic anemias, hematomas, and tissue hemorrhage Free haptoglobin assays are ordered to evaluate degree of intravascular hemolysis following transfusion reactions or hemolytic disease of the newborn
Alpha$_2$-macroglobulin	725,000	1.5-4.2	A protease inhibitor Binds some hormones (e.g., insulin) Increased serum values are found in nephrosis, during pregnancy, and with oral contraceptives
Ceruloplasmin	160,000	0.15-0.60	Binds copper for transport Has peroxidase activity Increased values occur in neoplastic and inflammatory states, copper intoxication, pregnancy, and with oral contraceptives Decreased values occur with Wilson's disease, nephrotic syndrome, and in some cases of advanced liver disease

Table 12-2 Selected plasma proteins: molecular weights, reference ranges, and interpretative comments—cont'd.

Protein	Molecular weight (D)	Reference range (g/L)	Interpretative comments
BETA-GLOBULINS			
Prebeta-lipoprotein (very low density lipoprotein)	250,000	1.5-2.3	Transports lipids, especially triglycerides Contains apoproteins B, CI, CII, CIII, and E Increased values are seen in primary and secondary hyperlipidemias Decreased values are associated with malabsorption, malnutrition, and severe hepatic dysfunction
Transferrin	76,500	2.52-4.29	Functions to bind and transport iron Increased values are seen in iron deficiency anemia, late pregnancy, with contraceptive therapy, and acute hepatitis
Hemoplexin	57,000-80,000	0.5-1.0	Functions to remove heme, ferriheme, and porphyrins circulating in the blood Increased values are seen in pregnancy, diabetes mellitus, Duchenne muscular dystrophy, and some malignancies
Beta-lipoprotein (low-density lipoprotein)	2,000,000	2.5-4.4	Serves to transport cholesterol Contains apolipoprotein B Increased values are seen in atherosclerosis, primary and secondary hyperlipidemias Decreased values are seen in malnutrition, severe hepatic dysfunction, and chronic anemias
Beta$_2$-microglobulin	11,800	0.003	Used in the clinical management of multiple myeloma Sensitive indicator of renal dysfunction Surrogate test for HIV-1 infection
Complement: C$_3$	185,000	0.55-1.80	An immune response protein Complement factor for coagulation Increased values occur in inflammatory disease, acute dermatitis Decreased values occur in autoimmune disease, respiratory distress syndrome, bacteremia, tissue injury, chronic hepatitis
Complement: C$_4$	200,000	0.8-1.4	An immune response protein Complement factor for coagulation Increased values occur in acute inflammatory processes and malignancies Decreased values occur in disseminated intravascular coagulation (DIC), acute glomerulonephritis, especially associated with systemic lupus erthymatosus, and chronic hepatitis
Properdin factor B (PFB)	94,000	0.12-8.0	A proenzyme of C$_3$ An acute-phase reactant protein Increased during inflammation and disseminated intravascular coagulation (DIC) Decreased values occur in dysfibrinogenemia and afibrinogenemia
GAMMA-GLOBULINS (IMMUNOGLOBULINS)			
IgG	150,000	8.0-12.0	Involved in secondary antibody response
IgA	180,000	0.7-3.2	Involved in antiviral antibody response
IgM	900,000	0.5-2.80	Involved in primary antibody formation
IgD	170,000	0.015-0.2	Involved in antibody formation
IgE	190,000	6×10^{-4}	Antibody involved in hypersensitivity reactions

DETECTION, IDENTIFICATION, AND MEASUREMENT OF PROTEINS IN BODY FLUIDS
Quantitation of total protein
Total protein in serum

Table 12-2 lists the major plasma proteins together with their reference ranges, molecular weights, and interpretative comments. Methods for identification of proteins can be divided into three main groups of analysis: (1) quantitation of total proteins and albumin, (2) separation and identifi-cation of proteins, and (3) quantitation of specific proteins.

The earliest approach to measurement of total protein in the serum was the determination of protein nitrogen. This first clinically useful technique for protein quantitation was Kjeldahl's method for determining the total nitrogen content in biological material (Table 12-3). Because of its precision and accuracy, it has been the long-standing reference method. This method is not used in the clinical laboratory, however, because it is time consuming and very tedious. It is useful for nitrogen balance studies, but is not specific or

Table 12-3   Selected methodologies for serum total protein quantitation

Method	Principle	Approximate time required (hours)	Sensitivity (g/dl)
1. Kjeldahl	Nitrogen-containing compounds in the serum are converted by oxidation to NH_4^+ then converted to NH_3 and titrated with a standardized solution of HCL. OR NH_4^+ is quantitated photometrically with Nessler's reagent. Correction for nonprotein nitrogen is required.	1	0.1
2. Biuret	Formation of a violet-colored complex when Cu^{+2} ions in alkaline solution bind with the peptide bonds of the protein; maximum absorbance occurs at 540 nm	<1	0.01
3. Lowry	Pretreatment of sample with an alkaline copper solution, followed by addition of Folin and Ciocalteu phenol reagent; reduction of phosphotungstic and phosphomolybdic acids produces a color, which is absorbed maximally at 750 nm	<1	0.001-0.0005
4. Refractometry	Measurement of the refractive index is proportional to the amount of dissolved solids	<0.01	0.1

Table 12-4   Proteins: specimen collection, storage, interference, and reference ranges

Proteins	Specimen	Collection	Storage stability	Interference	Reference range
Total protein	Serum	Red-top tube	1 wk @ 25°C 1 mo @ 4°C 2 mo @ 20°C	Hemolysis, venostasis	60-80 g/L
Total protein	Plasma	Green-top tube	1 wk @ 25°C 1 mo @ 4°C 2 mo @ −20°C	Hemolysis, venostasis	62-84 g/L
Total protein	Urine	12-24 hr specimen preferred	1 wk @ 4°C 2 yr @ 20°C	Varies, depending on the method employed	<150 mg/24 hr
Total protein	Cerebrospinal fluid	Cerebrospinal fluid tube	Stability is similar to serum if sterile	Traumatic tap causing blood in specimen, xanthochromia turbidity	30-170 mg/dL (0-3 mo), 30-100 mg/dL (3-6 mo), 15-50 mg/dL (adults)

sensitive to changes in protein content. Method 1 in Table 12-3 gives the principle of this test procedure, along with the approximate time required for the assay and its sensitivity. With this method, an assumption is made that 16% of the protein mass is nitrogen. In reality, the nitrogen content of proteins varies from 15.1% to 16.8%. Another assumption made with this procedure is that no proteins in significant concentrations are lost in the precipitation step.

The most frequently used method for serum total protein quantitation in the clinical laboratory is the biuret method (method 2, Table 12-3). This spectrophotometric method, recommended by the International Federation of Clinical Chemistry, has good specificity, accuracy, and precision, and has been proposed as the reference method.

Rarely is the Lowry spectrophotometric method used (method 3, Table 12-3). Although it is exquisitely sensitive, this method lacks specificity. Many substances found in body fluids interfere with this reaction. Interfering substances that must be removed before analysis include, but are not limited to, uric acid, ethylenediaminetetraacetic acid (EDTA), carbohydrates, K^+, and Mg^{+2}.

Refractometry is a useful method of choice when only a limited sample is available or if an answer is required immediately. This procedure (method 4, Table 12-3) is based

on the principle of total dissolved solids contributing to the refractive index. Refractometry is temperature-dependent, but most measuring devices are temperature corrected. The refractive index is determined by a refractometer, which must be calibrated with a serum of known protein conentration (certified bovine albumin is the calibrator of choice). Most refractometers are calibrated at 25°C. These hand-held instruments have an internal light source, or require the user to point the instrument at an external light source. A drop of serum is spread over a small glass plate and covered. One can then view the scale; a sharp line dividing the dark and light fields is the indicator line to read the protein concentration in g/dL. This method is most useful for stat analyses, thus it is the second most widely used method for serum total protein quantitation. It must be noted that protein concentrations less than 3.5 g/dL are frequently inaccurately determined by this method. Since other dissolved solids besides protein (e.g., glucose, electrolytes, and urea) contribute to the refractive index, when they are present in high concentrations, a positive error is introduced. Error is also introduced when the serum is lipemic or pigmented.

Certified (by the National Bureau of Standards, Washington, DC) bovine albumin has been adopted as the reference material for total protein assays. Conditions for spec-

Box 12-1 Clinical significance of alterations in serum total protein

CAUSES FOR LOW CONCENTRATIONS	CAUSES FOR HIGH CONCENTRATIONS
Excessive loss of protein (mainly albumin)	Polyclonal or monoclonal gammopathies (paraproteinurias)
Nephrotic syndrome	Certain chronic diseases
Severe burns	Chronic inflammatory conditions, cirrhosis of the liver, autoimmune disease, systemic lupus erthematosus, sarcoidosis
Protein-losing entropathy	
Decreased synthesis	
Severe dietary deficiency	
Severe liver disease (except in cases of concurrent rise in immunoglobulin)	
Severe malabsorption	

imen collection, storage, and stability appear in Table 12-4, along with interferences and reference ranges for both serum or plasma total protein analysis. Although serum or plasma may be utilized, serum is the preferred specimen. A fasting sample is not required; however, it may be the desired sample to decrease lipemia. Specimens are very stable at room temperature and at 2°C to 4°C. If frozen prior to analysis, the specimen must be thoroughly vortexed before assaying. More than one freeze-thaw cycle must be avoided to ensure full recovery of this analyte, and thus avoid falsely lowered values.

An alteration in serum total protein is a result of either a change in plasma water (relative change) or a change in the concentration of one or more specific plasma proteins (absolute change). Relative changes in plasma proteins result due to hemodilution, an increase in plasma water, which is reflected as a relative hypoproteinemia. Specific causes for a relative hypoproteinemia include: water intoxication, excessive salt retention, or massive intravenous fluid therapy. Individuals assuming a recumbent position will have a fluid shift of water from the tissues into the vasculature, thus a decreased serum protein value of approximately 3 to 5 g/L will result. Hemoconcentration, a decrease in the volume of plasma water, is reflected as a relative hyperproteinemia. Specifically, dehydration due to inadequate water intake, or excessive water loss due to vomiting or diarrhea, will cause a relative hyperproteinemia.

An absolute change in one or more plasma proteins can be mild, moderate, or severe depending on the proteins affected. Since albumin is in its highest concentration in the plasma, compared to the other proteins, low concentrations of this specific plasma protein alone will result in hypoproteinemia. General causes for a decreased or an increased serum total protein are summarized in Box 12-1.

Total protein in urine, cerebrospinal fluid, and other body fluids

Healthy adults excrete less than 150 mg of total protein per 24 hours. Approximately one third of this protein is albumin and two thirds are globulins. A normal 24-hour urine specimen contains approximately 70 mg of Tamm-Horsfall protein, a mucoprotein synthesized by epithelial cells in the distal tubule; 16 mg of albumin; 6 mg of immunoglobulins; 16 mg of acid mucopolysaccharides, 25 mg of blood group substances, and trace amounts of other proteins, including enzymes or hormones. Figure 12-2 repre-

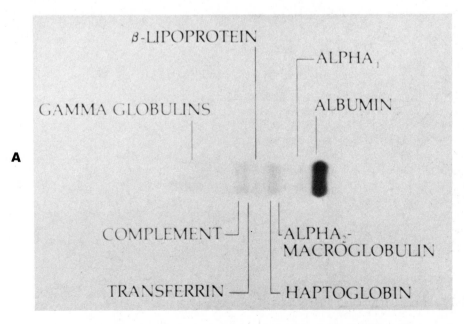

Fig. 12-2 Serum protein electrophoresis patterns. **A,** Normal (labeled). *Continued.*

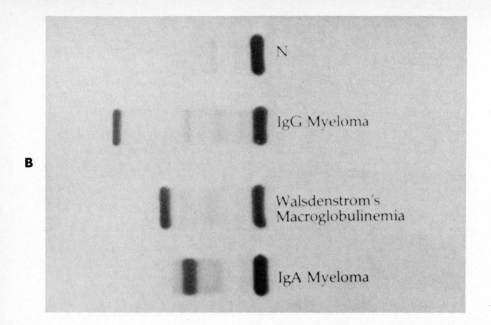

N

IgG Myeloma

Walsdenstrom's
Macroglobulinemia

IgA Myeloma

B

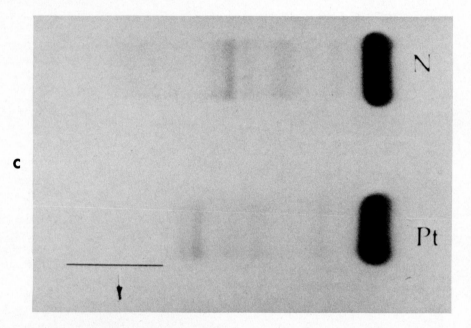

N

Pt

C

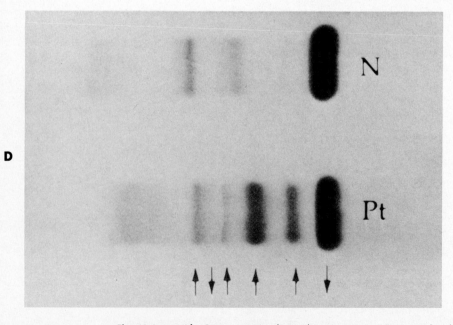

N

Pt

D

Fig. 12-2, cont'd Serum protein electrophoresis patterns. **B,** Monoclonalgammapathy. **C,** Hypogam-maglobulinemia. **D,** Acute phase reactants.

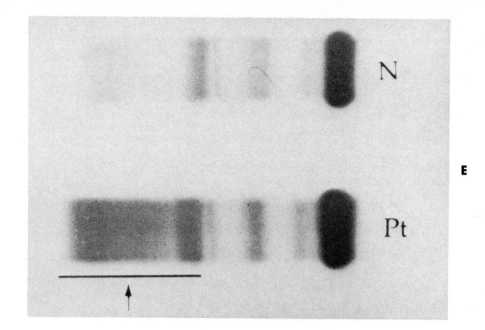

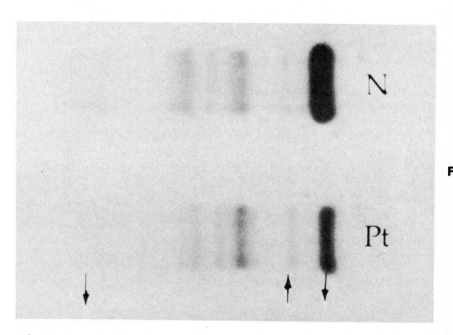

Fig. 12-2, cont'd   Serum protein electrophoresis patterns. **E,** Cirrhosis. **F,** Protein-losing enteropathy.

sents the characteristic excretion pattern of protein in urine.

Methods employed to quantitate protein in the urine usually differ from those to measure total protein in the serum. Quantitative analysis of urine total protein are based on four general properties of proteins: (1) the reaction of tyrosine and tryptophan residues on the amino acids with a phenol reagent, (2) characteristic absorption of ultraviolet light at 200 to 255 nm and 270 to 290 nm, (3) precipitation with measurement by turbidity or nephelometry, and (4) ability to bind colored dyes. These principles may be used for analysis of total protein in urine or cerebrospinal fluid.

There is no single, universally accepted method of urine or cerebrospinal fluid analysis. Both globulins and low molecular weight mass proteins are underestimated by most methods. This phenomenon results from a lack of calibrant that is sensitive to a wide variety of urinary proteins. Table 12-4 includes the specimen collection, storage conditions, interferences, and reference ranges for urine and cerebrospinal fluid protein (CSF).

The recommended reference method for total protein in urine is the modified biuret reaction. Although the color yield per weight of peptide is constant from protein to protein, the urine must first be concentrated when using this method (method 1, Table 12-5).

Because this method is time consuming, it is the least commonly used method for urine protein analysis. Another dye-binding method, developed by Bradford in 1976, is the Coomassie brilliant blue G-250 method (method 2, Table

Table 12-5 Methods for urine total protein quantitation

Method	Principle	Approximate time required	Sensitivity (mg/dL)
1. Biuret (modified)	Proteins are concentrated with TCA or ethanolic-HCL-phosphotungstic acid, and redissolved in biuret reagent (alkaline Cu^{+2} sulfate); the Cu^{+2} reagent in alkaline conditions forms a colored complex with the peptide bonds, which is detected at 540 nm.	1.0	10
2. Coomassie brilliant blue	The binding of the dye to the protein causes a shift of the absorption maximum from 465 nm (red) to 595 nm (blue).	0.01	2.5
3. Ponceau S	Precipitation of the dye with the protein forms a dye-protein complex that is redissolved in a dilute alkaline solution; the absorbance of the color produced is detected at 560 nm.	1.0	20
4. Folin-Lowry	Folin reagent consisting of an alkalinized solution Cu^{+2} in a phosphotungstic/phosphomolybdic acid solution; the Cu^{+2} binds to the peptide bonds and to the amino acid residues tyrosine and tryptophan. These complexes of Cu^{2+} with the peptide bonds and residues cause the formation of molybdenum blue and tungsten blue, which are measured at 650 nm.	1.0	5-10
5. Turbidimetry	Protein is denatured and precipitates out of solution; the resulting turbidity is measured spectrophotometrically at 450 or 620 nm.		
a. SSA*		0.05	10-25
b. TCA*		0.05	20
c. Benzethonium chloride		0.05	10
6. Indicator-Dye	Proteins, principally albumin, binds to a pH-indicator dye causing a color change (semiquantitate)	0.01	100

*SSA, sulfosalicyclic acid; TCA, trichloroacetic acid.

12-5). This rapid and inexpensive method has been adapted for automated analysis. It is very sensitive, especially to albumin, and forms a dye-protein complex that is stable for up to 1 hour. It must be noted that positive interferences have occurred in analyses of urine containing tolbutamide or high concentrations of urea. Conversely, very high concentrations of HCL, used to preserve urine specimens, cause a large negative interference.

Another dye-binding method developed in 1973 by Pesce and Strande is based on the formation of a protein-dye complex with Ponceau S (method 3, Table 12-5). The Ponceau S dye coprecipitates with the protein upon the addition of trichloroacetic acid (TCA). The precipitate is then redissolved in a dilute alkaline solution and the color produced is measured spectrophotometrically at 560 nm. Although an advantage of the Ponceau S method is that it is equally sensitive to both albumin and globulin, a disadvantage of this method is the time-consuming precipitation step. Not only does this step preclude the method from being adapted to automation, falsely low values may occur from loss of the precipitate during decantation of the supernatant. Interference by aminoglycosides, especially gentamicin, in the sample may cause falsely high values.

The Folin-Lowry method for protein quantitation has been used most extensively for research. It is seldom used in the clinical laboratory. This method (method 4, Table 12-5) involves the reaction of Folin reagent (phosphotungstic acid plus phosphomolybdic acid in an alkaline copper solution) with the tyrosine and tryptophan residues on the peptide bonds. The blue color produced is measured spectrophotometrically at 650 nm. Although this method is very sensitive, it is nonspecific and suffers from strong interfer-

ences. Interferents such as uric acid, guanine, xanthine, glycine, K^+, Mg^{2+}, EDTA, tris(hydroxymethyl)aminomethane (TRIS), and carbohydrates cause falsely increased or falsely decreased results. Standardization is also a problem since there is a wide variation in tyrosine and tryptophan residues in calibration materials.

The most widely used methods for quantitation of urine or cerebrospinal fluid protein are the turbidimetric methods. They are sensitive and easily performed. Sulfosalicylic acid (SSA), trichloroacetic acid (TCA), and benzethonium chloride have all been employed as precipitating agents (see methods 5 a, b, and c in Table 12-5). The fine suspension of precipitated protein resulting from the addition of any one of these acids is quantified turbidimetrically at 450 or 620 nm. There are variable degrees of precipitation depending upon the precipitating acid chosen. Temperature, rapidity with which the acid is added, duration of standing after the acid is added, and the presence of certain drugs can all potentially lead to variable results. The least sensitive acid is TCA; however, it estimates albumins and globulins equally if the temperature is controlled. Benzethonium chloride offers the advantage of being the least dependent on temperature. This method has been adapted to automation; however, an unevenly dispersed precipitate may occur if the protein concentration is markedly elevated, leading to falsely low values.

The most widely used technique utilized as a screening test to estimate urine protein concentration is the "dipstick" method. This semiquantitative method is based on a pH change of an indicator dye that is directly proportional to the amount of protein in the sample (see method 6 in Table 12-5). When the protein binds to a tetrabromol blue indicator dye, there is a change in the pH environment and a color change results. This test method is used to estimate the protein concentration of the urine.

The choice of method for quantitation of urinary total protein is difficult. Most clinical laboratories choose the turbidimetric or dye-binding methods because of their speed and simplicity. Often, urine samples must be diluted since these assays have limited linearity ranges; however, the urine protein concentrations can be estimated by the dipstick method first to determine the need to dilute. Unequal sensitivities for individual proteins is a problem that exists in most methods.

Although the intraindividual physiologic variation of urine protein is as high as 45% under carefully standardized conditions, the healthy range is 0 to 150 mg/day. Overt proteinuria is present at >300 mg/day in a nonexercising individual.

The reference ranges for total protein in cerebrospinal fluid is 15 to 50 mg/L. However, premature and full-term neonates have considerably higher values (30 to 170 mg/L; Table 12-4).

The specimen of choice for urine protein is a 24-hour sample; any timed urine sample has a higher predictive value for urine total protein than a random sample. However, as the time period shortens, the possibility of making volume errors by discarding samples increases. Since there is a great intraindividual variability because of nonuniform elimination of fluid and protein, the use of the total protein/creatinine ratio is advocated by some authors as an index that standardizes the excretion rate. Normally, this index is 0.1 or less. In a spot urine sample, this ratio correlates very well with total protein excretion in both healthy and unhealthy individuals. Although proteinuria may be incipient or persistent, it always deserves investigation when it persists (in 2 to 3 timed urine samples collected over a 2 to 3 month period). There are four categories of proteinuria: (1) glomerular (mainly albumin is detected); (2) tubular (usually normal low molecular weight proteins are detected); (3) overload proteinuria (resulting from an increased plasma concentration of certain proteins, such as immunoglobulin light chains); and (4) postrenal.

Glomerular proteinuria is associated with the presence of high molecular mass proteins such as albumin and IgA, which are not usually present in primary tubular disease. A major cause of glomerular proteinuria is diabetes. In fact, heavy proteinuria is one of the cardinal signs of diabetic nephropathy. Early in the course of diabetic nephropathy, the incipient proteinuria that occurs is associated with an increased excretion of albumin. One of the first clinical signs of diabetic nephropathy is proteinuria in the range of 30 to 300 mg/day.

Tubular proteinuria is associated with a host of specific proteins including, but not limited to, fibrin, polypeptide hormones, retinol-binding protein, alpha$_2$-microglobulin and B$_2$-microglobulin. Numerous proteins such as B$_2$-microglobulin, retinol-binding protein, N-acetyl-D-glucosaminidase, alpha$_2$-microglobulin, and leucine aminopeptidase have been proposed as markers of primary tubular dysfunction. Specific clinical causes of both glomerular and tubular proteinuria appear in Box 12-2.

Overload proteinuria is associated with hemoglobinuria, myoglobinuria, and Bence Jones proteinuria. Bence Jones proteins are immunoglobulin light chains that appear in the urine of patients with multiple myeloma.

Postrenal proteinuria arises from an infection, injury, or malignancy below the kidneys in the urinary tract. The presence of proteinuria along with pus cells, white cells, red cells, malignant cells, and/or urinary casts in the urine sediment offers valuable proof that the proteinuria is due to a postrenal cause.

In addition to pathologic causes for proteinuria, physiologic causes can result in benign proteinuria. Functional or benign proteinuria is associated with changes in blood flow through the glomeruli. Exercise, pyrexia, exposure to cold, congestive heart failure, hypertension, or arteriosclerosis have all been implicated with this type of proteinuria. Likewise, postural or orthostatic proteinuria is associated with an excretion of protein (>1 g/day) when in an upright position.

Examination of CSF for total protein is done primarily to detect increased permeability of the blood-brain barrier to plasma proteins or to detect an increased secretion of immunoglobulins. Box 12-3 summarizes causes for decreased or increased CSF total protein. Typically three, clean, sterile tubes are collected from the spinal tap. The three-tube collection allows for the clinical observation of a bloody tap. A traumatic tap will result in a bloody CSF specimen, which clears between the first and third tubes. In these cases, centrifugation of the specimens will yield a crystal-clear supernatant. A pigmented (xanthochromic) supernatant indicates a subarachnoid hemorrhage with lysis of red blood cells (RBCs), especially after these RBCs have resided in the CSF more than a few hours.

Methods for separation and quantitation of specific plasma proteins
Serum protein electrophoresis

Currently, over 100 serum proteins have been identified. One of the simplest techniques for assessing abnormalities of serum proteins is to perform serum protein electrophoresis (SPE). Electrophoresis is an analytic technique that is based on the principle of separation of proteins when subjected to an electromagnetic field. Since proteins are amphoteric and can carry either a positive or negative net charge, they migrate toward the cathode or anode in an electrophoretic system. The rate of migration depends upon the following factors: (1) net charge of the protein, (2) size and shape of the protein, and (3) electric field strength of the system. Movement of the protein is dependent on the degree of ionization of the protein at the pH of the buffer; thus, buffers serve both to fix the pH at which the electrophoresis is carried out and also to carry the applied current. Consequently, the buffer determines the direction of the electrophoretic migration to one of the two electrodes. The buffer ionic strength will determine both the rate of migration and the sharpness of the zones. As the ionic strength of the buffer increases, however, the proteins become more hindered in their movement through the buffer. The most widely used buffer systems that are used for electrophoresis are: (1) barbital, (2) TRIS, and (3) TRIS-boric acid-EDTA buffers.

Box 12-2 Causes of glomerular and tubular proteinuria*

GLOMERULAR PROTEINURIA	TUBULAR PROTEINURIA

GLOMERULAR PROTEINURIA

Systemic disease
Amyloidosis
Carcinoma
Hodgkin's disease
Leukemia
Lymphoma
Membranous glomerulonephritis (secondary forms)
Multiple myeloma
Polyarteritis nodosa
Poststreptococcal and other forms of parainfectious
    glomerulonephritis
Schönlein-Henoch purpura
Sickle-cell anemia
Systemic lupus erythematosus
Wegener's granulomatosis and other forms of vasculitis
Infectious disease
Hepatitis B
Malaria
Subacute bacterial endocarditis
Syphilis
Drugs and toxins
Gold salts
Heroin
Lithium
Mercury
Penicillamine
Trimethadione
Miscellaneous
Congenital nephrotic syndrome
Pre-eclampsia
Transplant rejection
Exercise

TUBULAR PROTEINURIA

Congenital anomalies
Bartter's syndrome
Familial asymptomatic tubular proteinuria
Fanconi's syndrome
Occulocerebrorenal dystrophy
Renal tubular acidosis
Renal dysplasia
Renal cystic disorder such as polycystic kidney disease
Systemic disease
Hereditary:
Cystinosis
Heritable fructose intolerance
Galactosemia
Glycogen storage disease
Oxalosis
Wilson's disease
Acquired:
Balkan nephropathy
Multiple myeloma
Sarcoidosis
Systemic lupus erythematosus
Acute renal disease
Acute renal failure
Acute tubular necrosis
Renal infarction
Transplant rejection
Infectious disease
Pyelonephritis
Viral- or bacterial-associated interstitial nephritis
Drugs and toxins
Acute hypersensitivity interstitial nephritis (penicillins,
    cephalosporins, sulfonamides, phenytoin)
Aminoglycoside toxicity
Analgesic nephropathy
Cyclosporin toxicity
Cd, Pb, As, Hg, ethylene glycol, CCl_4
Laxative abuse
Vitamin D intoxication
Miscellaneous
Exercise
Hemolytic disorders
Hypercalcemia
Hyperparathyroidism
Hypokalemia
Interstitial nephritis
Idiopathic muscle trauma (myoglobin)
Nephrocalcinosis
Obstructive uropathy
Pancreatitis
Renal ischemia
Renal tuberculosis
Vesicoureteral reflux

*From Waller KV, Ward KM, Mahan JD, and Wimsatt DK: Current concepts in proteinuria, Clin Chem 35:755, 1989.

Customarily, buffers of an alkaline pH (e.g., pH 8.6) are used for serum protein electrophoresis (SPE). At an alkaline pH, serum proteins separate into five bands or zones. In order of the fastest to the slowest moving fractions, the bands appear as albumin, alpha$_1$-globulins, alpha$_2$-glob-ulins, beta globulins, and gamma globulins. In recent years, application of high ionic strength buffers ($I = 0.075$ vs. 0.03 M) have been utilized for high resolution separations. Resolution of proteins into 13 or more zones is possible. Healthy individuals have shown 13 bands, while those in-

Box 12-3   Clinical significance of alteration in CSF total protein

CAUSES FOR INCREASED VALUES	CAUSES FOR DECREASED VALUES
Meningitis	Water intoxication
Encephalitis	CSF leak
Poliomyelitis	Hyperthyroidism
Brain tumor	
Spinal cord injury	
Cerebral hemorrhage	
Multiple sclerosis	
Tubercular meningitis	
Brain abscess	
Neurosyphilis	
After myelography	
Some cases of myx-edema	
Some neoplastic diseases	

dividuals with certain pathologic conditions will have one or more additional bands. Addition of calcium ions as a lactate salt aids in the resolution of the beta globulins, whereas high ionic strength buffers increase the resolution of albumin, alpha$_1$-globulins, and alpha$_2$-globulin fractions.

The earliest approach to the performance of SPE in the clinical laboratory involved the use of paper as a support medium. Later, cellulose acetate and agarose gel were employed as support media. Although cellulose acetate is the most commonly used support medium, agarose gel has increased in popularity. Illustrative SPE patterns are shown in Figure 12-2.

The procedure of electrophoresis involves placing the support medium containing the patient samples into an electrophoresis chamber, which contains the appropriate buffer. The electrophoretic strip undergoes electrophoresis and separation occurs while a constant voltage is applied for a predetermined period of time. The electrophoric strip is then removed and proteins are rapidly fixed, stained, and dried. The stains used to visualize and locate the separated protein fractions include: (1) amido black (i.e., naphthol blue black), (2) bromophenol blue, (3) Coomassie brilliant blue G-250, or (4) Ponceau S.

Visualization of proteins on the membrane are used to determine if there is an abnormal increase or decrease in any of the fractions and to determine if there is an atypical pattern. A scanning density spectrophotometer can be utilized to measure the light transmitted as a slit travels past each fraction. Most scanning densitometers will subsequently compute the percentage of total dye that appears in each fraction based on the absorbance record. Concentration of protein in each band is derived by multiplying the relative percent by the total protein quantitated previously by the biuret method.

Electrophoretic patterns yield both qualitative and quantitative information. Relative increases and decreases of each protein fraction can be noted, as well as the homogenicity of each band.

Immunoelectrophoresis

Immunoelectrophoresis (IEP) is a precipitation method that combines both electrophoresis and immunodiffusion. Following electrophoresis of either serum or urine, polyvalent (antitotal immunoglobulin) and monovalent antisera (anti-IgG, anti-IgA, anti-IgM, anti-kappa and anti-lamda) are separately added to individual troughs. The antigen and specific antibody diffuse toward each other and a precipitin band forms when the zone of equivalence is reached.

Immunoelectrophoresis is indicated when there is an apparent visual abnormality in the serum protein electrophoresis of the immunoglobulin quantitation. A monoclonal protein abnormality cannot be sufficiently differentiated by serum protein quantitation or electrophoresis alone. Immunoelectrophoresis is, therefore, useful in the diagnosis of multiple myeloma, macroglobulinemia, and other protein abnormalities. An SPE pattern should always be available when reading IEP patterns. Interpretation of IEP patterns requires considerable skill. Briefly, unknown bands are compared to normal control bands for each antisera. Monoclonal protein abnormalities are indicated when there is (1) an altered electrophoretic mobility, (2) an increased concentration evidenced by a broadening of the precipitation band, (3) a decrease or complete absence of a precipitin band, (4) an abnormal bowing or displacement of the precipitin band, and (5) an altered kappa:lambda ratio.

Immunoelectrophoresis is time consuming and costly, although the sensitivity of this method is 5 to 10 mg/dL. Immunoglobulins present in high concentrations often exhibit the prozone reaction and must be diluted to visualize the abnormality. Prozone reactions occur when the serum protein (antigen) is present in such high concentrations that optimal binding with antibody is inhibited and false-negative results occur. Monoclonal gammopathies of the IgM type present special problems. The IgM pentamer must be reduced to the monomeric form and the IEP repeated in order to identify the abnormality. Most monoclonal gammopathies can be identified by IEP, but occasionally a more sensitive procedure, immonofixation, is necessary to identify minor monoclonal proteins.

Immunofixation electrophoresis

Immunofixation electrophoresis (IFE) provides increased resolution to identify minor monoclonal proteins using a combination of electrophoresis followed by immunoprecipitation. Cellulose acetate strips are saturated with monospecific antisera and applied to serum protein, which has been separated by electrophoresis in the respective area of migration for that antigen. During incubation, immune complexes form that can be identified as distinct bands.

Although this method is sensitive at 5 to 10 mg/dL, there are several disadvantages. The monospecific antisera are expensive and a substantial amount is required to soak the cellulose acetate strips. The optimal antigen-antibody ratio must be estimated, and the proper dilution of serum often must be adjusted following electrophoresis. In addition, this procedure is time consuming and requires overnight incubation. Illustrative IEP and IFE patterns appear in Figure 12-3.

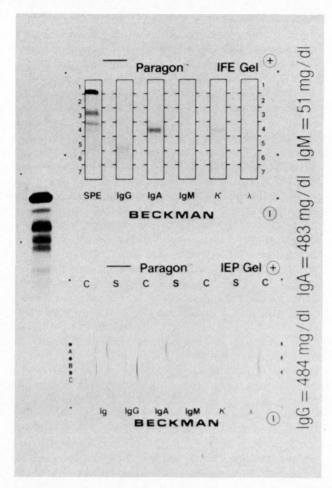

Fig. 12-3   Immunoelectrophoresis (IEP) and immunofixation electrophoresis (IFE) patterns.

Turbidimetry

Turbidimetry is one of two methods that involves the interaction of light with particles in solution. Turbidity is the diminution of light caused by reflection, scatter, and absorption by particles suspended in solution. Turbidimetry is the measurement of this decrease in light by passing a collimated beam of light through the suspension, and detecting the transmission of light by the photodetector. Thus, colorimeters, or spectrophotometers, are used to measure turbidity.

Turbidimetry is employed for specific protein applications, such as immune complexes that form as a result of the protein of interest, the antigen, binding with its specific antibody. Turbidimetry is chosen as a means of detecting particles in suspension if the solution has many dense, visibly turbid, particles. This technique is accurate and follows Beer's law over a wide range; however, if the suspension is very weak (i.e., % transmittance of light ⩾95%), then these small particles, or low concentration of particles, is better measured by nephelometry.

Nephelometry

A technique similar to turbidimetry is nephelometry. Light scatter occurring as a result of an antigen-antibody

reaction is quantitated via a nephelometer, which detects the scattered light at right angles to the incident light. The choice of technique to be used, turbidimetry or nephelometry, depends on the type of suspension to be measured. Dense, visibly turbid solutions are usually measured by turbidimetry in standard spectrophotometers. If weak scattering of light is present, or if very small particles are present, nephelometry is chosen. Nephelometry is, therefore, an extremely sensitive technique (e.g., a sensitivity of 0.6 to 1.0 mg/L). A sensitive nephelometer easily detects molecular aggregates in a solution that appears perfectly clear to the human eye. Nephelometry not only requires less time to detect, but also lends itself to automation. Because of the short measurement time, nephelometric methods can be used to analyze the kinetics of the antigen-antibody reaction.

How the light scatter is measured differs, depending on the instrument used. Most manufacturers have optimized the reaction conditions for each analyte kit they manufacture. Titering of the antisera to the human serum, urine, or cerebrospinal fluid proteins is an important step in the product development. Generally, the serum is diluted 100-fold. Approximately 60 µl of antiserum is mixed with the diluted serum. In rate nephelometry, kinetic readings are made as complexes form and increase in size. If the ratio of antigen to antibody (i.e., antiserum) exceeds the optimum titer, less scatter actually occurs. Thus, a limitation of rate nephelometry is the occurrence of excess antigen. Therefore, sensitive nephelometers must be able to differentiate the immune complex light scattering that results from all three phases—antibody excess, equivalence, and antigen excess. A second limitation of nephelometry is background scatter resulting from matrix effects. When serum or urine is centrifuged to remove lipoproteins or particular matter, sensitivity is improved.

In summary, the advantages to the nephelometric technique of protein quantitation are: (1) relatively short assay times, (2) rapid readout of results, adapted to automation, (3) simple, stable reagents requiring no label, (4) high sensitivity (<1 mg/L), and (5) excellent precision.

Radial immunodiffusion

Radial immunodiffusion (RID) is a method used to quantitate serum proteins using a reaction with single diffusion in one dimension. Reference sera, controls, and sera containing antigen are added to wells punched in an agarose medium containing monospecific antisera. The antigen diffuses radially through the gel and forms a precipitin ring with the antibody of the monospecific antiserum. Following a timed diffusion, the diameter of precipitin rings are measured and plotted on graph paper. In the Fahey and McKelvey, or early readout method, the precipitin ring is read before the zone of antigen-antibody equivalence is reached; thus, the log of the protein concentration is proportional to the ring diameter. In the Mancini or endpoint method, the precipitin ring is read after the zone of equivalence is reached; thus the serum protein concentration is proportional to the ring diameter squared when plotted on rectilinear graph paper.

Before the availability of nephelometry, RID was routinely used to quantitate immunoglobulins (IgG, IgA, and IgM) and other specific proteins in serum, urine, and cerebrospinal fluid. It is still used in smaller hospital laboratories or by laboratories with small numbers of requests for specific protein assays, and as a backup method for larger institutions. Although this method is easy to perform and economical, it lacks the sensitivity and precision of nephelometry and requires overnight incubation. The sensitivity of RID is approximately 1 mg/dL for most proteins, which makes the technique generally unsuitable for IgD and IgE determinations.

Various sources of error can affect the results. Time and temperature are critical factors in the assay. For serum immunoglobulins, this method was not affected by use of plasma, lipemic sera, hemolyzed sera, or aged sera, but icteric samples have been known to cause a slight elevation in IgG, IgA, and IgM. Samples containing IgM polymers and immune complexes yield falsely low results because of slower diffusion rates, whereas those with IgM monomers and individuals with antiruminant antibodies have falsely elevated results. Technical errors can also distort the accuracy and precision of the result. Serum proteins present in high concentrations must be diluted and retested, whereas serum proteins in low concentrations must be retested using plates containing high affinity antisera.

Radioimmunoassay and immunoradiometric assay

In the previously described techniques for quantitation of proteins, measurements are based on immune-complex formation. Thus, the final phase of the antigen-antibody complex is detected. In radioimmunoassay (RIA) or immunoradiometric (IRMA), only the primary reaction between the antigen (i.e., the hapten) and the antibody is measured.

The principles of RIA and IRMA are similar in that a radioisotope label such as iodine-125 or tritium is employed as a tag. In RIA, a competitive protein binding approach is employed. Labeled antigen (Ag*) compete for the same binding sites on the antibody (Ab). In this system, the avidity of the antibody for both Ag* and Ag must be the same. In order to quantitate the amount of protein (Ag) present, and thus detect the amount of Ag*, a means of separating the bound label Ag*-Ab from free label Ag* must occur.

There are three general methods used to separate free from bound label antigen. These include: (1) adsorption of free antigen (Ag* but not Ag*-Ab or Ag-Ab), (2) precipitation of bound antigen (Ag*-Ab and Ag-Ab), and (3) use of solid-phase antibodies to attract antibody (Ag*-Ab) and Ag-Ab). Adsorption of the free antigen can be accomplished with inert compounds such as fuller's earth, talc, charcoal, silicate, or with an ion exchange resin column. A disadvantage is that timing is critical, thus reproducibility is tenuous.

A second method, precipitation of the bound antigen-antibody complex, can be achieved by using a protein precipitant such as $(NH_4)_2SO_4$ or polypropylene glycol. Frequently, a second antibody is added to the test system to immunologically precipitate the antigen-antibody complex. Thus, if the first antibody source is from a rabbit, the source of the second antibody will be from a goat or a sheep that have formed anti-rabbit gamma-globulin antisera.

A third, and more recently employed method of accomplishing separation of bound from free label antigen, is use of solid phase antibodies. With this method the antibody has been previously polymerized, and an antibody is coated on the inside of a plastic tube.

After employing any of the separation techniques, the amount of radioactivity present as Ag*-Ab is detected by a scintillation counter. For a gamma-ray–emitting isotope tag, a crystal scintillation detector is chosen to detect the radiation. The crystal, usually a circular cylinder, is composed of sodium iodide. The gamma counter is capable of detecting gamma-emitting and X-ray emitting nuclides such as chromium-51, cobalt-57, iron-59, iodine-125, and iodine-131.

If a beta-emitter is chosen as the tag, a liquid scintillation detector must be used. This type of instrument (a beta counter) detects radioactivity occurring within a transparent vial containing a liquid scintillator. The liquid scintillator, or so-called scintillation cocktail contains both a primary and secondary scintillator. The solvent used for the primary scintillator is one of the aromatic hydrocarbons (e.g., xylene), which functions to absorb and to transfer the radiation energy to the primary scintillator, which converts the radiation energy into light energy. This primary scintillator is typically 2,5-diphenyl oxazole. A secondary solvent such as alcohol or dioxane is also added to the cocktail to improve solubility of the aqueous serum or urine samples. A secondary scintillator is necessary to shift the ultraviolet wavelength absorbed by the primary scintillator to a longer wavelength. Thus, the shifting of the wavelength allows the photomultiplier tube to detect the light emitted.

Although light is detected by these instruments, raw "counts per minute" (cpm) are quantitated by the instrument. In the clinical laboratory, these instruments typically have a computerized data reduction system interfaced with the scintillation counter.

Use of isotopes as labels can be adapted to two types of RIA techniques: (1) competitive protein-binding RIA, in which the antigen is tagged (i.e., a ligand) with an isotope, or (2) immunoradiometric assay (IRMA), in which the antibody is tagged with the isotope. In RIA, the ligand (e.g., the specific protein such as transferrin) and a constant amount of radioactively labeled ligand compete for a limited number of antibody binding sites. Therefore, the higher the concentration of the unlabeled ligand (e.g., the specific protein) in the sample, the less labeled protein is available to bind to the protein-specific antibody. The amount of bound antigen must be separated from the unbound antigen in this type of RIA. Frequently, a second antibody is added to the test system, which causes the bound antigen (both labeled and unlabeled) to precipitate out of solution. The precipitate is collected by centrifugation, and the pellet in the bottom of the tube is counted for radioactivity after the supernatant has been removed. Routinely, the best linear fitted standard curve is the log of bound (B)/maximum binding (B_o) vs. the log of the dose (i.e., standards). In this test system the higher the concentration of protein in the sample the lower the radioactivity. Table 12-6 summarizes various analytic characteristics of competitive-binding immunoassays.

Another type of RIA is the immunometric or IRMA assay. In this test system, radiolabeled antibody is utilized. With this assay system the ligand in the sample competes

Table 12-6   Analytic characteristics of various competitive-binding immunoassays

Method	Separation step	Detection limit	Low/high MW* proteins
RIA (radioimmunoassay)	Yes	1×10^{-12} to 1×10^{-14} M	Both
ELISA (enzyme-linked immunoabsorbent assay)	Yes	1×10^{-11} M	Both
EMIT (enzyme-multiplied immunoassay technique)	No	5×10^{-10} M	Low
FPIA (fluorescence polarization immunoassay)	No	5×10^{-9} M	Low
IEP (immunoelectrophoresis)	No	5-10 mg/dL	—
IFE (immunofixation electrophoresis)	No	5-10 mg/dL	—

*MW, molecular weight.

with the ligand attached to a solid surface (coated tubes or beads are frequently employed for this purpose) for the binding sites of the labeled antibody. There is a competition between the ligand bound to the solid surface and the ligand in the sample with the labeled antibody. The amount of labeled antibody bound to the solid surface is detected after excess label and sample have been removed. Again, there is an inverse relationship between the amount of radioactivity detected in the test tube and the concentration of the ligand in the unknown sample.

Enzyme-linked immunoabsorbent assay

The enzyme-linked immunoabsorbent assay (ELISA) is a useful tool in the diagnosis of infectious disease by detecting either antigen or antibody from an organism using a solid-phase and enzyme label. This method also requires the separation of the antigen-antibody complexes. Two common ELISA methods are the indirect method for the detection of antibody and the double antibody sandwich method for the detection of antigen.

In the indirect method, serum is incubated with a solid support media (i.e., bead or microtiter well) coated with the appropriate antigen. If antibody is present, it binds to the antigen and is available to bind the enzyme-labeled conjugate. The substrate is added and is acted on by the enzyme, producing a colored product. The amount of color is proportional to the amount of antibody present. This method is often used for the detection of antibodies to hepatitis, rubella, and herpes.

In the double antibody sandwich method the antigen in the serum, if present, is sandwiched between the antibody coated onto the support media and the enzyme-labeled conjugate. If the complex forms, substrate reacts and the amount of color produced is proportional to the amount of antigen present. This method is useful for the detection of hepatitis B surface antigen and IgE.

Radioimmunoassay has largely been replaced by the ELISA technique. The sensitivity of the ELISA method (less than 1 μg/dL) is similar to that for RIA, although the specificity is slightly lower. Radioactive reagents are replaced by stable enzyme reagents and results are easily read on a spectrophotometer.

In the past, total antibody concentration was measured, which did not differentiate an acute vs. chronic infection. To determine if the infection was acute or chronic, specimens were tested in parallel 10 days to 2 weeks apart. A two-tube or fourfold increase in antibody titer in the specimen of the convalescent (second) patient indicated an acute recent infection. Today, we can separate specific IgG from IgM and determine infectivity status at one point in time. The presence of IgM would indicate acute or recent infection, whereas an elevated IgG antibody titer without the IgM response would indicate prior infectivity. IgM capture techniques are also available to magnify the IgM response.

Enzyme-multiplied immunoassay technique

The enzyme-multiplied immunoassay technique (EMIT) is a homogeneous (does not require separation of the bound and free antibody or ligand) assay. This test system utilizes an enzyme-labeled ligand that competes with the unlabeled ligand in the sample. Binding of antibody to the enzyme-labeled ligand sterically hinders the enzyme and thus makes it unavailable to convert a substrate to product, which can be detected colorimetrically. As the concentration of ligand in the sample increases, less antibody is available to bind to the enzyme-labeled ligand; therefore, a direct relationship exists between the amount of substrate transformed and the amount of protein in the sample.

Fluorescence polarization immunoassay

The fluorescence polarization immunoassay (FPIA) has most recently been introduced in the clinical laboratory. This immunoassay technique is most suited to low molecular weight proteins. In this assay system the ligand in the sample and fluorophore-labeled ligand compete for a limited number of binding sites on an antibody. When antibody binds the fluorophore-labeled ligand, the fluorescence polarization is increased since the rotation of the labeled ligand-antibody complex is much slower than labeled ligands alone.

Currently, FPIA has been limited to the measurement of hormones and drugs that are small compounds. If a high molecular weight ligand were employed, no measurable change in polarization would occur since the molecule is already large.

Quantitation of specific plasma proteins
General considerations

Over 100 serum proteins have been identified and the major ones are classified by function. A functional classification would include immunoglobulins, complement factors, transport proteins (prealbumin, albumin, transferrin, haptoglobin, and ceruloplasmin), protease inhibitors (alpha$_1$-antitrypsin), and miscellaneous proteins (C-reactive protein, alpha$_1$-acid glycoprotein, alpha-fetoprotein, beta$_2$-microglobulin). Increases and decreases of these proteins are significant in various disease states.

Table 12-7   Methods for quantitation of albumin

Method	Principle	Comments
1. Electrophoresis	Albumin is separated from other proteins in an electrical field; quantitation is made by multiplying the percent of staining of the albumin fraction by the total protein value	Reference method; accurate, labor intensive, useful to detect qualitative defects (e.g., bisalbuminuria)
2. Immunochemical		
a. Electroimmunodiffusion (EID)	Migration of albumin in an electric field containing a specific antibody to albumin	Comparable to the reference method, labor-intensive
b. RID	Diffusion of the albumin through a medium containing a specific antibody to albumin	Long incubation time
c. Turbidimetry	Antigen-antibody complexes decrease light transmission more than free albumin	Involves expensive instrumentation, sensitive, specific
d. Nephelometry	Antigen-antibody complexes scatter light more than free albumin	Involves expensive instrumentation, sensitive, specific
3. Dye-binding	Albumin binds to a dye and changes the maximal absorbance of the dye	
a. Methyl orange	A_{1max} is 550 nm	Nonspecific for albumin
b. HABA (2-[4'-hydroxy-azobenzene] benzoic acid)	A_{max} is 485 nm	Specific for albumin; poor sensitivity; many drugs interferences
c. BCG (bromcresol purple)	A_{max} is 628 nm	Most often-used method; nonspecific for albumin
d. BCP (bromcresol purple)	A_{max} is 603 nm	Specific for albumin; albumins from animal sources will not bind equivalently to human albumin

Complement proteins function in the inflammatory response, opsonization, cell and bacterial lysis, anaphylaxis, and chemotaxis. Serum complement is measured to evaluate immunodeficiencies, autoimmune-like disorders, and the inflammatory response. Decreased serum complement is due to either decreased synthesis or increased catabolism. Decreased protein synthesis can be acquired and is associated with liver disease and malnutrition, or it can be congenital and is most commonly associated with C2 deficiency. Increased protein catabolism occurs in immune complex diseases such as systemic lupus erythematosus. Congenital complement disorders include deficiencies in individual components such as C3 and C1 esterase inhibitor. Complement levels are increased in acute inflammatory reactions; complement is one of the acute phase reactants (APR).

Although serum is the preferred sample, EDTA-anticoagulated plasma may be used. Methods for complement quantitation include RID (C1q, C1 esterase inhibitor, C3, C4, and properdin factor B), or nephelometry (C3 and C4). Although reference ranges are age- and method-dependent, Table 12-2 lists the average serum concentrations for C3, C4, and properdin factor B (PFB).

Prealbumin

Transport proteins carry proteins, amino acids, enzymes, drugs, and hormones throughout the body. Prealbumin is also known as thyroxine-binding prealbumin or transthyretin. Clinical interest in this protein has centered around its usefulness as a marker of nutritional status. Because of its short half-life of approximately 2 days, it is a sensitive indicator of any changes affecting protein synthesis and catabolism. Thus, prealbumin is frequently ordered to monitor the effectiveness of total parenteral nutrition (TPN). Prealbumin is significantly reduced in all cases of hepato-

biliary disease. It is a valuable indicator of liver function; serum prealbumin concentration reflects the severity of the liver injury more closely than albumin. Prealbumin is also a negative acute-phase reactant protein; the serum level falls in inflammation, malignancy, and protein-wasting diseases of the intestines or kidney. Since zinc is required for prealbumin synthesis, it decreases during zinc deficiency. Increased synthesis of prealbumin occurs in Hodgkin's disease and during chronic kidney disease, especially if tubular function is impaired. Measurement of prealbumin can be made by RID or nephelometry. The adult reference range appears in Table 12-2.

Albumin

The plasma protein in greatest concentration is albumin. In addition to its function as a transport protein, albumin serves to maintain the osmotic pressure of the intravascular fluid. Decreases in serum albumin occur as a result of an inadequate amino acid pool (malnutrition and muscle-wasting diseases), liver disease (infectious hepatitis and cirrhosis), gastrointestinal loss (inflammation of the intestinal mucosa), and loss in the urine (renal disease, especially glomerular kidney damage). Hyperalbuminemia is of little diagnostic significance, except in dehydration.

Methods for quantitating serum or plasma or urine albumin currently include electrophoresis, and immunochemical and dye-binding procedures. Table 12-7 outlines these principles. Electrophoresis is considered by many to be the reference method; however, electrophoretic assays tend to overestimate albumin quantities. Currently, automated nephelometers and turbidometers have gained in popularity. The immunochemical methods have similar sensitivity and specificity, and the precision is comparable from method to method.

Although serum is the specimen of choice, heparinized plasma may be used for all methods with the exception of the bromcresol green and bromcresol purple procedures. Reference ranges vary according to age. Table 12-2 lists the age-related ranges.

Alpha₁-antitrypsin

Alpha₁-antitrypsin (AAT), an inhibitor of trypsin and plasmin, is a serine protease that protects the body from autodigestion. Alpha₁-antitrypsin is synthesized in the liver. Values are increased in acute-phase reactions and pregnancy. Decreased values are seen in alpha₁-antitrypsin deficiency, which is characterized by pulmonary emphysema and hepatic failure in the homozygous state.

Alpha₁-antitrypsin, also known as alpha PI (protease inhibitor), has a high degree of genetic variability. About 80% of the population expresses the M phenotype (M₁ M₁). Variants include null, S, Z, and F. One in 2000 individuals will be homozygous, while the heterozygous state is found in approximately 1 in 20 individuals. Phenotyping should be performed on samples that have a decreased AAT. Genetic counseling is important in the management of AAT deficiency since serious hepatic and/or pulmonary pathophysiologic consequences are evident in AAT deficiency.

Presently, immochemical methods, mainly nephelometry, are employed to measure AAT, or more specifically, the M protein. A screen for AAT deficiency can be electrophoretic. Since AAT accounts for 90% of the alpha₁-globulin band on protein electrophoresis, a decrease in this fraction may be associated with ATT. If ATT is decreased <50 mg/dL, then phenotyping should be done by isoelectric focusing. Reference ranges for ATT can be cound in Table 12-2.

Alpha₁-acid glycoprotein

Alpha₁-acid glycoprotein (AAG) is an acute-phase reactant protein whose exact function is unknown. Clinically, this protein is used for monitoring the acute-phase reaction. The reference range for AAG can be found in Table 12-2. Immunochemical methods such as RID or rate nephelometry are used to quantitate AAG.

Alpha-fetoprotein

Serum alpha-fetoprotein (AFP) is a fetal protein that is elevated in approximately 80% of patients with hepatocellular carcinoma and 50% of patients with germ cell tumors, and in children with hepatoblastoma. This protein is frequently used to monitor tumor growth following treatment. Methods include RIA or ELISA. Values are generally less than 1×10^{-5} g/L (Table 12-2).

Haptoglobin

Haptoglobin is an acute-phase reactant protein that binds free hemoglobin in serum. Measurement of haptoglobin is frequently done using serial dilutions of serum to monitor acute-phase reactions and hemolytic states. Haptoglobin is increased in inflammatory disorders. Low serum values occur when there is increased hemoglobin turnover, such as transfusion reactions or hemolytic anemias.

Methods for total haptoglobin include nephelometry and RID. Haptoglobin phenotypes may be separated by starch gel or polyacrylamide gel electrophoresis.

Alpha₂-macroglobulin

Alpha₂-macroglobulin is a protease inhibitor that is capable of binding proteases as well as certain hormones. Although its role is not fully understood, it is increased in various inflammatory disorders. While not of particular clinical importance at present, AMG can be quantitated by nephelometry or RID. The reference range appears in Table 12-2.

Ceruloplasmin

Ceruloplasmin is an alpha₂-globulin that transports copper, which is increase in malignancies, inflammation, pregnancy, and with oral contraceptive use. Ceruloplasmin is decreased in Wilson's disease, where unbound copper is toxic to the body and is deposited in the eye, brain, liver, and kidneys.

The most common method for quantitating ceruloplasmin is nephelometry; however, RID may also be used. Ceruloplasmin varies with age; however, the average reference range appears in Table 12-2.

Transferrin

Transferrin is a beta globulin responsible for transporting iron. It also reversibly binds other cations such as copper, zinc, cobalt, and calcium. Plasma levels are regulated by the availability of iron. Since TRF is synthesized in the liver, it is decreased in liver disease, especially acute hepatitis. Low levels will also occur in chronic liver disease, malnutrition, and protein-losing enteropathies.

Plasma transferrin levels vary with specific anemias. In iron deficiency anemia or hypochromic anemia, a lack of iron causes an increased synthesis of TRF. Conversely, if the anemia is due to a failure to incorporate iron into the erythrocytes, the transferrin level is normal or low. In iron overload, transferrin is also normal, but saturation is very high. Elevated plasma TRF occurs in pregnancy and during administration of oral contraceptives.

The reference range for TRF is listed in Table 12-2. Transferrin may be estimated by the calculation: TRF mg/dL = 0.70 × TIBC (total iron-binding capacity) μg/dL. This calculation, however, overestimates the amount of TRF. Specific quantitation of TRF is performed by RID or, preferably, by nephelometry.

Beta₂-microglobulin

Beta₂-microglobulin is a light or beta chain of the human leukocyte antigen (HLA) on cell surfaces. This small protein passes easily through the glomerular membrane in the kidney; however, it is almost entirely reabsorbed by the proximal tubules.

Increased plasma levels occur in renal failure, inflammation, and neoplasms. Urine beta₂-microglobulin will, therefore, increase if renal tubular damage occurs. Tubular proteinuria is usually diagnosed by determining beta₂-microglobulin or other small proteins such as lysozyme or retinol-binding protein.

Table 12-2 gives the reference range for serum beta$_2$-microglobulin. Radioimmunoassay or ELISA are the currently used methodologies.

C-Reactive protein

C-reactive protein migrates in the fast gamma to slow beta region during electrophoresis. Increased values are seen in acute-phase reactions. C-reactive protein is used to monitor the acute inflammatory response to determine if a patient is improving or not. Within 2 hours of the inflammatory stimulus, the CRP concentration rises dramatically. Peak values occur within the first 48 hours. Because of the rapid response of CRP, this protein is a good monitor of post-surgical infections, chronic inflammatory states (e.g., rheumatoid arthritis), transplant rejections, and leukemia.

Table 12-2 lists the reference range for CRP. Methods employed for quantitation of CRP include RIA, RID, ELISA, and nephelometry.

Quantitation of immunoglobulins

Serum is the preferred sample to quantitate immunoglobulins and proteins. Immunoglobulins IgG, IgA, and IgM are quantitated by a nephelometric method or by radial immunodiffusion. Immunoglobulin E is quantitated by a more sensitive method such as ELISA. Immunoglobulin D is rarely quantitated, but can be done by nephelometry.

Serum immunoglobulin values are age-dependent. In the fetus, immunoglobulin synthesis begins at about 20 weeks of gestation. When the child is born, the IgG is maternal IgG that has crossed the placenta. The newborn value of IgG is higher than the maternal value because of the shift of fluid from the newborn. In the newborn, maternal IgG declines until about 5 or 6 months, when the newborn IgG begins to rise. Immunodeficiencies are often detected at this age since maternal antibody was protective until this time. Adult levels of IgG are reached around 2.5 to 3 years of age.

The newborn has low values of IgM (approximately 11 mg/dL). However, the newborn is capable of synthesizing IgM if an intrauterine infection exists. Adult values of IgM are reached around 1 to 2 years of age. The newborn has low values of IgA (approximately 2 mg/dL). Adult values are not reached until 10 to 11 years of age.

Serum immunoglobulins may be increased or decreased in a variety of diseases. Briefly, immunoglobulins are decreased in a variety of immunodeficiency diseases. Hypogammaglobulinemia or a decrease in total immunoglobulins is seen in Bruton's X-linked agammaglobulinemia, transient hypogammaglobulinemia of infancy, and combined variable immunodeficiency. A decrease in IgA only is seen in selective IgA deficiency, the most common immunodeficiency that affects 1 in 600 individuals.

Increased immunoglobulins are classified as either monoclonal or polyclonal by viewing the serum protein electrophoresis (SPE) and immunoelectrophoresis (IEP) separations. The presence of a monoclonal protein indicates a proliferation of one beta-cell type. Examples are multiple myeloma (IgG, IgA, IgD, and IgE) and Waldenström's macroglobulinemia (IgM). Polyclonal increases in immunoglobulins are present in infections, liver disease, and au-

toimmune disease. Immunoglobulin E can be elevated in allergic reactions, parasitic infections, and hyperimmunoglobulinemia E syndrome.

EVALUATION OF THE PATIENT
Immune disorders

Any investigation of immune dysfunction begins with a patient history to seek information on family history, repeated infections, allergies, diarrhea, eczema, joint stiffness, and fever. Initial blood work would include a complete blood count to evaluate anemia and relative and absolute white cell numbers, and quantitative immunoglobulin levels for IgG, IgA, and IgM. The SPE is not a good screening test because it is not sensitive to early detection of proteinopathies, but it is specific for certain diseases. It should be ordered to investigate the following conditions: the verification of quantitative immunoglobulins, proteinuria, and rouleaux formation on the peripheral blood smear; an acute inflammatory response or chronic liver disease; to define the cause of an increased CSF protein; and to investigate a lymphoma.

A decreased gamma region (hypogammaglobulinemia) on the SPE may be indicative of an immune deficiency and should be further investigated. Immunodeficiencies are academically classified as disorders of B cells, T cells, combined B and T cells, natural killer cells, phagocytosis, and complement, but often there is overlap between these categories. The most common immunodeficiency is selective IgA deficiency, which would be verified by a low to absent serum IgA level. The classical B-cell immunodeficiency is Bruton's agammaglobulinemia, in which all the serum immunoglobulins are decreased to absent, while cell-mediated immunity is intact. Five major consequences of immunodeficiency include infections, atropy, autoimmune disease, malignancy, and graft vs. host disease. Further testing that may be warranted when evaluating an immunodeficiency would include B- and T-cell subset quantitation, lymphoblast transformation, quantitative complement levels and hemolytic assays (CH$_{50}$), functional antibody tests, isohemagglutinins, and phagocytic assays.

An increased gamma region (hypergammaglobulinemia) will be polyclonal or monoclonal depending if all antibody clones are increased (polyclonal) or if one clone is proliferating (monoclonal). A normal polyclonal response is seen in infections. Individuals with allergies will have a polyclonal increase in the gamma region because of an increase in IgE, which will be verified by quantitation. The allergens are further identified by skin testing or the RAST (radioallergosorbent) test that identifies specific IgE.

Polyclonal hypergammaglobulinemia is also associated with disease states such as autoimmune disease and acquired immunodeficiency syndrome (AIDS). Systemic lupus erythematosus is an example of an autoimmune disease in which excess antibodies are produced against one's own tissue. The T-cell suppressor effect is depressed, allowing the antibodies to proliferate. Further tests to diagnose autoimmune disease include the antinuclear antibody test (ANA) and rheumatoid factor test. In AIDS patients, the increased antibodies are nonfunctional and hence these individuals succumb to infections.

A monoclonal increase in the gamma region may be indicative of a monoclonal gammipathies such as multiple myeloma or macroglobulinemia. Diagnosis is made from an SPE and IEP on serum and urine (and from the IFE, if needed), and by quantitating the serum immunoglobulins.

Another pattern seen on the SPE is the acute-phase response (APR) pattern found in patients with some acute inflammatory reaction. The C-reactive protein (CRP) band and the alpha$_1$-antitrypsin, haptoglobin, ceruloplasmin, and complement proteins will be increased (positive APR), while transferrin, albumin, and prealbumin will be decreased (negative APR). Since CRP increases within 24 hours of the inflammation and has a half-life of 24 hours, this protein can be quantitated daily to monitor the patient's response to the inflammation.

Renal disorders

Proteinuria has long been recognized as a sign of renal disease. Proteinuria may be classified as either glomerular or tubular in origin. If there is damage to the glomerulus and the filtration process is altered, albumin appears in increased amounts in the urine. Other macromolecules such as IgG and IgA may also appear in abnormal amounts. If a defect exists in the proximal tubule of the kidney nephron without an alteration in the glomerulus, smaller proteins such as beta$_2$-microglobulin or retinol-binding protein will appear in the urine. Causes of glomerular proteinuria and tubular proteinuria appear in Box 12-2.

Proteinura may also result from a prerenal cause. Overflow proteinuria can occur if there is excessive production of protein and if there is an increase in the filtered load (overflow). Excretion of excessive amounts of light-chain fragments will result from plasma cell dyscrasias, such as multiple myeloma. Inflammation can lead to a secretory type of proteinura. In this type of proteinuria, the predominant protein excreted in the urine is IgA. Thus, renal proteinuria

can be classified as primarily glomerular, tubular, overflow, or secretory.

The average healthy adult excretes less than 150 mg of total protein per 24 hours. The amount of albumin excreted is generally less than 15 mg/24 hours. Figure 12-4 shows the types and amounts of proteins found in a normal 24-hour urine specimen.

The major cause of glomerular proteinuria is diabetes. The clinical hallmark of diabetic nephropathy is proteinuria greater than 300 mg/24 hours. In the early stages of diabetic nephropathy, before there is a positive result on an Albustix, the urine albumin excretion may be 30 to 300 mg/day. This intermediate range of urine albumin excretion has recently been termed *microalbuminuria*. Quantitation of low levels of albumin excretion is done by immunochemical methods such as rate nephelometry, RIA, or ELISA. A patient is considered to have established microalbuminuria only when that level of albuminuria is present in at least two of three urine collections over a 6-month period. Current studies suggest that microalbuminuria is a risk factor that is highly predictive of diabetic renal disease.

Up to 50 different low molecular mass proteins have been identified in cases of primary tubular proteinuria. Various plasma proteins have been proposed as markers of renal tubular dysfunction. Beta$_2$-microglobulin, retinol-binding protein, and lysozyme are those low-molecular mass proteins that have been successfully employed.

In general, the evaluation of the proteinuric patient should (1) determine if significant proteinuria exists, (2) determine what size, type, and amount of protein is being excreted in a 24-hour period, and (3) determine if the proteinuria is associated with a prerenal, renal, or a postrenal (e.g., lower urinary tract infection) cause. If a proteinuric patient has no history, signs, or symptoms of renal disease, he or she should be evaluated for orthostatic (e.g., postural) proteinuria. Trace or negative results with urine dipsticks for morn-

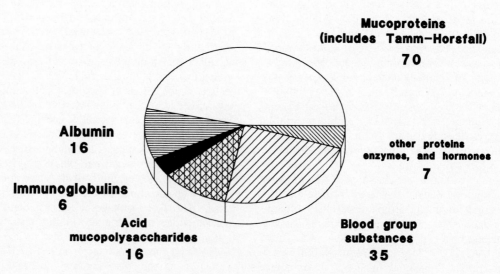

Fig. 12-4 Normal excretion patterns of protein in a 24-hour urine sample.

ing (supine) urine samples together with a 1^+ or greater reading occurring in an afternoon or evening (upright) sample indicates an orthostatic type of proteinuria. Generally, this condition is benign; however, patients should be monitored every 3 to 5 years in the unlikely event that the orthostatic proteinuria represents an early sign of future renal disease. Specific clinical conditions in which proteinuria occurs are summarized in Table 12-8.

Hepatic disorders

Since the majority of all serum proteins are synthesized in the liver with the exception of gamma globulin and hemoglobin, liver disorders will lead to changes in the pattern of serum proteins. Generally, serum total protein concentration is not altered until there is extensive liver damage.

Severe or chronic hepatic disease will lead to a decreased synthesis and, therefore, decreased plasma levels of albumin and other proteins. The electrophoretic patterns will vary depending upon the type, severity, and duration of the liver injury.

Albumin is decreased in chronic liver disease with a concomitant increase in the beta and gamma globulins. In chronic active hepatitis, there is a rise in IgG and IgM. In alcoholic or biliary cirrhosis, there is a rise in IgM and IgA. Various SPE patterns can be seen in liver disease. For example, fusion or bridging of the beta and gamma bands suggest an increase of IgA such as occurs in cirrhosis. An increase in the gamma band, with persistent, hypergammaglobulinemia, suggest active chronic liver disease (Figure 12-2). Oligoclonal bands are occasionally seen in chronic active hepatitis.

The alpha$_1$-fraction of serum protein is also decreased in chronic liver disease. If the alpha$_1$-fraction is absent, a primary alpha$_1$-deficiency exists and may be the cause of the liver disease.

Jaundice is also accompanied by an altered serum protein pattern. In obstructive jaundice, alpha$_2$-macroglobulin and beta globulin are increased. The alteration of these globulin fractions is associated with changes in the lipoproteins synthesized in the liver. Hepatic jaundice, as a result of acute viral hepatitis, is accompanied by an increase in the gamma globulin concentration. In the case of damage to the hepatic sinusoids, an immune response is elicited and increased antibody production occurs.

The liver responds to inflammation with an increase in acute-phase protein production. C-reactive protein, alpha$_1$-acid glycoprotein, alpha$_1$-antitrypsin, haptoglobin, complement C3 and C4, fibrinogen, and ceruloplasmin are increased.

In long-standing or severe liver disease, coagulation function may be impaired. Coagulation factors, produced in the liver, can decrease significantly in severe liver disease. The amount of fibrinogen will decrease, along with other coagulation factors produced in the liver. Because of the great functional reserve of the liver, however, altered hemostatic function is rarely seen unless the disease is long standing or of great severity.

Metabolic disorders

Certain metabolic disorders can result from genetic defects. Wilson's disease (hepatolenticular degeneration) is an autosomal, recessively inherited disorder involving copper metabolism. Copper accumulation occurs in the liver, brain, kidneys, and corneas. In addition, plasma ceruloplasmin is decreased. The laboratory diagnosis of Wilson's disease is determined by the finding of decreased serum ceruloplasmin, increased total serum copper, and increased urinary copper. Patient signs and symptoms include neurologic dysfunction, resulting in loss of cerebellar function and pseudosclerosis.

Various amino acid deficiencies can lead to metabolic disturbances. These include but are not limited to, the disease entities: phenylketonuria, maple syrup urine disease, homocystinuria, tyrosinemia, and alkaptonuria.

Phenylketonuria (PKU) refers to an increased urinary excretion of phenyl compounds. A genetic deficiency or complete absence of the enzyme phenylalanine hydroxylase causes an impaired conversion of phenylalanine to tyrosine. In a few cases (1% to 3%) the deficiency of tetrahydrobioterin causes PKU. In untreated patients with PKU, phenylalanine accumulates in the blood and cerebrospinal fluid, causing mental retardation; therefore, early diagnosis of PKU is essential. Neonatal screening is done by the Guthrie qualitative microbiologic test. Quantitative estimation of elevated serum phenylalanine can be done by spectrophotometric, fluorometric, or chromatographic methods. The ferric chloride test for phenylpyruvic acid in the urine is performed to monitor dietary therapy in PKU patients.

Table 12-8 Clinical conditions associated with proteinuria

Renal disorder	Cause	Amount of proteinuria
Functional proteinuria	Strenuous exercise, extreme cold, emotional stress, febrile disease	Minimal
Orthostatic (postural proteinuria)	Prolonged standing in susceptible individuals	Mild to moderate
Glomerulonephritis	Alteration of the glomerular basement membrane of the nephron	Mild to marked (nephrotic)
Nephrotic syndrome	Systemic lupus erythematosus, intercapillary glomerularsclerosis, or toxic or allergic reactions	Trace to marked
Pyelonephritis	Bacterial infection causing inflammation of the kidney	Mild
Polycystic kidney disease	Hereditary disorder in which the kidney becomes enlarged	Mild to moderate
Lipoid nephrosis	Fat globules deposit in the proximal tubules	Marked
Toxemia of pregnancy (eclampsia)	Unknown cause, associated with edema and hypertension of late pregnancy	Mild to marked

Maple syrup disease is an inherited defect caused by an accumulation of branched-chain amino acids and their corresponding alpha-keto acids in the blood, urine, and cerebrospinal fluid. The lack of the oxidative decarboxylation of leucine, isoleucine, and valine leads to acute ketoacidosis. In untreated cases individuals experience vomiting, lethargy, seizures, and coma. Mental retardation will be a consequence of survivors of the acute manifestations of the ketosis. The urine of these patients has a "maple syrup" odor. Neonatal screening is done by performing the Guthrie test. The urine of the neonate will also test positive for ketoacids with 2,4-dinitrophenylhydrazine.

Homocystinuria is usually caused by a deficiency of cystathione β-synthase. This condition results from a block in the conversion of homocysteine to cystine or back to methionine. The homocysteine that accumulates in the body fluids can lead to severe thrombosis or mental retardation. Although no skeletal or vascular symptoms appear in the newborn, neonatal screening for increased plasma methionine is performed. The presence of homocysteine in the urine can be detected by its reduction with silver nitroprusside plus sodium nitroprusside to yield a pink-purple color.

Tyrosinemia can be of one of two types. In either case, tyrosinemia leads to tyrosinuria and phenolic aciduria. Tyrosine is a precursor of thyroxine, melanin, and catecholamines. Inherited tyrosinemia may be due to defective fumarylacetoacetate (FAA) hydrolase, the enzyme that converts FAA formed from homogentisic acid to fumarate and acetoacetate. Liver damage and generalized renal tubular damage (Fanconi's syndrome) develop. These patients have elevated blood methionine, serum alpha-fetoprotein, and urine p-hydroxyphenylpyruvic acid (PHPPA). Another, rarer form of tyrosinemia is due to a defect in tyrosine aminotransferase, an enzyme responsible for the conversion of PHPPA to tyrosine. If tyrosinase, the enzyme responsible for converting tyrosine to melanin, is the cause for the tyrosinemia, then hypomelanosis, or albinism, results. Diagnosis of tyrosinemia can be made by measurement of tyrosine in the serum by fluorometric analysis or ion-exchange chromatography. Detection of PHPPA in the urine may also be done by chromatography. The more convenient, but nonspecific million reaction or nitrosonaphthol tests may

be used to detect a wide variety of phenolic compounds in the urine.

Alkaptonuria results from a deficiency of homogentisic acid oxidase, an enzyme responsible for the conversion of tyrosine to fumarate acetoacetate. Homogentisic acid accumulates, binds to collagen, and eventually causes degenerative arthritis and pigmentation of cartilage. Individuals with alkaptonuria will produce urine that darkens slowly on standing, on exposure to air or sunlight, or upon addition of alkali. Diagnosis of alkaptonuria may be more definitive by performing reduction tests for homogentisic acid in urine. Ammonical silver nitrate will react with homogentisic acid to form a brown-black to black precipitate of elemental silver. In addition, Benedict's qualitative glucose reagent will react with homogentisic acid after heating to form a dark supernatant with a yellow precipitate of cuprous oxide.

SUGGESTED READING

Bishop ML, Duben-Vol Laufen JL, and Fody EP: Clinical chemistry: principles, procedures, and correlations, St Louis, 1985, JB Lippincott.

Fahey JL and McKelvey E: Quantitative determination of serum immunoglobulins in antibody-agar plates, J Immunol 94:84, 1965.

Grant GH, Silverman LM, and Christenson RH: Amino acids and proteins. In Tietz NW (editor): Fundamentals of clinical chemistry, ed 3, Philadelphia, 1987, WB Saunders.

Jacobs DS and others: Laboratory test handbook, with DRG index, St Louis, 1984, Mosby–Year Book, Inc.

Koller A and Kaplan LA: Total serum protein. In Kaplan LA and Pesce AJ: Clinical chemistry: theory, analysis and correlation, ed 2, St Louis, 1989, Mosby–Year Book, Inc.

Mancini G, Carbonara AO, and Heremans JF: Immunochemical quantitation of antigens by single radial immunodiffusion immunochemistry, Immunochemistry 2:235, 1965.

Ritzman SE: Radial immunodiffusion revisited, part 2, application and interpretation of RID assays, Lab Med 9:27, 1978.

Stites DP and Channing-Rodgers RP: Clinical laboratory methods for detection of antigens and antibodies. In Basic and clinical immunology, 1987, Appleton and Lange.

Waller KV, Ward KM, Mahan JD, and Wimsatt DK: Current concepts in proteinuria, Clin Chem 35(2):755, 1989.

Ward KM: Microalbuminuria, Clin Lab Sci 2(4):212, 1989.

Wolf PL, Griffiths JC, and Lott JA: Interpretation of electrophoretic patterns of proteins and isoenzymes: a clinical pathologic guide, 1981, Marson Publishing.

13

Liver function and nitrogen metabolism

John E. Sherwin
Juan R. Sobenes

NORMAL PHYSIOLOGY AND METABOLISM OF THE LIVER

Anatomy and physiology

The liver is the largest gland in the body, weighing 1200 to 1600 g in an adult. It is located in the upper right portion of the peritoneal cavity and is composed of two principal lobes. The upper surface of the liver abuts the diaphragm, to which it is connected by five ligaments. The liver is soft, friable, and reddish-brown, with a specific gravity of 1.05. This organ is uniquely suited to exert significant metabolic control over the concentration of many materials in the body since the hepatic artery coming from the heart to the liver contains a significant blood flow from the internal circulation. The portal vein from the spleen and gastrointestinal tract contains many of the absorbed materials obtained from the ingestion of food and other exogenous materials. Thus, the liver can process both internal and external materials for the body. The majority of the metabolic functions of the liver are performed by the hepatocytes, which make up the bulk of the liver tissue.

The liver is also the principal organ for the metabolism of carbohydrates, lipids, porphyrins, bile acids, and proteins. It is also a major storage site for iron and other metals, glycogen, lipids, and vitamins, and plays a central role in nitrogen metabolism. It is involved with the metabolic in-terconversions of amino acids and synthesis of nonessential amino acids. The liver synthesizes most body proteins such as albumin, beta macroglobulin, and orosomucoid, but does not synthesize the immunoglobulins. Hemoglobin is synthesized in the liver of the neonate before birth but not in the liver of the adult. The liver is also largely responsible for the production of metabolic end products such as creatinine, urea, ammonia, and uric acid, which can be more easily excreted. The liver is the major organ involved with the detoxification of exogenous organic materials ingested by man. The metabolic reactions primarily are concerned with adding hydroxyl groups, glucuronic acid, or sulfate groups to the organic material to increase the aqueous solubility. These metabolites are usually more easily excreted in the urine or intestinal lumen as shown in Figures 13-1 and 13-2.

Bilirubin and liver function

The breakdown of heme-containing proteins, primarily hemoglobin, results in the production of about 250 mg of bilirubin per day. This occurs in the spleen as a result of hydrolysis of heme to release the iron and form the intermediate biliverdin, which is reduced to bilirubin. The iron is bound to transferrin and is reutilized for heme synthesis. The bilirubin is bound to albumin and is transported to the liver.

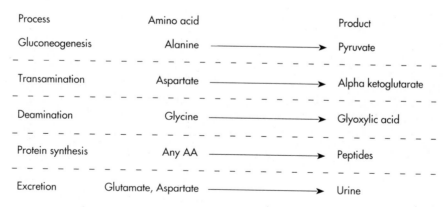

Process	Amino acid	Product
Gluconeogenesis	Alanine	Pyruvate
Transamination	Aspartate	Alpha ketoglutarate
Deamination	Glycine	Glyoxylic acid
Protein synthesis	Any AA	Peptides
Excretion	Glutamate, Aspartate	Urine

Fig. 13-1 Metabolic fate of amino acids.

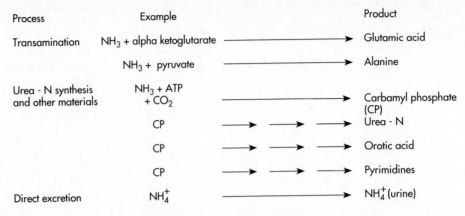

Process	Example		Product
Transamination	NH_3 + alpha ketoglutarate	→	Glutamic acid
	NH_3 + pyruvate	→	Alanine
Urea - N synthesis and other materials	NH_3 + ATP + CO_2	→	Carbamyl phosphate (CP)
	CP	→ → →	Urea - N
	CP	→ → →	Orotic acid
	CP	→ → →	Pyrimidines
Direct excretion	NH_4^+	→	NH_4^+ (urine)

Fig. 13-2 Metabolic fate of ammonia.

Table 13-1 Steady-state concentrations and changes in concentration of bilirubin and its metabolites

	Serum		Urine		
Condition	Total bilirubin	Conjugated bilirubin	Bilirubin	Urobilinogen	Feces pigment
Normal	2-14 mg/L	0-2 mg/L	Negative	0.5-3.4 mg/day	Brown
Prehepatic jaundice	Increased	Normal	Negative	Increased	Brown
Hepatic jaundice					
Hepatocellular disease	Increased	Increased	Positive	Decreased (normal)	Light brown
Gilbert's disease	Increased	Normal	Negative	Decreased (normal)	Brown
Crigler-Najjar syndrome	Increased	Decreased	Negative	Decreased	Light brown
Dubin-Johnson syndrome	Increased	Increased	Positive	Decreased (normal)	Light brown
Posthepatic obstructive jaundice	Increased	Increased	Positive	Decreased	Light brown

This serves to detoxify bilirubin during transport. In some instances bilirubin can become covalently bound to albumin, which is referred to as delta bilirubin. This complex is apparently nontoxic. Because it is covalently bound to albumin, delta bilirubin continues to circulate in the blood for a week or more after urine bilirubin has disappeared. Clinical studies show that during recovery from hepatocellular jaundice, the percentage of delta bilirubin may increase to 80% to 90% of total bilirubin. This suggests a role for delta bilirubin in monitoring the recovery phase of hepatic disease.

This binding of bilirubin to albumin occurs at 2 to 3 sites on albumin. One binding site has a high affinity for bilirubin and the other one or two binding sites are weak sites. This weakly bound bilirubin can be easily displaced by drugs such as salicylate. At high concentrations, the bilirubin that is released can cause nerve damage because it is highly lipid-soluble and somewhat toxic.

Once the bilirubin is transported to the liver it is released from albumin and reacts with one to two molecules of glucuronic acid. This increases the water solubility of bilirubin so that it can be excreted in the bile. The majority of bilirubin (about 85%) is excreted as diglucuronide and the remainder as monoglucuronide. Following excretion in the bile, the conjugated bilirubin is cleaved to bilirubin, which is converted by intestinal bacteria to a series of urobilinogens.

Overproduction of bilirubin, as in hemolytic anemia, increases the amount of urobilinogen formed in the intestine

and therefore the amount that is reabsorbed and excreted into urine. Hepatocellular disease may also increase urinary urobilinogen by interfering with its uptake and excretion into bile. Processes that reduce the flow of bilirubin into the intestine, as occurs in common bile duct obstruction, limit the formation of urobilinogen and thus the amount of urobilinogen in urine.

These metabolic steps result in steady-state concentrations in the blood and urine of bilirubin and its metabolites as indicated in Table 13-1.

Nitrogen metabolism in the liver

Metabolic pools of amino acids are present in the hepatocytes of the liver. From these pools amino acids are drawn for the synthesis of proteins. When a protein is degraded, the bulk of the constituent amino acids are returned to these intracellular pools. The released amino acids can also be used in gluconeogenesis, transamination, or deamination reactions, or they can be reincorporated into new proteins. Important transamination reactions are catalyzed by the enzymes alanine aminotransferase (ALT, or serum glutamate pyruvate transaminase [SGPT]) and aspartate aminotransferase (AST, or serum glutamic-oxaloacetic transaminase [SGOT]). In the normal person the amino groups of excess amino acids in serum are converted to ammonia or urea for excretion; the carbon skeletons are used for glycogen formation of gluconeogenesis. Some amino acids are also excreted unchanged in the urine, as shown in Figure 13-1.

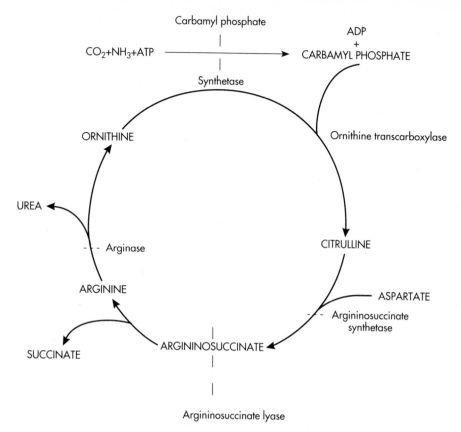

Fig. 13-3 The urea cycle describes the production of 1 mole of urea from 2 moles of ammonia in the liver.

Urea, creatinine, ammonia, and uric acid account for 70% to 75% of the serum nonprotein nitrogen; urea accounts for 60% of the total. Most of the metabolism of nonprotein nitrogen occurs in the liver. Urea is produced in the liver from ammonia via the Krebs Henseleit urea cycle given in Figure 13-3. Production of urea is restricted to the liver because arginase, the enzyme that converts arginine to urea and ornithine, is present only in the liver.

The majority of excess nitrogen is converted to urea. Since urea is the principal nitrogenous compound excreted by the body, the majority of this formed urea is eliminated in the urine.

Although blood ammonia concentration is normally quite low, less than 35 μm/L, ammonia is an important intermediate in amino acid synthesis. Sources of ammonia include hepatic oxidation of glutamate to α-ketoglutarate, the transamination and oxidative deamination of amino acids and catecholamines, and bacterial breakdown of urea in the intestines. The primary mechanism for the metabolic disposal of ammonia is the synthesis of glutamate, glutamine, and carbamyl phosphate. Glutamate and glutamine are both excreted into the urine when in excess. However, if required, they can be reabsorbed and returned to the amino acid pool. Carbamyl phosphate may be used to synthesize orotic acid and ultimately pyrimidines for nucleic acids or to synthesize urea.

In addition to being converted to urea, ammonia is also excreted in the urine as the ammonium ion (NH_4^+). This ammonium salt formation from ammonia serves as a significant mechanism for excretion of excess protons produced during metabolism. This acid-base balance function of ammonia becomes important particularly in diseases associated with acidosis.

Creatinine is formed by the dehydration of creatine. Creatine is produced by the reversible transamidination of the guanine group of arginine to glycine. The biochemical sequence of reactions is depicted in Figure 13-4. Creatine is produced in liver and muscle. It is phosphorylated with ATP to produce creatine phosphate, a reserve energy source. The irreversible dehydration of creatine to produce creatinine results in a metabolic end product that is filtered by the kidneys and excreted in the urine.

Creatinine concentration is relatively constant in the serum at 5 to 12 mg/L. The amount excreted daily is a function of individual body muscle mass. Therefore, women and children tend to have lower total urinary creatinine values than men. Serum and urine creatinine measurements are most useful in evaluating renal function. Calculation of a creatinine clearance by determining the ratio of serum to urine creatinine and correcting for body surface area is a good measure of kidney function, since, as noted earlier, creatinine does not vary appreciably with diet. The urea clearance is no longer used for this purpose because of dietary induced fluctuations in clearance results.

Uric acid is the end product of purine metabolism. As cells die and are replaced, a portion of the DNA and RNA

Arginine + Glycine $- - - - \xrightarrow{\text{Arginine}} - - - \rightarrow$ Ornithine + Guanidinoacetic acid

Guanidinoacetic acid $- - \xrightarrow[\text{Methyltranferase}]{\text{Guanidino acetate}} \rightarrow$ Creatine + S-adenosylhomocysteine
\+
S-adenosylcysteine

Creatine $- - - \xrightarrow[\text{dehydratase}]{\text{Creatine}} - - \rightarrow$ Creatinine + H_2O

Fig. 13-4   Production of creatinine from arginine.

Table 13-2   Reference ranges for selected nitrogenous metabolites in plasma

Age (years)	Ammonia (μm/L)	Urea (mg/L)	Creatinine (mg/L)	Uric acid (mg/L)
0-1	—	60-450	2-10	10-76
1-5	10-40	50-170	2-10	18-50
5-19	11-35	80-220	4-13	30-60
Adult male	11-35	100-210	5-12	40-90
Adult female	11-35	100-210	4-10	30-60

Table 13-3   Reference values for bilirubin

Age	Total bilirubin (mg/L)	Conjugated bilirubin (mg/L)	Delta bilirubin (mg/L)
Up to 1 week	1-126	0-12	Not detected
1 week to 1 year	2-12	0-5	3-6
Greater than 1 year	2-14	0-2	3-6

is degraded into the individual purines and pyrimidines. The purines are converted to uric acid as shown in Figure 13-5.

The production of uric acid in humans is relatively constant. However, dietary intake of foods high in purines such as liver and shellfish can increase serum uric acid concentrations. Men exhibit a higher concentration of uric acid than women and children because of their increased muscle mass. Continuous urinary excretion of uric acid is important, since uric acid is not highly water soluble and the normal concentration of 55 to 65 mg/L is near the solubility limit for uric acid. Therefore, increased dietary load or renal dysfunction can quickly result in crystallization of uric acid in the bladder and kidneys, resulting in stones, or in crystallization in the joints of the extremities, resulting in gout.

Table 13-2 lists the reference ranges for creatinine, ammonia, urea, and uric acid and the effect of age upon their concentrations. Blood ammonia decreases after the neonatal period because of the completion of the development of the hepatic portal circulation. Urea and uric acid increase be-

cause of dietary changes during development. Creatinine increases slightly because of growth, which increases muscle mass. This analyte is relatively independent of dietary influences and thus can be used as a measure of renal function.

Table 13-3 gives the changes in total bilirubin, conjugated bilirubin, and delta bilirubin with age. The most significant changes occur in the first week of infancy, prior to the development of the mature liver.

METABOLIC CHANGES IN DISEASE
Ammonia

Blood ammonia concentration is higher in infants than adults because the development of the hepatic circulation is not completed until after birth. Hyperammonemia results infrequently from congenital defects of the urea cycle. The most common of these inborn errors of metabolism is a deficiency of the enzyme ornithine transcarbamylase. A much more frequent cause of hyperammonemia in infants is hyperalimentation. Most hyperalimentation fluids contain amino acid concentrations above an infant's nutritional nitrogen

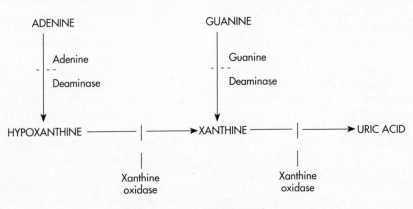

Fig. 13-5   Synthesis of uric acid.

Table 13-4 Changes of analytes in liver disease

Disease	Serum or plasma			Urine		
	NH$_3$	Urea	Uric acid	NH$_3$	Urea	Uric acid
Acute viral hepatitis	N, ↑	N, ↓	N	N, ↑	N, ↓	N, ↑
Alcoholic (drug) hepatitis	N, ↑	N, ↓	↓	N, ↑	N, ↓	N, ↑
Chronic hepatocellular disease	N, ↑	N, ↓	N, ↑	N	N	N, ↑
Cirrhosis	N, ↑	N, ↓	N, ↑	N	N	N
Reye's syndrome	↑ ↑	N, ↓	N	↑	N, ↑	N, ↑
Hepatomas	N	N, ↑	N, ↑	N	N	N
Cholestatic disease	N	N, ↑	N	N	N	N
Metabolic acidosis	N, ↑	N	↑	↑	N, ↑	N
Metabolic alkalosis	N, ↓	N	↑	↑	N, ↑	N
Urea cycle defects	↑ ↑	N, ↓	N	↓	↓	N
Gout with liver involvement	N	N	↑	↑	N	N
Malnutrition	N	N, ↑	↓	N	N, ↓	↑

requirements. The amino acids are used for energy and the excess ammonia excreted in the urine. Ammonia concentrations can be as high as 60 μm/L. Reye's syndrome is frequently diagnosed by an elevated blood ammonia in the absence of any other demonstrable cause. Reye's syndrome is usually seen in children rather than infants. This may be the result of maternally acquired immunity. Elevation of plasma ammonia above five times the normal levels is associated with significant mortality in Reye's syndrome.

Adult patients exhibit elevated blood ammonia in the terminal stages of liver cirrhosis, hepatic failure, and acute and subacute liver necrosis. This is due to the failure of the liver to produce urea. Ammonia is a toxin that acts as a central nervous system depressant and can cause coma. Urinary ammonia excretion is increased in acidosis and decreased in alkalosis, since ammonia salt formation is a significant mechanism for excretion of excess protons. Damage to the renal distal tubules, as occurs in renal failure, glomerulonephritis, hypercorticoidism, and Addison's disease all result in decreased ammonia excretion in the urine, in addition to the changes in liver disease as given in Table 13-4.

Urea metabolism in liver disease

Since urea is synthesized in the liver, liver disease without renal impairment results in a low serum urea nitrogen, though the urea-to-creatinine ratio may remain normal. Other causes of decreased urea include malnutrition, normal pregnancy, inappropriate antidiuretic hormone (ADH) secretion, and overhydration. An elevated serum urea nitrogen does not necessarily imply renal damage, since dehydration may result in a urea nitrogen as high as 600 mg/L. Infants receiving high-protein formula may exhibit a urea nitrogen level of 250 to 300 mg/L. Other causes of elevated urea during liver disease are given in Table 13-4. Causes not shown in Table 13-4 include congestive heart failure, hypotension, and renal diseases such as acute glomerulonephritis, chronic nephritis, polycystic kidney, and renal necrosis.

Blood urea nitrogen (BUN):creatinine ratio is normally between 15 and 24 to 1. The measurement of this ratio can be helpful in assessing the source of azotemia (elevated BUN). In cases of retention of urea because of prerenal causes such as intestinal bleeding, the ratio will be increased

Table 13-5 Changes in bilirubin metabolites with disease

Disease	Total bilirubin	Conjugated bilirubin	Urinary bilirubin
Hemolytic diseases			
Erythroblastosis fetalis	↑ ↑	N	N
Sickle-cell disease	↑	N	N
Physiologic jaundice	↑ ↑	N	N
Hepatocellular diseases			
Dubin-Johnson syndrome	↑	↑	↑
Wilson's disease	↑	N	N
Hepatitis (toxic or infectious)	↑	N	↑
Alcoholic cirrhosis	↑	N	↑
Gilbert's disease	↑	N	↑
Criglar-Najjar syndrome	↑	N	↑
Obstructive diseases			
Cholestasis	↑	↑	↑
Bile duct stones	↑	↑	↑
Carcinoma of the bile duct or external compressive tumors	↑	↑	↑
Cholangiolitis	↑	↑	↑
Biliary cirrhosis	↑	↑	↑
Drug-induced biliary statis	↑	↑	N ↑

sometimes as high as 40:1 since creatinine clearance is normal but the urea load is elevated. In cases of severe renal tubular damage the ratio will fall to as low as 10:1. However, in cases of postrenal obstruction the ratio will remain normal in the presence of elevated creatinine and urea.

Bilirubin

Increases in bilirubin result from either overproduction or impaired excretion. Overproduction is the result of hemolysis, whereas impaired excretion signals liver dysfunction. The distinction between these alternatives is accomplished by clinical assessment and laboratory evaluation; these possibilities are given in Table 13-5.

Increased production of bilirubin is the result of accelerated red cell hemolysis. Total serum bilirubin generally

Table 13-6 Methods of ammonia analysis

Method	Type of analysis	Principle	Usage	Comments
1. Ion-exchange chromatography	Adsorption of ammonia followed by colorimetric analysis by Berthelot reaction	$NH_3 + NaOCl \rightarrow H_2NCl$ (chloramine) $+ NaOH$ $[Fe(CN)_5H_2O]^{-3} + H_2NCl \rightarrow$ "Complex" "Complex" + Phenol $\xrightarrow{OH}$ Colored indophenol blue (560 nm)	Manual, not widely used	Good sensitivity and accuracy
2. Ion-selective electrode	Modified diffusion	Reaction of NH_3 at electrode surface; pH change measured potentiometrically	Automated	Good precision and accuracy
3. Enzymatic	Spectrophotometric	α-Ketoglutarate $+ NH_4^+ + NADPH \underset{\xrightarrow{GLDH}}{\rightleftharpoons}$ Glutamate $+ NADP^+ + H_2O$	Easily automated, most widely used	Good accuracy and rapid

does not exceed 50 mg/L in adults but may be higher in infants. It is virtually all unconjugated bilirubin. The laboratory analysis should include a complete blood count as a means of identifying the source of the hemolysis.

If the clinical features of the disease suggest liver dysfunction, bilirubin analysis can be helpful in differentiating the cause of jaundice. Prehepatic jaundice results in a large increase in unconjugated bilirubin because of the increased release and metabolism of hemoglobin after hemolysis. No increase or only a slight increase in conjugated bilirubin is observed because of the transport of bilirubin into the liver, and the formation of the glucuronide conjugate becomes rate limiting. Additionally, because of the increased levels of unconjugated bilirubin excreted by the liver, urinary urobilinogen and fecal urobilin concentrations are elevated, but urinary bilirubin (which is only the freely soluble, conjugated form) is absent. In contrast, posthepatic obstructive jaundice is characterized by large increases in serum-conjugated bilirubin. The accumulation of bilirubin in the serum is the result of decreased biliary excretion after the conjugation of bilirubin in the liver rather than the result of an increased bilirubin load caused by hemolysis. Excretion of bilirubin metabolites is low, and urinary bilirubin can usually be demonstrated. Hepatic jaundice presents an intermediate pattern wherein both conjugated and unconjugated serum bilirubin are increased to the same degree and conjugated bilirubin is present in the urine. However, the fecal concentration of urobilin is generally decreased.

Creatinine and uric acid in liver disease

The effect of disease upon creatinine is covered in Chapter 6 since this analyte is a good measure of renal function. Uric acid is also not a good measure of liver function but is useful in assessing cellular turnover and destruction, since uric acid is increased in idiopathic hyperuricemia, gout, chronic renal disease, tissue neurosis, metabolic acidosis, and hematologic conditions such as leukemia, lymphoma and anemia.

METHODOLOGIES AVAILABLE FOR ASSESSMENT OF NITROGEN METABOLISM
Ammonia

Ammonia may be quantitatively measured by several techniques (Table 13-6). The most commonly used technique is the enzymatic conversion of α-ketoglutarate to glutamate and the concurrent oxidation of NADPH with the consequent absorbance decrease at 340 nm. This reaction is readily automated. The College of American Pathologists' proficiency survey results indicate that the interlaboratory coefficient of variation (CV) for this method is less than 15%. The other method CVs are higher than this, showing greater imprecision. One potential problem with this method is that it is possible for other endogenous enzymes to compete for NADPH and adversely affect the accuracy of results. This does not appear to be a significant problem in this assay for ammonia.

Specimen collection and sample handling are the two biggest difficulties encountered when analyzing plasma ammonia. The specimen should be collected into fluoride and oxalate preservative tubes or into tubes containing heparin and transported to the laboratory on ice. The specimen should be separated quickly to minimize the deamination of red cell glutamate, which will artifactually increase the ammonia found in the specimen. Prompt separation of the plasma from the red cells and rapid analysis will minimize the possibility of the exposure of the sample to ammonia fumes. This may be a significant problem since many laboratory reagents and many cleaning agents contain ammonia. If specimens are collected into heparin, care should be taken to ensure that ammonium heparin is not used. Contamination of the sample with ammonium heparin will yield results of about 400 μM/L, far above what is usually found clinically.

Although ammonia is most commonly measured in plasma, it may also be measured in cerebrospinal fluid (CSF) for assessment of impending hepatic coma. This request has largely been replaced by measurement of CSF glutamine because it is more stable in the laboratory than CSF ammonia and it correlates well with the development of hepatic coma. Ammonia is also measured in urine to assess acid-base status and renal function (see Chapters 6 and 7). The methods of Table 13-6 can readily be adapted for this measurement.

Urea nitrogen

Urea is measured either colorimetrically with diacetyl monoximine or by a coupled enzymatic reaction using urease with subsequent measurement of ammonia (Table 13-7). Enzymatic methods using conductivity or coupled enzyme reactions are the most commonly used. They are sensitive and specific and can be used for analysis of either serum or urine. These methods measure ammonia produced from urea by the action of urease. The same pitfalls with regard to ammonia fumes as discussed in the ammonia section apply to these assays. Urea is stable in serum for up to 48 hours and deamination of glutamate is not a problem in these assays.

The diacetyl monoximine reaction is sensitive when used with color enhancers such as thiosemicarbazide, but this causes a loss of specificity. The diacetylmonoximine is hydrolyzed to hydroxylamine and diacetyl. The diacetyl condenses with urea to form a yellow-colored diazine. The use of this colorimetric assay is declining because of the fact that it uses caustic chemicals.

Increasingly, dye-binding assays are being coupled with urease to measure the ammonia produced from urea. This is particularly amenable to the dry chemical technology. Specificity is maintained by membrane separation of reactant layers and control of the medium. The coefficient of variation for these assays is generally below 5% in the analytical range of interest.

Creatinine

Creatinine is most commonly measured using a modification of the classic Jaffé reaction (Table 13-8). This assay is based upon the reaction of creatinine with an alkaline solution of sodium picrate to form a red Janovski complex. This reaction is difficult to control without automation since the absorptivity of the complex is quite temperature-sensitive. Additionally, the reaction is nonspecific if long reaction times, or very short ones, are used. Most automated analyzers use a kinetic measurement and a specific time window to reduce the effect of other reactants that will falsely elevate

the result. A variety of modifications of this method have been developed to enhance the specificity of the measurement of the creatinine/picrate complex. These have focused upon purification of creatinine before analysis using fuller's earth, ion-exchange chromatography, or high-performance liquid chromatography (HPLC). These methods are not widely used because they are technically difficult to perform and are not readily automated.

The Jaffé reaction suffers from several interferences depending upon the specific formulation. Hemoglobin and bilirubin are both negative-interfering substances, whereas ketones, ascorbic acid, glucose, and in some cases, cephalosporins (when creatinine is measured within 1 hour of the dose), are positive-interfering substances.

Enzymatic methods are gaining popularity in large part as a result of the dry reagent technology. The most common enzymatic method uses creatinine amidohydrolase in a series of coupled enzyme reactions to yield hydrogen peroxide, which oxidizes a dye to a colored product. This reaction is very specific but hemolysis interferes in some assays because of the nonspecific peroxidase activity of hemoglobin. Separation of hemoglobin from the reactants eliminates this problem when using the thin film technology.

The coefficients of variation for these assays are all generally below 5% in the range of interest. These assays can be used for either serum or urine creatinine measurement. However, urine samples must be diluted about 1:50 prior to analysis because of the concentration difference between serum and urine.

Uric acid

Uric acid is routinely measured using a uricase procedure that converts uric acid to allantoin and results in a decreased absorbance at 283 nm (Table 13-9). Traditionally, this reaction was performed on a protein-free filtrate. However, most methods in use today use detergents as protein solubilizers and carry out the reaction directly in serum. The advent of high-sensitivity stable spectrophotometers has made it possible to measure this uric acid conversion in the presence of protein that absorbs at 280 nm. A few laboratories still use the oxidation of uric acid to allantoin to reduce phosphotungstate to tungsten blue. This is a classic colorimetric method that has all but been replaced by the more specific enzymatic method. Nonetheless, the coefficients of variation for the two methods are similar at about 5%.

Bilirubin

Bilirubin is most commonly measured in serum or plasma by reaction with diazotized sulfanilic acid (Table 13-10). Conjugated bilirubin reacts in aqueous solution ("direct" bilirubin), whereas unconjugated bilirubin does not. Addition of an accelerator (alcohol or caffeine) that disrupts internal hydrogen bonding allows the unconjugated fraction to react as well, providing a value for total bilirubin. The unconjugated or "indirect" bilirubin is obtained by subtracting the direct from total bilirubin. Bilirubin is readily destroyed by light and heat; therefore, the analysis should be performed promptly in subdued light to avoid falsely low results.

Serum is preferred for the Malloy-Evelyn procedure, because the addition of alcohol in the analysis can precipitate

Table 13-7 Methods of urea analysis

Method	Type of analysis	Principle	Usage	Comments
1. Coupled enzymatic (urease/glutamate dehydrogenase [GLDH])	Quantitive, end-point kinetic, spectrophotometric	$Urea \xrightarrow{Urease} (NH_4)_2CO_3$ $NH_4^+ + \alpha\text{-Ketoglutaric acid} + NADH \xrightarrow[ADP,H^+]{GLDH} NAD^+ + Glutamic\ acid$	Most frequently used procedure	Very specific, rapid; easily automated urine samples must be prediluted
2. Conductimetric	Quantitative kinetic	$Urea \xrightarrow{Urease} (NH_4)_2CO_3 \rightarrow 2NH_4^+ + CO_3^{-2}$ Increased ions changed conductivity	Frequently used	Very specific rapid; easily automated
3. Diacetyl monoxime	Quantitative end-point, kinetic, colorimetric	$CH_3-\overset{O}{\overset{\|}{C}}-\overset{NOH}{\overset{\|}{C}}-CH_3 \xrightarrow[H^+]{H_2O} CH_3-\overset{O}{\overset{\|}{C}}-\overset{O}{\overset{\|}{C}}-CH_3 + HNO_2$ Diacetyl monoxime → Diacetyl → Hydroxylamine $NH_2-\overset{O}{\overset{\|}{C}}-NH_2 + CH_3-\overset{O}{\overset{\|}{C}}-\overset{O}{\overset{\|}{C}}-CH_3 \xrightarrow{H^+} CH_3-\overset{}{C}=\overset{}{N}\ \ \overset{}{N}=\overset{}{C}-CH_3 + 2 H_2O$ Urea Diacetyl → Diazine (yellow)	Less frequently used	Some nonspecificity of reaction; uses noxious, dangerous reagents
4. Indicatory dye	Quantitative end-point	$Urea \xrightarrow{Urease} (NH_4)_2CO_3 \rightarrow 2NH_4^+ + CO_3^{-2}$ $NH_4^+ + pH\ indicator\ dye \rightarrow Change\ in\ absorbance\ spectrum\ of\ dye$	Rarely used now, but will be used more frequently	Very specific; used with dry chemistry technology

Modified from Kaplan LA and Pesce AJ (editors): Clinical chemistry: theory, analysis, and correlation, ed 2, St Louis, 1989, Mosby–Year Book, Inc.

Table 13-8 Methods of creatinine analysis

Method	Type of analysis	Principle	Usage	Comments
1. Jaffé, kinetic	Spectrophotometric, quantitative, kinetic analysis during early color formation	$Creatinine + Picrate \xrightarrow{OH^-} Janovski\ complex\ (red)$	Serum, plasma, diluted urine	Requires automated equipment for accurate, precise absorbance measurements; most widely used
2. Creatinine amidohydrolase	Coupled enzymatic reactions leading to peroxidase indicator reaction	$Creatinine + H_2O \xrightarrow[amidohydrolase]{Creatinine} Creatine$ $Creatine + H_2O \xrightarrow[amidohydrolase]{Creatine} Sarcosine + Urea$ $Sarcosine + O_2 \xrightarrow[oxidase]{Sarcosine} Glycine + Formaldehyde + H_2O_2$ $H_2O_2 + Leukodye \xrightarrow{Peroxidase} Colored\ dye + H_2O$	Serum, urine	Automated on Kodak Ektachem; minimal interference from lidocaine metabolites

Modified from Kaplan LA and Pesce AJ (editors): Clinical chemistry: theory, analysis, and correlation, ed 2, St Louis, 1989, Mosby–Year Book, Inc.

Table 13-9 Methods of uric acid analysis

Method	Type of analysis	Principle	Usage	Comments
1. Phosphotungstic acid	Spectrophotometric	Oxidation of uric acid to allantoin and carbon dioxide with reduction of phosphotungstic acid to tungsten blue (A_{max}, 700 nm)	Serum, urine	Nonspecific; used on older, automated instruments
2. Uricase	Enzymatic	Oxidation of uric acid to allantoin, hydrogen, peroxide, and carbon dioxide	Serum, urine	
a. Colorimetric		Quantitation of hydrogen peroxide produced, especially when coupled to NAD/NADH		Specificity varies from method to method; NADH reaction; the most commonly used method
b. Differential absorption		Uric acid absorbs in the 290 to 293 nm (at pH $\geq$7) and 283 nm (at pH <7) region of ultraviolet spectrum, but allantoin does not		Basis for a candidate reference method; increased specificity

Modified from Kaplan LA and Pesce AJ (editors): Clinical chemistry: theory, analysis, and correlation, ed 2, St Louis, 1989, Mosby—Year Book, Inc.

Table 13-10 Methods of bilirubin analysis

Method	Type of analysis	Principle	Usage	Comments
1. Malloy-Evelyn	Kinetic, end point, with or without blank	Reaction shown in Fig. 13-6 performed at pH 1.2; azobilirubin measured at 560 nm	Very frequently used	Susceptible to significant hemoglobin interference
2. Jendrassik-Grof	Kinetic, end point, with or without blank	Reaction shown in Fig. 13-6 performed near neutral pH but chromophore measured at alkaline pH (approximately 13) at 600 nm	Most commonly used method	Has higher molar absorptitivity and thus is more sensitive and precise at low bilrubin concentrations than Malloy-Evelyn method
3. Bilirubinometer	Direct spectrophotometric	Bilirubin concentration directly determined by its absorbance at 454 nm; HbO_2 interference corrected by measurement of absorbance at a second wavelength (540 nm)	Not frequently used; primarily for neonatal analysis	Very simple to perform but very strong interference from carotinoids
4. High-performance liquid chromatography	Chromatographic separation	Methyl esters of conjugated and unconjugated bilirubin esters are detected at 430 nm	Research use only	May become future reference method

Modified from Kaplan LA and Pesce AJ (editors): Clinical chemistry: theory, analysis, and correlation, ed 2, St Louis, 1989, Mosby—Year Book, Inc.

proteins from plasma that interfere with subsequent analysis. Hemolysis falsely depresses the bilirubin result in most assays because of an increase in absorbance of the blank; therefore, samples used for analysis should not have any visible hemolysis and red blood cell contamination should be removed by centrifugation before analysis. Conjugated bilirubin may be determined in either serum or plasma, but serum is the usual sample because total bilirubin can be determined concomitantly.

The albumin-bound fraction of serum bilirubin (delta bilirubin) is included in the conjugated (direct) fraction of bilirubin when determined by conventional methods. Spe-

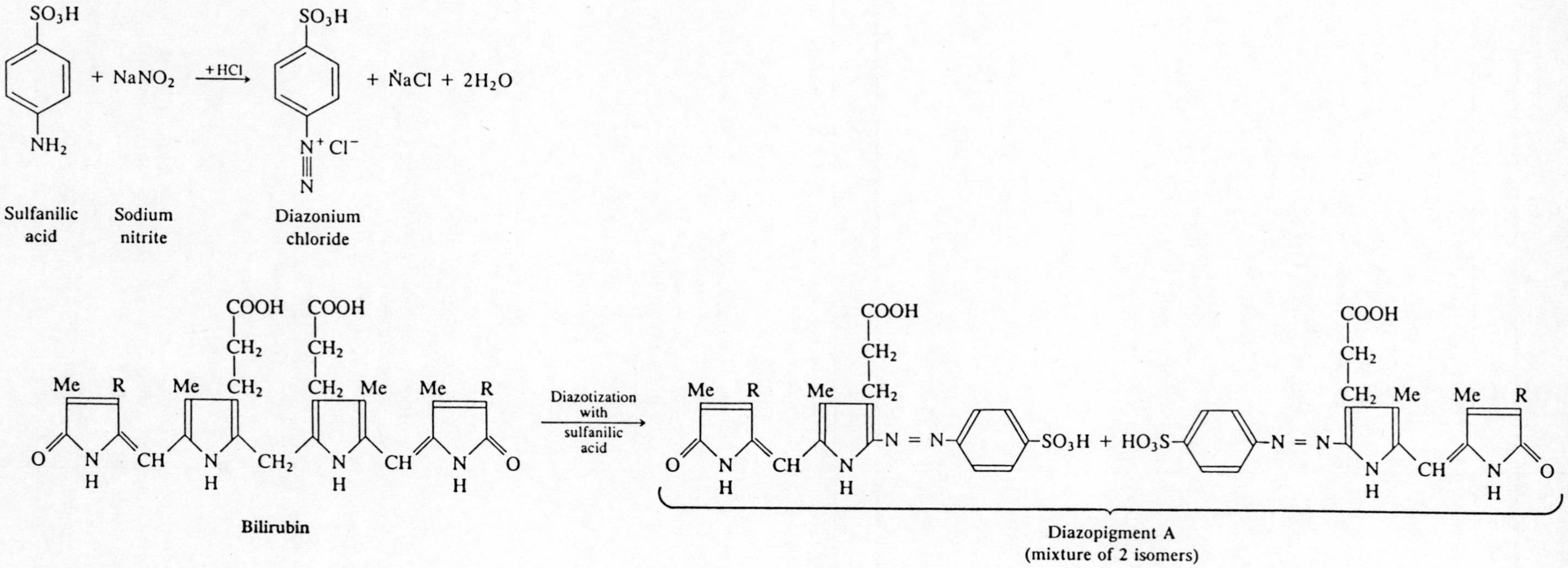

Fig. 13-6   Formation of diazotized sulfanilic acid and its reaction with esterified and nonesterified forms of bilirubin to form azobilirubin derivatives. *Me,—CH$_3$ group; R,—CH = CH = CH$_2$ group. From Sherwin JE and Obernolte R: Nonprotein nitrogenous compounds. In Kaplan LA and Pesce AJ: Clinical chemistry: theory, analysis, and correlation, ed 2, St Louis, 1989, Mosby–Year Book, Inc.*

cial techniques, such as high-performance liquid chromatography or a commercial thin-film system developed by Kodak, make it possible to measure delta bilirubin individually.

Urine bilirubin is derived from the conjugated bilirubin in blood, a portion of which is filtered by the kidneys and excreted in urine. One can easily test for urine bilirubin with commercial dipstick methods, and it is normally undetectable. The presence of bilirubin in urine indicates an elevation in the conjugated fraction of serum bilirubin. The normal excretion of urobilinogen in urine is 1 to 4 mg/day.

SUGGESTED READING

Kaplan L, and Pesce A (editors): Clinical chemistry: theory, analysis, and correlation, ed 2, St Louis, 1989, Mosby–Year Book, Inc.

Meites (editor): Pediatric clinical chemistry, ed 3, Washington, DC, 1989, American Association of Clinical Chemistry.

Tietz N (editor): Textbook of clinical chemistry, Philadelphia, 1986, Saunders.

14 Clinical enzymology

David C. Hohnadel

THE NATURE OF ENZYMES

Enzymes are biological materials with catalytic properties, i.e., they increase the rate of chemical reactions in cells and in vitro systems that otherwise proceed very slowly. Enzymes are large, naturally occurring proteins with molecular weights usually between 13,000 and 500,000. The study of these molecules has become a valuable diagnostic tool for the elucidation of various disease states and for testing organ function.

Tissues and cellular materials contain varying amounts and types of enzymes. The hundreds of enzymes in each cell are attached to the cell walls and membranes and are dissolved in the cytoplasm or sequestered in the nucleus and other specialized subcellular organelles including microsomes, mitochondria, and lysosomes. Often the identification of one or several enzymes in plasma indicates the tissue or cell type from which the enzymes have been derived. Different tissues—or even compartments within a single cell—can contain different forms of an enzyme that catalyzes the same chemical reaction. Assays for these different forms can sometimes determine an enzyme's source. A few enzymes are found in plasma or other extracellular fluids where they seem to perform a physiological function, but most enzymes catalyze reactions inside cells or in the lumen of various organs.

Composition and structure

All enzymes are proteins; that is, they are complex compounds of high molecular weight. They contain amounts of carbon, hydrogen, oxygen, nitrogen, and sulfur that are similar to amounts found in other protein materials. Hydrolysis with strong acid yields a mixture of amino acids and small peptides. Enzymes are distinguished from other proteins by their catalytic action.

The catalytic behavior of an enzyme depends on the primary, secondary, tertiary, and quarternary structures of the protein molecule. Changes to the primary amino acid sequence usually result in the differences in the three dimensional structure because the secondary and tertiary folding end up different. However, changes to any one of these structures can affect the enzymatic activity of the protein, usually reducing or abolishing it.

Apoenzymes and cofactors

An enzyme may have nonprotein substances that are needed for maximal activity. These other materials, called cofactors, may be either loosely or tightly bound to the protein portion of the enzyme. Loosely bound cofactors can often be removed by dialysis. These materials may be organic compounds such as nicotinamide adenine dinucleotide phosphate ($NADP^+$) and pyridoxyl-5-phosphate, which are called coenzymes, or inorganic ions like chloride (Cl^-) and magnesium (Mg^{+2}), which are called activators. Cofactors that are so tightly bound they are considered part of the enzyme structure are termed prosthetic groups. An example is the heme portion of peroxidase. Enzymes that have metal ions bound very tightly are called metalloenzymes. Two examples of metalloenzymes are ferroxidase, also called ceruloplasmin, an enzyme containing a relatively large amount of tightly bound copper, and carbonate dehydratase, also called carbonic anhydrase, an enzyme with a large amount of zinc.

The term "coenzyme" is often loosely used when referring to the compound NADH (or NADPH) in a reaction like the lactate dehydrogenase reaction.

$$\text{Pyruvate} + \text{NADH} + \text{H}^+ \xrightleftharpoons{\text{LD}} \text{Lactate} + \text{NAD}^+$$

In a formal kinetic sense, both pyruvate and NADH are substrates for the enzyme reaction and lactate and NAD^+ are products. In this case, pyruvate and NADH react with one another on a molar basis. The NADH that reacts is still called a coenzyme, i.e., a nonprotein organic material needed for maximal activity, perhaps for historic reasons, even though it should be called a second substrate or cosubstrate.

Since it is possible to dialyze away loosely held cofactors from some enzymes and still retain some activity, an enzyme without the associated cofactors is referred to as an apoenzyme, and the complete enzyme-cofactor complex is termed a holoenzyme. In the clinical use of enzyme assays, the enzyme assay mixture must contain an excess of all acti-

Some of the material in this chapter was taken from Hohnadel DC: Enzymes. In Kaplan LA, Pesce AJ: Clinical chemistry: theory, analysis, and correlation, ed 2, St. Louis, 1989, Mosby-Year Book, Inc.

vators and cofactors to ensure that the complete holoenzyme is being measured, rather than a mixture of apo- and holoenzyme forms.

Catalysts

Enzymes function as biological catalysts. They are proteins that accelerate specific chemical reactions toward equilibrium without being consumed in the process. The material an enzyme reacts with is called the **substrate.** A simple enzymatic reaction for one substrate and one product is listed below:

$$E + S \underset{k_{-1}}{\overset{k_{+1}}{\rightleftharpoons}} \{ES\} \underset{k_{-2}}{\overset{k_{+2}}{\rightleftharpoons}} P + E$$

EQ 14-1

In this case the enzyme is represented by E; the substrate on which the enzyme acts is S; $\{ES\}$ represents a postulated enzyme-substrate intermediate complex; and P is the product of the reaction. The forward reaction rate constants are represented by k_{+1} and k_{+2} while k_{-1} and k_{-2} indicate the reverse reaction rate constants. An example of a single substrate enzyme reaction is the action of the enzyme urease on the substrate urea. In this case two products are produced:

$$\underset{\text{Urea}}{H_2N - \overset{\overset{O}{\|}}{C} - NH_2} + E \underset{k_{-1}}{\overset{k_{+1}}{\rightleftharpoons}} \{Urea\text{-}E\} \underset{k_{-2}}{\overset{k_{+2}}{\rightleftharpoons}} \underset{\substack{\text{Ammonia} \quad \text{Carbon} \\ \text{Dioxide}}}{2\,NH_3 \quad + CO_2 + E}$$

Water also participates in the reaction but has been omitted for clarity. These biological catalysts are like other chemical catalysts in many respects, except that they function in biological systems. Enzyme catalysts, although unstable and easily destroyed, are similar to other chemical catalysts in terms of catalytic properties: they are effective in small concentrations; they are unchanged by the reaction; they affect the speed of attaining equilibrium but do *not* change the final concentrations of the substrates and products of the *equilibrium* state; and they demonstrate a much greater degree of specificity than the usual chemical catalysts for the reactions they accelerate.

It is the first property that makes enzymes such a valuable diagnostic tool. Since they are effective in small amounts, measuring changes in enzyme concentrations is a very sensitive way to follow changes that have occurred in various types of tissues.

In assays for plasma enzymes, the amount of enzyme involved is much smaller than the amount of glucose in an assay for glucose. A conventional chemical assay for enzyme material would be very difficult to produce and require large amounts of sample. Of the several thousand enzymes in plasma, the measurement of the concentration of a single enzyme, even if present at a very elevated value, is below the limit of detection for most chemical protein assays. Easier to measure—and biologically related to many clinical conditions—is the enzyme's catalytic activity and its changes with time.

The *activity* of an enzyme is the amount of substrate in an enzyme reaction that is converted to product per unit time under defined conditions. The use of activity as a concentration assumes that a given weight of enzyme has a fixed number of units of activity. The specific enzyme activity, in units per mg protein, remains constant even when the increase in enzyme activity during a particular disorder may come from a different tissue. The increased enzyme activity presumably results from the presence of more enzyme with the same specific activity rather than from the presence of another form of the enzyme with a higher specific activity. In practice, activity measurements of enzymes are used as if they were enzyme concentrations.

If the enzyme were acting as a catalyst it would be unchanged by the reaction, but due to the unstable nature of most enzymes this property is difficult to demonstrate. It is possible with many current assays to use very short analysis times to calculate enzyme activity early in an assay period and again after 10 to 15 minutes without showing a decrease in enzyme activity. The amount of substrate converted to product during this time might be 5% to 10% of the initial amount present. Since the enzyme activity determined at both times is unchanged, the enzyme does not participate in the reaction on a molar basis with the substrate and is acting as a catalyst.

Another aspect of the biological catalysts is that they accelerate the approach to equilibrium. One way of considering this process is to examine the effect of lactate dehydrogenase on the conversion of pyruvate to lactate. In the presence of the enzyme LD and the coenzyme NADH the conversion of pyruvate to lactate occurs rapidly, but without the enzyme, the process is so slow it can hardly be demonstrated.

$$\text{Pyruvate} + \text{NADH} + H^+ \overset{LD}{\rightleftharpoons} \text{Lactate} + NAD^+$$

$$\text{Pyruvate} + \text{NADH} + H^+ \overset{No}{\underset{Enz}{\rightleftharpoons}} \text{No detectable reaction}$$

In addition, this is not a one-way process but an approach to the equilibrium concentrations of pyruvate and lactate since the same enzyme converts lactate to pyruvate with the coenzyme NAD^+. The speed of the reaction and the conditions employed are not the same in both directions since they are related to the equilibrium constant. It is possible to measure the conversion from either direction and both methods are widely used to determine LD activity in the clinical laboratory.

Reactive sites

The Gibbs free energy change (ΔG) is the measure of the amount of work a chemical reaction can produce. All reactions that proceed from reactants to products have a net negative free energy $(-\Delta G)$. However, the reactants do not become products directly but must absorb enough energy to pass through an activated or transition state.

Enzymes lower the energy required for activation to the transition state. Without the enzyme, the reaction may not proceed to any appreciable extent, even if the reaction has favorable negative free energy, that is, with products having a lower ΔG than substrates. The reactants must gain the energy to overcome this activation energy barrier to enter the transition state and then pass on to products. Without a catalyst the reaction will occur only if enough heat or energy can be added to the reaction system. With an enzyme catalyst, the reaction may easily proceed at normal physiological temperatures. Equation 1 can be rewritten to account for this transition state in an enzyme catalyzed reaction,

EQ 14–2

$$E + S \underset{k_{-1}}{\overset{k_{+1}}{\rightleftharpoons}} \{ES \rightarrow ES^* \rightarrow EP\} \underset{k_{-2}}{\overset{k_{+2}}{\rightleftharpoons}} P + E$$

where ES* is the transition state form of the substrate and ES and EP are enzyme-substrate and enzyme-product forms with materials bound but not activated. Substantial reductions in the activation energy requirements are often found when enzymes are used as catalysts for the process. For example, the activation energy necessary for hydrogen peroxide to decompose is 18,000 cal/mol, but in the presence of the enzyme catalase the activation energy is less than 2,000 cal/mol.

One of the most difficult problems facing enzyme chemists is explaining how an enzyme can reduce the activation energy but remain unchanged by the reaction. Equation 2 shows one general possibility.

A wide variety of nonpolar hydrophobic and polar hydrophilic amino acids are present in enzyme proteins. The external surface of the enzyme is thought to be composed of mostly polar but generally unreactive side chains of amino acids for solubility reasons. The unreactive amino acid side chains may contain structures like methyl and isopropyl groups (i.e., R-CH$_3$ and R-CH-CH$_3$), found in alanine and leucine.
$$| \atop CH_3$$

Some of the enzyme surface areas are thought to contain amino acids with reactive side chains. The reactive amino acid side chains may contain charged groups like carboxyl and amino groups (i.e., RCOO$^-$ and RNH$_3^+$) found in aspartic and glutamic acids or lysine and arginine. Uncharged portions like the hydroxyl and sulfhydryl groups (i.e., ROH and RSH) found in serine, tyrosine, and cysteine, are also reactive. Other types of reactive groups are present in amino acids, e.g., histidine, which has an active nitrogen in a ring structure. It is thought that the reactive amino acids bind portions of the substrate through ionic and hydrogen bonds. These reactive areas of the enzyme may exist on the surface or in more hidden clefts or folds. These active areas are thought to be involved in the binding of substrates, products, activators, and inhibitors. They may be involved in the catalytic process itself.

Catalysis can take place in only a limited number of places on the enzyme. These areas are called active sites or active centers and may only involve five to ten amino acids out of a total of 200 to 300 in the entire enzyme. The active site with catalytic properties also serves to bind the substrate, thus facilitating the breaking and forming of new bonds. The substrate is positioned so other reactive amino acids at the active site cause this conversion from substrate to product.

The sites on the enzyme's surface that bind the substrate or product of the reaction are termed binding sites. Enzymes, particularly those of a complex structure composed of several subunits, often have binding sites far removed from the primary amino acid sequence at the active site but which affect enzyme activity. These sites are called allosteric sites or regulatory sites and much information about enzyme mechanisms has been derived from studies with inhibitors that affect these sites and consequently the enzyme activity. Although one would expect great diversity among the types of catalytic sites a number of common features have been observed.

The substrate of the reaction binds to the active site and is oriented so that a particular bond is subject to attack. The reactive side chain moieties of the enzyme interact with the group on the substrate so that the covalent bond to be altered weakens. This bond weakening decreases the activation energy needed for chemical reaction. The weakened bond then undergoes a chemical reaction that breaks the covalent bond and allows new ones to form. The product no longer has the same affinity for the active site as the original substrate and will be released from the enzyme.

Changes in the amino acid sequence of a protein could produce different enzymes presumably with different active and binding sites, or even similar proteins without catalytic activity. Such changes, caused by genetic mutations, are often the cause of inborn errors of metabolism and other diseases of genetic origin.

The chemical reactions in which these reactive amino acids take part not only define the enzyme's specific catalytic activity but also determine the sensitivity of the enzyme to losses of activity by such things as heavy metals, detergents, or even other reactive parts of the same protein molecule. Metals or detergents may bind to active groups and inactivate them. Changes in surface tension, i.e., vigorous shaking, may cause unfolding of the protein or denaturation. As a result, the spatial relationships of these reactive amino acids with each other are disrupted, preventing the usual reaction from taking place.

Specificity of reaction

Differences in enzyme specificity are thought to be related to physical differences at the active site. Some enzymes react with many related compounds and are said to have a broad specificity. Acid phosphatase, for example, exhibits a broad bond specificity, hydrolyzing several types of organic phosphate esters, e.g., beta-glycerol phosphate, thymolphthalein phosphate, para-nitrophenyl phosphate, and alpha-naphthyl phosphate. At an acid pH, the enzyme catalyzed reaction,

$$R\text{-}O\text{-}P + H_2O \underset{phosphatase}{\overset{Acid}{\rightleftharpoons}} R\text{-}O\text{-}H + Pi$$

produces an organic alcohol and inorganic phosphate.

Many enzymes that hydrolyze proteins also exhibit a broad bond specificity where a large number and variety of peptide bonds within a protein substrate are hydrolyzed. If the peptide bonds of the hydrolyzed substrate are located on the inside of the protein, the enzyme is called an endopeptidase, like pepsin A. Alternatively, carboxypeptidases are enzymes that act on protein substrates cleaving peptide bonds starting from the outside carboxyl end of the substrate and moving toward the middle of the protein. These enzymes are termed exopeptidases, and they also demonstrate a broad substrate specificity.

In contrast to the broad specificity of many peptidases, other enzymes are more specific in their action, in that they will only catalyze a definite reaction with a few substrates.

In extreme cases, an almost absolute specificity is demonstrated where only a single compound will serve as a substrate, e.g., phospho(enol)pyruvate, for the pyruvate kinase reaction.

$$\left.\begin{array}{c} \text{phospho(enol)pyruvate} \\ \text{(PEP)} \\ + \\ \text{Adenosine diphosphate} \\ \text{(ADP)} \end{array}\right\} \begin{array}{c} \text{PK} \\ \rightleftharpoons \end{array} \left\{\begin{array}{c} \text{pyruvate} \\ \text{(pyr)} \\ + \\ \text{Adenosine triphosphate} \\ \text{(ATP)} \end{array}\right.$$

Enzyme specificity should be described for each substrate involved in a reaction. In contrast to the absolute specificity shown for phospho(enol)pyruvate in the pyruvate kinase reaction, several natural and synthetic nucleoside diphosphates, e.g., UDP, IDP, GDP, and CDP, also serve as phosphate acceptors in the reaction in place of ADP. Thus, while an absolute specificity is shown for one substrate (PEP), an intermediate degree of specificity is shown for the other (ADP).

An intermediate degree of specificity for each substrate is shown by the hexokinase reaction, in which D-glucose and several other sugars may be phosphorylated, i.e., D-mannose, 2-deoxy-D-glucose, and D-glucosamine. However, D-galactose and 5-carbon sugars like D-xylose are not substrates. The enzyme can also use a variety of nucleoside triphosphates as phosphate donors, e.g., ITP and GTP as well as ATP.

$$\left.\begin{array}{c} \text{D-glucose} \\ + \\ \text{Adenosine Triphosphate} \\ \text{(ATP)} \end{array}\right\} \begin{array}{c} \text{HK} \\ \rightleftharpoons \end{array} \left\{\begin{array}{c} \text{glucose-6-phosphate} \\ + \\ \text{Adenosine diphosphate} \\ \text{(ADP)} \end{array}\right.$$

Many enzymes demonstrate a stereoisomeric specificity for either the L-form or the D-form of a pair of compounds. Hexokinase, for example, is absolutely specific for the D-form of glucose, but the L-form is not a substrate. Conversely, malate dehydrogenase acts only on the L-form of malate, not the D-form. However, stereoisomeric specificity does not necessarily mean that the enzyme is absolutely specific since some forms of lactate dehydrogenase act on hydroxybutyrate as well as lactate, and, as was mentioned above, hexokinase functions with several D-form substrates.

Subunit structure

Some enzymes occur in nature in several forms. That is, there may be several types of enzyme that catalyze the same reaction. These are known as isoenzymes or isozymes. In a few well-studied enzymes, different forms or isoenzymes occur because the enzymes are composed of two or more different polypeptide chains or subunits bound into an active form.

The subunits alone do not have the catalytic properties of the whole enzyme. The isoenzymes may have different kinetic or other physical properties that allow the different forms to be separated or measured. Many of these features have been used to differentiate and characterize the various enzyme forms and to assay for their presence in a sample. Other types or classes of isoenzymes can occur and will be considered in the section on isoenzymes, but clinically the most widely used forms are the subunit type of isoenzymes.

If an active enzyme is composed of two subunits and if there are two different types of subunits, i.e., A and B, then there are three possible types of isoenzymes: AA, AB, and BB. Creatine kinase (CK) is an example of this type of enzyme since it is a dimer composed of two types of subunits, M and B. The forms of CK are CK-MM, CK-MB, and CK-BB. Many normal samples from patients contain only the predominant CK-MM form.

If an active enzyme is composed of four subunits and there are two types of subunits, A and B, then there are five possibilities: AAAA, AAAB, AABB, ABBB, and BBBB. Lactic dehydrogenase (LD) is an enzyme with this type of structure. It is composed of the subunits H and M. The forms of LD are LD-HHHH, LD-HHHM, LD-HHMM, LD-HMMM, and LD-MMMM. For simplicity, these forms are designated: LD_1, LD_2, LD_3, LD_4, and LD_5. Most patient samples will contain all five forms in varying amounts.

Anabolism and catabolism

The synthesis of all enzymes is assumed to occur by intracellular protein synthetic pathways within the tissues that contain the enzymes. Extracellular enzymes like those involved in the coagulation process are synthesized in the liver and elaborated into the plasma. In some cases other organs, i.e., the kidney, lung, and pancreas, also contribute to the extracellular enzyme pool.

The large size and complex structure of enzymes results in molecular forms that are somewhat unstable and are therefore said to be labile. Many enzymes in vitro lose their catalytic activity with relatively slight changes in pH, temperature, or even salt concentration of the surrounding medium. It is presumed that similar processes occur intracellularly and that constant, although slight, synthesis of enzymes occurs in a steady-state fashion to maintain the amounts of intracellular enzymes required for intermediary metabolism.

A loss of enzyme activity can be either reversible and temporary or irreversible and permanent. Denaturation is a process where biological properties are lost by a protein, i.e., enzyme activity is lost. It has been suggested that the denaturation process is an unfolding or "melting" of tightly coiled peptide chains leading to a more disorganized structure. There is much experimental support for this idea, including increased reactivity of side chains, changes in viscosity, and changes in the sedimentation behavior of the "melted" protein solutions. Irreversible denaturation can occur when the enzyme protein chains unfold and are unable to refold to their biologically active form, or when a heavy metal ion (e.g., mercury or lead) or other material binds tightly at or near the active site. Many other factors and events can lead to denaturation and loss of activity including changes in temperature, the addition of strong acids or bases, exposure to high pressure, treatment with ultraviolet light, repeated freezing, and the addition of detergents, or organic solvents or the presence of high concentrations of urea or guanidine.

A reversible denaturation or loss of enzyme activity is called inactivation. For example, inactivation can occur if an enzyme solution remains for an extended time at room temperature and the enzyme partially loses activity. This temporary activity loss can have several causes including heat instability with the breaking of hydrogen bonds or oxidation of sulfhydryl groups. In both cases some loss of the natural structural form occurs. With some enzymes, reducing the temperature of the solution or the addition of a sulfhydryl reducing agent like dithiothreitol may allow the enzyme to refold to the original active form, with reformation of hydrogen-bonds or reduction of oxidized sulfhydryl groups, thus producing a reactivation of the enzyme and a restoration of lost activity.

Little is known about the mechanism of removal of enzyme proteins from the extracellular fluid compartment. Presumably, extracellular proteases hydrolyze the protein material, thus inactivating enzymes lost from cells. The degraded inactive proteins are then removed by one of several excretory routes: excretion in bile, the intestine, liver, kidney, or the reticuloendothelial system. In addition, various enzymes have different half-lives, which suggests there are several mechanisms of removal.

ENZYME CLASSIFICATION

Many enzymes were first named for their function (e.g., lactate dehydrogenase), but some were named for the type of substrate on which they act: urease hydrolyzes urea, lipase hydrolyzes lipids, and phosphatases act on organic phosphates. Many clinically important enzymes are still known by these trivial names, which arose from historic circumstances and will continue to pervade the literature because of their simplicity. But a more organized approach was needed because of the increasing complexity of names and the increasing number of enzymes. The Enzyme Commission (EC) of the International Union of Biochemistry (IUB) developed and proposed a systematic convention for the naming of enzymes.

IUB names and codes

The IUB systematic name describes the reaction catalyzed. The IUB also recognized that trivial names were important and assigned practical names (but no abbreviations) to many enzymes. For each individual enzyme the system provides a numeric code designation of four numbers separated by periods. The first number assigns the enzyme to one of six categories of reaction. The second number denotes the subclass, which is often based on the type of group (e.g., amino group or hydroxyl group) that takes part in the reaction. The third number of the EC code indicates the sub-subclass of reaction, often the acceptor group, and the last number is merely the serial number of the particular enzyme in the sub-subgroup. For the enzyme lactate dehydrogenase (EC 1.1.1.27), the first number, 1, indicates that the enzyme is an oxidoreductase; the second number, 1, indicates that the enzyme acts on the CH-OH group of donors; the third number, 1, indicates that the acceptor is NAD^+ or $NADP^+$; and the fourth number, 27, is the serial number of the enzyme in the EC 1.1.1.x group.

EC classification

All enzymes are divided into one of six general classes depending on the type of reaction they catalyze. A few clinically important enzymes, along with the EC codes and systematic names, are listed in Table 14-1.

The first class includes the oxidoreductases, enzymes that catalyze electron transfer or oxidation-reduction reactions,

which can be illustrated schematically as:

$$A_{red} + B_{ox} \rightleftharpoons A_{ox} + B_{red}$$

One enzyme of this category is lactic dehydrogenase (EC 1.1.1.27); others include dehydrogenases, reductases, oxidases, and peroxidases.

The second group of enzymes are the transferases, which catalyze the transfer of a group (e.g., an amino, carboxyl, glucosyl, methyl, or phosphoryl group) from one molecule to another. These reactions can be listed schematically as:

$$A\text{-}X + B \rightleftharpoons A + B\text{-}X$$

Alanine aminotransferase (EC 2.6.1.2) is an example of this group. Other common enzymes in this category include kinases and transcarboxylases.

A third group is the hydrolases, which catalyze the cleavage of C-O, C-N, C-C, and some other bonds with the addition of water. These hydrolysis reactions can be illustrated as:

$$A\text{-}B + H_2O \rightleftharpoons A\text{-}OH + B\text{-}H$$

An example of this group is acid phosphatase (EC 3.1.3.2). Common enzymes in this category include amylase, urease, pepsin, trypsin, chymotrypsin, and various peptidases and esterases.

A fourth group is the lyases, which hydrolyzes C-C, C-O, and C-N bonds by elimination, with the formation of a double bond or the reverse reaction, the addition of a group to a double bond. In cases where the reverse reaction is important the term *synthase* is used in the name. This type of reaction is illustrated as:

$$A + B \rightleftharpoons AB \text{ or } AB \rightleftharpoons A + B$$

As the EC listing shows, this and the subsequent groups contain relatively few enzymes used in clinical diagnosis.

The fifth group is the isomerases, which catalyze structural or geometric changes in a molecule. They may be called epimerases, isomerases, and mutases depending on the type of isomerism involved. This reaction can be illustrated as:

$$ABC \rightleftharpoons CAB$$

An example of this group is the enzyme glucose phosphate isomerase (EC 5.3.1.9).

A sixth and last group consists of the ligases or synthetases. In this case two molecules are joined, coupled with the hydrolysis of the pyrophosphate in ATP. Many ligases are involved in DNA, RNA, and protein synthesis; none are currently used in clinical diagnosis. The synthetic reaction type is illustrated as:

$$A + B + ATP \rightleftharpoons AB + ADP + Pi$$

An example of this reaction is the enzyme glutamine synthetase (EC 6.3.1.2), which is rarely used clinically.

Nonstandard abbreviations

A variety of simple abbreviations of four or fewer capital letters are used to represent enzymes that are routinely measured. These abbreviations, which have been suggested as a useful addition, are widely used in practice but are *not*

Table 14-1   Selected examples of enzyme nomenclature in common use

EC code	Recommended name (trivial)	Abbreviation*	Systematic name	Other name or abbreviation
OXIDOREDUCTASES				
1.1.1.27	Lactate dehydrogenase	LD	L-Lactate:NAD⁺ oxidoreductase	LDH
1.1.1.37	Malate dehydrogenase	MD	L-Malate:NAD⁺ oxidoreductase	MDH
1.16.3.1	Ferroxidase	—	Iron(II):oxygen oxidoreductase	Ceruloplasmin
TRANSFERASES				
2.3.2.2	γ-Glutamyl transferase	GGT	(5-Glutamyl)-peptide:amino acid 5-glutamyl transferase	—
2.6.1.1	Aspartate aminotransferase	AST	L-Aspartate:2-oxoglutarate amino-transferase	Glutamic oxaloacetic transaminase/SGOT
2.6.1.2	Alanine aminotransferase	ALT	L-Alanine:2-oxoglutarate amino-transferase	Glutamic pyruvic transaminase/SGPT
2.7.1.1	Hexokinase	HK	ATP: D-hexose-6-phosphotransferase	—
2.7.1.40	Pyruvate kinase	PK	ATP: pyruvate 2-O-phospho-transferase	—
2.7.3.2	Creatine kinase	CK	ATP: creatine N-phosphotransferase	CPK
HYDROLASES				
3.1.1.3	Triacylglycerol lipase	LPS	Triacylglycerol acyl hydrolase	Lipase
3.1.1.8	Cholinesterase	CHS	Acylcholine acyl hydrolase	Pseudocholinesterase
3.1.3.1	Alkaline phosphatase	ALP	Orthophosphoric-monoester phosphohydrolase (alkaline optimum)	—
3.1.3.2	Acid phosphatase	ACP	Orthophosphoric-monoester phosphohydrolase (acid optimum)	—
3.1.3.5	5'-Nucleotidase	NT	5'-Ribonucleotide phosphohydrolase	—
3.2.1.1	α-Amylase	AMS	1,4-α-D-Glucan glucanohydrolase	Diastase
3.4.11.1	Aminopeptidase (cytosol)	LAS	α-Aminoacyl-peptide hydrolase (cytosol)	Arylaminadase/LAP; leucine aminopeptidase
3.4.21.1	Chymotrypsin	—	None (preferred cleavage: Tyr, Trp, Phe, Leu)	Chymotrypsin A and B
LYASE				
4.1.2.13	Fructose-bisphosphate aldolase	ALS	D-Fructose-1,6,-bisphosphate:D-glyceraldehyde-3-phosphate-lyase	Aldolase
4.2.1.24	Porphobilinogen synthase	—	5-Aminolevulinate hydrolyase	—
ISOMERASES				
5.3.1.1	Triosephosphate isomerase	TPI	D-Glyceraldehyde-3-phosphate:ketol-isomerase	Triosephosphate mutase
5.3.1.9	Glucosephosphate isomerase	GPI	D-Glucose-6-phosphate:ketol-isomerase	Phosphohexose isomerase
LIGASES				
6.3.1.2	Glutamine synthetase	—	L-Glutamate:ammonia ligase (ADP-forming)	—

*Baron DN, et al: J Clin Pathol 24:656-657, 1971 (ref. 4) and Baron DN, et al: J Clin Pathol 28:592-593, 1975 (ref. 5) are not recommended by the International Union of Biochemistry but are in common use.

part of the IUB system. However they are so popular that discarding them would be difficult.

MEASUREMENT OF ENZYMES

The reaction rates of most enzymatic procedures are not constant. But by observing the rate of change of absorbance for a starting material or product at a specific wavelength, the reaction can be followed. When the reactants are mixed and reach thermal and kinetic equilibrium, a lag phase occurs with little change of absorbance per unit time. Then a linear phase of constant absorbance change per unit time occurs, and finally a substrate depletion

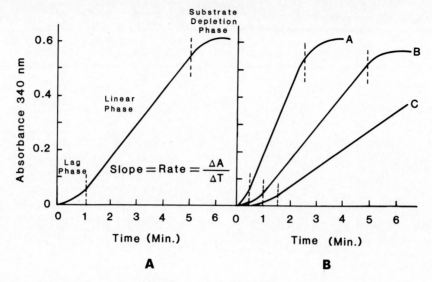

Fig. 14-1 Typical enzyme reaction with an initial lag phase, a linear change of absorbance, and a final phase of substrate depletion. The enzyme activity is the slope of the linear phase. As enzyme activity increases in an assay system, the lag phase decreases, the linear phase decreases, and substrate depletion occurs sooner. Δ A = change in absorbance; Δ T = change of time.

phase with little change of absorbance per unit time (Figure 14-1).

Enzyme assays must be performed during the linear phase of absorbance change, where a constant amount of activity can be determined for a period of time. Measurements do not start at zero time but after the lag phase has occurred. Measurements can be made at any time during the linear phase and can continue up to the substrate depletion phase.

Rather than changing the assay time, the most common way to handle samples with high activity is to dilute them two- or threefold with saline or water. However, not all enzymes demonstrate linearity on dilution, particularly if the enzymes are active at a lipid-water interface, e.g., lipase (EC 3.1.1.3), or if inhibitors are present in the sample (e.g., LD [EC 1.1.1.27] when measured in urine).

One of the more convenient methods of assaying enzyme activity is based on measuring spectral changes of either the substrates or the products. A number of enzyme systems involve the conversion of NAD^+ to its reduced form, NADH, or vice versa. NADH has a much greater absorption at 340 nm than does the oxidized form. Consequently, reactions that convert one form to the other can be conveniently followed by measuring the change in absorption at this wavelength. The difference between the absorption spectrum of reduced and oxidized compounds is shown in Figure 14-2.

Enzyme assays

Enzymes are measured by several techniques. The two most common are the one-point method at a fixed time, sometimes called an end-point method and multi-point fixed time assays, called kinetic methods.

The term "end-point methods" is also used to define assays that have come to an equilibrium or steady-state point, i.e., an assay used to measure the amount of an analyte after no further reaction is occurring.

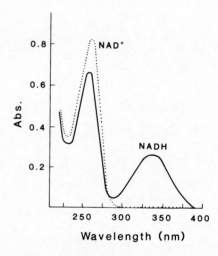

Fig. 14-2 Absorption spectrum, Abs., of 5×10^{-5} M NAD^+ in 0.1 M Tris buffer, pH 7.5 and the absorption spectrum of 4×10^{-5} M NADH in 0.1 M Tris buffer, pH 9.5.

End-point assays are still used in some cases, but in general, shorter time periods are employed. In these assays a reaction is started and allowed to incubate at a constant temperature for a fixed time period, e.g., 30 minutes. The reaction is then stopped, perhaps by adding another reagent, and the amount of product is measured. The assumption is that a constant amount of product is produced throughout the entire 30-minute assay period.

If the rate of reaction is followed continuously or with many points as a function of time, the assay is termed a kinetic assay. Usually the reaction time is short—a few seconds to a few minutes—and there is little danger of enzyme degradation. The term "kinetic assay" describes assays that form increasing amounts of product with time, whether they are one point end-point assays or multiple point assays. While this kinetic method terminology is not strictly correct, the continuous or multiple-point assays are superior to the single point fixed time assays since it is easier to demonstrate approximate linearity of the reaction over the entire measurement period.

Principles of kinetic analysis

Enzyme kinetics is the study of enzyme reaction rates and the factors that affect them. Initially, many experiments examine the effects of different assay conditions on measurements of enzyme activity. Eventually, a series of specific conditions are established that give rise to the maximum rate of enzyme activity.

The general enzyme reaction given previously for a single substrate reaction may be rewritten slightly for initial rates as Equation 3. In this case, the amount of product is very small and the reverse reaction of P combining with E and forming ES is ignored since initial rate measurements must be made. *Initial rate* refers to the rate at the start of the reaction, after the lag phase, and during the linear phase in Figure 14-3 but prior to substantial product formation.

$$E + S \underset{k_{-1}}{\overset{k_{+1}}{\rightleftharpoons}} \{ES\} \overset{k_{+2}}{\longrightarrow} P + E \qquad \textit{EQ 14–3}$$

For a given quantity of enzyme, the rate of activity increases with the amount of substrate, as shown in Figure 14-3. At low substrate concentrations, the rate is linearly dependent on the amount of substrate, i.e., first order, but at high substrate concentrations the rate is essentially independent of substrate concentration, i.e., zero order. A mathematical description of the reaction must explain how the reaction can be first order at low substrate concentrations and zero order at high substrate concentrations.

If the enzyme has a limited number of active sites, then at a low substrate concentration the rate will depend on the amount of substrate, since a large effective concentration of unfilled active sites will exist. However, since the total number of sites on the enzyme is limited and the amount of enzyme is constant, then as the amount of substrate is increased, the sites will become increasingly saturated with substrate until the reaction seems independent of the substrate concentration. At these high substrate concentrations all the enzyme active sites are filled and the reaction proceeds at maximal velocity. Small changes in the substrate concentration after saturation will not affect the enzyme rate.

The second step, product formation, presumably is the rate-limiting step, or the step that determines overall activity. The equilibrium for the formation of ES complex can be written as follows (the molar concentrations of all the reacting species are expressed in brackets):

$$K_{eq} = \frac{k_{+1}}{k_{-1}} = \frac{[ES]}{[E][S]}$$

The equilibrium constant, K_{eq}, is equal to the ratio of the forward over the reverse rate constants. From Equation 3, the rate of formation of the product P is the amount of [ES] times the rate, k_{+2}, at which the enzyme complex is converted to P. Thus, the rate of formation of product is

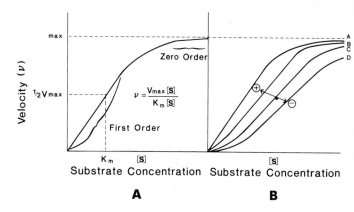

Fig. 14-3   Relationship of substrate, S, to velocity of reaction. At low substrate concentrations the rate is first order (linearly dependent) with respect to substrate concentration. At high substrate concentrations the rate becomes zero order (independent) with respect to substrate concentration. K_m, Michaelis-Menten constant; V_{max}, maximal rate of reaction.

velocity or rate = $[ES] \times k_{+2}$.

Since the rate is the amount of product formed for some period of time:

$$rate = \frac{\Delta P}{\Delta T} = [ES] \times k_{+2},$$

substituting $K_{eq}[E][S]$ for [ES] and rearranging gives

$$\Delta P = K_{eq} \times [S] \times [E] \times k_{+2} \times \Delta T.$$

The amount of product formed is proportional to the amount of enzyme present, the time of the assay, and the amount of substrate. When a proportionality constant is substituted for the rate constants, the equation becomes

$$\Delta P = K1 \times [S] \times [E] \times \Delta T,$$

where ΔP is the amount of product formed during the assay time, E is the amount of enzyme, S is the amount of substrate, ΔT is the assay time, and K1 is a proportionality constant. The enzyme activity or rate of product formation over time is then given by

$$Rate = \frac{\Delta P}{\Delta T} = K1 \times [S] \times [E]$$

Usually, enzyme assays are performed at a high substrate concentration for a time period short enough that the substrate concentration can be assumed to be constant. The value of this constant substrate concentration can be combined with K1 to produce a second proportionality constant K2, which is the product of K1 times the substrate concentration. The rate can then be expressed so that it depends only on the amount of enzyme present, i.e., a zero order reaction, independent of substrate concentration.

$$rate = \frac{\Delta P}{\Delta T} = K2 \times [E]$$

This rate of reaction or velocity is often listed as v or Vi or Vo in the enzyme kinetic literature.

Km and Vmax

The enzyme activity or rate or velocity depends on the substrate concentration when the amount of substrate is low relative to the amount of enzyme present in an assay. This relationship is shown in Figure 14-3, with the same enzyme concentration assayed at many different substrate concentrations.

At steady state, before much product is present, the rate of formation of the ES complex equals the rate of breakdown. This can be described with the following rate equation:

$$\underset{\text{formation}}{k_{+1}\,[E]\,[S]} \mid \underset{\text{breakdown}}{k_{-1}\,[ES] + k_{+2}\,[ES]}$$

By collecting terms and rearranging, the rate constants can be removed and a constant, Km, defined.

EQ 14–4

$$\frac{[E]\,[S]}{[ES]} = \frac{k_{-1} + k_{+2}}{k_{+1}} = Km$$

The rate or velocity of product formation, v, at any time, and free enzyme concentration, [E], are described by:

$$v = k_{+2}\,[ES] \text{ and } [E] = [Et] - [ES]$$

where [Et] is the total amount of enzyme and [ES] is the amount complexed with substrate. When all the enzyme is present in the form of ES (i.e., at very high [S]; zero order reaction) then the maximum rate, Vmax, is as follows:

$$Vmax = k_{+2}\,[Et]$$

Combining the above three equations gives:

$$[E] = \frac{Vmax}{k_{+2}} - \frac{v}{k_{+2}} = \frac{Vmax - v}{k_{+2}}$$

Since from Equation 4:

$$[E] = \frac{Km\,[ES]}{[S]} \text{ and } [ES] = \frac{v}{k_{+2}} \text{ then:}$$

$$\frac{Km\,[ES]}{[S]} = \frac{Vmax - v}{k_{+2}} \text{ or } \frac{Km \times v}{[S] \times k_{+2}} = \frac{Vmax - v}{k_{+2}}$$

Rearranging gives:

$$Km \times v = (Vmax - v)[S] \text{ or } v(Km + [S]) = Vmax[S]$$

When this equation is solved for v it gives the Michaelis-Menten equation, the equation for the rectangular hyperbola shown in Figure 14-3.

EQ 14–5

$$v = \frac{Vmax\,[S]}{Km + [S]}$$

[S] is the concentration of substrate, v is the velocity, Vmax is the maximal rate of reaction when the enzyme is saturated with substrate and Km, the Michaelis-Menten constant, is the substrate concentration that produces one half the maximal velocity.

At the fixed high substrate concentration found in the usual clinical laboratory assays, the velocity, v, approaches

Vmax and is proportional to the amount of enzyme present since all other factors are constant. The reaction is said to be zero order with respect to substrate, i.e., independent of the concentration of substrate. The common condition used for assaying enzyme activity is a high substrate concentration, where $[S] \simeq 10 \times Km$ or higher. The rate at a substrate concentration of $10 \times Km$ is given by the following equation:

$$v = \frac{Vmax\,(10 \times Km)}{Km + (10 \times Km)} = Vmax \frac{10 \times Km}{11 \times Km} = 0.91\,Vmax$$

Thus at $[S] = 10 \times Km$ the rate produced is greater than 90% of Vmax.

Another way to examine the Michaelis-Menten equation is to see if it is consistent with first-order kinetics at low substrate concentrations and zero-order kinetics at high substrate concentrations.

At low substrate concentrations, where $[S] \ll Km$, then:

$$v = \frac{Vmax\,[S]}{Km + [S]} \simeq \frac{Vmax\,[S]}{Km}$$

Since Km and Vmax are constants:

$$v = K1\,[S]$$

This shows that the rate depends only on the first power of the substrate concentration.

At high substrate concentrations, where $[S] \gg Km$, then:

$$v = \frac{Vmax\,[S]}{Km + [S]} \cong \frac{Vmax\,[S]}{[S]} = Vmax$$

showing that the rate (v) does not depend on substrate concentration.

As shown in Figure 14-3, the relationship of substrate concentration to enzyme activity is a curve that is often similar to a rectangular hyperbola. For multi-substrate enzyme reactions the kinetics are more complex. The presence of activators and inhibitors acting at allosteric or regulatory sites tends to make the curves less linear due to the complex kinetics.

Accurately determining Km and Vmax for each substrate or activator from Michaelis-Menten curves is very difficult, even if the curves are fairly linear. However, ascertaining these constants is necessary so that assays can be established using optimal conditions to correctly measure enzyme activity. If the curve is transformed into a straight line, then the Km and Vmax can be determined with greater accuracy. One may transform the Michaelis-Menten equation mathematically and obtain the equation of a straight line in several ways. The Km and Vmax can then be graphically determined from the line slopes and intercepts using these transformed equations. A common graph is shown in Figure 14-4, where 1/v is plotted against 1/s.

Calculation of enzyme activity

The results of an enzyme determination are expressed as an activity unit in terms of the amount of product formed per unit of time, under specified conditions, for a given volume

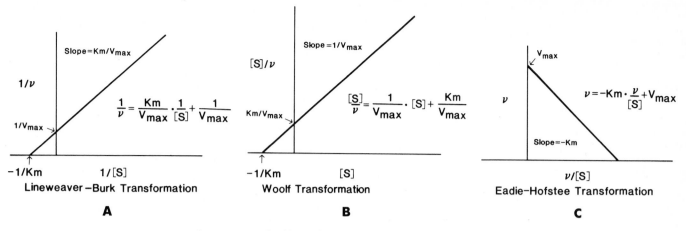

Fig. 14-4   Graph of linear form of the Michaelis-Menten equation.

of sample which is often serum. Thus one unit of enzyme activity might be the amount that would, under certain specified conditions, cause the formation of 1 mg of the product, P, per minute when 1 ml of the sample is used. In older procedures arbitrary units like these were often employed.

In 1961 the Enzyme Commission recommended the adoption of an international unit of enzyme activity. This unit was defined as the amount of enzyme that would convert 1 micromole of substrate per minute under standard conditions.

$$1\ IU = 1\ \text{micromole}/\text{minute}$$

If one molecule of substrate is transformed into a number of molecules of a product, the definition is per micromole of product formed.

This recommendation of an international unit was an attempt to standardize the units of assay and to reduce the large number of units in use. The international unit has been widely adopted, and in some respects it has standardized assay units. It has not reduced the number of reference ranges because if the standard conditions change, then the apparent enzyme activity changes. For example, if a new buffer were used in the assay, it may affect the enzyme rate and produce a different reference range.

The Systéme International d'Unités (SI), as originally adopted by the World Health Organization, established the katal (K) as the unit of enzyme activity. This is defined as 1 mole/sec of substrate changed. The katal is too large for clinical use, and, although it was recommended by the EC in 1972, it has had little acceptance in the United States.

To convert international units to katals:

$$1\ IU = \frac{\text{micromole}}{\text{min}} \times \frac{10^{-6}\ \text{mole}}{\text{micromole}} \times \frac{1\ \text{min}}{60\ \text{sec}} = 1.67 \times 10^{-8}\ K$$

Thus, 1.0 IU = 16.7 nK (nanokatals). Unlike the katal, international units (IU) have been widely accepted by clinical enzymology workers.

Pure human enzyme materials are not available, so enzyme assays cannot be standardized in each laboratory by calibration with pure materials. Other standardization methods must be used. Many enzyme assays are followed by making spectrophotometric measurements at a specific wavelength. With the spectrophotometric method, one usually assumes that at 340 nm, NADH has a molar absorption coefficient of

$$A/(b \times c) = 6.22 \times 10^3$$

where A is the actual absorbance of a solution, b is the light path in centimeters through the solution, and c is the concentration in moles per liter of the absorbing substance. For a 1 cm light path, rearranging for c:

$$c = A \times 10^{-3}/6.22$$

When the concentration is expressed in IU/L instead of moles/L the expression changes:

$$c = A \times 10^3/6.22$$

From the absorbance change that was measured and the volume of solution used, one can readily calculate the number of micromoles of NADH formed or used up during the enzyme measurement period.

$$c = \Delta A \times 10^3/6.22$$

For example, in the lactate dehydrogenase reaction above, if a change in absorbance of 0.06 A per minute was observed at 340 nm, and a 0.1 mL sample was used with a total assay volume of 3.0 mL then the calculation of activity would be as follows:

$$\text{international units}/L = \frac{0.06 \times 1000 \times 3.0}{6.22 \times 0.1} = 289\ U/L$$

Both enzyme units described express the activity in terms of units per volume of sample. This is a particularly convenient unit of measure when assaying enzymes in biological fluids like serum and plasma. If one is measuring an enzyme found in erythrocytes or in white blood cells, then another unit of measure is needed. In the case of RBC and WBC enzymes, the enzyme activity can be expressed as units per 10^{10} cells.

In biochemistry laboratories—where enzyme purification is important—the activity might be expressed per milligram of protein or per dry weight of cells or per microgram of DNA, but these units are not convenient for the clinical laboratory.

Analytical factors affecting measurement

The rate of reactions involving enzymes is markedly influenced by temperature, pH, concentration of substrate, and a number of other factors. Accordingly, all details of a given procedure must be followed exactly in order to produce precise and accurate results.

Assays of enzyme activity should be performed under optimal conditions of zero-order kinetics, so that the measured rate depends only on the amount of enzyme present. To optimize an assay (e.g., the lactate dehydrogenase reaction given earlier) a series of reaction assays are set up with increasing concentrations of lactate but at a fixed high NAD^+ concentration and a fixed amount of enzyme. The enzyme rates are then measured, and a graph similar to the one in Figure 14-2 is constructed. A second series of assays are then performed with increasing concentrations of NAD^+, but at the fixed high concentration of lactate determined from the first experiment, i.e., $[S] \simeq 10 \times Km$ for lactate, and the same amount of enzyme present. The enzyme rates are again determined and another graph created to determine the Km for NAD^+. This same type of experiment is performed for each item of the assay mixture (i.e., metal ions, pH, buffer) until all the variables had been evaluated for maximal enzyme activity. The final conditions determined from this set of experiments would be the optimal assay conditions. Experiments to determine optimal assay conditions have been performed for the current clinically important enzymes, and diagnostic kits are commercially available with all the materials at optimal concentrations.

pH

Changes in pH markedly affect enzyme reaction rates. For most enzymes there is a definite pH range where the enzyme is most active. A pH near the center of this range is usually specified for the measurement of that particular enzyme. The optimal pH varies from enzyme to enzyme. Reduced activity is observed at pH values greater to or less than optimal.

A typical pH curve of enzyme activity is given in Figure 14-5. The bell-shaped curve shows changes in enzyme activity vs. pH.

If pH values are not optimal, enzyme activity may be affected due to changes in enzyme structure. Changes may occur at the active site, or they may be due to conformational changes affecting the three-dimensional structure.

Since the active site of an enzyme often contains ionizable side chains of amino acids, i.e., $RCOO^-$ or RNH_3^+, a significant change in pH can lead to the gain or loss of a proton. The result is a substantial change in surface charge at the active site. The active site may therefore lose its ability to attract a substrate with an opposing charge. A similar loss of activity occurs when the change in charge is on the substrate molecule rather than on the enzyme. A change of pH might cause the enzyme to unfold and lose activity if pH change disrupts hydrogen-bonds and other intramolecular forces holding the enzyme in an active conformation.

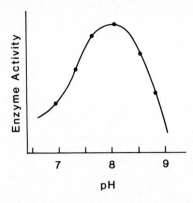

Fig. 14-5 Enzyme activity as a function of pH. Optimal pH range is 7.8 to 8.2; lower activities are observed at pH < 7.8 and pH > 8.2.

Buffer

In many cases, the enzyme reaction creates products that tend to alter the pH. Most assays include a buffer to maintain optimal pH range. The buffer should have a pKa within 1 pH unit of the enzyme's optimal pH in order to exert effective pH control.

Buffers not only serve to regulate an assay's pH, but they may take part in the reaction as well. For example, alkaline phosphatase (ALP, EC 3.1.3.1) assays with p-nitrophenol phosphate as a substrate use the buffer 2-amino-2-methyl-1-propanol (AMP) to maintain pH at 10.2. The enzyme hydrolyzes the substrate into p-nitrophenol and inorganic phosphate in a multistep process, part of which involves a temporary phosphorylation of the enzyme. The final and rate-limiting step includes hydrolysis of the enzyme-phosphate bond to regenerate free enzyme. At similar pH values, buffers that are phosphate acceptors in a transphosphorylation process with the enzyme produce higher rates of alkaline phosphatase activity than buffers that do not act as phosphate acceptors. Thus AMP buffer produces higher rates of alkaline phosphatase activity at pH 10.2 than glycylglycine buffer at pH 10.2 because AMP is a phosphate acceptor. When buffers do not participate in the reaction, the concentration of buffer that gives maximal enzyme activity at the optimal pH must also be experimentally determined.

The buffer and certain salts may have an unusual effect on the Km. When the buffer-to-substrate ratio is very large, the buffer and the substrate may compete for the enzyme and make the enzyme activity seem related to substrate concentration in a nonlinear way. This has been observed with NADH in the LD reaction. Here the buffer-to-substrate molar ratio is $10^4:1$ and the rate of reaction is affected by tris, phosphate, and NH_4HCO_3 buffers and certain salts (e.g., NACl and $(NH_4)_2SO_4$), which are often found in the coupling or auxiliary enzymes used to prepare assays. Buffer concentrations below 0.05 mol/L seem to have no effect on the Km. This is consistent with several recommendations for optimal assay conditions. It seems prudent to maintain the lowest possible buffer concentration without compromising pH stability or enzyme rate.

Cofactors

Many enzymes require a nonprotein—often dialyzable—material for maximal activity. Some of these materials are

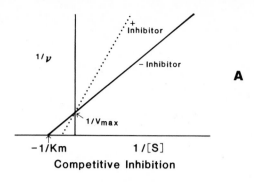

Competitive Inhibition

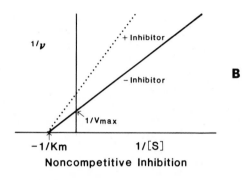

Noncompetitive Inhibition

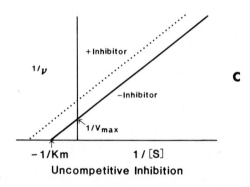

Uncompetitive Inhibition

Fig. 14-6   The three types of inhibition are shown. The Lineweaver-Burk graph demonstrates the effect of the type of inhibition on the K_m and the V_{max}.

related to vitamin structures. For example, thiamine (vitamin B_1) can be converted to thiamine pyrophosphate, a cofactor in many decarboxylation reactions. Niacin can be converted to nicotinamide adenine dinucleotide, and vitamin B_2 (riboflavin) can be converted to flavin adenine dinucleotide. Both of these compounds are involved in many dehydrogenation reactions. Pyridoxine, vitamin B_6, is modified to pyridoxal phosphate, which is used in many transamination reactions.

In analytical assays of transaminase activity, pyridoxyl-5-phosphate is an example of a tightly bound cofactor that is not a substrate. The optimal concentration of a cofactor is determined in the same way as a substrate so that assay conditions can be established with a cofactor concentration of approximately $10 \times K_m$ or higher.

Activators and inhibitors

Many enzymes require specific ions for maximal activity. All phosphate transferring enzymes (e.g., hexokinase) require magnesium ions (Mg^{+2}). Other common metal ion

activators are manganese (Mn^{+2}), calcium (Ca^{+2}), zinc (Zn^{+2}), iron (Fe^{+2}), and potassium (K^+). Amylase requires chloride (Cl^-) for maximal activity; other enzymes require several ions for maximal activity (e.g., pyruvate kinase requires magnesium [Mg^{+2}] and potassium [K^+]). In each case, the optimal concentration of the activator must be determined just as the optimal concentration of substrate is determined.

Inhibitors reduce an enzyme's catalytic activity. There are many types of inhibitors and several classes of inhibition. Inhibitors may act by removing an activator by chelation (e.g., Ca^{+2} and Mg^{+2} are removed by EDTA or oxalate to cause the inhibition of hexokinase). They may also act by binding to the active site to compete with the substrate or by forming a complex at a different allosteric site that may affect enzyme activity.

Inhibitors are divided into three main groups. Competitive inhibitors bind at the active site and compete with the substrate for binding sites. These materials demonstrate a reversible inhibition that can often be reduced by using a higher substrate concentration.

$$E + S \rightleftharpoons \{ES\} \rightarrow P + E$$
$$+$$
$$I \rightleftharpoons \{EI\}$$

If enough substrate is present, the maximum rate of reaction is not affected because of the irreversibility of the reactions. The binding of the substrate is affected and thus the apparent K_m is higher while V_{max} remains the same.

Noncompetitive inhibitors are a second group of materials that bind at an allosteric or regulatory site that may be far removed from the active site. Noncompetitive inhibitors cannot be reversed by adding more substrate, since they are believed to bind at a different location on the enzyme surface.

$$E + S \rightleftharpoons \{ES\} \rightarrow P + E$$
$$+ \qquad +$$
$$I \qquad I$$
$$\updownarrow \qquad \updownarrow$$
$$\{EI\} + S \rightleftharpoons \{ESI\}$$

Since the inhibitor does not compete with the substrate the K_m is unaffected but the amount of E or ES that converts substrate to product is reduced and the V_{max} is lessened.

A third group, uncompetitive inhibitors, are thought to bind with the enzyme substrate complex and not the free enzyme. In this case, at low substrate concentrations, adding substrate increases the inhibition, since it produces more enzyme-substrate complex to react with the inhibitor. As a result, the V_{max} is reduced and the K_m is increased.

$$E + S \rightleftharpoons \{ES\} \rightleftharpoons P + E$$
$$+$$
$$I$$
$$\updownarrow$$
$$\{ESI\}$$

The type of inhibition a substance exerts can be determined by examining the results of kinetic studies using a linear graph of enzyme activity with and without inhibitors, as shown in Figure 14-6.

Table 14-2 summarizes the effects of inhibitions on K_m and V_{max}.

Table 14-2   Kinetic effects of inhibition

Type of inhibition	Change in K_m	Change in V_{max}
Competitive	Increased	No change
Noncompetitive	No change	Decreased
Uncompetitive	Decreased	Decreased

Simple types of inhibition may be classified by examining the kinetic effect on Km and Vmax.

Coupling enzymes

Some enzyme reactions of interest (e.g., alanine aminotransferase (ALT) and aspartate aminotransferase (AST)) do not have substrates or form products that can be monitored directly. One may couple the initial enzyme reaction to a second indicating enzyme reaction that, for example, contains the $NAD^+/NADH$ conversion to make a convenient assay. The AST enzyme reaction can be coupled to the malate dehydrogenase reaction (MD, EC 1.1.1.37):

$$\text{L-Aspartate} + \alpha\text{-Ketoglutarate} \xrightleftharpoons{\text{AST}} \text{L-Glutamate} + \text{Oxaloacetate}$$

$$\text{Oxaloacetate} + \text{NADH} + \text{H}^+ \xrightleftharpoons{\text{MD}} \text{L-malate} + \text{NAD}^+$$

This gives the following net reaction:

$$\text{L-Aspartate} + \alpha\text{-Ketoglutarate} + \text{NADH} + \text{H}^+$$
$$\rightleftharpoons \text{L-Glutamate} + \text{L-malate} + \text{NAD}^+$$

In this case, the substrate for the second reaction, oxaloacetate, is supplied as the product of the first reaction. Oxaloacetate from the AST reaction serves as the substrate, with the cofactor NADH for the malate dehydrogenase reaction. This assay has L-aspartate, α-ketoglutarate, NADH, and the enzyme malate dehydrogenase (MD) in large excesses so the rate-limiting item in the assay would be the amount of AST in the added sample.

There are other enzymes (e.g., creatine kinase [CK, EC 2.7.3.2]) where the measurement of the first enzyme requires an intermediate auxiliary enzyme reaction and then an indicator enzyme. In the measurement of CK, hexokinase (EC 2.7.1.1) is used as an auxiliary enzyme and glucose-6-phosphate dehydrogenase (EC 1.1.1.49) is used as an indicating enzyme. Both additional enzymes must be present in large excesses to correctly measure CK. It is difficult to correctly produce optimum assays with more than two coupled reactions due to the large number of components in the assay system and the problems with maximizing all components without inhibiting the limiting reaction.

Temperature

There is no optimal temperature for enzyme assays. Most enzymes show increasing activity as the temperature is raised over a limited temperature range, i.e., 10° C to 40° C. An example is shown in Figure 14-7. To minimize loss of activity if the enzyme cannot be assayed immediately after collection, samples should be stored at refrigerator temperatures, 2° C to 6° C, or frozen (see Table 14-3). In a few cases, some forms of enzymes (e.g., LD$_4$ and LD$_5$)

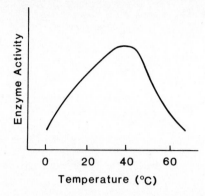

Fig. 14-7   Enzyme activity as a function of temperature of the assay. At low temperatures, the activity decreases. As the temperature rises, the activity increases until the rate of denaturation is greater than the increase in activity.

are more stable at room temperature than when refrigerated. Repeated freezing and thawing of a specimen often causes denaturation and loss of activity. Above 40° C, most enzymes rapidly denature and lose almost all activity. An exception is amylase, which seems to be stable up to about 60° C.

For many enzymes a 1° C change in temperature produces about a 10% change in activity. A tolerance of ±0.1° C for temperature control of an enzyme analyzer is recommended, since this would produce approximately a ±1% change in the activity which is small enough to ignore in most clinical work. A recommendation of ±0.05° C for temperature control has also been suggested. This reduces the change in activity to ±0.5%.

The apparent increase in activity with increasing temperature means that assays performed at higher temperatures, i.e., 37° C, are more sensitive to slight changes in the amount of enzyme. The common enzymes employed for clinical diagnosis are less stable at this temperature than at 25° C or 30° C and therefore assays at 37° C must be performed with relatively short assay times to minimize enzyme denaturation.

Arguments for both higher (i.e., 37°C) and lower (i.e., 25°C) temperatures are based primarily on scientific and technical reasoning. A reasonable compromise seems to be measurement at 30°C, the recommendation of the International Federation on Clinical Chemistry (IFCC). There is a very accurate Gallium standard melting point cell that is now available to all laboratories from the National Bureau of Standards. This material has a melting temperature plateau of 29.772°C and can be used to calibrate or check the assay temperature of a wide variety of instruments.

Assay type

Although an optimal set of conditions exists for the assay of an enzyme, not all assays are optimal. Differences between assays don't always appear significant, yet the results can be substantially divergent. The effect of various assay components on each other is even more significant when one considers a coupled assay. Coupled assays not only have the concentrations of substrates and activators of the primary reaction to consider but they must also have ex-

Table 14-3   Enzyme stability under various storage conditions (less than 10% change in activity)

Enzyme	Room temperature (about 25° C)	Refrigeration (0° to about 4° C)	Frozen (−25° C)
Aldolase (ALS)	2 days	2 days	Unstable*
Alanine aminotransferase (ALT, GPT)	2 days	5 days	Unstable*
α-Amylase (AMS)	1 month	7 months	2 months
Aspartate aminotransferase (AST, GOT)	3 days	1 week	1 month
Ferroxidase I (ceruloplasmin)	1 day	2 weeks	2 weeks
Cholinesterase (CHS)	1 week	1 week	1 week
Creatine kinase (CK)	1 week	1 week	1 month
γ-Glutamyl transferase (GGT)	2 days	1 week	1 month
Lactate dehydrogenase (LD)	1 week	1 to 3 days†	1 to 3 days†
Leucine aminopeptidase (LAP)	1 week	1 week	1 week
Lipase (LPS)	1 week	3 weeks	3 weeks
Phosphatase, acid (ACP)	4 hours‡	3 days§	3 days§
Phosphatase, alkaline (ALP)	2 to 3 days‖	2 to 3 days	1 month

*Enzyme does not tolerate thawing well.
†Depending on isoenzyme pattern in the serum.
‡Unacidified.
§With added citrate or acetate to pH ~ 5.
‖Activity may increase.

cesses of the auxiliary and indicating enzymes with their associated additional activators.

Alanine aminotransferase (ALT) is often measured by adding an excess of lactate dehydrogenase and NADH to a mixture containing L-alanine and α-ketoglutarate and buffer. Commercially available kits often specify that about 500 U/L of LD are present as an indicating enzyme and that the source of this enzyme perhaps is animal. This information is not sufficient to completely define the assay, since the Km of pyruvate varies with the isoenzyme type. About four times more units of M_4-LD_1 than H_4-LD_5 are required to achieve an equivalent reaction rate. A crude mixture of isoenzymes falls somewhere between these extremes. Even if the units of LD added are the same, the measured enzyme rates might vary with each lot of a kit if the indicating enzyme is added without regard to the isoenzyme content. This same kind of variability occurs between manufacturers with the same concentrations of substrates, activators, and units of LD if a different source (e.g., bacterial) of the indicating enzyme is used. For this reason a reference range should be checked by each laboratory, particularly when changing reagent manufacturers.

Enzymes as reagents

Substrate concentrations can be determined using many of the principles of enzyme kinetics applied in a slightly different way. The enzyme activity at low substrate concentrations is first order, i.e., linear, with respect to substrate concentration. In order to measure the concentration of pyruvate in a sample, a special assay mixture is prepared, with only a small amount of sample, so the amount of unknown pyruvate in the assay is low, that is, less than the Km. An assay mixture that contains an excess of LD, an excess of the coenzyme NADH, and a buffer is used. The reduction in the amount of NADH in this assay could be related to the amount of pyruvate from the millimolar absorption coefficient of NADH at 340 nm. Alternately, a series of pyruvate standards can be used to calibrate the assay. Other commonly used enzymatic assays include the determination

Table 14-4   Plasma half-lives for clinically important enzymes

Enzymes	Half-life (hours) (mean ± 2 SD)
LD_1	53-173
LD_5	8-12
CK	15
AST (GOT)	12-22
ALT (GPT)	37-57
AMS	3-6
LPS	3-6
ALP	3-7 days
GGT	3-7 days

of glucose, urea, ethanol, cholesterol, triglycerides, and uric acid.

Enzymes as markers

One unusual use of enyzme determinations is to quantitate some of them as an estimate of tumor mass. Excess specific proteins are sometimes found as antigenic markers that are elaborated into the plasma during tumor cell growth. In some cases, these specific proteins are enzymes, (i.e., prostatic acid phosphatase [PAP], or creatine kinase [CK]) and they can be conveniently measured to monitor response to therapy.

Storage of enyzmes

Most clinically used enzymes are stable at refrigerator temperatures from two to three days to about a week and at room temperature for a shorter time. Table 14-4 summarizes data for three temperatures. Several enzymes deserve particular comment. Acid phosphatase is particularly unstable at all temperatures unless the pH of the serum is reduced to about 5 to 6 with citrate or acetate. Alkaline phosphatase in human serum demonstrates a linear increase in activity dependent on temperature and time. At 96 hours (four days), there is a 6% increase at room temperature, a 4% increase at refrigerator temperature, and a 1% increase at $-20°C$. Enzymes in control materials are usually of nonhuman origin and are much more varied. Some are more stable and some are less stable than human serum.

The observed biological half-lives of several human enzymes in plasma are given in Table 14-4.

CLINICAL ENZYME MEASUREMENTS

A few enzymes have been used since the turn of the century to evaluate chronic diseases. But it wasn't until 1954 that LaDue, Wroblewski, and Karmen found a temporary increase in serum aspartate aminotransferase (EC 2.6.1.1) activity following an acute myocardial infarction. The measurement of changes in plasma enzyme activity gained importance as a means of following the course of a disease or to improve clinical diagnosis. Many investigators began to look for changes in enzyme activity specific for a disease state or reflected damage to a particular tissue.

Changes in enzyme activity in the plasma or serum are followed since enzymes are primarily intracellular constituents that are released after cell damage or cell death in a specific organ or tissue. The changes that occur with many diseases or in a particular organ can often be understood by examining the pattern of several enzyme or isoenzyme changes over a period of hours or days.

Extracellular vs. cellular enzymes

Enzymes in plasma are of two major groups: plasma-specific enymzes and non plasma-specific enzymes.

Plasma-specific enzymes have specific function in plasma. Plasma is their normal site of action and they are present in plasma at higher concentrations than in most tissues. Among these are the enzymes involved in blood coagulation, as well as ferroxidase, pseudocholinesterase, and lipoprotein lipase. Plasma-specific enzymes are synthesized in the liver and are constantly liberated into the plasma to maintain a steady-state concentration. These enzymes are of clinical interest when their concentration decreases in plasma. Some have historically been used as estimates of liver function.

Non plasma-specific enzymes have no known function in plasma. Their concentrations in plasma are usually lower than in most tissues. There may be a deficiency in activators or cofactors necessary for maximum enzyme activity. Non plasma-specific enzymes are divided into enzymes of secretion and enzymes of intermediary metabolism.

Some enzymes of secretion are from exocrine glands, that is, the pancreas and prostate, others are from the gastric mucosa and the bones. Enzymes in this group are clinically important when their concentrations are either higher or lower than normal. Elevated values appear when the normal mode of excretion is blocked or when the amount of enzyme produced is increased. Decreased values result when the tissue that normally produces the enzyme is damaged or necrotic. Common examples of enzymes of secretion are amylase, lipase, acid, and alkaline phosphatases.

The other major group of non plasma-specific enzymes are the enzymes of metabolism. The concentrations of these enzymes in tissues are very high, sometimes thousands of times higher than in plasma. Cellular damage resulting in leakage or necrosis allows a fraction of these proteins to escape into the plasma and causes a sharp rise in the concentration normally found. Some common examples are creatine kinase, CK, lactate dehydrogenase, LD, alanine aminotransferase, ALT, and aspartate aminotransferase, AST.

FACTORS AFFECTING REFERENCE VALUES

A number of factors affect the reference ranges for enzyme determinations. If these factors are not accounted for in the interpretation of results, misdiagnosis is possible.

Sampling time

Since enzymes do not undergo significant circadian rhythm, sampling time with respect to time of day is unimportant for determining enzyme normal or reference ranges. On the other hand, the sampling time with respect to the onset of a clinical condition may be important for detecting a variety of acute and chronic conditions if the changes observed are sufficiently rapid. The classic average time for maximum elevation for a series of enzymes in patients with a myocardial infarction was reported to be: CK-MB, 6 hours; CK, 18 hours; AST, 24 hours; and LD, 48 hours. Not all patients follow this pattern and a spread of several hours is seen for the rapidly changing analytes and several days for the slower changing analytes when a variety of patients are tested.

Age

Variations in the amounts of enzymes normally present in serum appear to be the result of differences in age between various subgroups in the population. There are perhaps three principle times to consider whether age is important to an assay: the first year of life, as various organs (e.g., liver) become functional; throughout puberty; and late middle age, when hormonal changes occur.

Some of the most dramatic changes are perhaps seen with the enzyme alkaline phosphatase. Using an alkaline phosphatase method with AMP buffer and p-nitrophenyl phosphate substrate at 30°C the following values are found: 135-270 U/L for children aged six months to 10 years; 90-320 U/L for children aged 10 to 18 years; and 40-100 U/L for adults.

Sex

Differences in assays are related to muscle mass, exercise, or hormone concentration. The assignment of the ultimate cause is difficult, but the difference is usually thought to be related to sex.

An example of these effects is seen with the enzyme creatine kinase, where males are reported to have higher reference ranges than females, most likely due to increased muscle mass. Alcohol dehydrogenase in gastric mucosa is also reported to be higher in males than in females, allowing males to metabolize ethanol more rapidly. A standard alcohol load would therefore not affect males as much as females.

Race

Race may also be a factor in a limited number of assays, but data are sparse. Black populations are reported to have higher reference ranges than comparable Caucasian populations for creatine kinase, but the effect may be an indirect result of several non race-related factors.

Exercise

Exercise and ambulation are important variables in the consideration of reference ranges for several enzymes. Patients at complete bed rest for several days have 20% to 30% lower values for creatine kinase than ambulatory patients. Normal amounts of exercise also elevate creatine kinase. The additional creatine kinase due to normal exercise is of the MM type, CK_3. Thus, the distinction between these elevations and those due to an acute myocardial infarction (the MB type, CK_2), is easily accomplished by determining the isoenzyme pattern. The increases after exercise usually disappear after 12 to 24 hours. This distinction is more difficult for extreme amounts of exercise. In ultra long-distance (races longer than 26 miles) runners, the normal CK_2 can be up to threefold higher than usual and the total CK can be up to fortyfold higher than usual. A runner with chest pain may be difficult to distinguish from a runner with chest pain and a myocardial infarct, even when CK isoenzymes are determined.

ISOENZYMES

The multiple natural forms of an enzyme catalyzing the same reaction in a single species are known as isoenzymes or isozymes. The Enzyme Commission of the International Union of Biochemistry has designated that this term apply only to forms of enzymes arising from genetically determined differences in amino acid structure. There is not complete agreement on this designation. Isoenzymes are to be distinguished on the basis of electrophoretic mobility and subscripted with the first form having the mobility closest to the anode (+). For example, CK-BB would be subscripted as CK_1, CK-MB as CK_2, and CK-MM as CK_3. Although many reports to the contrary exist in the literature, isoenzymes should not be labeled on the basis of tissue distribution (i.e., heart type, brain type) since some confusion may arise due to differences in the predominant form found in various species. There are three groups of multiple enzyme forms that have been defined as isoenzymes by the IUB. These are grouped as follows: genetically independent proteins, e.g., mitochondrial and cytosol forms of malate dehydrogenase; heteropolymers of two or more different subunits, e.g., CK and LD; genetic variants in protein structure, e.g., glucose-6-phosphate dehydrogenases, with more than 50 varieties known in man.

Some commonly encountered enzymes in the clinical laboratory are composed of subunits, but usually only the multiple subunit form has significant enzyme activity. The subunit structure of creatine kinase (CK) and lactate dehydrogenase (LD) have been studied most widely. Creatine kinase has two different subunits. These were historically designated M for muscle and B for brain after tissues that were rich sources of the enzyme that had these subunits as their predominant form. Both the M and B subunit forms are inactive alone and only enzyme containing the two subunits combined together as a dimer has enzyme activity. The three active polymeric forms are CK_3 (CK-MM), CK_2 (CK-MB) and CK_1 (CK-BB). These isoenzymes are from the cell cytosol.

Other forms of CK isoenzymes have also been found. The best characterized of the unusual forms are a) CK isoenzymes complexed with immunoglobulins or lipoproteins, called macro CK type 1 and b) mitochondrial CK, which has been called macro CK type 2.

Macro CK type 1 migrates on agarose electrophoresis between CK-MM and CK-BB so it can be confused with CK-MB. In a patient with a genuine CK-MB band, the unusual isoenzyme often migrates between CK-MB and CK-MM. Usually this is an IgG complex of CK-BB, but other types of immune complexes have been found as well. It is thought to be an auto-immune response, seems to occur in older patients, and is persistent. The band has been known to exist longer than a year, so patients with unchanging CK-MB bands may have isoenzymes that are macro CK type 1. Genuine CK-MB bands appear and disappear from the serum in a few days. The macro CK type 1 does not seem to be correlated with any specific disease process.

Macro CK type 2 migrates more cathodally than CK-MM, which has occasionally been called CK_4. This isoenzyme has been found to be a liver or tumor mitochondrial form of CK. It is usually found in sera of seriously ill patients, especially those with some type of carcinoma, and generally indicates a poor prognosis.

LD also has been found to have two different subunits. These have historically been termed H for heart and M for muscle. Unlike CK, where the active form is a dimer, the active LD enzyme is a tetramer. Since the LD enzyme is composed of four subunits, there are five possible active forms: LD_1 (H_4); LD_2 (H_3M); LD_3 (H_2M_2); LD_4 (HM_3); and LD_5 (M_4).

In a few unusual cases, an enzyme subunit may have catalytic activity by itself (e.g., glutamate dehydrogenase). In these cases, the natural enzyme form is made up of several subunits and has a greater activity than the sum of the activities of the separate subunits. In addition, the multiple subunit form of the enzyme often has activators and inhibitors that may more closely control the enzyme activity. A more complex biological structure exists in this case and the result is more exact control of enzyme activity.

The polymeric forms of glutamate dehydrogenase are not isoenzymes by the IUB definition, since they are polymers of a single subunit and do not differ in amino acid composition. A similar example is the polymeric forms of phosphorylase. Some additional forms of isoenzymes that do not fit the strict definition are enzymes with variations in molecular weight (or length). These forms may occur with the cleavage of different terminal segments of protein, which does not affect the enzyme activity, thus producing various isoenzymes. Hexokinase and carbonate dehydratase are examples of this type of isoenzyme.

Isoforms

The release of isoenzymes into the plasma causes an increase of these proteins that can often be used diagnostically, particularly in cases of cardiac injury. The isoenzymes released from tissue (CK-MM or CK-MB) are a single unmodified isoenzyme form. As a part of the normal clearance process of the body carboxypeptidases in serum cleave, the terminal lysine from the CK-M subunit and produce other isoforms of the isoenzyme with slightly different charges. High-res-

Table 14-5   CK Isoforms

Isoform	Subunit	Comment
MM₃	CK-M M	Unchanged isoenzyme
MM₂	CK-M M₋ₗ	End lysine removed from one M subunit
MM₁	CK-M₋ₗM₋ₗ	End lysine removed from both subunits
MB₂	CK-M B	Unchanged isoenzyme
MB₁	CK-M₋ₗB	End lysine removed from M subunit

Isoforms are numbered with the same convention as isoenzymes, with the band with the fastest electrophoretic mobility toward the anode (+) subscripted as the first form.

Table 14-6   Creatine kinase activity in various human tissues

Tissue	Isoenzyme distribution in U/g of wet tissue (% total activity)		
	MM	MB	BB
Skeletal muscle	3281 (100)	0-623 (0-19)	0 (0)
Heart	313 (78)	56-169 (14-42)	0 (0)
Brain	0 (0)	0 (0)	157 (100)
Colon	4 (3)	1 (1)	143 (96)
Stomach	4 (3)	2 (2)	114 (95)
Uterus	1 (2)	1 (3)	45 (95)
Thyroid	7 (26)	0.3 (1)	21 (73)
Kidney	2 (8)	0 (0)	19 (92)
Lung	5 (35)	0.1 (1)	9 (64)
Prostate	0.3 (3)	0.4 (4)	9.3 (93)
Spleen	5 (74)	0 (0)	2 (26)
Liver	3.6 (90)	0.2 (6)	0.2 (4)
Pancreas	0.4 (14)	0 (1)	2.6 (85)
Placenta	1.4 (48)	0.2 (6)	1.4 (46)

From Chapman J and Silverman L: Bull Lab Med (NCMH), no 60, pp 1-7, Jan 1982.

olution electrophoresis or isoelectric focusing can be used to demonstrate the presence of three CK-MM isoforms and two CK-MB isoforms, forming and disappearing with time. The CK-MM isoforms differ only in whether none, one, or two lysines have been removed from the CK-M subunits. The two CK-MB isoforms are the intact CK-MB and the CK-MB where the M subunit has had a lysine removed. These are of interest as possible early diagnostic markers of acute myocardial infarction. Examples of the CK isoforms are given in Table 14-5.

Distribution

Although all cells have most enzymes of intermediary metabolism, the distribution of isoenzyme patterns for CK and LD are quite different, depending on the tissue source of the two enzymes.

Adult skeletal muscle contains predominantly CK-MM, only a small amount of CK-MB, and no CK-BB. Myocardial muscle with 14% to 42% CK-MB is the only significant tissue source of this isoenzyme, the rest of cardiac CK is CK-MM.

Table 14-7   Lactate dehydrogenase activity in various human tissues

Organ	Isoenzyme distribution				
	H₄	H₃M₁	H₂M₂	H₁M₃	M₄
Heart	60	30	5	3	2
Kidney	28	34	21	11	6
Cerebrum	28	32	19	16	5
Liver	0.2	0.8	1	4	94
Skeletal muscle	3	4	8	9	76
Skin	0	0	4	17	79
Lung	10	18	28	23	21
Spleen	5	15	31	31	18

From Pfleiderer G, et al: In Schmidt E, et al, eds: Advances in clinical enzymology, Hanover, West Germany, 1979, S Karger AG.

Brain, colon, stomach, uterus, thyroid, and kidney all contain predominantly CK-BB, with traces of CK-MM and CK-MB. The distribution of these three CK isoenzymes is given in Table 14-6 for a variety of tissues. The distribution of CK isoenzymes found in plasma or serum under normal circumstances is 95% to 100% CK-MM and 0% to 5% CK-MB, with 0% CK-BB. This pattern is thought to occur due to normal cell turnover or cell leakage, since the predominant isoenzyme is CK-MM, the major form in many types of tissue. A variety of clinical conditions may cause tissues to release their cell contents. This can add other patterns of CK isoenzyme distribution to the isoenzyme pattern that may be present initially.

Lactate dehydrogenase is found in all tissues and has a distribution pattern in plasma or serum in which LD_2 is the predominant isoenzyme. In this pattern, LD_1 is about 50% to 75% of LD_2 and lesser amounts in order are LD_3, LD_4, and LD_5. All five of the isoenzymes are present in all clinical samples, although the absolute amounts of each isoenzyme varies.

Heart muscle has significant amounts of LD_1 and LD_2, with about twice as much LD_1 as LD_2. This is the only tissue with $LD_1 > LD_2$. Liver, skeletal muscle, and skin contain predominantly LD_5 with some LD_4 and traces of the other three LD isoenzymes. Lung contains a majority of LD_3 but it has large amounts of all the other isoenzyme fractions as well. The tissue distribution of LD isoenzyme activity is given in Table 14-7. Several other commonly measured enzymes have isoenzymes. Alkaline phosphatase, acid phosphatase, amylase, and lipase have shown promise as diagnostic markers. In these cases, however, the methods of isoenzyme analysis and clinical data are not developed to the same extent as CK and LD.

Clinical significance
CK and LD

Creatine kinase is found primarily in muscle tissue. Significant increases of CK occur in serum when either skeletal muscle or cardiac muscle has been damaged. Because the primary isoenzyme in the skeletal muscle is CK-MM, large increases in this isoenzyme occur in serum when damage occurs to the skeletal system (i.e., auto accidents). In contrast, significant amounts of CK-MB and CK-MM occur in

Table 14-8 Methods of isoenzyme analysis

Technique	Principles of analysis	Isoenzyme family
Electrophoresis	Subunits have different charges; isoenzymes separated in an electrical field	All
Immunoinhibition	Antibody reacts specifically with one subunit type; this property can be used to render an isoenzyme or isoenzymes catalytically inactive or be used to physically remove an isoenzyme or isoenzyme from solution	CK, LD, acid phosphatase
Immunoassay	Antibody reacts specifically with one subunit type; extent of reaction monitored by use of radioisotope, enzyme, or fluorescent tag	CK, LD, acid phosphatase

cardiac muscle and are released when the heart is damaged by anoxia, surgery, or myocardial infarction. Isoenzyme analysis is required to differentiate the tissue source of the increase of the CK present after injury to either skeletal muscle or myocardium. Large increases of CK may be from skeletal muscle if CK-MM is the predominant isoenzyme and CK-MB is present at less than 5%. Increases in serum of CK-MM with greater than 5% of CK-MB often occur when the heart has been damaged. There are some problems of interpretation since skeletal muscle has the CK-MB isoenzyme as well as myocardial tissue. The simple presence of CK-MB in the serum is not enough to indicate a cardiac problem. For example, certain muscle diseases, including Duchenne's muscular dystrophy, are associated with muscle regeneration, which increases the amount of CK-MB in muscle from less than 5% to between 5% and 15%. Damage to the muscle will therefore produce a pattern in the serum consistent with myocardial damage, not skeletal muscle damage.

Sometimes CK-BB isoenzyme is seen in patient samples. The presence of this isoenzyme is more rare than the finding of CK-MB. The CK-BB isoenzyme is found in serum from patients with tumors, particularly those of the gonads. An infarction of the intestine or kidney will also produce CK-BB in serum.

Lactate dehydrogenase is widely distributed in many tissues. The heart, however, contains an unusual distribution of LD isoenzymes, with an LD_1 concentration greater than LD_2. This LD result is similar to the finding of an unusual distribution of CK isoenzymes in this tissue. The combination of both CK and LD isoenzyme analyses is more powerful than either determination alone, since these results—which are somewhat independent measures of cardiac damage—tend to support one another. The timing of sampling after an event is important. For acute clinical events such as myocardial infarctions, obtaining several samples spread out in time is diagnostically significant. More information is obtained this way, since the pattern of the appearance of isoenzymes at various times in the serum is important. The average time for maximum elevation for a series of enzymes and isoenzymes in patients with a myocardial infarction has been reported as: CK-MB, six to 12 hours; total CK, 18 to 24 hours; and LD, 48 to 72 hours. LD_1 appears to be less than LD_2 in early samples, when CK-MB is rising. But as the total LD concentration increases, both LD_1 and LD_2 increase in serum. Eventually, the LD_1-to-LD_2 ratio flips so the LD_1 concentration is greater

than the LD_2. As the time after the clinical event increases, the LD_1 concentration eventually returns after several days to values lower than LD_2. Not all patients follow this classical pattern and a spread of several hours is seen for the rapidly changing analytes and several days for the slower changing analytes, if a variety of patients are tested.

Methods of analysis

Many older methods of analysis took advantage of slight differences in physical properties or of substrate specificity or inhibition patterns of some of the isoenzymes. These methods are rarely used today. The common methods of analysis either take advantage of differences in migration in electric fields or are based on immunologic differences in the isoenzyme subunits. These methods are given in Table 14-8.

The reference method for both CK and LD isoenzyme analysis is electrophoresis. This method is somewhat technique-dependent but generally is easy to use and is relatively inexpensive.

A large variety of different immunologic methods are also available. Because these methods are easy to use and because they are sensitive, they are gaining popularity. Some suffer from poor specificity and all are significantly more expensive than electrophoresis.

SUGGESTED READING

Baron DN, Moss DW, Walker PG, and Wilkinson JH: Revised list of abbreviations for names of enzymes of diagnostic importance: J Clin Pathol 28:592-593, 1975.

Bowers GN, Jr and Inman SR: The gallium melting-point standard: Its evaluation for temperature measurements in the clinical laboratory: Clin Chem 23:733-737, 1977.

Committee on Standards: Expert Panel on Enzymes: Provisional recommendation (1974) of IFCC methods for the measurement of catalytic concentrations of enzymes: Clin Chem 22:384-391, 1976.

Enzyme Nomenclature: Recommendations on enzyme nomenclature of the Commission on Nomenclature and classification of the enzymes of the International Union of Biochemistry, New York, 1979, Academic Press Inc.

Kaplan LA and Pesce AJ, Clinical chemistry: theory, analysis, and correlation, ed 2, St. Louis, 1989, Mosby-Year Book, Inc.

Pappas NJ, Jr, ed, Clinics in laboratory medicine: diagnostic enzymology 9:595-782, 1989.

Swaroop A:CK isoenzyme variants in electrophoresis, Laboratory Medicine, 305-310, 1989.

Wu AHB: Creatine kinase isoforms in ischemic heart-disease, Clin Chem 35:7-13, 1989.

Zilva JF, Pannall PR, and Mayne PD: Clinical chemistry in diagnosis and treatment, ed 5, Chicago, 1988, Mosby-Year Book, Inc.

15 Pancreatic and intestinal function

Michael D.D. McNeely

To continue functioning, the human body requires: (1) sufficient calories for its energy requirements, (2) basic substances such as carbohydrates, proteins, and fats, and (3) specific substances that the body cannot synthesize or upon which it is dependent (vitamins and essential trace metals). For this reason, a highly developed digestive system has evolved.

The overall purpose of the digestive system is to provide a means whereby the body can take in food, break it up in a series of steps until it is rendered into individual molecules, absorb these molecules in a selective fashion according to the body's needs, and eliminate excess and unwanted material.

Most diseases of the digestive tract are either anatomical disorders (tumors, ulcers, blockages), functional disorders (malabsorption, hyperacidity), or infectious processes. It is primarily in functional problems that clinical chemistry tests can be used as a diagnostic aid. In recent years, advances in techniques for directly visualizing the gastrointestinal (GI) tract with flexible fiberoptic scopes has provided a dramatic step forward in the diagnosis of GI tract disorders. There is much less need for clinical laboratory tests because of this newfound ability to actually look at virtually every part of the gastrointestinal tract and take biopsies at any time (Figure 15-1).

NORMAL PHYSIOLOGY
Mouth

The mouth is the initial part of the digestive system. It tastes the food, grinds it, adds enzymes to start the digestive process, coats the food with saliva to ease its transition into the stomach, and triggers the rest of the gastrointestinal tract to prepare for its digestive task (Table 15-1).

Taste is a neurologic response synthesized from a combination of input from receptors on the tongue and palate and the smell of food. The basic tastes are sweet, sour, salt, and bitter. Taste is important; it encourages eating and protects us from potentially harmful foods.

Food is ground and shredded by the action of the teeth into progressively smaller pieces that can safely pass through the esophagus and that are more readily attacked by digestive enzymes. This process is called mastication.

Another essential role of the mouth is to coat the food particles with a saliva layer. This renders the food slippery enough to be moved down the esophagus and into the stomach. The mouth has three salivary glands. The major

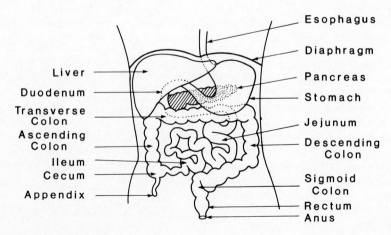

Fig. 15-1   Diagram of gastrointestinal tract. *From Kaplan LA and Pesce AJ: Clinical chemistry, ed 2, St. Louis, 1989, Mosby–Year Book, Inc.*

Table 15-1   Digestion

Food material	Digestive action	End product
Starch	Pancreatic amylase	Disaccharides (mainly maltose)
Disaccharides	Mucosal disaccharidases	Monosaccharides
Monosaccharides	None	
Protein	Gastric hydrochloric acid and pepsin	Partial degradation into large polypeptides
	Pancreatic trypsin, chymotrypsin, and carboxypeptidase	Polypeptides, dipeptides, and amino acids
Long-chain triglycerides	Emulsification with bile, hydrolysis by lipase	Fatty acids and glycerol

From McNeely MDD: Gastrointestinal function and digestive disease. In Kaplan LA and Pesce AJ: Clinical chemistry: theory, analysis, and correlation, ed 2, St Louis, 1989, Mosby−Year Book, Inc.

one is the parotid gland that is located in the cheek. The mandibular and sublingual glands are located beneath the tongue. These glands manufacture amylase in an alkaline bicarbonate buffer. This enzyme starts the process of breaking down complex carbohydrates (starches) into individual sugar molecules even as the food passes through the mouth cavity. The water and mucous excretion of these glands provides the essential lubrication already mentioned.

Esophagus

The esophagus is a strong muscular pipe that runs from the mouth to the stomach. The top third of this conduit is composed of voluntary muscle and the bottom third is made of involuntary muscle. Thus, we are able to voluntarily initiate a swallow in the upper end of our esophagus, but the swallow continues to completion on its own. The junction between the esophagus and the stomach is an important anatomic site. It is located immediately after the esophagus passes through the respiratory diaphragm. If the valve is damaged or ineffective, any stomach acid that enters the lower part of the esophagus can cause serious irritation and pain. When this occurs, the condition is known as "heartburn."

Another important anatomic feature of this part of the esophagus is its venous drainage. The veins in this region are able to drain blood from above and below the diaphragm. In situations where the natural drainage from below the diaphragm through the liver is blocked (i.e., cirrhosis of the liver), the blood will move backward through the esophageal veins. These veins swell up and become varicose. These distended, esophageal varices are susceptible to breaking and may result in massive blood loss into the stomach.

Stomach

The stomach is a muscular bag with a rough lining that is able to secrete a mixture of strong acid, enzymes, and mucus (Figure 15-2). When food enters the stomach via the esophagus, the stomach swells to accommodate its contents. This swelling is detected by stretch nerve fibers in the stomach wall. These detectors initiate the secretion of stomach acid and enzymes, and also close off the exit valve of the stomach, which is known as the pylorus.

There are four types of cells that line the inside of the stomach. The parietal cells secrete hydrochloric acid to the extent that the acidity of the stomach contents can be brought to a pH of less than 1. They also produce intrinsic factor, which is essential for vitamin B_{12} absorption. The chief cells produce an enzyme precursor called pepsinogen that can be activated to the enzyme pepsin, which breaks down proteins. Mucous cells are found throughout the stomach lining. They secrete a mucous layer to protect the stomach from attacking itself with its own acid and enzyme secretions. The surface epithelial cells comprise the actual stomach lining. They replace themselves very rapidly to ensure a continuing viable tissue layer.

The sight and smell (indeed, merely thinking about food) can trigger the stomach to begin the digestive process. This occurs via the vagus nerve, which can directly trigger the parietal cells to secrete acid. The vagus nerve also stimulates antral cells in the stomach outlet to produce the hormone gastrin. Gastrin further stimulates the parietal cells. Food in the stomach causes it to stretch. Stretching is the third stimulus of the parietal cells.

The outlet of the stomach closes down and traps the food, where a rhythmic muscular action renders the food into a fluid mixture. As the food breaks down even further, it is able to pass through the constricted stomach outlet and enter the duodenum. As more acid material enters the duodenum, the duodenum senses its presence and sends a reflex message that inhibits the stomach's activity.

The acid-grinding process of the stomach is very efficient. Whole food is rendered into a slurry of material in a matter of minutes. The pylorus, by opening slightly, is able to control the size of food particle that it releases into the rest of the intestinal tract.

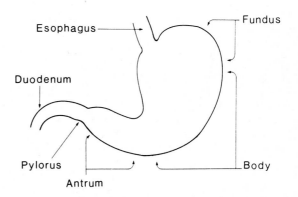

Fig. 15-2   Diagram of stomach. *From Kaplan LA, Pesce AJ: Clinical chemistry, ed 2, St. Louis, 1989, Mosby−Year Book.*

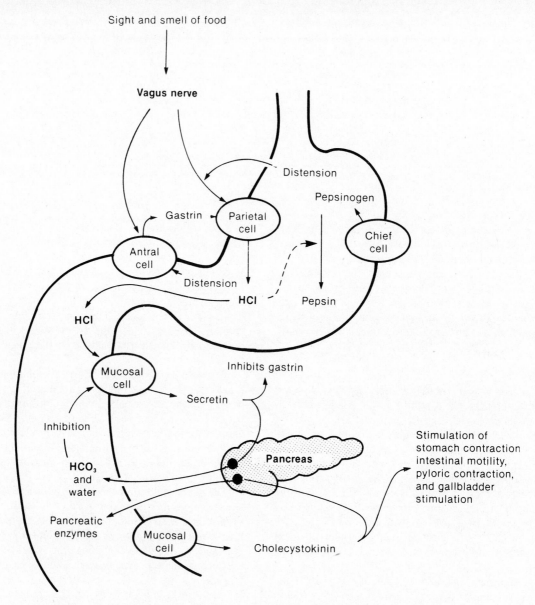

Sight and smell of food

Fig. 15-3 Schema demonstrating various stimuli of stomach and duodenum. *From Kaplan LA and Pesce AJ: Clinical chemistry, ed 2, St. Louis, 1989, Mosby–Year Book, Inc.*

Duodenum

The duodenum receives the food slurry from the stomach, bile from the gall bladder via the bile duct, and digestive enzymes from the pancreas via the pancreatic duct (Figure 15-3).

The bile duct is the drainage system of the liver. The liver synthesizes bile as a means of eliminating certain wastes from the body and to produce a material that is necessary for digestion.

Bile salts are essential for digestion. The main bile salts are conjugates of cholic and chenodeoxycholic acid. Bile is manufactured at a constant rate and is stored for use in the gall bladder.

The exocrine pancreas

The pancreas is a soft linear organ that lies across the midline of the abdominal cavity (Figures 15-4 to 15-6). It consists of a head, a body, and a tail. Running through the pancreas is a duct that has extended branches into all parts of the gland. At the end of each branch is a cluster of secretory cells called an acini. These secretory cells synthesize the potent digestive enzymes amylase, lipase, a precursor enzyme trypsinogen, and other proteolytic enzymes. The acini also produces an alkaline bicarbonate solution.

Duodenal activity

The acidic food slurry from the stomach is moved into the duodenum by peristaltic action. Peristalsis is a wavelike muscular action of the gastrointestinal tract by which it is able to move its contents.

As amino acids, fatty acids, hydrochloric acid, and food enter the duodenum they cause the duodenal cells to release the hormone cholecystokinin.

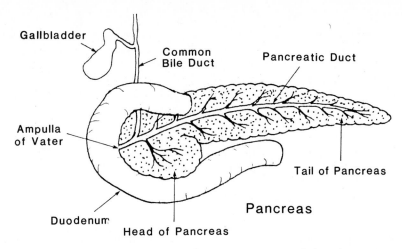

Fig. 15-4   Diagram of pancreas beside duodenum. Pancreatic duct extends throughout organ to convey exocrine enzymes into duodenum. Common bile duct enters duodenum beside or close to pancreatic duct. Endocrine islets are scattered throughout entire organ. *From Kaplan LA and Pesce AJ: Clinical chemistry, ed 2, St. Louis, 1989, Mosby—Year Book, Inc.*

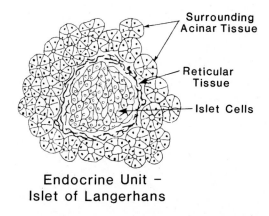

Endocrine Unit – Islet of Langerhans

Fig. 15-5   Islet cells are collected together in a cluster separated from acinar tissue by a thin layer of reticular tissue. On routine strains, islet cells appear to be similar but can be distinguished by special staining techniques. Islet cells release their hormones directly into circulation. *From Kaplan LA and Pesce AJ: Clinical chemistry, ed 2, St. Louis, 1989, Mosby—Year Book, Inc.*

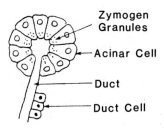

Exocrine Unit – Acinus

Fig. 15-6   Exocrine acinus terminates with a collection of acinar cells. They contain zymogen granules, which are loaded with proteolytic enzymes. Along wall of duct are located special cells that contibute fluid and bicarbonate. *From Kaplan LA and Pesce AJ: Clinical chemistry, ed 2, St. Louis, 1989, Mosby—Year Book, Inc.*

Cholecystokinin travels through the blood stream and causes the gall bladder to contract and the exocrine pancreas to secrete its digestive enzymes. the digestive solutions from these two organs then enter the duodenum to participate in the digestive process.

As the acid stomach contents enter the duodenum, the pH falls to less than 4.5. This causes the hormone secretin to be released by the duodenum. The secretion stimulates the pancreas to release bicarbonate and neutralize the acid.

Digestion of carbohydrates

Dietary carbohydrate is largely composed of starches, the disaccharides sucrose and lactose, and the monosaccharides glucose and fructose. To be absorbed, carbohydrates must generally be converted into monosaccharides.

Starches are long, branched-chain, polysaccharides built up by the linkage of glucose molecules through an α-1,4 linkage. Pancreatic amylase acts to break these α-1,4 bonds

at any point on the carbohydrate branches. The result of amylase action is a mixture of dextrins (polysaccharide chains), maltose (disaccharide consisting of two glucose units), and glucose. The fragments of starch breakdown join the dietary mono- and disaccharides as they are propelled further down the intestine.

Digestion of protein

The zymogen granules of the pancreatic acini produce a group of proteolytic enzyme precursors, including trypsinogen, chymotrypsinogen, proelastase, and procarboxypeptidase. These precursors must be kept in an inactive form until they reach the duodenum; otherwise they could digest the pancreas.

When secreted into the duodenum, an enzyme of the duodenal lining cells known as enterokinase causes trypsinogen to convert into the active enzyme trypsin. Enterokinase is released from the musocal cell as the result of direct stimulation from bile salts and proteases. The enterokinase splits a lysine-isoleucine bond in the trypsinogen molecule, leaving an active peptide that is known as trypsin. Trypsin, in turn, will convert chymotrypsinogen into chymotrypsin, proelastase into elastase, and procarboxypeptidase into carboxypeptidase. These newly activated enzymes may then attack proteins to yield polypeptides, dipeptides, and amino acids. Trypsin acts by hydrolyzing the protein chains at bonds of the carboxyl groups of L-arginine and L-lysine.

Digestion of fat

The breakdown of fats is the most complicated of all the basic food materials. The digestive environment of the duodenum is primarily water, but fats are not water-soluble. For this reason, pancreatic enzymes will not have an effect on fats without a physiochemical alteration. This is the role played by bile.

The bile acids chenodeoxycholic acid and cholic acid act as surfactants. They are able to surround tiny particles of fat and produce a microscopic-sized, water-soluble sphere called a micelle in which the nonpolar parts of the fat molecule are turned inward and the polar portions are turned outward. The surface polarity of the micelle causes it to be water-soluble and allows the water-soluble enzyme, pancreatic lipase, to act on it.

When the pH of the duodenal contents reaches 4.5, lipase attacks the triglyceride molecules and splits the fatty acid chains away from their glycerol backbone. The fatty acid chains may then be absorbed with specific mechanisms. Shorter fatty acids (C_1 to C_6) pass directly into the blood stream, the intermediate length (C_6 to C_{10}) may pass directly or may undergo re-esterification. The long chain fatty acids (C_{16} to C_{18}) require re-esterification into triglycerides before being linked to a lipoprotein and passed into the lymphatic system.

Jejunum and ileum (absorption)

Most of the absorption of food is accomplished in the part of the GI tract known as the small intestine, which is made up of the jejunum and ileum (Figure 15-7). At one time, absorption was thought to be a somewhat passive process in which the partially digested food from the duodenum became mixed with a slurry of enzymes from the GI tract called the succus entericus. This mixture was propelled down the intestine by peristalsis. The enzyme action allowed simple sugar molecules to be freed from complex carbohydrate chains, amino acids to be released from proteins, and fatty acids to be split from triglycerides. These food molecules were then thought to be absorbed by differential diffusion through the wall of the intestine, which was visualized as a semipermeable membrane.

It is now recognized that the action of pancreatic enzymes does indeed take place in the intestinal slurry, but additional enzyme activity occurs right on the surface of the intestinal cells. Absorption, rather than being the passive diffusion of small molecules, is an active, highly selective process that requires a specific mechanism for almost every different food molecule.

The efficient absorption task relies not only on general and specific enzyme and transport systems, but also depends on the anatomy of the intestine. The small intestine is approximately 4 m long with a 10-cm inside circumference. Its gross surface area is therefore slightly larger than 4 sq ft. However, the surface of the intestine is highly folded. These folds cause the surface area to be enlarged and provide assistance to the peristaltic action in moving the intestinal contents along the GI tract. The folds are covered by fingerlike projections known as villi. In turn, the surface of each villi is composed of thousands of microscopic projections known as microvilli. It is estimated that the total absorptive surface of the small intestine measures 5000 sq ft.

Thus, by a series of folds and projections, the surface area of the intestine is increased from the size of a floor mat to the floor space of an extremely large house! It is

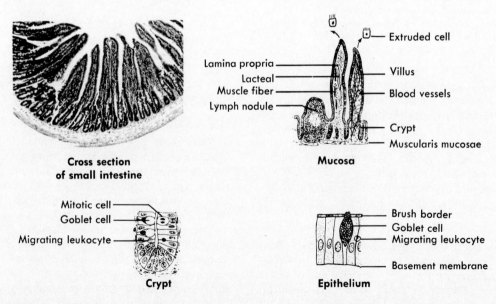

Cross section of small intestine

Mucosa

Lamina propria
Lacteal
Muscle fiber
Lymph nodule

Extruded cell
Villus
Blood vessels
Crypt
Muscularis mucosae

Mitotic cell
Goblet cell
Migrating leukocyte

Crypt

Brush border
Goblet cell
Migrating leukocyte
Basement membrane

Epithelium

Fig. 15-7 Structures of functional components of small intestine. *From Kaplan LA and Pesce AJ: Clinical chemistry, ed 2, St. Louis, 1989, Mosby–Year Book, Inc. In Arey LB: Human histology: a textbook in outline form, ed 4, Philadelphia, 1974, Saunders.*

easy to see how the digested slurry of a meal, when spread over such a large area, can be absorbed in less than 1 hour.

Another important anatomic feature of the small intestine is the speed with which its lining cells are replaced. The entire surface is replaced every 4 days. When food molecules are absorbed into an intestinal cell, they have 4 days to be passed further into the body or they will be shed. This is a protective mechanism that prevents overload of some nutrients (for example, trace metals). It also means that if the intestinal wall becomes infected or poisoned, it can shed its surface to get rid of the offensive agent and then quickly repair itself.

The small intestine is provided with a large blood supply into which newly absorbed nutrients can be delivered. The blood flow through the GI tract is greatly increased during and after a meal. The blood flow is considerably less between meals. The vascular supply may be almost stopped when blood is needed in other parts of the body (i.e., adrenaline rush, fainting, exercise), resulting in a charactistic queasy feeling. The blood flow from the intestine travels via the portal vein into the liver. This allows the liver the opportunity to detoxify or otherwise alter the newly absorbed molecules before they are released throughout the rest of the body. This is an efficient process that can metabolize over 90% of certain molecules on their first pass into the circulation. This is an important aspect of carbohydrate metabolism, amino acid absorption, ammonia absorption, and drug administration. Its significance is revealed dramatically in liver failure when many of these materials pass through the liver and into general circulation.

The intestine is also provided with an abundant lymphatic supply. This drainage system parallels the blood supply but eventually empties into the lymphatic duct. It allows water-insoluble materials, i.e., lipids, certain vitamins, to be carried away from the intestine and released into the circulation.

Absorption of carbohydrates

By the time they reach the intestine, carbohydrates will be either monosaccharides or disaccharides. Many will have been ingested in these forms; for example, as sugar in fruit (fructose, a monosaccharide), or milk (lactose, a disaccharide). Others will be the breakdown products resulting from amylase acting on complex carbohydrates such as starch.

Several of the monosaccharides (glucose, fructose) are absorbed by specific, active transport mechanisms. These molecules are identified, bound by the intestinal epithelium, and transported into the blood stream even though the concentration of the sugar in the blood is greater than in the intestine.

Other monosaccharides do not have a specific transport mechanism, for example, xylose, and must rely on passive diffusion down a concentration gradient to be absorbed. Some monosaccharides are very poorly absorbed or not absorbed at all and therefore cause abdominal distress when they eventually pass through the small intestine and are converted to gas by bacterial action in the large intestine.

Disaccharides are generally assimilated by breaking them into their component monosaccharides. The single-molecule sugars are then able to use the mechanisms described earlier. The cleavage of the disaccharides is undertaken by specific enzymes located on the surface of the microvilli. For example, the enzyme lactase reacts with lactose to produce the monosaccharides galactose and glucose, which both have active absorptive systems.

Absorption of protein

Protein must be absorbed as amino acids or small polypeptides. There are several different active transport systems located on the mucosal surface that act on different amino acid groups. In general, dipeptides are absorbed more rapidly than amino acids because of these mechanisms.

Absorption of lipids

When enzymatically broken down by lipase, lipids are rendered into glycerol, fatty acids, phospholipids and cholesterol. The absorption of each of these is slightly different.

Absorption of glycerol

Glycerol is water-soluble and readily absorbed into the portal blood supply.

Absorption of fatty acids

Fatty acids travel down the intestine as part of the micelles. They pass from the water-soluble micellar droplet through the epithelial cell wall where they become attached to a transport protein. The medium (eight to ten carbon atoms) and short-chain (six or fewer C atoms) fatty acids are then released directly into the blood stream, where they become immediately bound to albumin. The long-chain fatty acids (16 to 18 carbon atoms), which comprise the majority of the fat intake, must first be re-esterified into triglycerides by binding three fatty acids to glycerol. These triglycerides are then linked to an apolipoprotein molecule to form a material known as a chylomicron, a water-soluble microdroplet of otherwise insoluble material. The chylomicrons are then transported by the lymphatic system and enter the circulation via the lymphatic duct.

Absorption of cholesterol

Cholesterol is obtained equally from the diet and from endogenous sources (primarily bile). Because of the hydrolytic action of stomach acid, almost all the cholesterol is present in the unesterified form.

To be absorbed, cholesterol is made soluble by becoming part of the micelles. The cholesterol is absorbed primarily in the middle and terminal part of the ileum. Efficiency of absorption is limited by the integrity of the micelle. As the micellar components (fatty acids and cholesterol) are absorbed, the micelle degrades and further absorption is not effective. Between 30% and 70% of cholesterol is absorbed. The amount of cholesterol absorbed depends upon the amount of fat in the diet, because this is the factor that determines the nature of the micelle.

Absorption of other nutrients

There are many other nutrients which must also be absorbed.

Absorption of iron

To be absorbed, iron must be converted from the ferric to the ferrous oxidation state by gastric acid. Iron is then able to enter the mucosal cells at the crypt of the microvillus. A specific transport protein carries the iron across the mucosal cell and releases it into the circulation, where it is bound by transferrin. The transport system is rate-limiting and iron that is not absorbed in time will be re-released into the intestinal lumen when the epithelial cells are shed. By this means, iron overload is avoided. This protective mechanism can be overwhelmed by massive iron ingestion.

Absorption of trace metals

Trace metals are either essential (for example, zinc and copper) or nonessential (lead and aluminum). The essential metals are transported by protein carriers. It is not clear whether these carriers are unique or whether they are shared by groups of similar ions. In general, the absorption of essential metals is enhanced by intracellular transport mechanisms based on specific binding proteins. Nonessential metals have no such transport facilitation, but may compete with essential metals by using the same transport pathway. The ingestion of any metal in large quantitites may lead to overabsorption.

Absorption of calcium

Calcium is a very important nutrient in marginal supply. It is therefore important to have an efficient method of absorption in order to trap as much ingested calcium as possible. Because sudden increases in serum calcium may be fatal, the absorptive mechanism must have a delicate control system to avoid calcium overload. The fine tuning is accomplished by an absorptive protein known as calmodulin, which picks up the absorbed calcium as it enters the mucosal cell and controls its release into the circulation. The synthesis and activity of calmodulin is governed by vitamin D.

Absorption of vitamins

Vitamins can be divided into water-soluble and water-insoluble types. The water-insoluble variety (A, D, E, K) are absorbed in concert with lipids by being taken up into the micelles. Thus, they depend upon normal lipid absorption. Many water-soluble vitamins are passively absorbed. Others, such as vitamin B_{12}, have elaborate absorptive mechanisms that involve binding to intrinsic factor, which promotes absorption.

Absorption of electrolytes and water

Electrolytes such as sodium, potassium, and magnesium are required in abundance and can be eliminated from the body with incredible efficiency. For this reason, their absorption is encouraged and they are pumped vigorously by active transport into the blood stream. The electrolyte pump allows water to be co-absorbed. Most of the water that is ingested is taken into the blood stream. There is further control over water and electrolyte balance in the large intestine and the kidney (see Chapter 6).

Absorption of drugs

There are no specific mechanisms for the absorption of drugs. Drugs are therefore absorbed by the natural mechanisms that the body already has. To be effectively administered, the absorption of each drug must be understood.

Some must be taken with meals; some must never be taken with meals to avoid competing with food substances. In general, the smaller and more water-soluble the drug molecule is, the faster it will be absorbed.

Large intestine

The large intestine receives undigested and unabsorbable material. It gradually removes water, bioconverts some materials, and may add electrolytes. Eventually, it forms stool. Very little nutrient absorption other than water occurs in the large intestine. The small intestine is generally sterile. In contrast, the large intestine is extensively colonized by bacteria. These bacteria aid in the formation of feces by performing much of the bioconversion.

PATHOPHYSIOLOGY (Table 15-2)
Stomach

Disorders of the stomach can be classified as anatomical and physiological. There is considerable interrelationship between the two categories. The anatomic disorders include: (1) hiatus hernia and gastroesophageal reflux, (2) ulcers, (3) tumors, and (4) stricture of the pylorus. The functional disorders include: (1) hyperacidity, (2) the Zollinger-Ellison syndrome, and (3) pernicious anemia.

Hiatus hernia and gastroesophageal reflux

The esophagus passes through the left hemidiaphragm and enters the abdominal cavity to join the stomach. At their junction there is a valvelike structure known as the gastroesophageal sphincter. This valve is a muscular ring that tightens when the stomach is stretched with food. Its purpose is to prevent stomach acid and food from entering the esophagus. Abnormal backward movement of material from the stomach is known as gastroesophageal reflux. Should this happen, the strong acid will irritate, or even erode, the unprotected lining of the esophagus and cause a characteristic pain known commonly as heartburn. Mild heartburn is very common. Occasionally, the defect will be severe and will cause significant problems. The condition is aggravated by lying flat. It is treated symptomatically by raising the head of the patient's bed and by drugs. In serious situations, surgical correction may be needed.

Diagnosis of this disorder is primarily based on clinical features, with x-ray techniques being employed for confirmation. There is no role for the clinical laboratory in the diagnosis or follow-up of this condition.

Ulcers

Ulcers are erosions or holes that form in the stomach lining. There are two fundamental types of ulcer, gastric and peptic.

The exact reason why gastric ulcers develop is not known. However, it seems that these lesions form because the tissue of the stomach wall becomes abnormally weak. Gastric ulcers are often found in association with atrophic gastritis. This is a condition in which the stomach lining stops regenerating properly, leaving it susceptible to injury. Gastric ulceration is often associated with cancer of the stomach.

Peptic ulcers are quite different in origin. They form because of excessive production of stomach acid. This acid

Table 15-2   Change of analyte and function tests in disease*

Disease	Fecal fat	Lactose tolerance	S-carotene S-vitamin A	S-vitamin B_{12} S-folate	Schilling test	D-Xylose absorption	Stool occult blood	Carcinoembryonic antigen	5-Hydroxyindoleacetic acid (5-HIAA)	Pancreatic enzyme testing	Stool examination
Steatorrhea	↑↑	N	↓	N, ↓	AB	AB	Neg	N	N	AB	Foul smelling, greasy
Celiac disease	N, ↑	N	N, ↓	N, ↓	N, AB	N, AB	Neg	N	N	N	Variable
Lactose intolerance	N	AB	N	N	N	N	Neg	N	N	N	Loose in association with abdominal cramps
Carcinoid syndrome	N	N	N	N, ↓	N, AB	N	Neg, pos	N, ↑	↑↑	N	Loose in association with cutaneous flushing
Functional diarrhea	N	N	N	N	N	N	Neg	N	N	N	Loose
Bowel carcinoma	N	N	N	N, ↓	N	N	Neg or pos	N, ↑	N	N	Change in bowel habits
Inflammatory bowel	N	N	N	N, ↓	N	N	Pos	N, ↑	N	N	Loose, bloody

From McNeely MDD: Gastrointestinal function and digestive disease. In Kaplan LA and Pesce AJ: Clinical chemistry: theory, analysis, and correlation, ed 2, St Louis, 1989, Mosby–Year Book, Inc.
N, Normal; ↑ , elevated; ↓ , lowered; *AB*, abnormal; *S*, serum.

literally erodes the stomach lining. These ulcers are found in the lower part of the stomach, where the acid tends to pool. Or, very commonly, peptic ulcers will form in the first part of the duodenum, which receives the most concentrated flow of HCl.

The connection between the peptic ulcers and excess acid production has been recognized for decades. Treatment in the past consisted of taking bicarbonate or other antacids, or by manipulating the diet in an attempt to neutralize the corrosive agent. Surgery was a common form of therapy and most active hospitals would have two or more patients each week pass through their operating rooms for some type of ulcer surgery. There were many different operations. The simplest was a vagotomy and pyloroplasty. In this procedure, the surgeon destroyed the vagus nerve branches leading to the stomach. This reduced the neural reflex that caused acid production. Because the vagus nerve also controls the tension of the pyloric valve, it was always necessary to open this valve (by splitting it surgically) whenever a vagotomy was performed. Otherwise, food and acid would become trapped in the stomach.

More aggressive surgical techniques in which part of the stomach was removed were also used. These procedures involved the removal of portions of the acid-producing tissue. To compensate for the loss of stomach volume and control, various rerouting and reconnections of the duodenum and small intestine were generally required.

Although surgery does work, these are major procedures with a measurable risk. In addition, patients commonly suffer from eating problems such as bloating after meals, the dumping syndrome (a sudden loss of body fluid because of the osmotic force of a poorly digested meal in the intestine), vitamin B_{12} deficiency, and hypoglycemic attacks.

Because of these side effects, it was common in the past to use laboratory studies to assess whether surgery would be of benefit to the patient. Gastric analysis was employed for this purpose. This test employs a gastric acid stimulus (food, alcohol, histamine, or pentagastrin), followed by the removal of several timed samples of gastric juice via a nasogastric tube. The juice is tested for acid content. A patient with hypersecretion of acid is most likely to benefit from surgery.

In the 1970s, the drug cimetidine was developed. This is an H_2-receptor–blocking agent that dramatically reduces stomach acid production. The introduction of this class of drugs has virtually eliminated the need to perform ulcer surgery. Because of this change in therapy, there is little need to perform the gastric analysis.

Zollinger-Ellison syndrome

The Zollinger-Ellison syndrome is a condition in which the patient suffers from massive and recurrent peptic ulcers. The disorder is due to a tumor of the pancreas that secretes gastrin in excessive amounts. This excess gastrin causes overstimulation of the acid-secreting parietal cells with consequent hyperacidity. It can be diagnosed by measuring a fasting serum-gastrin concentration. The hyperacidity not only causes ulceration, but also interferes with the normal absorption of iron and fat.

Pernicious anemia

Once a fatal condition, pernicious anemia (PA) is now eminently curable. Patients with PA cannot absorb vitamin B_{12} and eventually become vitamin B_{12}-deficient. The pathogenesis of pernicious anemia is easily understood when the absorption of vitamin B_{12} is examined. When serious, vitamin B_{12} deficiency is characterized by atrophic epithelia, macrocytic red cells, and characteristic neurological damage of the spinal cord.

Vitamin B_{12}-containing food is broken down in the stomach and B_{12} is released. In the acid media of the stomach, the B_{12} becomes bound by intrinsic factor (IF), which is also secreted by the parietal cells. The IF-B$_{12}$ complex then travels the full length of the small intestine. When it reaches the terminal part of the ileum, the complex encounters specific receptors that are necessary for its absorption. In pernicious anemia, the stomach lining becomes atrophic and the parietal cells are unable to secrete HCl and intrinsic factor. The lack of intrinsic factor makes the absorption of vitamin B$_{12}$ impossible.

Small intestine

Because the small intestine is the primary site of food absorption, disorders of the small intestine manifest themselves as malabsorption states. These conditions can be roughly divided into: (1) defective intraluminal hydrolysis or solubilization, (2) mucosal cell abnormalities or inadequate mucosal surface, and (3) other disaccharidase deficiencies.

Defective intraluminal hydrolysis or solubilization

Pancreatic insufficiency. Deficient production of pancreatic exocrine secretion will prevent the normal breakdown of food. Most significantly affected is the hydrolysis of fat. The undigested fat is excreted in the feces. This condition is called steatorrhea. The feces of steatorrhea are extremely foul-smelling and foamy in consistency. Fat malabsorption is associated with deficiency of the fat-soluble vitamins A, D, E, and K, since these materials remain with the fat in the stool.

Vitamin D deficiency contributes to the hypocalcemia of malabsorption. Vitamin E deficiency is poorly characterized. Vitamin A deficiency in steatorrhea is rarely sufficient to cause blindness. It is associated with low serum levels of carotene, which becomes a rough screening test of fat malabsorption. Vitamin K deficiency leads to a prolonged prothrombin time and impaired blood coagulation.

Pancreatic insufficiency can be caused by pancreatitis (see following text). Occasionally, a single, severe episode of acute pancreatitis will destroy the pancreas. Usually, however, several acute episodes or a chronic disorder must occur before the pancreas is impaired to this extent.

Blockage of the pancreatic duct by a stone or tumor will prevent the normal release of pancreatic enzymes. The blockage will eventually lead to enzyme backup and destruction of the gland by these digestive enzymes.

Bile acid deficiency. Without a normal amount and composition of bile acid present, fat cannot be absorbed and steatorrhea will occur. Micelles can be prevented from forming by obstruction of the bile duct or by production of excess gastric acid.

Obstruction of the bile duct is usually due to blockage by a stone that has formed in the gall bladder and which has become dislodged to block the common duct. Tumors of the biliary system or intestine can also cause obstruction, but are much less common.

Excess acid from the Zollinger-Ellison syndrome or stomach surgery can cause a low pH in which the physicochemical requirements for micelle formation are not met.

Bacterial overgrowth. Normally, the small intestine is sterile. It can become colonized with bacteria in association with blind loops. Blind loops are anatomic disorders of the gastrointestinal tract in which pouches, channels with no outlet, or even circular pathways are formed. The cause is an abnormal connection due to surgery, fistulas due to infection or enzyme damage, or disease that causes weakness in the intestinal wall. Unable to be cleared by the normal motile activity of the intestine, bacterial colonies grow to an abnormal extent. The bacteria may biochemically degrade materials, rendering them nutritionally useless or unabsorbable.

Mucosal cell defects

Lactase deficiency. Milk contains lactose, which is a disaccharide composed of one molecule of galactose linked to one molecule of glucose. To absorb this "milk sugar," a specific intestinal brush-border enzyme known as lactase splits the molecule into glucose and galactose, which are then absorbed by their specific and selective active transport mechanisms.

All infants are born with brush-border lactase. The cultural groups of people that do not use milk as a dietary staple after weaning often do not retain intestinal lactase as adults. In contrast, groups that are exposed to milk products throughout their lives usually retain an active lactase enzyme. For this reason, northern Europeans and their descendants, having a long tradition of domesticating goats and cows, have an active lactase system. Orientals, in contrast, are often lactase-deficient. Other ethnic groups vary in their disposition to this condition.

When persons with lactase deficiency ingest lactose, the disaccharide is not split. The lactose cannot be absorbed and will travel through the intestinal lumen. It first causes cramping and discomfort by drawing fluid into the intestinal lumen by osmotic action. Large-bowel gas is produced when lactose provides an excessive carbohydrate substrate for the large-bowel bacteria. Fat may also be produced by the bacterial action. Diarrhea may be the end result of the process.

Most people with severe lactase deficiency are well aware of their condition and avoid milk products scrupulously. Mild deficiencies may not be clinically apparent since lactose (milk) is found in so many foods.

The diagnosis of lactase deficiency is made definitively by conducting enzyme assays on a biopsy of small intestinal mucosa. In practice, this is rarely done and a clinical challenge test is administered instead.

The clinical challenge (tolerance) tests are all conducted by administering an oral lactose drink containing 50 g of lactose. The most popular test employs serial measurements of plasma glucose to assess the absorption of the sugar. Since galactose is rapidly converted to glucose by the liver, this is quite satisfactory. An increase in glucose of 1.1 mmol/L during the first hour is considered normal. Less than 0.5 mmol/L with typical symptoms is considered diagnostic of lactase deficiency. Lactase deficiency, when diagnosed, is treated by avoidance of lactose-containing foods.

Galactose can also be measured but offers no diagnostic advantage and is analytically more difficult to perform than glucose. Breath-hydrogen measurements conducted at intervals after lactose ingestion is the best test, although special equipment is required. The principle behind this method is that, when the undigested lactose enters the large bowel (which it is able to do in 5 minutes), the gut bacteria metabolize it to form hydrogen among other gases. The hydrogen is rapidly absorbed into the blood stream and just as rapidly exhaled in the breath. Because the human body has no endogenous hydrogen production, any breath hydrogen can be attributed to the undigested lactose.

Other disaccharidase deficiencies

Other disaccharidase deficiencies have been reported. They have similar clinical presentations to lactase deficiency, but are very rare.

Small intestine disease

There are a number of specific disorders that cause a disruption of the intestinal mucosa. When this occurs, there is generalized malabsorption accompanied by diarrhea. When this condition is severe, laboratory studies show low calcium, iron-deficiency anemia, low albumin, decreased alkaline phosphatase, and decreased urea. Descriptions of the conditions that fall into this category follow.

Celiac disease

Celiac disease is a chronic malabsorption or chronic gastrointestinal discomfort caused by dietary gluten. The precise mechanism is not known but may be due to the absence of specific peptidases or an immunologic disorder. The result is villous atrophy and an ineffective intestinal absorptive surface. Laboratory studies show intestinal malabsorption. Treatment is the removal of gluten from the patient's diet.

Whipple's disease

Whipple's disease is an infiltration of the intestinal wall and lymphatics with macrophages filled with glycoprotein. Severe steatorrhea occurs. The diagnosis is confirmed by jejunal biopsy.

Allergic gastroenteritis

Allergic gastroenteritis is characterized by malabsorption, GI tract bleeding, protein-losing enteropathy with eosinophilic infiltrations. The patients usually have a history of other allergic disorders. Eosinophilia is always present.

Amyloidosis

Amyloidosis occurs in primary and secondary forms. Amyloid gains its name because of its resemblance to starch. However, it is actually an insoluble protein, resistant to proteolysis, that forms fibrils. There are various forms of amyloid. The protein stains with Congo red dye and biopsy is the diagnostic test of choice. An in vivo Congo red test is dangerous and of limited diagnostic utility, and is therefore no longer used.

Crohn's disease

Crohn's disease is an inflammatory condition of the small bowel that causes strictures, mucosal damage, and bacterial overgrowth. Malabsorption may be present.

Carcinoma

Adenocarcinoma of the bowel or rare tumors of the small intestine may cause obstruction and/or bleeding.

Pancreatic insufficiency

Pancreatic insufficiency results in an inadequate supply of pancreatic enzymes. This leads to an inability to digest food and thus, results in malabsorption.

Pancreatitis

Pancreatitis occurs in acute and chronic forms. Either variety may result in a decrease in pancreatic enzymes, which may then lead to pancreatic insufficiency.

Cystic fibrosis

Cystic fibrosis is an inherited condition that causes generalized destruction of the exocrine glands, causing life-threatening pulmonary disease. The disorder causes pancreatic destruction.

Pancreatic disease
Pancreatitis

Acute pancreatitis. Pancreatitis is a condition in which a sudden, noninfectious inflammation develops in the pancreas, causing extreme abdominal pain. The condition is often spontaneous, but may be brought on by alcoholic excess and hyperlipidemia.

Attacks may be mild, lasting for a few hours, or they may be fatal. The most severe attacks are accompanied by shock due to intra-abdominal fluid loss, hyperglycemia due to damage to the islet cells of the pancreas, hypocalcemia due to unknown reasons and retroperitoneal hemorrhage.

The time-honored laboratory tests for the diagnosis of pancreatitis are the measurement of serum and urine amylase and serum lipase. Treatment is supportive with intravenous fluids and analgesia being most important. Surgery is contraindicated. For this reason, accurate diagnosis is very important.

It is not known why amylase rises in pancreatitis, but several mechanisms have been suggested. The serum amylase rises rapidly after the onset of the attack in 1 to 2 hours. The extent of the elevation is roughly proportional to the severity of the pancreatitis. Ninety percent of persons with significant pancreatitis will exhibit increased amylase.

Milder cases of acute pancreatitis may have equivocal increases in the serum amylase level. It is often useful in these situations to collect timed urine samples and measure the amylase content of the urine.

In the early 1970s it became popular to compute the amylase clearance because it was thought that the clearance of amylase actually changed when pancreatitis occurred. This has not proven to be useful.

The serum concentration of the enzyme lipase also rises during pancreatitis. The diagnostic utility of lipase has been debated over the years. Using an appropriate lipase assay, the serum lipase rises with much the same pattern as amylase, though the increase is not as great. There is good evidence that lipase is increased in some of the pancreatitis patients who do not show elevated amylase values.

The lipase is more specific than amylase. Pancreatitis is the only entity that will cause an increase in lipase. In contrast, amylase levels will increase with parotitis, renal failure, ectopic pregnancy, perforated stomach, hepatitis, and a variety of intraabdominal catastrophes.

Carcinoid syndrome

Carcinoid syndrome is a serious, but curious, condition in which a tumor of the enterochromaffin cells of the small intestine produce large amounts of serotonin (5-hydroxytryptamine, 5-HT). Serotonin is a metabolic product of tryptophan that is converted into 5-hydroxytryptophan (5-HTP), then into serotonin or 5-hydroxytryptamine (5-HT), and finally into 5-hydroxyindole acetic acid (5-HIAA). If the tumor produces extremely large amounts of these substances, or if, because of secondary tumor deposits in the liver, there is no detoxification of the compounds to other metabolites, unusual amounts of circulating vasoactive substances will circulate through the blood stream. These will cause intermittent flushing, with irregular blush discoloration of the skin. The vasoactive materials cause dilation of the tricuspid valve of the heart. A bizarre feature of the disease is pellagra, which is caused by the diversion of the body's total reserve of tryptophan to the manufacture of serotonin with a simultaneous deficiency of tryptophan.

The diagnosis is assisted by measuring 5-HIAA in the urine.

Large intestine disease
Carcinoma of the large intestine

Colorectal cancer is the second most common adult malignancy in North Americans and causes 15% of all cancer deaths. Environmental factors (i.e., ingested carcinogens), low dietary fiber and heredity, preexisting diseases (i.e., polyps and ulcerative colitis), have all been implicated as causes of this condition.

The diagnosis is usually suggested by a history of obstruction, change in bowel habits, or blood in the stool. Diagnosis is made radiographically and by direct visualization (sigmoidoscope or colonoscope). Screening the stool for the presence of occult blood is widely used as a screening test for colorectal cancer.

Laboratory tests. Two laboratory tests are important: a test for stool occult blood and for carcinoembryonic antigen.

Test for occult blood in stool. The detection of trace amounts of blood in the stool is one sign that a carcinoma of the bowel is present; thus, the use of this test to screen for the presence of carcinoma of the bowel is valuable. It is important that the method used have an appropriate limit of detection. If the test is too sensitive, then false-positive results are overwhelming. It is also recommended that three samples be measured over a short period of time as this provides the optimum balance of cost and diagnosis.

Although it is a widely recommended practice, the routine screening of stool for the presence of occult blood has not been absolutely validated. At present, three randomized, controlled trials are in progress, two in North America and one in the United Kingdom. Each of the trials has over 10,000 subjects in their studies. The final result of these three trials will not be available until the mid-1990s.

The American Cancer Society recommends that persons over 50 years of age have annual tests for stool occult blood and digital rectal examination, with sigmoidoscopy every 3 to 5 years after two negative examinations are done 1 year apart.

The U.S. Preventive Services Task Force makes the following recommendation:

"Insufficient evidence exists to make a recommendation for or against fecal occult blood screening for individuals 45 years and older. Screening of individuals younger than 45 years is not recommended. Based on the higher expected prevalence in individuals aged 45 years and older with a family history of colorectal cancer in a first-order relative, a stronger a priori argument can be made for screening in this group. Individuals known to be unlikely to benefit if a cancer or adenoma is discovered should not be screened."

Test for carcinoembryonic antigen. Discovered by Gold of Montreal, carcinoembryonic antigen (CEA) was initially heralded as a diagnostic screening test for adenocarcinoma of the bowel. The test uses an antibody to measure the presence of a protein that is frequently produced by this cancer but is not found in normal tissue. The CEA can also be elevated in hepatitis, pulmonary infection, smokers, and inflammatory bowel disease, as well as with tumors of the stomach, lung, pancreas, and breast.

Carcinoembryonic antigen is found in 10% to 20% of persons with adenocarcinoma of the bowel. The concentration of CEA is usually correlated with the amount of tumor present. The CEA should not be used for diagnosis (see Chapter 21). It can, however, serve a useful role in monitoring the postoperative status of those who have been treated for colon-rectal cancer and who have had raised CEA preoperatively. A normal CEA following surgery is good evidence that the treatment removed the malignancy. A follow-up at monthly intervals can be used to determine whether or not a recurrence is appearing. Rising or falling changes in elevated levels of CEA after surgery can be used to monitor the effectiveness of chemotherapy. Assays are performed by both radioimmunoassay (RIA) and enzyme immunoassay (EIA) techniques.

ANALYTICAL METHODS
Measurement of gastrin

Gastrin is measured by radioimmunoassay. There is nothing particularly unusual about the assay if a suitable commercial reagent is used. Normal fasting serum gastrin concentrations range from 30 up to 100 pg/mL.

Minimal increases up to 150 pg/mL are not diagnostic and are found frequently in normal persons. Increases are also produced by the ingestion (or even smell) of food, insulin administration, malignant carcinoma of the stomach, pheochromocytoma, hyperthyroidism, hyperparathyroidism, peptic ulcer, gastritis, cirrhosis of the liver, renal failure, and rheumatoid arthritis.

Values betwen 500 and 1000 pg/mL are the result of food ingestion, insulin administration, pheochromocytoma, hyperparathyroidism, renal failure, pernicious anemia, and Zollinger-Ellison syndrome. Values over 1000 pm/mL are usually due to Zollinger-Ellison syndrome or pernicious anemia. Most cases of Zollinger-Ellison syndrome have values over 2000 pg/mL.

Low values of gastrin are common in normal persons with hypothyroidism, and after the administration of oral acid, streptozocin, and phenformin. Values less than 100 pg/mL in a truly fasting person essentially rule out Zollinger-Ellison syndrome.

Table 15-3 Schilling test

Group	Absorption of intrinsic factor–bound vitamin B_{12}	Absorption of unbound vitamin B_{12}	Ratio of bound to unbound
Normal	>15%	>15%	0.5-1.5
Gastric lesion group	>10%	<5%	>2
Pernicious anemia			
Gastrectomy			
Congenital absence of functional intrinsic factor			
Disorders of terminal ileum (see text)	<15%	<15%	0.5

From McNeely MDD: Gastrointestinal function and digestive disease. In Kaplan LA and Pesce AJ: Clinical chemistry: theory, analysis, and correlation, ed 2, St Louis, 1989, Mosby–Year Book, Inc.

Schilling test

The Schilling test provides a clear and almost definitive test of a patient's ability to absorb vitamin B_{12} (Table 15-3). The test requires radioactively tagged vitamin B_{12}, which is taken orally by the patient. The amount of radioactivity subsequently found in a urine collection is proportional to the amount of vitamin B_{12} absorbed by the GI tract and excreted by the kidney.

Fortunately, it is convenient to label vitamin B_{12} with a radioactive label because cobalt is an intimate part of its structure and both cobalt-60 and cobalt-57 are suitable gamma-emitting isotopes.

The classical procedure consists of two parts. In part 1 of the Schilling test, the labeled vitamin B_{12} in a capsule containing "cold" (not radioactive) vitamin B_{12} is consumed orally and a 1-mg intramuscular injection of cold vitamin B_{12} is administered. The injected B_{12} rapidly distributes itself through the body and fills up all the storage spaces for the vitamin. In normal persons, the labeled vitamin B_{12} passes through the stomach, where it is linked to intrinsic factor (IF) and is then absorbed by the terminal ileum. The intramuscular B_{12} injection (also known as the flushing dose) cannot be given too early or the excess vitamin B_{12} will pass into the bile and complete with the oral dose. If the flushing dose is not given, the oral dose, when absorbed, will be taken up by the depleted storage sites and will not pass into the urine. Urine is collected for 24 hours after taking the oral dose. Because vitamin B_{12} is filtered by the glomerulus of the kidney, but is not reabsorbed by the tubule, it passes readily into the urine. The amount of radioactivity in the urine collection is expressed as a percentage of the original dose. Normal persons will excrete a minimum of 7% of the dose, but usually, values over 15% will be obtained. Any impairment of vitamin B_{12} absorption will be revealed by low values in part 1 of the procedure. A normal value does not require part 2 of the procedure to be performed. A low value in part 1 should be followed up with the part 2 procedure no sooner than 1 week later.

In part 2, labeled vitamin B_{12} and intrinsic factor is administered orally to the patient. For the same reasons, the flushing intramuscular injection of nonradioactive vitamin B_{12} is administered. The rest of the test is identical to Part 1 of the procedure.

From these tests, the following combinations of results can be obtained: normal part 1, low part 1 with low part 2, low part 1 with normal part 2. The interpretations of these combinations are extremely diagnostic.

1. Part 1 normal: No impairment of vitamin B_{12} absorption. Any demonstrable serum vitamin B_{12} deficiency is due to low vitamin B_{12}-binding protein or to a chronic dietary deficiency of B_{12}.

2. Low part 1 with low part 2: Both parts less than 7%. There is significant impairment of vitamin B_{12} absorption, which is not corrected by the presence of intrinsic factor. These findings point to disease of the terminal part of the ileum where the specific IF-B_{12} receptors are located (e.g., Crohn's disease, surgery, or ulcerative colitis), to rapid transit through the small intestine (e.g., steatorrhea, diarrhea), or upper GI tract pathology, which prevents the administered IF and vitamin B_{12} from maintaining their bond (hyperacidity).

3. Low part 1 with normal part 2: This combination of results shows that vitamin B_{12} absorption abnormality can be corrected by the provision of intrinsic factor. This means that the subject or the environment is incapable of providing intrinsic factor necessary to encourage coupling. This is seen with pernicious anemia, gastrectomy, and some hyperacidity states.

Other approaches to the Schilling test have been attempted. Measurement of the radioisotope content of the blood or stool, or scanning the liver have all been abandoned as inconvenient and less accurate methods. A dual-isotope technique is popular. In this approach, vitamin B_{12} bound to intrinsic factor is administered in one capsule and vitamin B_{12} (without IF) is administered simultaneously in another capsule. The two preparations are labeled with different radioisotopes. One urine collection is obtained and both isotopes are counted. This is appealing because the test is completed in one step and, in theory, interpretation is possible even if the urine collection is incomplete. However, because vitamin B_{12} can be exchanged with the intrinsic factor and because the total load of vitamin B_{12} is not optimum, the results in practice are much more difficult to interpret. This approach is not recommended.

Measurement of fecal fat

Normally, even with very high fat diets, stool does not contain more than 20 g of fat per day. Two approaches to fecal fat measurement have been used: screening and quantitative methods.

Screening method

The screening method is useful when performed by skilled technologists who are able to maintain a very consistent technique. A single stool sample is collected. This sample is mixed very carefully. Part of the mixed sample is smeared on a slide. Sudan red fat stain is then applied, the slide is heated, and red fat droplets are observed if steatorrhea is present. The Sudan dye will stain intact triglyceride in the sample and when acidified, will also link with fatty acids. When the slide is heated with acid added to the sample, the triglyceride will be hydrolyzed and fatty acids soaps will be converted to the nonionized form. For this reason, the formation of stain-positive fat droplets after heat and acid treatment indicates the presence of fatty acid soaps. Experience is required to maintain accurate semi-quantitative standards. The test does not strictly correlate with the quantitative method because of the different mix of fats that are detected. This method is not sensitive but, if positive, is almost certain evidence of fat malabsorption.

Quantitative methods

Quantitative methods are generally carried out on a 3-day (72-hour) stool sample collected while the patient is on a high fat diet. A fat-restricted diet or one in which the fat is comprised largely of short- and medium-chain triglycerides will not reveal a malabsorption state. The easiest way to achieve the required fat load is to have the patient ingest a tablespoon of corn oil or olive oil with each meal, starting 48 hours prior to the collection.

The most successful collection technique is that developed by Jover, who recommended collection into pre-weighed, 1-gallon paint cans. When the collection is finished, the cans can be reweighed to determine the weight of the collection.

The mixing step is accomplished best using the approach described by Massion. After the sample weight is determined, a solution of alcohol and water is added to bring the weight up to 2 kg. The can is then placed on a commercial paint shaker and the sample is thoroughly homogenized. Before settling occurs an aliquot is removed for analysis.

There are various fat measurement techniques. Traditionally, fat was extracted into an organic solvent, taken to dryness and quantitated by weight measurement. This method has the disadvantage of working with dangerous solvents and is known to underestimate the fats that have been hydrolyzed in the bowel. Van de Kamer quantified the fat by liberating the fatty acids with an alkaline hydrolysis. The fatty acids were then titrated using a visual end point. Methods of fat measurement following hydrolysis and extraction include the use of a copper-soap reagent, a balanced indicator, and gas chromatography. The balanced indicator method is recommended.

Measurement of carotene

Carotene is the main precursor of vitamin A, and its concentration in the serum has a strong correlation with vitamin A absorption. The measurement of carotene involves mixing serum and alcohol to disrupt carotene-protein binding. An organic solvent such as petroleum ether is then used to extract the carotenoids, which are quantitated by direct spectrophotometry at 450 nm. This method will also measure other non-vitamin A carotenoids. Thin-layer chromatography (TLC) and high-performance liquid chromatography (HPLC) have been used to distinguish between the various carotenoids, but such methods are not needed for routine purposes because such information contributes nothing further to diagnostic utility.

A raised serum carotene level usually indicates a high vegetable diet (particularly carrots and leafy greens) with a high carotene content. Hypothyroidism may also cause carotenemia. Low serum carotene concentrations are due to low carotene diets and fat malabsorption. Normal values do not exclude fat malabsorption.

Measurement of vitamin A

Vitamin A depends on normal fat absorption for it to be taken up by the body. For this reason, its presence in serum is a reasonable estimate of the patient's ability to absorb fat. This is the same as the rationale for performing carotene measurements. Because vitamin A assays are much harder to perform and no additional information is derived when both are performed together, there is almost no reason to perform vitamin A assays.

Vitamin A is measured by mixing a small amount of serum with alcohol to disrupt protein binding. The vitamin A is then extracted into petroleum ether and the extract taken to dryness. Chloroform is added to put the vitamin A back into solution and a trifluoroacetic acid reagent is added. This reacts with the conjugated bonds of the molecule to produce an absorbance at 620 nm.

The earlier Carr-Price method uses antimony trichloride as the chromogenic agent. This method is susceptible to disruption by water in the reaction mixture and can be very difficult to perform.

The most reliable methods include HPLC methods, which are substantially more involved and require a high level of expertise.

Increased vitamin A concentrations in the serum are seen with high vitamin A diets and vitamin A administration. Low vitamin A concentrations reflect low vitamin A diets, fat malabsorption, or chronic liver disease.

Lactose tolerance test

The clinical protocol requires that the patient be in a fasting state. A drink, consisting of 50 g of lactose in approximately 200 mL of water, is consumed over a period of about 5 minutes.

Blood is traditionally collected at 5, 10, 30, 60, 90, and 120 minutes, and is analyzed for glucose content. It is also diagnostically correct to collect at 30, 60, and 90 minutes. An increase in glucose of more than 1.1 mmol/L in any collection when compared to the baseline, rules out lactose intolerance unless the patient is diabetic. If the glucose fails to increase more than 0.5 mmol/L at any point, then lactose intolerance should be suspected. If abdominal cramps and/ or diarrhea occur during the test and glucose increase is minimal, then a diagnosis of lactose intolerance is confirmed.

It has been shown that the measurement of hydrogen in the breath at intervals after oral glucose is administered is the most reliable indicator of lactose absorption. Hydrogen has only one possible source in the human body, from the breakdown of undigested carbohydrate by intestinal bacteria. A special gas chromatograph is required to perform these measurements.

Measurement of 5-hydroxyindoleacetic acid

The presumptive diagnosis of carcinoid syndrome rests on measuring excess 5-hydroxyindoleacetic acid (5-HIAA) in the urine of patients who are experiencing characteristic cutaneous flushing and diarrhea.

There are many screening tests for 5-HIAA, which are nonspecific and unreliable.

5-hydroxyindoleacetic acid has been measured spectrophotometrically with 1-nitroso-2-naphthol in nitrous acid and with Ehrlich's reagent. Methods have been published that employ gas liquid chromatography, column chromatography, fluorescence, RIA, and HPLC.

Modifications of the original nitroso-naphthol method are generally used. The difficulty with all of these procedures is the removal of the interferences. This is best done using 2-mercaptoethanol. In this approach, 5-HIAA is extracted from urine into an organic solvent. The 1-nitroso-2-naphthol is then added to form a blue color. The mercaptoethanol is then added to destroy the color produced by interferences and enhance the primary color.

Normally, up to 15 mg of 5-HIAA is excreted per 24 hours. In carcinoid syndrome more than 25 mg is usually measured. False-normal results are produced by a number of drugs, including p-chlorophenylalanine, ethanol, imipramine, isoniazid, monoamine oxidase (MAO) inhibitors, methenamine, methyldopa, and phenothiazines. Reduction of an elevated value is also seen in renal disease and in phenylketonuria.

In the carcinoid syndrome, results are usually between 25 and 1000 mg/day. False-positive results have been reported in nontropical sprue, intestinal obstruction, pregnancy, sleep deprivation, and oat cell carcinoma of the lung, and in ingestion of avocados, bananas, eggplants, pineapples, plums, and walnuts. Drugs that are known to cause an increase in 5-HIAA value are acetanilid, ephedrine, mephenesin, nicotine, phenacetin, phenobarbital, phentolamine, rauwolfia, reserpine, methocarbamol, and glyceryl guaiacolate cough medicines.

Measurement of fecal occult blood

A number of highly sensitive color reagents that are able to detect trace amounts of hemoglobin have been used to detect occult blood in stool. Most rely on the ability of hemoglobin and its derivatives to act as peroxidases and catalyze the reaction between hydrogen peroxide and a chromogenic, organic solvent. Benzidine has been used, but is carcinogenic and is not recommended as an in-laboratory reagent. The current standard reagent system is Hemoccult (SK and F, Philadelphia). This method is based on the guaiac-peroxide reaction and is not made positive by insignificant blood loss or meat ingestion.

SUGGESTED READING

Abramowitz A and others: Two-hour breath hydrogen test, J Ped Gastro Nutr 5:130, 1986.

Aleshire SL, Bradley CA, and Parl FF: The carcinoid syndrome: neuroendocrine and chemical considerations, Clin Lab Med 4:803, 1984.

Auricchio S and others: Toxicity mechanisms of wheat and other cereals in celiac disease and related enteropathies, J Ped Gastro Nutr 4:923, 1985.

Bond JH: Screening for colonrectal cancer: need for controlled trials, Ann Int Med 113:338, 1990.

Cooper AD and Young HS: Pathophysiology and treatment of gallstones, Med Clin N Am 73:753, 1989.

DiMagno EP: Early diagnosis of chronic pancreatitis and pancreatic cancer, Med Clin N Amer 72:979, 1988.

Eckfeldt JH and others: Serum tests for pancreatitis in patients with abdominal pain, Arch Pathol Lab Med 109:316, 1985.

Eddy DM: Screening for colonrectal cancer, Ann Int Med 113:373, 1990.

Eisenberg B and others: Carcinoma of the colon and rectum: the natural history reviewed in 1704 patients, Cancer 49:1131, 1982.

Feldman JM: Urinary serotonin in the diagnosis of carcinoid tumors, Clin Chem 32:840, 1986.

Fletcher RH: Carcinoembryonic antigen, Ann Int Med 104:66, 1986.

Hansky J: Gastrins and gastrinomas, Postgrad Med J 60:767, 1984.

Kelly DA and others: Rise and fall of coeliac disease 1960-85, Arch Dis Child 64:1157, 1989.

Khouri MR, Huange G, and Shiau YF: Sudan stain of fecal fat: new insight into an old test, Gastroenterol 96:421, 1989.

Knight K, Fielding J, and Battista R: Mass screening for colonrectal cancer: are we ready?, JAMA 261:586, 1989.

Littman A: Lactase deficiency: diagnosis and management, Hosp Pract 22:11, 1987.

Lott JA and Ellison EC: Amylase assay and diagnosis of pancreatic disease, Clin Chem 113:1263, 1985.

Mathews-Roth MM and Stamfer MJ: Some factors affecting determination of carotenoids in serum, Clin Chem 30:459, 1984.

Mulholland MW and Debas HT: Physiology and pathophysiology of gastrin: a review, Surgery 103:135, 1988.

Mylvaganam K and others: ^{14}C triolein breath test: a routine test in gastroenterology clinic?, Gut 27:1347, 1986.

Ranson JH: Etiological and prognostic factors in human acute pancreatitis: a review, Am J Gastroenterol 77:633, 1982.

Rosenberg JM and Welch JP: Carcinoid tumors of the colon: a study of 72 patients, Am J Surg 149:775, 1985.

Ryan ME and Olsen WA: A diagnostic approach to malabsorption syndromes: a pathophysiological approach, Clin Gastroent 12:533, 1983.

Sammons HG: Studies in the investigation of intestinal function: Experiences from the past and recommendations for the future, Ann Clin Biochem 19:1, 1982.

Targan SR and others: Immunologic mechanisms in intestinal diseases, Ann Int Med 106:853, 1987.

Watkins JB: Lipid digestion and absorption, Pediatrics 75:151, 1985.

Wenger J, Kirsner JB, and Palmer WL: Blood carotene in steatorrhea and the malabsorption syndromes, Amer J Med 22:373, 1957.

Wolfe MM and Jensen RT: Zollinger-Ellison syndrome: current concepts in diagnosis and management, N Engl J Med 317:1200, 1987.

Wolfe MM and Soll AH: The physiology of gastric acid secretion, New Engl J Med 319:1707, 1988.

16 Pituitary, hypothalmic, and adrenal hormones

Richard Kowalczyk

OVERVIEW OF ENDOCRINE FUNCTION

Each hormone covered in this chapter is considered the central or prime element in its own endocrine subsystem. In common with any system, each of these subsystems is composed of several interrelated elements that, taken together, define or describe the function of the system. For an endocrine system, these elements are the cellular site of origin of the hormone; its biosynthesis, storage, and secretion; its concentration and mode of transport in the blood and its distribution; its interaction with target tissue receptors; its alteration of target tissue function and ultimate effect on the whole organism; and finally, its metabolism, degradation, and excretion. For a complete understanding of the operation of an endocrine system, attention must be given to extraneous factors that modulate or alter any of these elements. Most importantly, the systems concept applied to endocrinology makes clear that dysfunction of any of the elements can lead to disease.

Each of the endocrine systems considered in this chapter is a regulator of cellular metabolic activity, which is integrated with the other major regulatory system of the organism, the nervous sytem. The operation of the hypothalamus and anterior pituitary and adrenal glands as an integrated functional unit (frequently referred to as the hypothalamic-pituitary-adrenal axis, or HPA axis) provides the most vivid example of the interplay of the neural and endocrine systems in medicine and indeed gave rise to the discipline of neuroendocrinology.

Other features of hypothalamic-pituitary-adrenal interplay lead to a further understanding of the scope and extensive influence of this multiorgan system on the whole organism. First, a large number of hormones are involved in its operation: growth hormone (GH or somatotropin), prolactin (PRL), luteinizing hormone (LH), follicle-stimulating hormone (FSH), adrenocorticotropic hormone (ACTH), antidiuretic hormone (ADH or vasopressin), oxytocin, all from the pituitary gland; cortisol and aldosterone from the adrenal cortex; and epinephrine from the adrenal medulla (Fig. 16-1). Second, the secretion of many of these hormones is in turn controlled by releasing factors from the hypothalamus, which are themselves hormones: growth hormone releasing factor (GHRF) and somatostatin (SRIF, or somatotropin release inhibiting factor), prolactin inhibiting factor (PIF) and prolactin releasing factor (PRF), corticotropin releasing factor (CRF), and gonadotropin releasing hormone (GnRH). Disturbances in the production of any of these releasing factors can lead to disease. Third, some of the hormones have what might be considered macroscopic or gross physiological effects, that is, effects extending far beyond the cellular, chemically mediated events. The effects of growth hormone on whole body growth; the effects of cortisol on protein, carbohydrate, lipid, and water metabolism throughout the body; and the effects of aldosterone on retention of salt and water are good examples of hormones that have a gross physiological effect. Fourth, some of the hormones, such as FSH and LH, are involved in the synthesis of estrogens and androgens, which also have widespread systemic effects. Finally, all of the activities of the hormones under review are influenced by the central nervous system through its control of the hypothalamic secretion of releasing factors.

A broad overview is presented for each hormone covered, to make the operation of its endocrine system understandable.

The thyroid hormones (thyroxine and triiodothyronine) and the estrogens and androgens are covered in separate chapters. Although the thyroid hormones are covered in Chapter 17, it should be noted that thyrotropin releasing hormone (TRH) is a hypothalamic hormone and thyroid stimulating hormone (TSH) is a pituitary hormone. The estrogens, whose activity is mediated by GnRH and luteinizing hormone releasing hormone (LH-RH) (both hypothalamic hormones) and the androgens, governed by this same set of trophic hormones, are covered in Chapter 18. The pituitary hormones LH and FSH are also discussed in Chapter 19.

Anatomy and physiology of the hypothalamic-pituitary adrenal system

The functional relationship of the hypothalamus to the pituitary and of the pituitary to the adrenal gland has its origin in the anatomical relationship between the hypothalamus and the pituitary (Fig. 16-2). The proximity of these two glands is a critical element in the interplay of the nervous and endocrine systems. Of the many target tissues and organs for the variety of hormones produced by these two

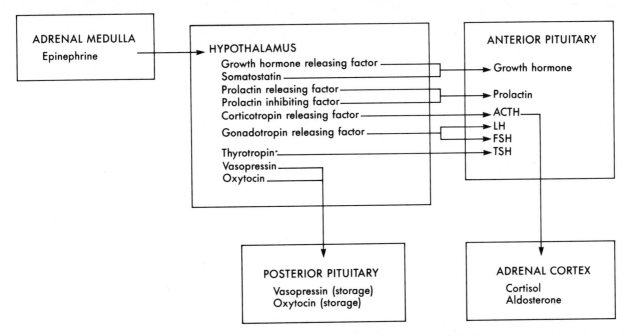

Fig. 16-1   Hormones involved in hypothalamic-pituitary-adrenal relationships.

glands, including the long bones, the thyroids, and the gonads, perhaps the most important are the adrenal glands. Through cortisol, the adrenals exert effects on carbohydrate, lipid, and protein metabolism as well as on water metabolism. Through aldosterone, the adrenals play a central role in the regulation of body water, blood pressure, and electrolyte homeostasis. Epinephrine, the main hormone of the adrenal medulla, affects carbohydrate, lipid, and protein metabolism.

The hypothalamus

The hypothalamus is a specialized area of the brain located below the third ventricle, directly above the pituitary gland. Thus, unlike other endocrine glands, its end organ, the pituitary, is in very close proximity to it. It is not a discrete area of the brain because it does not have a discernible anatomical boundary. The distal part of the hypothalamus that joins the pituitary stalk is called the median eminence.

These hypothalamic neurons are in every sense members of the nervous system; at the same time they may be described as endocrine glands because at their distal termini they secrete small polypeptide hormones. The hypothalamus has no blood-brain barrier so that circulating signals such as increased blood osmolarities or increased cortisol levels have direct access to the hypothalamus.

Secretions of the hypothalamus control the secretions of the anterior pituitary; in other words, they are hypophysiotropic. For most of the hormones secreted by the anterior pituitary, a tropic or releasing substance originating in the hypothalamus has been identified. These tropic substances are commonly referred to as releasing factors; once their chemical identity has been established, they are usually called releasing hormones. Release-inhibiting substances have also been identified: prolactin inhibiting factor (PIF) and somatostatin (SRIF, somatotropin release inhibiting factor) are two examples.

The hypothalamic trophic hormones controlling the secretions of the anterior pituitary are synthesized in cell bodies of neurons located throughout the hypothalamus; the distribution of these neurons in the hypothalamus is more widespread than that of the neurons synthesizing oxytocin and vasopressin. Once synthesized, the hormones are transported down axons that terminate in the median eminence of the hypothalamus. The terminals of these axons are in contact with the capillary tufts of blood vessels (known as the hypophyseal portal vessels), which then pass through the pituitary stalk to feed the anterior pituitary. When activated by a stimulus from the central nervous system, the axons of the hypothalamic neurons release their trophic hormones into the hypophyseal portal system, which then carries the hormones to the pituitary.

The pituitary gland

In humans, the pituitary gland has two lobes; each has a different embryological origin (Fig. 16-3). The anterior lobe (the adenohypophysis) arises fron non-neural tissue and develops upward to the pituitary stalk. The anterior pituitary has no direct nerve supply and receives the hypothalamic hormones in the blood delivered to it by the hypophyseal portal vessels. The posterior lobe of the pituitary (the neural lobe or the neurohypophysis) arises as a downgrowth of the hypothalamus, and is in fact an extension of it.

The posterior lobe of the pituitary only stores the hormones oxytocin and vasopressin, which have been identified as its secretory products. These two hormones are actually synthesized in cell bodies of neurons originating and located in primarily two areas of the hypothalamus. Once synthesized, the hormones are passed down the long axons of these neurons, which traverse the pituitary stalk to the axon terminals that are located in the neural lobe itself. In contrast to the transport system delivering tropic peptides to the anterior pituitary, no blood transport system is involved in

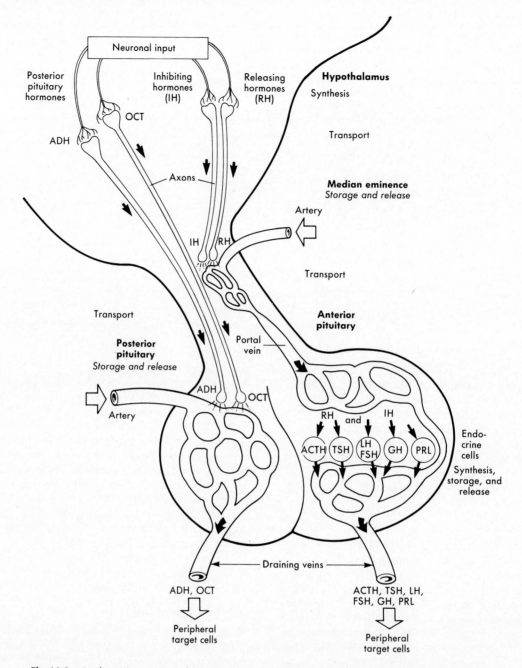

Fig. 16-2   A schematic overview of the anatomic and functional relationships between the hypothalamus and the pituitary gland. Note that the posterior pituitary gland is an extension of neural tissue that stores neurohormones and has its own arterial blood supply. In contrast the anterior pituitary gland is endocrine tissue with a blood supply derived from veins that first drain neural tissue in the median eminence. By this arrangement the endocrine cells are exposed to high concentrations of neurohormones originating in the hypothalamus and stored in the median eminence. The hormones exiting the posterior and anterior pituitary gland reach and act on peripheral target cells. *ADH,* antidiuretic hormone; *OCT,* oxytocin; *ACTH,* adrenocorticotropic hormone; *TSH,* thyroid-stimulating hormone; *LH,* leutinizing hormone; *FSH,* follicle-stimulating hormone; *GH,* growth hormone; *PRL,* prolactin. *From Berne RM, Levy MN: Principles of physiology, St. Louis, 1990, Mosby–Year Book.*

the delivery of hypophyseal hormones to the posterior pituitary. Like the neurons involved with the anterior pituitary, they are under nervous system control and respond to a variety of neurotransmitters such as norepinephrine, acetylcholine, and dopamine. In response to these neurotransmitters, they release the hormones oxytocin and vasopressin

from their terminals for further storage in the posterior pituitary. They are thus described as neurosecretory.

The adrenal glands

The adrenal glands are paired, pyramidal-like structures, weighing from 5 to 10 g each in an adult, sitting atop the

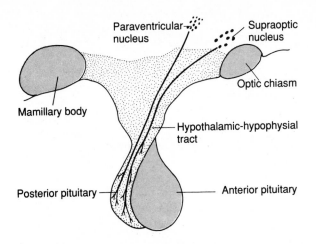

Fig. 16-3 Hypothalamic control of the posterior pituitary. *From Guyton AC: Textbook of medical physiology, ed 8, Philadeplhia, 1991, WB Saunders.*

adult, is fairly firm and golden-yellow in color. The inner portion, the medulla, is soft in contrast and reddish-brown in color.

In the adult adrenal, three zones of the cortex are histologically identifiable. The first is a very thin zone beneath the capsule, the zona glomerulosa, in which aldosterone synthesis takes place. Immediately below is the widest zone of the cortex, the zona fasciculata; it is composed of large, lipid-rich cells. Most of the cortisol synthesis in the adrenal occurs in this zone. The innermost zone, the zona reticularis, has cells similar to the cells of the zona fasciculata, but the cells have less lipid. The majority of adrenal androgens may be synthesized in the zona reticularis (Fig. 16-4).

Two types of cells make up the adrenal medulla: sympathetic ganglionic cells and large granular cells with chromaffin granules. Synthesis of epinephrine and norepinephrine takes place in the chromaffin cells.

In all three layers of the cortex, mitochondria, involved in steroid synthesis, are prominent. The granule cells of the medulla also have mitochondria, but they are less conspicuous.

Feedback regulation

An important operating characteristic of the endocrine systems to be discussed is feedback regulation. In general, feedback regulation involves a reciprocal relationship between two variables. In endocrine systems the relationship is usually between a hormone and its tropic hormone or between a hormone and a metabolite it controls. The concentration of one variable controls the concentration of a second variable, while at the same time the concentration of the second variable exerts an influence on the concentration of the first variable. Put another way, an effect pro-

superior pole of each kidney. In disease states associated with a chronic excess of ACTH, the size of the adrenals may be two to four times larger than normal; in disease states associated with a deficiency of ACTH, on the other hand, the adrenals may be smaller than normal.

The adrenals are richly supplied by a number of small arteries arising from several larger arteries, such as the aorta and the renal arteries. Venous drainage is through a central vein; the left adrenal drains into the left renal vein and the right adrenal drains directly into the inferior vena cava.

The outer portion of the adrenal, the cortex, which makes up approximate 80% to 90% of the gland by weight in the

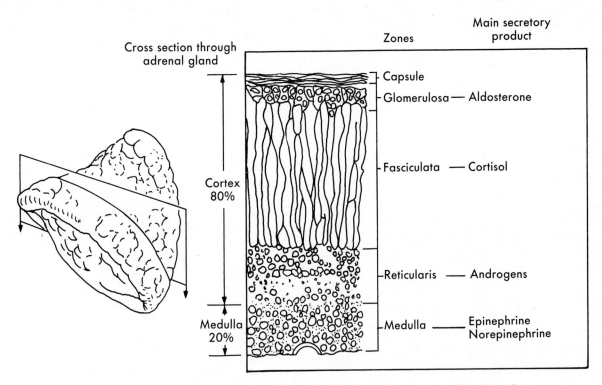

Fig. 16-4 Schematic representation of the adrenal gland and its main secretory products. *From Berne RM, Levy, MN: Principles of physiology, St. Louis, 1990, Mosby–Year Book.*

duced will influence the cause that was responsible for it. The most common type of feedback regulation in endocrine systems is negative feedback suppression of hormone secretion (Fig. 16-5).

The ability of rising blood cortisol concentrations to inhibit the pituitary's secretion of ACTH is a prime example of negative feedback. When cortisol values are low, the sensitivity of the anterior pituitary to CRF is high and it is stimulated to increase its output of ACTH. The increased ACTH acts on the adrenal cortex to stimulate its ouput of cortisol. When blood concentrations of cortisol rise, the sensitivity of the pituitary to CRF decreases, and less ACTH is secreted, thereby also decreasing the adrenal output of cortisol. The feedback system involving cortisol and ACTH also involves a direct effect of cortisol on the hypothalamic secretion of CRF.

Such feedback regulation modulates overproduction of hormone production and is a fine-tuning mechanism for maintaining hormone homeostasis.

GROWTH HORMONE
Characterization and biosynthesis

Of all the hormones found in the anterior pituitary, growth hormone (GH), also called somatotropin, is the most abundant and may account for as much as 8% to 10% of the dry weight of the gland. Some 90% of the growth hormone found in the pituitary is in the form of a 191-amino acid peptide, which occurs as a single protein chain with two intrachain disulfide bonds. The protein has a molecular weight of 21,500 daltons and no carbohydrate has been found to be associated with it.

The biological activity of the molecule resides in the amino terminal 123 amino acids; the amino acid sequence 150 to 153 is also required for biological activity. Both smaller and larger molecular fragments are attached to the biologically active portion, making up the remaining 10%. Such variants are also found in the serum and include a "big" and a "big big" GH. These larger types are believed to be aggregates of the hormone held together by interchain disulfide bonds and are not thought to be prohormones or precursors of GH. The primary structure (amino acid sequence) of GH is very closely related to that of human chorionic somatomammotropin, a hormone secreted by the placenta and less closely related to prolactin. Like GH, somatomammotropin is composed of 191 amino acids, of which the first 161 are identical to those of GH. Despite this extensive amino acid homology, somatomammotropin has little, if any, GH activity.

Prolactin, a more distant relative of GH, has 32 of its amino acids homologous to that of GH. The gene for GH and its variants is located on the long arm of chromosome 17. Because of the species specificity of the human growth hormone receptor, only primate GH is active in humans. For many years, only GH recovered from human cadaver pituitaries was available for administration. Synthetic human GH has been produced by recombinant DNA techniques and is now available.

Factors that affect secretion

Growth hormone is synthesized in specialized cells of the anterior pituitary that are identified as acidophilic somato-

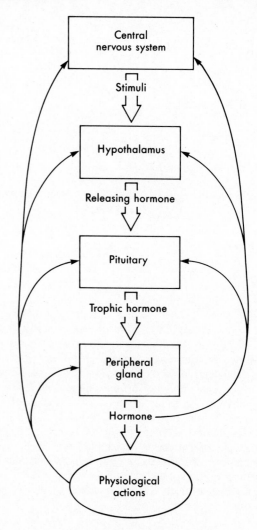

Fig. 16-5   Feedback of the H-P-A system.

tropes. The secretion of GH by the pituitary is episodic. The intermittent pulses of secretion are followed by periods of little or no secretory activity. The pattern of secretion and its magnitude varies among individuals and is affected by age. In children and young adolescents, pulses of secretory activity may occur every 3 to 4 hours; these pulses are less frequent and are of lower magnitude in adults. Once the adult pattern of secretory activity is reached, it does not change with age. In all groups, however, the maximum secretory activity appears to occur about 1 to 2 hours after the onset of deep sleep. If the sleep-wake cycle is altered, the association of maximum GH output with deep sleep persists.

The large array of physiological factors that affect GH secretion are presumed to act on the pituitary through the hypothalamus by modulating the release of either GH release stimulating or GH release inhibiting factors.

A GH release inhibiting factor from the hypothalamus has been identified, fully characterized chemically, and is known as somatostatin (SS or SRIF, somatotropin release inhibiting factor). Somatostatin is a peptide of 14 amino acids; it is distributed in other parts of the brain as well as in other tissues, including the gastrointestinal (GI) tract and pancreatic islet cells. It has biological actions in addition to its profound effect on GH release: it can block the release of GH from all physiological and pharmacological stimuli.

A long sought hypothalamic GH release stimulating factor (GHRF) has been finally characterized. A peptide, originally isolated from a pancreatic tumor, has been found to stimulate GH release from the pituitary and is identical to GHRF from the hypothalamus.

There is evidence that GH acts in a negative feedback manner, probably through a mechanism involving both GHRF and SS, to effect its own secretion. There is a reciprocal relationship between the blood glucose concentration and GH secretion. Hypoglycemia is a very powerful stimulus to GH release, and in turn, as glucose values rise, GH secretion is decreased. The rise in GH is very rapid and can be induced by as small a drop as 10 mg/dL in blood glucose. Insulin-induced hypoglycemia is used clinically as a dynamic test of GH secretion. Exercise and fasting also produce elevations of GH within 30 to 45 minutes. The hypoglycemia-induced elevations of GH are inhibited by corticosteroids and suppressed by the administration of glucose. Growth hormone in serum can also be elevated by stress, by the administration of glucagon, ACTH, ADH (vasopressin), and the infusion of amino acids. Arginine and/or leucine infusions are used most frequently. A high protein meal will also stimulate GH secretion. The serum concentration of GH also rises after oral administration of dihydroxyphenylalanine (L-dopa). The drug clonidine stimulates GH release and chlorpromazine inhibits GH release. The secretion rate of GH is elevated in hyperthyroidism and is decreased in hypothyroidism. Estrogen administration (oral contraceptives) has been found to increase basal GH secretion. A list of factors that have been found to affect GH secretion is presented in Box 16-1.

The secretion of GH amounts to about 500 μg per day. Growth hormone has a half life in blood of about 20 to 25 minutes, but its metabolic effects persist for a longer period of time. Children requiring treatment with GH usually receive GH injections only twice weekly.

Biological actions and pathophysiology

The physiological actions of GH are primarily anabolic. They are widespread both during childhood and adulthood, but are most pronounced on somatic growth during childhood.

In children absence of GH results in failure to grow, producing dwarfism; excess secretion of the hormone in children may produce gigantism and in adults, acromegaly. Excessive secretion of GH over a period of time produces gigantism if it occurs before epiphyseal closure, or acromegaly if excessive GH secretion occurs after epiphyseal closure. In its effect on skeletal growth, the activity of GH is mediated by a family of protein hormones known as somatomedins, which are synthesized in the liver. Growth hormone administration leads to an increase in tissue and organ weight, which results from an increase in mitosis, cellular hypertrophy, and hyperplasia. An increase in cellular water also occurs. Protein synthesis is stimulated and nourished by the increased uptake of amino acids into cells stimulated by GH.

Box 16-1   Factors that affect GH secretion

STIMULATORS	SUPPRESSORS
Deep (REM) sleep	Light sleep
Hypoglycemia	Hyperglycemia (glucose tolerance tests)
Stress	
Infusion of amino acids (arginine)	Elevated plasma-free fatty acids
Estrogens	Obesity
Vasopressin (in large doses)	Corticosteroids (in high doses)
Glucagon	Somatostatin
Norepinephrine	Acetylcholine
Dopamine	Corticotropin releasing factor
Serotonin	Chlorpromazine
GHRF	
Opiates	
TRH (in acromegalics)	
Clonidine	
ACTH	
Decreased plasma-free fatty acids	

In its actions on carbohydrate metabolism, GH opposes the effects of insulin; in other words, it is hyperglycemic. It is well documented that many acromegalics are diabetic.

In its actions on lipid metabolism, GH also opposes the effects of insulin: in other words, it is lipolytic. In response to GH, fat stores are mobilized and the serum level of free fatty acids increases. Growth hormone administration lowers serum cholesterol concentrations.

The second messenger involved in the cellular activity of GH is now known; activation of adenyl cyclose and cyclic AMP are not involved.

Deficient production of GH may be caused by either a deficient secretion of the hormone by the pituitary or it may arise as a result of a deficient secretion of GRF by the hypothalamus. Apparently, GH is not needed during fetal development, becuase the effects of a deficiency are not visible at birth. Deficiency becomes most prominent in infancy during the usually normal rapid growth period and the result is dwarfism. In the adult, although GH functions in the maintenance of carbohydrate and lipid metabolic homeostasis, there are no profound consequences of GH deficiency. A listing of some of the physiological actions of GH is presented in Box 16-2.

Analyte measurements and function testing

In either GH deficiency or GH excess, the value of a single measurement of serum GH by itself is very limited. The serum concentration, as might be expected from the intermittent pattern of secretion, is highly variable. The range of values found is subject to a large variety of stimuli.

In an unstressed, resting, and fasted individual, values of GH may be unmeasurable or up to 5 ng/mL in males and from 0 to less than 10 ng/mL in females. After any of the GH stimulation tests, levels may rise to as much as 15 to 35 ng/mL. In a resting state, most acromegalics will have serum values in this range or higher. The response to stimulation tests is greater in women than in men.

Box 16-2 Some physiologic actions of growth hormone

Increased cellular uptake of amino acids
Stimulation of new RNA synthesis
Stimulation of protein synthesis
Positive nitrogen balance
Decreased urea excretion
Increased collagen synthesis
Increased cellular proliferation
Increased intracellular retention of potassium, magnesium, and phosphate
Increased sodium retention
Stimulation of lipolysis
Increased lipid oxidation
Decreased body fat stores
Increased carbohydrate utilization
Increased intestinal calcium absorption
Increased urinary calcium excretion
Positive calcium balance
Increased tubular phosphate reabsorption
Antagonization of biological actions of insulin

The maximal output of GH, which occurs shortly after the onset of deep sleep, is measurable in most individuals. However, this requires that the patient be hospitalized and have an indwelling catheter inserted so that blood samples may be drawn about every 20 minutes. While asleep, the patient's sleep pattern should be ascertained by an EEG. Because extensive cost is involved, this procedure is used primarily in a research setting.

Exercise is an inexpensive stimulus of GH secretion and requires no hospitalization. Usually, the patient is required to do one-half hour of physical exercise such as vigorous walking, or use a bicycle ergometer just prior to the sample being drawn. Growth hormone values should rise above 20 ng/mL after exercise.

A variety of other methods are used to stimulate GH secretion, the most popular being insulin-induced hypoglycemia, amino acid infusion, or the use of drugs such as L-dopa, clonidine, or glucagon. Growth hormone releasing factor can also be used but it is more expensive.

Growth hormone can be measured either during a standard glucose tolerance test or 60 to 120 minutes after the ingestion of 75 g of glucose. In normal individuals the ingested glucose can be expected to suppress GH values to below 2 ng/mL; most acromegalics will not show this suppression.

Radioimmunoassay is the available method of choice to measure serum levels of GH. The sensitivity of these methods ranges between 0.5 to 1.0 ng/mL and is adequate to detect concentrations in normal serum. Growth hormone measurements are not done on urine, since the amount of GH that escapes metabolic degradation is very small and highly variable.

PROLACTIN

In many ways prolactin presents a contrast to the other pituitary hormones. Probably more functions have been ascribed to prolactin than to any other of the pituitary hor-

mones, but less in general is known about each of these suggested functions. Many of the actions attributed to prolactin have been observed only in other animal species and are presumed to occur similarly in humans. However, a clear demonstration of most of these actions remains to be shown.

In contrast to the other pituitary hormones, no stimulating factor secreted by the hypothalamus for prolactin release has been identified. If the pituitary stalk is severed to break all connections between the hypothalamus and the pituitary, the secretion of all of the pituitary hormones declines, with the exception of prolactin, which rises. Under normal circumstances prolactin is under inhibitory control of the hypothalamus; the inhibitor is the neurotransmitter L-dopamine. On a molar basis, TRH (thyroid releasing hormone) is as powerful a stimulator of prolactin release as it is of TSH (thyroid stimulating hormone) release. No significant biological importance is ascribed to such stimulation, as the stimulation of prolactin release is dissociated from TSH release. There have been many suggestions that a prolactin releasing hormone does indeed exist, but it has yet to be isolated in pure form and identified.

Unlike the other pituitary hormones, prolactin is widely distributed in a variety of body fluids and tissues, often in very high concentrations. In human semen, for example, prolactin is found at a value 1.5 times greater than that in plasma; in amniotic fluid the concentration may be some 10 times greater than in plasma.

As a further contrast, there is not a target organ for prolactin in the same sense that the other pituitary hormones have a target organ. Instead, a wide variety of tissues serve as target organs; specific prolactin receptors are distributed in tissues such as the liver, kidneys, adrenal glands, hypothalamus, pancreatic islet cells, and mammary glands.

A significant difference between prolactin and other pituitary hormones is the extraordinary growth of the pituitary during pregnancy, which is primarily due to the large increase in the number of lactotropes (cells producing prolactins). This occurs as the result of the profound stimulation of these cells in the pituitary by increasing concentrations of estrogen, particularly during the third trimester of pregnancy. In the normal pituitary of the nonpregnant female, 10% to 25% of the mass may be composed of lactotropes. During pregnancy, up to 70% of the mass may be occupied by these cells.

Characterization and biosynthesis

It has not been clearly established how many circulating forms of prolactin exist, nor what the relative biological activity is of the different circulating forms. Prolactin is considered to be a family of closely related proteins composed of both smaller and larger forms of the usual 198-amino acid prolactin molecule. The standard prolactin has a molecular weight of about 23,000 daltons and is glycosylated; the presence of three intrachain disulfide bonds is responsible for the molecule having three loops. In blood, in addition to the standard prolactin, at least two forms larger than the standard 23,000-dalton form have been identified: a "big" prolactin with a molecular weight between 48,000 to 56,000 daltons, and a still larger form with a molecular weight greater than 100,000 daltons. In addition, smaller cleavage forms of prolactin have been found. To add to the difficulty of defining the biological activity of these molecules, prolactin isolated from different tissues may be glycosylated to different degrees. Apparently, a series of post-transcription and post-translation events are responsible for the occurrence of a large family of related prolactin molecules.

Structurally, prolactin is so closely related in amino acid sequence to GH and chorionic somatomammotropin that all three hormones are considered to have evolved from the same ancestral gene. Prolactin has 32 of its amino acids homologous to that of GH. In the human, the gene for prolactin is located on chromosome 6.

Factors that affect secretion

Specialized acidophilic cells of the anterior pituitary called lactotropes, sometimes also called mammotropes, compose about 10% to 15% of the bulk of the anterior pituitary. These cells synthesize and secrete prolactin. Both the synthesis and secretion are under the control of the hypothalamus, like the other pituitary hormones. But unlike the other pituitary hormones, the hypothalamic effect of prolactin appears only to be an inhibitory one.

The neurotransmitter L-dopamine is considered to be the main PIF (prolactin inhibitory factor). The output of L-dopamine by the hypothalamus is high enough to account for almost all of the inhibitory activity on prolactin. The action of L-dopamine underscores the heavy influence of the nervous system on prolactin secretion. Secretion of prolactin quickly rises in response to an increase in stress. Through L-dopamine, prolactin is part of a short negative feedback loop involving both the pituitary and hypothalamus. Some of the prolactin secreted by the pituitary binds to prolactin receptors found in the hypothalamus; the binding of prolactin to these receptors stimulates the production of L-dopamine, which leads to the inhibition of prolactin synthesis and release by the pituitary.

The secretion of prolactin, like that of the other pituitary hormones, is episodic; plasma concentrations are highest just before waking and drop during the day. The lowest values are reached one to two hours after the onset of sleep. Day to day concentrations of prolactin remain relatively constant. The half-life of prolactin in the circulation is about 50 minutes. It appears that the liver and kidney are the major sites of prolactin removal.

Pregnancy appears to be the strongest physiological stimulus to prolactin release, resulting, as a consequence, in the rising estrogen concentrations that occur during pregnancy. Estrogens have a direct effect on the pituitary lactotropes; these cells increase in number and account for the increased size of the pituitary during pregnancy.

By term, prolactin values may be increased almost tenfold. During pregnancy prolactin values are even higher in amniotic fluid than in blood, but the concentration peaks between 18 to 25 weeks. During labor there is a dramatic drop in prolactin to roughly one-half of the prelabor value. About four weeks after delivery, prolactin concentrations return to normal if the mother does not nurse.

If the mother nurses, then lactational hyperprolactinemia ensues; high prolactin values are necessary to continue milk production by the breast. Prolactin values rise within 10 minutes after the beginning of suckling and peak during

---

Box 16-3 Factors that affect prolactin secretion

STIMULATORS	SUPPRESSORS
TRH (thyrotropin releasing hormone)	Hyperthyroidism
VIP (vasoactive intestinal peptide)	Dopamine
	L-dopa
Serotonin	Bromocriptine
GABA (γ-amino butyric acid)	Somatostatin
Histamine	
Melatonin	
Opioid peptides	
Morphine	
met-enkephalin	
β-endorphin	
Pregnancy	
Tactile stimulation of breast	
Stress	
Insulin hypoglycemia	
Exercise	
Hypothyroidism	
Lactation	
Oral contraceptives	
Sexual intercourse (in women)	
Sleep	
High protein meals	
Chlorpromazine	

---

nursing at about eight times the normal concentration. These high prolactin concentrations during nursing keep the mother in an anovulatory infertile state for a period of time. After a variable time, the suckling stimulus to prolactin secretion declines.

Chronic estrogen administration will stimulate prolactin release, whereas acute administration will not. In both non-lactating women and in men, stimulation of the nipple produces prolactin release. Prolactin values also rise after hypoglycemia, after severe physical exercise, and after sexual intercourse in women. Prolonged fasting leads to declining plasma prolactin levels. A listing of some of the factors that may affect prolactin secretion is presented in Box 16-3.

Biological actions and pathophysiology

Despite the wide distribution of prolactin receptors in many tissues and the occurrence of prolactin in some tissue at higher concentrations than in blood, the main known actions of prolactin are related to its role in the growth and development of the breast and in milk formation by that organ. In this role prolactin functions in an integrated fashion with insulin, estrogens, adrenal steroids, progesterone, and growth hormone.

A not-as-yet clarified role for prolactin in male reproduction has been suggested by the presence of prolactin receptors associated with male reproductive organs and the high concentration of prolactin in semen. In the testes prolactin may increase the sensitivity of that tissue to LH and thus help to maintain testosterone output.

A role for prolactin in female reproduction has been suggested by the frequent association of amenorrhea and/or galactorrhea in women with hyperprolactinemia. Prolactin may modulate the frequency with which the hypothalamus secretes GnRH, which in turn would effect LH release by the pituitary.

Increased prolactin concentrations have been found to be associated with a large variety of both hypothalamic and pituitary disorders and with other endocrine and nonendocrine diseases. The use of many drugs also affects prolactin concentrations, making the diagnosis of the etiology of the prolactinemia difficult.

Elevated prolactin values over a period of time may lead to gonadal dysfunction; in woman, such a state is evidenced by menstrual irregularities, amenorrhea, or infertility. In men, they may be associated with infertility. In both men and women, galactorrhea may or may not be associated with elevated prolactin values.

Both small (microadenomas) and large (macroadenomas) prolactin secreting tumors of the pituitary have been identified. Frequently, an elevated prolactin value is the only evidence of a pituitary abnormality that may not yet be radiographically discernible.

Prolactin concentrations may be increased by tumors of any kind that produce pressure on the pituitary stalk and reduce the amount of the PIF L-dopamine, which can reach the pituitary.

Prolactin values will rise after the use of drugs that interfere with L-dopamine synthesis or release. Among a wide variety of such drugs that affect the prolactin values are the neuroleptics such as chlorpromazine, haloperidol, and trifluoperazine; antihypertensives such as reserpine and α-methyldopa, and antidepressants such as amitriptyline and imipramine. Elevated prolactin levels are found in many patients with chronic renal failure and in patients with cirrhosis. Box 16-4 summarizes the known biological functions of prolactin. In Box 16-5, the effects of hyperprolactinemia in both men and women are presented.

Analyte measurement and function testing

Problems related to the determination of prolactin in serum arise from its pulsatile secretion, the multiple forms of the hormone present in serum, and the multitude of factors that can affect its secretion. Because serum values are altered significantly in most clinical cases, making small differences unimportant, these problems present no insurmountable barriers. Since its introduction and application to prolactin, radioimmunoassay (RIA) remains the method of choice for serum prolactin determination. Radioimmunoassay procedures utilizing polyclonal or monoclonal antibodies are available, cover a useful range, and usually have a sensitivity (usually about 1 ng/mL) more than sufficient for clinical application.

Although serum measurements are routine for clinical purposes, prolactin has also been detected in other body fluids, such as cerebrospinal fluid, amniotic fluid, ovarian follicular fluid, as well as in semen. Concentrations in amniotic fluid may be extremely high (greater than 2000 ng/mL); values in urine are usually about one-tenth those found in serum.

In men, normal serum prolactin values are 6 to 15 ng/mL; in women, values are slightly higher at 8 to 25 ng/mL. During sleep, values are approximately 50% higher than during wakefulness. Stress of any kind, even that caused by a venipuncture, may elevate the basal concentration to 50 to 60 ng/mL. Newborns have values 5 to 20 times normal for 4 to 8 weeks after birth; afterward, the serum concentration quickly declines and remains relatively constant for the rest of life. In women, there is no significant change during the menstrual cycle; values decrease somewhat after menopause. Serum concentrations increase during pregnancy, reaching 150 to 200 ng/mL at term. In nursing mothers serum values remain elevated for a short time after the cessation of nursing.

Radioimmunoassays based on monoclonal antibodies may not be able to detect all of the different isoforms of the hormone present in serum. In this regard there is evidence that ratio of the forms present may change during disease just as it does during pregnancy. The possibility also exists that the antibody used may detect prolactin degradation products as well as the intact molecule and that these may not be biologically active. In one study the ratio of biologically active prolactin (as determined by bioassay) to that determined by RIA ranged from 0.53 to 1.58. Again, because of the magnitude of serum prolactin changes associated with altered secretion of the hormone, these shortcomings of RIA procedures are of little consequence in a typical clinical setting.

Prolactin deficiency is infrequently encountered in clinical practice, generally in cases of Sheehous syndrome, anorexia nervosa, and total pituitary infarction. Prolactin values less than 2 ng/mL are indicative of deficiency, which carries no clinical sequelae with it. Deficiency can be confirmed by noting the absence of a prolactin response to a single intravenous injection of TRH (thyroid releasing hormone).

Hyperprolactinemia, on the other hand, is one of the most common hypothalamic-pituitary presenting disorders. In most cases a single serum prolactin determination on each of three consecutive days or three separate samples taken 30 minutes apart on the same day in a relaxed, unstressed

---

Box 16-4 Biological actions of prolactin

Stimulates synthesis of breast milk components
Necessary for initiation and maintenance of lactation
Not essential in adult life

Box 16-5 Effect of prolactin hypersecretion

IN WOMEN	IN MEN
Galactorrhea	Impotence
Oligomenorrhea	Decreased libido
Amenorrhea	Decreased GnRH
Infertility	Oligospermia
Menstrual irregularities	Gynecomastia
Anovulation	Galactorrhea
Decreased libido	

individual, is considered satisfactory to confirm hyperprolactinemia. The multiple sampling is recommended to obviate normal fluctuations and stress-induced elevations of prolactin. A concentration greater than 200 ng/mL is usually almost diagnostic of a prolactin-secreting tumor, although such tumors have been found in patients with concentrations less than 100 ng/mL. In patients with hyperprolactinemia of a nontumor origin, the hypersecretion of prolactin can usually be suppressed by an infusion of dopamine. Since this suppression test has not been helpful in distinguishing a hypothalamic or pituitary cause of the prolactinemia, it is not used frequently. Before any diagnostic importance is attached to an elevated prolactin value, pregnancy, hypothyroidism and drug ingestion should be excluded.

LUTEINIZING HORMONE AND FOLLICLE-STIMULATING HORMONE

There are many reasons to consider the pituitary hormones luteinizing hormone (LH) and follicle-stimulating hormone (FSH) together. There are many similarities in the amino acid structure of these hormones; they share a functional relationship as gonadotropins and in many actions, they appear to act in concert with each other. In addition, the secretion of both of these pituitary hormones is controlled by the same hypothalamic releasing hormone, gonadotropin releasing hormone (GnRH), although to a different extent. Throughout life, the secretion of both hormones varies with sex and age in an almost parallel fashion. Despite these close relationships, each hormone has unique properties and functions that clearly distinguishes it from the other.

Characterization and biosynthesis

Luteinizing hormone and FSH are both protein dimers, composed of an alpha and beta subunit with a total molecular weight of about 28,000 daltons. The alpha subunits of each hormone are identical to each other and to the alpha subunits of human chorionic gonadotropin (hCG) and thyroid stimulating hormone (TSH). The beta subunit of the dimer confers on each hormone its biological and immunological specificity; in LH, the beta subunit is made up of 116 amino acids and in FSH, this subunit contains 119 amino acids. Neither subunit has biological activity by itself. The hormones are both glycosylated, and removal of the carbohydrate from the molecule results in loss of biological activity. The genes for the alpha and beta subunits are located on different chromosomes, indicating they are synthesized separately and combined before release. Potentially, conditions could occur that would lead to an excess of either the free alpha or beta subunit if synthesis became unbalanced.

Factors that affect secretion

Specialized cells in the pituitary, called gonadotropes, that secrete either FSH or LH have been identified, although most gonadotropes secrete both hormones. The secretion of LH and FSH is under the control of a single hypothalamic hypophysiotropic hormone, GnRH, also referred to as luteinizing hormone releasing hormone (LH-RH). The response of LH to GnRH is independent of the response of FSH to GnRH. The difference in response is apparently the result of different negative and positive feedback effects of the gonadal estrogens and androgens on the hypothalamus and pituitary.

Gonadotropin releasing hormone is a stimulus for both the synthesis and secretion of LH and FSH. The function of the ovaries in females and the testes in males is influenced directly by FSH and LH and indirectly by GnRH. Subsequent sexual development at maturity in both sexes is considered to be under the control of GnRH.

Gonadotropin releasing hormone is a peptide of 10 amino acids synthesized by specialized neuronal cells in the hypothalamus. Once synthesized, GnRH is released into the vessels of the hypophyseal portal system, by which route it traverses the pituitary stalk to reach the anterior pituitary. The gonadoptropes of the pituitary have specialized high affinity receptors for GnRH.

Similar to other hormones, GnRH secretion by the hypothalamus is pulsatile or episodic, which in turn results in the pulsatile secretion of LH and FSH by pituitary gonadotropes. Pulsatile GnRH release is critical to normal LH and FSH stimulation; if GnRH (or its analogues) is given by constant infusion, LH and FSH secretion is inhibited. To stimulate LH and FSH, GnRH must be administered in pulses.

The pulsatile secretion of LH and FSH renders the determination of a single blood concentration of either of these hormones somewhat meaningless because they vary by 20% to 30% at any given time. The pulse intensity and frequency of both hormones also vary with age and sex, to further confound a single determination. In addition, LH has a short plasma half-life of about 50 minutes, whereas that of FSH is longer, about 3 to 4 hours. As a result, levels of FSH fluctuate less during the day than those of LH. Gonadotropin releasing hormone has a plasma half-life of about 10 minutes.

The responses of FSH and LH to GnRH vary greatly throughout life and are made complex by the way they are affected by sex and age. The FSH secretory response and the LH secretory response of the pituitary to pulses of hypothalamic GnRH differ somewhat from each other during gestation, childhood, puberty, adulthood, and old age. In addition, during the female menstrual cycle, the negative feedback effects of estrogens on the hypothalamus and the pituitary instead become positive feedback effects, so that the rising estrogen levels of the follicular phase now stimulate an increased production of LH and FSH.

In the fetus at mid-gestation, LH and FSH can be detected at very low values and both hormones remain low throughout gestation. Within 5 to 6 weeks after birth, there is a small but discernible increase in both hormones. Both hormones remain low throughout childhood. It is believed that during these early stages of childhood both the hypothalamus and the pituitary are highly sensitive to small changes in concentration of the gonadal steroids: estrogens in females and androgens in males. Although steroid concentrations are very low, they are still able to inhibit the secretion of LH and FSH by negative feedback, probably at the level of the hypothalamus.

With the onset of puberty, the LH secretory response to GnRH becomes greater than the FSH secretory response, but both LH and FSH concentrations begin to rise; FSH values rise first, LH values rise later but to higher concentrations. During puberty also, an increased secretion of both LH and FSH occurs during sleep, so that during this stage of development a circadian rhythm is imposed on the pulsatile secretory pattern. In men, this sleep-associated increase carries over into adulthood, but is not prominent.

By the later stages of puberty in females, the secretion of LH and FSH becomes cyclic and the menstrual cycle is established. In females, the increased LH and FSH concentrations stimulate ovarian production of estrogens. The higher concentrations of estrogens act on the pituitary to increase its secretion of LH and FSH by positive feedback. Estrogens in women, which up to puberty inhibited LH and FSH secretion, now have a stimulatory effect. This positive feedback is most evident in the preovulatory rise of LH and FSH stimulated by the rising estrogen levels that occur during this middle phase of the menstrual cycle.

The pattern of LH and FSH secretion during the menstrual cycle has been well established. During the preovulatory phase, both LH and FSH increase, the increase in LH being greater than that of FSH. Both increases are a result of the positive feedback effect of increasing estrogen concentrations during the preovulatory phase. Both hormone values peak about 24 to 36 hours prior to ovulation. After ovulation, if fertilization does not occur, both the LH and FSH values rapidly decline in response to the inhibiting effect of rising progesterone concentrations, which characterize the luteal phase of the menstrual cycle. The maturation of the corpus luteum and estrogen and progesterone synthesis by that structure require the presence of LH with the help of FSH. If fertilization occurs, the sustained progesterone levels are inhibitory and the secretion of both LH and FSH becomes minimal after a short period.

With the onset of menopause, ovarian estrogens regain their inhibitory effect on gonadotropin secretion, but since ovarian estrogen synthesis decreases, both LH and FSH are elevated in postmenopausal women.

In men, androgens have an inhibitory effect on LH and FSH secretion throughout life, so that a reciprocal relationship exists between testosterone secretion and LH/FSH secretion. Estrogens in men have only an inhibitory effect on gonadotropin secretion. With the decline of testicular function in men around the sixth decade, LH and FSH are released from the negative feedback effects of androgens and levels of both hormones rise.

In men, the seminiferous tubules produce a hormone, inhibin, which inhibits hypothalamic GnRH. In women, inhibin is produced in ovarian follicular fluid. The extent of the contribution of inhibin in controlling hypothalamic GnRH in concert with gonadal steroids is not yet clear.

Two aspects of LH and FSH physiology that have found practical clinical applications are in birth control and treatment of precocious puberty.

Estrogen-progesterone combinations are widely used as anovulatory drugs for birth control. A low dose of estrogen is given for 14 days followed by 7 days of a synthetic progesterone. This use of natural or synthetic steroids is based on the suppression of the mid-cycle surge of LH. Similar estrogen-progesterone combination medications are used to reduce LH secretion postmenopause, and therefore reduce phsiologic symptoms of aging.

Sustained administration of GnRH or of its analogues has been used as treatment for gonadotropin-induced precocious

puberty. On the other hand, the pulsatile administration of GnRH has been used to treat infertility in both men and women: in women, such treatment can restore a normal menstrual cycle; in men, it can lead to normal testosterone and sperm production.

Biological actions and pathophysiology

Luteinizing hormone and FSH have identifiable, singular activities on their target organs, the ovaries in women and testes in men (Box 16-6 and Box 16-7). In each of these activities the action of one hormone appears to require the activity or the presence of the other hormone.

In the female, LH and FSH are essential for ovulation. Normal growth and maturation of the ovarian follicle is maintained by FSH, with the help of LH and the estrogen produced by the granulosa cells of the ovary. An LH surge triggers ovulation. The development of the corpus luteum and steroid synthesis by that structure are stimulated by LH with the help of FSH.

Box 16-6   Biological actions of LH in men and women

IN WOMEN

Stimulates ovarian theca cell synthesis of androgens that serve as precursors of granulosa cell production of estrogens.

Mid-cycle surge induces maturation and release of ovum.

During fetal life, may play a role in sexual differentiation, especially in the male.

With FSH, promotes follicular luteinization.

Stimulates progesterone production by corpus luteum.

IN MEN

Stimulates Leydig's cell secretion of testosterone (which increases FSH binding to seminiferous tubules).

Stimulates testicular growth.

Stimulates testicular interstitial cell function.

Box 16-7   Biological actions of FSH in men and women

IN WOMEN

Stimulates estrogen secretion from ovarian granulosa cells.

Stimulates ovum maturation (along with estrogens and androgens).

Part of ovulatory surge.

Promotes growth and maturation of the primordial follicle cell.

IN MEN

Target is Sertoli's cell.

Enhances LH-induced testosterone secretion.

Important for spermatogenesis.

Stimulates development of LH receptors on Leydig's cells.

Increases tubular permeability to testosterone.

Stimulates testicular growth.

Enhances synthesis of androgen-binding protein by Sertoli's cells.

In men, the primary action of FSH is to stimulate spermatogenesis, but again this function requires the help of LH. Follicle stimulating hormone has little if any effect on androgen production by testicular interstitial cells. Luteinizing hormone stimulates the growth of testicular Leydig's cells and the testosterone production by those cells; in this function LH appears to require FSH.

The effect of an abnormality of FSH or LH secretion will depend on the age and sex of the individual with the defect. The hormonal abnormality will reflect the associated effect of gonadal steroids on sexual development that normally occurs at that age in that sex (Box 16-8).

During fetal life, for example, LH and FSH may play a role in sexual differentiation, particularly in the development of sexual genitalia in males, which requires androgen secretion by the testes. A deficiency of LH and FSH during fetal life may lead to stunted development of the external male genitalia.

In the years before puberty, excesses of LH and FSH may trigger precocious puberty; the earlier-than-normal maturation of the hypothalamic-pituitary axis that results in the earlier-than-normal development of sexual characteristics. Precocious puberty is seen more frequently in girls than in boys. By the same token, a deficiency of these hormones may lead to a partial or total failure of development of sexual characteristics. If sexual development during puberty does not occur because of a hypothalamic or pituitary defect, there is a deficient LH and FSH secretion. This condition is referred to as *hypo*gonadotropic *hypo*gonadism. If sexual development does not occur with normal LH and FSH values because of a primary gonadal deficiency, there is decreased estrogen and androgen production. This condition is called *hyper*gonadotropic *hypo*gonadism.

In adult life, deficiencies of the gonadotropic hormones affect aspects of fertility in both men and women. In women, the most prominent features are sterility due to anovulation. Amenorrhea, lack of menses, is also common. In men, the deficiency results in sterility and impotence.

Analyte measurement and function testing

The radioimmunoassays (RIA) and immunoradiometric (IRMA) assays that are available to measure LH and FSH in serum and urine present no significant technological problems. There are, however, a number of considerations that must be carefully weighed in association with the assays in order to make a serum or urine determination diagnostically meaningful.

It is clear from the influence of sex and age on both LH and FSH secretion that a patient serum or urine value must be compared to normal values obtained from individuals of the same sex and age, and in females, preferably at the same phase of the menstrual cycle. Further, in females, LH and FSH values obtained during menopause or postmenopause must be compared to those obtained from "normal" women in menopause or postmenopause, respectively. Because of the inhibitory/stimulatory effects of estrogens, and the inhibitory effects of testosterone and progesterone, the simultaneous measurement of these steroids along with LH and FSH is frequently indicated, particularly in cases of hypogonadism or infertility.

The pulsatile secretion of LH and FSH in both males and females, the cyclical secretion of LH and FSH during the female menstrual cycle, and the circadian pattern of secretion most prominently seen in adolescents, all contribute to the wide fluctuations over the entire normal range in serum which may be obtained from the same patient in different samples taken on the same day. Luteinizing hormone, because of its very short half-life, varies much more than FSH.

Box 16-8   Relationship between GnRH, LH, and FSH as affected by age and sex

FETAL: MALE AND FEMALE

Both LH and FSH detected at mid-gestation, both low.
LH higher in females than males.
FSH higher in females than males.
Low levels of androgens and estrogens: negative feedback on LH and FSH.

POSTNATAL: MALE AND FEMALE

At 6 weeks of life, small transitory rise in LH and FSH.

CHILDHOOD: MALE AND FEMALE

LH basal secretion and response to GnRH both low, similar in males and females.
Response of FSH to GnRH in females is highest in any period.
In males, FSH response to GnRH less than that of LH.
FSH levels greater than LH.

PUBERTY: MALE AND FEMALE

LH secretory response to GnRH increases.
FSH response to GnRH declines.
FSH response to GnRH greater in females than males.
Basal LH and FSH values increase during sleep.

PUBERTY: FEMALE

Increased estrogens during follicular phase have positive feedback on both LH and FSH release, responsible for mid-cycle LH surge.
LH values rise during follicular phase, peak at mid-cycle.
Serum FSH highest in follicular phase, declines before LH peak.
Secretion of LH and FSH becomes cyclical and synchronized.
Pulse frequency of GnRH increases.

ADULTHOOD: MALE AND FEMALE

LH response of GnRH greater than during puberty.
LH response to GnRH greater than that of FSH.
FSH response to GnRH declines further, similar in males and females.
In women, during luteal phase, LH response to GnRH still greater than that of male.

MENOPAUSE

Sharp increase in LH just before menopause.

POSTMENOPAUSAL WOMEN

Basal LH and FSH levels rise.
Sharp increase in FSH.
Estrogens have inhibitory effect on LH and FSH.

ELDERLY MEN

LH and FSH values gradually increase in men over 50.
LH and FSH response to GnRH increased in men over 65.

To obviate these fluctuations, many authorities recommend that multiple samples, three to four per hour, be taken instead of a single one. In addition, sampling should be carried out for 3 to 4 hours.

Urinary LH and FSH determinations have gained favor as a means of doing away with the drawbacks of serum testing. Standard 24-hour urine collections may be used to reflect integrated 24-hour serum levels; comparable results may be obtained with overnight urine collections or even with urine collections as short as 3 hours. In procedural modifications for urine, LH and/or FSH are first precipitated from urine with cold acetone; the dried residues are reconstituted and then assayed using serum reagents.

A very significant concern for anyone needing to interpret or compare LH and FSH values is the variations in these values for various normal and pathological states as reported in the literature. This variation arises from the number of different preparations of LH and FSH that are used as standards by kit manufacturers. While both LH and FSH concentrations are reported in either milli-international units per milliliter (mIU/mL) or in IU/L, the standards in kits may be based on different international standards or different international reference preparations supplied by the World Health Organization (WHO), or on different standards, and thus are not interchangeable. Most manufacturers supply conversion factors in their assay procedures, which may be used to compare one standard with another. It is clear that for comparison, one needs to know against which standards the values he or she is working with were standardized.

Frequently the clinician needs to determine which unit of the hypothalamic-pituitary-gonadal system may be malfunctioning in a particular patient. In these circumstances, basal LH and FSH levels, along with an estrogen determination in women or a testosterone determination in men, will generally indicate whether or not a disturbance is due to a gonadal deficiency or a deficiency in the hypothalamus-pituitary unit. For example, if LH and/or FSH values are normal to elevated and either estrogen or testosterone values are low, primary gonadal failure is indicated. On the other hand, if the gonadotropins and either estrogen or testosterone are low, the malfunction is probably in the hypothalamus-pituitary unit. To assess menstrual cycle function in women, a progesterone determination is frequently added to the other assays. Gonadotropin releasing hormone assays are also available.

Dynamic tests are used to assess whether or not the hypothalamus or the pituitary is at fault. Synthetic GnRH, given as a single intravenous bolus, is commonly used to directly stimulate the pituitary to release its pool of FSH and LH. Basal samples for FSH and LH assay are taken before the administration of the GnRH, as well as samples for either testosterone or estrodial. Samples again are taken from an indwelling catheter every 10 minutes after GnRH administration for gonadotropin measurement. Luteinizing values peak within 20 to 30 minutes then fall by 60 minutes. Follicle-stimulating hormone values peak at about 60 minutes. In interpreting results, consideration must again be given to the age and sex of the patient.

In another dynamic test, clomiphene, an estrogen antagonist, is administered. By binding to estrogen receptors in the hypothalamus, it negates the inhibitory effects of low levels of estrogens, allowing FSH and LH secretion to be increased. In this test, clomiphene must be administered daily for 7 to 10 days, and the effect of the administered clomiphene is sometimes not seen until day 4. If hypothalamic GnRH reserve is normal, both gonadotropins should increase, to an extent dictated again by sex and age.

In Box 16-9, LH values for serum are given in terms of mIU/mL, and for urine in terms of IU/24 hrs. These values are in terms of the second IRP-HMG (Second International Reference Preparations-Human Menopausal Gonadotropins) of the WHO. They should serve only as guides to comparative levels as related to age and sex.

In Box 16-10, FSH values for serum are given in terms of mIU/mL, and for urine in terms of IU/L/24 hrs. These values are in terms of the Second IRP-HMG. As for LH values, they should serve only as guides to comparative levels as related to age and sex.

The antibodies to LH used in both RIA and IRMA show considerable cross-reactivity with hCG (human chorionic gonadotropin) so that they are not reliable when hCG values are high, as in pregnancy. The cross-reactivity to hCG may be as high as 10%. Antibodies to FSH do not show this cross-reactivity to hCG.

Box 16-9   LH serum and urine values

SERUM

Prepubertal male and female:	up to 15 mIU/mL
Adult male:	up to 26 mIU/mL
Adult female	
Follicular phase:	up to 33 mIU/mL
Mid-cycle:	30 to 200 mIU/mL
Postmenopausal:	30 to 130 mIU/mL

URINE

Male and female	
Prepubertal:	up to 7 IU/L
Childhood:	up to 40 IU/L
Adult:	up to 45 IU/L

Box 16-10   FSH serum and urine values

SERUM

Prepubertal male and female:	up to 9 mIU/mL
Adult male:	up to 20 mIU/mL
Adult female	
Follicular phase:	up to 17 mIU/mL
Mid-cycle:	20 to 30 mIU/mL
Postmenopausal:	30 to 150 mIU/mL

URINE

Male

Up to 8 years:	<5 IU/24 hrs
	<22 IU/24 hrs

Female

Up to 8 years:	<5 IU/24 hrs
9-15 years:	<22 IU/24 hrs
>15 years:	<30 IU/24 hrs

Some concern has been expressed as to whether or not urine assays, even those based on acetone extraction, measure only biologically active hormones to the exclusion of immunologically active degradation products. This concern has not been adequately resolved.

ADRENOCORTICOTROPIC HORMONE
Characterization and biosynthesis

In specialized pituitary cells called corticotrophs, the 39-amino acid sequence of adrenocorticotropic hormone (ACTH), with a molecular weight of 4500 daltons occurs as part of a large precursor, proopiomelanocortin (POMC), with a molecular weight of 28,500 daltons. In humans, POMC is made up of 267 amino acids and undergoes subsequent glycosylation and multiple cleavages to give rise to a group of peptides with hormonal activity that are secreted in a one-to-one ratio with ACTH: these are β-lipotropin, (β-LPH), β-endorphin, and γ-MSH (melanocyte-stimulating hormone). Although ACTH is composed of 39 amino acids, full biologic activity resides in amino acid residues 1 to 24; amino acids 25 to 39 are not needed for biologic activity. Synthetic ACTH, used clinically for adrenal function testing, has the 1 to 24 amino acid sequence of native ACTH.

Factors that affect secretion

In a manner analogous to the control of the release of the other pituitary hormones, the release of ACTH is controlled by a hypothalamic factor, called corticotropin releasing factor (CRF). Both the synthesis and release of ACTH are mediated by CRF. Unlike the effects of the other releasing hormones, however, the effect of CRF on ACTH (and subsequently, on cortisol) is prolonged. After being stimulated by CRF, ACTH values remain elevated for hours rather than just minutes. The effect of CRF is most pronounced on the release of ACTH. As it exerts its effect on the pituitary, CRF probably does not act alone but is part of a complex that may include arginine, vasopressin, and other factors. Release of ACTH can be stimulated by the administration of neurotransmitters such as norepinephrine, serotonin, and γ-aminobutyric acid, or suppressed by the administration of dopamine.

Secretion of ACTH throughout the day is pulsatile. It also follows a circadian pattern, reaching peak values just before and after waking, then reaching a nadir in the early evening. The circadian pattern of cortisol secretion by the adrenal is in direct response to the circadian rhythm of ACTH secretion.

Stress serves as a powerful stimulus to ACTH secretion; the blood level of ACTH can be observed to rise within 1 minute after experiencing stress such as pain, trauma, surgery, severe depression, fever, or sharp, unexpected noise. Blood concentrations of ACTH during periods of stress are the highest seen under normal circumstances. Hypoglycemia is another powerful ACTH stimulus. Insulin-induced hypoglycemia is commonly used as a dynamic test of ACTH reserve. A list of factors affecting the secretion of ACTH is given in Box 16-11. The half-life of ACTH in the blood is short, ranging from 5 to 20 minutes.

The pituitary output of ACTH is modulated by adrenal steroids, primarily cortisol, through feedback effects exerted on both the hypothalamus and the pituitary. When circu-

---

Box 16-11   Factors affecting the secretion of ACTH

STIMULATORS

Vasopressin
Norepinephrine
Interleukin
Dopamine
Histamine
Serotonin
GABA (γ-aminobutyric acid)
Stress
Adrenolectomy
Metyrapone
Pyrogen administration
Glucagon

INHIBITORS

Glucocorticoids
Epinephrine

---

lating concentrations of cortisol decline, synthesis and release of CRF by the hypothalamus is stimulated; the increased CRF stimulates the pituitary to increase its synthesis and secretion of ACTH, which in turn stimulates adrenal cortical cells to synthesize and secrete more cortisol. The consequent rising cortisol values turn off CRF release by the hypothalamus and may directly affect ACTH output by the pituitary. This feedback system is also sensitive to exogenous steroids; the administration of a synthetic corticosteroid such as dexamethasone, for example, will lead to adrenal atrophy as a result of the inhibition of ACTH release and its effects on the adrenal. If exogenous steroids are administered over a period of time, ACTH secretion by the pituitary may be suppressed for as long as 6 to 9 months. By contrast, the administration of metyrapone, a drug that blocks the 11β-hydroxylation of cortisol, will increase ACTH secretion.

Biological actions and pathophysiology

The primary biological effect of ACTH is on the adrenal cortex, where it not only specifically increases both the synthesis and secretion of cortisol, but the synthesis of adrenal androgens as well. The enzymatic conversion of cholesterol to pregnenolone appears to be the step sensitive to ACTH (see page 238). At the cellular level, cyclic AMP acts as the second messenger for ACTH.

When given acutely, ACTH will stimulate aldosterone secretion by adrenal glomerulosa cells, but the effect is short lived; aldosterone secretion quickly becomes insensitive to continued ACTH administration.

In response to ACTH stimulation, blood flow to the adrenal gland is increased, adrenal corticotrophs increase in size (hypertrophy), and the adrenal gland itself increases in weight.

Adrenocorticotropic hormone has extra adrenal actions on carbohydrate and fat metabolism; it increases blood glucose and increases free fatty acid release from adipose tissue, but the quantitative contribution of these effects to overall carbohydrate and fat metabolism is unclear.

Adrenocorticotropic hormone is more powerful than γ-MSH in stimulating melanin production by melanocytes. This effect on melanin formation is prominent as increased pigmentation in those patients with Cushing's syndrome induced by high levels of ACTH. Some of the biological actions of ACTH are listed in Box 16-12.

A deficiency of ACTH secretion is evident by the features of hypoadrenalism produced by failure of stimulation of cortisol synthesis and secretion; these effects of cortisol are fully described in the following section of this chapter on cortisol. Primary ACTH deficiency is rare; patients with such a deficiency have a skin palor resulting from the lack of stimulation of melanocytes by ACTH. In patients with hypoadrenalism due to other causes, skin pigmentation is increased and serves as a clue that ACTH levels are high.

A pituitary tumor specifically involving corticotrophs is recognized (corticotroph cell adenoma); this tumor may be secretory, resulting in Cushing's disease or Nelson's syndrome, or it may be nonsecretory. The features of Cushing's disease are described in the next section of this chapter on cortisol. In Nelson's syndrome, excessive quantities of ACTH secreted by a corticotroph cell adenoma lead to intense hyperpigmentation. High plasma levels of ACTH are also found in Addison's disease; in this disease destruction of cells of the adrenal cortex results in absence of circulating cortisol to suppress pituitary output of ACTH.

Analyte measurement and function testing

Radioimmunoassay procedures for ACTH are available, but shortcomings of the blood collection methods required and of the assay have deterred these assays from increased popularity. Instead of measuring ACTH directly in patients suspected of hypopituitarism or specifically, of ACTH deficiency, assays of adrenal response are used instead to provide the necessary information. Insulin-induced hypoglycemia is commonly used to stimulate ACTH secretion; the response of the adrenal in increasing its output of cortisol is taken as a measure of pituitary ACTH reserve. The drug metyrapone, which blocks 11β-hydroxylation required as the final step in cortisol synthesis, can be used for the same purpose. The immediate precursor of cortisol, 11-deoxycortisol, accumulates and can easily be measured in blood by RIA methods or in urine as 17-hydroxycorticosteroids (17-OHCS).

In plasma used for RIA, ACTH is rapidly inactivated by proteolytic enzymes, so that blood collected for assay must be quickly chilled and kept chilled. To prevent binding of the ACTH to glass, samples must be stored in plastic vials before assay. Synthetic ACTH is used as the labeled species in the assay.

Because of the acute effects of stress and other factors, levels of ACTH show a wide normal range, from 10 to 80 pg/mL. Higher values are recorded in the early morning hours, and the lowest values occur at midnight.

CORTISOL

Over 20 different steroids have been identified in the venous effluent of the adrenal gland. The enzymes involved in steroid synthesis in the cortex are distributed in three different histologically identifiable zones: the glomerulosa (the outermost zone), the fasciculata (the middle zone), and the reticularis (the innermost zone). The practical result of this distribution is that certain enzymes are found only in one zone, so that the synthesis of an adrenal hormone requiring that enzyme will be limited to the zone that has that enzyme. Thus cortisol synthesis occurs primarily in the fasciculata zone but also in the other two zones, whereas aldosterone synthesis occurs only in the glomerulosa zone.

Of the steroids secreted by the adrenal cortex, two have a singular importance: cortisol and aldosterone. All of the physiological actions of the adrenal hormones necessary to sustain life can be ascribed to these two hormones; after adrenalectomy, for example, the physiological functions of the adrenal gland can be taken over by exogenously administered cortisol and aldosterone.

The effects of the adrenal steroids on metabolism have been traditionally classified as either glucocorticoid, if carbohydrate metabolism is primarily affected, or as mineralocorticoid, if mineral metabolism is primarily affected. In this schema, cortisol, having its most pronounced effects on carbohydrate metabolism, is the prime glucocorticoid. It has effects on protein and lipid metabolism as well. Aldosterone has only very minor glucocorticoid activity and is the adrenal glands' major mineralocorticoid. Corticosterone, another major secretory product of the adrenal gland in terms of the amount secreted, has both glucocorticoid activity, (but less than cortisol) and mineralocorticoid activity (but less than aldosterone).

Of the hormones secreted by the adrenal, cortisol is also secreted in the largest amount, from 5 to 30 mg per day. This can be compared to the 0.8 to 10 mg of corticosterone and the 0.05 to 0.25 mg of aldosterone secreted per day.

A singular, functional relationship between the adrenal steroids arises out of their sharing some common steps of the biosynthetic pathway. Although the amounts of the adrenal steroids, other than cortisol, corticosterone, and aldosterone, secreted by the cortex are relatively miniscule and the physiological effects of these other steroids relatively insignificant under normal physiological circumstances, perturbations may occur, as in disease. In some cases this leads to overproduction of these other adrenal steroids so that their physiological effects become significant. In a similar manner, ACTH, which affects cortisol and other adrenal steroids, when it is secreted by the pituitary or by an ectopic source in excessive amounts, can lead to production of these less important steroids in amounts that can have significant physiological effects.

The clinical importance of the increased output of these minor adrenal steroids outside of cortisol and aldosterone is that some of them, like dehydroepiandrosterone and androstenedione, have weak androgenic effects, but may be converted in the periphery to testosterone and estradiol. The recognition that in certain disease states the androgenic and/or estrogenic effects produced could be ascribed to the increased output of these minor steroids led to their descriptive classification as adrenal androgens or adrenal estrogens.

Characterization and biosynthesis

Cortisol shares with other steroids the cyclopentanoperhydrophenanthrene nucleus; its chemical name is 11-β, 17-α, 21-trihydroxy, delta-4, pregnene 3,20-dione (Figs. 16-6 and 16-7). Before its chemical structure was elucidated, cortisol was referred to as compound F, and reference to this name still appears in the literature. An alternate, less frequently used name for cortisol is hydrocortisone. Because of the conjugated double bond structure formed by the keto group on carbon atom 3 and the double bond between carbon atoms 4 and 5, cortisol absorbs ultraviolet light. The 11-beta hydroxyl group is held to be necessary for its glucocorticoid activity.

Cholesterol serves as the ultimate precursor for cortisol and the other steroids synthesized by the adrenal cortex. The first step in this synthesis, the conversion of the 27-carbon atom cholesterol to the 21-carbon atom pregnenolone by cleavage from cholesterol of a 6-carbon atom side chain, has been shown to be under ACTH control. Pregnenolone, the end product, becomes the common precursor of all of the C-21 adrenal steroids (Fig. 16-8).

Two pathways lead from pregnenolone to cortisol. In the first pathway, pregnenolone is hydroxylated by a 17 α-hydroxylase to 17 α-hydroxypregnenolone, which is then converted to 17 α-progesterone by the action of a 3-β-ol-dehydrogenase, δ-4,5 isomerase. In the alternate pathway, the isomerase can act directly on pregnenolone to yield progesterone, which in turn can be the substrate for the 17 α-hydroxylase, yielding the same product as the other pathway, 17 α-hydroxyprogesterone. The pathway that includes 17 α-hydroxypregnenolone is commonly referred to as the delta-5 pathway, the double bond is between carbon atoms 5 and 6, and is the pathway leading to the formation of the adrenal androgens and estrogens. The pathway from pregnenolone to progesterone is commonly referred to as the delta-4 pathway, the double bond is between carbon atoms 4 and 5, leading to the formation of cortisol, corticosterone, and aldosterone (Fig. 16-8).

The addition of two more hydroxyl groups is required for the synthesis of cortisol from 17 α-hydroxyprogesterone. The first hydroxyl is added by a 21-hydroxylase to yield 11-deoxycortisol; the second hydroxyl is added to 11-deoxycortisol by an 11 β-hydroxylase.

Changes in this pathway may occur as a result of genetic derangements and may lead to clinically recognizable entities. Partial or total absence of any of the enzymes involved in cortisol synthesis has been identified as leading to the group of clinical syndromes known as congenital adrenal hyperplasia. If an enzyme is missing or decreased in activity, steroids before the enzymatic block may accumulate and lead to the stimulation of the pathway leading to the production of adrenal androgens and estrogens. The syndrome-produced results from the biological activities of the steroids produced in excess, coupled to the deficient activity of the steroids whose synthesis is deficient or blocked; of these, cortisol is underproduced, while the overproduction of estrogens for androgens leads to symptoms of femininization or virilization, respectively.

Cortisone, an analogue of cortisol having a keto group on carbon 11 instead of an hydroxyl group, is found in barely detectable amounts in the blood and has been identified as a minor secretory product of the adrenal. Synthetic cortisone is frequently administered when cortisol is required; it is readily reduced to cortisol in vivo in the periphery, in which form it is biologically active.

The liver is the main site for the metabolic degradation of cortisol; some 75% of it is cleared from the blood by a single passage through the liver. The first step in the degradation, the reduction of the double bond between carbon atoms 4 and 5, is enough to terminate the physiological activity of the hormone. The further chemical modifications of the cortisol structure, by a series of enzymatic reductions, oxidations, hydroxylations, and conjugations, converts cortisol into more readily water-soluble metabolites that are easily excreted into the urine. A large portion of the metabolites of cortisol are excreted as glucuronides, with a lesser amount as sulfates. The large number of cortisol metabolites appearing in the urine, over 20 have been identified, arise in part from the formation of alpha and beta metabolites at asymmetric carbon atoms. Only about 1% of cortisol escapes metabolic inactivation and appears in the urine as unchanged cortisol. The determination of 17-hydroxycorticosteroids and 17-ketogenic steroids in the urine is based on these multiple metabolites of cortisol in the urine.

Factors that affect secretion

Of the cortisol that appears in the circulation, about 75% circulates tightly bound to a specific cortisol-binding glob-

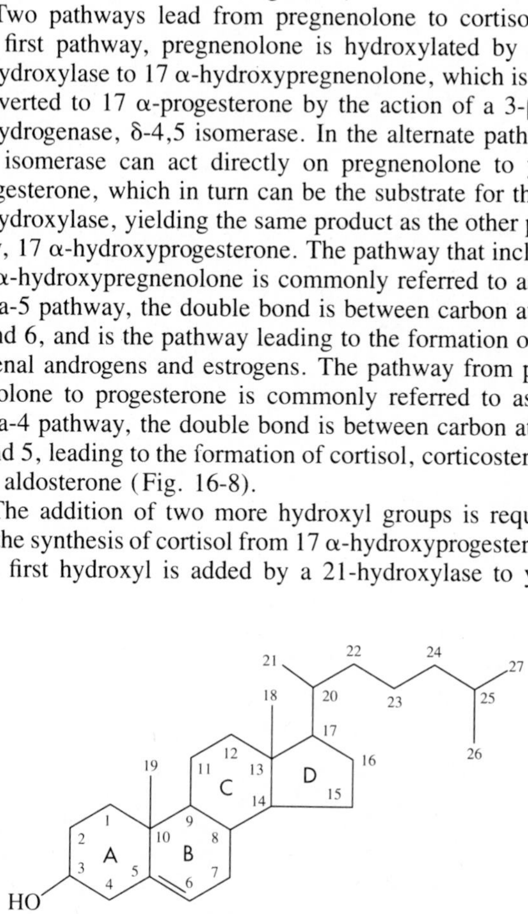

Fig. 16-6 Numbering of the basic steroid nucleus. Rings A, B, C, and D form the cyclopentanoperhydrophenanthrene nucleus.

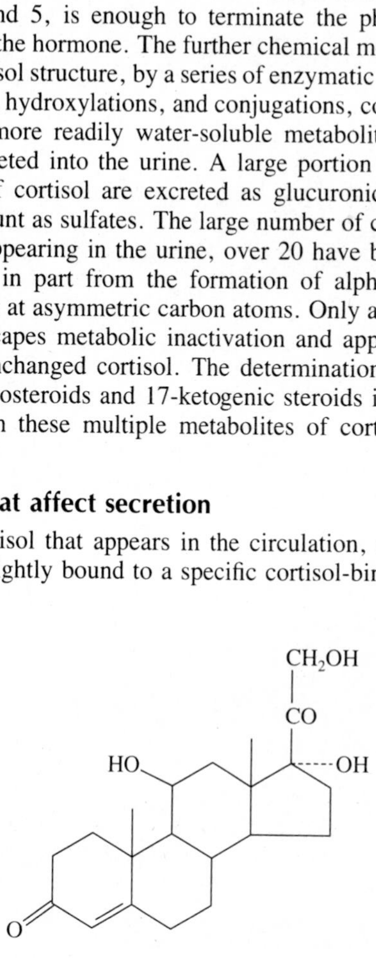

Fig. 16-7 The structure of cortisol.

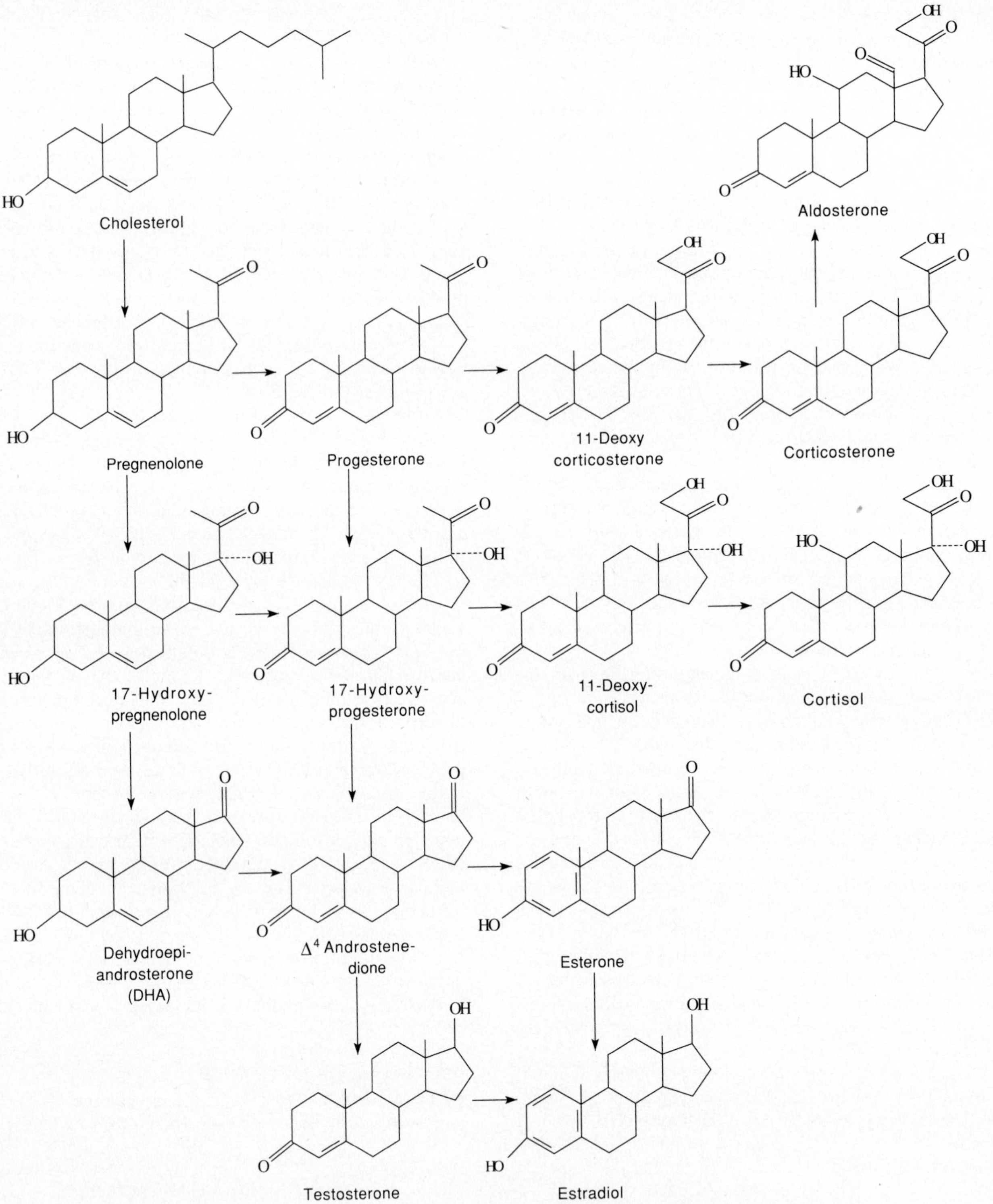

Fig. 16-8   The biosynthesis of cortisol from cholesterol and the biosynthetic pathways for the other adrenal steroids.

ulin, called corticosteroid-binding globulin (CBG) or transcortin. About 15% of the cortisol in the circulation is loosely and nonspecifically bound to albumin, whereas approximately 10% is unbound, that is, it circulates as "free" cortisol. It is this free cortisol that makes up the biologically active form of the hormone. The free form is in equilibrium with the protein-bound forms, so that as free cortisol enters

the tissues, it is replaced by cortisol, which dissociates from the protein-bound forms. The protein-bound forms thus not only represent a reservoir of available cortisol, but also prolong its stay in the blood, as protein-bound forms cannot be taken up by tissues such as the liver.

At normal plasma concentrations of cortisol, transcortin has unoccupied binding sites, so that despite slight elevations in total plasma cortisol, plasma values remain essentially unchanged and no effects of hypercortisolemia are evident. Increased estrogens produced during pregnancy, as well as exogenously administered estrogens, induce an increased synthesis of transcortin. Thus, during pregnancy, the increased amounts of transcortin easily bind the extra cortisol produced, so that the elevated total plasma cortisol does not result in an increase in the free, physiologically active form of the hormone.

The plasma half-life of cortisol is 80 to 90 minutes. The volume of distribution approximates the extracellular fluid volume (about 30 L) and the metabolic clearance rate is 200 to 250 L per day.

The secretion of cortisol by the adrenal cortex is subject to a diurnal rhythm; the amount secreted peaks at about 5 AM just before waking, then decreases throughout the day and night. On top of this diurnal variation, the secretion of cortisol is episodic; in other words, it is secreted in short bursts that are minutes apart, rather than in one continuous low concentration value from the adrenal. The practical effect of this episodic, diurnal secretion is a pronounced difference in the cortisol values in blood samples taken at different times during the day. A random sample has no diagnostic value. In most laboratories this problem is obviated by drawing samples for comparison at the same time each day. Usually, a sample is taken at 8 AM to reflect the peak plasma concentration, then another sample is taken late in the evening (6 PM to 8 PM) to reflect the trough of the plasma. Such a two-sample technique also confirms the presence of a diurnal rhythm; an elevated PM cortisol value would lead to suspicion of a persistent output of cortisol.

Biological actions and pathophysiology

The physiological effects of cortisol on the organism are widespread—almost every tissue/organ system in the body is affected—although the effects on some tissues are more direct and pronounced so that they may be more correctly referred to as target tissues. The varied effects of cortisol result from actions on carbohydrate metabolism, as well as protein, lipid, and nucleic acid metabolism. In addition, a number of less-defined effects such as the maintenance of cardiovascular tone and volume and the modification of emotional behavior are also seen (Box 16-13).

Cortisol is believed to enter cells by simple diffusion; specific receptors for cortisol, when they have been found, are located in the cytoplasm. After combining with its receptor, the cortisol-receptor complex is activated—a conformational change occurs that increases the affinity of the complex for DNA. The complex is transported to the nucleus, where it combines with an acceptor site on chromatin. This binding stimulates the activation of certain genes, leading to increased messenger RNA (mRNA) synthesis. Translation of the mRNA in the cytoplasm results in increased protein synthesis. The proteins whose synthesis is induced appear to be primarily enzymes, and it is through such modulation of enzyme activity that cortisol is believed to exert its biological effects.

Along with glucagon, growth hormone, and epinephrine, cortisol shares an anti-insulin activity resulting from its ability to promote increases in blood glucose. This is accomplished by promotion of the uptake and conversion of amino acids by the liver into glucose and by the simultaneous

---

Box 16-13 Biological actions of cortisol

STIMULATES

Liver and muscle glycogen depositions
Increase in blood glucose
Resistance to insulin
Lipolysis
Mobilization of amino acids to liver
Hepatic synthesis of selected enzymes
Skeletal muscle breakdown
Renal sodium retention
Renal potassium excretion
Glomerular filtration rate
Intestinal absorption of calcium

OTHER ACTIONS

Maintenance of cardiovascular tone and volume
Necessary for growth
Maintenance of normal renal hemodynamics
Redistribution of body fat
Modification of emotional behavior

INHIBITS

Peripheral utilization of glucose
Number of circulation lymphocytes (both T and B cells)
Circulating eosinophils

---

inhibition of the uptake and oxidation of glucose by cells. In tissues such as muscle, bone, skin, and connective tissue, cortisol promotes the breakdown of protein into amino acids and the mobilization of these amino acids to the liver. In these same tissues, protein synthesis and the uptake of amino acids is inhibited as well.

Whereas in the tissues just mentioned, protein synthesis and the uptake of amino acids is inhibited, in the liver, cortisol promotes the synthesis of some selective proteins, primarily enzymes. Tryptophan pyrrolase and tyrosine amino transferase are two enzymes whose synthesis is induced by cortisol. As part of this induction, the hepatic synthesis of mRNA is increased by cortisol, whereas in other tissues, this synthesis is inhibited.

The actions of cortisol on lipid metabolism are less understood; in some subtle way, cortisol affects lipid distribution. This affect on lipid distribution is seen in an exaggerated way in patients with profound Cushing's syndrome as truncal obesity and a characteristic "buffalo hump."

The anti-inflammatory effect of cortisol is taken advantage of clinically to suppress the undesirable side effects of inflammation that accompany many allergies and arthritis, as well as other diseases. A variety of synthetic glucocorticoids have been produced with the objective of enhancing the anti-inflammatory activity of these molecules at the expense of the glucocorticoid activity.

Patients with high cortisol values routinely show decreased resistance to infection. The explanation for this effect is not clear, but may arise from the ability of cortisol to modulate in some way, cell-mediated immunity and perhaps antibody production as well. Administration of cortisol or other glucocorticoids is known to produce a decrease in eosinophils and T-cells, while producing an increase in polymorphonuclear leukocytes.

Even with pharmacological doses of cortisol, the mineralocorticoid activity of cortisol is weak. In a generalized fashion, cortisol decreases water intake by cells and in the kidney it increases glomerular filtration. By this action it suppresses antidiuretic hormone secretion. Renal sodium reabsorption and potassium excretion are increased with pharmacological doses.

Some of the least understood effects of cortisol relate to stress and to its physiological and psychological effects. In the absence of cortisol, stress may produce hypertension that can be fatal. Either in the presence of excess cortisol, as in patients with Cushing's syndrome, or in its absence, as in patients with Addison's disease, cortisol can produce pronounced changes in mood and behavior.

Through its control of ACTH secretion by the pituitary by means of corticotropin releasing hormone (CRH), the hypothalamus integrates cortisol secretion by the adrenal according to the needs of the organism. When cortisol concentrations are high, the sensitivity of the pituitary to hypothalamic CRH is reduced, so that less ACTH is synthesized and secreted by the pituitary. When cortisol concentrations decrease, the pituitary sensitivity to CRH is increased and more ACTH is secreted. The secreted ACTH stimulates the adrenal cortex to increase its output of cortisol. Cortisol is thus a critical element in the feedback relationship between the hypothalamus, the pituitary, and the adrenal. There is some evidence that cortisol may have a direct feedback effect on the hypothalamus and may also affect higher nerve centers that affect the hypothalamus.

With respect to their production of cortisol, diseases of the adrenal cortex are conveniently categorized as resulting in either adrenal cortical hypofunction or adrenal cortical hyperfunction. These states are further described as primary, if the defect is in the adrenal cortex itself, or as secondary, if they result from a defect outside of the adrenal gland. They are further characterized as chronic, occurring over a period of time, or as acute, of sudden or short onset.

Primary adrenal insufficiency (hypofunction) results from the destruction of the adrenal cortex and is referred to as Addison's disease. A large variety of agents that can cause gradual or acute destruction of the cortex have been identified. Probably most common is autoimmune destruction, followed by tuberculosis. Hemorrhage, cytotoxic agents, metastatic tumors, fungal agents, and surgery may also be causative agents. Usually about 90% of the cortex has to be affected for clinical symptoms to appear. Cortisol concentrations in plasma may be at normal values up until almost complete destruction of the gland. Adrenocorticotropic hormone acts as a maximum stimulus to the decreasing amounts of tissue remaining. The destruction of the adrenal can occur over several months depending on the agent, or it can occur more quickly as a result of some direct insult (e.g., acute hemorrhage). In acute cases symptoms may be brought on by stress. In most patients a generalized hyperpigmentation resulting from the elevated ACTH is noted and is a diagnostic feature. Other symptoms include hypotension, weight loss, anorexia, weakness, and fatigue.

Primary adrenal insufficiency is much more common in females than in males.

Decreased production of ACTH by the pituitary, from whatever cause, will lead to secondary adrenal insufficiency. The use of exogenous steroids may lead to the suppression of ACTH output by the pituitary; their rapid withdrawal may precipitate symptoms of cortisol deficiency. Tumors of the hypothalamus or the pituitary may also lead to ACTH suppression. An important difference between primary and secondary adrenal insufficiency is provided by the blood ACTH concentration, which in primary insufficiency may be elevated; in secondary insufficiency, blood concentrations of ACTH may be significantly decreased. The hyperpigmentation routinely seen with primary adrenal insufficiency due to excess ACTH is not seen in secondary adrenal insufficiency.

Chronic oversecretion of cortisol by the adrenal with resultant hypercortisolemia leads to a group of related disease entities included under Cushing's syndrome. In patients with Cushing's syndrome the physiological effects of cortisol are frequently displayed in an exaggerated form. Many patients have an altered fat distribution evidenced by truncal obesity, a "moon face" and a buffalo hump. In females, menstrual disorders and hirsutism are common. Psychological changes, mainly altered mood, muscular weakness, and back pain are also common.

Only a small percentage, about 15% to 20% of the cases of Cushing's syndrome, can be traced to the adrenal cortex itself as the primary cause of the cortisol hypersecretion. Tumors secreting cortisol, both adenomas and carcinomas, are usually responsible. In patients with such adrenal tumors, blood cortisol concentrations, as well as urinary free cortisol, are elevated, whereas ACTH values are suppressed by the elevated cortisol.

A variety of tumors ectopically secreting ACTH have also been identified as a cause of some cases of Cushing's syndrome; tumors of the lung, such as oat cell carcinomas, are the most important. In patients with ectopic ACTH secreting tumors, the blood concentrations of both ACTH and cortisol are elevated, because the autonomously secreted ACTH is not suppressed by the elevated cortisol.

Pituitary tumors, primarily microadenomas, may also produce excess ACTH and overstimulate the adrenal to produce excess cortisol. When Cushing's syndrome is traceable to a pituitary tumor, it is referred to as Cushing's disease. Patients with Cushing's disease may have normal to elevated ACTH values with their elevated plasma cortisol concentrations and elevated urinary free cortisol values. Differentiation of Cushing's disease from the syndrome caused by ectopic ACTH secretion is usually based on the dexamethasone suppression test. In Cushing's disease, dexamethasone will usually suppress ACTH to less than 50% of the baseline value, whereas in Cushing's syndrome ectopic ACTH is not suppressed by dexamethasone.

Analyte measurement and function testing

Before the advent of RIA, a large clinical experience was gained with the use of chemical assays for steroids, which usually measured several related steroids as a group rather than as a single compound. Because of the clinical utility of this experience, reference is still made in the literature to values obtained by these methods, which are still available from most reference laboratories. A short description of the more common methods follows.

To assess either adrenal hypo- or hyperfunction, levels of urinary steroids bearing a 17-keto group (17-ketosteroids, or 17-KS) were measured by means of the Zimmerman reaction, which involved treating a urinary extract with a strongly alkaline solution of meta-dinitrobenzene. The 17-KS were frequently found to be low in adrenal insufficiency and high in Cushing's disease, but were unreliable diagnostic indices. The 17-KS measured by the Zimmerman reaction are derived primarily from steroids secreted by the gonads and only about 10% of the cortisol produced daily is metabolized to 17-KS. Thus measurement of 17-KS is not a good indicator of adrenocortical function. It is of value, however, in diagnosing patients with an adrenal tumor causing either Cushing's syndrome or the adrenogenital syndrome; in each case excessive amounts of 17-KS are excreted into the urine.

A number of urinary steroids possessing the dihydroxyacetone side chain can be similarly measured as a group by the Porter-Silber reaction, which involves treatment of a urinary extract with phenylhydrazine in strong sulfuric acid. The urinary steroids thus measured are referred to as 17-hydroxycorticosteroids (17-OHCS), or as urinary Porter-Silber chromogens. It has been estimated that about 30% of the urinary metabolites of cortisol are measured by this reaction. Despite drawbacks in the methodology due to low specificity and interferences from various drugs, measurement of 17-OHCS has proven most useful for diagnosing hypo- and hyperfunction of the adrenal. When applied to extracts of plasma, the reaction is specific and primarily measures cortisol and cortisone. The use of the Porter-Silber reaction to measure either plasma cortisol or urinary 17-OHCS has been largely supplanted by RIA.

A larger fraction of the urinary metabolites of cortisol than that measured by the Porter-Silber reaction can be measured by determining the level of 17-ketogenic steroids, or 17-KGS. For this determination urine extracts are first treated with periodate, which oxidatively cleaves off the side chain of C-21 steroids containing a hydroxyl group on carbon 17 and 20, to give 17-ketosteroids. The 17-KS produced are then measured by the Zimmerman reaction. To remove any preformed 17-KS, the urine extracts are treated with borohydride prior to oxidation with periodate. The measurement of 17-KGS is favored by some investigators over the measurement of 17-OHCS because a larger fraction of cortisol metabolites are measured, but the determination has drawbacks similar to those indicated for 17-OHCS.

Radioimmunoassay is the current preferred method for the measurement of plasma cortisol and is used as well for the measurement of urinary free cortisol. Radioimmunoassay procedures require no plasma or urine extraction and are straightforward to perform. Except for a cross-reactivity with cortisone, the antibodies used in the assays have no significant cross-reactivity with any other steroids. The convenience of RIAs makes them critical elements of the various function tests described shortly. Cortisol can also be measured by fluorescence polarization and by high-performance liquid chromatography (HPLC).

Since the adrenal gland functions as part of the hypothalamic-pituitary-adrenal axis, finding that a plasma cor-

tisol value is either elevated or depressed gives no indication as to which part of this system is malfunctioning. In addition, it must be kept in mind that because plasma cortisol values are subject to diurnal variation because cortisol is episodically secreted and because about 85% of the cortisol in plasma is transported bound to protein, either to transcortin or albumin, large variations in plasma cortisol concentrations occur and frequently overlap with normal values. Both suppression and stimulation tests are used to better pinpoint alterations in the component function of the hypothalamic-pituitary-adrenal axis.

The synthetic glucocorticoid dexamethasone (Fig. 16-9) is used in a suppression test to determine whether or not the inhibitory effect of glucocorticoids on CRF secretion by the hypothalamus or ACTH secretion by the pituitary is intact. Dexamethasone, a more potent glucocorticoid than cortisol so that it can be given in a small dose, has this inhibitory effect like cortisol. An added advantage is that it does not react in any of the RIAs for cortisol. In response to the dexamethasone, normal individuals will show a decrease in both plasma cortisol and ACTH and the urinary excretion of cortisol and its metabolites will fall as well. Several modifications of the test have been made to enhance the diagnosis of Cushing's syndrome and to help in differentiating between the different forms of the disease. Single-dose screening tests, low- and high-dose overnight tests, and multiple-dose suppression tests have been developed. Determination of the plasma cortisol value at specified times, as well as of urinary free cortisol, forms an integral part of the dexamethasone suppression test and its modifications.

The metyrapone test is a functional test used to evaluate adrenal reserve, that is, to measure the ability of the adrenal cortex to synthesize and secrete cortisol in response to an increased ACTH stimulus. Metyrapone (Fig. 16-10) is an inhibitor of the enzyme hydroxylating the 11 position of deoxycortisol, the immediate precursor of cortisol. Because

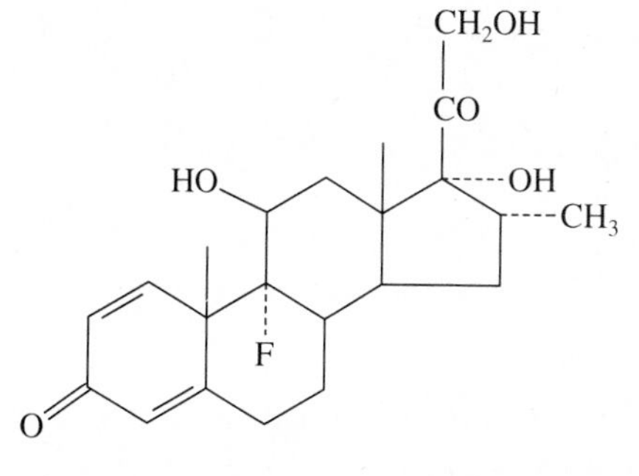

Fig. 16-9   Structure of dexamethasone.

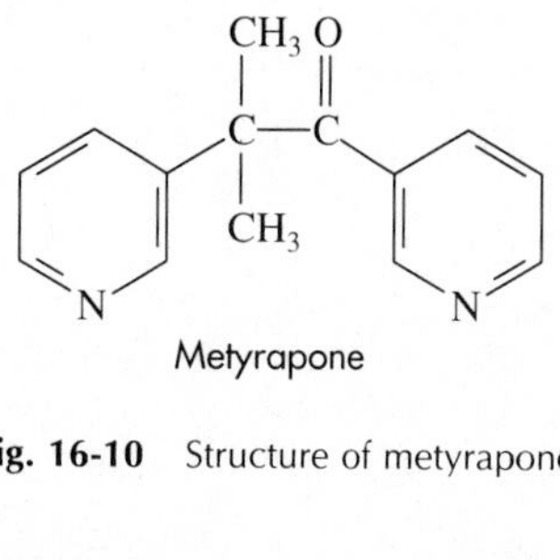

Metyrapone

Fig. 16-10   Structure of metyrapone.

this inhibition results in a lower value of plasma cortisol, ACTH secretion by the pituitary is enhanced. In turn, the increased ACTH stimulates the adrenal to produce more cortisol. Since cortisol synthesis is blocked by metyrapone, however, 11-deoxycortisol is produced instead in larger than normal amounts and concentrations in blood increase as do its urinary metabolites. 11-Deoxycortisol is easily measured in blood and urine by RIA.

A series of diagnostic algorithms have been developed to diagnose and differentiate between the enzyme defects in cortisol synthesis that give rise to the syndrome of congenital adrenal hyperplasia (CAH). Depending on the magnitude of the enzyme deficiency, cortisol secretion may be depressed or compensation may be provided by an increased secretion of ACTH, which stimulates the adrenal cortex to produce excessive amounts of steroids proximal to the enzyme defect. The algorithms developed make heavy use of various stimulation and suppression tests, coupled with plasma and urinary steroid determinations. A standard textbook of endocrinology should be consulted for a detailed description of these tests.

OXYTOCIN
Characterization and biosynthesis

Oxytocin is synthesized by the same cluster of neuronal cells in the hypothalamus, the supraoptic and paraventricular nuclei, that are responsible for the synthesis of vasopressin. Like vasopressin, oxytocin is cleaved from a larger precursor molecule, proneurophysin, and is stored in axon terminals in the posterior pituitary. Upon neural stimulation, oxytocin is readily released into the circulation in a one-to-one ratio with its binding protein, neurophysin I. In the circulation it is found in the free form, not bound to its neurophysin or to any other protein.

Structurally, oxytocin also resembles vasopressin, in that it is a peptide of nine amino acids, with two cysteine residues, residues 1 and 6, connected by a disulfide bond. The structure of oxytocin and vasopressin differ in the position of two amino acids; leucine makes up residue 3 in oxytocin (phenylalanine in vasopressin) and residue 8 is isoleucine (arginine in vasopressin).

Factors that affect secretion

Stimulation of the nipple area of the breast, such as by suckling, originates neural signals that reach the central nervous system (CNS) and result in the release of oxytocin from neurovesicles in the posterior pituitary into the circulation.

In the circulation oxytocin occurs in the free form, not bound to any protein, with a very short half-life of about 5 minutes. As with vasopressin, the liver (primarily) and the kidney are responsible for removing oxytocin from the circulation.

Biological actions and pathophysiology

The primary and perhaps only important physiological action of oxytocin appears to be exerted on the myoepithelial cells surrounding the mammary alveoli. Oxytocin causes contraction of these cells, resulting in milk ejection. During pregnancy, the sensitivity of the uterus to oxytocin increases, but there is no indication that oxytocin plays any role in either the onset or maintenance of labor.

Several biological actions, such as increasing the concentration of blood glucose, decreasing plasma free fatty acids, an antidiuretic effect, and the ability to constrict smooth muscle have been ascribed to oxytocin, but these have been observed only with doses of oxytocin that are far greater than physiological. For example, the antidiuretic effect of oxytocin is only 5% that of vasopressin. For this reason it is generally conceded that oxytocin under normal physiological conditions has no known biological activity outside of its effect on mammary myoepithelial cells.

Clinically, synthetic oxytocin is administered intramuscularly or by slow intravenous drip under prescribed conditions to initiate or augment labor. As a nasal spray (it is readily absorbed through the nasal mucosa), oxytocin is effective in promoting milk ejection if milk synthesis (promoted by prolactin) is not impaired.

Analyte measurement and function testing

Radioimmunoassay for oxytocin is available but has little if any clinical use outside of a research setting. Normal circulating levels appear to be less than 1 to 2 μU/mL.

ANTIDIURETIC HORMONE (VASOPRESSIN)
Characterization and biosynthesis

The posterior lobe of the pituitary serves as a storage organ for the hormones vasopressin (also called arginine vasopressin, AVP, or antidiuretic hormone, ADH) and oxytocin, which are synthesized in the hypothalamus, specifically in the neurons of the supraoptic and paraventricular nuclei. The axon terminals of these neurons extend down into the posterior pituitary and there are interwoven in a network with secretory granules and capillaries. Upon appropriate stimulation, the stored vasopressin and oxytocin are released from the storage granules into the capillaries and enter the systemic circulation.

Because the posterior pituitary is a neural extension of the hypothalamus, some authors question whether or not the posterior pituitary should be considered a separate endocrine gland. Because of its neural makeup, the posterior pituitary is referred to as the neurohypophysis.

Vasopressin is synthesized in cell bodies of neurons that are distinct from those synthesizing oxytocin. It is a peptide of nine amino acids that is first synthesized as part of a larger, inactive prohormone molecule, propressophysin, having a mass of 20,000 daltons. The propressophysin contains a signal peptide at its amino terminal joined to vasopressin, which in turn is joined to an approximately 10,000 dalton carrier protein called neurophysin II, followed by a glycosylated peptide at its carboxy terminal end (Fig. 16-11). Oxytocin originates in a similar molecule, except that its prohormone is not glycosylated and the carrier protein is different (neurophysin I).

Once synthesized, vasopressin is transported down the neuronal axons along with its carrier protein neurophysin II and is stored in the granules of the neurohypophysis along with it. For each molecule of vasopressin secreted into the circulation, one molecule of neurophysin II is also secreted, but in the plasma, vasopressin circulates in a free state unbound to the neurophysin II.

Six of the nine amino acids making up vasopressin are part of a ring structure formed by a disulfide bond formed between the two cysteine residues (Fig. 16-12). The three

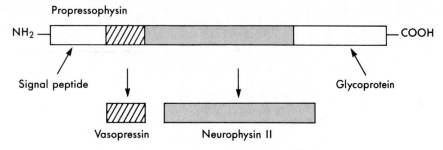

Fig. 16-11 Vasopressin and its precursor, propressophysin.

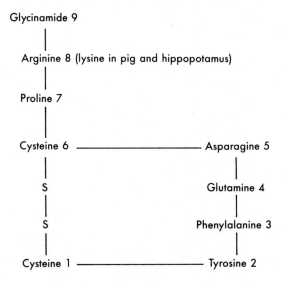

Fig. 16-12 Structure of vasopressin.

remaining amino acids may be visualized as forming a side chain on this ring structure. In humans and in all other species except the pig and hippopotamus, the amino acid in position 8 is arginine; this form is referred to arginine vasopressin (AVP). Lysine vasopressin, with a lysine substituting for the arginine, is the form of the hormone in the pig and hippopotamus.

Factors that affect secretion

Under physiological conditions, secretion of ADH is primarily and acutely sensitive to changes in the osmolality of the extracellular fluid that is in equilibrium with the plasma. The secretion of ADH is altered in response to small changes in plasma osmolality so that under normal physiological conditions, plasma osmolality is maintained within the rather narrow limits of 285 to 295 mOsmol/kg of body water. Changes in the osmolality around a given set point (which varies for each individual) are sensed by a group of osmoreceptors, which are specialized neurons located in the lateral hypothalamus. These receptors are anatomically close to, but separate from, the neurons that make up the supraoptic nuclei. These receptors are sensitive to changes in plasma osmolality as small as 1% to 2%. The percentage value varies among individuals. Infusions of hypertonic saline will quickly lead to an increase in ADH secretion, which suppresses renal water excretion, whereas infusions of hypotonic saline or water loading will suppress ADH secretion, leading to water diuresis.

Box 16-14 Factors affecting the secretion of vasopressin

STIMULI	INHIBITORS
Nausea	Alcohol
Nicotine	α-Adrenergic agents
Stress	Glucocorticoids
Pain	Lithium
Hypotension	Demeclocycline
Decreased blood volume	Hypoosmolality
Hyperosmolality	Blood volume expansion
Hot environment	Exposure to cold
Analgesics	Increased blood pressure
Diuretics	
Chlorpromazine	
Carbamazepine	
Barbiturates	
β-Adrenergic agents	
Morphine	
Clofibrate	
Angiotensin II	
Phenothiazines	
Prostaglandin E	
Vincristine	
Ferritin	

As plasma osmolality increases, secretion of ADH also increases, but at an osmolality of about 295 mOsmol/kg of water, the secretion of ADH becomes maximal and no further urine concentration is possible. The elevation of the plasma osmolality to this point triggers thirst receptors, specialized neurons located in the ventral hypothalamus. These thirst receptors, also in close proximity to the supraoptic and paraventricular nuclei but separate from them, send impulses to the cerebral cortex, which increases drinking behavior and water intake. The thirst receptors are different and separate from the osmoreceptors. In concert, the hypothalamus integrates the interplay of the osmoreceptors, the thirst receptors, and the secretion of ADH by the posterior pituitary to maintain water homeostasis.

The osmoreceptors do not respond equally to different osmotically active solutes. Sodium and chloride are potent stimulators of ADH release, as is sucrose, but glucose, urea, and glycerol are not. The reason for this difference is not clear.

As can be seen in Box 16-14, a large variety of other nonosmotic factors can influence ADH secretion, acting as either stimuli or inhibitors, some of which deserve special comment. Prominent among these factors are a decrease in total or effective blood volume and a decrease in blood pressure. It has been recognized for a long time that a change in posture from supine to upright results in increased ADH secretion and a decrease in urine flow. Under physiological conditions, blood volume and osmoreceptors are thought to act synergistically, but with the osmoreceptors being more sensitive than the volume receptors. A reduction of blood volume of about 10% and a fall in blood pressure of about 5% are needed to alter ADH release; both changes are greater than the percent change in osmolality needed to alter ADH secretion. Blood volume and blood pressure changes modify ADH release without changes in osmolality. The ability of some drugs, such as diuretics, isoproterenol, histamine, morphine, and nicotine to stimulate ADH is believed to reflect their ability to either lower the blood pressure or volume. Drugs such as alcohol, glucocorticoids, clonidine, and carbamazepine, which inhibit ADH release, also act through their effects on blood pressure and volume.

A most potent stimulus of ADH release is nausea; nausea with or without vomiting can quickly elevate the plasma ADH level more than a hundredfold. Cold exposure inhibits, whereas a hot climate stimulates ADH release. Stress, either emotional or physical, will also stimulate ADH release.

In the plasma ADH circulates in the free form, not bound to protein or neurophysin, but it circulates in equimolar amounts to neurophysin II. No biological activity has been found for neurophysin; it can be readily measured in plasma by immunoassay as an indirect measure of ADH. The volume of distribution of ADH approximates closely the extracellular fluid volume. The half-life of ADH in plasma is short, between 4 and 20 minutes. Most of the metabolic clearance of ADH from the plasma occurs in the liver, some in the kidney. A small percentage escapes metabolic degradation and appears unchanged in the urine. During pregnancy, the placenta gives rise to an active aminopeptidase, which rapidly degrades ADH.

Biological actions and pathophysiology

The primary and principal target organ for ADH is the kidney, specifically, the distal tubules and the collecting ducts. The primary function of ADH at these target sites is the conservation of water needed to maintain homeostasis. The efficiency of this system is such that humans can maintain water homeostasis despite the large number of factors that can alter ADH secretion, whether or not positively or negatively and despite the huge variation in water intake, which can range from as little as 500 mL to 20,000 mL per day.

In the absence of ADH the cellular membranes lining the distal tubule and collecting ducts are impermeable to water and solutes. In the process of urine formation after an intake of water, by the time the protein-free glomerular filtrate enters the distal tubule and the collecting ducts, solute reabsorption and secretion required to maintain the osmolality of plasma has already taken place along with the reabsorption of water, producing a slightly hypotonic urine.

In the presence of ADH, on the other hand, the water permeability of these membranes is increased in proportion to the plasma ADH concentration, so that water reabsorption can take place and the urine being formed can become hyperosmotic (concentrated) in relation to the plasma and

have a small volume. In humans, the maximum concentrating ability of the kidney is approximately 1200 mOsmol/kg body water, a threefold increase over plasma osmolality.

These actions of ADH on the renal tubule are apparently mediated through one specific type of receptor (V_2) and cyclic AMP. A second type of cellular receptor (V_1) is involved in the pressor response to ADH and is mediated by cellular calcium ion transport. However, the concentration of ADH needed to raise blood pressure by constriction of vascular smooth muscle is roughly 10 times that needed to produce maximal diuresis, so that no role in normal blood pressure regulation is ascribed to ADH.

Some axons of the cell bodies synthesizing ADH in the supraoptic and paraventricular nuclei do not reach the posterior pituitary; this ADH may be released into the portal circulation and thus reach the anterior pituitary instead. In this locale, ADH acts to enhance the activity of CRF on ACTH release.

Other minor activities of ADH not associated with the kidney include involvement in platelet aggregation and stimulation of hepatic glycogenolysis. The overall effect of these actions on homeostasis is not clear.

The narrow range of plasma osmolality is maintained by the hypothalamus integrating the secretion of ADH with signals from osmoreceptors and the thirst receptor. Either a primary defect in the operation of any one part of this system or a secondary effect produced on any part of it by an unassociated metabolic defect can lead to clinically recognizable hypoosmolar and hyperosmolar states.

Diabetes insipidus (DI), the classical example of a hyperosmolar state, is characterized by the excretion of large volumes of dilute urine, polyuria. This condition is usually associated with the intake of large volumes of water, polydipsia. Polyuria and DI are generally regarded as synonymous. To be classified as polyuria, urine output has to be greater than 2500 mL per day for at least two consecutive days. Three different types of DI, each presenting with the same symptoms of polyuria and polydipsia, and not distinguishable from each other on this basis, are differentiated instead on the basis of their differing origins.

Hypothalamic DI, also called neurogenic, central, or cranial DI, results from partial or complete failure of ADH secretion in the presence of normal osmotic stimuli. Many of these cases arise from trauma to the neurohypophysis, either from some sort of physical trauma, such as a blunt head injury, or from the trauma of neurosurgery in the region of the posterior pituitary. In most of the trauma-induced cases the DI is transient and may be as short as two or three days. Hypothalamic DI is frequently seen as a secondary result of some other disease capable of causing damage to the neurohypophyseal area, such as cranial tumors. In some patients with the disease, an autoimmune process may be operative, since in these patients antibodies to ADH have been demonstrated. In hypothalamic DI the plasma ADH concentration is low in relationship to the plasma osmolality; the thirst response is operative and responsible for the copious water intake needed to balance the copious water output of the kidney.

In the second type of DI, called nephrogenic or AVP- or ADH-resistant DI, circulating ADH values are normal or elevated. The kidney, because of a decreased sensitivity, fails to respond to ADH. Nephrogenic DI may be congenital;

when congenital, it is sex-linked and recessively inherited, but rare. It may also arise secondary to other diseases, such as polycystic disease or chronic renal failure, or it may result from the effects of certain drugs such as lithium, given for depression, or barbiturates. In patients with nephrogenic DI, the thirst response is normal.

In the third type of DI, also called primary or psychogenic polydipsia, the ingestion of large volumes of water by compulsive patients with no recognized defects of the neurohypophyseal system leads to large volumes of hypotonic urine. In these patients the large intake of water suppresses ADH release. The chronic ingestion of large volumes of water is known to lead to a decreasing responsiveness of the renal tubules to ADH.

A large number of diseases have associated with them disturbances of salt and water metabolism that leads to a hypoosmolar state with hyponatremia, plasma sodium ion concentration less than 125 mEq/L. In the majority of these cases, there is an increase in plasma ADH to which the lowered plasma osmolality can be ascribed. In turn, the increased secretion of ADH can be accounted for by the presence of some known stimulus of ADH secretion, so that the increased ADH is secondary to some other metabolic disturbance. This type of a hypoosmolar state is not infrequently seen in hospitalized patients. The secretion of ADH in these cases is described as inappropriate, because normally, even a slight lowering of plasma osmolality is sufficient to shut off ADH secretion.

In some 20% to 30% of these patients, however, there is a primary defect that directly leads to the increased ADH secretion. In this group of patients the extracellular fluid volume is normal despite the hypoosmolality, and urine osmolality is generally greater than that of the plasma. If other diagnostic criteria are fulfilled, these patients are classified as having the syndrome of inappropriate ADH secretion (SIAD or SIADH). The most common cause of SIADH is a neoplasm, most frequently an oat cell carcinoma of the lung that ectopically secretes ADH. This syndrome is also seen in some patients with inflammatory lung disease, such as pneumonia, or in patients with diseases of the central nervous system or with head trauma.

Analyte measurement and function testing

Before the availability of direct measurement of ADH by RIA, assessment of the ADH status of a patient was based on the evaluation of serum and urine osmolality, and the response of these two variables to tests that would stimulate ADH secretion, such as water deprivation or hypertonic saline injection. These tests would be immediately followed by an injection of desmopressin, a synthetic analogue of ADH, and again measurement of serum and urine osmolality. Along with a good clinical history, the physician could distinguish to some extent between hypothalamic DI, nephrogenic DI, and primary polydipsia, and gain some idea whether or not the secretion of ADH was inappropriate in some hypoosmolar states.

With the introduction of RIAs to measure ADH values, the diagnostic approach has not changed much. Since the assays are somewhat technically demanding, they have not become generally available even from large commercial laboratories and are still primarily used in research settings. In addition, the lower limit of sensitivity of these assays also

borders on, or is indistinguishable from, some of the low values seen in ADH deficiency states, making the assays of little value. However, when available, these assays give the clinician the means to relate ADH values to serum osmolalities in these dynamic tests.

In one modification of the standard 8-hour water deprivation test, from midnight on the day of the test the patient is allowed free access to water, but no coffee, tea, or cigarettes, all of which could stimulate ADH secretion. After a light breakfast, an indwelling catheter is inserted and for the following 8 hours the patient is not allowed any fluid intake. Serum osmolality is measured every hour; osmolality is also determined on urine collected every hour. At the end of 8 hours, the patient is given an intramuscular dose of desmopressin, then allowed free access to food and water.

In a normal patient in response to the water deprivation, serum osmolality will rise slightly, but not over 300 mOsmol/kg and the urine osmolality will generally be twice that of the plasma. In patients with DI, serum osmolality usually rises to a value greater than 300 mOsmol/kg, and the urine osmolality is less than that of the plasma.

After the injection of desmopressin, urine osmolality will increase in the patient with hypothalamic DI, since the kidney can react to the injected desmopressin. In the patient with nephrogenic DI, the kidney remains unresponsive to the injected desmopressin. Patients with primary polydipsia will have normal serum osmolalities at the beginning of the test, and will show no increase in urine osmolality after the desmopressin.

If assays for ADH are available, plasma samples are also assayed for ADH along with the osmolality. The plasma ADH value at a given serum osmolality is compared to the relationship between these two variables obtained from studies in normal individuals. Hypertonic saline infusion, which is a weaker ADH stimulus than water deprivation, may be used in similar tests to measure ADH responsiveness.

The normal range for plasma ADH determined by RIA is from 5 to 8 ng/mL. Blood is usually collected in chilled heparin tubes, and after precipitation of proteins with acetone and centrifugation, the supernatant is used for the assay. The lower limit of detection for these assays is about 1 pg/mL. Some patients who may have received a crude hypophyseal extract (Pitressin) for therapy may have antibodies to ADH that will interfere with the assay. Urinary assays of ADH are not useful to reflect plasma ADH variation because of the very large variation in the renal clearance of ADH.

ALDOSTERONE
Characterization and biosynthesis

Aldosterone shares with cortisol the steroid precursors cholesterol, pregnenolone, and progesterone from a common synthetic pathway (Fig. 16-8). Its biosynthesis diverges from that of cortisol by virtue of the fact that the cells of the glomerulosa do not contain the 17 α-hydroxylase needed for cortisol synthesis, and the cells of the fasciculata do not contain the 18-hydroxysteroid dehydrogenase needed for aldosterone synthesis. As a result of the physical separation of required enzymes, aldosterone synthesis is limited to the glomerulosa and cortisol synthesis does not occur there. By the same token, aldosterone is not synthesized in cells of the fasciculata.

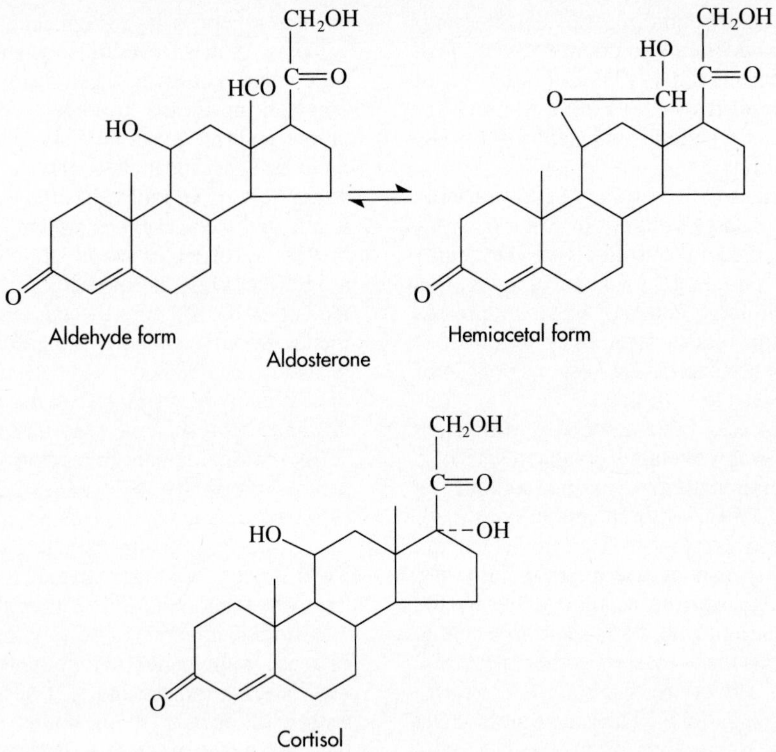

Fig. 16-13   The structure of aldosterone and cortisol.

Aldosterone shares with cortisol the 21-carbon atom pregnane nucleus but does not possess a 17 α-hydroxyl group like cortisol. Aldosterone is unique among naturally occurring steroids in having an aldehyde group in position 18 (Fig. 16-13). In solution (as in blood), the aldehyde group does not exist as the free aldehyde form but as a hemiacetal formed by reaction with the hydroxyl group on carbon 11.

Like cortisol, aldosterone is not stored in the adrenal cortex, but is synthesized and secreted in response to the stimulant action of angiotensin II. Once secreted into the circulation, most of the aldosterone is protein bound, primarily to transcortin, but it is not bound as firmly as is cortisol. About 5% to 10% of the aldosterone circulates in the free state, not bound to protein. As with the other steroid hormones, it is this free form that can diffuse into cells and is the biologically active form of the hormone.

The liver is the principal site of aldosterone inactivation, as it is for cortisol. The hepatic metabolism of aldosterone yields the same type of dihydro- and tetrahydro metabolites as does the metabolism of cortisol. These compounds are excreted into urine as glucuronic and sulfuric acid conjugates. Metabolism of aldosterone by the kidney produces a unique aldosterone metabolite, an 18-oxoconjugate. This compound, which is excreted in significant amounts, has proven to be a useful metabolite of aldosterone to measure in urine as an indicator of aldosterone secretion.

Factors affecting secretion

Aldosterone differs from the majority of the other hormones discussed in this chapter in that it is not primarily regulated by a trophic hormone secreted by the anterior pituitary. Aldosterone secretion can be enhanced by ACTH, but the effect of ACTH administration is transient and does not persist for more than a day. The primary control of aldosterone secretion is a function of the renin-angiotensin system.

Renin is a proteolytic enzyme secreted by renal juxtaglomerular cells in response to any reduction in blood flow to the kidney. In the circulation renin acts on angiotensinogen (also called renin substrate), an alpha globulin produced by the liver. The decapeptide angiotensin I is produced by cleavage. No physiological activity has as yet been ascribed to this peptide. Angiotensin I is rapidly converted to the octapeptide angiotensin II by a peptidase. This peptidase, angiotensin-converting enzyme is released into the circulation from the epithelial cells of the lungs. Angiotensin I is a very potent vasoconstrictor that acts on the adrenal cortex selectively to stimulate its production of aldosterone. The aldosterone produced acts primarily on the distal and collecting tubules of the renal nephrons to enhance sodium and chloride ion reabsorption and to simultaneously promote potassium and hydrogen ion excretion. As a result of the increased sodium reabsorption, a restoration of blood volume occurs and with it is associated an increased perfusion of the kidney, which counteracts the initial stimulus to renin secretion. Thus, aldosterone, once secreted, forms part of a negative feedback loop to inhibit renin release and further synthesis of angiotensin II.

Angiotensin stimulates aldosterone production by the glomerulosa cells of the adrenal cortex primarily by enhancing the conversion of cholesterol to pregnenolone and secondarily by enhancing the other steps of the pathway leading to aldosterone synthesis. The effect of angiotensin II on aldosterone synthesis is rapid and aldosterone synthesis ceases once the angiotensin II has been removed.

Any physiological occurrence that diminishes blood flow to the kidney, producing a decrease in renal perfusion pressure, will result in renin release and increased aldosterone synthesis. Mechanical occlusion of the renal vein as produced by a stenosis or a constriction brought on by disease will have such an effect. Blood flow to the kidneys can also be compromised by significantly decreased blood albumin levels, by loss of large volumes of blood as by hemorrhage, by entrapment of blood in the venous circulation as occurs in cirrhosis of the liver or in congestive heart failure, or by sodium depletion.

A rise in the plasma concentration of potassium has been shown to increase aldosterone secretion, as does hyponatremia. It has been demonstrated that the macula densa cells in the ascending limb of the loop of Henle are sensitive to bulk flow of sodium ions, a decrease of sodium ion bulk flow leading to aldosterone secretion.

Both plasma renin activity (PRA) and blood concentrations of aldosterone increase in pregnancy and in women taking oral contraceptives, but the increases have no consequences. The increased estrogen values in these cases lead to an increased production of angiotensinogen by the liver. Plasma angiotensinogen is also increased by glucocorticoid administration.

Assumption of an upright posture after a period of rest is a strong stimulus to aldosterone secretion. This must be taken into account when drawing blood samples for measurement of basal aldosterone values. A diurnal rhythm for aldosterone secretion has been demonstrated, with secretion being greater in the morning than in the afternoon. This pattern follows from the diurnal rhythm of PRA, which, like aldosterone, is greater in the morning than the afternoon.

The secretion rate of aldosterone ranges from 40 to 20 μg/day.

Biological actions and pathophysiology

Cortisol has a widespread influence on practically every body tissue, but aldosterone has as its target only a few selected tissues, the kidneys being the primary target. Aldosterone acts on the epithelial cells lining the distal and collecting tubules of the renal nephrons. Here it enhances the reabsorption of sodium and chloride ions and the simultaneous excretion of potassium and hydrogen ions. It promotes sodium conservation also in sweat glands, salivary glands, and in glands of the gastrointestinal tract.

The net affect of the enhancement by aldosterone of renal sodium retaining activity (along with the associated water retention) is an increase in total body sodium associated with an increase in extracellular fluid volume. The increase in extracellular fluid volume becomes an increase in blood volume and some increase in blood pressure. Whereas sodium is retained, the action of aldosterone also promotes the excretion of potassium and hydrogen ions by the renal tubules. The total body potassium and hydrogen ions are decreased as a result. If the action of the aldosterone is prolonged, hypertension, hypokalemia, and alkalosis may result.

When compared to cortisol, aldosterone is about 400 times stronger as a mineralocorticoid, but it has only one-tenth the glucocorticoid activity of cortisol. There is some indication that progesterone may act as an antagonist to

aldosterone with respect to its sodium-retaining activity, but the mechanism of this activity, if any, has not been clarified.

Like the other steroid hormones, aldosterone enters its target cells by diffusion and combines with its receptor in the cytoplasm. Transport of this aldosterone-receptor complex to the nucleus results in increased mRNA synthesis with eventual increased protein synthesis. The proteins induced by aldosterone are believed to be involved in the energy requiring processes that pump sodium ions out of cells.

The pathophysiology of aldosterone conveniently falls into two categories, that of primary and secondary aldosteronism.

Primary aldosteronism is defined by an abnormal increase in aldosterone secretion resulting directly from a defect in the secretion of the hormone by the adrenal cortex. It occurs most commonly as a result of autonomous secretion of aldosterone by an adrenal adenoma. In primary aldosteronism serum concentrations of aldosterone are elevated, whereas PRA is characteristically depressed because of the inhibitory effect of the elevated aldosterone. The clinical picture usually includes potassium depletion and sodium retention with an expansion of the extracellular fluid compartment and alkalosis. The expansion of the extracellular fluid volume may lead to edema and hypertension.

Secondary aldosteronism is defined as an increase in aldosterone secretion resulting from the stimulating activity of the renin-angiotensin system on the adrenal cortex. Any of the aforementioned factors that can diminish blood flow to the kidney or sequester blood in the venous circulation can lead to an increased activity of the renin-angiotensin system. In secondary aldosteronism, blood concentrations of aldosterone and renin as measured by PRA are both elevated. The clinical picture is similar to primary aldosteronism and usually clears with correction of the disorder causing the decreased renal blood flow.

Analyte measurement and function testing

Until the advent of RIA with its inherent sensitivity, aldosterone in serum was difficult to measure because of its low concentration in blood, about 10 ng/dL. With available RIA procedures, such low levels can be easily and accurately measured.

Values of free aldosterone in urine are about 1 μg/day. Advantage is taken of the fact that a urinary metabolite of aldosterone, the 18-oxo conjugate, is excreted in amounts of about 10 μg/day. Aldosterone can be cleaved from this conjugate by treatment of urine with acid. The aldosterone is then extracted with an organic solvent. The aldosterone can then be readily measured by RIA methods.

Because of the close dependency of aldosterone concentrations on sodium intake and on posture, baseline aldosterone values are usually determined on patients who have been on an adequate salt intake for at least 3 days and who have been supine for at least 3 to 4 hours before a blood sample is drawn.

To help distinguish primary from secondary aldosteronism, the measurement of the function of the renin-angiotensin system is a valuable adjunct to measurement of serum aldosterone and urinary aldosterone excretion. Of this system, the plasma renin activity (PRA) is most readily measured. Because under most conditions plasma concentrations of renin substrate are adequate, plasma is incubated under rigidly defined conditions of temperature, pH, and time. The generated angiotensin is then measure by RIA. To maximally stimulate renin output in patients, they are usually put on a sodium-restricted diet for 3 days prior to testing. On the morning of the test, blood is drawn from patients only after they have been upright (standing, sitting, or walking) for 3 hours. Under these test conditions, primary aldosteronism is indicated if the plasma renin activity is less than 1 ng of generated angiotensin per hour of incubation per mL of plasma, or if the aldosterone excretion is greater than 20 μg/day, or if the plasma aldosterone is greater than 20 ng/dL and the patient is hypokalemic and hypertensive.

CATECHOLAMINES

The cells of the adrenal medulla, because of their embryological origin from neural crest cells and because of their secretion of norepinephrine and epinephrine are part of the sympathetic nervous system. The classic neurotransmitters norepinephrine and epinephrine are active at sympathetic postganglionic neurons. Once secreted by the adrenal medulla into the circulation, these compounds function in every way as true hormones.

The adrenal medulla provides an interface between the nervous and endocrine systems in a manner very similar to that provided by the hypothalamus. The synthesis and secretion of the catecholamines can occur in concert with the activity of the sympathetic nervous system. The epinephrine released from the adrenal medulla reinforces the activity of the sympathetic nervous system, or the secretion of catecholamines can take place independently of it. The enzymes and pathways involved in catecholamine biosynthesis in the adrenal medulla are identical to those occurring in neuronal cell bodies of the sympathetic nervous system. The identification and consideration of these neurotransmitters as hormones becomes important when tumors develop from sympathetic nervous tissue. Large enough amounts of these hormones can be secreted so that their biological activity becomes manifested as a clinical syndrone.

Norepinephrine is generally considered in terms of its function as a neurotransmitter at sympathetic nerve endings. Its actions are limited to the local area in which it is released. The amount of norepinephrine secreted from the adrenal medulla does not significantly affect nervous activity because of the short half-life, about 2 minutes, of norepinephrine in blood. In contrast, epinephrine is considered the hormone of the adrenal medulla. Its release into the circulation is the basis for its peripheral effects as a hormone. Dopamine functions as a neurotransmitter in the central nervous system, but not in the periphery. It has functions other than being a precursor to norepinephrine and epinephrine, but its function, if any, as a hormone is not yet well defined.

Characterization and biosynthesis

Norepinephrine, epinephrine, and dopamine are amine derivatives of dihydroxybenzene, or catechol, and thus are conveniently grouped as catecholamines (Fig. 16-14).

In the chromaffin cells of the adrenal medulla, catecholamine synthesis begins with the hydroxylation of the amino acid tyrosine by the enzyme tyrosine hydroxylase to produce dihydroxyphenylalanine, DOPA (Fig. 16-15). This hydroxylation step has been demonstrated to be the rate-limiting step of catecholamine synthesis, and is subject to end-product inhibition by either norepinephrine or epinephrine. Dihydroxyphenylalanine is decarboxylated by the enzyme L-aromatic amino acid decarboxylase to produce dopamine. Both of these reactions occur in the cytoplasm of

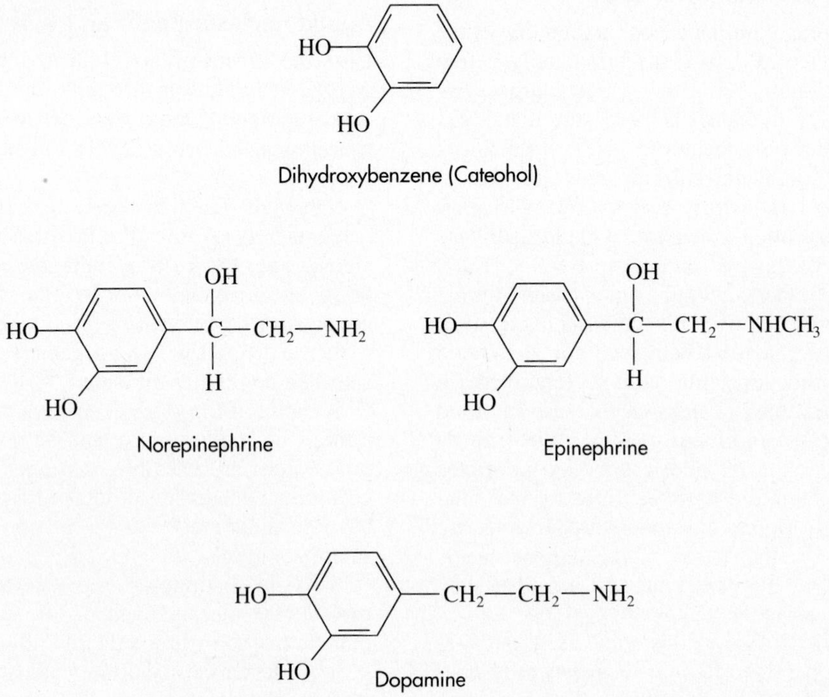

Fig. 16-14 Structures of the catecholamines.

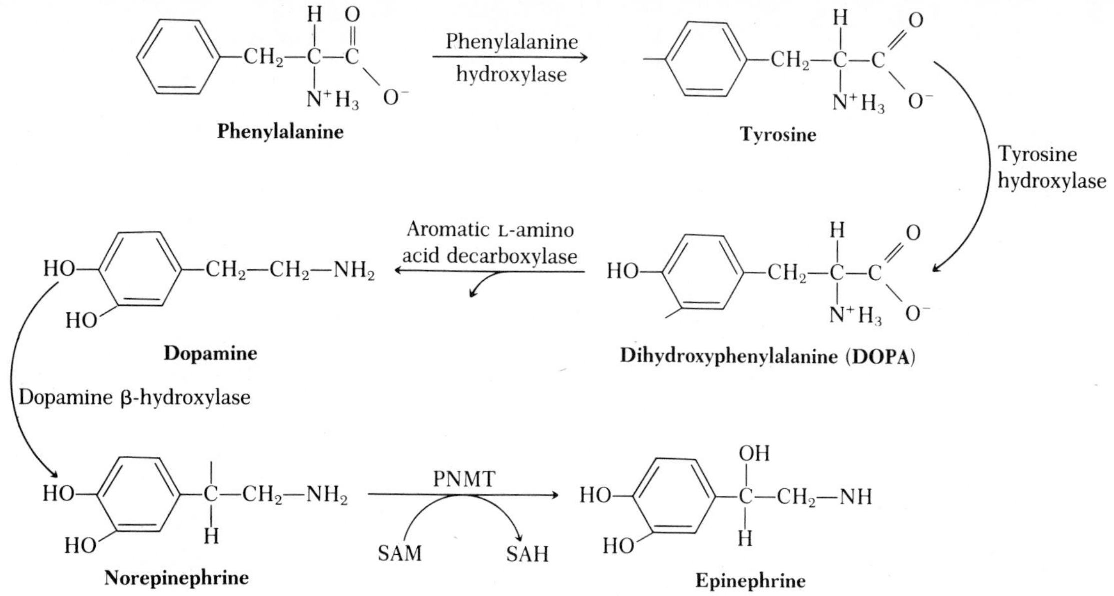

Fig. 16-15   Synthesis of catecholamines in the adrenal medulla. *Modified from Orten JM, Neuhaus OW: Human biochemistry, ed. 10, 1982, Mosby-Year Book.*

the chromaffin cells. Once formed, dopamine is transported from the cytoplasm into the chromaffin granules, where it is hydroxylated by the enzyme dopamine β-hydroxylase to norepinephrine, which then diffuses back out of the granules into the cytoplasm. There, its amino group undergoes methylation by the enzyme phenylethanolamine-N-methyl transferase to yield epinephrine, which then enters the chromaffin granules for storage. In the medulla, chromaffin cells have been identified that primarily store epinephrine, and in the CNS, sympathetic neurons store norepinephrine. The steps leading to the formation of norepinephrine are identical to those occuring in sympathetic neurons that release norepinephrine. These neurons lack the enzyme phenylethanolamine-N-methyl transferase needed for the final step in the synthesis of epinephrine, so they produce only norepinephrine. Besides the adrenal medulla, only some neurons in the brain have the capability of forming epinephrine.

In the adult, epinephrine accounts for some 80% to 85% of the catecholamines stored in the adrenal, whereas norepinephrine accounts for the majority of the remainder. In the chromaffin granules, norepinephrine and epinephrine are stored in concentrations that are up to 200 times greater than that in the cytoplasm. Only about 2% to 10% of this catecholamine content is turned over per day.

In the blood the catecholamines circulate loosely bound to protein, primarily albumin. Normal blood concentrations of the catecholamines are as follows: norepinephrine, 100 to 400 pg/mL; epinephrine, 25 to 50 pg/mL; and dopamine, 10 to 130 pg/mL.

Most of the norepinephrine and epinephrine released from the chromaffin granules into the circulation is metabolized by two enzymes, catechol-O-methyltransferase (COMT) and monoamine oxidase (MAO). Catechol-O-methyltransferase has a wide tissue distribution and is found in high concentrations in the liver and kidneys; it adds a methyl group to the meta-hydroxyl group, yielding normetanephrine from norepinephrine and metanephrine from

epinephrine (Fig. 16-16). These two products may be excreted as free metanephrines or conjugated as either glucuronides or sulfates. The metanephrines can be acted upon by the enzyme monoamine oxidase (MAO), which also has a wide tissue distribution, to yield 3-methoxy-4-hydroxymandelic aldehyde, which is either oxidized to vanillylmandelic acid (VMA) or reduced to methoxyhydroxyphenylglycol (MHPG). If either norepinephrine or epinephrine are first acted upon by MAO, 3,4-dihydroxymandelic acid is the intermediate product. When acted upon by COMT, 3,4-dihydroxymandelic acid is converted to 3-methoxy-4-hydroxy mandelic aldehyde, which is then either oxidized to VMA or reduced to MHPG. The major product of either pathway is VMA, MPHG being the minor product. Urinary analysis of VMA thus represents both norepinephrine and epinephrine metabolism. It is believed that COMT plays the more important role in the metabolism of circulating catecholamines, whereas MAO plays the larger role in sympathetic nerve endings.

Small amounts of both norepinephrine and epinephrine escape the aforementioned metabolism and appear in urine in microgram amounts. The determination of the metabolites, HVA and VMA, is easier due to the milligram amounts of these compounds that are excreted. Typical 24-hour urine excretion values are given in Box 16-15. The metabolism of dopamine by the same enzymes yields homovanillic acid (HVA) as the final product (Fig. 16-17).

Factors affecting secretion

There is a very close linkage between the secretion of cortisol by the adrenal cortex and the secretion of norepinephrine and epinephrine by the adrenal medulla. All of the products secreted by the adrenal cortex are carried to the chromaffin cells of the medulla by a portal blood system, so they are exposed to high concentrations of cortisol. The enzyme phenylethanolamine-N-methyl transferase is inducible by cortisol. Increased concentrations of the enzyme lead

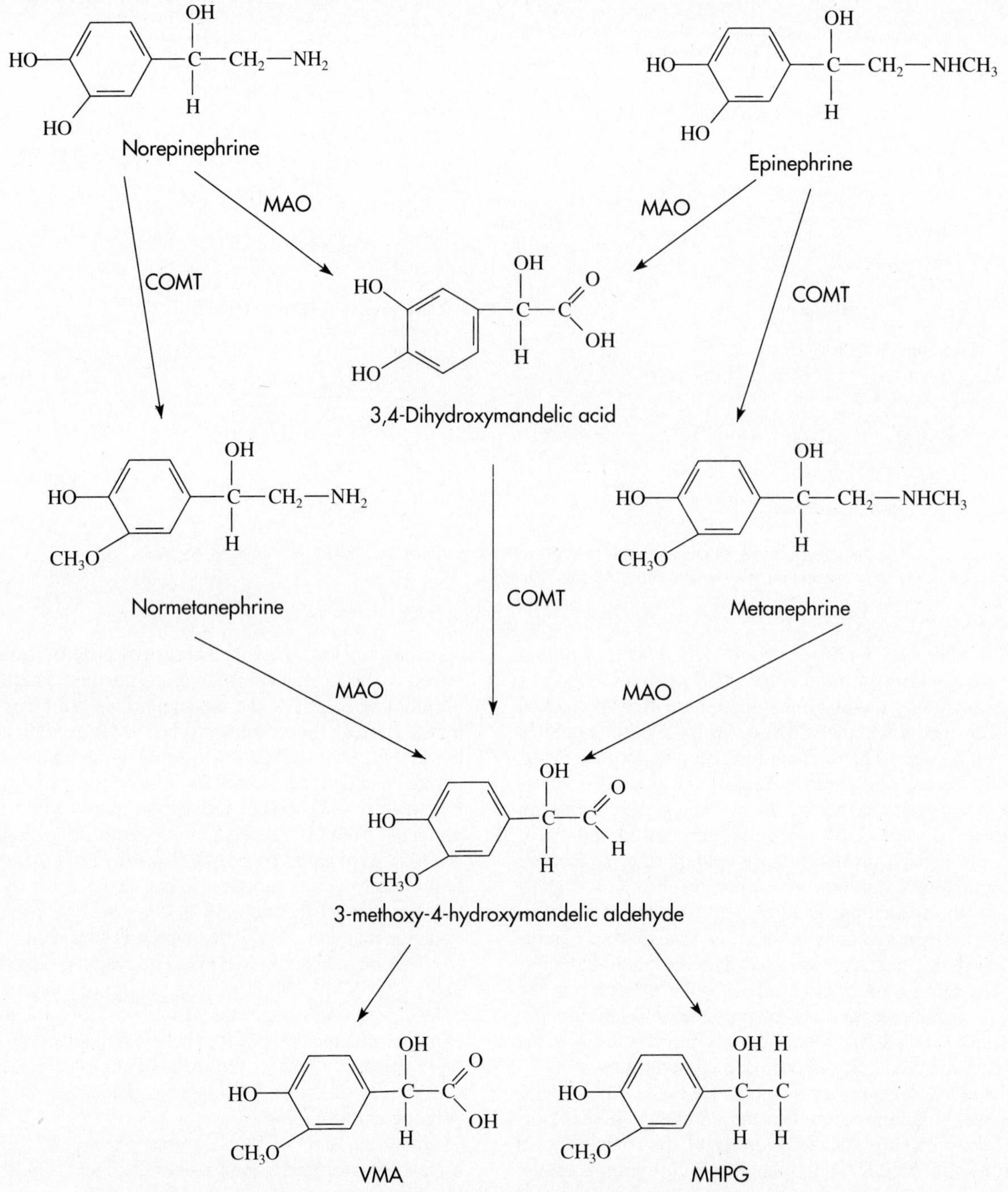

Fig. 16-16 Metabolism of the catecholamines. COMT, catechol-O-methyltransferase; MAO, monoamine oxidase; VMA, vanillylmandelic acid; MHPG, methoxyhydroxyphenylglycol.

Box 16-15 Urinary excretion of catecholamines	
Free norepenephrine	10-70 μg/24 hrs
Free epinephrine	0.5-25 μg/24 hrs
Metanephrine	0.2-1.3 mg/24 hrs
VMA	2-7 mg/24 hrs
Dopamine	60-400 g/24 hrs
HVA	<13 mg/24 hrs

VMA, vanillylmandelic acid; HVA, homovanillic acid.

to increased synthesis of epinephrine. As a result, any event that leads to an increased secretion of ACTH and thereby an increased synthesis of cortisol, also leads to an increased synthesis of epinephrine.

The release of norepinephrine and epinephrine from the storage granules (vesicles) of the chromaffin cells is initiated by the action of the neurotransmitter acetylcholine released from sympathetic nerve fibers on the chromaffin cells. Norepinephrine and epinephrine are released into the circulation by exocytosis.

Through the central nervous system, hypoglycemia is a most powerful stimulus to the secretion of epinephrine by

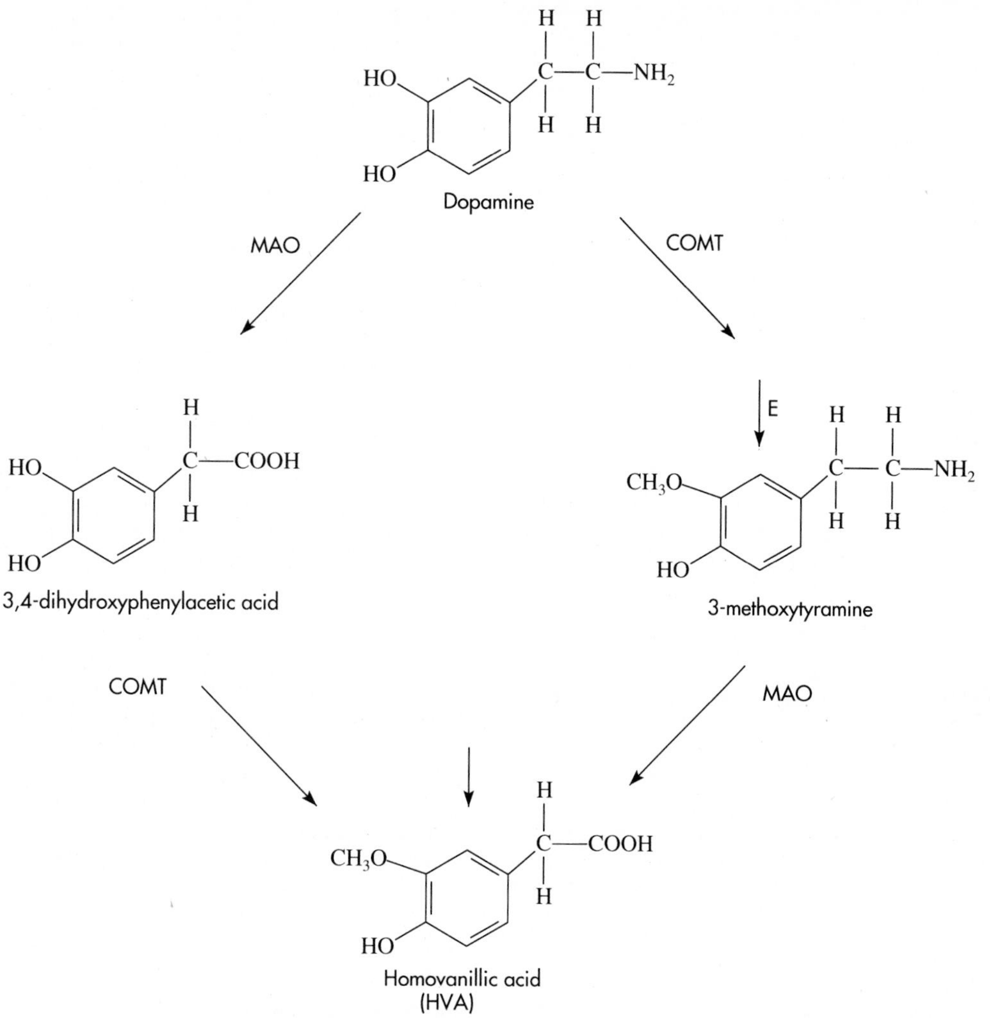

Fig. 16-17   Metabolism of dopamine. COMT, catechol-O-methyltransferase; MAO, monoamine oxidase.

the adrenal medulla. If the hypoglycemia is severe (below 50 mg glucose/dL), plasma epinephrine values may be elevated by as much as 50 times their baseline concentrations. Exercise, even of a mild form, also stimulates epinephrine release. Exposure to a cold environment affects the hypothalamus through the sympathetic nervous system and leads ultimately to an increased secretion of ACTH, followed by an increased secretion of cortisol and then epinephrine. The epinephrine acts to increase fuel utilization by tissues and increase heat production to counteract the effects of cold exposure.

Biological actions and pathophysiology

The majority of biological actions ascribed to the catecholamines result from their release as a result of stimulation of the sympathetic nervous system. Exposure to a cold environment provides one example; stress and hypoglycemia are other examples.

Norepinephrine and epinephrine have profound effects on smooth muscle contraction, which is explained on the basis of which catecholamine receptor type and which catecholamine are present. It was discovered early that administration of catecholamines could cause smooth muscle to either contract or relax; receptor sites at the contraction

or excitation that took place were called alpha receptors, whereas receptor sites where relaxation or inhibition of contraction took place were called beta receptors. The effects of either norepinephrine or epinephrine on smooth muscle become complex as some tissues, such as the gut, contain both alpha and beta receptors.

Norepinephrine acts primarily at alpha receptors, so its activity is mainly excitatory. Epinephrine can react with both alpha and beta receptors, but reacts more strongly with beta receptors, so its activity is more complex. The overall effect of a small dose of epinephrine on blood vessels, for example, is a vasodilation accompanied by a decrease in peripheral resistance and an increase in the cardiac rate and output. Norepinephrine, in contrast, produces a generalized vasoconstriction and a decrease in cardiac output. Both norepinephrine and epinephrine relax the gut. Epinephrine will relax bronchial smooth muscle; its action is most pronounced on bronchial muscle that is contracted due to disease, as in asthma.

Both norepinephrine and epinephrine have widespread biological effects, in addition to their effects on vascular smooth muscle. Both hormones inhibit insulin release from the pancreas and cause an elevation of blood glucose by increasing glycogenolysis. They increase lipolysis and cause

---

Box 16-16 Some biological effects of catecholamines (epinephrine)

STIMULATES	INHIBITS
Heart rate	Insulin secretion
Cardiac contractility	Intestinal smooth muscle
Cardiac output	Bronchospasm
Heat production	Histamine release
Lactic acid production	Anaphylaxis
Glycogenolysis in liver and muscle	
Adipose tissue lipolysis	
Hepatic gluconeogenesis	
Bronchodilation	
Aldosterone secretion	
Renin release	
Glucagon release	
Blood flow to skeletal muscle	

---

a rise in body temperature and an increase in oxygen consumption (Box 16-16).

There is general agreement that despite the profound physiological actions ascribed to the circulating catecholamines, particularly epinephrine (except in conditions of severe stress or when a secreting tumor is present), the catecholamines contribute little on a day-to-day basis to overall metabolism. This consensus is based on observations of persons with total adrenalectomy who generally survive well on corticosteroid replacement therapy alone. A supportive rather than a primary role is ascribed to the catecholamines in normal metabolism.

Pheochromocytomas are tumors that produce excess catecholamines; the most common forms are found in the adrenal medulla, where they may be singular or multiple, with up to as many as 20 in number. Other tumors are found associated with sympathetic ganglia, primarily in the abdominal and pelvic cavities. Most of these tumors are benign, but they may range in weight from less than 10 g to more than 1 kg. Interestingly, all of these tumors contain norepinephrine, but only about half also contain epinephrine. In most cases those synthesizing epinephrine can be traced back to the adrenal medulla. Hypertension is common in most patients with the tumor, but less than 1% of patients with hypertension have a pheochromocytoma. In most cases in which the tumor or tumors can be found, surgical removal results in a cure of about 90%.

Analyte measurement and function testing

Several factors combine to make the procedures available for the determination of free catecholamines in plasma and of their metabolites in urine nonroutine for the typical clinical laboratory. Some of these procedures, which involve isolation and purification by column chromatography and/or organic solvent extraction, are time consuming and technically demanding. Because of the low concentrations of the free catecholamines in plasma and urine, the analytical methods used must have a high sensitivity. Fluorescent methods of analysis are subject to nonspecific fluorescence

from interfering compounds. This presents a specificity problem. The need to control the many variables (drugs and stress) that can affect plasma catecholamine values has already been alluded to. Requests for plasma or urinary catecholamine determinations are infrequent, so that it is difficult for any laboratory to justify setting up a procedure or buying a chromatograph for this purpose. It is equally difficult to build up an experience with a methodology, if samples are run only infrequently. For these reasons, except in a research setting, most catecholamine determinations are done by large commercial laboratories.

High-performance liquid chromatography (HPLC) has proven useful for determining free catecholamines in plasma. The free catecholamines in plasma are first absorbed onto an alumina column, eluted, and then absorbed onto an Amberlite CG-50 column. The eluate from the Amberlite column is quantitated by means of HPLC with an electrochemical (amperiometric) detector. With minor modifications to remove interfering substances, this method can also be used to determine free catecholamines in 24-hour urine samples.

The amount of the metanephrines and VMA excreted in the urine is high enough to be easily determined by spectrophotometry. In one procedure the metanephrines are extracted from acidified urine with ethyl acetate, purified by absorption and elution from an Amberlite CG-50 column, then oxidized to vanillin with periodate. The vanillin produced is measured spectrophotometrically. A variety of other spectrophotometric, as well as gas chromatrographic and HPLC procedures have been developed to measure these compounds in urine.

Plasma catecholamine determinations, specifically of norepinephrine, are used primarily to assess the status of sympathetic nervous system activity in humans. To determine basal plasma values, because of the large variety of factors that influence plasma catecholamine concentrations, the blood sample is drawn from an indwelling catheter after the patient has been supine for at least 30 minutes. In response to a change of posture from supine to standing, the plasma norepinephrine concentration increases significantly; this feature has been used to measure the response of the sympathetic nervous system to this type of stress. Plasma epinephrine values change little in response to a change in posture, but rise significantly in response to mental stress or hypoglycemia.

The availability of methods to determine free catecholamines in urine as well as metanephrines and VMA has made urinary determinations the preferred methodology for verifying excess catecholamine secretion in patients with pheochromocytomas. Dynamic function tests that were used before reliable assay methods became available are no longer recommended. Because plasma values of epinephrine and norepinephrine are low and because they are subject to large variations, they are not recommended as a screening method for pheochromocytoma. In most patients with such a tumor, the increase in urinary excretion of catecholamines and catecholamine metabolites will be of a sizable magnitude, about twofold. The only precaution that needs to be observed is that the patient be hypertensive during the testing to obviate false-negatives.

17

Thyroid function

I-Wen Chen
Howard Smith

ANATOMY

The thyroid gland arises from endodermal tissue in the floor of the pharynx during embryological development and becomes functional by the end of the first trimester. During the second and third trimester, the fetus depends on its own thyroid hormone because very little maternal thyroid hormone crosses the placenta.

The thyroid gland is among the largest of the endocrine glands, weighing about 20 g in the adult, and is composed of two conical lobes joined by a narrow isthmus of tissue. The thyroid is located in the lower part of the neck, straddling the trachea and larynx. Typically, four small parathyroid glands are closely attached to the posterior surface of the thyroid gland, two in the upper portion and two near the lower portion of each of two lobes of the thyroid. The parathyroid glands are the source of parathyroid hormone involved in calcium homeostasis (Figure 17-1).

The functional units of the thyroid gland are individual thyroid follicles, which consist of cuboidal follicular cells arranged as a single layer surrounding a central core of amorphous colloid composed mainly of thyroglobulin, an iodinated glycoprotein. The follicular cells are responsible for the production and secretion of thyroid hormones. The other basic cell type is the parafollicular or clear (C) cells present in the follicles and in the interstitium. These cells produce and secrete calcitonin, a polypeptide hormone involved in the regulation of calcium metabolism (Figure 17-2).

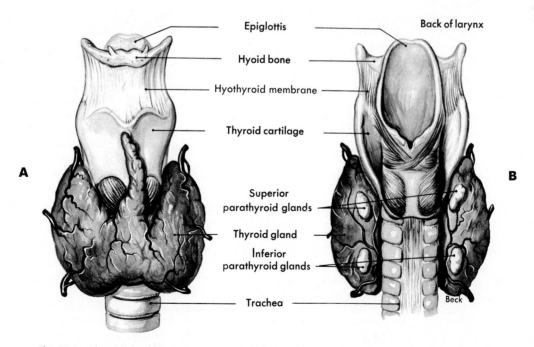

Fig. 17-1 Thyroid gland. **A,** Anterior view; **B,** Posterior view. *From Thibodeau GA: Anthony's textbook of anatomy and physiology, ed 13, St. Louis, 1990, Mosby–Year Book.*

253

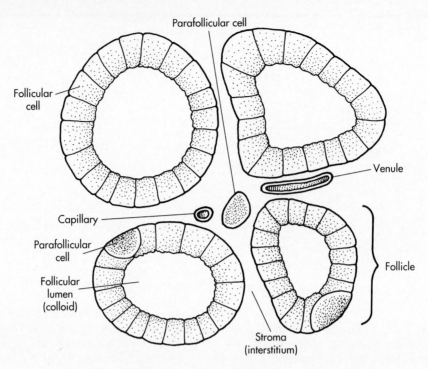

Fig. 17-2   Diagramatic histological representation of thyroid gland.

PHYSIOLOGY

The main functions of the thyroid gland are the synthesis, storage, and secretion of thyroid hormones. Each function is regulated through the action of thyroid-stimulating hormone (TSH) produced and secreted by the anterior pituitary gland. Two major hormones are produced by the thyroid gland, thyroxine (3,5,3′,5′-L-tetraiodothyronine, T_4) and triiodothyronine (3,5,3′L-triiodothyronine, T_3), which are indispensable for normal mental and physical growth and development. These hormones are involved in regulation of many cellular and metabolic processes. In addition, a small amount of biologically inactive reverse-triiodothyronine (3,3′,5′-L-triiodothyronine, rT_3) is also secreted by the thyroid gland (Figure 17-3).

Iodine metabolism and thyroid hormone synthesis

An extraordinarily high concentration of iodine is present in the thyroid gland, many hundreds of times more than that found in any other tissue. About 90% of all the iodine in the body is normally found in the thyroid. The daily intake of iodine depends on its content in the environment. In the United States, the typical daily intake is about 700 µg. Iodine in the diet is usually in the form of inorganic iodide and is absorbed mainly from the small intestine. The absorbed iodide is transported in the blood in loose attachment to plasma proteins, and removed from the circulation largely by the thyroid gland and kidneys. About two thirds of the ingested iodine is excreted primarily in the urine; the remaining one third is taken up by the thyroid. Iodide entering the thyroid cell from the plasma is very rapidly consumed in the synthesis of thyroid hormones. Therefore, the concentration of intracellular inorganic iodide in the thyroid is relatively low.

Biosynthesis of thyroid hormones involves the synthesis of thyroglobulin, trapping of iodide from the plasma by the thyroid, oxidation of iodide to iodine, incorporation of iodine into tyrosyl groups of thyroglobulin, coupling iodotyrosyl groups within the thyroglobulin molecules, and hydrolysis of thyroglobulin with subsequent release of thyroid hormones into the circulation (Figure 17-4).

Synthesis of thyroglobulin

Thyroglobulin is the major protein constituent of the thyroid, comprising 70% to 80% of the total protein of the gland. It is a large glycoprotein existing in multiple forms. The most prevalent form is a 19S iodinated molecule (MW 660,000 daltons) with four peptide chains. Thyroglobulin is the major protein in the follicular lumen colloid and serves as the precursor for all thyroid hormones. As with other proteins, thyroglobulin is synthesized on membrane-bound polyribosomes of the endoplasmic reticulum of follicular cells. After a complex sequence of protein synthesis steps, which include transcription, translation, and glycosylation, the matured protein is packaged into a secretory droplet in the Golgi apparatus. The secretory vesicles are transported to the microvilli of the apical (follicular) membrane and are iodinated at or near the membrane-lumen interface. They are released into the colloid space by exocytosis. Biosynthesis of thyroglobulin and its secretion into the follicular lumen are both controlled by thyroid-stimulating hormone (TSH).

Each thyroglobulin molecule contains about 123 tyrosine residues. Only a fraction of the tyrosyl groups that are closest to the surface of the globular molecule are available for iodination; the remaining tyrosyl residues are buried internally and not accessible to iodination. The propensity of

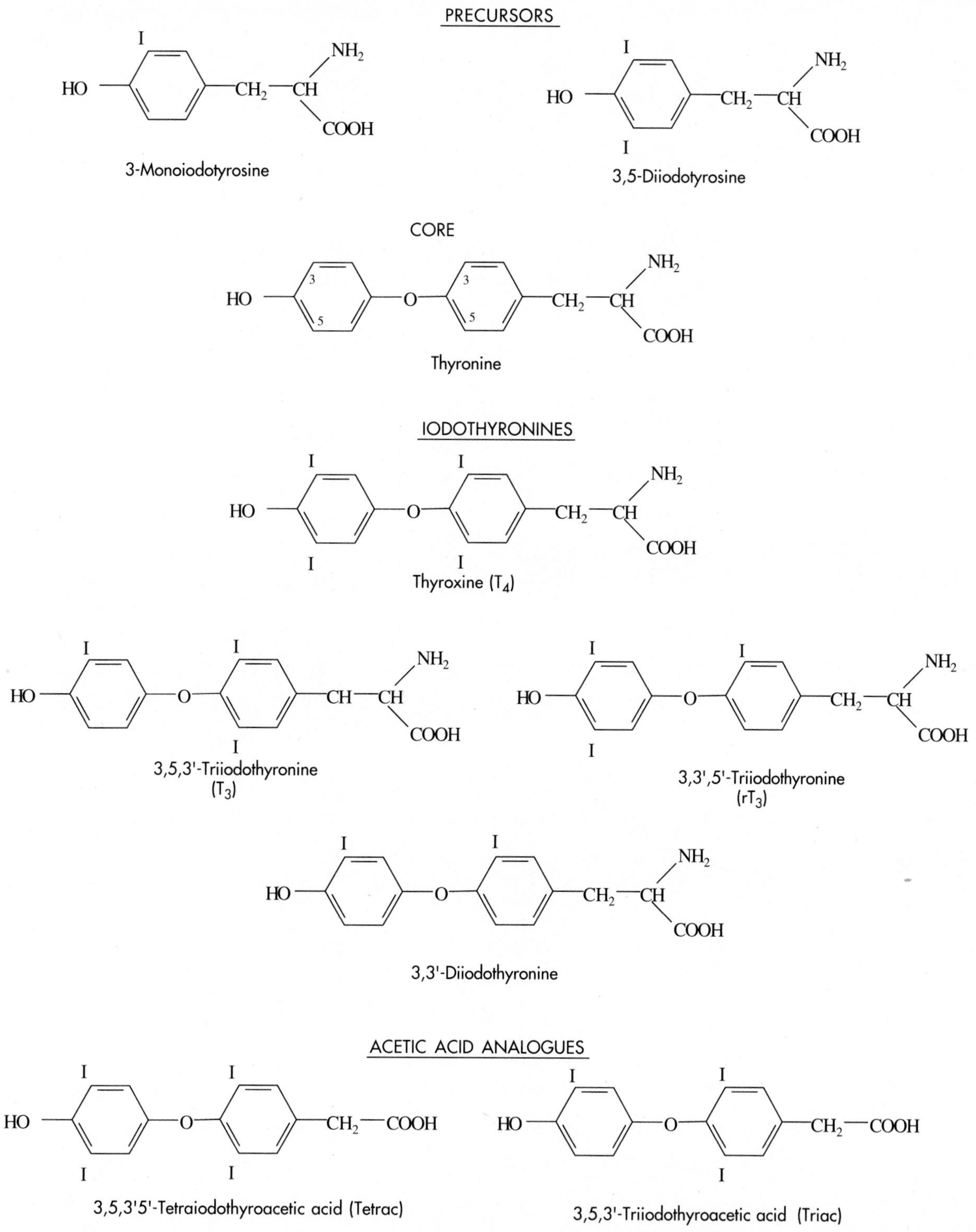

PRECURSORS

3-Monoiodotyrosine

3,5-Diiodotyrosine

CORE

Thyronine

IODOTHYRONINES

Thyroxine (T_4)

3,5,3'-Triiodothyronine
(T_3)

3,3',5'-Triiodothyronine
(rT_3)

3,3'-Diiodothyronine

ACETIC ACID ANALOGUES

3,5,3'5'-Tetraiodothyroacetic acid (Tetrac)

3,5,3'-Triiodothyroacetic acid (Triac)

Fig. 17-3 Structural formulas of various thyroid hormones and related compounds.

thyroglobulin for iodination depends on its proximity to the very efficient iodination system in follicular cells and on its tertiary structure, which may be favorable for iodination, but not on the total number of tyrosyl groups in thyroglobulin. In fact, the relative number of tyrosyl groups in thyroglobulin is not greater than in many other proteins.

Trapping of iodide

Iodide required in the iodination of thyroglobulin is actively transported ("trapped") from the plasma to the thyroid follicular cell against a strong electrochemical gradient across the cell. This process is energy dependent and is normally the rate-limiting step in the formation of thyroid

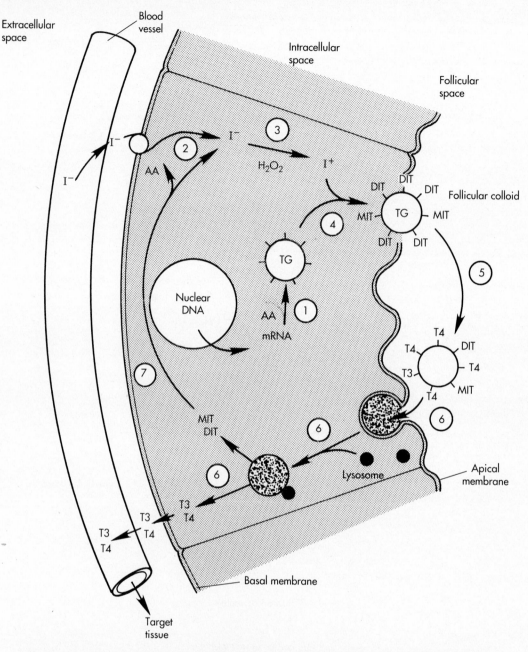

Fig. 17-4 Diagrammatic presentation of thyroid hormone biosynthesis and secretion (**A**) thyroglobulin synthesis; (**B**) trapping of iodide; (**C**) oxidation of iodide; (**D**) iodide organification; (**E**) coupling of iodinated tyrosyl residues; (**F**) reentry of thyroglobulin as colloid droplet by endocytosis, fusion of colloid droplet with lysosome, hydrolysis, and release of T_4 and T_3 to systemic circulation; (**G**) metabolic breakdown initiated by deiodinase. TG = thyroglobulin, AA = amino acids.

hormones. The iodide trapping ability of the thyroid cell can be represented by the ratio of inorganic iodide concentrations between the thyroid cell and the serum (T:S ratio). Because of the rapidity of diffusion of iodide and organification subsequent to trapping, it is difficult to get a true measure of the baseline T:S ratio in a normal human. The maximal steady-state T:S ratio, however, can be determined when iodination of thyroglobulin (iodide organification) is blocked by drugs of the thiouracil class such as propylthiouracil. A maximal T:S iodide ratio of about 25 has been observed in humans on a normal iodine diet and may rise as high as 200 or more in iodine deficiency.

Oxidation of iodide to iodine

Inorganic iodide trapped by the thyroid cell is rapidly oxidized by thyroperoxidase in the presence of H_2O_2 before it can be incorporated into thyroglobulin. Although tissues other than thyroid, such as gastric mucosa and salivary glands, are capable of trapping iodide, the thyroid is the only tissue that can oxidize iodide to a reactive intermediate for incorporation into the tyrosine residues of thyroglobulin. The exact nature of the reactive intermediate is unknown. Molecular iodine (I_2), free radical iodine ($I°$), and idoium ion (I^+) have been suggested. The site of iodide oxidation is most likely at or near the apical membrane where the enzyme activity of the membrane-bound thyroperoxidase is localized. A number of compounds inhibit iodide oxidation. Thiourea drugs such as thiouracil, propylthiouracil, and methimazole are antithyroid drugs used clinically for the treatment of hyperthyroidism. These drugs compete with iodide for oxidation by thyroperoxidase and thus inhibit formation of the active iodine intermediate and the subsequent thyroid hormone biosynthesis.

Incorporation of iodine into thyroglobulin (iodide organification)

The active iodine intermediate formed as the result of iodide oxidation reacts with tyrosyl residues in thyroglobulin. This reaction probably also involves thyroperoxidase and requires molecular oxygen. The third position of the phenolic ring of the tyrosyl residue is iodinated first and then the five position to form 3-monoiodotyrosine (MIT) and 3,5-diiodotyrosine (DIT), respectively (Figure 17-3). To date, 5-monoiodotyrosine has not been detected. This iodide organification process also occurs at or near the microvillous interface between the thyroid cell and the colloid as thyroglobulin leaves the cell.

Coupling of iodinated tyrosyl residues

Coupling usually involves the joining of two DIT molecules to form T_4 and of MIT and DIT to form T_3 and rT_3 within the thyroglobulin molecule. The thyroperoxidase involved in iodide oxidation and iodide organification also plays an important role in the coupling process. This finding is supported by the observation that all three biosynthetic steps for thyroid hormones are inhibited by thiourea drugs. Frequently, each molecule of thyroglobulin carries more than two T_4 residues whereas T_3 is present in some but not all thyroglobulin molecules. In iodide deficiency, the molar ratio of T_3 to T_4 in the thyroid gland increases. This step may represent a compensatory mechanism by which iodide is spared from making other T_4 residues in order to make a biologically more potent hormone, T_3. T_4 and T_3 remain an integral part of thyroglobulin and are stored in the follicular lumen in the form of colloid.

Hydrolysis of thyroglobulin and release of thyroid hormones

Since thyroglobulin containing T_4 and T_3 is stored extracellularly in the follicular lumen, it must reenter the thyroid cell and be hydrolyzed before thyroid hormones can be secreted into the systemic circulation. Under TSH stimulation, large colloid droplets enter the cytoplasm of the thyroid cell by endocytosis. The incoming colloid droplets are fused with lysosomes and hydrolyzed by lysosomal proteases to liberate T_4, T_3, rT_3, MIT, and DIT. T_4, T_3, and rT_3 diffuse, probably passively, through the basal membrane into the intracellular space and then into the systemic circulation. Most of the liberated iodotyrosines (MIT and DIT) are rapidly deiodinated, and the free iodide produced is reused in thyroid hormone synthesis. The de-iodination of

iodotyrosines and the reutilization of this iodide are very important in the efficient utilization of iodide by the thyroid because about 70% to 80% of the iodide in thyroglobulin is in the form of iodotyrosines, which can be rapidly metabolized and lost in the urine once released into the circulation. Pharmacological doses of iodide inhibit all states of thyroid hormone synthesis and secretion.

Transport and metabolism of thyroid hormones

Thyroid hormones are poorly soluble in plasma. They are therefore bound almost completely and reversibly to plasma proteins upon release from the thyroid to the blood stream and transported to the sites of their action. In normal individuals, only about 0.03% of the T_4 and 0.3% of the T_3 are present in the free or unbound state. Only the free thyroid hormones can penetrate the cellular membrane and enter the cells to exert their biological effects and then be metabolized. The free fraction of thyroid hormones also is responsible for the regulation of thyroid function through the pituitary feedback mechanism to be discussed in the next section. The large circulating pool of bound-thyroid hormones is metabolically inactive but can serve as a stable reservoir to replenish losses of free hormones that have been metabolized. This pool is in dynamic equilibrium with the plasma and hence with the intracellular free hormone pools. The protein binding also conserves thyroid hormones and limits the loss of the scarce element, iodine, because bound hormones do not pass through the renal glomerular membrane although free hormones do. There are three major thyroid hormone-binding proteins in plasma: thyroxine-binding globulin (TBG), thyroxine-binding prealbumin (TBPA), and albumin. TBG is the most important. Each molecule has a single binding site for T_4 or T_3. Its plasma concentration is the lowest (1-2 mg/dL, low capacity) among the three binding proteins, but it has a high affinity for T_4 (association constant, $K_A = 4 \times 10^{10}$ L/M) and a moderate affinity for T_3 ($K_A = 2 \times 10^9$ L/M). TBG therefore carries 70% to 75% of circulating T_4 and T_3 despite its low concentration. TBPA is about 20 times more abundant (about 25 mg/dL, intermediate capacity) than TBG and has a moderate affinity for T_4 ($K_A = 1 \times 10^9$ L/M), but does not bind T_3. Each TBPA molecule possesses a pair of T_4 binding sites, but they are located inside the molecule and thus are relatively inaccessible to the surrounding medium. Albumin is present in plasma at a very high concentration (about 3,500 mg/dL, high capacity) but its affinities for T_4 ($K_A = 1.6 \times 10^6$ L/M) and for T_3 ($K_A = 2.7 \times 10_5$ L/M) are very low. However, it binds significant amounts of T_4 (about 10%) and T_3 (about 30%).

In euthyroid individuals, alterations in the concentrations of thyroid hormone-binding proteins, particularly that of TBG, will result in significant changes in the total plasma T_4 and T_3 concentrations but will not affect the free fraction of these hormones, which are responsible for the metabolic effects of thyroid hormone. This regulatory process is achieved by the pituitary feedback mechanism. Since bound hormones and free hormones in plasma are in a dynamic equilibrium, increases in binding proteins will shift the equilibrium. This step increases the amount of bound hormones and transiently decreases the free hormone concentration. The decrease in free hormones stimulates TSH synthesis and secretion, resulting in thyroid hormone production to replenish the free hormone pool until the euthyroid level is normal. A transient decrease in the metabolic clearance rate of thyroid hormone is another contributing factor. The normal free hormone level is now in equilibrium with a larger pool of protein-bound hormone while the free hormone secretion, metabolism, and plasma concentration have returned to normal. The overall consequence of increases in binding proteins is an increase in the total (free and protein-bound) plasma hormone concentration.

Similarly, decreases in binding proteins will decrease the total plasma hormone concentration. Knowledge of possible changes in concentration of binding proteins is extremely important when total thyroid hormone measurements are used in the evaluation of thyroid hormone excess of deficiency states. Factors affecting the plasma concentration of protein-bound thyroid hormones are summarized in Box 17-1.

Thyroid hormone metabolism

The major thyroid hormone in human circulation is T_4. T_4 accounts for approximately 97%, T_3 about 2%, and rT_3 less than 0.5% of circulating thyroid hormones. Table 17-1 summarizes the production and circulating levels of thyroid hormones in a normal euthyroid individual. While all the T_4 originates from the thyroid gland, only about 20% of T_3 and less than 10% of rT_3 come from the thyroid gland; the rest is derived from monodeiodination of T_4 in the peripheral tissues, especially in the liver and the kidney. Under normal circumstances, about 35% of T_4 secreted by the thyroid gland is deiodinated to T_3 and about 45% to rT_3. The remaining 20% of T_4 is either metabolized through oxidative deamination to tetraiodothyroacetic acid (TETRAC) or excreted in the feces or urine in the free form or as glucuronide or sulfate conjugate.

Deiodination is the major metabolic pathway of T_4. rT_3 produced by removal of one iodine from the inner ring (5' deiodination, Figure 17-3) is metabolically inactive and is an end product of T_4 metabolism; T_3 produced by the outer-ring deiodination (5' deiodination) is biologically about five times more active than T_4. It is believed that a single microsomal enzyme is responsible for both deiodination reactions, and different physiological environments determine which reaction predominates. In acute illness or starvation, rT_3 is formed preferentially at the expense of T_3. A variety of pharmacologic agents such as propylthiouracil, glucocorticoids, propranolol, and amiodarone suppresses the rate of T_4 monodeiodination to T_3. The plasma T_3 concentration therefore is a poor indicator of thyroid function because it is influenced by many non-thyroid factors. The peripheral conversion of T_4 to T_3 or rT_3 is responsible not only for initiating the metabolic breakdown of T_4, but also for balancing hormone activation and inactivation. T_3 and rT_3 are both deiodinated further to diiodothyronines (T_2) and then to monoiodothyronines and rapidly cleared from the plasma.

Thyroid hormone actions

Only the free hormones can penetrate the cellular membrane and exert their effeects inside cells by binding to specific receptors in the cell nuclei. The thyroid hormones in plasma are in equilibrium with the thyroid hormones bound to the nuclear receptors, and the effects of thyroid hormones are related to the concentration of thyroid hormones bound to specific nuclear binding sites. T_3 is about five times more active biologically than T_4 because T_3 is not as tightly bound to the plasma-binding proteins and can more easily penetrate into the target cell to exert its biological effects. In addition, T_3 binds to specific high-affinity receptors in the target cell nucleus with approximately 10 times the affinity of T_4. A high correlation between binding affinity and ability to elicit biological effects of various thyroid hormone analogs has been demonstrated. It has therefore been suggested that T_3 is the physiologically active hormone and T_4 is the prohormone of T_3 although T_4 is known to have some intrinsic biologic activity.

Interaction of thyroid hormones with chromatin in the cell nuclei results in protein synthesis, e.g., stimulation of protein kinase activity. The thyroid hormone actions are not limited to the nucleus. Their direct actions on the plasma membrane and on the mitochondria have been demonstrated. For example, thyroid hormones stimulate the rapid

---

Box 17-1 Factors affecting the plasma concentration of protein-bound thyroid hormones

I. Increased protein-bound hormone due to rise in TBG
 1. Drugs (hyperestrogenic states caused by estrogen therapy, contraceptive medication, and other exogenous hormone; phenothiazines).
 2. Diseases (acute hepatitis, hypothyroidism, acute intermittent porphyria, estrogen-secreting tumor).
 3. Other (hyperestrogenic states in pregnancy, neonatal life, congenital TBG excess).
II. Decreased protein-bound hormone due to fall in TBG
 1. Drugs (androgens, anabolic steroids, glucocorticoids).
 2. Diseases (nephrotic syndrome, Cushings syndrome, protein malnutrition, hyperthyroidism, active acromegaly, cirrhosis).
 3. Other (congenital TBG deficiency, surgical stress).
III. Decreased protein-bound hormone due to competitive binding of drugs to TBG
 Salicylates, heparin, chlorpropamide, tolbutamide, diazepam, phenytoin (diphenylhydantoin, dilantin).

Table 17-1 Normal values of thyroid hormone production and circulating concentrations

	T_4	T_3	rT_3
Production from thyroid (ug/day)	80-100	3-7	<3
Peripheral production from T_4 (ug/day)	0	22-30	30-40
Mean plasma concentrations			
Total (µg/dL)	8.0	0.12	0.04
Free (ng/dL)	2.1	0.28	0.24
Plasma half-life (days)	6-7	1-2	<1
Relative biologic activity	1	5	0

uptake of amino acids into cells, and the uptake of adenosine diphosphate by mitochondria is stimulated by thyroid hormones. The net results of such thyroid hormone actions at the subcellular level are the effects of thyroid hormones on growth and development, on heat production, on neuromuscular activity, and on metabolic processes. Generalized effects of thyroid hormones are summarized in Table 17-2.

Regulation of thyroid hormone synthesis and secretion

Thyroid function is regulated by both extrathyroidal (hypothalmic-pituitary-thyroid axis) and intrathyroidal (autoregulatory) mechanisms.

Extrathyroidal mechanism

The primary components involved in the extrathyroidal mechanism of regulation of thyroid function consists of thyroid hormones T_4, T_3, the pituitary hormone TSH, and thyrotropin-releasing hormone (TRH).

Thyroid-stimulating hormone (or thyrotropin, TSH) of the anterior pituitary is a glycoprotein (28,300 daltons) consisting of two polypeptide subunits linked noncovalently. The alpha subunit is nearly identical to that of other pituitary glycoproteins (luteinizing hormone and follicle-stimulating hormone) and human chorionic gonadotropin (hCG); the unique beta subunit conveys the specific hormone action of TSH. Only the intact TSH molecule consisting of both subunits is biologically active. The plasma half-life of TSH is about one hour. TSH has a stimulatory effect on all aspects of thyroid metabolism (thyroidal uptake of iodide and synthesis and release of thyroid hormones). It also stimulates the thyroid cell reproduction and hypertrophy. TSH synthesis and secretion by the pituitary are modulated by a tripeptide (pyroglutamyl-histidyl-prolinamide) called thyrotropin-releasing hormone (TRH).

TRH is secreted by the hypothalamus and is transported to the anterior pituitary from the hypothalamus-hypophyseal portal system. TSH output, in turn, is regulated by free thyroid hormones in a negative feedback regulatory loop (Figure 17-5). T_3 produced in the pituitary by the monodeiodination of T_4 is primarily responsible for inhibiting TSH secretion. This is induced by an inhibitory protein synthesized as the result of intra-pituitary nuclear binding of T_3. It is believed that the pituitary acts as a "thyroidstat" to maintain the thyroid hormone production of the thyroid gland at the appropriate physiological level set by the hypothalamus (hypothalamus-pituitary-thyroid axis).

A significant inverse log/linear relationship exists between the serum TSH and free T_4 values (Figure 17-6). This log/linear relationship extends down to the subnormal TSH range. These data suggest that a doubling of the serum-free T_4 level is associated with an approximately 160-fold reduction in serum TSH, indicating the extreme sensitivity of the pituitary TSH production and secretion to minor changes in the circulating free T_4 status. This log/linear relationship also suggests that no clear-cut distinction exists between the normal and abnormal values for serum TSH and free T_4, and that there is a genetically determined pituitary set point for the serum TSH/free T_4 relationship (thyroidstat) for each individual.

Intrathyroidal mechanism (autoregulation)

Although thyroid hormone synthesis and secretion are regulated primarily by the extrathyroidal mechanism, the

Table 17-2   Basic physiological effects of thyroid hormones and their relationship with syndromes of thyroid dysfunction

| System | Thyroid hormone effects | Usual symptoms | |
		Hyperthyroidism	Hypothyroidism
Metabolic	Increased calorigenesis and O_2 consumption Increased heat dissipation Increased protein catabolism Increased glucose absorption and production (gluconeogenesis) Increased glucose use	Heat intolerance Flushed skin Increased perspiration Increased appetite and food ingestion Muscle wasting and weakness Weight loss	Cold intolerance Dry and pale skin Decreased appetite and food ingestion Generalized weakness Weight gain
Cardiovascular	Increased adrenergic activity and sensitivity Increased heart rate Increased myocardial contractility Increased cardiac output Increased blood volume	Palpitations Fast heart rate (tachycardia) Increased blood pressure, mainly systolic Bouncy, hyperdynamic arterial pulses Shortness of breath	Slow heart rate (bradycardia) Low blood pressure Heart failure Heart enlargement
Central nervous	Increased adrenergic activity and sensitivity	Restlessness, hypermotility Nervousness Emotional lability Fatigue Exaggerated reflexes	Apathy Mental sluggishness Depressed reflexes Mental retardation
Gastrointestinal (GI)	Increased motility	Hyperdefecation	Constipation

From Fernandez-Ulloa M and Maxon HR III. Thyroid In Kaplan LA and Pesce AJ Clinical Chemistry: theory, analysis, and correlation, ed 2, St. Louis, 1989, Mosby–Year Book, Inc.

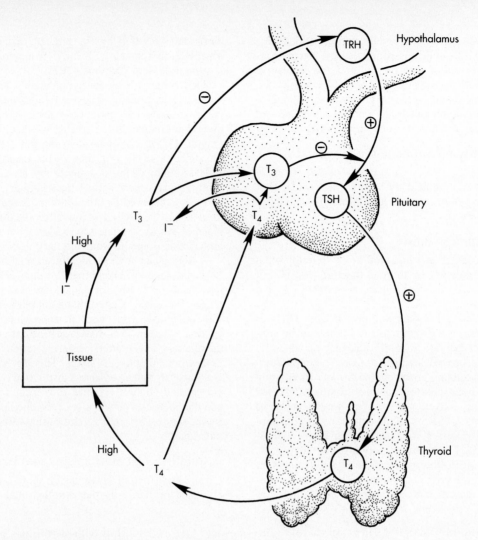

Fig. 17-5 Negative feedback regulation of thyroid function. T_4, T_3, TSH, and TRH are four primary hormones involved in the extrathyroidal regulation of thyroid function. + = stimulatory effects; − = inhibitory effects.

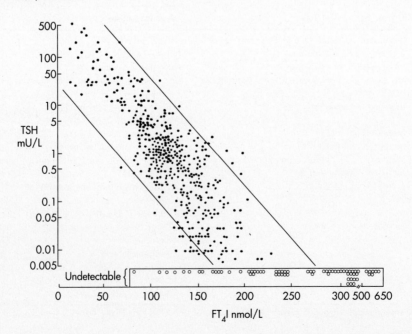

Fig. 17-6 Relationship between serum TSH and FT_4I values in 505 stable ambulatory patients. The open symbols represent undetectable TSH values (<0.005 mU/L). The solid lines represent the 95% confidence limits of the relationship (log TSH = 2.56 − 0.22 FT_4I r = −0.84; p <0.001). *Reproduced with permission trom Spencer CA, et al: Applications of new sensitive chemiluminometric thyrotropin assay to subnormal measurement, J Clin Endocrinol Metab, 70:456, 1990.*

importance of autoregulation of thyroid function is receiving increasing attention.

In iodide insufficiency, the iodide uptake by the thyroid becomes more active (independent of TSH) and accumulates the normal amount of iodide in the thyroid even though the plasma iodide concentration is subnormal. A decrease in an as yet unidentified intrathyroidal organic iodine intermediate is believed to be responsible for this autoregulation. Another compensatory mechanism plays an important role in iodide insufficiency. The ratio of T_3 to T_4 produced by the thyroid during a period of iodide deficiency is increased. Since T_3 is biologically more active than T_4, iodide is utilized more efficiently in the state of iodide deficiency. In this context, it is of interest to note that poorly iodinated thyroglobulin is more easily hydrolyzed to thyroid hormones than heavily iodinated thyroglobulin.

The thyroid is also capable of adjusting to an increased level of intrathyroidal inorganic iodide which would otherwise excessively increase thyroglobulin iodination and thyroid hormone synthesis. Above a certain critical level, the organic iodide production is inhibited. This is known as the Wolff-Chaikoff block. The normal thyroid gland is able to escape from the Wolff-Chaikoff block to prevent ensuing hypothyroidism because of intrathyroidal feedback inhibition of the iodide uptake mechanism. The diminished iodide uptake decreases the intrathyroidal iodide concentration, "escape" from the Wolff-Chaikoff block occurs, and the production of organic iodide resumes. In some thyroid disease, such as Hashimoto's thyroiditis, this escape mechanism does not occur, leading to hypothyroidism (iodide myxedema).

Test of thyroid function

The concentration of thyroid hormones in the systemic circulation in normal individuals is tightly controlled by extrathyroidal and intrathyroidal mechanisms and can be affected by various physiological and pharmacological factors. The evaluation of thyroid function therefore is not a simple procedure. In addition, a large number of laboratory tests for diagnosis of thyroid dysfunction have become available commercially in the last decade, and the selection of the most appropriate laboratory measurements from this bewildering array of tests is not a simple task even for the endocrinologist. However, a good history and sound examination of patients still play the most important role in the evaluation of thyroid dysfunction. The American Thyroid Association has published guidelines for use of laboratory tests in thyroid disorders to suggest to clinicians an approach to the laboratory diagnosis of the principal thyroid disorders.

Tests of thyroid function may be classified as 1) evaluating the function of the thyroid gland, 2) measuring the concentration of products secreted in the systemic circulation by the thyroid, 3) examining the hypothalmic-pituitary-thyroid axis, and 4) testing for other thyroid-related serum proteins.

Tests of thyroid gland

Several nuclear medicine procedures are used to evaluate the function of the thyroid gland. All utilize the unique ability of the thyroid gland to trap radioisotopes of iodine (^{131}I or ^{125}I) or technetium (99Tc). The radionuclide is administered intravenously or orally, and the amount of radioactivity taken up by the thyroid gland is determined qualitatively (thyroid imaging) or quantitatively (thyroid iodine uptake) at various specific times following administration by specially designed imaging and counting devices. In thyroid scanning using radionuclides, an image of isotope distribution within the thyroid tissue is obtained. The image fairly accurately represents the size of the thyroid gland and localizes palpable thyroid abnormalities. Ultrasonographic and, more recently, nuclear magnetic imaging techniques have also been used in thyroid imaging. In thyroid iodine uptake, the percentage of radioactivity taken up by the thyroid gland is usually determined 24 hours after radioiodine administration (^{123}I or ^{131}I), an uptake reflecting trapping and organification, or at five minutes after administration of radioactive technetium (99Tc), an uptake reflecting only trapping.

Tests for measuring thyroid products

Rapid development of commercial test kits during the last decade have made techniques for measuring thyroid hormones and related proteins in serum more complex and their nomenclature bewildering and sometimes misleading. In order to clarify and simplify the nomenclature of these assay techniques and to improve the understanding of the various tests and the communication between the clinicians and the laboratory, the American Thyroid Association has published guidelines for classification and nomenclature of tests for thyroid hormones and thyroid-related proteins in serum. Commonly used tests and their typical values given in these guidelines are listed in Table 17-3.

Immunoassays of thyroid hormones

Although T_4 is less biologically active than T_3, the serum T_4 concentration is a better indicator of thyroid secretion than that of T_3 because it is the main secretory product of the thyroid and is less susceptible to many nonthyroidal factors. In addition, the pituitary is more sensitive to serum T_4 than T_3 concentration because, as noted previously (Figure 17-5), most of the intrapituitary T_3 is derived from circulating T_4.

A variety of commercial kits are available for the determination of total serum T_4 and T_3 concentrations (Table 17-4). An immunoassay technique is used almost exclusively in these commercial kits. The principle of immunoassay is quite simple: the ability of the unknown, unlabelled antigen (analyte to be measured such as T_4 or T_3) to inhibit the binding of labelled antigen (isotopic labels such as ^{125}I or non-isotopic labels such as enzymes, fluorescent molecules, chemiluminescent molecules) is compared to that of known standards in the determination of the concentration of the unkinown antigen in biological samples. As late as 1982, both T_4 and T_3 were measured almost exclusively by radioimmunoassay (RIA) because of RIA's exquisite sensitivity and specificity achieved by combining the sensitivity of radiometry and the selectivity of immunochemistry. In RIA, the radioactivity produced by a radioactive atom through the radioactive decay process is the end-point signal measured and is not affected by the physicochemical environment. A separation step for antibody bound and free ra-

Table 17-3 Nomenclature and abbreviations for thyroid tests recommended by American Thyroid Association

Name of test	Abbreviation	Most common method	Representative midnormal values Present	SI units
Total thyroid hormone concentrations				
1. Thyroxine	T_4	Immunoassay	8 ug/dL	100 nmol/L
2. Triiodothyronine (3,5,3'-triiodothyronine)	T_3	Immunoassay	130 ng/dL	2.0 nmol/L
Free thyroid hormone concentrations				
1. Free T_4	FT_4	Immunoassay of ultrafil-	2.2 ng/dL	25 pmol/L
2. Free T_3	FT_3	trate or dialysate	0.4 ng/dL	6 pmol/L
Estimates of thyroid hormone binding in serum				
1. Thyroid hormone binding ratio	THBR	*	1.0 (unitless ratio)	same
Indirect estimates of free thyroid hormone concentration				
1. Free T_4 index	FT_4I	$T_4 \times THBR$	8 U	100 U
2. Free T_3 index	FT_3I	$T_3 \times THBR$	130 U	2.0 U
3. "Free" T_4 or T_3	FT_4 or FT_3	Many proprietary methods (analog, coated tube, etc.)	*	*
Other hormones				
1. Thyrotropin (thyroid stimulating hormone)	TSH	Immunoassay, immuno-metric	2 uU/mL	2 mU/L
2. Reverse T_3 (3,3',5'-triiodothyronine)	rT_3	Immunoassay	25 ng/dL	0.4 nmol/L

*See *"Estimates of thyroid hormone bindings and indirect estimates of free thyroid hormones"* section of the text from Larsen PR et al: J Clin Endocrinol Metab 64:1089-1093 (1987).

Table 17-4 Methods of T_4 and T_3 analyses

Methods	Signal measured	Automation	Marker	Comments
1. Radioimmunoassay (RIA)	Radioactivity	Full, manual	^{125}I	Heterogeneous assay requiring phase separation, most sensitive method
2. Enzyme-multiplied immunoassay technique (EMIT)	Light intensity	Full, manual	Enzyme, chromo-genic substrate	Homogeneous assay requiring no phase separation
3. Fluorescent polarization immuno-assay (FPIA)	Degree of polarization of fluorescence	Full	Fluorescein	Homogeneous assay requiring no phase separation
4. Fluorometric enzyme immunoas-say (FEIA)	Fluorescent intensity	Full	Enzyme, fluoro-genic substrate	Heterogeneous assay requiring phase separation, random access fully automated systems available commercially
5. Time-resolved fluorescence im-munoassay (TR-FIA)	Fluorescent intensity	Partial	Europium chelate	Heterogeneous assay requiring phase separation, fluorescent intensity measured after decay of back-ground fluorescence
6. Luminescence immunoassay (LIA)	Luminescent intensity	Manual	Luminescent labels	Heterogeneous assay requiring phase separation
7. Enhanced luminescence immuno-assay (ELIA)	Luminescent intensity	Partial	Horseradish perox-idase, H_2O_2, lu-minol	Heterogeneous assay requiring phase separation. Peroxidase converts H_2O_2 to O_2 and O_2 oxidizes lumi-nol to produce luminescence

diolabelled ligands therefore is always required in RIA (het-erogeneous immunoassay). Many different techniques are used in the phase-separation step. The most commonly used technique is the solid-phase separation procedure using the antibody chemically or physically bonded to solid support such as glass beads, plastic tubes, cellulose, or magnetic particles. Other separation methods involve the use of sec-ond antibodies or polyethylene glycol to precipitate the an-tibody-bound ligand.

Because of the problems associated with regulation of and licensing for the use of radioactive materials, waste disposal, record keeping, and relatively short shelf life, and because of the fear of radiation at any level by the general public, the use of non-isotopic alternatives in immunoassay has accelerated in the last several years. According to the basic ligand assay quality-assurance survey of the American College of Pathologists (CAP) in the last quarter of 1989, more than 55% (920 out of 1651) and 23% (197 out of 838) of the CAP survey participating laboratories used noniso-topic immunoassays for T_4 and T_3 measurements, respec-tively.

The enzyme-multiplied immunoassay technique (EMIT) for T_4 is a homogeneous immunoassay system that requires no separation step. In this technique, malate dehydrogenase chemically bound to T_4 is used as the tracer. The enzyme with bound T_4 is inactive because the active site of the enzyme is blocked by T_4. The enzyme becomes active in the presence of antibody specific for T_4 because T_4 binds to the antibody and is therefore displaced from the active site. Hence, the degree of binding of the enzyme-labelled T_4 to the T_4 antibody is directly proportional to the enzyme activity and can be measured without physical separation of bound and free T_4.

Fluorescent probes are also used in place of the radio-labels in T_4 and T_3 immunoassays. In the homogeneous fluorescence polarization immunoassay (FPIA), the label on the ligand (T_4 or T_3) is a fluorescent dye (fluorescein). When the ligand-fluorescein complex is excited by a polarized beam of light, it emits a polarized fluorescent light. The degree of polarization depends on the extent of rotation of the molecule during the period between excitation and emission (rotational relaxation time). The rotational relaxation time is proportional to the size of the molecule: the larger the molecule, the longer the rotational relaxation time and the larger the degree of fluorescence polarization. In FPIA, therefore, the quantity of antibody-bound ligand-fluorescein complex (a much larger molecule than the unbound complex) can be determined, in the presence of the unbound complex, by measuring the increase in the degree of polarization of the emitted fluorescence.

Both enzymatic and fluorometric techniques are utilized in the radial partition immunoassays for T_3 and T_4. This is a heterogeneous immunoassay in which the entire immunochemical procedure is conducted on a solid phase. An antibody specific for the ligand of interest (T_4 or T_3) is immobilized on a small area of glass-fiber filter paper (in $2'' \times 2''$ slides). Alkaline phosphatase-labelled ligand is used as the tracer. Ligands contained in the sample and the tracer are allowed to react sequentially with the immobilized antibody. After a suitable incubation period, a wash fluid that contains 4-methylumbelliferyl phosphate as the fluorogenic substrate of alkaline phosphatase is added. The substrate is dephosphorylated to 4-methylumbelliferone by alkaline phosphatase and, at the same time, the wash fluid allows the unbound labelled ligand to diffuse out of the area of fluorescence measurement (area with immobilized antibody). 4-methylumbelliferone generated by alkaline phosphatase is a fluorescent compound. A specially designed front-surface dichroic mirror fluorometer (365 nm light) excite and quantifies emission (450 nm light) from the fluorescence product. An aperture screens out the edge of the slide where the excess labelled ligand and serum proteins are now located. The rate of fluorescence development produced by the alkaline phosphatase-labelled ligand is viewed only in the specified area at the center of the slide. As with other immunoassays, the intensity or the rate of fluorescent signal produced by the antibody-bound enzyme labelled ligand is inversely proportional to the ligand concentration in the sample.

An enhanced luminescence immunoassay system (Amerlite) with a broad menu of tests is available now, including T_4, T_3, and FT_4. It is a solid-phase enzyme immunoassay using the luminescent intensity as the end-point signal that is measured. An antibody specific for the ligand is immobilized on the wall of a microtiter well, and horseradish peroxidase is used as a tracer molecule for labelling the ligand of interest. As in any coated-tube immunoassays, the labelled ligand and the ligand contained in a test specimen are allowed to compete for the binding sites on the solid-phase antibody. The microtiter wells are washed and the amount of antibody-bound peroxidase-labelled ligand, which is inversely proportional to the amount of ligand present in the test specimens, is determined by measuring the intensity of luminescence produced by addition of signal reagent to the wells. The signal reagent consists of a mixture of hydrogen peroxide, luminol, and a chemical enhancer of the phenol family. Horseradish peroxidase converts hydrogen peroxide to water and oxygen, and oxygen molecules in turn oxidize luminol to aminophthalic acid. The enhancer is capable of enhancing the light output from the oxidation of luminol by about 1000- to 1500-fold, significantly increasing the signal-to-noise ratio. In addition, the enhancer prolongs the luminescence signal up to 20 minutes, compared to the very short duration of light output (just a few seconds) in the conventional luminescence system. Therefore, this enhanced luminescence system requires no special luminometer for measurement of light emission immediately following addition of the signal reagent. In fact, the luminescence signal may be reread on the same sample any time during the period of stable maximum light output, which is reached about two minutes after addition of the signal reagents.

Total rT_3 in circulation is also measured by an RIA technique. rT_3 is biologically inactive and is known to form preferentially at the expense of T_3 production in acute illness or starvation. The test therefore may be helpful in defining the sick-euthyroid syndrome, but is of limited clinical use in the assessment of thyroid function. Only a few commercial kits are available at present.

The measurement of serum T_4 concentration is one of the most frequently ordered endocrine tests. Its automation is highly desirable from the standpoints of reproducibility and cost effectiveness. Both isotopic and non-isotopic immunoassays of total T_4 have been either partially or fully automated. The concept 4 and ARIA-HT are two fully automated RIA systems still in use in the United States. The concept 4 is a batch system using antibody-coated tubes to separate bound from free ligands, whereas the ARIA-HT is a sequential flowthrough system using a resin chamber for the phase separation. They are high capacity, high throughput systems especially suitable for reference laboratories with large test volumes.

A fully automated, high-throughput, high-capacity, non-isotopic immunoassay analyzer was developed recently by Tosoh Medics, Inc. In this system, all of the reagents needed to perform an assay are contained in a ligand-specific test cup. The reagents include magnetized microbeads coated with an antibody specific for the ligand to be measured and alkaline phosphatase-labelled ligand. When the diluent and sample are added to the test cup, the ligand (T_4 or T_3) competes with the enzyme-conjugated ligand for binding sites on the immobilized antibody. The unreacted sample and unbound enzyme conjugate are then washed away while the immune complex is retained by a magnetic force applied to the test cup. The enzyme activity remaining in the test cup, which is inversely proportional to the ligand concentration on the sample, is determined by measuring the rate of conversion of the substrate 4-methylumbelliferyl phosphate to a fluorescent compound, 4-methylumbelliferone. The self-contained, ligand-specific test cup with a bar code enables the analyzer to perform a broad range of assays in a random and continuous access fashion. This allows the operator to perform more than one test on a given sample and a variety of single tests on multiple patient samples simultaneously. It also permits the entry of additional tests or stat assays without interrupting the test in progress. The throughput of this analyzer is claimed to be 420 tests per three and a half hours.

The fluorescence polarization immunoassay and the radial partition immunoassay are the two fully automated, non-isotopic immunoassay analyzers receiving relatively wide acceptance in the United States for the measurements of serum T_4 and T_3 concentrations. They are batch systems with a relatively low capacity (20 to 30 samples) and thus are ideal for small-to-medium laboratories handling relatively low test volumes.

Since almost all circulating thyroid hormones are bound to plasma proteins, dissociation of the hormones from the binding proteins is required unless the hormones are extracted from serum prior to assay. In all of the assay methods described here, specific blocking agents such as salicylate, thimerosal, or 8-anilino-1-naphthalene-sulfonic acid (ANS) are used to inhibit the binding of thyroid hormones to TBG without affecting the binding to their specific antibodies in immunoassays. Plasma may also be used as a sample instead of serum but tends to form fibrin after freezing and thawing, which may mechanically interfere with the assay, especially in an automated system. Thyroid hormones are quite stable but it is recommended that serum samples be stored frozen if they will not be analyzed within 24 hours. Antibodies to thyroid hormones have been detected in some serum obtained from euthyroid subjects and patients with, for example, hypothyroidism, thyroid carcinoma, Hashimoto's thyroiditis, Graves' disease, and nontoxic goiter, and it is important to be aware of their potential interference in immunoassays of thyroid hormones. In the presence of the autoantibodies, the result may be falsely high when the bound fraction is a solid phase such as in double antibody or antibody-coated tube method, whereas the result may be falsely low when the bound fraction is a liquid phase such as in charcoal- or resin-phase separation method. As with all diagnostic tests, each laboratory should establish its own reference ranges, thereby allowing variability resulting from such factors as geography and assay techniques. There are conflicting reports regarding the age and sex dependency of serum thyroid hormone concentrations in adults, but these differences are small and can be ignored for routine testing. Although the age-dependent differences in serum thyroid hormone concentrations are of little significance in adults, they are important during childhood. Reference ranges for serum total T_4 and T_3 are summarized in Table 17-5. Reverse T_3 is elevated markedly while the T_3 level is decreased in the serum of newborns.

In patients without underlying systemic illnesses or conditions known to alter thyroid binding proteins, especially TBG, the total serum T_4 concentration is a specific and sensitive index of thyroid function and the first procedure in laboratory assessment of thyroid diseases. However, al-

Table 17-5 Age-dependent reference ranges of serum total T_4 and T_3 concentrations*

| Age | n | T_4 | | T_3 | |
		mg/dL	nmol/L	ng/dL	nmol/L
Cord blood	20	6.6-18.1	83-226	24-77	0.4-1.2
2-5 days	20	8.5-22.0	106-275	99-227	1.5-3.5
3-12 months	20	7.6-16.0	95-200	96-219	1.5-3.4
1-5 years	20	7.3-15.0	91-188	92-215	1.4-3.3
6-10 years	30	6.4-13.3	80-166	84-194	1.3-3.0
11-16 years	30	5.6-11.7	70-146	75-172	1.2-2.6
>16 years	100	4.5-11.5	56-144	94-168	1.4-2.6

*Established at University of Cincinnati Medical Center.

teration of plasma thyroid hormone-binding protein concentrations under a variety of conditions (Box 17-1) will result in altered total T_4 levels, while the metabolically active free T_4 concentrations remain almost constant. It is therefore more useful to directly or indirectly determine free T_4 concentrations.

Estimates of thyroid hormone binding and indirect estimates of free thyroid hormones

The free thyroid hormone concentration can be calculated from the total thyroid hormone concentration and the fraction (percent) of thyroid hormone which is free in serum. The free hormone fraction is traditionally determined by equilibrium dialysis or ultrafiltration of serum enriched with radioactive thyroid hormone. However, these procedures are cumbersome and too time-consuming for routine clinical use. The T_3-resin uptake test is more widely used for estimating the number of available unoccupied binding sites on thyroid hormone binding proteins in serum (Table 17-6). In this test, radiolabeled T_3 is added to serum followed by the addition of a resin and the distribution of radiolabeled T_3 between thyroid hormone binding proteins (endogenous binders, mainly TBG) and the resin (secondary binder) is determined. The percentage uptake of total radiolabeled T_3 by the resin (the T_3 resin uptake) is inversely proportional to the number of unoccupied binding sites on TBG in serum, which may be affected by total thyroid hormone concentrations (hyperthyroidism or hypothyroidism) and by TBG concentration in the test serum (Table 17-7). In addition to a resin, many other secondary binders are used in commercial T_3 uptake test kits (e.g., charcoal, solid phase anti-T_3 antibody, organic polymers (Sephadex), silicate, talc, and macroaggregated albumin). Although radiolabeled T_4 can theoretically be used for assessing the number of unoccupied binding sites on serum proteins, radiolabeled T_3 is preferred because of its relatively low affinity for TBG. The radioactive T_3 will fill the unoccupied binding sites but will not displace bound T_4. Further, T_4 binds to all thyroid hormone binding proteins. Thus the T_4 uptake values can be affected by the changes in any of the binding proteins. In the T_3 uptake test, the T_3 binding is affected primarily by the TBG concentrations since T_3 binds to neither prealbumin nor albumin under the conditions of most T_3 uptake tests. Nonradioactive labels are also used in the uptake test. A fluorescein-labeled T_4 rather than T_3 is used by the fluorescence polarization technique (TD_x) because fluorescein-

Table 17-6   Methods of estimate of thyroid hormone binding

Methods	Markers	Principle	Comments
T_3-uptake	^{125}I-labeled T_3	Distribution of marker between primary (TBG) and secondary (resin etc.) binder is measured by counting radioactivity	Heterogeneous system primarily measuring thyroid hormone binding sites in TBG, automated system available
	T_3	Amount of added T_3 bound to secondary binder (T_3-antibody) is measured by ELIA (Table 17-4)	Heterogeneous system primarily measuring thyroid hormone binding sites in TBG, partially automated
T_4-uptake	Fluorescein-labeled T_4	Amount of marker bound to thyroid hormone binding proteins is measured by FPIA (Table 17-4)	Homogeneous system measuring T_4 binding sites in TBG as well as prealbumin and albumin, fully automated
	T_4	Amount of added T_4 bound to secondary binder (T_4) antibody is measured by FEIA (Table 17-5)	Heterogeneous system measuring T_4 binding sites in TBG as well as prealbumin and albumin, fully automated

Table 17-7   Changes in total T_4 (bound T_4 + free T_4), unoccupied binding sites, and free T_4 under various conditions

	Free T_4	Bound T_4	Unoccupied binding sites	TBG	Unoccupied binding sites	(uptake)	Total T_4	Free T_4	FT$_4$I
A. Euthyroid normal				N	N	(N)	N	N	N
B. Euthyroid, increased TBG				↑	↑	(↓)	↑	N	N
C. Euthyroid, decreased TBG				↓	↓	(↑)	↓	N	N
D. Euthyroid, T_4 displaced by drugs		Drug		N	↓	(↑)	↓	N	N
E. Hyperthyroidism				N	↓	(↑)	↑	↑	↑
F. Hypothyroidism				N	↑	(↓)	↓	↓	↓

A. In healthy euthyroid individuals, 99.93% of T_4 is protein bound and about a third of the TBG binding sites are occupied by T_4.
B. An increase in TBG in euthyroid individuals (see Box 17-1) causes an increase in both bound T_4 and unoccupied binding sites, but their free T_4 and FT$_4$I are both normal.
C. A decrease in TBG in euthyroid individual decreases both bound T_4 and unoccupied binding sites, but their free T_4 and FT$_4$I are both normal.
D. Some drugs (Box 17-1) are bound by TBG and replace Bound T_4. Unoccupied binding sites and total T_4 are usually decreased but free T_4 and FT$_4$I are both normal.
E. In hyperthyroidism, bound T_4, free T_4, total T_4, and FT$_4$I are all increased. Unoccupied binding sites decreased but TBG levels are usually unaffected.
F. In hypothyroidism, bound T_4, free T_4, total T_4, and FT$_4$I are all decreased. Unoccupied binding sites increased but TBG levels are usually unaffected.

labeled T_3 loses almost all of its ability to bind TBG. The basic technology is the same as that used in the TD$_x$ thyroid hormone assay described previously except that no T_4-antibody is used. An increase in the degree of polarization of fluorescent light emitted from the fluorescein-labeled T_4 resulting from its binding to the T_4 binding proteins in serum is proportional to the number of unoccupied T_4 binding sites in serum T_4-binding proteins. The condition of this assay is such that it measures T_4-binding sites not only on TBG but also on prealbumin and albumin. In EMIT and Stratus systems described previously, the distribution of a fixed amount of added T_4 between thyroid hormone-binding proteins and the secondary binder (T_4-antibody) is determined by measuring the amount of T_4 bound to the secondary binder using an enzyme immunoassay with an enzyme-labeled T_4 as the tracer. A similar technique is used in the Amerlite system except that the amount of T_3, not T_4, bound to the secondary binder (T_3-antibody) is determined by the enhanced luminescence immunoassay as described previously. When the radioactive T_3 uptake test is used, uptake values are customarily expressed as the percentage of the total radioactivity that is taken up by the secondary binder

or that is not bound to TBG. For most assays, the reference range is 25% to 35%. However, the actual value depends on various assay conditions used, e.g., the specific activity of the radiolabeled T_3, the avidity of the secondary binder for T_3, the incubation time and temperature. Variation in the uptake values resulting from imprecise assay conditions can be minimized by using the T_3 uptake ratio, which is the T_3 uptake of the patient divided by the T_3 uptake of a pool of normal standard reference serum included in the same assay run. If the T_3 uptake value of the normal standard reference serum is 30%, the reference range of the T_3 uptake ratio will be 0.83 to 1.17. The T_3 uptake ratio can be calculated directly from the radioactivity taken up on the secondary binder (absorbent);

Patient T_3 uptake ratio =

$$\frac{\text{Absorbent counts for patient serum}}{\text{Absorbent counts for normal reference serum}}$$

The committee on Nomenclature of the American Thyroid Association (ATA) strongly recommends expression of the T_3 uptake as a ratio and considers it mandatory when calculating the free T_4 or T_3 index (FT$_4$I or FT$_3$I). The ATA committee also recommends that if the T_3 uptake is reported directly, it should always be reported with a serum total T_4 or T_3 concentration so that FT_4I or FT_3I can be calculated. In other words, the T_3 uptake test is useful only as a means of calculating FT_4I or FT_3I:

$$FT_4I \text{ or } FT_3I = (\text{total } T_4 \text{ or } T_3 \text{ concentration}) \times \\ (T_3 \text{ uptake ratio})$$

In order to reduce confusion caused by the similarity between the nomenclature used for a "T_3 uptake" and a total serum T_3 measurement, the ATA has recently recommended that the name of uptake tests be changed to Thyroid Hormone Binding Ratio (THBR) and that the results be calculated as the absorbent-bound counts divided by the residual serum protein-bound counts (or total counts less absorbent-bound counts), not as the absorbent-bound counts divided by the total count. This result for a patient's serum divided by that for the normal reference serum is the patient's THBR.

Thus patient's THBR = $(Ap/Bp) / (An/Bn) = (Ap/T-Ap) / (An/T-An)$

Ap = Absorbent counts for patient's serum

An = Absorbent counts for normal reference serum

Bp = Binding protein-bound counts for patient's serum

Bn = Binding protein-bound counts for normal reference serum

T = Total counts added

THBR is proportional to the free fraction of T_4 or T_3 and will be centered around 1.0 for healthy euthyroid subjects. A normal value of 1.0 ($\pm$ 0.1) can then be multipled by total T_4 or T_3 concentration to yield a free T_4 or T_3 index value with the same arithmetic range as that of the total T_4 and T_3 concentrations. The ATA committee recommends the use of "unit" (U) to express the free hormone index value in order to avoid confusion with measurement of hormone itself. Thus FT_4I or FT_3I = (total T_4 or T_3 concentrations) $\times$ (THBR) and the reference range will be 4.5 to 11.5 U (Table 17-5). The reference range is not necessarily identical for each method and may be affected by the type of exogenous thyroid hormones used in the assay. The ATA committee suggests specifying the labeled iodothyronine used in the assay as follows: THBR (T_3) or THBR (T_4).

A number of commercial kits are now available for measuring FT_4 and FT_3. Despite the implications of the term "free T_4 or T_3," most of the currently available kits measure this quantity indirectly. In these assays, the measured quantity (assay response) is converted to a free hormone concentration by using a standard curve calibrated independently with the free hormone values measured by equilibrium dialysis or ultrafiltration. These methods, therefore, fall more properly into the category of a free hormone index. Based on the technique used, these commercial kits can be classified by two major groups: one-step (analog) and two-step methods.

The one-step method is based on the assumption that a structurally modified labeled analog of thyroid hormone will not bind to serum thyroid hormone binding proteins, but will compete with free thyroid hormone for binding to a specific thyroid hormone antibody. In the two-step method, free thyroid hormone in serum is bound to the antibody-coated tube in an immunoextraction step. The serum is then decanted, and labeled thyroid hormone is added to saturate the antibody binding sites. The thyroid hormone binding proteins in serum in the one-step method make contact with the labeled thyroid hormone but not in the two-step method. Nonisotopic labels are also used in estimating free T_4 concentrations. In a one-step luminescent enzyme immunoassay, a horseradish peroxidase-labeled T_4 derivative is used, while an alkaline phosphatase labeled T_4 is used in a two-step radial partition immunoassay.

It has been reported that the currently available thyroid hormone analogs do bind to serum proteins, especially serum albumin, to an extent that a significant perturbation of the assay may occur and may give unreliable results whereas the results of two-step methods appear to correlate better with results by equilibrium dialysis.

Direct determination of free thyroid hormones

The most accurate and reliable methods presently available for measuring free thyroid hormone are the equilibrium dialysis and ultrafiltration methods. In both methods, thyroid hormone in the free fraction is physically separated and measured directly using a sensitive RIA procedure. Ultrafiltration can separate free thyroid hormone from bound thyroid hormone within one hour whereas equilibrium dialysis requires about 18 hours. These methods, however, are cumbersome and technically demanding and thus are not suitable for routine clinical use. They are used mostly as the reference method.

Tests for examining the hypothalmic-pituitary-thyroid axis

Immunoassays of serum TSH

Initially, TSH was measured using bioassays, and the measurement of serum TSH did not become a routine laboratory test for clinical evaluation of the thyroid until purified human pituitary TSH became available. The development of antibodies was then possible. Hormone was also available for radiolabeling and as a standard in an RIA procedure specific for human TSH. As with any immunoassay, the TSH RIA measures the immunological activity, not the biological activity, of circulating TSH, although the results are customarily expressed as milli-international units of biological activity per liter (mU/L) of serum. A TSH molecule can lose its biological activity without losing its immunological activity. However, all available data indicate that TSH concentrations measured by RIA methods correlate well with biological activity and are excellent indicators for the diagnosis of disorders of the hypothalmic-pituitary-thyroid axis. In addition to the conventional RIA, a solid-phase, two-site immunoradiometric assay (IRMA) has been used for measuring circulating TSH. In this method TSH is assayed directly by reaction with excess radiolabeled specific antibodies rather than by competition with a radiolabeled TSH molecule for a fixed number of binding sites on a limited amount of antibody. In general, samples containing TSH are reacted with a radiolabeled antibody directed toward a unique site on the TSH molecule and with an immobilized solid-phase antibody directed against a different antigenic site on the same TSH molecule. The radiolabeled antibody/TSH/solid-phase antibody complex formed is separated from the reaction mixture, washed, and counted. The radioactivity measured is directly proportional to the concentration of TSH present in the test sample. An assay of this type is also known as a "sandwich" assay because the antigen TSH becomes sandwiched between the labeled antibodies and immobilized antibodies.

A TSH IRMA kit using two high-affinity monoclonal antibodies is available, each specific to different antigenic sites on the same TSH molecule, to achieve a level of sensitivity and specificity impossible with traditional methods. One monoclonal antibody is labeled with ^{125}I, the second with fluorescein isothiocyanate (FITC), a highly immunogenic group. Patient samples are incubated with a liquid mixture of these two monoclonal antibodies to form a "sandwich." Anti-FITC linked to magnetizable particles is then added to the incubation mixture to achieve separation of excess ^{125}I-labeled antibodies from the labeled sandwich complex, which sediments rapidly in a magnetic field. In this assay method, since the interactions between TSH and antibodies proceed in a liquid phase, the diffusional and geometrical constraints encountered in the solid-phase, two-site IRMA are eliminated, resulting in a shortened reaction time. The minimum detectable level was claimed to be 0.1 mU/L. The assay turnaround time is three hours.

Immunometric assays of TSH using enzymes as labels have also been developed. Test serum is allowed to react with two different anti-TSH monoclonal antibodies. One antibody is affixed to a solid phase; the other is labeled with bovine alkaline phosphatase (AP), each antibody directed against a distinct antigenic site on the TSH molecule. The AP-labeled antibody/TSH/solid-phase antibody complex formed is separated, washed, and reacted with a chromogenic substrate, p-nitrophenylphosphate. The yellow color developed is measured spectrophotometrically at 405 nm. The concentration of TSH is directly proportional to the color intensity (enzyme activity). There is little, if any, detectable cross-reactivity between this TSH assay and hCG. FSH, or LH.

The use of a fluoroimmunoassay technique for measuring TSH has been described as well. This fluoroimmunoassay uses the TSH-antibody labeled with europium chelate as the tracer and time-resolved fluorescence as the detection method. The limited sensitivity of most fluoroimmunoassay methods results from the high background signal encountered in conventional fluorometric determinations. To minimize the high background fluorescence, serum samples are usually pretreated before they are used in the fluoroimmunoassay. The europium chelate used in the time-resolved fluoroimmunoassay of TSH has a much longer fluorescence lifetime (a half-life of decay in the range of 10^{-3} to 10^{-6} seconds) than that of fluorescence emitted from conventional fluorescent compounds including those causing the high background signal in serum (10^{-8} to 10^{-9} seconds), and thus its specific fluorescence can be measured after the background signal has decayed and no pretreatment step is needed. Two monoclonal antibodies directed against two separate antigenic determinants on the beta-subunit of the TSH molecule are used in this assay; one monoclonal antibody is labeled with europium as a nonfluorescent chelate,

and the other is immobilized on the surface of microtitration strip wells. After a four-hour incubation of the serum sample with the europium-labeled antibody at room temperature in the antibody-coated microtitration well, the well is aspirated and washed with water to remove the unbound europium-labeled antibody. The fluorescence of the europium ion in the solid-phase antibody/TSH/europium-labeled antibody complex is developed after the ion is released by dissociation. The dissociation is carried out in the presence of an enhancement solution containing energy-absorbing ligands required for the formation of a fluorescent chelate (tri-n-octylphosphine oxide and 2-naphthoyltrifluoroacetone). The light emission of the europium ion is measured in a time-resolving (400 usec) fluorometer. Europium concentrations as low as 5×10^{-14} M have been measured by this technique, and theoretically the assay sensitivity can be increased further because a number of europium ions can be coupled per antibody molecule. The sensitivity of this assay is claimed to be 0.3 mU/L.

An immunochemiluminometric assay employing an anti-TSH antibody labeled with a chemiluminescent molecule and a second anti-TSH immobilized on a plastic test tube has been developed. The chemiluminescent label bound to the tube through the formation of a sandwiched complex is activated by the addition of a hydrogen peroxide. The intensity of chemiluminescence proportional to the TSH concentration is determined. The kit manufacturer claims that the assay is capable of detecting a TSH concentration as low as 0.005 mU/L. The extreme sensitivity is said to be attributable to the high quantum efficiency of the luminescent compound used for labelling anti-TSH antibody.

Methods of TSH analysis described in this section are summarized in Table 17-8. Several fully automated systems capable of measuring subnormal levels of TSH are now available. All utilize a fluoroenzymometric technique in which an alkaline phosphatase-labeled anti-TSH-antibody, a solid-phase anti-TSH antibody, and a fluorogenic substrate of alkaline phosphatase, 4-methylumbelliferyl phosphate, are employed. Various methods separate the sandwiched complex from the unbound material. Since TSH secretion is relatively constant, useful clinical information can be obtained from a blood specimen drawn at any convenient time. Serum or plasma samples can be used, but some kit manufacturers recommend serum samples only. Although TSH in serum is stable for at least five days at 4°C, if the test is not administered within 24 hours, the serum should be kept frozen at -20°C. Repeated freezing and thawing of the sample should be avoided. The use of grossly hemolyzed or lipemic samples is not recommended.

Most of the older commercial RIA kits for TSH (first generation TSH assays,* sensitivity in the range of 1 to 2 mU/L) were not sensitive enough to detect TSH in all healthy subjects, but were able to statistically estimate the reference range of serum TSH to be about 0.51 to 5.75 mU/L (Tsay, et al, Clin Chem 25:2001, 1979). This range could

---

*This "generation" approach to the nomenclature of TSH assays was proposed by CA Spencer (Clinical Chemistry News, November 1989, p. 14) to help clarify the confusing terminology (i.e., used by commercial manufacturers of TSH assay kits "ultra sensitive," "supersensitive," and "highly sensitive") to market the new sensitive TSH immunometric assay kits.

Table 17-8 Methods of TSH analysis

Methods	Principle	Marker	Comments
1. Radioimmunoassay (RIA)	Competitive binding of radiolabeled TSH and nonlabeled TSH to limited binding sites on antibody	^{125}I	Not sensitive to measure subnormal TSH levels
2. Immunoradiometric (IRMA)	Binding of TSH to radiolabeled antibody	^{125}I	May be more sensitive and specific than RIAs; fully automated
3. Immunoenzymometric assay (IEMA)	Binding of TSH to enzyme-labeled antibody	Enzyme	May become an excellent alternative to radioassay as sensitivity is improved
4. Time-resolved immunofluorometric assay (TR-IFMA)	Binding of TSH to europium-labeled antibody	Europium chelate	Has potential of being very sensitive assay; available commercially
5. Immunoluminometric assay (ILMA)	Binding of TSH to luminescent molecule-labeled antibody	Luminescent labels such as luminol and luciferase	Has potential of being very sensitive assay; available for routine use

be confirmed by using second-generation TSH immunometric assays (sensitivity in the range of 0.1 to 0.2 mU/L). Third-generation TSH assays are now under development and are expected to detect TSH levels of 0.01 mU/L or lower. The availability of third-generation assays should help thyroid evaluation in sick patients and in thyroid patients requiring optimization of T_4 therapy.

No difference was found between TSH values in men and women 20 to 60 years of age. Men from 60 to 70 continue to have stable TSH levels, but women older than 60 show a significantly higher mean TSH level (3.4 ± 1.6 mU/L) than younger women (2.3 ± 1.3 mU/L). In neonates, serum TSH levels rise sharply within 10 minutes after delivery, reach a peak (10 to 24-fold increase) after 30 minutes, and then decline gradually and reach adult levels about five days after delivery.

Thyrotropin releasing hormone (TRH) stimulation test

Acute injection of TRH stimulates TSH release by the pituitary. Abnormally high circulating free T_4 levels can override the stimulatory effect of hypothalmic TRH and thus exogenous TRH has little or no effect on TSH secretion in patients with hyperthyroidism. The TRH stimulation test of pituitary TSH reserve is of clinical value in assessment of hyperthyroidism. It is also valuable in differential diagnosis of hypothalmic (tertiary) from pituitary (secondary) hypothyroidism. A TSH response to TRH is present in the former but not in the latter (Figure 17-7). In the TRH stimulation test, a baseline TSH sample is drawn before the test. Typically, 500 micrograms of TRH are given intravenously to the patient, and blood samples are drawn again 20, 30, and 40 minutes after TRH injection. Minor side effects caused by TRH injection include headaches, dizziness, nausea, and a momentary urge to urinate. The maximum increment of serum TSH from the baseline value (Δ TSH) after TRH injection is 2 to 20 mU/L in euthyroid subjects. Elderly men are less responsive to TRH stimulation than women and young men. Δ TSH is also normal in hypothalamic (tertiary) hypothyroidism, but the response is usually delayed (60 to 180 minutes versus 30 minutes for normal subjects). Δ TSH is less than 2 mU/L in pituitary (secondary) hypothyroidism and also in hyperthyroidism but is

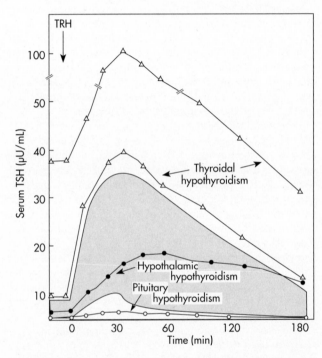

Fig. 17-7 Typical serum TSH responses to TRH in patients with thyroid (primary), pituitary (secondary), and hypothalamic (tertiary) hypothyroidism. The hatched area indicates the normal range. *From Werner's The thyroid, Ingbar SH and Braverman LE (eds), ed 5, 1986, Lippincott.*

greater than 20 mU/L in thyroidal (primary) hypothyroidism.

Tests for measuring other thyroid-related proteins
Measurement of thyroglobulin (TG)

Circulating TG can be measured by an RIA method. The presence of an excessive amount of circulating TG autoantibodies interferes with the assay. Samples containing such antibodies should be rejected for analysis. TG concentrations determined in 20 euthyroid-healthy volunteers at the University of Cincinnati Medical Center ranged from 3 to 18 μg/L with a mean value of 9 μg/L. Somewhat higher values are found in newborns and during the third trimester of pregnancy. The only source of circulating TG appears to be functioning thyroid tissue, whether normal or neoplastic. Accordingly, TG determinations are a valuable ancillary tool in diagnosing and managing residual and/or recurrent differentiated thyroid cancer. Excess thyroglobulin is also released into the general circulation when thyroid overactivity is present or when the follicular structure of the thyroid gland is damaged, as in subacute thyroiditis.

Measurement of thyroid autoantibodies

Antibodies against several components of thyroid follicles have been detected in the serum of patients with autoimmune thyroid diseases. They include thyroglobulin autoantibodies and thyroid microsomal autoantibodies. Thyroid microsomal antigen is an integral membrane protein and recent studies have shown it to be thyroid peroxidase. Traditionally, these two autoantibodies are measured by a hemagglutination technique. In this technique, tannic acid-treated sheep red blood cells with absorbed thyroglobulin or thyroid microsomal antigen are incubated with patient's serum. The presence of antibodies against these antigens agglutinates the cells. The test results are expressed as the antibody titers. Sera with titers greater than 1:10 are considered to be significant in patients with thyroid autoimmune diseases. An indirect fluorescent antibody technique has also been used to qualitatively or semi-quantitatively measure the thyroid autoantibodies. This technique employs monkey thyroid tissue substrate and fluorescein-labelled rabbit antihuman gammaglobulin. The tissue substrate is incubated with serially diluted sera, washed with a buffer, and then allowed to intereact with fluorescein-labelled antihuman gammaglobulin. The presence of thyroid autoantibodies will allow the fluorescein label to be absorbed at approporiate locations in the tissue substrate where thyroglobulin or microsomal antigen is located and produce apple-green staining, which is detected by a properly equipped fluorescence microscope assembly. This technique allows for the simultaneous detection of both thyroid autoantibodies in a single assay.

A sensitive direct radioligand assay system employing purified stable preparation of radiolabelled thyroglobulin or thyroid peroxidase as the tracer has also been developed. Calibrators used in this system have been standardized against the MRC Thyroglobulin or Microsomal Antigen Autoantibody First International Reference Preparation (code 65/93 or 66/387). The patient's serum is incubated with tracer and the thyroid autoantibody-tracer complex formed is precipitated by protein A and counted. The amount of radioactivity in the precipitate is directly proportional to the amount of thyroid autoantibodies contained in the calibrators and/or unknowns. A thyroid autoantibody concentration of 200 U/mL is approximately equal to a titer of 1:10 determined by a hemagglutination technique. The routine working range for these radioligand assays is 6 to 600 U/mL. Values greater than 20 U/mL indicate the presence of reactive thyroid autoantibody.

Measurement of thyroid-stimulating immunoglobulins (TSI)

The sera of many patients with hyperthyroid Graves' disease contain thyroid-stimulating activity quite distinct from TSH. This stimulator was initially termed Long-Acting Thyroid Stimulator (LATS) because of its prolonged course of action in the bioassay system used to measure it. Subsequent research suggested that LATS was an immunoglobulin with all the characteristics of a thyroid-stimulating autoantibody. These antibodies are now collectively called thyroid-stimulating immunoglobulins (TSI) and appear to induce hyperthyroidism in Graves' disease by binding to the TSH receptor in the thyroid and mimicking the action of TSH. Unlike TSH, TSI do not respond to the negative feedback system. The presence of TSI in the patient's serum can be tested by the ability of the serum to stimulate cAMP generation in human thyroid tissue or cells cultured in monolayers. These tests, however, are not practical enough for routine clinical use. A receptor-binding inhibition assay is a rapid and simple method for analyzing TSI in large numbers of specimens. This assay is based on the competition between TSI and radiolabelled TSH for a limited number of TSH-binding sites on TSH receptors. The radioactivity in the TSH-receptor complex is inversely proportional to the concentration of TSI in the patient's serum.

DISORDERS OF THE THYROID GLAND AND THEIR LABORATORY ASSESSMENT

As in most endocrine systems, disorders of the hypothalamic-pituitary system may result in hyperthyroidism (excessive thyroid hormone secretion), hypothyroidism (deficient thyroid hormone secretion), or no change in thyroid hormone secretion. Major physiological manifestations of hyperthyroidism and hypothyroidism are summarized in Table 17-2.

Hyperthyroidism (thyrotoxicosis)

Thyrotoxicosis is the clinical syndrome produced by sustained high levels of circulating thyroid hormone and may be recognized easily or in some cases may remain unsuspected for a long time. Thyrotoxicosis may be caused by over-activity of the thyroid gland itself (primary hyperthyroidism), excessive secretion of thyroid hormone from ectopic sites, excessive ingestion of thyroid hormone, or production of thyroid-stimulating immunoglobulins (TSI) in thyroid autoimmune diseases (secondary hyperthyroidism).

Graves' disease

The most common cause of thyrotoxicosis in the United States is Graves' disease (diffuse toxic goiter). It is an autoimmune disorder resulting in the production of TSI that has a TSH-like action on the thyroid. Women are involved about six times more commonly than men. The disease may occur at any age, but is more frequently encountered during puberty, pregnancy, menopause, or following severe stress. Any or all of the following clinical features have been observed in Graves' disease: 1) thyrotoxic goiter; 2) ophthalmopathy (bulging eyes); and 3) dermopathy (skin changes). Since TSI activates the TSH receptor and since the production of TSI is not under the feedback control of thyroid hormones, uncontrolled stimulation of the thyroid gland occurs in Graves' disease, causing a diffuse enlargement of the thyroid with resultant excess production of thyroid hormone. Circulating levels of both T_4 and T_3 are usually abnormally high, but the increase in T_3 levels usually become evident earlier than increases of T_4. Much of the circulating

T_3 is secreted directly by the thyroid. In addition, the TSH production is suppressed and the TSH response to TRH stimulation is blunted because of feedback mechanisms in the face of sustained excessive levels of circulating thyroid hormone (Figure 17-7). TSI are present in more than 90% of Graves' disease patients. The radioactive iodine uptake of the thyroid is elevated in these patients. Thus, the characteristic laboratory findings in Graves' disease are high levels of T_3 and T_4, subnormal levels of TSH, the presence of TSI, and an elevated radioactive iodine uptake by the thyroid gland.

Other common forms of thyrotoxicosis

Other forms of thyrotoxicosis include toxic adenoma, toxic multinodular goiter, hyperthyroid phase of thyroiditis, thyrotoxicosis factitia, and iatrogenic thyrotoxicosis. Toxic multinodular goiter tends to occur more commonly in older people. Cardiovascular symptoms such as tachycardia, palpitation, and shortness of breath are common clinical features of these diseases, but symptoms and signs do not suggest a particular etiology. The primary defect appears to be autonomous production of excess thyroid hormone without TSH stimulation. The thyroid tissue not located in the nodules becomes suppressed but always retains a small degree of function. The radioactive iodine or technetium scan reveals single or multiple functioning "hot" nodules. Laboratory investigations may show markedly elevated serum T_3 with less striking elevation of serum T_4. As in Graves' disease, TSH is suppressed by the negative feedback control.

Toxic multinodular goiter can occasionally be confused with Graves' disease. If the physical examination and radioactive iodine imaging are not helpful, features that favor toxic multinodular goiter include: longer onset of presentation, very large thyroid size, absence of TSI, older age at presentation, and lack of ophthalmopathy and dermopathy.

Thyroiditis is an inflammatory disorder of the thyroid gland. The inflamed and disrupted thyroid follicles may acutely release thyroid hormone and produce symptoms of thyrotoxicosis. Administration by a physician (iatrogenic) or intake by patients (factitious) of excessive amounts of thyroid hormone for whatever purpose may produce symptoms of thyrotoxicosis.

Rare forms of thyrotoxicosis

Ovarian struma and metastatic follicular carcinoma of the thyroid contain ectopic thyroid tissue that may become hyperactive and produce enough thyroid hormone to cause mild hyperthyroidism. Circulating levels of thyroid hormone are usually mildly elevated. A radioactive iodine whole-body scan after administration of ^{123}I will demonstrate the presence of ectopic thyroid tissue. Trophoblastic tumors such as hydatidiform mole, choriocarcinoma, or embryonal carcinoma of the testis produce human chorionic gonadotropin (hCG), which has minimal intrinsic TSH-like activity and may produce mild elevation of serum thyroid hormone and mild features of thyrotoxicosis if produced in great excess. Mild thyrotoxicosis and goiter may be present in patients with TSH-secreting pituitary tumors or selective pituitary resistance to thyroid hormone (impaired intrapi-

tuitary T_4 to T_3 conversion). Circulating levels of T_4 and T_3 are elevated. There is no response to TRH, but serum TSH levels, usually subnormal in Graves' disease, are elevated. Some patients with hyperthyroidism may have an elevated serum T_3 but normal T_4 (T_3 thyrotoxicosis). This phenomenon has been observed in patients with Graves' disease as well as other forms of thyrotoxicosis. An elevated serum T_4 with normal or only mildly elevated T_3 (T_4 thyrotoxicosis) has also been observed in patients with hyperthyroidism, most often in patients with an abnormality in conversion of T_4 to T_3 as a result of chronic debilitating disease or following an excessive intake of iodine.

After the diagnosis of hyperthyroidism is established, radioactive iodine ablation therapy, antibody drug therapy, or subtotal thyroidectomy may be used to lower thyroid hormone levels and control the hyperthyroidism on a long-term basis. Thyroid tests are useful not only for the diagnosis of thyroid disorders but also for monitoring antithyroid treatment in hyperthyroidism. As shown in Figure 17-8, a serum TSH measurement appears to be the most sensitive test for diagnosis of hyperthyroidism because the suppression of serum TSH value occurs considerably earlier than elevation of serum T_3 or T_4 value. During the early phases of antithyroid treatment (less than about 13 weeks), however, serum T_3 or T_4 concentrations appear to reflect the acute response to the treatment more accurately than serum TSH levels. During this early treatment phase, serum TSH levels remain suppressed even in the presence of a rapidly developing hypothyroid state due to the physiological lag (about six to eight weeks) in the pituitary reset of TSH secretion. Therefore, during this period of post treatment a low T_4 and low TSH should not prompt a search for secondary hypothyroidism. The TSH measurement again becomes the optimal test for detecting any subtle thyroid hormone excess or deficiency after a stable thyroid status has been restored. Laboratory findings in hyperthyroidism are summarized in Table 17-9.

Hypothyroidism

Hypothyroidism is a clinical syndrome resulting from inadequate secretion and/or insufficient amounts of thyroid hormones available at the tissues. Hypothyroidism is less common than hyperthyroidism but may occur at any time in life. The occurrence of hypothyroidism in infants (cretinism) results in developmental abnormalities and, without timely treatment, may cause mental retardation. Hypothyroidism later in life causes a generalized slowing of metabolic processes with a clinical picture involving myxedema resulting from tissue infiltration of mucopolysaccharides. Table 17-9 summarizes the major physiological manifestations of hypothyroidism.

Primary thyroid failure accounts for about 98% of hypothyroidism in the United States, and autoimmune chronic thyroiditis (Hashimoto's thyroiditis) is probably the single most common cause of hypothyroidism. In Hashimoto's thyroiditis, massive infiltration of lymphocytes into the thyroid gland cause destruction of normal thyroid architecture. The continued destruction of the gland eventually results in a decrease in serum thyroid hormone levels and a rise in TSH concentration.

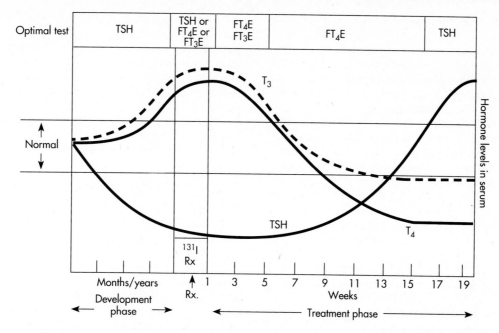

Fig. 17-8   Optimal tests for primary hyperthyroidism. *From Spencer CA, Thyroid status: trends in testing: selective test use cuts cost, Clinical Chemistry News, 1989, page 10.*

Table 17-9   Findings in thyroid function tests in various clinical conditions

Condition	T$_4$	FT$_4$I	T$_3$	FT$_3$I	TSH	TSI	TRH stimulation
Hyperthyroidism							
Graves' disease	↑	↑	↑	↑	↓	+	↓
Toxic nodular goiter	↑	↑	↑	↑	↓	−	↓
Pituitary TSH-secreting tumors	↑	↑	↑	↑	↑	−	↓
T$_3$ thyrotoxicosis	N	N	↑	↑	↓	+, −	↓
T$_4$ thyrotoxicosis	↑	↑	N	N	↓	+, −	↓
Hypothyroidism							
Primary	↓	↓	↓	↓	↑	+, −	↑
Secondary	↓	↓	↓	↓	↓, N	−	↑
Tertiary	↓	↓	↓	↓	↓, N	−	↓
Peripheral unresponsiveness	↑, N	↑, N	↑, N	↑	↑, N	−	N, ↑

N = Normal; ↑ = increased; ↓ = decreased; +, − = variable

Subacute thyroiditis during the late phase may also cause transient or, rarely, hypothyroidism. Unlike Hashimoto's thyroiditis, subacute thyroiditis is most likely caused by a viral infection.

Other common causes of primary hypothyroidism include iatrogenic factors (destructive therapy such as radioactive iodine therapy and subtotal thyroidectomy for Graves' disease or nodular goiter) and drugs (e.g., iodide-containing cough preparation, lithium carbonate used for the treatment of manic-depressive state, and antithyroid drugs propylthiouracil and methimazole). Secondary hypothyroidism caused by hypopituitarism may be due to pituitary adenoma, pituitary ablative therapy, or another pituitary destructive mechanisms. Tertiary hypothyroidism, caused by hypothalamic dysfunction, is quite rare.

Laboratory findings in hypothyroidism are summarized in Table 17-9. Primary hypothyroidism is characterized by a low-serum T$_4$ and elevated TSH because of the negative feedback relationship between serum thyroid hormone and TSH. The presence of antimicrosomal antibody and/or antithyroglobulin antibody suggests underlying chronic lymphocytic thyroiditis. At least one of these antibodies is usually present in roughly 90% of patients with Hashimoto's thyroiditis. The serum T$_3$ and FT$_3$I are normal in 20% to 30% of patients that are hypothyroid and thus are not helpful in the assessment of hypothyroidism. In patients with secondary or tertiary hypothyroidism, the T$_4$ and FT$_4$I are low, but their serum TSH is either normal or subnormal. The TSH response to TRH stimulation is most helpful in differential diagnosis of secondary from tertiary hypothyroidism; TSH response is absent in secondary hypothyroidism. A partial (delayed) or normal response of TSH to TRH is consistent with tertiary hypothyroidism. In patients with primary hypothyroidism, the basal TSH is elevated and the

TSH response to TRH stimulation is exaggerated (Figure 17-7).

Since secondary and tertiary hypothyroidism are rare entities, and since the second and third generation TSH assays are becoming sensitive enough to distinguish normal TSH levels from the depressed levels of patients with hyperthyroidism, the TRH stimulation test is now used relatively infrequently in the assessment of thyroid disorders. Laboratory measurements of serum T_4 and TSH are also useful in monitoring T_4 replacement treatment of hypothyroid patients. Figure 17-9 shows optimal tests for primary hypothyroidism and for monitoring T_4 replacement therapy for primary hypothyroidism. As is the case with hyperthyroidism (Figure 17-8), the serum TSH measurement is the most sensitive test for diagnosing primary hypothyroidism in stable ambulatory patients. In the early phases of initiating T_4 replacement treatment, however, a serum T_4 is a better indicator for thyroid status than TSH because serum TSH levels remain high during the initial treatment period due to the lag in the pituitary reset of TSH secretion. This lag period is considerably longer in neonates and therefore TSH should not be followed for neonates as indicative of proper replacement. After at least two months of replacement therapy with a stable T_4 dose, the TSH measurement again becomes the optimal thyroid test because a normal-range TSH value is the therapeutic end point for replacement treatment.

Neonatal hypothyroidism may be a result of thyroid dysgenesis, agenesis, or defects of thyroid hormone synthesis. Early detection and treatment are critical in preventing mental retardation and developmental abnormalities. Its incidence is about one in 4000 births. Due to this relatively high incidence, difficulty of early clinical diagnosis, and because early treatment of neonatal hypothyroidism may reduce attendant neurologic deficiencies, screening programs for neonatal hypothyroidism have been established in most of the United States. In large-scale screening, blood samples collected on filter paper are mailed to centralized screening laboratories such as State Health Department Centers. Blood samples on a punched-out filter paper spot are eluted and assayed for T_4. If T_4 is subnormal, TSH is measured using a second punched-out spot from the same filter paper for confirmation of neonatal hypothyroidism. If the TSH is elevated, thyroid hormone replacement is immediately started but it should be withdrawn transiently years later to recheck that the patient is truly, persistently hypothyroid.

Diseases of thyroid gland without hyper- or hypofunction

Thyroid disorders may be present without clinical and chemical features of thyrotoxicosis or of thyroid hormone deficiency. Nontoxic nodular goiter occurs in about 4% of the population. The term goiter represents enlargement of the thyroid gland usually from TSH stimulation. Iodine deficiency used to be the most common cause of nontoxic goiter (endemic goiter), but now is rare in developed countries due to widespread use of iodized salt. Iodine deficiency impairs T_4 synthesis, and the tendency of the serum T_4 to fall increases TSH secretion.

The thyroid cells continue to synthesize and secrete thyroid hormone to maintain normal circulating thyroid hormone levels at the expense of developing hyperplasia of thyroid cells. Graves' disease in younger patients may have symptoms and signs of ophthalmopathy without other abnormal thyroid function tests (euthyroid Graves' disease). Thyroid function in patients with thyroid cancer is usually normal, but hyperthyroidism may result. Excess thyroglobulin is often released into the circulation of thyroid cancer patients.

A serum thyroglobulin assay is a valuable aid in diagnosing and managing residual and/or recurrent differen-

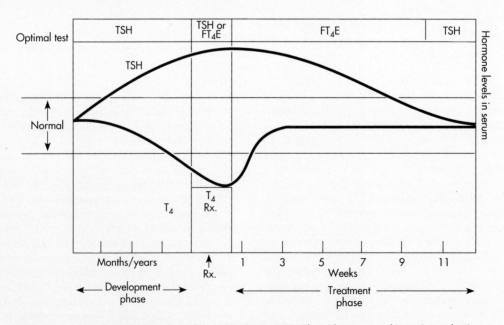

Fig. 17-9 Optimal tests for hypothyroidism. *From Spencer CA, Thryoid status: trend in testing: selective test use cuts cost, Clinical Chemistry News, 1989, page 10.*

tiated thyroid cancer. Establishing a baseline serum thyroglobulin is recommended for all patients with well-differentiated thyroid cancer and serum thyroglobulin assay should be used as an aid in the follow up of post-therapy thyroid cancer patients. T_4 suppression therapy is used in managing TSH-dependent thyroid cancer (well differentiated thyroid cancer). The objective is to suppress the serum TSH concentration to prevent trophic stimulation of differentiated thyroid tissue by TSH. It is important to monitor T_4 suppression therapy because insufficient T_4 doses may lead to recurrence of thyroid cancer while overreplacement may cause accelerated bone loss and cardiac arrhythmia. The second and third generation TSH assays capable of measuring subnormal levels of serum TSH are useful in monitoring T_4 suppression therapy. The current guidelines for adjusting the T_4 suppression dose suggest that the basal serum TSH be suppressed below 0.1 mU/L and that the T_4 dose chosen does not cause hyperthyroid symptoms. The third generation TSH assay with lower detection limit of 0.01 mU/L will allow physicians to titrate the degree of TSH suppression and minimize the potential adverse consequences of subclinical hyperthyroidism such as reduced bone density.

Abnormal laboratory thyroid test in the absence of thyroid disorders

Abnormal concentrations of circulating protein-bound hormones

Increases or decreases in protein-bound hormones due to a rise or fall in serum TBG concentrations and due to competitive binding of various drugs to TBG have been discussed previously (Box 17-1). Under such physiological and pathological conditions, concentrations of circulating total thyroid hormones (T_4 and T_3) are abnormal, but free thyroid hormone concentrations measured directly or indirectly (FT_4I and FT_3I) remain within the normal range (Table 17-6 and Table 17-10).

In individuals with familial dysalbuminemic hyperthyroxinemia, the total serum T_4 concentrations and free serum T_4 concentrations—determined indirectly by THBR (FT_4I)

or by radioimmunoassay methods that employ labelled T_4 analogues—are elevated. T_4 concentrations measured directly by equilibrium dialysis or ultrafiltration are normal (Table 17-10). The elevated T_4 concentrations in these individuals are caused by the presence of an abnormal high capacity, high affinity serum albumin.

The elevated FT_4I is attributable to the fact that use of THBR to calculate FT_4I is based on the assumption that TBG is the principle determinant of overall T_4 binding. This assumption is not valid when serum proteins other than TBG contribute substantially to T_4 binding. The elevated free T_4 concentrations measured indirectly by the analogue methods are due to binding of the analogue to serum albumin. Elevated thyroxine binding prealbumin (TBPA) also increases serum T_4 concentrations but serum T_3 concentrations remain normal because T_3 does not bind to TBPA.

The presence of autoantibodies to thyroid hormones occurs rarely in patients without thyroid disorders but occurs more frequently in patients with thyroid disease, especially with autoimmune disease. As with TBG, the presence of autoantibodies increases the concentrations of circulating total thyroid hormones, while free hormone concentrations are normal when measured directly by equilibrium dialysis or ultrafiltration. The free hormones are spuriously elevated when measured indirectly by the analogue method. As mentioned previously, the presence of the autoantibodies also interferes with the radioimmunoassay of thyroid hormones when unextracted serum samples are used.

Abnormal peripheral metabolism of T_4

As mentioned previously, T_4 in the peripheral tissue is monodeiodinated to either T_3 or rT_3. About 80% of T_3 and 90% of rT_3 in the systemic circulation are derived from peripheral monodeiodination of T_4. In acute illnesses such as myocardial infarction, febrile illness, trauma, burns, and surgery, or in chronic illnesses such as chronic liver disease, chronic renal disease, and advanced cancer, rT_3 is formed preferentially at the expense of T_3 production. These conditions are characterized by normal or slightly elevated T_4, increased rT_3, and normal TSH and are called the low T_3

Table 17-10 Causes of abnormal results of thyroid function tests in euthyroid state

Causes	T_4	FT_4I	Free T_4	T_3	F_3TI	Free T_3	TSH
Abnormal concentration of serum protein-bound hormones							
Altered TBG concentration*	↑, ↓	N	N	↑, ↓	N	N	N
Familial dysalbuminemic hyperthyroixinemia	↑	↑	N†	N	N	N	N
Increased T_4 binding to TBPA	↑	↑	N	N	N	N	N
Autoantibodies to thyroid hormones	↑, N	↑, N	N†	N, ↑	N, ↑	N†	N
Abnormal peripheral conversion of T_4 to T_3							
Nonthyroidal illness (low T_3 syndrome)	N, ↑	N, ↑	N, ↑	↓	↓	↓	N
Suppressed by drugs (glucocorticoids, propranolol, certain cholecystographic agents, amiodarone)	N, ↑	N, ↑	N, ↑	↓	↓	↓	N
Enhanced by drugs (phenytoin)	↓	↓	↓	N	N	N	N
Severe illness (low T_3, low T_4 syndrome)	↓	↓	↓	↓	↓	↓	N
Effects of drugs on hypothalamic-pituitary function							
Hypothalamic stimulation (amphetamine)	↑	↑	↑	N	N	N	↑
Inhibition of TSH secretion (glucocorticoids, dopamine)	↓	↓	↓	N, ↓	N, ↓	N, ↓	↓

*See Box 17-1 and Figure 17-5.
†See text.
N = normal; ↑ = increased; ↓ = decreased

syndrome or nonthyroidal illness (NTI). Systemic illness appears to have little effect on monodeiodination of T_4 to T_3 in the pituitary. Therefore, the pituitary is not aware of the peripheral low-circulating T_3 in systemic illness and so there is no resultant increased TSH secondary to feedback mechanisms. Consequently, the body maintains a condition of relatively reduced metabolic demands.

A low-T_3, low-T_4 syndrome has been reported in severely ill patients, usually in the intensive care unit, and has been associated with poor prognosis. As with the low-T_3 syndrome, the serum TSH is normal and serum rT_3 is elevated. It has been suggested that an inhibitor of T_4-binding to thyroid-binding proteins is present in these patients, resulting in the decreased serum total T_4 with normal or slightly elevated dialyzable T_4 (FT_4).

Familial elevations of total and free T_4 in healthy euthyroid subjects without detectable binding protein abnormalities have also been reported. These elevations could be caused by generalized resistance to thyroid hormone or by an elevated threshold for the serum T_4 level required to maintain adequate T_3 production from the peripheral monodeiodination of T_4.

Some drugs, such as glucocorticoids or propranolol hydrochloride in high doses, oral cholecystographic radioopaque agents (iopanoic acid, sodium ipodate); and amiodarone can inhibit peripheral conversion of T_4 to T_3. They all cause decreased levels of serum T_3 and free T_3, normal or elevated levels of serum T_4 and free T_4, and usually normal levels of serum TSH. Serum total and free T_4 concentrations are lowered in patients taking therapeutic doses of phenytoin, but serum total and free T_3 concentrations, as well as the serum TSH, are essentially unchanged. This may reflect the enhancement of the conversion of T_4 to T_3 by phenytoin. The decreased serum T_4 is accompanied by a lowered serum rT_3 concentration.

Effects of drugs on hypothalamic-pituitary function

Large doses of glucocorticoids may also cause decreased levels of serum TSH and decreased serum T_4 by depressing serum thyroid hormone-bnding proteins. The serum TSH also is suppressed by L-dopamine in doses used for the treatment of cardiovascular shock.

Increases in serum T_4, FT_4I and FT_4 levels observed in patients taking large doses of amphetamine may be explained by its effect on hypothalamic-pituitary function. The TSH secretory response to TRH is enhanced in these patients.

The effects of drugs described may cause transient abnormalities in thyroid function but the abnormalities usually disappear when the drug is withdrawn. Clinicians, however, should be aware of any medications taken by patients that may affect the results of thyroid function tests. Table 17-10 summarizes various abnormal results of thyroid function tests in euthyroid patients.

SUGGESTED READING

Fernandez-Ulloa M and Maxon HR III: Thyroid. In Kaplan LA and Pesce AJ: Clinical chemistry: theory, analysis, and correlation, ed 2, St Louis, 1989, Mosby–Year Book, Inc.

Greenspan FS and Rapoport B: Thyroid gland. In Greenspan FS and Forsham PH, eds: Basic & clinical endocrinology, ed 2, Los Altos, 1986, Lange Medical Publications.

Ingbar SH and Braverman LE: Werner's the thyroid, a fundamental and clinical test, ed 5, Philadelphia, 1986, JB Lippincott Co.

Larsen PR, Alexander NM, Chopra IJ, et al: Revised nomenclature for tests of thyroid hormones and thyroid-related proteins in serum, J Clin Endocrinol Metab 64:1089-1094, 1987.

Surks MI, Chopra IJ, Mariash CN, et al: American thyroid association guidelines for use of laboratory tests in thyroid disorders, 263:1529-1532, 1990.

18 Gonadal hormones

Paul T. Russell
R. Ian Hardy

THE GONADS—THEIR FUNCTION AND HORMONAL PRODUCTS
Anatomy and physiology

The gonads are the organs that produce the gametes, the egg and sperm, which are basic to the process of reproduction. In the human the ovaries, which produce the eggs, are paired structures in the abdomen that weigh from 4 to 8 g each at sexual maturity. Their weight varies with the phase of the menstrual cycle. In the male, the sperm-producing testes are contained in a sac outside the body called the scrotum. Each testis has an average weight of 15 to 19 g, with the right testicle usually 10% larger than the left.

The ovary

Ovaries are complex structures that change continuously as they perform their physiologic functions. They release a mature ovum every 28 to 30 days, and they secrete sex steroid hormones. The egg-producing function is closely tied to the formation of the hormones estrogen and progesterone, both of which are necessary for reproductive success. Estrogen is produced by cells that line the follicle as it matures. Progesterone is produced by derivatives of these cells after they have undergone a transformation following detachment of the egg during ovulation.

The ovary in cross section is composed of two parts: the outermost layer, called the cortex and the middle portion, the medulla (Figure 18-1). The thickness of the cortex varies with age, becoming thinner as a woman grows older. This outer layer contains the eggs, which are enclosed in graffian follicles. Each follicle contains a single egg. The inner medulla is composed of loose connective tissue containing arteries, veins, and muscle fibers. The ovary is innervated by both sympathetic and parasympathetic nerves.

A follicle in the early, primordial developmental stage (Figure 18-2) contains an oocyte, the development of which is arrested in the first of two meiotic divisions. This occurs early in the female's life, around mid-gestation. The oocyte remains at this stage until follicular maturation resumes prior to ovulation, which may be 12 to 40 years. How the ovary manages to keep the ova "on hold" for so many years is not known but is thought to involve inhibitors produced

within the follicle. Release from this inhibitory influence is believed to be initiated by luteinizing hormone (LH) action. How this happens to only some eggs each month is also unknown.

Throughout the course of a woman's life there is a dramatic decline in the numbers of germ cells, cells that can develop into ova (Figure 18-3). From a maximum of 7 million in each ovary at 15 to 20 weeks of fetal life to 2 million at birth, the numbers progressively decline until they reach about 400,000 at puberty. Over the next 30 to 40 years of reproductive life approximately 400 ova are lost because they undergo ovulation, others cease in their development and degenerate at intermediate stages of maturation. By menopause only a few thousand remain. It seems remarkably inefficient that only a few of the eggs originally present in germinal tissue (0.1%) will ever have the opportunity to participate in the procreative process.

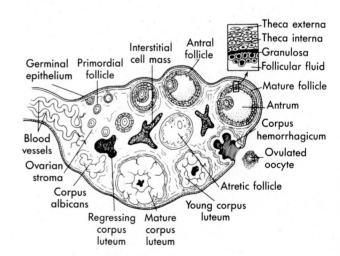

Fig. 18-1 Cross sectional diagram of an ovary showing the sequential development of a follicle, formation of a corpus luteum, and, in the center, follicular atresia. A section of the wall of a mature follicle is enlarged at the upper right. *Redrawn from Patten B and Eakin RM: Gonads and gonadal hormone. In Gorbman A and Bern HA: A textbook of comparative endocrinology, New York, 1962, John Wiley and Sons.*

275

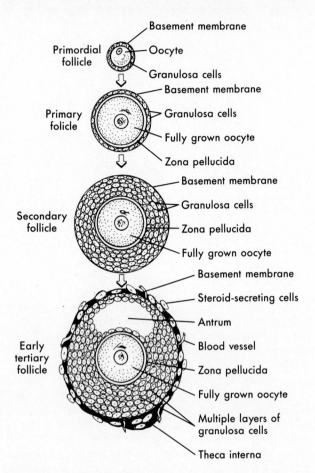

Fig. 18-2 Morphologic changes that occur in ovarian follicles during growth and development. *Redrawn from Erickson GF: Follicular growth and development. In Sciarra JJ, ed: Gynecology and obstetrics, vol 5, New York, 1981, Harper and Row.*

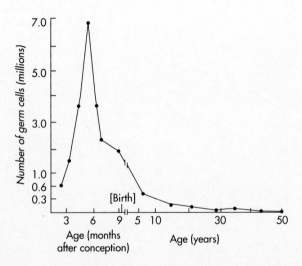

Fig. 18-3 Total number of germ cells in the human ovary at different ages. *From Baker TG: Oogenesis and ovulation. In Austin CR and Short RV, eds: Reproduction in mammals, vol. 1, New York, 1972, Cambridge University Press.*

The testis

The anatomical relationships of the testes and secondary sex organs are described in Chapter 31. Even though the sex of the embryo is genetically determined at fertilization, ovaries and testes develop similarly until about the fourth month of embryonic life. Testosterone is normally secreted by the fetal Leydig cells in the male by the seventh week of gestation, thus providing the hormonal stimulus for morphologic differentiation. Without androgen influence an ovary will be produced. This is an important physiologic concept to understanding sexual differentiation. Clinical examples of this phenomenon are given at the end of this chapter.

Hormones produced by the gonads: steroid pathways

Steroid hormone synthesis in both males and females is organized very efficiently. The sequence is such that the classes of steroid hormones are closely related chemically while their biological activities are quite varied. Cholesterol is the common precursor for all steroids and for this reason, the system of nomenclature relates to this steroid. The structure of cholesterol is shown below with the accepted convention for the number assigned to each carbon atom.

Cholesterol

Cholesterol and its products are made up of four rings attached to form the characteristic steroid structural pattern. Why the structural pattern is this way relates to the biochemical process that is responsible for steroid biosynthesis and is beyond the scope of this discussion. By convention, the rings are designated from left to right as A, B, C, and D. Rings A, B, and C are six-membered rings while ring D is five carbons.

Projecting from the steroid ring system are two methyl groups (—CH_3) attached to carbon atoms 10 and 13. These angular methyl groups are designated carbon 19, which is attached to carbon 10, and carbon 18, which is attached to

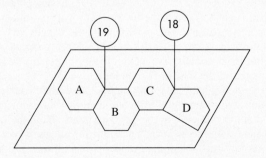

carbon 13. They are called "angular" because they stick up at right angles to the plane of the relatively flat ring system.

In cholesterol there is an aliphatic chain of eight carbons that is attached to carbon 17. This portion will be referred to in the subsequent discussion as the "side chain" of cholesterol.

In addition to the side chain (carbons 20 through 27) and the two angular methyl groups (carbons 19 and 18), additional features of the structure of cholesterol need to be recognized: two "functional groups," a hydroxyl group (—OH) at carbon 3 and a double bond ($\rangle C = C \langle$) between carbons 5 and 6.

The position of the double bond in ring A or B is useful in identifying steroids that can be grouped along similar pathways of formation. In general, the position of the double bond also helps identify biological activity within the steroids. The Greek letter delta (Δ) designates a double bond, and the superscript number that follows indicates the carbon atom that is first, or lowest, in numerical sequence. For example, a double bond that extends between carbons 4 and 5 is simply referred to as Δ^4 because the bond is between two carbons in numerical sequence. If a double bond is between two carbons not in numerical sequence, both numbers are cited (e.g., $\Delta^{5,10}$). Cholesterol—by these definitions—is referred to as a delta-5-steroid because the double bond extends between carbons 5 and 6.

Δ^4

Δ^5

$\Delta^{5,10}$

The type of oxygen function attached to carbon 3 changes with the position of the double bond. A 3-hydroxy (oxygen and hydrogen) function is usually associated with delta-5-steroids (except for estrogens), while delta-4-steroids generally have a ketone group (double-bonded oxygen) at position 3.

The estrogens differ from the steroid types that have just been described. Estrogens have a phenolic structure, a 3-hydroxy function on a benzene ring for ring A. Because of

this phenolic ring A they are referred to as aromatic, rather than aliphatic, compounds. This feature imparts physical, chemical, and hence biological properties to the estrogens that are quite different from the aliphatic steroid hormones.

Phenol

Estrogen structure

Because ring A of the estrogens has this characteristic aromatic bonding, no angular methyl group can be attached to carbon 10. Hence, estrogens possess one less carbon atom in their structure than their precursors, the androgens.

In humans there are six classes of steroids that are easily distinguished according to the number of carbon atoms in their structure.

STEROID	NUMBER OF CARBON ATOMS
sterols	27
bile acids	24
progestins	21
corticoids	21
androgens	19
estrogens	18

The biochemical routes of formation are referred to as "pathways" of formation. Since the sterol cholesterol is the "parent" of the steroids listed above, steroid hormone formation can be viewed as an enzymatically regulated, systematic loss of carbon atoms starting from cholesterol. Fewer and fewer carbons flow from cholesterol to the other steroids. Estrogens are the last stop along these pathways since, in mammalian systems, the enzymatic machinery to remove additional carbon atoms from the basic steroid ring structure is not present.

The corticoids (e.g., aldosterone and cortisol) have the same number of carbon atoms as do the progestins. The reason for this is that the corticoids are formed by sequential hydroxylations of progesterone.

Below is a brief outline of the biosynthetic relationships for the formation of the different classes of steroids:

$$\text{cholesterol} \rightarrow \text{progestins} \rightarrow \text{adrenal corticoids*}$$
$$\downarrow \qquad\qquad \downarrow$$
$$\text{bile acids*} \quad \text{androgens}$$
$$\downarrow$$
$$\text{estrogens}$$

To convert cholesterol to the progestins, six of the eight carbon atoms originally present in the side chain of cholesterol must be removed. This is accomplished by adjacent hydroxylation reactions at carbons 20 and 22 followed by a carbon—carbon bond cleavage between carbons 20 and

---

*included here only for completeness but not further discussed.

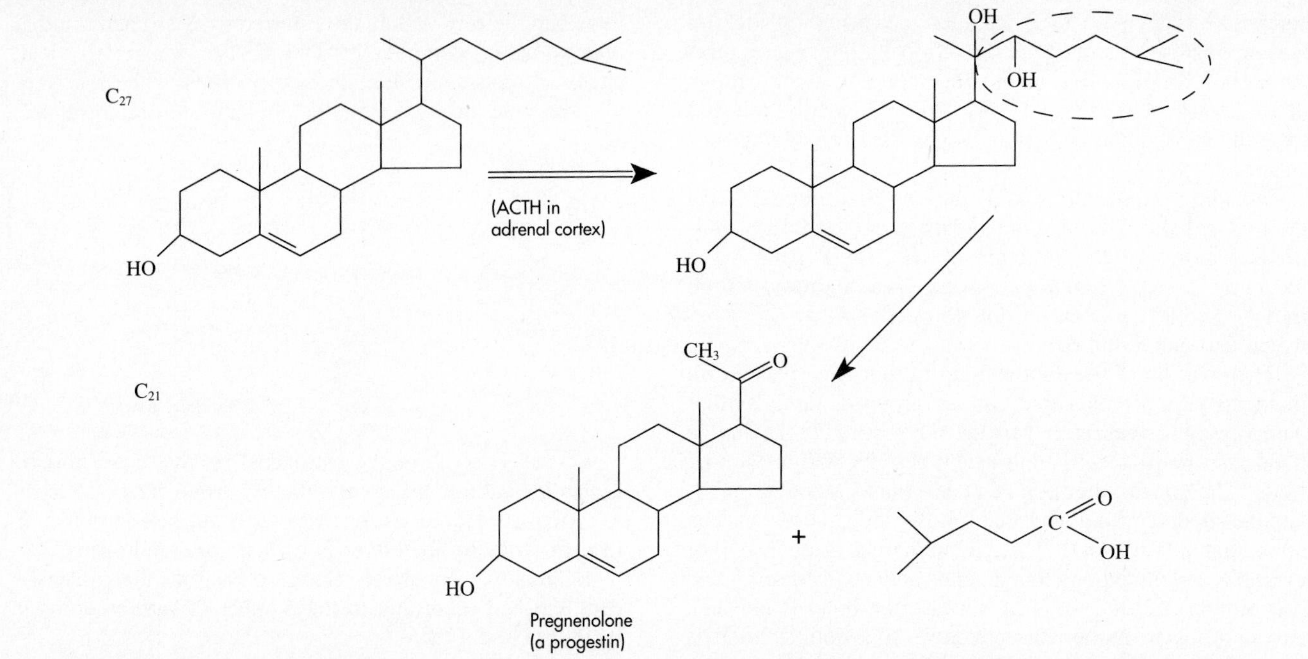

(ACTH in adrenal cortex)

C_{27}

C_{21}

CH₃

+

Pregnenolone
(a progestin)

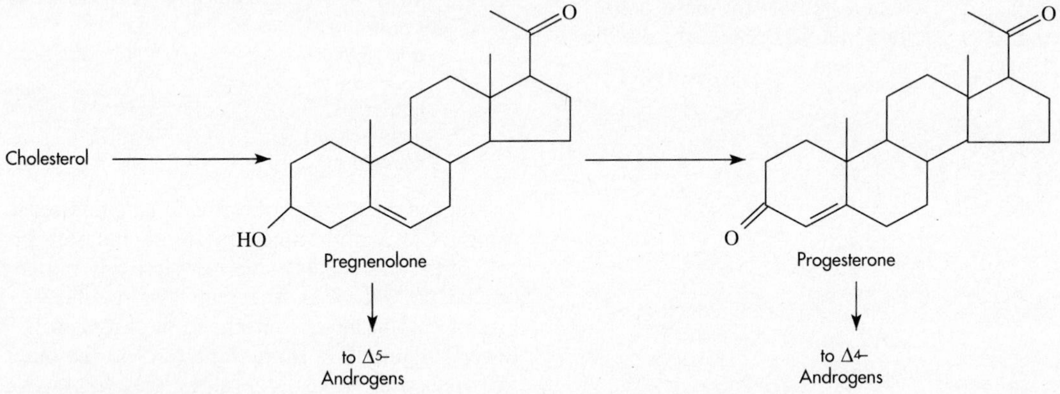

Cholesterol

Pregnenolone

to Δ⁵–
Androgens

Progesterone

to Δ⁴–
Androgens

22. The result is a 21-carbon steroid product and a 6-carbon byproduct. The carbon—carbon bond is broken by an enzyme called a "desmolase." This important step is under the control of the trophic hormones, LH in the gonads and ACTH in the adrenal cortex. Since cholesterol is a Δ^5-steroid, the progestin formed, pregnenolone, retains the Δ^5-bond.

Once pregnenolone is formed, two alternative pathways are available to form subsequent members of the steroids. One pathway follows a series of steroids that retain the Δ^5-steroid structure. The second pathway follows a parallel course but after pregnenolone is converted to its Δ^4-counterpart, progesterone.

The enzyme system that changes the Δ^5-steroids to Δ^4-steroids is the 3-beta-hydroxy steroid dehydrogenase-isomerase complex. This conversion is virtually unidirectional since Δ^5-steroids are not formed from Δ^4 steroids.

From progesterone and pregnenolone, hydroxylation reactions at carbon 17 form the 17-alpha-hydroxy derivatives. These hydroxylation reactions are obligatory steps in the formation of androgens from progestins.

With 17-hydroxysteroids formed, enzymes remove the 2-carbon remnant from the original side-chain of cholesterol. This converts C-21 progestins to C-19 androgens.

Two androgens are the products of these conversions, one from the Δ^5-steroid precursor and one from the Δ^4. The product from the Δ^5-pathway is dehydroepiandrosterone (abbreviated as DHEA or DHA); the product from the Δ^4-pathway is androstenedione. Both possess weak androgenic activity. Androstenedione is a major product of the ovarian stromal tissue while DHEA has two sites of origin, the gonad and the inner-most zone of the adrenal cortex (zona reticularis). In the female, the sulfated derivative of DHEA, DHEA-S, arises almost exclusively from the adrenal gland, and is therefore useful in determining whether gonadal or adrenal activity is responsible for abnormal androgen excesses. DHEA is also produced from the tissues of the fetus during pregnancy (see Chapter 19).

Testosterone is not a direct product of the pathways coming from the progestins, but instead is formed following the reduction of the ketone at position 17 of androstenedione. This conversion is reversible, subject to biologic conditions.

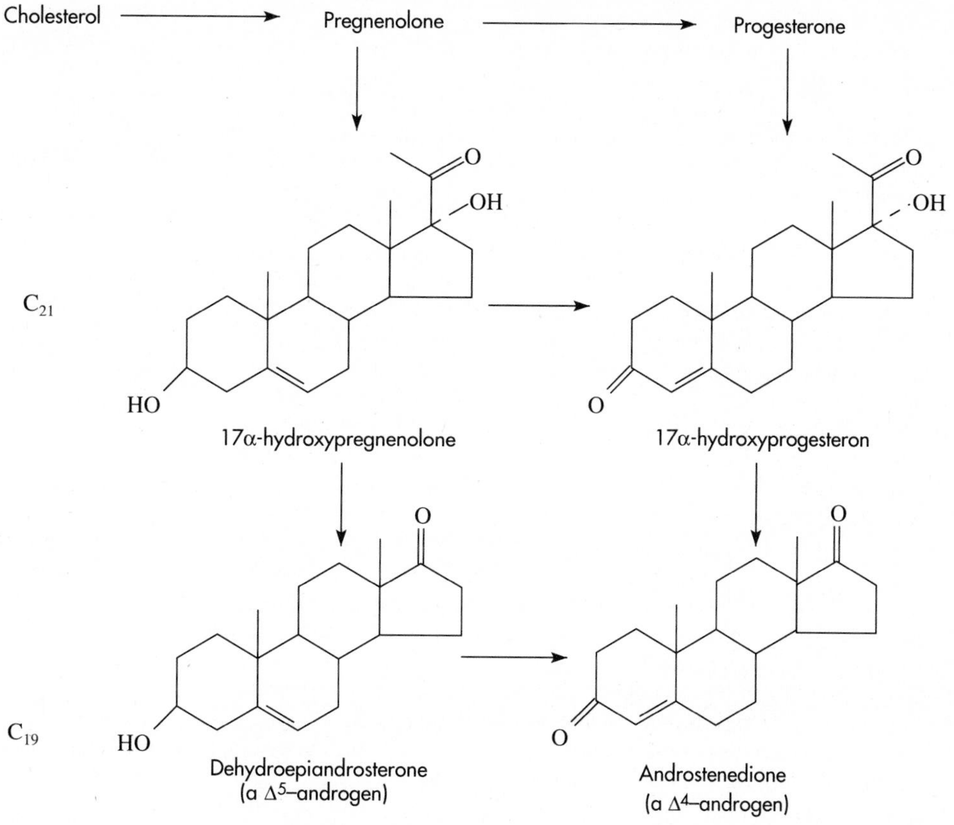

Cholesterol $\longrightarrow$ Pregnenolone $\longrightarrow$ Progesterone

C_{21}

17α-hydroxypregnenolone   17α-hydroxyprogesteron

C_{19}

Dehydroepiandrosterone
(a Δ^5–androgen)

Androstenedione
(a Δ^4–androgen)

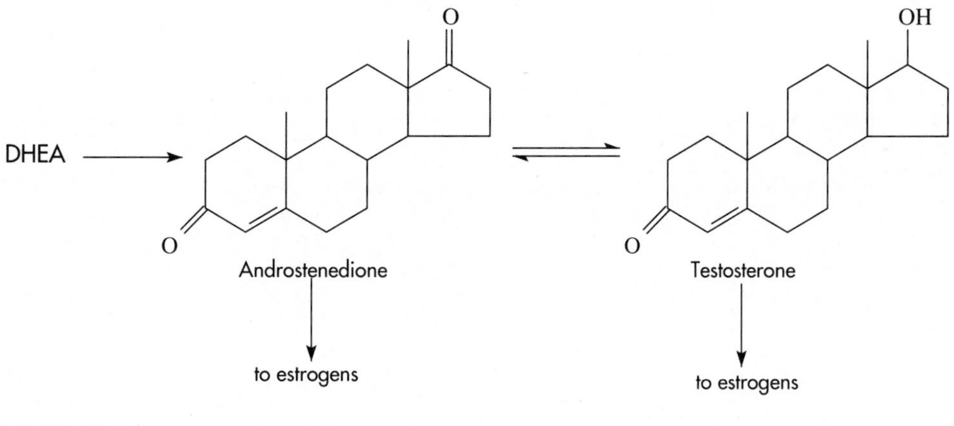

DHEA $\longrightarrow$

Androstenedione   Testosterone

to estrogens   to estrogens

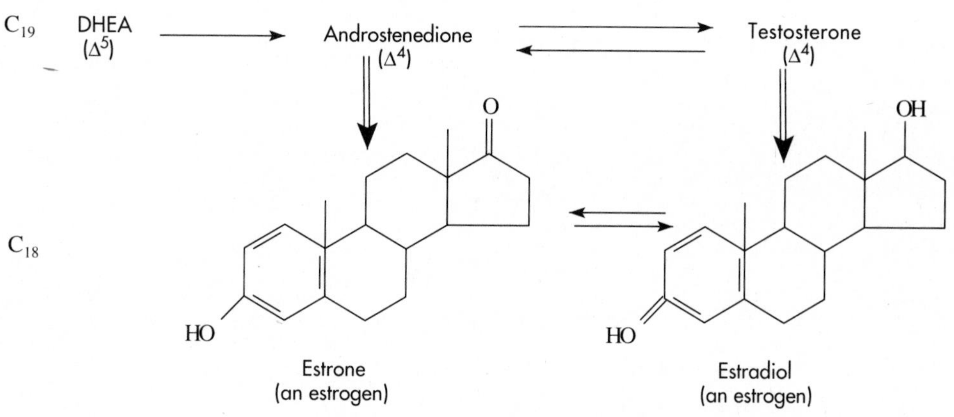

C_{19} DHEA $\longrightarrow$ Androstenedione $\longrightarrow$ Testosterone
       (Δ^5) (Δ^4) (Δ^4)

C_{18}

Estrone
(an estrogen)

Estradiol
(an estrogen)

Testosterone, like androstenedione, is a member of the Δ^4-pathway. This point becomes especially important as the conversion of androgens to estrogens is considered.

Estrogen formation from androstenedione and testosterone is by a complex series of enzymatic reactions collectively referred to as the "aromatase complex." Its name is derived from the fact that it converts aliphatic to aromatic steroids. Aromatase requires Δ^4-androgen substrates for its action, hence androstenedione and testosterone are the precursors.

Estrone is formed from androstenedione while estradiol comes from testosterone. In both cases the oxygen group at position 17 remains unchanged during the conversion from the respective androgen precursor. But once estrogens are formed this oxygen function can undergo oxidation-reduction similar to the androstenedione-testosterone interconversion. Estrone and estradiol are, therefore, interconvertible. Estradiol is biologically the most active estrogen of the natural estrogens. Its potency is about 10 times that of estrone.

In summary, there are two pathways for steroid hormone formation from cholesterol, the Δ^5- and the Δ^4-pathways. This type of organization is highly efficient and provides the opportunity for many subtle biologic control mechanisms. Steroids can act both as hormones and as intermediates or precursors to other hormones. Testosterone, for example, is an androgenic hormone with its own biological activity and it functions as a precursor to estradiol. However, because of the interdependence of each biosynthetically re-lated compound, a reduction in one type of steroid may lead to reductions in others.

Metabolism of gonadal hormones

Metabolism of the aliphatic steroids (the progestins and androgens) is by chemical reductions. Ketones are reduced to alcohols and double bonds are saturated with hydrogens to form the respective dihydro-derivative. Progesterone, for example, is metabolized from a delta-4,3-ketone structure to a tetrahydro derivative (i.e., four hydrogens are introduced). In addition, the ketone at C-20 is reduced to form an alcohol.

In principle the process seems simple, in practice the situation is complex.

This complexity is because of stereochemical considerations. When the ketone at C-3 is reduced, it can generate two possible hydroxy isomers, one oriented down (alpha-form), the other oriented up (beta-form) from the plane of the steroid ring system. The same is true for the reduction of the double bond at C-4. Hydrogen introduced at C-5 can be oriented alpha or beta. This means that four different metabolites are possible for any steroid possessing the delta-4,3-ketone structure. Each is not necessarily formed stoichiometrically with the others, but each can and probably will be formed.

The primary metabolite of progesterone is the 3-alpha-hydroxy-5-beta-structure. This product (with two hydroxy groups and a reduced double bond, 3-alpha-20-dihydroxy-5-beta-pregnane) goes by the common name of pregnanediol. About 10% to 20% of progesterone is excreted in this form.

Androgens such as testosterone and androstenedione also possess the delta-4,3-ketone structure, and these steroids are likewise metabolized through this reductive process. Testosterone generates two commonly encountered metabolites, androsterone and etiocholanolone. Both possess a ketone group at carbon 17 and, together with DHEA, constitute the bulk of the 17-ketosteroid metabolites for both men and women. They both possess a 3-alpha-hydroxy group but differ in the spacial orientation of the hydrogen at carbon 5.

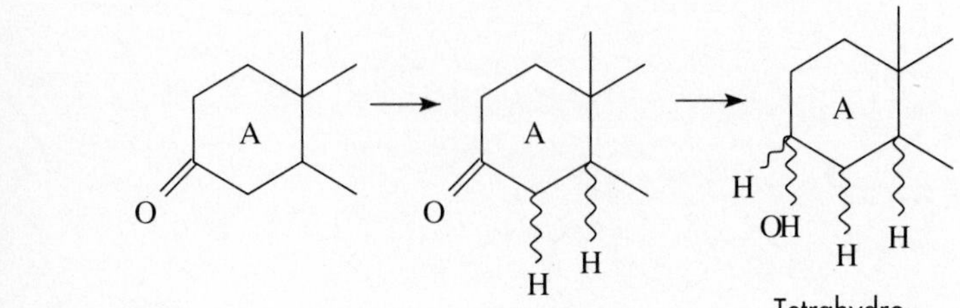

Dihydro–

Tetrahydro–

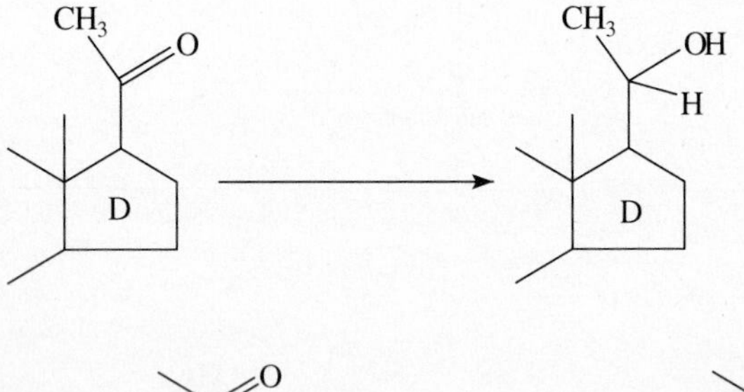

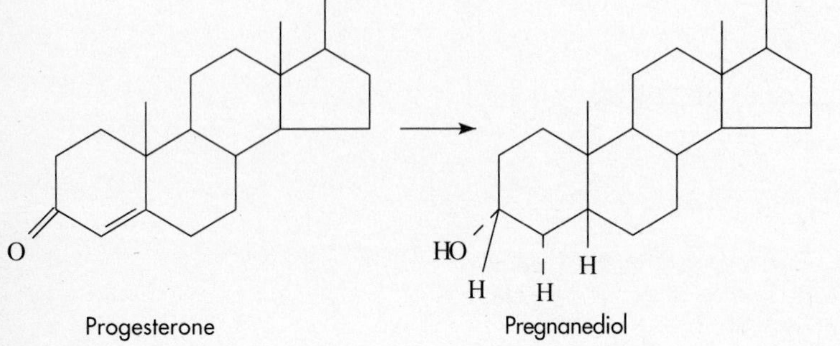

Progesterone

Pregnanediol

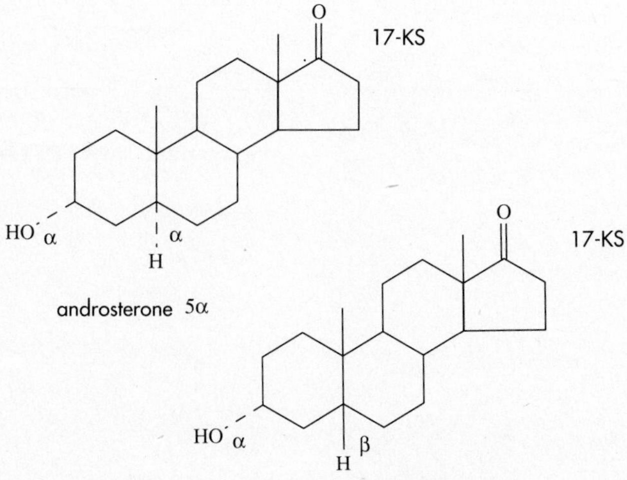

androsterone 5α

5β androsterone
(etiocholanolone)

The alpha or beta orientation of the hydrogen at C-5 may seem trivial but actually is profoundly significant. When the hydrogen at C-5 is oriented in the alpha orientation, the general shape of the steroid molecule remains planar. But in a beta orientation, ring A is bent at a sharp angle to the rest of the molecule, causing a severe change in its conformation.

Functionally, this distortion effectively eliminates biological activity since steroid molecules interact with receptors and enzyme sites from the underside of the molecule.

In specific target tissues, testosterone undergoes part of the process for metabolism, which eliminates the double bond but leaves the 3-ketone intact. The product, dihydrotestosterone (DHT), possesses a 5-alpha-hydrogen that retains the planarity of the ring system. DHT is a very potent androgen in a number of androgen-sensitive tissues (such as hair follicles). It undergoes its enzymatic formation from testosterone at its target site and expresses its biological activity through a receptor protein. The testosterone-to-DHT conversion follows the established pattern for metabolism (partial), but in the broader view it represents another example of the efficiency with which steroid reactions can be used for varied purposes.

Once reduction of the delta-4,3-ketone system occurs, the free hydroxy groups are usually conjugated at position 3 with either glucuronic or sulfuric acids. Both conjugation reactions and the steroid metabolism that precedes it occur in the liver. Conjugation is believed to facilitate excretion of these lipophylic molecules by increasing their water solubility.

Most circulating testosterone is converted to the metabolites androsterone and etiocholanolone. After conjugation with glucuronic or sulfuric acid, these metabolites are excreted into the urine as 17-ketosteroids (17-KS).

17-Ketosteroid
(17-KS)

However, only 20% to 30% of the urinary 17-KS are derived from testosterone metabolism. The majority are from the metabolism of adrenal steroids. For this reason 17-KS determinations do not reliably reflect testicular steroid secretion.

Estrogen metabolism differs in many ways from the metabolism of aliphatic steroids, progestins, corticoids, and androgens. Ring A of the estrogens remains unaltered because of the chemical stability of aromatic ring systems. Estrogens are generally conjugated with or without further hydroxylations. Hydroxylations that occur at carbon-2 of ring A impart a "catechol" nature to the estrogen, and for this reason these estrogens are referred to as catechol estrogens. The phenolic hydroxy group at C-3 is almost always conjugated with a sulfate group, whereas hydroxylations at C-16 and with most hydroxy groups on ring D are usually conjugated with glucuronic acid. In their conjugated forms, these water soluble compounds are readily excreted by the kidney.

Hormonal regulation of the gonads
Pituitary-hypophyseal-ovarian axis

Hormonal control of the gonads is from the pituitary by action of the gonadotropins, luteinizing hormone (LH, also called interstitial cell stimulating hormone, ICSH, in the male), and follicle-stimulating hormone (FSH). Two major parts—the anterior and posterior lobes—make up the pituitary. The anterior lobe (the adenohypophysis) synthesizes and releases the gonadotropins. It is functionally connected "downstream" from the hypothalamus by a vascular portal system through which the hypothalamic hormones, the releasing factors, gain access to the pituitary, which affects the release of the trophic hormones.

Control of the release of the gonadotropins by estrogen completes the circuit referred to as a "feedback loop." When estrogen diminishes the release of its initiating gonadotropin, the feedback is referred to as "negative." If the feedback augments gonadotropin release it is called "positive." The curious positive feedback phenomenon occurs during the menstrual cycle. At midcycle, a surge of estrogen causes the release of gonadotropins prior to ovulation. (See Chapter 19.)

The releasing factor for the gonadotropins, gonadotropin-releasing hormone (GnRH), is a small peptide of ten amino acid residues synthesized by the hypothalamus and secreted in pulses into the portal blood. After reaching the anterior pituitary, GnRH binds to receptors on cells that produce the gonadotropins and stimulates their release into the general circulation through which they reach and stimulate the gonads. Feedback controls also function between the gonads and the hypothalamus. The multiple feedback interactions that act to control the balance between the pituitary, hypothalamus, and gonads are very complex and illustrate the very intricate regulation that is possible. (See Chapter 16.)

Two-cell theory of estrogen formation by the ovary

Estrogens that appear in the blood stream during the first half of the menstrual cycle (follicular phase—see Chapter 19) are the products of the pathways that have already been described. In the ovary, the enzymes mediating the steps of the pathways are compartmentalized in adjacent cell types. The theca interna (see inset of Figure 18-1) houses the early parts of the pathways ending with the androgen, androstene-dione. Androstenedione then diffuses across the membrane barrier (basement lamina) to provide the substrate for the aromatase system to form estrogen.

Figure 18-4 shows how each cell type is under the control of one of the gonadotropic hormones, LH in the theca interna and FSH in the granulosa. Each cell type possesses receptors for its gonadotropin and each receptor-mediated event is processed through the cyclic-AMP messenger system. The ultimate product, the estrogen, is released into the blood stream and also appears in the follicular fluid where it can act on the theca to exert local feedback influences on the pathways of its formation. The rate of conversion of androgen to estrogen in the granulosa is directly related to the amount of androgen substrate made available by theca cells.

Blood concentrations and transport systems
Production rates and blood concentrations

Since little hormone is stored in the cells, the secretory activity of steroid-producing cells is closely coupled to their biosynthetic activity. The amount of steroid produced each day is considered its production rate. This includes not only the steroid a particular organ is producing but also steroids generated through peripheral conversions. For example, the adrenal cortex secretes relatively large quantities of the androgens, some of which ends up as estrogen. From all sources, the production of androstenedione is about 3 mg/day. In a nonpregnant female, about 1% of that (30μg) may be converted to estrogen peripherally. If estrogen is produced from all sources at the rate of 100 to 300 μg/day, 10% to 33% can be accounted for by the peripheral conversion from androstenedione. Estrogen production is the sum of ovarian secretion of estradiol and estrone plus the amount of estrogen formed by the peripheral conversion of androgens that can come from the ovary and from the adrenal.

Conversely, there is negligible peripheral conversion of steroid precursors to progesterone. The production rate for progesterone in the nonpregnant female is the sum of the secretion of progesterone from the adrenals and that from the ovaries. This amounts to about 2 to 3 mg/day during the preovulatory phase of the cycle and 20 to 30 mg/day after ovulation. Table 18-1 shows production rates, secretion rates, and blood concentrations in the female.

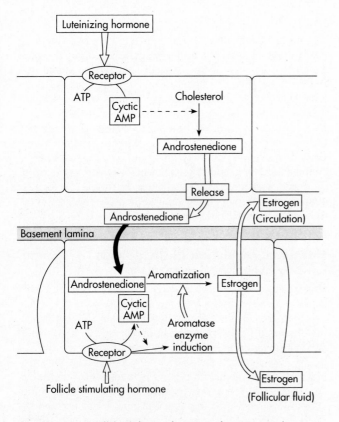

Fig. 18-4 Two-cell hypothesis of estrogen formation in the ovary. Luteinizing hormone stimulates androgen production in the thecal cells. Androgens then diffuse into the granulosa layer, where they are aromatized to estrogens. The aromatase enzyme system is induced by FSH.

Table 18-1 Concentrations, production rates, and ovarian secretion rates of steroids in blood

	Phase of menstrual cycle	Plasma concentration (μg/dL)	Production rate (mg/dL)	Secretion rate (both ovaries) (mg/d)
Estradiol	Early follicular	0.006	0.081	0.07
	Late follicular	0.033-0.07	0.445-0.945	0.4-0.8
	Midluteal	0.02	0.27	0.25
Estrone	Early follicular	0.005	0.11	0.08
	Late follicular	0.015-0.03	0.331-0.662	0.25-0.5
	Midluteal	0.011	0.243	0.16
Progesterone	Follicular	0.095	2.1	1.5
	Luteal	1.13	25	24
Androstenedione		0.159	3.2	0.8-1.6
Testosterone		0.038	0.26	0.2-0.3
Dehydroepiandrosterone		0.49	8	0.3-3
Dihydrotestosterone	. . .	0.02	0.05	0.01-0.02

From Lipsett MB: Steroid hormones. In Yen SSC and Jaffe RB (eds), Reproductive endocrinology, Philadelphia, 1978, Saunders.

The production rate of testosterone in the normal female is 200 to 300 µg/day. Approximately half arises from peripheral conversions of androstenedione. The adrenals and the ovaries contribute about equally to the circulating levels of testosterone, except at the midpoint of the menstrual cycle when the ovarian contribution is increased by some 10% to 15%.

For the male, steroids of primary interest are testosterone, dihydrotestosterone, and estradiol. Quantitatively, testosterone is the most important. More than 95% of the testosterone is secreted by the testicular Leydig cells; the remainder is derived from the adrenals. The testes secrete small amounts of the potent androgen, dihydrotestosterone, and the weak androgens, dehydroepiandrosterone (DHEA) and androstenedione. The Leydig cells also secrete small quantities of estradiol, estrone, pregnenolone, progesterone, 17-alpha-hydroxypregnenolone, and 17-alpha-hydroxyprogesterone. These steroids may be recognized as members of the pathways of steroid hormone formation. Normal ranges for gonadal steroids in men are given in Table 18-2. Dihydrotestosterone and estradiol are derived not only by direct secretion from the testes but also by conversion in peripheral tissues from androgen and estrogen precursors secreted by both the testes and the adrenals. About 80% of the circulating concentrations of these steroids is derived from peripheral sources (Table 18-3). Estradiol is formed locally in the hypothalamus from androgens and functions as the androgen messenger in the feedback loop from the gonads.

Transport systems

When released into the circulation, the gonadal steroids bind to plasma proteins. Estradiol binds strongly to a transport globulin called sex hormone-binding globulin (SHBG) and binds with less affinity to albumin. Progesterone binds strongly to corticosteroid-binding globulin (CBG) and weakly to albumin. Steroid carrier proteins are shown in Table 18-4. Concentrations of these binding proteins are increased by estrogen and thyroxine and decreased by androgens and progestins. SHBG, produced by the liver, is stimulated by estrogen and suppressed by androgen. For this reason, binding capacity is lower in men than in women. Even though the proportions of free and bound estradiol do not vary significantly during the menstrual cycle, differences in binding may occur after menopause or may assume clinical importance coincident with abnormal ovarian function.

Clearance

Only unbound (free) steroids are biologically active. For this reason, the function of plasma binding may be to provide a pool of circulating hormones with delayed metabolic clearances and favorable water solubilities to increase or decrease the free pool as needed.

Androgens are mostly converted by the liver to metabolites that are conjugated and excreted by the kidneys as 17-KS. Since most of the circulating androgen in both males and females is of adrenal origin, the vast majority of the 5 to 15 mg/day of 17-KS in women and 7 to 17 mg/day in men represent adrenal precursors. Dihydrotestosterone is cleared as 3-alpha-androstanediol and its glucuronide. This metabolite has a high correlation with clinical manifestations of androgens and is therefore of more practical value than the 17-KS for assessing androgen activities.

Table 18-2 Normal ranges for gonadal steroids in men

Testosterone	300-1100 ng/dL
Free testosterone	50-210 pg/mL
Dihydrotestosterone	60-300 ng/dL
Androstenedione	50-200 ng/dL
Estradiol	5-50 pg/mL
Estrone	30-170 pg/mL

From Braunstein GD: The testis in basic and clinical endocrinology, ed 2, Los Altos, Ca, 1986, Lange Medical Publications.

Table 18-3 Relative contributions (approximate percentages) of the testes, adrenals, and peripheral tissues to circulating levels of sex steroids in men

	Testicular secretion	Adrenal secretion	Peripheral conversion of precursors
Testosterone	95	<1	<5
Dihydrotestosterone	20	<1	80
Estradiol	20	<1	80
Estrone	2	<1	98
DHEA sulfate	<10	90	. . .

From Braunstein GD: The testis. In Greenspan FS (ed): Basic and Clinical Endocrinology, ed 3, Norwalk, Ct, 1991, Appleton and Lange.

Table 18-4 Total plasma concentration and percentage of steroid hormone that is free or bound to plasma transport proteins in normal women in the early follicular phase. During the luteal phase, the total concentrations of estradiol (0.72 nmol/L) and progesterone (38 nmol/L) are higher, but the distribution is the same.*

	Total plasma concentration (nmol/L)	Percentage distribution of steroid			
		Free	SHBG	CBG	Albumin
Estradiol	0.29	1.81	37.3	0.1	60.8
Estrone	0.23	3.58	16.3	0.1	80.1
Progesterone	0.65	2.36	0.63	17.7	79.3
Testosterone	1.3	1.36	66	2.26	30.4
Dihydrotestosterone	0.65	0.47	78.4	0.12	21
Androstenedione	5.4	7.54	6.63	1.37	84.5
Cortisol	400	3.77	0.18	89.7	6.33

*From Dunn JF, Nisula BC, Rodbard D: J Clin Endocrinol Metab 53:58, 1981.

Progesterone is rapidly cleared from the circulation demonstrating a half-life of about five minutes. It is metabolized in the liver to pregnanediol, which is subsequently conjugated with glucuronic acid. Twenty percent of pregnanediol glucuronide is excreted into the urine and may be used as an indirect index of progesterone production. The remainder is eliminated in the feces.

Laboratory steroid measurements

Current laboratory methodology includes specific and sensitive radioimmunoassays for individual steroids under study. This has not always been the case. For many years the best estimates of plasma steroid concentrations came from urine measurements of the metabolites of steroids, their chemical derivatives, and, in rare cases, the hormones themselves. These indirect approaches were necessary because radioimmunoassays for specific hormones of interest were not available. For example, instead of measuring testosterone directly, 17-keto steroid assessments were done to estimate the androgenic content of urine. The 17-KS method measured etiocholanolone, androsterone, DHEA, and other metabolites of testosterone or related androgens. Today these tests occasionally are encountered and still provide useful, but limited, clinical information.

When urine tests are performed, a 24-hour specimen is required. This averages in the various steroid excretions that occur throughout a day. A valuable adjunct to the urinary tests is a creatinine. This checks on the validity of the 24-hour collection. Creatinine values should remain relatively constant at approximately 1000 mg/24 hours.

Three classes of 17-keto steroids (17-KS) are present in urine. The first, the neutral 17-KS, includes the weak androgens and androgenic metabolites, DHEA, etiocholanolone, and androsterone. The second, the acidic 17-KS, is composed of estrone. The third are 17-KS that have an oxygen function (hydroxyl or ketone group) on carbon 11 of the steroid molecule. These 17-KS originate in the adrenal gland. The excretion of the 17-KS vary with age, which must be kept in mind when using them for diagnostic purposes.

Steroids that contain a hydroxyl group on carbons 17 or 20 can be converted to the respective ketone by chemical oxidation. These are referred to as ketogenic steroids and are prominent both as intermediates of the steroid pathways (e.g., 17 alpha-hydroxy progesterone) and as hormones themselves, such as cortisol, the glucocorticoid. As with the 17-KS, the ketogenics represent a mixture of a number of compounds.

Before radioimmunoassays, progesterone and estrogens were monitored in the urine through the metabolite pregnanediol for progesterone and as total estrogen for the estrogens. The pregnanediol method relied primarily on gas chromatographic techniques while colorimetric procedures could be used to assess total estrogens. In both cases the conjugated forms had to be cleaved by enzymatic or chemical hydrolysis to free the steroid before analysis could take place.

The introduction of specific and sensitive radioimmunoassay methods to the steroid field greatly facilitated the ease with which hormonal information could be obtained. These methods eliminated the problem of collecting a 24-hour urine sample because they provided the opportunity to measure the levels of "parent" steroids directly in blood. The old aphorism that "today's blood is tomorrow's urine" refers to the time advantage provided by these rapid, specific, and sensitive assays.

MECHANISMS OF ACTION
Hormonal receptors and messenger systems

There are two types of hormone actions at the cellular level. In one the action of the hormone is mediated to the cell by a messenger system since the hormone itself does not enter the cell. The second type is carried out by a hormone that does enter the target cell.

Glycoprotein (gonadotropic) hormones do not enter the cell. The message they carry is relayed through the cell membrane by receptors on the surface of the cell (Figure 18-5). These receptors transmit the message that leads to the formation of cyclic adenosine 3'5'-monophosphate (cyclic-AMP). Through subsequent phosphorylations of cellular proteins and enzymes, cellular functions are altered. The removal of cyclic-AMP by the action of the enzyme, phosphodiesterase, provides a means for cellular levels of cyclic-AMP to be regulated by the balance between its formation and removal. Because cyclic-AMP levels change rapidly and because its actions are intracellular in location, cyclic-AMP is not measured in most laboratories.

Steroid hormones act by entering target cells through passive diffusion and binding to specific receptor proteins (Figure 18-6). There are an estimated 5000 to 20,000 receptor sites per cell. Once bound with hormone, these hormone-receptor complexes proceed to bind to chromatin, resulting in a change in protein synthesis and cell function.

The cellular response to increasing concentrations of steroid hormones is gradual and increases proportional to hormone increase. Each receptor protein binds to a single molecule of hormone and each specific site on the chromatin binds to a single hormone-receptor complex. As the con-

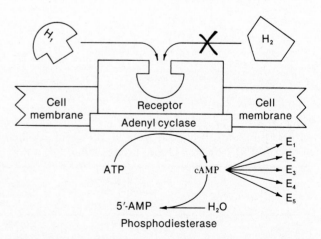

Fig. 18-5 Concept of hormone action by way of second messenger cyclic AMP. H_1 is a hormone recognized by specific membrane receptor sites, whereas H_2 is a hormone that is not sensed in the environment. E_1 to E_5, various metabolic effects of increased cAMP. *From Orten JM and Neuhaus OW: Human biochemistry, ed 10, St. Louis, 1982, Mosby–Year Book, Inc.*

centration of hormone increases, the concentration of hormone-receptor complexes increases proportionally, as does the number of complexes bound to specific sites on chromatin.

Estrogens induce the development of progesterone receptors, and the presence of estrogen can increase the affinity of the estrogen-receptor complex for its chromatin-binding site. The activation of estrogen binding sites lasts no more than six hours, after which they lose their binding capacity. The presence of estrogen is therefore an important factor for a continuing estrogen response. On the other hand, progesterone depletes estrogen receptors. Thus, the interplay between estrogen and progesterone at the receptor level shows not only that the presence of a hormone is important, but that the timing of its formation and release is critical.

There is also a practical laboratory use for the receptors of steroid hormones. When tissue samples taken from breast tumors are measured for estrogen and progesterone receptors, correlations between the presence of estrogen receptors and certain clinical characteristics of breast cancer can be made. The presence of estrogen receptors with the more slowly growing tumors implies that the chance of responding to endocrine therapy increases directly with the tumor's concentration of estrogen and progesterone receptors. Since it takes estrogen to make progesterone receptors, the fact that progesterone receptors are present proves that the estrogen receptor in the tumor is biologically active. The presence of progesterone receptors is, therefore, considered to be a good sign; the lack of progesterone receptors is foreboding.

For many androgen-sensitive tissues, androgen messages are transmitted to the target tissues by testosterone where testosterone binds to the androgen receptors. In hair follicles and other related tissues where testosterone acts through dihydrotestosterone (DHT), DHT is formed from testosterone after the testosterone arrives at the target cell (Figure

18-7). Whether testosterone acts through itself or through DHT is established during embryonic development. The purpose for the DHT mechanism may be to amplify androgen action since DHT binds to the androgen receptors more strongly than does testosterone.

Biological effects

Estrogens are responsible for the development of the female's secondary sex characteristics. This includes growth of the duct system of the breast, the uterus, and vaginal epithelium.

Androgens stimulate the development of male characteristics. In fetal life, the testis produces androgen, which promotes the development of the male genital organs. In adult life, androgens control spermatogenesis and the development and maintenance of the male secondary sex characteristics, including deepening of the voice, sexual hair, enlargement of the genitalia, and accessory glands. Androgens have an important anabolic affect on protein metabolism and influence sexual libido in the female, and aggression and libido in the male. The relative biologic activities of the androgens are given in Table 18-5.

Progesterone prepares the endometrium for implantation and provides the necessary support for pregnancy. It reduces the excitability of the myometrium. Together with estrogen it causes extensive growth and development of the lobular-alveolar system of the breast.

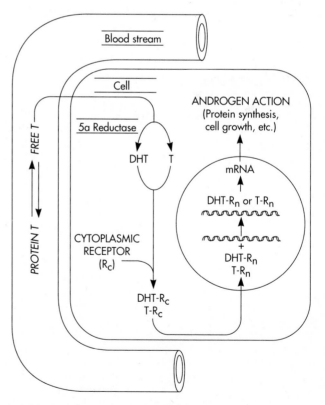

Fig. 18-7 Mechanisms of androgen action. T = testosterone; DHT = dihydrotestosterone; R_n = nuclear receptor; mRNA = messenger RNA. *From Braunstein GD: The testis. In Greenspan FS (ed): Basic and clinical endocrinology, ed 3, Norwalk, Ct, 1991, Appleton and Lange.*

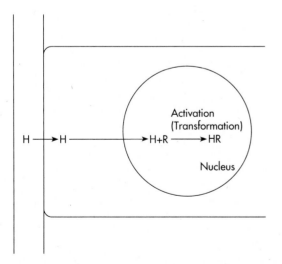

Fig. 18-6 Mechanism of action of steroid hormones. Hormone (H) enters the cell and binds to a receptor (R) in the nucleus. *From Speroff L, Glass RH, and Kase NG: Clinical gynecologic endocrinology and infertility, ed 4, Baltimore, 1989, Williams and Wilkins Co.*

Table 18-5 Hormone potency

Hormone	Relative androgenic activity*
Testosterone	100
Dihydrotestosterone (DHT)	250
Androstenedione	10-20
DHEA	5
DHEA sulfate	minimal

From Goldfien A and Monroe SE: The ovaries. In Greenspan FS and Forsham PH, eds: Basic and clinical endocrinology, ed 2, Los Altos, Ca, 1986, Lange Medical Publications.
*Testosterone has been assigned a value of 100.

Regulation of androgen action

The adult testis secretes mainly testosterone, although smaller amounts of androstenedione and DHEA are also produced. The ovary also secretes significant amounts of androgen, mainly androstenedione and DHEA, with very little testosterone. The secretion of these so-called weak androgens into the blood stream and their conversion to testosterone in target organs may be a means of providing high concentrations of androgen at specific tissues without a high concentration of testosterone in blood. In this way, inappropriate side effects, such as androgenization in women, may be avoided. The conversion of testosterone to dihydrotestosterone (DHT) in target tissues of the male (see Chapter 31). offers a way to direct varied degrees of androgen messages to androgen-sensitive tissues by providing a mechanism for amplification of the androgen signal at the end organ. In DHT-sensitive tissues, if DHT is regarded as the active hormone, DHEA, androstenedione, and testosterone can all be considered prohormones.

EXTRAGONADAL SOURCES OF GONADAL HORMONES

The adrenal androgens, DHEA and DHEA-sulfate, are produced in relatively large quantities by the innermost zone of the adrenal cortex (zona reticularis) although they have only minimal intrinsic androgenic activity, they contribute to androgenicity by their peripheral conversion to the more potent androgens (Tables 18-3 and 18-6).

Tumors can also produce steroidal products. Estrogens from estrogen-producing tumors in the female cause amenorrhea, often an early symptom of an ovarian tumor. Besides amenorrhea, estrogen-producing tumors can cause anovulatory bleeding in premenopausal women, irregular bleeding after menopause, and precocious puberty in children.

Androgen-producing tumors of the ovary can lead to virilization. With these tumors androgen production is independent of the normal mechanisms of control through feedback regulation. For this reason, plasma androgen levels cannot be suppressed by the administration of estrogens.

The most common of the testicular tumors, tumors of germ cell origin, do not produce steroidal products but rather present protein tumor markers of alpha-fetoprotein and hCG. The source of the alpha-fetoprotein is from embryonic cells that can occur in some types of this tumor. The hCG is the product of trophoblastic cells present in the tumor. The less frequently encountered testicular tumor, the Leydig cell tumor, can produce steroids. Urinary values of 17-KS

and serum DHEAS reflect increased androgen secretion, through serum testosterone is usually low or within the normal range. Estrogen concentrations may also be increased. In tumors that produce hCG, the hCG can stimulate the Leydig cells to produce increased estrogens such that an estrogen-androgen imbalance can occur.

Examples of clinical disorders and laboratory assessments

For the brain and the gonads to work together, the nervous system must be intact, the gonads must be functional, and the feedback loops must be operational. This permits balance and gives the system the ability to accommodate change. Underactivity or overactivity by individual components produces physiologic consequences that can alter sexual functions such as menstrual patterns, secondary sex characteristics, or body height. Body height can be affected since growth and height patterns relate to sex-steroid influences on the skeleton. The clinical identification of these under- and over-producing disorders requires laboratory support for classification and clarification.

Sexual maturity is initiated by pituitary function. Shortly after birth the gonads have the capacity to function and await hormonal stimulation from the pituitary. Early signs of puberty such as hair growth in the pubic and axillary regions are brought on by androgens from the adrenals, DHEA, DHEA sulfate, and androstenedione. These androgens increase progressively beginning in late childhood (around age six) to adolescence (ages 13 to 15, approximately). Because of this adrenal component, the early signs of sexual development are referred to as "adrenarche." In general, the beginning of adrenarche precedes by about two years the rise in gonadal steroids and gonadotropins of early puberty.

Since pituitary hormones are essential to the reproductive process, a loss in pituitary function for either sex before puberty results in gonads that fail to work. After puberty, gonads regress in size and deteriorate when pituitary function is lost. Classical studies have shown that following the removal of the pituitary gland, the gonadal function that is lost can be restored or maintained through injections or by implants of pituitary tissue.

When gonadal function is lost because of castration, pituitary and plasma gonadotropins increase significantly. This rise can be prevented or returned to normal by the administration of either estrogen or androgen. The quantity of androgen required to accomplish this is much greater because androgen must first be converted to estrogen in the central nervous system for it to be effective in this role.

A few clinical examples can illustrate why knowledge of gonadotropin and sex-steroid concentrations are important for the understanding of abnormal hypothalamic-pituitary-ovarian activity.

Precocious puberty in the female is generally regarded as pubertal changes that occur before the eighth year. Because the skeleton is very sensitive to even low concentrations of estrogen, girls with an abnormally early biologic transition between immature and adult reproductive function become adults of very short stature, even though they are tall for their ages when young. Increased growth often is the first change that accompanies the precocious maturing. About half of those with precocious puberty are less than

Table 18-6   Site of formation and serum concentrations of circulating androgens in women

Hormone	Serum concentration† (ng/mL)	Source of circulating hormone (Percentage of total)		
		Adrenal	Ovary	Peripheral conversion
Testosterone	0.2-0.7	5-25	5-25	50-70
Dihydrotestosterone	0.05-0.3	. . .	. . .	100
Androstenedione	0.5-2.5	30-45	45-60	10
DHEA	1.3-9.8	80	20	. . .
DHEA sulfate	400-3200	>95	<5	. . .

From Goldfien A and Monroe SE: The ovaries. In Greenspan FS and Forsham PH, eds: Basic and clinical endocrinology, ed 2, Los Altos, Ca, 1986, Lange Medical Publications.

5-feet tall as adults because of early fusion of the epiphyses caused by early estrogen production. Precocious puberty can happen when hormones are secreted by maturing gonads, such as in "true" precocious puberty, or when premature maturation of the hypothalamic-pituitary-ovarian axis produces gonadotropins that, in turn, stimulate sex-steroid secretion. Precocious puberty can also occur when the maturing normal gonads are not the source of the sex steroids.

Laboratory findings in disorders producing precocious puberty in the female may or may not show elevated values of gonadotropins, though estrogens are always elevated. In "true" precocious puberty, the early maturation of the hypothalamic-pituitary unit provides gonadotropin concentrations that are consistent with normal, functional activity. Only rarely will ectopic sources of gonadotropins cause sexual precocity, usually from tumors. When precocious puberty is from estrogens originating from a cyst or tumor of the gonad, the gonadotropins will be suppressed because of the role of estrogen in feedback control.

At the other extreme of the pubertal development spectrum, delay occurs in few individuals, but with those who are affected, it can occur for a number of reasons. Only 1% of females will not have started their periods by the age of 18. Some individuals have a family history of delayed onset of secondary sexual development. However, in many an initial rise in gonadal sex steroids has already begun. They may have a plasma LH response to intravenous GnRH that is typical of puberty (a rise in LH of greater than 15.6 mIU/ mL). Ovarian steroid production, while below normal in all cases of delayed puberty, may have gonadotropins above, below, or within normal range depending on the cause. The absence or decreased ability of the hypothalamus to secrete GnRH, or of the pituitary to secrete LH and FSH leads to a below normal functioning gonad caused by lack of gonadotrophic stimulation, or *hypo*gonadotropic *hypo*gonadism. On the other hand, elevated gonadotropins due to the absence of negative feedback control of the gonadal sex steroids is characteristic of the failure of the ovary to produce steroidal products. The most common causes for this *hyper*gonadotropin *hypo*gonadism (above normal gonadotropin activity with below normal gonad activity) usually is associated with genetic or somatic abnormalities.

Another example in the female comes from the polycystic ovary. The most common cause of ovarian androgen excess in women is the Polycystic Ovarian Syndrome. Women with this syndrome often have modestly elevated testosterone, DHEAS, and prolactin values, and frequently the LH to

FSH ratio is greater than 3:1. The consequence of the abnormal gonadotropin ratio is an LH-induced excess of androstenedione and testosterone from the ovarian thecal and stromal cells. Without the usual FSH values, granulosa cell aromatization of androstenedione and testosterone to estradiol is reduced. Androgens in the peripheral circulation are converted to estrogens. The many imbalances of both steroid and gonadotropic hormones in women with this syndrome result in the inability to cycle normally and to ovulate.

In the male, a disorder of sexual development can occur where the gonadal sex is not the same as the genital sex. These individuals have gonads that are exclusively testes, their karyotype is male (XY), but their phenotypic characteristics are, to varying degrees, female, showing varying degrees of failure to virilize. This condition is referred to as male pseudohermaphroditism.

Pseudohermaphroditism can develop from a number of causes, all with the common denominator that inadequate androgen is available to provide the appropriate end-organ responses. Causes of this condition include an inability to form androgen and a defect in response to androgen.

Inadequate androgen formation can be caused by defects at many levels of the steroid pathways (Figure 18-8). Certain defects can affect the adrenal gland as well as the testes. The enzymes involved include the enzyme complex that removes the side-chain of cholesterol (converting sterol to progestin, the 20,22-desmolase system), the enzyme that converts the Δ^5- to the Δ^4-steroids (the 3β-hydroxysteroid dehydrogenase system), and the enzyme that generates the obligatory intermediate in the formation of androgen from progestin (17 alpha-hydroxylase). The latter enzyme also catalyzes the first step of the pathway to cortisol formation. (See Chapter 16.)

In individuals afflicted by a deficiency of the enzyme that removes the side chain of cholesterol, the 20,22-desmolase, cholesterol cannot be converted to any of the steroid hormones. Among other developmental and metabolic changes, males demonstrate female external genitalia with a blind vaginal pouch and hypoplastic male genital ducts. The genitalia of affected females are normal, as might be expected since only androgen-dependent processes are involved. Diagnosis of this particular defect is confirmed by the absence of, or low values of, all steroid hormones in plasma and in urine.

With deficiency in the 3β-hydroxysteroid dehydrogenase (preventing conversion of the Δ^5- to Δ^4-steroids), males are incompletely masculinized, and females develop a mild en-

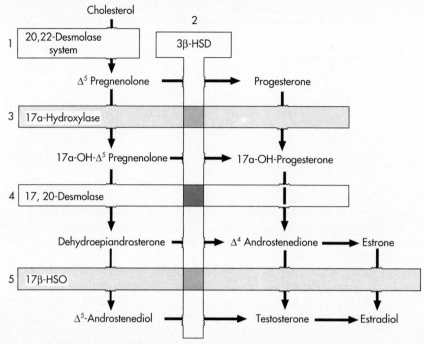

Fig. 18-8   Enzymatic defects in the biosynthetic pathway for testosterone. All five of the enzymatic defects cause male pseudohermaphroditism in affected males. Although all of the blocks affect gonadal steroidongenesis, those at steps 1, 2, and 3 are associated with major abnormalities in the biosynthesis of glucocorticoids and mineralocorticoids in the adrenal. OH = hydroxy; 3β-HSD = 3β = hydroxysteroid dehydrogenase; 17β = HSO, 17β = hydroxysteroid oxidoreductase. *From Conte FA and Grumbach MM: Abnormalities of sexual differentiation. In Greenspan FS and Forsham PH, eds: Basic and clinical endocrinology, Los Altos, CA, 1986, Lange.*

largement of the clitoris. These conditions occur because the Δ^5-androgens that are produced and impact the end organ have only weak, though significant, biological activities. Laboratory assessments show elevated concentrations of 17α-hydroxypregnenolone, DHEA, DHEAS, and other Δ^5-steroids in the plasma and urine.

With enzyme defects that prevent the conversion of progestins to androgens (17α-hydroxylase enzyme), males have a pseudohermaphroditism characterized by a lack of development of secondary sexual characteristics. Since testosterone synthesis is impaired from early fetal times in these males, genitalia is female or ambiguous. The extent of the physical abnormalities will reflect the severity of the enzymatic block. Females with this enzymatic block have normal development of the external genitalia and of the internal ducts, but show sexual infantilism with elevated gonadotropin concentrations at puberty. The elevated gonadotropins reflect a feedback control from androgen precursors instead of from estrogens. High concentrations of progesterone and pregnenolone are found in plasma and increased urinary metabolites of the steroids can be identified.

Other enzymatic defects of the gonads are more directly related to the production of testosterone and estrogens. Should an enzyme defect occur at the enzyme complex for the removal of carbons 20 and 21 of the steroid molecule, androgens cannot be formed from progestins, but the adrenal steroids, mineralocorticoids and glucocorticoids, are unaffected. A 17,20-desmolase (lyase) deficiency (the enzyme that cleaves the carbon to carbon bond between C-17 and

C-20, converting progestins to androgens) prevents the conversion of 17α-hydroxypregnenolone and 17α-hydroxyprogesterone to DHEA and androstenedione, respectively. With this deficiency, males are pseudohermaphroditic with either female or ambiguous genitalia and inguinal or intra-abdominal testes. These individuals have low-circulating concentrations of testosterone, androstenedione, DHEA, and estradiol. Circulating gonadotropins are increased, while testosterone and estradiol concentrations are low. With this type of defect, infantile physical characteristics of the androgen-sensitive organs can respond to the exogenous administration of testosterone.

A deficiency in the enzyme that regulates the reduction of C-17-ketones to C-17-hydroxy steroids (i.e., androstenedione to testosterone, estrone to estradiol), 17β-hydroxysteroid oxidoreductase, causes a deficiency in testosterone during male differentiation. This is manifest as female or mildly ambiguous external genitalia in males at birth. Testes are undescended. At puberty, progressive virilization with clitoral hypertrophy often is associated with breast development (gynecomastia). Plasma gonadotropins, androstenedione, and estrone are markedly elevated whereas testosterone and estradiol concentrations are relatively low. Stimulation with hCG (which mimics the action of LH) can produce increased ratios of plasma androstenedione to testosterone and estrone to estradiol.

A condition known as testicular feminization is the most common form of male pseudohermaphroditism. Androgens are produced by the testes but the chemical message is not received by the end organ. These individuals have circulating concentrations and production rates of testosterone that are the same as or higher than those of normal men. Enlarged breasts are presumably the result of the action of estrogen that is unopposed by androgen. This disorder occurs because the enzyme to reduce testosterone to DHT is missing or because of an absence of the cytoplasmic binding protein that is required for the initial step in dihydrotestosterone interaction with the cell (Figure 18-7).

Thus, knowledge of the overall patterns of steroid hormone formation permits one to predict to a large extent the sequelae that would result clinically when key steroids either cannot be formed or their biologic messages cannot be expressed.

SUGGESTED READING

Bernhisel MA and Hammond LB: Androgen excess. In Scott JR, DiSaia PJ, Hammond CB, and Spellacy WN, eds: Danforth's obstetrics and gynecology, ed 6, Philadelphia, 1990, JB Lippincott Co.

Braunstein, GD: The testis. In Greenspan FS and Forsham PH, eds: Basic and clinical endocrinology, ed 2, Los Altos, Ca., 1986, Lange Medical Publishers.

Conte FA and Grumbach MM: abnormalities of sexual differentiation. In Greenspan FS and Forsham PH, eds: Basic and clinical endocrinology, Los Altos, Ca., 1986, Lange Medical Publications.

Goldfien A and Monroe SE: The ovaries. In Greenspan FS and Forsham PH, eds: Basic and clinical endocrinology, ed 2, Los Altos, Ca., 1986, Lange Medical Publications.

Kicklighter EJ and Norman RJ: The gonads. In Kaplan LA and Pesce AJ: Clinical chemistry: theory, analysis and correlation, ed 2, St. Louis, 1989, Mosby–Year Book, Inc.

Lipsett MB: Steroid hormones. In Yen SSC and Jaffe RB, eds: Reproductive endocrinology, ed 2, Philadelphia, 1986, WB Saunders Co.

Liwnicz BH and Liwnicz RG: Endocrine function. In clinical chemistry: theory, analysis, and correlation; ed 2, St. Louis, 1989, Mosby–Year Book, Inc.

Ross GT and Schreiber JR: The ovary. In Reproductive endocrinology ed 2, Philadelphia, 1986, WB Saunders Co.

Speroff L, Glass RH, and Kase NG: Clinical gynecologic endocrinology and infertility, ed 4, Baltimore, 1989, Williams and Wilkins.

Styne DM: Puberty. In Greenspan FS and Forsham PH, eds: Basic and clinical endocrinology, ed 2, Los Altos, Ca., 1986, Lange Medical Publications.

Williams JA: Mechanisms in hormone secretion, action and response. In Greenspan FS and Forsham PH, eds: Basic and clinical endocrinology, ed 2, Los Altos, Ca., 1986, Lange Medical Publications.

19 Fertility, pregnancy, and fetal maturity

Paul T. Russell
R. Ian Hardy

FERTILITY
The menstrual cycle and ovulation

Child development is a complex process that can be traced to the release of an oocyte from an ovarian follicle during a woman's menstrual cycle. The first half of the cycle, the follicular phase, is when the follicle that will ovulate is developing. This part of the cycle is characterized by increasing concentrations of estradiol secreted by the developing Graafian follicle. Following ovulation, the second half of the cycle, the luteal phase, is dominated by increasing concentrations of progesterone. This occurs because cellular elements of the follicle, from which the egg is released, transform to form the corpus luteum (Figure 19-1). Progesterone, produced by the corpus luteum, prepares the endometrium for future implantation should pregnancy occur.

The cycle begins under the influence of follicle-stimulating hormone (FSH). Follicular development causes a coordinated proliferation of the lining of the uterus, the endometrium, because of rising concentrations of estrogens produced by the cellular elements of the follicle. During this time the egg contained in the maturing follicle progresses in development and is ultimately released from the follicle at ovulation through the action of luteinizing hormone (LH). The follicle destined to ovulate is identifiable by the sixth to eighth day of the cycle (the usual convention is to designate the first day of menstrual bleeding as the first day of the cycle) by its continuing enlargement. Cohort follicles, those starting to develop at the same time but not destined to provide the egg for that month, begin to regress by the sixth to eighth day.

Late in the follicular phase, rising estradiol levels stimulate the hypothalamus to release gonadotropin-releasing hormone (GnRH). This results in an abrupt peak of both LH and FSH (Figure 19-1). This preovulatory gonadotropin peak is the central endocrinological event in the menstrual cycle and precedes ovulation by 36 to 40 hours. Ovulation occurs 11 to 14 days before the next menstrual period (on or about the 17th day of a normal 28 day cycle).

During the preovulatory surge, LH initiates the process of ovulation and directs the egg to resume its development in preparation for fertilization. LH sets in motion a process that prepares the egg to become progressively isolated from the controlled, enclosed environment of the follicle. Shortly after the LH surge, the egg loses its nutritional support from the cells of the follicle and resumes its nuclear and cytoplasmic progress toward maturation. Only an egg prepared this way can become fertilized.

Following ovulation, the cycle becomes dominated by progesterone (Figure 19-1) produced by the rapidly developing corpus luteum. During this progestational, or luteal, phase, basal body temperature (Figure 19-1) rises with the increased production of pregnanediol, a metabolite of progesterone. The increase in temperature occurs when blood concentrations of progesterone exceed 2.5 to 4.0 ng/mL.

Toward the end of the two-week life span of the corpus luteum, progesterone values fall if fertilization has not taken place. This decline signals withdrawal of progesterone's effects on the endometrium and causes the onset of menstrual bleeding. The beginning of menstruation (and, by definition, the beginning of the next cycle) occurs approximately three days after plasma progesterone begins this precipitous decline, ultimately reaching concentrations below 1 ng/mL. As the new cycle begins, FSH values start to rise and several new follicles begin developing. If conception has occurred, the corpus luteum is kept active by human chorionic gonadotropin (hCG), which is produced by cells surrounding the early embryo.

The discovery that the gonadotropic hormones are released in rhythmic pulsations into the plasma introduced a new dimension to the understanding of the endocrine events of the menstrual cycle. Plasma LH concentrations oscillate with a period of approximately one hour and appear to be the result of brief releases of the hormone into the circulation. Apparently 92% of the total mass of the LH present in the circulation is the consequence of this pulsatile secretion.

During the beginning of the reproductive years in women, the first two years after menarche, as many as 55% to 90% of cycles are non ova-producing and these anovulatory cycles decrease to less than 20% within five years.

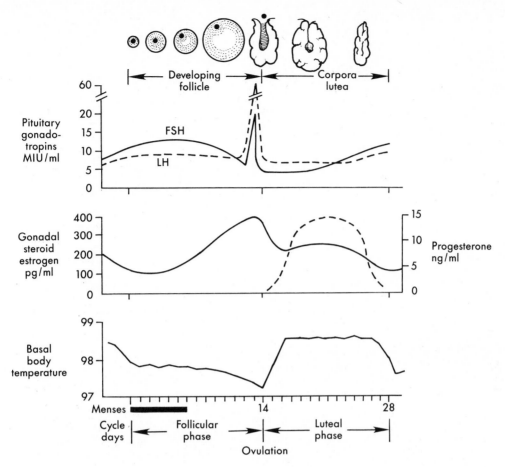

Fig. 19-1 Endocrinology of the menstrual cycle in humans. *From Haney AF: Effects of toxic agents on ovarian function. In Thomas JA, Korach KS, and McLachlan JA eds: Endocrine toxicology, New York, 1985, Raven Press.*

Although there is evidence for cyclic surges of LH during some of the anovulatory cycles in adolescence, the ovulatory mechanism as a unit seems unstable and immature, not yet attaining the fine tuning and synchronization required for maintenance of regular ovulatory cycles.

Toward the end of the reproductive years, menstrual periods cease. This phenomenon, referred to as the menopause, occurs in women as a natural course usually between the ages of 42 and 60. Its onset can be earlier if the ovaries have been surgically removed or irradiated, or if there are abnormalities of the ovaries. With normal aging, the changes leading to menopause are gradual and are identified endocrinologically by an increase in circulating concentrations of FSH and decreases in estradiol and progesterone. The ovary gradually becomes less responsive to gonadotropins several years before menses cease, and this may trigger the initiation of menopause.

Associated with the early manifestations of menopause are irregular cycles and anovulatory bleeding. The increase in FSH is greater than that of LH, a pattern that reflects a lack of feedback inhibition by estrogen. The average production rate of estradiol falls to 12 μg/24 hours, and the clearance rate is reduced. Serum concentrations of several hormones in pre- and postmenopausal women are shown in Table 19-1.

Table 19-1 Serum concentrations of steroids in premenopausal and postmenopausal women (mean ± SEM)

Steroid	Premenopausal* (ng/mL)	Postmenopausal (ng/mL)
Progesterone	0.47 ± 0.03	0.17 ± 0.02
DHEA	4.2 ± 0.5	1.8 ± 0.2
DHEA sulfate	1600 ± 350	300 ± 70
Androstenedione	1.5 ± 0.1	0.6 ± 0.01
Testosterone	0.32 ± 0.02	0.25 ± 0.03
Estrone	0.08 ± 0.01	0.029 ± 0.002
Estradiol	0.05 ± 0.005	0.013 ± 0.001

From Benson RC, ed: Current obstetric & gynecologic diagnosis & treatment, ed 5, Los Altos, CA, 1984, Lange.
*Follicular phase concentrations.

Fertilization

Ova usually are fertilized within 12 hours of ovulation. Fertilization typically occurs within the oviduct (Figure 19-2). After traversing the zona pellucida (Figure 19-1), the sperm head fuses with the oocyte membrane, and the sperm nucleus is incorporated into the egg cytoplasm. This process elicits changes in the oocyte membrane that prevent the entrance of additional sperm into the oocyte.

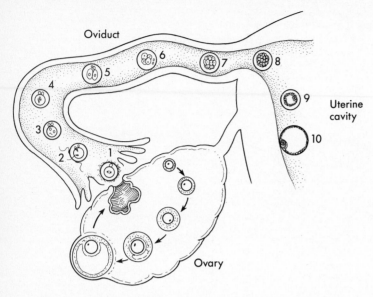

Fig. 19-2 Diagrammatic representation of follicular growth, ovulation, fertilization and preimplantation. 1 = egg released from ovary; 2 = sperm entry into egg; 3 = male and female pronucleus formation, sperm tail in egg cytoplasm; 4 = first cleavage metaphase spindle; 5 = 2 cell stage; 6 = 4 cell stage; 7 = 8 cell stage; 8 = morula; 9 = early blastocyst, blastocele cavity forming; 10 = blastocyst starting to implant. *Redrawn from Whittingham DG: Brit Med Bull 35:105, 1979.*

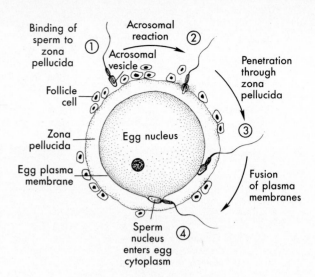

Fig. 19-3 Schematic illustration of events occurring as a sperm fertilizes an egg. Note that the sperm interact tangentially with the egg plasma membrane so that fusion occurs at the side rather than at the top of the sperm head. *Redrawn from Alberts B, et al: Molecular biology of the cell, ed 2, New York, 1989, Garland Publishing, Inc.*

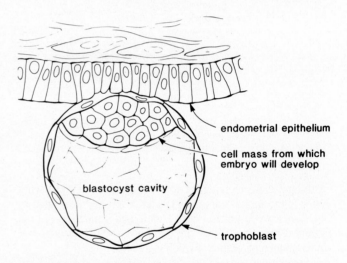

Fig. 19-4 Attachment of blastocyst to endometrial wall. *From Russell PT: Pregnancy and fetal function. In Kaplan LA and Pesce AJ: Clinical chemistry: theory, analysis, and correlation, ed 2, St. Louis, 1989, Mosby-Year Book, Inc.*

Freshly ejaculated sperm are incapable of fertilization. Changes that must occur in sperm usually begin in the lower part of the female reproductive tract and are completed upon contact with the egg (Figure 19-3). These changes, referred to as "capacitation" and "the acrosome reaction" are described in Chapter 31. Sperm can, however, acquire the ability to fertilize after a short incubation period in culture media without exposure to the female reproductive tract, thereby permitting in vitro fertilization. Of the 200 to 300 million sperm present in a normal ejaculate, less than 200 achieve proximity to the oocyte.

Cell division and tubal transport

After fertilization, mitotic division begins (Figure 19-2). The conceptus progresses through two-, four-, and eight-cell stages and then to a ball of cells, the morula. Fluid is secreted by the outer cells of the morula, and a single fluid-filled cavity, the blastocoel cavity, develops. An inner-cell mass (Figure 19-4) that eventually becomes the fetus develops and is attached eccentrically to the outer layer of flattened cells (trophoplast), which will become the placenta. Blastocyst formation begins about 5 days after ovulation. On the fifth or sixth day, the blastocyst enters the uterine lumen, where it continues a free-floating existence for at least 24 hours before implanting in the uterine lining.

Transport of the oocyte into and along the tube is facilitated by both muscular contractions and the movement of estrogen-dependent tubal hair-like structures, called cilia. Ciliary activity does not seem absolutely essential, however, since at least some women with immotile cilia become pregnant.

THE ENDOCRINOLOGY OF PREGNANCY
Conception and implantation

Implantation is the last step of conception and the first step of pregnancy. Implantation occurs some 150 hours after follicular rupture. The endometrium is only receptive to implantation over a one- to two-day period. Implantation starts on the sixth day and is complete by about the ninth. Human chorionic gonadotropin (hCG), produced by the trophoblastic cells surrounding the early embryo, can be detected in the circulation six to eight days after ovulation, just after vascular contact is established between the implanting embryo and the endometrium.

Fertilization normally occurs in the fallopian tubes. Under typical circumstances, the fertilized egg migrates down the tube and into the uterus, where it implants. Implantation, however, occasionally does not follow this pattern and occurs outside the uterus, commonly in the fallopian tube itself. An implantation that occurs outside the uterus is called an ectopic pregnancy. These outside-of-the-uterus implantations are thought to occur because of endocrine imbalances, residual effects stemming from tubal infections, or retrograde movements of the embryo from the uterus to the fallopian tube. Before rupture of the fallopian tube occurs, tubal pregnancies usually give a positive urine or serum pregnancy test and clinical symptoms of significant pelvic pain with abnormal uterine bleeding.

Serum values in an ectopic pregnancy are often considerably lower than those present in a uterine pregnancy. By four weeks the hCG concentrations fall off for the ectopic pregnancy, especially after a fallopian tube ruptures. Thus, after four to eight weeks of ectopic gestation, serum hCG values can range from less than 20 to 20,000 mIU/mL, whereas for normal pregnancies the serum hCG concentrations are two to two-and-a-half times higher.

Serial measurements of quantitative serum hCG are used to predict abnormal or ectopic pregnancies. Normal pregnancy β-hCG values rise by at least 66% within a 48-hour sampling period. The rate of rise of β-hCG in an ectopic pregnancy is less than one half of that in intrauterine pregnancies. Normal pregnancy is not associated with falling β-hCG measurements.

Polypeptide hormones
Human chorionic gonadotropin (hCG)

Human chorionic gonadotropin (hCG) is a glycoprotein hormone secreted by the trophoblast and eventually the chorionic villi of the placenta. The presence of hCG in urine and serum of pregnant women provides the basis of tests for the diagnosis of pregnancy. Specific and sensitive analytical methods for the whole molecule or the β-chain subunit of hCG permit the detection of pregnancy as early as one day after implantation. HCG reaches a peak high about nine to 10 weeks after the first missed menstrual period when conception has occurred. After this peak, the blood and urinary titers drop to lower values with a nadir being reached at about 20 weeks of gestation. HCG concentrations remain easily detected and fairly constant until a few days after parturition (Figure 19-5).

The chemical structure and properties of hCG are similar to LH. HCG converts the corpus luteum of the menstrual cycle into the corpus luteum of pregnancy, thereby prolonging the luteal production of progesterone until the placenta is capable of secreting the high amounts of gonadal steroids required for the continuation of pregnancy.

Since hCG is secreted by placental tissue, its presence in the urine or blood has formed the basis for many tests of pregnancy. A wide array of tests, both qualitative and quantitative, are available for the monitoring of hCG (Table 19-2). Qualitative tests have important utility because they provide quick and inexpensive methods for determining an established pregnancy. These tests include "slide tests," "tube tests," and immunoenzymatic concentration tests. The first two types use the agglutination- (flocculation-) inhibition principle. The last type is an ELISA procedure that is optimized for rapid answers but lacks sensitivity for quan-

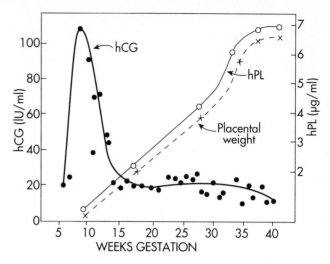

Fig. 19-5 Concentrations of chorionic gonadotropin (hCG) and placental lactogen (hPL) in serum of women throughout normal pregnancy. *From Cunningham FG, MacDonald PC and Gant NF: The placental hormones. In Williams Obstetrics, ed 18, Norwalk, CT, 1989, Appleton and Lange.*

titative use. This type of test has supplanted the stat pregnancy testing previously performed by slide and tube methods since it gives sensitivities of 20 to 50 mIU/mL in about five minutes of assay time.

Quantitative hCG information can be obtained through both radioimmunoassay (RIA) and more sensitive ELISA methods. RIA has sufficient sensitivity to detect serum hCG valves (over 20 mIU/mL) by one to two and a half weeks of gestation.

The absolute amount of hCG present in the serum during pregnancy varies greatly with gestational age and from patient to patient. Table 19-3 gives hCG values for the first trimester of pregnancy. During this trimester hCG doubles approximately every two days. A slower rate of rise can be associated with a higher prospect for miscarriage.

In normal pregnancies, serum contains intact hCG and little, if any, free alpha- or beta-hCG subunits. In urine, intact hCG is present, and, depending on the gestational time, both free alpha- and beta-hCG may appear along with fragments of hCG. The relative concentrations of intact and subunit hCG have been found to vary greatly in patients with trophoblastic disease and ectopic pregnancies. The proportion of fragments and subunits can also vary with many types of tumors.

Human chorionic somatomammotropin (hCS or hPL)

Human chorionic somatomammotropin (hCS) is a product of the placenta. It is a single chain polypeptide, very similar to pituitary growth hormone (96% homology) and to human prolactin. Maternal serum concentrations parallel placental weight, rising throughout gestation to maximum levels in the last four weeks (Figure 19-5). At term, hCS accounts for 10% of the protein produced by the placenta. Since hCS antagonizes the cellular action of insulin and decreases glucose utilization, its function may be to shift glucose availability toward the fetus.

Table 19-2 Methods for hCG measurements

Method	Type of analysis	Principle	Use	Comments
QUALITATIVE ASSAYS				
1. Slide tests	Agglutination inhibition	Colored latex or other visible particles (red blood cells) coated with hCG, antibodies to hCG, and urine are mixed with particles. Negative urine results in visible agglutination; presence of hCG in urine inhibits agglutination (or protein flocculation).	Was frequently used as stat urinary pregnancy test; urine	Least sensitive of all hCG methods; most rapid (2-3 min)
2. Tube tests	Same as method 1	Same as method 1; reaction occurs in tube.	Was sometimes used for stat urine pregnancy tests; urine	More sensitive than slide; some approach upper limit of sensitivity of RIA methods; 45-120 min per assay
3. Immunoenzymatic concentration tests	Sandwich immunometric assay	Solid-phase, double-antibody sandwich ELISA in which hCG binds to antibody. Enzyme-labeled antibody added, and residual activity directly related to hCG concentration.	Has become assay of choice, has speed of "slide" and sensitivity of "tube" with a colored end point; urine and serum	Reported sensitivity 20-50 mU/mL, 5- to 15-min assay; many forms: membrane, bead, paddle, dipstick, coated tube
QUANTITATIVE ASSAYS—SERUM AND URINE				
4. Radioimmunoassay (RIA)	Competitive inhibition	Radiolabeled (radioactive iodine, ^{125}I) hCG competes with sample analyte for binding to anti-hCG. Increased hCG in sample, decreased bound radioactivity.	Infrequently used as stat procedure; serum or urine	Most sensitive hCG assay available; 40-60 min per assay
5. Enzyme-linked immunosorbent assay (ELISA)	Sandwich immunometric assay	Enzyme-labeled anti-hCG reacts with sample hCG bound to solid-phase anti-hCG. Amount of bound enzyme activity directly proportional to amount of hCG in sample.	Most frequently used assay; serum and urine	Reported sensitivity of 2-10 U/mL; assay time 1-3 hr

From Hohnadel DC and Kaplan LA: Hormones and their metabolites. In Kaplan LA and Pesce AJ, Chemistry: theory, analysis, and correlation, ed 2, St Louis, 1989, Mosby-Year Book, Inc.

Table 19-3 Serum hCG values with gestational age

Gestational age	hCG (mU/mL)
0.2-1 week	5-50
1-2 weeks	50-500
2-3 weeks	100-5000
3-4 weeks	500-10,000
4-5 weeks	1,000-50,000
5-6 weeks	10,000-100,000
6-8 weeks	15,000-200,000
2-3 months	10,000-100,000

From Hohnadel DC and Kaplan LA: Hormones and their metabolites. In Kaplan LA and Pesce AJ, Chemistry: theory, analysis, and correlation, ed 2, St Louis, 1989, Mosby-Year Book, Inc.

HCS can be found in the urine and serum in both normal and molar pregnancies. Values of 7 to 10 ng/mL are present in the maternal circulation by 20 to 40 days of gestation. By the last four weeks of pregnancy, concentrations of 5 µg/mL can be achieved, a 1000-fold increase. Low values correlate with threatened abortion and intrauterine fetal growth retardation. HCS is also found in the urine of patients harboring trophoblastic tumors and in men with choriocarcinoma of the testis.

Oxytocin

Oxytocin is a cyclic polypeptide containing eight amino acids. Its primary function is in the ejection of milk from

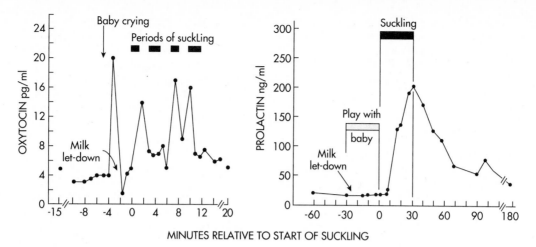

Fig. 19-6 Plasma oxytocin (left) and prolactin (right) concentrations in response to the anticipation of nursing and suckling in lactating women. Milk "let-down" occurred in association with acute release of oxytocin but not prolactin. *Modified from Noel GL, et al: J Clin Endocrinol Metab 38:413, 1974; McNeilly AS, et al: Br Med J 286:257, 1983.*

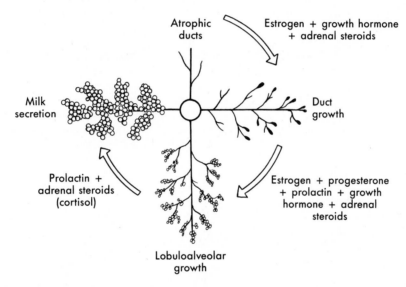

Fig. 19-7 Schematic representation of the multihormonal interaction on the growth of the mammary gland and in the initiation of milk formation and lactation.

the breast during nursing. Oxytocin is released in response to suckling, mediated through impulses generated at the nipple (Figure 19-6). Oxytocin is also released by olfactory, visual, and auditory pathways. To a nursing mother, the cry of her baby often brings milk let-down in the breasts.

Oxytocin is also a potent uterine stimulant used in obstetrics and perinatal medicine for the induction and augmentation of labor, for antenatal fetal assessment (oxytocin challenge test), and for the control of postpartum hemorrhage.

Prolactin

The prolactin molecule is a single polypeptide containing 198 amino acid residues which shares 16% homology with human growth hormone and 13% with hPL. It is secreted by the anterior pituitary.

Prolactin is the key hormone controlling milk production. Prolactin works in concert with estrogen, progesterone, growth hormone, insulin, and cortisol in this function. Growth of the duct system, in preparation for lactation, depends on estrogen, synergized by the presence of growth hormone, prolactin, and cortisol (Figure 19-7). Development of the lobulo-alveolar system requires both estrogen and progesterone in conjunction with prolactin. The synthesis of milk protein and fat is regulated principally by prolactin and is facilitated by insulin and cortisol.

In pregnancy, serum prolactin begins to rise in the first trimester and increases progressively to about 200 ng/mL by term. This is about 10 times the concentration found in nonpregnant women. An approximate linear increase with time is seen. As with several other hormones, there is a pulsatile nature to the release of prolactin and its release is higher with sleep and with food ingestion.

In nonpregnant females, normal prolactin levels are less than 20 ng/mL. Elevations above this may be caused by pituitary microadenomas, hypothyroidism, or dopamine-inhibiting medications. Elevated prolactin has an inhibitory effect on GnRH and, hence, may cause anovulation and infertility.

Steroid hormones

Large quantities of progesterone and estrogens are produced during pregnancy and there is an integrated role and constant interaction between the fetus, placenta, and mother in the formation of these steroids. Since the placenta is incapable of forming androgens from progestins, it must rely on precursors reaching it from the fetal and maternal circulations. The formation of progesterone by the placenta is in large part derived from circulating maternal cholesterol. Production of progesterone is massive and approximates 250 mg/day by the end of pregnancy. Circulation values can exceed 150 ng/mL.

Progesterone is essential for the maintenance of pregnancy. Its primary roles seem to be to support the uterine lining in a state that will support embryo development and to maintain the uterine myometrium in a quiescent mode during the term of the pregnancy. All hypotheses that explain the onset of labor have a common denominator: some mechanism to diminish the quieting effect of progesterone, thereby producing myometrial activity leading to expulsion of the fetus. Some speculate that progesterone is responsible for inhibiting T-lymphocyte cell-mediated responses involved in tissue rejection, thereby permitting the presence of the "foreign" fetus.

The placenta has an active aromatizing capacity, utilizing available androgens. But in order for estrogen formation by the placenta to occur, androgen precursors must reach it from both the fetal and the maternal compartments. A major androgenic precursor in placental estrogen formation is DHEA-S (dehydroepiandrosterone sulfate). This compound comes mainly from the fetal adrenal gland. Once in the placenta, DHEA-S is converted to free DHEA, then to androstenedione and testosterone and, finally, to estrone and estradiol.

In human pregnancy, an interesting variation of this system produces another estrogen. This estrogen is neither estrone nor estradiol but rather estriol (16-alpha-hydroxy-estradiol). The unique formation of estriol is the consequence of the interdependence of fetus, placenta, and mother. This interdependence is commonly referred to as the "feto-placental unit" (Figure 19-8). DHEA-S is the steroid of interest in this relationship. DHEA-S of either fetal or maternal origin undergoes 16α-hydroxylation, primarily in the fetal liver. When the 16α-hydroxy-DHEA-S reaches the placenta, placental sulfatase acts to remove the sulfate side chain. The resulting unconjugated 16α-hydroxy-DHEA is aromatized to form estriol which is then secreted into the maternal circulation and voided into the urine.

Estriol is not a product of the ovary to any appreciable extent in nonpregnant women. By contrast, estriol constitutes more than 90% of the known estrogens in pregnancy urine, into which it is excreted as its sulfate and glucuronide conjugates. Concentrations increase tremendously (more than 1000-fold) with advancing gestation and range from approximately 2 ng per 24 hours at 16 weeks to 35 to 45

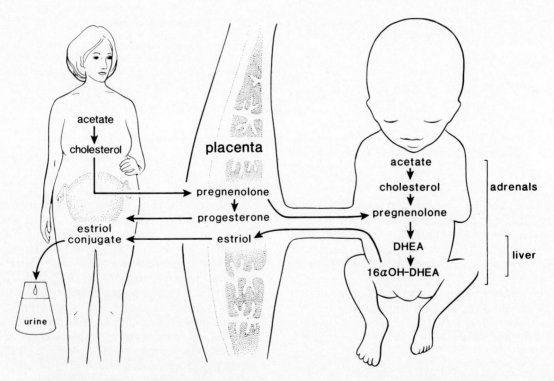

Fig. 19-8 Schematic representation of the fetoplacental unit. DHEA, Dehydroepiandrosterone; 16α-OH-DHEA, 16α-hydroxydehydroepiandrosterone. *From Russell PT: Pregnancy and fetal function. In Kaplan LA and Pesce AJ: Clinical chemistry: theory, analysis and correlation, ed 2, St. Louis, 1989, Mosby-Year Book, Inc.*

mg/24 hours at term. At term, the concentration of estriol in the maternal circulation is between 8 and 13 ng/dL. Estriol is also found in high concentrations in amniotic fluid.

According to standard assays that measure uterine weight increases in ovariectomized mice, estriol is a weak estrogen. Its activity is 0.01 times the potency of estradiol and 0.1 times the potency of estrone based on a per weight basis. Estriol, however, is more active than the other two estrogens in increasing uteroplacental blood flow. Thus, the function of estriol may be related to its ability to augment uterine perfusion during pregnancy.

Maternal adaptation to pregnancy

Most maternal organ systems change because of pregnancy. Some changes clearly support a pregnancy or the period of lactation that follows, but the benefit of other changes is not so evident. A few of the maternal adaptations to pregnancy are related to the effects of an enlarging uterus and its conceptus, but the majority appear to be responses to ovarian and placental hormones, either directly or through secondary effects on maternal regulatory mechanisms.

The cardiovascular system adapts to pregnancy with major changes in cardiac output and differences in regional blood flow distribution. Cardiac output increases by 30% to 40%. An increased uterine blood flow is another prominent change that develops with pregnancy. Estriol may be responsible for this augmented flow. There is a progressive decrease in uterine vascular resistance as pregnancy advances, since blood flow is increased without much change in maternal blood pressure. Expansion of the vascular beds undoubtedly is an important factor in this adaptation.

A number of changes occur in the vascular compartment. Plasma volume increases from about six weeks of gestation to term, as does the total volume of red blood cells. Both the hemoglobin concentration and hematocrit tend to fall. This is a dilution effect, because the proportional increase in plasma volume is greater than the increase in red cell mass. This trend is reversed in the last six to eight weeks as hemoglobin and hematocrit rise by about 0.5 g and 1% to 2%, respectively. The total white cell count increases to about 10,500 per mm³ in late pregnancy. This is accounted for predominantly by a rise in the number of polymorphonuclear leucocytes. The platelet count is reduced somewhat, also as the result of hemodilution. The large increase in fibrinogen concentration is probably brought about by the action of estrogens on the liver.

The total serum lipid concentration rises progressively from the end of the first 12 weeks and is 40% to 50% above nonpregnant values at term. All components of the serum lipids are increased, with the triglyceride fraction showing the largest proportionate rise.

Most of the commonly measured endocrine function tests are radically changed with pregnancy. These are summarized in Table 19-4. In some cases, true physiologic alteration occurs. In others, the changes result from an increase in the production of specific serum binding proteins by the liver or to decreases in serum levels of albumin.

Glucosuria is common in healthy, pregnant women. Glucose excretion occurs early in pregnancy, peaking between eight and 11 weeks of gestation. The degree of glucosuria varies thereafter. The cardinal feature of the glucosuria of pregnancy is a conspicuous variability both from day to day and during the course of a day. This glucosuria appears to be caused by a reduced efficiency of the kidneys to reabsorb glucose.

The endocrine stresses of pregnancy are potentially diabetogenic and diabetes mellitus may be aggravated by pregnancy. Clinical diabetes may appear in some women only during pregnancy. The frequent appearance of clinical glycosuria and the necessity to differentiate "renal glycosuria" from pregnancy-aggravated diabetes mellitus is very important because of the potential for negative effects on the fetus. Pregnant diabetic women should be monitored by serum glucose testing because of the many variables associated with an altered renal physiology in pregnancy. Perhaps because urine glucose testing can yield misleading values, screening for gestational diabetes by a glucose challenge test has become routine. It is important to maintain normal serum glucose concentrations during pregnancy to prevent perinatal morbidity that can occur with gestational hyperglycemia.

The maternal thyroid gland enlarges during pregnancy and although many laboratory tests for thyroid function are

Table 19-4   Effect of pregnancy on endocrine function tests.

	Test	Result
Pituitary		
FSH, LH	GnRH stimulation	Unresponsive from third gestational week until puerperium.
GH	Insulin tolerance test	Response increases during the first half of pregnancy and then is blunted until the puerperium.
	Arginine stimulation	Hyperstimulation during the first and second trimesters, then suppression.
	TRH stimulation	Response unchanged.
TSH		
Pancreas		
Insulin	Glucose tolerance	Peak glucose increases, and glucose concentration remains elevated longer.
	Glucose challenge	Insulin concentration increases to higher peak levels.
	Arginine infusion	Insulin response is blunted in mid to late pregnancy.
Adrenal		
Cortisol	ACTH infusion	Exaggerated cortisol and 17-hydroxycorticosterone responses.
	Metyrapone	Diminished response.
Mineralocorticoids	ACTH infusion	No DOC response.
	Dexamethasone suppression	No DOC response.

From Martin MC and Hoffman PG: The endocrinology of pregnancy. In Greenspan FS (ed): Basic and clinical endocrinology, ed 3, Norwalk, CT, 1991, Appleton and Lange.

altered during pregnancy, the pregnant woman appears to remain euthyroid. Estrogen-induced increases in serum thyroxine-binding globulin (TBG) occurs, thus increasing total thyroxine (T4). Basal metabolic rate is increased 15% to 20% due to an adaptation related to the presence of the fetus, increased uterine size, and increased cardiac output.

Fetal endocrinology

Many components of the hypothalamo-pituitary-target organ axis of the fetus develop and become functional relatively early in gestation. Of the hypothalamic hormones, the production of the neurotransmitters, dopamine, norepinephrine, serotonin, the peptides, vasopressin and oxytocin, and the releasing- and inhibiting-factors, including GnRH, begin during intrauterine life. The rising profile of FSH and LH in the fetal circulation at mid-gestation probably reflects developmental processes taking place in the fetus prior to birth. The presence of steroid hormones and metabolites in both fetal blood, fetal urine, and amniotic fluid (derived in large part from fetal urine) attest to the presence of the steroid pathways in fetal tissues, with the biologically less active delta 5-pathway steroids being the most prominent.

A unique feature of the fetal endocrine system is the "fetal" zone of the adrenal cortex. This tissue constitutes about 80% of the gland and actively produces large quantities of DHEA-S. The mean concentration of DHEA-S in the fetal circulation at term is about 130 μg/dL. Production of this androgen in the fetal adrenal cortex appears to be controlled by hCG during the early half of pregnancy and by ACTH during the latter half. Much of the fetal zone has regressed by the first two to three months after birth, and is almost completely gone by the end of the first year.

The corticosteroids, particularly cortisol, produced by the definitive zone of the adrenal cortex, have a variety of important functions during fetal life. They induce the development of a variety of enzyme systems in the liver of the fetus: they play a role in the switch from fetal to adult type of hemoglobin; and they induce the formation of surfactant in fetal lungs.

Thyroid hormone synthesis in the fetus begins at 10 to 12 weeks, remains low through the second trimester, and finally increases in the last three months of pregnancy. High values of reversed T_3 (3,3',5'-triiodothyronine) are found in the amniotic fluid between 15 and 30 weeks. At the end of the first trimester, the fetus develops its own hypothalamic-pituitary-thyroid axis, which remains independent of the mother's thyroid status. T_4, T_3 and TSH do not cross the placental barrier.

The pituitary gland of the human fetus is able to synthesize, store, and secrete prolactin early in gestation. The physiologic role of fetal prolactin is unknown. Its highest concentration is found in amniotic fluid, where it is five- to tenfold greater than in maternal serum.

In the early embryonic period, the internal sexual structures develop as female unless exposed to androgens (See Chapter 18.). Testosterone production by the fetal testis, consequently, plays a key role in sexual development in the male. Testosterone itself is probably responsible for the development of the internal genital structures while dihydrotestosterone, a reduced product of testosterone, brings about the development of the external genital structures.

Since the maximal production of testosterone by the fetal testis corresponds to the time of maximal production of hCG by the placenta, it is likely that hCG plays a key role in regulating fetal steroidogenesis during the first half of pregnancy. If this is the case, then hCG governs the production of both DHEA-S in the fetal zone of the adrenal gland and of testosterone in the testis.

The human fetus exhibits an extensive ability to add sulfate to steroids in many tissues. The placenta has active sulfatase activity (i.e., the ability to remove steroid sulfates). Thus, when steroid sulfates reach the placenta, the sulfate is rapidly and efficiently removed. Sulfatase activity is essential for estrogen formation by the feto-placental unit.

When placental sulfatase is lacking (as in the placental sulfatase deficiency syndrome), maternal estriol excretion is approximately 5% of that found in normal pregnancy while estrone and estradiol are about 15% of normal. At the same time, pregnanediol excretion remains at normal values. Patients with this syndrome can metabolize DHEA but not DHEA-S. Thus, in pregnancies where estriol values are low throughout pregnancy, the values may be related to a sulfatase deficiency rather than to anencephalic development of the fetus, a distinction that can be made by ultrasound.

Endocrinology of the puerperium and lactation

By breaking contact between placenta and uterus at parturition, hormonal concentrations change rapidly in the postpartum woman. Whether or not the mother chooses to breast-feed sets the stage for the next set of hormonal adaptations.

Development of the breast alveolar lobules occurs throughout pregnancy. This preparation requires the participation of estrogen, progesterone, cortisol, prolactin (PRL), and growth hormone (Figure 19-7). PRL concentrations, which increase from less than 20 ng/mL before pregnancy to approximately 250 to 300 ng/mL at term, fall with the onset of labor. Prolactin values exhibit variable patterns of secretion depending on whether the mother breast-feeds. A surge in PRL accompanies delivery, and in women who do not breast-feed, PRL values return to pre-pregnant concentrations by four to six weeks post partum. In nonlactating women, the return to normal cycles and ovulation may be expected as soon as the second post partum month, with resumed ovulation occurring about nine to 10 weeks post partum.

Milk secretion does not take place until after delivery because of the blocking effect of high concentrations of estrogen. During each breast-feeding episode, oxytocin release causes myoepithelial cells in the breast to contract, and milk is ejected from the alveolus into the adjacent ducts. Bursts of PRL also take place (Figure 19-6). The more frequent and intense the suckling, the higher the PRL concentrations. Prolactin prepares the mammary glands for milk production for the following feeding period.

In lactating women, PRL usually prevents ovulation. Surges of PRL are believed to act on the hypothalamus to inhibit GnRH secretion and estradiol values remain low despite an increase in FSH. Only after PRL values start to fall to normal do LH and estradiol concentrations begin to rise. The average time before ovulation resumes in women who have lactated for at least three months is about 17 weeks.

Endocrine disorders and pregnancy

Pituitary

In women of reproductive age, small tumors of the anterior pituitary are not uncommon. While most are nonfunctional and without symptoms, when symptoms do occur the most common is amenorrhea, frequently accompanied by galactorrhea. Without therapy, most patients with prolactinomas are anovulatory and infertile. Hyperprolactinemia interferes with reproductive function at several levels, but the primary site is probably at the hypothalamus where it interferes with the normal pulsatile secretion of GnRH. The use of bromocriptine, a dopamine agonist, lowers plasma prolactin values and restores menses and ovulation in over 80% of these patients.

Post-partum pituitary necrosis, or Sheehan's syndrome, is the most common cause of anterior pituitary insufficiency. During pregnancy, the pituitary, because of its hypertrophied state, is more vulnerable to a compromised blood supply. Classically, the patient initially is unable to breast-feed. This is accompanied with breast involution, amenorrhea, loss of axillary and pubic hair, skin depigmentation, hypothyroidism, and adrenocortical insufficiency. The diagnosis is suspected in patients who fail to develop a normal increase in serum growth hormone (GH), PRL, and cortisol following an insulin-induced hypoglycemic episode.

Thyroid

Pregnancy mimics hyperthyroidism. There is a steady increase in serum thyroxine-binding globulin (TGB) that results in increased serum concentrations of total thyroxine (T_4) and total triiodothyronine (T_3), which remain elevated during pregnancy. Pregnant women are usually euthyroid, however, since serum free T_4 (FT_4), free T_3, and TSH concentrations remain within the normal range.

It is often difficult to distinguish the clinical signs and symptoms of hyperthyroidism from those of normal pregnancy. Heat intolerance, increased appetite, warm skin, full pulse, and increased pulse pressure may be found in both conditions. Weight loss during pregnancy should strongly suggest hyperthyroidism.

Hyperthyroidism during pregnancy is most often due to Grave's disease. Since the fetus does not have a thyroid gland until 14 weeks of gestation, before this time radioactive iodine-uptake measurements are feasible without harm to the fetus.

Molar pregnancy, choriocarcinoma, hydatidiform mole, and other gestational trophoblastic neoplasms which secrete large quantities of hCG, can all cause biochemical hyperthyroidism. On a molar basis, hCG demonstrates about 1/4000 the thyrotropic activity of pituitary TSH. For this reason, the high concentrations of hCG attained in molar pregnancies are believed to be the reason maternal hyperthyroidism is often associated with molar pregnancies. Biochemical and clinical hyperthyroidism occurs when hCG serum values exceed 100,000 mIU/mL.

Clinical hypothyroidism or hyperthyroidism due to an underlying thyroid disorder may appear when the immune tolerance of pregnancy disappears postpartum. The immune tolerance of pregnancy may ameliorate autoimmune diseases such as autoimmune hypothyroidism and Hashimoto's thyroiditis.

Adrenal cortex

Cushing's syndrome, resulting from excessive glucocorticoids, is rare during pregnancy. Many of these cases are secondary to benign or malignant ACTH-producing neoplasms. Pregnancy exacerbates the clinical picture of Cushing's syndrome since both pregnancy and hyperadrenocortisolism are characterized by increased unbound plasma cortisol. Diagnosis of Cushing's syndrome during pregnancy can be made from routine screening tests. An overnight dexamethasone suppression test is followed with measurement of 24-hour, urinary-free cortisol (UFC). A normal cortisol suppression (<5 mg/dL) virtually rules out Cushing's syndrome. An elevated UFC (>100 mg/24 hours) is highly correlated with Cushing's syndrome. In pregnant patients with Cushing's syndrome, UFC values have ranged from 225 to 885 mg/24 hours. Part of the plasma ACTH may be of placental origin and subsequently unresponsive to dexamethasone suppression. Therefore the measurement of plasma ACTH may be helpful. Low values suggest adrenal neoplasia; a very high value (>200 pg/mL) suggests an ectopic source.

Primary adrenal insufficiency (Addison's disease) is also rare. The more common secondary adrenal insufficiency may be due to chronic steroid use, pituitary tumors, irradiation, trauma, or vascular insufficiency due to postpartum necrosis. The clinical picture of secondary adrenocortical insufficiency is similar to primary adrenal insufficiency except for the absence of skin pigmentation (ACTH levels are not elevated) and less severe electrolyte and water disturbance (aldosterone is much less affected).

In diagnosing adrenocortical insufficiency, baseline values in plasma cortisol or urinary corticoids are inadequate because they largely overlap the normal values. A low or low normal plasma cortisol concentration does not diagnose adrenal insufficiency. An abnormal ACTH stimulation test with a high plasma ACTH (400 to 2000 pg/mL) suggests Addison's disease. A normal ACTH stimulation test rules out Addison's disease but not secondary adrenocortical insufficiency. A blunted response to insulin-induced hypoglycemia supports the diagnosis of secondary insufficiency, but this is usually not performed during pregnancy. An ACTH concentration inappropriately low or normal (0 to 50 pg/mL) for the decreased cortisol value suggests secondary insufficiency.

Trophoblastic disease

HCG is helpful in identifying and following the course of treatment of trophoblastic disease. Trophoblastic disease has very high β-hCG values (three to 100 times higher than in normal pregnancy). As early as three weeks, and usually by six weeks after the missed menstrual period, an abnormal hCG titer (a titer greater than 500 mIU/mL) can be seen. Once the abnormal tissue has been removed or destroyed, hCG concentrations decrease and return to baseline within 12 to 16 weeks. The sensitivity of the currently available antibody methods for detecting hCG and its subunits permits close monitoring for the presence of remaining trophoblastic tissue.

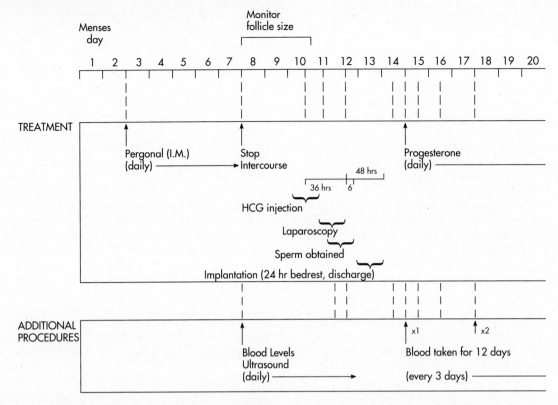

Fig. 19-9   Protocol for the induction and monitoring of an ovarian stimulation cycle for assisted reproduction. *From Laufer N and Navot D: Human invitro fertilization. In DeCherney A, ed: Reproductive
failure, New York, 1986, Churchill Livingstone.*

INFERTILITY

Infertility is defined as one year of unprotected intercourse
without conception. Infertility affects nearly one sixth of
couples in the reproductive years, and its incidence doubles
for women 35 to 44 years compared to those 30 to 34.

Ovarian stimulation is a common clinical approach to
the infertile woman. A number of protocols for ovarian
stimulation are used worldwide with success. One such protocol for the induction of follicular growth is shown in
Figure 19-9. Human menopausal gonadotropin (hMG [Per-
gonal]—a mixture of FSH and LH) is given by injection
until the most rapidly growing follicle, as observed by ul-
trasonography, reaches 18 mm in size and serum estradiol
concentrations are in excess of 400 pg/mL. Twenty-four
hours after the last dose of hMG, a single injection of hCG
(5000-10,000 IU) induces ovulation. The eggs are harvested
from the follicles 34 to 36 hours after the hCG. Spontaneous
ovulation would normally occur 38 to 39 hours after the
hCG, so intervention takes place prior to spontaneous ovulation.

Serum estrogen measurements are used to monitor the
progress of the stimulation protocol and to assist in defining
the correct moment to administer the ovulatory dose of hCG
(Figures 19-9 and 19-10). The likelihood of establishing
pregnancy in an in vitro fertilization/embryo transfer cycle
can be predicted by the pattern and height of the serum
estradiol response to the hormonal stimulation. The best
success occurs in patients whose estradiol increases continuously up to the day of hCG administration, equaling or

exceeding 400 pg/mL and continuing to rise thereafter. In
general, three patterns of estradiol response to stimulation
have been recognized: patients with low, intermediate, and
high responses (Figure 19-10). Very high estrogen responses
may not be as successful because of endometrial abnormalities associated wth elevated estradiol values in stimulated cycles. The low response group is least likely to con-
ceive for reasons that are not understood.

Ovulatory disorders

Ovulatory disorders fall into three categories: 1) failure of
the ovary to respond to gonadotropic stimulation (primary
ovarian failure); 2) inadequate hypothalamus or pituitary
production or release of the gonadotropins or their controlling agents (central failure); and 3) asynchronous production
of gonadotropin and estrogen that leads to anovulation (anovulatory dysfunction).

Failure to ovulate is the major problem in approximately
40% of infertile women. Several diagnostic tests are useful
in the clinical evaluation of ovulatory disorders. Monitoring
of FSH and LH can be very helpful in making the distinction
between ovarian failure and central failure. FSH is elevated
to values greater than 40 mIU/mL in women with ovarian
failure because of the loss of estrogen feedback control. By
contrast, FSH is reduced to chronically low concentrations
of less than 5 mIU/mL in women with hypogonadotropism
due to hypothalamic-pituitary dysfunction. LH values elevated to greater than 30 mIU/mL for a short time at mid-
cycle are used as an estimate of the timing of the LH surge.

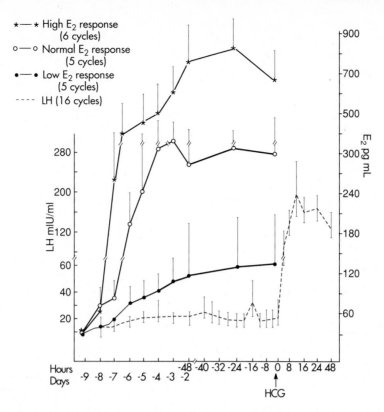

Fig. 19-10   Serum luteinizing hormone during ovulation induction with human menopausal gonatropin for *in vitro* fertilization in normally menstruating women. *From Ferraretti AP, Garcia JP, Acosta AA, and Jones GS: Fertil Steril 40:742, 1983. Reproduced with permission of the publisher, The American Fertility Society.*

LH is chronically elevated with ovarian failure or polycystic ovarian disease. LH concentrations of less than 5 mIU/mL can be found in women with hypogonadotropism due to hypothalamic-pituitary dysfunction.

Progesterone is elevated to values greater than 2.5 ng/mL after ovulation, reaching the 10 to 30 ng/mL range at the mid-luteal phase and dropping to low values just before menses. Progesterone values are conveniently used as an indication that ovulation has occurred.

Infertility in the presence of ovulation

Approximately 30% to 50% of infertile women have disease of the fallopian tubes, and although they may ovulate, fertilization and/or oocyte transport deficits may preclude pregnancy. Another 10% of infertile women may have a cervical barrier to fertility. About 10% of infertile couples are categorized as idiopathic or unexplained infertility. In any one of these conditions the chances of a pregnancy can be improved by the help of washed intrauterine insemination techniques or through methods of assisted reproduction.

Methods of assisted reproduction

In vitro fertilization (IVF), also known as extracorporeal fertilization because it takes place outside the body, was originally applied for the relief of uncorrectable tubal disease. With time, however, the uses of IVF have expanded to provide potential benefits for many causes of infertility. IVF is used primarily in patients with mechanical infertility (78%), infertility of unknown origin (13%), and endometriosis (9%). Other indications include male infertility or subfertility, immunologic infertility, and infertility related to cervical factors.

Tubal damage is the major cause of mechanical infertility. The reasons for tubal damage may be previous pelvic inflammatory disease (PID), sterilization procedures, or prior tubal pregnancies. Extensive endometriosis with multiple pelvic adhesions can also be a cause of mechanical infertility.

In 10% of infertile patients the cause of infertility remains unknown even after thorough investigation. In these patients the oviduct, which may seem normal in appearance, may have subtle functional or morphologic alterations that prevent sperm or ovum transport. Failure of the oocyte to be released at ovulation is another possible cause of unexplained infertility.

Approximately half of infertility is because of male reproductive dysfunction. Male infertility can be related to decreased total sperm counts, decreased sperm concentrations, decreased motility, and abnormal morphology (see Chapter 31). Because of the advantage that culture methods offer by placing sperm in the immediate vicinity of the egg (IVF), fertilization is possible with as few as 10,000 motile sperm.

In general, IVF is done by fertilizing eggs with previously capacitated sperm in a culture dish. The eggs are harvested from hyperstimulated ovaries either through the abdominal wall with a laparoscope or by inserting a long, ultrasound-guided needle through the vagina to the ovaries. The fertilized eggs are maintained in culture for approximately 48 hours where they developed to 2- to 4-cell stage early embryos. These are transferred through the cervix to the uterus by means of a small plastic catheter. Implantation occurs within the next few days as pregnancies are established.

A variety of options for this procedure have been developed to meet specific needs. The most common variation is the gamete intrafallopian tube transfer (GIFT) method. With this procedure the eggs are (as with IVF) obtained from hyperstimulated ovaries. But instead of adding sperm to the eggs in culture, the eggs, together with sperm, are placed, by way of a catheter through the laparoscope, directly into the fimbriated end (ovarian end) of the fallopian tube. Therefore fertilization takes place in the usual location of the fallopian tube. Idiopathic infertility is usually treated using the GIFT procedure as long as at least one tube is functionally patent and the sperm is of good vitality. A limitation to the GIFT procedure is that fertilization cannot be directly visualized as it can with IVF.

Other procedures are being developed rapidly. Zygote intrafallopian tube transfer (ZIFT) places an early embryo or zygote into the fallopian tube after culturing for 24 hours or more. Transvaginal sperm intrafallopian tube transfer (SIFT) permits sperm to be introduced directly into the fallopian tube to fertilize eggs that have undergone normal ovulation. Other variations on the general theme will undoubtedly appear as specific needs arise.

A most important factor in determining the success of any assisted reproduction procedure is an optimal system for ovulation induction. Natural and induced cycles are different in many ways and each may affect embryo development and implantation differently. Follicular growth during a natural cycle is linear with time and is paralleled by an increase in circulating estradiol. In these cycles ultrasonic follicular measurements correlate well with serum estradiol levels. Thus both are equally useful in monitoring follicular growth. With induced cycles follicular maturation occurs in a different pattern from that of the normal cycle. There is a disparity between follicular volume (as monitored by ultrasound) and estrogen secretion that suggests that follicular growth and functional maturity do not occur together. Consequently, it is particularly important to monitor serum estradiol values to estimate follicular functional maturity and to assess the degree of target organ stimulation.

Serum progesterone values during the immediate preovulatory period can provide useful additional information. A significant rise in plasma progesterone in the presence of a stable or falling pattern of estradiol suggests that luteinization has already occurred (prematurely), and that it is too late to administer hCG. Premature luteinization is a cause for cancelling a scheduled oocyte aspiration.

The pattern of estradiol the day after the hCG can correlate with success of the assisted reproductive procedure. When serum estradiol concentrations increase following hCG administration the highest rate of pregnancy per transfer is obtained. This correlation supports the premise that the physiologic events around the time of ovulation are critical to the success of these assisted reproductive procedures.

FETAL GROWTH AND DEVELOPMENT

The fetus grows and develops from the nutrition provided by the mother. Unlike the infant, whose diet is a compelx mixture of carbohydrates, fats, and proteins, the fetus' diet consists largely of glucose. The source of this glucose is maternal blood and the amount available depends on its concentration. Since the fetus depends solely on the mother for its glucose, fetal values mirror the fluctuations in the mother but will always be somewhat lower because of utilization by the placenta during the course of its passage to the fetus.

In pregnancies complicated by diabetes, maternal hyperglycemia is followed by elevated blood glucose in the fetus. This increase elicits the release of fetal insulin that can promote fat deposition and excessive weight gain. This can lead to an undesirably large baby at the time of birth.

One of the unfavorable complications of excessive glucose transfer to the fetus occurs after delivery when the glucose source is removed. High insulin levels in the fetus prompt accelerated metabolism of the glucose, which leads to hypoglycemia in the newborn. This hypoglycemic crisis, if recognized early, can be corrected by the exogenous administration of glucose to the newborn until a proper glucose-insulin balance is regained.

Early fetal assessments

Pregnancy is monitored with chemical tests that obtain information about the functional, or metabolic, status of the fetus. The information desired and the physiological pattern of growth and development determine the time in which a particular test must be performed. Figure 19-11 shows the occasions that tests for fetal-maternal monitoring are usually requested.

The earliest and most common tests determine whether pregnancy has occurred. These tests rely on the capacity of the early trophoblast to secrete chorionic gonadotropin. Human chorionic gonadotropin can be detected in maternal blood as early as eight days after ovulation and continues to increase, reaching maximum values of 50,000 to 100,000 mIU/mL near 10 weeks of gestation.

Other clinical uses of blood hCG titers include the detection and monitoring of trophoblastic disease and the confirmation of an ectopic pregnancy.

At the end of the first trimester or the beginning of the second trimester (14 to 20 weeks), under appropriate indications, amniocentesis can detect the presence of neural tube defects or genetic disease (chromosomal abnormalities). The neural tube defects are the most frequently encountered central nervous system malformations, and their prenatal diagnosis relies on the measurement of alpha-fetoprotein (AFP) and acetylcholinesterase (CHE) in the amniotic fluid. AFP reaches a peak in fetal serum between the thirteenth and sixteenth weeks of gestation when it measures 3 mg/mL. Concentrations in amniotic fluid follow a curve similar to that of fetal serum but at a hundredfold lower value. Acetylcholinesterase in amniotic fluid is also associated with neural tube defects, and this enzyme serves as a definitive "second marker"; that is, its presence will confirm the elevated AFP result.

AFP crosses the placenta to the mother and can be detected in the maternal circulation. AFP concentrations rise to a peak of about 250 μg/mL in maternal serum at 32 weeks and then slowly decline. Screening for neural tube defects (elevated maternal serum AFP values) or chromosomal abnormalities, as in Down's syndrome (low maternal

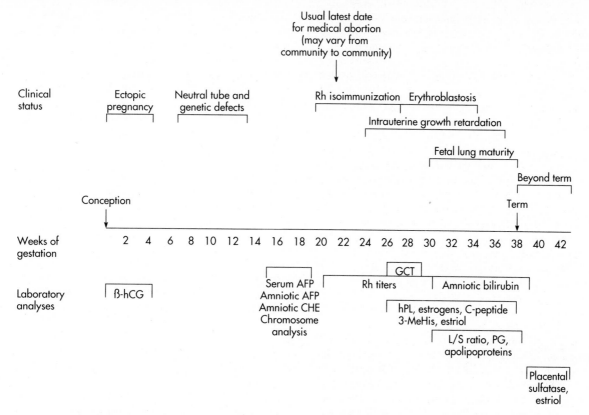

Fig. 19-11 Time periods in pregnancy for fetal-maternal monitoring. AFP = α-fetoprotein; CHE = Cholinesterase; β-hCG = Human chorionic gonadotropin; hPL = Human placental lactogen; L/S ratio = Lecithin/sphingomyelin ratio; 3-MeHis = 3-methyl histidine; PG = Phosphatidylglycerol; GCT = glucose challenge test.

serum AFP values), is usually performed between 15 and 20 weeks of gestational age. Because the maternal serum AFP increases rapidly from five to 24 gestational weeks, an accurate determination of gestational age is crucial for diagnostic purposes. All positive maternal serum AFP results (elevated and low) must be confirmed by amniotic fluid AFP testing, for confirmation of gestational age or ruling out multiple gestations.

The timing of amniocentesis for genetic assessment is determined by both practical considerations and by the legal and societal time limits set for the performance of therapeutic abortions. Obtaining amniotic fluid in the first trimester requires a transvaginal approach and is associated with a significant risk of uterine infection and spontaneous abortion. Most clinical programs perform amniocentesis for prenatal diagnosis at 16 to 18 weeks. This practice allows time for a second amniocentesis if there is a culture failure and often allows the diagnosis to be made before the legal limit for termination of a pregnancy. Chorionic villus sampling is an alternative to amniocentesis for prenatal diagnosis and can be performed between eight and 12 weeks gestation.

Advanced maternal age is the most common indication for prenatal analysis. The age-specific risk that the fetus will have an abnormal chromosomal constitution (trisomy) rises from 0.9% at 35 to 36 years to 7.8% at 43 to 44 years. In addition, the sex of the fetus can be determined when the mother is known or suspected to be heterozygous for a deleterious X-linked gene. The prenatal diagnosis of metabolic disorders is made by measurement of the gene products; that is, the proteins synthesized. Additional information is available from amniotic fluid by determining the concentrations of metabolites that accumulate secondary to an enzymatic block. More than 90 genetic disorders are potentially detectable by early amniocentesis.

Later fetal assessments

Near the end of the second trimester (28 to 30 weeks), tests for intrauterine growth retardation (IUGR) and fetal well-being can be peformed if problems are suspected. Growth-retarded neonates whose birth weight is at or below the tenth percentile for gestational age are more frequently affected by perinatal mortality, intrapartum asphyxia, neonatal acidosis, hypoglycemia, hypocalcemia, and polycythemia than infants whose birth weight is normal for gestational age. Ultrasound techniques are often used to diagnose intrauterine growth retardation, but maternal human placental lactogen, maternal urinary estrogens, amniotic fluid C-peptide values, and the molar ratios of 3-methyl histidine to creatinine in amniotic fluid have also been used as biochemical markers for intrauterine growth retardation. All presently available techniques for the diagnosis of IUGR suffer from high frequencies of false-negative or false-positive diagnosis. Many of the techniques require knowledge of the patient's gestational age or repeat studies, or both.

Several problems exist in the management of a pregnancy complicated by Rh isoimmunization. It is necessary to identify the erythroblastic infant, particularly the one destined to become hydropic in utero. It is important to predict when hydrops will occur and to be sufficiently confident of that prediction to delay delivery until there is a reasonable chance for infant survival. It is important that a blood sample for blood grouping and antibody screening be obtained at the first prenatal visit in every pregnancy.

To assess the risks that hydrops might develop when the pregnant patient is Rh isoimmunized, close attention should be directed to the amniotic fluid spectrophotometric readings used to detect the presence of bilirubin (Figure 19-12). Although single amniotic fluid assessments after 29 weeks are reasonably accurate in the prediction of the severity of disease, serial-fluid examinations give a more accurate index of severity of erythroblastosis. In very severe cases fetal transfusions may be required. Serial amniotic fluid spectrophotometry has increased the accuracy of prediction of severity of erythroblastosis to a range of 90% to 95%. If an isoimmunized woman has had a previous stillborn infant or an infant requiring an exchange transfusion, amniocentesis is indicated at 20½ to 21 weeks of gestation. Repeat amniocenteses are carried out at five- to 21-day intervals depending on the absorbance of the preceding test. In many instances, amniocentesis done weekly may be necessary for five to six weeks or even longer before the frequency of the procedure can be reduced or definitive treatment undertaken.

Most clinicians agree that estriol measurements are not clinically useful. They are currently considered to be of little value in clinical management.

Fetal maturity indices

Not too many years ago, it was not uncommon for fetal death to occur late in the pregnancies of diabetic mothers from causes unknown (but probably metabolic). Thus, a number of methods to assess the development of the fetus for the purpose of an early delivery were developed. Am-

niocentesis provided amniotic fluid from which tests for creatinine, bilirubin, and cytological staining for fetal cells could be done. These approaches gave helpful information but did not address the organ system most responsible for the problems associated with premature delivery.

Not only did these tests not provide information about the pulmonary system, but to make matters worse, creatinine, a by-product of protein metabolism, tended to run higher than appropriate for fetal age in amniotic fluids that involved a large-for-gestational-age fetus. Amniotic fluid values could approach mature values in a large fetus while the fetus was still functionally immature. Creatinine was therefore a potentially misleading indicator in the diabetic patient. Some other approach to correctly estimate fetal maturity was needed. This problem was addressed through basic studies that identified the chemical nature of pulmonary surfactant. From these studies came the L/S ratio and the use of pulmonary phospholipids to assess the developmental status of pulmonary function.

At birth an abrupt physiological transition requires the newborn infant to assume vital functions previously handled by the mother and/or placenta. Respiration is one of these functions as the lung shifts from a fluid filled sack to a gas exchange system in a matter of a few minutes. This transition is possible only if sufficient maturation of the fetal lung has occurred.

Fetal lung maturation is closely related, in a functional sense, to the presence of surfactant. Surfactant facilitates pulmonary function in at least two ways: It maintains alveolar stability by preventing collapse of the lungs, and it reduces the pressure needed to inflate the lungs. Infants who lack surfactant exert more effort to breath in, and the excessive effort leads to fatigue. Without adequate surfactant, mechanical ventilation is often required to assist with lung expansion.

Surfactant identified as lecithin is composed principally of phospholipid containing fatty acids that are highly saturated (Table 19-5). In nature, this unusual lecithin functions as surfactant in animals from fish to man. It has physical properties ideally suited to its function. Other important constituents of the surface-active system include phosphatidyl glycerol and a protein component.

Surfactant is formed in the large alveolar epithelial cells known as the type II pneumocytes, which comprise about

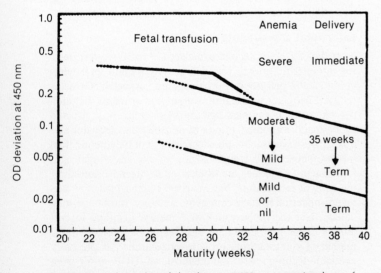

Fig. 19-12   Relationship of absorbance at 450 nm, gestational age of amniotic fluid associated with fetal anemia, and suggested clinical management. *From Liley AW: Am J Obstet Gynecol 86:485, 1963.*

Table 19-5   Surfactant composition

Constituent	Percent
Phospholipids	85
Saturated phosphatidylcholine	60
Unsaturated phosphatidylcholine	20
Phosphatidylglycerol	8
Phosphatidylinositol	2
Phosphatidylethanolamine	5
Sphingomyelin	2
Others	3
Neutral lipids and cholesterol	5
Proteins	10

From Russell PT: Pregnancy and fetal function. In Kaplan LA and Pesce AJ, Clinical chemistry: theory, analysis, and correlation, ed 2, St Louis, 1989, Mosby–Year Book, Inc.

10% of the lung cells. Surfactant produced by these cells washes into the fluid, filling the alveolar spaces during the fetal period. This alveolar fluid mixes with the amniotic fluid as a consequence of fetal respiratory movements. By this mechanism, surfactant moves into the amniotic fluid and, with amniocentesis, can be assessed by a variety of methods.

What is present in the amniotic fluid is the result of a dynamic balance between the materials entering the fluid and their removal from the fluid. About 200 to 450 mL of amniotic fluid per day flow out from the amniotic cavity by fetal swallowing, accounting for about one half of the daily urine production of the fetus. Because of the dynamic nature of the amniotic fluid compartment, a sample of fluid drawn at any time provides a reasonable indication of the current status of metabolic analytes or pulmonary surfactant.

The lecithin-sphingomyelin ratio (L/S) is the most-used test for assessing fetal pulmonary maturity. Measuring just lecithin concentrations in amniotic fluid proves unsatisfactory because of the wide range of normal volumes observed for amniotic fluid. The phospholipid sphingomyelin, unrelated to the events of lung maturation, is used as a reference lipid, or as a biologic internal standard. It is present in amniotic fluid in rather constant amounts, it is extracted as a typical phospholipid with organic solvents, and it is readily separated from lecithin with standard chromatographic methods. The L/S ratio therefore offers a practical way of following the changes in amniotic fluid lecithin without having to correct for differences in amniotic fluid volumes or extraction losses (Table 19-6). Figure 19-13 presents the values of lecithin, sphingomyelin, and the L/S ratio as they typically appear throughout the course of pregnancy. Table 19-6 gives an example of the clinical correlation that justifies the use of the L/S ratio in assessing the prospects for developing respiratory distress.

A number of methlogic considerations are relevant to any discussion of the use of the L/S methods. A major factor that will change the L/S ratio is the initial centrifugation of the amniotic fluid. Most of the surfactant in amniotic fluid is present as a suspension of large aggregates that will be removed at higher centrifugal forces resulting

in a low and incorrect L/S ratio. Centrifugation at 500 × g is high enough to remove cellular debris but not high enough to remove surfactant. The test result can also be affected by whether or not an acetone precipitation step is used in the isolation methodology; it is suggested that the step be included. High values of L/S may be obtained without this step due to the presence of other lipid materials that chromatograph with the area of the lecithin. The effectiveness of the separation and quantitation methods employed may also affect the results obtained. Because so many modifications and options are possible for the L/S procedure, each hospital should establish its own standards and evaluate the predictability of the test for respiratory distress gleaned from their own experiences.

Surfactant from the mature lung contains not only saturated phosphatidylcholine, but also phosphatidylglycerol, another phospholipid, which accounts for about 10% of the weight of surfactant lipids. Phosphatidylglycerol is absent from fetal lung fluid early in gestation, making its appearance at the time of normal lung maturity—about 35 weeks of gestation. The presence of phosphatidylglycerol in amniotic fluid helps to pinpoint the time of lung maturation (Table 19-7). Thin-layer and immunologic agglutination methods can both detect phosphatidylglycerol near 0.5 μg/mL, a sensitivity that makes their use valuable. Phosphatidylglycerol can also assist in assessing the risk of respiratory distress from amniotic fluid samples contaminated with blood or meconium. These two problem contaminants create false positive and false negative results for the L/S method.

Since surfactant has unique surface properties, it can be used to assess surfactant in amniotic fluid. While elaborate measurements of surface tension and surface properties are possible, these methods often require extensive equipment and exacting methodologies. However, the simple, easily performed "shake test" has gained considerable popularity.

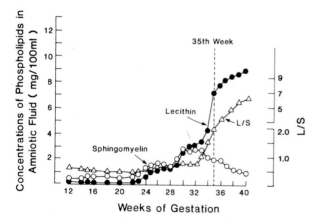

Fig. 19-13 Lecithin, sphingomyelin, and lecithin/sphingomyelin ratios in amniotic fluid during normal pregnancy. *From Gluck L and Kulovich MV: Am J Obstet Gynecol 115:539, 1973.*

Table 19-6 Relationship of lecithin/sphingomyelin ratio to development of respiratory distress

L/S ratio	Number of infants	Respiratory distress (%)	
		All cases	Deaths
<1.5	162	73	14
1.5-2.0	223	40	4
>2.0	1596	2.2	0.1
>2.5	543	0.9	0

From Harvey D, Parkinson CE, and Campbell S: Lancet 1:42, 1975.

Table 19-7 Phosphatidylglycerol (PG) with L/S ratio less than 2

	Respiratory distress syndrome	
	No RDS (%)	RDS (%)
PG present	91.6	8.4
PG absent	20.0	80.0

From Bent AE, Gray JH, Luther ER, et al: Am J Obstet Gynecol 139:259-263, 1981.

Table 19-8   Fetal lung maturation in relation to disorders

Accelerated fetal lung maturation with:	Delayed fetal lung maturation with:

Maternal hypertension
  Renal
  Cardiovascular
  Severe, "chronic" toxemia
	Diabetes mellitus
	  Classes A, B, C
	  Hydrops fetalis

Hemoglobinopathy—sickle
  cell disease
	Infections
	  Chorioamniotitis
	  Fetal infections, viral

Narcotics addiction (heroin,
  morphine)
	Placental conditions
	  Chronic abruptio placentae

Diabetes mellitus, classes
  D, E, F
	Prolonged rupture of mem-
	  branes

From Gluck L: In Lung maturation and the prevention of hyaline membrane disease, Proceedings of the 7th Ross Conference on Pediatric Research. Columbus, Oh, 1976, Ross Laboratories.

This test relies on the ability of surfactant to stabilize bubbles generated in dilute alcohol solutions for periods of several minutes. Its simplicity, convenience, and speed make it a useful adjunct to methods of assessing fetal lung maturity or as an initial screening test since the "shake test" can be performed at any time and requires only a few minutes to complete.

Although a test that offers accurate predictions for all circumstances of fetal lung maturity has yet to be developed, amniotic fluid analyses can provide important information about fetal lung maturity. Where the clinical evidence indicates poor fetal development or in pregnancies that are inadequately documented for gestational age, amniotic fluid analyses provide strong adjuncts to clinical assessment and intervention. Under most circumstances, test indices can be correlated to predict fetal maturity by the 35th week of gestation. However, a number of clinical conditions can accelerate or retard the process of fetal lung development (Table 19-8). Although methodological considerations must be taken into account, indices of 2.0 for the L/S ratio, 0.5 μg for phosphatidylglycerol/mL of amniotic fluid, and a phosphatidyl glycerol concentration of greater than 3% of the phospholipids present in the fluid sample all represent common minimal criteria for pulmonary maturity. The measurement of certain apolipoproteins that contribute to surface activity may eventually become an additional analyte that will help improve the reliability of predicting lung maturity, particularly in the diabetic pregnancy.

SUGGESTED READING

Bardin CW: Pituitary-testicular axis. In Yen SSC and Jaffe RB, eds: Reproductive endocrinology: physiology, pathophysiology, and clinical management, ed 2, Philadelphia, 1986, W.B. Saunders Company.

Brody SA and Kent U, eds: Endocrine disorders in pregnancy, San Mateo, Ca, 1989, Appleton and Lange.

Jaffe RB: Endocrine physiology of the fetus and fetoplacental unit. In Yen SSC and Jaffe RB, eds: Reproductive endocrinology: physiology, pathophysiology and clinical management, ed 2, Philadelphia, 1989, WB Saunders Co.

Jobe A: Amniotic fluid tests of fetal lung maturity. In Creasy RK and Resnik R, eds: Maternal-fetal medicine: principles and practice, ed 2, Philadelphia, 1989, WB Saunders Co.

Jobe A: Development of the fetal lung. In Creasy RK and Resnik R, eds: Maternal-fetal medicine: principles and practice, ed 2, Philadelphia, 1989, WB Saunders Co.

Kicklighter EJ and Norman RJ: The gonads. In Kaplan LA and Pesce AJ, Clinical chemistry: theory, analysis, and correlation, ed 2, St Louis, 1989, Mosby-Year Book, Inc.

Laufer N and Navot D: Human in vitro fertilization. In De Cherney, A, ed: Reproductive failure, New York, 1986, Churchill Livingstone.

Martin MC and Hoffman PG Jr: The endocrinology of pregnancy. In Greenspan FS and Forsham PH, eds: Basic and clinical endocrinology, ed 2, Los Altos, Ca., 1986, Lange Medical Publications.

Russell PT: Pregnancy and fetal function. In Kaplan LA and Pesce AJ, Clinical chemistry: theory, analysis and correlation, ed 2, St Louis, 1989, Mosby-Year Book, Inc.

Speroff L, Glass RH, and Kase NG: Clinical gynecologic endocrinology and infertility, ed 4, Baltimore, 1988, Williams and Wilkins.

Yen SSC: Endocrinology of pregnancy, in maternal-fetal medicine: principles and practice, ed 2, Philadelphia, 1989, WB Saunders Co.

20 Vitamins

Marge A. Brewster

Vitamins are compounds essential for life, primarily serving as cofactors for enzymatic reactions. They are obtained directly or in precursor form from a combination of diet and the actions of intestinal bacteria. Inadequate supplies of a vitamin results in vitamin deficiency, whereas excessive demands not met by the usually adequate intake, such as are present in cancer, pregnancy, infection, or other stresses, result in vitamin insufficiency. Symptoms vary with the degree of vitamin deficiency; mild deficiencies often produce subtle clinical signs that are difficult to diagnose.

Vitamins occurring together in foodstuffs, e.g., the B vitamins, will be simultaneously deficient if intake of those foodstuffs is inadequate, and will produce a variety of symptoms. Those vitamins whose chemical structures make them fat-soluble can also be simultaneously deficient in disease states altering fat absorption. It is thus common to separate the vitamins into two groups according to their solubility: fat soluble or water soluble. This chapter will discuss the major vitamins in each of these two solubility groups, focusing upon dietary abnormalities or clinical conditions most likely leading to deficiency or insufficiency. This distinction is perhaps a subtle point, as the patient's symptoms, chemical findings, and therapies would be the same. Although it is improbable to overdose on vitamins via dietary intake alone, an excess of therapeutic vitamins can, in some instances, be toxic. Recommended dietary allowances (RDA) are given in Table 20-1. These recommendations from the Food and Nutrition Board are for intakes that should meet the daily needs of "healthy persons." Intake requirements are increased by stresses, pregnancy, lactation, and many disease states.

It is desirable to learn from laboratory measurements whether there is a biochemical dysfunction resulting from inadequate vitamin intake, inadequate absorption, defective conversion to active forms, or defective mechanisms to deliver the active forms to their proper tissue and intracellular site of action. As the site of action is often not accessible for analysis, liver cells for instance, judgments must be made about that status from measurements made more remotely from the site of action. For many of the vitamins, therefore, there are multiple indirect approaches to the assessment of vitamin status, and it is often desirable to employ data obtained from several indirect approaches to come to a decision about the true vitamin status. These approaches include: (1) measurement of the active vitamin form within an accessible tissue, e.g., blood cells, (2) measurement of the active vitamin form or its precursor(s) in circulating plasma or urine, (3) measurement of the vitamin's metabolite(s) in urine, (4) measurement of an enzymatic reaction, usually in erythrocytes, needing the vitamin cofactor with and without in vitro addition of this cofactor, (5) measurement of the vitamin or its metabolites in urine after giving an oral loading test, and (6) giving an oral loading test of a substance whose metabolism requires the vitamin, then measuring that substance's metabolites in urine. Reduced serum concentrations of a vitamin do not always indicate that the patient is deficient—namely, has decreased function of a biochemical pathway in a tissue—conversely, normal serum concentrations of a vitamin do not always indicate that the patient has adequate vitamins functioning at the tissue level. These points will often be restated for particular vitamins, as the clinical laboratorian must understand the complexity of inferring tissue activity from remote measurements.

FAT-SOLUBLE VITAMINS

This group includes vitamins A, D, E, and K (Hint: remember a mnemonic such as "A Dear Earnest Kiss"). They are absorbed by the intestine along with triglycerides in the chylomicron complex. Any condition involving long-term malabsorption of lipids can result in deficiency of all four of these vitamins. Short-term deprivation through malabsorption often doesn't create a deficient state, since these fat-soluble vitamins are stored in body fat. Such chronic malabsorptive states include cystic fibrosis, biliary tract diseases, obstruction of the small intestine, and alcoholic liver disease. Although all four vitamins are fat soluble, they are stored for different lengths of time—vitamins D and K become deficient much quicker than do vitamins A and E, namely, weeks vs. months. This ability to accumulate in body fat makes excessive intake, and resultant toxicity, quite possible.

Vitamin A

This vitamin occurs in three biological forms, as shown in Figure 20-1, each with somewhat different biologic activity.

Table 20-1 1989 Recommended dietary allowances for vitamins

Age (years)	Vitamin A (µg RE*)	Vitamin E (mg α-TE†)	Vitamin D (µg‡)	Vitamin K (µg)	Thiamine (vit B₁) (mg)	Riboflavin (vit B₂) (mg)	Pyridoxine (vit B₆) (mg)	Niacin (mg NE§)	Vitamin C (µg)	Vitamin B₁₂ (µg)	Folate (µg)
INFANTS											
0-6 mo	375	3	7.5	5	0.3	0.4	0.3	5	30	0.3	25
6-12 mo	375	4	10	10	0.4	0.5	0.6	6	35	0.5	35
CHILDREN											
1-3	400	6	10	15	0.7	0.8	1.0	9	40	0.7	50
4-6	500	6	10	20	0.9	1.1	1.1	12	45	1.0	75
7-10	700	7	10	30	1.0	1.2	1.4	13	45	1.4	100
MALES											
11-14	1000	8	10	45	1.3	1.5	1.7	17	50	2.0	150
15-18	1000	10	10	65	1.5	1.8	2.0	20	60	2.0	200
19-24	1000	10	10	70	1.5	1.7	2.0	19	60	2.0	200
25-50	1000	10	5	80	1.5	1.7	2.0	19	60	2.0	200
51+	1000	10	5	80	1.2	1.4	2.0	15	60	2.0	200
FEMALES											
11-14	800	8	10	45	1.1	1.3	1.4	15	50	2.0	150
15-18	800	8	10	55	1.1	1.3	1.5	15	60	2.0	180
19-24	800	8	10	60	1.1	1.3	1.6	15	60	2.0	180
25-50	800	8	5	65	1.1	1.3	1.6	15	60	2.0	180
51+	800	8	5	65	1.0	1.2	1.6	13	60	2.0	180
Pregnant	800	10	10	65	1.5	1.6	2.2	17	70	2.2	400
Lactating											
1st 6 mo	1300	12	10	65	1.6	1.8	2.1	20	95	2.6	280
2nd 6 mo	1200	11	10	65	1.6	1.7	2.1	20	90	2.6	260

From Food and Nutrition Board, National Academy of Sciences-National Research Council, 1989.
*One retinol equivalent (RE) = 1 µg of retinol or 6 µg of β-carotene; 3 µg of retinol = 10 U.
†One mg of α-tocopherol equivalent (TE) = 1 mg of d-α-tocopherol.
‡As cholecalciferol; 10 µg of cholecalciferol = 400 U.
§One mg of niacin equivalent (NE) = 1 mg of niacin or 60 mg of dietary tryptophan.

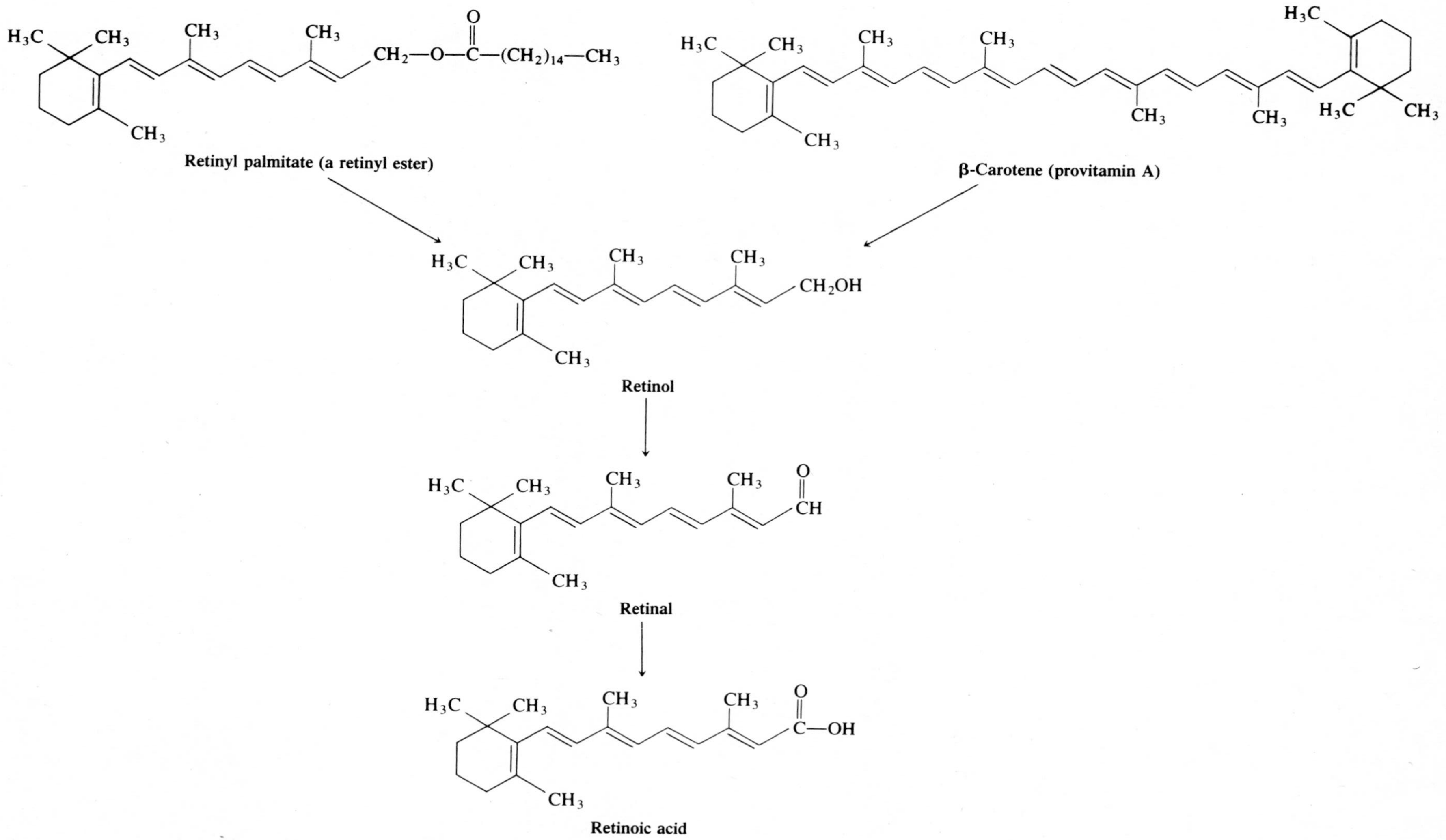

Fig. 20-1 Structures of vitamin A (retinol) with its precursors and metabolites. *From Brewster MA: Vitamins. In Kaplan LA and Pesce AJ: Clinical chemistry: theory, analysis, and correlation, ed 2, St Louis, 1989, Mosby-Year Book, Inc.*

Retinol is the predominant form (an alcohol), whereas its oxidized derivatives, retinal (an aldehyde), and retinoic acid (an acid form), occur in much smaller amounts. The major precursor of all these forms is β-carotene, a yellow pigment found in carrots and other pigmented vegetables and fruits. Carotenes and chemical relatives are termed "carotenoids." Animal products contain retinol esterified to a fatty acid, namely, its -OH group has formed a bond with a -COOH group. These compounds are termed retinyl esters. Ingestion of food therefore supplies some of both—carotene precursor and, after intestinal hydrolysis of the ester bond, the retinol itself. Intestinal mucosal enzymes convert the carotene precursor to retinol; this retinol and the retinol absorbed directly from the diet end up in liver cells where they are esterified for storage.

For target tissues to obtain some of this stored esterified retinol, it must be hydrolyzed, the free retinol moved to the circulation, and further transported to the target tissue. Each of the transport steps involves a specific protein. Retinol-binding protein (RBP) is synthesized within the liver, complexes with retinol, and moves into the circulation to complex further with prealbumin, making a retinol:RBP:prealbumin complex. Target tissues have a receptor that recognizes this complex by its RBP. Once bound, the retinol is transferred into the target cell where it complexes to another transport protein, cytosolic RBP (CRBP), to travel to the intracellular site. The importance of these specific proteins is that if they are not in sufficient supply, the target tissues are deprived of retinol even though there may be plenty of retinol stored in the liver. The major circumstance reducing the supply of these proteins is protein deficiency.

Retinol is involved in the visual process. In the rods of the eye, it is oxidized to retinal, which in turn complexes with opsin to form rhodopsin, a compound necessary for

Table 20-2 Common assay methods for fat-soluble vitamins

Vitamin	Approach	Description	Comments	Deficiency value
Vitamin A	HPLC	Organic solvent extraction of retinol plus esters from serum spiked with internal standard, retinyl acetate; separation on reverse-phase column; absorbance measured at 292 nm	Allows simultaneous assay of vitamin E and of retinyl palmitate; therapeutic ingestion of retinyl acetate requires alternate internal standard	<0.1 mg/L
	Fluorometric	Organic solvent extraction of retinol plus esters from serum; fluorescence measured with 340 nm excitation and 480 nm emission	Major interference from the plant pigment phytofluene, which must be removed from the extract by column absorption, or corrected for by multiwavelength spectrofluorometry	
Vitamin E	HPLC	Organic solvent extraction of tocopherols from serum spiked with internal standard, tocopheryl acetate; separation on reverse-phase column; absorbance measured at 292 nm	Allows simultaneous assay of vitamin A; tocopherol isomers can be separately quantitated; therapeutic ingestion of tocopheryl acetate requires alternate internal standard	<5.0 mg/L
	Fluorometric	Organic solvent extraction of tocopherols from serum; fluorescence measured with 295 nm excitation and 340 nm emission	Total tocopherol is measured; same extract can be assayed for vitamin A as above	
Vitamin D	Competitive protein binding	Extraction from serum or plasma of 25-OH-D and 1,25-$(OH)_2$-D; prepurification of 1,25-$(OH)_2$-D by HPLC competition with ^{3}H-labeled vitamins for binding to tissue or serum binding protein; separation of bound and free ligands by dextran-charcoal; bound radioactivity in supernatant measured	1,25-$(OH)_2$-D concentration is much lower than 25-OH-D, requiring extra steps to quantitate; tissue-binding protein for 1,25-$(OH)_2$D is unstable; high concentrations of 25-OH-D requires preliminary chromatography	25-OH-D: <4 μg/L 1,25-$(OH)_2$-D: <20 ng/L
Vitamin K	HPLC	Organic extraction of vitamin K from serum or plasma; prepurification from lipid by normal-phase HPLC using ^{3}H-phylloquinone for recovery correction; reverse-phase HPLC separation; quantitation by: (1) absorbance at 248, 254, or 270 nm, (2) reduction, then fluorescence with 340 nm excitation and 430 nm emission, (3) amperometric detection during reduction	Amperometric detection is most sensitive; absorbance method is least sensitive; not routinely performed, as prothrombin time determination is usually sufficient	<0.5 μg/L

vision in dim light. It is thought that retinol also functions by maintaining epithelial cells, and is involved in reproduction. Retinoic acid's function is poorly understood; it is important for growth and epithelial cell maintenance, but not for vision or reproduction. Deficiency symptoms include night blindness, growth retardation, loss of appetite, reduced taste, recurrent infections, dermatitis, and dry mucous membranes. More severe deficiency can result in failure of bone growth, lack of sperm production, abnormal eyes, such as xerophthalmia or conjunctivitis with atrophy and lack of normal secretions, and blindness. Signs of acute toxicity are skin desquamation and raised intracranial pressure, whereas chronic toxicity can result in skin changes, liver damage, and exotose, which are bony growths on bone surfaces.

Direct measurement of plasma retinol is the approach most often employed to assess adequate supplies. Values below 0.1 mg/L are generally associated with deficiency symptoms; values above 0.2 mg/L are not considered deficient, whereas values between 0.1 and 0.2 mg/L are questionable. Low values that do not improve with vitamin A therapy suggest a deficiency of a transport protein or a more complex problem. Excessive intake of vitamin A results in high concentrations of plasma retinyl esters.

Both retinol and retinyl esters are best determined by HPLC. Plant pigments β-carotene and phytofluene do not interfere. For laboratories without HPLC capability, the flu-

orescence methodology is recommended over the spectrophotometric method in common use, the Carr-Price method, as sensitivity is greater and it avoids the problems of instability of colored end product and unstable reagents. As indicated in Table 20-2, fluorescence methodologies must include a mechanism to avoid phytofluene interference; physical removal by column chromotography or two wavelength corrections are the two major approaches to this inference.

Vitamin E

This vitamin's modern name is tocopherol; it is comprised of several biologically active isomers. Whether these different isomers possess separate activities is unknown; α-tocopherol is the predominant isomer in plasma and has the greatest activity in current biologic assays. Other isomers, shown in Figure 20-2, are denoted by Greek letter prefixes to tocopherol. These compounds vary in number and ring placement of methyl groups and in which of two hydrocarbon side chains are present.

Vitamin E occurs in fresh leafy vegetables, vegetable oils, margarine, legumes, peanuts, and egg yolk. Insufficient intake of these foodstuffs can lead to deficiency; other causes of deficiency are fat malabsorption disorders, as discussed earlier for vitamin A.

The major known activity of vitamin E is in protecting unsaturated fats from oxidation, thus, it is an antioxidant.

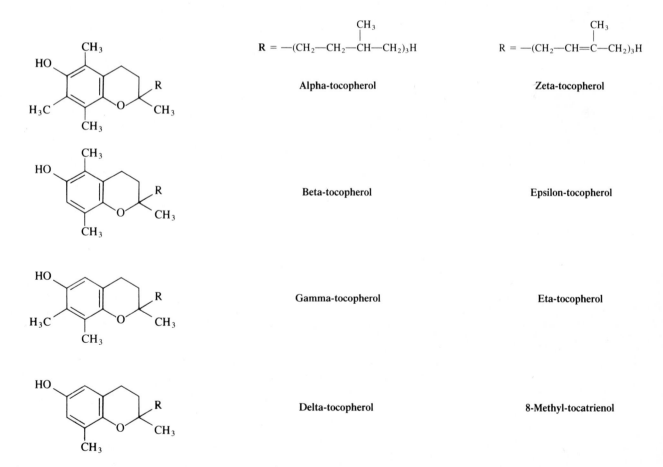

Fig. 20-2 Vitamin E isomers. *From Brewster MA: Vitamins. In Kaplan LA and Pesce AJ: Clinical chemistry: theory, analysis, and correlation, ed 2, St Louis, 1989, Mosby-Year Book, Inc.*

It is also thought to function in prevention of several problems of the newborn including retrolental fibroplasia and intraventricular hemorrhage, and to reduce infant mortality. Diets high in unsaturated fats can lead to vitamin E deficiency as the vitamin performs its antioxidant role by being itself oxidized. A recognized sign of deficiency is hemolytic anemia, secondary to the lack of erythrocyte membrane protection from oxidation. Its deficiency is thought to be responsible for the neurologic dysfunction sometimes seen in infants with chronic cholestasis. Other neurologic states thought to result from deficiency include ataxia, loss of tendon reflexes, and pigmentary retinopathy.

Toxicity has not been well established, but may be associated with excess excretion of creatine, decreased platelet aggregation, impaired wound healing, hepatomegaly, impaired fibrinolysis, and coagulopathy. Adequate supplies of this vitamin are usually assessed by direct measurement of plasma concentrations of individual isomers, or all isomers together, by HPLC. Plasma concentrations are to some extent dependent upon the level of plasma lipids, so that it has been recommended that vitamin E assessment include plasma lipid assessment. Plasma concentrations of α-tocopherol below 5 mg/L are associated with hemolysis of erythrocytes when they are challenged by the oxidant, hydrogen peroxide; thus, this level is often quoted as being "deficient." Elevation of plasma lipids above 15 g/L can allow hemolysis in this in vitro test, presumably by solubilizing vitamin E out of the erythrocyte membrane. Thus, "deficiencies" diagnosed by hydrogen peroxide in the presence of elevated plasma lipids are invalid.

Monitoring is most often performed on patients receiving synthetic diets, to assure that intake of vitamin E is sufficient and not at toxic levels. High-performance liquid chromatography is the recommended method as it allows measurement of individual tocopherol isomers; many HPLC methods allow simultaneous quantitation of retinol, retinyl esters, and individual tocopherol isomers. Fluorescence methods are recommended if HPLC technology is not available; only total tocopherols can be assayed without chromatography. Erythrocyte fragility in the presence of hydrogen peroxide is a direct assessment of intracellular stores of vitamin E, but results correlate poorly with serum tocopherol; this assay is rarely performed.

Vitamin D

This vitamin, required to prevent rickets (muscle hypotonia and skeletal deformities), occurs in multiple forms. Vitamin D_3, cholecalciferol, is produced in the skin from ultraviolet activation of 7-dehydrocholesterol. It is a prohormone, converted in the liver to 25-hydroxycholecalciferol, or calcidiol, which is further hydroxylated in the kidney to the hormone 1,25-dihydrocholecalciferol, or calcitriol. Vitamin D_2, calciferol, is the primary dietary form, because of milk supplementation, and is similarly hydroxylated. Discussion of physiology and assessment of these hormone forms of vitamin D is included in Chapter 10.

Vitamin K

This vitamin includes several compounds having antihemorrhagic properties with a structure similar to menadione, shown in Figure 20-3. Major dietary sources are cabbage, cauliflower, spinach and other leafy vegetables, vegetable oils, soybeans, liver, and pork. It is required for the synthesis of clotting factors VII, IX, and X, so that assessment is usually performed by tests of coagulation rather than by direct assay.

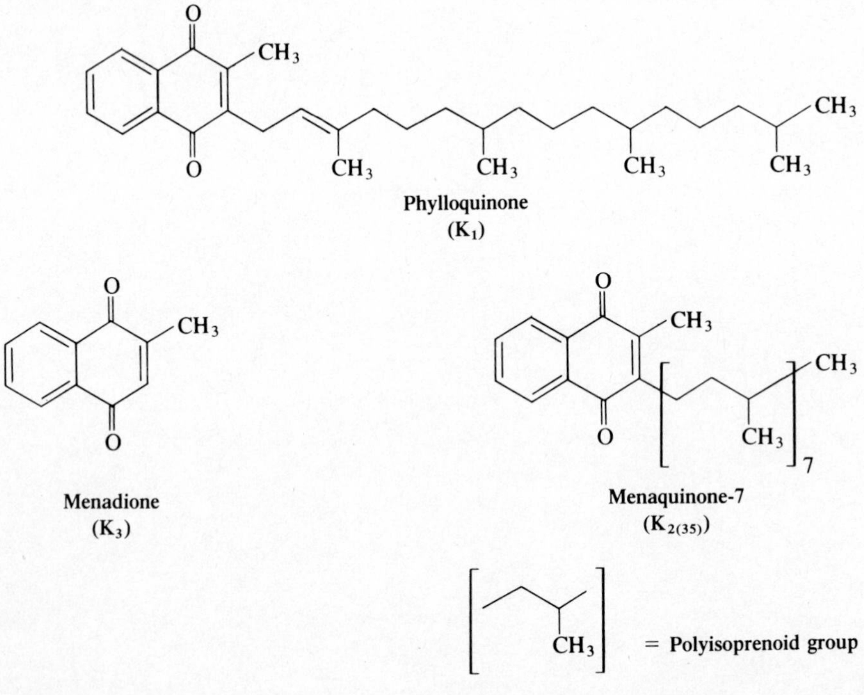

Fig. 20-3 Structures of vitamin K forms. *From Brewster MA: Vitamins. In Kaplan LA and Pesce AJ: Clinical chemistry: theory, analysis, and correlation, ed 2, St Louis, 1989, Mosby-Year Book, Inc.*

WATER-SOLUBLE VITAMINS

By virtue of their water solubility, excess intake of any of these vitamins does not generally lead to toxicity. The excess vitamin is rapidly excreted in the urine. This water solubility also creates circumstances for deficiency to develop fairly rapidly if intake is decreased, as there is little storage of these vitamins. Most of the nine water-soluble vitamins can be stored for about 2 months; thiamine storage is only sufficient for 2 weeks. Vitamin B_{12}, although classified as a water-soluble vitamin, is the exception, being stored in the liver for several years. These water-soluble vitamins occur in foods in inactive, precursor forms, requiring metabolic conversion to other compounds before they become biologically active. In the active forms, they function as coenzymes, facilitating enzymatic reactions. Deficiency of a vitamin precursor thus leads to deficiency of active cofactor forms, and reduced activity of the specific enzymatic reactions in which these vitamins normally participate.

Thiamine

This vitamin, historically known as vitamin B_1, contains a pyrimidine amine group and a sulfur thia group. It is enzymatically converted to two active cofactor forms, thiamine pyrophosphate (TPP) and thiamine triphosphate (TTP), as shown in Figure 20-4. Dietary sources of thiamine include cereals, yeasts, wheat, whole grains, breads, nuts, most vegetables, potatoes, and peas. Deficiencies of this vitamin were originally discovered in people eating polished rice; modern circumstances of deficiency occur mostly in alcoholics, in the elderly, in patients with vomiting, diarrhea, anorexia, or in postoperative states.

The TPP active form participates in decarboxylation reactions, pyruvate and α-ketoglutarate decarboxylation, oxidative decarboxylation by α-ketoacid dehydrogenases, and in the formation of ketols. These reactions are central in the metabolism of carbohydrates and amino acids; lowered enzyme activities result in accumulation of pyruvate and lac-

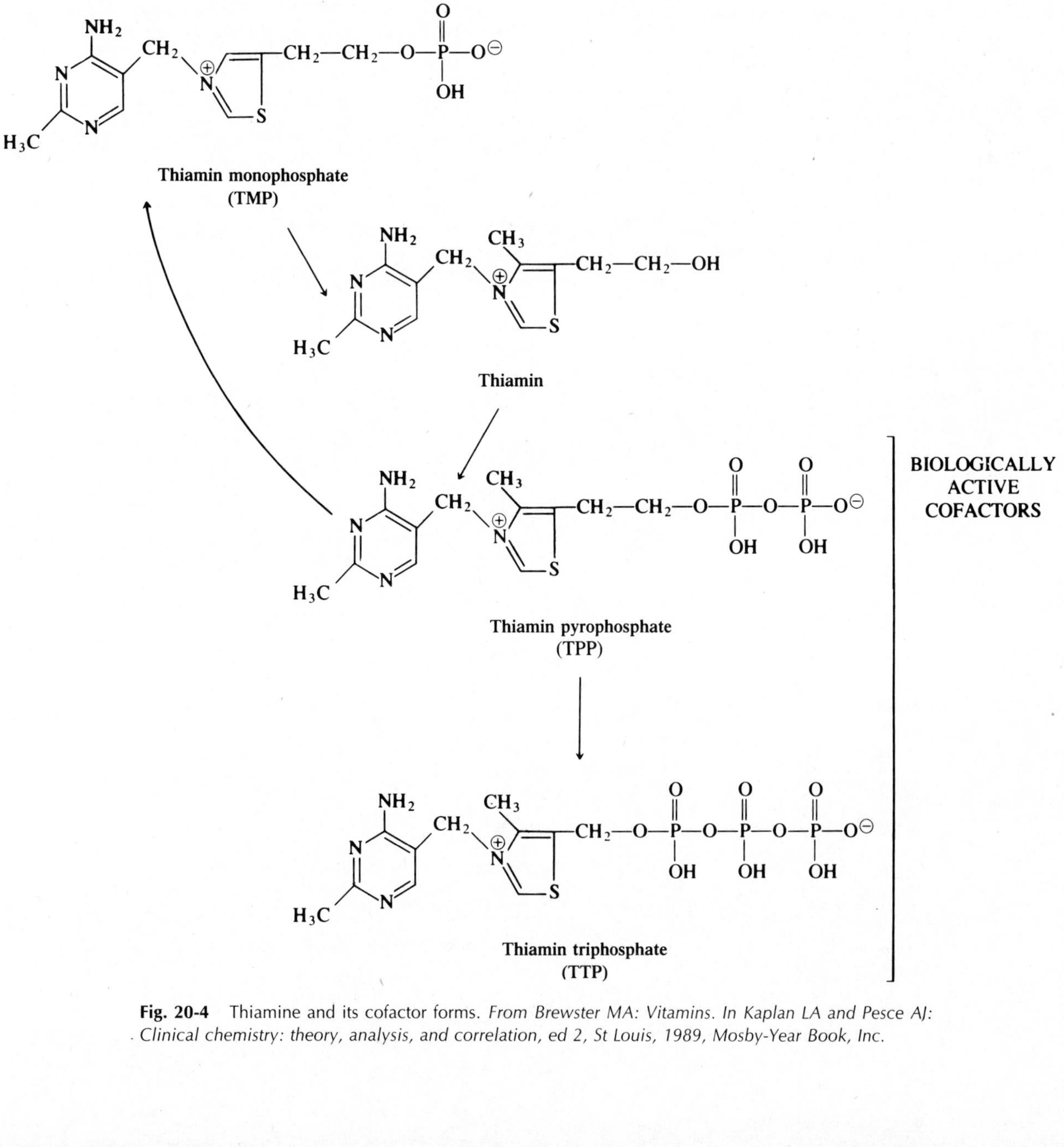

Fig. 20-4 Thiamine and its cofactor forms. *From Brewster MA: Vitamins. In Kaplan LA and Pesce AJ: Clinical chemistry: theory, analysis, and correlation, ed 2, St Louis, 1989, Mosby-Year Book, Inc.*

tate in physiologic fluids. The TTP active form is thought to function in neurotransmitter metabolism. Mild deficiency of thiamine can lead to impaired memory and other subtle neurological signs. More severe deficiency produces two groups of symptoms, although generally only one is present, known as "dry beriberi" or "wet beriberi." Beriberi is a polyneuritis; symptoms of dry beriberi include poor appetite, fatigue, and peripheral neuritis, whereas symptoms of wet beriberi include edema and cardiac failure. Some patients develop the Wernicke-Korsakoff syndrome, which is loss of recent memory, drooping eyelids, double vision, apathy, ataxia, nystagmus, and intelligence disturbance.

No one single chemical measurement of thiamine status has emerged as a clear favorite. The transketolase enzyme of erythrocytes, ETK, catalyzes a reaction requiring TPP as a cofactor. Deficiency is commonly assessed by measuring ETK with and without in vitro addition of TPP—a large boost in activity in the presence of this added cofactor, the ETK index, signaling its deficiency in tissues. Correlation of this test with clinical and dietary status is not always satisfactory. A promising newer assay involves the activation of yeast apopyruvate decarboxylase. Other measures include simple measurement of ETK without added TPP, and measurement of urinary thiamine. These latter methods are seldom employed. Thiamine toxicity is rare—symptoms include trembling, anxiety, headache, weakness, convulsions, and neuromuscular collapse.

Riboflavin

This vitamin, originally known as B_2, contains a ribose moiety and flavin, a yellow fluorescent isoalloxazine ring structure, shown in Figure 20-5. Its two active cofactor forms are flavin mononucleotide (FMN), which is riboflavin-5-phosphate, and flavin adenine dinucleotide (FAD), which is riboflavin phosphate plus adenosine monophosphate. Dietary sources of riboflavin include milk, liver, eggs, meat, and some green leafy vegetables. The FMN and FAD active cofactors function as prosthetic groups of flavoprotein enzyme systems, catalyzing removal of hydrogen (oxidation). These oxidations include substrates involved in respiration, peroxidation protection, metabolism of foreign compounds, granulocyte superoxide generation, and metabolism of iron, pyridoxine, and folate. Clinical signs of deficiency include smooth tongue, mouth lesions,

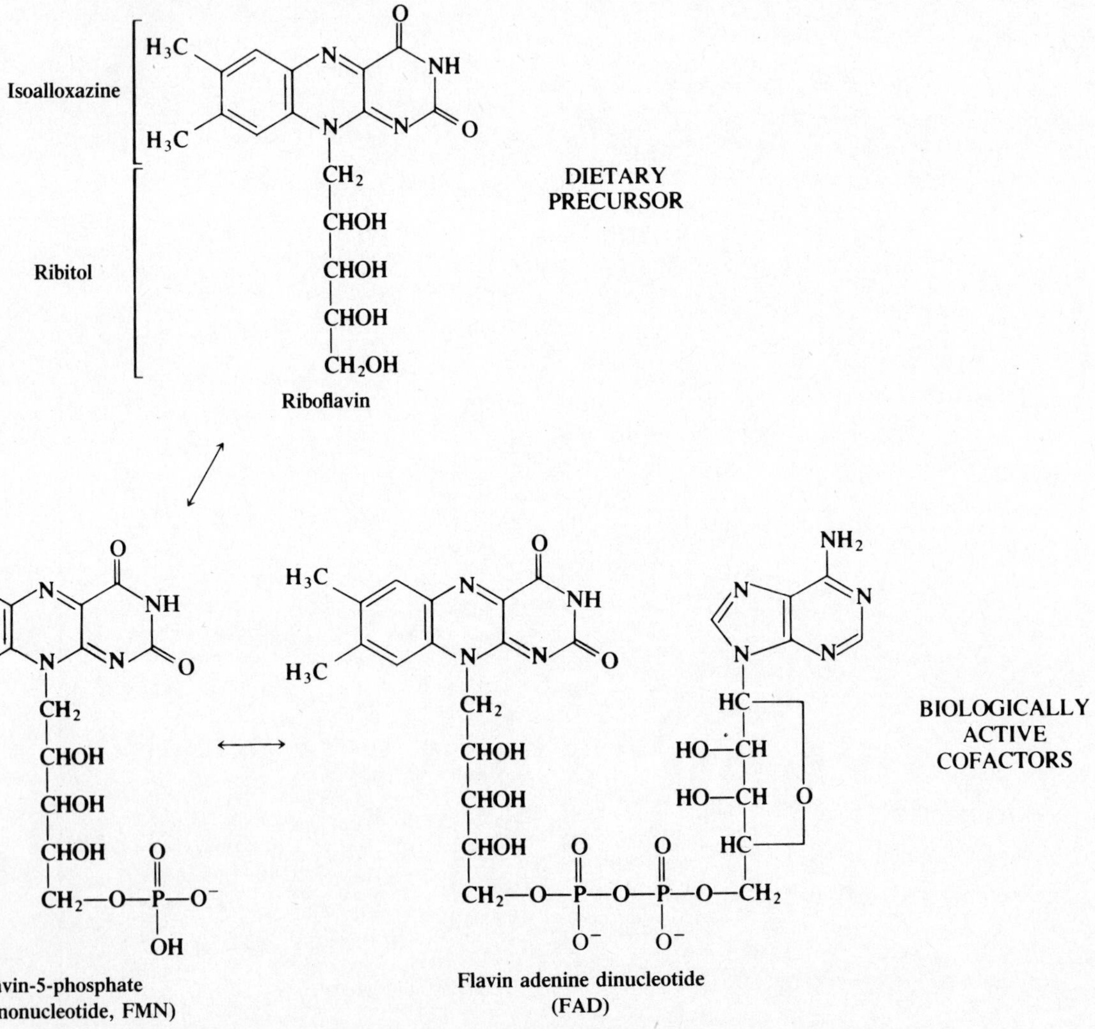

Fig. 20-5   Riboflavin and its active cofactor forms. *From Brewster MA: Vitamins. In Kaplan LA and Pesce AJ: Clinical chemistry: theory, analysis, and correlation, ed 2, St Louis, 1989, Mosby-Year Book, Inc.*

photophobia, ocular changes, dermatologic changes, reticulocytopenia, anemia, and neurologic changes, including burning feet, decreased hand grip, and behavior abnormalities. Riboflavin deficiency, or ariboflavinosis, is common in adolescents and in the elderly, in poverty states, and in pregnant females. It can also be expressed in numerous disease states, including diabetes mellitus, gastrointestinal disorder, malignancies, hyperthyroidism, and febrile illnesses. Alcoholism usualy involves deficiency of this vitamin as well as others. Toxicity is low, with no clincial signs described.

The most commonly measured parameter is an activation index similar to that described for thiamine—in this case the enzyme measured is erythrocyte glutathione reductase (EGR), with and without added FAD. Stimulation of EGR activity with FAD, the EGR index, signifies its tissue deficiency. Other measures include urinary or plasma riboflavin, and erythrocyte concentrations of riboflavin, FMN, or FAD. These latter parameters decrease late in the deficiency process, but correlate better with tissue status than do concentrations in plasma or urine. The extreme photolability of riboflavin is a critical factor in assaying this vitamin form.

Pyridoxine

This vitamin and two related compounds, pyridoxal and pyridoxamine, are dietary precursors for the two active cofactor forms, pyridoxal phosphate (PLP) and pyridoxamine phosphate. All these forms are collectively termed vitamin B_6, which are shown in Figure 20-6. Dietary sources of this vitamin include vegetables, potatoes, fish, meat, and poultry. Vitamin B_6 functions as a cofactor mostly in amino acid metabolism with the transaminases, racemases, decarboxylases, deaminases, and also phosphorylases. Clinical signs of deficiency in infants include vomiting, irritability, weakness, seizures, ataxia, anemia, and abdominal pain; adults have facial seborrhea. Deficiency is often seen in pregnancy, during lactation, in alcoholic states, epilepsy, ulcerative colitis, celiac disease, renal calculi, paranoia, and schizophrenia.

Chemical indices of deficiency include decreased pyridoxine or PLP in plasma and erythrocytes, decreased pyridoxine or pyridoxic acid (a pyridoxal metabolite) in urine, and increased xanthurenic acid in urine following an oral tryptophan load. Pyridoxal phosphate is required to metabolize tryptophan; PLP deficiency stops the normal pathway, allowing an alternate path to xanthurenic acid. Possibly the most commonly measured parameter is stimulation of erythrocyte aspartate (or alanine) aminotransferase activity (AST or ALT), before and after the addition of PLP. This is called the EAST (or EALT) index. As for thiamine and riboflavin, the stimulation of enzymatic activity by an added cofactor indicates a tissue deficiency of that cofactor. As plasma PLP concentrations in fasting patients correlate with

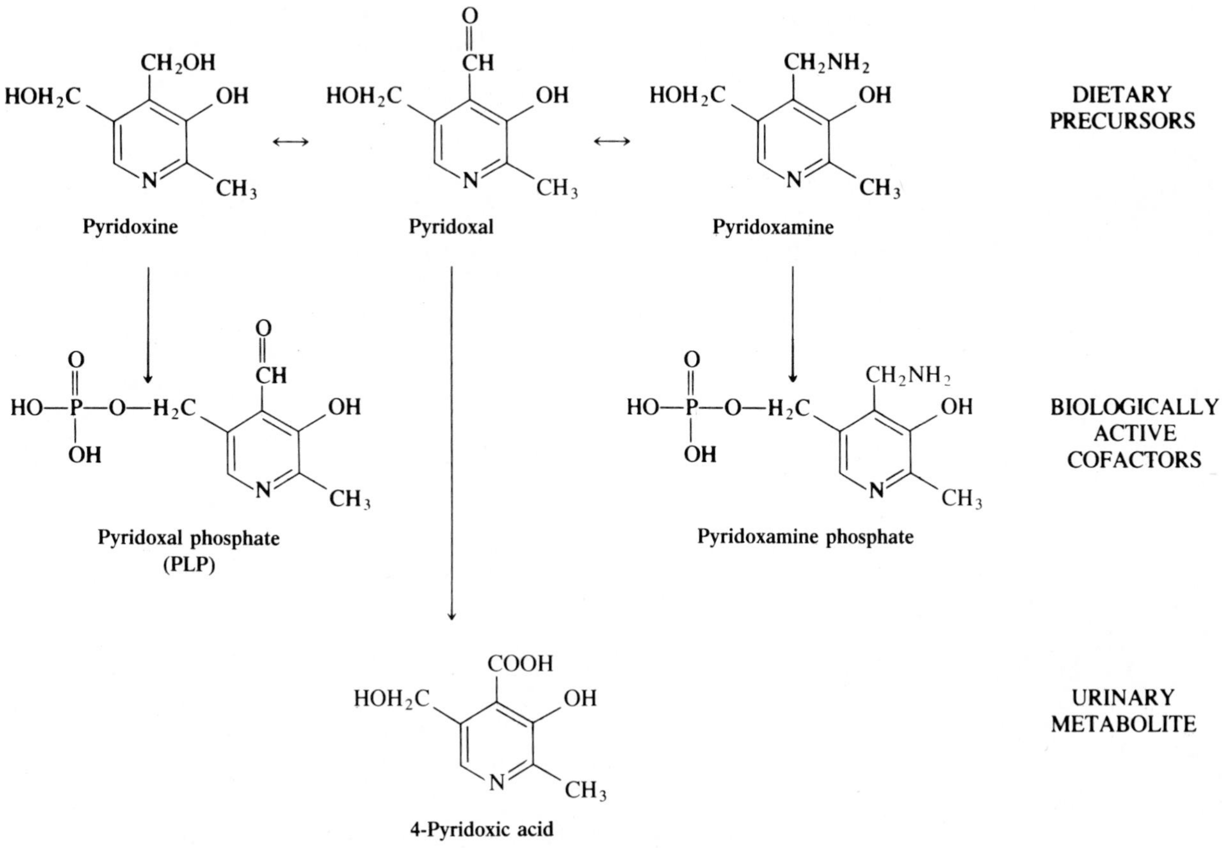

Fig. 20-6 Vitamin B_6 forms and major metabolites. *PLP*, Pyridoxal phosphate. *From Brewster MA: Vitamins. In Kaplan LA and Pesce AJ: Clinical chemistry: theory, analysis, and correlation, ed 2, St Louis, 1989, Mosby-Year Book, Inc.*

amounts stored in muscle, measurement of this form is recommended for assessment of tissue stores.

Pyridoxal phosphate methods include HPLC and enzyme activation. High-performance liquid chromatography methods are not commonly employed as they are complex; one method requires postcolumn reaction with bisulfite, whereas the other method requires two columns at two temperatures, both utilizing fluorescence detection. Of the enzyme activation methods, the one most widely used employs purified tyrosine apodecarboxylase, as described in Table 20-3. This methodology requires purification of the enzyme (until it is commercially available) and trapping/counting of $^{14}CO_2$.

Table 20-3   Common assay methods for water-soluble vitamins

Vitamin	Approach	Description	Comments	Deficiency value
Pyridoxal phosphate (B_6)	Enzyme activation	Conversion of ^{14}C-tyrosine to tyramine plus $^{14}CO_2$ by purified tyrosine apodecarboxylase is measured in the presence of PLP from standards or plasma; $^{14}CO_2$ is trapped and radioactivity is measured	PLP form is quantitated by this method; hydrogen bonds to albumin are broken by acid; very sensitive method; standards are unstable	<15 nM
Thiamine (B_1)	Apoenzyme stimulation	Patient erythrocyte transketolase activity is measured before and after addition of TPP; ETK index is calculated as the stimulation of activity by TPP	Tissue deficiency of TPP is detected by this method	ETK index >1.25
Riboflavin (B_2)	Apoenzyme stimulation	Patient erythrocyte glutathione reductase activity is measured before and after addition of FAD; EGR index is calculated as the stimulation of activity by FAD	Tissue deficiency of FAD is detected by this method	EGR index >1.4
Niacin	Metabolite ratio	Urinary metabolites N'-methyl-nicotinamide and N'-methyl-2-pyridone-5-carboxylamide are measured by HPLC; ratio is calculated	Both metabolite concentrations decrease in deficiency, but disproportionately	Pyridone: methylnicotinamide ≥1.0
Ascorbic acid (C)	Spectro-photometric	Ascorbic acid in serum (or leukocytes) is oxidized by copper then reacted with 2, 4-dinitrophenylhydrazine to form colored phenylhydrazone complexes that absorb at 520 nm	Method measures both oxidized (dehydroascorbic acid) and reduced (ascorbic acid) forms of the vitamin; serum quantitation is most commonly performed for convenience; it reflects recent intake more than tissue stores	<2.4 mg/L serum
Vitamin B_{12} (cobalamins)	Competitive protein binding	Cobalamins in serum or plasma compete with ^{57}Co-B_{12} for binding to purified IF* ("true" B_{12}) or to crude IF ("total" B_{12}, including analogs); separation of bound and free forms by a variety of techniques; radioactivity of bound form is measured in supernatant	Heparin anticoagulant should not be used as it can bind B_{12}; endogenous serum-binding proteins must be inactivated, usually by boiling or by alkali denaturation; most methods allow simultaneous assay of folate	"True" B_{12}: <100 ng/L "Total" B_{12}: <200 ng/L
Folate	Competitive protein binding	Folates in serum, plasma, or erythrocytes compete with tritiated (or ^{125}I-) pteroylglutamic acid for binding to milk proteins; separation of bound and free forms by dextran-charcoal binding of free; radioactivity of bound folate in supernatant is measured	Endogenous folate binders must be inactivated, usually by boiling; milk protein binder can be an impure mix or lactoglobulins; other folate binders have been employed; erythrocyte folate measurement requires liberation of folate from cells, usually done by freeze/thaw methods	Serum <3.0 μg/L RBC <140 μg/L

*IF, Intrinsic factor.

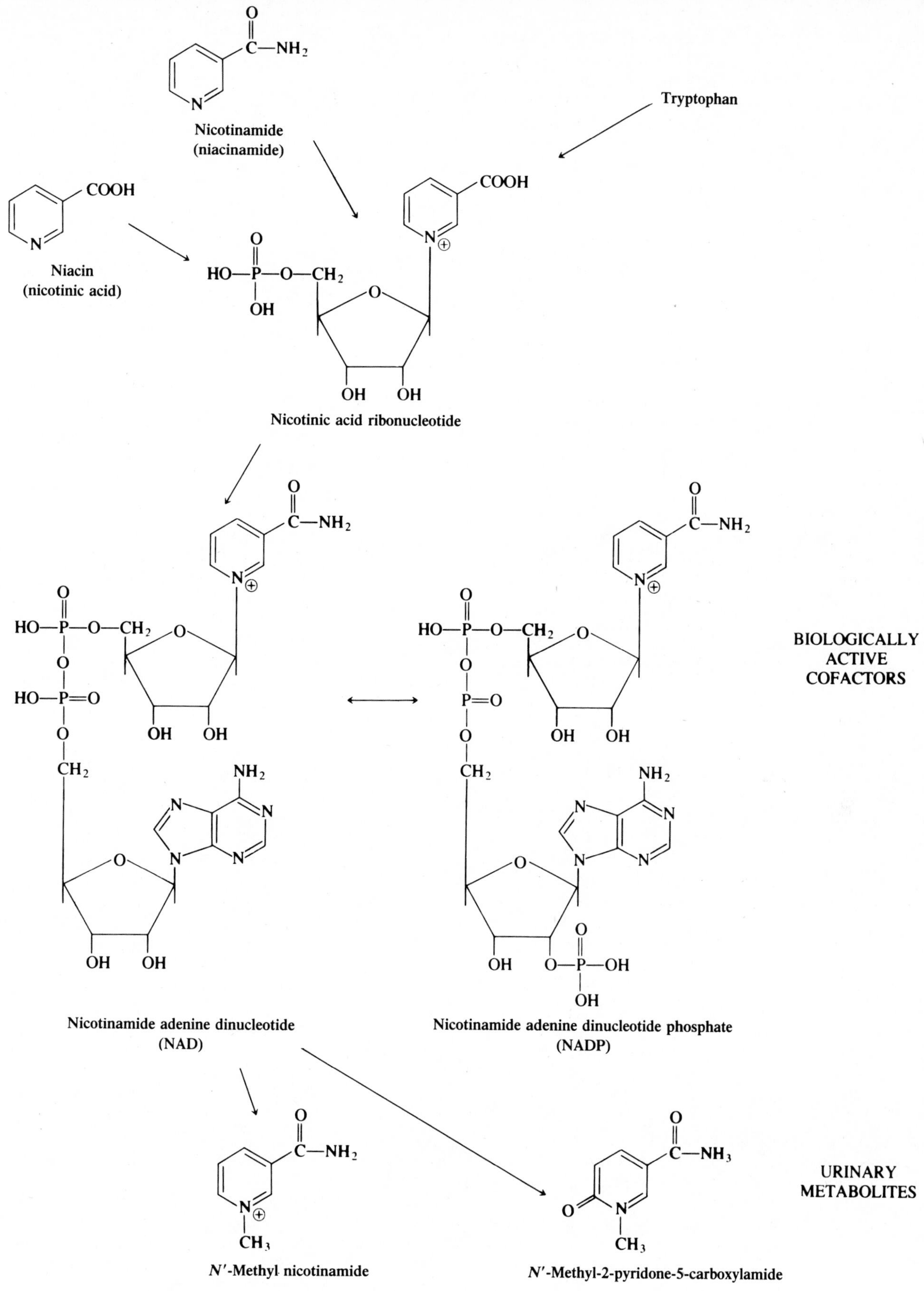

Fig. 20-7   Cofactor forms and metabolites derived from niacin or tryptophan. *From Brewster MA: Vitamins. In Kaplan LA and Pesce AJ: Clinical chemistry: theory, analysis, and correlation, ed 2, St Louis, 1989, Mosby-Year Book, Inc.*

4-Pyridoxic acid, the major urinary metabolite of vitamin B_6, may be a valid index of B_6 nutritional status; HPLC determination of this metabolite is not complex. There is much argument as to whether some chemical indicators of deficiency are true clinical indicators. For example, plasma PLP is decreased during the acute phase of myocardial infarction, but B_6 deficiency does not appear to play a role in increased risk for ischemic heart disease.

Niacin

This vitamin occurs naturally in meats and grains; many manufactured food products, especially cereal, are supplemented with it. Its two active cofactor forms, nicotinamide adenine dinucleotide (NAD) and nicotinamide adenine dinucleotide phosphate (NADP) can be synthesized from niacin or from nicotinamide, and also from the amino acid tryptophan. These compounds are shown in Figure 20-7. Nicotinamide adenine dinucleotide and NADP function in oxidation-reduction reactions catalyzed by dehydrogenases, serving as either donors or acceptors of hydrogen. The reduced forms, NADH and NADPH, absorb light strongly at 340 nm, a property often followed in assays for the dehydrogenase enzymatic activities and in assays for substrates or products of those enzymes.

Clinical signs of niacin deficiency include weakness, lassitude, anorexia, anxiety, irritability, depression, and digestive disturbances. Severe deficiency results in pellagra, which is a form of dermatitis, mucous membrane inflammation, weight loss, disorientation, delirium, and dementia. Plasma concentrations of niacin and its nucleotide derivatives are thought to be poor indices of tissue status. The most common assay employed to detect niacin deficiency is measurement of its two metabolites in urine, N'-methylnicotinamide and N'-methyl-2-pyridone-5-carboxylamide. Adults normally excrete 20% to 30% of their niacin as the methylnicotinamide and 40% to 60% as the pyridone, with an excretion ratio (pyr:me) of 1.3 to 4.0; in deficient states the ratio of the pyridone metabolite to the N'-methylnicotinamide is reduced; that is, a ratio of less than 1 is seen along with a decrease in concentration of both metabolites. Deficiency is most suspect in persons with corn and/or cereals as their main food staple, an uncommon situation today in the United States, so that assessment of this vitamin is seldom requested in clinical settings. Most types of corn are low in tryptophan, which is metabolized to the nicotinamide adenine dinucleotide cofactors, and in addition, part of the niacin required for cofactor synthesis is not absorbed. The leucine in cereals interferes with niacin metabolism to the cofactor forms (NAD, NADP).

Ascorbic acid

This vitamin, commonly known as vitamin C, was isolated from citrus fruits as the agent that prevented scurvy. Swollen gums with loss of teeth, skin hemorrhages, and pain and weakness in the lower extremities are symptoms of this condition. The name *ascorbic acid* is derived from its being an antiscorbutic agent. Ascorbic acid is a very strong reducing compound by virtue of its ene-diol group; its oxidized form dehydroascorbic acid, is metabolized to oxalic acid, which has no vitamin activity. The structure of these com-

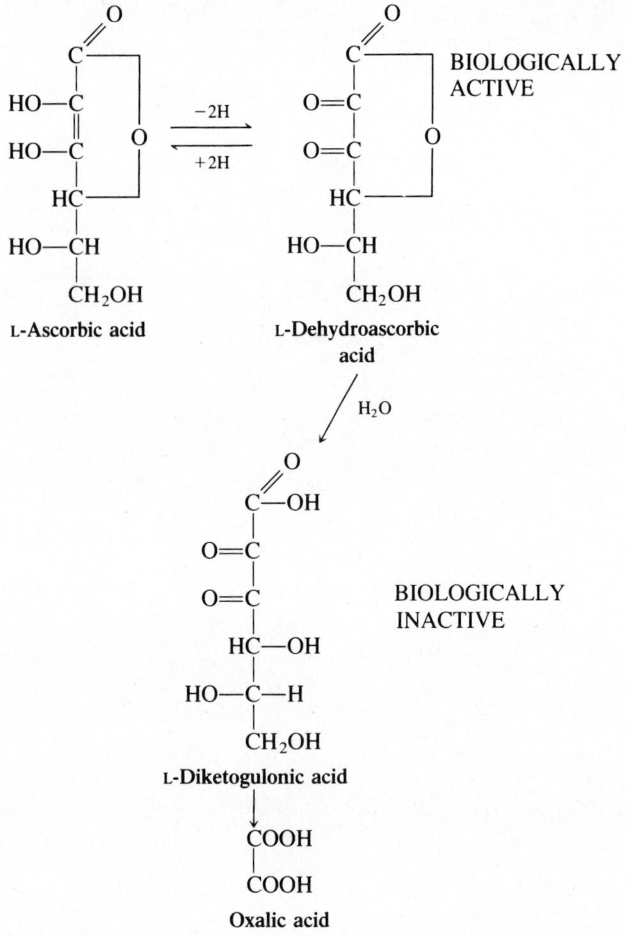

Fig. 20-8   Structures of ascorbic acid and metabolites. *From Brewster MA: Vitamins. In Kaplan LA and Pesce AJ: Clinical chemistry: theory, analysis, and correlation, ed 2, St Louis, 1989, Mosby-Year Book, Inc.*

pounds is given in Figure 20-8. Most plants and many animals can synthesize ascorbic acid, but humans cannot, making its dietary intake essential.

Aside from citrus fruits, other sources include vegetables (tomatoes, green peppers, cabbage, leafy greens) and potatoes. It is very unstable in the presence of oxygen and heat. Deficiencies are suspected in persons not ingesting adequate fresh fruits or vegetables and in infants exclusively ingesting cow's milk. Ascorbate functions in collagen formation by hydroxylation of proline and lysine during cross-linking, in catecholamine synthesis as a dopamine-β-hydroxylase cofactor, in cholesterol catabolism with hydroxylation to bile acids, in other hydroxylations, including steroid synthesis and metabolism of foreign organic compounds, and as an antioxidant protecting against lipid peroxidation; it is possibly involved in heme synthesis. Deficiency signs prior to frank scurvy include weakness, lassitude, irritability, vague aches and pains.

Ascorbate status has been assessed by its measurement in urine, serum, and leukocytes. Measurement of urinary ascorbate is not generally recommended as it reflects only very recent intake and may not reflect tissue status. Serum ascorbate below 2.4 mg/L or whole blood ascorbate below 3 mg/L are associated with clinical symptoms of scurvy, but transient low values may not be accompanied by clinical symptoms. Leukocyte ascorbate is considered more reflective of tissue levels, but its assay is technically more difficult as the leukocytes must be rapidly isolated from plasma to obtain a true measure. Table 20-3 lists the 2,4-dinitrophenylhydrazine method for assessment of vitamin C status. This method, which is most commonly used, measures the sum of ascorbic acid and its oxidized form, dehydroascorbic acid. Several other colorimetric and fluorometric methods have been described; none of these methodologies could be stated to have distinct advantages over others. High-performance liquid chromatography methods exist and will probably become the preferred approach in the future; ultraviolet absorption is insensitive and electrochemical detection is recommended for the HPLC approach. Electrochemical detectors are not yet commonly available in clinical laboratories.

Vitamin B$_{12}$ and folic acid

These two vitamins are discussed together as their functions are intertwined; in fact, the disorder known as pernicious anemia was found to be corrected by two different dietary therapies in different people. One form responded to liver extract, while the other responded to yeast extract, leading to the isolation of each of these vitamins. As shown in Figures 20-9 and 20-10, these two vitamins are entirely different structurally. Vitamin B$_{12}$ is a complex substance similar to chlorophyll and porphyrins—with a corrin ring containing pyrroles. Folic acid, however, is pteroylglutamic acid. Many forms exist by addition of one-carbon fragments to the pteroyl portion and there are polyglutamate forms as well. As symptoms of deficiency for both B$_{12}$ and folic acid are similar, they are usually assessed together.

Vitamin B$_{12}$ occurs primarily in meat, milk, and eggs; total vegetarian diets can create a deficiency. Absorption requires complex formation with intrinsic factor (IF), a protein secreted from cells in the stomach lining. Antibodies to these gastric parietal cells can develop, as in one cause of pernicious anemia. The IF-B$_{12}$ complex attaches to specific receptors in the ileum, where absorption takes place. Blocking antibodies can occur, which prevent binding of IF to B$_{12}$; binding antibodies can attach to free IF or to the IF-B$_{12}$ complex, preventing their absorption. Disease states accompanied by production of any of these antibodies can therefore lead to intracellular deficiency of B$_{12}$ and pernicious anemia symptoms. Once absorbed, the B$_{12}$ is released from its IF complex and circulates in plasma bound to specific transport proteins called transcobalamins.

The dietary form of B$_{12}$, hydroxycobalamin (OH-cbl), is converted to two active cofactor forms. Deoxyadenosylcobalamin (Ado-cbl) is required for metabolism of odd-numbered carbon chain fatty acids needed for formation of myelin sheath. A deficiency of B$_{12}$ results in the accumulation of methylmalonyl-CoA and the excretion into urine of methylmalonic acid. Methylcobalamin (Me-cbl) functions in methyl group transfers; a deficiency results in blockage of DNA synthesis and megaloblastic anemia. Dietary deficiency of OH-cbl thus leads to neurologic abnormalities

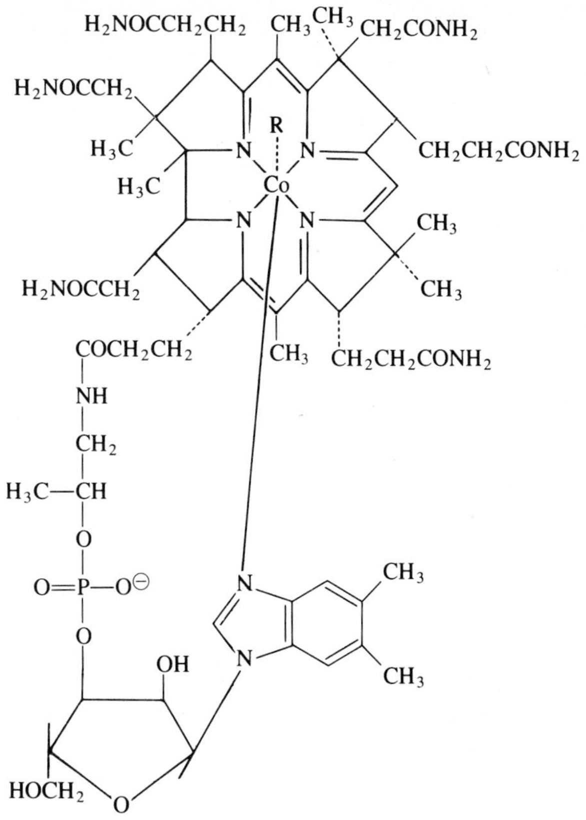

	R		
(Me-B$_{12}$)	CH$_3$	Methylcobalamin	ACTIVE COFACTOR FORMS
(Ado-B$_{12}$)	5'-Deoxy-adenosine	Deoxyadenosyl-cobalamin	
(OH-B$_{12}$)	OH	Hydroxocobalamin	DIETARY FORMS AND THERAPY
(CN-B$_{12}$)	CN	Cyanocobalamin	

Fig. 20-9 Vitamin B$_{12}$ forms. *From Brewster MA: Vitamins. In Kaplan LA and Pesce AJ: Clinical chemistry: theory, analysis, and correlation, ed 2, St Louis, 1989, Mosby-Year Book, Inc.*

(paresthesias progressing to spastic ataxia, and possibly to cognitive impairment in early stages) from lack of Ado-Cbl, and to megaloblastic anemia from lack of Me-Cbl. Genetic disorders of enzymes in these conversion pathways can lead to alterations of one cofactor without alteration of the other.

Plasma B$_{12}$, primarily Me-Cbl, has been assessed by microbiologic and by competitive protein binding methodologies. The microbiologic assays, labor-intensive and subject to a variety of interferences, are seldom performed in clinical laboratories; their advantage lies in their specificity for biologically active derivatives. A variety of competitive protein-binding assays have been developed, differing as to source and purity of the binding protein, approach to inactivation of endogenous binding proteins, separation of free- from bound-ligand, and quantitation of one ligand form. Several of these assays are commercially available; selection is primarily a matter of laboratory preference as to methodology, and whether the capability for simultaneous folate assay is needed. Nonradioisotopic immunologic meth-

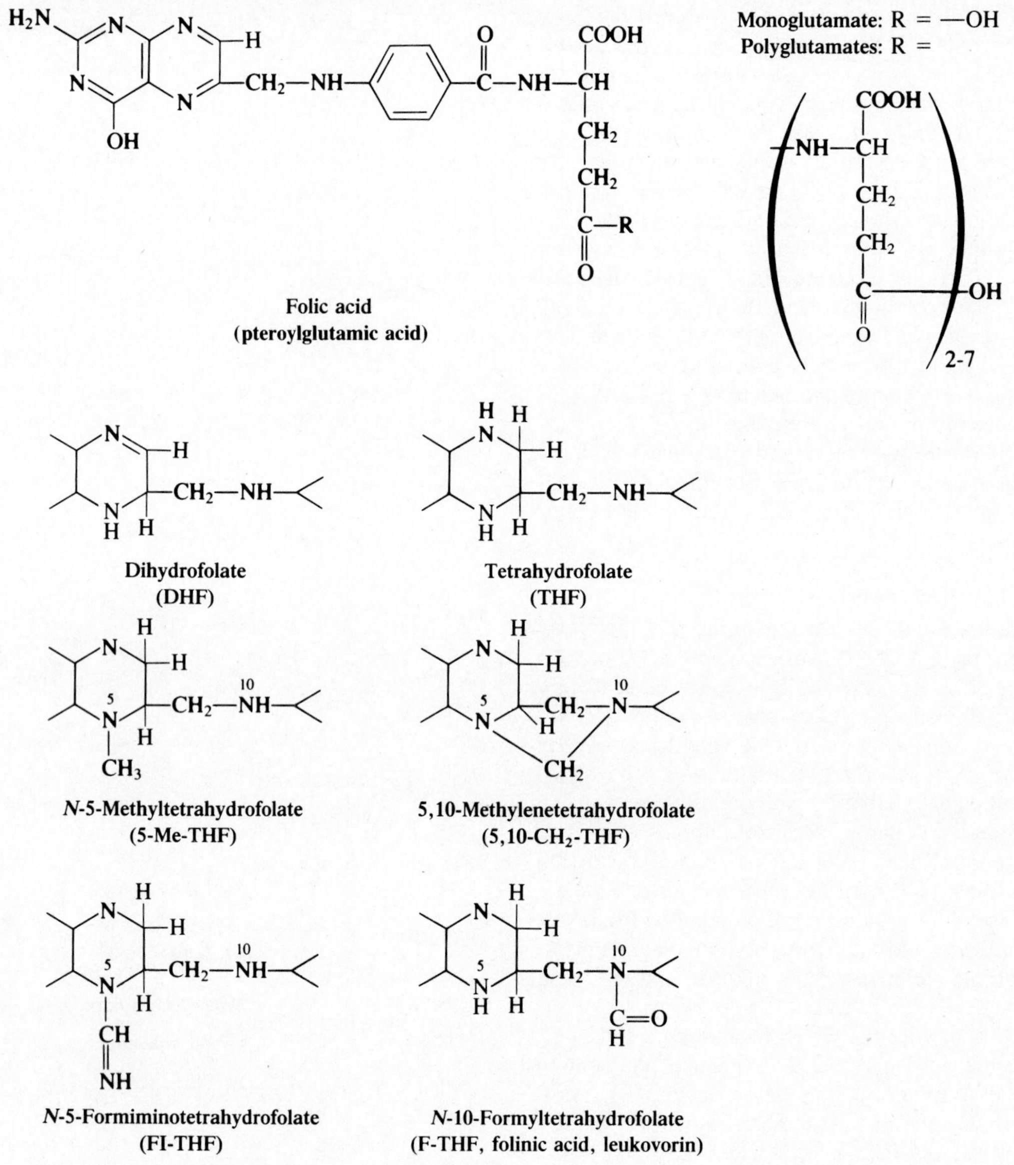

Monoglutamate: R = —OH
Polyglutamates: R =

**Folic acid
(pteroylglutamic acid)**

**Dihydrofolate
(DHF)**

**Tetrahydrofolate
(THF)**

**N-5-Methyltetrahydrofolate
(5-Me-THF)**

**5,10-Methylenetetrahydrofolate
(5,10-CH₂-THF)**

**N-5-Formiminotetrahydrofolate
(FI-THF)**

**N-10-Formyltetrahydrofolate
(F-THF, folinic acid, leukovorin)**

Fig. 20-10 Structures of folic acid forms. *From Brewster MA: Vitamins. In Kaplan LA and Pesce AJ: Clinical chemistry: theory, analysis, and correlation, ed 2, St Louis, 1989, Mosby-Year Book, Inc.*

ods have recently been introduced and will likely replace radioisotopic ones. Other measures include assays of serum or urinary methylmalonic acid; the latter is most often applied as a spot test of urine. The Schilling test involves determination of radiolabeled B_{12} appearing in urine following its oral ingestion with and without intrinsic factor; this test is utilized to determine whether deficiency is due to poor absorption, and if so, if it is due to lack of IF. Other tests that may be required include specific assays for antibodies or for transport proteins (not widely available), or the deoxyuridine suppression test (in vitro test of incorporation of thymidine into bone marrow DNA).

Folic acid and its relatives, all termed *folates*, are primarily derived from green leafy vegetables and fruits. Dietary deficiency is common in adolescents and in elderly individuals avoiding these food items; because of high fetal

demand, intake during pregnancy may be insufficient without supplementation. The dietary folates contain up to eight glutamate residues; these polyglutamate forms are hydrolyzed in the intestine to monoglutamate, which is absorbed. Liver enzymes resynthesize the polyglutamate forms, presumably a storage form. Serum folate is primarily N5-methyltetrahydrofolate (Me-THF). As shown in Figure 20-10, Me-THF is a cofactor involved in one-carbon transfers. Its conversion to tetrahydrofolate (THF) requires Me-Cbl, thus lack of this B_{12} form can trap folate in the Me-THF form and produce symptoms of folate deficiency even though dietary intake may be sufficient. The major known result of folate deficiency is megaloblastic anemia. Genetic disorders of folate interconverting enzymes are described, one resulting in mental retardation associated with the inability to transfer folates into cerebrospinal fluid. Deficiency can be secondary to disease (malabsorptive states, cardiac failure, uremia, systemic infections), or drugs (dilantin, alcohol, methotrexate, and possibly, oral contraceptives).

Serum folate is often measured and is reduced early in the deficient state. However, as low values can be obtained despite adequate tissue stores, erythrocyte folate is considered a more accurate measure of tissue stores. As folate and B_{12} are so intertwined metabolically, deficiency work-ups often require multiple tests of both vitamins to pinpoint causes other than dietary insufficiency. Microbiological methods for folate assessment, of historical importance, are seldom used today. Most commonly, competitive protein binding (CPB) is the measurement approach employed, usually utilizing commercial methods. The multiple folate forms are variably detected by different CPB methods and not all methods utilize the same standard.

21 Tumor markers

Lawrence W. Bond

NEOPLASIA

Tumor markers are analytes that are associated with neoplasia or cancer. *Neoplasia* is the medical term used for new growth, which results in a neoplasm or tumor. Willis provided a widely accepted definition: "A neoplasm is an abnormal mass of tissue, the growth of which exceeds and is uncoordinated with that of the normal tissues and persists in the same excessive manner after cessation of the stimuli which evoked the change." The growth process is often benign, but it could be malignant and possess the ability to metastasize within the host and invade other sites or tissues, ultimately leading to death of the host. Tumors of this type are generally referred to as cancerous. Understanding tumor markers and the role they play in the diagnosis of cancer and its management requires a basic comprehension of neoplasia. The reader is strongly encouraged to review a fundamental chapter on the subject; several reviews are listed in the Suggested Reading at the end of this chapter.

DEFINITION OF TUMOR MARKERS

Ideally, tumor markers are biochemical analytes that are found in blood, urine, or other specimens from patients with a type of neoplasia, for example, carcinoembryonic antigen (CEA) with cancer of the liver. In addition, this associative relationship would indicate by the tumor marker's quantitation above a specified background concentration that the tumor was present. Finally, the quantity of tumor marker should indicate how much tumor was present or to what stage the tumor has progressed. Not all tumor markers fulfill both criteria of the definition.

CLINICAL LIMITATIONS OF TUMOR MARKERS

Unfortunately, most tumor markers are not specific for a given type of cancer, nor are they necessarily quantitatively related to the physical mass of the cancer. This limitation applies for most tumor markers. Each marker's specificity and sensitivity delineates whether or not it can serve as a "screening test" or as a quantitative indicator of the amount of cancer present. Years of evaluation may be required until there is a statistically significant body of knowledge concerning a marker's clinical and analytical performance. The U.S. Federal Drug Administration (FDA) stipulates how commercial assay kits for tumor markers should be used, namely, for research only, or for designated diagnoses or prognoses.

A physician may order the quantitation of a marker such as CEA in a patient suspected of having cancer. Carcinoembryonic antigen has a normal range of approximately 0 to 10 µg/L in most patients, but is not considered a good screening test since it may be elevated above 10 µg/L because of any one of a variety of other conditions, such as smoking, alcoholic cirrhosis, inflammatory bowel, or chronic pulmonary disease. Thus, although a value of 15 µg/L would be above the reference interval established for a healthy, nonsmoking population, such a value could reflect a patient with an underlying chronic condition in the liver, intestine, or lung, instead of the presence of cancer. This limitation has lead to the recommendation that CEA not be quantitated as a tumor marker to screen for cancer of the gastrointestinal tract. A patient with a previously diagnosed cancer and with a demonstrated elevation of CEA may be clinically observed by CEA measurements. If the cancer goes into remission because of treatment, then the CEA level will usually go down; if it climbs higher, then this is tentative evidence that the cancer is continuing to increase in size and the patient's prognosis would be considered "poor" (Fig. 21-1).

LABORATORY TESTING FOR TUMOR MARKERS

Although tumor markers may be detected qualitatively for their presence or absence, most are measured quantitatively and considered elevated when compared to a baseline from a noncancerous reference population. The biochemical techniques used to measure these analytes vary considerably. They may range from traditional enzyme rate measurements, to immunoassays, to cytogenetic techniques. The biochemical class and the concentration range of the marker usually determine the methodology required for its measurement.

Currently, immunoassay is the predominant method to quantitate tumor markers. Historically, radioimmunoassay (RIA) was the first immunoassay in common use for measuring these analytes. This method used radioactivity as the property to quantitate the antibody-antigen association.

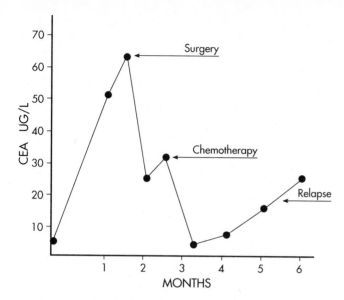

Fig. 21-1 Utilization of CEA to monitor a hepatic tumor. The tumor marker may decrease in response to therapy, or increase when therapy is failing.

More recently, a variety of other properties have been commercially developed to avoid the problems associated with RIA, such as handling radioactive reagents, requirements of documentation, and short expiration dates for kits. The newer methods utilize spectrophotometric enzyme rate measurements (EIA), fluorescence, polarized fluorescence, time-resolved fluorescence, and luminescence to quantitate the antibody-antigen equilibria. Most of the tumor markers listed in this chapter are quantitated by the following: RIA, using kits with beta-emitting radionuclides detectable in a gamma counter; fluorescent markers, detectable in fluorometers; or chemiluminescent markers, detectable in ultrasensitive spectrometers. In this chapter, the abbreviation FIA is used to incorporate all forms of fluorescent immunoassays, such as standard fluorescence, polarized fluorescence, and time-delayed fluorescence. Some markers are not commercially available to clinical laboratories and their availability to patients is limited to obtaining access to the research laboratory performing the assay.

CLASSIFICATION OF TUMOR MARKERS

One approach to the categorical organization of tumor markers suggests there are only two types—those markers produced by the tumor and those produced by the host tissue in response to the tumor. A second approach is to separate "normally present" markers (which rise in concentration) from those which are detectable only after the cancer is present. For example, the tumor marker can be either a biochemical substance, which is normally found in vivo, or a genetically repressed substance. The latter is seen when a gene for the marker produces very little, if any, of the marker in the normal adult stage of development, but is now present in a large quantity due to the cancer process, which allows the uncontrolled genetic transcription of DNA. An example of this is alpha-fetoprotein (AFP), the prefix "feto" indicates that the protein is usually synthesized primarily in the fetal stage of growth. It is believed that the essentially

uncontrolled cellular growth results in expression of many gene products that are not synthesized in any significant quantity in normal adult tissue.

TUMOR MARKERS BY CATEGORY

Another approach to categorical organization of tumor markers is to classify the marker by using more traditional biochemical classifications such as "enzyme" or "hormone" as shown in (Box 21-1). This approach is difficult, as it suffers from inadequate biochemical knowledge of many of the markers and the fact that many of these are detected by their antigenic properties, not their structural or biochemical properties. However, the genetic aspects of neoplasia are brought into focus when one classifies markers as genes, chromosomes, and oncogenes. The latter term, oncogenes, is frequently mentioned when discussing tumor markers. These are a family of genes that have the potential to produce tumors, but may be a normal component in the genetic control of growth regulation. In spite of somewhat arbitrary designations, the biochemical approach is used in this chapter to organize most of the currently known tumor markers as this may present the reader with a more familiar association. *The Tumor Marker Reference Guide* (Herberman) listed in the Suggested Reading is an excellent source for the clinical laboratorian to keep abreast of current markers.

Proteins
Enzymes

Cathepsin D (cath-D). This glycoprotein (molecular weight [MW] = 52,000) is an enzyme, lysomal aspartyl protease (Enzyme Commission [EC] 3.4.23.5), that functions in lysosomes as a proteolytic agent at an acidic pH and as a mitogen, a substance that promotes cell growth by division and multiplication. In the latter role, cathepsin D may facilitate cellular actions such as migration, metastasis, and invasion of other tissues. Estrogen has been shown to stimulate the secretion of this tumor marker in certain hormone-dependent breast cancer cell lines. This antigen has been found to have potential application in breast cancer prognosis as its concentration appears to be related to the patient's overall chance for survival. Cathepsin D is assayed by an immunoenzymatic (alkaline phosphatase) assay using a monoclonal antibody (M2E8), which is approved in the United States for research use only.

Neuron-specific enolase (NSE). This is an enzyme, EC 4.2.9.11, that is glycolytic and contains three subunits (alpha, beta, gamma), MW = 100,000. The gamma subunit is associated with neurons and consequently is found to be elevated in tumors of neuroendocrine origin, such as neuroblastoma, carcinoid, thyroid medullary carcinoma. It is also associated with small cell lung cancer and seminoma. It is used only as an investigational tool in the United States at this time.

Prostatic acid phosphatase (PAP). PAP is a glycoprotein that is one of a group of enzymes, of which all are capable of catalyzing the hydrolysis of organic phosphate esters in the presence of an alcohol to a new alcohol and phosphate ester at a pH of less than 7.0. All of these enzymes are unstable at a pH greater than 7.0, and all are heat denatured above 37°C. These various enzymes are located in lysosomes, which are present in almost all cell lines (except possibly erythrocytes) and thus are found in almost all human tissues. In addition, acid phosphatase proteins are present as extra lysosomal enzymes, which probably accounts for their high concentration in liver, spleen, erythrocytes, platelets, bone marrow, and the prostate gland. Specifically, only the acid phosphatase found in prostatic tissue, PAP, is of clinical utility regarding the staging of prostatic cancer. It is approved for accessing metastasis, prognosis, and monitoring therapy, as serum values generally reflect the extent of these conditions.

Traditionally, PAP has been quantitated by its enzymatic activity by utilizing certain chemical properties, such as substrate specificity, which is unique to PAP. Interference by related enzymes that may be present in the specimen, for example, red cell acid phosphatase, is removed by using select inhibitors of enzyme activity. Detailed reviews of many of these assays may be found in other texts. An example of a selective substrate assay as used by the DuPont ACA analyzer is considered here:

$$\text{Thymolphthalein monophosphate} \xrightarrow[\text{pH 5.6}]{} \text{Thymolphthalein} + PO_4^{-3}$$
$$\text{Thymolphthalein} + NaOH \rightarrow \text{Product that absorbs at 600 nm}$$

NaOH is added after the fixed period of reaction and the thymolphthalein product forms a strongly absorbing species that is monitored at 600 nm. The final concentration of thymolphthalein is proportional to the activity of PAP in the specimen. The sensitivity of this chemical assay is enhanced by immediate processing of serum specimens upon arrival at the laboratory to minimize the effects of the lability of this enzyme's activity at room temperature and a normal serum pH range.

Terminal deoxynucleotidyl transferase (TdT). This is an enzyme, EC 2.7.7.31, that is a DNA polymerase that catalyzes the elongation of DNA. This approved marker is specific to immature lymphocytes and is used to classify and monitor leukemias.

Glycoproteins or polypeptides

Alpha-fetoprotein (AFP). An oncofetal glycoprotein with a MW = ~70,000, AFP is synthesized in fetal liver, fetal yolk sac, and the developing gastrointestinal tract. It is remarkably similar to albumin in its physical size and amino acid composition. Its biological function is unknown, but it is speculated to act as a carrier or transport protein (similar to albumin in a child or adult), as a modulator of immunologic functions, or as a growth regulator. The level of AFP is normally <15 μg/L in an adult. It becomes progressively elevated in the serum of pregnant females, peaking at a gestational age of ~16 weeks with a concentration of 2 to 3 G/L. The origin of this AFP is from the fetus, which excretes the AFP in its urine and thus into the amniotic fluid. Eventually, this AFP is transported or diffuses across the extraembryonic membranes into the mother's serum. Certain fetal abnormalities such as neural tube defects (NTD) often result in gross elevations of AFP in the amniotic fluid and subsequently the mother's serum. In addition, certain fetal defects may be associated with an unusually low concentration of AFP in the amniotic fluid and mother's serum, for example, Down's syndrome. Assays for AFP in pregnant females between their 15th and 21st weeks of gestation are expressed as multiples of the median (MOM units) for a normal, single fetus pregnancy. In order to compare all pregnant female serums to the same data base, in other words, a normal, single fetus, adjustments to MOM units are made for multiple fetuses (which produce more AFP), insulin-dependent diabetics, and the mother's race and weight. An AFP value >2.5 MOM (or 2.0 in some laboratories) is considered elevated, whereas an AFP value <0.5 MOM is considered low.

Male and nonpregnant female adults may exhibit elevations of AFP with cirrhosis, hepatitis, cytomegalovirus infections, ataxia-telangiectasia, and chronic hepatic conditions. As a tumor marker, AFP is often elevated with either primary hepatocellular carcinoma or nonseminomatous testicular cancer. In the latter type of cancer, it is used to aid in the differential diagnosis of differentiating seminomas (non-AFP secreting) and nonseminomatous germ-cell tumors. It is approved for the diagnoses of primary hepatocellular carcinoma or nonseminomatous testicular cancer in the United States. Quantitation is done with RIA, EIA, and FIA procedures and most large clinical laboratories offer an AFT test in routine batches. In general, most serum AFP levels are <15 μg/L in healthy subjects. Elevations in nonmalignant conditions may range up to approximately 350 μg/L, whereas malignant diseases may exhibit even greater elevations of AFP.

Beta₂-microglobulin (B₂-M). Beta₂-microglobulin is a relatively small protein, MW = 11,800 daltons, that was reported on in 1968 by Berggard and Bearn. The protein is present on the surface of most nucleated cells, especially lymphocytes, and is the light chain part of the histocompatibility leukocyte antigen (HLA). It is found in both serum and urine with respective reference intervals of 1000 to 2600 μg/L and 30 to 370 μg/day. It is easily passed through the glomerular membrane and is reabsorbed in the proximal tubule. Dysfunctions in the proximal tubule result in elevated urine concentrations. Serum concentrations are influenced by both the clearance of the protein and its release into the serum pool. Consequently, B₂-M is sometimes used to monitor renal function and the glomerular filtration rate in renal transplant patients. Beta₂-microglobulin is elevated in patients with multiple myeloma and is used in staging and prognosis of the disease. It is also elevated in patients with inflammatory disorders such as Crohn's disease, systemic lupus erythematosus, and rheumatoid arthritis. It is authorized for investigational use only in the United States.

Current methods for assay include FIA and nephelometric procedures, which are used to detect the relatively low concentration of this protein.

*CA 15-3 (cancer antigen 15-3).** A glycoprotein, MW = 300,000 to 450,000, that was first identified in 1984 in the serum of women with metastatic breast cancer. It appears to originate in alveoli and ducts of mammary glands. It is to be used for research purposes only in the United States for monitoring breast CA metastasis and chemotherapy. Quantitation is by RIA and EIA. A normal reference interval is <30 units/mL.

*CA 19-9 (cancer antigen 19-9).** A glycoprotein, MW = 210,000, that has an unknown physiological function and is found on the surface of carcinoma cells. Serum elevations are seen in pancreatic, colorectal, and gastric carcinomas. Its most frequent utilization is in the diagnosis and monitoring of adenocarcinoma of the pancreas, however, it is only approved for research in the United States. Measurement is by RIA and EIA with a reference interval of <37 units/mL.

CA 50 (cancer antigen 50). A glycoprotein that has unknown physiological function, but is associated with large molecular weight glycoproteins and gangliosides. The antigen is similar to the tumor marker CA 19-9, but it is immunologically distinct. It is elevated in the serum of patients with pancreatic and gastrointestinal cancers, but its utilization is limited to research in the United States as an investigational tool. Procedures for measurement are limited to a monoclonal antibody directed against the CA 50 antigen with quantitation by RIA. Reference intervals for normal serum is <17 U/mL. However, with this reference interval, significant numbers of patients with pancreatitis, benign biliary disease, and hepatocellular jaundice also have elevated CA 50 (up to 170 U/mL). Patients with extrahepatic cholestasis (caused by stones) can exhibit even higher levels of CA 50 (up to 250 U/mL). Patients with pancreatic CA may have dramatic elevations up to 68,000 U/mL.

*CA 125 (cancer antigen 125).** A glycoprotein, MW = 200,000, that is found on the surface of ovarian cells that arise from carcinoma. Although this protein is not usually found with normal ovarian cells, its serum value is affected by pregnancy and the menstrual cycle. It is approved in the United States to assess tumor size and recurrence, and to monitor therapy. Quantitation by RIA and EIA procedures indicates a reference interval of ≤35 U/mL. Approximately 10 individuals per 1000 will have a value >35 U/mL, giving a false-positive result. Approximately 60 individuals per 1000 will have a value >35 U/mL when these individuals have a nonmalignant disease. Up to 80% of patients with ovarian cancer have elevated values of this tumor marker that may range up to 10,000 U/mL. In these cases, serial measurements often correlate with the progression or regression of the disease.

CA 195 (cancer antigen 195). This antigen of unknown function binds to the Lewis blood group antigens. It is elevated in the serum of patients with pancreatic and colorectal cancers. This tumor marker has also been reported to be elevated in cancer of the lung and prostate. It is mea-

sured by an RIA procedure and is approved only for investigational use in the United States.

CA 549 (cancer antigen 549). A complex, acidic glycoprotein that may occur in two forms, one of MW = 400,000, the other of MW = 512,000. The antigen has been located in breast, kidney, and colon tissue, and is elevated in the serum of advanced breast cancer patients. Quantitation by a double monoclonal antibody technique (RIA) has established a reference interval of <11 kU/L in healthy females. The antigen is more sensitive to detecting metastasis of primary breast cancer than carcinoembryonic antigen. It is found to be elevated in nonmalignant disease, such as various forms of liver disease, and in malignant disease other than breast tissue, for example, endometrial, lung, prostatic, and ovarian cancers. It is approved only for investigational use in the United States.

Carcinoembryonic antigen (CEA). This antigen is a glycoprotein with a molecular weight of ~200,000. The protein is normally found on the cell surface of embryonic fetal tissue and its biochemical function is unknown. Carcinoembryonic antigen is elevated in adults with cancer or carcinoma of the lung, liver, breast, pancreas, and colon. It is approved in the United States for use as a method to assess colorectal cancer with respect to its prognosis and recurrence (if surgically removed). In general, the higher the serum value of CEA in a patient with colorectal cancer, the poorer the prognosis. Clinical resection of the tumor will result in the protein returning to baseline values. Usually if there is a recurrence, CEA will again begin to rise several months prior to any clinical symptoms or signs of the returning tumor. If the tumor was inoperable, then serial measurements of CEA can be used to monitor the success of chemotherapy. Unfortunately, this tumor marker is also elevated in patients with some benign tumors and a variety of other conditions such as emphysema, cirrhosis, ulcerative colitis, Crohn's disease, hepatitis, and pulmonary infections. Smokers generally have slightly higher baselines than nonsmokers. Many laboratories routinely offer CEA analysis using RIA and FIA procedures. The reference interval for nonsmokers is <2.5 µg/L, for smokers, it is <5.0 µg/L. Patients with certain carcinomas may have elevations up into the thousands; in general, the higher the value, the greater the extent of the tumor volume.

Prostate-specific antigen (PSA). A glycoprotein reported in 1977 by Wang and others, PSA's biochemical function is unknown. This single-chain protein does not appear to be related to prostatic acid phosphatase as it exhibits unique immunochemical and functional properties. Physiologically, it appears to be located in the epithelia of prostatic ductal cells. It is not approved as a screening tool for cancer of the prostate as it is also elevated in the serum of patients with inflammatory conditions in the prostate area and in benign prostatic hypertrophy (a condition commonly seen in males over the age of 50). Over 97% of males over 40 years old have a serum level of <4.0 µg/L. Prostate-specific antigen is approved for monitoring established cases of prostatic CA as serum levels tend to correlate with surgical staging of the cancer and metastases. The test is often used in tandem with prostatic acid phosphatase to monitor patients with adenocarcinoma of the prostate for residual disease or metastases after prostatectomy. Prostate-specific an-

*CA 15-3, CA 19-9, CA 72-4, and CA 125 are registered trademarks of Centocor, Inc.

tigen appears to be more sensitive than prostatic acid phosphatase (PAP) in monitoring prostate cancer, especially in the early stages of the disease, but PAP appears to be equally or slightly more specific for prostatic carcinoma. Both tests are subject to similar interferences from prostatic massage (digital examination), prostatic infarction, or the presence of nonmalignant genitourinary inflammations. The assay is usually performed by either EIA or RIA.

Squamous cell carcinoma antigen (SCC). A glycoprotein antigen that is a subfraction of a tumor-associated antigen, TA-4. TA-4 is a glycoprotein that has been found in the cytoplasm of squamous cell carcinomas of the uterine cervix and tumors of the head and neck (especially large-cell, nonkeratinizing carcinoma). Squamous cell carcinoma antigen may be elevated in the serum of patients with squamous cell carcinoma of the uterus, cervix, neck, and head. Measured by RIA, SCC antigen has a reference interval of <2.5 μg/L (however, at this value, up to 5.5% of a normal population may exhibit false-positive elevations). Greater than 50% of patients with cervical squamous cell carcinoma will exhibit values greater than 2.5 μg/L. Despite its poor correlation to detect early cases of cervical carcinoma, once SCC antigen is elevated, the serum concentration of this antigen will increase with advancement of the disease. The majority of patients with stage II to III squamous cell carcinoma of the cervix will range between 5 and 20 μg/L, with elevations up to 150 μg/L. Used to evaluate prognosis and detection of metastases in cervical and uterine cancers, the marker is limited to research only in the United States.

Tissue polypeptide antigen (TPA). This is an oncofetal antigen that is found in the cytoplasm of epithelial cells as a single chain polypeptide. Serum elevations are found with urological, breast, lung, gastrointestinal, and gynecological cancers. Tissue polypeptide antigen is limited to research use only in the United States.

Alpha-transforming growth factor (alpha-TGF). Alpha-TGFs are polypeptides ranging in molecular weight from 6,000 to 30,000 that bind to epidermal growth factor receptors and are involved in the maturation of cells. This marker appears to be excreted from both normal and cancerous cells. Quantification by RIA on pleural effusions from cancer patients has shown a positive correlation of 42% with malignant disease and an 18% positive rate for nonmalignant diseases. A reference interval of <2 μg/L has been established with values of 2 to 50 μg/L reported for cases of malignancy. Elevations are seen with breast, colon, and ovarian cancers. Alpha-TGF is also found in the urine of patients with glioma and melanoma. The marker is limited to research use only in the United States.

Tumor-associated antigen-72 (TAG-72). This mucin-like glycoprotein tumor marker was derived from tissue extracts of epithelial-derived cancers (ovarian, pancreatic, gastric, esophageal, non–small-cell lung carcinomas, and colonic adenocarcinomas). It is one of several known large molecular weight antigens that are found on the surface or are secreted by human carcinoma cell lines. It is classified as an oncofetal antigen as monoclonal antibodies against TAG-72 react with fetal colon and stomach tissues, but not corresponding normal adult tissues. This tumor marker is quantitated by RIA using a monoclonal antibody, but no reference intervals for blood have been established. TAG-

72 is currently used as an immunohistochemical marker in a research capacity for cancers from breast, stomach, colon, lung, and ovarian tissues.

Mucin or filament-type proteins

Cytokeratins. Filamentous structural proteins are found in the cytoplasm of most cells. Keratins are one family of five known subsets of these structural proteins. All five groups are tissue-specific in distribution and are expressed in neoplasms arising from their tissue of origin. They are biochemically and immunologically distinct. The cytokeratins range in molecular weight from 40,000 to 68,000 and are often found in pairs, one acidic, the other basic.

Nineteen different keratins have been identified and all epithelial cell lines contain a subset of these 19 proteins. Thus, monoclonal antibodies that are developed for specific keratin subgroups are used as immunohistochemical tools to assist in identifying undifferentiated tumors that may arise from epithelial tissue, for example, bladder, prostate, or cervical tumors. These tumor markers are limited to research use only in the United States.

Receptor-site proteins

Epidermal growth factor receptor (EGF-R). A glycoprotein, MW = 170,000, located in the cell membrane receptor site for epidermal growth factor (EGF). Epidermal growth factor is a potent mitogenic protein that binds to its receptor site (EGF-R) and initiates intracellular responses. A receptor assay for EGF-R has been developed using radiolabeled EGF. Tissue values from breast cancers may be prognostic for patient survival. Tissue values are also elevated in cancers from bladder, renal, head, neck, glial cells, and non–small-cell lung tumors. There are no established reference intervals for EGF-R and it is limited to research use only in the United States.

Estrogen receptor (ER). It has been observed since 1896 that some breast tumors were stimulated by hormones within the patient. In 1971 it was shown that a receptor site protein, MW = 70,000, that binds estradiol and is found in the nuclei of cells from uterine and mammary tissues was partly responsible for this hormonal response. By measuring the amount of estrogen receptors per gram of breast tissue, oncologists can determine which patients are most likely to respond to antihormone therapy. Uterine tissue also contains estrogen receptors and may be used to access endometrial carcinoma prior to the initiation of therapy. Reference intervals are affected by race, sex, age, day of menstrual cycle, pregnancy, and histologic tumor cell differentiation. Quantitation is based on a titration assay using radiolabeled estrogen in the presence of various concentrations of unlabeled inhibitors. Estrogen receptor is reported in units of femtomoles (fmol)/mg of cytosol protein. For breast tissue, significant ER values are ≥10 fmol/mg; <3 fmol/mg are insignificant; values between 3 to 9 fmol/mg lie in a gray zone.

Interleukin-2 receptor (IL-2 receptor, Tac antigen). T-cell growth factor or interleukin-2 is an inducible lymphokine that is synthesized and secreted by T-lymphocytes following activation with an antigen or mitogen. This glycoprotein (MW = 15,000) has a specific T-cell receptor that is also a glycoprotein, MW = 55,000. Normal resting

T-cells and most leukemic T-cell populations do not exhibit IL-2 receptors on their cellular surface. However, studies have shown that patients with human T-cell lymphotropic virus-associated adult T-cell leukemia usually have this tumor marker.

The assay for T cells expressing Tac antigen is carried out using a specific monoclonal antibody directed toward the IL-2 receptor. Peripheral blood mononuclear cells are analyzed using immunofluorescence and fluorescence-activated flow cytometry. The method is limited to research use only in the United States and there are no established reference intervals.

Progesterone receptor (PR). The steroid progesterone, analogous to estrogen, was found to have a protein receptor by which it initiated its hormonal action. Two molecular forms appear to exist within the nucleus of human mammary and uterine cells, MW = 94,000 and 120,000, respectively. Clinical studies have clearly established that endometrial carcinoma tissue that has elevated values of PR is more probable to be responsive to endocrine therapy (progestins). Although estrogen and progesterone receptors appear to be independent prognostic markers for breast and endometrial cancers, they are usually assayed in tandem, which increases the predictability for hormonal therapy.

The assay for PR is similar to ER. A radiolabeled progesterone is used to titrate aliquots of tissue protein in the presence and absence of unlabeled inhibitor. Currently, PR is approved only as a clinical investigatory tool in the United States. Reference intervals are: negative, <3 fmols/mg cytosol protein; positive, ≥10 fmol/mg cytosol protein.

Lipid-associated

Lipid-associated sialic acid (LASA-P)

Lipid-associated sialic acid is a general tumor marker that is the acylated derivative of neuraminic acid found in many glycoproteins and glycolipids. It appears to increase in plasma as the surface membrane of neoplastic cells is altered. Although this tumor marker may be elevated (ranging from 20 to 50 mg/dL) in the plasma of patients with lung, Hodgkin's disease, melanoma, leukemia, lymphoma, breast, or gastrointestinal tract cancers, clinically, it is most beneficial when used in conjunction with other tumor markers, such as CA-125 or CEA.

LASA-P is quantitated by an organic extraction and partition method developed by Katopodis and Stock. The suggested reference interval is <20 mg/dL. The marker is approved only as an investigational assay in the United States.

Hormones

Beta-core human chorionic gonadotropin (B-core HCG)

The beta core HCG is a fragment of the normal beta chain portion of the HCG molecule. It is comprised of two separate polypeptides of approximately 10,000 daltons and is linked by two disulfide bonds. B-core HCG is immunologically different than beta-HCG. It may be uniquely synthesized by trophoblast tissue, or it may simply be a catabolic residue from normal HCG. Serum concentrations are increased in cervical, ovarian, testicular, and endometrial cancers. No commercial test is currently available and the test is not approved for routine clinical usage in the United States.

Calcitonin (hCT)

Calcitonin is a 32 amino acid peptide hormone that is found in heterogeneous forms, with molecular weight ranging from 3,500 to 20,000. Biochemically, hCT inhibits bone resorption by blocking bone osteoclastic activity and increasing urinary calcium excretion. It acts to decrease serum concentrations of total calcium, ionic calcium, and inorganic phosphate.

Calcitonin is secreted into the serum from C-cells in the thyroid gland, where it is synthesized. Secretion is regulated by the serum ionic calcium concentration. Most gastrointestinal hormones stimulate the synthesis of calcitonin, and the intravenous infusion of pentagastrin will release hCT from the thyroid.

Elevated serum concentrations of hCT are primarily found in patients with medullary carcinoma of the thyroid. It may also be elevated in carcinoid tumors as well as in cancer of the breast, lung, liver, and renal tissues.

This tumor marker is quantitated by an RIA method. Reference intervals are: males, <40 ng/L; females, <20 ng/L.

Human chorionic gonadotropin (HCG)

This is a glycoprotein, MW = 45,000 that is composed of two subunits, an alpha and beta chain. The intact molecule is secreted by the placenta and functions to regulate other hormones. Serum assays using monoclonal antibodies directed toward either the beta subunit or intact molecule (usually double antibody or "sandwich" antibody assays) are clinically used to determine the presence of pregnancy, the presence of hydatidiform moles, trophoblastic (or germ cell) tumors, breast cancer, choriocarcinoma, and testicular cancer. The beta-subunit assay is used to monitor choriocarcinomas and testicular germ cell neoplasms, whereas the intact-HCG assay is more frequently used to determine if female patients are pregnant. Many laboratories now have the instrumentation to routinely quantitate beta-HCG using EIA or FIA procedures. Beta-HCG reference intervals for males and nonpregnant, premenopausal females is <5 IU/L and is <7 IU/L for postmenopausal females.

Urinary gonadotropin peptide (UGP)

Human chorionic gonadotropin (HCG) is found in urine in the form of the whole molecule (alpha + beta subunit), as individual alpha and beta subunits, and as fragments of the two subunits. A specific fragment (beta 6-40 residues linked by disulfides to beta 55-92 residues) termed UGP has a very short half-life in blood and is rapidly cleared to urine.

This fragment of HCG (MW = 10,000) is apparently produced intracellularly (probably as a cleavage by-product of beta-hCG) in nontrophoblastic cancers and is secreted into the blood and then into the urine. Radioimmunoassay for this fragment has shown that approximately two thirds of women with ovarian, endometrial, or cervical cancers had elevated urine values of this tumor marker. A reference interval of <8 nmol/L has been proposed for screening and differentiating between malignant and benign neoplasias (sensitivity = 46%, specificity = 99%).

Virus
Human papilloma virus (HPV)

Papilloma viruses are found in humans and are classified into 50 genotypes based upon their DNA nucleic acid sequence. Studies of genital cancer (cervical, vulval, and penile) and benign genital warts have found that HPV types 6, 11, 16, 18, 31, and 35 may be associated with these clinical lesions. Several of these variants are associated with sexually transmitted diseases and may be indicators of increased risk for the development of a genital cancer. Tissue biopsy specimens are assayed for HPV using Southern blot hybridization techniques to a cloned HPV DNA. No reference intervals are established and the assay is approved only as an investigatory tool in the United States.

Oncogenes/genes/chromosomes
c-erb B-2 (or HER-2/neu)

The c-erb B-2 or neu oncogene is located on human chromosome 17 and is responsible for a 185,000 dalton protein with tyrosine kinase activity. This glycoprotein is believed to be a membrane receptor site for an unidentified ligand. It is structurally similar to epidermal growth factor receptor (EGF-R, already described).

Alterations in either the structure, amplification, or expression of this gene may play a role in adenocarcinomas of various tissues and breast cancer. Breast cancer tissue that is positive for this tumor marker indicates a poorer patient prognosis.

The assay for the neu oncoprotein is based upon immunohistochemical staining of tissue specimens. No reference intervals have been established and the marker is limited to research use only in the United States.

myc (c-myc and N-myc)

Myc is a family of oncogenes that produces phosphoprotein (MW = 64,000) found in the cell nucleus. This protein may be involved with RNA processing, DNA synthesis, or transcription.

The c-myc proto-oncogene is similar to the virus MC29, which causes accelerated development of cancers in birds. In humans, c-myc has been found to occur in elevated concentrations in 68% of primary adenocarcinoma cancers of the colon (38 cases studied).

Similarly, elevated levels of the N-myc oncogene have been shown to indicate prognostic value in predicting survival of patients with neuroblastomas.

The assay for these oncogenes is carried out on tissue specimens using the Southern blot hybridization technique. No reference intervals or commercial assay for this tumor marker is available. Studies are limited to research use only in the United States.

p53 gene

The p53 gene contains the DNA for the transformation-associated protein p53. It is located on the short arm of chromosome 17. The normal role of p53 gene product may be to interact with either DNA or specific proteins in order to suppress neoplastic growth of certain epithelial cell lines. However, since mutations in the DNA code of the p53 gene have been found in 75% of colorectal tumors, the altered p53 gene product may not be successful in controlling neo-plasms, in other words, it is no longer a functional "suppressor" protein. It is available only in some research centers as clinical assay is not available.

Philadelphia chromosome (Ph^1)

The Philadelphia chromosome arises from a translocation of the c-abl gene from chromosome 9 to chromosome 22. The protein synthesized by the Ph^1 gene has tyrosine kinase activity that is altered from the normal c-abl gene located on chromosome 9. Over 90% of chronic myelogenous leukemia patients have been found to have the Philadelphia chromosome. The presence of Ph^1 in cases of chronic myelogenous leukemia has significant implication in the prognosis and therapy of this disease. Patients who are positive for Ph^1 have a median survival time of 40 months, whereas Ph^1 negative cases have 10- to 20-month survival times.

The tumor marker is detected in karotypes of chromosomes isolated from cultures of the patient's bone marrow cells. A reference interval is either present or absent. This is an approved tumor marker in the United States.

ras

These markers make up a ubiquitous gene family that is found in all mammals, birds, and insects, whose protein products appear to play a fundamental role in cell division. The proteins produced by these genes have an approximate molecular weight of 21,000 and are located on the inner plasma membrane.

When mutations are found in certain regions of these DNA markers, they become oncogenic and are often found associated with carcinomas of breast, lung, colon, and bladder tissues, as well as in several types of leukemia. Ras oncogenes have been found in approximately 10% to 40% of most neoplasias, which is the most frequent oncogene family now known in human cancer. Assays for the ras oncogenes are limited to research use only in the United States. No reference intervals have been established.

Retinoblastoma gene product (RB gene)

Retinoblastoma is the most common ocular cancer in children and it occurs in both a hereditary and nonhereditary form. The RB gene product has been identified as a nuclear phosphoprotein, MW = 110,000, that inhibits cellular division. When the RB gene has a partial loss or deletion of its DNA, then the gene product is altered and retinoblastoma or other types of cancer may develop. Prostate, bladder, breast, small-cell lung cancers, and osteosarcomas are examples of other types of cancer. Apparently both normal RB gene alleles must be altered to allow tumor production to occur.

Alteration of the RB gene is determined using the Southern blot analysis. No reference intervals have been established and the procedure is limited to research use only in the United States.

Antigenic material (biochemical class unknown)
Ki-67 antigen

This is an antigen located in the nucleus of proliferating cells. Immunocytochemical assays using a monoclonal antibody to this marker in breast cancer specimens have shown that the antigen increases in concentration in this malignancy and may be correlated to the degree of tumor differentiation, vascular invasion, and the occurrence of lymph node metastases. There is also a correlation of elevated levels of Ki-67 in breast tumors having low values of estrogen and progesterone receptor sites. This tumor marker is limited to research use only in the United States and no reference intervals have been established.

SUGGESTED READING

Bast RC, Hunter V, and Knapp RC: Pros and cons of gynecologic tumor markers, Cancer 60:1984, 1987.

Garrett PE and Kurtz SR: Clinical utility of oncofetal proteins and hormones as tumor markers, Med Clin North Am 70:1295, 1986.

Hansen M and Pedersen AG: Tumor markers in patients with lung cancer, Chest 89S:219S, 1986.

Herberman RB (editor): Tumor marker reference guide, Alameda, Calif, 1990, Triton Biosciences, Diagnostics Division.

Lieberman MW and Lebovitz RM: Neoplasia. In Kissane JM (editor): Anderson's pathology, ed 9, St Louis, 1990, Mosby–Year Book, Inc.

Statland BE and Winkel P: Neoplasia. In Kaplan LA and Pesce AJ; Clinical chemistry: theory, analysis and correlation, ed 2 St Louis,1989, Mosby–Year Book, Inc.

Torosian MH: The clinical usefulness and limitations of tumor markers, Surg Gynecol Obstet 166:567,1988.

Virji MA, Mercer DW, and Herberman RB: Tumor markers in cancer diagnosis and prognosis, Cancer 38:104, 1988.

Wills RA: The spread of tumors in the human body, London, 1952, Butterworth.

22 Laboratory investigation of sexual assault

Charles G. Massion

The terms *rape* and *sexual assault* are not medical, but legal definitions, and they are not synonymous. An adequate investigation of alleged sexual assault is a complex social and medical affair in which the clinical laboratory can occasionally play a significant or even decisive part. A significant percentage of assailants experience sexual dysfunction so that the absence of prostatic fluid may not be germaine to the total legal and medical evaluation and treatment. On the other hand, the presence of any of the constituents of semen is indicative only of recent sexual activity and may have nothing to do with a criminal offense. The victim of sexual assault who presents herself (sometimes, himself) at an emergency medical department may have injuries and emotional needs that require treatment before laboratory testing is appropriate.

Relatively few hospital emergency services are adequately prepared to carry out the steps necessary to protect the interests of all concerned in cases of suspected sexual assault. However, some cities and states require every emergency service to perform an examination at the request of the police or of an alleged victim. It is also in the best interests of good patient care that every laboratory have in place policies and procedures to support the medical and nursing staffs in the investigation of alleged sexual assault.

Prepackaged kits containing specific instructions, swabs, envelopes, vials, and combs should be available to aid in the thorough examination of supposed victims. Ideally, these kits should be tailored to the needs of each institution so that appropriate samples are taken for the laboratory of that institution. Table 22-1 is an example of the contents of one type of kit used in Ohio.

DEFINITIONS

Rape is defined as "unlawful carnal knowledge of a woman by a man forcibly and against her will." *Unlawful* means that the woman and man are not married, and carnal knowledge refers to any penetration of the penis into a woman's genitalia. *Forcibly and against her will* refers not only to physical force, but to threats of violence, impersonation of her husband, or while the woman is under the influence of alcohol or other drugs.

The recent trend in state legislatures has been to vastly expand this definition to cover sexual abuse of children,

homosexual assault, and any sexual activity without consent. For example, the Minnesota legislature in 1975 defined four degrees of criminal sexual conduct ranging from penetration (rape) to intentional touching of intimate parts including breasts and buttocks. Higher degrees of force are required for first- and second-degree offenses.

GENERAL LABORATORY INVESTIGATION

The help of the clinical laboratory is integral to the diagnosis of sexually transmitted disease or pregnancy that may have resulted from an assault. This medical testing is a part of the routine laboratory work as is the quantitation of prostatic proteins. The latter tests, along with microscopic examination of body fluids for spermatozoa, are currently the primary clinical laboratory tests used in alleged rape cases. In most cases, samples will be taken from the vagina or rectum, but swabs of the vulva or other skin surfaces may be pertinent for testing. Lesser degrees of alleged sexual assault are, for the most part, beyond the purview of the clinical laboratory, although the impact of the act on the victim may be as great.

In the recent past, elaborate protocols for the immunologic typing of many genetic markers present on red blood cells, and in seminal fluid and saliva, have been advanced as aids in the identification of suspect assailants. That is, blood stains from the victim's clothing or crime scene do not match the victim, but are the same type and with similar antibody specificity to an alleged assailant. While somewhat specific, these tests only indicate that someone with a similar blood type may have caused the assault. Even this type of laboratory testing is difficult for the average clinical laboratory to perform and is best left for crime laboratories that are set up to run such tests.

These blood type and antigenic markers are rapidly being replaced by DNA "fingerprinting" techniques that, unlike the immunologic tests, are much more specific for the individual. Since the DNA in each person's cells is unique and identical in all cells from that individual, blood samples are not necessary to carry out an identification. Any cellular material, for example, buccal cells from mouth washings, can be sufficient.

The DNA fingerprinting methods are technically difficult, time-consuming, and expensive. They must be carried

Table 22-1 Contents of sexual assault kit

Item	Amount
Swabs	6
Test tubes, capped, containing 2.5 ml broth*	2
Slides	4
Combs	2
Plastic bags	3
Envelopes	6
Marking pen	1
Clothing bag	1
Specific instructions regarding the conduct of the medical examination and the preparation of laboratory smears and samples	
Chain-of-custody forms	Several sets

From Lantz RK and Eisenberg RB: Preservation of acid phosphatase activity in medico-legal specimens, Clin Chem 24:486, 1978.
*Broth contains: 50 g bovine albumin and 0.2 g sodium azide diluted to 1L with 10 mmol/L phosphate buffer, pH = 7.4, containing 9 g/L sodium chloride.

Table 22-2 Stability of samples (before collection)*

Material	No.	Percent of samples	Time (hours)
Motile sperm	15	50	At 3
Whole sperm	15	All	18
Sperm heads	15	All	24
Identifiable sperm	15	50	72
Prostatic acid phosphatase (PAP)	15	50	9
	15	None	>36
Prostatic specific antigen (PSA)	48	All	27 (range, 13-47)
PSA positive (PAP negative)	48	25	Variable
PAP positive (PSA negative)	48	2	Variable

*Data are from samples obtained from consensual couples and may or may not represent material from alleged assaults.

out with especially rigorous quality control and a chain-of-custody formality to avoid legal challenge. In this technique, multiple DNA fragments are matched with those taken from samples obtained from a victim of sexual assault. The DNA fragments must match an alleged assailant and not match a victim's DNA fragments. Many such DNA matches may identify the assailant with a high degree of certainty, but much research needs to be done to establish exactly how certain these identifications are. Although such certainty may be preferred from a legal point of view, it is difficult to obtain the assays. For the foreseeable future, the performance of such technically demanding analyses will be limited to a few highly specialized laboratories.

The role of the clinical laboratory in defining an alleged rape, as noted earlier, is usually limited to examination of fluid from the body orifices, most particularly the vagina, as obtained by the examining physician. The tests that demonstrate sexual activity are:
1. Detection of spermatozoa
   a. Wet mount
   b. Stained smear
2. Assay of prostatic proteins
   a. Prostatic acid phosphatase (PAP) activity
   b. Prostate specific antigen (PSA) quantitation

The presence of identifiable sperm in either a wet mount or on stained smears is, of course, conclusive medical evidence that vaginal intercourse has occurred fairly recently. It does not define that rape, including penetration without seminal fluid emission, has occurred. It does not rule out that consensual intercourse occurred within hours or days before the assault. Prostatic acid phosphatase and prostatic specific antigen, when present in vaginal fluid with several cells, would be corroborative findings, although presence of these proteins identifies seminal fluid with near certainty. In the presence of sperm, PAP and PSA will usually both be at high levels, but the presence of these proteins without sperm cells will occur if the man has been vasectomized or is cytologically infertile.

STABILITY OF SAMPLES

The absence of spermatozoa does not prove that vaginal intercourse did not take place in the recent past since the detection time is variable, as shown in Table 22-2. Data obtained from examination of vaginal fluid after consensual intercourse showed that only 50% of the fluid contained motile sperm after 3 hours. Whole sperm were present in the vaginal fluid of all volunteers for up to 18 hours and heads for up to 24 hours. At 72 hours, sperm were identifiable in about 50% of the volunteers. Depending on the stain and technique used, sperm can be demonstrated in some cases considerably longer than 72 hours, but the limit is uncertain.

Prostatic acid phosphatase is normally present in small amounts (2 to 6 IU/L at 30°C) in vaginal fluid so that the demonstration of relatively high activity (>50 IU/L) is necessary to prove the presence of seminal fluid. Prostatic acid phosphatase is an unstable protein that rapidly disappears from samples, swabs, and other materials. Because of its unstable nature, it is usually recommended that the analysis of prostatic acid phosphatase should be completed in as short a time as possible after the sample has been obtained. However, samples can be maintained for up to a month at room temperature without loss of activity when collected in a preservative broth at pH = 7.4. In contrast, prostatic specific antigen is a relatively stable protein found only in prostatic fluids and, when detected in vaginal fluid, demonstrates recent vaginal intercourse.

As with spermatozoa, if not preserved, the length of time that these proteins are detectable is quite variable, ranging from 8 to 40 hours with a mean of 24 hours for PAP, and 13 to 47 hours with a mean of 27 hours for PSA. Of the two, PSA has been reported to be present in about 25% of the samples in which PAP activity was negative. The presence of both proteins should probably be analyzed for confirmatory purposes. This data obtained after consensual intercourse may or may not represent assault conditions.

LEGAL ASPECTS

Ideally, laboratory facilities for the preparation and microscopic examination of a wet mount should be readily available to the examining physician for his or her direct use. This eliminates the necessity for chain-of-custody forms and lockbags for these smears, which are critical to legal proceedings in the case of positive findings. Fluid samples and/or smears taken by pelvic, anal, and oral examination need to be uniquely identified by the examining physician.

Since the chemical assays are not performed by the examining physician, they do require chain-of-custody forms and proper treatment. These materials are placed in a sealed container and passed to each successive person on route to the laboratory with a series of acknowledgments noted on the form that attest to the sealed condition and indicate when and who had the material until the material reaches the person who actually performs the test. That person then becomes legally responsible for recording the test result(s) and, if necessary, testifying in court. (For a more extensive explanation of chain-of-custody processes, see Chapter 28.)

SPECIFIC LABORATORY INVESTIGATION

The diverse laboratory testing done in all cases of alleged rape include some testing for medical reasons and some testing for legal reasons. Such testing does not necessarily need to be completed for lesser degrees of sexual assault. The medical tests include:

- Blood or urine for pregnancy testing (beta-human chorionic gonadotropin [beta-hCG]) initially to establish whether the victim was pregnant at the time of assault. About 1% of victims become pregnant as a result of sexual assault. Repeat 7 to 14 days later if results were initially negative to establish whether pregnancy was the result of the assault.
- Urine tests for drug and alcohol screening.
- Cultures for *Neisseria gonorrhoeae,* and *Chlamydia trachomatis* from the cervix and, when indicated, from the throat and rectum. These should be repeated several days later to indicate if infection was the result of the assault.
- Serological tests for syphilis, hepatitis B and, more recently, hepatitis C and human immunodeficiency virus (HIV).
- The initial samples establish/eliminate preexisting infection. The later testing is done to be sure no infection has occurred as a result of the attack.

In theory, the common sexually transmitted diseases should be tested for by culture or by immunological procedures. The effectiveness of doing this is a function of the population served by a particular institution. As shown in Table 22-3, incubation times are quite variable among the transmissible diseases. Thus, if initial cultures and tests are negative, repeated blood sampling may be necessary over a 6-month period to truly rule out particular transmissions via the assault.

Procedures done primarily for legal reasons or to support criminal charges include the following:

- Wet mounts make intact spermatozoa readily identifiable, especially when still mobile.
- Dried smears of vaginal fluid are fixed and stained with either Papanicolaou's or Wright's stain, the former being preferred by most microscopists. Intact spermatozoa are distinctive and easily seen, but positive identification becomes progressively more difficult in smears with time as the sperm cells lose their tails and deteriorate in vivo.

Table 22-3 Guidelines for laboratory testing

Reason for test	Procedure	Initial incubation time	
		Initial	Subsequent
MEDICAL			
	Cervical cultures		
	Gonorrhea	X	+1 week
	Chlamydia	X	+1 week
	Blood samples		
	Syphilis	X	+1 month
	Hepatitis B	X	+2 months
	Hepatitis C	X	+6 weeks
	HIV-I	X	+6 weeks and 6 months
	Blood and urine		
	beta-hCG	X	+7-14 days
LEGAL			
	Urine		
	Drugs	X	—
	Alcohol	X	—
	Swabs/vaginal fluid/clothing		
	Sperm	X	—
	Prostatic acid phosphatase	X	—
	Prostatic specific antigen	X	—

- Fluid samples can be made by soaking swabs in the fluid of the vagina, mouth, or rectum, or sometimes by rubbing broth-moistened swabs over skin possibly coated with seminal fluid. Dried seminal fluid fluoresces brightly under an ultraviolet (Wood's) light, making areas to sample readily visible. The swabs are placed into tubes containing broth and are stable at this point. These samples are used for preparation of wet mounts, if not already done, and for the assay of PAP and PSA. They must be carefully handled and refrigerated until the tests are done. They must also be tracked by chain-of-custody procedures.

Table 22-2 summarizes sample stability before collection as shown from limited studies of voluntary couples. It appears that spermatozoa can be identified from samples taken from the uterine cervical canal after both prostatic proteins are undetectable, and that PSA is present, on the average, longer than PAP.

SUGGESTED READING

Geer JH: Proceedings of a forensic science symposium on the analysis of sexual assault evidence, FBI Academy, July 1983.

Hochbaum SR: The evaluation and treatment of the sexually assaulted patient, Emerg Med Clin N Am 5(3):601, 1987.

Keller E (editor): Sexual assault: a statewide procedure manual for law enforcement, medical, human services, and legal personnel, Minnesota Program for Victims of Sexual Assault, 1981.

Marx JL: DNA fingerprinting takes the witness stand, Science 240:1616, 1988.

Ricci LR and Hoffman SA: Prostatic acid phosphatase and sperm in the post-coital vagina, Ann Emerg Med 11:530, 1982.

PART THREE

TOXICOLOGY, HEAVY METALS, AND THERAPEUTIC DRUG MONITORING

23 Basic pharmacokinetics

Ann Warner

Drugs contribute much to modern life. Among their positive contributions are the means to control such previously debilitating and life-threatening conditions as asthma, epilepsy, cancer, diabetes, and infection. In fact, the discovery of antibiotics in the 1940s was probably the most significant factor in increasing longevity in the history of man. The dark side of drugs is their increasing use and abuse for recreational reasons or as a response to the stress of modern life. This negative use results in high costs to our society due to an increased crime rate, decreased productivity of our work force, and increased health costs for individuals suffering the physical effects of drug abuse. This is not a new phenomenon, since many of these drugs have been abused since ancient times. However, the problem appears to be growing.

TYPES OF TESTING

In recent years, in response to the greater use of drugs for both therapeutic and nontherapeutic reasons, the clinical laboratory has become increasingly involved in drug testing. This testing can be roughly divided into two main types: quantitative serum or blood analysis (therapeutic drug monitoring or TDM) and qualitative urine analysis. Urine testing is further divided into clinical testing for diagnostic purposes (toxicology) and legal testing for drug use in the context of employment (drug abuse testing).

Urine testing

Toxicological testing in the clinical setting involves testing urine to detect and identify drugs that may be contributing to the patient's symptoms. Often this type of testing is requested as part of evaluating patients in emergency rooms. Patients, such as those with a history of overdose or those exhibiting bizarre behavior, sedation, or coma, may also be tested for the presence of drugs. Such testing may involve simple procedures to identify the presence of a few agents or may include extensive, sophisticated testing for a hundred or more drugs.

The other type of urine testing, drug abuse testing, applies some of the technology used in toxicological testing but for a nonclinical reason, namely to identify workers and job candidates who have used certain drugs in their recent past. This type of testing is increasing for a variety of rea-

sons. Thus clinical laboratories are finding themselves engaged in legal as well as medical testing.

Blood and serum testing

Therapeutic drug monitoring (TDM) developed when easy-to-perform immunoassay methods for quantifying drugs in serum and occasionally whole blood became widely available. TDM has been combined with pharmacokinetic calculations in order to more effectively dose drugs used for therapy. Since the number of drugs routinely monitored is small compared to the thousands used, this area will continue to expand.

An understanding of the principles and factors affecting the presence of drugs in urine and serum is needed to correctly interpret assay results. This chapter will cover the principles of drug pharmacokinetics from this standpoint.

PHARMACOKINETICS
Pharmacodynamics versus pharmacokinetics

Drugs and biological systems (i.e., man) interact in two ways: pharmacodynamically and pharmacokinetically. What the drug does to the body is pharmacodynamics. This includes the therapeutic effect, which is the reason the drug has been used. Examples of pharmacodynamic effects include: lowering blood pressure, preventing seizures, and improving mood. Toxicity, like kidney damage, is also a pharmacodynamic effect, although not a desired one.

It is generally accepted that drugs exert their effects through various interactions with structures in the body called receptors. For example, a receptor might be a particular enzyme and the drug effect might be to inhibit that enzyme. The drug allopurinol, used in the treatment of gout, inhibits the enzyme that has a key role in the production of uric acid, the precipitating factor in gout attacks.

What the body does to the drug is pharmacokinetics. The pharmacokinetic processes determine what pharmacodynamic effect will be achieved.

Pharmacokinetic principles are used in overdose situations to determine how much drug is in the body (particularly if an antidote is available) and also to evaluate how well the person is clearing the drug in order to guide clinical treatment.

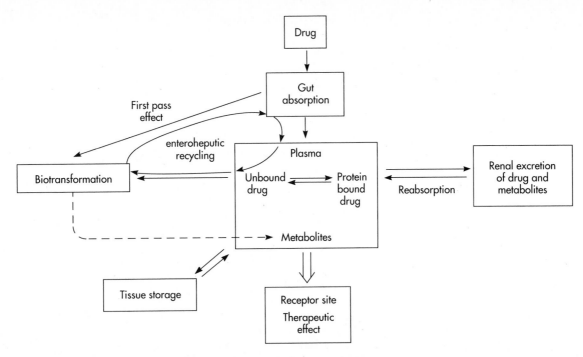

Fig. 23-1   Interactions of pharmacokinetic processes.

In TDM, pharmacokinetics' greatest utility is providing the means to individualize the use of a drug in a particular person so that the therapeutic effect is maximized and toxicity is avoided.

Pharmacokinetic processes/CLADME

The easiest way to remember which body processes make up pharmacokinetics is through use of an acronym, CLADME: *C*ompliance, *L*iberation, *A*bsorption, *D*istribution, *M*etabolism, *E*limination. Figure 23-1 illustrates the interactive nature of these processes.

Compliance

Compliance is a pre-pharmacokinetic factor, which refers to the patient taking the drug as ordered. This must occur in order for all of the other processes to take place. Particularly in the case of therapeutic drug use, lack of patient compliance has been shown to be a major cause of therapeutic failure. Studies have shown that as many as 60% of patients fail to take drugs as prescribed, either by taking too much or too little or at different time intervals than prescribed.

Liberation

Liberation refers to the release of the drug from whatever form in which it has been administered. This applies primarily to oral preparations. When a tablet or capsule is ingested, it must first break up and dissolve in gastrointestinal contents. This, along with absorption, will be the rate-limiting steps for the appearance of drug in the blood.

The formulation of drug products affect their liberation and dissolution. Some drugs are formulated for rapid release (i.e., minor analgesics such as acetaminophen), others for release over long periods (i.e., the "tiny time capsules" of Contac®).

Some of the factors affecting this process include:
1. Types and quantities of excipients mixed with the drug.
2. Compression pressure used to form the tablet.
3. Presence of enteric coatings, which prevent the dissolution of the tablet at acidic pH (i.e., in the stomach).

Liberation can occur in whole or in part in the acidic environment of the stomach. Many preparations, however, are designed to remain intact until they enter the more basic milieu of the ileum. The location of liberation will often be dictated by the chemical nature of the drug: acidic drugs are best absorbed in the stomach, while basic drugs absorb better in the duodenum. Since the drug must be in an un-ionized form for absorption to occur, the pKa of the drug must be considered when designing its formulation.

Figure 23-2 illustrates the various chemical environments to which an orally ingested drug will be exposed during the processes of liberation and absorption.

Substantial research effort is currently directed at novel designs for more effective drug delivery systems, and formulation plays a key role in these developments.

Absorption

Drugs that are ingested, smoked, used sublingually or as suppositories or intramuscular injections will all have to be absorbed, crossing cell membranes, in order to reach the blood stream. This process is relatively rapid in the case of smoked or sublingual drugs but slower for drugs which must cross the gastrointestinal barrier.

Before absorption can occur, the drug must pass to the portion of the gastrointestinal tract where it can be dissolved in its un-ionized form. Since most drugs are absorbed after they pass into the small intestine, one of the rate-limiting steps is gastric-emptying time. Gastric emptying, and, there-

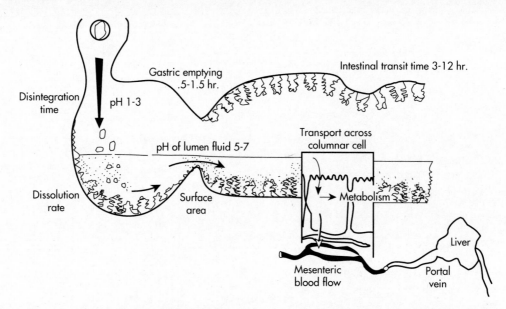

Fig. 23-2 Aspects of the gastrointestinal environment that affect liberation and absorption of drugs. *Redrawn from Barr WH: Am J Pharm ED 32:958, 1968.*

fore drug absorption, is retarded by meals high in fat or bulk, lying on the left side, gastroenteritis, and gastric ulcer.

Factors which facilitate drug absorption in the duodenum include:

1. pH (basic)
2. presence of bile to help solubilize lypophilic drugs
3. presence of active transport systems
4. high blood perfusion

Absorption can occur through passive diffusion and facilitated or active transport. These processes are briefly described in Table 23-1. The main factors affecting passive diffusion are the lipid solubility of the drug and the concentrations of the drug on the two sides of the separating membrane. Lipid solubility is important since membranes have a major lipid component that may retard the passive diffusion of polar molecules. The concentration gradient for drugs being absorbed from the gastrointestinal tract will favor absorption into blood, since the drug is carried away and diluted in the blood. Theoretically this means that drugs can be almost totally absorbed.

Facilitated and active transport are similar processes in which protein carriers in the membranes combine with the specific drug on the cell surface and carry it into the cell. The main difference between the two processes is that active transport can take place against a concentration gradient with the expenditure of energy, thus concentrating the drug within the cell, while facilitated transport cannot.

Absorption will be further affected by such factors as presence or absence of food, motility of the gut, and malabsorption syndromes. Food has mixed effects, increasing the absorption of some drugs, while hindering others. Often the patient will be instructed to take a drug with food in order to decrease the possibility of irritation and nausea and to aid absorption.

The absorption of some drugs is specifically inhibited by the presence of certain foods. For example, the widely used tetracycline antibiotics will be poorly absorbed if any cal-

Table 23-1 Major drug transport mechanisms

Mechanism	Characteristics
Passive diffusion	Affected by lipid/water partition coefficient and the concentration gradient
Facilitated transport	Specific carrier which can be saturated; competitive inhibition possible, does not operate against a concentration gradient.
Active transport	Carrier works against both concentration gradients and electrochemical potentials; saturation and competitive inhibition possible.

cium is present, since it forms an insoluble salt with the drug, thus preventing absorption. Therefore, anytime a prescription for these drugs is filled it comes with the warning to avoid dairy products and antacids close to the time the drug will be taken.

Gastrointestinal motility also affects absorption. If a person is suffering from diarrhea, the drug may pass through too rapidly to be effectively absorbed. Decreased motility may delay the onset of drug activity if the drug cannot move to the portion of the gut where absorption is optimal. Absorption when it occurs, however, may be more complete.

Some drug overdoses are particularly dangerous because the drug slows the motility of the gut, and absorption will continue unless aggressive measures are taken to remove the drug from the gut. Patients can appear to be getting better and subsequently die because this possibility was overlooked. Tricyclic antidepressants are known to cause this type of effect.

Drug bioavailability

The U.S. Food and Drug Administration's official definition of bioavailability is "the rate and extent to which the active drug ingredient or the therapeutic moiety is absorbed from a drug product and becomes available at the site of drug action."

Factors that affect the bioavailability of drugs include the composition of the dosage form, differences in manufacturing procedures, and the physiology of the patient.

Comparisons of two or more dosage forms in the same patient can provide the relative bioavailability of the different preparations. Bioequivalent dosage forms do not differ significantly in their rate and extent of absorption when compared with a standard.

Distribution

Distribution of the drug, which begins after the drug reaches the blood stream, is the key process initiating drug action, since this results in the drug reaching its site of action. Drugs administered intravenously bypass the liberation and absorption steps since they are introduced directly into the blood stream. Once the drug reaches the blood, either directly through injection or indirectly after absorption, the drug is rapidly distributed first through the plasma volume (3 L). If the drug crosses the red blood cell membrane, then its distribution volume will increase to 6 L. It takes about a minute for the entire blood volume to circulate so that the initial distribution of an intravenous bolus is complete in a few minutes. Drug distribution is affected by conditions that affect blood flow such as hemorrhage or shock.

As the drug circulates in the blood, it has opportunities to enter interstitial water, cells of various organs, the brain, and adipose or skeletal tissue. The extent and the tissues to which a drug distributes are a function of the drug's chemical nature, and also depend on patient-specific factors such as body composition (obese, lean, edema) and physiologic state (level of activity, pregnancy).

More polar drugs will preferentially remain in an aqueous phase (blood, lymph, interstitial fluid), while less polar drugs may pass through a number of membranes and enter the adipose tissue. They may accumulate in large amounts, as does delta⁹-tetrahydrocannabinol, the active ingredient in marijuana. Un-ionized lipid-soluble drugs with a molecular weight below 600 will very rapidly cross membranes.

The extent of distribution or volume to which the drug is distributed is referred to as the volume of distribution or V_d and is expressed in units of L/kg.

In practical terms, the V_d of a given drug can be determined by measuring the blood concentration of an intravenous dose of the drug after equilibration has occurred. The following equation is used:

$$V_d = \text{Total dose (mg)}/\text{Blood concentration (mg/L)}$$

The result is expressed in liters and can be further divided by the patient's weight to give a result in L/kg which can be universally applied to patients of varying weights. This illustrates part of the reason drugs are often dosed based upon the patient's weight. The desired blood concentration is the total dose divided by the amount of "space" available. For example, a six-foot, 250-pound man will have more space and require a larger dose to achieve the same blood concentration as a four-foot, 85-pound woman.

Drugs accumulated in deep tissues such as the adipose tissue (i.e., THC) or skeletal tissue (i.e., digoxin) will have extremely high V_d values, often of several hundred liters, which translates into $>1 - 10$ L/kg.

This has a number of practical consequences such as determining drug dosage for an obese patient. If the drug distributes into lipid tissue, the dose for the obese patient must be larger than for the lean individual. On the other hand, drugs primarily distributed in the aqueous phase are dosed based on the obese patient's ideal weight. In this latter case, doses based on actual weight would lead to toxicity.

Distribution has other implications as well. The more widely distributed throughout the body, the more likely the drug will be slowly eliminated and, consequently, accumulate in a particular tissue (i.e., adipose) if taken over a long period. The example already mentioned, delta⁹-tetrahydrocannabinol, distributes into lipid tissues and may be gradually excreted in urine for a month or more after its last use.

Protein binding. An equilibrium exists in the blood between drug bound to protein and unbound, or "free," drug. Protein-bound drug is not able to cross membranes, either to exert its therapeutic effect or to be metabolized and excreted. The active portion of the drug is the unbound amount. Drugs can also enter cells of various tissues and become bound in those tissues. Some drugs are so highly protein bound (85% to 95%) that conditions that affect the fraction of the total bound drug can profoundly affect the pharmacokinetics and pharmacodynamics of the drug.

One of the processes affected by protein binding is the volume of distribution of the drug. As a drug's binding to plasma proteins increases, the drug's V_d decreases. Also affected is the body's ability to remove the drug through metabolism and excretion, both of which may be increased as free drug increases. This will depend, however, on whether the drug is rapidly ("high extraction") or slowly ("low extraction") cleared by the liver.

The two plasma proteins primarily involved in drug binding are albumin and alpha₁-acid glycoprotein. Albumin binds acidic drugs, some basic drugs, and many endogenous hormones; alpha₁-acid glycoprotein binds most basic drugs and some hormones.

Since the binding process is in equilibrium, any factor that shifts that equilibrium can potentially alter the fraction of unbound drug. Such factors as competition between two drugs or between a drug and an endogenous compound such as bilirubin or fatty acid can shift this equilibrium. A decrease in plasma proteins results in fewer total binding sites and increased unbound drug. Albumin can be decreased by aging, burns, cancer, cardiac failure, trauma, liver disease, nephrotic syndrome, pregnancy, and surgery. Alpha₁-acid glycoprotein is an acute phase reactant protein that increases during physiological stress and decreases as a result of many of the same conditions that decrease albumin.

Blood concentration versus time curves. In order to evaluate the pharmacokinetics for a particular drug in an individual, a series of blood samples are taken over a period of time, usually several hours, and the concentration of drug in these samples is plotted as a function of time (Figure 23-3).

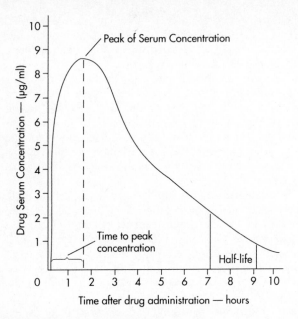

Fig. 23-3 Drug concentration in blood versus time curve for an orally administered drug. *Redrawn from Koch-Weser J: NEJM 291:234, 1974.*

BLOOD LEVEL
Semilog paper

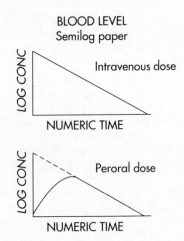

Fig. 23-4 The open one compartment model for intravenous and oral dosing. *From Ritschel WA: Handbook of basic pharmacokinetics— including clinical applications, ed 4, Hamilton, IL, 1992, Drug Intelligence Publications, Inc.*

Several pharmacokinetic aspects of drugs are readily apparent from the plot. Among these aspects are the time it takes a drug to reach peak level (i.e., an intravenous dose peaks immediately after infusion while an oral dose takes longer). The shape of the curve as it descends from the peak provides information about the distribution of the drug, and the final linear portion of the curve represents the elimination phase, during which metabolism and excretion occur. This linear portion also allows for calculation of drug elimination half-life.

The shape of the curve relates to how the drug is distributed in the body and therefore indicates the mathematical model that will most accurately predict the pharmacokinetics.

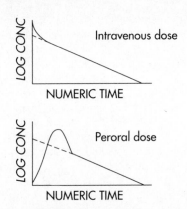

Fig. 23-5 The open two compartment model for intravenous and oral dosing. *From Ritschel WA: Handbook of basic pharmacokinetics— including clinical applications, ed 4, Hamilton, IL, 1992, Drug Intelligence Publications, Inc.*

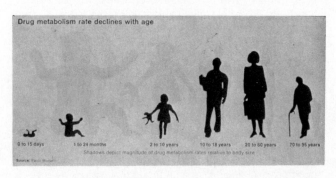

Fig. 23-6 Drug metabolizing capacity as a function of age.

Compartment models. The two primary mathematical models used to determine the pharmacokinetic parameters involve the use of compartments. Compartments are a way of mathematically handling an extremely complex physiological process through arbitrary division of the body into a series of fluid-filled containers into which the drug can move. In the open one compartment model, the body is considered to be a single container with the drug distributing simultaneously throughout. When this happens the logarithm of the blood concentration versus time curve, as shown in Figure 23-4, gives a straight line from the peak blood level to the point where the drug becomes nondetectable.

In the open two compartment model, the drug undergoes a longer distribution phase because it is moving into an additional compartment. As a result, the blood concentration versus time curve demonstrates two phases after the peak blood level is reached: an initial slow distribution phase followed by a linear elimination phase (Figure 23-5).

Metabolism

As the drug distributes, it comes in contact with a number of plasma and tissue enzymes, which may cause chemical changes in the parent drug. Drugs ingested orally may undergo some metabolism by the bacterial flora even before absorption. The principal site of metabolism is the liver. However, some metabolism occurs in the kidney, muscle, and gut wall. In the liver, metabolic enzymes are variously

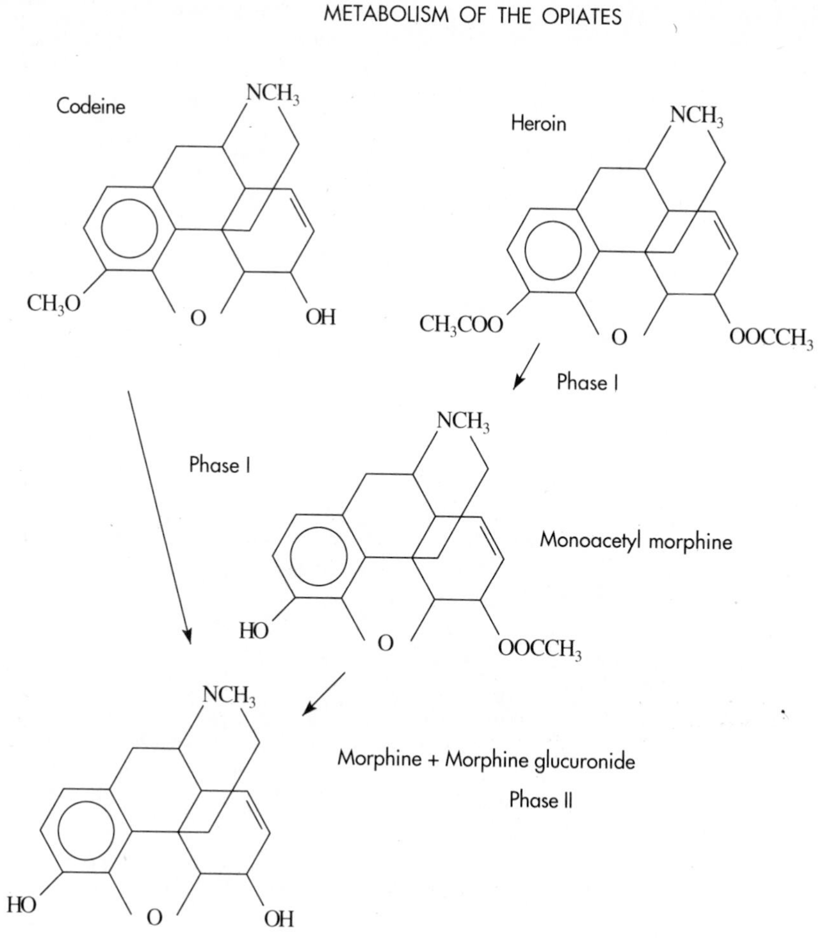

METABOLISM OF THE OPIATES

Fig. 23-7 Example of drug metabolism reactions illustrated by morphine.

present in the microsomal, mitochondrial, and soluble cell fractions.

First pass metabolism. Drugs ingested orally and therefore absorbed across the gastrointestinal tract enter the portal vein and pass directly into the liver before reaching any other part of the body. Some drugs are so efficiently extracted and metabolized by the liver that little parent drug exits this organ to be distributed to the rest of the body. Drugs that undergo extensive first pass metabolism must be dosed in an alternate fashion, usually intravenously.

Hepatic metabolism. Metabolism in the hepatocytes is of two main types: non-synthetic, or Phase I, reactions and synthetic, or Phase II, reactions. The purpose of the liver's metabolic efforts is to transform the nonpolar parent drug into a more polar, and thus water soluble, metabolite. With increasing water solubility, the body is able to more efficiently excrete the drug through the kidney. Usually, metabolites are less active and less toxic than parent drug, although this is not always the case. Both primidone and procainamide are metabolized to active metabolites, phenobarbital and N-acetylprocainamide, respectively, which also need to be considered when these drugs are used therapeutically.

Phase I reactions introduce or uncover polar groups through oxidation, reduction, and hydrolysis reactions. This is often followed by a Phase II reaction which results in a conjugation of the polar group (i.e., acid or hydroxy) with glycine, glucuronic acid, or a sulphate group. Glucuronidation is the major conjugation reaction by which humans deal with drugs as well as endogenous substrates.

Some drugs will have a stimulating effect on the hepatic-metabolizing enzymes. An example of this is phenobarbital, an anticonvulsant, which induces the enzyme responsible for glucuronide formation. After a few weeks of phenobarbital use, the patient may require an increased dose of phenobarbital and possibly an increased dose of other drugs they are taking.

The body's capacity to metabolize drugs, environmental chemicals, and natural substrates varies with age (Figure 23-6). During the first two weeks of life, this capacity is very low. This is probably because the neonate enzyme systems are not functioning at full capacity, and/or because enzyme concentrations are decreased. After the first two weeks, the infant, for the first year, develops a metabolic capacity that greatly exceeds that of an adult, and it remains high until puberty.

The decrease in metabolic activity at puberty may be due, in part, to the increasing competition for the metabolic systems by the natural substrates of these enzymes, in particular the steroid hormones. The change from rapid to slower metabolism for some drugs may be comparatively sudden so that a child well maintained on a particular dose of, for example, anticonvulsant, may begin to develop signs of toxicity and thus require a reduced dose.

Adult metabolic rates decrease with age due to the interplay of a number of processes occurring in the individual.

Drugs are frequently metabolized by several reactions or combinations of Phase I and Phase II reactions so that a number of metabolites are formed (Figure 23-7). Enough is known about drug metabolism so that the structures of these metabolites can be predicted. It should also be mentioned that some drugs are administered as *prodrugs*, which require metabolism to the active drug. Compounds chosen to be dosed as prodrugs are usually chemically unstable, not readily soluble, or poorly absorbed.

Elimination

Drugs are eliminated through a number of routes including tears, saliva, bile, feces, expired air, sweat, and breast milk. However, by far the most important route of elimination is through the kidney into the urine. Whether a drug is excreted unchanged as the parent drug or transformed into one or more metabolites, or a combination of the two, depends on the chemical nature of the drug.

In drug testing where urine is the specimen, the analyst must know the chemical structure of the major metabolite of the drug of interest so that an assay can be designed to identify that metabolite.

Drugs excreted into bile undergo recycling, since the bile empties into the gut and the drug can then be reabsorbed into the blood stream. Such recycling can have important consequences when a drug that undergoes such recycling is taken in overdose. A therapeutic approach would be to have the patient drink a suspension containing charcoal in order to bind the drug as it reenters the gut and prevent its reabsorption. Charcoal is also frequently used when ingestion of a large amount of unknown drug is suspected. Charcoal lessens absorption of the drug as much as possible.

Drug clearance. Clearance of drugs involves either metabolism or excretion or both. The major clearance mechanisms—whether hepatic, renal, or a combination of the two—must be known for drugs given to patients with kidney or hepatic failure. For example, a drug mainly cleared by the liver may be affected by liver perfusion, which is decreased in congestive heart failure and shock. Intact drugs or metabolites cleared by the kidney will require much lower doses in patients suffering renal failure.

The rate of clearance of drug from the blood can be determined during the terminal elimination phase. This rate is referred to as half-life, which is the time required for the blood concentration of drug at equilibrium to decrease by one half. Half-life is important in establishing or adjusting dosing schedules for therapeutic drugs. Half-life determinations are also important for the physician treating an acetaminophen overdose. By determining the drug concentration in two timed specimens, the half-life can be calculated from semi-log graph paper, as illustrated in Figure 23-8.

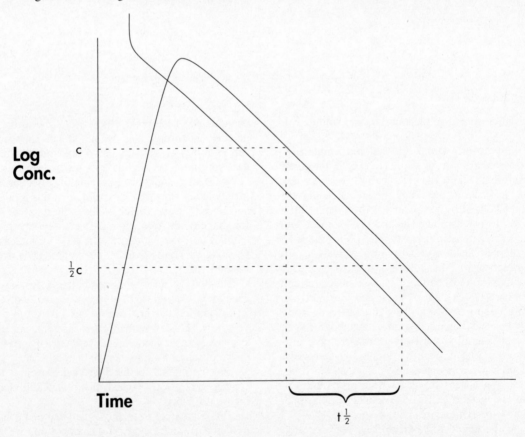

Fig. 23-8 Example of a half-life calculation for acetaminophen elimination. As blood drug concentrations obtained at various times fall, the time difference for each halving of concentration gives the elimination t½ (half-life).

Kinetics of drug elimination. Most of the pharmacokinetic processes—absorption, distribution, metabolism, and excretion—can be described by either zero- or first-order kinetics. In a first-order, or linear, reaction, the rate of change of concentration of the drug in blood is proportional to the concentration of drug (Figure 23-9). A constant percentage of drug is eliminated per unit of time. In zero-order reactions, a constant amount, rather than a constant percentage, of drug is eliminated per unit of time (drug concentration does not affect rate) (Figure 23-10).

Since nearly all the metabolism of drugs is catalyzed by enzymes with a limited capacity, the kinetics of metabolism are best described by Michaelis-Menton kinetics, which are affected by concentration. At low drug concentrations, the process will follow first order, with a constant percentage of the drug metabolized. At high concentrations of drug, the capacity of the enzyme will be exceeded and the process will become pseudo-zero order, with a constant amount of drug metabolized per unit of time.

When drugs are taken in overdose, their elimination may change from first order to zero order as large amounts of drug saturate the capacity of hepatic enzymes. The impact of the type of kinetics operating can be readily seen in the dosing of the anticonvulsant, phenytoin. This drug is eliminated by first-order kinetics at low concentrations. However, as the concentration increases, the kinetics demonstrate saturation elimination kinetics. This can result in rapid increases in drug concentration in blood with the appearance

of toxicity. The amount of dose causing this change varies dramatically from patient to patient, as illustrated in Figure 23-11.

APPLICATION OF PHARMACOKINETICS TO THERAPEUTIC DRUG DOSING
Steady state

A drug can be used in the intermittent treatment of occasional problems. Examples include over-the-counter medications such as acetaminophen for headache and antihistamines for allergic reactions. In these situations, a single dose of the drug may suffice, unless symptoms persist. However, in many treatment situations, a drug is prescribed over a long period to prevent problems (i.e., seizures) or to ameliorate a chronic condition (i.e., hypertension). The physician must determine the dosage regimen; that is, the size and frequency of the drug dose.

As multiple doses of drug are taken by the patient, the blood concentration curve shown in Figure 23-3 is replaced by a series of curves. As shown in Figure 23-12 the blood level after each dose is higher than the previous one, until a steady blood concentration or steady state is achieved. "Steady state" means drug intake is balanced by the clearance of the drug from the body. The patient will have a relatively constant concentration of drug in the blood.

Therapeutic range

Steady state blood concentrations high enough to be effective and low enough to avoid toxicity are said to be in the therapeutic range. The purpose of the dosage regimen is to achieve concentrations within the therapeutic range. If the level is below the range, the patient cannot be expected to respond clinically to the drug. If the dose results in levels which exceed the range, the patient may accumulate potentially toxic amounts. If the time between doses is too long, widely fluctuating concentrations of the drug may leave the patient above or below the therapeutic level for a portion of each dosing interval. If the time between doses of an

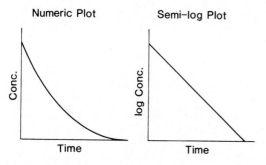

Fig. 23-9 Concentration verus time curves in first order and zero order kinetics. *From Ritschel WA: Therapeutic drug monitoring. In Kaplan LA and Pesce AJ: Clinical chemistry: theory, analysis, and correlation, St. Louis, 1984, Mosby-Year Book, Inc.*

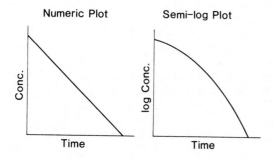

Fig. 23-10 Concentration versus time curves zero order kinetics. *From Ritschel WA: Therapeutic drug monitoring. In Kaplan LA and Pesce AJ: Clinical chemistry: theory, analysis, and correlation, St. Louis, 1984, Mosby-Year Book, Inc.*

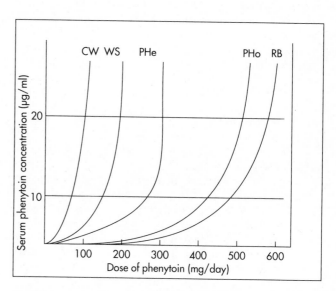

Fig. 23-11 Examples of the variety of individual responses to phenytoin dosing. *From Richens A and Dunlop A: Lancet 2:247, 1975.*

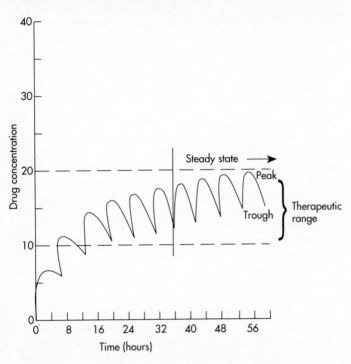

Fig. 23-12 Attainment of steady state drug concentrations with multiple dosing.

Table 23-2 Effect of half-life on drug elimination and attainment of steady state

Half-life number	% Concentration remaining	% Steady state attained
0	100.0	0
1	50.0	50.0
2	25.0	75.0
3	12.5	87.5
4	6.3	93.8
5	3.1	96.9
6	1.7	98.4
7	0.8	99.2

Rule 1. Drug concentrations must always be interpreted in the context of the clinical status of the patient.

Rule 2. Everyone is different.

Pharmacokinetics are an individual set of processes affected by genetics and such physiological variables as age, sex, weight, health habits, and health status. Identical twins have very similar pharmacokinetics. However, fraternal twins and the general population have greater differences.

The need for individualized dosing for phenytoin is illustrated in Figure 23-11 and theophylline in Figure 23-13. These figures show the individual response to various dosing regimens.

Therapeutic drug monitoring

With the increasing use of drugs in medical treatment, misadventure with drugs may be more common than is recognized. Drug toxicity or drug interactions, particularly among the elderly, who often take a number of medications at once, may masquerade as physical and mental illness.

In the millenium before blood concentration monitoring of drugs became readily available, drugs were used in conjunction with careful observation of the patient's condition, whether by medicine man, witch doctor, or physician. The easiest drugs to use were those for the treatment of a constant condition. For example, drugs used to treat high blood pressure can be monitored by measurement of blood pressure. Anticoagulant medication can be checked by measuring the clotting of the patient's blood. When a drug is used to treat an intermittent condition, physiologic or indirect monitoring becomes much more difficult. A good example is the treatment of seizure disorders. Since seizures occur intermittently, drug therapy can only be presumed to be working if the patient remains seizure free over a period of time. The main difficulty is giving enough drug to keep the patient free of seizures, but not so much that it will cause toxic side effects. In the past, this type of treatment was very much a trial and error process that sometimes required extended periods of time and experimentation with various drugs, combinations, and dosage regimens before the patient was comfortably controlled. In this type of situation, pharmacokinetics has a great deal to offer the patient and clinician.

In an ideal world, pharmacodynamic evaluation, combined with measuring the concentration of the drug at its receptor, would be the best way to determine the most effective way to dose drugs. Such sophisticated technology has yet to be developed, and study of receptors is a fledgling

antibiotic or an anticonvulsant is too long, the appearance of drug resistant organisms or seizures, respectively, may result.

Elimination half-life

The time required for a patient to reach steady state varies with the drug and the person and is related to the elimination half-life of the drug. As discussed earlier, drug half-life ($t_{1/2}$) is the time required for the blood concentration of the drug to decrease by one half. Drug half-life is calculated from the final linear portion of the blood concentration curve. How rapidly the patient gets rid of the drug also dictates the amount of time needed to reach steady state. The half-life table (Table 23-2) shows that the steady state will be attained in approximately five to seven half-lives. After a dosage change, the patient will require another five to seven half-lives to reach a new steady state.

Conversely, if the drug is discontinued after steady state is attained, the drug will require five to seven half-lives to disappear from the blood.

Through the use of a loading dose, a patient can achieve a therapeutic concentration without waiting for steady state. This is why at the beginning of therapy, the patient may be given a large amount of the drug, followed by a smaller maintenance dose. The patient will achieve steady state more rapidly after an appropriate loading dose, since it results in more rapid accumulation of the drug.

Some drugs have extremely short half-lives, and steady state may be achieved in a few hours. Others have half-lives of days, and steady state may require weeks.

Differences in pharmacokinetics

Below are two rules that need to be remembered by anyone involved in therapeutic drug dosing and monitoring:

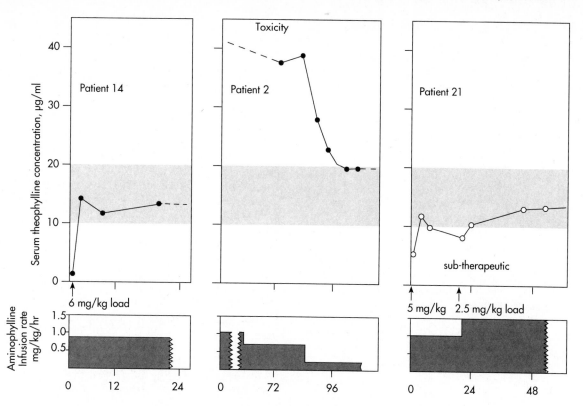

Fig. 23-13 Examples of individual response to dosage regimens for theophylline. *From Wernberger M, et al: JAMA 235:2110-2113, 1976.*

science. In the meantime, TDM is based on the next best thing: blood concentration determination. It is apparent that there are difficulties with this choice. One reason so few drugs are monitored routinely is that either the relationship between that drug's blood concentration and its effect has not been established or the two have not been found to correlate.

Even with correlation, blood concentration is only an indirect indication of what is happening pharmacodynamically at the drug's receptor. In many cases, this is good enough.

Urine specimen testing is a very limited pharmacokinetic process. This is mainly due to the differences in excretion patterns from one random sample to another due to the effects of activity, fluid intake, and cyclical changes on urine constitution. In order to relate anything found in urine to the entire organism, at the very least a timed specimen is needed. A random specimen of blood, on the other hand, is under tighter homeostatic controls and thus can yield a great deal of information although, in the case of drug assays, timing factors need to be considered. Urine concentrations in random samples cannot, therefore, be related to blood concentrations and subsequently to drug effect. This is why urine is not used for TDM and, when used for toxicological or drug abuse testing, urine results are not reported as quantitative values.

Unbound drugs

Measuring the total amount of drug in blood is not always the best choice. In some situations, total drug concentration can be misleading, and the unbound drug level is needed to understand the patient's response. This applies to drugs that are ~85% or greater in bound form.

Drugs are primarily bound to albumin and alpha$_1$-acid glycoprotein. Conditions that alter the amount of serum proteins or the number of binding sites will affect the amount of unbound drug in the plasma.

For example, at a therapeutic concentration of 10 mcg/mL, and 90% binding, the concentration of free drug will be 1 mcg/mL. If for some reason the binding of the drug is decreased at the same total drug concentration, the amount of unbound drug can increase several fold. A decrease in binding to 80% at the same total concentration of 10 mcg/mL would increase unbound drug from 1 to 2 mcg/mL. The unbound concentration has been doubled by a 10% decrease in binding.

Unbound drug concentrations are monitored only when the easily measured total concentration is not good enough. This is because unbound drug concentrations are technically harder to measure.

Typically, measuring unbound drugs requires removing protein-bound drug from the sample prior to analysis. This is most easily done with an ultrafiltration device that retards the passage of the proteins and provides an ultrafiltrate containing only unbound drug. Free drug concentrations will be much lower than the total drug measurements, and thus more sensitive analytical methods may be required.

Guidelines for therapeutic drug monitoring

A number of criteria must be met for the most effective application of TDM. These criteria explain why particular drugs have been chosen for monitoring.

1. Blood concentrations of the drug correlate with therapeutic and/or toxic effects, and blood concentrations vary from patient to patient on similar dosage regimens.

This is the most important criteria since, if no relationship exists between blood level and drug effect, then TDM will not be effective in evaluating patient response to the drug. All drugs which are currently routinely monitored have been studied, and therapeutic ranges have been established. These studies further revealed that different patients responded to different dosage regimens. Timing of the blood sample so that it correlates best with patient response was also determined.

For example, the cardiac drug digoxin undergoes an extremely long distribution phase of at least six hours, during which the drug distributes into skeletal and heart muscle. Only after this distribution do blood levels correlate (indirectly) with the amount of drug in the target organ, the heart. If blood levels are drawn too soon after the dose, the erroneous impression that a toxic amount of the drug is present could result in a lowered dosage, leaving the patient without effective therapy.

2. The drug has a low therapeutic index (TI). This means that the dose providing the therapeutic effect is very close to the dose that causes toxicity.

$$TI = \text{Toxic Dose}/\text{Therapeutic dose}.$$

The closer this ratio is to 1, the more difficult the drug is to use. General anesthetics have a TI of 1 because the therapeutic dose that produces anesthesia will also cause death if supportive measures, such as respiratory assistance, are not used. However, these drugs are not monitored since the patient's vital signs are followed and supported.

On the other hand, for drugs with low therapeutic indices used outside the hospital setting, monitoring can be very important. Digoxin and theophylline are two such drugs.

If a drug has a high therapeutic index and, therefore, a toxic dose many times greater than the therapeutic dose, there will be little need for monitoring since, if the patient doesn't respond, more drug can be safely given. Penicillin is an example of this type of drug. It can be used in massive doses, with no toxic effects. This may seem a strange example since extremely small doses of penicillin have resulted in death. However, this "toxicity" is due to an anaphylactic allergic reaction to the drug and is unrelated to dose or pharmacokinetics. In sensitive individuals, no amount of penicillin is safe.

3. The drug is being used to treat an intermittent condition. The resulting pharmacodynamic effect of the drug is hard to evaluate.

As already mentioned, anticonvulsant drugs fall into this category along with theophylline, which is used to treat asthma and is the most frequently monitored drug in most laboratories. Measuring the blood concentrations of these drugs rapidly ensures that the patient is receiving sufficient drug to achieve a steady state in the therapeutic range without going through extended periods of trial-and-error dosing.

This will provide the patient with the confidence that his/her condition is being controlled, and it can prevent toxic side effects by helping to establish the smallest amount of drug needed to achieve the therapeutic range.

4. It must be determined whether patient symptoms are due to drug toxicity. Reasons for failure of therapy must be evaluated.

A common reason for therapeutic failures is the patient not taking the drug. This, along with identifying situations where the dose needs to be increased, are possible by measuring blood concentrations.

Blood concentration information can also assist the physician when the patient has problems. It can be rapidly determined, for example, whether seizures are occurring because of a subtherapeutic drug level, inadequate dose, patient noncompliance, or a toxic reaction. If a therapeutic level is found, it may indicate that the patient is resistant to this drug and needs either a higher-than-usual dose or another drug.

A number of drugs cause toxic reactions similar to the condition for which the drug is being used to treat. For example, tricyclic antidepressant toxicity can result in a return of depression. Hence, it is difficult at times to determine whether the drug is subtherapeutic or toxic from a clinical assessment. Blood concentrations are a great help in sorting out these situations.

5. The effects of other drugs or diseases on the drug concentration must be assessed.

An example of drug interaction that can be identified with TDM is the effect of quinidine on digoxin. If patients on digoxin have quinidine added to their regimen, the digoxin concentration in 90% of patients will increase within two to three days, sufficient to cause toxicity. The usual decrease in digoxin dose required to counteract this effect is 50%. Affected patients can be readily identified by a check of their digoxin concentrations 24 to 48 hours after quinidine is started.

A second example is the interaction of two anticonvulsants, phenobarbital and valproic acid. When valproic acid is given to a patient taking phenobarbital, the phenobarbital levels increase after 24 to 26 days.

Drug interactions causing changes such as these can be due to a number of factors such as competition between the two drugs for metabolic enzymes, resulting in decreased metabolism of one of the two; the displacement of one drug from binding sites in plasma or cellular proteins; effects on absorption; or unidentified effects. Drug interaction studies are increasingly important as the population ages, since the elderly are frequently treated with several drugs which, if not carefully monitored, can result in significant problems. Effects on mental functioning may be difficult to differentiate from deterioration occurring because of the aging process. In the next few years the elderly patient will become a major focus of pharmacokinetic studies.

6. Evaluate the patient on chronic drug treatment so the dosage regimen can be adjusted in response to physical changes.

Children who receive anticonvulsant or cardiac drugs, like theophylline or digoxin, need their blood concentrations checked on a regular schedule so that doses can be increased in response to growth. Since drug doses are based on patient weight, a growing child will need gradual increases in dosage.

In addition, as already mentioned, at puberty, monitoring is needed to identify when the child should be changed to adult dosage schedules due to the slowdown of metabolism.

In adult patients, routine monitoring will detect changes due to lifestyle or health changes. For example, smokers metabolize theophylline faster than nonsmokers. A person on theophylline who stops smoking will require a downward adjustment in dose.

Other health factors that require reassessment of drug therapy include weight changes, pregnancy, and kidney or liver disease.

Most drugs that are monitored fulfill one or more of these criteria. Table 23-3 lists the categories and specific drugs that are currently routinely monitored.

Patient information needed for therapeutic drug monitoring

Unlike most of the blood components which are usually collected whenever convenient, samples for drug concentrations must be collected at specific times in order for results to yield useful information.

The following information will be required in addition to the laboratory value in order to apply pharmacokinetic calculations to a particular patient.

1. Time of last dose
2. Amount of last dose
3. Dosing regimen
4. Dosing route (i.e., intravenous, oral)
5. Time of dosing regimen
6. Time of phlebotomy
7. Patient age, weight, and sex
8. Other concurrent medications

Recommendations have been developed for commonly monitored drugs with regard to when blood concentration monitoring will be most useful. For a large number of drugs, the recommended timing is immediately prior to the next dose, or trough level. Trough level is when the drug concentration is at its lowest (Figure 23-12). Trough levels are best for routine checking to ensure that the patient has achieved the therapeutic range and remains in that range. From a timing standpoint, trough levels are also the easiest samples to obtain reliably, since the patient can be scheduled for phlebotomy based on their drug-taking schedule, and since the patient can be instructed not to take medication until after blood is drawn.

Peak concentrations are recommended for some drugs, and these are slightly more problematic. If a drug is being given intravenously, it is a simple matter to sample for the drug assay at the end of the infusion. However, it becomes more difficult to assess peak levels of drugs taken orally, since time to peak will vary among patients, and timing of the phlebotomy may be more difficult.

Sampling is also recommended at the time a patient exhibits toxic symptoms or lack of therapeutic effect (i.e., sampling at the time of an asthmatic attack or seizure).

Regardless of sampling time, it is extremely important that the time of the blood sample in relation to the time of the last dose is documented for each sample, so that any changes from the ideal timing can be considered when using the data for dosage adjustment.

The individual evaluating the patient also must establish how long the patient has been on a particular dosage regimen in order to determine if the patient is at steady state. Dosage changes require five to seven half-lives before the new steady state is achieved. In the past it was recommended that all monitoring occur only after steady state was achieved. Today, however, computer programs can predict, on the basis of how the patient handled the initial doses, the steady state level. Such programs can further suggest alternative dosing regimens if the predicted steady state level is sub-therapeutic or toxic.

Such calculations, combined with the laboratory's ability to rapidly and accurately analyze drugs, can be very effective in providing better patient care. Numerous studies have shown that proper use of this type of patient evaluation will result in faster, more effective therapy and thus more rapid discharge of patients from the hospital which, in this day of managed care and reimbursement limitations, can be an effective way for a hospital to decrease costs.

SUGGESTED READING

Katzung BG: Basic and clinical pharmacology, ed 2, Los Altos, Ca, 1984, Lange Medical Publications.

Ritschel WA: Handbook of basic pharmacokinetics, ed 3, Hamilton, Ill, 1986, Drug Intelligence Publications.

Ritschel WA: Therapeutic drug monitoring (TDM). In Kaplan LA and Pesce AJ: Clinical chemistry: theory, analysis and correlation, ed 2, St. Louis, 1989, Mosby–Year Book, Inc.

Yesavage JA, Leirer VO, Denari M, and Hollister LE: Carry-over effects of marijuana intoxication on aircraft pilot performance: a preliminary report, Am J Psychiatry 142:1325-1329, 1988.

Table 23-3 Drugs commonly monitored in blood

Drug class	Drug name	Drug class	Drug name
Antibiotics:	Amikacin	Cardiac drugs:	Digitoxin
	Gentamicin		Digoxin
	Tobramycin		Lidocaine
	Vancomycin		Procainamide*
			Quinidine
Anticonvulsants:	Carbamazepine	Other:	Caffeine
	Ethosuximide		Cyclosporine
	Phenobarbital		Lithium
	Phenytoin		Methotrexate
	Primidone*		Salicylate
	Valproic acid		Theophylline

*Metabolites are also monitored.

24

Techniques of drug analysis

Louis Steinert
Norman Coffman

The reasons for the analysis of drugs are varied and the techniques for measuring them are almost as numerous as the drugs themselves. Proper matching of need and technique demands that one first have a clear understanding of the reasons the test is being performed, and secondly that the tentatively chosen technique can meet those needs. Thus, a properly functioning laboratory will work with those who use the test results to provide a product or answer which is both timely and appropriate. It is also mandatory that the specimens chosen are those which will contain the drug of interest and in which the drug concentrations will be related to the clinical conditions.

Thus, the analysis of drugs demands an understanding of the needs of the recipient of the test results and of the available technologies. The correct mixing of clinical requirements and analytical methods can result in laboratory answers which are very useful.

COLORIMETRIC TEST METHODS

Colorimetric test methods usually include all the analytical techniques in which the analyte either absorbs electromagnetic radiation in the range of 185-800 nm or can be made to undergo a chemical reaction where a reaction product will absorb light in that range. This includes both spot tests and the more sophisticated ultraviolet or visible spectrophotometry. Methods requiring chromatographic separations are explained later in this chapter, even though colorimetric or spectrophotometric techniques are often used as the detection techniques of the instruments utilized.

COLORIMETRIC METHODS THEORY

Electromagnetic radiation, or photons, can be absorbed by a molecule or ion only if that molecule or ion has an electron in the lower of two electron orbitals separated by an energy identical to the energy of that photon. Electron orbitals also have symmetry (shape), and absorption is more or less probable depending upon the relative compatibilities of the symmetries of the two orbitals involved in the photon's absorption. This latter requirement is the reason some materials absorb light readily and have high extinction coefficients while others absorb light poorly and have low extinction coefficients.

Table 24-1 Effect of conjugation upon absorption maxima

Molecule	Major structure	Maximum absorption (nm)
$CH_3CH_2 = CH_2$ (1−butene)	lone pi bond	185
$CH_2 = CHCH = CH_2$ (1, 3−butadiene)	conjugated pi bonds	217
C_6H_6 (benzene)	conjugated pi bonds	256
C_6H_5OH (phenol)	conjugated pi— lone pair	270
$C_{10}H_8$ (naphthalene)	extended conjugated pi	312

In practice, orbitals which are conducive for the absorption of uv and visible light are commonly found only on organic chemicals with pi bonding (unsaturated) electrons or lone pairs of electrons, or on metal ions. In general, these types of materials can be analyzed by colorimetric tests. It is also found that conjugation of double bonds, that is, the alternation of single and double bonds, such as is found in butadiene or in aromatic compounds such as benzene, results in shifting of the absorption to longer wavelengths (lower energies). For example, 1-butene has an absorption maximum at 184 nm while 1,3-butadiene has the corresponding absorption maximum at 217 nm. It is also found that the longer the chain of conjugation in a given series, the longer the wavelength of maximum absorption. (See Table 24-1.)

SPOT TESTS

The simplest colorimetric tests are qualitative and rely on the analyst's eyes for detection. In general, these tests are referred to as spot tests. Spot tests are simple in design, and it is this simplicity which makes them valuable.

Spot tests need to be sensitive. False negative results are to be rigorously excluded. The tests need to be sensitive enough that positive patients are always identified. Since spot tests usually screen for a class or a broad category of compounds, a positive result is usually considered to be presumptive only.

Table 24-2 Spot tests commonly used for drug/toxin analyses

Drug/toxin	Test principle	Remarks
1. Acetaminophen	Reaction with α-naphthol and nitrite produces a red color.	This analysis tests for p-aminophenol, a metabolite of acetaminophen and phenacetin.
2. Alcohols	Sample is delivered directly to the bottom of a stoppered test tube. Glass wool with dichromate solution is placed in tube above sample. Volatile alcohols, etc. diffuse to wool and cause yellow dichromate to turn greenish.	This is a general test for volatile reducing substances including alcohols, aldehydes and ketones. Sensitivity to alcohols and aldehydes <50 ppm; ketones <100 ppm.
3. Barbiturates, glutethimide, ethchlorvynol	Residue from acid chloroform extract of sample is reacted with mercurous nitrate. Blue-purple color indicates barbiturates, etc.	General test for a number of acid hypnotic drugs. Sensitivity varies with drug.
4. Carbon monoxide in blood	Diluted blood is alkalinized with NaOH. The more stable carboxyhemoglobin remains red while the other hemoglobins turn brownish or straw colored.	The limit of detection is approximately 20% carboxyhemoglobin. Smokers can have concentrations up to 10%.
5. Oxidizing agents	The sample is reacted with acid diphenylamine. A blue color shows the presence of oxidizing compounds.	Detects a wide variety of oxidizing compounds such as bromate, chlorate, nitrate, and nitrite.
6. Phenothiazines	Ferric-perchloric-nitric (FPN) reagent is added to urine. A pink violet color indicates the presence of phenothiazines.	Good sensitivity but poor specificity. Light pink-orange color appears with dose of 5-20 mg/day. About 125 mg/day gives deep purple.
7. Salicylates	Blood or other fluid is mixed with mercurous chloride, ferric nitrate (Trinder) solution. Centrifugation leaves a purple supernatant.	Very sensitive but not very specific. Color appears at about 1-5 mg/dl.

Rigorous quality control of spot tests is absolutely essential. Since rapid decisions regarding courses of therapy can be based on spot test results, the validity of test results must be determined by the inclusion of both positive and negative controls in the testing protocol. The analyst must have experience with the test since the interpretation of spot tests often requires judgments based on shades of color and rates at which colors develop and/or fade. Color blindness in the analyst can invalidate the test results.

The real advantages of spot tests are:

Simplicity—they usually require little apparatus or instrumentation.

Convenience—they can often be performed near the patient.

Economy—costs per test are usually low.

Reliability—experience in interpretation is usually more important than great technical skill.

A wide variety of spot tests have been developed. Examples of tests used as screening procedures for common drugs or toxic materials are given in Table 24-2.

ULTRAVIOLET/VISIBLE SPECTROPHOTOMETRY

Prior to the development of immunochemical mediated analysis techniques, uv/visible spectrophotometric methods were commonly used for quantifying drugs. These methods are still important where immunochemical probes are not available.

The utility of spectrophotometry comes from the fact that each substance has an absorption spectrum determined by its own structure. The absorption spectrum of any substance is therefore unique to it and can be used for its identification. Furthermore, if a substance follows Beer's Law, the absorbances of solutions of that substance will be linearly related to concentration. Thus the quantity of that substance in unknown samples can be determined.

It is often found that a drug can have multiple forms and this property can be used in its analysis. For example, secobarbital has one un-ionized and two ionized forms. Usually only the name of the parent, un-ionized form is used to represent a drug, with the understanding that all forms of the drug are included. Each form is a unique chemical compound with its own individual solubility, melting point, molecular weight, acidity, and absorption spectrum. The spectra of the singly and doubly ionized forms of secobarbital are shown in Figure 24-1, *A* and 24-1, *B*. The superimposition of these is shown in Figure 24-1, *C*.

These types of spectra can be used to derive qualitative identification of specimens possibly containing secobarbital. In a manner readily suggested from the data shown in Figure 24-1, an aliquot of the unknown is first extracted into a buffer at a pH = 9.9, and an absorption spectrum of the solution is obtained from about 200-400 nm. Next, the solution's pH is adjusted to pH = 14, and a second absorption spectrum is obtained over the same wavelength interval. The two spectra are then overlapped and examined. If the unknown is indeed secobarbital, maxima and minima of the spectra will be found at those wavelengths characteristic of secobarbital. Isosbestic points (the points a and b, where the spectral curves cross because the molar absorptivities of the two forms are identical at those wavelengths) will be found at the previously known characteristic wavelengths. Relative heights of the two curves will be those typical of secobarbital, and the familiar "figure eight on its side" seen in Figure 24-1, *C* will be observed. Very careful work will allow secobarbital to be distinguished from other barbitu-

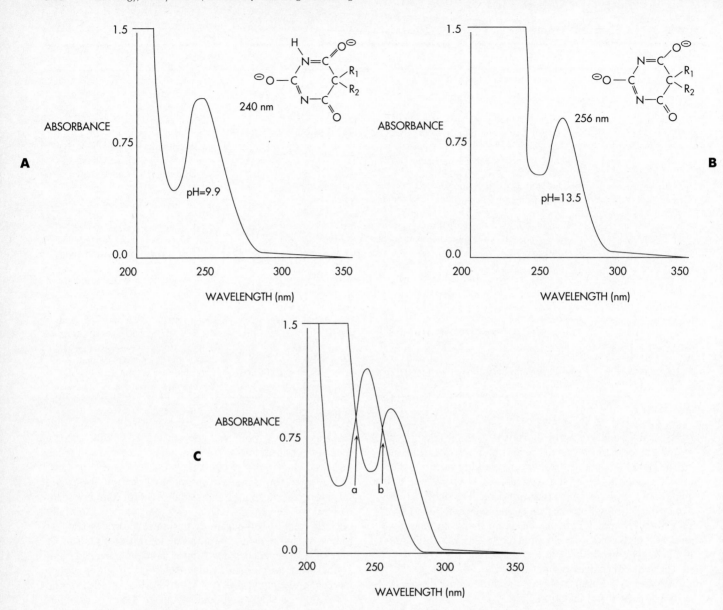

Fig. 24-1   Structures and spectra of **A)** secobarbital^{-1}, and **B)** secobarbital^{-2}, and **C)** the superimposed spectra from **A** and **B** showing isosbestic points *a* and *b*.

rates, many of which have quite similar spectral characteristics. Spectra for many drugs in various solvent systems are available for reference, and can be used to determine a drug's identity. However, it must be recognized that these techniques are only useful with pure substances or with mixtures in which overlapping and interfering absorbances from multiple chemical species in the mixture can be eliminated.

In addition, quantitation can be accomplished or approached in two slightly different ways using these same absorption spectra. First, one could choose to work at either pH = 9.9 or at pH = 14 and simply relate the absorbance at a given wavelength to the Beer's Law curve determined for pure secobarbital at that same wavelength and pH. Alternatively, one could extract secobarbital from a specimen aliquot at pH = 9.9 and determine the absorption spectrum. Next, that same extract would be adjusted to pH = 14 and

again its absorption curve would be obtained. Overlaying the two spectra and measuring the distance between the curves (i.e., determining the absorbance difference at a wavelength where the two curves are widely separated) would allow quantitation by comparison of this difference with a standard curve similarly obtained using pure secobarbital. This second approach will effectively eliminate interferences in many cases where the potentially interfering substance(s) contained in the mixture absorbs light equally whether at pH = 9.9 or at pH = 14.

IMMUNOCHEMICAL MEDIATED ANALYSES

Immunochemical methods of analysis have grown rapidly in recent years and continue to expand. This growth can be attributed to the availability of more specific antibodies, including monoclonals; to the development of more versatile detection methods, and to increasing governmental regulation of the use and disposal of radioactive materials. The latter has been indirectly beneficial as the increased regulation of radiochemicals has spurred the development of better alternative detection methods. This in turn has increased the usefulness of immunological techniques.

Scrutinizing the components of any immunological testing procedure reveals that these methods have certain common functional parts. First, all have an interaction between the analyte (antigen) and an antibody. Second, all have some method of distinguishing, isolating, or separating this antigen-antibody complex from the rest of the reaction mixture. Third, there must be some way in which this uniquely isolated complex can be detected and—if quantitation is desired—accurately measured. Another feature that may be operationally important is whether the reaction components are homogeneous (all contained within one physical phase) or are heterogeneous (distributed between at least two physical phases).

All immunological drug analysis methods start with the association of the drug with an antibody directed against that drug or drug class. In general, free drug molecules (less than 4-5K Daltons) are too small to directly induce antibody production within the immune system of an animal. But these small molecules can act as haptens to elicit the production of antibodies when combined with an immunogen such as a protein. The resultant antibodies can combine with the free drug molecules (haptens) in an antigen-antibody reaction.

The specific part of an antigenic molecule which associates with an antibody is called an epitope. The uniqueness of the epitope determines the specificity of the antibody and thus the specific analytical method. For example, if the epitope for an anti-phenobarbital antibody is the heterocyclic ring (see Figure 24-2), which is constructed of both carbon and nitrogen atoms and is common to all barbiturates, then that antibody will cross-react with any barbiturate. On the other hand, if the epitope includes both the heterocyclic ring and the benzene ring, which is unique to phenobarbital among common barbiturates, then that antibody will be specific for phenobarbital.

The degree of specificity of a given immunologically mediated technique will depend on the uniqueness of the antibody in that assay. Specificity is aided by the use of monoclonal antibodies, while the identification of a class of drugs is aided by the use of polyclonal antibodies or a mixture of monoclonal antibodies. A high degree of specifity is not always desirable. For example, in tests for drugs of abuse, when screening is done for an entire drug class or for those therapeutic drugs where both the parent drug and its metabolites have significant pharmacological activities.

The first stage of an immunological analysis is an antigen-antibody interaction. Antigen-antibody reactions may be either competitive or endpoint. In competitive techniques a limited amount of antibody is present in the reaction mixture. This small amount of antibody is mixed with analyte (antigen) from the patient sample and also with some exogenous, tagged antigen. These three substances are allowed to react competitively until an equilibrium state is reached. (See Figure 24-3A.) If little patient analyte (antigen) is present, then much of the tagged antigen will be bound by the antibody. Conversely, if the concentration of patient

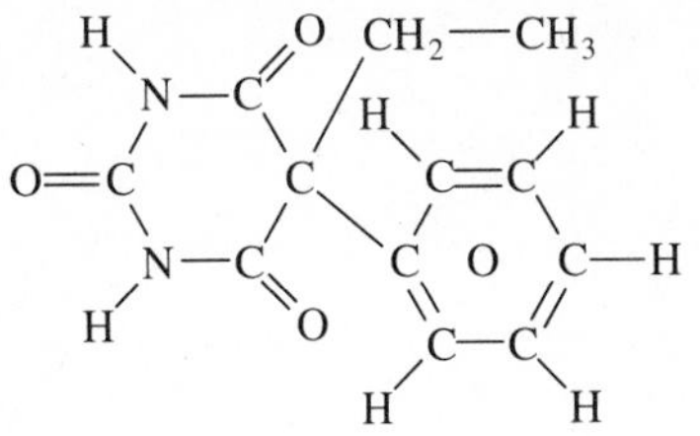

Fig. 24-2 The structure of phenobarbital.

analyte is high, then most of the tagged or labeled antigen will still be free in the reaction mixture. An alternate end-point approach is to use a high avidity antibody in relatively large amounts and therefore to bind all of the analyte in antigen-antibody complexes. (See Figure 24-3, *B*.) With analyses using end-point techniques, the label is often introduced late in the analytical sequence of operations and the label is added in such a fashion that the amount of bound label is directly proportional to the analyte concentration. Measurement of the amount of bound labeled antigen then gives a quantitative measure of the amount of analyte present in the original sample.

The second stage of an immunological analysis is bound antigen versus free antigen discrimination. At some point in the analysis procedure, a process must be employed which will, in effect, separate antigen-antibody complexes from free antigen and/or free antibody. This separation may be either an actual physical separation or alternatively, the reaction mixture may contain a label which has its properties altered upon being incorporated into an antigen-antibody-label complex. This latter approach is usually employed in homogeneous assays. In many assays, sample antigen is allowed to react in solution with antibody. In some early techniques, various organic polymers such as polyethylene glycol (PEG) were added to aid complex formation and precipitation. Centrifugation then caused "insoluble" antigen-antibody complexes to be precipitated onto the bottom of the reaction tube; free fractions were removed by pouring off the supernatant. In another early technique, free antigen was removed by absorption into dextran-coated charcoal. More recently, antibody has been bound to the inner surface of the reaction tube or onto the surface of a bead or other solid support placed into the reaction tube. After the antibody-antigen reaction takes place, unbound molecules are discarded by simply pouring off the liquid from the reaction tube. The competitive, homogeneous EMIT® technique effects the characterization of free versus bound antigen in a quite different manner. This technique mixes a limited amount of antibody with an approximately equivalent amount of a manufactured antigen-enzyme complex. If this complex is bound to antibody, the enzyme is inactivated. As the added sample contains more and more antigen, more antigen-enzyme complex is freed from the antibody and becomes active. Measurement of the reaction mixture's enzyme activity thus is a measurement of the amount of an antigen such as phenytoin or digoxin present in the original standard or unknown sample. Another competitive, homogeneous technique, fluorescence polarization immunoassay (FPIA), relies on the fact that small molecules in

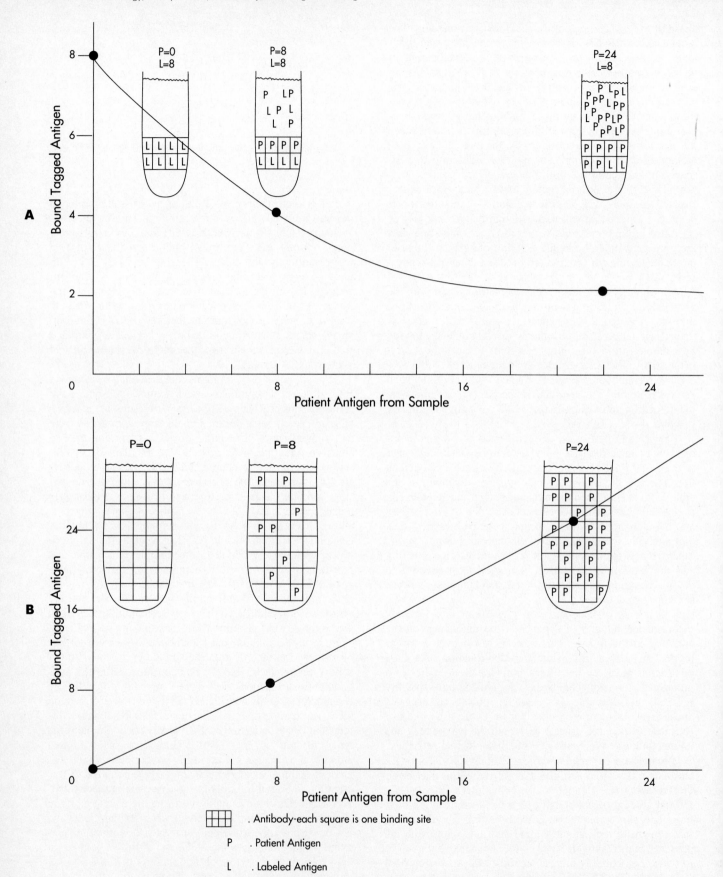

Fig. 24-3 **A,** Binding pattern of tagged antigen in a competitive binding analysis. **B,** Binding pattern of tagged antigen in an endpoint analysis.

solution rotate rapidly while more massive ones rotate more slowly. As small fluorescene-drug complexes are forced from huge antibody-drug-fluorescene complexes by the presence of drug from a patient sample, the amount of fluorescene which is spinning rapidly is increased. FPIA instrumentation detects this shift as increasing scatter (decreasing polarization) of fluorescent light.

The third stage of an immunological analysis is the measurement itself. Detection techniques are just as varied as are separation methods. The first to be widely used was the detection of radiation produced by an unstable isotope incorporated into the exogenous antigen added to the analytical reaction mixture. ^{3}H, a beta radiation emitter with a half-life of 12.3 years, and ^{125}I, which produces gamma radiation and has a half-life of 60.2 days, have been commonly utilized. The main advantage of radioactive isotope labeling is that it allows very sensitive detection limits to be achieved since, theoretically, the distintegration of a single radioactive nucleus can be detected. However, the actual limit for the sensitivity of any radioimmunoassay is a function of the avidity (binding) of the antibody for antigen. Increased avidity gives lower limits of detection or increased sensitivity. This limit of detection must be experimentally determined for each assay. Disadvantages of the use of radioactive labels are radiation hazards and short lifetimes for many reagents.

A second type of label which has achieved very widespread use is enzymes with measurement of their activity. Alkaline phosphatase and glucose-6-phosphate dehydrogenase are two of the more widely used enzymes. After isolation of the desired immunoglobulin-enzyme fraction, the enzyme activity of that fraction is measured. The limit for the sensitivities of enzyme labeled immunoassays has been the relatively low activity of enzymes. Research for more

active enzymes and for enzyme activity multiplication techniques is continuing. Fluorescing molecules have also been used as labels. The theoretically higher sensitivity of fluorescence is well recognized and appealing for use as a probe. However, quenching from many sources has sometimes limited its usefulness.

The fourth stage of an immunological analysis is data reduction. In general, only end point methods incorporating excess antibody give linear responses of reading versus concentration. Other techniques generally produce non-linear responses. Data reduction is usually accomplished utilizing empirically derived mathematical transformations of the data. The transformation that gives the most nearly linear fit of concentration versus response is then used for data reduction. Logarithmic and logit transforms have been found to have especially widespread utility. Statistical tools should be employed to verify the validity of the mathematical analysis of each set of data.

The result is a wide variety of test procedures that are available commercially for many types of analytes. Yet only a few techniques have become widely used for the analysis of drugs. The popularity of these specific methods seems to derive from the concurrent development of instrumentation which allows these methods to be used easily and reliably in clinical and toxicological laboratories. Some of the most widely used techniques are outlined in Table 24-3.

MISCELLANEOUS METHODS

There are several techniques which may not immediately come to mind as methods for drug analysis, but which nevertheless have found widespread use — especially for toxicological work. Among these techniques are Conway

Table 24-3 Common immunological methods for drug analysis

Method	Antigen-antibody interaction	Characterization of bound versus free antigen	Detection method
1. RIA Radioimmunoassay. (Heterogeneous)	Sample antigen plus radioactive nuclide labeled antigen compete for limited antibody binding sites.	Bound antigen is separated from free by binding with second antibody. Alternatively, antibody is bound to test tube walls, bead, or magnetic particles. Free antigen is removed by rinsing.	Bound radioactive label is measured by gamma ray, for ^{125}I, or scintillation, for ^{3}H, detector. See Note 1.
2. EMIT® Enzyme Multiplied Immunoassay Technique. (Homogeneous)	Sample antigen plus enzyme labeled antigen compete for limited amount of antibody in the reaction mixture.	Binding of antibody to antigen inhibits the activity of the enzyme label.	Uninhibited enzyme label is detected by enzyme activity measurements. See Note 2.
3. FPIA Fluorescence Polarization Immunoassay. (Homogeneous)	Fluorescein labeled antigen and sample antigen are mixed with and compete for antibody.	Large antigen-antibody complexes have decreased rates of rotation compared to the rotation rates of the free antigen.	The change in amount of rapidly rotating labeled antigen is detected as a change in polarization of fluorescent light. See Note 3.

Note 1. Since the bound phase is usually counted, increased levels of sample antigen lead to decreased counts. Data is often evaluated by plotting some mathematical function, such as the logit transform, of the counts versus log concentration.
Note 2. Increased sample antigen leads to decreased inhibition of enzyme label and thus to greater measured enzyme activities. Glucose-6-phosphate dehydrogenase is a commonly used enzyme label. Enzyme activity versus concentration is non-linear.
Note 3. An increase in sample antigen concentration leads to decreased polarization.

diffusion, fluorometric and infrared spectroscopy, and melting point determinations. These analytical tools can be of great help in the analyses of certain drugs.

Conway diffusion

The Conway diffusion technique has found widespread use in methods for the analysis of drugs which are either volatile or can be transformed into a volatile reaction product. At the heart of the technique is the Conway diffusion cell. This is a small covered dish partitioned into two concentric circular compartments. Sample is placed in one compartment, reagent in the other. The plate is covered and sealed in such a manner that gas(es) can diffuse between compartments. The analyte is allowed to elute as a gas from the sample and to diffuse into a colorimetric reagent in the other compartment. After a period of time any change in the appearance of the colorimetric reagent is noted. This method has been widely used to detect alcohols and carbon monoxide in blood. It is also valuable for the detection of substances which can be volatilized, such as cyanides and fluorides.

Fluorometry

Fluorometric techniques depend on the ability of certain molecules to absorb light and then to emit most of that energy as light of a longer wavelength. (The remaining energy is dissipated as heat.) Conservation of energy demands that the emitted (emission) light be of longer wavelength than the absorbed (excitation) light.

The specific wavelengths of excitation and emission are properties of the substance being investigated. This pairing of wavelengths imparts specificity to fluorometric testing. Since emitted light is being detected, baseline light intensities are zero. Therefore, fluorometric analytical methods can be very sensitive. Unfortunately, when an excited molecule collides with another molecule, the excited molecule can lose all its energy as heat. This process is called quenching and causes a loss of fluorescent intensity. Quenching effects are so common and serious in liquid and solid phases that the utility of fluorometric techniques has been significantly limited.

Infrared spectroscopy

Infrared spectroscopy covers the 12,800 to 10 cm^{-1} (reciprocal centimeters) range of the electromagnetic spectrum, which is the same as 780 nm to 1,000,000 nm. This range is often subdivided into the near, middle, and far infrared regions with the near region being closest to the visible light spectrum. Most infrared absorption bands derive from transitions between vibrational modes (patterns) of a molecule. Molecular vibrational modes depend on the exact geometrical configuration of a given molecule. Thus, infrared spectra contain excellent information about molecular architecture. Isomers can often be easily distinguished by infrared spectroscopy.

Infrared spectroscopy is very useful for the identification of pure compounds. Absorption spectra in the infrared region tend to be very complex with many minima and maxima. This complexity imparts uniqueness to any compound's spectrum and provides an excellent "fingerprint" for its identification. For this reason infrared measurements can be very useful in determining the identity of powders found during forensic or clinical investigations if the powders are pure compounds. However, mixtures can produce very complex spectra which are difficult to interpret. In fact, this difficulty has severely limited the application of infrared spectroscopy in clinical and toxicological laboratories, where analytical samples are usually complex mixtures of many different compounds.

Melting point determinations

Melting points are properties of compounds and can be used to confirm a compound's identity. Tables of the melting points for many compounds have been published and various instruments are commercially available for melting point measurements. Melting points are very sensitive to change with inclusion of impurities. In fact, experimentally determined melting points can be used to establish and document the purity of products. The validity of a pure drug standard can be ascertained in part by a melting point determination. However, since most samples of clinical and toxicological interest are mixtures rather than pure compounds, the application of melting point determinations is severely limited in laboratories engaged in drug testing. Still, melting point determinations can be useful adjuncts to infrared data for the identification of pure compounds (powders).

CHROMATOGRAPHY METHODOLOGIES

In addition to utilizing immunoassay methodologies, toxicology laboratories usually employ a variety of chromatographic techniques and instruments for the identification and quantification of drugs in biological samples. The techniques most often utilized include Thin Layer Chromatography (TLC), Gas Liquid Chromatography (GLC, often abbreviated GC) and High Performance Liquid Chromatography (HPLC).

Chromatography overview

Chromatography can be described as a separation process or technique that involves a sample mixture containing two or more substances requiring separation. This sample mixture is introduced into a mobile or moving phase that is flowing through or across a bed of stationary phase. As the mobile phase, which contains the sample mixture (solute), moves through (or across) the stationary phase, the individual solute molecules are distributed so that they spend part of their time in each phase. Depending on the characteristics of the solute molecules and the mobile and stationary phases, the solute molecules will preferentially spend time in either the mobile phase or on the stationary phase. If the components of the mixture have sufficiently different characteristics in any particular system, the mixture will separate because of the different preference of each component for the two phases. After separation, a technique must be employed which will permit the detection of the separated components of the mixture.

Chromatographic methods can be classified according to the physical state, either liquid or gas, of the solute carrying mobile phase. Using this classification criteria, two broad categories result—liquid chromatography (LC) and gas chromatography (GC). These two classifications and their subclassifications are shown in Figure 24-4. Not all of the analytical methods shown, are commonly used. TLC and

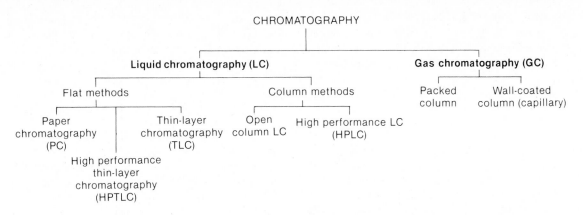

Fig. 24-4   Branches of chromatography according to mobile phase and physical apparatus. *From Tabor MW: Chromatography: theory and practice. In Kaplan LA and Pesce AJ: Clinical chemistry: theory, analysis, and correlation, ed 2, St. Louis, 1989, Mosby-Year Book, Inc.*

HPLC are often utilized as LC methods and both packed column and capillary column are often used for GC.

In addition to classification based on the state of the mobile phase, classification can be done according to the characteristics of the solid or stationary phase. The stationary phase can be either a solid or a solid support which is coated with an extremely thin layer of a very high boiling liquid. With packed column techniques the solid support for the liquid is a very small particle-sized material such as diatomaceous earth or silica. For capillary columns the inside column surface itself is the solid support.

Separation occurs in these chromatographic methods by one of two mechanisms—adsorption or partition. Adsorption chromatography, either gas-solid or liquid-solid, is a process where the components within a sample are separated because of the differences in their attraction to the stationary versus the mobile phase. Techniques utilizing this mechanism are TLC, HPLC and Gas-Solid Chromatography, which is rarely used. Partition chromatography, either liquid-liquid or gas-liquid, utilizes differences in the distribution or solubility of solute molecules between two liquid phases or between a gas and a liquid phase for its separating power. Those GLC and HPLC techniques that utilize the partitioning phenomenon are extensively used.

When establishing a chromatographic technique, some of the parameters that must be considered include quantitative versus qualitative results, compound volatility, polarity, molecular size, thermal lability, detection characteristics, and the ability of the unknown compounds to form derivatives that enhance detectibility.

If only qualitative information is desired, any of the three methodologies, TLC, GC or HPLC, would be a potential candidate. However, for reasons of cost and simplicity, TLC would probably be the method of choice. A drawback to TLC is that it is difficult, without photography, to obtain a permanent record of the chromatographic results. Although GC and HPLC are more expensive and complex, both techniques can be utilized for qualitative identification and both are more commonly employed when quantitative results are required.

The choice between GC or HPLC as a separation technique is often not clear cut and in many situations is a matter of the analyst's preference. However, several considerations may dictate a particular choice. If, as with forensic drug testing, it is necessary to use mass spectrometry as the identification methodology, then GC would be the required separation technique since currently the coupling of an HPLC to a mass spectrometer is not available to most laboratories. If mass spectrometry detection is not required then the factors mentioned previously become important. Several factors would quickly rule out GC. Since GC employs high temperatures, any compound that is thermally unstable would not be compatible with GC. Conversely, if the compound can not be volatilized at a reasonable temperature (200° C or less), GC analysis would be difficult. Since volatility is related to molecular weight, the larger compounds would be those excluded from GC analytical techniques.

With the development of bonded phase HPLC columns and the reverse phase technique, HPLC has grown to be an extremely popular separation technique. It is especially useful for moderately to highly polar compounds because they elute rapidly in this type of system and because many polar compounds do not chromatograph well in GC systems. Another HPLC advantage is that the analyte can be recovered. HPLC detection is nondestructive while GC detection is not. There are no hard and fast rules that dictate the use of one technique over the other. In many situations either technique provides very satisfactory results.

Sample preparation

Unfortunately, samples which require analysis are usually complex mixtures in which the compounds of interest are present in low concentrations. For example, the most common specimens, urine and serum, involve biological-sample matrices that make direct sample analysis extremely difficult. Before analysis, the sample must often be processed through a "clean-up" procedure which separates the components of interest from the biological matrix. Direct analysis can be a problem for a variety of reasons: sample impurities can interact with the stationary phase, thereby reducing the resolving power of the system; saturation of the detector system can occur and this tends to reduce sensitivity; interaction of the components of interest with the matrix can make the analysis irreproducible from sample to sample; components within the matrix may chromatograph with nearly identical characteristics to the component of interest, thus making identification and quantitation impossible.

The most commonly used separation techniques are either chromatographic or extraction methods.

Chromatographic methods

A common chromatographic technique for removing an analyte from its matrix is accomplished with the use of XAD-2[R] resin. The resin, which is polydivinylbenzene, is packed into a small vertical plastic or glass extraction tube and the urine or serum is allowed to pass slowly through the resin bed. This resin, which is nonionic with a large surface area, is capable of absorbing many classes of organic compounds. However, for absorption to occur properly it is necessary for the compounds of interest to be in a neutral rather than ionic state. Therefore, if the compounds being extracted are either acids or bases the pH must be appropriately adjusted to assure that these compounds are not charged. After absorption, the compounds are eluted from the XAD-2[R] resin with organic solvents such as methanol, methylene chloride, diethyl ether, hexane, acetone or combinations of these solvents.

In addition to XAD-2[R] resin, other solid phases, such as silica or octadecylsilyl-bonded phase, have also been employed for isolating analytes from their biological matrix. As with XAD-2[R] resin, the analytes are absorbed onto the surface of the solid phase and are then eluted with a small amount of an appropriate polar organic solvent.

While a laboratory may pack its own extraction columns, it is expensive, time consuming, and sometimes difficult to produce columns which provide reproducible results. Fortunately, there are several vendors that market sample extraction columns for toxicological applications.

Extraction methods

Liquid-liquid extraction methods have been widely used for sample clean up prior to analysis. For liquid-liquid extraction to be effective, several requirements must be met.

Since the partitioning of an analyte between two liquids (solvents) is a function of the polarity of the analyte, an estimate of the analyte polarity must be possible. Once polarity is determined, a solvent of comparable polarity must be selected as the extracting solvent. It is important to remember the axiom "likes attract likes." That is, a polar solute will preferentially partition itself into a polar solvent and vice-versa.

A second requirement for liquid-liquid extraction is that the two solvents must be immiscible. If the two partitioning solvents are soluble in each other, no separation is possible. Additionally, the extracting solvent and the analyte must not react with each other. After extraction, it is usually necessary to remove all or nearly all of the extracting solvent in order to concentrate the analyte into a small volume. Therefore, it is also necessary for the solvent to be volatile enough for easy evaporation. This criteria is also necessary for the solid phase extraction procedures. One must be careful to use pure solvents so that contaminants contained within the solvent are not introduced into the analytical process. A simple partition of a solute is shown in Figure 24-5.

Proper pH adjustment of the sample matrix is important and necessary for the effective extraction of organic acids and bases. In addition to pH adjustment, one other technique is sometimes used to enhance the extraction of organic compounds from an aqueous environment. An increase in the ionic strength of the aqueous (more polar) phase will cause the neutral solute to favor the organic (less polar) phase. It is possible to increase the ionic strength by adding a neutral salt, such as sodium chloride, to the aqueous phase prior to extraction.

The extraction process itself is relatively simple. The appropriate volumes of the aqueous phase, after proper pH and ionic strength adjustment, and the selected extraction solvent are combined in a screw cap culture tube and shaken for an appropriate length of time (typically five to 15 minutes). The two liquid phases are then allowed to separate by either standing or centrifugation. After phase separation, the aqueous part is discarded and the organic phase saved for analysis.

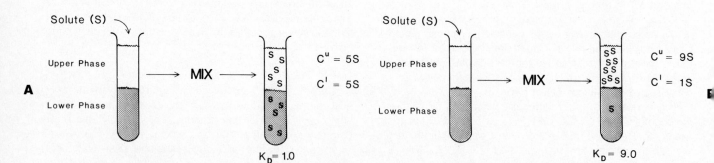

Fig. 24-5 Separation of a solute, S, by partition into two different solvent systems. In the first system, **A,** solute has a distribution coefficient, K_D, of 1.0, indicating an equal partitioning between upper and lower phases after mixing. In second system, **B,** solute has a K_D of 9.0, indicating a partitioning of nine parts of the solute in the upper phase and one part of the solute in the lower phase after mixing. C_u, Upper-phase concentration; C_l, lower phase concentration. *From Tabor MW: Chromatography: theory and practice. In Kaplan LA and Pesce AJ: Clinical chemistry: theory, analysis, and correlation, ed 2, St. Louis, 1989, Mosby-Year Book, Inc.*

An individual laboratory can either make its own liquid extraction system or it can purchase extraction tubes. These tubes, which contain both the extracting solvent and pH buffers, can be used to isolate drug analytes from a urine or serum matrix. The Toxilab company markets two types of tubes. Style A tubes are used to extract basic and neutral drugs while style B tubes extract principally the acidic drugs. Although these tubes are designed to be part of a complete TLC drug identification system, they can be utilized with other drug analysis techniques as well. And while these extraction tubes may be more expensive than "home-made" tubes, their convenience and ease of use probably compensates for the greater expense.

Thin-layer chromatography

Of the many chromatographic techniques, thin-layer chromatography (TLC) and the related paper chromatography are among the oldest. Age, however, has not diminished their utility as toxicological tools. The TLC technique is practical in multiple drug screening programs. Although generally less sensitive than immunoassay techniques, TLC is not restricted to the detection of only 10 to 12 drugs or drug groups. Literally hundreds of drugs can be detected and identified with TLC.

In TLC, a stationary phase or absorbent, such as silica gel or alumina, is applied in a very uniform and thin layer (about 0.25 mm) to a physical support such as a glass plate or plastic film. Although it is possible for a laboratory to prepare these plates, they are usually purchased since uniform plate production is difficult and time consuming and reproducible drug separation depends on uniform plates.

Separation

After the drugs have been extracted and concentrated from the original specimen, the extraction residue is reconstituted in a small volume (50 μL or less) of a volatile solvent such as methanol or methylene chloride. This is then applied, as a very small spot, approximately one-half inch from the bottom of the TLC plate and allowed to dry. The plate is then stood on edge, with the application spots down, in a closed container which contains just enough solvent to wet the bottom of the plate and remain below the sample application point. The solvent or mobile phase, which moves up the plate by capillary action, is allowed to travel up the plate until it reaches a predetermined point close to the top of the plate. As the solvent moves up the plate, the substances contained in the sample spot are partly dissolved and moved by the solvent. The relative solubilities of sample materials between the solvent and the stationary phase determines how far each of the various substances contained in the sample will travel up the plate. Those substances that are more soluble in the mobile phase will travel farther up the plate while those substances that prefer the stationary phase will tend not to travel as far. In order to obtain the desired separation of the analytes of interest, a mobile phase of the appropriate polarity and pH must be selected.

In any particular TLC separation system, the distance traveled by a particular compound is characteristic for that compound and, if the experimental procedures are consistently repeated, the migration distance will not vary from one run to the next. However, since the experimental conditions cannot be completely controlled, a relative migration factor, termed the R_f factor, is calculated for each compound (See Figure 24-6.) The use of the R_f factor, which is the ratio of the distance the compound travels divided by the distance the solvent travels, compensates for slight variations in experimental technique over time. A more practical and convenient approach to dealing with slight changes in migration distance from one run to the next is to include, with the unknowns being analyzed, a sample which contains a mixture of the compounds being studied. In this way the known standard components can be directly compared with the unknowns.

Detection

After the separation step, the TLC plate is heated slightly to dry the plate. Visualization of the compounds of interest is the next step. This involves spraying or dipping the plate with one or more color-developing reagents that react with the compounds to produce characteristic colors. It is the combination of migration distance and color development that permits the identification of drugs and/or their metabolites.

Advantages of TLC include low cost, relative rapidness, the ability to identify a large number of drugs and their metabolites at one time. One disadvantage is a lack of sensitivity and specificity, especially when compared to the immunoassay methods. More importantly, the technique is highly dependent on the technician's skill and experience. In the hands of an inexperienced technician, TLC is often of little value.

Fortunately for the clinical laboratory that processes a relatively small number of samples, the Toxilab Company of Irvine, California, has developed a complete TLC drug identification system. The system includes buffered extraction tubes, pre-prepared standards, specially designed TLC plates, standardized reagents for color development and most importantly a very extensive colored compendium detailing the migration and color development of hundreds of drugs and drug metabolites.

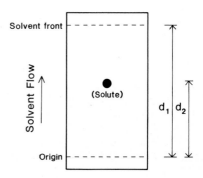

Fig. 24-6 Calculation of R_f (solvent-front ratio) value for a sample component from a paper or thin-layer chromatogram. The distance d_1 from origin to solvent front and distance d_2 from origin to center of spot of separated component are measured, as shown, in terms of same units; that is, length (centimeters or inches). Resulting R_f value, d_2 divided by d_1 is unitless. *From Tabor MW: Chromatography: theory and practice. In Kaplan LA and Pesce AJ: Clinical chemistry: theory, analysis, and correlation, ed 2, St. Louis, 1989, Mosby-Year Book, Inc.*

Gas chromatography

Gas chromatography is a separation process by which a mixture of compounds, in a volatilized state, is separated into its component parts by carrying the vaporized mixture with an inert gas through a stationary phase. As in all chromatographic systems, gas chromatography is a two-phase system. The mobile phase can be one of several inert gases, usually helium, argon, or nitrogen, and the stationary phase can be one of two types. If the stationary phase consists of a thin layer of nonvolatile liquid held to a solid support, the technique is termed gas-liquid chromatography (GLC). However, if the stationary phase consists only of a solid sorbent, then the technique is termed gas-solid chromatography (GSC). Regardless of the stationary phase, separation of a mixture is achieved by a difference in the partitioning of the various molecules between the two phases.

Instrumentation

A gas chromatograph basically consists of six parts or components: (1) a pressurized carrier gas with the appropriate pressure and flow regulators, (2) a sample injection port, (3) a column, (4) a detector, (5) an electrometer and recorder, and (6) thermal compartments that enclose the injection port, column and detector. (See Figure 24-7.)

For efficient and reproducible chromatography, it is important that the carrier gas flow at a very constant rate. To achieve constant flow, the gas pressure and flow rate are maintained by high-precision flow meters and pressure regulators. Carrier gas, in addition to the requirement of constant flow, must also be inert, dry, and pure. Inertness is achieved by using nonreactive gases such as nitrogen or helium (Table 24-4). Dryness and purity can be achieved by purchasing only ultra-pure gas and then passing the gas through a molecular sieve trap before the gas enters the instrument.

The sample injection port is located at the beginning of the column just before the point where the carrier gas enters the column. Samples are injected with a microliter syringe into the hot injection port through a silicone rubber septum. Once in the injection port, the sample is immediately vaporized and swept by the carrier gas into the column, where separation occurs. In order to obtain rapid and complete vaporization, the injection port temperature is often set 25 to 50° C higher than the boiling point of the highest-boiling component in the sample. Because many drugs can be degraded on hot, metal surfaces, it is commonplace to either have the injection port equipped with a glass liner or to have the end of the glass column fit into the injection port region so that the sample is injected directly into the beginning of the column.

Separation

The columns used in clinical and toxicological separations are usually one of two types, both of which are made of glass. The more conventional columns are constructed of glass tubing with a 2 to 4 mm inside diameter. These columns are packed with a variety of stationary phases depending on the analysis being performed. In drug analysis, it is common to use finely powdered silica coated with one of several high-boiling silicone oils. These oils are available with varying degrees of polarity so that the polarities of the samples can be matched. The column material is held in

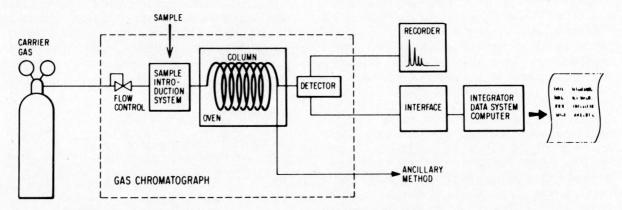

Fig. 24-7   Basic components of a gas chromatographic system. *From Ettre, LS: Practical gas chromatography, Norwalk, Conn, 1973, Perkin-Elmer Corp.*

Table 24-4   Detectors and appropriate gases

Detector	Carrier gas	Detector gas
Thermal conductivity (TCD)	Helium, hydrogen	—
Flame ionization (FID)	Helium, nitrogen	Air and hydrogen
Nitrogen-phosphorus (NPD)	Helium, nitrogen	1. Air and hydrogen
		2. Air and 8% hydrogen in helium
Electron capture	Nitrogen	5% methane in argon
	5% methane in argon	—

From Poklis A: Gas chromatography. In Kaplan LA and Pesce AJ: Clinical chemistry: theory, analysis, and correlation, ed 2, St. Louis, 1989, Mosby-Year Book, Inc.

place with small plugs of glass wool at each end of the column.

The other column type is the capillary column, which is rapidly gaining in popularity. Instead of packing the column with a coated stationary phase, the inside column wall is directly coated with the liquid phase.

Although there are a large number of liquid and solid stationary phase materials available for gas chromatographic applications, only a few are necessary to satisfy the requirements of most clinical and toxicological applications.

Table 24-5 indicates phases most often used in the clinical setting.

The column of a gas chromatograph is enclosed in an oven that controls the column temperature. Precise temperature control (within 0.1° C) is required in order to obtain reproducible results. A GC analysis can be performed in one of two temperature modes. In the isothermal mode, a constant oven temperature is maintained during the complete separation process. In the temperature-programming mode, oven temperature is increased at a constant rate during the

Table 24-5 Examples of commonly used stationary phases and their applications

Stationary phase	Structures	Temperature (°C min/max)	Application	Specific compounds
Silicone OV-1 (100% methyl)	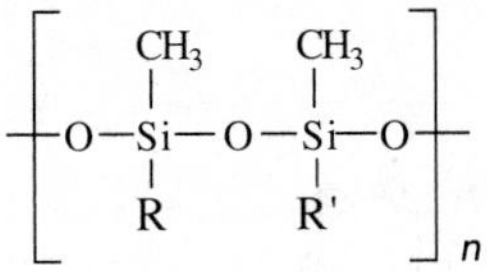 (silicone polymer structure) R and R′ = CH$_3$ in above structure	100/350	Bacteria, drugs	Fatty acid methyl esters, benzodiazepines
Silicone OV-17 (50% phenyl)	R and R′ = phenyl in above structure	20/350	Drugs, steroids	Tricyclic antidepressants, barbiturates, cholesterol
Silicone OV-210 (50%, 3,3,3-trifluoropropyl)	R and R′ = -CH$_2$-CH$_2$-CF$_3$ in above structure	20/300	Drugs, pesticides	Basic drugs, lindane, aldrin, DDT
Silicone OV-225 (25% cyanopropyl, 25% phenyl)	R = phenyl, R′ = -CH$_2$-CH$_2$-CH$_2$-CN in above structure	20/275	Steroids	TMS derivatives of 17-ketosteroids
10% Apiezon L 2% KOH	Undefined mixture of high-boiling hydrocarbons	50/225	Amines	Amphetamine
NPGS (neopentyl glycol succinate)	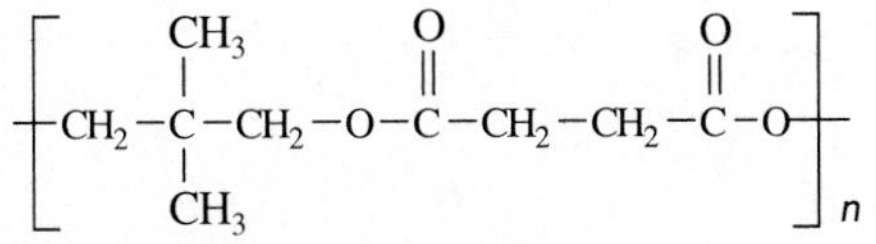 (polymer structure)	50/240	Volatile fatty acids	Acetic through caproic acids
Carbopack B/5%	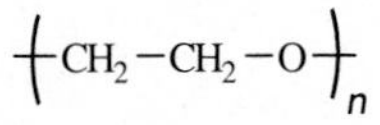 -CH$_2$-CH$_2$-O-		Alcohols, aldehydes, ketones	Methanol, ethanol, acetaldehyde acetone
DEGS (diethylene glycol succinate)	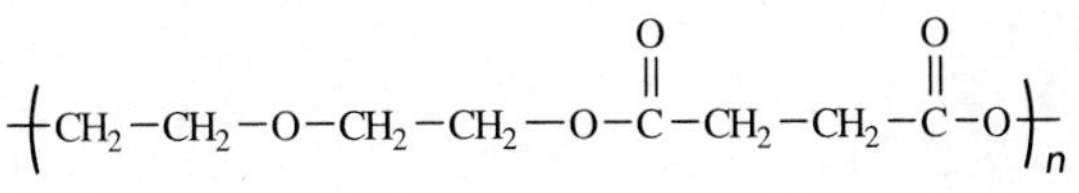 (polymer structure)	20/200	Bacteria	Fatty acid methylesters
EGA (ethylene glycol adipate)	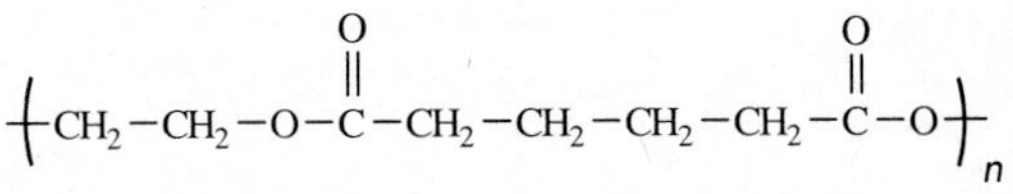 (polymer structure)	100/210	Amino acids	NBTFA* derivatives of amino acids
Chromosorb 102 (styrene divinyl benzene polymer)	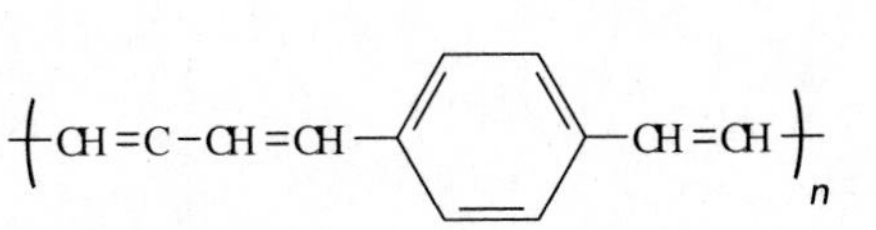 (polymer structure)	<250° C	Alcohols, aldehydes	Methanol, ethanol, acetaldehyde
Porapak Q (ethylvinyl benzene + divinyl benzene polymer mixture)	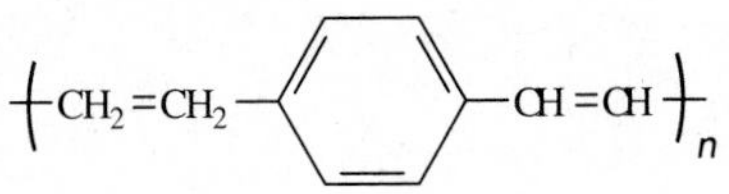 (polymer structure)	<250° C	Low molecular weight	Chlorinated hydrocarbons

Modified from Poklis A: Gas chromatography. In Kaplan LA and Pesce AJ: Clinical chemistry: theory, analysis, and correlation, ed 2, St. Louis, 1989, Mosby-Year Book, Inc.
*NBTFA, Nitroblue tetrazolium fatty acid.

analysis. Temperature programming is highly advantageous for mixtures that contain compounds of widely varying separation characteristics since, through temperature programming, analysis time can be shortened. Shorter analysis times are desirable since sharper, less diffuse sample peaks result.

Detection

As the carrier gas exits the column, a detector senses the separated components of the sample mixture and produces an electrical signal that is proportional to the amount of material entering the detector. Although a variety of detectors have been designed for GC application only a few types are routinely utilized in the clinical setting. Those of general applicability to the clinical laboratory are shown in Figure 24-8.

The flame ionization detector (FID) is a widely used, general purpose detector. The FID (Figure 24-8, *A*) is simple to operate and it can detect and quantify a wide variety of organic compounds. The FID utilizes a flame produced by the burning of hydrogen in air. Few ions are formed until an organic compound elutes from the column into the flame. When this occurs, ion formation is greatly increased. These ions, which are collected on a charged collector electrode, cause a flow of current within the detector. This flow of current is proportional to the amount of sample compound in the flame. The FID responds to all organic compounds except those which do not burn or ionize in a hydrogen/air flame. There is little or no response for H_2O, CO_2, CO, N_2, or CS_2. Also, heavily halogenated compounds produce a very small response.

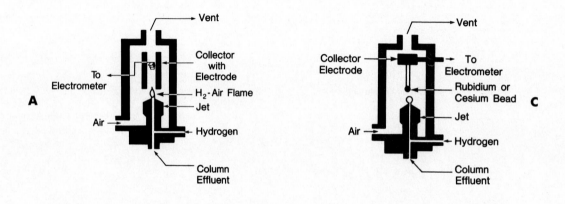

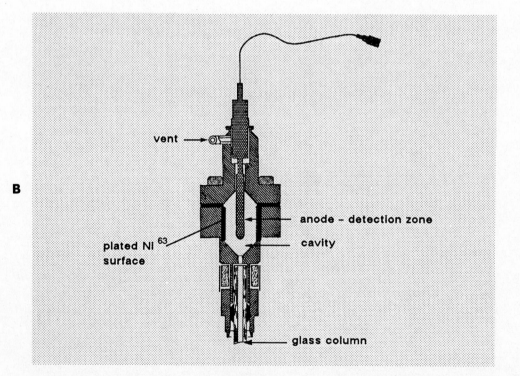

Fig. 24-8   **A,** Schematic diagram of flame ionization detector. **B,** Design of a commercially available electron capture detector. **C,** Schematic diagram of alkali-metal flame detector. **A** and **B** from Werner M, Mohrbacher RJ, and Riendeau, CJ: In Baer DM and Dito WR: Interpretation of therapeutic drug levels, Chicago, 1981, American Society of Clinical Pathologists. **B** from Buffington Rand Wilson MK: Detectors for gas chromatography: a practical primer, Avondale, Pa, 1987, Hewlett-Packard Co.

The special-purpose electron capture detector (ECD) is selectively sensitive to halogen atoms (Figure 24-8, *B*). Its use is therefore limited to analyses involving compounds, such as pesticides, which contain multiple halogen atoms. The ECD principle arises from the phenomenon that electronegative species can react with thermal electrons to form negatively charged ions. In order to produce capturable thermal electrons, the carrier gas is ionized by beta particles from a radioactive source placed in the detector. This electron flow produces a small measurable current. When sample molecules eluting from the column are introduced into the detector, electrons that would have been measured are instead captured by the sample, which results in a decrease in current flow. The current decrease is quantitatively related to the amount of sample entering the detector.

Another special purpose detector used extensively in drug analysis is the nitrogen phosphorus detector (NPD) (Figure 24-8, *C*). This detector is somewhat similar to a FID with the additional feature that alkali metal ions are introduced into the flame. The introduction of these metal ions, coupled with modified flame characteristics, causes the detector to selectively ionize compounds containing nitrogen and/or phosphorus. The NPD is both highly sensitive and selective for organic compounds containing these atoms. Since many drugs contain nitrogen atoms, the NPD detector is specially suited for drug analysis.

The electrical current output from the detector passes through an electrometer which converts the change in current to a voltage change. These voltage changes are then recorded on a strip chart recorder and appear as one or more peaks depending on the number of compounds detected. The elapsed time from sample injection to peak detection is termed the "retention time." This time is a function of both the compound in question and the experimental conditions. Through the use of experimentally determined retention times for known compounds, it is possible, through the matching of retention times for knowns and unknowns, to identify unknown compounds within a sample.

Quantitation

Quantitative results can be obtained through the use of peak-area measurements. This is possible since the area of a peak is directly proportional to the amount of material that produced the peak—that is, the concentration of the material in the original sample. In the quantitative applications encountered in the clinical setting, an internal standard procedure is utilized. With this technique, the same amount of a compound (internal standard) structurally similar to the unknown but not present in the specimen is added at the beginning of the analytical process to each of the standards, controls, and unknowns. Then, in the preparation of a calibration curve, the ratio of the peak area of the compound being quantitated to the area of the internal standard is plotted versus concentration. Quantitative results for controls and unknowns are determined by using this same ratio and the established calibration curve. Typically, internal standard techniques offer significantly better precision than do techniques that do not incorporate an internal standard. Performance is improved because any inadvertent losses or variations within the analytical procedure will affect the analyte and the internal standard equivalently, causing the peak-area ratios to remain unchanged. With today's technology, microprocessor units are available that automatically perform sample identification, quantitation, and report generation.

Mass spectrometry detection

Although the detectors described above have been utilized with great success in the toxicology laboratory, they are being replaced for forensic and legal applications by mass spectrometer detectors (MS). By using a mass spectrometer, it is possible, in most cases, to obtain a definitive identification of an unknown compound in addition to determining the amount of the unknown compound. This is in contrast to other detectors which do not permit definitive identification. Prior to the mid 1980s, mass spectrometer detectors were very expensive and difficult to operate. As a result, they were not utilized for clinical or many forensic applications. However, it is now possible to purchase, from at least one vendor, compact, affordable, and easy to operate low resolution GC/mass spectrometers that are suitable for most clinical/toxicology applications. The price of these instruments can be as low as $65,000 to $70,000 depending on the features purchased.

Interfacing a GC to a mass spectrometer has, historically, presented a significant design problem. The problem results from the differences in the operating pressure environments of the two components. A gas chromatograph operates at atmospheric pressure with high flow rates while the mass spectrometer typically operates at a 10^{-5} torr vacuum. The interface devices developed to allow the two components to operate together are known as molecular separators. The function of these separators is to remove the unwanted helium carrier gas while allowing the analyte molecules to enter the mass spectrometer. With the advent of small bore (<0.2 mm id) capillary columns, it is possible to bypass the difficulties of GC/MS interfacing since the gas flow from these columns does not overload the capacity of the vacuum pumping system. With small-bore columns, a direct coupling can be made between the capillary column and the mass spectrometer source. Direct coupling results in greater sensitivity since none of the sample is lost in the separation process.

The generation of a mass spectrum by the mass spectrometer involves three steps: ionization of the analyte molecules, mass filtration, and detection. Currently, three modes of ionization are available for the analysis of biological specimens: electron impact, chemical ionization, and negative chemical ionization. In the electron impact (EI) mode, the sample molecules are bombarded with high-energy electrons to produce negatively charged molecules or molecular fragments. In the chemical ionization (CI) technique, the sample molecules are mixed with an ionized gas such as methane. A positive charge is transferred to the sample molecule as a result of the ion-molecule collision. This produces a positive M + 1 ion. By controlling the experiment conditions, it is possible to limit the fragmentation of the sample molecules and thus yield a spectrum that is predominantly the M + 1 ion of the sample molecule. In negative chemical ionization (NCI), oxygen or hydrogen is mixed with the sample molecules to produce a dominant negative ion of M − 1. The detection of compounds containing halogen atoms may be greatly enhanced by NCI. Of the three ionization techniques, electron impact (EI) has had the largest acceptance. However, chemical ionization is growing in popularity principally because of the much simpler spectra produced and also because the prices of these instruments are becoming competitive with EI instruments.

As stated previously, when using the EI mode, sample molecules, in the gas phase, are bombarded with high energy electrons which produces a negatively charged molecule (molecular ion) and usually multiple ionic molecular fragments. The resulting charged particles are separated (mass filtered) and then detected according to their respective molecular masses. The mass spectrum that results displays both the masses of the various fragments and the abundance of each fragment. This spectrogram, which is characteristic of the molecule in question, provides virtually unequivocal identification of the unknown material. In addition to identification, the same spectrum can be used to quantitate the unknown material provided a calibration curve has been prepared from standards of known concentrations. Because of the complexity of mass spectrometer operation and the time needed for mass spectral data interpretation, mass spectrometers are connected to computerized systems for operation, data collection, library searching for compound identification, and compound quantitation.

High performance liquid chromatography

One branch on the liquid chromatography side of Figure 24-4 refers to two types of column methods—open and high performance. Typically, open column liquid chromatography has no application in the toxicology setting for identification or quantitation. However, it is often used as a sample extraction technique.

The high-performance branch can be subdivided into several classifications depending on the nature of the stationary phase: liquid-solid chromatography, liquid-liquid or partition chromatography, bonded phase chromatography, ion exchange chromatography, and exclusion chromatography. Of these subdivisions only one, bonded phase chromatography, has found a significant place in the toxicology laboratory.

Instrumentation

Modern HPLC requires relatively sophisticated instrumentation which contains four basic components (see Figure 24-9): a solvent (mobile phase) delivery system, a sample introduction system, the column, and a detector.

The solvent delivery system is commonly based on some type of reciprocating piston pump. One of the shortcomings of a reciprocating pump is that the solvent moves in pulses rather than in a continuous stream. Since pulsing is not acceptable for chromatographic purposes, manufacturers have devised a variety of techniques, such as sophisticated pulse suppressors or a multiple pump system that operates with two or three pumps 180° or 120° out of phase to eliminate the pulsing effect. For any particular test method, mobile phase may be delivered in one of two modes—isocratic or gradient. In the isocratic mode, the solvent composition remains constant during the chromatographic separation while in the gradient mode, the composition will change as the analysis progresses. Depending on the sophistication of the HPLC instrumentation, gradient chromatography may or may not be possible. In a typical HPLC system the mobile phase will flow at a rate of 0.5 to 2.0 ml per minute at a pressure of 100 to 300 atmospheres.

Sample introduction is achieved through the use of a fixed-loop injection valve. With this valve an aliquot of sample is loaded into an external loop of tubing. The valve is then rotated so that the sample is flushed into the column by the mobile phase.

Separation

HPLC columns for analytical applications typically range in length from 10 to 30 cm with internal diameters of 3 to

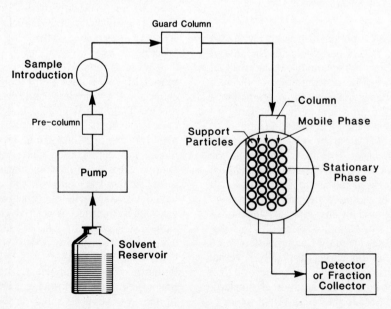

Fig. 24-9 Schematic diagram of a column liquid chromatographic system. *From Bowers LD and Carr PW: Quantitative Aspects of HPLC Workshop, Minneapolis, Minn, 1983.*

4 mm. Most often the columns, which are made from precision bore stainless steel, are packed with a very small diameter bonded phase 5 to 10 μm particles which produce very high-column efficiencies. These high efficiencies make very difficult separations possible.

Bonded phase stationary phase is prepared by reacting the surface SiOH groups on very small silica particles with a silane such as octadecyl-dimethylchlorosilane. The resulting nonpolar surface contains octadecyl groups bonded to the surface by siloxone (Si-O-Si) bonds. Although octadecyl bonded stationary phase is very common and versatile, a variety of other bonded phases are also available (see Table 24-6). Chromatography utilizing a nonpolar stationary phase with a polar mobile phase, is termed reverse phase chromatography. The opposite, polar stationary phase and nonpolar mobile phase, is termed normal phase since

in the early years of chromatography, this represented the normal situation.

Detection

In clinical/toxicology laboratory applications the detectors most often used are either photometers or fluorometers. However, success has been achieved recently using a mass spectrometer as a HPLC detector. Refer to Table 24-7 for the operating characteristics of the more common detectors.

Photometers can operate in either the uv or visible regions of the spectrum. A typical photometric detector is a 254 nm fixed wavelength detector. This detector is simple and inexpensive but it is not selective since most compounds that contain aromatic rings absorb energy at this wavelength. Variable wavelength detectors are available for those analyses that require wavelengths other than 254 nm. Fluores-

Table 24-6 Sample of HPLC usage in the clinical laboratory

Analyte	Sample matrix	Chromatographic mode	Mobile phase*	Detection system†
Antiarrhythmic drugs (procainamide, lidocaine, quinidine, disopyramide, propranolol)	Serum	Reversed phase	I	UV (254), fluorescence
Anticonvulsant drugs (phenobarbital, phenytoin, ethosuximide, primidone, carbamazepine)	Serum	Reverse phase	I	UV (200)
Amino acids	Urine	Reversed phase	G	Fluorescence, dansyl derivatives
Bile acids	Serum	Reversed phase	G	Fluorescence, enzyme reduction of NAD to NADH
Bilirubin	Serum	Reversed phase	I	Vis (403)
Carbohydrates (from fungal infections)	Serum	Normal bonded phase (NH$_2$)	I	UV (200)
Chloramphenicol	Serum	Reversed phase	I	UV (278)
Cholesterol	Serum	Reversed phase	I	UV (205)
Cortisol	Serum	Reversed phase	I	Fluorescence
Creatinine	Serum	Reversed phase	I	UV (238)
Creatinine kinase isozymes	Serum	Ion exchange	G	Chemiluminescence
1,25-Dihydroxyvitamin D	Plasma	Normal bonded phase (NO$_2$)	G	CPB
Epinephrine	Plasma, urine	Reversed phase	I	Electrochemical
Estriol	Urine	Reversed phase	I	Fluorescence
Gentamicin	Serum	Reversed phase	I	Fluorescence, o-phthalaldehyde derivative
Hemoglobin A$_{lc}$	Red blood cell hemolysate	Ion exchange	G	Vis (403)
Homovanillic acid	Urine	Reversed phase	I	Fluorescence, o-phthalaldehyde derivative
5-Hydroxyindole acetic acid	Urine	Reversed phase	I	Electrochemical
17α-Hydroxyprogesterone	Serum	Reversed phase	I	UV (254)
Metanephrines	Urine	Reversed phase	I	Fluorescence, o-phthalaldehyde derivative
Norepinephrine	Plasma, urine	Reversed phase	I	Electrochemical
Porphyrins	Urine	Reversed phase	G	Fluorescence
Prednisone, prednisolone	Serum	Reversed phase	I	UV (254)
Proteins	Serum	Ion exchange	I	UV (254), p-bromophenacyl derivative
Serotonin	Serum	Reversed phase	I	Electrochemical
Tricyclic antidepressants	Serum	Adsorption	I	UV (254)
Vitamins A and E	Serum	Reversed phase	I	UV (290)

From Bowers LD: Liquid chromatography. In Kaplan LA and Pesce AJ: Clinical chemistry: theory, analysis, and correlation, ed 2, St. Louis, 1989, Mosby-Year Book, Inc.
*Type of elution system used; I, isocratic; G, gradient.
†CPB, Competitive protein binding; UV, Ultraviolet photometry; Vis, visible light; numbers in parentheses indicate wavelength.

Table 24-7 Performance characteristics of commonly used detectors

Ideal detector characteristic	Fixed wavelength	Variable wavelength	Fluorescence	Electrochemical	
				Oxidation	Reduction
Selective?	No	No	Yes	Yes	Yes
Sensitivity to flowrate changes?	Possibly	Possibly	No	Yes	Yes
Limit of detection?	10^{-10} g/L	10^{-9} g/L	10^{-11} g/L	10^{-12} g/L	10^{-9} g/L
Cell volume?	8-10 μL	8-10 μL	20 μL	≤1 μL	
Compatible with gradient?	Yes	Yes	Yes		

From Bowers LD: Liquid chromatography. In Kaplan LA and Pesce AJ: Clinical chemistry: theory, analysis, and correlation, ed 2, St. Louis, 1989, Mosby-Year Book, Inc.

cence detection is more selective as well as more sensitive than absorbance detection but fluorescence detection suffers from the drawback that not all compounds are fluorescent or can be made to fluoresce through derivative formation. The output from these detectors is most often plotted on a strip chart recorder. As with other types of chromatography, the retention time of the peak is related to the compound and the area of the peak is a function of the concentration of the compound that produced the peak. Therefore, both quantitation and identification is possible with HPLC techniques.

SUGGESTED READING

Jaffe HH and Orchin M: Theory and applications of ultraviolet spectroscopy, New York, 1962, John Wiley and Sons, Inc.

Kaplan A and Pesce J: Clinical chemistry: theory, analysis, and correlation, ed 2, St. Louis, 1989, Mosby-Year-Book, Inc.

Levine IN: Physical chemistry, ed 3, New York, 1988, McGraw-Hill Book Co.

Morrison RT and Boyd RN: Organic chemistry, ed 5, Boston, 1987, Allyn and Bacon, Inc.

Rodbard D et al: Computer analysis of radioligand data: advantages, problems, and pitfalls, In Rapaka RS and Hawks, RL, eds: Opioid peptides: molecular pharmacology, biosynthesis, and analysis, Rockville, Maryland, 1986, National Institute on Drug Abuse.

Skoog DA: Principles of instrumental analysis, ed 3, Philadelphia, 1985, Saunders College Publishing.

Sunshine I, editor-in-chief: CRC handbook series in analytical toxicology, section A: general data, vol 1, Boca Raton, Fla, 1969, CRC Press.

25 Heavy metal analysis

Donald J. Cannon

Exposure to metals is a continuous, daily process. Metals can be found in the workplace, in drinking water, in food, and in the air. Metals can exist in many forms and some are essential for life. Many metals can produce toxic reactions usually by combining with reactive ligands that are part of essential biochemical processes. Because of their ubiquity, toxicity, and incidence of poisoning, arsenic, lead, mercury, and aluminum are frequently encountered in toxicological presentations. Less frequently observed but potentially toxic are cadmium, nickel, and thallium.

The laboratorian should be familiar with all aspects of metal analysis, from proper sample collection to the interpretation of results. An appreciation of the clinical effects and treatment of metal poisoning completes the necessary cycle of information that will maximize patient care.

In addition to the potentially toxic metals there are a number of trace metals whose biochemical role is very important and whose deficiency in the human body produces physiological impairment. The assessment of these trace metals is a continuing challenge to laboratory personnel.

In the sections that follow, normal or reference values for many different metals in different specimens are presented. Also presented are values consistent with either chronic or acute toxicity. Analysis of any metal must be performed under rigorous conditions to prevent exogenous contamination. In addition, the collection of samples must be performed under careful conditions to prevent contamination. Because of these caveats, reference levels should be used as guidelines and laboratory staff whose objective is to analyze a considerable number of samples for trace metal analysis should establish their own reference ranges. In general, reference ranges higher than those cited here are probably a reflection of sample or process contamination.

As a general rule blood samples should be drawn through a stainless steel needle (except for nickel analysis) into a disposable plastic syringe. The first 2 to 3 ml is discarded, and the sample for analysis is then collected into a certified metal-free tube. These can be purchased (e.g., Peel-A-Way, Becton Dickinson), prepared in the laboratory, or provided by a reference testing laboratory. If other types of blood collection tubes are used, there will be trace metal contamination. Heparin and ethylenediamine tetraacetic acid (EDTA) are acceptable anticoagulants for whole blood, although the former can be contaminated with trace metals.

When collecting a 24-hour urine specimen, it is important to use acid-washed plastic containers. Any aliquot should be stored or transported in acid-washed containers. Urine should not be collected in an area that could contribute metal-laden dust to the sample. Some metals must be collected under acidic conditions to prevent loss of metal in urinary sediments. This can be accomplished by the addition of acetic (10 mL glacial), hydrochloric (10 mL, 6 N), or nitric acid (20 mL, 6 N) at the start of collection and by placing a warning label on the collection container. No preservative should ever be added to urine collected for metal analysis; the best preservation step would be to refrigerate the sample during collection. Prior to aliquoting from a 24-hour urine collection, the sample should be thoroughly mixed.

The use of hair samples for the analysis of potentially toxic heavy metals is well established. The analysis of trace metals in hair samples is less well established and is burdened with tremendous variability in baseline values among laboratories and lack of uniform procedures for the collection and analysis of samples. Scattered reports in the literature indicate promising potential for trace metal hair analysis in diagnostic and epidemiological studies. The use of hair analysis for nutritional counseling studies has been heavily criticized.

The collection of hair samples for metal analysis should follow some basic rules: (1) collect sample from a standardized anatomical location; the back of the head (posterior vertex) is preferred because of less variability in hair growth rate and less influence on hair growth by age and sex; (2) collect sufficient sample (minimum of 50 mg); (3) collect sample at a uniform distance from the scalp; this is especially important if sectional analyses of hair strands will be performed since levels of trace metals vary with distance from the scalp; (4) prevent contamination of sample; and (5) thoroughly document all steps in the collection process, including accurate identification of the sample. Since hair is not a usual sample in the laboratory, a thorough knowledge of the biology of hair, the technological analysis of hair samples, and the potential pitfalls of hair analysis should be established.

INDIVIDUAL METALS
Arsenic
Sources and exposure

Arsenic (As) is a common environmental toxicant and the elemental form is produced as a by-product of ore smelting using the minerals arsenopyrite and loellingite. It is found in soil, water, and air, and is a common ingredient of a wide range of products, including pesticides and insecticides (Box 25-1). Arsenic drugs were used in the treatment of syphilis and are one of the more effective treatments for trypanosomiasis.

There are three major forms of arsenic; inorganic arsenic (usually arsenite with arsenic in the $+3$ oxidation state), organic arsenic (usually arsentate with arsenic in the $+5$ state), and arsine gas (AsH_3). Arsine gas is the most toxic form of arsenic followed by the inorganic arsenites and then the organic arsenates. The colorless, nonirritating arsine gas can be generated from arsenic salts on the addition of an acid.

Arsenic can be absorbed through the gastrointestinal tract via inhalation through the lungs and by penetration of the skin. Arsenic trioxide, which can be absorbed through the lungs and intestines, is fatal at a dose of 120 mg. The exposure limit to arsine gas is 0.05 ppm; death can occur in 30 minutes at 25 to 50 ppm. The threshold limit value for inorganic arsenic is 0.2 mg/m^3. Average adult intake is 2 to 3 mg/day, and more if the diet is heavy in seafood (lobster can contain 10 mg arsenic per pound). In general, adults handle these amounts without difficulty, but children are more susceptible to the toxic effects of arsenic.

Clinical effects and mechanisms

Absorbed arsenic combines with hemoglobin and after 24 hours it is distributed chiefly to the liver, spleen, lungs, and kidneys. Within 2 to 4 weeks following ingestion and absorption, arsenic is incorporated into hair, nails, and skin via the binding of arsenic to the sulfhydryl groups of the protein keratin. Prior to this, arsenic salts are biotransformed by methylation to methylarsenic and dimethylarsenic acids.

The latter is the major form of arsenic that is excreted, and excretion is mainly in urine; however, arsenic can be eliminated in feces, sweat, and hair. The half-life for urinary arsenic excretion is 3 to 5 days. Arsenic crosses the placental barrier and is a teratogenic agent.

The clinical effects of arsenic poisoning are a reflection of this compound's biochemical effects. These include reversible combination of arsenites with protein sulfhydryl groups, in particular, protein coenzymes that are necessary for the oxidation of pyruvic and succinic acid. The net effect of this action is to reduce oxidative phosphorylation and ATP energy production. Arsenic as an arsenate can substitute for phosphorus in biochemical reactions, also preventing ATP formation.

Symptoms of toxicity

Arsenic is so quickly absorbed that symptoms of acute poisoning can occur within minutes to hours of exposure. Because of this rapid distribution, a wide range of organs are involved. Table 25-1 is a summary of selected symptoms of acute and chronic arsenic poisoning. No single symptom is exclusively associated with arsenic poisoning, although the garlic breath odor and the transverse white lines of the nails (Aldrich-Mees lines) are unique.

Exposure to arsine gas is different than exposure to inorganic or organic arsenic in that there is a variable delay of up to 24 hours in the onset of symptoms (Box 25-2). Patients exposed to the gas have severe hemolysis and compromised oxygen-carrying capacity.

Laboratory analysis

Because arsenic is cleared so rapidly (half-life = 7 hours) urine is the more useful specimen for the determination of arsenic exposure. Blood can be analyzed if exposure has

---

Box 25-1 Arsenic exposure

OCCUPATIONAL

Coal dust
Insecticides
Herbicides
Rodenticides
Fungicides
Paints

HOUSEHOLD

Wallpaper
Ceramics
Glass

ENVIRONMENTAL

Fruits
Water
Shellfish
Livestock feed additives

Table 25-1 Symptoms of arsenic poisoning

Acute*	Chronic
Vomiting	Nausea
Bloody diarrhea	Vomiting
Garlic breath odor	Diarrhea
Abdominal pain	Jaundice
Cardiac abnormalities	Hyperpigmentations
Shock	Proteinuria
Convulsions	Anemia
Tremor	Neuropathy
Coma	Loss of hair
Mees' lines	Edema (local)

*0.5–2.0 hours post ingestion; acute fatal dosage is 120 mg.

Box 25-2 Arsine gas exposure

Latent period
Abdominal pain, nausea, vomiting
Headache, weakness, numbness
Hemolysis (hyperkalemia)
Renal failure (hemoglobinuria)
Pulmonary edema

been very recent. Hair and nails can be analyzed for arsenic to confirm chronic toxicity. For blood analysis of arsenic, trace metal–free tubes using an oxalate anticoagulant are preferred, although heparin is acceptable. Normal whole blood concentrations are usually 5 to 60 μg/L, but should be determined by each laboratory since values are affected by arsenic in the water supply and dietary intake of the local region. Blood concentrations of 100 to 500 μg/L are indicative of chronic exposure, and levels greater than 600 μg/L are indicative of acute exposure (Table 25-2).

For urinary arsenic detection, a 24-hour specimen is acceptable. The sample should be collected in an acid-washed, metal-free container with no preservative and should be stored refrigerated prior to analysis. Normal urine arsenic concentrations are usually 0 to 100 μg/L (ng/mL). At values of 100 to 200 μg/L, chronic arsenic exposure is probable unless there is heavy consumption of seafood. Urine concentrations above 200 μg/L are indicative of acute arsenic exposure.

Following exposure to arsenic, urine values can remain elevated for up to 6 to 8 weeks, although within 4 to 5 days the less toxic methylated arsenic forms are predominant in urine.

Arsenic can also be measured in hair and in nails as noted earlier. Care must be taken to avoid exogenous surface contamination. For this reason, in a suspected industrial exposure, it is desirable to use pubic hair or toenails, since these samples are more difficult to contaminate. A sample of 200 to 500 mg is collected in a small, clean, plastic bag. Normal values in hair range up to 65 μg/100 g, with values greater than 100 μg/100 g indicative of chronic exposure. In nails, the comparable normal values are 90 to 180 μg/100 g; greater than 200 μg/100 g indicates chronic exposure.

Arsenic can be qualitatively detected in urine by the Gutzeit test, in which the test tube generation of arsine gas discolors silver nitrate paper, or by Reinsch's test, in which arsenic, when heated, forms a black deposit on a copper wire. The preferred methods for arsenic determination are by atomic absorption spectrometry either via the generation of arsine gas or through the use of electrothermal atomization.

Treatment

Treatment for acute arsenic exposure involves emesis and/or lavage within 6 hours of exposure, followed by

administration of activated charcoal and a cathartic. Chelation therapy with dimercaprol should be instituted until urine arsenic values drop to 30 to 50 μg/L. Dimercaprol (British anti-Lewisite, BAL) itself can cause adverse reactions, and if it is not tolerated, D-penicillamine can be used.

In cases of exposure to arsine gas, chelation therapy is not useful. Treatment is directed at the management of severe hemolysis, which may include transfusions, and supportive care for renal failure. Hyperkalemia should be monitored closely and urine should be alkalinized.

Lead
Sources and exposure

Lead (Pb) occurs widely in the environment and is extremely hazardous because its effects are both severe and cumulative. It is mined throughout the world and sources of exposure include occupational, household, and general environmental. Examples are given in Box 25-3. Children are most susceptible to the toxic effects of lead. There does not appear to be any biological role for lead and the majority of toxic cases arise from chronic exposure.

For all practical purposes, exposure is mainly to lead in its inorganic form as a lead salt. Organically bound lead is almost exclusively associated with leaded gasoline and its combustion. Occupational exposure is chiefly the inhalation of lead dusts generated in a variety of industries (Box 25-3). The major household exposure route for lead is drinking water, especially where lead pipes are used and the water is soft. The concentration of lead in water should not exceed 50 μg/L; this may be decreased to 5 μg/L by the federal government. In addition to moonshine whiskey (distilled in lead-lined car radiators), certain wines may be high in lead. Smoking cigarettes is a source of lead exposure. On the average, respiratory tract exposure to lead results in the absorption of 30% to 40% of the dose. Inhalation of auto exhaust and leaded gasoline fumes is the principal exposure route to organic-bound lead. Included in the latter source

Table 25-2   Reference values for arsenic

Specimen	Concentration	Comment
Whole blood	5-60 μg/L	Normal
	100-500 μg/L	Chronic exposure
	>600 μg/L	Acute exposure
Urine	0-100 μg/L	Normal
	100-200 μg/L	Chronic exposure
	>200 μg/L	Acute exposure
Hair	0-65 μg/100 g	Normal
	>100 μg/100 g	Chronic exposure
Nails	90-180 μg/100 g	Normal
	>200 μg/100 g	Chronic exposure

Box 25-3   Lead exposure

OCCUPATIONAL

Batteries
Refineries
Printing
Smelting
Shipbuilding
Welding
Paint and pigments

HOUSEHOLD

Water (lead pipes)
Herbal medicines
Moonshine whiskey
Burning color magazines
Paints
Pottery glaze

ENVIRONMENTAL

Gasoline
Auto exhaust

would be intentional gasoline-sniffing by adolescents. Lead is a major toxic metal to children because they absorb and retain more than adults and have less capacity for excretion than adults. They have a high frequency of accidental exposure through oral ingestion of lead-based paints since young children have a tendency to consume nonfood items.

Lead is initially distributed to soft tissues, especially the kidneys and liver. With time, the metal is redistributed to bone, teeth, and hair, with 95% of the body burden found in bone. The remainder of body lead is found in blood, chiefly in erythrocytes. Unabsorbed lead is excreted in feces and absorbed lead is excreted in urine.

Clinical effects and mechanisms

The toxicity of lead is due to the ability of the metal to bind with a number of amino acid ligands, especially sulfhydryl groups. This is significant because sulfhydryl groups are at the active sites of enzymes, which are crucial to normal cell energy output and to oxygen transport. Amino acids with strong metal-binding groups include cysteine (sulfhydryl) and histidine (imidazole). The major cellular site of lead toxicity is in the mitochondrion. Lead toxicity results in structural changes in this organelle and in many biochemical perturbations. A list of specific hematopoietic effects of lead is contained in Table 25-3. Lead also prevents the catabolism of ribonucleic acid (RNA), resulting in the accumulation of aggregates of incompletely degraded ribosomes, which are observed as basophilic stippling. This condition is not specific to lead poisoning.

Symptoms of toxicity

Lead toxicity affects many systems as seen in Table 25-4. The effects of lead are dependent on the chemical form of lead and the duration of exposure. With inorganic and elemental lead, and acute exposure, the triad of colic, anemia, and encephalopathy are observed. Chronic exposure may not produce typical symptoms. Organolead compounds, which are lipid-soluble, volatile, and rapidly absorbed, have major effects on the central nervous system. Both neurologic and psychiatric symptoms are manifested.

The symptoms of acute lead poisoning can include metallic taste, abdominal pain, vomiting, diarrhea, black stools, behavioral changes, convulsions, and coma. Chronic symptoms are nonspecific and vague. A partial list of the effects of chronic lead intoxication is given in Table 25-4.

Table 25-3 Hematopoietic effects of lead*

Site	Effect
Aminolevulinic acid (ALA) synthetase	Increased ALA in urine
Delta ALA dehydratase	Decreased porphobilinogen
Coproporphyrinogen decarboxylase	Increase coproporphyrin in urine
Ferrochelatase	Increased protoporphyrin in erythrocytes (FEP)†
Na-K pump and erythrocyte membrane	Increased fragility of erythrocyte

*Net effect is decreased heme synthesis and anemia.
†FEP, free erythrocyte protoporphyrin.

Laboratory analysis

Clinical or other evidence of exposure to lead can be buttressed by laboratory findings. Whole blood lead is the most reliable indicator of exposure. Since lead binds so extensively to erythrocytes, serum and plasma concentrations are not useful. Blood should be drawn by venipuncture, never by fingerstick because of surface contamination, and drawn into trace metal–free containers containing either heparin or EDTA (blue or brown top). Samples should be refrigerated within 48 hours if not analyzed immediately. Lead can also be measured in urine, but because values do not correlate as well as whole blood with total body burden, urine is not the specimen of choice to screen for inorganic lead toxicity. Lead is frequently measured in urine to assess organolead poisoning, as part of a urinary heavy metal screen, and to monitor lead excretion following chelation therapy. For urinary lead determination, a 24-hour collection should be performed using acid-washed polycarbonate containers. The collected sample should be acidified to pH 2.0 or below and refrigerated prior to analysis. Blood lead values are usually measured by anodic stripping voltametry (ASV) or by electrothermal atomic absorption spectrophotometry (EAAS) and urine concentrations by EAAS. Guidelines for normal and elevated values are presented in Table 25-5.

Other tests that are sometimes used as a method of screening for lead exposure are based on lead's interference with the synthesis of heme and include whole blood free erythrocyte protoporphyrin (FEP). Tests for this analyte are excellent methods for detection of chronic lead exposure. Free

Table 25-4 Chronic lead exposure symptoms

System	Symptoms
Gastrointestinal	Constipation, metallic taste, abdominal pain, loss of appetite
Hematopoietic	Anemia, basophilic stippling
Neurologic	Peripheral neuropathy, wrist or foot drop, lead encephalopathy
Other systems affected	Protein and casts in urine; possible gingival lead line; abnormal ovarian cycles and menstrual disorders; increased infertility; increased spontaneous abortions; fetal malformations

Table 25-5 Reference values for lead

Specimen	Concentration	Comments
Whole blood	0-200 μg/L	Normal*
	200-700 μg/L†	Chronic exposure, subclinical to mild symptoms
	>700 μg/L	Acute exposure, severe symptoms
Urine	0-80 μg/24 hr	Normal
	80-120 μg/24 hr	Possible exposure, inconclusive
	>120 μg/24 hr	Excessive levels associated with toxicity

*Concentrations should be lower (1/3 to 1/2) in pregnant women.
†The Centers for Disease Control has defined an elevated blood lead level = 100 μg/L for children younger than 6 years old.

erythrocyte protoporphyrin values are also elevated in iron deficiency anemia, but values of FEP over 350 μg/L, coupled with whole blood lead concentrations greater than 200 μg/L, should be investigated further as should any blood lead results >500 μg/L in children. Erythrocyte zinc protoporphyrin is a test that sensitively reflects lead absorption over the preceding 3 months. The presence of elevated zinc porphyrin (whole blood: normal <1000 μg/L) indicates that the presence of lead has prevented iron incorporation into heme and zinc has substituted for iron. Tests performed less frequently include urinary and blood aminolevulinic acid (ALA) values, and the enzymes, aminolevulinic acid synthetase and delta ALA dehydratase, which are reduced in activity beginning at about 100 μg/L of blood lead. Because of potential contamination, lead analysis in hair has not proven useful.

Treatment

The treatment of lead poisoning will be dictated by the level of presenting symptoms, but will in general include some form of chelation therapy. The guidelines for therapy can be complex and can include chelation with a single agent or with multiple agents (usually dimercaprol, BAL, and/or calcium-disodium EDTA).

Mercury

Sources and exposure

Mercury (Hg), like arsenic, was an important therapeutic agent in years past. Today, contact with mercury and its salts is most likely to occur in an occupational setting or through the environment (Box 25-4). Elemental mercury is a liquid at room temperature and the forms of the metal most often encountered are mercury vapor (elemental mercury), inorganic mercurous and mercuric salts, and organic aryl (phenyl), and alkyl (methyl) mercurial compounds.

Mercury enters the body via the respiratory system through the inhalation of elemental mercury vapors, through the gastrointestinal tract via ingestion of inorganic or organic mercury compounds, and through the skin via absorption of organic alkyl mercury compounds. The absorption of elemental mercury is poor.

Mercury exists in inorganic compounds as the monovalent mercurous or divalent mercuric salts. The latter is the more toxic. Mercuric nitrate salt that was used in the manufacture of felt hats was a common industrial hazard that produced profound behavioral and neurologic changes in exposed workers (mad hatters). Organic mercury compounds (alkyl and aryl salts) are absorbed in the gastrointestinal tract and are quite toxic. The most common organic form is methylmercury, which was identified as the causative agent in a toxic epidemic in Minimata, Japan, in the 1950s. Inorganic mercury, dumped into the ocean, was converted by bacteria to methylmercury, which was concentrated in fish and consumed by the local population.

After absorption, inorganic mercury is distributed to a number of tissues within 2 to 3 hours, with the highest concentration found in the kidneys (proximal tubules). Organic mercurials, which are more completely absorbed than the inorganic forms (90% of oral dose absorbed), are distributed uniformly in the body (liver, hair, skin, blood, brain). The major clinical effects of organic alkyl mercury occur in the central nervous system. Non-alkyl organic mercurials undergo biotransformation to produce inorganic mercury. Therefore, their toxicity is similar to inorganic mercury poisoning. All forms of mercury can cross the blood-brain barrier. Inorganic mercury is chiefly eliminated in the urine and feces; organic forms of mercury are excreted in the bile.

Clinical effects and mechanisms

Mercury readily reacts with protein sulfhydryl groups to form mercaptides, thus inhibiting a wide range of enzymes and protein transport mechanisms. Mercury can also react with other ligands (e.g., amine, carboxyl, and phosphoryl groups) to further interfere with metabolism. The high concentrations of mercury in the kidneys, reached during excretion, can lead to severe damage of the glomeruli and tubules.

Symptoms of toxicity

Symptoms of mercury poisoning will differ depending on the route and form of the mercury exposure. Table 25-

---

Box 25-4 Mercury exposure

OCCUPATIONAL

Mining (gold)
Dental labs
Manufacturing (paper, chlorine, plastics, thermometers, lamps, batteries)
Photoengraving
Fungicides

HOUSEHOLD

Broken fluorescent bulbs and thermometers
Antiseptics
Mercury switches

ENVIRONMENTAL

Seafood
Dental analgams

Table 25-6 Acute mercury exposure symptoms

Route	Compound	
Inhalation	**Vapors**	
	Cough	
	Dyspnea	
	Nausea	
	Pulmonary	
	Oral burning	
	Salivation	
	Vomiting	
Ingestion	**Inorganic**	**Organic**
	Abdominal pain	Ataxia
	Bloody diarrhea	Convulsions
	Metallic taste	Speech problems
	Thirst	Tremors
	Vomiting	Visual field constriction

6 lists some of the signs and symptoms of acute mercury exposure. The symptoms of chronic exposure to mercury (inorganic, elemental, non-alkyl organic) include disorders associated with the oral cavity, involuntary tremors, a broad range of psychological disturbances, renal edema and proteinuria, and a number of nonspecific symptoms (weakness, weight loss, gastrointestinal problems). Chronic exposure to alkyl mercury compounds affects the central nervous system with symptoms of intoxication that include headache, numbness, ataxia, tremor, and hearing loss. In severe poisonings paralysis and coma have been observed.

Laboratory analysis

To confirm suspected mercury poisoning, both whole blood and urine mercury can be analyzed. In cases of recent exposure to mercury, whole blood is the specimen of choice. Samples should be drawn into a trace-element–free tube containing either heparin or EDTA. The normal range is 0 to 5 µg/L; toxicity symptoms are evident at 20 to 30 µg/L (Table 25-7). Chronic exposure to mercury may be confirmed by mercury analysis through a 24-hour timed urine collection. Urine should be collected in an acid-washed plastic (polycarbonate) container and the sample acidified to pH 2.0 with concentrated hydrochloric acid. A 24-hour urine sample from an unexposed individual should have 0–20 µg Hg/24 hours collection. Values ≥100 µg/24 hours may indicate exposure to organic mercury and values ≥200 µg/24 hours may indicate exposure to inorganic or elemental mercury. There is variation between symptomatic patients and even in an individual patient over time. Urinary or blood concentrations do not correlate with clinical signs. Urinary values of mercury are useful for monitoring chelation therapy. Blood is a better specimen for the assessment of alkyl mercury exposure since less than 10% is excreted in urine. The erythrocyte/plasma ratio of organic mercury is 5 to 20 and is 1.0 for inorganic mercury. Separate measurement of plasma and erythrocytes may distinguish between these two types of exposure.

Hair can be analyzed for mercury; however, sample collection must be done carefully as external contamination may be a problem and the results may be unreliable.

Treatment

Acute mercury poisoning is treated with gastric lavage or emesis and catharsis. Other methods of elimination enhancement are not useful. Dimercaprol is an excellent chelator of inorganic mercury and is useful in severe inorganic

exposure and in aryl organic exposure (aryl mercury compounds are biotransformed to inorganic mercury). Penicillamine has also been used when chelation is indicated; however, chelation therapy does not aid alkyl organic mercury poisoning.

Aluminum
Sources and exposure

Aluminum (Al) is the most abundant metal and represents the third most common element in the earth's crust (exceeded only by oxygen and silicon). Aluminum does not occur in nature in the metallic state, but rather exists in combination with other elements in rocks, clay, soils, gems, and minerals. Aluminum as a silicate or oxide occurs in high concentrations in dust particles and air conditioner exhausts. Aluminum is found in all types of soil, in natural and fluorinated waters, and in plants. The major sources of aluminum in the normal human diet are from plant sources and processed foods. Compounds of industrial importance that contain significant amounts of aluminum include bauxite, alum, cryolite, corundum, and kaolin. Bauxite, the only major commercial source of aluminum, contains 45% to 60% aluminum oxide (alumina).

Aluminum compounds are added to many processed foods as buffering, neutralization, firming, and leavening agents. Aluminum-containing products are extensively employed as cooking ware, eating utensils, food storage containers; in the manufacturing of abrasives, cements, and ceramic products; and as a filler in plastic products. The petroleum industry utilizes aluminum extensively for the removal of moisture from vapors, liquids, and natural gas, and as a catalyst in refining processes. The United States, Great Britain, and most developed nations use alum (aluminum sulfate) as a coagulant (flocculant) in their water purification plants.

Medicinally, aluminum compounds have been used most extensively for their antacid and phosphate-binding capacties and as adjuvants in a number of vaccines. Salts of aluminum are employed as astringents, styptics, and antiseptics. The principal therapeutic use of aluminum-containing compounds is as antacids for the treatment of ulcers and other gastrointestinal disorders. Because of aluminum's prevalence in the environment, it is virtually impossible to avoid an almost continual exposure to aluminum compounds.

Aluminum enters the human body via oral ingestion of food and drink, as well as by inhalation of atmospheric dusts (Box 25-5). The normal daily oral intake ranges from 10 to 100 mg, and the total body content of aluminum is approximately 30 mg. Means values (mg/L or mg/kg dry weight) of aluminum in adult humans not taking aluminum-containing drugs are as follows: bone, 3.9; muscle, 1.2 to 1.55; brain, 1.1 to 1.4; and serum, 0.024 to 0.34. The biological role of aluminum has not been demonstrated, nor has an aluminum deficiency state been characterized in animals. Aluminum is primarily removed from the body in the urine and feces.

Clinical effects and mechanisms

Insoluble aluminum compounds (e.g., mixtures of aluminum phosphate and pyrophosphate) appear to be devoid

Table 25-7 Reference values for mercury

Specimen	Concentration	Comments
Whole blood	0-5 µg/L	Normal
	20-30 µg/L	Toxic
Urine	0-20 µg/24 hr	Normal
	≥100 µg/24 hr	Exposure to organics
	≥200 µg/24 hr	Exposure to inorganic or elemental
WBC*/Plasma ratio	5-20	Organic exposure
	1.0	Inorganic exposure

*WBC, white blood cells.

of acute toxicity by all routes of administration (with the exception of transient skin irritation). By contrast, soluble salts of aluminum are acutely toxic (Box 25-6).

Chronic exposure to high doses of aluminum via all routes of administration (i.e., topical, oral, parenteral, inhalation) causes small but detectable toxicity symptoms. Aluminum toxicity is most commonly associated with pulmonary toxicity in industrial workers, resulting from inhalation of aluminum as dust. This toxicity has also been observed to involve the nervous system. In fact, the first suspected aluminum encephalopathy in man—characterized by mental deterioration, focal neurological signs, general convulsions, and death—was associated with the inhalation of aluminum dust. At postmortem, the brain contained 17 times the normal concentration of aluminum. Aluminum has been strongly implicated in several clinical neurotoxicities, including dialysis encephalopathy, Alzheimer's disease, and anterior horn cell disorders such as Guamanian amyotrophic lateral sclerosis. Aluminum has been reported to affect membrane lipids, decrease respiration, reduce sugar phosphorylation, interfere with the uptake and utilization of calcium, phosphorus, and other elements, alter energy metabolism, and inhibit acetylcholine esterase activity. However, of greatest interest is that a primary site of aluminum action appears to be in cellular events associated with cell division and genetic processes.

Symptoms of toxicity

Symptoms of toxic exposure to aluminum usually develop over a long period of time and include hypercalcemia, anemia, osteodystrophy (refractive to vitamin D), and encephalopathy. Pulmonary fibrosis has been reported in industrial exposure cases. Patients on long-term hemodialysis treatment have experienced dialysis dementia due to exposure to elevated aluminum-containing dialysis fluids. Initial behavioral changes and speech disorders progress to dementia and sometimes convulsions in these patients.

Laboratory analysis

In addition to the usual laboratory support to assist in the diagnosis of symptoms associated with aluminum toxicity, analysis of aluminum can be of assistance, for example, in the monitoring of exposure of dialysis patients to aluminum in dialysis fluid. Normal individuals should have serum aluminum values of 0 to 10 μg/L; patients on chronic hemodialysis can have results up to 60 μg/L with minimal symptoms (Table 25-8). Serum concentrations exceeding 100 μg/L would be consistent with potential toxic symptoms. Since aluminum is highly protein bound, serum values do not reflect total body burden but can be used to monitor aluminum exposure, especially that associated with hemodialysis. Serum samples should be drawn into trace-metal–free tubes, centrifuged as rapidly as possible, and stored in acid-washed plastic tubes. Analysis is by electrothermal atomic absorption spectrometry and great care must be taken to avoid contamination. Patients on chelation therapy with desferrioxamine may exhibit very high post-dosage aluminum concentrations. Urine has been used (24-hour timed collection, collected in acid-washed plastic containers) to monitor occupational exposure and chelation therapy (normal = 0 to 30 μg Al/24 hour). The analysis of aluminum in hair is too variable to be clinically useful.

Treatment

Dialysis encephalopathy and osteomalacia have been treated with the chelating agent desferrioxamine. The procedure is usually initiated when serum aluminum concentrations reach 100 to 200 μg/L. Desferrioxamine has also been used in the diagnosis of aluminum-related osteodystrophy. In one study an increase of 200 μg Al/mL serum following a challenge with the chelator identified 95% of biopsy diagnosed osteodystrophy cases.

OTHER TOXIC METALS
Cadmium

Cadmium is a nonessential, toxic, carcinogenic, trace metal. Cadmium is an important industrial metal that is used in electroplating, as a pigment in paints and plastics, and in the cathodes of nickel-cadmium batteries (Box 25-7). Exposure to cadmium is mainly occupational in industries associated with the aforementioned uses, as well as in welding and smelting industries. Cadmium occurs in nature in association with zinc and lead. Environmental exposure to

---

Box 25-5   Aluminum exposure

OCCUPATIONAL
Bauxite mining
Plastics
Ceramics

HOUSEHOLD
Antacids
Astringents
Cookware
Processed Foods

ENVIRONMENTAL
Water
Dusts

Box 25-6   Symptoms of aluminum toxicity

Hypercalcemia
Pulmonary symptoms
Encephalopathy
Convulsions
Anemia
Osteodystrophy

Table 25-8   Reference values for aluminum

Specimen	Concentration	Comments
Serum	0-10 μg/L	Normal
	<60 μg/L	Dialysis
	>100 μg/L	Chronic exposure
Urine	0-30 μg/24 hr	Normal
	>50 μg/24 hr	Toxic?

Box 25-7	Cadmium-nickel-thallium exposure
Cadmium (Cd)	Electroplating
	Paint manufacturing
	Battery cathodes
	Welding
	Smelting
Nickel (Ni)	Mining
	Refineries
	Electroplating
	Alloys
	Batteries
Thallium (Th)	Medicinals
	Insecticides
	Jewelry manufacturing

Table 25-9 Cadmium-nickel reference values

Specimen	Cadmium	Nickel
Whole blood (N)*	0.5-1.1 μg/L	0-1.05 μg/L
(T)*	>7-10 μg/L	
Urine (N)	<1 μg/L	0-7 μg/L 24 hr
(T)	>10 μg/L	>20 μg/L
Serum	—	0.05-1.1 μg/L

*N, normal; T, toxic.

cadmium includes smelting fumes, cigarette smoke, and contaminated foodstuffs. A striking example of cadmium-contaminated food occurred in Japan when the effluent from a cadmium-lead-zinc mining operation contaminated rice fields. Ingestion of the rice resulted in severe rheumatic and myalgic pain, especially among middle-aged women.

Cadmium accumulates in the body throughout life (estimated half-life in man is 19 to 38 years), and the average body burden in the United States is around 30 mg. Cadmium can enter the body via the lungs and gastrointestinal tract, with about 25% and 10%, respectively, of an available dose being absorbed. Once absorbed, cadmium is bound to the plasma proteins metallothionein and albumin. A majority of absorbed cadmium is stored in the kidneys, and to a lesser extent in the liver. The dominant excretory route for cadmium is in urine.

Acute respiratory exposure to cadmium results in fever, headache, chest pain, sore throat, and cough, which develop 6 to 12 hours after exposure. Acute oral exposure causes severe gastroenteritis. In chronic exposure the kidney is the main target organ, and renal dysfunction (proteinuria) and renal hypertension are symptoms. The incidence of emphysema and chronic bronchitis are significantly elevated in cadmium workers.

Cadmium's toxic effects result from enzyme inhibition via binding to key ligand groups, including cysteinyl sulfhydryls. Cadmium inhibits alpha$_1$-antitrypsin, which may account for its pulmonary symptoms.

Recent exposure to cadmium is best assessed by the measurement of whole blood cadmium concentrations by electrothermal atomic absorption. Normal whole blood cadmium values range from 0.5 μg/L in nonsmokers to 1.0 to 1.1 μg/L in smokers. Values greater than 7 to 10 μg/L would indicate excessive exposure to cadmium (Table 25-9). Chronic exposure to cadmium can be monitored by using serial urine cadmium concentrations. Normal urine cadmium values in nonsmokers are usually less than 1 μg/L and most of the cadmium is bound to metallothionein. Urinary cadmium values in excess of 10 μg/L indicates toxic exposure. Chronic exposure usually increases concentrations two- to threefold. Serial monitoring of urinary values is the usual procedure to detect occupational exposure. Because chronic cadmium exposure targets the kidneys, re-

sulting in proteinuria, a number of biological markers have been measured to detect exposure. The most sensitive appears to be beta$_2$-microglobulin, which is analyzed by immunoassay techniques. Normal urine concentrations are usually less than 120 μg per 24 hours. Elevated values are directly related to years of exposure. Increased results are also observed in acquired immunodeficiency syndrome (AIDS), systemic lupus erythematosus, and rheumatoid arthritis, among other conditions.

The treatment of chronic cadmium exposure involves removal from all sources of contamination; chelation therapy is ineffective. Acute exposure is treated with supportive care for pulmonary edema, and although chelators can increase cadmium excretion, the complexes dissociate easily in the kidneys and their use can increase renal toxicity.

Nickel

Nickel is a ubiquitous, carcinogenic trace metal found in mining operations, refineries, and certain manufacturing industries (electroplating, alloys, batteries). Severe toxicity has been observed following inhalation of nickel carbonyl. This compound is a key intermediate in the refining of nickel. Following exposure to nickel carbonyl, immediate symptoms include dizziness, headache, epigastric pain, nausea, and vomiting. Some individuals only develop symptoms following a latent period of 1 to 5 days. Nickel can produce a severe contact dermatitis.

The majority (90%) of ingested nickel is excreted unabsorbed in the feces. Absorbed nickel accumulates in the connective tissue, kidneys, and lungs, but the majority of absorbed metal is excreted in the urine.

The analysis of nickel is most often performed by electrothermal atomic absorption spectrometry. Normal (unexposed) urinary values are 0 to 7 μg/24 hour collection, and in general, values can exceed 20 μg/L in cases of chronic exposure. Nickel has been measured in serum, plasma, and whole blood. Normal serum concentrations are 0.05 to 1.1 μg/L and serum values up to 100 μg/L have been observed in nickel refinery workers. Monitoring of chronic exposure is best accomplished with urine analysis since nickel concentrations are higher in urine than serum in both nonexposed and exposed individuals, and nickel contamination from stainless steel needles is avoided. Plastic cannulae are recommended for blood collection for nickel analysis. Acute nickel poisoning can be treated with the chelating agent diethyldithiocarbamate (Dicarb). This compound has also been successfully used in reversing symptoms of chronic exposure among affected workers.

Thallium

Thallium was discovered in the mid-nineteenth century and was used to treat syphilis, ringworm, and dysentery, and was also used as a depilatory paste. Thallium is used in a number of industries, including the manufacture of jewelry, optical lenses, pigments, low-temperature thermometers, glass, and semiconductors. Until banned by the government, thallium was used in insecticides and rodenticides.

Thallium may be one of the most toxic metals known. It is quickly adsorbed from the gastrointestinal tract, has a high volume of distribution, and is extensively distributed intracellularly, where it attaches to protein sulfhydryl groups and inhibits many enzymatic reactions. Thallium has a much greater affinity than potassium for Na^+/K^+ ATPase, and subsequently disrupts oxidative phosphorylation. Thallium can substitute for potassium in physiologic reactions (depolarizing membranes), and is soluble at physiological pH and thus does not deposit in bone. Thallium crosses the blood-brain barrier and is stored in axons.

The symptoms of thallium poisoning are most evident in the gastrointestinal tract and in the central nervous system. Symptoms in the gastrointestinal tract occur within 4 hours of ingestion and include nausea, vomiting, and diarrhea. Effects on the nervous system may develop hours to days following exposure and include lethargy, coma, convulsions, neuromuscular symptoms and hypertension, sweating and fever. Late symptoms (2 to 4 weeks) include alopecia, Aldrich-Mees lines across the nails, kidney and liver damage.

Thallium is best analyzed by electrothermal atomic absorption in blood and urine. Urine analysis can be a problem because thallium is excreted mainly in feces; hair analysis is useless because thallium is not incorporated into hair. Normal concentrations of thallium should be zero, so the presence of any metal would indicate exposure. The presence of thallium lowers serum potassium levels and creates a mild hypochloremic metabolic alkalosis.

There is really no safe, efficient treatment or any compound that neutralizes thallium exposure.

NUTRITIONAL TRACE METALS
Chromium

Chromium is an essential metal that functions as a component of glucose tolerance factor (GTF). Glucose tolerance factor is a naturally occurring complex of nicotinic acid, chromium, glycine, glutamate, and cysteine, which enhances the effects of insulin presumably by facilitating insulin binding to receptor sites.

The recommended daily allowance (RDA) for chromium is 50 to 200 µg and less than 25% is absorbed by the gastrointestinal tract. The average consumption in the United States is about 60 µg/day, chiefly from meat, cheese, whole grain, brewer's yeast, and molasses. The range of chromium intake is very wide and there is no good evidence of cases of chromium deficiency. Deficiency assessment is further confused by the fact that certain individuals can synthesize GTF from its components, whereas other individuals depend on preformed GTF in the diet. The distribution of GTF in natural foods is not known. Most, but not all, diabetics do not respond to either chromium or GTF treatment.

Table 25-10   Trace metal reference values

Metal	Specimen	Reference range	SI conversion
Chromium (Cr)	S*	0.2-0.5 µg/L	19.2 (nmol/L)
	WB*	0.7-2.8 µg/L	19.2 (nmol/L)
	U*	<1.0 µg/d	19.2 (nmol/d)
	H*	0.1-3.6 µg/g	19.2 (nmol/g)
Cobalt (Co)	S	0.2-2.0 µg/L	17.0 (nmol/L)
	WB	2.0-2.8 µg/L	17.0 (nmol/L)
	U	0.7-10 µg/d	17.0 (nmol/d)
	H	0.2-1.0 µg/g	17.0 (nmol/g)
Copper (Cu)	S	700-1400 µg/L (M)	0.0157 (µmol/L)
		800-1550 µg/L (F)	0.0157 (µmol/L)
	U	15-60 µg/d	0.0157 (µmol/d)
	H	10-40 µg/g	0.0157 (µmol/g)
Manganese (Mn)	S	1-3 µg/L	18.2 (nmol/L)
	WB	<10 µg/L	18.2 (nmol/L)
	U	<1.0 µg/d	18.2 (nmol/d)
	H	0.1-2.1 µg/g	18.2 (nmol/g)
Molybdenum (Mo)	S	0.1-6.0 µg/L	10.4 (nmol/L)
	WB	1-15.0 µg/L	10.4 (nmol/L)
	U	10-16 µg/L	10.4 (nmol/L)
	H	0.06-0.20 µg/g	10.4 (nmol/g)
Selenium (Se)	S	78-320 µg/L	0.0127 (µmol/L)
	WB	100-340 µg/L	0.0127 (µmol/L)
	U	15-100 µg/L	0.0127 (µmol/L)
	H	0.60-2.6 µg/g	0.0127 (µmol/g)
Zinc (Zn)	S	700-1500 µg/L	0.0153 (µmol/L)
	U	0.15-1.0 mg/d	15.3 (µmol/d)
	H	100-280 µg/g	0.0153 (µmol/g)

*S, serum; WB, whole blood; U, urine; H, hair.

Chromium is used in a number of industries and exposure is usually by inhalation of dust or fumes. Some chromite(ate) compounds are carcinogenic. Hexavalent chromium salts are more toxic than trivalent forms.

Unexposed, healthy individuals have serum chromium values of 0.20 to 0.50 µg/L and urinary values less than 1.0 µg/d (electrothermal atomic absorption spectrometry) (Table 25-10). Exposed workers have demonstrated urine values of 30 to 200 µg/L. Chromium has been assayed in hair, and normal adult values (0.1 to 3.6 µg/g) increase twentyfold in workers exposed to chromium salts (15 to 17 µg/g).

Cobalt

Cobalt is an essential element found in vitamin B_{12}. Vitamin B_{12} (cobalamin, extrinsic factor) is an obligatory cofactor in the synthesis of methionine and in the catabolism of branched-chain amino acids. Vitamin B_{12} deficiency is manifested by megaloblastic anemia associated with neurological deterioration. Vitamin B_{12} is found in a wide range of foods of animal origin; a deficiency in this vitamin or in cobalt is rare. There is no RDA for cobalt and average intake is 250 to 300 µg/day.

Industrial exposure to cobalt dust and fumes in the steel and paint industries produces an allergic dermatitis and pulmonary fibrosis. In uremic patients cobalt accumulates in the serum and is cardiotoxic. When cobalt was an additive in beer productions, it was implicated in the heart disease and polycythemia of chronic beer drinkers.

Normal urinary cobalt output can range from 0.7 to 10 μg/d, and whole blood cobalt ranges from 2.0 to 2.8 μg/L (Table 25-10).

Copper

Copper is an essential metal contained in a number of important metalloenzymes, for example, cytochrome c oxidase, dopamine β-hydroxylase, superoxide dismutase, lysyl oxidase, and ferroxidase (ceruloplasmin). Thus, copper is essential for proper iron metabolism (ferroxidase) and connective tissue (collagen and elastin) synthesis (lysyl oxidase).

The RDA for copper is 2 to 3 mg for adults. Approximately 35% of an ingested dose is absorbed, and of this, 80% is excreted in the bile, 18% in feces, and 2% in urine.

Adequate copper should be available from the diet; however, absorption via the gastrointestinal tract can be variable. The major factors affecting absorption include the amount ingested, bioavailability, dietary constituents, and disease state.

Copper deficiency has been observed in malnourished infants and in infants on hyperalimentation in which trace metal levels were inadequate. As indicated earlier, copper is essential for the integrity of ceruloplasmin. Since this metalloprotein converts ferrous ion to ferric ion, which then binds to transferrin, a deficiency in copper will result in an iron-deficiency anemia. This condition can be corrected by iron *and* copper supplementation.

Excessive intake of copper, leading to copper toxicity, can arise from accidental ingestion of copper salts. Copper sulfate was once (but no longer) used as an antiemetic in drug overdose cases; accidental and nonaccidental overdose with this salt is common in India. Other sources of copper poisoning include food contamination from copper utensils or industrial (refining and welding) exposure to copper fumes or dust. Acute copper toxicity is marked by nausea, vomiting, bloody diarrhea, hypotension, and hemolytic anemia. Acute inhalation of copper can cause metal fume fever, central nervous system disturbances, and respiratory distress. Chronic exposure is characterized by loss of appetite, vomiting, and hepatomegaly. The most effective management of copper poisoning is the use of the chelating agent, penicillamine.

There exist two rare inherited disorders of copper metabolism. The first is Wilson's disease, which is associated with an accumulation of copper in tissues and is characterized clinically by neurological abnormalities, liver cirrhosis, and rings of discoloration in the cornea (Kayser-Fleischer rings). Ceruloplasmin levels in most, but not all cases, will be decreased and urinary copper levels may be increased. The disease can be treated with penicillamine.

The second inherited disease of copper metabolism is Menkes' syndrome, also known as kinky hair disease. This disorder is an x-linked recessive disease in which there is a defect in copper transport. Serum copper and ceruloplasmin levels are low and there is no treatment.

The majority of absorbed copper is stored in the liver (90%); in blood, copper is bound to ceruloplasmin and albumin (10%). Copper can be measured in blood (serum or plasma) or urine, most commonly by flame or flameless atomic absorption spectrometry. Blood is usually drawn into a trace-metal–free tube with no anticoagulant. Normal values are approximately 700 to 1500 μg/L, slightly higher in women and much higher during pregnancy. Estrogens and estrogen-contraceptives increase serum copper concentrations. In suspected toxic exposure cases, serum copper values can range from 3000 (mild) to 8000 (severe) μg/L. For urine copper concentrations, a 24-hour collection (in plastic, no preservative) should be made, then acidified to pH 2.0. Normal values are 15 to 60 μg/24 hours.

Manganese

Manganese (Mn) is a trace essential metal that is a cofactor in a number of biochemical reactions. It is a component of pyruvate carboxylase and superoxide dismutase, a required cofactor in fatty acid and cholesterol synthesis, and is involved in the digestion of nucleic acids and in the synthesis of polysaccharides and glycoproteins.

Manganese intake is approximately 3 to 8 mg/d. There is no well-documented manganese deficiency state. Exposure to manganese fumes and dust in foundries, battery production, welding, and mining can result in a systemic toxicity. The effects of toxic exposure are mainly central nervous system disturbances, and specific therapy includes administration of antiparkinsonian drugs.

Manganese, like many trace metals, concentrates in erythrocytes. Whole blood, drawn in metal-free containers, is the specimen of choice for analysis of exposure. Whole blood values of less than 10 μg/L are found in unexposed individuals. Serum manganese concentrations in normal adults are usually 1 to 3 μg/L. Manganese has been measured in urine (24-hour collection in an acid-washed plastic container), but only a very small percentage is excreted in urine. In one study unexposed individuals had values less than 10 μg/L and asymptomatic manganese workers had values 25 to 125 μg/L. Atomic absorption spectrometry and neutron activation analysis are the analytical techniques of choice for manganese determination. With careful collection and if analytical precautions are followed, less than 1.0 μg/d of manganese is observed in unexposed individuals (Table 25-10).

Molybdenum

Molybdenum is an essential trace metal necessary for normal growth. The average daily intake is 200 to 400 μg. Deficiencies of molybdenum are unknown in humans. High levels of this nutrient can be found in shellfish, and it is found in many plants because of its necessary role in plant nitrogen fixation.

Molybdenum is an essential component of the enzyme xanthine oxidase. There are two atoms of molybdenum per enzyme molecule, one on each enzyme monomer. Xanthine oxidase plays a major role in purine metabolism and is the target of the drug allopurinol in the treatment of gout. Molybdenum is also an essential cofactor in the hepatic enzymes sulfite oxidase and aldehyde oxidase. Sulfite oxidase converts sulfite to sulfate in liver mitochondria and contains two molybdenum atoms per enzyme molecule. Aldehyde oxidase is an hepatic enzyme that plays a key role in both tryptophan metabolism (formation of indoleacetic acid) and in ethanol metabolism (formation of acetate from acetaldehydes).

Molybdenum can be measured in whole blood, serum, plasma, or urine (24-hour collection). The sample is usually preconcentrated, then analyzed by neutron activation analysis or atomic absorption spectrometry. Reference values are 1 to 15 μg/L (whole blood); 0.1 to 6.0 μg/L (plasma or serum); and 10 to 16 μg/L (urine).

Selenium

Selenium is an essential trace metal whose main biological role is its incorporation into the enzyme glutathione peroxidase. This enzyme is part of the body's antioxidant defense system. The enzyme destroys hydroperoxides and thus protects membrane lipids and other tissues from oxidation damage.

Seafood, milk products, and grain are the major sources of dietary selenium and the safe dietary intake for adults is 50 to 200 μg/d. The food content of selenium and the subsequent intake can vary depending on geographical area. In selenium-poor rural areas of China, there exists an endemic cardiomyopathy (Keshan disease) that is accompanied by very low blood selenium levels and which has been successfully treated with oral sodium selenite.

Chronic selenium toxicity usually associated with selenium mining and exposure to dust is similar to arsenic toxicity, producing a characteristic "garlic breath," dizziness, nausea, metallic taste, anemia, hair loss, and fingernail streaking. Urine selenium levels are the best indications of toxicity.

Acute toxicity is frequently fatal, producing major central nervous system effects, which include convulsions, within hours of ingestion.

Selenium is used in many industries, including electronics, glass, refining, copper, ceramics, and pigment manufacturing. Selenious acid (the most toxic form) is found in gun blueing solutions.

Selenium can be measured by spectrofluorometry, electrothermal atomic absorption, and by neutron activation analysis. Whole blood selenium concentrations are preferred for nutritional status studies since the major portion of blood selenium is in erythrocytes. Samples should be drawn in acid-washed or certified trace metal–free plastic tubes (heparin). Normal adult values can vary with diet and geography, but in general, range from 100 to 340 μg/L. Values over 400 μg/L are considered toxic. Urinary selenium values from an aliquot of a 24-hour specimen collected in metal-free containers should be below 100 μg/L. Higher concentrations would indicate toxic exposure, although values ranging from 1 to 5000 μg/L have been observed in exposed individuals. Selenium has also been measured in hair; in healthy adults, the range is 0.67 to 2.6 μg/g hair.

Zinc

Zinc is an essential trace metal and a critical component of a broad range of metalloenzymes (Box 25-8). Zinc is necessary for both structural stability and catalytic function in these enzymes.

Zinc is ubiquitous in food products and its content is high in meat, fish, and dairy products. Zinc absorption is inhibited in the presence of phytates (inositol phosphates), which are found in cereal grains and vegetables. The RDA for zinc in adults is 15 mg/day, lower for new-

---

Box 25-8 Zinc enzymes

Alcohol dehydrogenase
Alkaline phosphatase
Carbonic anhydrase
Carboxypeptidase
Polymerases (DNA and RNA)
Superoxide dismutase
Thymidine kinase

---

borns and infants, and higher for pregnant and lactating women. Zinc absorption in the gastrointestinal tract is an active, energy-dependent process, and is dependent on the protein metallothionein.

Zinc deficiencies are marked by poor growth, impairment of sexual function, and poor wound healing. Deficiencies are usually seen in children and have been documented in young Middle Eastern males as directly related to a low zinc-high fiber (phytates) diet. Zinc is also a necessary component of the salivary polypeptide gustin, which is necessary for the normal development of taste buds. In the United States the only symptom of marginal dietary zinc deficiency is a decrease or loss of taste acuity.

Severe zinc deficiencies have been observed in alcoholic patients, in particular those with cirrhosis. This condition is accompanied by increased infection susceptibility, impaired wound healing, sores and ulcers, dermatitis, and diarrhea. Severe deficiencies have also been observed in patients with chronic renal disease, severe malabsorption syndromes, and occasionally in individuals on long-term total parenteral nutrition. Zinc deficiency is associated with the genetic disorder acrodermatitis enteropathica and with sickle cell anemia; both diseases are treatable with zinc supplementation.

Overexposure to zinc is most common in situations in which zinc salts are ingested, or by inhalation of zinc oxide fumes. Inhalation results in metal fume fever syndrome (sudden thirst, fever, chills, and headache). Metal fume fever can arise from exposure to the fumes of copper, magnesium, aluminum, antimony, iron, manganese, and nickel. Welding, metal cutting, and zinc alloy smelting are areas that produce zinc oxide fumes. Rubber workers, embalmers, and dental cement makers are exposed to zinc salts.

Zinc is usually measured in serum, hair, or urine, and in research settings in erythrocytes and saliva. All blood should be drawn into metal-free glass tubes (e.g., dark blue BD Vacutainer, or use an acid-washed syringe), using stainless steel needles. A 24-hour urine sample should be collected in an acid-washed polyethylene container without preservative. Avoid contact with any rubber and keep the sample refrigerated. Analysis of urine samples usually requires acidification with hydrochloric or nitric acid to pH 1.5 to 2.0, followed by analysis or transport of an aliquot to the testing laboratory.

Zinc can be analyzed by colorimetry, fluorimetry, and anodic stripping voltammetry, or by the more sensitive and specific methods of atomic absorption spectrometry (flame or flameless) and neutron activation analysis.

Normal adult serum zinc concentrations are 700 to 1500 µg/L; 24-hour urine values are 0.15 to 1.00 mg/24 hours; hair (15- to 20-mg sample) values are 100 to 280 µg/g.

SUGGESTED READING

Arena JM and Drew RH: Poisoning, ed 5, Springfield, Ill, 1986, Charles C Thomas.

Baselt RC and Cravey RH: Disposition of toxic drugs and chemicals in man, ed 3, Chicago, Ill, 1990, Mosby–Year Book, Inc.

Bryson PD: Comprehensive review in toxicology, ed 2, Rockville, Md, 1989, Aspen Publishers.

Ellenhorn MJ and Barceloux DG: Medical toxicology, New York, 1988, Elsevier.

Gerson B: Clinics in laboratory medicine, 10:2,3, 1990.

Goldfrank LR and others: Goldfrank's toxicological emergencies, ed 3, Norwalk, Conn, 1986, Appleton-Century-Crofts.

Haddad LM and Winchester JF: Clinical management of poisoning and drug overdose, ed 2, Philadelphia, 1990, WB Saunders.

Henry JB: Clinical diagnosis and management by laboratory methods, ed 18, Philadelphia, 1991, WB Saunders.

Jacobs DS and others: Laboratory test handbook, Hudson, Ohio, 1990, Lexi-Comp.

Kaplan LA and Pesce AJ: Clinical chemistry: theory, analysis, and correlation, St Louis, 1984, Mosby–Year Book, Inc.

Klaassen CD, Amdur MO, and Doull J: Casarett and Doull's toxicology, ed 3, New York, 1986, Macmillan.

Noji EK, Kelen GD, and Goessel TK: Manual of toxicological emergencies, Chicago, 1989, Mosby–Year Book, Inc.

Pesce AJ and Kaplan LA: Methods in clinical chemistry, St Louis, 1987, Mosby–Year Book, Inc.

Tietz NW: Textbook of clinical chemistry, Philadelphia, 1986, WB Saunders.

26 Therapeutic drug monitoring and antibiotics

Victor Mondy

Therapeutic drug monitoring (TDM) as it is currently practiced has existed for barely two decades. Its emergence coincides with the development of more numerous and more effective drugs with therapeutic potential. The application of technological processes that allow accurate and specific detection of small amounts of substances has produced sensitive assays, down to microgram and picogram levels. Gas liquid chromatography (GLC) in the 1970s was followed in rapid succession by radioimmunoassay (RIA), homogeneous enzyme immunoassay (EMIT), high-performance liquid chromatography (HPLC), and fluorescence polarization immunoassay (FPIA). These methods led to an increasing ability to provide timely plasma levels of therapeutic drugs as a direct adjunct to drug therapy.

Historically, therapeutic effectiveness was largely a trial and error process. Generally, a standard dose was given and if the patient failed to achieve therapeutic relief, the dose was increased until either symptoms were eliminated or signs of toxicity began to develop, in which case the dose was decreased or a new drug substituted, and the process was repeated.

The clinical value of TDM was introduced in very early studies of Henn Kutt and Bernard Brodie. These investigations identified the great variability of drug utilization patterns among different individuals and concluded that pharmacologic effectiveness was better related to drug plasma levels than to drug dosage.

Therapeutic drug monitoring has become a routine part of laboratory testing. The advances in instrumentation allow for rapid, accurate results for almost any drug that requires monitoring.

RATIONALE FOR THERAPEUTIC DRUG MONITORING

Over the previous two decades the development of more numerous and effective drugs having potential therapeutic application has led to more requests for plasma drug concentrations (Table 26-1). Many situations present themselves in which therapeutic drug monitoring may be useful. These include situations in which:

1. There is a wide pharmacokinetic variation among individuals taking the compound

2. Zero-order kinetics apply, as with phenytoin and salicylate
3. The difference between the minimum effective concentration (MEC) and the minimum toxic concentration (MTC) is small; this is referred to as the therapeutic index of the drug
4. It is difficult to recognize toxicity clinically
5. Physiologic factors exist that may alter pharmacokinetics
6. The presence of illness or disease states may affect drug pharmacokinetics
7. The standard dose does not achieve expected results
8. Noncompliance is suspected
9. Surreptitious use is suspected
10. Drug interaction with co-administered drugs is suspected

For TDM to be of value, certain prerequisites must also exist. Most important is that the analytical method involved be specific, sensitive and accurate with results available in the appropriate time frame. The assay must also be able to measure the active drugs and important metabolites. It is also important that the concentration of drug in the serum accurately reflects the concentration of drug at the receptor site and that the development of a tolerance for the drug at the receptor site does not occur. The therapeutic range should be well defined and there should be good correlation between serum concentration and drug efficacy.

PHYSIOLOGIC VARIABILITY

The pharmacokinetics pattern of a given drug is a complex set of processes, any one of which may be affected by a multitude of factors. If a random portion of the population was given a standard dose of a drug based on mg/kg body weight for a specified period of time and plasma drug values were determined, a Gaussian or bell-shaped curve would result, with a portion of the population in the therapeutic range and the remainder either subtherapeutic or toxic. The ability of the clinician to adjust drug dosage for these extremes is the reason why therapeutic drug monitoring is valuable.

Many factors can affect the disposition of a drug in the body. These include:

Table 26-1 Therapeutic and pharmacologic data

Drug	Therapeutic range (µg/ml)	Toxic levels (µg/ml)	% Protein binding	Half-life (hours)	Vol. Dist. (L/kg)	Time to peak (hours, oral dose)
Anticonvulsants						
Carbamazepine	5-12	>15	75-90	10-60	1.2	2-8
Ethosuximide	40-100	>100	<10	24-72	0.62	4
Phenobarbital	15-40	>50	20-45	84-108	0.7	8-12
Phenytoin	10-20	>25	95	12-36	0.65	1.5-3.0
Valproic acid	5-12	>100	80-95	6-18	0.8	1-4
Cardiac glycosides						
Digoxin	0.5-2.0*	>2.0*	20-30	40	6.3	6-8
Antiarrhythmics						
Disopyramide	3-5	>5	50-65	4-10	0.45-0.7	2.5
Flecainide	0.2-1.0	>1	40-50	11.5-16	10	2-3
Lidocaine	1.5-5	>5	60-80	1.8	1.5	
Procainamide	4-10	>12	14-23	2.5-5.0	2.0	0.75-2.5
Quinidine	1.5-4	>5	60-80	63	3.0	1-2
Antiasthmatics						
Theophylline	10-20	>20	56	3-12.8	0.3-0.7	1-2
Immunosuppressants						
Cyclosporine	100-300	>400	90	19-27	1.3	3.5
Aminoglycoside antibiotics						
Amikacin	20-30†	>30	<10	2-3	0.5-0.7	0.75-2.0‡
Gentamicin	6-10†	>12	0-30	2-3	0.15-0.25	0.5-1.5‡
Tobramycin	6-10†	>12	0-30	2.0	0.15-0.25	0.5-1.5‡
Tricyclic glycopeptide antibiotics						
Vancomycin	10-30	>30	52-60	4-6	—	—

Compiled from McEvoy, GK and Retschel, Wolfgang: Therapeutic drug monitoring (TDM). In Kaplan LA and Pesce AJ: Clinical chemistry: theory, analysis, and correlation, St Louis, 1984, Mosby–Year Book, Inc.
*ng/ml.
†Peak concentration.
‡Intramuscular dose.

1. Age
2. Pregnancy
3. Disease states
4. Concomitant use of other drugs

Effect of age on drug disposition

The aging process brings with it a variety of physiologic changes that affect drug disposition. From birth, the body experiences a slow but steady decline in renal function, cardiac output, levels of plasma albumin, lean body mass, and total body water. The density of various tissue receptors and the ability of those receptors to bind drug is reduced. The enzyme activity responsible for metabolism of drugs and endogenous compounds is also reduced. Often, these changes are combined with disease states or the use of several drugs concurrently to complicate the situation even further.

Pharmacokinetics in the child

Even today, information remains sparse relating age to drug disposition in children between 1 and 15 years of age. Generally, children are divided into groups based on stage of development.

1. Neonates (birth to 1 month)
2. Infants (1 month to 5 years)
3. Prepubescent (6 to 10 years)
4. Pubescent (10 to 14 years)
5. Adolescent (15 years and up)

The biologic response that is observed after a given dose of drug is a reflection of the concentration of that drug at the receptor site. This drug concentration is affected by alteration of numerous processes, such as rate of absorption, protein binding, and drug metabolism and excretion. These alterations can occur as a normal consequence of physiologic changes during aging.

Neonate. The rapid maturation in body and organ functions in the neonate present a unique picture of drug disposition. The neonate does not absorb, metabolize, and excrete as if it were a small adult. These developmental changes can be further complicated by additional factors such as gestational age (term vs. premature) birthweight (small for gestational age), and various pathologic conditions.

Absorption. Gastrointestinal absorption is dependent on pH, gastrointestinal motility, and gastric emptying time. The newborn has a highly alkaline pH for the first 12 hours of life, after which there is a marked increase in gastric acidity. A relative achlorhydria exists until the eighth to tenth day of life. The changing pH in the gastrointestinal (GI) tract results in highly variable patterns of absorption.

Gastrointestinal motility is reduced for the first 6 months or more. This allows more time for drug absorption. Prolonged gastric emptying time, on the other hand, may lead to a decrease in overall absorption, particularly of basic drugs, which are poorly absorbed in the stomach.

The interplay of these factors will determine whether or not a greater or lesser amount of drug is absorbed at a given time. The rapid developmental changes occurring during this time may make the prediction of drug concentration for dose difficult.

Protein binding and distribution. Drug distribution is affected by the following:

1. Protein binding
2. Water content of various body compartments
3. Body fat content
4. Vascular perfusion of the target organ

Protein binding is dependent on quantity of protein, quantity of drug, and the presence of competitive binding substances such as other drugs for binding sites on the plasma proteins. Protein binding is also affected by the type of protein and the protein's affinity for the drug.

Plasma protein binding in the newborn is less than in children or in adults. The newborn albumin is qualitatively different with a different affinity for drugs. There is generally greater competition for bindings sites with the presence of bilirubin and fatty acids. The lower pH of the blood of the newborn changes the binding affinity.

Total body water in neonates is greater than in adults and ranges from 70% to 78% of total body weight. It is even higher in premature infants. Extracellular water content is also higher than in adults, ranging from 45% to 47% of total weight. Intracellular water is a relatively low 32% to 34%. These differences will tend to dilute hydrophilic drug concentrations when compared to adult values and result in variations of volume of distribution.

Percentage of body fat in newborns is also decreased relative to adults, especially in low birth weight premature infants. The change in the lipid/water partition coefficient also alters the distribution of drugs.

There are major changes in cardiovascular anatomy. The switch from fetal to neonatal circulation results in changes in blood flow to different organs. Vascular perfusion of the target organ is critical to effective therapeutic use of the drug.

Metabolism. The metabolic function of the liver is to make lipid-soluble drugs more water-soluble so they can be excreted in the urine. This process is generally described as a two-phase process. Phase I converts a drug to a more polar compound by the addition of, or removal of, certain functional groups. Generally, hydroxyl or carboxyl groups are added or produced and methyl or other nonpolar groups are removed. Phase II involves the coupling of phase I metabolites or parent compounds with an endogenous substance like sulfate or glucuronic acid. In this form a drug conjugate is generally therapeutically inactive and more water-soluble, making it easily cleared by the kidneys.

Both phase I and II activities are depressed in the neonate. This results in an increased half-life of drugs that require metabolic alteration for their elimination.

There is evidence to indicate that the two systems can be induced to more efficient performance, for example, by the administration of phenobarbital, either postnatally or prenatally, by treating the mother.

Excretion. Renal excretion is the major route for elimination of drugs. Water-soluble drugs are removed from the system by glomerular filtration or tubular secretion. Glomerular filtration removes free drugs of small size, whereas bound drugs and larger molecules are removed by active secretion into the renal tubules. Neonates have a glomerular filtration rate (GFR) of only about 30% of the normal adult values and renal blood flow of only 25% of the adult level.

Substantial increases in function occur within 5 days, with normal adult values achieved within 1 year.

The lower GFR is a result of the small number and size of glomeruli. Reduced tubular secretion is due to the smaller number of functioning tubular cells; blood flow is not yet sufficient and the tubules are not yet developed.

Infants (1 month to 5 years). During infancy, drug disposition rates achieve the highest value they will throughout life. The reduced physiologic processes of the neonate have matured. These processes reach and, in some instances, exceed normal adult rates.

Prepubescent (6 to 10 years). Drug utilization in this age group is as much as twice that seen in adults. In fact, drug dosage, in mg/kg of body weight, is usually twice the adult dose. It is in this age group that the gradual decrease in rate of drug disposition begins to occur that will continue throughout the rest of life.

Pubescent (10 to 14 years). It is during the early teen period that childhood drug utilization patterns become adult patterns. Many sex- and age-dependent changes occur rapidly with the onset of puberty. Changes in drug utilization are directly related to these changes. Evidence indicates utilization changes are directly attributable to increased concentrations of sex hormones. The competition between the sex hormones and drugs for metabolic sites within the microsomal enzyme system is one explanation given for decreased drug metabolism.

Because of these rapid and significant changes, therapeutic drug monitoring in this group is essential, especially when symptoms of toxicity are present.

Adolescent (15 years and up). For all practical purposes, drug disposition after age 15 is identical to that of adults. The appearance of the physical secondary sex characteristics generally marks this change.

Drug utilization in the elderly

Changes in many physiologic functions occur with aging, including decreases in:

1. Cardiac output
2. Renal function
3. Plasma albumin
4. Lean body mass
5. Metabolic enzyme activity
6. Quantity and quality of various tissue receptors
7. Total body water

These changes, along with the effects of disease or the presence of concurrently administered drugs, present a problem in predicting drug effects and utilization in the elderly. The incidence of adverse drug reactions occurs three times more frequently in the elderly than in the young adult population.

Absorption. Many changes occur in the gastrointestinal tract with aging. They include decline in gastric acid output with associated pH changes; delayed gastric emptying time; changes in the small bowel, which result in decreased mucosal surface area; and decreased mesenteric blood flow, resulting from decreases in cardiac output. In spite of these changes, recent studies have indicated little change in the rate or extent of drug absorption.

Protein binding and distribution. Drug distribution is affected by a number of factors, most notably:

1. Cardiac output

2. Number and quality of protein binding sites
3. Changes in body composition

Systemic blood flow, albumin concentrations, lean body mass, and total body water all decrease with age. There is a 30% to 40% decrease in cardiac output, resulting in decreased blood flow to the liver and kidneys. Serum albumin levels have been found to be decreased by as much as 15% to 25% in patients over 60 years of age. This could significantly affect the use of medications that are highly protein-bound. Aging is associated with significant changes in body composition. Total body water decreases as does lean body mass with a significant increase in body fat. The lipid/water partition coefficient will have an effect on the volume of distribution of drugs. Drugs distributed mainly in the body water will have a decreased volume of distribution, whereas more lipophilic drugs will have increased distribution along with the increased elimination half-life that would be expected.

Metabolism. Drugs are metabolized more slowly in the elderly, resulting in longer half-lives and increased steady-state concentrations. Drug metabolizing capacity is influenced by hepatic perfusion, liver mass, and cellular activity. The effects of all three conditions have been documented in this age group. The decrease in cardiac output in the aged is reflected by a decreased blood flow to the liver up to as much as 40% by age 65. Liver mass also shows a reduction of about 20%, accompanied by a reduction of microsomal enzyme activity in phase I metabolism. Although phase II conjugation reactions appear generally unaffected by age, the phase I activities of hydrolysis, oxidation, and reduction have shown a reduced capacity to metabolize drugs.

Excretion. The most widely studied and best understood aspect of drug disposition in the elderly is that of renal excretion. Studies have found significant changes occurring in the kidney and in kidney function, including:

1. Reduction in renal blood flow
2. Decline in kidney size and weight
3. Decline in the glomerular filtration rate (GFR), resulting from glomerular and tubular function reductions

Reduction in renal blood flow seems to be, in part, due to sclerotic events in the walls of intrarenal vessels. Renal blood flow decreases by almost 50% by age 80. Morphologic changes in the kidney affects the cortical region rather than the medullary area and results in a loss of total glomeruli.

It is believed that the reduction in the GFR and in tubular secretion result from the loss of nephron units because the clearance ratio between the two functions remains fairly constant. Aging also results in a reduction of glomerular surface area and reduction in the length of the proximal tubule.

It has been reported that overall, a 50% reduction of normal renal function can occur by age 80. This results in a significant accumulation of parent drug and of potentially active metabolites in the vascular system.

Pregnancy and pharmacokinetics

Pregnancy brings with it a number of physiologic changes and an increase in the number of prescribed drugs taken. The average pregnant woman takes three to four different drugs during pregnancy, including those given during labor and delivery, making therapeutic drug monitoring extremely important in this group of individuals.

Absorption

Changes in gastric emptying time, intestinal motility, pH of the GI tract, along with changes in blood flow have an impact on drug absorption. An increase in gastric emptying time and a prolongation of intestinal exposure time, a delay of up to 30% to 40%, can affect the rate and time of absorption. An increase in pH due to reduced gastric acid secretion has a substantial impact on absorption of acid drugs in the stomach. An increased blood flow due to increased cardiac output and regional vasodilation also affects absorption.

Distribution

The volume of distribution of a compound is altered by changes in body size and composition, blood flow patterns, protein binding, and tissue permeability.

During pregnancy there is an increase of approximately 8 L in total body water, with extracellular water accounting for 90% of the increase. There is an overall increase in plasma volume of nearly 50% above that of a normal, nonpregnant female.

Pregnant women demonstrate increased blood flow to various organs. Cardiac output triples during the first two trimesters and remains high until delivery. The most significant increases in blood flow occur in peripheral, renal, and uterine blood supplies.

Research indicates a reduction in albumin by as much as 25%, which reduces binding capacity of acidic drugs. At the same time, increased concentrations of lipoproteins occur along with decreases in α-1-acid-glycoprotein. These substances are associated with binding of alkaline drugs. There is also some evidence that indicates qualitative changes in albumin may affect binding patterns.

Metabolism

Drug clearance is affected by hepatic perfusion, liver function, including phase I and phase II metabolic processes, and protein binding patterns. Recent evidence indicates an increase in the blood flow during pregnancy to the liver. Since a drug's clearance is proportional to blood flow, the increase in perfusion should cause xenobiotic compounds to be removed more rapidly.

High levels of circulating progesterone during pregnancy are known to stimulate the liver's microsomal mixed function oxidase system. At the same time, estrogens act as strong inhibitors of the same system. The rate of drug metabolism thus depends on the rates of these endogenous hormones.

Hepatic drug metabolism is dependent on the free drug concentration and the ratio of free to bound drug is affected by plasma protein changes occurring in the pregnant patient.

Excretion

The two main determinants of renal excretion rate are renal blood flow and glomerular filtration rate, both of which increase during pregnancy. The increased function begins during the first 15 weeks and continues throughout pregnancy, falling slowly during the months before delivery.

Of importance to clinicians is the fact that these changes are temporary, some declining slowly during the last trimester, others returning to nonpregnant levels rapidly postpartum. It is imperative that TDM be utilized consistently throughout pregnancy and immediately postdelivery until it is determined that drug disposition parameters have returned to a nonpregnant level for the individual patient.

The effect of disease on drug disposition

Creating probably the highest need for therapeutic drug monitoring is the presence of disease. The widest variabilities in pharmacokinetics is brought about by the presence of disease. The severity of a disease state, the presence of more than one pathologic condition, and the need for multiple drugs in the treatment of disease all complicate the treatment picture.

Cardiac disease, pulmonary disease, and thyroid disease, along with malnutrition and burns all have an impact on drug therapy. The most important factors are changes in liver and kidney function because of their direct role in drug disposition. Neoplastic disease is also important because of its incidence today and its varied and difficult treatment.

Diseases of the liver

The liver plays a central role in the elimination of drugs from the body. Drugs and other foreign substances presented through the portal blood flow are made water-soluble for easy elimination by the kidneys. The major reactions that occur to make compounds more polar and less active are oxidation, reduction, hydrolysis, and conjugation. These reactions occur in two phases.

Phase I metabolism works by introducing, unmasking, or removing certain functional groups. The enzymes employed in this activity are located in the smooth endoplasmic reticulum of hepatocytes. This system is referred to as the microsomal mixed function oxidase system (MFO) and requires oxygen and reduced nicotinamide adenine dinucleotide phosphate (NADPH). Cytochrome P-450 is the main enzyme employed in this system. The main function of phase I metabolism is to render substances more polar and less toxic. Some active metabolites, however, may be formed, which react with tissue macromolecules with toxic effects. Phase I reactivity has been found to be inducible or restricted by the presence of certain substances.

Phase II reactions involve the coupling of parent drug or phase I metabolic products with endogenous materials. Phase II reactions that use glucuronic acid and glutathione conjugation occur in the smooth endoplasmic reticulum of hepatocytes. In cell cytosol, conjugation with acetate, glutathione, or sulfate occurs, whereas in the mitochondria, conjugation with glycine is the predominant reaction. The products of phase II metabolism are polar acids that are inactive and are easily excreted in urine or bile.

Any liver dysfunction that alters either one or both of the two phases of metabolism will result in an accumulation of drug in the body. Impairment of hepatic blood flow would also produce similar results.

Patients with liver dysfunction also may show altered nutritional status, may be receiving multiple drugs concurrently, and also may have multiple organ pathologies. Therapeutic drug monitoring is clearly indicated to ensure that appropriate drug concentrations are achieved.

Diseases of the kidney

Renal elimination of drugs and their metabolites occurs through two processes: filtration of unbound small molecular weight drugs through the glomerulus and active secretion of bound drugs in the proximal tubule. About 25% of the blood pumped from the heart enters the renal artery, which branches into the one million nephrons of each kidney. The nephron is composed of the glomerulus, the proximal tubule, the loop of Henle, the distal tubule, and the collecting duct.

The glomerular filtration rate is only about 20% of renal plasma flow. Tubular secretion, in addition to filtration, is important for elimination of drugs. Drug protein binding plays an important role in tubular secretion because the affinities of renal receptors involved in transtubule transport for drug must be greater than the protein binding the drug.

As the tubular fluid moves through the nephron, the drug concentration increases, favoring passive reabsorption back into the body. Factors that influence reabsorption include pH of the fluid, the disassociation constant of the drug, and the urine flow rate.

As with liver disease, any pathologic renal condition may create altered elimination. Generally, renal dysfunction results in an accumulation of drug and metabolites in the body. Many factors must be considered when evaluating these patients. Drug accumulation may include many inactive metabolites, which, in high concentration, could cause problems or which may cross-react with methods employed to analyze blood concentrations. Interpretation of results must be based on the patient's overall condition, other drugs being given concurrently, and how long the therapy has been applied.

Neoplastic diseases

One of every five deaths in the United States is cancer related. Cancer's effect on drug disposition occurs through one of two mechanisms. The primary tumor or its metastasis can affect any stage of drug disposition—absorption, distribution, metabolism, or excretion. The treatments used for cancer patients—chemotherapy, radiation therapy, and surgery—also have a significant effect on drug disposition.

Absorption. Absorption is dependent on the GI tract mucosal permeability and the surface area available for absorption. It is also affected by quality of GI blood supply and motility of the GI tract.

Malignancy can affect any of these physiologic factors. Surgical removal of portions of the stomach or bowel substantially affect absorption. Some cytotoxic drugs used in the destruction of cancers can cause changes in absorption properties of intestinal epithelial cells. Primary liver carcinomas or metastatic conditions involving the liver could reduce the "first pass" elimination of some drugs, creating increased bioavailability.

Distribution. Drug distribution through the body is a function of protein binding. Albumin concentration is reduced in cancer patients because of both poor nutritional intake and loss of the tissue responsible for albumin synthesis, especially in patients with primary liver cancer. This decrease often results in increased concentrations of free drug, with the accompanying toxic effects, especially in drugs normally highly protein-bound. These difficulties can often be compensated for by lowering the drug dose. Frequently, drugs employed in cancer treatment will compete for binding sites on this reduced level of albumin, causing free concentrations of some drugs to increase.

Metabolism. There is increasing evidence of reduced activity in the microsomal enzyme system of tumor-bearing individuals. The lower enzyme activity results in increased toxicity. The reduction seems to be related to tumor size and can apparently be reversed upon tumor removal.

Excretion. Most drugs are eliminated into the bile or through renal excretion pathways. Renal dysfunction due to cancer is not frequently seen. Primary renal carcinoma is uncommon. Renal dysfunction can occur, however, due to physical obstruction from abdominal tumors. Some drugs used in cancer therapy are nephrotoxic. The by-products of cellular destruction by chemotherapeutic agents may cause nephropathy. Predictions of the effects of cancer on drug disposition are seldom reliable. The overall clinical picture and consideration of concurrent medications must be considered.

Drug interactions

Any time a patient is taking two or more medications, the possibility exists for drug-drug interaction. These interactions may occur at any phase of disposition—absorption, distribution, metabolism, or excretion. Seldom do these interactions have a significant impact on patient health, but occasionally, serious harm to the patient can occur. Not all drug interactions are harmful, and some present benefits to the patient.

Absorption

Two mechanisms account for most drug interactions during the absorption process. One drug may significantly alter the pH of the gastrointestinal contents, such as an antacid, which can have an impact on the absorption of another drug. Sometimes a chelate may form by the interaction of two compounds as when tetracycline chelates the divalent cations, Ca^{2+}, Mg^{2+}, Al^{2+}, of an antacid. The chelate formed is poorly soluble and therefore poorly absorbed.

Absorption drug interactions can generally be managed by spacing out administration of the different compounds, although this may create a difficult dosing schedule for the patient.

Distribution

Interactions in the distribution process generally involve competitive binding incidents, both on plasma protein and at the receptor site. When one drug is displaced from protein binding sites by another, concentrations of free drug will increase, leading potentially to toxicity, even though total plasma drug concentrations may be within normal therapeutic limits.

At the receptor site beneficial interactions can occur. For instance, naloxone displaces analgesic narcotics from their receptor sites, proving valuable in overdose situations. But in many situations harmful interactions also occur. The antihypertensive effects of the drug guanethidine are reduced when tricyclic antidepressants such as amitriptyline are given concurrently.

Metabolism

Alterations in metabolism can affect drugs by either increasing or decreasing metabolism. If administration of a drug induces the microsomal enzyme system to increase its capacity, the result may be a reduction in concentration to below the therapeutic range for another drug.

Just as the metabolic pathways can be stimulated to more rapid production, they can also be inhibited to slow the metabolism of some drugs. In methanol poisoning, ethyl alcohol can be given to slow the metabolism of methanol to its toxic metabolites, formic acid and formaldehyde. This inhibition occurs because the same enzyme system is responsible for metabolizing both alcohols. The enzymes bind more readily to the ethanol, effectively shutting down methanol breakdown.

Excretion

Urinary elimination of drugs occurs through two routes—glomerular filtration and renal tubule secretion with reabsorption. Secretion and reabsorption are more commonly involved in drug-drug interactions. A compound may block either secretion, resulting in prolongation of the drug's half-life, or reabsorption, resulting in a shortening of the half-life.

FREE DRUGS

Free-drug concentrations are those drug concentrations measured when the pharmacologic agent is not bound to other molecules, particularly proteins. Certain criteria must be met when considering whether or not free-drug measurement should be undertaken:

1. Drugs should have the free-drug concentration–clinical effect relationship that is well understood and defined.
2. Drugs should have a narrow therapeutic range in which small variations can result in toxic or subtherapeutic effects.
3. Drugs should be extensively protein bound, 60% to 70% or more. Drugs with minimal binding need not be evaluated.
4. Drugs should have a free-drug fraction that does not remain constant with changes in dose or concentration.

Many physiologic variables affect drug disposition, including protein binding. Age, disease, pregnancy, and concurrent administration of several drugs all make the normal total drug concentrations misleading and unreliable in certain circumstances. Because free-drug values are more directly related to efficacy and toxicity, their measurement under the following conditions is warranted:

1. When the concentration of drug is high relative to the number of binding sites; saturation of sites may occur, resulting in higher free-drug values
2. When drug is displaced from protein binding sites by other drugs or endogenous substances such as free fatty acids or bilirubin

3. When binding protein concentrations are reduced; acidic drugs are bound mainly to albumin and basic drugs to α_1-acid-glycoprotein
4. When qualitative changes in albumin, as is seen in chronic renal failure, result in increased affinity for certain drugs

Several methods of analysis exist for free-drug measurement. The two most frequently used are equilibrium dialysis (ED) and ultrafiltration (UF). In equilibrium dialysis, plasma is equilibrated with an isotonic buffer solution across a membrane with a specific pore size. The type of membrane chosen is dependent upon the size of binding protein to be excluded. It is also important that the membrane not nonspecifically bind the drug of interest. At equilibrium, the concentration of free drug in the dialysate equals the concentration of free drug in the retentate. Each solution is tested and the free-drug percentage determined. Using the original total drug concentration, the free concentration can be determined.

Ultrafiltration forces serum or plasma through a semipermeable membrane into a filtrate collection cup by centrifugation. The filtrate is then tested for the concentration of the drug of interest.

It is imperative that the sources of variability in each of these procedures be rigorously controlled. In equilibrium dialysis, the temperature, pH of the sample, concentration of drug, composition of dialysate, and in vitro release of free fatty acids all affect the free-drug concentration. Ultrafiltration has fewer variables to control, but still must be standardized so the analytical conditions of analysis are identical.

The final testing process is also important. The procedure used to determine final free-drug concentration must be accurate and sensitive enough to determine the very low concentrations of drug recovered.

Only a few drugs meet the criteria for measurement. Most commonly they are carbamazepine, phenytoin, and valproic acid. It is often the case that total drug concentration will correlate with the clinical condition. Only under the aforementioned conditions will the free-drug measurements provide more reliable information than total drug values.

ACTIVE DRUG METABOLITES

Generally, the processes involved in phase I and phase II metabolism of a drug produces metabolites that are inactive or substantially less active than the parent compound. In some cases, however, metabolites with significant pharmacologic activity are produced. Ultimately, the pharmacologic response of the patient is a result of both parent drug and active metabolite(s). Several of the major active metabolites assayed in the clinical laboratory are discussed briefly.

Procainamide

N-acetyl-procainamide is the principle metabolite produced from procainamide and it has antiarrhythmic activity similar to the parent compound. In the patient with normal kidney function, 50% of procainamide is excreted unchanged. In uremic patients, lower doses of procainamide will result in similar antiarrhythmic activity because higher concentrations of N-acetylprocainamide are present.

Quinidine

There is little known about active metabolites of quinidine. Dihydroquinidine is a pharmacologically active contaminant that is present in the pharmaceutical preparations of the parent compound. (3S)-3-hydroxyquinidine has been found to be more toxic but less potent than the parent compound. The 2'-oxoquinidine has some antiarrhythmic activity.

Lidocaine

Lidocaine is de-ethylated to monoethylglycinexylidide (MEGX) and glycinexylidide (GX). Both compounds have antiarrhythmic activity but are less potent than the parent. Monoethylglycinexylidide is now being marketed as a sensitive measure of liver function when a standard dose of lidocaine is administered to a patient. Samples tested under standard conditions for this metabolite provide an extremely rapid way to evaluate liver function.

Other drugs

The 10-11 epoxide of carbamazepine is an active metabolite but is generally present in concentrations lower than that of the parent. Phenobarbital is a metabolite of primidone, possessing anticonvulsant activity. Prednisone must be metabolized to its active metabolite, prednisolone, before it can exert its pharmacologic effects.

THERAPEUTIC DRUG DATA
Anticonvulsants

Anticonvulsant drugs are used in the prevention of recurrent seizures in patients with epilepsy. Bromide was introduced as the first anticonvulsant agent in 1857. Phenobarbital was introduced in 1912 and phenytoin in 1937. The appropriate choice of medication is based on the most frequent type of seizure demonstrated by the patient.

The main principles followed in seizure control therapy are:

- Use single drug therapy, if possible; 75% of patients can be controlled using only one drug.
- Drug build up should be slow to minimize side effects, increasing the drug until seizure control is achieved or toxicity develops.
- Elimination of drugs should be done slowly to minimize withdrawal seizures.
- Patients who remain seizure-free for 2 years can be considered candidates for elimination of medication. One study found 75% of children who were seizure-free for 2 or more years remained seizure-free after cessation of medication.
- When multiple drugs are used for treatment, particular attention must be paid to drug interactions. These interactions can affect absorption, protein binding, metabolism, and elimination. Multiple drug therapy can result in altered therapeutic ranges and dosage requirements.

Classification of seizure disorders

I. Partial (localized, focal): These involve a relatively small area of the brain.
   A. Simple (no loss of consciousness): Depending on the area of the brain, these can be manifested in motor, sensory, psychic, or emotional signs.

B. Complex (loss of impairment of consciousness): These tend to originate in the frontal or temporal lobe.
C. Localized leading to secondary generalized seizures.

II. Generalized: These involve both cerebral hemispheres or large areas of the brain.

A. Absence (petit mal): Seizures are expressed as periods of staring, without convulsive movements. Patients have brief periods, lasting seconds, during which they appear to be asleep or day dreaming, or not aware of their surroundings.

B. Tonic clonic (grand mal): These seizures are the ones most frequently associated with epilepsy. They involve tonic contraction and flexion of muscles, followed by clonic jerking movements. Tonic and clonic seizures can occur individually as can myoclonic seizures, which are small, quick, jerking movements, or atonic seizures, which involve falling without loss of consciousness. All these individuals seizure types are believed to be fragments of an interrupted tonic clonic seizure, most often in a patient on drug therapy.

Aminoglycosides

The aminoglycosides inhibit protein synthesis of bacterial organisms. This group of drugs includes gentamicin, kanamycin, streptomycin, netilmycin, tobramycin, and amikacin. Their use is generally for treatment of serious gram-negative bacilli infections.

The principle behind antibiotic therapy is to establish a minimal inhibitory concentration that destroys the organism without harmful side effects to the host. Because this group of drugs is polar, absorption is poor. The problem of inadequate absorption can be overcome with intravenous or intramuscular injection. The elimination half-life usually is only 2 to 3 hours for these drugs. Usually, peak and trough samples are collected on the patient, although it is felt the trough specimen provides the best monitoring information.

Therapeutically effective concentrations are listed here:

	PEAK	TROUGH	TOXIC (μg/mL)
Amikacin	20-30	5-10	>30
Gentamicin	6-10	1-2	>12
Tobramycin	6-10	1-2	>12

The use of aminoglycosides must be weighed against their adverse effects. The dosages and concentration required for maximum efficacy are also associated with nephrotoxicity and ototoxicity. The use of aminoglycosides to treat infection in patients with a high risk of mortality also means there is a high risk of toxicity. When combined with the narrow therapeutic index of most antibiotics, the requirement for effective monitoring becomes imperative.

Antiarrhythmic drugs

This class of drugs is used to treat disorders in the electrical conduction system of the heart. This system is composed of a network of simple and efficient fibers. The system provides two functions. The first is the production of an electrical signal that will direct heart muscle contraction at the appropriate interval. The sinus node that provides this signal is equipped with receptors, allowing the heart to be responsive to physiologic needs of the body. The second function is to provide a low resistance pathway that will lead to a homogenous distribution of the signal. One last aspect of the process that bears mentioning is the presence of an electrical filter, the atrioventricular node, which helps to slow conduction between the atria and the ventricles. Disorders in this system have a significant impact on the ability of the heart to maintain adequate blood flow to the body.

Abnormalities of the electrical conduction system can occur in the generation, conduction, or origin of the electrical wavefront. These disorders are generally referred to as arrhythmias.

A variety of drugs are available to treat the many disorders that can occur. These drugs are classified according to mechanism:

• Class I drugs depress phase 0 of action potential, tend to prolong repolarization, and slow conduction. This class of drugs includes procainamide, quinidine, lidocaine, disopyramide, and flecainide.
• Class II drugs block beta-adrenergic receptors. This group includes propranolol; they are effective in the treatment of supraventricular and ventricular arrhythmias.
• Class III drugs increase repolarization time.
• Class IV compounds block slow channels (calcium) and includes verapamil. These drugs inhibit the influx of calcium ions into cells of the myocardium and atrioventricular and sinus nodes, and vascular smooth muscle.

Antiasthmatics

Asthma is a disorder of diverse etiology resulting from an obstruction to airflow as a result of constriction of the central air passage of the trachea and bronchii. Accompanying this muscular constriction is swelling of the mucosa and the secretion of mucus into the lumen.

There are two theories about the causes of this process. One is the belief that neurological control of the bronchial smooth muscle is abnormal. The second states that chemical mediators, such as histamine, are released by mast cells when stimulated by such factors as the presence of allergens or irritants.

There are generally considered to be five classes of antiasthmatic medications: methylxanthines (including theophylline), beta-adrenergic agonists, cholinergic antagonists, cromolyns, and corticosteroids.

Theophylline, the most commonly used drug, inhibits phosphodiesterase leading to increased 3'5'-adenosine monophosphate, which inhibits the release of histamine, and results in bronchodilation.

Immunosuppressants

These drugs, primarily cyclosporine and azathioprine, are used to suppress host vs. graft rejection in organ transplant patients. Cyclosporine acts by inhibiting the proliferation of lymphocytes, thereby suppressing humoral and cellular immunity. Its main use is in the prevention of rejection in kidney, liver, and heart allogenic transplant patients.

Cardiac glycosides

Cardiac glycosides are used to increase the force, as well as the velocity of heart contractions. They are used in the treatment of congestive heart failure. The most common drug in the group is digoxin. The drug improves contractibility by altering transport of Na^+, K^+, and Ca^{2+}. When the force of contraction is increased in patients with failing hearts, there is an increase in cardiac output, systolic emptying is more complete, and diastolic heart size is decreased.

SUGGESTED READING

Baugh-Bookman C, Friel P, and Ojemann LM: Epilepsy I: anatomy, physiology, and epidemiology, TDM/TOX InService Training and Continuing Education, 9 (3):15, 1987.

Cawthorn DF: Epilepsy III: drug treatment, TDM/TOX InService Training and Continuing Education 9 (8):7, 1988.

Chapron DJ: Drug disposition and response in the elderly, Part 1, TDM/TOX InService Training and Continuing Education 10 (1):7, 1988.

Hanyok JJ: Cardiac arrhythmias, Part II: clinical pharmacology and therapeutic uses of antiarrhythmic drugs, TDM/TOX InService Training and Continuing Education 8 (9):1, 1987.

LeGrys VA: Drug disposition and response in the elderly, Part II, TDM/TOX InService Training and Continuing Education 10 (3):7, 1988.

McEvoy GK (editor): ASHP drug information 90, Bethesda, Md, 1990, American Society of Hospital Pharmacists.

27 Emergency overdose toxicology

Michael Hassan

POISONS AND POISONINGS

If the age-old dilemma of the clinical toxicologist is that the only distinction between a poison and a nonpoison is the dosage, then almost any chemical becomes a potential problem. The analytical toxicologist's dilemma lies with subsequent requests to identify and quantify this vast array of possible toxicants. This insurmountable task asked of the laboratorian becomes even more of a formidable challenge when the time constraints of hospital emergency testing are added. In this case, the laboratory data may be used as an aid in the treatment and clinical management of the poisoned patient. For laboratory personnel to develop an expertise in testing for suspect poisons, they must first expand their knowledge of the clinical problem of poisoning, have a working understanding of the classification of poisons, and finally, have the ability to integrate this knowledge into analytical applications.

The poisoned or overdosed patient will be characterized as an individual who comes to the acute care facility (i.e., hospital emergency room) with symptoms, signs, and clinical findings indicative of potential undue exposure to a chemical. This living patient is in contrast to the dead on arrival cases addressed by the coroner's laboratory. The terms *poisoned* and *overdosed* will be used synonymously, although overdose generally implies overmedication with a drug, while poisoning denotes a broader chemical definition not necessarily restricted to drugs. Both terms may indicate either self-inflicted or accidental poisoning.

Poisons are generally classified according to either their chemical properties and/or structures, their pharmacological or physiological mechanisms, their functional use, or to their origins. These classifications tend to overlap but are useful in a variety of circumstances. The following poisons are grouped according to functional use, which helps to define the scope of the laboratory problem in supporting the emergency room staff.

Medicinal poisons

Drugs, derived from both natural and synthetic sources, are defined as any chemical agent used "therapeutically" to affect a living system. These compounds represent the most widely recognized potential poisons because of the prevalence of acute incidents of toxicity associated with their use.

The presence of many of these compounds can be tested for in serum or urine.

Household poisons

Common everyday household products, because of their ubiquitous nature, raise cause for concern, especially as they pertain to ingestion by children. These poisons may account for as many as 25% of the inquiries directed to drug and poison information centers, and are represented by soaps, detergents, cleaners, bleaching agents, cosmetics and toiletry articles, and hobby supplies. These compounds are usually not tested for directly, but evidence of their presence may be obtained by indirect means (odor, pH, color changes).

Industrial poisons

As evidenced by the latest and voluminous listings of "toxic substances" as they relate to the Toxic Substances Control Act, the number of industrial chemicals and compounds has become categorically massive. Subcategories of poisons in this group include radioactive compounds; gases and gaseous by-products (carbon monoxide, hydrogen cyanide, hydrogen sulfide); metals (lead, arsenic, mercury); volatiles and solvents (glycols, hydrocarbons); and corrosives. Some compounds, namely, metals and carbon monoxide, may be tested for directly, whereas others may be tested indirectly, such as through radioactivity or pH changes.

Agricultural and vermin poisons

This group includes commercial products used for the control of unwanted plants or animals, and may be divided into pesticides (warfarin, fluoride, barium, thallium, strychnine); insecticides (chlorinated hydrocarbons, organophosphates, carbamates); herbicides; fumigants; and fungicides.

Poisons from animals and plants

Poisonings or toxic reactions attributed to animals most often occur because of toxic venoms produced by reptiles (pit vipers); arachnids and insects (spiders, scorpions); and marine animals (jellyfish, stonefish, shellfish). Various houseplants (ornamentals such as the poinsettia) and those found outdoors (amanita and muscaria mushrooms, poison ivy, jimsonweed) contain select toxins. Most of the

384

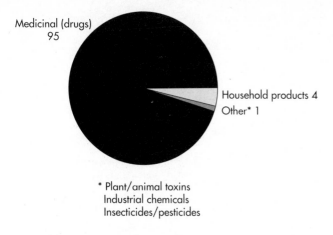

Medicinal (drugs)
95

Household products 4
Other* 1

* Plant/animal toxins
Industrial chemicals
Insecticides/pesticides

Fig. 27-1 Involvement of poisons in acute care cases.

Table 27-1 Antidotes and reversing agents for select poisons

Drug/poison	Antidotes/antagonist
Acetaminophen	N-Acetylcysteine
Anticholinergic drugs (antidepressants, atropine)	Physostigmine
Carbon monoxide	Oxygen
Cyanide	Sodium nitrite
Digoxin	Digoxin antibody fragments
Ethylene glycol	Ethanol
Heavy metals (Hg, Ar)	Chelaters (BAL*, EDTA)*
Methanol	Ethanol
Nitrites, chlorates	Methylene blue
Organophosphate insecticides	Atropine, pralidoxime
Opiate narcotics (codeine, morphine)	Naloxone
Snake bite (Pit vipers)	Select antivenin
Stimulant drugs (amphetamine, methamphetamine)	Chlorpromazine

*BAL, dimercaprol; EDTA, ethylenediamine tetraacetic acid.

compounds in this class of poisons cannot be tested for directly.

As can be seen in Figure 27-1, although each of the previously mentioned poisons contribute to the patient population treated in the emergency room, medicinal compounds dwarf the others in frequency, due largely to their availability and widespread use.

THE LABORATORY'S ROLE IN THE MANAGEMENT OF THE POISONED PATIENT

Upon arrival at the emergency room, management of the poisoned patient will generally involve supportive therapy, which is the maintenance of life-support systems such as cardiac and respiratory functions. In addition, poison-specific treatments may be undertaken, such as the administration of antidotes or antagonists, or of removal enhancers such as diuretics or chelating agents. Supportive therapy is given as required, based upon acute patient needs, and is initiated quite often without knowledge of the specific poison involved. Special treatments may also be initiated based upon a patient's verbal acknowledgment of the poison, or after witnessing definitive signs or symptoms associated with specific poisons. In the absence of a reliable patient history, or when patient symptoms are unremarkable and nonspecific, the laboratory may play a significant role in decisions related to patient management. Even when histories are provided, they must be used cautiously as they are quite often incorrect. In the author's laboratory, approximately 40% of patient histories are either only partially correct, or completely incorrect and misleading. Laboratory analyses may serve to: (1) aid the physician in confirming the diagnosis of poisoning, (2) enable the physician to follow the clinical course of the poisoning, and (3) aid the physician in developing a prognosis.

In order for the laboratory to confirm the diagnosis, it must first choose which poison groups, and which specific compounds in the groups, to include in its testing schemes. Constituents of the testing regimen will be chosen by: (1) highlighting those compounds frequently responsible for poisonings, (2) highlighting compounds for which there may be a specific antidote or treatment, (3) assessing the time alloted to the laboratory staff for the testing process, and

(4) assessing the analytical instrumentation, techniques, personnel, and budget available.

As noted in Figure 27-1, the majority of poisonings involve medicinal compounds, with the other poison groups contributing only slightly to the overall patient population. Therefore, drugs are an obvious group for which the laboratory should develop testing expertise, and indeed, a plethora of methods exist to aid the analyst in accomplishing this task. It should be noted that the availability of antidotes or antagonists used by the physician are quite limited, that they will generally be administered immediately to the patient upon any indication of the specific poison's involvement, and that quick, reliable tests for many of the poisons are not readily available to the analyst. Table 27-1 lists some of the more common reversing agents utilized. Analysis for select drugs, as well as for such compounds as methanol, ethylene glycol, metals, and carbon monoxide, are the most feasible for the laboratory to provide with a reasonably rapid turnaround time.

Having emphasized the need for capabilities to test for the drug groups, the physician's expectations relating to testing turnaround time will influence which and how many drugs to include in the process. For test data to be useful in the management of the patient, physicians anticipate results to be available within 1 to 3 hours after receipt of the specimen. Within this alloted time, the laboratory staff will now limit their testing to specific qualitative and quantitative assays for indicated poisons, or to somewhat abbreviated qualitative screening panels for prescribed groups of drugs. This development of relatively limited testing capability does not preclude laboratory staff from setting up additional methodical testing schemes, to include more poisons or quantitative tests that are not feasible to offer on a rapid basis, and which may provide useful prognostic information.

The laboratory's role in the management of the poisoned patient will be to provide an analytical search for as many poisons as is technically feasible in a relatively short period of time.

SPECIMENS OF CHOICE FOR ANALYSIS

The success of any analytical endeavor is dependent upon the proper selection of the sample or specimen to be tested, the timeliness of the specific sample collection as it pertains to the reason for testing, and the proper processing and storage of the specimen until time of testing. With these factors in place, toxicological testing to assess poisoning may proceed with some confidence.

The toxicologist's most direct approach to the quick identification of a potential poison involved in an overdose is to actually have in hand a sample of the suspect compound, whether it be a pharmaceutical preparation, a near-empty container of cleaning solution, or any other actual material that may have accompanied the patient to the emergency room. The suspect poison may be recognized by distinctive characteristics or markings, by odor, or by employing minimal analytical endeavors. Therefore, all suspect materials should be submitted to the laboratory as they become available. Unfortunately, in reality actual suspected poisons accompany the overdosed patient in less than 5% of the cases seen, making it imperative that the proper patient specimens be submitted to the laboratory.

Biological samples most readily available and useful to the analyst include urine, blood, and stomach contents. The choice of one specific specimen over another is dictated by several factors, including: (1) the specific poison or class of poison sought, (2) whether parent drug/poison or only significant metabolites of the poison are anticipated to be found, (3) the available analytical testing schemes, and whether a single specific poison will be tested for, or a more comprehensive pursuit for many compounds will be undertaken, (4) the route of administration of the poison, (5) the time since the exposure to, or ingestion of, the poison, and (6) the compatability of the analytical technique and instrumentation to the various specimens.

Urine (20 to 50 ml) is the specimen of choice for many qualitative and select quantitative analyses. Specifically, qualitative testing to identify most drugs (or drug classes) or their metabolites will most often employ urine. Of importance to the success of urine testing is having a strong working knowledge of normal urinary constituents, and of the excretion patterns of parent drugs and their related metabolites. Table 27-2 notes several examples of prevalent drugs often encountered and the analytes of interest as they pertain to urine testing. In general, urine specimens should be submitted as spot samples, collected during the acute phase of toxicity when the patient is admitted to the emergency room. No preservatives should be added to the sample. Refrigeration of the specimen is recommended if there is to be a lengthy delay in testing (>6 hours), but due to the immediate nature of most test requests, initial storage is of no consequence. Occasionally, a second collection may be requested if a negative urine test result is questioned. A urine analysis deemed negative, in which suspect poisons are not identified, may require repeat testing. This may be due to sample matrix problems, such as unusual pigmentation or discoloration, a dilute specimen, or a suspicion that the potential poison has not had enough time to reach the urine. For some quantitative urine testing, especially that relating to the assessment of undue exposure to industrial or environmental poisons such as the heavy metals, 24-hour, timed collections may be necessary.

Table 27-2 Drugs and metabolites of analytical interest*

Parent drug	Analytes of interest
Hypnotic sedatives	
Amobarbital	Amobarbital, OH-amobarbital
Ethchlorvynol	Ethchlorvynol, OH-ethchlorvynol
Flurazepam	Flurazepam, OH-ethylflurazepam, desalkylflurazepam
Anticonvulsants	
Carbamazepine	Carbamazepine, di-OH-carbamazepine, epoxy-carbamazepine
Phenytoin	Phenytoin, OH-phenytoin
Antidepressants	
Amitriptyline	Amitriptyline, OH-amitriptyline, nortriptyline, OH-nortriptyline
Desipramine	Desipramine, OH-desipramine
Narcotics/Analgesics	
Acetaminophen	Acetaminophen, acetaminophen sulfate, acetaminophen glucuronide
Codeine	Codeine, norcodeine, morphine
Morphine	Morphine, morphine glucuronide
Propoxyphene	Propoxyphene, norpropoxyphene
Tranquilizers	
Chlordiazepoxide	Chlordiazepoxide, demoxepam, norchlordiazepoxide, nordiazepam
Diazepam	Oxazepam glucuronide, nordiazepam
Carisoprodol	Carisoprodol, meprobamate, OH-meprobamate
Chlorpromazine	Chlorpromazine, OH-chlorpromazine, sulfoxides, N-oxide
Miscellaneous	
Diphenhydramine	Diphenhydramine, diphenmethoxyacetic acid
Methamphetamine	Methamphetamine, amphetamine, OH-methamphetamine
Cocaine	Cocaine, benzoylecgonine, ecgonine methyl ester

*OH represents hydroxylated metabolites, some of which subsequently form conjugated compounds.

Stomach contents are provided as emesis fluid, derived after administration of an emetic such as syrup of ipecac to induce vomiting. Alternately, stomach contents may be provided as gastric lavage fluid, derived from washings of the stomach via intubation. Qualitative analysis of gastric fluid may be beneficial in that parent drug or poison, vs. metabolite, may be present, aiding the analyst further in rendering a specific identification of the poison instead of a simple class distinction. Gastric analysis may also detect compounds that may have been missed in urine testing because of delayed excretion of the poison. On the other hand, substances that are quickly absorbed in the stomach, such as secobarbital, may be missed by a gastric screen. And obviously, poisons that are not orally ingested, but instead injected, absorbed through the skin, or inhaled, will not be detected in this type of specimen. When available, 20 to 50 ml of gastric fluid should be submitted to the laboratory.

Blood and its products, serum or plasma, have been of most use to the analyst when a specific poison is indicated for testing by clinical condition or history, or after the poison has been previously detected in either the urine or gastric fluid. Most often, testing of the blood involves a direct quantitative assay and, unlike the urine or gastric testing, will generally provide data regarding the concentration of the poison. In choosing between various whole blood samples (varying by type of anticoagulant used), serum, or plasma, the most significant factors include: (1) whether the poison of interest is found predominantly in the red blood cells (RBCs) or in the serum/plasma, (2) the stability of the poison in blood, (3) which specimen was used to establish accepted standard therapeutic ranges or normal values, and (4) the compatibility of the various matrixes to analytical techniques and instrumentation. Poisons that distribute significantly into the RBCs include lead, carbon monoxide, and cyanide, and therefore require the submission of whole blood for testing. Certain compounds, such as cocaine and ethanol, may require the addition of a preservative, namely, sodium fluoride, to ensure stability. For the purposes of most emergency testing, the differences between using serum or plasma are deemed insignificant. All blood samples should be obtained during the acute phase of toxicity, with approximately 10 ml collected into the appropriately preserved or anticoagulated container. It should be noted that collection containers with serum separator gels should not be employed, since the potential for absorption of the drug into the gel is a possibility. Care should be exercised when choosing collection tubes to avoid minimum interferences from butylphthalate plasticizers. Inappropriate selection of collection tubes may result in a lowering of the drug concentration, a redistribution of the drug to the red blood cells, or direct interference with the test procedure. Processed specimens should be stored at 4°C until the time of testing.

Table 27-3 lists specimens of choice for prevalent tests. At the present time other biological specimens, such as hair, nails, and saliva, have not been widely accepted as useful samples with regard to emergency poisoning testing schemes. In the case of hair and nails, these samples are most useful in the reconstruction of potential chronic exposure to toxins, rather than acute poisoning. Saliva, if it can be properly collected, can often be used as an alternate to serum or plasma for the quantitation of select analytes.

ANALYTICAL PROCEDURES

Having chosen general categories of compounds to include in the laboratory's regimen of testing, the analyst must next address specific analytes. As noted previously, these compounds will be largely composed of select drugs. Figure 27-2, which shows agents involved in poisonings in the author's laboratory, indicates a need to concentrate analytical endeavors for detection of sedatives and hypnotics, benzodiazepines, phenothiazines and other tranquilizers, narcotics and other analgesics, stimulants, lithium, antihistamines and sympathomimetics, cardiac depressants, iron, and antidepressant drugs, as well as non-drugs such as alcohols, carbon monoxide, and ethylene glycol.

The laboratory will attempt to assemble, when symptoms and/or history do not indicate a specific poison, testing panels comprised of the aforementioned compounds, which may be matched to general clinical conditions. These panels are somewhat nonstandardized, and panel names and constituents will vary among different testing facilities. As examples, three emergency testing panels are presented, the acidosis screen, the stimulant panel, and the coma panel. Boxes 27-1 to 27-3 note compounds included in each panel, along with clinical indications for their use. Obviously, when specific poisons are suspected, the laboratory staff will begin direct qualitative or quantitative analysis. Direct quantitative testing will, in general, employ a single, relatively specific analytical procedure. Quite often a quantitative test result is not verified by a second confirmatory test. In contrast, qualitative, and somewhat less specific, testing will utilize an initial screening test procedure, followed by a more specific confirmation. Unlike forensic testing programs, these confirmatory methods for emergency testing do not necessarily need to employ gas chromatography/mass spectrometry, and therefore may consist of other chromatographic, spectrophotometric, or immunoassay techniques.

The choice of test procedure will be dictated by both technical and economic concerns. Volume of testing, experience of personnel, turnaround time expectations, and staffing patterns will all influence analytical decisions. Historically, laboratory testing evolved from spectral techniques (ultraviolet, visible, and fluorometric), through early chromatographic (conventional thin-layer chromatography, flame ionization detector gas chromatography), and immunoassay (radioimmunoassay, enzyme immunoassay) methods, to more specific or user-friendly techniques (commercial thin-layer chromatography, nitrogen-phosphorous detector gas chromatography and mass spectrometry, high-performance liquid chromatography, and fluorescence polarization immunoassay). Table 27-4 lists these general procedures, noting advantages and disadvantages of each. Table 27-5 relates these techniques to the individual analyses and panels of interest.

At this time many of the standard qualitative spot test procedures (Table 27-6) have been replaced by direct and specific quantitative analyses. This is especially true of those compounds in which quantitative test data correlate to a

Table 27-3 Specimens of choice for toxicological analysis

Poison/poison class	Specimen	Amount	Comments
Alcohols	Whole blood	2 mL	NaF
Carbon monoxide	Whole blood	2 mL	EDTA*
Cyanide	Whole blood	5 mL	Heparin
Drugs			
Specific (known)	Serum	5 mL	No preservatives
Acidosis panel	Serum	5 mL	No preservatives
Stimulant panel	Urine	20 mL	No preservatives
Coma panel	Urine	20 mL	No preservatives
	Gastric	20 mL	Filter before use
	Serum	5 mL	No preservatives
Ethylene glycol	Serum/Urine	5 mL	No preservatives
Metals			
Arsenic/Mercury	Urine	30 mL	No preservatives
Lead	Whole blood	5 mL	EDTA
Iron	Serum	5 mL	No preservatives
Organophosphate insecticides	Whole blood	5 mL	EDTA

*EDTA, ethylenediamine tetraacetic acid.

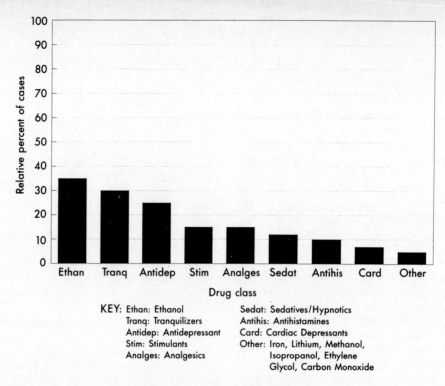

Fig. 27-2 Drugs identified in overdose.

KEY: Ethan: Ethanol Sedat: Sedatives/Hypnotics
Tranq: Tranquilizers Antihis: Antihistamines
Antidep: Antidepressant Card: Cardiac Depressants
Stim: Stimulants Other: Iron, Lithium, Methanol,
Analges: Analgesics Isopropanol, Ethylene
Glycol, Carbon Monoxide

Box 27-1 Acidosis screen

Constituents of the serum screen utilized to assess a patient showing signs of acidosis.
Methanol
Salicylate
Ethylene glycol

Box 27-2 Urine stimulant panel

Constituents of the urine drug screen used when a patient exhibits hyperactive behavior.
Amphetamine
Cocaine
Ephedrine
Methamphetamine
Phencyclidine
Phenmetrazine
Phentermine
Phenylpropanolamine

Box 27-3 Urine coma panel

Constituents of the urine/gastric drug screen used when a patient is comatose (hypoactive)

ALCOHOLS

Ethanol
Isopropanol
Methanol

ANALGESICS/NARCOTICS

Acetaminophen
Codeine
Hydromorphone
Meperidine
Methadone
Morphine
Pentazocine
Propoxyphene
Salicylate

ANTICONVULSANTS

Carbamazepine
Phenobarbital
Phenytoin
Primidone

ANTIDEPRESSANTS

Amitriptyline
Amoxapine
Cyclobenzaprine
Desipramine
Doxepine
Fluoxetine
Imipramine
Loxapine
Maprotiline
Nortriptyline
Trazodone
Trimipramine

ANTIHISTAMINES

Brompheniramine
Chlorpheneramine
Diphenhydramine
Doxylamine
Promethazine
Pyrilamine

CARDIAC DEPRESSANT

Disopyramide
Lidocaine
Procainamide
Propranolol
Quinidine

HYPNOTICS/SEDATIVES

Amobarbital
Butalbital
Pentobarbital
Secobarbital
Ethchlorvynol
Ethinamate
Flurazepam
Glutethimide
Methaqualone
Methyprylon

MISCELLANEOUS

Atropine
Benzotropine
Theophylline

TRANQUILIZERS

Benzodiazepines*
Phenothiazines*
Carisoprodol
Haloperidol
Hydroxyzine
Meprobamate

*Designated by class only.

Table 27-4   Analytical procedures (general)

Test	Advantages	Disadantages
Spot test/Visible spectroscopy	Rapid turnaround, economical, technically undemanding	Limited tests available, may identify "class" only, poor sensitivity, poor specificity
Ultraviolet spectroscopy	Economical, suitable for many compounds	Fair sensitivity, fair specificity, technically demanding
Thin-layer chromatography (conventional)	Economical, screens for many drugs simultaneously	Fair sensitivity, fair specificity, technically demanding, lengthy turnaround
Thin-layer chromatography (commercial: Toxi-Lab)	Screens for many drugs simultaneously, technically less demanding than conventional TLC, applications and R/D support, rapid turnaround	Relative cost, fair sensitivity, fair specificity
Gas chromatography	Screens for many drugs simultaneously, good sensitivity, good specificity	Relative cost of instrumentation, technically demanding, lengthy turnaround
Gas chromatography/Mass spectrometry	Screens for many drugs simultaneously, excellent sensitivity, excellent specificity	Cost of instrumentation, technically demanding, lengthy turnaround
High-pressure liquid chromatography	Good sensitivity, good specificity	Cost of instrumentation, technically demanding, fair turnaround
Enzyme immunoassay	Good sensitivity, good specificity for select analytes, technically undemanding, excellent turnaround	Cost of instrumentation, reagent costs, limited number of tests
Fluorescence polarization immunoassy	Good sensitivity, good specificity for select analytes, technically undemanding, excellent turnaround	Cost of instrumentation, reagent costs, limited number of tests
Atomic absorption spectroscopy	Excellent sensitivity, excellent specificity	Cost of instrumentation, technically demanding, limited number of tests

Table 27-5   Analytical procedures (specific)

Test/panel	Analytical procedure*
Acidosis panel	
Methanol	GC
Ethylene glycol	GC
Salicylate	Spot, FPIA, HPLC
Stimulant panel	EMIT, FPIA, TLC, GC, GC/MS
Coma panel	TLC, GC, GC/MS, HPLC
SPECIFIC QUANTITATIVE ANALYSIS	
Acetaminophen	EMIT, FPIA, HPLC, Spec
Alcohols	GC, Spec
Anticonvulsants (select)	EMIT, FPIA, HPLC
Antidepressants (select)	HPLC
Barbiturates	GC, HPLC
Carbon monoxide	Spec, GC
Cardiacs (select)	EMIT, FPIA, HPLC
Cholinesterase	Spec
Cyanide	Spec, GC
Heavy metals	AAS
Iron	Spec
Lithium	AAS, FES

*Analytical procedure key: GC, gas chromatography; Spot, colorimetric spot test; FPIA, fluorescence polarization immunoassay; HPLC, high-pressure liquid chromatography; EMIT, enzyme immunoassay; TLC, thin-layer chromatography; GC/MS, gas chromatography/mass spectrometry; Spec, spectrophotometric; AAS, atomic absorption spectroscopy; FES, flame emission spectroscopy.

Table 27-6   Spot tests*

Analyte	Specimen	Test	TAT	Comments
Acetaminophen	U	o-Cresol	15	Fair specificity
Alcohols	U, B, S	Microdiffusion	60	Fair specificity
Ethchlorvynol	U, S	Diphenylamine	15	Good specificity
Heavy metals	U, G	Reinsch's	60	Fair specificity
Iron	S	Bathophenanthrolene	15	Good specificity
Phenothiazines	U, G	FPN	2	Fair specificity, poor sensitivity
Antidepressants (imipramine)	U	Forrest	2	Fair specificity, good sensitivity
Salicylates	U, S	Trinder's	1	Good specificity

*Specimen, test, key: U, urine; B, blood; S, serum; G, gastric; FPN, Ferric-perchloric-nitric-reagent, TAT, turnaround time min

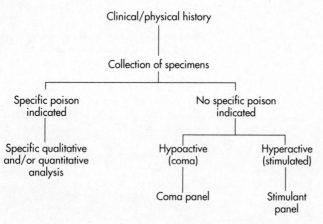

Fig. 27-3   General emergency drug detection scheme.

PATIENT NAME: _____

PATIENT ID #: _____

PATIENT LOCATION: _____

PHYSICIAN: _____

GENERAL INFORMATION:

SPECIMENS SUBMITTED _____

DATE/TIME _____

DRUGS/POISONS SUSPECTED _____

SUSPECTED ROUTE OF ADMINISTRATION: ____ORAL   ____INJECTION   ____INHALED   ____OTHER _____

PHYSICAL CONDITION: ____ RATIONAL & ALERT   ____ DEPRESSED   ____ STIMULATED/HYPERACTIVE
____ SEDATED   ____ COMATOSE   ____ HALLUCINATING

PUPILS: ____ DILATED ____CONSTRICTED

UNUSUAL BREATH ODOR ____ NO ____ YES (DESCRIBE) _____

OTHER INFORMATION: _____

TELEPHONE TEST RESULTS TO:

Fig. 27-4   Emergency patient toxicology history and information form.

great degree with the clinical condition or severity of toxicity, including carbon monoxide, alcohols, ethylene glycol, acetaminophen and salicylate, lithium, theophylline, iron, and select anticonvulsant and cardiac depressant drugs. Thin-layer chromatography remains a standard method to screen for a vast array of drugs simultaneously, as does gas chromatography and high-performance liquid chromatography. Utilization of the mass spectrometer as a gas chromatographic detector has increased the structural elucidation power of the analyst, and is sometimes found in the clinical laboratory in conjunction with forensic drug screening programs. Whereas radioimmunoassays have not played a major role in emergency testing, enzyme and fluorescence polarization immunoassays for specific compounds are commonplace.

The overall testing scheme developed by laboratory personnel (Figure 27-3) encompasses a review of the clinical history either by verbal discussion with the examining physician or via written history (Figure 27-4), collection of appropriate specimens, and choice of either direct quantitative or qualitative test methods, or screening panels.

INTERPRETATION OF QUALITATIVE RESULTS

Results of emergency overdose or poisoning analysis simply indicating the presence of a specific drug or poison may be difficult to interpret, especially in the absence of a definitive drug usage history, or without unusual physical or clinical examination findings. If nontherapeutic compounds are identified, such as ethylene glycol or methanol, their presence in any concentration is cause for concern and may be associated with the patient's condition. Positive qualitative findings for other poisons or drugs may also be deemed significant if the sensitivity or cutoff concentration of the employed test method is set to only detect abnormal amounts of the compound of interest. Examples would include spot tests for carboxyhemoglobin set to react at >20%, or Reinsch's test for selected heavy metals, detecting only clinically significant concentrations.

When drugs used in therapy are detected and reported, the task of relating the qualitative finding to clinical impairment becomes more difficult, since the patient may be undergoing treatment with the drug that has been found. If the patient is being treated therapeutically, one would expect to find the drug or its metabolites in the urine. In this case the presence of the drug may only be significant in situations in which distinct signs and symptoms of toxicity can be matched to the drug. For example, if a patient is exhibiting classic systemic anticholinergic signs of toxicity, namely, tachycardia, dry mucous membranes, and dilated pupils, and a tricyclic antidepressant drug such as amitriptyline is found in the testing process, the physician may readily attribute the toxicity to the antidepressant.

When the symptoms of toxicity are relatively vague or minor, or if the patient is asymptomatic but with a history of overdose, then qualitative test results may not provide the attending physician with enough information to confirm the diagnosis of poisoning. At these times, subsequent quantitative analysis may be indicated and required.

INTERPRETATION OF QUANTITATIVE RESULTS

The need to provide a quantitative drug or poison concentration may be necessary if the physician's goal is to objectively associate the poison with the clinical state of the patient. Quantitative drug data may also be used to predict the course of the toxic episode. The task of providing quantitative data is accomplished by selectively testing for a specific compound. In order to accomplish this, laboratory staff must utilize a preferred analytical method and an appropriate biological specimen. Test data can be interpreted by comparison to established lists, noting normal endogenous concentration ranges or anticipated therapeutic ranges of administered drugs. These expected concentration values are derived from studies and case reports designed to provide the laboratorian and the physician with standards by which their test data may be compared. Table 27-7 is a listing of selected drugs and poisons most often encountered in emergency poisoning and overdose cases, and their respective normal or expected therapeutic concentration values. Concentrations greater than stated values should be considered as potentially abnormal. Specific toxic or lethal concentration values are not given because of the extreme variation in concentrations necessary to produce toxicity or death.

Indeed, caution should be applied when interpreting all quantitative test data. Many factors will influence the patient's tolerance to a given poison, and will be somewhat independent of the quantitative concentration found. These factors include age, general health, body mass, duration of exposure to the poison or medication, as well as the presence of other drugs or synergistic compounds. Table 27-8 highlights the need for cautious interpretation of quantitative data. In the example shown in this table, three women were treated for overdose of the sedative hypnotic methaqualone. No other drugs or ethanol, aside from methaqualone, were detected in the testing process. There was no direct correlation between serum drug concentration and level of consciousness, or duration of toxicity in the patients.

The interpretation of toxicological test findings is a complex matching of qualitative and quantitative data with the clinical history and condition of the patient. Negative findings for specific poisons are objective indicators of a lack of involvement of that specific poison in the case of interest. However, negative findings from comprehensive drug and poison screens cannot completely rule out poisoning, since it is not technically feasible for any laboratory to detect all of the potential poisons available to the patient.

The hospital clinical laboratory has played a major role in upgrading analytical methodology and services related to the needs of the clinical toxicologist and the emergency room physician. Although requiring sophisticated technology and experienced personnel, rapid testing, at least for major drug groups, has become commonplace. Turnaround times for panel-specific poisons have improved immensely over the past decade, and with the advent of simpler operating mass spectrometers, the accuracy of test findings has become less suspect. With newer technologies come the challenge to expand and broaden the scope of testing to include additional environmental poisons, and to continue to establish a data base of quantitative test data, with subsequent improvement of existing quantitative analyses.

Table 27-7 Therapeutic drug concentrations

Analyte	Therapeutic/normal concentration*	Analyte	Therapeutic/normal concentration*
Acetaminophen	10-20 mcg/mL; <50 mcg/mL 10 hours postingestion	Ethylene glycol	None detected
Alprazolam	20-60 ng/mL	Fluoride	<0.5 mcg/mL (blood)
Amitriptyline	125-300 ng/mL (amitriptyline plus nor-triptyline)		<1 mcg/mL (urine)
Amikacin	15-30 mcg/mL	Fluoxetine	<1200 ng/mL
Arsenic	<2 mcg/mL (whole blood)	Flurazepam	<20 ng/mL
	<100 mcg/24 hr (urine)	Glutethimide	<10 mcg/mL
Barbiturates		Haloperidol	<15 ng/mL
Amobarbital	1-10 mcg/mL	Imipramine	150-300 ng/mL (imipramine plus desi-pramine)
Butabarbital	1-10 mcg/mL	Iron	0.5-1.6 mg/dL (blood); 10-250 mcg/24 hr (urine)
Butalbital	1-10 mcg/mL		
Pentobarbital	1-6 mcg/mL	Isopropanol	None detected
Phenobarbital	15-40 mcg/mL	Lead	<40 mcg/dL (blood)
Secobarbital	1-6 mcg/mL		<80 mcg/24 hr (urine)
Thiopental	<4 mcg/mL	Lidocaine	1.2-5 mcg/mL
Benzene	None detected	Lithium	0.5-1.3 mcg/mL
Bromide	500-1500 mcg/mL	Maprotiline	120-300 ng/mL
Caffeine	<15 mcg/mL	Meperidine	<1 mcg/mL
Carbamazepine	4-12 mcg/mL	Mephenytoin	5-16 mcg/mL
Carbon monoxide (carboxyhemoglobin)	Smokers: <8% (whole blood); nonsmokers: <2%	Meprobamate	<20 mcg/mL
		Mercury	<0.05 mcg/L (blood); <5 mcg/L (urine)
Cholinesterase (pseudo)	1800-4800 mIU/mL	Methanol	None detected
Chloral Hydrate (trichloroethanol)	<10 mcg/mL	Methaqualone	<5 mcg/mL
		Methyprylon	<10 mcg/mL
Chloramphenicol	<40 mcg/mL	Morphine	<200 ng/mL
Chlordiazepoxide	<1 mcg/mL	Nortriptyline	50-150 ng/mL
Chlorpromazine	<0.5 mcg/mL	Oxazepam	<500 ng/mL
Cocaine	Not established	Phenytoin	10-20 mcg/mL
Cyanide	<0.1 mcg/mL (whole blood)	Primidone	5-12 mcg/mL
Desipramine	150-300 ng/mL	Procainamide	4-10 mcg/mL
Diazepam	0.2-2.0 mcg/mL	Propoxyphene	<0.5 mcg/mL
Digoxin	0.5-2.2 ng/mL	Propranolol	<100 ng/mL
Digitoxin	<35 ng/mL	Quinidine	2-5 mcg/mL
Disopyramide	2-4 mcg/mL	Salicylate	<300 mcg/mL
Doxepin	75-200 ng/mL (doxepin plus desmethyl-doxepin)	Sulfa	<250 mcg/mL
		Theophylline	10-20 mcg/mL
Ethanol	None detected	Toluene	None detected
Ethchlorvynol	<10 mcg/mL	Trazodone	<1600 ng/mL
Ethosuximide	40-100 mcg/mL	Valproic acid	50-120 mcg/mL

*Concentration units: mIU/mL, milli-international units per milliliter; ng/mL, nanograms per milliliter; mcg/mL, micrograms per milliliter; mcg/dL, micrograms per deciliter; mcg/L, micrograms per liter; mg/dL, milligrams per deciliter.

Table 27-8 Quantitative drug analysis

Subject	Clinical condition	Serum methaqualone*
A	Grade IV coma; sedated; unresponsive to stimuli for 36 hours	11 mcg/mL
B	Grade II coma; sedated; responsive to verbal stimuli	12 mcg/mL
C	Grade I coma; lethargic	18 mcg/mL

*Serum methaqualone concentrations reported in micrograms per milliliter. Optimal therapeutic values generally do not exceed 5 mcg/mL. Subject A: First time use of the drug. Subject B: Occasional use (weekly). Subject C: Daily addictive use for 2 years.

SUGGESTED READING

Basselt R: Biological monitoring methods for industrial chemicals, Davis, Calif, 1980, Biomedical Publications.

Basselt R: Disposition of toxic drugs and chemicals in man, ed 2, Davis, Calif, 1982, Biomedical Publications.

Ellenhorn MJ and Barceloux DG: Medical toxicology, diagnosis and treatment of poisonings, New York, 1988, Elsevier.

Haddad LM and Winchester JF, editors: Clinical management of poisoning and drug overdose, Philadelphia, 1983, WB Saunders.

Kaye S, editor: Handbook of emergency toxicology, ed 3, Springfield, Ill, 1977, Charles C Thomas.

Moffiat AC, editor: Clarke's isolation and identification of drugs, ed 2, London, 1986, Pharmaceutical Press.

Sunshine I and Jatlow PJ, editors: Methodology for analytical toxicology, vols I and II, Boca Raton, 1982, CRC Press.

28 Legal aspects of drug screening

Amadeo J. Pesce

In drug testing some of the variation in the approach to the problem of laboratory analysis arises from the legal definition that some drugs are illegal, that is, their possession or use is against the law. The presence of such drugs or agents in the body fluid of an individual is considered an illegal act. Therefore, the individual who tests positive for their presence may be subject to certain legal sanctions. The gathering and use of information to administer civil penalties and perhaps criminal punishment then places this drug testing evidence subject to legal dispute.

It should be emphasized that any specimen collected for analysis and used for medical treatment and diagnosis has a well-defined legal status. Because medical and legal actions vary, they may be challenged in a court of law. In this sense, every specimen is a legal one. Thus all systems of specimen handling and analysis have elements that are designed to ensure that the analysis is done in a proper manner, and the data are restricted to properly designated individuals. Similarly, sample handling, analysis, and documentation for legal purposes should be done in a way that is not contrary to good laboratory practice or that would not jeopardize the health and safety of the patient. It is, in part, the sample handling and degree of analytical documentation required that often distinguishes the legal aspects of medical testing for the presence of drugs from ordinary medical testing. The legal aspects of drug screening reflect the use to which the results are put, that is, the civil or criminal penalties associated with the illegal drug use vs. the medical treatment of most results obtained in a hospital laboratory. The laboratory results obtained for legal purposes almost certainly will be challenged in court. Every aspect of specimen handling, analysis, documentation, security, and verification will be questioned usually by the defense attorney. In all cases, the usual questions of good laboratory practice apply: (1) Was the specimen collected properly? (2) Was the specimen labeled properly? (3) Was the specimen transported properly? (4) Were the analyses done with proper controls and calibrators? (5) Were the analytical procedures and instruments functioning properly? (6) Were the results confirmed? (7) Were the results validated by a technologist or certifying scientist? (8) Were the results consistent with the patient's expected symptoms or behavior? (9) Were the results reviewed in a medical context? (10) Was the laboratory

secure so that no tampering of samples, reagents, or reports could occur or no unauthorized individual could gain access to them? (11) Were the results acted upon in an appropriate manner? The documentation of these issues is usually sufficient to support the legal and scientific aspects of the drug analysis.

SPECIMEN COLLECTION

The question of whether or not the specimen was collected properly has implications in addition to whether or not the correct body fluid was collected. The specimen must be collected with knowledge of the individual, labeled properly, and be prepared for transportation so that sample tampering will be evident. For drug screening, most often the body fluid of choice is urine because the drug concentrations are higher than in blood, and it is usually simple to collect the volume needed for testing and confirmation. In addition, the collection is noninvasive, and the patient is not at risk for any other medical consequence of the test procedure.

Proper collection of a specimen for legal purposes means that: (1) a consent form was read, understood, and signed by the individual giving the specimen; (2) the specimen was collected properly, with or without witnessing; (3) the specimen was placed in a tamper-proof container that will not affect the specimen during transportation and storage. An example of a consent form is presented in Fig. 28-1. This form contains patient identification, information including the subject's home address, and identification such as driver's license, social security number, or employer's number. Often the subject must provide identification with a photograph. Sometimes two photographic identifications are required to validate the identity of the individual before a specimen is collected. The type of specimen, for example, blood or urine, that is to be analyzed and which tests are to be performed are clearly defined on the form. This information is to be read and understood by the subject. The subject's signature, date, and time are recorded. The signing of this form is witnessed. Instructions for collection and handling of the specimen are also included. To make certain that the specimen was a proper one and not tampered with or substituted by another one, the collection is witnessed or collected in such a way as to prevent possible misrepresentation. If the individual objects to someone watching him

APPLICANT DRUG TESTING CONSENT & RELEASE OF LIABILITY

I have voluntarily agreed to take a urinalysis or other similar substance screen test used to detect the presence or absence of illegal drugs. I have further voluntarily agreed that the results of such a test may be furnished to those agents of The Christ Hospital as may be designated by The Christ Hospital.

Accordingly, I hereby authorize The Christ Hospital to conduct through its designated medical examiner(s)/laboratory a urinalysis or other similar substance screen test for Amphetamines, Barbiturates, Methadone, Opiates, Benzodiazepines, Cannabinoids (THC), Cocaine, Phencyclidine and Propoxyphene. I authorize that designated medical examiner(s)/laboratory to release the results of the substance screen test(s) to those agents of The Christ Hospital as may be designated by The Christ Hospital. I hereby release The Christ Hospital and its related entities, their directors, employees and agents and also release The Christ Hospital's designated medical examiner(s)/laboratory from any and all claims and/or legal responsibility in any way arising out of the administration of the substance screen test or any action taken based upon the information obtained from the substance screen test.

I understand that it is a condition of employment that I satisfactorily complete the substance screen test and that if the results of the substance screen test indicate the presence of any illegal drug, I will not be eligible for further consideration for employment for six months after being advised of rejection.

I am currently taking the following over-the-counter and/or prescription drugs (birth control drugs need not be listed):

_____   _____

_____   _____

I certify that I have read this form, that I understand its contents and that I have signed this of my own free will.

Driver's License #: _____

_____   _____/_____
Signature   Date/Time

Address: _____

_____

_____   _____/_____
Signature of Witness   Date/Time

┌─────────────────────┐
│   │   Specimen Number
└─────────────────────┘

Fig. 28-1 Example of a consent form for drug testing.

or her give a urine specimen or if NIDA (National Institute of Drug Abuse) guidelines are being followed, then the collection is taken in a carefully designed and supervised facility. A carefully designed facility, such as that recommended by NIDA, usually has the following features: (1) only a toilet bowl that contains water with a blue dye or other marker to prevent sample dilution; (2) access to a sink with water only in the presence of a witness; (3) a dressing area in which the subject is undressed and gowned for a physician's examination. No cleaning supplies or other chemicals are stored under the sink or in other places of access. Finally, the subject is not allowed to bring purses or other packages into the rest room. Additional verification procedures are often used to ensure that the specimen did come from the proper individual. Immediately after collection (within 4 minutes), the temperature of the urine is taken to be certain that another urine was not substituted by the patient. NIDA guidelines require that the temperature be between 32.5°C to 37.7°C (90.5°F to 99.8°F). For some specimens, the laboratory may also check the creatinine concentration, pH, color, smell, and specific gravity.

In one particular circumstance of drug testing, the consent and collection are unique, that is, the obtaining of a blood alcohol content. In the state of Ohio, for example, it is considered that "any person who operates a motor vehicle upon the public highways in this state shall be deemed to have given consent to a chemical test or test of his blood, breath, or urine for the purpose of determining the alcoholic or drug content of his blood, breath or urine if arrested for the offense of driving while under the influence of alcohol or drugs." Thus, in legal terms, it is presumed that blood may be drawn under these circumstances without a consent form. However, it must be noted that two restrictions apply: "Only a physician, a registered nurse or qualified technician or chemist may withdraw the blood; these individuals may refuse to withdraw blood if, in their opinion, the procedure

PRESS FIRMLY — YOU ARE MAKING MULTIPLE COPIES

METHODIST MEDICAL CENTER
Toxicology Laboratory
221 N.E. Glen Oak
Peoria, Il. 61636

URINE CUSTODY AND CONTROL FORM

I. TO BE COMPLETED BY EMPLOYEE OR APPLICANT PROVIDING SPECIMEN

SOC. SEC. NO OR EMPLOYEE NO.   EMPLOYER NAME

EMPLOYER ADDRESS

II. TO BE COMPLETED BY EMPLOYER REPRESENTATIVE/OR COLLECTOR

REASON FOR TEST (check one)
☐ PRE-EMPLOYMENT   ☐ POST ACCIDENT   ☐ RANDOM   ☐ PERIODIC MEDICAL   ☐ REASONABLE CAUSE

MEDICAL REVIEW OFFICER (M.R.O.) & ADDRESS

NAME & ADDRESS   PHONE

LAB — PLEASE RETURN 2ND ORIGINAL & RESULTS TO M.R.O. AT THIS ADDRESS

III. INDICATE WHICH DRUGS SPECIMEN IS TO BE TESTED FOR:

INDICATE WHICH DRUGS SPECIMEN IS TO BE TESTED FOR:
☐ Only THC and Cocaine   ☐ THC, Cocaine, PCP, Opiates, and Amphetamines   ☐ Other (Specify): _____

IV. TO BE COMPLETED BY EMPLOYER REPRESENTATIVE/OR COLLECTOR

TEMPERATURE OF SPECIMEN HAS BEEN READ WITHIN 4 MIN.   ☐ YES   ☐ NO   TEMPERATURE IS WITHIN RANGE OF 32.5-37.7°C/90.5°-99.8°F   ☐ YES   ☐ NO - IF NOT, RECORD ACTUAL TEMP.

V. TO BE INITIATED BY THE PERSON COLLECTING SPECIMEN AND COMPLETED AS NECESSARY THEREAFTER

PURPOSE OF CHANGE	RELEASED BY - Signature - Print Name	RECEIVED BY - Signature - Print Name	DATE
Provide Specimen for Testing	DONOR		

VI. TO BE COMPLETED BY EMPLOYEE OR APPLICANT PROVIDING SPECIMEN

FEDERAL REGULATIONS PROHIBIT DISCLOSURE OF THE DONOR'S IDENTITY TO THE LABORATORY. DONOR SHALL COMPLETE INFORMATION IN SECTION V ON COPIES 2 THROUGH 5 ONLY.

VII. TO BE COMPLETED BY PERSON COLLECTING SPECIMEN **AFTER** DONOR HAS COMPLETED SECTION VI — (SEE COPY 2 OF FORM)

COLLECTOR'S NAME - PRINT (first, m.i., last)   DATE OF COLLECTION

COLLECTION SITE ADDRESS: PHONE

REMARKS CONCERNING COLLECTION: Split sample collected in accordance with applicable Federal requirements.   ☐ Yes   ☐ No

I certify that the specimen identified on this form is the specimen presented to me by the employee providing the certification above, that I have certified that it bears the same identification number as that set forth above, and that it has been collected, labeled and sealed as required by the instructions provided.

SIGNATURE OF COLLECTOR

VIII. TO BE COMPLETED BY THE LABORATORY

I certify that the specimen identified by this accession number is the same specimen that bears the identification number set forth above, that the specimen has been examined upon receipt, handled and analyzed in accordance with applicable Federal requirements, and that the results attached are for that specimen.   ACCESSION NO.

LABORATORY   ADDRESS   PHONE

(PRINT) Certifying Scientist's Name (Last, First, Middle)   Signature of Certifying Scientist   Date

THE RESULTS FOR THE ABOVE IDENTIFIED SPECIMEN ARE IN ACCORDANCE WITH THE APPLICABLE SCREENING AND CONFIRMATION CUTOFF LEVELS ESTABLISHED BY THE HHS MANDATORY GUIDELINES FOR FEDERAL WORKPLACE DRUG TESTING PROGRAMS (found only on copies one and two)

☐ NEGATIVE   ☐ POSITIVE, for the following:
☐ Cannabinoids as Carboxy—THC
☐ Cocaine Metabolites as Benzoylecgonine
☐ Phencyclidine
☐ Opiates
　☐ Codeine
　☐ Morphine
☐ Amphetamines
　☐ amphetamine
　☐ methamphetamine
☐ _____

IX. TO BE COMPLETED BY MEDICAL REVIEW OFFICER

I have reviewed the laboratory results for the specimen identified by this form in accordance with applicable Federal requirements. My final determination/verification is: (Check one)   ☐ NEGATIVE   ☐ POSITIVE

SIGNATURE OF MEDICAL REVIEW OFFICER: _____   DATE: _____

COPY 1—ORIGINAL—MUST ACCOMPANY SPECIMEN TO LABORATORY—LABORATORY RETAINS

Fig. 28-2   Example of a chain of custody form for specimen transportation.

would endanger the physical welfare of the driver." Thus, the blood must be withdrawn in an appropriate manner. In addition, there are restrictions as to how the blood can be analyzed before the evidence is admissable. "The blood must be analyzed in accordance with the methods promulgated by the Director of Health." In this regard, for example, alcohol or phenol may not be used as a skin antiseptic to cleanse the venipuncture site. Thus, there are restrictions as to who can draw the blood, methods of analysis, and

how the blood is drawn in order to meet the specifications required by law.

SPECIMEN LABELING AND TRANSPORTATION

Labeling of a forensic specimen requires special attention. In addition to the usual label with the patient's demographic information, the label is initialed by the subject. Sealing tape is placed on the container and initialed to validate the specimen was delivered intact. From a legal point of view, transport of the specimen to the laboratory is a process during which the specimen could be tampered with or substituted. The transportation and sample handling is therefore validated by a chain of custody form. This form documents who had custody or control over the specimen from the time it was collected until the time it was opened in the laboratory. The form, an example of which is given in Fig. 28-2 (note that because the drug testing purposes are different, the drugs being tested in Figs. 28-1 and 28-2 are different), contains information including the subject's name or identification number, date, time of collection, the number and type of specimen, and the witness who will verify the history of the specimen. The names of the individuals sending the specimen, the individual receiving the specimen, and the condition of the specimen, particularly the seals, are noted when control of the specimen is transferred from one individual to the next. The transporting package may be a locked container that may only be opened by the designated laboratory personnel. In such a case, the courier may not be required to sign the forms. The name of the individual who opened the specimen as well as the time are recorded. Both the condition of the transporting package and the inner package are recorded.

SPECIMEN TESTING AND CONFIRMATION

The testing itself must be done according to good laboratory standards. Quality control samples must be analyzed at the same time as the unknown sample, and the calibration of any instruments used must be documented. The analytical results obtained on the quality control specimens must be within accepted limits. If a positive result is obtained on a specimen, a known negative specimen must be analyzed before and sometimes after the positive specimen to validate that no sample-to-sample carryover of drugs occurred. The term *carryover* is applied to the process in which material from one analysis can be transferred into subsequent analyses or analytical runs. This carryover phenomenon can occur with automated instruments or with manual methods where proper washing and rinsing between samples is not performed. To eliminate this possibility, some laboratories perform all analyses in duplicate on positive specimens to demonstrate the second result is the same as the first. Other laboratories analyze a blank or negative sample between presumptive positive specimens.

Single-blind proficiency specimens are included with every run in addition to quality control specimens. The single-blind proficiency specimens are samples that contain known values that are unknown to the analyst. Preferably, they should also be blind to the certifying scientist until results are reviewed. Some agencies require 10% or more of all specimens to be of this single-blind type. Blind specimens are different from the usual quality control specimens because the usual quality control specimens have values that are known by the analyst and are used as part of the validation of the analytical assay. Therefore, they may be assayed in duplicate or handled in a manner different from those of the patients. The blind specimen eliminates this bias of treating proficiency testing specimens differently. Furthermore, double-blind specimens are also necessary as part of some proficiency evaluations. In this case, the spec-

imens appear as actual patient samples whose identity as blind specimens is not known.

All positive drug screening tests are corroborated by a second confirmation procedure. The second procedure must use a different analytical principle from the initial screening procedure. Thus, in current practice, an immunoassay is often used to detect the presence or absence of a drug. The principle of this assay is that an antibody reacts specifically with the drug and that this interaction is measured by a particular type of detection procedure, either enzymatic, fluorescent dye, or radioimmunoassay. The confirmation procedure cannot be one that uses an antibody reaction, even though it may be a different antibody and different detection system, in other words, radioimmunoassay cannot be confirmed by a fluorescence polarization immunoassay. The confirmation procedure may be thin-layer chromatography (TLC), gas chromatography (GC), or gas chromatography/mass spectroscopy (GC/MS). All of these methods are fundamentally different from immunoassay. They do not use an antibody reaction and rely on separation and detection by chemical or physical means.

The legal system prefers GC/MS as a confirmation method, and this method of analysis is specified in NIDA guidelines. The reason for this acceptance of GC/MS analysis is that the procedure is considered to yield an analytical fragmentation pattern of various molecular weight materials that is specific for the drug at a particular retention time. Of the millions of compounds tested in GC/MS systems, no two chemicals have been shown to have the same retention times and ion fragment patterns. Thus it can be stated unequivocally in court that, to date, no drug other than the one stated could give the specific pattern observed in the analysis. However, it must be demonstrated in court that the GC/MS was functioning properly. The controls, standards, and other measures of instrument validity have to be shown to be accurate. Recordings of the instrument parameters for that day may be requested and examined in court. Items such as injection temperature and fragmentation pattern of the standard must all be recorded and kept on file.

There are two possible problems with using GC/MS as the legal confirmation method of choice. First, not all compounds to be tested can be vaporized to pass easily through a gas chromatograph without decomposition. In these cases, more volatile derivative compounds must be made before using chromatography.

A second problem with the low resolution mass spectrometers used in most laboratories for legal drug testing is that some materials, for example, alcohols and amphetamines, have such low molecular weights that there is not enough of a fragmentation pattern to be absolutely diagnostic of the original compound.

Both sets of data, the initial screening information and the confirmation of results by GC/MS or by any second procedure, should be reviewed by a certifying scientist. This individual reviews all the foregoing information including the consent forms, chain of custody document, quality control, and instrument data as well as the analytical result to verify that the result is correct. This individual, in part, bears the legal responsibility of the analytical results and must defend them in court. Usually, considerable experience in toxicology and forensic testing is required. NIDA guidelines specify a bachelor's degree in chemical or biological sciences or medical technology with training and experience in quality control and drug testing.

One of the most important analytical decisions of the drug testing laboratory is the establishment of cutoff levels for the positive detection and identification of drugs. Two factors determine cutoff levels, one is the legal definition and the other is the analytical process itself.

An example of how a legal definition is derived is given by the NIDA cutoff level for delta-9-cannabinoid. It has been argued in court, and accepted, that levels of delta-9-tetrahydrocannabinol carboxylic acid (Δ 9-THC-COOH) of 20 ng/mL in urine could be present as a result of passive inhalation of marijuana smoke; that is, an individual could be in a room with other people smoking marijuana and inadvertently inhale the smoke. Therefore, the cutoff level for the excretion of Δ 9-THC-COOH in urine is set at 100 ng/mL, because at this level it has been successfully argued that it must have been due to smoking with active inhalation of marijuana. The second consideration of analytical cutoff level is the simple consequence of the limits of the analytical sensitivity and reproducibility in proficiency surveys. The confirming method must be able to verify the screening results 100% of the time if the drug is truly present. From the point of view of proficiency surveys, once the cutoff limits are stated by a laboratory for its practice, all true positive values above a cutoff limit must be verifiable. Therefore, for a laboratory, a level is chosen for a cutoff value in which both the screening and confirmatory analytical procedures can achieve the level of reliability of 100% in proficiency surveys. Recently, NIDA has set cutoff guidelines for several drugs, which are listed in Table 28-1.

In court, the laboratory must defend its cutoff criteria, that is, the drug concentration above which a result is considered positive. It must be able to demonstrate that a concentration above the specified amount will reproducibly yield the same answer and be confirmed 100% of the time.

Table 28-1   NIDA drug cutoff levels*

	Initial screening test (ng/mL)
Marijuana metabolite	100
Cocaine metabolite	300
Opiate metabolite	300
Phencyclidine	25
Amphetamines	1000

	Confirmatory test
Marijuana metabolite	15
Cocaine metabolite	150
Opiates	
Morphine	300
Codeine	300
Phencyclidine	25
Amphetamines	
Amphetamine	500
Methamphetamine	500

*Procedures for transportation workplace drug testing programs: final rule and notice of conference, Federal Register, December 1, 1989, 54(230): 49854–49884.

Thus analytical procedures are not set at the lowest measurable concentration, the limit of sensitivity, but rather at a higher concentration that is 100% reliable. In terms of sensitivity and specificity, the assay cutoff limits are set so that sensitivity is much less than 100% and therefore a significant portion of specimens with low concentrations of drugs are reported as negative. However, the specificity is set at a concentration at which virtually all true positives observed by the screening procedure can be confirmed by the second procedure. For example, if a value of 100 ng/mL for cannabinoid metabolites is set as the cutoff limit for the screening procedure, then in an ideal situation with no bias but with the usual analytical variability, 50% of the values above 100 will be reported as positive and 50% as negative. If the standard deviation for the test method is 10 ng/mL, then if a specimen is received by the laboratory with a true value of 100 ng/mL, one-half the time the value would be recorded as positive and one-half the time it would be recorded as negative. If the same laboratory receives a specimen with a true value of 80 ng/mL, then 97.5% of the time (-2 SD) it will report the value as negative, while 2.5% of the time the value will be reported as positive. This calculation comes from multiplying the 10 ng/mL SD by the number of standard deviations between 100 ng and 80 ng (-2 SD). Similarly, if the true value were 120 ng/mL, then 97.5% of the time the screening result would be recorded as positive and 2.5% of the time as negative ($+2$ SD). If the true value is 70 ng/mL, then it will be judged positive about 0.3% and judged negative 99.7% of the time. For a value of 70, the likelihood of this occurrence is calculated by assuming that a value 3 SD from the true value ($70 + 3 \times 10$) occurs only 3 times in 1000. The confirmatory cutoff is usually set at a lower concentration so that nearly all of the time any of the values recorded as positive on screening, including the 70 ng value, will be confirmed. Therefore, the confirmatory value is set so that the mean and standard deviation of a positive are well below the screening procedure. For example, if the confirmatory test is set as positive at 40 ng $\pm$ 10 ng, the probability of 70 ng not being confirmed would also be 0.3% ($+3$ SD). This is calculated using the same probability estimate, mean $+3$ SD, as mentioned earlier. The possibility of not confirming a true positive with a value of 100 ng/mL at 6 SD above 40 ng/mL is very low, about 1/500,000,000. Thus, the initial screening procedure may miss some true positives, but all those observed can be confirmed.

The length of time between sample acquisition and the analytical determination can sometimes be significant. The deterioration of the drug and its metabolites can be important if this time is significant. For practical and sometimes legal reasons, specimens are usually analyzed within 48 hours of receipt. NIDA guidelines require that a written report be produced within 5 working days. Because of the disputes that may surround a legal case, specimens should be stored for later re-analysis. Positive specimens are treated differently from negative ones. The negative specimens are not further tested to confirm they are negative. Only the initial result is used and the specimens discarded. Positive specimens are preserved for possible reconfirmation. NIDA guidelines require preservation of samples by freezing for 12 months. Some samples, because of litigation contesting the result, may be kept until the legal dispute is settled, which may be for many years. In some drug screening contracts, a specimen is split so that the analyses may be performed in a second laboratory.

PATIENT HISTORY

Very often, urine or serum specimens are given to the laboratory without any patient history. In these circumstances it is not possible to establish if the results are consistent with the behavioral or pathophysiological pattern of the patient. Urine concentrations of drugs do not correlate with behavior physiology, which further complicates the usual interpretation patterns done on clinical specimens. While these samples only rarely correlate well in demonstrating impaired behavior, they can be used to indicate the presence of the drug. Blood drug concentrations, particularly alcohol, do tend to correlate with the patient's physiological condition. Therefore, if very high blood alcohol concentrations are observed, these should roughly correlate with patient condition.

MEDICAL REVIEW OF THE RESULTS

The analytical results should be submitted to a responsible physician, and the organization requesting the analysis should have a policy of action on the results that is legally defensible and nondiscriminatory. In some cases, results of preemployment testing are sent to personnel directors of the employer for implementation of some process, namely, probation (or discharge). It is preferred, because of the complexities of interpretation, that drug testing results be sent to a medical review officer. This individual is charged with reviewing the patient's medical and drug history to establish if there was any potential that a positive result was due to ingestion of medication or from dietary intake, and not due to illegal drug use. Poppyseed ingestion from bagels, rolls, or poppyseed cakes can cause positive opiate test results. This is just one example of the care needed to interpret this type of information. Patient behavior or other history and physical findings should be integrated with the laboratory result for proper interpretation.

It is considered an invasion of privacy if information other than that agreed to by the subject is obtained and released. For example, the patient may be epileptic and on medication to control the condition. If the laboratory detects a drug such as phenytoin in the urine of such a subject, it should not be disclosed to the interested party if consent for the analysis of phenytoin was not given.

LABORATORY SECURITY

In the usual hospital setting the laboratory should be unaccessible to unauthorized personnel. In the legal setting, this procedure must be strictly enforced. The design and operation of the laboratory facility must be such that only authorized individuals can actually enter the facility. Ideally, a list of authorized individuals is kept, as well as a log of the names and times of occupancy. The facility must be constructed so that security is controlled by physical barriers and entrance possible only with such devices as cipher-coded cards or keys. All entrances are kept locked at all times. Similarly, the specimens and preferably all the reagents are kept in locked storage areas. Access to these areas is restricted to only those individuals processing the drug specimens, including the laboratory staff. Other support staff, such as janitorial personnel, are escorted when present in the facility. The use of reagents and specimens is recorded to make certain no substitutions could have occurred.

Reports are kept in a secure manner so that only the assaying technologist and certifying scientist know if a specimen was positive. Access to reports is only given on a "need to know" basis. Laboratory data, if stored in a computer even with restricted access, should be coded so casual examination will not allow viewing or tampering with results. Physical reports must be kept in a secure area with no possibility of tampering. The laboratory procedures must include a trash disposal system designed and operated to be certain no data leaves the facility.

Confidentiality of data is a theme that is common to all patient records, including all laboratory data. Failure to observe confidentiality and release of patient data can result in loss of job, civil, and possibly criminal suits. This concept cannot be overemphasized. Virtually every state and municipality have laws that regulate patient medical data. These same laws extend to drug testing. The information is confidential and is to be released only to authorized individuals.

ACTION BASED ON THE LABORATORY RESULT

One area with which the laboratory does not usually involve itself is the consequence of what happens to the patient based on laboratory results. Since the results obtained are often used for discipline or other legal recourse, it is important that the results be used in a responsible manner. If a company or organization does not have a policy of action to take in the event of a positive drug test, then they may be liable for damages for discrimination, and the laboratory performing the test may be liable as well.

It is very important to delineate in advance which drugs are to be tested and what cutoff levels will be used. A corollary issue is the extent to which information is restricted. In theory, only one individual should know the individual's drug testing results. The potential for blackmail, slander, and other actions is great with a widespread availability of such information. Therefore, before any testing is done, there should be restrictions of such data if it is to be used for forensic purposes.

IMPAIRMENT

Drugs such as cocaine and marijuana are different from the historic drug, alcohol. The legal system has not yet defined the blood drug concentration for these newer drugs, over which an individual is considered impaired. In the case of alcohol, an individual is legally described as impaired, for example, drunk or intoxicated, when the blood concentration exceeds a given amount; in the state of Ohio, this is greater than 1000 μg/mL (0.1%, 0.1 gm/100 mL). Blood concentrations are not commonly obtained for cocaine and marijuana, but because these substances are illegal for possession and use, their presence in urine can be used for legal sanctions. If a driver demonstrates erratic behavior and urine tests positive for cannabinoid metabolites, the erratic behavior cannot definitely be proven to be due to the marijuana since no evidence exists to correlate the presence of the drug in urine at this concentration or any concentration with impairment to drive. The same can be said for cocaine. Therefore, civil punishment is due to both improper driving of a motor vehicle and possession and use of an illegal substance.

In addition, in many states the possession and use of a driver's license implies consent to be tested for alcohol or drugs. Refusal to agree to be tested implies that the subject is drunk. Not all states have such laws, and it is important to understand what can be and cannot be tested in an individual state without additional permission.

TESTIMONY

In general, laboratory personnel such as the medical technologist will be called as witnesses only to validate the fact that they performed a particular assay for drugs or that there was a specimen that was applicable to that particular patient. The technologist must be able to identify that specimen as being unique to that patient. In addition, the technologist should be able to testify that the instrument was performing properly, all controls were within accepted limits, and that the result was valid. In rare cases, the technologist may be called as an expert witness to interpret the values, but this is quite different from the usual circumstance in which only the validation of the data is checked.

Very often, physicians and staff in the hospital emergency units are asked to obtain blood levels on individuals who are not patients at the institution. Because of the legal requirements related to sample handling and transport, and the time commitment required for participation in court cases, it is not to be entered into casually. It is best for an institution to provide an individual with information on where he or she can obtain such laboratory results in a manner that would meet the standards of the court and refer individuals to these laboratories rather than to perform the analyses on site. If requested by a law officer, the staff should have the appropriate subpoena and should ensure the proper chain of custody by giving the specimen directly to the requesting law officer.

SUGGESTED READING

Chamberlain RT: Drug screening in the workplace: medicolegal implications. American Association for Clinical Chemistry, TDM-T, no. 12, 1986.

Cowan MS: Workers, drinks and drugs: can employers test? Univ Cincinnati Law Rev 55,129–151, 1986.

Hoffman A and Silvers J: Steal this urine test: fighting drug hysteria in America, New York, 1987, Penguin Books.

Mandatory guidelines for federal workplace drug testing programs, Federal Register, Monday, April 11, 1988, 53(69):11970–11989.

Ohio Revised Code (ORC) §4511.191 (Deals with issues related to implied consent.)

Ohio Revised Code (ORC) §3701.143 and Ohio Administrative Code (OAC) §§3701-53-01 et seq (Deals with how to analyze blood alcohol levels.)

Pickard NA: Collection and handling of patient specimens. In Kaplan LA and Pesce AJ: Clinical chemistry: theory analysis and correlation, ed 2, St Louis, 1989, Mosby–Year Book, Inc.

Warner A and Stinson M: The legal issues in urine drug screening in substance abuse: meeting the challenge for laboratories, employers, University of Cincinnati Department of Pathology and Laboratory Medicine, Cincinnati, Ohio 45267-0714.

PART FOUR

URINALYSIS, CLINICAL MICROSCOPY, AND FLUIDS

29 Urinalysis

Michael D.D. McNeely
Malcolm L. Brigden

Routine urinalysis is one of the oldest clinical laboratory tests. One can imagine the primitive shaman making observations about a patient's urine in order to gain prognostic information. Certainly, ancient Greek physicians (later known as Pisse prophets) routinely examined the urine as part of their test repertoire. Early physicians were able to observe the appearance of urine and thereby detect the presence of bilirubin or blood, indicating liver disease or glomerulonephritis, respectively. Tasting urine or pouring it on the ground to see if insects were attracted were techniques employed to assess for the presence of sugar. Protein was identified by the coagulum that appears when urine is boiled. More sophisticated ancients apparently used sulfur to suggest the presence of bile in the urine.

Unfortunately, in spite of its distinct value, the humble urinalysis has fallen into a state of semi-disrespect. Today's physicians sometimes neglect the proven value of the urinalysis for the diagnosis of liver abnormalities, urinary tract diseases, or metabolic diseases such as diabetes, given its effectiveness in both monitoring chronic problems or screening for asymptomatic conditions. The knowledgeable laboratory director will attempt to raise the urinalysis technique to a position where it receives the attention that it deserves.

ROUTINE URINALYSIS
What is a routine urinalysis?

Routine urinalysis has been defined by the National Committee for Clinical Laboratory Standards (NCCLS) as "the testing of urine with procedures commonly performed in an expeditious, reliable, and cost effective manner in clinical laboratories." The term "routine" is not meant to suggest the indiscriminate performance of urinalysis because this investigation, like any test, should be used in a cost-effective manner. Although individual laboratories should customize their own protocols, today's routine urinalysis commonly consists of a visual examination of the urine to note its color and consistency. This may be followed by a measurement of specific gravity. Next, a series of semi-quantitative chemical screening tests are conducted on the urine. This is most conveniently done using "dipsticks." Dipsticks are thin, plastic strips on which are fixed chemically impregnated

squares of porous material. These chemicals are able to react with various components of the urine. With chemical tests completed, the urine is centrifuged and the heavier particulate matter is concentrated and isolated onto a microscope slide. This is then examined microscopically to identify the specific nature of the particulate matter and determine whether or not it is made up of cells, casts, or debris. Typical values for the normal urinalysis are provided in Table 29-1. A synthesis of the facts provided supplies a vast amount of information at a very low price.

The routine and microscopic urinalysis therefore consists of:
1. Macroscopic observation (color, clarity, odor)
2. Physical measurements (volume, specific gravity)
3. Dipstick or tablet chemical analysis
4. Microscopy of the centrifuged solid debris

Purposes for which a urinalysis is performed include:
1. To aid in the diagnosis of specific diseases.
2. To monitor disease progress.
3. To monitor therapy (effectiveness or complications).
4. As a population screening for congenital, hereditary, or asymptomatic diseases.

Facilities

Urinalysis should be carried out in a clean, well-illuminated, well-ventilated space. At least one sink with running water should be close at hand. A separate area for microscopic work should be available with a conveniently centered centrifuge capable of holding the number of tubes appropriate for the laboratory workload and spinning them at a relative centrifugal force (RCF) of 400 to 450 for 5 minutes. Relative centrifugal force rather than revolutions per minute (rpm) is used as this value can be corrected for differences in centrifuge rotor radius. The formula for the calculation is:

$$RCF = 1.118 \times 10^{-5} \times radius\ (cm) \times (rpm)^2$$

A regular cleaning routine must be employed in the laboratory. This should involve disposing of completed urine samples down the drain, followed by flushing with copious amounts of water, and the disinfection of bench tops and sinks. Freshly voided urine is usually almost odorless and

Table 29-1   Typical urinalysis results*

Assay	Findings
Specific gravity	1.003-1.040
pH range	4.8-7.5 (mean, 6)
Protein	Negative to trace
Glucose	Negative
Ketones	Negative
Urobilinogen	Less than 1 mg/dL
Bilirubin	Negative
Occult blood	Negative
WBC esterase	Negative
Nitrite	Negative

MICROSCOPIC EXAM

RBC	0-3/HPF
WBC	0-5/HPF
Bacteria	Few/HPF or less than 1+
Epithelial cells	Renal tubular, 0-1/HPF; transitional, 0-2/HPF; squamous variable/HPF
Mucus	Less than 1+
Crystals	Few calcium oxalate, few amorphous urates or phosphates
Casts	0-2 Hyaline casts/LPF
	0-1 Granular casts/LPF
Spermatozoa	May be present in both men and women
Yeast	Negative
Trichomonas	Negative

*WBC, white blood cell; RBC, red blood cell; HPF, high power field; LPF, low power field.

therefore a disagreeable smell emanating from the urinalysis area may indicate a lack of hygiene (see "Specimen Collection").

Specimen collection

Urinalysis is ideally carried out with an aliquot of a single voiding of urine within 2 hours of collection. The minimum sufficient quantity to permit adequate macroscopic and microscopic exam is considered to be 12 mL, but a volume of 50 mL is preferable. The first morning specimen is considered the most valuable diagnostically because it is standardized and also reflects the kidney's ability to concentrate urine after an overnight period.

The ideal specimen is collected as a clean-catch midstream urine. This is obtained by having the patient begin to void, then interrupt the stream to catch the midportion. The first portion of the voiding is undesirable as it may contain surface debris from the genitalia, such as degenerated epithelial cells that can provide a false result. Providing the urine is collected in a sterile container, it is possible to follow up the routine urinalysis with a culture if initial tests warrant this procedure. A variety of other urine specimens are sometimes collected, including random samples and timed, 24-hour collections.

All urine samples should be collected into absolutely clean, though not necessarily sterile, containers. Features of a desirable collection container (NCCLS recommendations) are listed in Box 29-1. The responsible laboratory will ensure that any containers used are biodegradable.

Urinalysis samples should be examined within 2 hours. If they cannot be examined within this timeframe, they

Box 29-1   Desirable features for urine collection devices (NCCLS recommendations)

1. The container should be labeled with: patient's name, identification code, location, time and date of collection. (The label should be on the side, not on the lid, and should adhere to the container even if the specimen is refrigerated.)
2. Collection devices should be free from interfering chemicals (e.g., detergent).
3. Sterile containers should be used (if culture specimen).
4. Sufficient volume (approximately 50 mL is preferred).
5. Collection devices should have a wide opening (minimum 4.0 cm) to facilitate collection yet avoid contamination.
6. There should be a leakproof closure that is easily applied and removed.
7. Collection devices should have a wide base to avoid accidental spillage.
8. Specialized smaller containers should be available for pediatric specimens.
9. The reuse of collection containers is not recommended.

should be refrigerated at 4°C. Unfortunately, refrigeration may precipitate amorphous urates or phosphates, which can obscure subsequent microscopic examination. Undue delay in performing urinalysis may also allow bacteria to proliferate, cells and casts to degenerate, the pH to change, certain chemical substances (glucose and ketones) to disappear, and other substances (bilirubin, urobilinogen) to degrade. Even with refrigeration, microscopic examination should still be carried out within 4 hours of collection. Samples that have been maintained for 24 hours are only suitable for albumin, and hemoglobin testing.

Although the use of chemical preservatives is not recommended by the NCCLS, the Metropolitan Life Insurance Company has developed a unique preservative tablet (potassium-acid-phosphate, 100 mg; sodium benzoate, 50 mg; benzoic acid, 65 mg; methenamine, 50 mg; sodium bicarbonate, 10 mg; and red mercuric oxide, 1 mg). The use of this tablet is said to allow the preservation of urine for routine chemical tests for a period of weeks at room temperature.

Unacceptable specimens should be rejected rather than tested. Criteria of unacceptability are:

1. Sample age
   - Unrefrigerated samples older than 2 hours
   - Refrigerated samples older than 4 hours
2. Collection container used
   - Unclean specimen containers (e.g., pickle jars); containers supplied by the laboratory are preferred.
3. Sample volume
   - Less than 2.5 mL. In the case of children or elderly patients, satisfying this criterion may be difficult. Patients with urinary tract infections often produce very small volumes. In this instance, the sample should be accepted. Volume should always be recorded.
4. Sample label
   - Improperly labeled samples should be rejected.

Dipsticks

Until the late 1950s, chemical tests were carried out on urine specimens using a variety of liquid chemical reagents. Current urinalysis depends on the use of the dipstick. The dipstick is a thin strip of plastic with one or more cellulose pads affixed. Each pad is impregnated with buffer and certain chemicals. The specific combination of materials in the dipstick pad is activated when water from the urine sample soaks into the pad. Reagents in the pad are then able to react with components of the urine sample. By this means the presence of various substances in the urine can be detected and their relative amounts can also be estimated. There are a number of important considerations involving the successful use of dipsticks.

1. The expiration date on the bottle is vital and materials must never be used beyond this date.
2. The container should be stored in a cool, dark place but not in the refrigerator.
3. Moisture must be avoided in the storage area as this may inactivate the pads.
4. Contamination of the test area by fumes or chemicals must be avoided to prevent false interpretation of the strip.
5. The lid of the container should be screwed on tightly when dipsticks are not in use. The potency of many of the chemical reagents in the pads declines with air exposure.
6. Reagent strips from different containers should never be combined. When strips are removed from a container but not used, they should not be placed back in the container.
7. The test strip should be applied to the sample briefly, but completely, so that the cellulose pads are completely immersed. If the immersion period is too long, chemicals may be allowed to dissolve or wash out of the pads. Following immersion, the dipstick is generally tapped lightly to remove excess moisture.
8. The clinical test sites on reagent strips should not be physically touched.
9. The developed color must be read at exactly the time specified by the manufacturer for the individual dipstick pad. A timing device with a second hand is required for visual reading. If used, automated strip readers should be adjusted to read the reaction pads at the times specified by the manufacturer.
10. All color readings should be conducted in a quiet, well-lit (illumination 500 lux) room where the light has a color temperature corresponding to that of daylight.
11. The instructions for dipsticks are all somewhat similar but sufficient differences exist such that the product monograph should be carefully reviewed for each product used.
12. The specificity and limitations of each test must be understood.
13. Quality control procedures must be incorporated.

There are a variety of different commercial products available for use in urinalysis. Because these undergo constant evolution, only the basic principles of individual tests will be reviewed in detail. A summary of the different dipstick reactions is provided in Table 29-2.

Automation

There are a number of instruments that have been developed to mechanize part or all of the routine urinalysis examination. The most common and most useful of these are relatively inexpensive devices that automate the reading of the dipstick. When using such a system, the dipstick is immersed in urine in the usual fashion, excess urine is removed, and the stick is placed on or in the machine. The machine then reads the pads at the appropriate times, utilizing reflectance photometry.

These instruments are supposed to offer increased precision over visual reading, but studies have not always proven this to be the case. Depending on the instrument, the work throughput may be no greater than (and may actually be less than) a manual/visual approach. The machines do offer a convenient way to perform stat analyses because timed readings can be performed without waiting. Significant time and labor savings can be realized when it is possible to interface these instruments with a laboratory computer system. At least one manufacturer has developed an instrument that performs routine urinalysis, chemical testing, and specific gravity in a totally "walkaway" mode.

Developments currently underway that allow semiautomated microscopic examinations to be performed show excellent promise. To date, because of the expense of this technology, any potential labor saving (particularly if microscopic examinations are performed selectively) has inhibited widespread introduction.

Quality assurance

A quality assurance program for urinalysis should incorporate continuous monitoring of every aspect of this procedure. Quality control represents only a single aspect of quality assurance. Quality assurance programs involve coordination and communication between the patient, the laboratory, and the clinician. According to NCCLS recommendations, components of urinalysis quality assurance should include specimen collection and handling, recordkeeping, technical competence, standardization, continuing education, and a scheduled, documented review process.

Recordkeeping

Recordkeeping is a fundamental part of quality assurance and all records must be reviewed on a daily basis by the urinalysis supervisor or designee. Records, controls, and instrument checks should be available for each shift. Written procedures for detection and correction of errors, out-of-control results, and review of test results are required. Patient results should be reported accompanied by reference ranges.

A workbench record or log book should be available with the following information:

1. Reagent strip lot number and expiration date
2. Date of opening of reagent strip containers (should also be written on the bottle)
3. Patient and control results
4. Specimen collection time and laboratory time of arrival
5. Identification of technical staff who performed the test(s)

Table 29-2 Summary of dipstick reagent testing

Test	Principle	Reaction interference		Correlation with other tests
		False-positive	False-negative	
Specific gravity	pK change of polyelectrolyte	Protein	Alkaline urine	None, extremes may affect some pad results
pH	Double-indicator system	None	None	Microscopic exam, nitrite
Protein	Protein error of indicators	Highly alkaline urine, quaternary ammonium compounds, detergents	High salt concentration, very dilute urine, does not detect Bence Jones protein	Blood, leukocytes, nitrite, microscopic exam
Glucose	Glucose oxidase, double sequential enzyme reaction	Peroxide, oxidizing detergents, and hypochloride	Ascorbic acid, 5-HIAA, homogentisic acid, aspirin, levodopa, ketones, high specific gravity with low pH	Ketones
Ketones	Sodium nitroprusside reaction	Levodopa, phthalein dyes, phenylketones	—	Glucose
Blood	Pseudoperoxidase activity of hemoglobin	Oxidizing agents, vegetable and bacterial peroxidases	Ascorbic acid, nitrite, protein, pH below 5.0, high specific gravity	Protein, microscopic exam
Bilirubin	Diazo reaction	Medication color	Ascorbic acid, nitrite	Urobilinogen
Urobilinogen	Ehrlich's reaction	Ehrlich-reactive compounds (Ames), medication color	Nitrite, formalin	Bilirubin
Leukocytes	Granulocytic esterases reaction	Oxidizing detergents	Glucose, protein, high specific gravity, oxalic acid, gentamicin, tetracycline, cephalexin, cephalothin	Nitrite, protein, microscopic exam
Nitrite	Griess's reaction	Medication color	Ascorbic acid	Protein, leukocytes, microscopic exam
Ascorbate*	Tilmann's reaction	Pad is sensitive to ascorbate concentrations 10 mg/dL or greater. Approximately 2.5% false-positive reactions occur	—	Glucose, blood
Micro albumin*	Conjugated antibodies and enzyme	Pad is sensitive to micro albumin concentrations 10 mg/dL or greater, no known substances		Glucose, microscopic exam

Modified with permission from: Strasinger SK: *Urinalysis and body fluids*, ed 2. Philadelphia, 1989, FA Davis.
*Available as special dipstick pad or separate dipstick.

Procedure and instrument manuals

Urinalysis procedure and instrument manuals, including test directions, should be available at the workbench and include the following:

1. Acceptability and rejection criteria for specimens
2. Reference ranges
3. Panic values
4. Information regarding controls
5. Procedures for confirmatory testing

Instruments and other mechanical equipment should have:

1. A written procedure manual and manufacturer's instructions manuals
2. A written maintenance routine and regular maintenance schedule
3. Service and repair records

Proficiency testing

Some type of external proficiency testing program should be employed with results recorded on a regular basis. The 35-mm transparencies included with some external proficiency surveys are useful to assess technologists' recognition capacities but do not check urine handling or slide preparation. In-house and commercial controls for microscopic examination should only serve as precision checks.

Continuing education and training

Only qualified, properly trained personnel should perform a complete urine microscopic examination. Workshops and self-study programs for technical personnel should be provided. All technical personnel should have regular skill updates. Up-to-date reference texts, atlases, charts, and posters should be readily available. In-house conferences and seminars should be periodically held and any changes in procedures or reference ranges must be published and circulated to all appropriate staff and clients.

Quality control

Quality control is an important element of quality assurance and constitutes an accepted absolute requirement for the performance of clinical laboratory tests. For some reason, this principle is often less rigorously implemented in the area of urinalysis. There are four fundamental methods for establishing quality control in the urinalysis laboratory:

1. Maintaining an awareness of the daily distribution of positive results

2. Recognizing internally inconsistent results on a given patient's sample and following up results that strongly suggest improper collection or some form of unusual sample
3. Using quality control materials designed to mimic abnormal urines
4. Organizing repeat samples and introducing split samples into the laboratory

Urinalysis technologists should be well acquainted with possible combinations of abnormalities so that they will be alerted when illogical results occur.

Quality control of the chemical urinalysis

Multiconstituent controls to validate the performance of each chemical test at two distinct levels are recommended. Controls should be tested each day a test is performed, and whenever a fresh bottle of reagent strips is opened. When dipsticks are changed, parallel testing with old and new lots on controls and patient specimens is desirable. Commercial materials may be used as multiconstituent controls. However, commercial lyphilized materials are often very expensive. It is this expense that frequently prohibits the routine use of these materials. It is easy for any laboratory to prepare its own control samples. One formulation is as follows:

To make 300 mL of solution:

pH: Use phosphate buffers to create the desired pH
Protein: 0.3 g Bovine albumin (100 mg/dL)
Glucose: 750 mg Dextrose (0.014 m/L or 14 mmol/L)
Specific gravity: 15.0 g NaCl per 300 mL (1.022)
Ketones: 0.09 g Acetoacetic acid per 300 mL (pinch)
Nitrite: Sodium nitrite (one minute grain)
Color: Clayton yellow (small pinch)
Method:
Add phosphate buffer solutions in required amount.
Add remaining reagents in amounts required.
Add demineralized water to bring volume to 300 mL.
Add small stirring bar and mix until all reagents are dissolved.
Dispense into 7.0-mL serum tubes labelled "Urine QC."

The supervisor may split several samples each day and reintroduce them into the analytical area on a blind basis during each shift. After results are recorded, the supervisor is then able to identify the samples and access consistency.

Some important points to consider regarding quality control of the chemical urinalysis are: (1) if confirmatory chemical tests are carried out after dipstick analysis, these should be consistent with dipstick results; (2) brown urine should usually test positive for bilirubin, (3) bloody appearing urine or urine with erythrocytes on the microscopic examination should test hemoglobin-positive; (4) in most instances, urine with a large number of white cells on microscopic examination should test positive for esterase and nitrite; (5) urine with a high glucose content should have an increased specific gravity.

Freis has defined overall goals for quality control samples in chemical urinalysis. He has suggested that not more than 50% of positive results be more than one color block away from the assigned value. Obviously, a negative result is not acceptable for a positive control. Similarly, a negative reaction is the only acceptable result for a negative control. Participation in an external urinalysis proficiency survey to

evaluate the performance of the chemical urinalysis is also desirable.

Quality control of refractometers and specific gravity determinations

A quality control program for refractometers and specific gravity reagent strips must include the daily use of reference solutions or commercial control urine. Specific gravity (SG) standards can be created to calibrate this measurement.

Result:	Amount of sodium chloride
SG 1.009:	1 g NaCl per 100 mL
SG 1.014:	3 g NaCl per 100 mL
SG 1.022:	5 g NaCl per 100 mL

Make up in 1 L amounts and store refrigerated.

Refractometers can be checked with deionized or distilled water (SG = 1.000) and with the aforementioned solutions. The calibration and daily performance checks of refractometers and specific gravity reagent strips must be documented and retained.

Quality control of the microscopic examination

During the microscopic portion of the urinalysis, all personnel should follow the same procedure using the identical equipment and report results in a standard format using the same terminology. Commercial control products are not generally available for all sediment elements. However, controls containing red blood cells (RBCs) and white blood cells (WBCs) are commercially available. Replicate testing of fresh patient specimens can establish the reproducibility of microscopic analysis of casts, renal cells, and other formed elements, both within the laboratory and between several laboratories. For any microscopically detected element, the result should agree within ± 1 reporting range.

If a disagreement exists regarding the presence or quantity of a microscopic element, the examination must be repeated. When necessary, the urinalysis supervisor or laboratory director should resolve discrepancies. Each laboratory should establish appropriate criteria for reviewing abnormal sediment results.

QUALITATIVE CHEMICAL EXAMINATION
Physical appearance

Normal urine is usually a pale, straw-yellow color due to the presence of the pigment urochrome and small amounts of uroerythrin and urobilin. Urochrome is a product of endogenous metabolism, and under normal conditions it is produced at a constant rate. Urochrome production increases in thyroid conditions or when urine stands at room temperature. However, normal urine may also appear deep amber to almost colorless secondary to the wide variation possible in urine fluid volume. When reporting urinary color, a good light source should be used and the specimen should be examined against a white background.

Whereas normal urine may be almost any color, the presence of certain colors may be the result of pathology or may be secondary to the presence of a drug or food. It is important to be able to recognize a possible cause of urine color change because, besides constituting a disconcerting symptom for the patient, it may be mistaken for a pathological process. In addition, the intensity of the color change may obscure the ability to read dipstick results properly. This is especially true in the case of the drug phenazopyridine (Pyridium), which is frequently used as a urinary antiseptic.

Orange urine

Orange urine may very rarely be due to bile pigments. Their detection is outlined later in this chapter. Usually, anisindione, gantrisin (azogantrisin) ethoxazene, indanediones, mannose, phenothiazines, nitrofurantoin, phenazopyridine (Pyridium), rifampin, rhubarb, carrots, or senna is the cause.

Yellow urine

Yellow urine may also be due to bilirubin or urobilin but is probably the result of carrots, rhubarb, cascara, fluorescein, nitrofurantoin, phenacetin, picric acid, or quinacrine.

Green, blue-green, or blue urine

Bilirubin may become oxidized to biliverdin and generate green urine. Bacteria may also tinge the urine green, as will acriflavine, amitriptyline, methocarbamol, anthraquinone, azuresin, creosote, Doan's pills, Clorets, methylene blue, nitrofurans, phenols, phenyl salicylate, resorcinol, tetralin, thymol, tolonium, triamterene, and vitamin B complex. Blue or blue-green urine is exclusively due to medications such as dithiazanine, Doan's pills, Evans blue, methylene blue, and nitrofurans.

Red urine

Urine may be red as a result of the presence of red cells, hemoglobin or myoglobulin. Each of these substances can activate the dipstick's hemoglobin pad. Myoglobin can be identified using the special tests indicated later in this chapter. Porphyrins may also, on occasion, produce a red hue. Other reported causes of red urine include acetophenetidin, acrolein, aminopyrine, anisindione, antipyrine, beets, rhubarb, benzene, bromsulfophthalein (Bromsulphalein), cascara, chincophen, chrysarobin, Congo red, crayon pigment, danthron, deferoxamine, emodin, ethoxazene, indanediones, merbromin (Mercurochrome), methyldopa, phenazopyridine, phenindione, phenolphthalein, phenothiazines, phenolsulfonphthalein (PSP), phenytoin, and senna.

Brown or black urine

Biliary pigments, hematin, and myoglobin (positive hemoglobin on dipstick) color the urine brown. In addition, brown urine may be due to aloin, cascara, chloroquine, cresol, furazolidone, iron salts, metronidazole, nitrobenzene, nitrofurants, nitrofurantoin, rhubarb, sulfamethoxazole, and sulfonamides. The discovery of black urine is often an ominous sign. Of particular interest is a clear or dark urine that becomes even darker when left to stand. This phenomenon is observed in the presence of homogentisic acid, indican, melanin, metranidazole, and urobilinogen. Other nonpathologic causes are cascara, iron-sorbitol-citric acid complex, methyldopa, levodopa, methocarbamol, nephthol, phenols, and pyrogallol.

A summary of a number of the most common agents that cause different colored urines is provided in Table 29-3, along with possible additional tests that may facilitate identification.

Turbidity

Turbid urines are very common and are usually due to crystal formation in the bladder secondary to concentration or pH changes. Turbidity may also occur in the collection vessel as urine cools to room temperature. Acid urine will encourage the formation of uric acid crystals, whereas amorphous phosphates form in alkaline urine. Besides amorphous crystals, other common causes of turbidity in the urine are the presence of white blood cells, epithelial cells, and bacteria. Other possible causes include the presence of lipids, semen, mucus, yeast, fecal material, or possible extraneous contamination with substances such as talcum powder or X-ray contrast material. The presence of turbidity on the macroscopic examination of the urine should be followed up during the microscopic examination. The degree of turbidity should correspond with the types and amounts of material observed under the microscope.

Odor

Fresh urine has a mild but characteristic odor. The breakdown of urea in the urine is responsible for the characteristic ammonia odor. A pungent aroma may be the result of urinary tract infections, a high ammonia concentration, failure to deliver the specimen to the laboratory in a fresh state, or an unclean collection vessel. Some unusual conditions may be associated with very characteristic odors. For example, maple syrup urine disease is often first detected by a maple-syrup–like smell observed in a patient's urine. Other metabolic diseases that can result in a characteristic urine odor include phenylketonuria, isovaleric acidemia, and methenamine malabsorption. The ingestion of particular foods (such as asparagus) may impart a characteristic smell from the amino acid asparagine.

Evaluation

The clarity of the urine should be reported as clear, slightly cloudy, or cloudy. Other descriptive words can be used but should be employed sparingly.

Next, the color should be stated. Acceptable terminology includes colorless, pale yellow, dark yellow, amber, brown, red, or green. Words such as straw, dark, coffee, and so forth should be avoided if possible.

When present, other unusual findings should be mentioned (blood clots, fatty layers, or mucous clots). Any unusual odor should also be noted on the report form.

In some instances it may be impossible to read the dipstick because of the presence of Pyridium, other chemical contamination, or dark-colored urine samples. In this case, report: "Unable to read because of color interference on dipstick."

Specific gravity
Clinical significance

Specific gravity is the weight of a measured volume of a substance expressed in relation to the same volume of pure water. The specific gravity of urine increases as the concentration of material dissolved in it increases. In normal urine the main constituents that lead to an increase in specific gravity are salts (such as sodium and chloride) and nitrogenous wastes (such as urea and creatinine). In abnormal situations glucose or protein may be excreted in large

Table 29-3 Potential factors affecting urine color

Color	Possible cause	Laboratory correlations
Dark yellow Amber orange	Concentrated specimen	May be normal after strenuous exercise or in a first-morning specimen
	Bilirubin	Dehydration from fever or burns; yellow foam when shaken; and positive chemical tests for bilirubin
	Acriflavine	Negative bile tests and possible green fluorescence
	Carrots or vitamin A	Soluble in petroleum ether
	Phenazopyridine (Pyridium)	A drug commonly used for urinary tract infections; may have orange foam and thick orange pigment that can obscure or interfere with dipstick readings
	Nitrofurantoin	An antibiotic used for urinary tract infections
Yellow-green	Bilirubin oxidized to biliverdin	Colored foam in acidic urine and negative chemical test for bilirubin
Yellow-brown	Rhubarb	
		Seen with acidic urine
Green/blue-green/blue	*Pseudomonas* infection	Positive urine culture
	Amitriptyline	An antidepressant
	Methocarbamol	A muscle relaxant
	Clorets	Breath freshener
	Indican	Confirm with Obermayer's test
	Phenol	When oxidized
	Methylene blue	None
Pink/red	Red blood cells	Cloudy urine with positive chemical tests for blood and RBCs visible microscopically
	Hemoglobin	Clear urine with positive chemical tests for blood; plasma may be red
	Myoglobin	Clear urine with positive chemical tests for blood; plasma will be colorless; specific tests are available
	Porphyrins	Negative chemical tests for blood; confirm with Watson-Schwartz screening test or fluorescence under ultraviolet light
	Beets	With alkaline urine in genetically susceptible persons
	Phenolsulfonphthalein	With alkaline urine after *PSP test for renal function
	Bromsulphalein	With alkaline urine after *BSP test for liver function
	Rhubarb	Seen with alkaline urine
	Phenindione	An anticoagulant
Brown/black	Red blood cells oxidized to methemoglobin	Seen with acidic urine after standing; positive chemical test for blood
	Myoglobin	Positive chemical test for blood
	Homogentisic acid (alkaptonuria)	Seen with alkaline urine after standing; specific tests are available
	Melanin or melanogen	Urine darkens upon standing and reacts with nitroprusside and ferric chloride
	Phenol derivatives	Interfere with copper reduction tests
	Argyrol (antiseptic)	Color disappears with ferric chloride
	Methyldopa	An antihypertensive
	Levodopa	An anti-Parkinson drug
	Metronidazole (Flagyl)	Urine may darken on standing

Modified with permission from Strasinger SK: *Urinalysis and body fluids,* ed 2. Philadelphia, 1989, FA Davis.
*PSP, Phenolsulfonphthalein; BSP, Bromsulphalein.

amounts. These substances can have a significant influence on urinary specific gravity. Also, contaminants in the urine may cause an increase in the specific gravity. In general, however, the specific gravity is a reflection of the state of the patient's hydration, combined with the functional ability of the kidney tubules. A normal individual who has been deprived of water for a period of time will concentrate urine, resulting in a high specific gravity. Large amounts of fluid given to a normal individual will naturally result in a dilute urine with a low specific gravity.

The normal spectrum of urinary specific gravity results for random specimens ranges from 1.003 to 1.040. The highest values are found with first-morning specimens following an overnight fast. The lowest values are observed

several hours after a large amount of water has been consumed.

Very high values (greater than 1.040) are almost always secondary to the presence of a contaminant in the urine. One of the most common causes is the presence of high molecular weight radiopaque dyes given for radiographic imaging of the kidneys. Another possibility is sucrose (table sugar) added to the urine by individuals attempting to mislead their physicians. Very high values may be seen in diabetes mellitus when large amounts of glucose are present. Serious proteinuria will also cause a raised specific gravity. The specific gravity of a first-morning specimen should be greater than 1.015. An inability to concentrate the urine above this value after fasting overnight provides strong evidence that kidney tubules are losing their ability to concentrate urine, that the body is greatly overloaded with fluid, that antidiuretic hormone is not being released (diabetes insipidus), that a diuretic is being administered, or that early glomerular disease is leading to an excess of fluid in the tubules.

Very dilute urine with specific gravity between 1.001 and 1.005 may be associated with extremely high fluid intakes, diuretic administration, and diabetes insipidus. In general, the urinary specific gravity is lower in persons on low-protein diets.

Measurement of specific gravity

Traditionally, specific gravity measurements were performed by using a modified hydrometer known as a urinometer. This consists of a glass vial with a thin top and weighted bottom. The urinometer is floated in the urine in such a way that the higher the specific gravity of the urine, the higher the device will rise. A dilute urine will allow the flotation device to float very low in the sample. The specific gravity is read directly from a calibrated scale fixed to the urinometer.

Currently, the specific gravity is usually evaluated using a commercial refractometer or total solids meter (TS meter). Two basic types of refractometers are commonly used; a hand-held model requiring only a single drop of urine and pour-through models (often incorporated with automated instruments). The principle involved with refractometry is the measurement of the refractive index. Refractive index is a comparison of the velocity of light in air to light velocity in a solution (urine). The velocity depends on the concentration of dissolved particles in the solution, which in turn affects the angle at which light passes through the solution. With different urine densities (different specific gravities), light will be bent to different degrees in an ocular device and this deflection can be calibrated using an appropriate scale.

Recently, a dipstick pad has been developed that approximates the specific gravity. This strip contains a polymeric acid that releases hydronium (H^+) ions when reacting with positive ions in the urine. The released hydronium ions cause a pH change, which in turn results in a color change. The higher the acidity, the higher the ion-concentration, and thus the higher the specific gravity result. This evaluation should be repeated using a refractometer if there is any amount of glucose or protein present when the dipstick pad is used for specific gravity measurements.

Cleaning, calibration, and maintenance of the refractometer is important and should be carried out carefully as follows:

1. Always check calibration daily. Raise the daylight plate and place a few drops of distilled water on the prism face.
2. Close the daylight plate gently. Look through the eyepiece and bring the scale into focus by turning the eyepiece. If the scale is correct, the boundary line should fall on the Wt and UG line. If it does not, adjust the boundary line to make it coincide with the zero line by turning the scale-adjusting knob. If the zero reading is correct for distilled water, it is unnecessary to check the instrument with the three specific gravity standards.
3. Wipe off the refractometer with a soft tissue. Place a few drops of urine on the prism and read the results on the UG scale.
4. Wipe off the sample with a soft tissue. It is important that the face of the prism is not scratched during cleaning.
5. It is important to keep all areas near the hinges and adjusting screws clean and dry at all times.

Interfering substances

As noted earlier, dipstick determinations of specific gravity depend on hydronium ion generation. High concentrations of nonionic substances such as glucose, protein, or X-ray contrast media may result in an elevated true specific gravity but will not affect the dipstick result.

When to perform specific gravity measurements

The choice of which specific gravity measuring technique to employ or, indeed, whether or not this measurement should be performed at all is a topic of debate. Physiologically, the only specimen that has clinical significance is one in which the hydration of the patient is well known prior to collection of urine for specific gravity measurement. In most routine instances, only a first-morning urine specimen will provide any valuable clinical information. Specimens collected randomly and without knowledge of the patient's state of hydration probably do not warrant performing urine specific gravity measurements. However, there is additional useful information obtained from urine specific gravity that can be helpful in the interpretation of other dipstick pad results. For example, a very dilute urine could cause a dilution of substances such as protein and glucose, rendering the detection of trace values of these substances clinically significant.

It is widely considered that specific gravity measurements performed by an accurate device, such as a TS meter, should use the first-morning voided specimen. The dipstick pad, which estimates the specific gravity, is all that is necessary under other clinical circumstances.

Ultimately, it must be remembered that in complex solutions such as urine, there is only a very general relationship between specific gravity and osmolarity. When more elaborate hydration studies need to be carried out, the formal measurement of urinary osmolality is a far more accurate tool.

pH
Clinical significance

The human body produces acid as a by-product of metabolism. A portion of the acid is volatile and can be eliminated through the lungs as CO_2. Some acid remains in the form of fixed organic acid (phosphoric, citric, oxalic), which must be removed by the kidneys. In general, urinary pH reflects the status of the pH of the blood. Under normal circumstances, urine is slightly acidic with a pH ranging from 4.8 to 7.5 (mean, 6.0). This pH is a function of the need to eliminate fixed acids.

A strongly acidic urine may be found in patients with systemic acidosis, when the body has an undue burden of hydrogen ions to remove. If there is acidemia, but the urine is neutral or just barely acidic (pH greater than 6), then a condition known as renal tubular acidosis must be considered to be present. In this condition the ability of the kidneys to secrete hydrogen ions into the urine is impaired.

An alkaline urine is seen in patients with systemic alkalosis as the body attempts to conserve hydrogen ions and remove fixed base. Following meals, all patients will experience a certain degree of alkalosis as a result of the stomach's production and secretion of hydrochloric acid. Vegetarians tend to have a more alkaline urine than persons who ingest meat. This is because ingested meat contributes to the fixed acid load that must be removed by the kidneys. With urinary tract infections, microorganisms in the urine may, through enzymatic action, split urea into ammonia. This will cause a distinct increase in urinary pH. Thus, with severe urinary tract infections or if urine is allowed to sit resulting in bacterial overgrowth in vitro, there will be a high pH. Increased alkalinity of the urine may destroy red blood cells and casts, especially if the specific gravity is also low. A knowledge of urinary pH is helpful for the identification of crystals noted during microscopic exam.

As part of the therapy for certain conditions, there may be a need to manipulate urinary pH to affect the solubility of inorganic substances that may be precursors of crystals and calculi. For instance, an acidic urine may be beneficial in the prevention of calcium carbonate and magnesium-ammonia-phosphate kidney stones. Maintaining an acidic urine may also benefit the treatment of certain urinary tract infections, because urea-splitting organisms cannot multiply as readily at an acidic pH. An alkaline urine may be induced to prevent stones due to oxalate, uric acid, and cystine. Alkalinization of the urine is occasionally used for the treatment of drug overdose (such as salicylate) or hemolytic transfusion reactions. Alkalinization of the urine also encourages the optimum action of some antibiotics.

Measurement

The most accurate measurement of urinary pH is performed using a pH meter. This degree of accuracy is seldom clinically necessary but may be useful as part of the formal evaluation of suspected renal tubular acidosis.

For patients who need to maintain their urine at either an acidic or alkaline pH, there are a variety of pH papers that can be used for frequent monitoring purposes. The dipstick pad that is part of routine urinalysis generally combines indicators such as methyl red and bromthymol blue. This provides a visual range of between pH 5 to 9. Urinary pH should be reported to the nearest whole number.

The routine measurement of urinary pH has little clinical significance. Its most important role is that, if very alkalotic, it may suggest that the specimen was not stored properly prior to testing. This observation suggests that bacteria may have been allowed to proliferate in urine left to stand too long at room temperature or at warmer temperatures. A strongly acid urine may suggest contamination of the collection vessel. Because several of the pads on the dipstick depend upon some aspect of pH, it is important that other dipstick pad results from urine specimens with extremes of pH be interpreted with caution.

Reaction interference

No known substances interfere with pH measurements performed by using dipsticks. However, care must be taken that no runover takes place between the adjacent highly acidic protein testing pad, or false acidic results may be reported.

Follow-up testing

A follow-up test is generally not required for urinary pH. As noted earlier, if very high or very low values are discovered, then it may be wise to collect another specimen and ensure its integrity before other dipstick measurements are recorded. A neutral or alkaline urinary pH observed in a patient with known acidemia merits consideration of possible renal tubular acidosis and may prompt a formal work-up for this condition.

Protein
Clinical significance

Although the kidney glomerulus may be considered to be an efficient filter, in reality, the situation is considerably more complex. As a result of hydrostatic pressure, serum proteins below a certain molecular weight routinely pass through the glomerulus and into the proximal tubule. Tubular proteins are mostly reabsorbed. Some protein, however, normally passes through the tubules and enters the urine in trace amounts. A normal individual may be found to have between 50 and 150 mg of protein in the urine each day. Between 20% and 50% of this protein is albumin. The remainder consists of high molecular-weight, uromucoid, Tamm-Horsfall proteins emanating from the renal tubular cells; small amounts of serum and tubular microglobulins; and proteins from vaginal, prostatic, and seminal secretions.

There are five different categories of proteinuria that should be considered when evaluating protein found in the urine. These are prerenal, glomerular, tubular, lower urinary tract, and asymptomatic proteinuria.

Prerenal proteinuria is caused by disorders that occur elsewhere in the body rather than in the kidneys themselves. They can be further divided into two different types. In the first type, an abnormal low molecular-weight protein finds its way into the circulation and, because of its small size, easily passes through the glomerulus into the urine. This is the case with myoglobinuria (seen after crush injury or with inflammatory myopathy), hemoglobinuria, or the light chain proteinuria associated with multiple myeloma. The other form of prerenal proteinuria is secondary to a change in hydrostatic pressure in the kidney glomerulus. Following an increase in pressure, proteins that would normally not be filtered are forced through the filtration bed and into the urine. For this reason, a mild degree of proteinuria in the absence of primary kidney disease may be associated with hypertension, congestive heart failure, or dehydration.

Proteinuria due to glomerular disease represents the most common pathological form. A wide variety of agents, including toxins, infections, vascular disorders, and immunological reactions, may produce damage to the glomerular filtration device. This allows an excessive protein leak to occur. In the earliest stages of glomerular damage, proteinuria is selective and the urinary proteins are primarily the lowest molecular weight proteins found in the bloodstream, such as albumin and transferrin. Later, if glomerular damage progresses, virtually all of the proteins found in the serum may appear in the urine in approximately the same distribution as they occur in the bloodstream. When very severe, proteinuria can lead to nephrotic syndrome. In this situation, so much albumin is lost via the urine that the liver cannot keep up with synthesis and serum albumin concentration is ultimately reduced. This results in a variety of hydrostatic problems throughout the body, producing tissue swelling and edema. Generally, for the nephrotic syndrome to be present, there must be a minimum of 2 g of proteinuria a day. However, in severe cases, 10 g or more of protein may be present in a 24-hour urine collection.

Tubular proteinuria is generally mild, resulting in less than 2 g of proteinuria per day. In this situation, the proteins are low molecular weight (between 14,000 and 50,000 daltons). Thus, it may be possible to distinguish tubular proteinuria from glomerular proteinuria by using electrophoretic techniques to segregate the proteins on the basis of size. Tubular proteinuria is usually secondary to damage to the proximal tubules, which prevents the normal reabsorption of some of the smaller proteins. Some causes of tubular proteinuria include heavy metal intoxication, phenacetin damage, vitamin D intoxication, hypokalemia, Wilson's disease, galactosemia, Fanconi's syndrome, post-transplantation syndrome, pyelonephritis, acute tubular necrosis, and polycystic kidney disease.

Lower urinary tract diseases may result in exudation of protein through the mucosal layer of the lower urinary tract. This is almost always secondary to infection of either the ureters or bladder.

Asymptomatic proteinuria is generally discovered by accident. The most curious variant is orthostatic proteinuria. Individuals with this condition do not excrete protein into the urine after they have been lying down (first-morning specimen) but, after standing for 2 hours or more, will routinely display a small amount of proteinuria. About 50% of such individuals will be found to have minor glomerular disorders if subjected to kidney biopsy. The long-term significance of asymptomatic proteinuria is not fully known. However, it is recognized that a few of these individuals progress to more serious disorders, while the majority remain without any subsequent renal problems.

Another form of asymptomatic proteinuria is exercise proteinuria. Following severe exercise, many individuals will excrete a small amount of protein. This is of limited clinical significance providing it does not continue during times of rest.

Measurement

The first-line measurement of proteinuria is via the dipstick. Methods for measuring protein by a dipstick rely on a well-known phenomenon called the "protein error of indicators." In this situation, pH indicators change color in the presence of protein as ion transfer with the positive and negative groups on the protein molecule takes place. This protein error effect has been exploited to determine the amount of protein present in a sample. It should be recognized that only proteins that are capable of producing this phenomenon will participate in a measurement. For this reason, urine proteinuria determined by dipstick is almost entirely due to albumin. In general, dipsticks will not detect abnormal proteins such as myeloma light chains.

Typical reagent combinations for dipstick technology include: a citrate buffer (pH 3), tetrabromophenol blue, and a protein absorbent. Another combination uses tetrabromophenolphthalein ethyl ester.

There are other tests for performing semiquantitative measurements of protein in the urine, which include the heat-and-acid method. With this technique, the combination of heat and acid denatures protein and allows the semiquantitation of values down to 25 mg/dL. Phosphates and a variety of drugs may interfere with this technique. A somewhat more specific approach uses sulfosalicyclic acid. This method is sensitive to protein concentrations down to 20 mg/dL. Some antibiotics have been reported to interfere with this method. The protein area of the dipstick is one of the most difficult to interpret, especially in regard to "trace readings."

Protein should be reported as trace, 0.3 g/L, 1 g/L, 3 g/L, 20 or more g/L, or some other number as provided by the individual strip. "Plus" values should not be used. If the protein concentration is greater than 3.0 but less than 20 g/L, report "greater than 3.0 g/L." When the SG is greater than 1.025, trace protein results should be reported as negative.

Reaction interference

False-positive dipstick reactions may occur when urine is highly concentrated (specific gravity >1.030), whereas alternatively false-negative reactions may be associated with very dilute specimens (specific gravity <1.010). However, the major source of error with protein dipstick pads results when highly alkaline urine overrides the buffer system, producing a rise in pH and color change that is unrelated to protein concentration. The technical error of allowing the reagent pad to remain in contact with the urine over a prolonged period can strip the buffer, producing a false-positive reaction. Container contamination with quaternary ammonium compounds and detergents may also cause false-positive reactions.

Follow-up testing

If protein is discovered in the urine as part of a routine urinalysis or on a random specimen, it is generally superfluous to evaluate another urine specimen using a different semiquantitative method. It is far better to proceed directly to a 24-hour urine collection with quantitation of total protein and protein electrophoresis. This will provide an accurate quantitation of the amount of protein in order to properly assess the severity of the proteinuria. The electrophoresis will also help by indicating the specific nature of the disorder. In patients strongly suspected of excreting small amounts of Bence Jones proteinuria, either an early morning specimen or 24-hour specimen for concentration and protein electrophoresis may be used. However, both should ultimately be performed if either is initially negative because there are individual patients who will be negative by one collection technique but positive by another.

Microalbumin

The introduction of radioimmunoassay (RIA) methods for the measurement of albumin in urine has resulted in an awareness that urinary albumin excretion in amounts below the usual limit of detection (<200 mg/L) can have clinical significance especially in diabetes mellitus. The range for microalbuminuria has been defined as 20 to 200 μg/min (30 to 300 mg/day) or >20 but <200 mg/L in a random sample. Subclinical albumin excretion in this range has been given the misnomer "microalbuminuria." It has been noted that the detection of microalbuminuria precedes the onset of clinical proteinuria associated with diabetic retinopathy and nephropathy. For example, insulin-dependent diabetics who excrete more than 15 μg of albumin per minute have been recognized to have an almost 90% chance of developing diabetic retinopathy, while those producing less than 15 μg per minute have less than a 4% chance of developing this complication. Trials are currently underway in diabetic patients with microalbuminuria to see if aggressive management of diet, blood sugar, and arterial blood pressure can reverse microalbuminuria and prevent progression to full-blown retinopathy or nephrotic syndrome with proteinuria. It is likely that measurement and monitoring of microalbuminuria will become an integral part of the assessment and management of diabetes mellitus.

There is much debate as to the best urine sample to test for microalbumin. Most data have been collected using 24-hour specimens or timed overnight samples. The actual measurement of microalbuminuria can be performed by radio-immunoassay or enzyme-linked immunoassay. For screening purposes, random urine samples may be tested. Recently, a manufacturer has developed a dipstick with good sensitivity for screening for microalbuminuria. Other companies are certain to follow.

Sugar
Clinical significance

Sugars are a normal component of urine. As small molecules, glucose (and other sugars) is easily filtered through the glomerulus, following which they enter the proximal tubule. In order to prevent the loss of valuable carbohydrate energy, the body ordinarily reclaims this filtered glucose. For this purpose, an active transport reabsorptive mechanism is located in the cells of the proximal kidney tubule. This transport mechanism is very efficient and removes almost all of the glucose originally filtered at the glomerulus. When the plasma glucose concentration exceeds 10 mmol/L, the reabsorptive capacity of the tubules is exceeded and unabsorbed sugar passes into the urine. Even with normal concentrations of blood glucose, some sugar may be found in urine because it is not possible for the proximal tubules to be 100% efficient in reabsorption.

Significant amounts of glucose will therefore be detectable in the urine when there is a high concentration of glucose in the bloodstream, as occurs in diabetes. Glucose will also be found in the urine in the case of certain proximal tubular diseases that can impair the ability of the reabsorptive mechanism.

Measurement

Dipstick. The dipstick measurement of glucose utilizes the enzyme glucose oxidase, which is highly specific for glucose. When mixed with atmospheric oxygen (a normal component of urine), glucose is acted upon by glucose oxidase to produce gluconic acid and hydrogen peroxide. The

hydrogen peroxide thus generated can then be coupled with an oxygen-accepting indicator with an associated color change. The color change is proportional to the amount of glucose present. This enzyme is highly specific and will not react with other sugars such as galactose, lactose, levulose, maltose, or pentose. However, contaminants such as bleach or peroxide in the collection vessel can cause a false-positive reaction by producing the indicator color.

Glucose dipstick results should be reported as: negative, 6 mmol/L, 15 mmol/L, 30 mmol/L, or greater than 100 mmol/L rather than using the + designations.

Reducing substances. Another technique for estimating the amount of glucose present is to measure reducing substances. This test is begun by heating alkalinized urine. Any glucose present under these conditions will reduce metal ions. This process is nonspecific and any reducing substance present in urine can potentially cause this color change.

An elegant example that utilizes this approach is the Clinitest tablet. This tablet is a combination of cupric sulfate, citric acid, sodium carbonate, and anhydrous sodium hydroxide. When urine is added to one of these tablets in a test tube, a heat-generating reaction that also liberates carbon dioxide occurs as the sodium hydroxide and citric acid are combined. The carbon dioxide generated protects the tablet from room air and allows the reaction to proceed in an anaerobic environment. If reducing substances are present in the urine, the cupric ion is changed to cuprous ion, producing a bright orange color.

Benedicts' reaction is similar in principle to the chemical changes involved with the Clinitest tablet.

Reaction interference. **Dipsticks.** As noted earlier, the glucose oxidase method is specific for glucose and false-positive reactions will not occur from other sugars. However, false-positive reactions may occur when the specimen container has been contaminated with peroxide, hypochlorite, or strong oxidizing detergents. Similarly, substances that interfere with the enzymatic reaction or reducing agents that prevent oxidation of the chromogen will produce false-negative results. Such substances include ascorbic acid, aspirin, levodopa, and homogentisic acid. Bacteria metabolize glucose so specimens that are allowed to sit at room temperature for several hours may also have false-negative results. High levels of ketones may inhibit the dipstick test pad when accompanied by low urinary glucose concentrations.

Clinitest and copper reduction tests. The copper reduction test is relatively nonspecific and a variety of reducing substances that may be present in the urine can produce false-positive results. These include aspirin, vitamin C, levodopa, probenecid, and a variety of antibiotics such as the cephalosporins, tetracyclines, and nalidixic acid.

Sugars other than glucose. Sugars other than glucose may also be found in the urine. The most common is fructose. Fructose will appear in the urine after the ingestion of large amounts of fruit. It can also be found in the urine in a harmless condition known as essential fructosuria, which results from an inability to efficiently remove fructose. Another condition, hereditary fructose intolerance, due to a deficiency of fructose-1-phosphate aldolase deficiency, is more severe. With this enzyme deficiency excess fructose distorts the normal glycolytic pathway, resulting in hypoglycemia, vomiting, jaundice, amino-aciduria, cirrhosis of the liver, and renal tubular acidosis.

Pentoses (five-carbon sugars) may also be present in the urine following massive fruit ingestion. Ribose can be found in the urine of individuals with muscle-wasting conditions. A benign variant known as essential pentosuria has also been described.

Galactosuria is an inherited condition resulting in liver disease secondary to a deficiency of the enzyme galactose-1-phosphate-uridyl-transferase. Infants with this condition fail to thrive and eventually develop cataracts due to the unusual deposition of the converted sugar alcohol, galactol, in the lens.

Mannoheptulose has been noted in the urine of people who have eaten large amounts of avocado. Lactose may be detected in the urine during the latter part of pregnancy and is also seen in lactating women as a result of the production of breast milk.

Sucrose can be found in urine following massive ingestive of cane sugar. However, a more common cause of sucrosuria follows its factitious addition to urine samples by individuals attempting to cause a false-positive result who are unaware that this sugar will not be identified by routine urinary dipstick analysis.

The best approach for measuring an unusual sugar in the urine is to perform a quantitative reducing method to determine the amount of material present. This should be followed by thin-layer chromatography to actually identify the nature of the individual sugar.

There are some methods that can be used to specifically identify sugar, such as Seliwanoff's fructose test, which utilizes resorcinol and heat. There is little call to perform these tests in the routine clinical laboratory.

Ketones
Clinical significance

Ketone bodies are short-chain organic acids produced as an end-product of fat breakdown. Fat metabolism will occur in starvation and in insulin-deprivation. Therefore, when a person starves or follows a severe diet, ketones will routinely appear. Indeed, after a 14-hour fast, many persons will show a small amount of urinary ketone. Insulin-deprivation (diabetes mellitus) prevents normal metabolism of glucose, so the body must metabolize fat stores to provide energy. An end-product of this process is the production of ketones.

There are three main ketones. With human ketosis, 78% is comprised of β-hydroxybutyric acid, 20% is acetoacetic acid, and 2% is acetone. These ratios may vary slightly but are usually relatively constant. It is important to recognize that analytical methods that detect a single species correlate well with total ketones present, but, to truly quantitate the total amount of ketones, the distribution between species must be taken into consideration.

Measurement

The dipstick measurement of ketones employs sodium nitroprusside, glycine, and buffer incorporated into a reagent pad. This chemical combination is very sensitive to the presence of acetoacetic acid, producing 15 times as much color with this material vs. acetone. The combination does not react at all with β-hydroxybutyric acid. There are other tests available for the measurement of ketones, such as Gerhardt's ferric chloride reagent. This reagent acts in the presence of acetoacetic acid but it is neither sensitive nor specific. Urinary ketones should be reported as negative, trace (0.5 mmol/L), small (1.5 mmol/L), moderate (4 mmol/L), or large (8 or 16 mmol/L).

Reaction interference

False-positive results have been reported with levodopa, phenazopyridine, phenformin, and with paraldehyde ethanol combinations. Specimens collected after diagnostic procedures employing phthalein dyes can generate an interfering red color in the alkaline test medium. Ketones are volatile and will disappear from a sample over time. Thus, false-negative results may occur if the urine sample is allowed to stand for any length of time, particularly in a warm environment. Aspirin has also been reported as a cause of false-negative results. Paradoxically, aspirin in large amounts may also cause the body to produce ketones.

Follow-up

The presence of ketones in the urine can be accepted at face value and will usually correlate with the patient's clinical condition. Therefore, there is little need to follow up with any further urinary tests, although, depending on the patient's condition, a variety of blood measurements for glucose may be required.

Hemoglobin
Clinical significance

Hemoglobin can be present in the urine following intravascular hemolysis, as the result of red cells being filtered through the glomerulus, or secondary to red cells entering the lower urinary tract. There are many possible causes of hemolysis (see Chapter 11). When an intravascular hemolytic disorder occurs, hemoglobin is released from red cells into the bloodstream. Here, it is picked up by hemopexin and haptoglobin and recycled to the liver. When the capacity of these proteins to bind and remove hemoglobin is exceeded by the rate of hemoglobin release, the free hemoglobin is left to pass through the glomerulus and into the urine.

Red cells may pass through the glomerulus as a component of glomerular disease. In this case the hemoglobinuria may be associated with the presence of red cells and red-cell casts in the urine.

Bleeding from the lower urinary tract (particularly the bladder) is a frequent cause of hemoglobinuria. Such bleeding can be accompanied by red cells but never red-cell casts.

When small amounts of hemoglobin are detected in the urine of an asymptomatic person, follow-up is often required to determine if this finding is clinically significant. It has been shown that almost half of all patients with asymptomatic hematuria have no discernible cause for this condition. However, the degree of diagnostic yield on follow-up is definitely age- and sex-related. For instance, the incidence of pathology found may be as low as 2% in persons under the age of 30 years. In the older age group, investigation of asymptomatic hematuria in individuals (especially males) over the age of 60 has revealed significant pathology in up to 50% of the cases. Diseases found in this population include prostatic disease, urinary tract infections, or renal calculi. Urinary tract tumors are rarer but obviously constitute a very significant finding. A cost benefit analysis for all ages showed that the large increase in life expectancy for younger vs. older patients to some extent balanced out the lower prevalance of disease discovered in the younger group. Thus, the repeated detection of hematuria probably warrants a thorough investigation of the urinary tract regardless of a patient's age.

Measurement

Hemoglobin is a peroxidase and this chemical feature is exploited for its detection capability. The peroxidase effect is used to catalyze O-toluidine to form a blue complex. Myoglobin will also cause a positive reaction with this enzyme system.

A recent feature in dipstick technology has been the inclusion of red cell lysing agents with the hemoglobin pad. These agents cause the lysing of intact red cells. The lysed red cells in turn cause compacted or scattered green dots on the pad. Without the lysing agents, it is theoretically possible for red cells to remain intact, preventing a positive hemoglobin reaction from occurring on the dipstick pad. Whereas most cases of hematuria are accompanied by some degree of spontaneous red cell lysis and hemoglobinuria, this phenomenon is still occasionally observed.

Hemoglobin should be reported as: negative, trace, small, moderate, or large rather than using the (+) designation.

Reaction interference

Excessive urinary nitrate levels associated with severe urinary tract infections may induce false-negative results. Vitamin C-induced false-negative reactions for both hemoglobin and glucose may represent a significant problem of unsuspected magnitude. For instance, a recent study of routine urinalysis results in a West Coast population documented a 23% incidence of significant urinary ascorbate levels. Since few published studies of individual dipstick performance have included checks for urinary ascorbate, unsuspected urinary contamination with vitamin C may have been responsible for many of the false-negative reactions for hemoglobin and glucose noted in published dipstick evaluations.

Manufacturers have devised two potential solutions to this problem. One has been the development of a vitamin C-resistant dipstick that utilizes an iodate-impregnated mesh layer to resist ascorbic acid interference. Another manufacturer has actually incorporated a vitamin C test pad onto its dipstick. Any urine testing positive for vitamin C with this pad can be followed up with a careful microscopic exam and consideration can be given to alternative testing for glucose and hemoglobin.

False-positive reactions owing to menstrual contamination may be seen and will also occur if strong oxidizing detergents are present in the specimen container. False-positive reactions may also be caused by bacterial or vegetable peroxidases, including *Escherichia coli* peroxidase. For this reason, sediments containing bacteria should be followed up closely on microscopic exam for the presence of red blood cells.

Myoglobin
Clinical significance

As myoglobin will be detected by the dipstick hemoglobin pad, it is important to be aware of potential causes of myoglobinuria. Myoglobin is a muscle protein responsible for oxygen transport. It is very similar to hemoglobin in nature. Myoglobinuria may occur following crush injuries, heavy exercise (particularly in the untrained), grand mal seizures, comas (particularly those resulting in decreased oxygen supply to the periphery of the body), and a variety of myopathies. The clinical picture of myoglobinuria usually includes one of the aforementioned clinical scenarios associated with a positive dipstick hemoglobin test, reddish-gold urinary pigment, granular casts on urinary microscopic exam, and an increased creatinine kinase in the serum.

Measurement

Whereas the existence of myoglobinuria may be suspected following the detection of the triad of findings noted earlier, its presence can be verified by a variety of different techniques. Electrophoresis has been used as an analytic technique. Spectrophotometry is also possible as myoglobin demonstrates characteristic absorption wavelengths. However, spectrophotometry is not a definitive test. Filtration techniques have been devised, capitalizing on the smaller size of the myoglobin molecule, which allows it to be filtered through an ultrafiltration membrane and thereby distinguished from hemoglobin. This filtrate will continue to test positive on the hemoglobin pad of the dipstick. Hemoglobin and myoglobin can also be distinguished by differential solubility. However, none of the above techniques is easy to perform or completely reliable. For routine use, an immunological technique using immunodiffusion is probably best.

Reaction interference

Contamination of urine with povidone iodine (Betadine) used as a skin decontaminant for surgical procedures can produce a positive chemical test for blood secondary to the strong oxidizing properties of iodine. Following micturation postsurgery, if iodine contamination is not considered, there may be a concern that the surgery has caused muscle damage and myoglobinuria.

Bilirubin
Clinical significance

After 120 days, as red blood cells reach the end of their natural life span, they undergo lysis by the body and their components are broken down either to be removed from the body as waste or recycled for the formation of new red cells. It is from this breakdown of the heme group in hemoglobin that bilirubin is formed (see Chapter 11). Bilirubin is not soluble in plasma and must be transported bound to albumin. When it arrives at the hepatocyte, it is removed from albumin and, conjugated through a series of enzymatic steps, with glucuronic acid. In its conjugated form bilirubin is soluble and is secreted into the biliary tract for removal from the body. Bilirubin and urobilinogen metabolism is summarized in Box 29-2. Normally, almost none of the conjugated bilirubin enters the circulation. With biliary tract obstruction (stone or tumor) or obstruction involving the

Box 29-2   An outline of bilirubin and urobilinogen metabolism

1. Synthesis from heme
   a. From hemoglobin
      • Senescent red cells
      • Ineffective erythropoeisis
   b. From other heme containing compounds
      ↓
2. Transport in plasma bound to albumin
   ↓
3. Uptake by liver
      Dissociation from albumin—entry into hepatocytes
      ↓
4. Conjugation with glucuronic acid
   ↓
5. Excretion of conjugated bilirubin into bile
   ↓
6. Degradation in gut—formation of urobilinogen—fecal excretion
   ↓
7. Enterohepatic circulation of some urobilinogen
   a. Mostly recycled by liver
   b. Small amount excreted into urine

passage from the hepatocyte into the biliary system, conjugated bilirubin will reflux back into the circulation and appear in the bloodstream. Since conjugated bilirubin is water soluble, it easily passes through the glomerulus and into the urine. Thus, the appearance of conjugated bilirubin in the urine is strong evidence for some type of obstruction lesion in the liver or biliary system.

Measurement

Bilirubin degrades quickly in the urine and must be measured within a few hours. An ancient assessment of bilirubin involved the shake test. Following a vigorous agitation of urine, the visual detection of yellow foam was taken as strong evidence for the presence of bilirubin.

Today, dipstick detection of bilirubin relies on the diazotizing of bilirubin to a complex organic molecule, which changes color in the process. For example, diazotized 2,4-dichloroaniline in an acid buffer has been employed as a stable diazonium salt, 2,6-dichlorobenzene-diazonium fluoroborate, used to detect bilirubin.

There are a variety of additional tests for measuring bilirubin in the urine. However, even if carried out with accuracy and precision, the urinary measurement of bilirubin has limited diagnostic utility. It is far better to proceed with specific serum tests of liver function, such as serum bilirubin, aspartate transaminase (AST), alkaline phosphatase, and γ-glutamyl transpeptidase than to waste time with the further quantifying of urinary bilirubin. Urine bilirubin should be reported as positive or negative.

Reaction interference

The most frequent problem area associated with bilirubin testing is false-negative results caused by the testing of specimens that are not fresh because bilirubin is an unstable compound rapidly destroyed following light exposure. Exposure to air causes oxidation of bilirubin to biliverdin, which does not react in standard test systems. False-negative results will also occur following the hydrolysis of bilirubin diglucuronide to free bilirubin because this substance is less reactive in reagent strip tests. High concentrations of ascorbic acid and nitrate have also been noted to lower the sensitivity of this test pad reaction.

Urobilinogen
Clinical significance

Once bilirubin enters the biliary tract it ultimately passes into the intestinal lumen. After traversing the small intestine and reaching the large intestine, the action of various bacteria break bilirubin down through a series of steps to a number of metabolites, including urobilinogen. Highly converted forms of bilirubin can be absorbed in the large bowel to a minimal degree. Ordinarily, minute amounts of urobilinogen find their way back into the bloodstream and are then re-excreted through the liver and into the biliary system. Various disorders of the liver or biliary system have the potential to impair this enterohepatic circulation. Significant amounts of urobilinogen will then be excreted in the urine. For this reason, increased urobilinogen can be found in the urine of those suffering from either obstructive liver disease or hepatocellular liver disease. In addition, persons with a hemolytic process will have an increased enterohepatic circulation of bilirubin by-products such that increased amounts of urobilinogen will appear in the urine.

Urobilinogen disappears very quickly from urine following degredation by oxidation. Initially, the molecule is colorless, but after standing for a few hours the urine may be rendered dark.

Measurement

Dipstick measurement of urobilinogen depends upon linkage with complex organic molecules. One manufacturer's product uses a buffered p-dimethylaminobenzaldehyde. When this material combines with urobilinogen it produces a pink color. There are other methods for the measurement of urobilinogen such as the Wallace-Diamond test or Watson's quantitative test. As in the earlier discussion of bilirubin, further specific measurement of urobilinogen is usually not worth the effort. Following its initial detection, investigation should proceed using well-established serum tests of liver function. An approach to the simultaneous use of bilirubin, urobilinogen, and liver enzymes in defining hemolytic, hepatic, and biliary causes of jaundice is outlined in Table 29-4. Urinary urobilinogen should be reported as normal (3 to 17 μmol/L) or positive (34, 68, 135 μmol/L).

Reaction interference

The dipstick pads that test for urobilinogen using p-dimethylaminobenzaldehyde are susceptible to false-positive results from compounds such as p-aminosalicylic acid, antipyrine, apronalide, chlorpromazine, phenazopyridine, phenothiazine, sulfadiazine, and sulfonamide. The utilization of p-methoxybenzene-diazonium-fluoroborate as a reagent on the Chemstrip dipstick produces a more specific test. However, false-negative results may occur when large

Table 29-4 Helpful tests in the evaluation of jaundice

	Hemolysis	Acquired hepatocyte disorder	Biliary tract obstruction
Urine test			
Bilirubin	−	+	+
Urobilinogen	↑	↑	− or ↓
Serum enzyme activity			
Alkaline phosphatase	±	Variable	↑
Alanine and/or asparate aminotransferase	±	↑	+ or ↑
γ-Glutamyl transpeptidase	±	Variable	↑

quantities of nitrite are present and highly pigmented urine samples may also interfere with the detection of this color reaction.

Leukocyte esterase

Clinical significance

Many white cells (particularly granulocytes) contain an enzyme known as leukocyte esterase. Detecting the presence of this esterase provides strong evidence that white cells are present in the urine. The inclusion of the esterase test on the dipstick allows the detection of the presence of white cells without necessarily requiring a visual search. It should be recognized that not all white cells produce leukocyte esterase and therefore it is possible to have white cells in the urine without a positive dipstick leukocyte esterase. In general, this pad is 90% to 95% sensitive and over 95% specific.

Measurement

The leukocyte esterase test requires up to 2 minutes (or longer) for the resulting color change. Manufacturers are currently working on developing faster reagent combinations. Test timing is critical, otherwise reduced sensitivity is obtained. The sensitivity of this test also varies with the number of leukocytes present. While positive reactions may be noted at 5 to 15 WBC/HPF, many dipsticks only give 80% to 90% positive results with greater than 15 WBC/HPF. However, beyond a general indication of leukocyturia, the esterase test has only a limited ability to predict the number of leukocytes that will ultimately be found on microscopic examination of the urinary sediment. Urine containing large amounts of yellow pigment may generate a green rather than purple color with the esterase reaction. The observation of this color also constitutes a positive test. Dipstick leukocyte esterase should be reported as positive or negative.

Reaction interference

Taking too early a reading is the most common cause of a false-negative leukocyte esterase test. False-negative results may also be noted with high specific gravity urine because crenation of leukocytes can prevent release of their esterases. Other conditions that have been reported to cause reduced leukocyte esterase reactions include elevated glucose (>3 g/dL), cephalexin, cephalothin, high concentra-

tions of oxalic acid, tetracycline, and boric acid. Formalin can cause a false-positive reaction.

Nitrite

Clinical significance

Occult urinary tract infections can be devastating disorders that ultimately result in chronic renal failure. The detection of urinary tract infection has traditionally involved either performing a culture or at least identifying white cells and bacteria in the formed elements of the urine. Recently, a dipstick test has been introduced that attempts to identify the presence of bacteria without the need for a visual search.

Normal human beings excrete a certain amount of nitrate in their urine. This nitrate is converted to nitrite by certain species of bacteria. A positive dipstick pad to detect the presence of nitrite will therefore, by inference, provide strong evidence for the presence of certain types of bacteria.

For the test to be positive, the patient must first have nitrate in the urine. The production of urinary nitrates is largely associated with the consumption of vegetables, so therefore, individuals must be consuming adequate amounts of these foodstuffs to start off with.

In addition, only certain bacteria have the ability to produce the nitrate-nitrite conversion. *Escherichia coli, Proteus, Klebsiella, Enterobacter, Citrobacter,* and *Salmonella* are very aggressive nitrate reducers. *Enterococcus, Staphylococcus,* and *Pseudomonas* are only partial converters. Other bacterial species do not promote this conversion.

Furthermore, the production of nitrite will increase if the urine is held in the bladder for a period of hours. Since this is often not feasible, the reliability of the test is only about 50% positive in random samples. For all the aforementioned reasons, a first-morning specimen is certainly the best sample for nitrite testing.

Obviously, a negative nitrite test does not exclude the presence of a urinary tract infection. However, a positive test provides strong evidence for a urinary tract infection and should be followed up via appropriate culture.

Measurement

The presence of urinary nitrite is detected by linking an aromatic amine with nitrite to produce a diazonium compound with a characteristic color. The pink color reaction is not directly quantitative in relation to the number of bacteria present. However, any degree of color should be interpreted as a positive nitrite test and is suggestive of 10^5 or more organisms/mL. A negative test result is not proof that significant bacteriuria does not exist. The sensitivity of the nitrite test is also reduced in urine with a high specific gravity. Urinary nitrites should be reported as positive or negative.

Reaction interference

Ascorbic acid concentrations of 25 mg/dL or greater may cause false-negative results when specimens contain small amounts of nitrite ion (0.06 mg/dL or less). Other causes of false-negative results include the inhibition of bacterial metabolism by antibiotics and ongoing reduction of nitrate to nondetectable nitrogen, which may occur if large numbers of bacteria are present in the bladder. False-positive results may be obtained if nitrite testing is not performed on fresh samples as a multiplication of contaminant bacteria can rapidly generate measurable amounts of nitrite.

MICROSCOPIC EXAMINATION
General

A traditional part of urinalysis is the performance of a microscopic examination. This is generally carried out by taking a standard amount of urine, centrifuging the specimen for a fixed period of time, removing the supernatant fluid, resuspending the sediment in a standard volume (usually 1 mL), and finally examining this sediment under the microscope. For the microscopic exam, commercially available slides with incorporated counting chambers of a constant volume have been available since the early 1970s. Their use is highly desirable because they offer a standardized sediment analysis that eliminates many of the variables inherent in "drop on slide" techniques.

Standardized sediment analysis enables the observer to observe and quantitate cells (red cells, white cells, bacteria, yeast, epithelial cells, and tumor cells), crystals, which are formed from the precipitation of salts; and casts, which are formed in the kidney tubules. Each of these substances may be a valuable indicator of pathology. Whether or not to routinely stain urine sediment is a question of some debate as is the necessity for phase or interference contrast microscopy. Given a proper level of professional expertise and good equipment, bright field microscopy of unstained urine should identify all clinically important and relevant sediment. However, polarization of the sediment may be helpful in some circumstances, especially in identifying crystals and lipids. For instance, six-sided cystine crystals that are non-birefringent can be differentiated from six-sided urate crystals that are birefringent. Doubly refractile lipids show a typical "Maltese cross" pattern under polarized light. Many foreign contaminants such as talc or starch granules are birefringent, whereas most noncrystalline human sediment elements are not.

When to perform the microscopic examination

It has been argued that, under routine circumstances, microscopic examination of the urinary sediment is not necessary. This argument is based upon the rationale that the only features of the urinary sediment that are not detected by the dipstick in asymptomatic individuals are certain bacteria and/or some white cells. The presence of other urinary constituents such as red cells or casts will be heralded by positive dipstick reactions for hemoglobin, esterase, or protein. Whereas some investigators advocating a "dipstick only" screening approach have claimed a false-negative detection rate for significant urinary constituents of only a few percent, other studies have demonstrated false-negative rates as high as 30%.

Most clinicians would generally agree that an important advantage of the microscopic examination performed on an asymptomatic patient is the possible detection of occult urinary tract infection. However, with the recent development of the nitrite and leukocyte esterase pads, the ability to detect occult infections has increased. Some studies have found that the diagnostic efficiency of the esterase-nitrite combi-

nation is similar to that of sediment microscopy in detecting or excluding urinary tract infections. However, the impact of the pretest probability of infection on the overall test reliability and infection detection rates has also been emphasized. Proponents of the "dipstick only" approach would still argue that the chances are very small of finding an occult infection in an asymptomatic individual with an otherwise normal urinalysis. In addition, the high labor costs associated with performing additional microscopic procedures further detract from cost effectiveness.

These arguments will continue to be debated in the literature. In the interim, each laboratory should develop an individual approach that ideally would be based on a survey of the false-negative dipstick results in their own urinalysis patient population. However, at the present time, whenever a positive pad is detected on the dipstick it is necessary to complete the urinalysis by performing a microscopic examination.

Clinical significance of the formed elements of urine
Red blood cells

Whereas more than 0 to 3 RBC/HPF in the urine is considered abnormal, some authors have suggested that 8 RBC/HPF is an appropriate level dividing normal and abnormal hematuria. RBC are found in the urine after passing through the glomerulus in glomerulonephritis. In addition, they may enter the urine following direct bleeding into the lower urinary tract as may occur with urinary infections, tumors, or renal calculi. Hematuria may also follow trauma or exposure to toxic chemicals or drugs. In female patients, the possibility of menstrual contamination must also be considered. On microscopic examination red blood cells are noted as uniform, colorless disks. However, in concentrated urine red cells may shrink and appear crenated. In dilute alkaline urine RBC can lyse rapidly, releasing hemoglobin so that only the red cell membrane remains as a "ghost cell." Ghost cells may be missed unless specimens are reviewed under subdued light.

Recent attention has been directed to urinary red blood cell morphology in the form of "dysmorphic red blood cells" as an indicator of glomerular bleeding. Dysmorphic red blood cells vary in size and are fragmented or have cellular protrusions. Although the exact number of dysmorphic RBC necessary to represent significant renal pathology has been disputed, one study has suggested that an incidence of 14% or greater of dysmorphic RBC is highly suggestive of an intrarenal source. The presence of less than 14% dysmorphic red cells suggests an extrarenal bleeding site. Urine samples stored up to 5 hours at 4°C to 20°C did not show any apparent change in the percentages of dysmorphic RBC present. It should be noted however, that other studies have been unable to demonstrate a clear correlation between the presence of dysmorphic red cells and the site of bleeding. Intraobserver discrepancy in the intrepretation of red cell morphology has also been a problem.

As explained earlier, the presence or absence of red blood cells noted on microscopic examination does not always correlate with the results of the dipstick pad test for hemoglobin. Urinary tract hemoglobin loss secondary to intravascular hemolysis can produce a positive dipstick pad result for hemoglobin with no RBCs noted on microscopic examination. Similarly, occasional specimens will be found with significant numbers of RBCs on microscopic examination but a negative dipstick pad result for hemoglobin. In this instance, possibilities include the failure of red cells to lyse, releasing hemoglobin, or the presence of significant amounts of urinary ascorbic acid or another oxidant, providing false-negative dipstick pad results.

White blood cells

White cells present in the urine at more than 3 to 5 HPF point to an infectious or inflammatory process somewhere within the urinary tract. White blood cells are larger than red blood cells and are easier to identify because of the presence of cytoplasmic granules and nuclei. Although neutrophils are the most commonly seen white cells in the urine, on occasion, other leukocytes such as eosinophils, lymphocytes, or monocytes may be noted. Supravital staining may be used to enhance white cell nuclear detail and Hansel's or Wright's stain should be used if eosinophiluria is suspected. Degenerated neutrophils called "glitter cells" are sometimes found in the urinary sediment. The nuclear lobes of these cells are no longer clearly delineated and in dilute urine their cytoplasmic granules display Brownian movement, resulting in a glittering phenomenon. Although glitter cells are most commonly associated with pyelonephritis, they may also be noted when the urinary specific gravity is low.

Epithelial cells

The three major types of epithelial cells that may be found in the urine are squamous, transitional, and renal tubular cells. There may be no medical significance to the presence of moderate numbers of squamous or transitional cells in the urine as they are derived from the normal lining of the genitourinary system. When large numbers of epithelial cells are present, this may point to poor specimen collection, signifying that the first part of the voided sample was taken rather than a midstream portion.

Microorganisms

Bacteria are not normally present if the urine has been collected under sterile conditions. However, urine allowed to stand at room temperature may contain noticeable numbers of bacteria following the multiplication of contaminants. Bacteria will appear either as rods or cocci in the urine. Providing contamination or overgrowth has not occurred, the presence of bacteria correlates strongly with the presence of urinary tract infection, especially when seen in association with white blood cells. Yeast in the form of *Candida albicans* may also be present in the sample as a contaminant. Yeast may be confused with red cells but may be distinguished by the observation of budding forms and an ovoid rather than a round shape.

Casts

Casts represent a collection of protein and cellular debris that have gathered together in the kidney tubule, particularly where there has been low fluid flow. The coalescence of these materials forms a structure molded by the tubule itself, which subsequently appears in the urine as a tapered tube.

The ends of the tubule may be pointed rather than round, in which case it traditionally has been called a cylindroid rather than a cast. Cylindroids have the same clinical significance as casts. The size of the cast depends on its site of origin and the length of time it remains in the kidney tubule. Casts formed in the earliest parts of the nephron tend to be the thinnest. The material that makes up the cast can cause it to differ in physical appearance. Whereas the actual chemical constituents of casts have not been completely analyzed, their major component is a glycoprotein called Tamm-Horsfall protein, derived from the renal tubular cells. Tamm-Horsfall protein is not detected by the urinary protein dipstick pad and, consequently, is not responsible for any increased urinary protein noted in urine containing casts.

Casts are best seen and examined utilizing low-powered microscope fields (LPFs). On occasion, phase microscopy may be helpful.

1. Hyaline casts: These are pale and transparent. Their presence can be nonspecific and may be due to an increased concentration of solid materials in the renal tubules.
2. Red blood cell casts: Red blood cell casts vary greatly in appearance. The presence of true red blood cell casts indicates bleeding at the level of the nephron. Whereas red blood cell casts are primarily associated with glomerulonephritis they may also be seen with any condition that damages the glomerulus, tubules, or renal capillaries. RBC casts can usually be recognized because they are refractile and colored. The color of RBC casts ranges from a brown-yellow to red.
3. White blood cell (WBC) casts: WBC casts are rarely true casts. They are, instead, conglomerations of white cells that have been packed closely together in a tubelike formation. White blood cell casts exhibit granules and nuclei unless disintegration has begun. Staining to show nuclear detail or phase microscopy may be necessary to distinguish white cell casts from epithelial casts. The finding of white cell casts usually suggests the presence of a urinary tract infection.
4. Epithelial casts: The finding of significant numbers of epithelial casts suggests the presence of an acute inflammatory process such as glomerulonephritis or pyelonephritis in the kidney. Epithelial casts can be distinguished from white blood cell casts by the fact that epithelial cells have a round, centrally located nucleus.
5. Granular casts: The mechanism responsible for the formation of granular casts is not well understood. They may represent a further evolution of epithelial cell casts in which the cells themselves have degenerated, leaving only a rough, granular appearance. On occasion, white WBC cells may also be embedded in granular casts, forming part of the component structure. The presence of granular casts generally indicates a chronic disorder as they are rarely seen in acute inflammation.
6. Waxy casts: Waxy casts are refractile, lack differentiated structures, may have serrated borders, and often display cracked or broken ends. Waxy casts are not made of wax. Scanning electron micrograph studies

have shown they represent an advanced stage of hyaline casts. Waxy casts are most commonly associated with severe chronic renal disease.

7. Fatty casts: Fatty casts represent a breakdown product of epithelial casts that contain fat bodies. These casts may contain a few fat droplets within a hyaline matrix or may be completely filled with fat globules of different sizes. Fat is best recognized via polarized microscopy, which gives lipid globules a distinctive Maltese cross configuration and a doubly refractile appearance. Alternatively, fatty casts may be positively identified with the use of a Sudan III stain. The presence of fatty casts is usually associated with severe renal disease and nephrotic syndrome.

8. Broad casts: Broad casts are formed in the collecting ducts when urine flow is low. As such, broad casts have been called "renal failure casts." All types of casts may be present in broad forms.

9. Pseudo casts: Fibrin, epithelial cells, mucous strands, white blood cells, red blood cells, and bacteria from time to time may coalesce together, giving the appearance of a cast. Mucous strands usually have a much less structured morphology vs. true casts and frequently exhibit longitudinal striations.

A summary of various casts with their clinical correlations is provided in Table 29-5.

Crystals

Crystals form as a result of the precipitation of inorganic salts contained in the urine. Any fresh urine sample may contain crystals, especially if concentrated. Unfortunately, refrigerated specimens or those allowed to stand for any length of time frequently contain large numbers of crystals that may interfere with the microscopic detection of other urine elements. Whereas some crystals will dissolve on warming, others may require acidification of the urine.

Although crystals vary in appearance and are sometimes entrancingly beautiful to look at, most do not have clinical significance. The main reason to attempt to classify urinary crystals is to identify the few types that may be associated with systemic illness, such as inborn errors of metabolism or liver disease. Abnormal crystals of primary concern include cystine, leucine, tyrosine, and some drug crystals. Hexagonal cystine crystals may be noted in patients with hereditary cystinosis and may predispose to renal calculi. Leucine crystals that appear as spheres with concentric striations and tyrosine crystals that appear as bundles of needles may occasionally be seen together in cases of serious hepatic damage. When either is seen in isolation, they may signify a rare hereditary metabolic disorder. A variety of drug crystals may be present in the urine. Sulfa crystals, ampicillin crystals, and some crystals associated with radiographic dyes may produce renal tubular damage in certain clinical conditions, especially if associated with dehydration.

To properly identify crystals it is important to be aware of urinary pH. For instance, uric acid and calcium oxalate crystals are frequently found in acidic urine, whereas phosphates and calcium carbonate constitute the most common crystals noted in alkaline urine. The appearance of crystals under polarized light is also helpful and there are various confirmatory chemical tests that may be performed for individual species of crystals. However, many problems associated with the identification of specific crystals may be simply resolved by inquiring about patient medications. A summary of the appearance and other identifying features of various crystals is provided in Table 29-6. In most circumstances, it is a mistake for the technologist to spend an inordinate amount of time trying to specifically identify the wide variety of crystals that may, on occasion, be present in a urine sample.

Method of performing the microscopic examination

A commercial system is recommended.

1. Mix the sample and pour off a standard amount into a disposable tube. (Always note volume if it is impossible to collect the full amount.)

2. Centrifuge for 5 minutes at 400 RCF (relative centrifugal force). This will generally be 1500 to 2000 rpm but must be determined for each centrifuge.

3. Remove the tubes from the centrifuge and place in an appropriate plastic rack. Remove lids. Turn the whole rack completely upside down to drain the supernatant liquid. Dry the lip of the tube by wiping

Table 29-5   Urinary cast summary

Type	Origin	Clinical significance
Hyaline	Tubular secretion of Tamm-Horsfall protein	Glomerulonephritis, pyelonephritis, chronic renal disease, congestive heart failure, stress and exercise, 0-2/HPF normal
Red blood cell	Red blood cells enmeshed in, or attached to, Tamm-Horsfall protein matrix	Glomerulonephritis, strenuous exercise
White blood cell	White blood cells enmeshed in, or attached to, Tamm-Horsfall protein matrix	Pyelonephritis
Epithelial cell	Tubular cells remaining attached to Tamm-Horsfall protein fibrils	Renal tubular damage
Granular	Disintegration of white cell casts, bacteria, urates, tubular cell lysosomes, protein aggregates	Stasis of urine flow, stress and exercise, urinary tract infection, 0-1/HPF normal
Waxy	Evolution of hyaline casts	Stasis of urine flow
Fatty	Renal tubular cells, oval fat bodies	Nephrotic syndrome
Broad casts	Formation in collecting ducts	Marked stasis of urine flow
Pseudo casts	Mucus, fibrin, or contaminants	May be mistaken for true casts

Modified with permission from Strasinger SK: *Urinalysis and body fluids*, ed 2, Philadelphia, 1989, FA Davis.

Table 29-6 Major characteristics of urinary crystals

Crystal	pH	Color-shape	Solubility	Appearance
Uric acid	Acid	Yellow-brown	Alkali	
Amorphous urates	Acid	Brick dust or yellow brown	Alkali and heat	
Calcium oxalate	Acid/neutral (alkaline)	Colorless (envelopes)	Dilute HCl	
Amorphous phosphates	Alkaline Neutral	White-colorless	Dilute acetic acid	
Calcium phosphate	Alkaline	Colorless	Dilute acetic acid	
Triple phosphate	Alkaline	Colorless (coffin lids)	Dilute acetic acid	
Ammonium biurate	Alkaline	Yellow-brown (thorny apples)	Acetic acid with heat	
Calcium carbonate	Alkaline	Colorless (dumbbells)	Gas from acetic acid	
Cholesterol	Acid	Colorless (notched plates)	Chloroform	
Cystine	Acid	Colorless (hexagonal shapes)	Ammonia, dilute HCl	
Leucine	Acid/neutral	Yellow (concentrically ribbed spheres)	Hot alkali or alcohol	
Tyrosine	Acid/neutral	Colorless-yellow (bundles of needles)	Alkali or heat	
Bilirubin	Acid	Yellow	Acetic acid, HCl, NaOH, ether, chloroform	
Sulfonamides	Acid/neutral	Green	Acetone	
Ampicillin	Acid/neutral	Colorless	Refrigeration produces bundles	
Radiographic dyes	Acid	Colorless	10% NaOH	

Modified with permission from Strasinger SK: *Urinalysis and body fluids*, ed 2. Philadelphia, 1989, FA Davis.

with absorbent tissue. This should leave a uniform volume of sediment in all tubes. (Flush sink with dilute bleach after dumping urine samples down the drain.)

4. Resuspend the sediment by agitating the tube contents with a Pasteur pipette.
5. Draw out the resuspended sediment. Deliver one drop onto the side chamber.
6. Examine preparation immediately before evaporation occurs.
7. Inspect the slide generally over a wide area using low power.
8. Reduce the light intensity to a minimum and scan several fields searching for casts. Alternatively, phase contrast microscopy can be used. Note: Casts are reported as number per low power field.
9. Turn to the high power lens and increase the light intensity. Scan several fields to evaluate cells. Discard slides into dilute bleach.

Examine and report microscopic findings

The following terminology should be valid if the high-powered field consists of a X10 eyepiece and a X40 objective lens. This results in a 0.375 mm diameter field, which is the standard field for reporting numbers per high-powered field. The standard low power field consists of a X10 eyepiece and a X10 objective lens, providing a field of 1.5 mm.

Using the average number of cells observed in four or five fields, the microscopic examination is reported using the following terminology (WBC is used as an example):

1. For small numbers of cells in which some high power fields do not contain any cells, report "0 to 2 WBC/HPF."
2. When a countable number of cells per high power field are present, count four to five fields, average, and report "5 to 10 (or 5 to 8 or 10 to 15) WBC/HPF."
3. When large numbers of cells are present, count one quarter of a field and report this number times four (rounded to the nearest ten) per HPF. Suppose that 24 cells are counted, $24 \times 4 = 96$. Report "about 100 WBC/HPF."
4. If there are too many cells to count, report "fields packed."
5. Note the presence of clumping, in other words, "WBC clumps present."
6. Red blood cells are reported using the same system as for WBCs.

Report epithelial cells as:

Occasional	0-2 per HPF
Few	3-4 per HPF
Moderate	5-10 per HPF
Many	10-15 per HPF
Gross	Packed field

Microorganisms. The discovery of bacteria in a properly handled specimen indicates that a second collection should be made with a midstream portion collected and immediately examined. Report as: few, moderate, many, or field packed.

Yeast must be distinguished from red blood cells, which they resemble. They tend to be ovoid, variable in size, and often demonstrate budding. If any question exists, a drop of 2% acetic acid added to the sediment will destroy red cells but will leave yeast intact.

Casts/cylindroids. Casts are best detected by using, on occasion, lower power fields and varying illumination; phase-contrast microscopy or staining may be helpful. Casts should be counted per low power field, but initial identification is sometimes easier using high power.

When reporting casts, it is permissible to use the terms "rare" or "occasional" when there is less than one cast in two or three low power fields. As is practical, report different types of casts separately. For example, "0 to 1 hyaline casts per low power field, 1 to 2 fine granular casts per low power field, and rare waxy cast."

Mucous strands or fibers. Mucous strands appear normally in small numbers, particularly in male patients. Increased numbers may be found in chronic inflammation of the urethra and bladder. Mucous strands may be difficult to distinguish from casts and phase-contrast microscopy allows for easier discrimination.

Crystals. When the type of crystals cannot be clearly identified but are not of a clinically significant variety, they should be reported as "nonpathologic unidentified crystals present."

Report crystals as few, moderate, or many.

Report amorphous sediment as light, moderate, or heavy.

Report mucus as light, moderate, or heavy.

Report spermatozoa when present.

Report yeast cells, trichomonas, parasites, or ova.

SUGGESTED READING

Akin BV and others: Efficacy of the routine admission urinalysis, Am J Med 82(4):719, 1987.

Berg B and others: Guidelines for evaluation of reagent strips: exemplified by analysis of urine albumin and glucose concentration using visually read reagent strips, Scand J Clin Lab Invest 49:689, 1989.

Bolann BJ, Sandberg S, and Digranes A: Implication of probability analysis for interpreting results of leukocyte esterase and nitrite test strips, Clin Chem 35(8):1663, 1989.

Bradley M: Urine crystals: identification and significance, Lab Med 13(6):348, 1982.

Brigden ML and others: The optimum urine collections for the detection and monitoring of Bence Jones proteinuria, Am J Clin Pathol 93(5):689, 1990.

Britton JP, Dowell AC, and Whelan P: Dipstick haematuria and bladder cancer in men over 60: results of a community study, Br Med J 299:1010, 1989.

Cannon DC: The identification and pathogenesis of urine casts, Lab Med 10(1):8, 1979.

Carel RS and others: Routine urinalysis (dipstick) findings in mass screening of healthy adults, Clin Chem 33(11):2106, 1987.

Carlson DA and Statland BE: Automatic urinalysis, Clin Lab Med 8(3):449, 1988.

Ferris JA: Comparison and standardization of urine microscopic examination, Lab Med 14:659, 1983.

Finney J and Baum N: Evaluation of hematuria, Post Grad Med 85(8):44, 1989.

Haber MH: Pisseprophesy: a brief history of urinalysis, Clin Lab Med 8(3):415, 1988.

Haber MF: Quality assurance in urinalysis, Clin Lab Med 8(3):431, 1988.

Hurlbut TA and Littenberg B: The diagnostic technology assessment consortium: the diagnostic accuracy of rapid dipstick tests to predict urinary tract infection, Am J Clin Pathol 96:582, 1991.

Kiel DP and Moskowitz MA: The urinalysis: a critical appraisal, Med Clin North Am 71(4):607, 1987.

Komaroff AL: Urinalysis and urine culture in women with dysuria, Ann Int Med 104(2):212, 1986.

Lawrence VA, Gafni A, and Gross M: Unproven utility of the preoperative urinalysis: an economic evaluation, J Clin Epidemiol 42(12):1185, 1989.

McEwan RT and others: Screening elderly people in primary care: a randomized controlled trial, Br J Gen Pract 40(332):94, 1990.

NCCLS: Routine urinalysis: proposed guidelines. Document GP-16, July 1991.

Newall RG and Howell R: The principles and practice of urine testing in the hospital community, Clin Urin Ames Division, Miles Limited.

Pels RJ and others: Dipstick urinalysis screening of asymptomatic adults for urinary tract disorders II: bacteriuria, JAMA 262(9):1221, 1989.

Pezzlo M: Detection of urinary tract infections by rapid methods, Clin Microbiol Rev 1:268, 1988.

Pillsworth TJ Jr and others: Differentiation of renal from non-renal hematuria by microscopic examination of erythrocytes in urine, Clin Chem 33(10):1791, 1987.

Pradella M, Dorizzi RM, and Rigolin F: Relative density of urine: methods and clinical significance, CRC Crit Rev Clin Lab Sci 26:195, 1988.

Strasinger SK: Urinalysis and body fluids: a self-instructional test, ed 2. Philadelphia, 1989, FA Davis.

US Preventive Services Task Force: Recommendations on screening for asymptomatic bacteriuria by dipstick urinalysis, JAMA 262:1220, 1989.

Woolhandler S and others: Dipstick urinalysis screening of asymptomatic adults for urinary tract disorders. I. Hematuria and proteinuria, JAMA 262(9):1214, 1989.

Zweig MH and Jackson A: Ascorbic acid interference in reagent-strip reactions for assay of urinary glucose and hemoglobin, Clin Chem 32(4):674, 1986.

30 Serous, cystic, and synovial fluid analysis

Gordon Hoag
Michael McNeely
Malcolm Brigden

Although body fluids are usually meant to reflect only blood, cerebrospinal fluid, and urine, the body has many potential spaces that may also contain fluids. The pleural cavity is such a potential space that lies between the membrane that surrounds the lungs and the lining of the thoracic cavity. The potential space between these two cell linings is the pleural space (pleural cavity) and normally contains minute amounts of fluid. The lining of the pericardial sac and the surface of the heart also create a potential space referred to as the pericardial space. The peritoneal cavity consists of a group of organs surrounded by a lining mesothelium and the abdominal wall, which has an inner mesothelial lining. Cysts and pseudocysts may also contain fluids and these may represent either birth anomalies or pathological processes. Various birth anomalies may include cystic changes in liver, kidneys, pancreas, and lungs. Cyst and pseudocyst formation of the pancreas and ovaries may occur as a pathological change. Fluids may accumulate in a cyst and be sent to the laboratory for analysis.

BACKGROUND

Serous fluid is an ultrafiltrate of plasma that occurs in all potential spaces, such as the pleural cavity. There is a continuous process of formation and reabsorption of serous fluid in these body spaces. Various factors contribute to the normal formation, including plasma oncotic pressure, capillary permeability, and hydrostatic pressure in the vascular system. Reabsorption of serious fluids occurs through the lymphatic system. These processes are normally in equilibrium; however, either excess formation or decreased reabsorption will lead to accumulation of excess fluid, which is referred to as an effusion.

Cystic fluid is the fluid that is present in a cyst. It frequently consists of the breakdown products of an organ, or is produced by anomalous tissues, or by activation of the formation processes in an unusual location. Cystic fluids may be reabsorbed very slowly or may require drainage in order to facilitate removal of the fluid in the cyst. The role of the laboratory in the analysis and examination of cystic

fluids is frequently to establish the possible origin of the fluid.

Synovial fluid is found in the enclosed space surrounding the joints. The fluid is derived from lining cells and from sera. It is present in the joint space and allows for the smooth movement of the two cartilaginous surfaces against each other without much friction. The amount of fluid in the joint space is determined by formation and reabsorption processes. When these processes are impaired, excess fluid accumulates within the joint space. In order to establish the underlying cause, whether an arthritic condition, infectious agent, or crystal disease, a portion of the fluid is analyzed in the laboratory.

SPECIMEN COLLECTION AND HANDLING

Fluids from cystic formations and synovial fluids should be withdrawn into a heparinized syringe. If laboratory personnel could be present at the time that the collection is made, this will ensure that a specimen is properly labeled, collected, and handled.

Proper collection of the fluid is a prerequisite for satisfactory laboratory assessment. Serous fluid evaluation requires both a specimen from the site and a serum tube for comparative analysis. An ethylenediaminetetraacetic acid (EDTA) tube is required for a hematological profile and etiological assessment; a heparin tube is used for total protein and enzymes, and for bacteriologic stains and cultures; and a heparinized syringe is used for pH, if required. Other tubes may be collected depending upon the specific analysis required, such as cytological and immunochemical assessment.

SEROUS FLUIDS

Serous fluids are classified as either transudates or exudates. It is important to categorize them when diagnosing the underlying cause of an effusion. Transudates and exudates are distinguished from each other by specific gravity and total protein (Table 30-1). A transudate has a specific gravity of less than 1.015, and a total protein less than 30 g/L. Ex-

Table 30-1 Laboratory characteristics of transudates and exudates

Parameter	Transudate	Exudate
Specific gravity	<1.015	>1.015
Total protein	<30 g/L	>30 g/L
Fluid total protein: Serum total protein	<0.5	>0.5
Fluid LDH: Serum LDH	<0.6	>0.6

udates have a specific gravity of 1.015 or greater, and/or a total protein of 30 g/L or greater. As with any precise cutoff values, there are features that cause overlap and make precise determinations of a transudate or exudate ambiguous. To add further precision to the classification of the transudate or exudate, there should be simultaneous measurement of the serous fluids and serum for total protein and lactate dehydrogenase (LDH). A transudate is a fluid in which the ratio of serous fluid total protein:serum total protein is less than 0.5 and the corresponding LDH ratio is less than 0.6. Exudates have a corresponding total protein ratio greater than 0.5 and/or an LDH ratio greater than 0.6. Again, there is overlap between the two, and therefore, there is no absolute group of laboratory tests that defines each specimen.

Even if the precise etiology is not known of a transudate, it can be assumed that further laboratory investigation will be required only rarely as it is affiliated with benign conditions such as nephrotic syndrome, congestive heart failure, cirrhosis, sepsis, peritoneal dialysis, and postoperative sequela. In most instances, exudates require further, more detailed examination. Cytological examination with immunochemical analysis is necessary to define whether cells are malignant or not. The origin of malignant cells in fluids must be determined. The lung and bowel should be considered in patients of both sexes and, in addition, metastatic ovarian tumors (Krukenberg's tumor) and breast tumors are to be considered in female patients. Culturing of the specimen or other testing is required to assess the presence of bacterial, viral, fungal, and parasitic etiologic agents.

Other conditions associated with exudates include the collagen vascular diseases such as rheumatoid arthritis, systemic lupus erythematosus (SLE), and mixed connective tissue disease. A history consistent with severe trauma is supportive of an exudate. Acute or chronic pancreatitis, or infarction of the bowel or lung, both of which have a single blood supply, are consistent with an exudate. On occasion, it may be evident that there is a chylous effusion with obvious lipid droplets. This is especially true in a clinical setting after a postoperative event that may have involved trauma to the lymphatics. A chylous effusion may also be associated with a metastatic malignancy or lymphoma.

Cystic fluid collection into aerobic and anaerobic blood culture systems may be of benefit for microbiological identification. Syringe collections, if promptly transported to the laboratory (within 10 minutes), are satisfactory. With infectious diseases, cystic fluids may be dealt with by various techniques, including culture, review of wet mounts, gram's stain preparations, acid-fast stains, DNA hybridization, enzyme-linked immunosorbent assay (ELISA), and other highly specialized techniques. Cystic fluids may also be

evaluated for various enzymes, lipids, total protein, and tumor markers. The enzymes include amylase and lactate dehydrogenase. Other chemical determinations include glucose and total protein. Triglycerides may be used to estimate whether or not the fluid is chylous. This may further be confirmed by lipoprotein electrophoresis, demonstrating the presence of chylomicrons. Useful tumor markers are epithelial membrane antigen (EMA), carcinoembryonic antigen (CEA), alpha-fetoprotein, and CA-125.

Synovial fluid evaluations include glucose, total protein, and specimen collection suitable for bacteriological investigation. The same procedures apply as to a cystic fluid, in that consultation with a laboratory physician prior to collection will allow optimization of laboratory assessment. EDTA tubes, blood culture, and anaerobic collection tubes may facilitate differentials, and white blood cell, red blood cell, and cytological evaluations. If a specific etiologic agent is sought and identified, it makes directed therapy possible. Cytological assessment may provide information whether or not there is a primary lesion of the pleural mesothelioma or a metastatic lesion. The information may suggest a specific site biopsy, further medical imaging, or a treatment modality (surgery, chemotherapy, radiation therapy).

Tumor markers may be performed on serous fluids in which a cytological preparation is either not performed or is equivocal. Carcinoembryonic antigen is indicative of a metastatic lesion in the patient who has had a previously diagnosed CEA-producing tumor. Elevated CEA values (greater than 10 ng/mL) are supportive of a malignant pleural effusion and malignant ascites. If an ovarian carcinoma in a patient has been noted to produce CA-125, assessing the presence of CA-125 in peritoneal washings or ascites fluid may demonstrate tumor recurrence in the patient. Obtaining fluid or washings may be associated with a laparotomy or simply as an alternate to laparotomy in specific cases. CA 15-3, a breast tumor marker, may be of assistance in the case of a pleural effusion. If the primary tumor was CA 15-3 producing, it is logical that the metastatic lesion would produce CA 15-3 if there is a serous effusion. CA 15-3 testing may add to cytological evaluations and increase the sensitivity of identifying a malignant effusion. Prostatic specific antigen (PSA), is a tumor marker that is elaborated by the prostate in the male. This tumor marker would be a useful adjunct in assessing any patient in whom a serous effusion was identified and a stage C or D prostatic tumor was previously diagnosed. The role of tumor markers in many instances is hypothetical, but the previous studies do support a role in evaluating serous fluids for specific markers with the appropriate clinical setting.

Amylase values are also elevated in pleural effusions. There are essentially three major categories of increased amylase results. The first includes pancreatitis with or without pseudocyst information or a direct pancreatic-pleural fistula. Rupture of the esophagus is the second condition, and finally, malignant effusions may have elevated amylase values. It has been estimated that left-sided pleural effusions occur in about 10% of cases of acute pancreatitis, and these fluids have amylase concentrations twice the reference values in sera. The most common neoplasms associated with pleural effusion are carcinoma of the lung, ovarian tumors, and gastrointestinal tumors. The fluid-to-serum ratio of amylase is highest for carcinoma of the lung and carcinoma of the ovary. It is useful in the differential diagnosis as mesotheliomas of the lung are not reported as secreting amylase. If isoenzyme separations are available, the pancreatic isoamylase is the most commonly seen isoenzyme associated with these tumors.

Other assays also may be employed to distinguish the origin of an effusion. These include triglycerides to determine whether the fluid is chylous or not, mucopolysaccharides to assess whether mesothelioma is present, and organic acids, which may represent a specific bacterial infection.

SYNOVIAL FLUID ANALYSIS

Hematological, biochemical, and cytological parameters are useful in the assessment of synovial fluids. Biochemical analyses are related to defining inflammatory processes, or infectious and systemic disease. The vital part of the examination is the microscopic analysis for crystals. The various entities that must be considered include uric acid (gout), pyrophosphate (pseudogout), hydroxyapatite (Milwaukee shoulder syndrome), and drugs. It is most important to obtain a well-documented history in order to establish previous interarticular joint administration of drugs. This will greatly enhance the ability of the laboratory physician to assess and interpret the microscopic findings.

Monoarticular joint involvement is classically seen in bacterial infections. It is important that a culture be taken under optimal conditions. Consideration should be given to *Staphylococcus aureus, Nisseria gonorrhoeae, Haemophilus influenza,* and *Mycobacterium tuberculosis,* depending on the age of the individual, culture, and socioeconomic status.

Symmetrical arthritis or polyarticular joint involvement is most consistent with systemic disease that is probably not infectious in origin, although exceptions do exist. It is important to have available any history of trauma, recent use of antibiotics, and any previous radiographs or computerized tomography (CT) scans to assess joint damage.

The assessment of clot formation is useful and the procedure is simple. The analysis permits an assessment of whether or not a process is inflammatory or noninflammatory. Glucose analysis is also of value. The comparison of serum glucose to serous fluid glucose may be useful in establishing an infectious etiology, since reduced serous fluid glucose values are obtained. The precise infection cannot be quantitated but low glucose values provide further support for careful processing of the culture specimen.

Cytological assessment is useful to determine if there is a primary tumor that involves the joint space itself (villonodular synovitis), or if there is an extension of a cartilaginous tumor into the joint space or a bony tumor. These require careful assessment and must be correlated to the medical imaging findings. With the advent of arthroscopy, some of these tests will become redundant, whereas others will be increasingly utilized to evaluate the pathological processes.

CYSTIC FLUIDS

Many of the comments that apply to serous fluids also apply to cystic fluids. The most important aspects are proper sample collection and site of the cyst. A lesion in the neck region may be questioned as to whether or not it is of salivary gland origin or thyroid gland origin. The cystic lesion may be evaluted cytologically, but in some instances a biochemical analysis may also provide further documentation about its origin. In such instances, amylase and thyroxin assays would be of merit. Increased amylase would point to a salivary gland origin, whereas increased thyroxine would indicate a thyroid origin.

Cystic regions of the breast are frequently aspirated and cytological assessment is performed. Very rarely are these cystic lesions evaluated for biochemical or infectious etiologies. With the increased availability of tumor markers such as CA 15-3, it is possible that cystic fluids will more frequently be submitted for analysis. A history of trauma (sharp, blunt, or insect bite) may assist in the interpretation as the cyst is likely to represent a benign inflammatory process as opposed to malignant breast disease.

The advent of aspiration cytology is markedly changing the approach to the diagnosis of many lesions. Combined with medical imaging, these techniques are very powerful tools. In the future, cystic lesion analysis may be directly proportional to the incorporation of newer, effective, analytical methodologies such as monoclonal antibodies that will support cytological evaluations.

Peritoneal cysts are rarely aspirated. Any abdominal cyst that is aspirated should have an amylase test performed to determine whether or not it is of pancreatic origin. Although pseudocyst formation is uncommon, and ectopic pseudocyst formation is even less common, the possibility of such formations cannot be excluded and elevated amylase is a positive finding consistent with pancreatic origin.

SUMMARY

Serous fluids, cystic fluids, and synovial fluids are useful in establishing diagnoses, providing a baseline for therapy, and as an adjunct to other modalities.

SUGGESTED READING

Duffy MJ: New cancer markers, Ann Clin Biochem 26:379, 1989.

Ende N: Studies of amylase activity and pleural effusion in ascites, Cancer 13:283, 1960.

Esteban JM and others: Immunocytochemical profile of benign and carcinomatous effusions, Am J Clin Pathol 94:698, 1990.

Kjeldsberg CR and Knight JA: Body fluids: laboratory examination of amniotic, cerebral spinal, seminal, serous, and synovial fluids, ed 2, 1986, American Society of Clinical Pathologists.

Kramer MR and others: High amylase levels in neoplasma: related pleural effusion, Ann Int Med 110:567, 1989.

Light RW: Pleural effusions: symposium on pulmonary disease, Med Clin N Am 61:1339, 1977.

Permanetter W and Wiesinger H: Immunohistochemical study of alpha-anti-chymotrypsin, tissue polypeptide antigen, keritin, carcinoembryonic antigen in effusion sediments, Acta Cytol 31:104, 1986.

Peterman TA and Speicher CE: Evaluating pleural effusions: a 2-stage laboratory approach, JAMA 252:1051, 1984.

Rudolph RA, Marguerite PM, and Bernstein LH: Measuring decision values for CEA and CA-125 in effusions, Lab Med 21:574, 1990.

Wroblewski F and Wroblewski R: The clinical significance of lactate dehydrogenase activity in serous effusions, Ann Int Med 48:813, 1958.

31 Seminal fluid analysis

William Daniel Follas
John K. Critser

The analysis of semen dates back as early as the 17th century with the observations of Leewenhoek and other scientists. Although Leewenhoek's drawings of sperm cells appeared more in line with today's morphological observations, other scientists of his time provided more colorful explanations. One such view was that the sperm cells, known as "humunculi," were fully formed (albeit tiny) humans who, when nurtured in the confines of the female uterus, simply grew until they were born Mister or Missus Baby.

With an estimated 2.4 million married couples affected by infertility, the importance of semen analysis as an evaluation tool for male infertility has brought to the forefront the importance of standardization of current analytical procedures. Serious attempts have begun to standardize the basic analytical parameters such as morphology, motility, kinetics, and count. How semen is collected and multiple specimen analysis are now recognized as being as important as the actual analytical parameters measured. Even though our knowledge is expanding, science has not yet identified the elusive answer to the question of what constitutes a sperm cell that has the capacity to fertilize an egg.

Not only is it important to know how to perform semen analysis accurately and reproducibly, but also how to prepare semen, whether fresh or cryopreserved, for use in various reproductive procedures. Other procedures finding increased utilization in infertility assessment include testing for anti-sperm antibodies, acrosomal status, cervical mucous testing, zonafree hamster ova penetration tests, and various biochemical analyte measurements. As standardization and understanding of sperm-fertilizing factors develop, new assays will be implemented in the laboratory with more meaningful clinical interpretation available for these methods.

ANATOMY AND PHYSIOLOGY

At six weeks of gestation, the undifferentiated gonad morphologically consists of a medulla, cortex, and primordial germ cells. During the seventh week of gestation, gross morphologic differentiation of the testes occurs under the influence of testosterone secreted by the fetal Leydig cells.

A schematic diagram of the fully matured human testis and paratesticular structures is shown in Figure 31-1. The major component of the testis, both structurally and functionally, are the seminiferous tubules. The seminiferous tubules lie within the testes as convoluted tubules separated by interstitial tissue comprised primarily of blood and lymph vessels and islands of Leydig cells. These are luteinizing hormone stimulated cells which are the primary androgen-producing cells in the testis. The organization of this separation of interstitial tissue and the seminiferous tubules is structured in such a manner that the seminiferous tubules are not freely accessible to the circulatory system. Rather there is a blood-testis barrier formed by tight junctions between the Sertoli cells of the seminiferous epithelium which markedly restricts permeability. The mature seminiferous tubule epithelium, site of spermatogenesis, is composed of Sertoli cells and the germ cells proper.

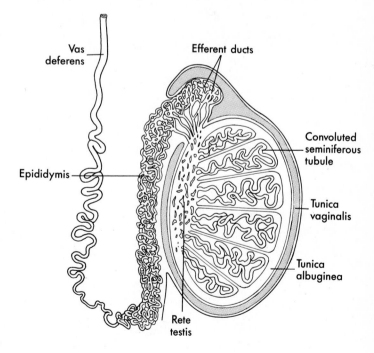

Fig. 31-1 Testis and paratesticular structures. *Redrawn from Weiss L, ed: Histology: cell and tissue biology, New York, 1983, Elsevier Science Publishing Co., Inc.*

425

The Sertoli cells line the seminiferous epithelium which provide the necessary structural and functional milieu in which spermatogenesis, spermiogenesis, and spermiation occur (Figure 31-2). The Sertoli cells are responsive to both follicle stimulating hormone (FSH) from the pituitary and testosterone from Leydig cells. Androgens are essential for most stages of spermatogenesis. To sequester testosterone from the Leydig cells, Sertoli cells produce androgen-binding protein which has high affinity for both testosterone and its reduced product, dihydrotestosterone. There are separate, structurally unique, androgen receptors in these cells which bind testosterone. The binding of testosterone and its reduction (by 5-alpha-reductase) is a prerequisite for the biological action for all androgen-induced responses. In addition to the production of androgen-binding protein and androgen receptors, which have intracellular roles to play, the Sertoli cells also synthesize and secrete a protein hormone called inhibin. Inhibin has systemic effects primarily at the level of the pituitary, where it provides negative feedback, lowering the circulating concentrations of FSH.

The epididymis is located on the testis and is comprised of the ductuli efferentes (efferent ducts) and the ductus epididymis (epididymis) (Figure 31-1).

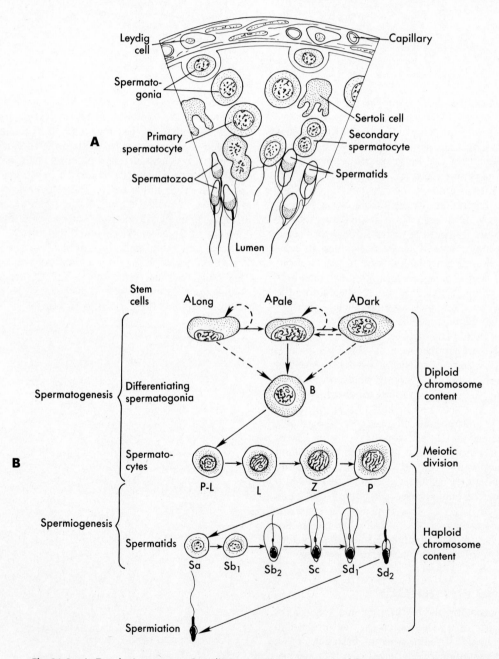

Fig. 31-2 **A,** Developing gametes. **B,** A diagrammatic representation of the process of spermatogenesis, spermiogenesis, and spermiation, during which the developing germ cells undergo mitotic and then meiotic division to halve their chromosome content. *Redrawn from Lipshultz LI and Howard SS, eds: Infertility in the male, Edinburgh, 1975, Churchill Livingstone.*

The epididymis serves multiple purposes. Spermatozoa are transported from the testis to the ejaculatory duct via the epididymis. Spermatozoa mature and acquire motility and the capacity to participate in fertilization during their transit through the epididymis. Subsequently, sperm are stored in the cauda epididymis and vas deferens. During this storage phase, if the frequency of ejaculation is low, the epididymis serves to eliminate "old" spermatozoa by phagocytosis and reabsorption.

The vas deferens is essentially a tube which extends from the epididymis to the ejaculatory duct. At its terminal end, the vas deferens dilates to form the ampulla of the vas deferens. Here, at the base of the prostate, the vas deferens fuses with the neck of the seminal vesicle to form the ejaculatory duct. The ejaculatory duct passes through the prostate and opens into the prostatic urethra.

The primary functions of the vas deferens are the transport and storage of spermatozoa. Congenital absence of the vas deferens or acquired obstruction should be considered in cases of observed azoospermia or oligospermia during semen analyses. Absence of occlusion at the level of the ejaculatory duct may be investigated by the measurement of fructose concentration in the semen as a measure of seminal vesicle contribution.

The seminal vesicles appear as convoluted glandular tubules. However, each seminal vesicle actually consists of a single tube which is folded back upon itself over and over again. The proximal end of this tube fuses with the ampulla of the vas deferens. The fluid which forms accumulates in the lumen of the tube. This fluid is eliminated during ejaculation and comprises approximately 60% to 70% of the total ejaculate volume. These seminal vesicle secretions are classically characterized as having high fructose concentration (200-500 mg/dL). In fact, it is common laboratory practice to use fructose as a biochemical marker to monitor seminal vesicle function (see Table 31-1). In addition to high fructose concentrations, seminal vesicle fluid in man includes the presence of large amounts of ascorbic acid and very low sodium concentrations with correspondingly high concentrations of potassium. The high concentrations of fructose and ascorbic acid are thought to serve as energy sources to the spermatozoa at the time of ejaculation.

Because the seminal vesicles arise from the same embryonic tissue as the vas deferens, the congenital absence of the vas deferens is often associated with the absence of the seminal vesicles. In cases of azoospermia, upon routine semen analyses, it is important to consider this possibility and to measure fructose concentrations to distinguish testicular dysfunction from the absence (or occlusion) of the ejaculatory duct components.

The prostate is the largest secondary sex gland, consisting of 30-50 secular glands and 16-32 excretory ducts. In the adult man, the secretory function of the prostate is continuously producing 0.5-2 ml of fluid/day which account for approximately 20% to 30% of the total ejaculate volume. Prostatic fluid is characterized by its high concentrations of citric acid, acid phosphatase, and zinc. Functionally, the prostatic fluid contributes components of the seminal coagulation-liquefaction process.

NORMAL METABOLISM OF THE SPERMATOZOON
Spermatogenesis

Spermatozoa are produced within the seminiferous epithelium, which is composed of the Sertoli cells, progenitor spermatogonia, and the developing germ cells. The entire process of development from the spermatogonia to fully morphologically differentiated spermatozoa and their subsequent release into the lumen of the seminiferous tubules, involves the processes of spermatogenesis, spermiogenesis, and spermiation. Spermatogenesis involves meiosis of the progenitor cells resulting in primary (initial mitotic division) and secondary (meiotic or reduction division) spermatocytes. Spermiogenesis is the process of morphological change from an essentially round cell type (secondary spermatocyte) to a flagellated cell with greatly reduced cytoplasmic volume (spermatids and spermatozoa). Finally, the morphologically modified spermatozoa are released from the surrounding Sertoli cells into the lumen in a process termed spermiation. This process is represented schematically in Figures 31-2, *A* and *B*, and microscopically in Figures 31-3 and 31-4.

The spermatogenic cycle

Early investigation of the histologic nature of the seminiferous epithelium in model species such as the rat found that sperm development does not occur in a continuous manner. All developmental stages involved in spermiogenesis are not present at one time in a specific location. Rather, only certain developmental stages occur together in time and space, creating stages of maturity. It should be noted that while this

Table 31-1   Biochemical changes that may be seen in the semen of men with a variety of different causes of infertility

Genital tract lesion causing infertility	Sperm concentration	pH of semen	Seminal volume	Seminal fructose	Seminal acid phosphatase/citrate
Bilateral epididymal obstruction	Azoospermia	Normal	Normal	Normal	Normal
Congenital absence of vasa deferentia	Azoospermia	Normal, or reduced	Reduced	Absent	Raised
Ejaculatory duct obstructions	Azoospermia	Normal, or reduced	Reduced	Absent	Raised
Polyzoospermia	Raised (>350 × 10⁶)	Normal	Normal	Reduced	Normal

From Jequier A.: Semen analysis: a practical guide, 1986, Blackwell Scientific Publications.

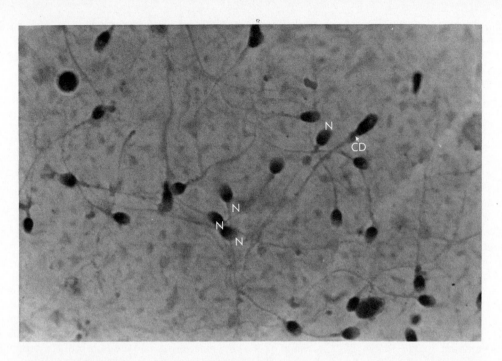

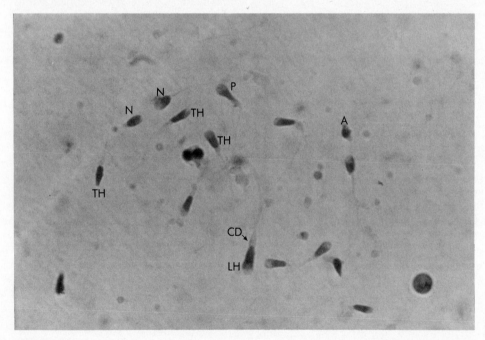

Fig. 31-3 Morphological features of spermatozoa. *N*, Normal; *A*, Amorphous; *CD*, Cytoplasmic Droplet; *CT*, Coiled Tail; *LH*, Large Head; *SH*, Small Head; *TH*, Tapered Head; *P*, Pyriform (Tear Drop) Head.

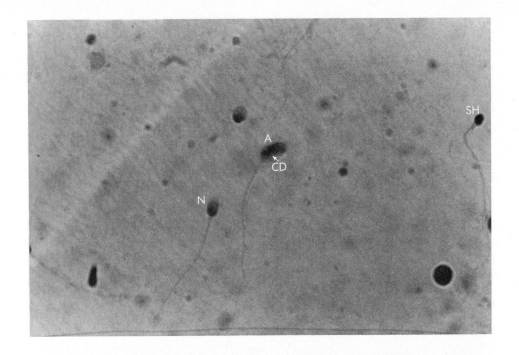

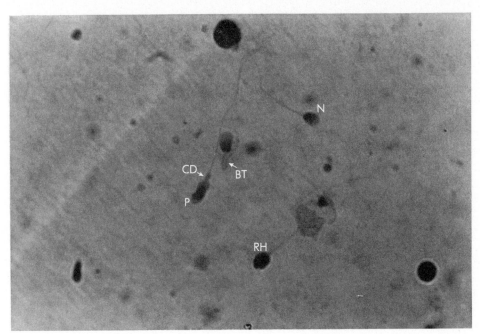

Fig. 31-3, cont'd.   Morphological features of spermatozoa. *N,* Normal; *A,* Amorphous; *CD,* Cytoplasmic Droplet; *SH,* Small Head; *BT,* Bent Tail; *RH,* Round Head; *P,* Pyriform (Tear Drop) Head.   *Continued.*

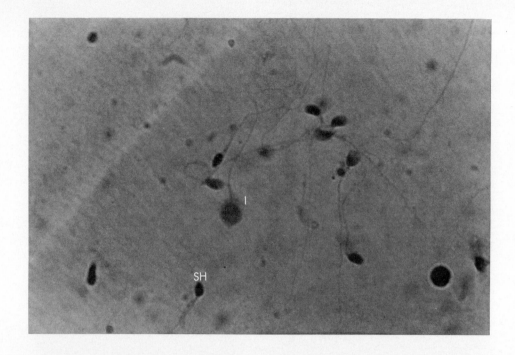

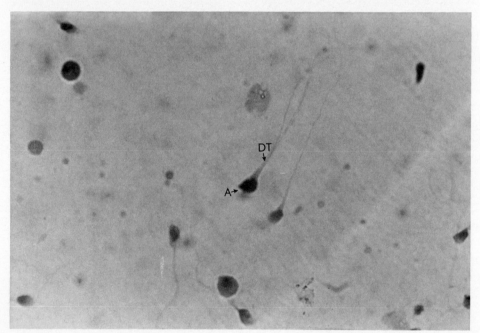

Fig. 31-3, cont'd. Morphological features of spermatozoa. *A,* Amorphous; *SH,* Small Head; *DT,* Duplicate Tail; *I,* Immature Germ Cell.

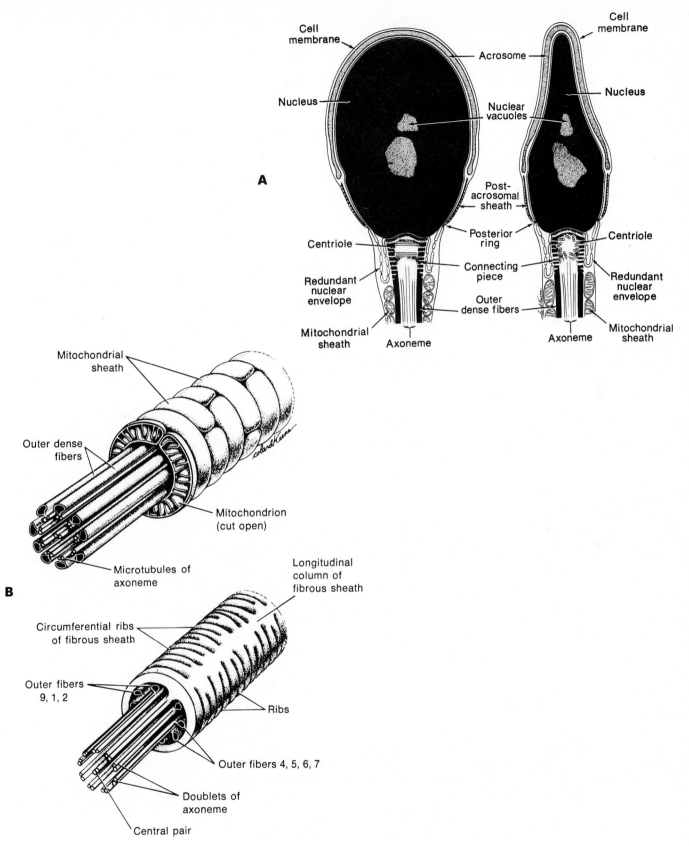

Fig. 31-4 **A,** Longitudinal section parallel *(left)* and perpendicular *(right)* to axis of proximal centriole of human spermatozoon. **B,** Organization of midpiece *(above)* and principal piece *(below)* of human sperm tail. *From Pedersen H and Fawcett DW: Functional anatomy of the human spermatozoon. In Hafez ESE, ed: Human semen and fertility regulation in men, St. Louis, 1976, Mosby–Year Book.*

is clearly evident in nonhuman species, it is less dramatic in the human. The entire series of stages in their chronological order generate the cycle of the seminiferous epithelium. This cycle is composed of various numbers of stages in different species. In the rat, there are 14 stages. In man, there are six stages. In the human, stage one is characterized by the presence of round spermatids. In stage two, the spermatids characteristically have so-called residual bodies or cytoplasmic droplets and the nuclei are essentially round but not morphologically distinct. Stage three is denoted by the lack of spermatozoa and the spermatids have clear, round nuclei. Stage four seminiferous epithelium also has no spermatozoa, but unlike stage two, the spermatid nuclei are more oval in shape and more dense. In stages five and six, there are no early spermatids. However, the sixth stage is characterized by a higher frequency of cells in the final stage of meiotic prophase (diakinesis) in which the chromosomes condense and thicken, and each bivalent chromosome, if clearly seen, contains four separate chromatids.

The formation of mature spermatozoa from spermatogonia requires four complete cycles of the seminiferous epithelium and takes between 64 and 80 days in the human. This entire process (64 to 80 days) constitutes one spermatogenic cycle. This concept is important for semen analysis since a disruption (e.g., thermal, pharmacologic, physical) in this spermatogenic cycle might be observed in sperm counts during this period. However, if the alteration was acute, semen analyses after the start of a new cycle might well show a very different (and improved) result. Therefore, it is important to conduct multiple semen analyses over a time exceeding approximately one full spermatogenic cycle to insure representative results.

Capacitation

Upon ejaculation, epididymally matured spermatozoa have the ability of motility but not fertilization. Historically, it was observed that sperm acquire the ability to fertilize only after residing in the female reproductive tract for some time. This phenomenon is termed capacitation, and the time required for sperm to capacitate is called the "capacitation-time." Capacitation is not required to occur in vivo but under appropriate conditions can occur in vitro. Such in vitro capacitation techniques are now routinely used and provide the basis for many of the more applied aspects of in vitro fertilization (IVF). Because sperm are able to acquire fertilizing capacity in vitro, some investigators suggest that capacitation is not a necessary prerequisite for fertilization. However, freshly ejaculated sperm placed into in vitro conditions do not fertilize oocytes immediately. There is always some time elapsed between insemination and fertilization.

Therefore, capacitation has been described in phenomenological terms as "a series of physiologic changes in sperm that render the spermatozoa capable of fertilizing eggs"; or as "the process in the female (or in vitro) that prepares the spermatozoon to undergo the acrosome reaction and also quite probably develop a whiplash or hyperactivated motility that may enhance ability to penetrate the zona pellucida."

Acrosome reaction

The acrosome forms a cap-like structure at the apical portion of the sperm head. The acrosome contains a large number of hydrolytic enzymes such as hyaluronidase, proacrosin (acrosin), neuraminidase, acid phosphatase, and phospholipase. These enzymes, when released during the process of the acrosome reaction into the vicinity of the oocyte, are believed to aid the sperm in obtaining passage to and through the zona pellucida via enzymatic digestion. Indeed, it is generally held that capacitation and the acrosome reaction are, at least under normal physiologic conditions, continuous phenomena, with the acrosome reaction following completion of capacitation directly.

Fertilization

The site of fertilization, under normal conditions, is in the ampullary-isthmus junction of the oviduct. Spermatozoa are transported from the site of semen deposition (vagina) to the oviduct over time, with the so-called "rapid transport" mechanism moving the vanguard sperm there within minutes after ejaculation. This rapid transport mechanism is thought to involve the propulsion of sperm through the cervix and uterus, into the oviduct via strong uterine musculature contractions. However, these vanguard sperm are not thought to be capable of fertilization (due to mechanical damage during the rapid transport). Relative to the number of sperm in the ejaculate (10^8), few sperm populate the oviduct at any one time (10^1-10^2). Subsequent to the initial rapid transport of sperm, sperm continuously move first from the vagina into the cervix (where they may reside for an extended period of time [approximately three to four days] providing a "sperm reservoir") to the uterus and finally into the oviduct.

PATHOPHYSIOLOGY OF THE MALE REPRODUCTIVE PROCESS

Abnormalities in the male reproductive process which contribute to infertility are often termed "male factor(s)." Such male factors reportedly account for between 25% and 50% of all cases of infertility. The physiologic basis for male reproductive disorders are diverse and, as one would expect, originate most commonly with the dysfunction of either the hypothalamic-pituitary-gonadal axis, the spermatogenic function of the seminiferous tubules, or ejaculatory failure (including both impotence and obstruction of the male reproductive tract duct system through which spermatozoa and seminal fluid pass during the ejaculatory process). Additionally, there are a number of disorders which do not fit into these categories such as the presence of a varicocele, antisperm antibodies, and genitourinary infections.

Endocrine dysfunction

In the area of endocrine dysfunction, pathophysiology of either the hypothalamus, resulting in altered gonadotrophin releasing hormone (GnRH) release, and/or altered responsiveness of the gonadotropes (LH and FSH producing cells) within the anterior pituitary, can result in abnormally low circulating concentrations of gonadotrophins (LH and FSH) (hypogonadotropism) causing a resultant reduced level of testicular function (hypogonadism). Because the altered testicular function resulting from low circulating gonadotropin concentrations would produce low testosterone levels, patients often seek medical treatment for androgen deficiency rather than for infertility. Such so-called hypogonadotropic-hypogonadism syndromes may be the result of varied etiology from either congenital (i.e., GnRH deficiency-Kallmann's syndrome) or acquired (e.g., pituitary adenomas) conditions. Although more rare, conditions resulting in elevated circulating concentrations of gonadotropins (hypergonadotropic syndromes (can also impair male reproductive function via alterations in either androgen synthesis or the development of androgen insensitivity. The most common example of this type of endocrine dysfunction is Klinefelter's syndrome (XXY genotype) with elevated circulating concentrations of gonadotropins and an associated azoospermia.

Testicular dysfunction
Congenital

A number of congenital disorders are known to produce testicular dysfunction. These include genetic abnormalities such as Klinefelter's syndrome (the most common genetic abnormality affecting testicular function) with its characteristic karyotype of 47X, X, Y (an extra X chromosome) or its more rare form of 46X, Y/47, X, X, Y (a mosaic condition with some cells having a normal (46, X, Y chromosomal complement while other cells have the abnormal 47, X, X, Y genome). While these types of disorders are relatively rare in the general population (e.g., 0.2% have Klinefelter's), there is a significantly higher frequency in the male factor population. Approximately 4% of men with infertility and 11% of azoospermics are diagnosed with Klinefelter's. An additional 1% to 2% have some other type of chromosomal abnormality.

Another fairly common disorder leading to testicular dysfunction is cryptorchidism or the failure of the testes to descend from the abdomen to the scrotum during fetal development. Testes retained within the abdomen are exposed to core body temperature (37°C) while intrascrotal temperatures are approximately (34-35°C). Spermatogenic function is impaired at temperatures exceeding 35°C resulting in markedly reduced sperm quality.

Acquired

Factors resulting in acquired testicular dysfunction are diverse. Some examples include: testicular trauma; inflammation (orchitis, notably from mumps or epididymitis/epididymo-orchitis, for example from sexually transmitted diseases); malignancies (leukemia, lymphoma); torsion (resulting in an occlusion of the testicular blood supply with an associated testicular atrophy); varicocele (enlarged blood vessels surrounding the testes thought to increase intratesticular temperature); drugs (prescribed, e.g., chemotherapeutic agents; recreational, e.g., alcohol, opiates, tetrahydrocannabinol); elevated scrotal temperature (high environmental temperatures, e.g., hot baths). It is important to note for proper interpretation of semen analyses, that many of the factors listed above are reversible. Exposure to drugs or elevated temperatures may acutely and dramatically impact upon a given spermatogenic cycle or simply a cohort of

stored epididymal sperm. This may be observed in the resulting quality of a man's particular series of ejaculates. However, when these causative factors are removed and given sufficient time the individual may well revert to producing "normal" ejaculates. Again, these potential situations underscore the importance of 1) communicating with the patient to determine if such factors may be affecting sperm quality and 2) the need to perform multiple semen analyses several months (64 to 80 days) apart, covering a time period greater than a single spermatogenic cycle.

Genital tract obstruction

The complete absence of sperm in an ejaculate (azoospermia) may be the result of the presence of an obstruction in the male reproductive tract. In the infertile male population the presence of such an obstruction is fairly common (3-13%). Congenital absence of the vas deferens of the ejaculatory duct segment are often involved. It is important to recognize that azoospermia may be the result of an occlusion and to measure fructose concentrations in the semen of such samples to determine whether the seminal vesicle components are entering the ejaculate. This is because the ejaculatory duct is formed anatomically when the distal segment of the vas deferens fuses with the urethra at the point where the neck of the seminal vesicles also fuse. Therefore, an occlusion at the level of the ejaculatory duct will result not only in an azoospermia but also abnormally low concentrations of fructose in the semen. This information can be important when attempting to determine the etiology of the azoospermia.

Immotile sperm syndrome

Immotile-cilia syndrome is characterized as a defect in the axoneme of the cilia in the respiratory tract and may be present as a defect in the flagellum of the spermatozoa. Individuals with this disorder produce semen samples which characteristically have normal sperm concentrations and morphology, but the sperm are immotile.

SEMEN ANALYSIS
Collection techniques

Before collection of a semen specimen, the patient should be given clear instructions (see Box 31-1) for proper specimen collection. An overview of the effects of drugs should be explained as well as the physiologic and psychological influences on semen characteristics. This information will increase the likelihood of receiving a good semen sample for analysis.

A period of sexual abstinence from two to five days is ideal before the collection of a semen sample. For an initial evaluation, at least two semen samples should be collected with a time interval of between seven days (to address acute affects) and three months (to address chronic affects). However, the spermatogenic cycle is approximately 74 days. Therefore, semen samples would have to encompass this period of time to evaluate any aberrations in the normal physiological cycle. It is best if these samples are produced in a suitably private room at the laboratory. If the specimen is produced outside the lab, the specimen should be protected from temperature extremes and transported to the lab

Box 31-1 Instructions for collection of a semen specimen

Prior to submission of a specimen, the patient should contact the laboratory to set up an appointment.

Abstinence of two days but not more than five days is recommended. Ideally, the total number of days of abstinence should reflect the person's usual sexual pattern (i.e., if two days between intercourse is the usual pattern, then two days of abstinence should be allowed).

The laboratory should be notified of any medications the patient is taking.

The specimen is collected in a sterilized container. The entire specimen is needed for an accurate analysis.

Once the specimen is collected, it should be kept next to the body (e.g., inside a shirt) to keep it warm and to avoid temperature fluctuations. Transport the specimen to the lab as soon as possible. If driving time from home to the lab exceeds one hour, the specimen must be collected at the laboratory.

If you have any questions please contact the laboratory.

within one hour. It is of importance to note that while human spermatozoa are not classically sensitive to abrupt changes in decreased temperatures above freezing (cold-shock sensitivity), elevated temperatures are clearly detrimental and temperature fluctuations in either direction may alter motion characteristics measured during a routine semen analysis.

Semen specimens should be collected in clean, wide-mouth glass or non-toxic plastic containers. Due to the large number of manufacturers of plastic containers, one should examine specimens collected in any proposed collecting device and determine potential sperm toxicity prior to placing them into use. Collection by masturbation is preferred. The use of specially manufactured condoms free of spermicidal agents can be obtained through physicians and laboratories when masturbation is circumstantially objectionable. Coitus interruptus can be used but is least preferable due to the potential loss of the sperm-rich first fraction of the ejaculate and possible interference of vaginal secretions.

Obtaining sperm-rich fractions of semen for analysis and use in artificial insemination is aided by split-specimen analysis. This is used to determine the characteristics of the first and second fractions of an ejaculate separately. The first fraction usually contains the majority of sperm cells without the seminal vesicle secretions. Therefore, this fraction is usually of low volume (0.5 mL), contains citric acid from the prostate, and is in a non-coagulating medium. The second fraction will have an increased fructose level due to seminal vesicle secretions. However, the majority of the spermatozoa may be found in the second fraction approximately 6% of the time.

General characteristics of human semen

Human semen is ejaculated as a viscous, gray-yellow fluid which forms a fairly solid gel-like clot immediately after ejaculation. This clot usually liquefies spontaneously and completely within 5 to 60 minutes either *in vitro* and some-

what more rapidly *in vivo* (5 to 10 minutes). The entire seminal coagulum represents a thorough mixture of coagulated seminal plasma and spermatozoa trapped in the matrix. The spermatozoa within the coagulum are effectively immobilized until liquefaction is completed.

The coagulating and liquefying properties of an entire ejaculate differ markedly when compared to semen collected in different portions (split ejaculate samples). In the human, the first fraction of the ejaculate consists of spermatozoa, epididymal fluid and prostatic fluid; while the second fraction contains primarily seminal vesicle fluid. In human semen collected as split-ejaculates, the first fraction usually does not coagulate or if it does clot, liquefaction occurs immediately. In contrast, the second fraction forms a firm coagulum which liquefies over 20 to 60 minutes and then often incompletely. Addition of the first fraction to the second speeds up the liquefaction process. This has been shown not to be due to the large numbers of spermatozoa in the first fraction and is not different between vasectomized or intact males. In men who congenitally lack seminal vesicles, the semen does not coagulate. These observations suggest that in the human, 1) the coagulum-forming substrate originates in the seminal vesicles, and 2) the liquefying properties of the ejaculate originate in the prostate.

Analytical parameters
Physical measurements

Viscosity. The human ejaculate forms a coagulum rapidly after ejaculation which, under normal conditions, liquefies after 5 to 60 minutes. From the laboratory point of view, this process is of practical importance simply because the semen sample is not amenable to laboratory procedures until it undergoes the liquefaction process. This degree of liquefaction is measured in the laboratory in terms of the viscosity of the semen. Viscosity is measured after sufficient time has elapsed for liquefaction to occur. There are various approaches to estimating viscosity. One method commonly employed is to simply aspirate a small volume of semen into a Pasteur pipette and the relative ease or difficulty of flow noted. Additionally, the length of the thread formed when the pipette is removed from the semen may be estimated. The longer the thread that is formed, the more viscous the sample. It is useful to observe a thread length of three to five cm even after complete liquefaction. Utilization of these methods provides a subjective estimate of viscosity. The information is most often recorded on the semen analysis report in descriptive terms such as: normal, more viscous than normal, or very viscous. An alternative method which provides more quantitative data is to draw a small volume of semen into a pipette and then record the time it takes for the first drop of semen to flow back out of the pipette. Pipettes used for this assay are of 100 uL volume and a length of 12 cm. The pipettes routinely used for this procedure are standardized by using silicone oil (MS 200, viscosity 20 cST). Using this standard approach, with the pipette in a vertical position, three drops of oil will flow out of the pipette in approximately 5 seconds. If it takes more than 5 seconds for a single drop of semen to flow out of such a pipette, the sample is classified as abnormally viscous.

Coagulation and liquefaction. The biochemical processes of seminal coagulation are not clearly defined in the human. Current collective data suggest that coagulation of human semen is a result of processes different from those involved in blood coagulation. The current hypothesis regarding human semen coagulation is that the HMW-SV (high molecular weight-seminal vesicle) protein constitutes the major structural component of the seminal clot and that the association of these molecules is noncovalent. There are a number of approaches for processing samples which do not liquefy or liquefy incompletely. Among these are to draw the viscous sample in-and-out of a pipette in an attempt to physically decrease the viscosity. This procedure, while common, has the potential to damage the spermatozoa in the sample and thereby adversely affect the resulting semen analysis. Another, more elegant approach is to add enzymatic reagents (e.g., alpha-amylase) to the sample to biochemically decrease the sample viscosity.

Volume. The measurement of semen is most easily performed by the use of disposable plastic pipettes. With the semen in a suitable container, select a pipette until all the specimen is collected into the pipette. By carefully allowing the semen to fill the lower portion of the pipette, one can then measure the volume by subtracting the value found at the meniscus from the total pipette volume. Volumes are normally reported to the closest 0.1 mL. The normal range is between 2 and 6 mL.

pH. Hydrogen ion concentration is an important factor in motility, viability, and metabolism of spermatozoa. Generally, pH values greater than 7.0 provide optimal survival of spermatozoa and have been observed to enhance the movement up to pH 8.5 and above. Below the optimal pH, both motility and metabolism decline. Measurement of pH can be performed by using pH paper provided its accuracy has been ascertained by reference to a glass electrode.

Sperm concentration. The total number of sperm cells in an ejaculate should be counted so as to yield accurate

and reproducible results. Various authors present differing normal ranges for sperm counts but most agree that a count of 20×10^6 sperm cells per mL and below is considered subfertile. However, this is only a guideline, and fertilization can occur at this level given that the fertilizing capacity of semen encompasses other factors such as motility, and viability.

Two commonly used manual counting methods are the Neubauer hemocytometer and the Makler counting chamber. Use of the hemacytometer is described in many hematology textbooks and involves appropriate dilution of the sample (approximately 1:20) prior to placing the specimen on the hemocytometer. The sperm cells, when diluted with an isosmotic (approximately 300 mOsm) buffered formalin solution, are immobilized for counting. It should be noted that while it is common to use water as a diluent prior to counting sperm, placing the cells in an extremely hypoosmotic environment will cause the sperm tails to coil and/or lyse.

Use of the Makler counting chamber requires no dilution. However, the semen must be pre-treated to immobilize the spermatozoa prior to counting. This is accomplished by placing an aliquot of the well-mixed, liquified ejaculate into a small tube and heating at 57°C for ten minutes. Although more convenient to use, the Makler is more expensive than a hemocytometer.

Motility. Estimates of the percent of spermatozoa which are motile in an ejaculate (motility or percent motility) may be made subjectively by placing a drop of semen onto a prewarmed (37°C) microscope slide and observing the specimen at 100 to 400X. Using this approach, it is essential to ensure that a sufficient number of microscopic fields are examined to avoid non-representative sampling errors. It is common to examine at least four and often eight fields to address this issue. Additionally, it is equally important to observe a sufficient total number of spermatozoa, usually a minimum of 200. While it is common to determine sperm motility only during the initial semen analysis, significant additional information regarding the characteristics of the spermatozoa can be obtained by examining the sample for motility at various later time intervals. Such time intervals often employed are some combination of two, four, six, 12, or 24 hours after liquefaction. This approach is of particular importance in analyzing samples suspected of containing anti-sperm antibodies or frozen-thawed sperm which often demonstrate marked "latent" immobilization which cannot be observed initially.

The data which can be collected using this technique are: 1) a subjective estimate of the percent of the spermatozoa which are motile (defined as showing any signs of flagellar activity); this is essentially a visual estimate of (the number of motile sperm/the total number of sperm) × 100. Note: It is often helpful to record this value for each field and after all fields have been examined, take the average value as the reported value. 2) The percentage of spermatozoa which are demonstrating progressive motility (the number of spermatozoa actually changing their location/the number of motile sperm) × 100. 3) A subjective score of the velocity (sometimes called forward progression score) of the motile spermatozoa (usually using a scoring system ranging from 0 to 4 where 0 represents no progressively motile sperm

Table 31-2 Normal values of semen variables

Volume	2.0 mL or more
pH	7.2-7.8
Sperm concentration	20×10^6 spermatozoa/mL or more
Total sperm count	40×10^6 spermatozoa or more
Motility	50% or more with forward progression (i.e. categories (a) and (b): Section 2.4.2) or 25% or more with rapid linear progression (i.e. category (a)) within 60 min after collection
Morphology	50% or more with normal morphology
Viability	50% or more live, i.e. excluding dye
White blood cells	Fewer than 1×10^6/mL
Zinc (total)	2.4 micromol or more per ejaculate
Citric acid (total)	52 μmol (10 mg) or more per ejaculate
Fructose (total)	13 micromol or more per ejaculate
MAR test	Fewer than 10% spermatozoa with adherent particles
Immunobead test	Fewer than 10% spermatozoa with adherent beads

World Health Organization: WHO laboratory manual for the examination of human semen and semen-cervical mucous interaction, pg 27, 1987.

and 4 indicates that all sperm are vigorously moving forward).

Morphology. The human spermatozoa, once fully differentiated, appears at the light microscopic level as a highly elongated cell, with a marked reduction in cytoplasmic volume (see Figure 31-4). Sperm morphologic characteristics include the HEAD region (approximately 4 to 5 μm in length, 3 μm in width, and 1 to 2 μm in depth) with the Acrosome (a modified Golgi apparatus which covers the apical aspect of the head) and the post acrosomal region (the area of the head not covered by the acrosome); the MIDPIECE (5 to 7 μm long and 1 μm in diameter), consisting of the spiraling mitochondrial sheath which terminates at the annulus; the PRINCIPAL TAILPIECE (approximately 45 μm in length with a tapering diameter) consisting of an axial core with two central microtubules surrounded by nine double microtubules surrounded again by an outer ring of nine dense fibers (a modification on the common theme of the 9 + 2 configuration of mammalian cilia and flagella); and lastly the ENDPIECE (approximately 5 μm in length with a diameter of 0.1 μm) which is formed with the termination of the fibrous sheath near the tip of the cell. not pass; while dead cells do not have intact membranes

The two most popular stains used for assessing sperm cell morphology are the Papanicolaou and the hematoxylin/eosin stains. Sperm cells can exhibit morphologic aberrations in either the head or tail. The most common head abnormalities include acrosomal aberrations (absence or abnormal shape), vacuolation, bicephalis (double-headed sperm), nuclear abnormalities, micro (small), and megalo (large) cephalic sperm. Tailpiece abnormalities include coiled tailpieces, kinked midpieces, lengthened neckpieces, cytoplasmic extrusions, tailpiece length variations and multitailed spermatozoon. Other abnormal forms observed are immature spermatocytes and/or spermatids. Examples of normal sperm and various abnormal forms are depicted in Figures 31-3 and 31-4.

Viability. Spermatozoa viability may be determined using one of a variety of supravital staining techniques. These techniques are based on the principle that live cells possess intact plasma membranes through which these stains will and will allow passage of the macromolecular sized stain. Many of these procedures utilize eosin or a combination of eosin and nigrosin as the supravital stain. Alternatively, supravital stains such as trypan blue may be used. For complete protocols, refer to the World Health Organization laboratory manual for the examination of human semen and cervical-mucus interaction.

In general, it is important to examine and classify 100 to 200 spermatozoa per sample to obtain accurate estimates of the number of viable cells. It is useful to compare the results of such an estimate of sperm viability with percent motility information. The percentage of nonviable sperm should not significantly exceed the percentage of nonmotile sperm. However, if the percentage of nonmotile sperm exceeds the percentage of nonviable sperm, there may be more subtle pathology occuring such as a motile apparatus defect resulting in an intact membrane but immotile cells.

After completing the semen analysis, laboratory personnel must report the findings to the clinician. All report formats should incorporate the normal ranges for the laboratory performing the analyses. Various report formats are commonly used and an example is shown in Figure 31-5.

Biochemical measurements

Fructose. Fructose is the primary energy source for sperm. It is required for spermatozoa survival in an anaerobic environment and it stimulates sperm motility. Spermatozoa which are subjected to centrifugation and thus separated from the seminal plasma will not survive anaerobically unless seminal plasma or a carbohydrate source is added back to separated spermatozoa.

Seminal plasma fructose is produced by the seminal vesicles. Fructose production is stimulated by testosterone. Since the seminal vesicles do not have a large storage capacity, collection of several ejaculates within a few days will yield decreased fructose values. It takes about two days for fructose levels in the seminal vesicles to be replenished.

Fructose measurements are useful diagnostically in men with low-volume ejaculates. The absence of fructose can indicate the congenital absence of the seminal vesicles and/or vasa deferentia. Obstructions or infections that affect the seminal vesicle secretions will also result in absent or reduced fructose concentration.

Men with polyzoospermia and low motility may have a fructose deficiency. Fructose measurements are useful in confirming this diagnosis. Fructose values have been found to respond indirectly to insulin via the blood glucose concentrations. Seminal plasma fructose values in diabetics are elevated above the normal range to 650 to 1230 mg/dL.

Two common methods of measuring seminal plasma fructose are the resorcinol test of Seliwanoff and the indole test of Karvonen and Malm. The Karvonen and Malm procedure requires deproteinization of the seminal plasma with zinc sulfate and sodium hydroxide. The resulting supernatant is then incubated at 50°C with an indole reagent and a colored product read at 470 nm. This procedure, as outlined by the World Health Organization laboratory manual for semen testing (now available in kit form), can be performed in most clinical laboratories.

Citric acid. In the human, citric acid is a useful biochemical marker for prostatic function. In this regard, it is commonly used to determine the relative contribution of the prostate to the seminal plasma as a whole. Although the andrological interest in citric acid historically has been limited to its use as a prostatic marker and its role remains enigmatic, there are data suggesting a correlation between seminal citric acid concentrations and circulating testosterone levels.

Acid phosphatase. There are a number of seminal phosphatases described to date, which include 1) monophosphatases (acid and alkaline); 2) pyrophosphatase; and 3) ATPases (acid, alkaline, and pyrophosphate-forming ATPase). Among these the monophosphatase called the acid (prostatic) phosphatase is the best known and best characterized. Like citric acid, acid phosphatase is a useful biochemical prostatic marker and in this regard is commonly used to determine the relative contribution of the prostate to the seminal plasma. Additionally, because of the heterogeneity of the forms of acid phosphatase found among

			PHYSICIAN OR LABORATORY			
LAST FIRST	PATIENT NAME MIDDLE	DATE OF SPECIMEN	DATE OF PROCESSED	SEX	AGE
ACCOUNT NUMBER	SPECIMEN NUMBER	ADDITIONAL INFORMATION			

RESULT

TIME SPECIMEN COLLECTED: _____   TIME SPECIMEN DELIVERED TO LAB: _____

TIME SPECIMEN TESTED: _____   METHOD OF COLLECTION: _____

DAYS OF ABSTINENCE: _____   POST VASECTOMY: _____

<table>
<tr><td></td><td></td><td></td><td colspan="2">RESULTS
NORM ABN</td></tr>
<tr><td>TIME OF LIQUEFACTION:</td><td>_____</td><td>(5–60 minutes)</td><td>_____</td><td>_____</td></tr>
<tr><td>VISCOSITY OF SPECIMEN:</td><td>_____</td><td></td><td>_____</td><td>_____</td></tr>
<tr><td>TOTAL VOLUME:</td><td>_____</td><td>(2–6 ml)</td><td>_____</td><td>_____</td></tr>
<tr><td>CONCENTRATION OF SPERM:</td><td>_____</td><td>(greater than 20×10^6/ml)</td><td>_____</td><td>_____</td></tr>
<tr><td>TOTAL COUNT:</td><td>_____</td><td>(60–300 million)</td><td>_____</td><td>_____</td></tr>
<tr><td>LEUKOCYTE CONCENTRAION:</td><td>_____</td><td>(less than 2,000/ml)</td><td>_____</td><td>_____</td></tr>
<tr><td>MOTILITY:</td><td>_____</td><td>(greater than 50%)</td><td>_____</td><td>_____</td></tr>
<tr><td>MORPHOLOGY:</td><td>_____</td><td>(greater than 60% normal)</td><td>_____</td><td>_____</td></tr>
</table>

PRINCIPLE CELL TYPES
   PRESENT (if abnormal specimen): _____

   ADDITIONAL COMMENTS:

REPORTED BY: _____   DATE: _____

Fig. 31-5   Sample semen analysis reporting form.

different individuals, this enzyme provides a powerful tool in the forensic detection of semen stains and in vaginal contents. Yet another clinically important aspect of the determination of acid phosphatase is in the area of diagnosis of prostatic cancer. It is well documented that serum acid phosphatase activity reaches abnormally elevated levels among patients with metastatic cancer of the prostate.

Zinc. Seminal plasma contains approximately 140 μg/mL of zinc, which comes primarily from the prostate. In a manner similar to citric acid and acid phosphatase, zinc may be used to determine the relative prostatic contribution to the seminal plasma as a whole.

Transferrin/lactoferrin. The iron-binding proteins ferritin, transferrin, and lactoferrin are biologically ubiquitous and their potential role in male reproductive biology is not clear. Elevated concentrations of ferritin in seminal plasma suggest that this protein is either produced in the male reproductive tract or sequestered from the circulation and are thought to play a role in protection against lipid peroxydation. Transferrin is produced by the Sertoli cells and is useful as a marker of spermatogenic function. Seminal concentrations of transferrin correlate well with seminal sperm cell concentration and are reported to correlate with sperm-fertilizing ability *in vitro*. In the male reproductive tract, lactoferrin is produced primarily by the seminal vesicles and may be used to determine the relative vesicle contribution to the seminal plasma in a manner similar to fructose. However, the physiological role of seminal lactoferrin is not understood.

Other measurements

Acrosome status. This phenomenon is of fundamental importance to the normal physiology of the spermatozoon. The ability of the andrology laboratory to determine the frequency of sperm in a semen sample which has undergone the acrosome reaction is often of clinical importance. The human has a relatively small acrosome for which the presence or absence (acrosomeal status) can only be determined using either electronmicroscopic or light microscopy in combination with special staining techniques. It is important to note that dead sperm undergo a spontaneous "shedding" of the acrosome. Therefore, it is important to utilize techniques which allow the distinction between cells which are alive and underwent the acrosome reaction versus sperm which are dead and shed their acrosomal membranes.

Historically, the first approach to determination of acrosomal status was the use of electronmicroscopy. This method is still considered the "gold standard"; but is inherently time consuming, expensive, and does not allow for the distinction of true acrosomal loss versus shed acrosomes. Subsequent staining techniques have made this determination more efficient. The triple stain developed by Talbert utilizes trypan blue as a viability stain; rose bengal to stain the acrosome, if it is present; and bismarck brown as a contrast stain. This approach has been widely used and addresses the issue of nonviable sperm shedding the acrosome. However, this staining approach is still fairly time consuming. More recently, techniques using fluorescenated plant lectins which bind specifically to sites on the acrosome region of mammalian sperm, in combination with a flu-

orescent supervital stain (e.g., propidium iodide or Hoechst 33258) have provided more efficient methods for this determination.

Antisperm antibodies. There are many reports indicating a relationship between the presence of either circulating or seminal anti-sperm antibodies and infertility. Additional studies have developed several lines of evidence implicating immunity to sperm as a cause of reproductive failure. However, there are contrasting data which indicate that infertility patients diagnosed with circulating anti-sperm antibodies may be relatively common among fertile individuals.

Some patients with seminal plasma anti-sperm antibodies will exhibit agglutination of sperm within 10 to 15 minutes after ejaculation. Since it is difficult to enumerate the number of sperm involved in agglutination, the approximate percentage of the total spermatozoa involved can be reported. There are a variety of methods used to detect anti-sperm antibodies.

To measure antibodies on the sperm cells' surface, our method is the mixed antiglobin reaction (MAR). This method uses sensitized red blood cells for detecting IgG or IgA class antibodies. The MAR test was adapted for routine use by Hendry and Stedronska and is described in various texts. Another common approach to measuring anti-sperm antibodies is the Immunobead Test (IBT). In this assay anti IgG, IgA or IgM molecules are bound to polystyrene beads which, when mixed with sperm, adhere to any sperm cells that are antibody coated. The immunobead test is now commercially available. Further examination of this area of reproductive immunology is required before a useful clinical interpretation of these data can be made. Current investigation of specific sperm antigen-antibody interactions are likely to provide a more thorough understanding of the complex nature of this problem.

Cervical mucus penetration. The presence of anti-sperm antibodies in the cervical mucus is another cause of infertility. Although these antibodies are generally IgA or, less commonly, IgG class, they may impair the movement of semen through the mucus. Semen, when allowed to come into contact with cervical mucus containing anti-sperm antibodies will remain motile yet do not exhibit forward progression resulting in a "shaking phenomenon."

Special techniques

Sperm washing. For many clinical procedures such as intrauterine insemination or many of the assisted reproduction techniques, it is desirable to remove the majority of the seminal plasma constituents from the spermatozoa. One common method for this is simply to "wash" the sperm by diluting the semen with tissue culture media (e.g., Tyrode's or a modified Tyrode's medium) between 1:1 and 1:3 (semen:media) and centrifuge the diluted sample at forces between 200 and 600 × g. This washing process is often repeated twice and the final pellet resuspended in a small volume (often 500 uL) of medium.

Swim-up technique. The use of the "sperm rise" technique in its original form involved the initial washing of the semen sample via dilution and subsequent centrifugation. Instead of resuspending the sperm pellet, the pellet is overlaid with fresh media and the centrifuge tube is incubated at 37°C for 1 hour. During this time, the progressively motile sperm "swim" out of the pellet, into the media. After the incubation period, the upper portion of the media is harvested yielding a population of spermatozoa with increased percent motility and decreased abnormal morphology. There are several modifications of this technique using various washing methods (or not washing at all) and incubation times, but the same basic principles are used among all of these so-called swim-up procedures.

Cryopreservation

While cryopreserved human spermatozoa has been used clinically since the mid-1950s, there has been a recent marked increase in the use of frozen sperm. During the past few years, it has become essential that only frozen-thawed human sperm be used for donor insemination. Although there are many advantages to using cryopreserved material, including the convenience of shipping and increased diversity of donor characteristics, the primary benefit is that the use of cryopreserved semen provides the opportunity to maintain samples over a period of time sufficient to retest donors for sexually transmissible diseases. This is particularly important for pathogens such as HIV and hepatitis B and C. Because of this advantage and the increased frequency of sexually transmissible pathogens in the general population, it is now considered clinically irresponsible to use nonfrozen-thawed/screened semen for donor insemination. Indeed the use of such semen is mandatory in many areas (e.g., New York and Indiana). In addition to donor insemination, the use of semen cryopreservation in the areas of assisted reproduction (e.g., IVF) and pre-iatrogenic loss of fertility (e.g., chemotherapy) is also rapidly increasing. Collectively, these developments increase the probability that andrology laboratories will be involved with the initial cryopreservation of semen or will be faced with processing previously frozen samples. Therefore, an understanding of what semen cryopreservation is and how frozen samples should be handled is essential to andrology laboratory personnel.

Historically, it is of interest to note that spermatozoa were the first cell type to be successfully cryopreserved. This was due to the serendipitous discovery of the cryoprotective properties of glycerol. Cryopreservation involves the cooling and storage of cells at a temperature low enough to prevent biological activity. This must be done in such a way that upon warming, at least some of the cells retain viability. When cells are cooled below approximately −5°C, water in the extracellular medium freezes, removing liquid water and increasing the solute concentration (osmolality). This in turn increases the chemical potential of the water inside the cell and water flows out of the cell into the surrounding media where it freezes. This process continues until the cells within their suspending medium reach a temperature at which they freeze intracellularly (intracellular freezing point).

During the cooling process, there are primarily two types of damage which can affect subsequent cell survival: 1) if cooling is too rapid, the cell will remain relatively hydrated and the ice formed within the cell (which will expand) will cause damage; 2) if cooling is too slow, the cell will become excessively dehydrated and the intracellular solute concentration will rise to damaging levels. To avoid these potential damaging effects, two solutions are commonly applied. To avoid intracellular freezing, the cooling rate must be adjusted to be slow enough to allow the cell to dehydrate prior to reaching its intracellular freezing point. For human spermatozoa, this rate is between 1 and 100°C/minute with an approximate optimum of 10°C/minute. To avoid the problem of increased intracellular and extracellular solute concentrations, cryoprotectant compounds, such as glycerol, dimethylsulfoxide or propylene glycol, are commonly utilized. These compounds are highly water soluble and act to reduce solute concentrations in the face of ice formation. Current methods for cryoprotectant of choice, use concentrations of approximately 0.5 to 1.0 Molar. It is also common to include macromolecular components which are unique to sperm cryopreservation and which putatively act as cryoprotectants. These are most often chicken egg yolk proteins and lipoproteins at concentrations of 5% to 20% v/v. Once cooling has occurred, storage is typically at a temperature of −196°C (in liquid nitrogen).

Warming or thawing frozen semen involves the removal of the samples from the liquid nitrogen storage device and allowing the sample to warm. Thawing is currently performed in a variety of ways (ice-water bath, bench top, warm-water bath) and is directly related to the manner in which the sample was frozen and the thermal properties of the vessel type used (e.g., plastic straw, vial, ampule). As the temperature of the cell suspension is increased and the existing ice crystals begin to liquefy, the ice may undergo a process called recrystallization in which partially liquefied areas fuse and form larger ice structures (analogous to the fusing of ice cubes in a glass of water). Formation of these larger ice structures can be damaging just as the formation of disruptive ice during the cooling process. Therefore, in general, the more hydrated the cell at the point of intracellular freezing point (cooling step), the more rapid the corresponding thawing rate should be (to minimize the recrystallization process). Conversely, the more dehydrated the cell during the cooling step, the slower the warming process should proceed. This phenomenon is termed the cooling rate/thawing rate interaction and has been demonstrated for a variety of cell types.

Computer-aided semen analysis

A major advancement in the area of Andrology generally and semen analyses specifically, has been the recent development of computer-aided semen-analysis systems or CASA. The CASA systems utilize computer-aided image analysis techniques to objectively measure motion characteristics of the spermatozoa. Among these motion characteristics is the commonly evaluated aspect of percent motility as described previously. However, using CASA, this value is obtained from actual counts of motile and nonmotile sperm, theoretically resulting in a percent motile value that is more accurate than the approach of simply subjectively estimating the motility. In addition to percent motility, most CASA systems quantitatively measure the velocity of the sperm (an objective value analogous conceptually to forward progression described above); the linearity or straightness

Table 31-3 Computed assisted analysis normal ranges (Cell Soft)

	Normal range (min-max) n = 61
Concentration (Million/mL)	22.79— 330.8
Volume (mL)	1.2 — 8.5
% Motility	38.35— 93.69
Conc. Motile (Million/mL)	9.41— 299.3
Total # Motile Cells (Million)	55.28—1100.
Mean Velocity (Microns/Sec)	25.02— 89.98
Mean Linearity	3.87— 7.07
Maximum	1.65— 5.7
Amplitude of Lateral Head Displacement (Microns)	
Mean	1.42— 4.88
Amplitude of Lateral Head Displacement (Microns)	
Beat/Cross Freq. (Hz)	11.11— 17.93
Morphology (% Normal)	> 50%

Table 31-4 Nomenclature for semen variables

Normozoospermia	Normal ejaculate as defined above
Oligozoospermia	Sperm concentration fewer than $20 \times 10^6/$mL
Asthenozoospermia	Fewer than 50% spermatozoa with forward progression (categories (a) and (b)) or fewer than 25% spermatozoa with category (a) movement (see Section 2.4.2)
Teratozoospermia	Fewer than 50% spermatozoa with normal morphology
Oligoasthenoterato- zoospermia	Signifies disturbance of all three variables (combinations of only two prefixes may also be used)
Azoospermia	No spermatozoa in the ejaculate
Aspermia	No ejaculate

World Health Organization: WHO laboratory manual for the examination of human semen and semen-cervical mucous interaction, pg 28, 1987.

of the sperm motion; the amplitude of lateral head displacement (how far the sperm head moves from side to side); and an estimate of flagellar beat frequency (Hz). In practice it is important to note that the true accuracy obtained using CASA methods depends heavily on the parameter settings used and the sperm concentration. These aspects of validating CASA systems for appropriate parameter settings and sperm concentration require careful attention just as any clinical assay.

Quality control

There is a growing need and concern for the application of more stringent quality control/quality assurance measures to be applied to the clinical andrology laboratory. Issues which need to be addressed are essentially those required for most other areas of the clinical laboratory. These include: 1) a clear description of laboratory services provided and written protocols for those procedures, 2) participation in a standardized proficiency testing program, 3) clear documentation of quality control measures in conjunction with an appropriate review process, 4) establishment and compliance with minimum educational and training requirements for laboratory personnel including laboratory directors, and 5) compliance with requirements of appropriate accrediting agencies regarding physical facilities and safety-related issues.

Safety

It should be noted that a variety of pathogens have been isolated from semen including Cytomegalovirus, Herpes, HIV, *Neisseria gonorrheae, Hycoplasma, Ureaplasma,* chlamydia, and others. Therefore, it is important to follow safe laboratory practices and universal precautions when handling semen.

SUGGESTED READING
Adelman MM and Cahill EM: Atlas of sperm morphology, Chicago, 1989, ASCP Press.

Hafez ESE: Techniques of human andrology, United Kingdom, 1977, Elsevier/North-Holland Biomedical Press.

Jequier AM and Crich UP: Semen analysis: a practical guide, Great Britain, 1986, Blackwell Scientific Publications.

Mann T: The biochemistry of semen and of the male reproductive tract, Great Britain, 1964, Butler & Tanner Ltd.

Mann T and Lutwak-Mann C: Male reproductive function and semen, Great Britain, 1981, Springer-Verlag Berlin Heidelberg.

Siebel MM: Infertility: A comprehensive text, Norwalk, Conn, 1990, Appleton and Lange.

World Health Organization: WHO laboratory manual for the examination of human semen and semen-cervical mucus interaction, New York, 1987, Cambridge University Press.

32

Gastrin and gastric fluid analysis

Stanford Marenberg

GASTRIN

Gastrin was one of the first hormones described in medical literature, with references dating back to the early 1900s. However, it was not until 1964 that gastrin was isolated and its structure elucidated by Gregory and Tracy. They showed that gastrin was a linear polypeptide of 17 amino acids. It has since been shown that gastrin is present in tissues and in the circulation in a variety of molecular species, as listed in Table 32-1.

The two most important molecular forms are G-17 (I and II) and G-34 (I and II). The alpha-numeric abbreviations refer to the number of amino acids in the particular gastrin (G) species, and the Roman numerals (I, II) refer to the absence or presence, respectively, of a sulfated tyrosine residue in the polypeptide chain. Sulfation apparently does not affect the physiologic activity of gastrin. In contrast, sulfation does affect immunologic recognition, resulting in significant differences among commercial antisera in their ability to accurately measure the various sulfated gastrin species. The majority of tissue gastrin (antral and duodenal) is non-sulfated, whereas gastrins in serum are both non-sulfated and sulfated.

Approximately 90% of tissue gastrin is G-17, whereas greater than 60% of serum gastrin, in the fasting state, is G-34. Postprandial blood samples contain about equal proportions of G-17 and G-34. The increased levels of G-34 in the fasting state are due to the longer half-life of the larger gastrin species. The half-life of G-34 is about five to six times longer than that of G-17.

Other molecular forms of gastrin occur in blood and in tissues. They include the major gastrin precursors, component I and big-big gastrin, and the smaller gastrin fragments, G-14 and N-terminal G-13, given in Table 32-1. Of the various gastrin species, G-17 has the greatest biologic potency and is five to six times more effective than G-34 as a stimulant of gastric acid secretion. The biologic potency of G-14 is similar to that of G-17. The four carboxyl-terminal amino acids (actually, the tetrapeptide amide) are considered the biologically active portion of the natural gastrin species. N-terminal G-13, the amino-terminal tridecapeptide, is unable to stimulate gastric acid secretion. Pentagastrin, a synthetic pentapeptide, contains the four carboxyl-terminal amino acids responsible for gastrin activity,

Table 32-1 Gastrin, molecular species

	Trivial name	Molecular weight (daltons)	Relative potency
G-17 I	Little Gastrin non-sulfated	2098	100%
G-17 II	Little Gastrin sulfated	2178	100%
G-34 I	Big Gastrin non-sulfated	3839	20%
G-34 II	Big Gastrin sulfated	3919	20%
G-14 I	Mini-Gastrin non-sulfated	1647	95%
G-14 II	Mini-Gastrin sulfated	1727	95%
NT-13	NH2-terminal fragment of G-17	1331	0%
C-I	Component I	12,000 (approximate)	?
BBG	Big-Big Gastrin	20,000 (approximate)	?

and is used as a diagnostic agent for the evaluation of gastric acid secretion.

Gastrin is synthesized and stored in the specialized endocrine G-cells. These cells are interspersed among the pyloric glands in the antrum and are also present in the duodenum, but to a lesser extent. Extracts of vagus nerve fibers supplying the stomach and duodenum have also been shown to contain gastrin.

Physiology of gastrin secretion

The major physiologic role of gastrin is stimulation of parietal-cell gastric acid secretion, as listed in Box 32-1. Gastrin also exerts a trophic effect on gastric and duodenal mucosa. Hyperplasia of the gastric mucosa is often observed in patients with Zollinger-Ellison (Z-E) syndrome. These changes are secondary to the chronic hypergastrinemia that is characteristic of this syndrome. In contrast, atrophy of the gastrointestinal mucosa is a common sequela to gastric resection and the resultant gastrin deficiency.

Gastrin release is stimulated by the thought, sight, and/or smell of food. This cephalic phase of gastrin stimulation is mediated by the brain via the vagus nerve. The gastric

Box 32-1   Physiologic actions of gastrin

Stimulation of gastric acid secretion
Stimulation of gastric and pancreatic enzyme secretion
Stimulation of gastric and pancreatic water and electrolyte
    secretion
Stimulation of gastric mucosal growth (body and fundus of
    stomach)
Stimulation of intrinsic factor secretion
Stimulation of contraction of lower esophageal sphincter,
    stomach, small intestine, gallbladder

**Box 32-2   Hypergastrinemia and decreased
gastric acid secretion**

Chronic Atrophic Gastritis
Pernicious Anemia
Gastric Carcinoma
Gastric Resection
Vagotomy

**Box 32-3   Hypergastrinemia and increased
gastric acid secretion**

Zollinger-Ellison Syndrome
Antral G-Cell Hyperplasia
Renal Failure
Gastric Outlet Obstruction
Pheochromocytoma
Hypercalcemia

phase of digestion is initiated by the introduction of food into the stomach. Of the various food groups, products of protein digestion, especially the amino acids tryptophan and phenylalanine, are the most potent stimuli of gastrin release. Carbohydrates and lipids, on the other hand, are weak stimulants of gastrin secretion. Inhibition of food-stimulated gastrin release occurs when acidification of the contents of the gastric lumen reaches pH 2.5.

Specimen collection and reference ranges

The methods employed for collection and storage of samples have been shown to have an effect on the observed gastrin value. Values from heparinized plasma may be as much as 33% lower, and those from EDTA plasma, 15% lower than comparable serum values. Temperature of sample storage is also an important consideration. Gastrin samples are unstable at room temperature, declining in value by as much as 50% after 24 hours. Gastrin values from serum samples stored at 4°C and at −6°C also decline over time. Blood samples for serum gastrin determinations should be collected on ice, centrifuged at 4°C, and stored at or below −40°C.

The upper limit of normal serum gastrin in fasting individuals ranges from 50 pg/mL to 300 pg/mL. Considerable variation exists with regard to normal ranges and observed patient values, which can be attributed to differences in antibody specificity, antibody cross-reactivity, and assay standardization. Depending on the gastrin species present, and the corresponding antibody specificity, up to a sixfold difference in apparent gastrin value can be observed for the same serum sample when assayed with different commercial antisera. As mentioned previously, gastrin is present in the blood in a variety of molecular species. The major circulating forms are G-17 and G-34. G-34 is the predominant fraction in the serum of normal fasting individuals, of ulcer patients, and of patients with Zollinger-Ellison syndrome, whereas G-17 is the major form present in the blood following a meal. In addition, both of these species exist as non-sulfated (G-17 I, G-34 I) and sulfated (G-17 II, G-34 II) forms. Unfortunately, commercial antisera often do not recognize the various gastrin species equally.

Clinical significance

The most common cause of increased gastrin levels is diminished gastric acid secretion, as shown in Box 32-2. An inverse relation exists between fasting serum-gastrin levels and gastric acid output. Modest hypergastrinemia is often observed in older patients, secondary to gastric mucosal atrophy and reduced gastric acid secretion. Markedly elevated levels of serum gastrin have been reported in patients with pernicious anemia. One of the hallmarks of pernicious anemia is achlorhydria.

Hypergastrinemia can also be associated with increased levels of gastric acid secretion, as listed in Box 32-3. One of the major indications for measuring serum gastrin is confirmation of a diagnosis of Zollinger-Ellison (Z-E) syndrome. Z-E syndrome is characterized by a gastrin-producing tumor(s), hypersecretion of gastric acid, ulcer disease, and/or diarrhea. Except for the symptoms resulting from possible tumor metastases, the clinical manifestations of this disorder are almost entirely due to the effects of the hypergastrinemia.

The diagnosis of Z-E is generally established by demonstration of increased levels of serum gastrin in the fasting state, of greater than 500 pg/mL, and by hypersecretion of gastric acid, with BAO greater than 15 mmol/hour, in the appropriate clinical setting. However, approximately 50% of gastrinoma patients show non-diagnostic fasting gastrin levels, with values between 200 pg/mL and 500 pg/mL. Since hypergastrinemia is a non-specific finding, gastric analysis should be performed on all patients in whom the diagnosis of Z-E syndrome is suspected. Gastric analysis will help rule out the more common causes of elevated gastrin levels, which are secondary to hypo- or achlorhydria.

The diagnosis of Z-E syndrome may be further substantiated with the aid of provocative testing. The most useful of these is the secretin-stimulation test. The protocol calls for the intravenous injection of secretin (2 C.U./kg body weight) and frequent blood sampling over a 30-minute interval, including a pre-secretin level, and sampling at 2½ minutes, 5 minutes, 10 minutes, 20 minutes, and 30 minutes. In normal individuals, intravenous administration of secretin has little effect on serum gastrin levels, whereas an increase over baseline of 200 pg/mL or more is consistent with the diagnosis of gastrinoma. Peak gastrin levels usually occur as soon as 5 or 10 minutes after the administration of secretin.

Studies have shown that the major molecular species of gastrin in the serum of patients with Z-E syndrome is G-34, as shown in Table 32-2. However, in 20% of these patients, big-big gastrin accounts for the major molecular form present, and in 10%, G-17 is the major molecular species. As such, normal levels of serum gastrin can be observed in some patients with gastrinoma if antiserum utilized for the gastrin determinations does not cross-react with the major gastrin species. The antiserum employed for these determinations should react not only with G-17, but also with G-34 and with big-big gastrin.

Unlike patients with Z-E syndrome, fasting serum-gastrin levels in patients with duodenal ulcer disease are not increased. However, these patients are more sensitive to the stimulatory effects of gastrin than normal individuals. The negative feedback mechanism by which acid in the stomach inhibits further gastrin release may also be blunted in duodenal ulcer patients. Overall, gastrin determinations contribute little to the evaluation and diagnosis of patients with commonly encountered ulcer disease.

GASTRIC ANALYSIS
Normal anatomy of the stomach

The stomach is a complex organ with muscular, glandular, and endocrine components each contributing, in an integrated fashion, to the process of digestion. Anatomically, the stomach is divided into four major regions, the cardia, fundus, body, and antrum, which are shown in Figure 32-1.

The most proximal portion of the stomach is the cardia, an area rich in mucus-secreting cardiac glands. Adjacent to the cardia are the fundus and body, which account for the largest portions of the stomach and in which the oxyntic glands, pictured in Figure 32-2, are found. The oxyntic glands are the secretory units of the gastric mucosa and contain parietal cells, which secrete HCl as well as intrinsic factor, important for vitamin B_{12} absorption. The oxyntic glands also contain chief cells, which secrete pepsinogen-I and -II. The most distal portion of the stomach is the antrum, which contains mucus-secreting pyloric glands.

Scattered among the glandular elements of the stomach, from the cardia to the antrum, are a variety of endocrine cell types, which are listed in Table 32-3. One type in particular, the G-cell, secretes the hormone gastrin, and is found in the antral portion of the stomach and in the duodenum. The secretory products of the endocrine cells act as

Table 32-2 Molecular forms of gastrin in patients with Zollinger-Ellison Syndrome

Major gastrin species	Frequency
G-34	70%
G-17	10%
Big-Big Gastrin	20%

From Johnson J, Fabri P, and Lott J: Serum gastrins in Zollinger-Ellison Syndrome: identification of localized disease. Clin Chem 26:867-870, 1980.

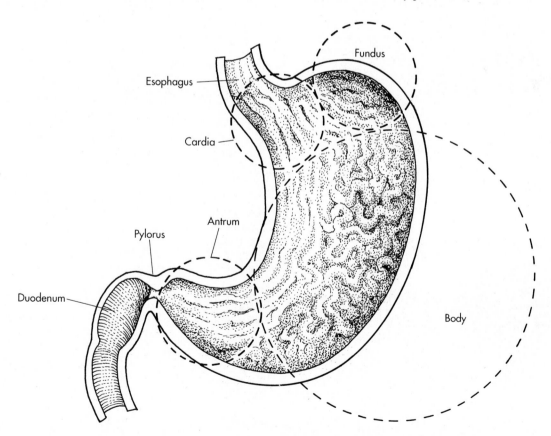

Fig. 32-1 Normal anatomy of the stomach.

chemical messengers, modulating normal digestive processes by a combination of endocrine, paracrine, and neurocrine mechanisms.

The mucosal surface of the stomach, as well as the lining of some of the glands, is composed of "surface cells," which secrete an alkaline mucus. This mucus provides the stomach wall a layer of protection from the acidic and digestive products of the oxyntic glands. Defects in the mucosal barrier are thought to be responsible for the development of gastric ulcers.

Physiology of acid secretion
Basal acid secretion

Both basal and stimulated acid secretion vary considerably among individuals, with secretion being greater in men than in women. Basal acid secretion appears to follow a circadian rhythm, reaching its peak around midnight and its nadir in the early morning hours. Between meals, the stomach secretes only a small volume of gastric juice, composed almost entirely of mucus, with little or no acid. Gastric secretions during this interdigestive period may actually be slightly alkaline, containing moderate quantities of bicar-

bonate. However, emotional stress can markedly increase the volume of interdigestive secretions up to 50 mL or more. The increased secretions caused by emotional stimuli may be an important factor contributing to the development of peptic ulcers.

Meal-stimulated acid secretion

The capacity to secrete HCl is directly related to the parietal cell mass of the stomach. The most important physiologic stimulus to these cells is the presence of food in the stomach, the mechanism being mediated by both neurologic and hormonal stimuli. Gastric secretion is traditionally divided into three separate phases—cephalic, gastric, and intestinal. As mentioned previously, the cephalic phase is initiated by the thought, sight, or smell of food. This phase of secretion accounts for between one third and one half of the total acid-secretory response associated with eating a meal. Acid secretion during the cephalic phase is largely mediated by direct vagal stimulation of parietal cells.

Once food enters the stomach, it initiates the gastric phase. Distention of the stomach wall activates stretch receptors, causing vagovagal reflexes that pass to the brain and return. These reflexes result in the release of acetylcholine and the stimulation of parietal cells. In addition to mechanical stimuli, chemical stimuli also play an important role in this phase of digestion. Gastrin release is stimulated by increased intraluminal pH and by food, especially protein hydrolysates. Fat and glucose are weak stimuli of gastric acid secretion. The gastric phase accounts for approximately 50% of the total gastric acid-secretory response to a meal.

The intestinal phase begins when digested food enters the duodenum. This phase accounts for only 5% of the total acid-secretory response. Only a small amount of gastrin is found in the upper small intestine. However, several other secretory products and hormones have been detected in this region of the intestine, which contribute to the intestinal phase of gastric acid secretion.

Mechanisms of hydrogen ion secretion

The oxyntic (parietal) cells secrete an electrolyte solution that can contain up to 160 mmole of HCl per liter. The hydrogen ion concentration of this solution would be equivalent to a pH of less than 1.0! The mechanisms involved in parietal-cell hydrogen-ion secretion are complex, but three different pathways have been described: a neurocrine pathway involving acetylcholine release from nerves in the stomach wall; an endocrine pathway involving gastrin release from the antral G-cells; and a paracrine pathway, involving local histamine release.

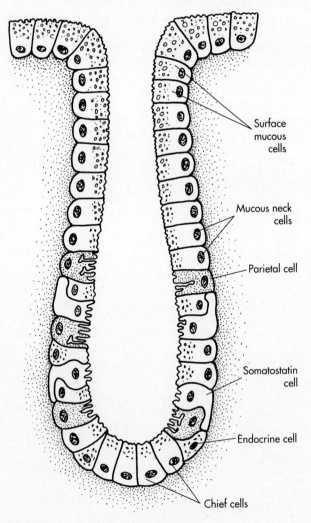

Fig. 32-2 Schematic diagram of an oxyntic gland in the body of the stomach.

Surface mucous cells

Mucous neck cells

Parietal cell

Somatostatin cell

Endocrine cell

Chief cells

Table 32-3 Endocrine cell types in the stomach

Cell type	Secretory product	Location
G	Gastrin	Antrum
D	Somatostatin	Fundus, Body, Antrum
EC₁	Substance P	Fundus, Body, Antrum
P	Gastrin-releasing peptide	Body, Antrum
?	Glicentin	Antrum
?	Vasoactive Intestinal Polypeptide (VIP)	Fundus, Body, Antrum

Acetylcholine and gastrin appear to stimulate the parietal cells by increasing cytosolic calcium ion, whereas parietal cell stimulation by histamine is mediated by cyclic AMP. Unique to the parietal cell is *hydrogen*-potassium ATPase, which exchanges hydrogen ion for potassium ion across cell membranes. In addition, a separate cotransport mechanism for potassium and chloride ions has also been described, which promotes secretion of both potassium and chloride ions. Potassium ions, thus secreted by the cotransport mechanism, are available for exchange with hydrogen ions via hydrogen-potassium ATPase.

Gastric analysis, laboratory aspects

The laboratory study of gastric acid secretion is usually expressed as the amount of acid secreted in the basal state (Basal Acid Output, BAO) and after maximal chemical stimulation (Maximal Acid Output, MAO). The test is performed in the morning, after an overnight fast. It is important that all medications that interfere with gastric acid secretion, particularly H_2-receptor antagonists, be discontinued 24 to 48 hours prior to testing.

Following fluoroscopic placement of a nasogastric tube, specimens are collected at 15-minute intervals for one hour. Pentagastrin is administered, intramuscularly, at a dose of 6 μg/kg, and specimens are subsequently collected at 15-minute intervals, for a total of 90 minutes. Volume, pH and titratable acidity, against 0.1 N NaOH, are measured on each 15-minute specimen. BAO is the sum of the acid secretion of the four 15-minute samples collected prior to the administration of pentagastrin. MAO is the sum of the acid secretion of the four highest consecutive 15-minute samples after pentagastrin is injected.

Gastric analysis, interpretation of results

Values for basal acid secretion are greater for males than for females, as shown in Table 32-4; values decline with advancing age. A diurnal variation has been observed for basal acid secretion. Basal secretory rates are lower in the morning and higher in the afternoon and evening. Considerable variability exists among individuals. Basal rates as high as 17 mmol/hour have been observed in apparently healthy individuals. Emotional stress is a significant factor contributing to elevated secretory rates.

The volume of basal acid secretion ranges normally from 50 mL/hour to 100 mL/hour. Decreased volume and/or decreased acid secretion in the basal state have little diagnostic significance. In contrast, BAO greater than 10 mmol/hour is suggestive of a hypersecretory state, possibly con-

tributing to duodenal ulcer disease. In addition, 66% of patients with Zollinger-Ellison syndrome (gastrinoma) have basal secretory rates greater than 10 mmol/hour; 50% have values greater than 15 mmol/hour. However, a small percentage of patients with duodenal ulcer disease also have BAO values greater than 15 mmol/hour.

Maximal acid output (MAO) reflects the number of parietal cells, that is, the parietal cell mass. Reference ranges (normal ranges) for both men and women are shown in Table 32-4. The upper limit of normal for MAO is approximately 48 mmol/hour for men and 30 mmol/hour for women. These values may appear elevated compared to values mentioned in the literature. Some publications list statistical *mean* values of BAO and MAO, rather than upper limits of normal.

One of the major indications for gastric analysis is confirmation of gastric acid hypersecretion in patients suspected of having Zollinger-Ellison syndrome, as listed in Box 32-4. Z-E syndrome is characterized by ulcer disease and marked hypersecretion of gastric acid in association with a non-beta islet cell tumor of the pancreas. The hypergastrinemia and concomitant gastric acid hypersecretion are responsible for the majority of the clinical manifestations. Almost 90 percent of Z-E syndrome patients develop ulcers during the course of their disease.

The diagnosis of Z-E syndrome is usually established by demonstration of markedly elevated fasting gastrin values and BAO values greater than 15 mmol/hour, in the appropriate clinical setting. Following pentagastrin stimulation, the BAO/MAO ratio is often greater than 0.6, owing to gastrin-induced HCl hypersecretion in the basal state. In contrast, patients with common duodenal ulcer disease typically have BAO/MAO ratios less than 0.6. However, these values need to be interpreted with caution, since fewer than 50% of Z-E syndrome patients have BAO/MAO ratios greater than 0.6. Laboratory evaluation of a patient for Z-E syndrome usually includes measurement of BAO, fasting serum-gastrin levels, and studies of secretin-stimulated gastrin release.

Acid secretory studies contribute little, if anything, to the diagnosis of common ulcer disease. Although about 50% of patients with duodenal ulcers show increased rates of gastric acid secretion, the remaining 50% demonstrate normal acid secretory rates. Therefore, measurement of acid secretion is usually not helpful in differentiating between patients with duodenal ulcers and normal individuals.

Gastric acid secretion diminishes with age, more so in men than in women. For individuals over the age of 60, acid secretion is decreased in approximately 45% of men, and in 35% of women. In this age group, achlorhydria following pentagastrin stimulation occurs with a frequency

Table 32-4 Reference ranges for basal and maximal acid output*

	Basal acid output (BAO) mmole/hour	Maximal acid output (MAO) mmole/hour
Men	0—10	7—48
Women	0— 6	5—30

From Feldman M: Gastric secretion in health and disease. In Sleisenger M and Fordtran J, eds: Gastrointestinal Disease, Philadelphia, 1989, WB Saunders, 717-734.
*95% Confidence Limits

Box 32-4 Indications for gastric analysis

Zollinger-Ellison Syndrome (diagnosis; assessment of medical therapy)
Evaluation of Hypergastrinemia
Estimation of Parietal Cell Mass (prior to gastric surgery)
Assessment of Completeness of Vagotomy

of about 25% for men and 10% for women. Diminished acid secretion is commonly observed in patients with chronic atrophic gastritis and gastric atrophy. Chronic gastritis, which increases with age, is probably the main cause of hypo- and achlorhydria observed in the elderly.

Nearly 20% of patients with gastric carcinoma demonstrate achlorhydria following pentagastrin administration. Historically, gastric secretory studies were sometimes utilized to help differentiate between gastric carcinoma and benign disease. However, these studies are currently not recommended because of the low incidence of achlorhydria in gastric carcinoma patients. In addition, 20 to 30% of normal individuals over the age of 60 will also demonstrate achlorhydria. Radiologic studies, especially endoscopy, are considered to be more sensitive and specific for diagnosis of gastric and duodenal ulcer disease.

SUGGESTED READING

Feldman M: Gastric secretion in health and disease. In Sleisenger M and Fordtran J eds: Gastrointestinal Disease, Philadelphia, 1989, WB Saunders 717-734.

Heise C and Richter J: Clinically significant differences in serum gastrin concentrations as measured with commercial RIA reagents, J Clin Immunoassay 10:173-177, 1987.

Johnson J, Fabri P and Lott J: Serum gastrins in Zollinger-Ellison syndrome: identification of localized disease, Clin Chem 26:867-870, 1980.

Kubasic N, Ricotta M, Hunter T, and Sine H: Effect of duration and temperature of storage on serum analyte stability: examination of 14 selected radioimmunoassay procedures, Clin Chem 28:164-165, 1982.

Spindel E, Harty R, Leibach J, and McGuigan J: Decision analysis in evaluation of hypergastrinemia, Am J Med 80:11-17, 1986.

Wolfe M and Jensen R: Zollinger-Ellison Syndrome, N Engl J Med 317:1200-1209, 1987.

Wolfe M and Soll A: The physiology of gastric acid secretion, N Engl J Med 319:1707-1715, 1988.

PART FIVE

IMMUNOLOGY

33

Immunobiology, immunochemistry, and immunopathology

Mario R. Escobar

This chapter is intended to serve as an introduction to immunology. A basic approach will be used with particular emphasis on those areas of human immunology considered to be most appropriate to the practice of clinical laboratory medicine, irrespective of laboratory size. Although the chapter title implies a vast scope of subject matter, space will allow only the presentation of major concepts regarding the biological (i.e., immunobiology) and clinical (i.e., immunopathology) relevance of the molecular nature (i.e., immunochemistry) of the interacting elements of the immune response. Hopefully, the up-to-date references at the end of this chapter will satisfy readers who need greater detail.

Any compartmentalization of the immune system is made chiefly for didactic purposes and may not always be functionally real. In practice it is difficult to identify an infectious agent that does not challenge multiple-host defense mechanisms. In fact the concept of overlapping host defenses is basic to our understanding of susceptibility to infection because immunological redundancy may be crucial to the preservation of health, even though an apparently significant host immune defect might be present.

IMMUNOBIOLOGY
Host-parasite interactions

Infection, the process by which a parasite enters into a relationship with its host, turns out to be a harmful event in only a minority of cases. Most host-parasite interactions do not result in disease, since the infection is eradicated or remains latent or subclinical. The outcome of this relationship is determined by characteristics of the parasite that favor its establishment—with resulting damage to the host—and by the various host mechanisms that oppose these processes. If the parasite injures the host to a significant degree, disturbances will occur in the host that manifest themselves as disease. The host defense systems and operational factors that determine resistance to microorganisms are presented in Table 33-1. These systems include the first line of external defense, innate (or natural) immunity and adaptive (or acquired) immunity. They are modulated by a number of factors, which can be separated into three groups.

The first two groups consist of nonspecific factors that operate against a variety of parasites at the portal of entry. These factors consist, in part, of nonspecific anatomic barriers (e.g., skin and mucous membranes), biochemical tissue products (e.g., lysozyme, proteolytic enzymes, basic polypeptides, fatty acids, etc.); and physiologic reactions (e.g., fever, acid pH, etc.); as well as cellular components (e.g., phagocytes and natural killer cells) and acute-phase proteins, which mediate the inflammatory response (e.g., complement, C-reactive protein, interferon, cytokines, prostaglandins, leukotrienes and thromboxanes).

The third group consists of specific factors (e.g., antibodies and T lymphocytes) involved with immunologic responses (i.e., humoral and cellular) toward specific agents. The protection conferred on the host may range from almost total susceptibility to complete resistance. Therefore, "resistance" and "immunity" are relative terms implying simply that one host is more or less susceptible to a given infection than another host (e.g., due to race, age, physiologic state, or genetic differences). In general, immunity and predisposition toward specific disease states have a genetic component. Disease susceptibility is related to genes closely associated with the major histocompatibility complex (MHC), particularly the HLA-D region located in chromosome 6 in humans, which is believed to carry the immune response (Ir) genes.

Natural immunity is not acquired through previous contact with the infectious agent (or with related species), but is largely genetically determined (e.g., species immunity). On the other hand, passively acquired immunity may be induced either temporarily (i.e., a few weeks) by administering antibodies against an infectious agent (e.g., immune and hyperimmune globulins) preformed against that agent in another host, or by the *in utero* transfer of antibodies from the mother to the fetus. The latter protects the newborn child—at least during the first three to four months of life—against some common infections and can be reinforced by antibodies through the mother's milk (i.e., mainly colostrum). Actively acquired or adaptive immunity is a state of resistance built up in an individual as a result of an effective contact with foreign antigens (e.g., microorganisms or their products). An effective contact may consist of clinical or subclinical infection, injection with live or killed microorganisms or their antigens, or absorption by bacterial products (e.g., toxins, toxoids). Active immunity (i.e., humoral

Table 33-1 Host defense systems and operational factors

First line of defense (external)	Innate (natural) immunity	Adaptive (acquired) immunity*
Normal Bacterial Flora (lactobacilli)	Acute Phase Proteins Complement	Naturally Acquired Active (infection)
Anatomic Barriers (skin, mucosae, cilia)	C-reactive Protein Interferon	Passive (transplacental) Artificially Acquired
External Secretions (mucus, tears, sweat)	Cytokines Arachidonic Acid Metabolites	Active (vaccination) Passive (γ-globulin)
Antimicrobial Substances (lysozyme, fatty acids)	Inflammatory Response (edema, fever)	
	Cellular Components	
	Granulocytes	
	Monocytes and Macrophages	

*Humoral (B lymphocytes, plasma cells, antibodies) and cellular (T lymphocytes)

or cellular) develops slowly over a period of days or weeks but tends to persist, usually for years.

Anatomic contributions to the development and function of the immune system

Many organs participate in host defenses and are either involved with the activity of the immune system or affected by it. Some of the interactions between certain organs—such as the thymus, spleen, lymph nodes, bone marrow and regional lymphoid tissue (e.g., Peyer patches, tonsils, appendix)—and the immune system are well known. Other interactions are known to exist but are not well defined (e.g., interactions connected with the central nervous system, liver, skin, etc.). The spread of infection by simple extension may be prevented by anatomic barriers between and within the organs. For example, the fibrous capsules around most organs are more resistant to penetration than the soft tissues they surround. Hematogenous, lymphatic dissemination of infectious agents, or possible erosion of the capsule are the means by which these barriers may be overcome.

Available evidence suggests that the human immune system begins to develop *in utero* during the second and third months of gestation. The earliest site of development for blood cell precursors may be in the para-aortic mesenchyme of the embryo. These embryonic cells migrate into the yolk sac, where they form blood islands. Cells destined to perform both nonspecific and specific immunologic functions are believed to have a common ancestral origin. Both cell types appear to differentiate from a population of progenitor cells referred to as stem cells or hemocytoblasts. These are found in the hematopoietic tissues of the developing embryo (yolk sac, fetal liver, and bone marrow). Depending on the characteristics of the microchemical environment surrounding these cells, their maturation will proceed along at least two different pathways: the hematopoietic and the lymphopoietic. The former leads to proliferation and differentiation of nonlymphoid stem cell hematopoietic precursors. The products of these cell lines are the hematopoietic elements of the peripheral blood and tissues and include the erythrocytes, granulocytes, platelets and monocytes. The progenitor cells that differentiate along the second pathway are the stem cell lymphoid precursors. These cells can follow one of two different routes. The first, under the influence

of the thymus, perhaps within the substance of the gland itself, consists of a population of small lymphocytes (thymic dependent or T lymphocytes) that are assigned the role of cell-mediated immunity. The second route, which is under the influence of the bursal equivalent in humans (e.g., the bone marrow), produces, as a result of further differentiation, a population of lymphocytes (B lymphocytes) and plasma cells involved with humoral immunity or antibody synthesis.

The biological role of this two-compartment system is of major relevance to clinical laboratory medicine since it lays the foundation on which rests our understanding of immunologic deficiency disorders (See Chapter 36.). The type of infectious agent against which the host is unable to defend itself depends on which of the two compartments is affected and at what point the impairment has occurred. For example, selective deficiencies within the thymic-dependent compartment will render the host susceptible to fungal and viral infections; whereas individuals who present with deficiencies affecting the bursa-equivalent tissues will suffer from recurrent bacterial infections. Individuals with profound abnormalities in both compartments will therefore experience the most severe sequelae of all the immunologic deficiency syndromes and frequently will succumb to a diversity of infections.

In addition to the anatomic relationships already described, it is also important to mention the immunologic relevance of maternal-fetal relationships, as well as the interactions between the neuroendocrine and the immune systems.

One of the most significant steps in the evolution of vertebrates was the emergence of multilayered placenta in the viviparous species. On the one hand, the placenta acts as a mechanical barrier against the paternal antigens from the fetus during pregnancy and separates the formed elements of the mother's blood from those of the fetus. On the other hand, certain substances (e.g., IgG immunoglobulins) purposely pass from the maternal circulation to the fetus' circulation, providing protection to the fetus and newborn infant during at least the first three months of life. This is accomplished by an active transport mechanism of IgG antibodies by virtue of a receptor located on the Fc fragment of the molecule. Thus the fetus receives a library of preformed maternal antibodies, reflecting most of the mother's experiences with infectious agents. Despite this awesome teleologic design, occasionally fetal cells or certain proteins escape into the maternal circulation. This unusual process may then actively sensitize the mother to the paternal allotypes (antigen) associated with these transgressors.

The immune system is by no means isolated from other control systems of the body; indeed, many possibilities exist for communication between the nervous, endocrine, and immune systems. This can be deduced from morphological evidence of the innervation of lymphoid tissues. The fibers connect not only to blood vessels, which modulate cellular traffic, but also to neuroendocrine cells which release hormones that can influence lymphocytes. Lymphocytes themselves have receptors for a wide variety of hormones, including corticosteroids, insulin, catecholamines, growth hormone, and met-enkephalin. Furthermore, virtually every hormone investigated has some effect on the immune system, although not necessarily direct effects. Evidence shows that the thymus may play a central role both in receiving nervous and hormonal signals and in relaying them to the immune system via its own hormones. The physiological manifestations of neuroendocrine control of the immune system can be observed in the effects of stress on the immune responses. For example, an immunosuppressive effect, which is mediated mainly by corticosteroids, endorphin, and met-enkephalin has usually been noted. This may represent a general effect resulting from degradation of the integrity of the body's control systems by stress. Interestingly, when the challenge posed by the stressing agent is met by an adequate coping response, the immune system may be unaffected or even stimulated to respond stronger than usual. This coping response may also be mediated by the nervous system, since the pineal hormone melatonin can reverse the immunosuppressive effect of stress on the immune system of animals responding to a virus infection. Although it is unlikely that the neuroendocrine system can process information directly related to immunological specificity, there are many instances where it can control the intensity, modality, kinetics, and localization of immune responses. Conversely, lymphoid cells themselves can produce immunoreactive hormones such as adrenocorticotropic hormone (ACTH), follicle stimulating hormone (FSH), and thyroid stimulating hormone (TSH), which may have further modulating effects on the immune response.

Cells involved in nonspecific immune responses and their effector mechanisms

The so-called "Lymphoreticular System," which consists of various types of cells distributed strategically throughout the tissues as well as lining lymphatic and vascular channels, is ubiquitous among the vertebrates. The cells of the internal secretory component of this system are housed within the blood, tissues, thymus, lymph nodes, and spleen; whereas those of the external secretory component are in certain areas of the body exposed to the external environment, such as the respiratory, gastrointestinal, and genitourinary tracts.

The tissues contain a variety of cell types, each performing a separate function either directly or through the elaboration of soluble products (e.g., cytokines). The system can be activated by a variety of stimuli that have the common

characteristic of being recognized as foreign by the host. These stimuli may be presented to the host either exogenously (e.g., microorganisms) or endogenously (e.g., effete cells or transformed neoplastic cells). Following activation, a spectrum of cellular and humoral events occurs as a part of the nonspecific and specific immune responses.

Initially, the body will react to injury through the nonspecific process of inflammation comprising the following events:

1. blood supply to the infected area is increased;
2. capillary permeability caused by the retraction of endothelial cells is also increased to permit larger molecules (i.e., soluble mediators of immunity) to traverse the endothelium and reach the site of infection;
3. leukocytes, particularly neutrophils and to a lesser extent macrophages, migrate out of the capillaries and into the surrounding tissue.

The cells then move from the tissue toward the site of infection by a process called "chemotaxis." Once at the site of injury phagocytosis by the so-called professional phagocytes (macrophages, monocytes, neutrophils and, to a lesser extent, eosinophils) ensues as part of the nonspecific response, thus representing the body's initial confrontation with foreignness.

A few terms should be clarified before describing the biological properties of the cells involved with inflammation. Endocytosis is a rather general term which includes both phagocytosis (i.e., ingestion of particles) and pinocytosis (i.e., uptake of nonparticulates or fluid droplets). In humans, these functions are carried out primarily by the professional phagocytes, which are able to recognize and ingest particles and soluble ligands through receptors on their cell surfaces and to digest these substances within lysosomal compartments. Mononuclear phagocytes, however, show much greater diversity in function and response than polymorphonuclear leukocytes. This diversity of structure and function is the result of the progressive maturation of monocytes and macrophages from their bone marrow precursors, their experiences with endocytosis, and their interactions with T lymphocytes.

Further details on the molecular biology of these nonspecific effector mechanisms, including phagocytosis and chemotaxis, are beyond the scope of this discussion. For in-depth discussions of these areas, use the references at the end of this chapter.

Mononuclear phagocytes

The mononuclear phagocytes include both monocytes of the circulating blood and macrophages found in various tissues of the body. They are produced in the bone marrow, undergo proliferation, and then are released into the blood after a period of maturation through the stages of monoblast, promonocyte, and monocyte. One to two days later, they migrate from the blood to the tissues where they differentiate further into macrophages. On the basis of their common origin from a hematopoietic stem cell, morphologic features, and observed functions, these cells have been grouped together into one system: "The Mononuclear Phagocyte System." Despite the unifying concept of this classification scheme, mononuclear phagocytes are also heterogeneous since different cell subpopulations acquire and display diverse functional properties depending on the environment of the organ system in which they home, including the lymphatic organs and connective tissues.

Macrophages are highly specialized to perform their function in the ingestion and destruction of all particulate matter. Thus, they remove and destroy certain bacteria, damaged or effete cells, neoplastic cells, colloidal materials, and macromolecules. The phagocytic process is sometimes facilitated by antibodies (or opsonins) for easier ingestion. Complement may also assist as an amplifier of phagocytosis. The circulating monocytes are attracted to an area of injury by chemotaxis. A number of chemotactic factors exist, some of which are derived from the complement system or secreted by the T lymphocytes. Besides their functions of defense and surveillance, mononuclear phagocytes play a role in the initial recognition and processing of antigen, leading to the induction of specific immunologic responses.

Neutrophils or polymorphonuclear leukocytes

In humans, circulating granulocytes include three varieties of morphologically identifiable cells involved in a number of immunologic reactions in tissue: the neutrophil, the eosinophil, and the basophil. Of these, only the neutrophil and, to a lesser extent, the eosinophil are primarily phagocytic. Unlike the macrophage, the neutrophil is an end cell of myeloid differentiation and does not divide. The neutrophils also arise in the bone marrow from common ancestral stem cells and, after a series of divisions, undergo maturation through the phases of myeloblast, promyelocyte, metamyelocyte, band cell, and mature polymorphonuclear leukocyte. After remaining in the blood for 12 hours, the mature neutrophils enter the tissues, where they complete their life span of only a few days.

Eosinophils

Eosinophils mature in the bone marrow in three to six days before delivery into the circulation. In the circulation they have a half-life of approximately 30 minutes. In tissues, where they fulfill their major function, eosinophils have a half-life of 12 days. Like the neutrophil, they do not return from tissues to the circulation but are eliminated through the mucosal surfaces of the respiratory and gastrointestinal tracts. Unlike the neutrophils, the granules of the eosinophil do not contain lysozyme and phagocytin but are rich in acid phosphatase, peroxidase, and eosinophilic basic protein.

Although eosinophils can phagocytose a variety of particles, including microorganisms and soluble antigen-antibody complexes, the process appears less efficient than that of neutrophils. In addition to their well-established association with allergic and parasitic diseases, research suggests that eosinophils ingest immune complexes, limit inflammatory reactions by antagonizing the effects of certain mediators (e.g., aryl sulfatase B from eosinophils inactivates SRS-A released by mediator cells); direct cytotoxicity by the release of toxic components (e.g., eosinophilic basic protein); and direct antibody-mediated cytotoxic reactions involved in the clearance of certain parasites (e.g., Schistosoma). The regulation of eosinophils involves a complex set of mechanisms, including products of T lymphocytes, complement components, and mast cell products (e.g., eo-

sinophilic chemotactic factor A or ECFA, as well as a variety of arachidonic acid metabolites).

Mediator cells

These cells may participate in immunologic reactions through the release of chemical substances (mediators) that have a variety of biologic activities, including increased vascular permeability, contraction of smooth muscle, and enhancement of the inflammatory response. They consist of a heterogeneous collection of morphologic types, including mast cells, basophils, platelets, enterochromaffin cells, and certain phagocytic cells (e.g., neutrophils and macrophages participating in the allergic response are major sources of SRS-A leukotrienes, prostaglandins, and kinins). The major mediator cells in the circulation are basophilic granulocytes and platelets, which have been shown to contain a variety of vasoactive amines (e.g., histamine and serotonin). The granules of basophils contain acid mucopolysaccharides (e.g., heparin). Although basophils and mast cells resemble each other morphologically, they differ in several ways (e.g., the ultrastructure of their granules). There are two kinds of mast cells. One is mucosa associated (MMC) and the other is found in the connective tissue (CTMC). MMCs appear to depend on T cells for their proliferation. On the other hand, the CTMCs are T-cell independent.

Cells involved in specific immune responses and their effector mechanisms

The cells responsible for specific immune responses are distributed in organs and tissues, which collectively are known as the lymphoid system. This system is composed of various subpopulations of lymphocytes, as well as plasma, epithelial, and stromal cells. It is structured into either discretely encapsulated organs or accumulations of diffuse lymphoid tissue. The lymphoid system may be envisioned in two compartments. One includes the primary or central lymphoid organs, which are the major sites of lymphopoiesis and provide the appropriate microenvironment for the maturation and differentiation of T and B lymphocytes into functional immunocytes. Accordingly, in humans, these organs are the thymus; where T lymphocytes are produced, fetal liver; bone marrow; and an area yet to be fully identified (i.e., the bursa-equivalent tissue). Islands of hematopoietic cells can be found in the fetal liver, as well as in the fetal and adult bone marrow, which give rise directly to B lymphocytes. Interestingly, the adult bone marrow serves not only as a site of B cell generation, but also as an important secondary lymphoid organ that contains many mature T lymphocytes and plasma cells.

The second compartment includes the secondary or peripheral lymphoid organs, where lymphocytes can interact with each other and with antigens, thus serving to disseminate the immune response once it has been elicited. These functions are executed by phagocytic macrophages, antigen-presenting cells, and mature T and B lymphocytes. The differentiation of lymphocytes in the peripheral compartment is antigen dependent; whereas the maturation of these cells in the central compartment can occur in the absence of antigen.

Lymphocytes and plasma cells differ from mononuclear phagocytes and granulocytes, as previously described, by their ability to react specifically with antigen and to elaborate specific cell products. Once sensitized, these cells become committed and are also referred to as "immunocytes." An immunocyte is a cell of the lymphoid series which, when reacting with antigen, can produce antibodies or a cell-mediated event. Differentiation of the two types of lymphocytes found in the peripheral lymphoid tissue depends on their respective sites of maturation in the central lymphoid system.

Phenotype identification and enumeration of the various T and B lymphocyte subpopulations have been made possible by the presence of a number of surface markers, or antigens, on these cells. Each antigen is detected with monoclonal antibodies and is expressed on a molecule(s) that plays an important role in the differentiation and function of these cells (Table 33-2).

Additional information on the structure of the primary and secondary lymphoid organs is provided in the reference sources found at the end of this chapter.

T cell functions

T lymphocytes, which develop in the thymus and differentiate into small lymphocytes, mediate two types of immunological functions: effector and regulatory. Effector functions include reactivity, such as delayed hypersensitivity, allograft rejection, tumor immunity, and graft-versus-host reactivity. These effector functions represent two general properties of T lymphocytes: the secretion of soluble mediators of immunity (e.g., lymphokines) and cytotoxicity (i.e., the ability to kill other cells). Regulatory functions include the amplification of cell-mediated cytotoxicity by other T cells and immunoglobulin synthesis by B cells. The regulatory functions also require the production of lymphokines. The α/β heterodimer represents the T lymphocyte antigen receptor (Ti). The receptor does not recognize soluble antigen alone. Instead, the T cell antigen receptor recognizes antigen in conjunction with products of MHC genes (i.e., Class I and Class II molecules). In the case of soluble antigens, recognition occurs in the context of Class II molecules; whereas, for viral antigens, recognition takes place in connection with Class I antigens. Moreover, large, soluble antigens must be processed by an appropriate accessory cell (e.g., macrophage or dendritic cell). There appears to be a mechanism whereby a binding site is generated from an associative determinate represented by antigen plus MHC as a result of the interaction between the α and β chains of the T cell receptor. The final confirmation of this mechanism would provide another similarity between the T cell antigen receptor and antibody molecules where the combination of light and heavy chains produce the best binding to antigen when compared to the binding of isolated light and heavy chains.

B cell functions

There is evidence that in humans, all types of hematopoietic cells, including B lymphocytes, develop from a pluripotential stem cell. The evidence is that individuals with chronic myelogenous leukemia and a marker Philadelphia

Table 33-2 Cluster designation of leukocytes by identification of their cell surface markers

Antigen	Mol. wt. (KD)	Monoclonal antibodies	Cell distribution	Identity/function
CD1	43-49	Leu 6, T6, OKT6	Thymocytes	
CD2	50	Leu 5B, T11, OKT11	T cells, NK cells	Sheep erythrocyte receptor
CD3	20-26	Leu 4, T3, OKT3	Mature T cells	Part of T cell antigen receptor complex
CD4	60	Leu 3, T4, OKT4	Helper-inducer T cells, monocytes	MHC class II restricted immune recognition
CD5	67	Leu 1, T, T101	T cells, B cell subset	Lymphoblastic lymphoma, chronic lymphocytic leukemia, pre-lymphocytic leukemia
CD6	120	T12	T cells	
CD7	40	Leu 9, 3A1	T cells	? IgM Fc receptor
CD8	32	Leu 2, T8, OKT8	Suppressor-cytotoxic T cells	MHC class I restricted immune recognition
CD9	100	BA-2		Lymphoid leukemia associated antigen
CD10	160	CALLA, J5	Pre-B cells, granulocytes	Pre-B leukemia cells
CD11	150	CR3/Leu 15, OKM1, MO1, Mac-1	Monocytes, granulocytes	1 subset: Complement C3bi receptor
CD15	50-80	Leu M1	Monocytes, granulocytes	Carbohydrate hapten
CD16	50-70	Leu 11	Granulocytes, NK cells	Low affinity Fc receptor (FcγRIII)
CD18	95		Leukocytes	β-chain of LFA-1, CR3
CD19	40-80	Leu 12, B4	Pan-B cells	
CD20	35	Leu 16, B1	B cells, dendritic cells	
CD21	140	CR2, B2	Mature B cells, dendritic cells	Complement C3d receptor (CR2)
CD22	135	Leu 14, B3	B cells	
CD23	45	Blast-2, B6	Activated B cells	Low affinity IgE receptor
CD24		BA-1	Pre-B cells	
CD25	60	IL-2 receptor	Activated T cells, B cells, macrophages	IL-2 receptor (low affinity polypeptide chain), α-chain
CD28	44		T cell subset	
CD33	67	My9	Monocyte precursors, monocytes	
CD35	220		Various types of cells	Complement receptor CR1

chromosome in their malignant cells possess the same chromosomal abnormality in all hematopoietic cell lines, including both B and T lymphocytes. Also, early divergence of blood cell development along at least two pathways has been suggested based on the finding that individuals with polycythemia vera manifest an aberrant development of erythrocytes, platelets, and myeloid cells but relatively normal lymphoid elements. Experimental studies in rodents, using marker chromosomes or radiation-induced chromosome lesions, have similarly provided evidence for a common origin of lymphoid, myeloid, erythroid, and megakaryocytic cells, followed by an early separation of lineages along two branches: the lymphoid versus the hematopoietic precursor cell populations. Thus, despite their common cell origin, T and B cells appear to diverge from other hematogenous elements and from each other early in their developmental history.

The stages in the natural history of B cells include the antigen-independent development of stem cells into pre-B cells followed by the antigen-dependent development of B cells into plasma cells. These stages in B lymphocyte differentiation can be defined by both phenotypic markers and functional properties. Monoclonal antibodies can be used to identify cell surface markers on human B lymphocytes. Such antibodies may react with all cells of B lineage or with surface molecules expressed only at certain points in B cell differentiation. For instance, monoclonal antibodies to the C3d receptor, which also serves as the EBV receptor, are reactive with mature B cells in both resting and activated states but appear unreactive with pre-B and mature plasma cells. Antigens detected on B cells may also be expressed by cells of other lineages, such as monocytes or T cell populations, but may still provide useful markers for functional B lymphocyte subpopulations. An example is the T10 glycoprotein expressed by some B cells and non-B cells. Within the B lineage, expression of this antigen is restricted to pre-B, immature B, and plasma cells. Mature B cells do not express detectable T10 antigen.

After antigen or mitogen stimulation, B lymphocytes can proceed along one of two pathways: They can either differentiate (with or without cell division) into plasma cells and secrete large amounts of immunoglobulin, or they can divide and return to a resting state as small, postmitotic B lymphocytes that function as memory B cells. The latter can rapidly differentiate into plasma cells after a second exposure to the homologous antigen.

Plasma cell functions

Plasma cells represent the terminally differentiated state of high-rate antibody synthesis and secretion toward which all B cells aspire. It has been calculated that more than 40% of the total protein synthesized and secreted by plasma cells may be immunoglobulin. Thus a single plasma cell can release thousands of antibody molecules per second. A cell type known as plasmablast can be described both morphologically and functionally as existing between the activated lymphocyte (or B lymphoblast) and plasma cell stages. Unlike activated B cells, they actively secrete immunoglobulin, albeit at a lower rate than mature plasma cells. Such plasmablasts contribute a large proportion of the antibody-secreting cells during the early phases of antibody responses.

Few plasmablasts and plasma cells can be found in the circulation; most are present in lymphoid tissues, such as the medullary cords of lymph nodes, red pulp areas of the spleen, lamina propria of the intestinal and respiratory tracts, and bone marrow sinusoids.

The role of the complement system in the immune response

The complement system, an integral component of the host's defenses, has evolved primarily for protective functions, and is essential to maintaining health. The complement system offers three major functions in host defense:

1. coating pathogenic microorganisms or immune complexes with opsonins, resulting in removal by phagocytes;
2. activating inflammatory cells; and
3. killing target cells.

These three functions can be performed by the classical or alternative pathway. Both pathways have a similar molecular organization consisting of three operational phases: recognition, amplification, and membrane attack. Understanding the modulating mechanisms operating in the two pathways—which regulate the activation of the complement cascade and control the synthesis of biologically active split products—is important for diagnosing and managing patients who present with recurrent infectious allergic diseases and autoimmune disorders. This system's vital role is illustrated by the onset of recurrent infections or immune complex diseases in patients with congenital defects of one or more of at least 20 proteins comprised by this system.

The classical pathway

The binding of C1q to the altered Fc of two IgG or one IgM molecule(s) in complex with antigen, which results in the activation of C1r and C1s, represents the recognition phase of the classical pathway. The outcome of this process is the generation of the enzymatically active component C1s that activates C4 and C2, and thereby initiates the amplification phase. In this phase, C4 is cleaved by C1s into C4a (one of the anaphylatoxins that promotes vascular permeability and smooth muscle contraction) and C4b, which binds to the target surface. In addition to C4, C1s also cleaves C2 in complex with C4b. The products are C2b, which is released, and C2a, which remains bound to C4b. The bimolecular complex C4b,C2a (also known as C3 convertase) is a protease that cleaves C3 into C3a (another anaphylatoxin) and C3b. C3b is recognized by macrophage receptors, attaches to target cell surfaces, and binds to C5. C5, when in complex with C3b, can be cleaved by C3 convertase (also known at this point as C5 convertase) generating C5a (another anaphylatoxin) and C5b. The formation of C5b marks the initiation of the membrane attack phase. Nascent C5b binds to C6, producing the stable C5b,6 complex. This complex reacts with C7 to generate the trimolecular complex C5b,6,7, which binds to the target cell membrane. Next, binding of C8 to the C5,6,7 complex takes place at the cell membrane, which causes the transposition of C9 from the plasma into the target cell membrane by inducing polymerization of C9. The poly C9 with the attached C5b,6,7,8 complex is conventionally referred to as the membrane attack complex (MAC).

The alternative pathway

Binding of a molecule of C3b to a target cell and its combination with the plasma protein Factor B (a zymogen) represents the recognition phase of the alternative pathway. Factor B, when combined with C3b, splits into Ba and Bb upon activation by another plasma protein, Factor D. Fragment Ba is a small peptide with an uncertain function. On the other hand, fragment Bb (which contains the active enzymatic site) attaches to C3b to form complex C3b,Bb. This complex, like C4b,2a in the classical pathway, is also a C3 convertase that is stabilized by properdin (another plasma protein). The Bb fragment is also chemotactic for both neutrophils and monocytes. A formidable amplification results from the positive feedback loop where only a single molecule of Bb can generate many molecules of C3b,Bb and C3b. C3b,Bb acts as a C3 convertase which can split C3 into C3a and C3b. C3b combines with other molecules of Bb to produce more C3b,Bb, which can in turn cleave more molecules of C3. From this point on the activation cascade is the same as that for the classical pathway. Attachment of many C3b molecules to the target cell will allow binding of C5 and its cleavage into C5a and C5b by C3b,Bb (C5 convertase), and so on to the end.

Regulatory mechanisms

Activation of the complement cascade results in a complex series of molecular events with powerful biological effects on the host and/or the parasite.

The host

In the human host, modulating mechanisms regulate complement activation and control the production of biologically active split products. These mechanisms consist of the following:

1. spontaneous decay because of the transient stability of the activated thioester bond in C3b and C4b and the short half-life of the enzymatically active complexes C4b,2a and C3b,Bb;
2. the inactivation of certain components of the complement system by proteolytic enzymes (e.g., Factor I with certain cofactors, serum carboxypeptidase N, chemotactic factor inactivator); and
3. the regulatory function of certain plamsa proteins: Factor H and Factor I.

Factor H (formerly called B1H) competes with Factor B for binding to C3b and, in addition, dissociates C3b,Bb. Factor I (formerly called C3b inactivator) cleaves C3b, which is bound to Factor H or similar proteins present on the host cell surface, to generate iC3b (which cannot produce a C3 convertase).

The parasite

Microorganisms such as bacteria can activate complement via the classical or alternative pathway leading to their opsonization and/or lysis. However, an important determinant of pathogenicity of many bacterial strains is their ability to resist complement-mediated destruction. The following mechanisms against the bactericidal activity or complement have been proposed:

1. the orientation of C3b and MAC deposition to sites on the bacterial surface where they cannot facilitate opsonization and lysis;
2. the complex structure of bacterial cell walls, coupled with efficient means of membrane repair and rapid division, confers considerable resistance to complemented-mediated damage;
3. the presence on the bacterium of surface molecules that resist alternative pathway activation and amplification of C3 deposition.

For example, the presence of a capsule rich in carbohydrate moieties (e.g., sialic acid) differentiates some pathogenic Gram positive bacterial strains from their nonpathogenic counterparts. This is due to the preferential binding on such a capsule as Factor H, rather than Factor B, to C3b. This event leads to catabolism of C3b.

On the other hand, a sort of "suicide" may occur when the surface of a number of target cells, including bacteria and other microorganisms, protect C3b,Bb from inactivation by Factor H and Factor I. This action allows the positive feedback loop to proceed, leading ultimately to the death of the target cell. Selectively, only "foreign" substances—or the surface of target cells—can restrict the activity of Factor H and Factor I, allowing the positive feedback loop to continue.

Complement seems to be less important in host defense against viral infections, where T lymphocytes play a more important role. This is consistent with the observation that complement deficiency is not associated with undue susceptibility to viral infections. Nonetheless, there are many links between viruses and the complement system. The most remarkable is the use of the CR2 by Epstein Barr virus as the receptor for gaining intracellular access. Experimental work with mice has shown that some viruses (e.g., flaviviruses) may enter cells indirectly via immunoglobulin and C3 fixed to the virus (e.g., antibody enhanced uptake of dengue virus via macrophage Fc receptors and CR3-mediated uptake of West Nile virus by C3 fixed to virus particles). Molecules with Fc receptor activities have been known to exist on a number of microorganisms, including certain bacteria and viruses (e.g., staphylococcal Protein A and the Fc receptor present on members of the Herpes virus group). A recent discovery shows that herpes simplex virus can express a surface molecule with complement receptor activity. Such molecules may protect these microorganisms from the normal effects of the binding of antibody and complement proteins to their surfaces; that is, the bound IgG or C3 may be blocked from recognition by opsonic receptors on host phagocytes.

The cytokine network

The term "cytokine" designates a group of protein cell regulators, variously called lymphokines, monokines, interleukins, and interferons. Cytokines share a number of features: they are secreted by a wide variety of cells; they play an important role in many physiological responses and in the pathophysiology of a number of diseases; and they offer therapeutic potential. These proteins often are gycosylated and have a low molecular weight (<80,000). As a group cytokines:

1. regulate the amplitude and duration of immunological and inflammatory responses;
2. are produced transiently and locally;
3. act on a paracrine or autocrine, rather than endocrine, manner;

4. are active at picomolar concentrations; and
5. interact with high affinity cell surface receptors (10-10,000 per cell) with specificity for each cytokine or cytokine group.

At least five of these receptors have been characterized, including IL-1α and β, IL-2, IL-6, IFN γ and macrophage colony stimulating factor (M-CSF). IL-1 and IL-2 receptors are members of the immunoglobulin gene superfamily and are related to integrin receptors. The M-CSF receptor is coded for by the proto-oncogene *c-fms*. Their cell surface binding ultimately leads to a change in the pattern of cellular RNA and protein synthesis, and to altered cell behavior.

Individual cytokines have multiple overlapping regulatory activities, in such a way that the response of a cell to a given cytokine depends on its local concentration, the cell type, and other cell regulator to which it is concomitantly exposed. Cytokines interact in a network by inducing each other, transmodulating cytokine cell surface receptors, and participating in cell functions which involve synergistic, additive, or antagonistic interactions. These interactions may be very complex, with different cell types or subsets producing a distinct spectrum of cytokines. For example, although IL-4 and IFNγ have similar or synergistic functions with respect to the activation of T cells, their actions on immunoglobulin isotype selection or MHC class II expression are differential or antagonistic. In murine T cell clones TH1 cells produce IL-2, IL-3, and IFNγ; whereas TH2 cells produce IL-4 and IL-5. Recent *in situ* hybridization studies in human T cells, following polyclonal activation, have revealed that IL-4 mRNA can be detected in <5% of CD4 + T cells, while 60% of CD4 + T cells express IFNγ and IL-2 mRNA.

Growth factors, such as epidermal growth factor (EGF), platelet-derived growth factor (PDGF), and transforming growth factor α (TGFα) could also be called cytokines, and links between these and other peptide regulatory molecules are being discovered. For example PGDF and M-CSF are linked *in tandem* and exhibit similar organization and encoded amino acid sequence.

On the basis of very recent studies, the following preliminary conclusions (listed below) can be drawn about the cytokine network:

1. All the cytokines so far investigated have growth factor activity, but the growth inhibitory or cytocidal activity is limited to IFNs, tumor necrosis factor (TNF), lymphotoxin (LT), IL-1, and TGFβ.
2. Most cytokines, if not all, act on B and T cells at some stage of their responses, except for CSFs and IL-5 in humans. Their actions on B and T cells are overlapping; that is, two or more cytokines are often necessary to achieve a response. However, the regulation of immunoglobulin isotypes seems more specific. For instance, IFN regulates IgG2a, IL-4 regulates IgE and IgG1, and IL-5 and TGF-β regulate IgA.
3. Cytokine regulation of MHC expression seems to be more restricted, with IFN and TNF/LT found to upregulate MHC class I. IFNγ is the major regulator of MHC class II (IL-4 upregulates this in B cells).
4. Action of cytokines on macrophages, granulocytes, natural killer cells, and eosinophils also, at this time, have been reported to be more restricted. IL-2 and

potentially IFNγ are the only cytokines that can induce lymphokine-activated killer (LAK) activity in cells. Other cytokine activities that seem to be restricted to a few of the presently available cytokines are stimulation of osteoclastic bone resorption, activation of vascular endothelium, the establishment of a cellular antiviral state, and induction of chemotactic migration.
5. The only cytokine that so far appears to have a very restricted activity is human IL-5. Species differences have been observed, such that human IL-5 acts only on eosinophils, but murine IL-5 can also modulate B cell responses. IL-4 is a powerful stimulator of LAK activity in murine cells, but not in human cells, where it can be inhibitory.

Briefly, the recent availability of recombinant cytokines, or their inhibitors, and molecular probes for their genes have presented a number of opportunities for successful clinical applications. Accordingly, these advances have led to the development of newer therapeutic strategies for the management of patients with neoplastic, infectious, or autoimmune diseases.

IMMUNOCHEMISTRY
External physical and biochemical barriers against host infection

The first lines of host defense are represented by the external host system, which is present outside the physiological milieu of the body. The major anatomic components of this system are the skin and the mucous membranes that can be penetrated by relatively few pathogens, unless they can escape through accidental breaks (e.g., wounds, scratches, etc.) or natural portals of entry (e.g., digestive, genitourinary and respiratory tracts). The skin is protected by antibacterial substances (e.g., the lactic acid in sweat and long-chain saturated and unsaturated fatty acids). Even though the mucous membranes appear to be structurally more susceptible to penetration by microorganisms than the skin, they are protected by antimicrobial agents, such as the mucous secretion itself which overlays ciliated tissue. The cilia constantly sweep the mucus upward toward the oropharynx at the rate of 10 to 20 mm/minute. Other mucous surfaces depend on somewhat different mechanisms. In the genitourinary system, for example, urine, which is normally slightly acidic, provides both a mechanical and chemical protection. In the reproductive tract of the mature woman, the thick underlying cell bed is responsible for the synthesis and storage of glycogen. Glycogen is degraded to lactic acid when cells die, creating a bacteriostatic environment in the vagina. The mucosal surface of the eye is protected by tears, which have an effective cleansing action. Tears have a high concentration of lysozyme which, due to its isoelectric point (near pH 11), is attracted to Gram-positive bacteria (i.e., most have acidic isoelectric point).

The efficiency of lysozyme against Gram-positive bacteria is greater than that of Gram-negative bacteria, since the substrate for lysozyme in the latter is shielded by a lipid coat. This is consistent with the observation that pinkeye and common urinary tract infections are caused by the lysozyme-resistant, Gram-negative bacteria.

The digestive system, like the genitourinary and respiratory systems, is especially protected at the level of the stomach where the pH may be as low as 1.0, lethal for a number of microorganisms. Rhinoviruses, for instance, are unable to survive at this low pH in contrast to enteroviruses, to which they are closely related. Hence, rhinoviruses cause upper respiratory infection in lieu of enteroviral infection. Conversely, acid-resistant microorganisms pass to the ideal growth environments of the small and large intestines, but fail to establish themselves because of competition or interference from the heavily colonized normal flora. The many species of basically noninvasive bacteria that constitute this flora generate a number of beneficial products (acids, antibiotic-like substances, vitamins, etc.).

Immunochemical aspects of innate or natural immunity

Successful pathogens, which are able to circumvent the external host defense system, can penetrate the host's true physiologic interior 1) by virtue of their own invasive properties; 2) by the opportunity to gain access through wounds or scratches; or 3) by being ingested in food, milk, water, etc. Once inside the host, the intruder must still overcome a series of defense forces before it can establish an infection. The innate (nonspecific) immune system consists of a variety of cells and their biochemical products, which are distributed throughout the body.

Inflammation is initiated by trauma, tissue necrosis, infection, or immune reactions. It can be induced, maintained, or limited by signaling molecules or chemical mediators that act on smooth muscle, endothelial or white blood cells. The acute phase of inflammation spans a series of sequential events that begin with temporary vasoconstriction. Temporary vasoconstriction is believed to be mediated by the sympathetic nervous system. The first agents in the sequence affect smooth muscle cells of precapillary arterioles to produce dilatation and increased blood flow. Increased vascular permeability proceeds in two phases: an early phase, which occurs within minutes and is mediated by histamine and serotonin, and a late phase, which occurs in six to 12 hours and is mediated by various molecules derived from different sources. These sources include arachidonic acid metabolites; breakdown products of the coagulation system (fibrin split products); peptides formed from blood or tissue proteins (bradykinin); and activated complement components; as well as factors released from bacteria; necrotic tissue; neutrophils (inflammatory peptides); lymphocytes (lymphokines); and monocytes (monokines). The cellular elements that play an important role in the acute inflammation process include mast cells, neutrophils, platelets, and eosinophils, which act in sequence. They are activated by a variety of chemical processes and in turn produce and release a number of chemical mediators.

Mast cell mediators

Most manifestations of the early acute vascular response are mediated by histamine and serotonin, which are released immediately after the degranulation of mast cells, leading to vasodilatation and increased vascular permeability. Later vascular events, occurring six to 12 hours after the onset of inflammation, are mediated by prostaglandins and leukotrienes. The latter are the metabolic products of phospholipids from membrane-like material released from mast cell granules. Chemotaxis of neutrophils and eosinophils is af-

fected by leukotrienes and by platelet-activating factor. Enzymes activated by solubilization of granular material may also contribute to tissue damage and/or repair.

Histamine is the major preformed mast cell mediator with powerful biological effects. It acts through two sets of receptors, H1 and H2. Effects mediated through H1 receptors are the classic acute vascular inflammatory events. Anti-inflammatory effects, as well as vasodilatation, are mediated through H2 receptors. Hence, histamine may activate acute vascular reactions, yet inhibit acute cellular inflammation. Acute cellular inflammation is mediated by the products of arachidonic acid.

Arachidonic acid is derived from membrane phospholipids by the enzymatic action of phospholipases. In humans, membrane phospholipids are released from mast cells and other cell membranes in the early phase of acute inflammation. The metabolism of arachidonic acid is believed to occur in macrophages, but metabolites may also be synthesized by most, if not all, cells that participate in inflammation, including the mast cell. Metabolism of arachidonic acid proceeds via two major pathways, cyclooxygenase and lipooxygenase, which produce prostaglandins and leukotrienes, respectively.

Prostaglandins PGE2 and PGD2 are the most active and are responsible for vasodilatation and increase in vascular permeability, as well as causing hyperalgesia. Although prostaglandins are responsible for some of the late vascular effects of anaphylaxis, they may also modulate anaphylaxis by increasing cyclic nucleotide levels of mast cells and inhibiting histamine release. In addition to prostaglandins, the cyclooxygenase pathway also gives rise to thromboxane A2, albeit the primary source of this mediator is platelets. Thromboxane A2 is active in vasoconstriction and platelet aggregation. Prostaglandins and thromboxanes are rapidly metabolized to their inactive forms by further oxygenation. Nonsteroidal anti-inflammatory drugs (e.g., aspirin) inhibit cyclooxygenase and therefore block the formation of these mediators.

Leukotrienes are generated by leukocytes and mast cells. Each leukotriene is identified individually by a numeral that indicates the number of double bonds present in that particular molecule. The activity of leukotrienes C4, D4, and E4 is believed to be consistent with that of a factor previously called SRS-A (slow reacting substance of anaphylaxis). Leukotriene B4 is chemotactic for eosinophils and neutrophils.

Neutrophilic polymorphonuclear leukocytes and their mediators of inflammation

These cells constitute the major cellular component of the acute inflammatory response. They have at least three types of cytoplasmic granules that store highly destructive hydrolytic enzymes:

1. primary or azurophil granules, which consist of lysosomes and contain acid hydrolases and other enzymes (e.g., lysozyme, elastase, cathepsin G, and other cationic proteins);
2. secondary or specific granules, which contain lactoferrin and lysozyme; and
3. a third granule compartment which has gelatinase.

Neutrophils may be attracted to inflammation sites by a variety of chemotactic factors and may display cell surface receptors for some of these factors, such as activated fragments of complement and formylmethionyl tripeptides. Acute inflammatory reactions are frequently elicited by non-immune mechanisms, such as bacterial infections (e.g., streptococcal or staphylococcal) or traumatic tissue injury. Under these circumstances, neutrophils are attracted into sites of inflammation by chemotactic factors released by the incumbent infectious agent (f-Met peptides); by products of damaged tissue (e.g., fibronectin, fibrin, collagen degradation products); or by factors derived from other inflammatory cells. In antigen-antibody (immune complex) reactions, neutrophils are attracted by the formation of activated complement components subsequent to antibody-antigen reactions in tissues. Once at the site of inflammation, neutrophils engulf and digest complexes consisting of bacteria coated with antibody and complement. Nonetheless, phagocytosis by neutrophils is generally coupled with the release of lysosomal acid hydrolases into tissue spaces (especially when the neutrophil has difficulty ingesting the antigen), thus causing local tissue digestion at the site of the reaction. The characteristic lesion is fibrinoid necrosis. Reactive oxygen metabolites, primarily involved in bacterial killing, may also damage infiltrating neutrophils and adjacent tissues contributing to the production of pus.

Platelets and inflammatory mediators derived from the coagulation system

Although the role of platelets in the inflammatory response is not well defined, platelets release heparin and serotonin, which may contribute to the acute vascular phase of inflammation. Platelets also produce oxygen radicals, which may induce tissue damage. Nonetheless, the primary role of platelets is to block damaged vessel walls and prevent hemorrhage. Platelets react at sites of vascular damage via a receptor for a tripeptide—arginine-glycine-asparagine—which is present in fibrin, fibronectin, and vitronectin. At these sites, the extracellular matrix proteins fibronectin and vitronectin are exposed, and fibrin is formed through activation of the clotting system. Thus, platelets bind to these molecules, forming aggregates that plug up leaks in the vascular system.

Several components of the coagulation system may also serve as mediators in the inflammatory reaction as a result of a significant degree of inflammation. Coagulation products that participate actively in inflammation include fragments of the Hageman factor and of thrombin, as well as fibrin split products. Peptides that are active as mediators of inflammation may be generated from a number of cells and tissue products. Of these, the most active is the kinin system.

In summary, the complement, coagulation, kinin, and mast cell systems, as well as bacterial products, contribute to vasodilation, increased vascular permeability, and chemotaxis of the primary cellular mediator of inflammation, the neutrophil. Consequently, the neutrophil and its lysosomal enzymes have a microbicidal role as well as the potential to cause tissue necrosis.

The major inflammatory mediators derived from complement are C3a and C5a. Cells destroyed by the activation of complement may contribute indirectly through the release of intracellular contents that may generate further tissue destruction (enzymes) or activate the extrinsic coagulation system. Activation of the intrinsic coagulation system generates a series of active fragments. Activated factor XII (Hagemen factor) contributes to the formation of three inflammatory mediators:

1. bradykinin,
2. Hageman factor fragments, and
3. fibrin split products.

Mast cells contribute directly by release of mediators such as histamine and serotonin and indirectly by providing arachidonic acid precursors for the production of leukotrienes, prostaglandins, and other factors. These systems are responsible for the increase in blood flow and vascular permeability leading to edema, in addition to attracting neutrophils and eosinophils to sites of inflammation. Neutrophils kill infectious agents following phagocytosis and digestion, but in the process also release lysosomal enzymes that may cause tissue damage. Eosinophils, on the other hand, are believed to modulate inflammatory responses by deactivating mast cell mediators.

Immunochemical aspects of adaptive or acquired immunity

Unlike innate, or natural, immunity, which is a broad-spectrum resistance not directed against any particular pathogen, acquired immunity is expressed most typically against a specific pathogen and develops following exposure to that pathogen. The specificity of antibody and specifically sensitized T effector cells provides for the identification of the target—the infecting foreign organisms—against which the immune effector mechanisms augmented by accessory inflammatory processes can be effectively directed.

The first attempt to classify the immune reactions according to mechanism was made by Gell and Coombs in 1963. However, more recently, Stewart Sell proposed six immune effector mechanisms as follows:

1. inactivation (e.g., via neutralization) or activation (e.g., of complement components)
2. cytotoxic or cytolytic
3. immune complex (Arthus)
4. atopic or anaphylactic
5. delayed hypersensitivity and
6. granulomatous

The first four types are mediated by antibodies. The characteristics of the reactions are not only defined by the properties of the immunoglobulin molecules involved, but also depend on the nature and tissue location of the pathogen and on the accessory inflammatory systems that are called into play. The last two mechanisms, delayed hypersensitivity and granulomatous reactions, do not depend on antibodies but on the reaction of antigen with specifically sensitized T lymphocytes. Delayed reactions are typically elicited by soluble degradable antigens. In contrast, granulomatous reactions are brought about by poorly degradable antigens.

Immunochemistry of the antigen recognition process

Foreign antigen recognition is the hallmark of specific acquired or adaptive immunity. There are two types of molecules which determine the specificity of the recognition process: immunoglobulins and T lymphocyte antigen receptors. Both types of molecules undergo extensive gene rearrangements in order to generate different immunoglobulins or cell surface receptors capable of recognizing many different antigens. Heterogeneity (e.g., isotypic, allotypic, and idiotypic variations) and diversity (e.g., different forms and types of antibodies) are characteristics of each type. Both types of molecules are probably derived from a common ancestor and both belong to the immunoglobulin supergene family. Circulating immunoglobulins are structurally identical to B cell antigen receptors but lack the transmembrane and intracytoplasmic sections. The T cell receptor has an antigen-binding portion consisting of an α and a β chain (or a γ and a δ chain), which are associated with three other transmembrane polypeptides (γ, δ and ε), structurally distinct from the chains of the receptor.

Immunoglobulins

Immunoglobulin molecules are a family of proteins with the same basic molecular architecture; yet they are extremely heterogeneous in terms of their enormous diversity of antigen-binding specificities and different biologic activities. With the possible exception of natural antibodies, these specific proteins are produced in response to foreign substances in the body. Immunoglobulin molecules are a heterogeneous group of glycoproteins that account for 20% of the total plasma proteins. In serum electrophoresis, most of the immunoglobulins migrate to the zone designated γ-globulin, but significant amounts are also found in the β-globulin zone. These glycoproteins are composed of 82% to 96% polypeptide and 4% to 18% carbohydrate. The polypeptide moiety has most of the biologic properties ascribed to antibody molecules. Different populations of immunoglobulins are also found in varying proportions in extravascular fluids, in exocrine secretions, and on the surface of some lymphocytes. Immunoglobulins are bifunctional molecules that bind antigens and, in addition, initiate other biologic phenomena independent of antibody specificity.

Five major immunoglobulin classes—including IgM, IgG, IgA, IgD, and IgE—and 10 subclasses have been identified in humans (Table 33-3). The basic structural unit of each immunoglobulin class consists of two pairs of polypeptide chains joined by disulfide bonds that may be reduced by mercaptoethanol. Treatment with denaturing agents (e.g., acid, urea) produces four polypeptide chains, two L (light) and two H (heavy) chains. Each antibody molecule contains two identical L chains and two identical H chains. The entire molecule can be digested by proteolytic enzymes to yield other fragments (Fc and Fab fragments). The L chains are shared by immunoglobulins of the different

classes and can be divided into two subclasses, kappa (κ) and lambda (λ), on the basis of their structures and amino acid sequences. These two types are mutually exclusive in the sense that a given immunoglobulin molecule has either two κ or two λ chains but not a mixture of both. Approximately 60% of the serum immunoglobulin molecules contain κ-type L chains and 40% λ-type L chains. The H chains are unique for each immunoglobulin class and are designated by the Greek letter corresponding to the capital-letter designation of the immunoglobulin class (α chains for the H chains of IgA, γ chains for the H chains of IgG). IgM and IgA have a third chain component, the J chain, which joins the monomeric units.

The five classes of immunoglobulins differ in their biological properties (Table 33-4). The structure responsible for the biological properties of each class is located in the part of the molecule that is unique for that class (i.e., the Fc portion of the H chain). In addition to the five major classes of immunoglobulins in humans, subclasses of IgG, IgA, and IgM have also been identified.

IgM. This is the first immunoglobulin class produced by the maturing fetus and does not normally cross the placenta from mother to fetus. It may be the first class representing a given antibody specificity after immunization (i.e., primary response). It has a molecular weight of 970,000, 12% carbohydrate, and a half-life of 10 days. It occurs as five H_2L_2 units joined to each other by disulfide bonds located on the Fc portion of the molecule and to the J chain. It is found mainly in the intravascular fluids (80%). Although both IgG and IgM fix complement, the latter is the most efficient immunoglobulin class in this regard; hence, it is very active in cytotoxic and cytolytic reactions.

IgG. Each IgG molecule consists of one H_2L_2 unit with a molecular weight of 146,000, 2% to 3% carbohydrate, and a half-life of 23 days. Actively transported across the placenta, IgG is responsible for passive immunity in the newborn infant. IgG is widely distributed in the tissue fluids and is about equally divided between the intravascular and extravascular spaces.

IgA. IgA is the predominant immunoglobulin class in body secretions, where it exists as two 4-chain basic units and one molecule each of secretory component and J chain. Secretory IgA has a molecular weight of approximately 400,000, 10% carbohydrate, and a half-life of six days. It provides the primary defense mechanism against certain local infections because of its high level in saliva, tears, bronchial secretions, nasal mucosa, prostatic fluid, vaginal secretions, and mucous secretions of the small intestine.

Table 33-3 Physicochemical characteristics of immunoglobulin classes* and subclasses

	IgG1	IgG2	IgG3	IgG4	IgM	IgA1	IgA2	sIgA	IgD	IgE
Heavy Chain Designation	γ_1	γ_2	γ_3	γ_4	μ	α_1	α_2	α_1 or α_2	δ	ε
Light Chain Type	κ or λ	κ or λ	κ or λ	κ or λ	κ or λ	κ or λ	κ or λ	κ or λ	κ or λ	κ or λ
Molecular Weight ($\times 10^3$)	146	146	170	146	970	160	160	385	184	188
Sedimentation Coefficient	7S	7S	7S	7S	19S	7S	7S	11S	7S	8S
Electrophoretic Mobility	γ	γ	γ	γ	Between γ and β	Slow β	Slow β	Slow β	Between γ and β	Slow β
Carbohydrate Content (%)	2-3	2-3	2-3	2-3	12	7-11	7-11	7-11	9-14	12

*IgG and IgA have three constant domains and four disulfide bonds; IgM and IgE have four constant domains and five disulfide bonds.

Circulating IgA is normally present in serum in both monomeric and polymeric forms and accounts for approximately 15% of the total serum immunoglobulins.

IgD. This immunoglobulin class is normally present in serum at very low levels (0.2% of total serum immunoglobulins). It has a molecular weight of approximately 180,000, 13% carbohydrate, and a half-life of three days. IgD is also found on the surface of a high proportion of immature human B lymphocytes, possibly serving as a cellular receptor for antigen and playing a role in the differentiation of these cells. There are isolated reports indicating that IgD has antibody activity for certain antigens, including insulin, penicillin, milk proteins, diphtheria toxoid, nuclear antigens, and thyroid antigens.

IgE. This immunoglobulin is present in very low concentrations in serum (only 0.004% of the total immunoglobulins) and tissue fluids. It has a molecular weight of 190,000 to 200,000, 10% carbohydrate, and a half-life of two-and-a-half days. It binds with very high affinity to mast cells via a site in the Fc region. Upon reacting with certain specific antigens (allergens), IgE antibodies trigger the release of pharmacologic mediators (e.g., histamine and serotonin) from mast cells. Like IgG and IgD, IgE only exists in monomeric form.

T cell receptors

These recognition molecules are expressed exclusively on the membrane surface of T lymphocytes and there is no comparable production of soluble molecules analogous to the circulating antibodies. T cell recognition of antigen through the T cell receptor is the basis of a range of immunological phenomena including T cell helper and suppressor activity, cytotoxicity, and possibly NK (natural killing) activity. T cell receptors can be divided into two main groups defined by the nature of the heterodimeric receptor chains (γ/δ or α/β) expressed. A provisional designation of TCR1 and TCR2 has recently been proposed since the γ and δ genes are rearranged and expressed before the α and β genes in ontogeny. The most recent data suggest that cells expressing the α/β receptor and those expressing γ/δ are on separate lineages.

The TCR2 subunit is relatively well characterized. It has a molecular weight of 90,000 and consists of a heterodimer of α and β peptide chains. Each peptide chain comprises a constant region and a variable region with sequence homology to the immunoglobulin domains. The α and β chains are disulfide-linked near the membrane. The amino acid sequences of the T cell receptor α and β chains places the TCR2 subunit in the immunoglobulin superfamily, although there are some differences between the TCR2 subunits and immunoglobulins.

The characterization of the TCR1 subunit and the organization of the relevant genes are still the subject of intensive research. However, the overall protein structure of the γ/δ TCR1 heterodimer is believed to be similar to that of the α/β TCR2 heterodimer. A precise functional role for cells bearing the TCR1 subunit has yet to be defined but may include regulation of the differentiation of T cells with the TCR2 receptor.

Both helper and cytotoxic T cells express their T cell antigen receptor in a molecular complex involving three other polypeptide chains, γ, δ and ϵ, which comprise the CD3 subunit (previously identified with monoclonal antibodies as T3 and Leu4) in humans. The three chains of the CD3 subunit are noncovalently associated with each other and the α/β heterodimer of the T cell antigen receptor. Each chain is a transmembrane peptide and approximately one third of the γ chain is intracytoplasmic. All appear to have an extracellular domain. It has been suggested that they may be members of the immunoglobulin supergene family.

IMMUNOPATHOLOGY

The aspects of the immune system discussed thus far have dealt mostly with immune effector mechanisms amplified by accessory inflammatory processes that protect against specific infections. These mechanisms, which direct the defenses of the host against the foreign invaders, involve specific antibodies (generally most effective against bacteria or bacterial products) and T lymphocytes (primarily operative against viral and mycotic agents). However, specific situations are increasingly recognized in which the host immune response functions in an exaggerated or unconventional way, producing tissue injury and therefore disease. It may thus be said that the immune response is being used for the wrong purpose. Yet the very same processes responsible for the immunopathogenesis of that particular disease are also essential for the protection required for preserving health. Teleologically, one could then ask: Why a "double-edged sword?" At least a partial answer to this complex and loaded question will be provided in this section by discussing the role of immunopathologic mechanisms in disease. This discussion will be based on the same six immune effector mechanisms activated by the reaction of antibodies or sensitized cells with antigens in vivo. Immunodeficiency disorders and autoimmune diseases will not be covered in this chapter, but will be presented elsewhere in this book.

Effector mechanisms of atopic diseases, anaphylaxis, and urticaria

A number of terms that originated at the beginning of this century are still used today, albeit somewhat inconsistently, to describe the various allergic disorders included under the Gell and Coombs Type I reaction. The term "anaphylaxis" was originally coined by Porter and Richet in 1902 to indicate adverse reactions to horse serum injected for passive

Table 33-4   Biological properties of immunoglobulins

	IgG	IgM	IgA	IgD	IgE
Serum concentration (mg/dl)	1000	120	200	3	0.05
Serum half-life (days)	23*	10	6	2-8	1-5
Intravascular distribution (%)	45	80	42	75	50
Placental transfer	Yes	No	No	No	No
Reaginic activity	?†	No	No	No	Yes
Complement fixation	+	++++	0	0	0
Antibacterial lysis	+	+++	+	0	0
Antiviral activity	+	+	+++	?	?

*IgG3 has a half-life of only seven days.
†IgG4 may have reaginic activity.

therapy of certain infections. This term implies a damaging effect and is antonymous to prophylaxis. The term "allergy" was introduced by von Pirquet in 1906 to describe the two opposite sides of the altered state of host reactivity to exogenous antigens. The beneficial response was called "immunity" and the harmful response, "hypersensitivity." Today, however, the term "allergy" has become synonymous with the adverse effects of hypersensitivity, and the broader responses to antigens are termed "immunity." The first description of the mechanism of the allergic reaction was made by Prausnitz and Kustner in 1921 and demonstrated that a serum factor (termed "reagin") could mediate the reaction on passive transfer to the skin of a nonsensitized subject. Some 45 years later, Ishizaka and colleagues determined that this "atopic reagin" was a new class of immunoglobulin (IgE). The term "atopy," derived from the Greek term "atopia," meaning strangeness, was applied by Coca and Cooke in 1923 to a variety of strange reactions in humans. The term "allergy," or "immediate hypersensitivity," is now used interchangeably to designate atopic or anaphylactic reactions. With the advent of modern concepts in many areas of immunobiology, Gell and Coombs in 1963 introduced a new classification system that included Types I, II, III, and IV allergic reactions. Although still widely used, modifications to this classification system have been proposed. The Gell and Coombs system is not all-inclusive, and any given pathologic process may comprise overlapping mechanisms for more than one or all of these groups of reactions. This section, however, will focus on the Type I reaction.

A number of parameters determine the resulting type of lesion, such as the dose of antigen, the route and frequency of exposure to the allergen, and the tendency for a given organ to react (shock organ). The patient's degree of sensitivity is also an important determinant and may be genetically controlled or altered by the environment (e.g., temperature); an unrelated episode of illness (e.g., viral upper respiratory infection); or psychological stress.

During the last several years, many reports have suggested that allergic disease is caused by quantitative and functional lymphocyte abnormalities. It appears most probable, however, that the atopic condition brings about those lymphocyte abnormalities. In turn, a genetic determinant predisposes to the development of atopy. The capacity to produce IgE antibodies to specific antigens is inherited in connection with specific transplantation alloantigens. For example, HLA-Dw2 is an almost perfect genetic marker for the IgE and IgG immune responses to short ragweed pollen antigen Ra5. HLA-MB3 is found in 100% of Japanese subjects with an IgE response to antigens of the house dust mite *Dermatophagoides farinae*. Interaction between HLA-linked immune response genes and a non-HLA IgE regulating gene exists. Allergy to an antigen is the result of the HLA-D-determined genetic predisposition for an antigen-specific IgE response, which is regulated by antigen-specific suppressor T cells. Regulatory aspects of this IgE antibody response may indeed result in measurable abnormalities in OKT4+ helper cell function or in the types of cellular effects observed after activation in the autologous mixed lymphocyte reaction. Conversely, it is very unlikely that the vast number and variety of abnormalities associated with allergic disorders represent primary or basic immunological defects. Most defects can be attributed to allergic-mediator induced deactivation, desensitization, or direct agonist effects. Obviously, findings of decreased numbers of total T cells or suppressor T cells cannot explain a very selective elevation of the concentration of one class of antibodies to one or a few antigens.

The inhalation, ingestion, or injection of an "allergen" (i.e., the antigen involved in an allergic reaction) by a previously sensitized and genetically predisposed host can, under appropriate conditions, produce an atopic or anaphylactic reaction within minutes. This reaction is called "immediate" as opposed to slower reactions, which are called "delayed." Anaphylaxis refers to the most rapid or acute hypersensitivity reactions (wheal and flare and systemic shock) of the immediate type, whereas atopy refers to the chronic recurring reactions (e.g., hayfever). However, this distinction is not always made, and there is considerable overlap in the use of terms. Anaphylaxis is characterized by an explosive response occurring within minutes of the challenging dose, and it can be either "systemic" (generalized) or "localized" (cutaneous).

Contrary to popular belief, IgE-mediated inflammatory reactions can last not just a matter of minutes but many hours. Accordingly, the concept of biphasic responses induced by IgE antibodies was established. The initial phase is the typical immediate hypersensitivity reaction, classically demonstrated in the skin by the wheal and flare response. This develops rapidly after exposure to antigen, peaks in 10 to 20 minutes, and then subsides within one to two hours. The second phase is designated as a "late" reaction to distinguish it from the "delayed" hypersensitivity or cell-mediated reaction. It represents a continuation of the initial phase but with greater intensity. Typically, the early reaction begins to fade after two hours, but after three to four hours the site undergoes renewed inflammation, which reaches its greatest intensity at eight to 12 hours and then gradually resolves over 24 to 48 hours. The characteristics of this late-phase response are quite different from the well-circumscribed, pruritic wheal of the initial reaction. The lesion is characterized by diffuse erythema, warmth, edema, and tenderness and is usually more extensive in area and results in much greater discomfort than the early-phase lesion.

The effects produced by atopic or anaphylactic reactions are initiated by mediators released by the reaction of antigen with effector cells (mast cells) passively sensitized by IgE antibody. Upon reacting with antigen, these mediator cells release a number of pharmacologically active substances including histamine, heparin, and serotonin (early phase). Also released is arachidonic acid, which is converted by other cells into prostaglandins and leukotrienes responsible for the later phase inflammatory reaction. The early phase is characterized by smooth muscle constriction or dilation, which occurs within minutes of the challenging dose. In one case, the smooth muscle of arterioles is stimulated to dilate by reaction of histamine with H-2 receptors (blocked by cimetidine). In the other case, the smooth muscle of the pulmonary bronchi, the gastrointestinal tract, and the genitourinary system, in addition to endothelial cells, is stimulated by the action of histamine on H-1 receptors (blocked by antihistamines).

Among the principal mediators of immediate hypersensitivity, prostaglandin E is a potent dilator of bronchial smooth muscle and prostaglandin F is a potent constrictor. Leukotriene E4 (slow-reacting substance of anaphylaxis) causes later vasoreactions, and leukotriene B4 is chemotactic for acute inflammatory cells. The late phase takes place six to 12 hours after antigen exposure and is characterized by a more prolonged reaction with infiltration of neutrophils, eosinophils, and basophils in addition to lymphocytes and macrophages. This late phase is typified by an indurated, erythematous, painful reaction in the skin.

This causes a more prolonged deterioration in air flow than asthma, where a rapidly reversible bronchoconstriction occurs in the immediate or early phase. The effects of these agents include contraction of smooth muscle, increased vascular permeability, early increase in vascular resistance leading to collapse (shock), and increased gastric, nasal, and lacrimal secretion.

Although cell surface receptors with high affinity for IgE are present only on mast cells, basophils, and neoplastic counterparts of these cells, receptors that bind monomeric IgE with lower affinity are present on the surface of many other cell types (e.g., eosinophils, macrophages, and monocytes, B and T lymphocytes). Since monomeric IgE dissociates rapidly from those low-affinity receptors, it is presumed that usually an antigen-IgE complex is formed initially. Subsequently, the complex binds via multipoint attachment to multiple lower-affinity receptors and activates the cell. Lower-affinity Fc_E receptors appear to be involved in cellular cytotoxicity against parasites and in regulation of IgE synthesis.

While the role of phagocytic cells in the development of adverse reactions such as serum sickness has been extensively explored, the most impressive hypersensitivity reaction certainly is Type I. The clustering of the surface receptors for IgE triggers the anaphylactic discharge of the pharmacologically active mediators of mast cells or basophils. In this process, it has been shown that small oligomers of IgE, at least dimers, can provide a signal for mast cell degranulation. However, nonreaginic antibodies belonging to one of the IgG subclasses (IgG4 in humans) can also be involved in immediate type reactions. Human allergy usually develops in two steps. The first is the binding of free monomeric IgE antibody to Fc_E receptors on mast cells or basophils. The second is the triggering of the cell on the interaction of a multivalent antigen with the surface-bound IgE. Circulating immune IgE complexes have, however, been characterized in allergic patients, which might induce mast cell degranulation directly. The fact that many mediators of anaphylaxis are also produced by phagocytic cells, and the characterization on their surface of receptors for anaphylactic antibodies or immune complexes suggest that phagocytic cells can participate in immediate-type reactions not only as recruited inflammatory cells, but also as direct effectors of allergy. But in infections by helminths, the sustained release of circulating antigens and the mass production of anti-parasite IgE lead to the formation of the largest amount of circulating immune complexes of ana-

phylactic antibodies. Interestingly, this does not result in dramatic anaphylactic reactions. Instead, immune complexes of anaphylactic antibodies have been shown in host defense against helminths.

Finally, a functional role for antibodies of the IgE class has been implicated in antibody-dependent cell-mediated cytotoxicity reactions associated with helminthic infections and allergic disorders. For example, it has been demonstrated that monocytes incubated with IgE-containing immune complexes were able to kill schistosomula of *Schistosoma mansoni*. This is consistent with the subsequent finding that selected immune sera contained high levels of antiparasite IgE antibodies.

Among the reactions that the clinician sees most frequently are urticaria (wheal and flare, hives), hay fever, asthma, eczema, angioedema, and anaphylaxis. The reader should consult the references at the end of this chapter for specific details on these clinical disorders.

Antibody-mediated cytolytic or cytotoxic reactions

Cytolytic or cytotoxic (Gell and Coombs Type II) reactions occur when IgG and/or IgM antibodies react with either an antigenic component of a cell membrane or an antigen that has become passively attached to a cell. The binding of antigen and antibody may activate all nine components of the complement system through the classical pathway and/or may interact with a variety of effector cells (e.g., neutrophils, eosinophils, platelets, and mononuclear phagocytes) to bring about the lysis or destruction of the target cells. The result of these reactions (e.g., hemolytic anemia, agranulocytosis, thrombocytopenia, and vascular purpura) depends on several factors including: type of cell involved, antibody characteristics, number of antigen sites per cell, and amount of antibody available.

The target cells usually involved in these reactions are erythrocytes, leukocytes, platelets, and vascular endothelium. These reactions are mediated by IgM or those IgG immunoglobulin subclasses able to activate complement. Selected IgG subclasses, such as IgG1 and IgG3, bind complement better than IgG2 or IgG4. Only one IgM antibody molecule reacting with a cell is sufficient to activate complement, in contrast to two IgG molecules in close apposition. In fact, antibodies of the IgM class are approximately 600 times more efficient in producing lytic reactions than antibodies of the IgG class. The number of antigen sites on the surface of the target cell must be relatively high for IgG to be able to fix complement.

Antibodies interact with complement by activating the C1 component of the classical pathway. Alternatively, they may cross-link the antibody-sensitized tissue to the Fc receptors of effector cells. The complement system can act in two ways in these reactions:

1. antibody-sensitized cells can be lysed by activation of the classical and lytic pathways, resulting in the deposition of the C5b-C9 membrane attack complex on the target cells; and
2. C3b can be deposited onto target tissues by activation of the classical pathway and amplification loops. This sensitizes the target cells for interaction with effector cells, such as macrophages and neutrophils, which

carry receptors for complement components (CR1, CR3).

These Type II cytotoxic reactions proceed according to the following mechanisms: the antibodies bound to the membrane antigens on the target cells facilitate their opsonization by the phagocytes. Cross-linking of the Fc receptors results in:

1. activation of a membrane oxidase complex generating oxygen radicals (e.g., O_2^-, H_2O_2). Although these reactive oxygen intermediates increase the effector cell capacity to destroy pathogens, they also increase their capacity to produce immunopathologic damage in hypersensitivity reactions;
2. increased protein phosphorylation and hence cellular activation;
3. increased arachidonic acid release from membrane phospholipids mediated by phospholipase A, providing the precursor for production of prostaglandins and leukotrienes, which are involved in the development of inflammation.

Immune complexes induce complement C3b deposition, which can also interact with opsonic adherence receptors on phagocytes. Activation of the lytic pathway leads to the assembly of the membrane attack complex by complement components C5-C9.

In addition to their ability to activate the complement classical pathway, antibodies can interact with cells carrying Fc receptors. These include macrophages, neutrophils, eosinophils, and K cells. Antibody subclasses vary in their ability to interact with the various effector cells and with the C1q fragment. This is because of the diversity of binding characteristics among the different kinds of Fc receptors. For instance, C1q binds to a site in the $C\gamma2$ domain of IgG1; whereas macrophages bind to a site in the $C\gamma2$ and $C\gamma3$ domains.

Antibodies also mediate hypersensitivity by cross-linking K cells to target tissues. K cells are mainly found in the population of large granular lymphocytes and bind sensitizing antibody via their high affinity Fc receptors. Cytotoxicity then appears to follow the same mechanisms used by cytotoxic T cells. Although K-cell activity can be demonstrated in vitro against a number of different cell types, their role in hypersensitivity reactions cannot be ascertained because of a number of variables (e.g., the amounts of particular antigens expressed on the target cell's surface and the inherent ability of different target cells to sustain damage). For example, an erythrocyte may be lysed by a single active C5 convertase site; whereas it takes many such sites to destroy most nucleated cells. The latter are particularly susceptible to K cell-mediated damage, and chick erythrocytes, which are nucleated, are frequently used as the standard target to test K cell activity.

Immunohematologic disorders may arise from the immune destruction of eythrocytes that leads to:

1. the loss of erythrocyte function,
2. damaging effects of the released cell contents, and
3. cytotoxicity.

These disorders include transfusion reactions, erythroblastosis fetalis, acquired autoimmune hemolytic diseases, and drug-induced hemolytic reactions.

Antibody effects may also occur with polymorphonuclear leukocytes, resulting in loss of neutrophils or agranulocytosis. However, most of these cases are secondary to a lack of proliferation of granulocytes in the bone marrow on a metabolic basis. Many drugs are known to inhibit granulocyte production. The outcome of leukocyte destruction is an impaired ability to fight infection.

Immune reactions to platelets may cause destruction of platelets with resulting purpura and other hemorrhagic manifestations. Since one function of platelets is to prevent such hemorrhages, loss of platelets permits purpuric lesions to develop. An antiplatelet antibody can be found in approximately 60% of affected individuals. Recent reports indicate that in certain disorders, antigen-antibody complexes cause thrombocytopenia. Sensitive immunoassays are now under evaluation for the detection of antiplatelet antibodies. Thrombocytopenia may also occur congenitally (e.g., neonatal thrombocytopenic purpura) or secondarily as a result of hypersplenism or some other nonimmune abnormality.

Immunosuppression of blood cell production may occur when antibody to blood cell precursors injures proliferating cells in the bone marrow, thus producing an aplastic anemia or agranulocytosis. This immunosuppressive activity may involve one or all cell lines, depending on whether the antibody is directed against differentiation antigen(s) or common antigen(s). Antibodies to stem cells have rarely been detected spontaneously in humans. Such antibodies to erythrocyte or leukocyte precursors have been associated with aplastic anemia, red cell aplasia, profound panleukopenia, and systemic lupus erythematosus. Therefore, although rare, patients with antibodies to blood cell precursors may present with a clinical picture similar to that associated with a metabolic defect in blood cell maturation.

Therapeutic drugs can elicit allergic and autoallergic reactions against blood components, including erythrocytes and platelets. Usually, the antibody activity is directed to the drug or its metabolites that adsorb to cell membranes. Thus antibodies to the drug will bind to the cell, leading to complement-mediated lysis. Alternatively, immune complexes of drug and antibody may adsorb to the target cell. The latter appears to be mediated by the immune adherence receptor (CRI) and/or the immunoglobulin Fc region. It is uncertain whether Fc-dependent binding is specific. In this case, damage also occurs by complement-mediated lysis. Instead of the reaction between the antibody and the drug, cytolytic antibodies may be produced against certain blood group antigens on the cell surface. In this case, the drug, which is presumably adsorbed onto cell membranes, induces a breakdown of self-tolerance, possibly by stimulating CD4+ lymphocytes. Occasionally, drugs may induce allergic reactions where autoantibodies directed against the erythrocyte antigens are produced.

Vascular purpura is characterized by hemorrhagic phenomena due to the destruction of vascular endothelium. The phenomenon of anaphylactoid purpura may correspond to this category. Clinically, urticarial and hemorrhagic lesions are the most prominent features and tend to occur around joints. The immunopathogenic mechanism of vascular purpura is not necessarily direct cytolysis. In fact, most cases are believed caused by focal deposition of immune complexes and activation of complement leading to cell lysis and inflammation with infiltration of polymorphonuclear leukocytes. Thus vascular purpura may be caused by antibody to vascular epithelium or by a particular form of immune complex reaction. In either case, the clinical manifestation is focal bleeding due to a loss of the integrity of small vessels.

Other cytotoxic reactions based on autoimmune or autoallergic processes exist. However, the primary mechanism of these diseases is delayed hypersensitivity. This group of disorders will be covered in another chapter of this book.

Immunopathology of immune complex diseases

Like Type II, type III hypersensitivity reactions are also caused by IgG and IgM antibodies. The major difference between them is that Type II reactions are due to antibodies directed against antigens on the surface of specific cells or tissues; whereas in the Type III reactions the antibodies bind to widely distributed antigens, or soluble antigens in serum. Accordingly, the damage produced in type II reactions is localized to a particular tissue or cell type, while damage caused by Type III reactions affects organs where antigen-antibody complexes are deposited. Although immune complexes are usually removed by the reticuloendothelial system, occasionally their formation can lead to a hypersensitivity reaction. In this case, activation of the complement system by these immune complexes results in the accumulation of neutrophils, leading to the release of lysosomal enzymes and reactive oxygen metabolites that cause destruction of the elastic lamina of arteries (e.g., serum sickness); basement membrane of the kidney glomerulus (e.g., glomerulonephritis); walls of small vessels (e.g., Arthus reaction); or articular cartilage of joints (e.g., rheumatoid arthritis).

The alternative pathway of complement activation plays a role in the pathogenesis of some types of lesions that may resemble immune complex-mediated lesions. Activation of this pathway also results in formation of C3a and C5a, accumulation of polymorphonuclear cells, and tissue destruction. Complement mediators such as anaphylatoxins may induce endothelial cell contraction and open cell junctions so that soluble immune complexes can deposit in basement membranes or inflammatory cells can enter into tissue spaces.

The introduction of new and more sensitive methods of detecting immune complexes has generated a large catalog of diseases associated with circulating immune complexes. Yet the purely diagnostic role attributed to the detection of immune complexes has lost some of its clinical significance. Nevertheless, the detection of immune complexes is still a useful tool in clinical medicine. For example, identification of the antigen in the complex may help determine the cause of the disease; e.g., drugs and infectious (viral, bacterial, parasitic) agents. In addition, study of the molecular composition of immune complexes may give an insight into their pathogenic potential. That is, the pathogenicity of immune complexes depends on the physicochemical and biological properties of the antigen, antibody, and their product; i.e., the molecular weight and antigenic valency of the antigen; the class, subclass, and affinity of the specific an-

tibody; the relative ratio of antigen to antibody within the complex; the ability of the complex to activate complement by the classical or alternative pathway, through the antigen or through the antibody, and its ability to react with rheumatoid factors or with various cellular receptor systems. The demonstration in the patient's specimen of the presence of soluble immune complexes coupled to any evidence of disequilibrium in the normal homeostasis of the complement system strongly indicates their pathogenic role.

On the other hand, immune complex formation may often be a desirable phenomenon effecting fast antigen removal. This process is mediated, at least in part, by Fc receptors present on lymphocytes, macrophages, Küpffer cells, hepatocytes, platelets, and cells of the human glomerulus. Formation of high-affinity IgG antibody during the secondary immune response should accelerate antigen removal when compared to formation of low-affinity IgM antibody during the primary immune response. Moreover, immune complex formation allows for prolonged contact of the immune system (e.g., in the lymphoid organs) with antigen, thus leading to extensive immune recognition of the antigen. This notion is consistent with the possibility that insufficiency of Fc receptors in systemic lupus erythematosus may favor the prolonged circulation of immune complexes. Another mechanism for antigen removal is the clearance of immune complexes through filtering membranes, provided they are small enough to leave the circulation. This is possible when the antigen is small and the immune complexes are formed in large antigen excess. By this mechanism, however, there is a risk of producing localized tissue damage due to immune complex trapping that leads to complement activation. Several mediators can influence the pathogenic effect of immune complexes. Rheumatoid factors, complement components, and immunoconglutinin are the most efficient humoral receptors for modulating certain characteristics of immune complexes, such as size, solubility, and tissue affinity.

Rheumatoid factors can react with the Fc portion of altered immunoglobulins, including IgG, or they may alter the binding of immune complexes or aggregated IgG via the C3b receptor present in renal glomeruli. IgM-rheumatoid factor has also been found to inhibit complement binding by red cell-bound aggregates.

The complement system is probably the most important humoral receptor that can affect the pathogenicity of immune complexes. Clearly, complement activation by immune complexes is the hallmark and initial event in immune complex-induced tissue injury; that is, the generation of anaphylatoxins C3a and C5a leads to increased vascular permeability by triggering mast cell degranulation and histamine release. It has been suggested that immune complex-induced hypercatabolism of complement can be dampened by an amplification pathway that in itself is attenuated by control proteins.

Immunoconglutinin antibody, primarily of the IgM class, is directed at activated complement components (e.g., C3b and activated C4). It reacts in vitro with antigen-antibody-complement complexes, markedly enhancing their clumping. In humans, it is produced in response to immunization during certain infections as well as in patients with rheumatic diseases. Immunoconglutinin may have an important bearing on immune complex metabolism, distribution, and target organ effects. For instance, it could either enhance complement fixation, or inhibit C3b binding to membrane receptors. The role of immunoconglutinin in promoting aggregation of complement-containing complexes may be a balance to the recently reported solubilization of complexes by C3b. Whether the net effect of immunoconglutinin is harmful or beneficial to the host may actually depend on the delicate balance of a number of specific factors.

The major allergic disorders with pathogenesis mediated by Type III hypersensitivity reactions will be discussed briefly in the remainder of this section.

Arthus reaction

This is a dermal inflammatory response caused by the reaction of precipitating antibody with antigen placed in the skin. Histologically, this reaction consists of vascular fibrinoid necrosis and emigration of neutrophils and eosinophils. Extension of the response reveals thrombosis with subsequent ischemic necrosis. Immune complexes forming microprecipitates in vessel walls or in adjacent tissue spaces, along with the activation of complement, contribute to the development of the lesion. Infiltration by polymorphonuclear leukocytes and the release of lysosomal enzymes following phagocytosis of immune complexes result in damage to the vascular endothelium. Clumping of cells and activation of the clotting system may produce occlusion of small vessels and ischemic necrosis.

Serum sickness

This was a common disorder when heterologous antiserum was used as passive immunization in the treatment of a number of infectious and toxic conditions in the preantibiotic era. This clinical approach is limited now to a very few toxic diseases and the use of antilymphocyte or antithymocyte globulin for immunosuppressive therapy. Other drugs may occasionally cause a mild serum sickness response, particularly sulfonamides, penicillin, and cephalosporins. The pathogenesis of the human disease is based on the brisk IgG or IgM antibody response, which is elicited upon exposure to a high-dose protein antigen. Thus, when newly formed antibody reacts with residual antigen in the circulation to form immune complexes in moderate antigen excess, the circulating immune complexes are deposited on vascular endothelium in various organs. Activation of complement via the classical pathway generates chemotactic factors that localize inflammatory cells in and around blood vessels. Failure of mononuclear phagocytes to efficiently remove immune complexes leads to tissue damage. If further antigen exposure is prevented, the disease is self-limited because complement activation is much less efficient in the presence of antibody excess complexes. Certain manifestations of serum sickness may be due to activation of complement-derived anaphylatoxins, vasoactive peptides, or coincidental IgE antibody response.

Goodpasture's syndrome

This hypersensitivity reaction is clinically manifested by a combination of pulmonary hemorrhage and glomerulonephritis. In severe cases there is extensive intraalveolar hemorrhage and marked proliferative glomerulonephritis. The disease is caused by antibodies to basement membrane antigens shared by the lung and kidney. Immunoglobulin and complement may be identified in the basement membrane of pulmonary alveoli and renal glomeruli. Experimental Goodpasture's syndrome has been produced using passively transferred antibody to Type IV collagen and/or laminin, both components of the basement membrane.

Other immune complex diseases

In addition to the renal glomerulus, other organs of the body contain capillary basement membrane exposed to circulating blood, such as the synovial capillaries (e.g., in arthritis); the choroid plexus of the brain (e.g., in systemic lupus erythematosus); and the uveal tract of the eye (e.g., in uveitis). These organs are susceptible to anti-basement membrane antibody attack and deposition of immune complexes.

Finally, connective tissue (collagen-vascular) disorders include a number of conditions believed to be caused primarily by immune complex mechanisms. These diseases include polyarteritis nodosa, systemic lupus erythematosus, dermatomyositis, progressive systemic sclerosis (scleroderma), thrombocytopenic purpura, rheumatic fever, and rheumatoid arthritis. The shared lesions include fibrinoid necrosis, glomerulonephritis, and vasculitis. Other immune effector mechanisms (e.g., neutralization, cytotoxic, delayed, and granulomatous reactions) play a pathogenic role in some lesions seen in these diseases, but the major manifestations may be attributed to immune complex reactions. The causes of these diseases are quite variable.

Cell-mediated immune reactions

The immune reactions included under this heading are only those that involve specific cell-mediated cytotoxic effector mechanisms. These must be distinguished from reactons mediated by nonsensitized lymphocytes and hence are "nonspecific." The nonsensitized lymphocytes involved in the latter group of reactions are either null cells activated by antibodies bound to their Fc receptors (i.e., antibody-dependent cell-mediated cytotoxicity or ADCC) or natural killer (NK) cells, which react directly with target cells. Activated macrophages can also produce direct cytotoxicity. In addition, other cell types such as polymorphonuclear leukocytes or macrophages may function as killer cells via cytophilic antibody. Macrophages may also be activated by nonspecific stimulators such as phorbol esters or polynucleotides.

In contrast to nonspecific cell-mediated reactions, the original classification of hypersensitivity proposed by Gell and Coombs in 1963 included within Type IV (delayed hypersensitivity) only those specific reactions that take more than 12 hours to develop. Since then, much more has been learned about the mechanisms underlying Type IV reactions. Originally, four subtypes of delayed hypersensitivity were identified depending on the type of reaction observed when antigen was directly applied to the skin or injected intradermally: the Jones-Mote reaction, contact hypersensitivity, tuberculin-type hypersensitivity, and granulomatous response.

These four subtypes (Type IV reactions) differ from types I, II, and III, as originally described by Gell and Coombs, in at least three ways:

1. all four subtypes of this immunologically-specific, delayed inflammatory reaction are not mediated by antibodies but by specifically sensitized T lymphocytes bearing a variety of surface phenotypes,
2. each subtype occurs within at least 12 to 72 hours, and
3. their gross (e.g., erythema and induration) and microscopic (e.g., composed predominantly of lymphocytes and macrophages or mononuclear cells) appearances are different.

The four subtypes of delayed hypersensitivity response are associated with T-cell protective immunity but do not necessarily run parallel to it. Although sensitized T cells do initiate the response, they often perform their task by recruiting other cell types to the reaction site. The Jones-Mote reaction is maximal at 24 hours. Contact and tuberculin-type hypersensitivities, which have a similar time course, are maximal at 48 to 72 hours. In certain situations, tuberculin-type reactions may develop at 21 to 28 days into a granulomatous hypersensitivity response that may continue for several weeks (e.g., skin testing in leprosy).

Again, the four immunopathologic types of cell-mediated specific immune reaction are not clear-cut or mutually exclusive. In fact, they may overlap to some extent, or occur sequentially following a single antigenic challenge. Therefore, many of the hypersensitivity reactions encountered in practice do not fit into one category alone. Histologically, one can observe an infiltration of cells, initiated with a perivascular accumulation of lymphocytes and monocytes at the site of antigen deposition. Experimental studies using labeled, specifically sensitized lymphocytes transferred to normal donors have demonstrated that only a few infiltrating cells are actually sensitized. These cells were found to be responsible for the large numbers of unlabeled cells that infiltrated the reaction site and produced tissue damage. The inflammatory response is induced and maintained by soluble mediators derived from macrophages (monokines) or from T lymphocytes (lymphokines). Activated macrophages secrete interleukin 1 along with a variety of other inflammatory mediators and enzymes. These mediators may stimulate proliferation of fibroblasts, digest tissue components, or activate other inflammatory systems that participate in the later phases of the delayed hypersensitivity response ending up with resolution and healing. Tissue destruction may be brought about by T cytotoxic lymphocytes or lymphokine activated macrophages.

As with the in vitro antigen-antibody reaction, the reaction of specifically sensitized lymphocytes with antigen may also be measured in vitro. Primary reactions involve direct effects of antigens on sensitized cells (e.g., antigen binding or induction of proliferation of reacting cells); whereas secondary reactions are the result of the effects of immune activated cells on other cells (e.g., killing of target cells by sensitized lymphocytes), or of the effects of products released from cells (i.e., lymphokines). The effect of cell-mediated immunity in vivo is represented by the delayed hypersensitivity and granulomatous reactions. Duplication of these reactions in vitro has yet to be accomplished. None-

theless, in many situations a correlation has been established between the in vitro and in vivo activity of effector cells (predominantly T lymphocyte subpopulations) or their cell products as measured by in vitro tests and by in vivo responses. The immune specific delayed hypersensitivity reactions are mediated by T_D (delayed hypersensitivity) or T_K (killer or cytotoxic) cells.

Sensitized T_D lymphocytes are activated to proliferate in the presence of antigen and to produce and release a variety of lymphocyte mediators (lymphokines). Their activity correlates in vitro with antigen-induced blast transformation. Lymphokine production may be measured by determining a variety of effects on other cells, some of which may be measured in vitro. For example, lymphokines may activate macrophages to produce damage to cells not bearing the specific antigen recognized by the T_D effector cell ("innocent bystander" effect). In this way, reactions of T_D cells with antigen on one cell may ultimately cause damage to an antigenically unrelated cell if a severe inflammatory response is generated. Another in vitro technique employed to measure the effects of antigen on T_D cells is macrophage migration inhibition.

Target cell killing by specifically sensitized T_K lymphocytes is an immune-specific, strictly cell-mediated, effector function that does not require antiserum or complement to be effective. It is active against foreign MHC class I antigens (graft rejection), viral antigens expressed on cell surfaces, or tumor antigens. Upon second contact with antigen in vivo, this population of cells is available to kill cells expressing the antigen (memory).

It has been demonstrated that interleukin 2 has the capacity to expand and activate a new class of cytolytic cells, lymphokine-activated cells (LAK). These cells are potent killers of fresh tumor cells both in vitro and in vivo. In contrast to the lytic activity of T_K cells, lysis by LAK cells in vitro is not antigen specific, i.e., more than one type of tumor can be lysed, and killing is not self restricted. However, on the basis of cell surface markers, interleukin 2 acts on a precursor cell that differentiates into the activated killer, LAK. This finding has great potential in the clinical application of cancer immunotherapy.

This section has focused more on the efferent limb, or effector phase, of cell-mediated immunity than on the afferent limb, or induction phase, because of the paucity of knowledge available regarding the induction phase.

There are a considerable number of chronic diseases in humans, whose pathogenesis is mediated by delayed hypersensitivity. Most are due to infectious agents such as mycobacteria, protozoa, and fungi (e.g., tuberculosis, leprosy, leishmaniasis, listeriosis, deep fungal infections, and helminthic infections). The threat posed by these diseases is met by lymphocytes and macrophages. Although these diseases have a protective immune response, protective immunity and delayed hypersensitivity do not necessarily coincide.

SUGGESTED READING

Adams DO and Hanna Jr MG: Contemporary topics in immunobiology, macrophage activation, vol 13, New York, 1984, Plenum Press.

Barrett JT: Basic immunology and its medical application, ed 2, St. Louis, 1980, Mosby–Year Book, Inc.

Bellanti JA: Immunology III, Philadelphia, 1984, WB Saunders Co.

Bellanti JA and Herscowitz HB: The reticuloendothelial system: a comprehensive treatise. In Friedman H, Escobar MR, and Reichard SM, eds: Immunology, vol 6, New York, 1984, Plenum Press.

Escobar MR and Friedman H: Macrophages and lymphocytes: nature, functions and interaction part A and part B, vols. 121A and 121B, New York, 1980, Plenum Press.

Nahmias AJ and O'Reilly RJ: Comprehensive immunology. In Good RA and Day SB, eds: Immunology of human infection—Part I: bacteria, mycoplasmae, chlamydiae, and fungi, vol 8, New York, 1981, Plenum Publishing Corp.

Nahmias AJ and O'Reilly RJ: Comprehensive immunology. In Good RA and Day SB, eds: Immunology of human infection—Part II: viruses and parasites; immunodiagnosis and prevention of infectious diseases, vol 9, New York, 1982, Plenum Publishing Corp.

Parker CW: Clinical immunology, vols I and II, Philadelphia, 1980, WB Saunders Co.

Paul W: Fundamental immunology, ed 2, New York, 1989, Raven Press.

Phillips SM and Escobar MR: The reticuloendothelial system: a comprehensive treatise. In Friedman H, Escobar MR, and Reichard SM, eds: Hypersensitivity, vol 9, New York, 1986, Plenum Press.

Roitt IM, Brostoff J, and Male DK: Immunology, ed 2, St. Louis, 1989, Mosby–Year Book, Inc.

Rose NR and Siegel B: The reticuloendothelial system: a comprehensive treatise. In Friedman H, Escobar MR, and Reichard SM, eds: Immunopathology, vol 4, New York, 1983, Plenum Press.

Salinas FA and Hanna Jr, MG: Contemporary topics in immunobiology. In Hanna Jr, MG, ed: Immune complexes and human cancer, vol 15, New York, 1985, Plenum Press.

Sell S: Immunology, immunopathology and immunity, ed 4, New York, 1987, Elsevier Science Publishing Co, Inc.

Stites DP, Stobo JD, and Wells JV: Basic and clinical immunology, ed 6, Los Altos, Ca 1987, Appleton and Lange.

34 Antibody detection for the diagnosis of infectious disease

Thomas J. Tinghitella

The latter half of the nineteenth century saw great advances in man's ability to identify and culture many microorganisms, particularly those that cause disease in man or animals. At the same time the first agglutination reactions were observed when serum and whole microorganisms were mixed together. This observation led to the realization that serum contained substances which caused clumping of bacteria and potentially could be used to identify microorganisms.

The early bacteriologists demonstrated that in both animals and man the appearance of these "agglutinins" occurred after naturally acquired disease or experimental inoculation. The molecular identity as well as other properties of these "agglutinins" did not occur until many decades later during the blossoming of what has come to be known as immunochemistry. We know today that phenomenon observed is due to immunoglobulins with either specific interaction for antigens of the microorganism or nonspecific for a microorganism but measurable during infection with that microorganism.

Since the first observation of agglutination, many other methods have been devised for the detection and specific-quantitation of antibody. This review will focus on those methods that currently enjoy the most popularity in clinical laboratories and provide the most clinically relevant information.

ROUTINE METHODS TO DETECT SPECIFIC ANTIBODY

A wide range of methods have been developed to detect antibody. Some, such as latex agglutination, do not require instrumentation, are simple to perform, are relatively fast, and are less sophisticated in principle. Others require or use instrumentation and require an increased level of sophistication by the technologists. The most common methodologies presently in vogue, with examples of current usage are listed in Box 34-1.

Agglutination

These are among the earliest methods used to detect antibody to soluble antigens. Bentonite flocculation and later agglutination tests mimic the agglutination or clumping of particulate antigens such as bacteria.

Box 34-1 Some common laboratory methods for the detection of specific antibody

METHOD	EXAMPLE OF USAGE
Bentonite Flocculation	Syphilis screen
Latex Agglutination	Rubella
Passive Hemagglutination	Heterophile antibody
Complement Fixation	Influenza A and B
Radioimmunoassay	Strep *pneumoniae*
Enzyme linked immunoabsorbent assay (ELISA)	HIV-1, hepatitis B
Indirect Immunofluorescent Microscopy	Measles, Varicella-Zoster *Toxoplasma*
Microparticle Immunoassay	Rubella
Precipitation in Agarose Gels	Fungal antibodies
Particle-Enhanced Immunoassay	Rubella antibody

Soluble antigens adhere to bentonite carbon or red cell particles by electrostatic forces. In the presence of antibody the particles agglutinate, showing macroscopically visible clumping after rotation or rocking the system. A semi-quantitative estimate of the amount of antibody present can be obtained by making serial (generally twofold) dilutions of the fluid being examined.

Whether or not agglutination occurs is affected principally by the variables of pH, salt, and protein concentration. Most commercially available agglutination methods perform best in serum (not plasma) and cerebrospinal fluid. Other fluids such as synovial, urine, or sputum, because of their nature (including changed viscosity), often require some chemical pretreatment before testing.

These tests are generally easy to perform and require only brief periods (10 minutes) of incubation after mixing the components.

Reading and interpretation, however, requires experience. Appropriate controls are required particularly to pre-

467

vent the interpretation of nonspecific findings as a positive result. This is often accomplished by utilizing particles to which *no* antigen has been attached. This is a very important control when the particle is a biological substrate (e.g., a red blood cell) having its own antigens.

Agglutination tests of all types have found widespread use in clinical laboratories particularly since no additional instrumentation is required.

These tests are most often performed on slides (glass or waxed cardboard) but can also be accomplished in test tubes or plastic trays with wells (microdilution format).

One significant disadvantage of agglutination assays is that they are susceptible to the prozone phenomenon. At very high concentration of antibody the crosslinking of antigen does not take place, producing a falsely negative result. Diluting the specimen for screening reduces the incidence of this problem.

There remains little place for methods which utilize direct agglutination of whole microorganisms to detect antibody. The so-called "Febrile agglutinins" are an example which have been replaced by more clinically relevant tests. Detection of antibody to *Brucella* organisms is the only exception to this.

Inhibition of agglutination, whether latex particles or red blood cells, is an alternative method for the detection of antibody. In many systems this appears to have increased sensitivity. In agglutination inhibition reactions, patient serum and antigen (attached to particle) are reacted together first. If antibody is present in patient sera then subsequent addition of indicator antibody will not result in agglutination. A variation of this makes use of virus receptors on red blood cells for Influenza and Rubella virus which directly agglutinate red cells. In the past, this methodology was most useful for detecting antibody to Rubella.

Precipitation assays

Another early test method for detection of either antigen or antibody is precipitation of immune complexes. Many variations of this have been used over time but the basic principle of a soluble antigen complexing with antibody to form a visible precipitate is the same. This method has been performed in a fluid phase or a semi-solid phase such as agar gel, in tubes, and in plates. It has been most widely used in immunodiffusion systems which extend the utility of this test to determination of antigen/antibody identity or nonidentity.

Conversely, precipitation requires a great deal more antigen and antibody for visualization; hence, its sensitivity is significantly less than agglutination assays. This limits the utility of precipitation in clinical assays to disease states in which extremely high levels of antibody are diagnostic. This method is most useful to detect antibody to clinically important fungi.

Complement fixation (CF) assays

A previous generation of "serologists" relied heavily on the method known as "Complement Fixation." Although somewhat cumbersome and tedious, it routinely made possible a degree of sensitivity not formerly observed. This method has been used for a large variety of analysis, both for antigen and antibody. The assay is simply a competition for complement, usually guinea pig, between the antigen-antibody interaction being measured and an indicator system of red blood cells and anti-red blood cell antibody (referred to as Hemolysin). If complement is bound by the antibody being sought, none remains to be bound by the red blood cell/anti-red blood cell antibody complex and the cells remain intact. If little or no antibody is present, then the indicator cells bind the complement proteins and are lysed. Results are reported as a serial dilution end point (titer). Unfortunately, bacterial contamination, high levels of lipoprotein, and immune complexes also bind complement, so that some specimens are inherently anticomplementary. Likewise, sera in which severe hemolysis has occurred is unsuitable for testing. CF tests do not distinguish the class of antibody present (all IgG, IgM, and some IgA) and therefore have little value in the diagnosis of acute infection unless performed on acute and convalescent sera. For the most part, this test has been abandoned in favor of EIA and other new methods.

The "sandwich assays": RIA, EIA, and IFA

Some of the most popular assays used in clinical laboratories are radioimmunoassay (RIA); enzyme-linked or enzyme immunoassay (EIA, ELISA); and indirect immunofluorescence (IFA). In detecting and quantitating antibody, these three methods are similar in concept, differing only in the type of signal that is generated and how it is observed or measured. Each assay begins with some form of a solid support such as polystyrene beads, plastic tube, microtiter trays, or paper disks for EIA and RIA. Glass slides are used for IFA. Attached chemically or absorbed onto the surface of these supports are the antigen(s) of the test system. Bovine serum albumin or another protein (e.g., casein) is used in EIA and RIA as a blocking agent to decrease any nonspecific attachment of antibody at unoccupied sites. Sera to be tested is added to the test system and allowed to interact with the antigens on the solid support. This interaction or incubation is usually performed at room temperature or 37°C for a period (often 15 minutes to one hour) determined empirically by the manufacturer or researcher to obtain optimal results. Once incubation is complete, a washing step is performed to remove any immunoglobulin that has not attached specifically to antigen. Washing agents are usually a combination of buffer, such as phosphate buffered saline (PBS), and a surfactant like Tween 20. Wash steps are most crucial in all these assays for precise and reproducible results. Mechanical washers are most often used to achieve this goal although manual methods can produce the same result. The attached antibody is then detected by the addition of antisera to human immunoglobulin. This antisera, whether polyclonal or monoclonal, has a detectable marker attached. RIA uses a radioactive element such as 125_I. EIA systems use an enzyme, the most popular being alkaline phosphatase or horseradish peroxidase. IFA uses a molecule such as fluorescein or rhodamine which emit a particular wavelength of visible light after stimulation by ultraviolet light. After incubation of this marker immunoglobulin, additional washing removes any nonspecifically attached immunoglobulin. At this point, the test system consists of solid support with antigens, specific antibody from the patient serum, and detecting antibody, with marker, in effect a sandwich of reagents.

At this point, both RIA and IFA methods can be read. The RIA requires quantitation of the total amount of radioactive material usually by using a gamma counter. IFA tests require the use of a fluorescent microscope with a wavelength of excitation light that meets the requirement for the particular fluorochrome chosen. This is generally read and interpreted visually but has been adapted in some systems to be read by instrumentation (fluorometer).

EIA tests require an additional step. A substrate for the marker enzyme is needed for development of a colored reactant. This becomes the end point for observation and measurement is often by spectrophotometer and is analogous to the radioactivity of RIA and the fluorescence of IFA.

DETECTION OF ISOTYPIC SPECIFIC ANTIBODY

All three of the "sandwich" assays described can be designed to detect a particular isotypic antibody. Most commonly these are for IgG specific antibody and IgM specific antibody. Specific IgA can also be detected but the clinical relevance of this molecule for infectious disease diagnosis is at present of limited importance.

In order to detect class specific antibody, one can utilize as the signal or marker immunoglobulin (i.e., radiolabelled, fluorescein labelled, or enzyme labelled) either a polyclonal or monoclonal antibody to the heavy chain of IgG or IgM.

Detection of IgG-specific antibody is by far the simplest since in most patient specimens the quantity of this far exceeds other immunoglobulins. In addition most IgG will be of high affinity for the antigens present on the solid support.

Detection of IgM is much more problematic. A variety of reasons account for the high incidence of false positive and false negative findings when using the systems outlined in this section. The presence of rheumatoid factor, for example, may produce false positive results, while competition for antigenic sites with higher concentration and higher affinity IgG may result in false negative findings. In some infections the IgM response is relatively weak, making more sensitive assays those of choice over those with a high percentage of false negatives.

Methods have been developed to surmount the problems associated with the detection of IgM-specific antibody. Essentially they all involve a physical separation of IgM from other immunoglobulins and other serum proteins prior to the use of the marker anti-IgM. These methods are either extrinsic or intrinsic to the procedure. Extrinsic procedures separate IgG from IgM prior to performing the usual routine assay. An intrinsic procedure is typified by the method called "reverse capture." In this method, IgM in the patient serum is "captured" by anti-IgM coated onto microdilution plates. In theory, washing removes all other serum proteins so that only the patient's IgM remains. The captured antibodies are then reacted with antigens which are conjugated to a marker enzyme such as alkaline phosphatase. In a fashion similar to the generalized EIA method described previously, the amount of bound antibody is measured directly by the amount of colored product from the enzyme substrate interaction. The amount of bound antibody is directly proportional to the amount of specific patient IgM originally bound to the microtiter wells.

Separating IgG from IgM prior to testing is achieved by some form of column chromatography, centrifugation, or an adsorbent process (see Table 34-1) such as incubating patient serum with aggregated IgG to remove rheumatoid factor, or with *Staphylococcus aureus* protein A, or streptococcal protein G to remove most of the IgG present. Commercially available columns with protein G appear to be the most suitable for the clinical laboratory because of speed and efficiency.

Advantages and disadvantages of "sandwich assays"

Sensitivity

Collectively, the group of assays described are significantly more sensitive than previously used methods like agglutination, hemagglutination inhibition, and complement fixation. Sensitivity among these varies with the analysis. RIA in general is believed to be somewhat more sensitive than either EIA or IFA. Steric hindrance of large enzymes is often cited as reducing the sensitivity of EIA when a comparable RIA is performed. IFA and EIA have very similar sensitivities but IFA is heavily dependent on the quality of the fluorescent microscope or fluorometer used. Since, at present, there is no standard for fluorescence, a given IFA assay will at the same time be more or less sensitive than the equivalent EIA.

Specificity

Specificity depends most heavily on a combination of the antisera or antibodies used in the detection signal and the purity of the antigen in the test system. Spurious or nonspecific findings can occur particularly when the signal (i.e., positive finding) to noise (i.e., background) is very low. Each particular analysis for detection of specific antibody must undergo extensive analysis with clinical comparisons and other methodologies to determine its sensitivity. Reconfiguration of first generation tests regardless of whether they are in-house or commercially available kits is often needed to improve specificity and sensitivity.

Results

Any of the sandwich methodologies described can be constructed to provide qualitative, semi-quantitative, or quantitative results. IFA methods are most often semiquantitative or qualitative although quantitative results can be produced if one uses a fluorometer. Qualitative results are

Table 34-1 Methods to separate IGM immunoglobulins from other serum proteins

Method	Ease of use	Efficiency
Gradient Centrifugation	Difficult	Excellent
Protein A*	Easy	Good
Protein G*	Easy	Excellent
Sieving Chromatography	Moderate	Very good
Affinity Chromatography*	Easy	Very good

*Commercially available products

those which are constructed to give an interpretation of reactive, nonreactive, immune, or nonimmune. Semiquantitative results are those obtained as a traditional titer from a serial twofold dilution scheme. IFA results are most often and most easily constructed to obtain semiquantitative results although both EIA and RIA methods which have an established quantitative analytical curve can be reinterpretated in a semiquantitative manner.

Endpoint determinations

The greatest difficulty in each of those assays is in establishing a valid endpoint determination, i.e., 1) the ability to distinguish a positive finding from a negative finding if the results are reported in a qualitative manner or 2) in determining the point at which the level of antibody is reduced to zero in a semiquantitative or quantitative assay.

Qualitative assays

In both RIA and EIA procedures, the discriminator between a positive and negative finding is usually determined by establishing a cutoff produced by either a ratio or a subtractive method between known negative and a reference standard positive. In order to increase specificity, one may choose to add a fraction obtained by experience to establish the cutoff or one may use a number of multiples or standard deviations from the result. The variation inherent in these assays makes it necessary to consider a grey zone, i.e., neither positive or negative in establishing the cutoff. Common practice and the need for specificity often dictate a 10% to 20% margin of error for interpretation of endpoint.

In the IFA procedure, interpretation is much more subjective and usually obtained by grading the intensity or degree of fluorescence to that of a known positive specimen. The use of a fluorometer eliminates the subjectivity of this determination and becomes essentially similar to the EIA and RIA procedure.

Semiquantitative assays

The endpoint of those assays which are performed with serial twofold dilutions (principally microscopically read IFA) is obtained by using the principle outlined previously in that one dilution visually appears to the reader to be the endpoint. The intensity of reaction in that dilution is compared to the endpoint result of a known positive specimen which is performed at each testing time. This is the same as that performed for other assays like complement fixation or latex agglutination.

Quantitative assays

Regardless of the assay used one can quantitatively determine the amount of specific antibody by construction of a standard curve using manufacturer-provided or other standard references. Whether the results are obtained in International Units (IU) or direct quantitation depends on the historical development of the assay or work done by organizations such as The World Health Organization to standardize the results.

These assays generally have a limit of sensitivity, the reliability of which varies from assay to assay. Laboratorians must be aware of this limit in order to make appropriate clinical decisions. Likewise these assays generally have a plateau of reactivity so that results at the high end of the standard curve generated will also give inaccurate results. Dilution and retesting of patient specimen may be necessary to obtain accurate results.

Quality control

All assays should incorporate a known negative and positive specimen. This may be commercially available or may be an in-house product. It is imperative that for all EIA and RIA testing this be done with each assay run. Negative controls examine the specificity of testing while positive controls determine the accurate performance of the testing and consistency in test sensitivity.

Which type of test to use

In addition to sensitivity, specificity, and endpoint results, a number of other factors determine the type of method one may choose to perform for a given analysis. RIA tests appear to have the advantage of sensitivity: they are able to detect quantities of protein in the picogram range. RIA methods also appear to have a greater degree of reproducibility for some analysis. Most clinical analysis for antibody to infectious agents rarely requires this degree of sensitivity or reproducibility. EIA methods have the advantage of generally having greater storage potential and do not require the worrisome aspect of disposal of radioactive material.

EIA, RIA and the use of a fluorometer remove the subjectivity of analysis inherent in IFA methods using microscopy. However, the specificity of IFA testing may be greater for some analyses if the test visualizes specific components (e.g., intranuclear inclusions of viruses like CMV) for a positive finding.

The choice of a method for a particular analyte requires an evaluation of all these parameters as well as a cost effectiveness analysis for a particular laboratory setting.

CONFIRMATORY TESTS FOR THE PRESENCE OF ANTIBODY

As the methods outlined previously are applied to specific detection of antibody, it is clear that for most analysis the issue of specificity is still at question. This is so principally because the precise antigenic nature of the antigen(s) is not known or if it is known, the possibility of cross-reactivity and other interfering substances can be raised. The use of recombinant antigens in theory increases specificity since other antigens are not present, although some cross-reacting antibodies may occur.

The methods outlined previously are for the most part, considered to be screening tools particularly with assays utilizing crude or uncharacterized antigens. The simplest way to confirm RIA or EIA results is by neutralization of patient antibody activity by competing specific antibody. The confirmatory reagent is specific antibody, usually of human origin, which results in a blocking of patient antibody reaction with the antigen. This blocking results in a reduction of signal when compared to the nonneutralized specimen. A result is usually considered confirmed if a reduction in signal of at least 50% is attained. Neutralization is a useful method but it has its disadvantages. Results of weakly reactive specimens may be so close to the assay cutoff that it is impossible to reliably achieve a 50% reduction. Further, cross reactive results, because of their similarity, may also result in a significant signal reduction.

The most reliable method (greatest sensitivity) for confirming antibody reactions is by visualization of the antigen antibody reactions.

Western blotting is a method for analysis of proteins which is similar to the method of Southern (hence the name) for analysis of DNA. In this method, protein antigens are treated with an ionic detergent such as sodium dodecyl sulfate, and then subjected to electrophoresis through a polyacrylamide gel. Proteins are separated by their molecular weight resulting in bands of antigens migrating through the gel. Mirror images of these bands are transferred to a solid support such as nitrocellulose during a second electrophoresis. Most frequently the solid support is cut into strips for ease of handling. The remainder of the assay is similar to the sandwich EIA tests described previously. Patient sera is incubated with the separated antigens, then washed and incubated with polyvalent or isotypic specific antibody that is conjugated to an enzyme. The final procedure—after washing to remove any nonspecifically bound antibody—is visualization of the specific antigen and antibody reactants by incubation with a substrate for the particular conjugated enzyme. The results are read visually or by densitometer. Most often the presence of specific molecular weight bands for a particular pathogen are needed for a positive interpretation. Visual interpretation makes the method somewhat subjective, particularly if the band patterns are weak. Standardized interpretations are rare and thus, interlaboratory discrepancies exist.

Indirect immunofluorescence, because of its visual nature, can also be utilized as a confirmatory test. This is particularly true if specific fluorescent structures or patterns, such as the intranuclear inclusions of virus replication, can be used as the standard.

Finally, the use of highly specific recombinant antigens with little or no cross-reactive epitopes are ideally suited as confirmatory tests. If they are inexpensive and simple enough to produce, they can simply replace current screening methods.

NEWER METHODS
Chemiluminescent assays

Many of the assays described previously can be tailored into a chemiluminescent assay. The final marker or signal, be it a radioactive isotope or an enzyme which effects a substrate, can be readily replaced by the enzymes luciferase (and others) and the substrates necessary for bursts of light to be produced. Manual methods introduced in the 1970s were the major disadvantages. The need for precise and accurate manual manipulations made this method impractical for daily clinical use. The development of fully automated methods, however, has solved these problems. Theoretically, these assays offer the sensitivity of radioimmune assays without the inherent problems. In addition, those assays which require photographic development, such as autoradiography, significantly speed up the process. Many chemiluminescent assays are on the horizon for use in clinical laboratories but have not yet made a great impact principally because of the need for capital investment.

Particle enhanced immunoassays

As antigen and antibody complexes increase in size, the light-scattering properties change. This change can be monitored by spectrophotometry or nephelometry. The sensitivity of this method can be increased by attaching an inert support particle to a reagent such as antigen. This method can achieve sensitivity and specificity comparable to RIA and EIA. If not performed carefully, however, this method is prone to nonspecific agglutination of the particles. This relatively new method has been explored for detection and quantitation of anti-streptolysin O and C-reactive protein.

Membrane associated and microparticle EIA

These two tests are reconfigurations of the standard EIA sandwich methodology and are suitable for either individual tests (membrane associated EIA) or for high-volume fully automated systems (microparticle EIA). Both are enjoying increasing utilization in the clinical laboratory.

In the configuration of the membrane-associated test, a plastic cartridge containing absorbent material has a plastic membrane across the top. A capture antigen is attached to the plastic membrane, often in the configuration of a line or circle. As a serum specimen passes through the filter, specific antibody attaches to the membrane at the site of the antigen. Enzyme-tagged antibody and substrates are filtered through in successive steps.

A color change takes place on the surface of membrane denoting a positive reaction. The results obtained by this are qualitative only. While the sensitivity and specificity of this method is comparable to standard EIA methods, interpretation of low levels of antibody can often be subjective.

The microparticle enzyme immunoassay (MEIA) technology uses submicron particles as the solid phase to which antigen is attached. These assays are faster because of the smaller diffusion distances. The antigen-antibody complexes formed are passed over a glass fiber matrix to which the microparticle binds irreversibly. Further EIA reagents are then rapidly passed through this matrix as the final steps in the assay. This assay is somewhat more sensitive than traditional EIA procedures and certainly more rapidly accomplished.

BASIC PRINCIPLES OF SEROLOGY

Many clinicians often consider serological testing to be rarely rewarding, often confusing, bothersome at best, and totally irrelevant at worst. This is often because they do not know how to ask the appropriate questions for the tests they request. Laboratories need to not only help educate clinicians in the use of serological tests as an adjunct to clinical judgment, they also must establish protocols and practices which will aid the clinician seeking answers.

Rationale for testing

Detection of antibody to infectious agents requires asking the question, "Why is this test being performed?" There are five basic answers to this question. 1) Is antibody present? If so, this establishes exposure or possibly a past infection if only IgG is being measured. Concurrently this may be used to determine immunity to further infection. 2) Is this an acute infection? This requires demonstration of change in the quantity of antibody over time or in some cases the demonstration of IgM specific antibody. 3) Can detection of antibody provide an answer that culturing for a particular microorganism cannot? Growing some microorganisms is either difficult or requires long periods of time. Therapy for some infections requires immediate action. Therefore, culture becomes at best a confirmatory answer to clinical judgment. 4) Can detection of antibody differentiate infection from colonization? Certain microorganisms may be part of the normal flora or may be colonizers of superficial surfaces. The presence of *aspergillus* in sputum is not necessarily an indicator of invasive aspergillosis. The presence of antibody to this organism, however, supports systemic involvement. 5) Can the presence or absence of antibody determine the need for a more invasive procedure such as biopsy? A panel of antibodies for Hepatitis B, for example, can establish chronic infection as the etiology of chronic liver disease, thus eliminating or reducing the need to biopsy that organ.

Establishing the right questions before testing allows the appropriate test or panel of tests to be performed. Often times the laboratory test requisition is the appropriate starting point to guide the clinician to ask the appropriate question. Further consultation may be necessary on occasion.

Collection and storage

All specimens should be collected aseptically into sterile tubes to prevent bacterial contamination and growth. This is not a problem in specimens which are analyzed immediately but can become critical in stored specimens. Grossly lipemic specimens can be a problem in all the methods discussed above. Hemolyzed specimens generally will effect complement fixation assays but rarely will effect other assays unless there is little dilution of the original serum and the results are read colorimetrically.

All specimens should be aliquoted and stored according to the length of time before testing. It is appropriate to refrigerate at 2 to 4°C if storage is at most four to five days. Antibody concentration remains stable at −20°C for several weeks, and can be stored indefinitely at −70°C. Dilution of serum to very low levels of protein concentration, however, decreases stability regardless of the temperature at which it is stored.

Repeated freezing and thawing results in the aggregation of immunoglobulins (i.e., the formation of immune complexes). This should be avoided since it may interfere with the performance of some assays.

Contamination of cerebrospinal fluid with blood or serum is problematic because it, in effect, becomes more or less a reflection of antibody concentration in serum. Interpretation of results obtained are highly suspect.

Save the sera principle

It has always been a basic tenet of serologists that all serum samples be saved. The rationale is 1) to repeat controversial or questionable results; 2) to test acute and convalescence sera at the same time; 3) to confirm in retrospect originally unsuspected infectious agents; and 4) that it may be useful in the development of new assays.

How long frozen specimens should be maintained is often a matter of space. A good rule of thumb is the fact that it often takes two to three weeks to demonstrate a significant change in antibody level and it takes time for physicians to

see patients and order additional testing. Keeping these ideas in mind, a period of six to eight weeks is most useful. Specimens needed in development or in retrospective analysis for a new agent can be kept indefinitely at the appropriate temperature.

Antibody detection in various body fluids:

Traditionally, the detection and measurement of specific antibodies has been performed using serum. This still remains the most significant fluid for analysis of systemic illness. Analysis of other fluids, particularly cerebrospinal fluid, has often been attempted for diagnosis of local or systemic illnesses. Testing synovial, urine, and pericardial fluid are examples of attempts which, for the most part, do not provide any additional information.

Cerebrospinal fluid, on the other hand, may be helpful in the diagnosis of CNS disease when the manifestations of neurological complications are the result of local infection and a result of local inflammatory response. However, in order to do so one must also examine a concomitant serum specimen for the same antibody. Examination of only the CSF does not distinguish between the antibody present by passive transfer and the antibody which may be locally produced. Comparison of the amount (either semiquantitatively or quantitatively) in both types can determine whether or not antibody is locally produced. Ancillary tests determining the percentage of IgG in CSF, or those which establish a ratio between the amount of albumin and IgG in both CSF and serum (termed the IgG Index), or determine the rate of CNS synthesis of IgG, are also useful tools.

Since the much larger IgM molecule does not normally penetrate the blood brain, it would appear that it could also be used as a marker of CNS infection. However, its utility in this regard has not been widely studied and is complicated by the fact that during many infectious diseases, the integrity of the blood brain barrier is compromised.

BASIC GUIDELINES FOR INTERPRETATION
Detection of IgG specific antibody

Detection and measurement of this class of antibody is best used for determining immune status (as in the case of rubella infection), or exposure to a particular microorganism. High levels of IgG antibody when compared to that found in the general population are at best only suggestive of a recent infection or exposure.

Acute and convalescent sera

Ideally, demonstrating a change in the quantity of specific IgG or specific total antibody in a specimen taken at the onset of disease compared to a specimen taken two to three weeks later still represents the best serological evidence for an acute infection. Any demonstration of a single reproducible change in specific antibody provides significant evidence for acute infection. In order to accurately demonstrate any change in antibody, both specimens must be tested in the same analytical run.

A significant change in test methods which employ a twofold dilutional scheme is generally considered to be a fourfold rise in titer. The same concept can be utilized for EIA tests with a significant difference demonstrated if a ratio between the two specimens is greater than 1.5, provided that the results of at least one of the specimens is within the portion of the curve which indicated the presence of antibody.

IgM specific antibody

Since the IgM isotype is generally the first class of antibody to be produced after antigenic stimulation, its presence theoretically provides good evidence of acute infection. During the course of disease, the concentration of IgM peaks and then rapidly falls as the isotype of antibody being produced is switched to IgG. The time sequence of this is variable but usually IgM falls to undetectable levels in four to six weeks.

In some infections and in some individuals IgM persists for greater periods of time, obviating its effectiveness as a marker of acute infection. Quantitative measurements of IgM and IgG from a single specimen can often resolve the issue.

Detection of IgM-specific antibody in neonates provides the strongest support for an acute or congenital infection since any IgM found is solely the product of the neonates immune system. IgM is not transplacentally passed like IgG.

DETECTION OF SPECIFIC ANTIBODY IN BACTERIAL, VIRAL AND PARASITIC DISEASES

This section will review the current status of detecting antibody to a few selected specific microorganisms. Table 34-2 presents an overview of the utility of detecting antibody to clinically important infectious agents. The emphasis is on microorganisms that because of either the nature of the organisms or the pathogeneses of the disease makes detection of antibody rather than culture or histological examination the method of choice for diagnosis of infection. While we have previously established general principles for the performance and interpretation of tests, it is important that they are viewed in the context of the idiosyncrasies of specific microorganisms.

Treponema pallidum

Serological diagnosis of syphilis in all of its stages and manifestations depends on those antibodies called reagin. The standard flocculation test for both IgM and IgG antibody to an antigen composed of cardiolipin, cholesterol, and lecithin is known as the VDRL (for Venereal Disease Research Laboratory). This has been the most commonly employed screening method, although a similar method known as the RPR (Rapid Plasma Reagin) is fast becoming the most popular. RPR, however, is not useful when the specimen is cerebrospinal fluid and used in the diagnosis of neurosyphilis. Both tests are biologically nonspecific and therefore prone to false positive and occasionally false negative results. False positives can occur during pregnancy, exacerbations of autoimmunity, and in chronic infectious diseases. When false positive results occur the titers are generally low (1:8), but not all low titers are false positive, since low titers often occur. Most commonly this occurs in autoimmune diseases.

The VDRL and the RPR, because they are both quantitative tests and detect IgM, can be used to monitor therapy. In general, with adequate treatment there should be at least a fourfold drop in titer within three months.

Table 34-2 Clinical utility of some infectious disease antibody studies

Antibody to	Method	Clinical significance	Comments
Salmonella	Agglutination	Poor	Culture preferable
Brucella	Agglutination	Excellent	IgM antibody confirms diagnosis faster than culture.
Treponema pallidum	Agglutination/IFA	Good	See text.
Rickettsia	Agglutination	Poor	
Chlamydia trachomatis	IFA/EIA	Poor	Demonstration of organism is preferable.
Fungi (*Aspergillus, Blastomyces, Coccidioides*)	Immunodiffusion	Good	Correlates well with current systemic disease.
Toxoplasma gondii	IFA/EIA	Good	See text.
Cysticerca	EIA	Fair	Requires CSF.
Cytomegalovirus	IFA/EIA	Excellent	See text.
Epstein-Barr virus	Agglutination IFA/EIA	Excellent	See text.
Herpes simplex virus	IFA/EIA	Poor	Extensive cross-reactivity between types 1 and 2. Culture or direct smear preferable.
Influenza	CF/EIA	Excellent	
Rubella	Agglutination/EIA	Excellent	Most useful for immune status.
Rubeola	IFA/EIA	Excellent	"
Varicella Zoster	IFA/EIA	Excellent	"

All positive results from nontreponemal tests must be confirmed by treponemal specific tests. There are both indirect fluorescent tests and hemagglutination tests used for this purpose. The most commonly used are the FTA-ABS (fluorescent treponema antibody with absorption) and the MHA (microhemagglutination assay). The correlation of these tests is quite good since they both detect specific IgG. EIA tests are currently available but field experience with this method is limited. The value of these qualitative tests is that they differentiate false positives from true positives. The specificity of these tests has been found to be about 99%, therefore some false positives do occur principally in autoimmune disease.

There is still a need for a good serodiagnostic test for congenital syphilis. Current literature has suggested a renewed interest in the use of the FTA-ABS detecting specific IgM as a useful diagnostic tool. This remains to be seen. More sensitive and specific tests are also needed for neurosyphilis. Major breakthroughs in technology may be required to achieve this.

Lyme disease

Like syphilis, Lyme Disease caused by *Borrelia burgdorferi* can be manifest acutely or months to years after initial infection. Serological detection is complicated apparently by the weak immune response elicited as well as by the prominent crossreactions to treponemes and other *Borrelia* species. The methods predominantly used are commercially available IFA and EIA procedures. Sensitivities are comparable although some researchers give the edge to the EIA method. Since so many variables exist in these methodologies, definitive comparative studies have not been accomplished.

Specificity of these tests appears to be quite variable with some relying on high-screening dilutions or absorptions with treponemal antigens to improve specificity. This is all complicated by the fact that a standard strain or strains of *B. burgdorferi* are not in use, although it is not certain that this is necessary.

While most screening tests detect IgG and IgM antibody simultaneously, recent evidence suggests that testing IgM separately may be useful in diagnosing acute disease.

Western blot analysis is currently the best way to confirm serological findings, although criteria for interpretation are not currently standardized.

Epstein-Barr virus

The most common cause of the mononucleosis syndrome is Epstein-Barr virus (EBV). Detection of a nonspecific, nonviral antibody, referred to as heterophile antibody, has been the most commonly used diagnostic tool. Detecting the presence of this antibody is the first and usually the most useful step in making a diagnosis of mononucleosis. The recently available EIA methods which include a nonspecific absorption antigen are more sensitive and probably will become the test of choice.

Individuals who are heterophile negative but are suspected of having EBV infection might require a repeat heterophile test. Delayed development of heterophile antibody is documented in a significant number of individuals. In others it never develops. This is particularly true in the very young population (less than four years old). In these cases detection of EBV specific antibody is generally recommended. These include detection of IgM to the virus capsid (VCA) and transient antibody to early antigens (EA) which generally are indicative of acute infection. Antibody to the nuclear antigens (EBNA) occurs predominantly during convalescence. The presence of IgG to these antigens occurs weeks to months after infection and is generally thought to exclude recent infection but indicative of past infection. More recently EIA methods to detect antibody to a particular EBNA (EBNA-1) have been found to correlate with acute infection. This antigen crossreacts with Cytomegalovirus antigens and hence is best used as a screening procedure.

Cytomegalovirus

Current methods for culturing this agent are quite good and readily available. Isolation of this virus should be the method of choice in making a diagnosis although it does not differentiate infection and disease. When this is not possible, however, IFA and EIA serological methods are useful. Using these methods, antibody prevalence in a population over 30 years old ranges from 40% to 100%.

Detection of IgM in neonates by this method is helpful in diagnosing congenital CMV disease. This assumes that appropriate techniques for avoiding false positives due to rheumatoid factor are used. Individuals, however, who have heterophile positive mononucleosis may demonstrate low level false positive IgM antibody to CMV. This reactivity may be due to the polyclonal antibody stimulation by Epstein-Barr virus.

The demonstration of a fourfold rise in titer whether by complement fixation, EIA, or IFA is only suggestive of recent infection. Postnatal disease can be primary or a reactivation of latent infection, hence the demonstration of a rising titer may be due to the antigenic stimulation of reactivation or due to a primary infection.

Toxoplasma gondii

The high prevalence in some populations as well as the many manifestations of infection with this organism make diagnosis extremely challenging. Serological tests have changed from the Sabin-Feldman methylene blue dye test used in research centers to commercially available IFA and EIA formats. Useful and accurate interpretation of these tests varies with the clinical state; i.e., congenital infection, primary infection acquired during pregnancy, congenital infection particularly in the immunosuppressed host, and adult disseminated cerebral disease.

Determination of immune status by detecting specific IgG antibody is simple and accurate. As with other infections it reflects exposure or past infection and therefore immunity to the organism. The diagnosis of congenital infection by serological tests, however, requires careful and accurate measurement of IgM-specific antibody. Antinuclear antibodies as well as rheumatoid factor can give false positive results. Infant sera must be tested in parallel with maternal sera for both IgM and IgG antibody. The diagnosis of toxoplasmosis in a newborn then requires a positive IgM and an IgG equivalent in maternal serum.

The level of serum antibody in ocular disease is generally quite low. Therefore a diagnosis of ocular toxoplasmosis is generally based on clinical grounds. Serology at best is only confirmatory. If, however, the patient is not immunocompromised, then the absence of antibody indicates that the likelihood of disease is nil.

Cerebral toxoplasmosis, a rare clinical entity until the appearance of acquired immune deficiency syndrome, is also difficult at present to diagnose by serological testing. Comparative examination of CSF and serum as well as determination of intrathecal synthesis of IgG may be useful in some cases. The reference test for acute toxoplasmosis is a reverse capture IgM method.

Hepatitis viruses

The commercially available third generation tests for antibody to Hepatitis A and B are highly specific and sensitive with excellent precision and ease of performance. Both RIA and EIA tests provide comparable results although the edge once again appears to be with RIA method. The advantages of the EIA methods are numerous and, therefore, they are the most popular tests. Detection of IgM specific antibody to Hepatitis A is straightforward with its presence being highly specific for acute infection with this virus. Specific IgM antibodies can be detected six to 16 weeks after infection.

Hepatitis B infection, on the other hand, requires a panel of tests for detection of surface antigen and antibody to the viral core and the surface antigen. Other markers, such as the presence of "e" antigen, are useful only under limited circumstances. While the methods are highly specific and sensitive, interpretation may be complex, requiring an understanding of the immune response to this virus. Laboratories should establish schema for evaluating patients that are both clinically useful and cost effective.

Recently, tests for the detection of Hepatitis C antibody have become available. This agent appears to be responsible for most of what has been called Non-A, Non-B hepatitis. In these tests, the product of molecular research requires significant study and improvement. Confirmation of EIA test results requires the use of immunoblot assays. These confirmatory tests also require improvement. At present the incidence of nonspecific or poorly understood results requires significant clinical judgment.

Mycoplasma pneumoniae

Serological confirmation of respiratory disease due to infection with mycoplasma pneumoniae has relied on non-specific tests such as those antibodies known as cold agglutinins. Since these tests also lack sensitivity, more specific methods have been sought. The complement fixation test using whole organisms or extracted lipid antigen has been shown to effectively detect antibody in some pneumonia patients. However, since the lipid antigen is a relatively simple glycolipid, it is not strongly immunogenic. This antigen is also relatively widespread in nature, hence, the test is not sensitive and is prone to false positives. Currently available EIA tests also use lipid antigens so that their problems are little different from the complement fixation assay. They do have the advantage of being able to distinguish IgG and IgM antibody. Clinical laboratories need to perform both specific and nonspecific assays. More importantly, clinical laboratories must make the clinician aware of the problems inherent in these assays.

SUGGESTED READING

Balows, Hausler, Herrmann, Isenberg, and Shadomy, eds: The Manual of Clinical Microbiology, ed 5, Washington, D.C., 1991, The American Society for Microbiology.

Kemeny DM and Challacombe SJ, eds: Elisa and other solid phase assays, Chichester, UK, 1988, John Wiley and Sons Ltd.

Rose, Friedman, and Fahey, eds: The manual of clinical laboratory immunology, Washington, D.C., 1986, American Society for Microbiology.

Stites DP, Stobo JP, and Wells JV, eds: Basic and clinical immunology, ed 6, Los Altos, Ca, 1987, Appleton and Lange.

35 The human leukocyte antigen system

Petrina Genco

The function and purpose of the Major Histocompatibility Complex (MHC) has been an area of intense investigation for the last 25 years. Data collected over the years has revealed the far-reaching effects of MHC in the areas of immunogenetics, immune responses, and organ transplantation.

HISTORY OF THE MAJOR HISTOCOMPATIBILITY COMPLEX

The concept of the MHC evolved from work done in the mid-1930s by Peter Gorer, who was investigating tumor transplantation and survival in several strains of mice. Early trials showed that matching for red cell antigens, as suggested by Landsteiner, did not promote engraftment. From the data collected, Gorer concluded that a system additional to red cell antigens was important in the survival of tumor allografts. He called the antigen which determined the acceptance or rejection of the tumor tissue Antigen II.

In 1948, George Snell published a paper in which he introduced the term "histocompatibility" gene. Snell had performed several grafting experiments in mice and concluded that graft rejection was not controlled by a single gene, but by several. A combination of Gorer's Antigen II and Snell's "histocompatibility" gene (H) gave rise to the title for the *H-2 system of the mouse*.

In 1952, Jean Dausset reported finding leukoagglutinins in the sera of patients who had received multiple transfusions. Further studies showed that these agglutinins were also found in 20% to 30% of multiparous women. The identification of these leukoagglutinins was the first major step in defining the *Human Leukocyte Antigen (HLA) System in man*.

Figure 35-1 compares the H-2 and HLA systems. The H-2 system is coded by genes located on chromosome 17 and the HLA system is controlled by genes located on the short arm of chromosome 6. Over the past 33 years, investigators have identified probable relationships between the H-2 complex and HLA system. Understanding of the H-2 complex has been advanced through the use of inbred mouse strains and extensive grafting experiments. These animal studies have given researchers greater insight into unraveling the MHC in man.

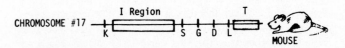

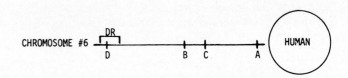

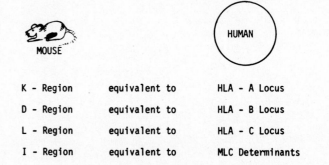

MOUSE		HUMAN
K - Region	equivalent to	HLA - A Locus
D - Region	equivalent to	HLA - B Locus
L - Region	equivalent to	HLA - C Locus
I - Region	equivalent to	MLC Determinants

Fig. 35-1 Comparison of H-2 mouse to HLA-human complex.

NOMENCLATURE ASSOCIATED WITH THE MHC
Defining the major histocompatibility complex

The *Major Histocompatibility Complex* is defined as that region of the short arm of chromosome 6 which contains an undetermined number of genes which are known to code for multiple factors including the HLA antigens and the immune response genes. The MHC is composed of loci and alleles. A *locus* is the specific site of a gene on a chromosome such as the location of HLA-A, B, C, or D locus sites. An *allele* is an alternate gene found at a given locus. In terms of the HLA system, the expression of the different

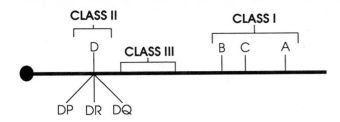

SEROLOGICALLY DEFINED ANTIGENS

HLA - A
HLA - B
HLA - C
HLA - DR
HLA - DQ

LYMPHOCYTE DEFINED ANTIGENS

HLA - D
HLA - DP

Fig. 35-2   Short arm of chromosome #6. The MHC is controlled by the short arm of chromosome #6. The HLA-A, B, and C antigens are Class I genes. The HLA D, DR, DQ, and DP antigens are Class II genes. The Class III genes are composed of C2, C4A, C4B, Factor B, and P.450 21 hydroxylase.

alleles at a specified locus would be the alternative alleles such as HLA-A1, A2, or A3. Figure 35-2 shows a simplified version of the short arm of chromosome 6. The major loci of the system and some of the important gene products of the D locus are shown.

HLA nomenclature

The HLA complex is a highly polymorphic system. Each locus is composed of multiple alleles as seen in Table 35-1. The "w" prefix stands for a workshop antigen and implies a conditional characterization of the antigen. The terms "private" and "public" can be used in reference to the HLA antigens. The term "private specificity" indicates that the HLA antigen is the only specific product of that given allele and has determinants which are restricted to that antigen. "Public specificity" describes antigenic determinants which are commonly shared by various HLA antigens which manifest recognizable private antigens. It had been found that certain HLA antigens that were considered to be private were really a group of two or three closely related antigens that shared common determinants. The term "broad specificity" is given to the initially identified HLA "private" antigen and the term "split" is given to the antigens in the group of closely related antigens. For example, in Table 35-1, the HLA A29, A30, A31, A32, and A33 are the splits of the Aw19 broad specificity.

In the HLA system, certain antigens are grouped in cross reactive groups or CREGS. This means that an antibody to a specific antigen reacts to a lesser degree with other HLA antigens within a defined group. For example, HLA-A1, A3, A11, and Aw36 are part of the HLA-A1 CREG; HLA Bw62, Bw63, Bw57, and Bw58 are part of the B15 CREG. This indicates that the antigens within the specific CREG group show a common molecular determinant which the antibody recognizes.

Table 35-1   Currently recognized HLA specificities

A	B	B	C	D	DR	DQ	DP
A1	B5	Bw50 (21)	Cw1	Dw1	DR1	DQw1	DPw1
A2	B7	B51 (5)	Cw2	Dw2	DR2	DQw2	DPw2
A3	B8	Bw52 (5)	Cw3	Dw3	DR3	DQw3	DPw3
A9	B12	Bw53	Cw4	Dw4	DR4	DQw4	DPw4
A10	B13	Bw54 (w22)	Cw5	Dw5	DR5	DQw5 (w1)	DPw5
A11	B14	Bw55 (w22)	Cw6	Dw6	DRw6	DQw6 (w1)	DPw6
Aw19	B15	Bw56 (w22)	Cw7	Dw7	DR7	DQw7 (w3)	
A23 (9)	B16	Bw57 (17)	Cw8	Dw8	DRw8	DQw8 (w3)	
A24 (9)	B17	Bw58 (17)	Cw9 (w3)	Dw9	DR9	DQw9 (w3)	
A25 (10)	B18	Bw59	Cw10 (w3)	Dw10	DRw10		
A26 (10)	B21	Bw60 (40)	Cw11	Dw11 (w7)	DRw11 (5)		
A28	Bw22	Bw61 (40)		Dw12	DRw12 (5)		
A29 (w19)	B27	Bw62 (15)		Dw13	DRw13 (w6)		
A30 (w19)	B35	Bw63 (15)		Dw14	DRw14 (w6)		
A31 (w19)	B37	Bw64 (14)		Dw15	DRw15 (2)		
A32 (w19)	B38 (16)	Bw65 (14)		Dw16	DRw16 (2)		
Aw33 (w19)	B39 (16)	Bw67		Dw17 (w7)	DRw17 (3)		
Aw34 (10)	B40	Bw71 (w70)		Dw18 (w6)	DRw18 (3)		
Aw36	Bw41	Bw70		Dw19 (w6)			
Aw43	Bw42	Bw72 (w70)		Dw20	DRw52		
Aw66 (10)	B44 (12)	Bw73		Dw21			
Aw68 (28)	B45 (12)	Bw75 (15)		Dw22	DRw53		
Aw69 (28)	Bw46	Bw76 (15)		Dw23			
Aw74 (w19)	Bw47	Bw77 (15)		Dw24			
	Bw48			Dw25			
	B49 (21)	Bw4		Dw26			
		Bw6					

W = Specificities not sufficiently defined.

Box 35-1   HLA antigen inheritance*

FATHER'S PHENOTYPE		MOTHER'S PHENOTYPE	
HLA-A1, A2, B8, B44		HLA-A24, A30, B13, B14	

FATHER'S HAPLOTYPES		MOTHER'S HAPLOTYPES	
a) HLA-A1, B8		c) HLA-A24, B13	
b) HLA-A2, B44		d) HLA-A30, B14	

CHILD 1	CHILD 2	CHILD 3	CHILD 4
a) HLA-A1, B8	a) HLA-A1, B8	b) HLA-A2, B44	b) HLA-A2, B44
c) HLA-A24, B13	d) HLA-A30, B14	c) HLA-A24, B13	d) HLA-A30, B14

*HLA-C, D, and DR antigens were eliminated to simplify the chart.

Linkage disequilibrium

It has been found that certain HLA alleles are inherited more commonly together than would be expected by random mating. The term associated with this phenomenon is called "linkage disequilibrium." A primary example of this linkage is seen in the increased frequency of the occurrence of HLA-A1 and B8 on the same haplotype of North American whites. The gene frequency of HLA-A1 is 0.138 while the gene frequency of HLA B8 is 0.090. The calculated frequency of HLA-A1 and B8 occurring on the same chromosome would be the cross product of the two known frequencies (0.138 × 0.090 = 0.0124), but population studies have shown that the actual occurrence of the these two alleles in combination is greater then the calculated value (0.0609). The most common linkages are found between the HLA-B and C antigens and several have been determined for approximately eight of the HLA-A and B alleles. The reason for this linkage in the MHC is not understood. One theory maintains that linkage may occur as a natural selection which allows for "survival of the fittest."

HLA CLASS I, CLASS II, AND CLASS III ANTIGENS
Inheritance and distribution of the antigens

The HLA antigens, as well as other MHC genes, are inherited in simple Mendelian fashion and the characteristics are codominant traits. The combination of alleles is inherited as one unit called a haplotype. As seen in Box 35-1, two distinct haplotypes are inherited because one HLA-A, B, C, D, and DR allele is received from each parent. Due to the codominant characterization of the alleles, both HLA antigens at a given locus can be expressed and detected during testing.

The Class I antigens (HLA-A, B, and C antigens) are found on all cells in the body. On some cellular components, like brain and red cells, the antigens are in low concentrations. The highest concentration of Class I antigens are found on lymphoid cells, including T and B cells.

The Class II antigens (HLA-D, DR, DQ, and DP) have a restricted distribution. The highest concentrations are found on B cells, macrophages, and dendritic cells. Lower-density occurrence of these gene products is found on epidermal Langerhans cells, sperm, and intestinal epithelium. Resting T cells do not have the Class II antigens present on their cell surfaces, but activated T lymphocytes express these antigens after stimulation by foreign antigens.

The molecular structure of class I and class II antigens

Figure 35-3 is a schematic representation of the Class I and Class II molecules. The Class I antigens are composed of two non-covalently linked polypeptide chains. The glycoprotein-heavy chain has a molecular weight of 44,000. It is coded for by genes on chromosome 6 and is polymorphic. The Beta 2 microglobulin is the light chain, only 1,200 daltons. It is coded for by genes on chromosome 15 and is a non-polymorphic protein. The heavy chain carries the specificity of the antigen and its hydrophobic region is anchored into the cell membrane.

The Class II antigens are also composed of two non-covalently linked glycoproteins. The heavy chain of 34,000 daltons is called the alpha chain and the lighter 29,000 dalton chain is called the beta chain. The antigen is anchored into the cell membrane by the hydrophobic regions of both chains. Recent data have shown little variability between the alpha chain of DR antigens. However, there is a high degree of variability between the beta chain. The antigenic determinants for the DR antigens therefore reside on the beta chain.

Class III antigens

The MHC codes for proteins other than the classic HLA antigens. The Class III region is composed of the complement components C2, C4A, C4B, Factor B, and two genes for cytochrome P.450 21 hydroxylase. The HLA locus which codes for these molecules lies between the area which controls the expression of the Class I and Class II gene product. The Class III region genes are not considered part of the histocompatibility antigen network.

Antibodies to the HLA antigens

Unlike the ABO red cell system, antibodies to the white cell antigens are not naturally occurring. The formation of leukocyte antibodies is in response to three known specific immunogenic stimuli. Immunization to HLA antigens can occur through pregnancy. The expression of the paternal HLA antigens on the fetal tissue can act as an immunogen and cause the antibody production. Nineteen percent of women with four or more pregnancies have detectable antibodies to HLA-A, B, and C antigens in their sera.

Blood transfusions are also known to initiate HLA antibody formation. Red cell and platelet transfusion products contain leukocytes which express the HLA antigens on their

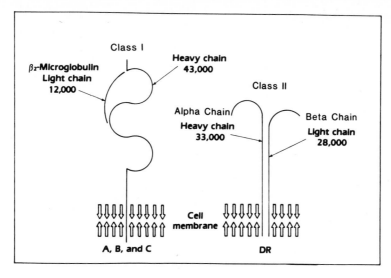

Fig. 35-3 Molecular structure of HLA antigens.

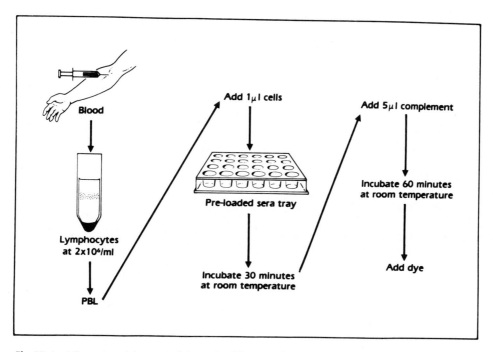

Fig. 35-4 Microcytotoxicity assay. Schematic of the procedures involved in the microcytotoxicity assay. Peripheral blood lymphocytes (PBL) are the cells used in this test to identify serologically defined HLA antigens.

surfaces. Multiple exposures to these blood products can cause formation of HLA antibodies. Dialysis patients and leukemics are known to have a higher incidence of HLA antibodies than other patient groups. This finding is related to the number of transfusions this population receives as part of their clinical therapy.

An allograft will also stimulate the formation of white cell antibodies. After transplant, primary, nonsensitized, renal graft recipients have a high incidence of antibodies. Fifty-five percent of these patients make antibodies to the disparate antigens of the allograft and these donor-specific antibodies play a role in graft rejection episodes.

LABORATORY EVALUATION OF HLA ANTIGENS
Serological testing

As shown in Figure 35-2, the HLA antigens fall into two broad categories: a) Serologically Defined (SD) and b) Lymphocyte Defined (LD). The HLA-A, B, C, DR, and DQ antigens are detected by a serological technique called the microcytotoxicity assay. The principle of this complement-dependent procedure is shown in Figure 35-4. The initial step is to separate lymphocytes from the peripheral blood. The separation technique most often used is a ficoll-hypaque density gradient. Diluted whole blood is layered on top of the gradient and then centrifuged. Four distinct layers can be seen after the centrifugation step. The lymphocytes are found at the interface between the top layer of plasma and the density gradient. The granulocytes and red cells are found at the bottom of the gradient. The separated lymphocytes are then tested against a battery of sera containing antibodies specific for each known HLA antigen. One ul of the lymphocyte suspension is incubated with 1 ul of each typing sera. Complement is added to each cell and sera combination followed by a 60-minute incubation period. If there is an antigen/antibody recognition, the complement causes lysis of the cell membrane as shown in Figure 35-4. To detect membrane damage, a vital dye such as eosin red is added to the test system. If lysis has occurred, the cells take up the dye and appear red under the microscope. The viable cells exclude the dye and remain unstained. By determining the cell lysis seen in each cell and sera combination, antigen assignments can be made for the HLA-A, B, and C series.

Because of the restricted distribution of the HLA-DR and DQ antigens, several procedures have been developed to aid in the identification of these antigens. One of the earliest methods developed was to isolate B cells from a ficoll-hypaque separated lymphocyte preparation by using a nylon wool column. The B cells adhere to the nylon wool and the T cells are easily flushed off the filaments. The B cells washed off the column can then be used in the microcytotoxicity assay.

The use of fluorescent microscopy has also been used to type for the HLA-DR and DQ antigens. A two-color fluorescence technique's advantage is that the B cells do not have to be separated from the T cells. A lymphocyte preparation is incubated with a FITC labelled anti-globulin. The B cells form a distinctive fluorescent cap while the T cells fail to react with the tagged antibody. The FITC-treated cells are then used in the standard cytotoxic assay. B cells that test positive for the specific antigens present on their cell surface are indicated by a red fluorescence following the addition of ethidium bromide.

Crossmatching

White cell crossmatches are carried out in an attempt to prevent hyperacute rejection of allografts. The purpose of this assay is to detect preformed cytotoxic antibodies that a patient may have which are reactive with the potential organ donor's antigens.

The crossmatch is an extension of the microcytotoxicity assay (Figure 35-5) and the serum of the patient can be tested against the T and/or B cells of the prospective donor. A positive T cell crossmatch indicates antibodies against the Class I antigens and a positive B cell crossmatch detects antibodies not only against the Class II antigens but other antigenic moieties of this cell. T cell cytotoxic antibodies are well recognized as mediators of allograft destruction, and their presence precludes a transplant. The significance of B cell specific antibodies is not well defined. There have been many controversial reports of either successful or failed grafts with positive B cell crossmatches. These findings imply that positive reactions for different antigen-antibody interactions may have different interpretations and suggest that all positive crossmatches may not be a contraindication to transplantation.

Lymphocyte defined testing

The mixed lymphocyte culture (MLC) is the method by which HLA-D antigens are defined. Observations by Herschorn, Bach, and others demonstrated that blastogenic transformation occurred when lymphocytes from nonrelated individuals were cultured together. Further studies concluded that this stimulation was due to antigens coded for by the HLA-D locus.

In an MLC, the lymphocytes from two individuals are placed in culture. The cellular interactions in an MLC are shown in Figure 35-6. The stimulator population consists of the B cells that express the Class II antigens. The T cells are the responder cells that recognize the disparity of these determinants. In a classic one-way MLC, the cells from the

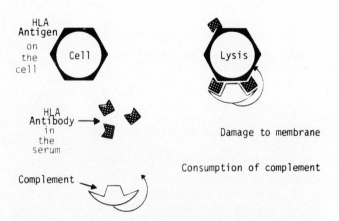

Fig. 35-5 Antigen and antibody recognition. Schematic of the principle of a microcytotoxicity assay. The antigens reside on the cells and the antibodies are found in the test serum. If recognition occurs, there is complement consumption and damage to the cell membrane. This immunological recognition can be applied for serological testing for both HLA antigens and antibodies (crossmatches).

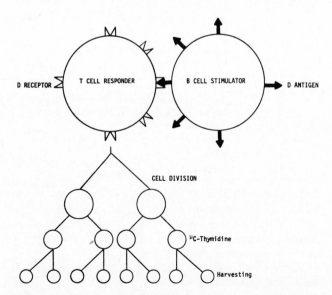

Fig. 35-6 The immunological principles of mixed lymphocyte culture. The B cells have the HLA-D antigens on their surfaces and the T cells have the receptors. If the T cells recognize disparity with the HLA-D antigens presented to them, they respond by blastogenesis.

stimulator individual are treated with irradiation or mito-mycin C. This is done to prevent the T cells in the sample from responding to the Class II antigens of the other individual and proliferating.

The treated and untreated cell samples are placed in culture and on the fifth day tritiated thymidine is added. The MLC is allowed to incubate for an additional 18 hours and then harvested. To determine the degree of blastogenesis in the responding T cells, the uptake of thymidine is measured. A high uptake of the radiolabeled nucleotide indicates disparity between the individuals' D antigens. MLCs are done in family studies to help determine the plausibility of transplantation based on the compatibility of the HLA-D alloantigens found on the patient's cells and those of the possible donors.

For actual D locus typing, homozygous typing cells (HTC) are used as the stimulators in the MLC. Through extensive studies, HTC are known to express the same HLA-D antigens on both haplotypes. The irradiated HTC are cultured with cells of unknown HLA-D expression in an MLC procedure. Lack of response to the HTC suggests that the cells carry the same HLA-D antigens expressed on the HTC.

Primed lymphocyte typing (PLT) is used to define HLA-DP antigens. A PLT is a dual stage MLC. In the initial phase, response cells are exposed to stimulator cells whose HLA-D- or D-related determinants are known. These response cells form a clone of memory which have an accelerated response or an anamnestic response to those antigens which they have been exposed to in this culture. These primed lymphocytes may be used immediately or be frozen in aliquots for future cultures. In the second phase of the test, the primed memory cells are cultured with irradiated test cells of unknown HLA-DP determinants for only 40 to 42 hours. After this short incubation, tritiated thymidine is added and its uptake is measured as in an MLC. If the unknown cells stimulate the primed lymphocytes, tritium will be incorporated into the response cells. The presence or absence of stimulation in this assay system allows for the identification of the HLA-DP antigens on the test cells.

Molecular genetic techniques

Advances in molecular biology have allowed for the study of HLA Class I and Class II antigens at the genomic level. A detailed description of the techniques used for DNA and RNA analysis is beyond the scope of this chapter, but a brief description of the basic steps will follow.

The Southern Blot and Restriction Fragment Length Polymorphisms (RFLPs) are methods to analyze DNA while Northern Blot techniques study mRNA and pre-mRNA. (Western Blot assays are used for protein analysis.) There are several basic steps common to nucleic acid hybridization studies. Initially the DNA or RNA must be extracted from cells or tissue and purified. The purified RNA molecules or DNA fragments generated by restriction enzyme digestion are separated by size using agarose gel electrophoresis. The gel-separated molecules are denatured and transferred to a solid support such as nylon or nitrocellulose filters. After transfer, a labeled nucleic acid probe is hybridized (bound) to the filter-bound nucleic acid. The hybridized probe is specific for the molecules or genes under study. The final step is detection of the labeled probe to determine quanti-

tative and qualitative information concerning the gene of interest.

DNA analysis has given researchers new insights into the function and structure of both Class I and Class II antigens. The subregions of the Class II genes and the polymorphisms of these molecules have been extensively defined using these techniques. The use of RFLPs is now being applied in conjunction with HLA antigen typing for parentage testing. Molecular techniques are also being used in the study of HLA and disease association to better understand the possible mechanisms involved in disease susceptibility.

Pitfalls in HLA typing

When trying to identify HLA antigens, several problems can be encountered. Many problems can arise from the blood sample itself. During blood component therapy, lymphocytes are transfused along with the red cells or platelets. These contaminating lymphocytes are separated along with the patient's cells and can cause problems not only with the identification of the HLA phenotype but also with determining a true stimulation response in an MLC. To eliminate this problem, an attempt should be made, if it is clinically feasible, to keep the patient transfusion free for 48 hours to clear transfused white cells. The disease state of a patient may also present difficulties in typing. The patient may not have enough normal lymphocytes to perform a typing. In order to do typings in these cases, larger volumes of blood are needed and special clean-up techniques can be attempted. Several trouble-shooting methods have been devised over the years. These range from a double ficoll-hypaque separation on the cells to using enzymes to remove unwanted dead cell debris. One method devised over the last few years has been the use of monoclonal antibodies to selectively remove any contaminating cellular components. The separated cells are incubated with the specific monoclonal antibody and then washed to remove the cellular debris. This technique has proven successful in many laboratories. Another problem may be encountered while attempting to type patients on massive drug therapy. Some chemotherapeutic agents and steroids are cytotoxic to circulating lymphocytes and make the separation of these cells very difficult. Typing these patients may be almost impossible while they remain on the drug therapy.

Many technical problems can be encountered while performing a microcytotoxicity assay or an MLC. Stringent quality-control measures can help eliminate many of these problems. One of the most prevalent difficulties is the presence of nonspecific cytotoxic antibodies or agents in the complement, serum, and/or media used in any of the assays. These contaminants may cause problems ranging from inability to retrieve viable lymphocytes to inability to interpret test results. The best way to avoid these technical mishaps is to test all new reagents in parallel with those reagents which have been found to give reliable results.

CLINICAL APPLICATION OF THE HLA SYSTEM
Paternity testing

The HLA antigens have become an important genetic marker in Paternity Testing. The main reasons this system has become valuable are 1) the antigens are fully expressed at birth; 2) the techniques used in the identification of the markers are accurate and highly reproducible; and 3) the antigens have a high degree of polymorphism associated with them. Another aspect that makes this system an important tool is the fact that the antigens are highly stable. If separated lymphocytes are stored at −80°C, the surface HLA antigens are stable for a six-month period and can be retested if the need arises.

The American Bar Association and the American Medical Association have recommended that both red cell and HLA antigens be used for testing, but this does not exclude the use of other genetic systems. Red cell enzyme and serum protein analysis have also been applied to the problems of disputed parentage. From a statistical standpoint, the HLA complex is an excellent system for both inclusion and exclusion in paternity testing. If a man is falsely accused of being the father, he has a 91% chance of exclusion by use of HLA testing. On the other hand, if a child has inherited antigens identical to those found in the putative father's phenotype, there is a probability of greater than 90% that he will be decreed the biological father. It stands to reason that the more antigen systems used in testing this problem, the greater the certainty of parentage. But even using all the presently accepted genetic markers does not provide 100% inclusion. However, the new technology of DNA analysis is affording the medical community a new tool with which to test for paternity. Several hundred restriction fragment length polymorphisms (RFLPs) have been characterized and reports have shown that these polymorphic RFLPs give exclusion as good as, and sometimes better than, HLA antigens. As DNA "fingerprinting" techniques advance, they will revolutionize the area of paternity testing because of the indisputable results obtained.

Blood component therapy

Antibodies directed against HLA and other antigens situated on the surface of leukocytes are implicated in the causation of febrile transfusion reactions and rarer cases of non-cardiogenic pulmonary edema associated with transfusion. In addition, since HLA-A and B antigens are present on the surface of platelets, repeated transfusion of leukocyte containing blood products often results in immunization of the transfusion recipient and induction of a refractory state associated with non-survival of transfused platelets. Finally, such sensitization has been found to seriously jeopardize the survival of bone marrow allografts in patients with aplastic anemia requiring transplantation. These issues will be explored in great detail in Part XI.

HLA and disease association

Many investigators have evaluated the association of HLA and disease. The products of the MHC have been studied to determine their effect on the inheritance of disease susceptibility and on the interaction of these gene products on disease pathogenesis. In order to understand the genetic control of disease, it is important to comprehend the difference between an association and a genetic linkage. When studying a specific disease, genes or gene products may be found in a higher frequency in the patient groups than found in the normal controls. The term "association" is used when the gene responsible for the disease and the marker gene do not reside on the same chromosome. The term "linkage"

is applied when the two genes reside on the same chromosome and are in close proximity to each other. The term presently used for the role the MHC play as markers in disease is "association."

There are an increasing number of diseases associated with the HLA antigens. HLA-associated diseases appear to have several common characteristics: 1) The cause of the disease and the pathophysiological mechanisms are poorly understood or not known; 2) The causative agents for many of these disease entities are thought to be viral agents; 3) There is a tendency to find these diseases in families and an inheritance pattern can be identified; and 4) Certain groups of these diseases are associated with autoimmune mechanisms.

Disease association research uses both family and population studies. Family studies are often difficult to carry out because of the small number of family members who may have inherited the disease. The data gathered from successful family studies establishes linkage between HLA antigens and other genes. The "other" genes are referred to as the disease susceptibility genes.

Population studies investigate the frequency of HLA antigens found in a patient population as compared to the frequency found in a normal control group matched for ethnic origin. The strength of the association is called the Relative Risk (R.R.). The R.R. indicates how many times more frequently the disease occurs in the group having the antigen. If the antigen is present in an individual's phenotype, it does not mean that the individual will contract the disease, rather it suggests a higher susceptibility to the disease in those individuals who possess the antigen.

Several hypotheses have been brought forth in an attempt to explain HLA and disease association. One hypothesis is that the HLA antigens are markers for undefined determinants which may confer disease susceptibility. Another postulant is that the HLA antigens may act as receptors for viruses, toxins, or other substances which may cause the disease process. Studies have shown that both the Class I and Class II antigens do play a significant role in the disease process. The use of DNA sequencing has contributed to the further understanding of how these associations effect the development of disease, but the exact mechanisms of disease susceptibility are still not understood.

Many diseases have been associated with antigens coded for by the HLA loci. Ankylosing spondylitis' association with HLA-B27 was one of the first disease associations reported. It has been found that 90% of patients with the clinical diagnosis of ankylosing spondylitis have HLA-B27

Table 35-2 Association between HLA and disease

Disease	Antigen	Relative risk
Ankylosing spondylitis	B27	87.4
Acute anterior uveitis	B27	14.6
Chronic active hepatitis	DR3	13.9
Graves' disease	DR3	6.0
Hematochromatosis	A3	8.2
Multiple sclerosis	DR2	5.0
Myasthenia gravis	DR3	3.4
Reiter's disease	B27	37.0

in their phenotype. Table 35-2 represents a brief list of diseases which are reported to have an association with either Class I or II antigens.

Immune response

The regulation of the immune response is one of the most complex phenomena of the immunological repertoire. If the major cellular interactions involved in this process were fully understood, the therapy to treat autoimmunity could be developed and the successful induction of tolerance could be achieved for transplant recipients. The MHC has aided science in understanding these problems and it plays a pivotal role in immune regulation.

Using inbred strains of both mice and rabbits, it became evident that the MHC antigens were linked to the immune response. McDevitt and his colleagues showed that the response to specific antigens was genetically controlled. The gene or the gene product that controlled the interactions of macrophages, T cells, B cells, and other immunological components was called the immune response gene (Ir gene). This Ir gene has been defined more extensively in the mouse than in the human system, but it is felt that the D locus of the HLA system is the Ir gene in man.

The possible role of the Class II antigens in immunoregulation has been defined over the past 10 years. These antigens are responsible for modulating cell-to-cell interaction and are important in the recognition of antigens by helper T cells (CD4+). T cell interactions during an immune response appear to be mediated by the presence of Class II antigens on accessory cells like macrophages or antigen presenting cells (APC) as seen in Figure 35-7. If an antigen is presented to a T helper cell in conjunction with the Class II antigens, it can then stimulate the helper cell to produce a variety of lymphokines. These mediators can aid B cells in the production of antibody and help regulate cells like natural killer cells, macrophages, and other effector cells.

Not only do the Class II antigens of the MHC have immunoregulatory functions, but the Class I antigens of the system are able to modulate specific recognition. The Class I antigens are responsible for the regulation of the cytotoxic T cells (CD8+) in the recognition of virus-infected cells. Lilly was the first to demonstrate that cell surface presentation of viruses in association with the Class I antigens was necessary for recognition by cytotoxic T cells. This dual recognition by primed T cytotoxic cells was an absolute condition for cell killing. This recognition network has been called haplotype restricted killing and a schematic of this is shown in Figure 35-7. The scope of the immune modulation mechanisms of the MHC is not fully understood. The information available has made us more knowledgeable about many aspects of the immune response, but the genetic control of this regulation needs further clarification.

Transplantation

In any transplantation, the entire focus is the induction of tolerance between the recipient and the graft. In the 1970s, it was thought that the HLA antigens may hold the key to the induction of tolerance. Early results showed that transplants occurring between HLA identical siblings had a better graft survival than non-matched grafts. Over the past 20 years the debate concerning the importance of matching for HLA antigens continues, and the development of better immunosuppressive drugs has not helped to clarify this important issue.

In the area of bone marrow transplantation, matching for both the HLA Class I and II antigens is an accepted standard. The selection of suitable HLA-matched family members allows for a lower rate of graft rejection and a decrease in the presence of significant graft versus host disease (GVHD). Many patients do not have HLA-identical family members and the use of non-HLA identical donors has been evaluated by several transplant programs. Data collected has shown that the use of family members who are only mis-

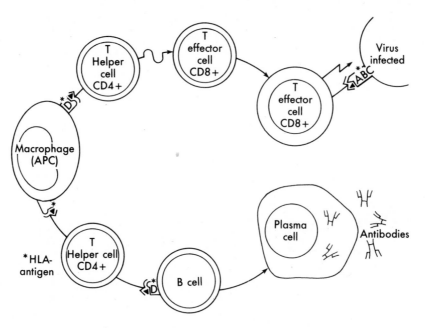

Fig. 35-7   HLA system and the immune response.

matched for one HLA antigen or the use of nonrelated donors who are phenotypically identical yield the same results as those seen in transplants from HLA-identical siblings.

Of all the solid organ grafts, renal transplantation is the one area where the significance of matching for HLA antigens has been extensively studied. It is well documented that grafts from HLA identical siblings have excellent survival rates, and this is due to the effect of matching for the Class I and Class II antigens. During the era of azathioprine/prednisone immunosuppressive therapy, it became evident that matching for the Class II DR antigen showed an increase in graft survival rate by 15% for the first year in cadaveric recipients. With the incorporation of cyclosporine as part of the immunosuppression regime, the controversy about the importance of matching for the HLA antigens has again emerged. Transplant Registry studies in both this country and Europe have reported that even in the age of cyclosporine, matching for HLA-A, B, and DR separately or in combination increases graft survival by approximately 10% for the first 12 months.

Matching for HLA antigens for solid organ transplantation does not have any set coding system. Transplant programs will identify the HLA compatibility between the recipient and donor by the number of antigens matched or mismatched. The best match would be a six-antigen match or a zero-antigen mismatch, which would indicate that the HLA-A, B, and DR antigens of both the donor and the recipient were identical. A-four antigen match or a two-antigen mismatch would mean that the patient did not have two antigens found in the donor's phenotype.

Data collected over the past 20 years has shown that the MHC does have an effect on graft survival. The exact mechanism of this influence is not known, and the ability to use this system to its full advantage has not yet been accomplished. Only through trial and error and continued investigation into the area of tolerance will we be able to define the best way to use the HLA antigens as an immunological tool.

SUGGESTED READING

Bell JJ, Todd JA and McDevitt HO: Molecular bases of HLA-disease association. In Harris H and Hirschhorn K (eds): Ad Hum Genet 18:1-41, 1989.

Borowsky R: HLA and the probability of paternity, Am J Hum Genet 42:132-134, 1988.

Calne RY: Transplantation immunology, clinical and experimental, 1984, New York, Oxford University Press.

Crumpton MJ, ed: HLA in medicine, Med Bull 43:1-240, 1987.

Dick HM and Kissmeyer-Nielsen F, eds: Histocompatibility techniques, Amsterdam, 1979, Elsevier/North Holland Biomedical Press.

Heise ER, ed: Paternity testing data analysis and management in the immunogenetics laboratory, New York, 1983, AACHT.

Helminen P, Ehnholm C, Lokki ML, et al: Application of DNA "fingerprints" to paternity determinations. Lancet 1:583-585, 1989.

Kahan DB: The impact of cyclosporine on the practice of renal transplantation, Transplant Procedure 21(Suppl):63-69, 1989.

Leivestad T, Albrechsten D, Bratlie A, et al: The role of HLA compatability in renal transplantation from living donors: an analysis of 379 grafts, Transplantation Procedure 22:153-154, 1990.

Levinsky RJ: Recent advances in bone marrow transplantation, Clinical Immun Immunopath 50:5124-5132, 1989.

Mehra NK and Taneja V: HLA, immune response and disease, Indian J Pediatr 56:171-179, 1989.

Rodey GE: Prevention of alloimmunization in thrombocytopenic patients. In Smith D and Summers S, eds: Platelets, Arlington, AABB, 1988.

Sanfilippo F, Thacker and Vaughn WK: Living-donor renal transplantation in SEOPF: the impact of histocompatibility, transfusion, and cyclosporine on outcome, Transplantation 49:25-29, 1990.

Smouse PE and Chakraborty R: The use of restriction fragment length polymorphisms in paternity analysis, Am J Hum Genet 38:918-939, 1986.

Sullivan KM: Current status of bone marrow transplantation, Transplant Proc 21, Supp 1:41-50, 1989.

36 Immunodeficiencies and autoimmune disorders

Gayle B. Jackson

IMMUNODEFICIENCY DISORDERS

Understanding the immune system is essential to understanding the immunodeficiency syndromes and autoimmune disorders. A concise review of the immune system is found in Chapter 33. Before acquired immunodeficiency syndrome (AIDS), defects in immunity were considered rare. It has been estimated that agammaglobulinemia occurs with a frequency of 1:50,000 and severe combined immunodeficiency (SCID) with a frequency of 1:100,000 to 1:500,000 live births. Selective IgA deficiency is the most common disorder, with incidences ranging from 1:500 to 1:3,500. Conversely, more than 200,000 cases of AIDS have been reported to the Centers for Disease Control in Atlanta since 1978. One hundred thousand cases have occurred since 1989.

Immunodeficiency disorders are the result of the impaired function in one or more of the components of the immune system, including lymphocytes, phagocytes, and the complement system. The disorders are classified as acquired or congenital. The acquired immunodeficiencies include the many clinical conditions associated with secondarily depressed cell mediated immunity such as viral and fungal infections and malignancies. Hypogammaglobulinemia is often seen as secondary to B cell malignancies. However, the most significant acquired deficiency is AIDS.

Acquired immunodeficiency syndrome (AIDS)
Etiology and pathogenesis

AIDS is a highly lethal epidemic immunodeficiency disease that was unknown prior to 1978. Although first noted in homosexual males, AIDS is also found in intravenous drug users, recipients of blood transfusions or products, and infants born to mothers with AIDS. The disease is transmitted by either hetero- or homosexual activity or intravenously. There has been a 50% increase in heterosexually acquired AIDS in 1991. AIDS is caused by infection with the human immunodeficiency virus (HIV), also known as the lymphadenopathy-associated virus (LAV). There are at least two serotypes of HIV (HIV-1 and HIV-2). Patients with this syndrome present with life-threatening opportunistic infections and/or Kaposi's sarcoma. *Pneumocystis carnii, Candida albicans, Mycobacterium avium-intracellulare*, herpes simplex virus, *Toxoplasma gondii*, hepatitis B,

cytomegalovirus, and *Cryptococcus* lead the list of infectious agents.

Until 1979, Kaposi's sarcoma was a rare tumor occurring only in persons 50 or older, and it responded well to chemotherapy or irradiation. During the past nine years, a rapidly fatal form has been found in young homosexual men in the United States. The overall mortality rate from AIDS is higher than 40% and will probably approach 100%. Although many vaccines are currently being evaluated, there is no known cure for AIDS.

The natural history of HIV infection begins with exposure to the virus, resulting in rapid replication in susceptible cells. The CD4 receptor on helper T lymphocytes is a major molecule used for viral entry. The HIV envelope glycoprotein, gp 120, (Figure 36-1) binds to the cell surface receptor which, in most cases, is CD4. However, the CD4 receptor is apparently not the only material required for viral at-

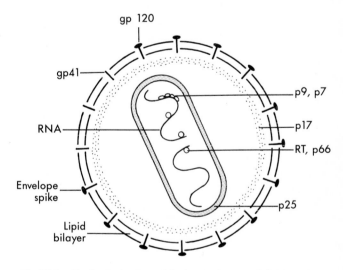

Fig. 36-1 The basic structure of the human immunodeficiency virus. The location of the envelope glycoproteins (gp120 and gp124) are shown, as are the major viral core proteins (p25, p17, p9, and p7). The core protein, p17, is found outside the viral nucleoid and forms the matrix of the virion. RT indicates reverse transcriptase. *Redrawn from Levy JA: JAMA 261:2997-3006, 1989.*

tachment and penetration. Brain-derived cells and human fibroblasts devoid of CD4 can be infected in vitro by HIV. In addition to the CD4 binding, another HIV envelope glycoprotein, gp 41, binds to the cell surface. Gp 41 apparently binds with a receptor on the cell surface that fuses the virus to the cell membrane. In cells lacking the CD4 antigen, the fusion receptor alone may be the site for virus entry. The viral nucleoid (core) then enters the cell cytoplasm and reverse transcriptase within the core initiates transcription. The transcription events lead from viral RNA to a DNA copy (cDNA) that eventually integrates into the host cell chromosomal DNA. (See Figures 36-1, 36-2.) At this point, the cell may enter a latent period when little viral protein or DNA is produced. When the cell enters a productive state, two types of RNA, mRNA and virion RNA, are produced. The mRNA codes for proteins necessary for replication of the infectious virions. The virion RNA is encapsulated into a particle and the progeny human immunode-ficiency viruses are released from the infected cell by a budding process.

Laboratory tests for HIV

Enzyme immunoassay (EIA)

Routine laboratory tests for HIV-1 infection detect specific retrovirus antibody. The EIA is the most widely used serological test for HIV in the world. The first kit (Abbott) was licensed in March of 1985 and there are now numerous products available. The FDA approved EIA's use as an antigen source partially purified viral lysate derived from either the NIH H-9 cell line or the CEM-F line from the Pasteur Institute. Most kits detect only IgG antibodies, but some detect IgG and IgM by using a mixture of heavy- and light-chain antibody.

Both sensitivity and specificity of the currently available EIA kits are >99% when an immunoblot is used as the reference standard. The value of a test, that is the predictive

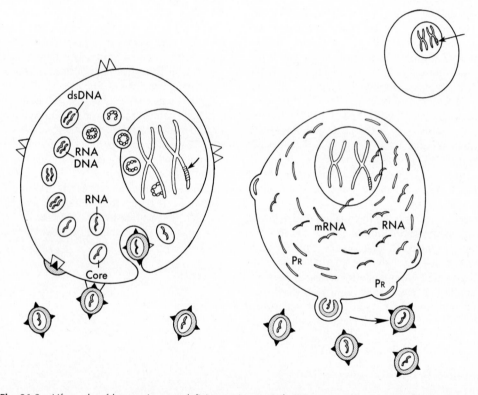

Fig. 36-2 Life cycle of human immunodeficiency viruses. **Left,** Retrovirus infection of cells. Human immunodeficiency virus attaches to a specific receptor on the cell surface. In many cells, this binding involves the envelope gp120 and the cell surface CD4 molecule. Subsequently, virus entry takes place most likely by fusion of the virus to the cell membrane. In some cases, endocytosis may be involved. The human immunodeficiency virus gp41 probably participates in the virus-cell fusion. The intact viral nucleoid (core) then enters the cell cytoplasm and reverse transcriptase within the core begins the transcription events that lead from viral RNA to RNA/DNA hybrids and the double-stranded DNA (dsDNA) that is a copy (cDNA) of the viral RNA. This cDNA in a circular but noncovalently bound form enters the nucleus and integrates into the cell chromosome (arrow) using the endonuclease enzyme coded for by the viral *pol* region. **Right,** retrovirus replication in cells. Following viral infection, the cell may enter a latent (shown on top) or productive state. In the former, the viral cDNA as an integrated proviral copy (arrow) is present in the infected cell and very little viral protein or RNA is made; no infectious virions are produced. In the latter situation, the proviral DNA produces RNA in two species, mRNA and virion RNA. The mRNA codes for the proteins (PR) required for replication of infectious virions. The progeny human immunodeficiency virus, formed by encapsulation of the virion RNA into a particle, is produced at the cell surface by a process of budding. Maturation of some of the viral proteins takes place at this time. *Redrawn from Levy JA: JAMA 261:2297-3006, 1989.*

value of a positive or negative result, is highly dependent on the incidence of the disease in the population. However, in tests for HIV antibody in a population with an incidence of <.25%, the predictive value may be very low. This is why mass screening of a "normal" population for HIV antibody, even with excellent tests such as those available, is risky. Box 36-1 outlines some test characteristics.

As will be further discussed in the section on clinical application of HIV tests, all EIA's must be repeated if positive and then confirmed with another test using a different procedure such as Western blot.

While the majority of EIA tests use whole or partially purified viral lysates on the capture antigen, there are recombinant polypeptide-based products available. Some are licensed in Europe, but until recently, experience with these tests has been limited in the United States. The recombinant tests use either envelope or core proteins as capture antigens.

Western blot (immunoblotting)

Western blotting is a commonly used tool to distinguish a specific antibody response to different molecular weight proteins. Initially an antigen preparation is electrophoresed in a gel matrix. Then the separated proteins are transferred (blotted) on a nitrocellulose membrane. The membrane is incubated with patient sera and positive and negative controls. An enzyme labelled antibody conjugate is added followed by substrate. If antibodies to specific molecular weight proteins are present, they will appear as colored bands on the membrane. Figure 36-3 depicts a Western blot for HIV antibodies.

Table 36-1 shows the viral source of the major bands encountered in patients with AIDS.

A key issue in the use of Western blots (WB) for confirmation of an EIA assay is interpretation. There are currently four interpretive criteria. The one most commonly used (up to 65% of respondents to a 1991 CDC survey) was published by the Association of State and Territorial Public Health Directors (ASTPHLD) and the CDC. Table 36-2 lists the various criteria for WB interpretation.

Radio immuno precipitation assay (RIPA)

Relatively few laboratories—primarily research facilities—offer this cumbersome test. HIV infected cells are incubated with ^{35}S-methionine. The cell lysates are exposed to a patient's serum preabsorbed to Protein A-Sepharose. The precipitates are electrophoretically separated. The results resemble a WB, but RIPA is more sensitive and specific. RIPA is often used when the WB is indeterminate.

Latex agglutination

A latex agglutination test for HIV antibody was developed for use primarily in developing countries. The kit (Cambridge Biotech, Worcester, MA) is now available in

---

Box 36-1   Characteristics of HIV antibody tests by EIA

Sensitivity (%)	—	98-100
Specificity (%)	—	99.6-100
Predictive value positive		
° High risk	—	>99%
° Low risk	—	5-100%
(blood donors)		

False positives: HLA antibodies, heat inactivated sera, contaminating X-reactive antigens from cell lines used to cultivate HIV. Cross-reactions seen in alcoholics and patients with hepatitis and hemophilia.

False negative: Late seroconversion in infected individuals, infection with different HIV strains (HIV-2).

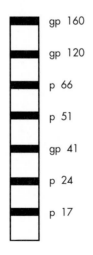

Fig. 36-3   Western blot (HIV)

gp 160
gp 120
p 66
p 51
gp 41
p 24
p 17

Table 36-1   Source of HIV Antibody

Antigen	Source
gp 160	envelope (env) gene product
gp 120	env fragment
gp 41	transmembrane fragment
gp 31	
gp 51	polymerase (pol) gene product
p 66	
p 24	core protein (gag)

gp	=	glycoprotein
p	=	protein
p17	=	core (gas) protein
p14	=	TAT protein

Table 36-2   Interpretive criteria for Western blot tests

Organization	Minimum band requirements for Western blot "reactive" pattern
American Red Cross	At least one band from each gene product group: gag AND pol AND env
ASTPHLD/CDC	Any two of p24, gp41, or gp120/160
Consortium for Retrovirus Serology Standardization	p24 OR p31 AND one of GP41 or GP120/160
DuPont	p24 AND p31 AND gp41 or gp120/160

the United States. Although rapid, the particle agglutination is very fine and equivocal results may be very difficult to read.

HIV-1/HIV-2 combined tests

While there have been few cases of HIV-2 disease in the United States, it has been suggested that donated blood be screened for both HIV-1 and HIV-2. A number of companies offer combination tests and it is likely that combination HIV-1/2 testing will become the standard.

Indirect fluorescent antibody microscopy (IFA)

IFA for HIV antibody detection is a confirmatory test equivalent in sensitivity and specificity to WB. Slides with both HIV infected and uninfected cells are overlaid with the serum, washed, and then stained with an antihuman fluorescein conjugate. The slides are examined microscopically and positives are determined by the fluorescent intensity of the infected cells. The advantage of IFA over WB is time (>2 hours), but reading an IFA is more subjective than viewing bands on WB.

HIV antigen detection

There are at least two commercial sources for HIV antigen detection kits: Abbott Laboratories and Coulter, Inc. Both kits detect the specific p24 antigen of HIV-1 by EIA. Serum, CSF, and cell-free supernate can be used to detect HIV antigen. Because some patients may show low levels of nonspecific reactivity, neutralization of positive tests is necessary before the reactive result can be confirmed. The HIV p24 antigen test is used to:

a. monitor treatment—p24 antigen has been shown to decrease in some AIDS patients as a function of antiviral therapy
b. diagnose neonatal HIV infection—p24 antigen testing has been used to detect infection in infants born of HIV positive mothers
c. detect HIV prior to seroconversion—It is possible to detect p24 antigen in some patients prior to seroconversion. However, this test is not recommended for routine HIV screening due to its reduced sensitivity.
d. determine progression to AIDS—Some have suggested that the appearance or reappearance of p24 antigen can be used as a marker for progression to active disease. Beta 2–microglobulin tests have been similarly used, but the total CD4 lymphocyte count is a better predictor of progression to AIDS.

HIV culture

HIV-1 can be cultured using a co-culture of peripheral mononuclear leukocytes (PML) and phytohemagglutinin stimulated PML's. The presence of HIV in this co-culture can be determined by electron microscopy, p24 antigen detection, or specific HIV reverse transcriptase activity. This co-culture procedure grows other HIV strains as well as other retroviruses. HIV culture can be used for the same clinical situations as p24 antigen. It is more sensitive than p24 antigen detection, but much more time consuming and expensive.

Molecular detection of HIV nucleic acid

Southern blots can be used to detect HIV DNA directly in tissues or body fluids, but this technique is insensitive. Of much greater promise is an amplified DNA probe for HIV. Although a number of amplification methods exist, the polymerase chain reaction (PCR) is the best. PCR for HIV DNA is commercially available from at least one private laboratory and has been used extensively in research protocols.

Clinical use of HIV testing

The issue of HIV testing is politically explosive. It is not the intent of this chapter to detail the reasons for or against mass HIV screening tests, premarital HIV testing, and screening of health care workers. Of importance, however, is the fact that HIV tests can, at a minimum, (1) effectively protect the blood supply and (2) detect high-risk patients who are HIV positive. An HIV antibody test that is positive does not diagnose AIDS, but only indicates that the patient has been infected with the virus and has mounted an antibody response to it.

Presently, it is possible to routinely test patients or blood for transfusion for HIV-1, HIV-2, and HTLV I and II. With HIV-1/2 testing, most states require a consent form indicating that the patient has been informed of the test procedure, its risks, and benefits. Figure 36-4 shows Connecticut's consent form. Results must be kept confidential, given only to designated individuals, and kept in a secure place in the laboratory. Computer data must be protected from unauthorized persons. Phone reporting of HIV test results should be discouraged. The laboratory must also recognize that all reactive EIA tests must be repeated and that all EIA tests reactive X2 must be confirmed with either WB, IFA, or RIPA.

If a WB test is "indeterminate," most authorities suggest retesting in two to three months. If the WB is still indeterminant and there is no clinical evidence of disease, then a RIPA should be ordered.

As the numbers of requests for HIV tests increase and the variety of kits increase, the laboratory must ensure that results are well controlled, secure, and handled expeditiously.

The primary immunodeficiency disorders

The 1985 revision of the World Health Organization lists 24 separate conditions related to primary immunodeficiency disorders, some of which have only a few examples. The immune deficiency disorders may be caused by defects in lymphocytes, the phagocytic system, or the complement system. (Figure 36-5) Most patients have a history of recurrent infections or a history of treatment failure. However, some individuals—such as those with selective IgA deficiency or infants with transient hypogammaglobulinemia—may have few infections.

B cell deficiency disease

The ultimate product of the B cells is immunoglobulin. Any abnormalities in the transition of the B lymphocyte from the stem cell level to the plasma cell may affect immunoglobulin synthesis. The earlier the rupture in the de-

REQUEST FORM ADDENDUM FOR HIV RELATED TESTING
(must included with Test Request Form)

Patient: _____

Date: _____

<   >   This test is being performed WITH the informed consent of the above-mentioned patient, pursuant to Connecticut Public Act No. 89-246.

<   >   This test is being performed WITHOUT the informed consent of the above-mentioned patient, pursuant to Subsection E of Section 2 of the Connecticut Public Act No. 89-246.

_____ a. Blood or body part donations

_____ b. Court order

_____ c. Post occupational exposure

_____ d. Other

_____
Signature of ordering clinician

Fig. 36-4   Consent form for HIV testing

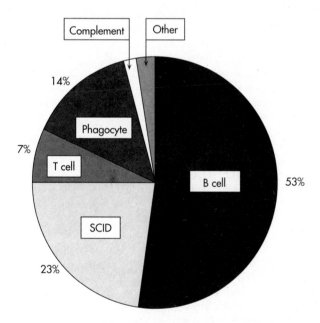

Fig. 36-5 This pie diagram illustrates that pure B cell deficiencies represent 53% of the human immunodeficiencies, T cells only 7%, SCIDs 23%, and phagocytic deficiencies 14%. Complement and undeciphered deficiencies represent less than 3%. *From Barret JT: Textbook of Immunology, ed 5, St Louis, 1988, Mosby—Year Book, Inc.*

velopmental pathway, the more extensive the loss in antibody-forming capacity. However, in addition to breaks in the transition chain of B lymphocytes, losses of T helper cells or an overabundance of T suppressor cells can also lead to impaired immunoglobulin performance. Table 36-3 presents a classification of primary immunodeficiency diseases. Although the term "agammaglobulinemia" is often used, in this classification traces of gamma globulin, 5-500 ug/mL, can usually be found. "Hypogammaglobulinemia" is a more exact term.

Transient hypogammaglobulinemia of infancy. This condition appears to be a prolongation and accentuation of the decline in serum immunoglobulin seen during the first three to seven months of life. The disease is rare. Patients usually can synthesize antibodies to diphtheria and tetanus toxoids by six to 11 months of age, well before immunoglobulin concentrations become normal. The different lymphocyte subpopulations are present in normal percentages. The condition is self-correcting.

X-linked (Bruton's) agammaglobulinemia. Infantile sex-linked agammaglobulinemia is a disease transmitted by the mother to her male children. The disease becomes apparent around six months of age after the immunity derived from maternal IgG has waned. Thereafter, infections with high-grade extracellular pyrogenic organisms such as pneumococci, streptococci, and hemophilus are acquired unless given prophylactic antibiotics or gamma globulin therapy.

All classes of immunoglobulins are absent or extremely low in X-linked agammaglobulinemia. The total number of T cells is usually increased and the percentages of T cell subsets are normal in most of these patients. B cells are

Table 36-3 Classification of primary immunodeficiency diseases

Disorder	Functional deficiencies	Presumed cellular level of defect
Transient hypogammaglobulin-emia of infancy	Low IgG and IgA	Delayed T helper cell maturation
X-Linked (Bruton's agamma-globulinemia)	All immunoglobulins markedly de-creased	Failure of pre-B cells to differentiate and mature
Common variable hypogamma-globulinemia	Various isotype combinations de-creased	Defective B cell switch, excess T suppressor
DiGeorge's Syndrome	T cells decreased	Embryonic failure to complete 3rd & 4th pharyngeal arch
Nezelof's Syndrome	T cells markedly decreased	Block in cellular development
Severe Combined Immunodefi-ciency (SCID)	Absence of all immune function	Unknown
Ataxia telangiectasia	B cells often normal, decreased T cells	Defect in T cell maturation and DNA repair enzymes
Wiskott-Aldrich	Decreased IgM, progressive T cell loss, accompanied by platelet defects	Uncertain
Chronic Granulomatous Disease (CGD)	Neutrophils phagocytize but do not kill organisms	Failure of neutrophils to form toxic forms of oxygen
Chediak-Higashi Disease (CHD)	Endocytosis is normal but organ-isms are not killed	Failure to release myeloperoxidase

absent or present in very low numbers. However, normal numbers of pre-B cells are found in the bone marrow. Hypoplasia of adenoids, tonsils, and peripheral lymph nodes is the rule. Cell mediated immune responses can be detected in vitro and in vivo and the capacity to reject allografts is intact. These children respond normally to most viral diseases of childhood (i.e., measles, mumps, and chickenpox) and develop a lasting immunity.

The prognosis is good if antibody replacement therapy is instituted early. A few unfortunate patients develop polio, persistent enterovirus infections, and lymphoreticular malignancy.

Common variable hypogammaglobulinemia (CVH). Far more common than generalized hypogammaglobulinemia is selective or variable hypogammaglobulinemia (dysgammaglobulinemia). In this disorder, only one or a combination of immunoglobulins is missing or present in much lower than normal concentrations. Recurrent bacterial infections are usually not a problem, except when IgG is the deficient immunoglobulin. When IgG is involved, the level is often less than 500 mg/dL, but not as low as in sex-linked agammaglobulinemia. IgG levels greater than 250 mg/dL are adequate for protection against most bacterial infections.

Selective IgA deficiency is the most common form of dysgammaglobulinemia. The incidence is estimated at 1 in 500 to 3500 persons. The patients may have noninfectious diarrhea and/or sinopulmonary disease (loss of secretory IgA). While some individuals with the disorder are healthy, the majority have ill health with infections predominantly in the respiratory, gastrointestinal, and urogenital tracts.

Patients with IgA deficiency frequently have IgG antibodies against cow's milk and ruminant serum proteins. There is a high incidence of autoantibodies and a frequent association with collagen, vascular, and autoimmune diseases. Forty-four percent of IgA deficient individuals have antibodies to IgA in their serum. IgA deficient persons with anti-IgA have had severe or fatal anaphylactic reactions after receiving IgA-containing solutions intravenously. For this reason, blood bank products containing the plasma proteins are contraindicated.

Immunoglobulin quantitation by radial immunodiffusion (RID) or nephelometry is the main diagnostic test for common variable hypogammaglobulinemia. In selective IgA deficiency, the serum IgA concentration will be below 10 mg/dL. Serum protein electrophoresis is not a good screen since, if only one immunoglobulin class is deficient, the other two may be present in normal or increased amounts, thus masking the deficiency. B lymphocytes are present in normal or near normal numbers, but these cells are unable to mature to plasma cells. In some cases, an exaggerated activity or an excessive number of T suppressor cells may lead to the disorder.

Immunodeficiency disorders involving T lymphocytes

In general, individuals with partial or absolute defects in T cell function have infections or clinical problems for which there is no effective treatment. The T cell disorders are more severe than the B cell disorders and these patients rarely survive infancy or childhood.

DiGeorge's syndrome (thymic hypoplasia). DiGeorge's syndrome is not a genetic disease. Its cause is unknown. The syndrome is the result of dysmorphogenesis of the third and fourth pharyngeal pouches during early embryogenesis, leading to hypoplasia or aplasia of the thymus and parathyroid glands. Abnormalities of the aortic arch, the mandible, and the ear may be present since these tissues have a common embryonic origin. Some children have little trouble with life-threatening infections and grow normally. Such patients are referred to as having partial DiGeorge's syndrome. Those with complete DiGeorge's syndrome are susceptible to infections from low-grade or opportunistic pathogens and to graft-vs-host disease from nonirradiated blood.

Concentrations of serum immunoglobulins are usually normal, although IgA may be diminished and IgE elevated. There is a decrease in total T cell number, although there is a normal proportion of helper and suppressor cells. After birth, the infant may progress toward hypocalcemia since the parathyroid gland is hypoplastic or aplastic.

Nezelof's syndrome. Nezelof's syndrome is caused by a recessive trait which prevents normal lymphoid development. The lymphoid development of the paracortical and medullary regions of lymph nodes, the T cell regions, are markedly restricted. Patients are athymic. The block in cellular development resides in or near the stem cell level. Infants have recurrent or chronic pulmonary infections, failure to thrive, oral or cutaneous candidiasis, recurrent skin infections, chronic diarrhea, and severe progressive varicella.

The laboratory findings include lymphopenia, neutropenia, and eosinophilia. Occasionally, selective IgA deficiency or markedly elevated IgE or IgD values are observed. However, serum concentrations of the five immunoglobulin classes are usually normal or increased. Since the defect is cellular, these individuals show delayed cutaneous anergy and low to absent in vitro lymphocyte responses to mitogens and allogeneic cells. Total T cells are profoundly deficient. However, the normal helper (C D4) to suppressor (C D8) cell ratio is usually normal.

Severe combined immunodeficiency diseases (SCID)

The syndromes of SCID are the most severe of the recognized immune deficiency disorders. Unless the patient is kept in gnotobiotic isolation, transplanted with immunocompetent tissue or given enzyme replacement, death from infection usually occurs during the first year and invariably during the second year. The patients suffer from congenital absence of all immune function and have genetic, enzymatic, hematologic, and immunologic disease features.

Autosomal recessive severe combined immunodeficiency disease (Swiss type) was the first described of the SCID syndromes. Within the first few months of life, affected infants present with frequent episodes of otitis, sepsis, diarrhea, pneumonia, and cutaneous infections. Extreme wasting develops and death from opportunistic organisms frequently follows.

Despite the uniform lack of B and T cell function, the lymphocyte subpopulations show a marked heterogeneity among SCID patients. Many patients have elevated percentages of B cells. The T cell and T cell subset percentages are extremely low. The T cells lack CD6, an antigen present on immature cortical thymocytes. Thus, the lymphocytes appear to have acquired surface markers characteristic of a mature T cell. A phenotype of SCID has been reported where virtually all lymphocytes were natural killer (NK) cells.

Approximately 40% of SCID patients with the autosomal recessive form of SCID have an absence of the enzyme adenosine deaminase (ADA). As with other forms of SCID, ADA deficiency can be cured with bone marrow transplant. Clinical improvement has been noted in some patients by enzyme replacement with irradiated, packed, normal erythrocytes or polyethylene glycol-modified bovine ADA. Since the entire ADA gene has been cloned, the defect is a leading candidate for gene insertion therapy.

Immunodeficiency with other defects

Ninety-three percent of immunodeficiency disorders are either B cell, T cell, or combined deficiencies. Phagocytic deficiencies comprise about 14% of the remaining disorders and complement other deficiencies represent less than 3%.

Wiskott-Aldrich syndrome. This is a sex-linked recessive disease with combined loss of B and T lymphocytes. The total immunoglobulin level may be normal because of elevated IgA and normal or elevated IgG. However, the IgM level is decreased, suggesting that the B cell deficit is related primarily to polysaccharide antigens. The true locus of the defect is unknown but may actually be in the macrophages that process the polysaccharide antigens for the B cells rather than in the B cells themselves.

The thymus is normal and only the peripheral organs demonstrate losses in T cells. Patients suffer innumerable bacterial, viral, fungal, and protozoan infections. The disease is progressive and associated with the thrombocytopenia and eczema.

Ataxia telangiectasia. This is an autosomal recessive disease with progressive loss of muscle coordination (ataxia) accompanied by blood vessel dilation (telangiectasia) combined with deficits in IgA production and T lymphocytes. All patients have an aplastic or hypoplastic thymus. Patients have a defect in DNA repair enzymes, which makes them very sensitive to irradiation and may account for a 10% malignancy rate. The low IgA levels may not reflect a loss of IgA lymphocytes but may be the result of faulty T cell-B cell interaction.

Chronic granulomatosis disease (CGD). This is a sex-linked disease of males; although a second, less severe form is found in females and probably is an autosomal recessive trait. Infants with CGD have normal or elevated immunoglobulin levels, respond normally to vaccines, normal B and T lymphocyte functions and complement levels. Nevertheless, these patients are victims of numerous bacterial infections and frequently virulent yeasts and fungi. The defect in CGD patients is in the neutrophils. The neutrophils phagocytize bacteria normally but after phagocytosis do not shift to the HMP shunt as their energy source. The HMP shunt results in the production of H_2O_2. Normally hydrogen peroxide functions in cooperation with lysosomal myeloperoxidase to iodinate and kill intracellular bacteria. The nitroblue tetrazolium (NBT) reductase test is based on the metabolic shift of normal phagocytes to oxidative metabolism. Neutrophils in the act of phagocytizing latex spheres are incubated in a solution of NBT dye. The dye acts as a hydrogen acceptor as oxidative metabolism ensues. The reduced dye is insoluble and is seen as distinct blue intracytoplasmic granules in normal neutrophils. Neutrophils from CGD patients are not engaged in active oxidative metabolism and thus cannot reduce NBT.

Chediak-Higashi disease (CHD). This disease results in faulty phagocytic destruction of parasites. All phagocytic cells in CHD victims have abnormally large granules in the cytoplasm. The central defect lies in the inability to form normal primary granules (lysosomal) in cells of the granulocytic series. Retarded intraphagocyte killing is not the result of depressed H_2O_2 formation, but rather the inability of cells to degranulate normally and deliver myeloperoxidase to the phagocytic vacuole. Therefore, CHD victims suffer from recurrent infections and have a mean survival of six years of age. Physically, the victims have a partial albinism, extreme sensitivity to light, and rapid involuntary eye movements.

LABORATORY TESTING

The clinical laboratory evaluation of the primary immunodeficiency disorders begins with quantitative techniques and, if warranted, may progress to the more esoteric functional tests.

Most clinical laboratories can screen for immunoglobulin deficiency. Nephelometry is the most common method used for quantitation of serum IgG, IgM, and IgA. A light is passed through a solution containing immunoglobulin and its specific antibody. The light is scattered as immunoprecipitate is formed in the tube and the amount of light scatter measured by the nephelometer is proportional to the concentration of immunoglobulin.

Immunoglobulin E is quantitated by radioimmunoassay (RIA) or by enzyme immunoassay (EIA). In these tests the immunoglobulin reaction with antibody replaces radiolabeled or enzyme labeled immunoglobulin.

Quantitation of B, T, and NK cells and subsets can be performed with flow cytometry. The cells are reacted in suspension with fluorescent labeled monoclonal antibodies. The antibodies are specific for surface antigens. In the flow cytometer, the labeled cells pass, single file, through a laser beam. The energy of the laser excites the fluorochrome attached to the cells. The light intensity is measured by photodiodes and the resulting electrical signals are amplified and passed to a computer for further processing, storage, and analysis. The percentage of cells with a specific marker is then determined.

A panel of monoclonal antibodies is used to ascertain the total T cell population (CD3, CD2); the total B cell population (CD19, CD20, CD22); helper and suppressor cell populations (CD4, CD8); and ratio of natural killer cell (CD56, CD57) population. Further testing for lymphocyte subsets and maturation markers might be performed if clinically warranted.

Table 36-3 is a summary of immunoglobulin concentrations and B and T cell deficiencies in the primary immunodeficiency disorders.

Flow cytometry can be used to monitor the absolute number of CD4 lymphocytes in patients infected with the HIV viruses. The total T cell population can be determined with the monoclonal antibody to CD3. Antibodies to the CD4 and CD8 receptors are used to determine the absolute number of CD4 and CD8 lymphocytes and to determine a CD4/CD8 ratio. Since monocytes may mark dimly with the monoclonal CD4 antibody, it is preferable to use a two or three color methodology. CD4 antibody is paired with CD3 in the same tube (one antibody is marked with fluorescein isothiocyanate, a green fluorescence, and the other with phycoerythrin, a red fluorescence). The true CD4 lymphocytes will be dual stained with CD3 and CD4 antibodies. The absolute number of CD4 lymphocytes will decrease as patients progress into a severe acquired immunodeficiency disorder (AIDS).

Another quantitative test that monitors patients with the HIV virus is beta-2-microglobulin. Beta-2-microglobulin is the light chain component of human leukocyte antigens (HLA). A high-circulating concentration of beta-2-microglobulin, in the absence of renal failure, indicates a large amount of lymphocyte turnover and suggests in HIV seropositive subjects, that the virus is killing lymphocytes. A radioimmunoassay method is used to quantitate serum beta-2-microglobulins.

Functional testing for immunodeficiency syndromes usually is outside the capability of the clinical laboratory. The laboratory tests are difficult to perform and the demand is too low to warrant setting up the testing. This type of testing is handled best in reference centers.

The nitroblue tetrazolium (NBT) test has been used to assess neutrophil phagocytic dysfunction in chronic granulomatous disease. The defect in this disease is the failure of neutrophils to form toxic forms of oxygen and subsequently kill phagocytized microorganisms. Patient polymorphonuclear cells are incubated with opsonized zymosan (C3 deposited on the surface). During ingestion of zymosan particles, superoxide anions are formed. When NBT (a yellow reducible compound) is present in the extracellular medium, it is swept into the phagocytic vacuole with the ingested particle, where it is reduced by the superoxide anions. The reduction product of NBT is a purple insoluble formazan. The formazan can be extracted from the washed cell button with pyridine. The absorption of the extract is then determined in a spectrophotometer at 550 nm using pyridine as the blank control. Cells from patients with chronic granulomatous disease fail to reduce the NBT compound.

A newer assay to measure the oxidative burst in neutrophils uses flow cytometry. This assay depends on the incorporation of $2',7'$-dichlorofluorescin diacetate (DCFH-DA) into the hydrophobic lipid regions of the cell, where the acetate portions are cleaved by hydrolytic enzymes to the nonfluorescent molecule $2',7'$-dichlorofluorescin (DCFH). This compound is trapped within the cell due to its polarity. PMA (phorbol myristate acetate) is used to stimulate an oxidative burst in the neutrophils. The H_2O_2 and peroxidases produced oxidize the trapped DCFH to $2',7'$-dichlorofluorescein (DCF), which is fluorescent at 530 nm. The green fluorescence produced is proportional to the amount of H_2O_2 generated. This method is more accurate than the NBT test.

AUTOIMMUNE DISORDERS
General concepts of autoimmunity

The current concepts of autoimmune disease reflect the evolution in our understanding of the immune response itself. Autoimmunity can be defined as the production of circulating immunoglobulins or sensitized lymphocytes that react with autoantigens. Ehrlich referred to autoimmune disease as "horror autotoxicus," a condition in which a self-destructive process occurs directed by one's own immune system. In the 1950s Burnet proposed the clonal deletion theory. This theory proposes that potential clones of self-reactive lymphocytes are deleted during fetal or early postnatal life as a result of exposure to self antigens. Forbidden clones of autoantibody-producing cells might arise later in life through somatic mutation in other antibody-forming cells.

The newer concept of "clonal balance" proposes that self-tolerance resides in the preferential production of T cells with a suppressive or regulatory function, so that the body normally remains in a negative (suppressed) balance. It has been proposed that T cells with primarily suppressor function exit the thymus slightly earlier than the corresponding helper population of T cells. In the case of self antigens, the antigen-specific suppressor T cells are continually stimulated and are normally slightly more prevalent than their helper counterparts. Suppressor T cells that are not antigen-specific are readily demonstrated in normal animals.

In addition, two antigen-specific regulatory mechanisms have been described: antigen-specific suppressor T cells and antiidiotypic antibodies. Idiotypes (Ids) represent structural sites located on the Fab fragment of antibodies. These are combining sites for antigenic determinants. However, these unique sites are also antigenic, generating anti-Ids which act as suppressive agents for the further production of antibody. Ids are present on immunoglobulins whether they are free antibodies or surface receptors of B-lymphocytes and on T-cell receptors. Experiments and clinical evidence show an inverse relationship between serum levels of anti-Ids and autoimmune disease activity.

B cells responsive to most self-antigens are found in normal individuals. They produce naturally occurring antibodies, are usually of the IgM class, and may be involved in a housekeeping role for the removal of damaged cells and tissues. These antibodies are rarely involved in autoimmune disease, which depends on a T cell-dependent switch to IgG antibody or to the development of cell-mediated immunity.

Inheritance plays a role in the risk for autoimmune disease. The occurrence of autoimmune disorders is greater in females, suggesting that steroid hormones may play a role. Autoimmune disorders run in families and some autoimmune diseases show association with specific HLA antigens, i.e., HLA-B27 and ankylosing spondylitis. The expression of class II major histocompatibility complex (MHC) antigens on cells is critical in the presentation of antigen to and in the interactions of immunologically active cells. The MHC class II genotype often influences the susceptibility of an animal to autoimmune disease. Genes associated with the heavy chain of the immunoglobulin, such as the human Gm, also influence the occurrence of autoimmunity in humans. Immune complex disorders, such as systemic lupus erythematosus, are associated with genetic complement deficiencies.

However, while inheritance plays a role in the risk of acquiring an autoimmune disease, an initiating factor also seems necessary for developing disease. Bacteria and viruses may simulate self-antigens (molecular mimicry). A cross reaction between antibodies to myosin heavy chain and a membrane determinant of *Streptococcus* has been demonstrated. Chemicals, including heavy metals, may alter self-antigens. Also, an increased expression of class II MHC antigens on target tissue has been shown in many autoimmune disorders. Gamma interferon resulting from virus infection could be responsible for the increase of class II MHC antigens. Haptens complexing with native protein can provide a mechanism for T cell recognition. Drugs, such as alpha-methyldopa, can complex with red cell membrane structures and stimulate the production of autoantibodies,

resulting in a hemolytic anemia. Lymphoproliferative disorders may trigger autoimmunity. B cell malignancies are accompanied by autoimmune hemolytic anemia, connective tissue disease, and even thyroiditis with higher than expected frequency.

In summary, autoimmune disease is the result of dysregulation of the T cell and/or of the anti-idiotype system. (Figure 36-6) An imbalance of controlling functions, such as ineffective T cell suppression or failure of anti-idiotypic antibody against idiotypes of autoantibodies, may lead to autoimmune disease. Suppressor and helper T cells may influence or balance each other to achieve a net regulation on B cells.

T cell lymphokines directly affect B cells. Interleukin-3 (IL-3) activates bone marrow pre-B cells; B cell growth factor (BCGF) acts on B cells; and B cell differentiation factor (BCDF) helps convert B cells to antibody producer (plasma) cells. Auto-antibodies are then produced and may act directly on target tissue or on red blood cells, leukocytes, or platelets. They may complex with autoantigen to form circulating immune complexes, which cause injury to kidneys, lungs, joints, skin, and other tissues.

Other lymphokines may injure host cells directly or may activate macrophages, which can inflict tissue damage. Natural killer (NK) cell activity may be increased by T cell production of interleukin 2.

Autoimmunity is not a single condition. Animal models have shown a large variety of genetic predispositions and processes leading to autoimmune manifestations.

NON-ORGAN SPECIFIC DISEASES

The autoimmune disorders may be divided into (1) non-organ specific disease with systemic manifestations and (2) organ-specific disease, which mainly affect one organ. The term "collagen" disease was used when grouping the non-organ specific diseases because the extracellular components of the connective tissue seemed to be primarily affected. The term "connective tissue" disease is also used. The non-

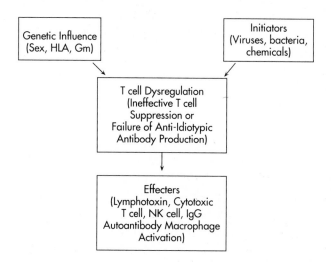

Fig. 36-6 Overall scheme for autoimmunity. An initiating factor such as a virus or bacteria acts on a genetically susceptible host resulting in T cell dysregulation. The self-reactive T cells produce lymphotoxin, activate macrophages with macrophage activating factor (MAF), stimulate cytotoxic T cells with IL-2 and NK cells with interferon, and stimulate self-reactive B cells with B cell stimulating factor.

organ specific diseases include systemic lupus erythematosus (SLE), rheumatoid arthritis, Sjogren's syndrome, polyarteritis nodosa, polymyositis and dermatomyositis, progressive systemic sclerosis (scleroderma), and mixed connective tissue disease.

Systemic lupus erythematosus

Systemic lupus erythematosus (SLE) is a chronic inflammatory disease which may affect the skin, joints, kidneys, lungs, nervous system, serous membranes, and/or other organs of the body. The disease course is characterized by periods of remission followed by chronic or acute relapses. The term lupus, Latin for wolf, is used because the red rash that sometimes occurs across the nose and upper cheeks resembles a wolf's mask.

The prevalance rate of SLE is one in 2000. However, the prevalance is one in 700 for women between the ages of 20 and 64 years and one in 245 for black women. The disease is more common in urban than rural areas.

Clinical features

The most common manifestations of lupus are fatigue, arthritis and arthralgia, fever, and weight loss. Swollen glands, nausea and vomiting, headaches, depression, easy bruising, hair loss, edema, and swelling are other symptoms frequently reported either prior to diagnosis or coincident with a disease exacerbation.

Eighty percent of patients have skin involvement, which may include a butterfly rash (greater than 50%), photosensitivity, mucous membrane lesion, alopecia, Raynaud's phenomenon (cold sensitivity), purpura, and urticaria. Discoid lupus refers to a condition involving only the skin as distinguished from systemic lupus. However, discoid lesions (discrete, round erythematous plaques) may develop years before other manifestations of systemic disease. Approximately 50% of lupus patients develop renal disease. Pulmonary manifestations include pleuritis, effusion, and pneumonia. Pericarditis, murmurs and ECG changes are seen with cardiac involvement. Lymphadenopathy, splenomegaly, and hepatomegaly may be present.

Some 25% to 75% of patients have disorders of the central nervous system. These disorders range from depression to psychosis and/or convulsions.

Etiology and pathogenesis

At present, no etiology has been found for systemic lupus erythematosus. SLE may not be a single disease, but a constellation of signs and symptoms produced by a variety of etiologic agents. Viral, genetic, environmental, and hormonal influences have been proposed as etiologic factors for SLE. However, the development of SLE probably requires an interaction between a pathogen, the environment, and a predisposed host. Viral antibodies have been found in serum from SLE patients but they are directed against apparently unrelated viruses, including measles, rubella, parainfluenza, mumps, and Epstein-Barr. These antiviral antibodies may be the result of nonspecific B-lymphocyte activation. Viruses have not been directly isolated from SLE patients.

Genetics seems to play a part in the development of lupus. Relatives of patients with SLE develop lupus with a frequency of between 0.4% and 5%, representing a several hundred-fold increase over the incidence in the general population. Fifty percent of monozygotic twin pairs are concordant for the disease; whereas the frequency of SLE in dizygotic twins is the same as with other first-degree relatives. HLA-DR3 and DR2 show only a weak genetic predisposition to SLE suggesting that genes outside the major histocompatibility locus may be involved. Homozygous deficiencies of C2 and C4 are frequently associated with SLE. Lupus patients show a reduced number of erythrocyte complement receptor type 1 (CR1), suggesting a possible defect in the clearance of immune complexes. Drug-induced SLE, a milder form with no associated renal and CNS disease is most commonly induced by procainamide, hydralazine, anticonvulsants, and chlorpromazine. Since SLE has a propensity for women in their childbearing years, hormonal influences are thought to play a role in disease expression. Female patients excrete excessive amounts of material with high estrogenic activity.

While the etiology of SLE remains unclear, much of the tissue damage is caused by antigen-antibody complex deposition. Systemic lupus is considered the prototype of human immune complex disease. Antigen-antibody complexes are demonstrable in renal glomeruli, blood vessels, skin, and the choroid plexus of the brain.

Studies of the complement system, immunofluorescent and electron microscopic studies of renal biopsies, and identification of the immunoreactants eluted from kidneys strongly suggest that immune complexes mediate the renal injury in SLE. Lupus nephritis is found in approximately 50% of lupus patients.

The immunologic features of lupus include the following: lupus erythematosus (LE) cell, antinuclear antibodies (ANA), immune complexes, complement level depression, tissue deposition of immunoglobulins and complement, circulating anticoagulants, and other autoantibodies.

Diagnosis and laboratory findings

Anemia, which may reflect inflammation, renal insufficiency, blood loss, dietary insufficiency, medications, or immune mechanisms, is found in approximately 50% of patients. Suppressed erythropoiesis from chronic inflammation and/or uremia may cause a normocytic, normochromic anemia. Serum iron may be low even though bone marrow stores are adequate. The reticulocyte count may be relatively low for the degree of anemia. Red cell aplasia has been observed, probably caused by antibodies against erythroblasts.

Ten to forty percent of patients have a hemolytic anemia with a positive direct antiglobulin test. Leukopenia (WBC less than 4500) has been noted in 50% to 60% of patients; lymphocytopenia (less than 1500/mm^3) has been observed in 84%. Suppressor T lymphocytes and/or CD4$^+$ cells are depressed.

Cytotoxic antibodies to lymphocytes are associated with lymphopenia. Less than 10% of patients have a platelet count of less than 50,000. However, mild thrombocytopenia (50,000 to 100,000) is seen in 25% to 50% of patients.

The lupus anticoagulant is found in 25% of SLE patients. This antibody is associated with thrombotic episodes but not with bleeding, except when thrombocytopenia is present. The lupus anticoagulant may be recognized by a prolonged PTT. Its presence may be confirmed with the platelet neutralization test or the tissue thromboplastin inhibition test. Cardiolipin antibodies may also be present and lead to a false positive test for syphilis. Antibodies to a number of clotting factors, including VIII, IX, XI, and XII have been noted in SLE.

Virtually all patients with SLE have an elevated erythrocyte sedimentation rate. Decreases in CH 50, C3 and C4 may correlate with disease exacerbation.

Autoantibodies are a hallmark of systemic lupus. Ninety-five to one hundred percent of patients with SLE will have antinuclear antibodies (ANA). Therefore, a negative ANA test is useful in ruling out SLE. Specific antinuclear antibodies such as Sm and double stranded DNA (dsDNA) antibodies are highly specific for SLE and are found in 25% and 49% respectively. Titers of dsDNA rise with disease activity and fall during remission and are therefore useful in monitoring disease.

Antibodies to SSA and RNP are found in 35% and 34% respectively of SLE patients. Sera from patients with drug-induced lupus usually contain antibodies to histones (96%). In contrast, only 5% of patients with idiopathic SLE have histone antibodies. Sera from patients with idiopathic SLE contain a heterogeneous mixture of nuclear antibodies, i.e., native DNA, histones, Sm, nRNP; whereas sera from patients with drug-induced lupus are less heterogeneous and contain primarily histone antibodies. The LE cell test, which detects antibodies to deoxyribonucleoprotein, was found positive in 60% to 70% of acutely ill SLE patients.

Lymphocytotoxic antibodies are found in the sera of approximately 80% of patients with SLE. Normal numbers of B lymphocytes are found in SLE. T lymphocytes numbers, particularly suppressor T lymphocytes, are decreased.

The diagnostic criteria listed in Table 36-4 can aid in establishing a diagnosis of SLE. A patient with four or more of the 11 criteria present, serially or simultaneously during any interval, can be said to have SLE.

Rheumatoid arthritis

Rheumatoid arthritis (RA) is a chronic inflammatory disease affecting multiple joints with varying degrees of systemic involvement. Prevalence increases with age, peaking at 35 to 45 years.

Clinical features

Lymphadenopathy, weight loss, low-grade fever, morning stiffness, and fatigue may be present early in the onset of RA. Initial presentation may be insidious or rapid and may involve one or many joints. Muscle contractures and joint deformities are present in advanced cases. Subcutaneous modules may be present.

In addition, nail-fold thrombi, pleurisy, pulmonary fibrosis, pericarditis, nerve entrapment syndromes, scleritis, Sjogren's syndrome, and vasculitis may also be present.

Etiology and pathogenesis

The etiology of rheumatoid arthritis is unknown. Genetic factors probably play a role as indicated by the prevalence of HLA-DR4 positive patients. The prevalence is higher in females (hormonal influence) and stress is known to precipitate and aggravate disease activity. Epstein-Barr virus (EBV) has been implicated, since patients with RA have a high frequency of precipitating serum antibody which reacts

Table 36-4 Criteria for diagnosis of SLE

Criterion	Definition
1. Malar rash	Fixed erythema, flat or raised, over the malar eminences, tending to spare the nasolabial folds.
2. Discoid rash	Erythematous raised patches with adherent keratotic scaling and follicular plugging; atrophic scarring may occur in older lesions.
3. Photosensitivity	Skin rash as a result of unusual reaction to sunlight, by patient history or physician observation.
4. Oral ulcers	Oral or nasopharyngeal ulceration, usually painless, observed by a physician.
5. Arthritis	Nonerosive arthritis involving two or more peripheral joints, characterized by tenderness, swelling or effusion.
6. Serositis	a) Pleuritis - convincing history of pleuritic pain or rub heard by a physician or evidence of pleural effusion, or b) Pericarditis - documented by electrocardiogram or rub or evidence of pericardial effusion.
7. Renal disorder	a) Persistent proteinuria greater than >0.5 g/dl or >3+ if quantitation not performed, or b) Cellular casts - may be red blood cell, hemoglobin, granular, tubular, or mixed.
8. Neurologic Disorder	a) Seizures - in the absence of offending drugs or known metabolic derangements, eg, uremia, ketoacidosis, or electrolyte imbalance, or b) Psychosis - in the absence of offending drugs or known metabolic derangements, eg, uremia, ketoacidosis, or electrolyte imbalance.
9. Hematologic Disorder	a) Hemolytic anemia - with reticulocytosis, or b) Leukopenia - less than 4.0×10^9/L (4000/mm³) total on two or more occasions, or c) Lymphopenia - less than 1.5×10^9/L (1500/mm³) on two or more occasions, or d) Thrombocytopenia - less than 110×10^9/L ($\times 10^3$/mm³) in the absence of offending drugs.
10. Immunologic Disorder	a) Positive lupus erythematosus cell preparation, or b) Anti-DNA antibody to native DNA in abnormal titer, or c) Anti-Sm - presence of antibody to Sm nuclear antigen, or d) False-positive serological test for syphilis known to be postive for at least six months and confirmed by negative *Treponema pallidum* immobilization or fluorescent treponemal antibody absorption test.
11. Antinuclear antibody	An abnormal titer of antinuclear antibody by immunofluorescence or an equivalent assay at any point in time and in the absence of drugs known to be associated with drug-induced lupus syndrome.

The 1982 Revised criteria for the classification of systemic lupus erythlmatosus: Tan Eng M, et al: Arthritis and rheumatism, 25:1271-1277, Nov 1982.

specifically with nuclear antigens from the EB virus. EBV is a polyclonal stimulator of B cells and can lead to the in vitro production of rheumatoid factor by human B cells.

A virus may be the inciting agent acting in a genetically susceptible host. Synovial lymphocytes then produce an altered IgG. The altered IgG may stimulate a local immune response within the joint with the production of rheumatoid factors. Immune complexes, composed of altered IgG and the anti-IgG rheumatoid factors in the synovial fluid, activate the complement system, resulting in histamine release, production of chemotactic factors, and an influx of neutrophils into the joint fluid. The neutrophils release lysosomal enzymes, such as elastase and collagenase, which are capable of inducing tissue injury. Further tissue injury may be induced by mediators of inflammation released by lymphocytes, plasma cells, mast cells, and macrophages within the synovium.

Laboratory findings

The most common laboratory findings with rheumatoid arthritis are rheumatoid factors, antinuclear antibodies, immune complexes, and characteristic complement levels. Rheumatoid factors are immunoglobulins with specificity for the Fc fragment of IgG.

While most rheumatoid factors are of the 19S IgM class, 7S IgM, IgG, and IgA rheumatoid factors may be present. Eighty percent of patients who fit the American Rheumatism Association criteria for classic or definite rheumatoid arthritis have a positive latex agglutination test. Thus, a negative result does not rule out rheumatoid arthritis.

High titers of rheumatoid factor are associated with the presence of subcutaneous nodules and extra-articular manifestations, especially vasculitis. The rheumatoid factor test is not specific for rheumatoid arthritis. A positive test may be seen in chronic infections, idiopathic pulmonary fibrosis, sarcoidosis, chronic active hepatitis, mixed cryoglobulinemia, hypergammaglobulinemia purpura, and other collagen-vascular disorders.

Antinuclear antibodies are found in 14% to 28% of patients with rheumatoid arthritis. There are no differences in disease manifestation between ANA positive and ANA negative patients. However, ANA positive patients often have more advanced disease.

Immune complex tests, which utilize monoclonal rheumatoid factors and C1q binding assays, are positive most frequently in patients with RA. RA patients with positive tests for mixed cryoglobulins often have extra-articular manifestations, particularly vasculitis.

Serum complement levels are usually normal in patients with rheumatoid arthritis. Low complement levels are usually associated with very high levels of rheumatoid factors and immune complexes.

Low complement levels are characteristic in synovial fluid. Synovial fluid complement levels, (less than one third of the serum complement levels) may be indicative of in situ complement fixation. Thus, complement levels should be measured simultaneously in serum and joint fluid.

Other forms of rheumatoid arthritis

Felty's syndrome. Felty's syndrome is the association of RA, splenomegaly, and leukopenia. Ninety-five percent of patients are positive for HLA-DR4 and have high titer rheu-

matoid factor and rheumatoid nodules. ANA tests are usually positive. The leukopenia increases the risk of bacterial infection. Leg ulcers, pleuritis, neuropathy, and episcleritis are often present.

Juvenile rheumatoid arthritis. Juvenile rheumatoid arthritis (JRA) occurs in children under 16. It is believed to be more than one disease. The patients suffer from morning stiffness, rash, fever, pericarditis, uveitis, cervical spondylitis, and rheumatoid nodules. Arthritis in one or more joints for six weeks may be sufficient for diagnosis if trauma and other causes are ruled out.

Twenty percent of patients experience a spontaneous and permanent remission by adulthood. Antinuclear antibodies are positive in approximately 13% of all patients with JRA. A positive rheumatoid factor by the latex fixation method is found in 20% of patients. A high titer rheumatoid factor is associated with more unremitting, disabling disease. Immune complex testing is not useful in the diagnosis, prognosis, or monitoring of patients.

Sjogren's syndrome

Sjogren's syndrome is a chronic inflammatory disease involving the lacrimal, salivary, and other excretory glands. The main clinical manifestations are dry mouth, dry eyes, and recurrent salivary gland pain and swelling. A primary (1°) form is not associated with other diseases. A secondary (2°) form is associated with RA and other connective tissue diseases.

The etiology of Sjogren's syndrome is unknown. Since there is a strong association with the histocompatibility antigens HLA-B8 and HLA-DR3, genetic factors are thought to play a role in the disease. The strong association with RA and SLE suggests that immunologic processes play a role.

Hypergammaglobulinemia is seen in 50% of patients. The pattern is usually polyclonal, but an occasional patient will develop an IgM paraprotein with resulting hyperviscosity syndrome and hypergammaglobulinemic purpura. Ninety percent of both 1° and 2° cases are positive for rheumatoid factors. Antinuclear antibodies are observed in 65% of patients, frequently directly against SS-B antigen. Other autoantibodies differ in frequency between 1° and 2° Sjogren's syndrome. Mitochondrial antibodies are seen in 10% of patients with 1° Sjogren's and in only 4% and with 2° Sjogren's.

Antibodies to salivary duct antigens are usually seen in 2° Sjogren's. Patients with 1° Sjogren's have a higher level of antibodies to the thyroid gland, gastric parietal cells, pancreatic epithelial cells, and smooth muscle. Elevated levels of salivary beta-microglobulin may be observed with the level correlating to the number of lymphocytes observed on the lip biopsy of labial salivary glands.

Definitive diagnosis depends on the characteristic histological changes present in biopsied labial salivary glands. Indirect measurement of ocular secretion by the Shirmer's test may aid in diagnosis. In this test, a strip of filter paper is placed in the lower palpebral fissure. Less than 10 mm of wetting in five minutes indicates an abnormal result.

Progressive systemic sclerosis (scleroderma)

Progressive systemic sclerosis is characterized by fibrosis in the skin and internal organs and by arterial occlusions with a distinct proliferative pattern. Raynaud's phenomenon (cold sensitivity) occurs prior to the onset of other manifestations in approximately 50% of cases. The skin manifestations follow three consecutive stages:

1) a non-painful pitting edema phase
2) a sclerotic "hidebound" stage, during which the skin folds disappear and patients develop atypical faces and "sausage" digits; and
3) a third and final stage with atrophy or softening and a return toward normal. Muscle wasting, due to disuse, is a common feature.

The disease course is usually slow and chronically disabling. However, it can be rapidly progressive and fatal. The etiology is unknown.

Low titers of antinuclear antibodies are found in 40% to 90% of patients with scleroderma. When an ANA antibody producing a nucleolar pattern is the only antibody present, the finding is highly specific for scleroderma. However, nucleolar patterns are found in approximately 20% of patients with other rheumatic diseases, along with other autoantibodies. Antibodies producing a nucleolar pattern are rarely seen in patients with early features of scleroderma, thus limiting its diagnostic usefulness.

The CREST syndrome is a variant of scleroderma with *c*alcinosis, *R*aynaud's phenomenon, *e*sophageal dysfunction, *s*clerodactyly, and *t*elangiectasia. These patients have a limited scleroderma that progresses slowly and rarely develop renal disease. The disease is associated with a centromere antibody, which is an ANA directed against the mitotic plate region of the dividing HEP-2 cells. The centromere antibody may be present early in the disease, when the only clinical manifestation is Raynaud's phenomenon. Scl-70 antibody is seen in 25% of patients with scleroderma and is highly specific, but occurs relatively late in the course of the disease, when the diagnosis is usually obvious.

Polymyositis and dermatomyositis

Polymyositis and dermatomyositis are a group of inflammatory diseases of skeletal muscle. All of the diseases have skeletal muscle that has been damaged by a lymphocyte inflammatory process resulting in symmetrical weakness, predominantly of proximal muscles. The presentation of dermatomyositis is similar to polymyositis except for the presence of skin lesions.

Roughly 32% of patients have a positive ANA test by routine immunofluorescence using Hep-2 cells. The pattern is often speckled and associated with antibody to the non-histone nuclear PM-1 antigen.

Evidence for myositis is obtained from the presence of increased levels of creatine kinase (CK) and transaminase in the serum of a patient with proximal muscle weakness. The diagnosis is confirmed by biopsy. Patients who are regenerating muscles manifest an increased percentage of myocardial CK, which does not indicate cardiac muscle involvement but reflects regeneration of skeletal muscle.

Mixed connective tissue disease and overlap syndromes

Many patients have diffuse connective tissue disease (DCTD), which does not fall into the classic descriptions of systemic lupus erythematosus, scleroderma, polymyositis, dermatomyositis, or rheumatoid arthritis. These patients have clinical features which overlap several diseases. Furthermore, 25% of patients with "classic" disease evolve with features more commonly associated with another disease. A common finding in the overlap syndromes is the frequent occurrence of Sjogren's syndrome. This has been associated with RA, SLE, PM, mixed connective tissue disease, primary biliary cirrhosis, necrotizing vasculitis, autoimmune thyroiditis, chronic active hepatitis, mixed cryoglobulinemia, and hypergammaglobulinemia purpura.

A syndrome with an overlap of SLE, PSS, and PM has been described. In most cases antibodies were present in the serum to a ribonuclease-sensitive extractable nuclear antigen. This syndrome is called mixed connective tissue disease (MCTD). MCTD has not been universally accepted as a distinct disease entity.

Clinically, patients with MCTD have a sequential evolution of overlap features over the course of several years, including Raynaud's phenomenon, serositis, gastrointestinal dysmotility, myositis arthritis, sclerodactyly and skin rashes. Severe renal disease and severe CNS involvement are absent.

Patients with MCTD have a positive ANA with a high-titer speckled pattern. The titer is often greater than 1:1000 and sometimes greater than 1:10,000. This finding should prompt the measurement of antibodies to extractable nuclear antigen (ENA), double-stranded DNA (dsDNA), Sm, and histones. Patients with MCTD have high titers of antibodies to ribonucleoprotein (RNP) only. Patients with antibodies to dsDNA, histone, and Sm usually best fit the clinical description of classic SLE. Low titers of anti-RNP have been described in many conditions other than MCTD and are nondiscriminatory. Sometimes antibodies to double-stranded DNA are reported as positive in MCTD sera. In most cases, this is due to the frequent presence of antibodies to single-stranded DNA (ssDNA) reacting with a DNA preparation that contains single-stranded contamination of the test DNA. If sensitive enzyme-linked immunosorbent assays are employed, low levels of other antibodies are sometimes found in MCTD as well as in normal individuals. Thus, anti-RNP is really the predominant antibody in MCTD rather than the sole antibody.

Chronic fatigue syndrome (CFS)

Chronic fatigue syndrome (CFS) has been previously known as "chronic mononucleosis," low natural killer cell syndrome, myalgic encephalomyelitis and "yuppie flu." CFS is a complex illness characterized by extreme fatigue, lethargy, and a variety of symptoms resembling at one time or another infectious mononucleosis, Lyme disease, AIDS-like illness, multiple sclerosis, post-polio syndrome, and autoimmune diseases such as lupus. All age groups appear to be at risk, but women under the age of 45 are the most susceptible. The Center for Disease Control in 1988 developed the following case definition for CFS:

1) "New onset of persistent or relapsing, debilitating fatigue or easy fatigability in a person who has no previous history of similar symptoms, that does not resolve with bedrest, and that is severe enough to reduce or impair average daily activity below 50% of the patient's premorbid activity level for a period of at least six months."

2) Exclusion of other plausible disorders "by thorough evaluation, based on history, physical examination, and appropriate laboratory findings."

Most clinicians base their diagnosis on this case definition.

The etiology of CFS is not well understood, having been attributed to Epstein-Barr virus, human Herpes virus 6 (HHV6), and a retrovirus. Most recently, reports have suggested a role for HHV6, a retrovirus resembling HTLV-I or II or a retrovirus known as human spumavirus or "Foamy" virus.

CFS is now believed to be an immune disorder. CD8 lymphocytes are infected with either a retrovirus or other virus such as HHV6. Cells are stimulated to produce a variety of cytokines, including interleukin 2 (IL-2). While in most patients with a viral infection the immune response is eventually "turned off," patients with CFS seem to have prolonged immune stimulation. The production of cytokines causes unpleasant symptoms. Treatment of cancer patients with IL-2 causes a CFS-like illness. Other investigators have noted that while IL-2 is elevated, gamma interferon production is suppressed.

Laboratory diagnosis

There is no single laboratory test for CFS. At one time, antibody to Epstein-Barr virus early antigen was considered diagnostic. This has proven to be an unreliable test. At this time, neither antibody to HHV6 or HTLV-I/II appears to be the test of choice. Most CSF patients have markedly elevated IL-2 levels. IL-2 assays have been proposed as an aid in diagnosing CFS.

Some recently published results indicate that CFS patients have altered levels of certain brain hormones. This adds weight to the argument that CFS is an elaboration of a psychiatric disorder.

LABORATORY TESTING FOR NON-ORGAN SPECIFIC DISEASE
Antinuclear antibody testing

The first test for antinuclear antibodies is the lupus erythematosus (LE) cell test published by Hargraves in 1948. The LE cell test consists of the following: antigen is provided in the form of the nuclei of leukocytes, with membranes that have been damaged by mixing the cells with glass beads or by passing them through a wire mesh. Antibody is provided by the patient serum. The antigen-antibody reaction alters the nuclear material. Polymorphonuclear leukocytes then phagocytize the altered nuclear material, which appears as inclusion bodies within the polymorphonuclear leukocytes (LE cells, see Plate A). The LE cell test has positive results in 60% to 70% of cases of acutely ill patients with SLE. The test detects antibodies to deoxyribonucleoprotein, which appear to react with a DNA-histone complex. The LE cell test is not specific for SLE. The test is labor intensive and subject to observer bias. In most clinical laboratories, antinuclear antibody testing has replaced the LE cell test.

Ideally, testing for antinuclear antibodies is done in two steps. A screening test using either indirect immunofluorescence or an immunoenzyme test is first performed. If the screening test is positive, specific identification of the nuclear antigens may be performed using immunoprecipitation or hemagglutination techniques.

The indirect immunofluorescent test (IF-ANA) is performed as follows:

Fixed tissue culture cell or tissue substrate mounted on microscope slide
↓
Overlay with patient serum
| incubate and
↓ wash off excess

Overlay with fluorescein-conjugated antihuman immunoglobulins
| incubate and
↓ wash off excess

Mount cover slip with buffered glycerol and read with fluorescent microscope

The immunoenzyme technique is similar except that an enzyme-conjugated anti-human globulin is used instead of the fluorescein conjugated antibody. An enzyme substrate color product rather than fluorescence is used for localizing serum autoantibodies over the nucleus. The immunoenzyme method produces a permanent slide which can be read with a conventional microscope. The disadvantages are the difficulties of standardization and reproducibility with different batches of reagent.

A number of substrates have been used in the IF-ANA test. The substrates include chicken erythrocytes, human leukocytes, human skin tissue, rat or mouse kidney and liver, and tissue culture cells (HEp-2 and KB-cells). Chicken erythrocytes are poor in detecting certain antibodies, such as Sm and RNP. False positives, such as interference with blood group antibodies, are a problem with human leukocytes and human skin tissue. Two thirds of patients who were "ANA negative" using mouse or rat tissue are ANA positive with HEp-2 substrate. The HEp-2 substrate is more sensitive to nuclear antibodies, such as SSA/Ro, which are missed with the rat or mouse substrate.

A review of the 1991 diagnostic immunology surveys for the College of American Pathologists (CAP) shows that 84% of the participants used human tissue culture cells and an IF-ANA method for antinuclear antibody testing. Only 5% used an immunoenzyme technique. Ninety-nine percent used commercial kits. The human cell lines, particularly HEp-2 cells, offer many advantages. The monolayers of cell lines allow better recognition of the distinct nuclear staining patterns since the cells are undamaged and have large nuclei in contrast to the presentation of the nuclei in tissue sections. The fluorescent patterns allow, to some extent, characterization of the antigenic specificities of ANA. The presence or absence of nuclear staining in mitotic cells aids in pattern identification. In addition, certain nuclear antigens such as anti centromere and anti Ro (SS-A) are expressed preferentially in the cell lines. These antibodies may be overlooked when using tissue substrates. Two thirds of "ANA negative" SLE patients produce SS-A/Ro antibodies. Since anti SS-A/Ro produces a speckled ANA pattern on the HEp-2 cell line, many "ANA negative" SLE patients have a positive ANA when using this substrate. A reference preparation is available through the College of American Pathologists for testing each new lot number of HEp-2 cells for the presence of SSA/Ro antigen. The reference serum has a positive range of titer of 1:4 to 1:32. In addition, the reference serum has an assigned value of positive immunodiffusion antibody to SSA/Ro and can be used for specific identification of unknown anti-SSA/Ro by immunodiffusion analysis. The centromere antibody is an ANA which is directed against the mitotic plate region of the dividing HEp-2 cells. Centromere antibody correlates highly with the CREST syndrome.

Clinical significance

Since approximately 96% of patients with systemic lupus erythematosus (SLE) have a positive fluorescent antibody test, the ANA test is useful in ruling out SLE. False positive reactions to the HEp-2 substrate are more common than with animal tissue. Weak positives (titer $\geq 1:80$) are found in 5% of well individuals over 40 years and in as many as 10% of those over 60 years, decreasing the usefulness as a screening procedure in older people. Each laboratory should establish a range of reference values for 95% of the population with representative patients from age groups younger than 40 and older than 40. ANA immunofluorescent titers do not correlate with the clinical treatment of disease.

The ANA test screens for a number of nuclear antibodies. Some of these antibodies and their frequency in clinical disease are listed in Table 36-5.

The patterns observed in the ANA screening procedures are indicative of certain types of nuclear antibodies, see Plates B to I. Table 36-6 shows the ANA patterns produced by the specific ANA antibodies.

ANA specific assays. The IF-ANA and the immunoenzyme ANA tests have limited value in the quantitation and identification of various specific antinuclear antibodies. A positive ANA should be followed by specific testing. The IF-ANA tests may have negative results in patients with certain disease (Sjogren's syndrome, progressive systemic sclerosis, and polymyositis) even though "marker" antibodies may be present. In general, antibodies to dsDNA are detected by an indirect IF assay with the hemoflagellate substrate *Crithidea luciliae;* antibodies to histones are detected by an indirect IF procedure on a "histone-reconstituted" substrate; and Sm, U1-RNP, SS-A/Ro, SS-B/La, RANA, and ScL-70 antibodies are assayed either by Ouch-

Table 36-5 The presence of various ANA in defined disorders

Disorder	Percentages of positive sera against mentioned antigens													
	ANA	RANA	dsDNA	ssDNA	ENA	Sm	RNP	SS-A	SS-B	Histones	Centromeres	Scl-70	PMI	Jol
RA	56	93	2	4	7	5	1	4	1	10	—	—	—	—
RA + 2" Sjogren's syndrome	56	60	—	—	—	—	—	15	8	—	—	—	—	—
(I") Sjogren's syndrome	—	30	—	—	—	0	5	70	60	—	—	—	—	—
Felty's syndrome	75	—	0	100	—	—	—	—	—	—	—	—	—	—
Juvenile RA	57	8	5	3	—	0	3	0	0	—	—	—	—	—
SLE	100	2	49	42	—	23	34	35	5	46	—	—	—	—
Drug-induced LE by														
Procainamide	90	—	0	24	—	0	0	—	—	94	—	—	—	—
Acetylprocainamide	17	—	—	0	—	—	—	—	—	—	—	—	—	—
Hydralazine	44	—	—	—	—	—	—	—	—	—	—	—	—	—
MCTD	—	—	25	—	—	8	100	—	—	—	—	—	—	—
Scleroderma (PSS)	58	—	0	14	—	0	5	33	6	—	10	23	—	—
CREST-syndrome	100	—	0	0	—	0	2	—	0	—	77	10	—	—
Polymyositis	28	—	—	—	—	—	0	—	—	—	—	—	—	—
Dermatomyositis	—	—	25	—	—	0	0	—	—	—	—	—	60	45

Antinuclear antibody determination: the present state of diagnostic and clinical relevance: Smeenk R, Westgeest T, Swaak T: Scand J Rheumatology, suppl 56:78-92, 1985.

Table 36-6 ANA patterns produced by the specific ANA antibodies shown in Table 36-5

Diffuse or homogeneous	RIM or peripheral	Speckled	Nucleolar
1. anti-deoxyribonucleic acid (anti ds-DNA) 2. anti-histone 3. antideoxyribonucleo-protein (LE cell factor) (also sNP or DNA-histone)	1. anti ds-DNA 2. anti-deoxyribonucleoprotein	saline extractable; acidic 1. anti-Sm 2. anti-RNP 3. anti-Scl-70 4. anti-SS-B 5. anti-SS-A	1. anti-4-6S nucleolar RNA

ANA clinical significance chart: Kallestad diagnostics, Ref No 4, Feb 1988.

terlony double immunodiffusion or by microhemagglutination techniques.

DNA antibody testing

Screening techniques. Antibody to native doubled stranded DNA (dsDNA) is highly specific for SLE; whereas anti single stranded (ss-DNA) is found in a variety of diseases. DNA antibody testing is performed either by using a radioactively labeled DNA or by the *Crithidia luciliae* assay.

An example of a radioimmuno binding technique is the Farr (ammonium sulfate) assay using ^{125}I-DNA. Radioactive DNA is incubated with serum to allow the DNA to complex with antibody. Saturated ammonium sulfate is then added. DNA bound to anti DNA is precipitated, whereas free DNA is soluble and remains in the liquid phase. The radioactivity in the precipitate is a measure of the DNA-binding activity of the serum. The DNA-binding value of a serum (%P) is the percentage of the DNA that was in the ammonium sulfate precipitate of the serum. The raw result may be reported along with the upper limit of the normal serum binding. Since dsDNA tends to denature very easily to ss-DNA, the specificity of this test is difficult to control.

An indirect immunofluorescent test using the hemoflagellate, *Crithidia luciliae,* is a low-cost, simple assay for detecting DNA antibodies. The organism contains a kinetoplast, a giant mitochondrion, which is composed of a single, large network of N-DNA. If DNA antibody is present, the kinetoplast will fluoresce. In the presence of antibodies other than anti-DNA, the organism's nucleus may also fluoresce. Therefore, it is important to only examine the kinetoplast to detect the presence of anti dsDNA.

Studies comparing the *Crithidia luciliae* assay to the radioimmunoassays have had variable results. Some authors have found the radioimmunoassays to be more sensitive, but less specific than *C. luciliae;* whereas others have found *C. luciliae* to be as sensitive and some more sensitive and specific than radioimmunoassays. The *C. luciliae* test is low cost and simple to perform.

Clinical significance of anti dsDNA. The presence of antibodies to dsDNA correlates highly with SLE. Although IFA titers of ANA are not useful for following the course of SLE; titers of anti dsDNA are quite useful. In response to prednisone and immunosuppressive agents, the level of dsDNA antibody in SLE patients will decrease and eventually disappear.

Rheumatoid factors

Rheumatoid factors are immunoglobulins (autoantibodies) with antibody activity for IgG antibody activity for IgG class immunoglobulins. Most rheumatoid factors are IgM and are directed against the Fc portion of the IgG molecule. IgG and IgA rheumatoid factors exist, but are not detected by the most commonly used screening methods since they do not readily agglutinate.

Screening techniques

The original test for rheumatoid factors is the Waaler-Rose test. This test utilizes sheep erythrocytes (SRBC) coated with rabbit anti-SRBC. The test is considered positive if the patient's serum agglutinates the coated SRBC. Most tests for rheumatoid factor involve the presence of a particulate indicator system containing a large number of IgG molecules to which the rheumatoid factor binds. Either human or rabbit IgG is bound to the particulate carrier and the presence of rheumatoid factor is recognized by agglutination or flocculation. The carrier particles utilized include erythrocytes, latex, charcoal, and bentonite. The most common test is the latex slide test based on the method of Singer and Plotz. More recently, detection methods for rheumatoid factor by nephelometry have become readily available. These methods use aggregated human IgG as the antigen. The light scattering produced by antigen-antibody complexes is then measured by the nephelometer.

Clinical significance. Rheumatoid factor is found in 75% of patients with rheumatoid arthritis. It is present in SLE (18%), progressive systemic sclerosis (20%), mixed connective tissue disease (45%), and in less than 5% of patients with polymyositis and polyarteritis nodosa. Rheumatoid factor may be detected in a significant titer in 5% to 10% of healthy persons. High titers do not present a problem in interpretation, but titers of 1:20 to 1:80 raise questions. Early rheumatoid arthritis as well as many other conditions associated with chronic stimulation of the immune system may fall in this titer range.

Cryoglobulins

Cryoglobulins, immunoglobulins that precipitate in the cold, may precipitate as monomeric immunoglobulin or, when bound to antigen, as an immune complex. The following precautions must be taken, when testing for cryoglobulins, to ensure valid results: 1) blood should be transported at 37°C and incubated at 37°C until it clots; 2) serum should be separated by centrifugation at 37°C; and 3) serum should be kept at 4°C for at least three to five days and inspected for the presence of precipitate or gel that dissolves on rewarming. Some cryoprecipitates form at 32°C and will be lost if clotting takes place at room temperature or lower. Detection of cryoglobulins is facilitated if large amounts of blood are used; however, from a practical standpoint, 20 ml are often used.

A relative quantitation of the cryoglobulin may be done by performing a cryocrit (serum precipitated in a hematocrit tube at 4°C), or a simple Biuret test for protein.

The cryoprecipitate should be dissolved and the components identified by immunoelectrophoresis or immunofixation.

Clinical significance. The cryoglobulins may be divided into the following three classes: Class I cryoglobulins are monoclonal immunoglobulins associated with the plasma cell dyscrasias including Waldenstrom's macroglobulinemia, and multiple myeloma. A single monoclonal immunoglobulin is usually present and the cryoprecipitate is copious (greater than 5 mg/mL). Class II cryoglobulins are usually IgM-IgG, with a monoclonal component (usually IgM rheumatoid factor). These cryoglobulins can induce arthralgias, purpura, and glomerulonephritis. Deposition of cryoglobulin in vessel walls initiates inflammation. Class III is a mixed polyclonal-polyclonal cryoglobulin (usually IgG-IgM but occasionally IgG-IgM-IgA). These cryoglobulins are found in very low levels (less than 1 mg/mL). This class is associated with a wide variety of immune-complex diseases, including infections with *Streptococcus* and hepatitis B, systemic lupus erythematosus, and occasionally in association with tumors.

Immune complex assays

None of the methods available for measuring immune complexes is satisfactory for all types of complexes. Ideally, the presence of circulating immune complexes should be sought by several different assays. In addition, these assays cannot distinguish between antigen-antibody complexes and nonspecifically aggregated gamma-globulin. Physical techniques, such as ultracentrifugation and gel filtration, are relatively insensitive and are used more for separation than for detection of immune complexes. Assays using purified C1q, a subunit of the trimolecular first component of complement, can be used to detect and quantitate immune complexes in serum. In a solid-phase assay, C1q is attached to polystyrene tubes and the patient's serum is incubated in the tube. After washing, ^{125}I- labeled anti-human immunoglobulin antiserum is added to detect immune complexes that are bound to C1q. The amount of radioactivity bound to the polystyrene tube reflects the amount of immune complex present. The Raji cell assay utilizes a tissue culture cell (Raji) that has membrane receptors for complement (C3b and C3d) and receptors for the Fc portion of IgG. The patient's serum is incubated with Raji cells and, if immune complexes containing C3c or C3d are present, they are bound to the cell. After washing, ^{125}I- labeled antihuman IgG is added and binds to the immune complexes on the Raji cell surface. The radioactivity detected in the cell pellet is proportional to the amount of immune complexes in the patient's serum. IgG antilymphocyte antibody interferes with the Raji cell assay. Since patients with SLE may have this antibody in their serum, the Raji cell test may not be useful.

ORGAN SPECIFIC DISEASES

The organ specific immune diseases generally affect one organ, as opposed to the previously described systemic diseases, which affect many. The organ specific diseases and associated autoantibodies are outlined in Table 36-7.

Blood

The autoimmune hemolytic anemias are a group of diseases with autoantibodies to red blood cells. Warm autoimmune disease is the most common and is associated with IgG antibody with optimal activity at 37°C. The antibody is often directed against an Rh antigen. Usually there is limited complement-fixing ability and little intravascular hemolysis. In 50% to 75% of the cases, the cause is unknown; these are the so-called idiopathic acquired hemolytic anemias.

In the remainder, the condition develops secondary lymphoproliferative diseases, tumors, viral diseases, sarcoidosis, and drugs.

Cold autoantibodies are usually of the IgM class and react primarily against the I blood group. These antibodies react best at 4°C and fix complement. They are frequently associated with atypical pneumonia (*Mycoplasma pneumoniae*), infectious mononucleosis, and cold agglutinin disease.

Cold autohemolysins (Donath-Landsteiner type) are associated with paroxysmal cold hemoglobinuria. These autoantibodies are biphasic in that antibody is bound in the cold and lysed at warmer temperatures. After extreme cold exposure, these patients suffer a severe hemolytic episode. The antibody is of the IgG class, avidly binds complement, and is specific for the P antigen of the human red blood cell. Paroxysmal cold hemoglobinuria was originally associated with tertiary syphilis. However, the antibody may be seen following viral infections, particularly measles and mumps.

Endocrine

The autoimmune endocrine diseases include thyroiditis, Addison's disease, hypoparathyroidism, and diabetes. The thyroid diseases are fairly common. Hashimoto's thyroiditis (hypothyroiditis) is found in 1% or 2% of autopsies in the United States. Incidence increases with age and is found

Table 36-7 Organ specific diseases and associated serum autoantibodies

Organ	Disease	Autoantibody
Blood	Autoimmune hemolytic anemia, leukopenia, thrombocytopenia	IgG class antibody to formed elements of the blood
Endocrine	Hashimoto's thyroiditis (hypothyroidism)	Antithyroglobulin, Antithyroid microsomal antibody
	Grave's disease (hyperthyroidism)	Thyroid-stimulating antibodies (TSI)
	Addison's disease	IgG antibodies against the microsomal fraction of adrenal tissue
	Insulin-dependent Diabetes Mellitus, type I	Antibodies to pancreatic islets
Central Nervous System	Multiple sclerosis	Antibodies to myelin basic protein
Gastrointestinal	Pernicious anemia	IgG class antibodies to intrinsic factor, parietal cells
Hepatobiliary	Chronic active hepatitis	Smooth muscle antibodies
	Primary biliary cirrhosis	Mitochondrial antibody
Kidney	Goodpasture's syndrome	Glomerular basement membrane antibody
Muscle	Myasthenia gravis	Antibodies to acetylcholine receptors
Skin	Dermatitis herpetiformis	IgA deposition in perilesional area
	Bullous pemphigoid	IgG antibasement membrane antibody in skin
	Pemphigus vulgaris	Antibody to intercellular squamous epithelium

four times more frequently in women than in men. Goiter and disturbances of thyroid function dominate the clinical picture. Two autoantibodies, antithyroglobulin (anti-Tg) and antithyroid microsomal (anti-M), are useful for diagnosis. The antibodies are usually assayed by hemagglutination method. Anti-Tg titers of 1:10 or greater are found in approximately 60% of patients. Ninety-four percent have anti-M titers of 1:100 or greater. Titers of anti-Tg of greater than 1:1,280 or anti M greater than 1:6,400 are inconsistent with any diagnosis other than Hashimoto's or Grave's disease.

Grave's disease (hyperthyroidism) is associated with diffuse thryoidal hyperplasia and by the presence in the serum of one or more immunoglobulins (TSI) that stimulate the function of thyroid disease. These TSI's are unique to Grave's disease. The thyroid-stimulating antibodies are listed in Box 36-2.

Autoimmune adrenalitis (Addison's Disease) is the most common form of adrenal insufficiency. IgG autoantibodies, directed toward one or more microsomal fractions may be detected by immunofluorescence using human or monkey adrenal tissue. Approximately 60% of patients have these serum antibodies at diagnosis, but the incidence declines later.

Hypoparathyroidism may occur alone or in association with autoimmune adrenalitis, thryoid disease, and pernicious anemia. It is also associated with microcutaneous candidiasis and with developmental failures of the thymus-dependent immune system, such as DiGeorge's syndrome. Serum antibodies specific for normal parathyroid tissue have been identified by immunofluorescence.

Both diabetes mellitus and insulin resistant diabetes are autoimmune in nature. Insulin-dependent diabetes mellitus (IDDM), Type I, is associated with antibodies to pancreatic islets and certain HLA types. The genetic predisposition includes having HLA DR3 or DR4. Approximately 70% have islet cell antibodies, which can be assayed by immunofluorescence on unfixed sections of normal human pancreas.

Insulin resistant diabetes is a rare disorder usually occurring in black women with diabetes. Thousands of units

of insulin per day have been used in some patients. Many patients have antinuclear antibodies or other evidence of autoimmunity. The disorder is due to insulin receptor antibodies that physically prevent the insulin from binding with the appropriate receptors.

Central nervous system

Multiple sclerosis is a disease of unknown etiology that primarily affects young people (15 to 45 years). The disease results in active demyelinating lesions of the brain and spinal cord, which contain lymphocytes, plasma cells, and macrophages. Multiple sclerosis follows an unpredictable pattern of progression and remission, sometimes remaining in remission for years.

CSF IgG levels increase in multiple sclerosis. It appears that the increased IgG is attributable to increased synthesis in the CNS and is not a plasma filtration product. The oldest method for quantitation of CSF IgG is by calculating the protein level from the height of the gamma globulin peak on the protein electrophoresis scan, since the gamma portion is composed almost entirely of IgG. However, immunochemical methods for quantitating CSF IgG offer a more accurate method of quantitation.

A ratio of CSF IgG to CSF albumin is used since albumin is synthesized only in the liver and thus CSF albumin must be derived from blood. The clinical interpretation of the CSF IgG/CSF albumin ratio assumes that an increase in permeability of the blood-brain barrier allows for a proportional increase of both IgG and albumin, thus showing no real change in the ratio. With increased CNS IgG production, the percentage of CSF IgG to CSF albumin would increase.

In addition to CSF IgG levels, the presence of oligoclonal bands and myelin basic protein in CSF are used in the diagnosis of multiple sclerosis. Oligoclonal bands are discrete and are seen in the gamma region of a CSF agarose electrophoresis separation. The oligoclonal band represents IgG restricted heterogeneity.

A radioimmunoassay can detect myelin basic protein in cerebrospinal fluid. Myelin basic protein is present in CSF during periods of active demyelination.

Myelin basic protein is present in CSF in 90% of patients with multiple sclerosis within one week after an acute episode. The value returns to normal after two weeks. Approximately 70% of patients with multiple sclerosis have elevated CSF IgG and approximately 90% have oligoclonal bands.

Gastrointestinal and hepatobiliary

The autoimmune gastrointestinal diseases include pernicious anemia, ulcerative colitis, and regional ileitis. Pernicious anemia is characterized by an atrophy of the gastric mucosa with inability to secrete hydrochloric acid, intrinsic factor, or pepsin. Eventually, megaloblastic anemia develops. Ninety-five percent of patients have IgG class antibody against instrinsic factor. It is not known if these antibodies are the result or the cause of the disease. Circulating antibodies to colonic tissue can be found with ulcerative colitis and regional ileitis.

Autoimmune chronic active hepatitis is a rare form of chronic hepatitis of unknown etiology. Unlike viral hepa-

---

Box 36-2 Thyroid-stimulating antibodies

Long-acting thyroid stimulator (LATS)
  Release of iodine 131 from labeled mouse thyroid (McKenzie assay).
Thyroid-stimulating immunoglobulin
  Release of adenosine 3':5'-cyclic phosphate from human thyroid cells or from the rat thyroid cell line, FRTL-5.
Thyrotropin-binding inhibitory immunoglobulin
  Inhibition of the binding of labeled thyroid-stimulating hormone (usually bovine) to human or porcine thyroid membranes or guinea pig fat membranes.
Thyroid growth immunoglobulin
  Increased DNA synthesis by human thyroid cells assayed by cytochemical bioassay on human thyroid slices or with the rate thyroid cell line, FRTL-5.

Beall GN: Immunologic aspects of endocrine diseases: JAMA, 258:2952-2956, Nov 27, 1987.

titis, it responds to corticosteroid treatment. About half of these patients have autoimmune syndromes including thyroiditis, rheumatoid arthritis, and Sjogren's syndrome. Patients have elevated serum transaminase levels and hypergammaglobulinemia.

Autoantibodies, including smooth-muscle antibodies and antinuclear antibodies, can be demonstrated by indirect immunofluorescent methods.

Primary biliary cirrhosis is characterized by inflammation and necrosis of intrahepatic bile ducts. The disease primarily affects middle-aged women and is often associated with other autoimmune disorders such as Sjogren's syndrome, thyroiditis, and progressive systemic sclerosis.

Laboratory features include elevations of liver enzyme and serum bilirubin levels, cholesterol and lipoprotein abnormalities, and increased copper/ceruloplasmin levels. Serum IgM is usually elevated and mitochondrial antibody titers are found in more than 90% of patients.

Kidney

Goodpasture's syndrome is characterized by antibodies to glomerular basement membrane (anti GBM) and pulmonary hemorrhage. The attack of kidney antibodies against kidney antigens leads to local activation of complement. Linear deposition of antibody and complement along the GBM can be shown by direct immunofluorescence.

Acute poststreptococcal nephritis is caused by deposition of immune complexes in the glomerular capillary wall. Antibodies against the streptococci combine with streptococcal antigens to form immune complexes. Direct immunofluorescence reveals a "lumpy-bumpy" pattern in the capillary wall, rather than the smooth, linear fluorescence observed with anti-GBM.

Muscle

Myasthenia gravis is a neuromuscular disease characterized by muscle weakness. Functional postsynaptic acetylcholine receptors (AChRs) are depleted by an immune-mediated destruction. Over 90% of patients with myasthenia gravis have anti AChR antibodies. Antinuclear antibodies are seen in 25% to 40% and rheumatoid factor, antithyroid and some other organ-specific antibodies are seen in about 20% of patients, even when there is no clinical expression of associated disease.

Skin

Dermatitis herpetiformis, bullous pemphigoid, and pemphigus vulgaris are autoimmune diseases of the skin. Dermatitis herpetiformis is characterized by grouped vesicles surmounted on an erythematous base involving predominantly the extensor surfaces of the back and arms. Patients

have a burning pruritis as well as a patchy duodenal-jejunal atrophy indistinguishable from celiac disease.

Granular deposition of IgA in the perilesional skin is seen in 95% of the patients and can be demonstrated by direct immunofluorescence. In addition, C3, C5, properdin, and properdin factor B have been noted along the dermal-epidermal junction, suggesting activation of the complement pathway by the alternative pathway.

Bullous pemphigoid lesions are characterized by tense subepidermal blisters on the flexural areas of the body, including the neck, axillae, and inguinal area. A linear homogeneous IgG deposition along the basement membrane zone is demonstrable by direct immunofluorescence; although all classes of immunoglobulins and early and late components of complement may be seen. IgG anti-basement membrane may be demonstrated by indirect immunofluorescence in the serum of approximately 80% of patients.

Pemphigus vulgaris is a blistering disease characterized by the presence of flaccid bullae arising in the mouth and scalp but rapidly disseminating over the entire body. Direct immunofluorescence of the perilesional skin lesions reveals IgG, C1q, C3, properdin, and properdin factor B in the squamous intercellular spaces. A circulating antibody to intercellular squamous epithelium has been demonstrated by indirect immunofluorescence in approximately 90% of patients.

SUGGESTED READING

Barrett JT: Autoimmunity and immunodeficiency. In Textbook of immunology, ed 5, St. Louis, 1988, Mosby–Year Book, Inc.

Bauman GP and Hurtubise P: Anti-idiotypes and autoimmune disease, Clinics in Lab. Med. 8 (2):399-407, 1988.

Bennett RM: Mixed connective tissue disease and other overlap syndromes. In Textbook of rheumatology, ed 3, Philadelphia, 1989, WB Saunders Co.

Buckley RH: Immunodeficiency diseases. JAMA, 258:20:2841-2850, 1987.

De Shazo RD, et al: Use and interpretation of diagnostic immunologic laboratory tests. JAMA, 258:20:3011-3031, 1987.

Feldmann M: Regulation of HLA Class II expression and its role in autoimmune disease. In Autoimmunity and autoimmune disease, Ciba Foundation Symposium #129:88-108, 1987.

Jackson G: Cerebrospinal fluid proteins—fractionation. In Pesce AJ, and Kaplan LA: Methods in Clinical Chemistry, St. Louis, 1987, Mosby–Year Book, Inc.

Levy JA: Human immuno deficiency viruses and the pathogenesis of AIDS, JAMA 261:20:2997-3006, 1989.

Rose NR: Current concepts of autoimmune disease, Transplantation Proc 20(3):3-10, 1988.

Schur PH: Clinical features of SLE. In Textbook of Rheumatology, ed 3, Philadelphia, 1989, WB Saunders Co.

Schwartz JS et al: Human immunodeficiency virus test evaluation performance and use, JAMA 259:17:2574-2578, 1989.

PART SIX

CLINICAL MICROBIOLOGY

37 Contemporary approaches to clinical microbiology

Albert Balows

In societies throughout the world infectious diseases remain one of the major causes of morbidity, and in many areas they are a major cause of mortality. Microbial agents are increasingly involved directly or indirectly in both acute and chronic diseases, for example, arthritis, diabetes, cancer, gastrointestinal disease, diseases of the central nervous, hematopoietic, and respiratory systems, and in pregnancy and infant mortality. It has become increasingly difficult to define a pathogenic agent without explicity including the host. What is pathogenic for one host may not be for another. This is further complicated by changes that may occur in the host (e.g., age, nutritional and immunological state) or the microbial agent (e.g., antibiotic resistance, invasive attributes, and antigenic changes).

In each of the major scientific disciplines embodied in laboratory medicine the dynamic state of the patient must be recognized and considered when laboratory analyses are made. In clinical chemistry, for example, we may initially look for deviations from what we regard as normal and subsequently test again to determine if the previously measured analyte has increased, decreased, or has returned to normal. Clinical microbiological analyses usually involve two dynamic systems, the patient (host) and the microbial agent. Changes in one usually affect the other. Clinical microbiology tests also differ from chemical determinations in that most clinical chemistry tests yield a quantitative result, whereas most microbiology test results are qualitative. This distinction is real because qualitative results are different in terms of reproducibility, interpretation, control, verification, and occasionally, correlation with the patient's clinical presentation.

From 1985 through 1989, specifically collected and analyzed data indicated that approximately three quarters of a billion cases of infectious diseases occurred annually in the United States. While not all of these cases of infectious diseases required hospitalization, an annual utilization of 52 million hospital days was required at a total *direct* cost that exceeded $35 billion—and growing. In spite of the present trends in the annual number of chronic and acute infectious disease cases, there is mounting pressure to contain, if not decrease, the total direct costs involved in the diagnosis and treatment of disease. It is the obligation of every microbiologist to be aware of the direct costs of laboratory medicine, and in particular of clinical microbiology, and be able to institute cost-saving measures where possible without compromising the quality of test results. Contemporary approaches to the conduct of clinical microbiology include not only the close cooperation with the medical and nursing staff of the institution, but an awareness of the entire process by which specimens are collected, delivered to, and accessioned by the laboratory; once in the laboratory, test procedures are initiated, followed through to an acceptable completion, and a report issued . . . all in a timely, meaningful, and cost-effective manner. This is not an easy task; it requires skill, technical expertise, and knowledge of the principles of clinical microbiology.

Specimens are submitted to the clinical microbiology laboratory for one or more of the following purposes: (1) Screening test(s) for one or more specific infections. This is usually done because the patient is asymptomatic or shows vague or general signs but no clear indication of an infectious process. (2) Directed tests to assist the clinician by providing laboratory test data to confirm or direct the decision in making a diagnosis. (3) In vitro antibiotic susceptibility tests to support the therapeutic administration of one or more antibiotics. (4) Immunologic tests to establish the status of an infectious disease. (5) Specific tests to detect microbial cell fragments or metabolic products that may be useful in the diagnosis of an infectious disease in one or more individuals. (6) Epidemiologic tests for the diagnosis and control of an outbreak of an infectious disease in the community or in the hospital. Irrespective of the purpose for specimen submission, the diagnosis of an infectious disease and the determination of which antibiotics to use or not to use for therapy or the immune status of the host is not unilaterally accomplished by the clinical microbiology laboratory. Rather, it is an integrated effort that utilizes the knowledge and expertise of the microbiologist, the clinician, and many others whose professional roles contribute to health care.

Although the microbiology laboratory is best located in an area of minimal traffic and should not be used for meetings and social events, the staff should maintain high visibility and availability to all others for information exchange, consultation, and assistance with interpretation of laboratory test results. Likewise, the director of the microbiology laboratory and delegated members of the laboratory staff should be active participants in various institutional committees and activities that relate to microbiology and infectious diseases.

There are a number of important practical considerations that should be incorporated into the overall operational plan and activities of the clinical microbiology laboratory, irrespective of size and volume of work. The remainder of this chapter will focus on these practical issues and concerns that must be addressed by the microbiologist(s) and should be either integrated into the flow of work or incorporated into the overall responsibility of the microbiology laboratory.

TRAINING AND EDUCATION

Acceptable levels of education and training of the clinical microbiology staff is a mandate from which there should be no exception. Minimally, a microbiologist should have a bachelor's degree from an accredited institution. The American Medical Association's Committee on Allied Health Education and Accreditation can provide information on the more than 450 medical technology programs in the United States. The American Society for Microbiology has information on 375 colleges and universities in the United States and Canada that offer undergraduate and/or graduate degrees. There are innumerable 2-year programs that offer associate of arts degrees for laboratory technicians. In pursuing any of these programs it is important to recognize the important distinctions between education and training. The educated microbiologist has the ability to think critically, understand the dynamics of biology, make value judgments, and effectively communicate, whereas the trained clinical microbiologist has acquired a body of factual information and developed technical skills to perform a variety of simple or complex technological procedures. Because clinical microbiology is dynamic, it is very important to participate in an ongoing continuing education program that provides the opportunity to become educated in new advances in the science and to be trained in the technical know-how by which scientific advances are applied and used in the diagnosis or therapy of disease.

REGULATORY REQUIREMENTS

In 1967 the Congress of the United States passed a law titled the Clinical Laboratories Improvement Act (CLIA-67) that led to the development of rather stringent federal regulations that touched virtually every activity in the clinical laboratory—from laboratory licensure, personnel qualifications and standards, to quality control, quality assurance, proficiency testing, control of commercially available reagents and instruments to test procedures, and payment of laboratory charges by Medicare and Medicaid. Subsequently, additional legislation was passed that created a new and controversial approach to reimbursement of physicians and hospitals (including the clinical laboratory) for their service fees. A series of categorized diagnostic related groups (DRG) were established and a fee structure for the various groups was put in operation. These federal laws were augmented and supplemented in many instances by state and local enactments. All of these were designed to improve the quality of health care, which included, but was not limited to, diagnostic radiology and clinical laboratory tests, improvement of the quality and purpose of all medical devices, instruments, equipment, and reagents, and to effect cost-containment measures to reduce (or at least control) the increasing cost of medical care. In 1988 the Congress passed the Clinical Laboratory Improvement Amendments (CLIA-88). Officials within the Department of Health and Human Services (HHS) have developed regulations to implement the meaning and intent of the law. In general, the regulations contain rules pertaining to licensing of laboratories; revisions in proficiency testing, design, and enforcement of quality control and quality assurance programs; standards for ranking diagnostic tests in terms of difficulty in performance and possible risk to patients who rely on the diagnostic accuracy of the tests; and standards for the site (laboratory or elsewhere) where tests may be performed. Additional federal legislation became law toward the end of 1990, when the president signed the Safe Medical Devices Act, which, when fully implemented over the next 3 to 5 years, should have a far-reaching and profound effect on those who produce, use, and benefit from the use of medical devices. The Food and Drug Administration (FDA) has the lead responsibility in the enforcement of the rules and regulations, and the major impact will likely be upon manufacturers of devices—particularly those that are placed within the patient (heart valve, prosthesis) or those used on the patient for diagnosis (tomography) or to monitor vital signs (pulse, blood pressure). However, laboratory devices are very likely to come under the jurisdiction of this law as full implementation takes place. While it is not expected that clinical microbiologists become experts in law, it is nonetheless important that they know of the existence of these and other state and federal legislative matters that relate to the conduct of laboratory testing, patient privacy, biosafety in the workplace, proper disposal of infectious waste, and safe handling and containment of corrosive or dangerous chemicals and radioactive materials. The laboratory director, the institutional library, and professional societies are usually reliable sources for current legal information and approved practices.

LABORATORY PROCEDURE MANUAL

One of the federal, state, and private agency requirements of all laboratories that are engaged in interstate testing of specimens or receive federal money in payment for laboratory testing is that a complete procedure manual be developed in-house and be readily available for use at the bench by all technical staff performing analytical procedures. Further, the manual must spell out in reasonable detail the evaluation of the specimen, the stepwise test procedure, the source of reagents and instruments (where purchased or how made, stored, and used), conditions of testing, controls required, reading and interpreting the test results, and how to report results to the referring physician. The procedure manual must not consist of a compilation of photocopied pages of other manuals, manufacturers' package inserts, or pages removed from books or journals. It must be a tailor-made manual that is individualized for each laboratory. The manual should be developed by the head of the microbiology laboratory with input from supervisors, section heads, and so on. The use of existing published procedures, approved commercial reagents, kits, media preparation, instructions, use and care of instruments, test controls, and the like are very appropriate and should be used and followed to the fullest extent possible. Alternate procedures, where available, should be included. The designated laboratory staff should be familiar with and able to do the procedures in the manual. The procedure manual should be used to indoctrinate new additions to the technical staff and they should be monitored to make certain they understand each procedure. The manual is intended to serve as a guide for all personnel in the microbiology laboratory and should be updated with new or revised procedures as they are introduced into the laboratory. A total review of the manual should be undertaken on an annual basis. The College of American Pathologists (CAP) requires that methods in the manual follow the NCCLS format.

CONTINUING EDUCATION PROGRAMS

One of the benchmarks of a good, dynamic clinical microbiology laboratory is the concerted effort given to continuing education. This can be approached in several ways—encourage informal, in-house discussion groups, establish journal reviews and brief lectures by senior staff members, encourage membership in regional or national organizations that sponsor continuing education programs, and promote attendance at short-term courses or workshops that introduce theory and practice of new technology. Participation in a continuing education program is one of the best ways to stay abreast of the increasing number of new technological advances and the expanding applications of older methods.

NEW TECHNOLOGICAL APPLICATIONS

Advances in basic research over the past 10 to 15 years have resulted in the development of many new and different applied technologies. Biology no longer exists as a separate science. Contemporary microbiology is bursting with a rapid influx of applied molecular biology, protein and nucleic acid biochemistry, and biophysics. These applications, coupled with newly recognized or emerging pathogens, the ability to obtain specimens for testing that were previously unobtainable, and the increased interest in rapid diagnostic methods are all indicative of the broadening horizons of clinical microbiology. A brief overview of some of these newer advances follows. More information and greater detail are found in the specific chapters in Part 1 and Parts 5 to 8.

Monoclonal antibodies were first prepared on a large scale in 1975 as a result of the research of Kohler and Milstein, who developed a hybrid clone of mouse spleen cells fused to multiple myeloma cells that were capable of producing high titer sensitive and specific antibody. The antibody was also monoclonal (specific for a specific antigen determinant) and virtually eliminated cross-reactions and lot-to-lot variation in antibody content that were found in antiserum produced by conventional methods. The number and variety of commercially available monoclonal antibody (MAb) reagents are rapidly increasing, and with their use in the laboratory, the time required to issue a useful report is rapidly diminishing. Soluble or particulate microbial antigens can be detected in body fluids, exudates, transudates, and tissue preparations for a large number of infectious diseases. The techniques vary from the simple microscopic observation of antigen-antibody clumping to a microscopic search for fluorescence resulting from the reaction of a fluorescein-conjugated MAb with its specific antigen. Similarly, MAb have been incorporated into commercially produced kits for use outside of the clinical laboratory as a screening test for several infectious diseases. The overall success of these screening kits is variable and a careful judgment should be made on each particular kit. The intended use should be evaluated by parallel cultures or other definitive tests.

Probes, blots, and immunoblots are similar, yet different diagnostic applications of earlier basic research. The Southern blot technique takes its name from E.M. Southern, the developer of the procedure. The technique is very useful in identifying organisms or determining how closely or distantly related two organisms are by comparing or matching designated chromosomal deoxyribonucleic acid (DNA) sequences. Extracted DNA preparations are treated with one or more restriction enzymes to cut or disassociate the chromosome strand at specific sites. The preparation is then placed on a thin layer or slab of agarose gel (a gel made from special high-grade agar) and subjected to an electric current. The DNA fragments move in this electric field in a pattern governed by their size and molecular weight. Following this process, called electrophoresis, the agarose gel is carefully placed over a nitrocellulose or nylon membrane and again subjected to an electric current, which causes the small DNA fragments to adhere or bind to the membrane. Next, a radiolabeled or biotinylated probe—a tagged or labeled single segment of DNA with the specific nucleic acid sequence being sought—is introduced into the membrane. The probe seeks the complementary sequence in the bound DNA fragments. Hybridization between the nucleic acid base pairs takes place in direct proportion to their level of complementary matching. The degree of matching is determined by developing the tag. Autoradiography is used in the case of radiolabeled DNA and an enzyme immunoassay is used for biotin labeling. The hybridized bands stand out clearly on the membrane whereas the nonhybridized bands do not develop because their DNA failed to match with that of the probe.

The Northern blot technique (so named merely to distinguish it from the Southern blot) employs an almost identical technique as the Southern blot except the Northern blot technique is used to detect and identify either intact or denatured ribonucleic acid (RNA). Both Southern and Northern blotting techniques can be used to identify bacteria, viruses, and virtually all other sources of DNA and RNA. As our ability to employ known probes to identify or detect the presence of specific microorganisms increases, the commercial availability of the necessary blot reagents will increase and the test procedure will become less complex.

The Western blot technique (so named to distinguish it from Southern and Northern blots) is a very sensitive and specific technique for detecting and characterizing microbial antibodies. It is not only possible to detect antibodies related to a specific antigen or antigenic fragment, but this technique is very useful in detecting the class of immunoglobulin to which the antibody belongs. The technique employed is similar to the other blotting methods. In the Western blot technique the focus is on amino acids and proteins rather than nucleic acids. The primary gel used to electrophoretically separate the proteins in a microbial extract is a polyacrylamide gel that contains sodium dodecyl sulfate (SDS-PAGE). The electric current causes the proteins to separate and migrate at rates proportionate to their molecular weights. These proteins (or amino acid complexes) are deposited in different places on the gel and are referred to as protein bands. These bands are transferred from the SDS-PAGE to a solid-phase membrane of nitrocellulose, where they are fixed. The membrane can now be exposed to serum to detect antibodies specific for the fixed protein(s). This is easily accomplished by cutting the nitrocellulose sheet into strips and immersing and incubating a strip in each of the serum specimens being tested for antibody. Following incubation each strip is developed to make the antigen-antibody reaction bands visible. This can be done by using radiolabeled antihuman-goat serum or biotin-labeled antihuman-goat serum to give a color or visibility to the antigen-antibody bands. By using antihuman-goat serum for any of the antibody classes or subclasses, a complete qualitative and quantitative spectrum of a given individual's immune response to an infectious agent can be determined.

Despite the sensitivity and specificity of the various nucleic acid blotting techniques, one of the major difficulties encountered is the inability of the probe to detect very small amounts of DNA in the sample to be tested. In 1985 an in vitro method was described that made it possible to amplify a specific gene sequence such that picrograms of a DNA (or RNA) sequence could be amplified to micrograms, thus providing more than enough for organism identification or other analyses. The amplification technique is known as the polymerase chain reaction (PCR). In this reaction a designated sequence of DNA or RNA can be replicated in vitro tenfold or more in 3 to 4 hours. The synthesis of the DNA is initiated by the enzyme DNA polymerase in the presence of a known existing sequence of single-stranded DNA that serves as a template. This template is obtained by denaturation at high temperature of a double strand of DNA that contains the desired DNA sequence. Also needed is a piece of double-stranded DNA at one end of the template to serve as primer. The initial reaction takes place at a high temperature (about 95°C) at which the template is denatured. Next, the resulting oligonucleotides are annealed at a low temperature (35°C) to the denatured template. This gives rise to enzymatic extension (polymerase) of the primer and the process repeats 25 to 30 times with a 10^5 or 10^6 increase in the targeted DNA. There are now available several instruments that can be programmed to perform the temperature changes and incubation automatically over a given time span. The PCR technique has been applied to several areas of laboratory medicine that require specific DNA sequence detection and identification.

In the intervening years since the discovery of the PCR, other methods for amplifying designated DNA sequences and the direct detection of specific nucleic acids have been described. The ligase chain reaction (LCR) and the transcription-based amplification system (TAS) are two additional assays that amplify designated DNA sequences. A third assay, using an RNA polymerase known as Q-beta replicase has been described in which a single molecule of RNA will yield 10^{12} progeny strands in about 10 to 15 minutes. As reagents become available and procedures are standardized, the probe techniques will be used with increasing frequency in the diagnostic laboratory and is clear indication of the need for a good basic knowledge of molecular biology.

Instruments for performing complete blood cell counts by flow cytometry and white blood cell differential counts by image analysis are frequently found in hematology laboratories. (See Part 1.) These technologies are also being used in several research and applied areas of microbiology with some applications in clinical microbiology.

Assays using flow cytometry and light-scattering instruments have been described that determine antibacterial and antiviral activity of various therapeutic drugs, microbial counts in body fluids, microbial detection and identification. Other instruments provide videolike images of clinical specimens and cultures that can be further processed to yield rapid microbial identification and antimicrobial susceptibility results.

THE CONTROL AND PREVENTION OF INFECTIOUS DISEASES

In a very real sense the entire staff of the clinical microbiology laboratory has a major goal, the control and prevention of infectious diseases. All of the chapters in Part 1 and Parts 5 to 8 deal with achieving this goal. However, this goal goes far beyond the patients whose specimens are brought to the laboratory for testing. The head and technical staff of the microbiology laboratory should be active in the infection control program of the hospital. This is accomplished by participating in the following institutional programs:

1. Careful instruction of all nursing and technical hospital staff who have patient contact on the proper collection, handling, and transport of specimens, surgical tissues, exudates, secretions, and the like, obtained from patients for testing or discarding.
2. Active participation in selection of germicides and disinfectants to be used in various areas of the hospital. This may be accomplished by serving on an institutional committee that reviews and recommends the various agents and procedures used for sterilization and disinfection. The laboratory should cooperate in the routine sterilization testing of autoclaves and dry heat sterilizers, and be prepared to conduct periodic microbiological sterility assays of medical devices such as hemodialysis systems, arterial pressure transducers, and selected endoscopic instruments.
3. Active participation in institutional committees responsible for providing scientific and technical information on the management of radioactive, chemical, and infectious waste. Waste management is a major responsibility of all institutions and is subject to various federal and state regulations. The clinical laboratory plays a major advisory role in waste management and should have staff members knowledgeable in the regulatory, scientific, and technical aspects of all types of waste management. Close liaison with regional offices of responsible federal agencies and corresponding state officials is recommended.

4. Active participation in the institution's program to monitor, control, and prevent hospital-acquired infections. This requires close collaboration with the medical and nursing staff, and especially with the epidemiologist in tracking down the source and extent of nosocomial infections. This includes among other laboratory tests, the determination of exogenous vs. endogenous infection and performance of one or more of the recognized typing systems for determining relatedness of the isolates obtained during an investigation.

5. Establish good working relationships with appropriate members of the state health department laboratory and state epidemiologist. Solicit their assistance in the investigation of incidents important to the public's health, such as food- or water-borne illness in patients or hospital staff, isolation of agents likely to be involved in public health outbreaks, or with antibiotic resistance patterns that may be a problem in other patients with the same organism. Proper communication of appropriate microbiologic information can and should be done without damaging patient confidentiality and ensuring the public's health.

SUGGESTED READING

Balows A, and others: Manual of clinical microbiology, ed 5, Washington, DC, 1991, American Society for Microbiology.

Balows A, Hausler WJ Jr, and Lennette EH: Laboratory diagnosis of infectious diseases: principles and practice, vols 1 and 2, New York, 1988, Springer-Verlag.

Baron EJ and Finegold SM: Bailey and Scott's diagnostic microbiology, ed 8, St Louis, 1990, Mosby-Year Book.

Finlay BB and Falkow S: Common themes in microbial pathogenicity, Microbiol Rev 53:210–230, 1989.

Garcia LS and Bruckner DA: Diagnostic medical parasitology, New York, 1988, Elsevier Science.

Howard BJ, and others: Clinical and pathogenic microbiology, St Louis, 1987, Mosby–Year Book.

Macario AJL and deMacario EC: Gene probes for bacteria, San Diego, 1990, Academic Press.

Cumulative techniques and procedures in clinical microbiology (Cumitechs), Washington, DC, American Society for Microbiology, (new additions annually).

Rose NR, Friedman H, and Fahey JL: Manual of clinical immunology, ed 3, Washington, DC, 1986, American Society for Microbiology.

Smith JW: The role of clinical microbiology in cost effective health care, Skokie, Ill, 1985, College of American Pathologists.

Turgeon ML: Immunology and serology in laboratory medicine, St Louis, 1990, Mosby–Year Book.

Washington JA: Laboratory procedures in clinical microbiology, ed 2, New York, 1985, Springer-Verlag.

38 Quality assurance in clinical microbiology

Ron B. Schifman

The objectives of a quality assurance program in the clinical microbiology laboratory are to improve reliability, efficiency, and utilization of laboratory services. The elements of quality assurance consist of structure, process, and outcome. Structure is the aspect related to adequacy of the workplace and the provisions required to do the job. Process describes the proficiency with which the work is done, whereas outcome reflects the consequences of work performed. Quality is measured by specifying indicators and setting thresholds for acceptable performance. This spans a wide spectrum; from monitoring reagent performance to assessing test usage. Limits may be set so that action is taken only when the number of deficiencies exceeds a specified threshold, or it may be defined as a sentinel event that requires review and action whenever encountered. Although monitoring is important, the most effective results are achieved by employing strategies to prevent problems rather than by detecting and correcting defects after they have occurred.

Passage of the 1967 Clinical Laboratory Improvement Act marked the beginning of systematic laboratory quality assurance. Since then, most attention has focused on quality control. This includes monitoring the dependability of reagents, procedures, and equipment, and checking the adequacy and appropriateness of specimens. Less consideration has been given to other components of quality that deal with the issue of why tests are ordered and how results are utilized. Recognition of this latter concern is being driven, in part, by the need to meet new requirements originating from regulatory and accreditation bodies, as well as the growing perception that quality is ultimately determined by how laboratory practice affects patient outcome.

BASIC COMPONENTS

Documentation is an essential requirement. All methods, policies, quality control results, and corrective actions need to be described in writing and made available to those working in the microbiology laboratory and those responsible for its management.

Procedure manual

The procedure manual is a reference document describing all established methods, materials, and policies. Its purpose is to standardize the performance of laboratory operations. It includes procedures for collecting, transporting, and rejecting specimens; methods for processing samples, and reporting results; quality control procedures for reagents, media, and equipment; as well as schematic procedures to follow when quality control data indicate unacceptable performance. Pertinent hospital and laboratory policies, including guidelines for safety and waste disposal, are also included. The manual should have a consistent format for method descriptions and include appropriate citations. Another manual describing specimen and requisition requirements, storage and transport conditions, laboratory policies, and safety precautions must be available to physicians, nurses, and anyone else responsible for ordering tests, collecting specimens, and delivering them to the microbiology laboratory. The required manual on laboratory safety is yet another requirement that must be available in all laboratories (see Chapter 2).

Quality control logs

The quality control (QC) log is a form for documenting quality control results and corrective action. It contains the date and time that testing is performed, the person doing the test, the test results, acceptable limits, result interpretation (pass or fail), and, when necessary, comments on corrective actions. A place to document periodic review and a description of procedures to follow when deficiencies are identified should also be included. Figure 38-1 is an example of a QC form for equipment.

Worksheets

Worksheets are used daily to document all observations made during specimen processing. Documentation includes specimen descriptions, growth on specific media, and flow diagrams of biochemical results, susceptibility tests, and any other observations that are pertinent to the specimen, test results, or interpretation. The worksheet can be employed to detect and evaluate potential problems either before or after specimens and culture plates are discarded. It also organizes the evaluation of culture findings and helps with processing partially completed examinations with pending tests.

	Month _____ Year _____
INCUBATOR	
Unit No. _____	
Temperature, Humidity, CO$_2$ Record	

Date	Range 34-36 Temp °C	Range 30%-50% Humidity	H$_2$O Level*	Range 4%-6% CO$_2$	Init.	Corrective action
1						
2						
3						
4						
5						
6						
7						
8						
9						
10						
11						
12						
13						
14						
15						
16						
17						
18						
19						
20						
21						
22						
23						
24						
25						
26						
27						
28						
29						
30						
31						

* Water level adequate in humidity pan (fill with sterile deionized water)

Date	Reviewed by	Comments/ Actions

Fig. 38-1   Sample quality control equipment form.

QUALITY CONTROL OF THE MICROBIOLOGY SPECIMEN

Quality microbiology results are achieved when proper specimens are collected for appropriate reasons and tested by a well-trained staff working in a suitably equipped laboratory. Examining an unsuitable specimen, responding to a clinically inappropriate request, is not only inefficient, but the results can be misleading. Ongoing instruction of those collecting and ordering tests, as well as those performing the tests is the most effective method for reducing this source of error. In addition, specific monitors of specimen quality and test usage are useful for identifying distinct problem areas requiring more intensive control.

Test ordering and the requisition form

The microbiology requisition form should provide enough information to evaluate a specimen's suitability for processing. It must include the patient's name and identification, requesting physician, date, and time of collection; examination requested (including special requests); and specimen source. It is also very beneficial to provide information about antibiotic therapy since this may influence processing or affect how results are reported. For example, information about antimicrobial therapy can be used to decide if immediate physician notification is warranted when an isolate is resistant to the specified antibiotic. The requisition form also serves to communicate information from the laboratory staff about specimen requirements. This may include a statement about specimen transport, container requirements, volume for blood cultures, or the need to submit multiple specimens (e.g., sputum specimens for *Mycobacterium* spp. culture).

It is important to establish guidelines for rejecting a specimen, or questioning its value when there is incomplete information (e.g., swab from unknown site), an improper submission, (e.g., delayed specimen transport), an inappropriate test request (e.g., anaerobic urine culture), or poor quality collection (e.g., expectorated sputum containing numerous epithelial cells). The guidelines must also cover the procedures for handling specimens that are unacceptable but may be difficult or impossible to recollect (surgical biopsy, cerebral spinal fluid). An unacceptable specimen may have to be processed, with appropriate caveats stated in the report.

Test selection

Evaluating the appropriateness of test ordering is an important quality assurance task. Sometimes, distinctive clinical circumstances other than the specimen's characteristics prevail when making this decision. For instance, ova and parasite examinations on inpatients, or tests for *Clostridium difficile* toxin in patients not receiving antibiotics are usually nonproductive. However, clinical correlations for evaluating test usage usually require information from outside sources (e.g., chart audits). This is a formidable challenge since monitoring is labor-intensive and interventions to modify test usage when standards are not met requires multidepartmental cooperation, is difficult to implement, and its effectiveness is transient without ongoing effort.

Microbiology testing that is done primarily for diagnosis differs from testing in other laboratory sections where tests are done primarily for monitoring. This makes it easier to assess appropriateness of test usage since outcome directly relates to the timeliness and accuracy of diagnosis. An interesting consequence of this is that test underutilization is often identified. For example, although it is well established that two or more separate blood culture specimens per febrile episode are needed to achieve maximum sensitivity and to properly interpret results, approximately 25% of blood cultures collected nationwide are solitary. This may have serious consequences if the diagnosis of bacteremia is missed. Procedures to resolve this problem include sending reminders to physicians about previously established and agreed upon blood culture procedures, or giving instructions to a phlebotomy team to collect multiple specimens per agreed upon policy when a blood culture is ordered. Other examples of underutilization include failures to obtain sufficient sputum samples when tuberculosis is suspected; order blood cultures in cases of suspected pneumonia; or obtain urine cultures in patients with suspected nosocomial urinary tract infections. Excessive culturing or overutilization can also be a problem. Most laboratories will not be aware of these utilization problems unless they are monitored, and even when detected, solutions are difficult to achieve.

The clinical relevance of examining a specimen must also be considered. Material from a decubitus ulcer, periodontal lesion, nose, perirectal abscess, or Foley catheter tip rarely provides clinically useful information, and these specimens should be processed only after consultation with the requesting physician, or not at all. Communication is important when a poor-quality specimen is determined unsuitable for processing. The reasons for rejecting the sample are explained and, when possible, an alternative procedure or corrective action is recommended. Since opinions about specimen quality differ, the rejected specimen should be held at 4° C until a final decision is made. It bears repeating that processing poor-quality specimens should be done when another would be difficult to collect (i.e., cerebrospinal fluid). However, a comment about the apparent problem must be included on the final report to avoid the possibility of a misinterpretation.

Specimen collection and transportation

Adherence to standard collection and transportation procedures improves specimen quality. It is helpful to structure collection guidelines by anatomic site and pathogen. Indications for obtaining a specimen should be described. Instructions for transporting specimens to the microbiology laboratory should specify time limits, transport media, and type of container. Materials for transporting specimens should be specified by the laboratory.

The most effective approach for getting good specimens is to prevent problems before they happen. It is beneficial to schedule regular meetings with medical and nursing staffs to review procedures and address concerns. Written instructions need to be readily available in all clinical areas, and direct communication with the clinical microbiology laboratory staff should be encouraged. Monitoring tends to be most effective when data are stratified by specific hospital location. Hospital wards are generally organized according to certain medical specialties, with particular needs and concerns and each ward is likely to have the same nursing and support staff who are responsible for collecting speci-

Table 38-1   Example of data from sputum quality monitor*

Ward	Sputum samples submitted	Poor collections (>25 epithelial cells/ low power field)	% with 4+ epi's
A	12	2	17
B	29	7	24
C	6	3	50†
D	71	18	25
E	33	4	12
F	9	7	78†
G	11	1	9
Total	171	42	24.6

*Survey of sputum quality, first quarter, 1989.
†These wards may need more intensive instruction on specimen collections or indications for sputum culture.

mens. When monitoring is done, indicators such as transport times and sputum quality are useful. It then becomes easy to identify wards that show a greater-than-average specimen transport time or that submit proportionately large numbers of sputum samples with excessive epithelial cells (Table 38-1). In these circumstances more intensive educational activities or other corrective measures are warranted. Likewise, continued monitoring will demonstrate the success or failure of attempts to correct the problem. When improvement is noted or performance is consistently good, a complimentary statement or note to the responsible ward personnel is helpful.

SPECIMEN PROCESSING

Evaluation of a microbiology specimen is technically complex and labor-intensive. The extent of processing depends on evaluating the probable clinical significance of information obtained from the exam and affects the interpretation of final results.

Gross and microscopic examination

Gross examination helps determine a specimen's suitability for processing. An inadequate sample volume, nonsterile container, or improper collection technique may be grounds for possible rejection. A sample should not, however, be rejected on the basis of its gross appearance alone (e.g., sputum specimen that macroscopically appears like saliva). Gross examination is also useful by making smears or culturing from the most promising portions of specimens that contain mucus, pus, or blood. The sample's description or volume in the case of blood or fluid should be indicated on the worksheet and laboratory report.

Examination and quantitative evaluation of direct smears are beneficial for assessing specimen quality, checking culture results, and possibly establishing a preliminary diagnosis. An expectorated sputum sample that contains excessive epithelial cells indicates oropharyngeal contamination and has dubious value, whereas the etiologic diagnosis is more likely to be determined if the sputum specimen contains inflammatory cells.

Turnaround time of the smear report

The genuine stat tests in microbiology that require prompt reporting are the smear examination and those tests that require a very short time to demonstrate the presence of an antigen. A rapid, presumptive, etiologic diagnosis in life-threatening infections is critical. A survey of over 400 clinical laboratories, conducted as part of a quality-assurance program, showed that the median turnaround time for processing, examining, and reporting cerebrospinal fluid (CSF) Gram's smears was 45 minutes. The target turnaround time that laboratories established for this procedure was set at <60 minutes for 45% of all responders, 60 minutes for 47%, and >60 minutes for 8%. The survey demonstrated that these goals were met, on average, 62% of the time, and 15.3% of the laboratories met the goal 100% of the time. Another important quality assurance goal is making sure that, in serious infections, smear results are properly reported, interpreted, and utilized. Although microbiologists may not be accustomed to pursuing this objective, a plausible monitor would involve checking for an appropriate clinical response to the report. For example, reporting "pleomorphic gram-negative rods and numerous inflammatory white blood cells" in a CSF specimen would invoke a procedure to verify that the patient is receiving appropriate therapy.

Preparation of the primary culture

Guidelines for preparing primary cultures are based on the specimen source. Instructions should specify media and incubation requirements. Streaking agar plates should be standardized to include the number of times the loop is struck back into the primary inoculum. To some extent, this improves the reproducibility of quantitative interpretations and is monitored simply by examining primary culture plates for adequate numbers of well-isolated colonies.

The accuracy of delivering specific urine sample volumes with a calibrated loop is affected by the angle at which the tip is withdrawn from a urine sample, as well as the diameter of the container being sampled. It is important that these variables be standardized since error rates may approach 100%.

Evaluation and reporting of culture results

A worksheet is used to document all smear and culture observations, and test results. Culture plates should be retained for at least 2 to 3 days in the event that reexamination is necessary after the final report. This can happen when there is a concern that results are erroneous or when additional assessments are needed. Likewise, it is worthwhile to save isolates from appropriately identified specimens since they may occasionally be needed for further testing in an epidemiologic investigation. Most bacteria can be stored for prolonged periods in bovine serum at −40° C, or in tightly stoppered tubes of sterile, distilled water at room temperature.

Quality assurance of the final report

Decisions about what to report depend on the specimen source, clinical relevance, primary smear, identification, and number(s) of colony(s), and sometimes on direct communication with the physician. Tests performed to produce the final result may be reliable but of questionable quality if the report's significance is misunderstood. Making decisions about the extent of work to perform on specimens obtained from nonsterile sites that yield mixed flora of un-

Table 38-2 Common predictable susceptibility patterns

Susceptibility result	Organism
Ampicillin susceptible	*Proteus mirabilis* (tetracycline resistant)
	E. coli (tetracycline susceptible)
Ampicillin and carbenicillin resistant	*Klebsiella* spp,
	Citrobacter diversus
Ampicillin and cephalothin resistant	*Enterobacter* spp
	Citrobacter freundii
	Serratia spp
Ampicillin, cephalothin, and tetracycline resistant	*Providencia* spp
	Proteus vulgaris
	Morganella morganii

Table 38-3 Example of classification scheme for evaluating errors made in the final report

Category A error	The primary provider has responded to the result by ordering the next test, repeating the test, changing treatment or diagnosis.
Category B error	A serious error, but unlikely to affect patient care; similar to category A error, but primary care provider has not yet been notified or acted on the reported erroneous error.
Category C error	Minor clerical error in reporting and "cosmetic" corrections to report.

determined significance present a challenge, since in many cases the results provide no useful information. Complete testing and antibiotic susceptibility testing of all isolates are unnecessary, misleading, and inefficient. It is counterproductive and misleading to identify and report every isolate detected in mixed cultures from specimens originating from nonsterile sites. For example, reporting all organisms detected in an expectorated sputum specimen that is known to be contaminated with upper respiratory flora can be misinterpreted and is not appropriate. In this circumstance it is better to report predominate growth, or simply indicate the presence of mixed flora. Similarly, decisions about performing susceptibility tests on isolates from mixed cultures should be given careful consideration since susceptibility testing of all isolates is wasteful and may result in unnecessary or incorrect antibiotic usage. The information gained from the examination of the primary smear and clinical circumstance helps in the evaluation of specimens with mixed flora.

Daily review of final reports is an important quality control procedure. Direct microscopic examinations should be compared with culture results. Poor correlation between smear and culture results occur from inaccurate readings, poor technique, unsatisfactory media, inappropriate growth conditions, or the presence of dead organisms. The smear, culture, and worksheet should be reviewed when discrepancies are detected. Results should also correlate with specimen source. For example, *Enterococcus* spp. are generally not recovered from sputum specimens, whereas *Streptococcus pneumoniae* is not an expected urinary tract pathogen. Susceptibility results should be consistent with the organism's identification (Table 38-2). Any inconsistencies may indicate errors in either test and should be investigated before the final report is issued.

When an error is detected after the final report goes out, a second revised report should contain the corrected results and should indicate that the initial results were erroneous. An ongoing system should be in place to actively search for errors in reported results. This can be done by retrospective comparison of results on worksheets, instrument logs, and the like, with results reported on the chart. The clinical significance of errors discovered after the report is available for patient care should be classified and periodically reviewed to determine if modifications in procedures or policies are needed (Table 38-3).

QUALITY CONTROL OF MATERIALS AND PROCEDURES

Accurate and reproducible results are obtained when tests are performed by qualified personnel in a consistent manner with dependable materials. Reaching a final result generally involves numerous procedural steps and the interpretation of many pieces of information. While this creates a challenge to ensure that all materials are under quality control, it also provides an opportunity to evaluate the consistency and interrelationships of method results. A single unexpected or inappropriate finding may identify a problem without necessarily producing an inaccurate result. Thus, each microbiologic study provides its own internal quality control checks to identify procedural errors and material defects.

Reagents and stains

Reagents must be dated when received and when first used. Expiration dates and storage requirements must be indicated on all reagent containers. A standardized label and log helps ensure consistency (Fig. 38-2).

The in use performance of reagents and stains is evaluated by demonstrating appropriate reactivity by stock control organisms. There is generally a wide tolerance for errors since most reactions are interpreted as positive or negative. Furthermore, a single discrepancy may not affect the accuracy of a final result since bacterial identifications are usually determined by multiple tests with variable reactivities. Errors are detected when a reagent does not show an expected reaction when compared to other test results. For example, a reagent defect is suggested when an isolate that is clearly an *Escherichia* also yields a negative indole reaction.

Regulatory and accreditation agencies specify how the performance of certain reagents and stains are to be evaluated. However, these expectations have been challenged as excessive and inefficient because there is inconsistency between checklists. Requirements often fail to consider the wide variability in performance between materials, and checklists do not always conform with published, state-of-the-art consensus recommendations. The frequency and methods for monitoring reagent reliability should depend on their performance characteristics, manufacturers' recommendations, frequency of use, and user's experience. As a general rule, reagent performance is evaluated when first prepared or whenever a new lot is placed in service. The need for additional monitoring can be determined by assessing the frequency of deficiencies found with regular use. Reagents that demonstrate a potential to fail or are seldom

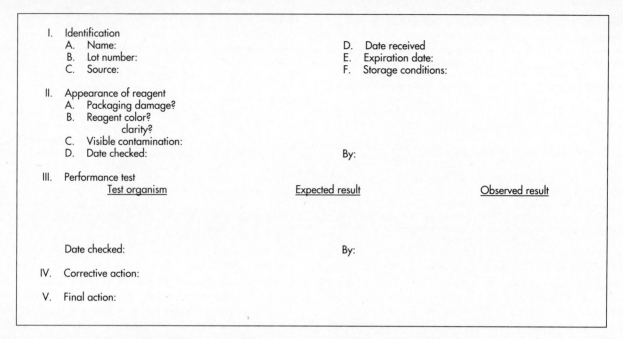

I. Identification
   A. Name:
   B. Lot number:
   C. Source:

   D. Date received
   E. Expiration date:
   F. Storage conditions:

II. Appearance of reagent
   A. Packaging damage?
   B. Reagent color?
          clarity?
   C. Visible contamination:
   D. Date checked: By:

III. Performance test
          Test organism   Expected result   Observed result

     Date checked: By:

IV. Corrective action:

V. Final action:

Fig. 38-2 Quality control worksheet for commercial reagents.

employed should be monitored with each use. Likewise, reagents that prove to always perform as expected can be evaluated with less intensity. Interpretation of reagent performance by review of quality control documentation provides a rationale for accepting or modifying procedures and helps demonstrate compliance with regulatory agency expectations.

Media

All media must be labeled with lot number, preparation date, expiration date, and constituents or medium name. A medium should be marked with the date when first placed into service and stored according to the manufacturer's recommendations. The performance of each new lot or shipment of each medium must be evaluated before it is used. This includes visual inspection, sterility checks, and checks of performance characteristics. Gross inspection should check for proper clarity and color. Turbidity suggests the presence of a precipitate and the medium should be used only if turbidity disappears after incubation. A change in color between lots may indicate improper pH or the presence of other constituents (e.g., concentration of red blood cells). The surface of all plated media should be smooth and flat, and should not contain excessive moisture or cracks. A pitted or cracked medium suggests improper preparation or storage conditions.

Culture media must be tested for contamination before being placed into service by incubating a proportion of each new lot overnight. It is recommended that 5% of small batches (<100) and 10 samples from large lots be tested. Inhibitory media that may not show contamination by this method can be tested by incubating a sample from each new batch in sterile broth. Appropriate stock control organisms are employed to check for expected positive and negative reactions and growth requirements. A light, standardized inoculum should be used (1:10 dilution of a McFarland 0.5

standard bacterial suspension with a 0.001-ml calibrated loop) and provides semi-quantitative results that can be employed to evaluate between-lot performance. Examples of expected growth patterns and reactions to control organisms are shown in Table 38-4.

Deficiencies may also be detected during routine processing. For example, sheep blood agar may support the growth and show expected hemolytic reactions for *Streptococcus pneumoniae* and *Streptococcus pyogenes* in control tests, but fail to produce an accurate CAMP (Christie, Atkins, Munch-Petersen) test. This type of problem will only be identified if a high index of suspicion is maintained, and if performance of all media is continuously cross-checked with expected culture and identification findings.

Many types of commercially available media are consistently reliable because extensive quality control testing is performed before distribution, and it has been shown that reevaluation in the clinical laboratory is unnecessary. Regulatory agencies accept a recent National Committee for Clinical Laboratory Standards (NCCLS) consensus recommendation that certain types of bacterial and fungal media do not require intensive monitoring if sterility (<5% contamination) and performance has been checked and documented by the manufacturer (Table 38-5).

Antisera and antigens

Monitoring the performance of serologic tests with positive and negative controls is similar to quality control practices described for other reagents. However, these materials tend to be more labile and susceptible to contamination. Exposure to room temperature for prolonged periods should be avoided. Antisera should be grossly inspected before tests are performed, and contamination should be suspected when a clear solution becomes turbid. It is generally necessary for antisera to be monitored each time a test is performed. Controls not only ensure proper reactivity, but also aid in

Table 38-4 Examples of performance standards for media*

Medium	Test organisms†	Incubation conditions	Expected results
TRANSPORT MEDIA			
Culturette^R swab	*Haemophilus influenzae* 10211	Pick one colony on swab. Re-insert swab into tube and crush vial. Hold tube at room temperature for 24 hr. Use swab to inoculate chocolate agar. Incubate plate at 35° C in CO_2 for 24 hr.	Good growth
	Streptococcus pneumoniae 6305	Pick one colony on swab. Re-insert swab into tube and crush vial. Hold tube at room temperature for 24 hr. Use swab to inoculate sheep blood agar. Incubate plate at 35° C aerobically for 24 hr.	Good growth
GROWTH AND SELECTIVE/DIFFERENTIAL MEDIA			
Sheep blood agar	*Streptococcus pyogenes* 19615	Incubate at 35° C aerobically or in CO_2 for 24 hr	Good growth, beta hemolysis
	Staphylococcus aureus 25923		Good growth
	Streptococcus pneumoniae 6305		Good growth, alpha hemolysis
	Escherichia coli 25922		Good growth, beta hemolysis
MacConkey agar	*Escherichia coli* 25922	Incubate aerobically for 24 hr	Good growth, rose-red colonies
	Proteus mirabilis 12453		Good growth, colorless colonies, inhibition of swarming
	Salmonella typhimurium 14028		Good growth, colorless colonies
	Enterococcus faecalis 29212		Inhibition, partial
BIOCHEMICAL DIFFERENTIAL MEDIA‡			
Triple sugar iron agar (TSI)	*Salmonella typhimurium*	Incubate at 35° C aerobically for 24 hr	Alkaline slant, acid butt, with gas, H_2S positive
	Shigella flexneri		Alkaline slant, acid butt
	Pseudomonas aeruginosa		Alkaline slant, no change in butt
	Escherichia coli		Acid slant, acid butt, with gas

*Full listing of performance standards may be found in NCCLS, 1987; Schifman, 1987; Weissfeld, 1987.
†Number is American Type Culture Collection identification.
‡Standardized reference strains have not been established.

Table 38-5 Commercially prepared, ready-to-use media that do not require retesting*

Solid media	Liquid media
Blood, aerobic and anaerobic	Thioglycolate
MacConkey	Tryptic digest casein soy
Eosin-methylene blue	Gram-negative
Colistin-nalidixic acid (aerobic)	Enterococcus, selective
Löwenstein-Jensen	Thiol
Phenylethyl alcohol (aerobic)	Brain-heart infusion
Hektoen enteric	Selenite
Sabouraud dextrose	
Xylose-lysine-deoxycholate	
Mannitol salt	
Middlebrook 7H10	
Mycology, selective	
Salmonella-Shigella	

*Retesting not required if manufacturers can document reliability by meeting NCCLS performance criteria.

the interpretation of reactions. Before a new lot is placed into service, its performance should be tested in parallel with the expiring lot to check for between-test consistency.

QUALITY CONTROL OF ANTIMICROBIAL SUSCEPTIBILITY TESTS

In the late 1950s, the Food and Drug Administration (FDA) began to monitor and regulate the production of antibiotic-containing disks utilized for susceptibility testing. In the early 1970s, progress was made in standardizing susceptibility test procedures, and since 1975, the National Committee for Clinical Laboratory Standards has published a series of ongoing standards for the performance, surveillance, and interpretation of broth dilution and agar diffusion procedures.

The quality control of antimicrobial susceptibility tests consists of monitoring the precision and accuracy of results, performance of materials, and execution of manual and automated procedures. Monitoring is done by testing genetically stable reference strains with the same materials and procedures that are employed for routine testing. While this practice eliminates the need to evaluate each component of the assay separately, it has the potential to fail if two deficiencies occur that simultaneously cancel each other and provide apparently accurate results (e.g., light inoculum tested against low potency antibiotic disks). Furthermore, this method is not as effective for testing the performance of broth dilution methods.

Quality assurance of susceptibility testing should extend beyond the limits of methodological performance. Susceptibility test results may have a profound impact on therapy and ultimately, patient outcome. Procedures for ensuring that susceptibility test results are reported in a timely fashion and are appropriately utilized are important considerations.

Selection of antibiotics and method of reporting

A decision to perform susceptibility tests should be based on the clinical relevance of culture findings. Testing is usually unnecessary for organisms that have predictable susceptibility patterns (e.g., *Streptococcus pyogenes* against penicillin G). In some cases one test result will influence the interpretation of another. Methicillin-resistant *Staphylococcus* spp. may show false susceptibility to cephalothin and should always be considered as resistant to this antibiotic. Tests for certain antibiotic-organism combinations are unreliable with routine methods (e.g., erythromycin/ *Haemophilus influenzae*, *Enterococcus* spp./cephalosporin), or do not reliably predict clinical outcome (e.g., cephamandole susceptibility in *H. influenzae* meningitis). The choice of antibiotics to test depends on the bacterial isolate and culture site. Recommendations for selecting the proper antibiotic-organism combination are published by the National Committee for Clinical Laboratory Standards (Villanova, PA 19085), but the final decision should be made after consultation with the pharmacy, medical staff, infectious disease specialists, and the published literature.

Routine susceptibility tests should only be performed on rapidly growing aerobic organisms. Methods for testing slow-growing, fastidious organisms with the exception of *Haemophilus influenzae*, *Neisseria gonorrhoeae*, *Branhamella* spp, and *Streptococcus pneumoniae* are not standardized and may yield invalid results. In these cases therapy is guided by expected results based on published studies from reference laboratories.

The laboratory should record and tabulate cumulative hospital susceptibility patterns and make this information available to the medical staff. This aids in the empiric selection of antibiotics, formulary development by the pharmacy, and trend analysis of endemic resistance by infection control practitioners. Use of this information may be improved by participating in programs that provide interinstitutional statistical comparisons of cumulative susceptibility data (Table 38-6).

Control strains

Quality control reference organisms must be available to monitor the precision and accuracy of susceptibility tests. They may be stored for long periods at −40°C in 50% calf serum. Tests should be performed from fresh subcultures that have been incubated for at least 18 hours. Subcultures should be checked for contamination and good growth before use. Tests performed directly from stored stock cultures may produce unreliable results.

Escherichia coli ATCC 25922, *Staphylococcus aureus* ATCC 25923, *Pseudomonas aeruginosa* ATCC 27853, and *N. gonorrhoeae* ATCC 49226 are recommended for use in test monitoring. *Staphylococcus aureus* ATCC 29213 is a weak β-lactamase producer that is specifically recommended for broth dilution assays. *Pseudomonas aeruginosa* ATCC 27853 may spontaneously develop resistance to carbenicillin when repeatedly subcultured. A new subculture should be prepared from stock cultures when this occurs. High levels of thymidine in Mueller-Hinton medium that may adversely affect trimethoprim-sulfamethoxazole susceptibility testing can be detected by *Enterococcus faecalis* ATCC 29212 or 33186. β-Lactamase producing *E. coli* ATCC 35218 has been selected to test the performance of disks with a combination of β-lactam antibiotic and β-lactamase inhibitor (e.g., augmentin). Additional control organisms may be selected by individual laboratories for spe-

Table 38-6 College of American Pathologists Interhospital Antimicrobial Susceptibility Program, susceptibility report for *Escherichia coli*

Antibiotic/methodology	Six-month time period	Your hospital		All teaching hospitals				
		Percent susceptible	Number tested	Percent susceptible	Number tested	Number of hospitals	Your percentile	Central 90th percentile range
Amikacin	Jul-Dec 1986	98.0	277	99.3	2,601	5	16	98.0-100.0
	Jan-Jun 1987	98.0	240	99.6	2,738	5	16	98.0-100.0
Inpatients and outpatients	Jul-Dec 1987	99.0	292	99.6	3,791	7	37	97.0-100.0
Urine & non-urine sources	Jan-Jun 1988	97.0	207	99.4	6,301	9	10	97.0-100.0
Abbott MS-2	Jul-Dec 1988	98.0	232	99.1	7,690	12	12	98.0-100.0
Usage level: LOW	Jan-Jun 1989	100.0	190	99.5	6,836	11	79	98.9-100.0
Formulary antibiotic: NO								
	Jan-Jun 1989	ALL HOSPITALS		99.5	12,603	28	72	96.1-100.0
Ampicillin	Jul-Dec 1986	67.0	277	70.3	2,601	5	33	36.9- 84.0
	Jan-Jun 1987	68.0	240	66.0	2,535	6	42	18.0- 72.2
Inpatients and outpatients	Jul-Dec 1987	67.0	292	70.1	4,334	9	40	34.0- 76.0
Urine & non-urine sources	Jan-Jun 1988	70.0	207	70.1	7,238	11	37	57.0- 78.0
Abbott MS-2	Jul-Dec 1988	73.0	232	69.0	10,246	14	66	52.8- 83.0
Usage level: HIGH	Jan-Jun 1989	62.0	190	67.0	9,110	13	28	49.4- 79.0
Formulary antibiotic: YES								
	Jan-Jun 1989	ALL HOSPITALS		69.9	17,652	37	15	54.7- 80.0

cific purposes. For example, methicillin resistance in some strains of *Staphylococcus aureus* may be difficult to detect by standard and automated methods. Laboratories that encounter these strains may wish to periodically test a well-characterized strain of methicillin-resistant *S. aureus* as part of routine quality control activities.

Antibiotics

Prior to the standardization of antimicrobial susceptibility methods, commercially prepared antibiotic disks were not uniform and many had unsatisfactory potency. This prompted the Food and Drug Administration at one time to require batch certification and standardization of all lots of disks and specified control limits between 67% and 150% of labeled activity. This has improved the accuracy of diffusion susceptibility tests but does not ensure reliability under routine laboratory conditions. Substantial variability may occur from inactivation during transport and normal use. β-Lactam antibiotics are especially labile in the presence of excess humidity and high temperatures. Antibiotic disks must be periodically evaluated. This is done by monitoring zone diameters produced by reference strains that indicate antibiotic potency. Recommended control limits are established for these strains from collaborative studies, but tend to be wider than what is generally achieved with interlaboratory monitoring. In fact, it has been shown that 91% of disks with marginal potency (67% of labeled activity) pass recommended control limits. This underscores the need for each laboratory to determine its own working control mean and precision limits by repeated testing of control strains. A precision control value for disk diffusion tests is calculated from the five previous susceptibility determinations performed on reference strains. A maximum range of allowable values, as well as cumulative mean zone diameters, are used to monitor intra-assay precision (Table 38-7). A single value that significantly deviates below the control range suggests deterioration of antibiotic, and the batch of disks should be discarded. Values that are consistently above or below the control means suggest a deficiency in inoculum preparation or inoculation technique. A deteriorating lot of antibiotic disks may be detected by a trend toward declining control zone diameters. Control values that deviate in opposite directions when testing aminoglycosides and tetracycline suggest unsatisfactory medium pH.

Acceptable limits for precision may also be considered as method reproducibility that will yield the least tolerable interpretive error. That is, the consistency of disk diffusion results should be sufficient to minimize false-susceptible and false-resistant interpretations to 1% or less of all results. This theoretical precision limit can be determined for each antibiotic-organism combination by the formula:

$$\text{Standard deviation (SD)} = S_{min} - R_{max}/2.33$$

where:

SD = maximum allowable limit to minimize interpretive errors
S_{min} = Smallest zone size interpreted as susceptible
R_{max} = Largest zone size interpreted as resistant
2.33 = SD that includes 98% of expected determinations

Quality control limits for broth dilution procedures are also established for control reference strains. However, these tests are often not configured to contain appropriate dilution schemes to properly check accuracy and precision because the lowest dilution is higher than the minimum inhibitory concentration of the reference strain. A similar problem is encountered with certain types of automated methods that use disk elution techniques. Reference strains produce scant turbidity that is measured at the extreme of the instrument's interpretive scale, making it difficult to detect significant deterioration of antibiotic by monitoring with control organisms. In this case, antibiotic activity can be monitored by periodically testing disks with a standard agar diffusion method. Achievable precision with this procedure is about ±3 mm.

Expected precision for broth dilution tests is plus or minus one twofold dilution from the modal minimum inhibitory concentration (MIC) level. The precision of automated and commercially prepared broth dilution methods tends to be better than the reference broth dilution assay. Because broth dilution control ranges may vary between commercial methods, control limits determined from reference methods

Table 38-7 Control limits for monitoring antimicrobial disk susceptibility tests*

| Antibiotic (disk content) | E. coli ATCC 25992 | | S. aureus ATCC 25923 | |
	Zone diameter limits (mm)†	Maximum zone diameter range (mm)†	Zone diameter limits (mm)	Maximum zone diameter range (mm)
Amikacin (30 μg)	19-26	6	20-26	6
Cefazolin (30 μg)	23-29	8	29-35	8
Chloramphenicol (30 μg)	21-27	10	19-26	10
Trimethoprim/sulfamethoxazole (1.25/23.75 μg)	24-32	10	24-32	10

*Partial list, see NCCLs, ed 4, 1990.
†Daily quality control. Corrective action is required when; (1) more than 1 of 20 consecutive tests exceed zone diameter limits, (2) any single value is above or below 4 SD (i.e., midpoint ±maximum minus minimum zone diameter limits), or (3) any consecutive series of 5 tests exceed the allowable zone diameter range (largest minus smallest zone diameter).
Weekly quality control. To perform weekly quality control; (1) no more than three consecutive tests must be outside zone diameter limits during 30 test periods, (2) none should exceed 4 SD, and (3) none in each group of six zone diameter ranges (of 30 performed) should exceed allowable maximum range. When these conditions are satisfied, quality control can be performed weekly until a test fails by exceeding allowable zone diameter limits. When a deficiency is detected, weekly quality control may continue after five consecutive tests of the organism/antibiotic combination that failed show no value beyond the allowable zone diameter limits and the range of the five tests is within the maximum zone diameter range.

may not conform when commercial and automated dilution assays are monitored.

Inoculum

The preparation of standardized inoculum is a critical component of susceptibility methods and must be done precisely. Inoculum is prepared by adjusting the turbidity of a bacterial suspension to a McFarland 0.5 standard that has been vigorously shaken before use. The McFarland 0.5 turbidity standard—equal to about 2×10^8 CFU/ml—is prepared by adding 0.5 ml of 0.048 M $BaCl_2$ to 99.5 ml of 0.18 N H_2SO_4. After preparation, the accuracy of the standard should be verified by testing with a spectrophotometer (McFarland 0.5 standard optical density for a 1-cm light path at 625 nm should be between 0.08 to 0.10). The standard is generally stable for 6 months when tightly sealed and stored at room temperature in a dark container.

Bacterial suspensions should be made with the aid of a lightbox or photometer. Inoculum preparation without comparison to a turbidity standard is discouraged. The accuracy of inoculum preparation techniques should periodically be determined by performing quantitative colony counts from standardized inocula. Accurate susceptibility results can be obtained with inoculum in either stationary or log phase growth.

Broth dilution tests must include a growth control (inoculation of broth media without antibiotics) used to determine inoculum viability and as a control to interpret endpoints. The inoculum for broth dilution and automated susceptibility tests should also be tested for purity by making a subculture from the bacterial suspension and observing for pure growth after overnight incubation.

Media

Mueller-Hinton medium is recommended for susceptibility testing of aerobic organisms. Control limits and interpretive criteria have not been validated for alternative media. Mueller-Hinton medium is not uniform from batch to batch and changes in composition have the potential to adversely affect results. Three major constituents have been identified that influence the test: cation concentration, pH, and thymidine concentration. These factors must be carefully monitored and adjusted when necessary to obtain satisfactory results.

Mueller-Hinton medium must have adequate levels of magnesium (25 mg/L) and calcium (50 mg/L) to reliably detect aminoglycoside resistance in some strains of *Pseudomonas aeruginosa*. Deficient quantities of these cations most commonly occur with broth medium. Cation deficiencies are not identified by testing the reference *P. aeruginosa* strain because this organism is susceptible to aminoglycosides. The calcium and magnesium concentration of each batch of Mueller-Hinton medium should be specified by the manufacturer or determined in the laboratory. Alternatively, a control strain of *P. aeruginosa* with a moderately resistant MIC (8 to 16 μg/ml) may be tested with each new lot of medium. A cation deficiency should be suspected if this organism fails to demonstrate aminoglycoside resistance. Amikacin is less sensitive to the effects of cation deficiencies. A cation deficiency should be suspected when amikacin is tested in conjunction with other aminoglycosides and shows resistance while the others show susceptibility.

The pH of Mueller-Hinton medium should range between 7.2 and 7.4. This should be documented by the manufacturer or measured in the laboratory. Media pH can be determined with a surface pH electrode or a standard pH electrode placed into mashed agar pieces. When preparing Mueller-Hinton agar medium, the pH can be measured by allowing media to solidify around a pH electrode. Susceptibility results are affected by media pH. The activity of penicillin, aminoglycosides, and erythromycin is decreased and tetracycline is increased when tested with a low pH medium. Unsatisfactory pH may be suspected when mean zone diameters of control organisms tested against tetracycline and gentamycin deviate in opposite directions.

The thymidine concentration in Mueller-Hinton medium affects susceptibility tests with trimethoprim and sulfa antibiotics. Excess thymidine and thymine levels may produce false-resistant results. A decreased zone diameter and inner colonies, or increased MIC observed when testing *Enterococcus faecalis* ATCC 29212 against trimethoprim-sulfamethoxazole suggests an inappropriately high level of thymidine.

Performance and interpretation

Unsatisfactory technical performance is the most common source of error associated with susceptibility testing. In one study, 3.9% of diffusion susceptibility results performed with control strains were inaccurate. In nearly all cases, errors were linked with performance failures, whereas material deficiencies were detected in only 0.06% of all control tests. Technical problems included unsatisfactory inoculum (most common), improperly placed disks, and rarely, misreading of zone diameters. Errors may also occur when tests are correctly performed but results are misinterpreted or inaccurately reported. This problem is well illustrated by an interlaboratory proficiency survey conducted to assess the accuracy of detecting a strain of penicillin-resistant *Streptococcus pneumoniae*. Nearly all participants accurately performed the test, but less than 15% reported a correct result because proper criteria for interpreting the result were not applied.

Errors may also occur when methods are not standardized or controlled. For example, in vitro susceptibility testing has demonstrated that some strains of *Staphylococcus aureus* are killed only with penicillin or methicillin concentrations that are significantly higher than inhibitory levels of these antibiotics. This phenomenon, referred to as tolerance, has been implicated as a cause for treatment failures in patients with serious infections. However, the significance of this finding has been seriously questioned because the performance and interpretation of bacteriocidal assays are not standardized and results can be markedly affected by uncontrolled variables such as growth phase, mode of inoculation, and antibiotic carryover.

Frequency of quality control testing

Guidelines for diffusion susceptibility testing include daily quality control of reference strains. However, it is apparent that many laboratories can achieve acceptable results with less frequent testing. Weekly quality control testing is acceptable if a laboratory can document adequate daily performance for 30 days. This is accomplished by observing no more than three out of control values for each antibiotic during this time period. Daily quality control testing must resume when weekly surveillance demonstrates an accuracy control problem, and should continue until the problem is identified and corrected. While this approach appears to be more efficient than daily checks, it may be unrealistic for testing multiple antibiotics. It becomes impractical to isolate one antibiotic from all the others for daily quality control checking since disks are generally dispensed as a group on to plated medium, and when testing many different antibiotics, there is a high likelihood of relative frequent quality control problems. For these reasons, some laboratories find it convenient to perform daily quality control. Nevertheless, reference strains should always be tested with all new lots of medium and antibiotics. Daily quality control of reference strains is recommended for broth dilution and automated methods.

Quality assurance of utilizing the susceptibility test result

One of the key ingredients for improving susceptibility test reporting is knowledge of the patient's current antibiotic therapy. After all, the patient's culture and susceptibility test results are first available to the microbiologist. Laboratory staff are therefore placed in an ideal position for initially correlating this information with the patient's antimicrobial therapy. For example, one study demonstrated that the mean interval between completing a susceptibility test and acting on the results could be reduced from 26 hours to 2.4 hours when knowledge of the patient's antibiotic therapy was used for reporting results to the physician.

Unfortunately, many laboratories report susceptibility results without any appreciation of their significance within the context of the patient's therapy. As laboratory and hospital computer systems become more sophisticated, methods for correlating pharmacy and laboratory data will likely become available. Linking these data, in combination with procedures for swift intervention when potentially inappropriate treatment is identified, promises to be an important future, outcome-related quality assurance activity.

REFERENCE LABORATORY

A referral clinical laboratory is a valuable resource for checking the accuracy of results and is essential for providing assistance when difficult culture, identification, susceptibility, or serologic problems are encountered. This is particularly important if an unusual result is obtained or a test is infrequently performed. Confirmation of results provides confidence in the regular laboratory's procedures and materials. New findings or discrepancies serve to resolve potential problems and enhance the education and experience of laboratory personnel.

EXTERNAL QUALITY ASSURANCE PROGRAMS
Proficiency testing

An important component of quality control in the clinical microbiology laboratory is the processing of unknown specimens with defined constituents. Results obtained from these specimens are compared with expected results to evaluate the quality of laboratory performance. Internal proficiency testing is conducted by processing test specimens that are disguised as routine samples. This exercise provides the advantage of evaluating all procedures and materials that are routinely employed to process specimens (i.e., transport, smear, culture, timeliness of reporting). More commonly, external proficiency testing is conducted by outside laboratories and agencies to evaluate interlaboratory performance. One of the largest clinical microbiology proficiency surveys that evaluates identification and susceptibility procedures is conducted by the College of American Pathologists (CAP). This program has important benefits in assessing the performance of specific methods. These include: identification of individual laboratory deficiencies, detection of inadequate or improved methods, continuing education, and standardization of methods and materials. External proficiency challenges have demonstrated that most laboratories can achieve acceptable results with standardized disk diffusion methods. Q-Probes is another CAP program, oriented toward interlaboratory assessment of other quality assurance standards.

QUALITY CONTROL OF EQUIPMENT AND THE ENVIRONMENT

The performance of laboratory equipment must be properly monitored to identify problems that will affect test results. This should include written instructions for preventive maintenance, performance checks, and calibration procedures. All maintenance and performance activities, as well as equipment failures and repairs, must be documented and periodically reviewed. Suggested performance monitoring schedules for general laboratory equipment and tolerance limits for common laboratory equipment are published elsewhere (See August, 1990 Suggested Reading).

Temperature-sensitive equipment must be constantly monitored, preferably with a recording thermometer that can identify unacceptable drifts in temperature. An alarm system can be employed for critical control when it is necessary to have prompt recognition of temperatures that exceed tolerance limits. This is important for some tests that can be severely affected by improper incubation temperatures. Thermometers employed to monitor temperatures above freezing should be placed in water. Incubators with added CO_2 should be tested daily for CO_2 content with an indicator such as Fyrite. Environmental chambers should be tested for proper atmospheric conditions with chemical indicators (e.g., methylene blue for anaerobic conditions) or control strains (e.g., *Campylobacter jejuni* for microaerophilic conditions). The performance of autoclaves should be periodically checked with spore strips or spore solutions. Temperatures should be recorded with each use. Autoclave times should be established and monitored for assuring total decontamination of waste materials in a fully loaded chamber. Autoclaves should have attached recording thermometers that operate with each run.

The accuracy of calibrated loops and pipettes should be periodically inspected. Centrifuges should be checked at least once a year for proper speed (with tachometer), calibration, and braking. This should also include inspection of brushes and bearings. Microscopes should be kept clean and periodically adjusted and lubricated. Ocular micrometers must be calibrated for each microscope. Dustcovers should be used when microscopes are not in service.

Biologic safety cabinets should be inspected for the proper amount and pattern of air flow. Smoke sticks can be employed to determine the pattern of air flow. A paper strip attached to the cabinet opening will ensure that the air stream is maintained and flowing in the proper direction. A schedule should be followed for replacing HEPA filters. Safety cabinets should be decontaminated before filters are removed. Ultraviolet (UV) lights should be periodically checked for light intensity with a UV light meter. It is recommended that a UV lamp be replaced when light intensity drops below 70% of initial readings.

The laboratory environment must be kept clean and well ventilated. A minimum of at least 100 square feet should be available per full time employee (FTE). Incandescent lighting should be used, when possible, for reading culture plates and tubes. Cultures should be processed in one area to avoid the potential hazard of transporting potentially harmful pathogens. Policies for handling infectious and hazardous waste should be developed. See Chapter 2.

SUGGESTED READING

August MJ and others: Cumitech 3A, Quality control and quality assurance practices in clinical microbiology. AS Weissfeld, coordinating editor, Washington, DC, 1990, American Society for Microbiology.

Bachner P: Quality assurance: an accreditation perspective, Lab Med 20:159–162, 1989.

Bartlett RC: Making optimal use of the microbiology laboratory. I. Use of the laboratory. II. Urine, respiratory, wound and cervicovaginal exudate. III. Aids of antimicrobial therapy, JAMA 247:857, 1982.

Bartlett RC: Cost effective quality control in microbiology, Clin Microbiol Newsletter 7:3, 1985.

Bartlett RC, Rutz CA, and Knopacki N: Cost effectiveness of quality control in bacteriology, Am J Clin Path 77:184, 1982.

Berwick DM: Continuous improvement as an ideal in health care, N Engl J Med 320:53, 1989.

Biosafety in microbiological and biomedical laboratories, US Dept of Health and Human Services document NIH 88-8395, Washington, DC, 1988, US Government Printing Office.

Fuchs PC: Microbiology proficiency testing in the care of patients. In Lorian V, editor: Significance of medical microbiology in the care of patients, ed 2, Baltimore, 1982, Williams & Wilkins.

Howanitz PJ and Steindel SJ: Intralaboratory performance and laboratorians' expectations for stat turnaround times. A College of American Pathologists Q-Probes study of four cerebrospinal fluid determinations. Arch Pathol Lab Med 1991;115:977-983.

Hyams KC: Inappropriate urine cultures in hospitalized patients receiving antibiotic therapy, Arch Intern Med 147:48, 1987.

Laffel G and Blumenthal D: The case for using industrial quality management science in health care organizations, JAMA 262:2869, 1989.

Lorian V, editor: Antibiotics in laboratory medicine, ed 2, Baltimore, 1986, Williams & Wilkins.

Makadon HJ and others: Febrile inpatients: house officer's use of blood cultures, J Gen Intern Med 2:293, 1987.

National Committee for Clinical Laboratory Standards: Tentative standard, quality assurance for commercially prepared microbiological culture media, Doc M22-T, Villanova, Pa, 1987, NCCLS.

National Committee for Clinical Laboratory Standards: Tentative standard, methods for dilution antimicrobial susceptibility tests for bacteria that grow aerobically, Doc M7-A2, Villanova, Pa, 1990, NCCLS.

National Committee for Clinical Laboratory Standards: Tentative standard, performance standards for antimicrobial disk susceptibility tests, ed 4, Doc M2-A4, Villanova, Pa, 1990, NCCLS.

Schifman RB: Quality assurance in microbiology. In Howanitz P and Howanitz J, editors: Laboratory quality assurance, New York, 1987, McGraw-Hill.

Schifman RB and Bachner, P: Blood culture utilization (Q-Probes) Northfield, Ill, 1990, College of American Pathologists.

Smith JW, editor: The role of clinical microbiology in cost-effective health care, Skokie, Ill, 1984, College of American Pathologists.

Soo Hoo GW, Palmer DL, and Sopher RL. Reducing tuberculosis detection costs, Chest 86:860, 1984.

Tardio JL and Westhoff D: Suitability of the ASM-2 standard test of the National Committee for Clinical Laboratory Standards for evaluation of antimicrobial disk potency, J Clin Microbiol 19:783, 1984.

Taylor PC and others: Determination of minimum bacteriocidal concentrations of oxacillin for Staphylococcus aureus: influence and significance of technical factors, Antimicrob Agents Chemother 23:142, 1983.

Trenholme GM and others: Clinical impact of rapid identification and susceptibility testing of bacterial blood culture isolates, J Clin Microbiol 27:1342, 1989.

Walker K and Howanitz PJ: Reporting error (Q-Probes), Northfield, Ill, 1989, College of American Pathologists.

Von Seggern RL: Culture and antibiotic monitoring service in a community hospital, Am J Hosp Pharm 44:1358, 1987.

Weissfeld AS and Bartlett RC: Quality control. In Howard B: Clinical and pathogenic microbiology, St Louis, 1987, Mosby–Year Book, Inc.

39 Specimen collection, transport, and initial processing*

Richard C. Tilton

GENERAL PRINCIPLES

Certain general principles apply to all specimen collections, no matter what the source. They are as follows:

1. The quality of the microbiological result is only as good as the specimen collected. A poorly collected specimen will often result in an inferior result. While adequate collection does not ensure quality work, it is one less variable with which to be concerned.
2. The specimen must be representative of the area infected, in other words, the causative agents of bacterial pneumonia must be isolated from sputum, not saliva.
3. An adequate amount of specimen must be collected for the analyses requested. If sufficient specimen is not received, then a consultation on test priority must be requested with the ordering clinician.
4. Treatment of the patient with antimicrobial agents must be noted at the time of specimen collection. In some situations, such as blood cultures, antibiotics can be removed with resins.
5. The stage of the disease must be considered as well as the likelihood of a microorganism being present in a particular specimen. *Salmonella typhi* is initially found in the blood of a patient with typhoid fever early in the disease process, but is found in the stool a week later. A search for blood-borne viruses, with a few exceptions, may be an inappropriate use of laboratory resources.
6. Geography and season may be a factor. Respiratory syncytial virus is uncommonly isolated in the summer and *Vibrio cholerae* is rarely isolated in the Midwest or New England states.

The foregoing six principles are based on valid assumptions, but laboratory personnel must be willing to discuss them with the medical staff in light of conflicting clinical information or unusual circumstances.

Common general questions often arise concerning numbers of specimens from the same site and for the same tests to be collected. Repeat daily specimens should be discouraged unless there is a marked change in the clinical course or other such clinical event, such as nonresponsiveness to therapy, to warrant repetitive specimens. Rarely is septicemia diagnosed by collecting more than 4 to 5 pairs of blood cultures over the course of the septic event. On the other hand, blood cultures should be collected in pairs, not in single bottles or vials. Greater than three fecal specimens for either bacteriology or parasitology is contraindicated. Pooled, 24-hour urine, feces, or sputum specimens for microbiological examination should be discouraged and not tested without prior arrangements.

GUIDELINES FOR SPECIMEN TRANSPORT

This section can be summarized by stating that once a clinical specimen is collected, it should be transported to the laboratory for processing as fast as possible under the appropriate environmental conditions. All laboratorians recognize that the organisms present in some specimens survive better than others. In general, however, "fresh is best" is a good rubric.

The simplest and most accessible collection and transport device for specimens best obtained by aspiration is needle and syringe; their use should only be encouraged when appropriate. If a fairly large volume is collected in a syringe (2 ml or more), anaerobic bacteria and most but not all aerobes usually survive for 24 hours at room temperature. Following collection, excess air is carefully expressed and the needle is capped by sticking it into a rubber stopper. The syringe is labeled and delivered to the laboratory as soon as possible.

Adhering to universal precautions and exercising good judgment, syringes and needles must be handled with *extreme* caution. The contents of the syringe must be carefully transferred to an appropriate sterile container and the specimen processed as requested. The syringe and needle must be discarded into an appropriate biosafety container for disinfection and disposal.

Specimens such as sputum or urine require a leakproof sterile container. Many such containers are commercially available, ranging from simple screw-capped cups to more complex devices. They should be obtained from a reputable source.

*Credit is given to the late SJ Rubin, author of the chapter from which this chapter is derived, in Howard BJ, et al: Clinical and pathogenic microbiology, St Louis, 1987, Mosby–Year Book.

Although generally undesirable, many specimens are collected on sterile swabs. Swabs consist of wooden sticks, plastic, or wire rods with cotton, rayon, Dacron, or calcium-alginate tips. Cotton is the least desirable material because it may contain oils that are toxic to some microorganisms. Swabs without a transport medium should not be used be-

cause most bacteria are susceptible to drying and may not survive transport. (A notable exception are throat swabs for beta hemolytic streptococci.) A number of transport media are available including Amies and Stuart transport media for facultative bacteria, and prereduced, anaerobically sterilized (PRAS) carrier media for anaerobic bacteria. A trans-

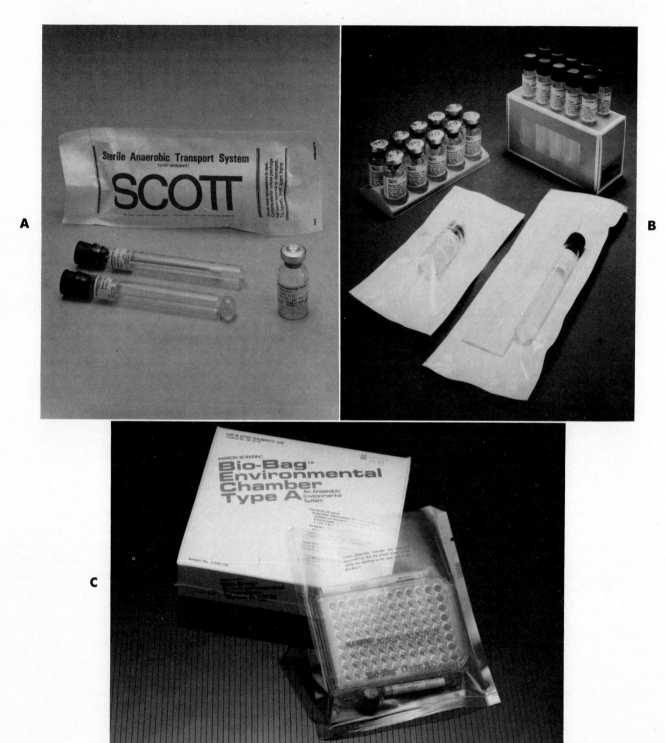

Fig. 39-1   Anaswab system consisting of two rubber-stoppered tubes with oxygen-free CO_2. One tube has swab attached to stopper. *From Rubin SJ: Specimen collection and processing. In Howard BJ and others: Clinical and pathogenic microbiology, St Louis, 1987, Mosby–Year Book, Inc.*

port medium is used to maintain pH, prevent drying, and most important, preserve the different types of organisms in the ratio collected, which is critical when specimens are collected from contaminated sites such as the throat or cervix, or from a mixed infection. Many combined swab-transport medium devices are commercially available, including those designed for preservation of anaerobic bacteria.

Most swab-transport systems for facultative bacteria consist of a sterile, single or double dry swab and a vial of transport medium. The medium is released by breaking the vial or by inserting the swab through a seal.

Several anaerobic transport systems are available: Anaswab (Adams Scientific Co., West Warwick, RI), Porta-Cul and Anaerobic Culturette (BBL Microbiology Systems, Cockeysville, Md.). All provide a reduced oxygen environment for the specimen. Another system is the Bio-Bag (BBL Microbiology Systems). Any specimen container can be placed in this plastic bag, which contains an anaerobic indicator, catalyst, and a H_2-CO_2 generator. The ampule is crushed after the bag is sealed (Figure 39-1).

Specimens should be delivered to the laboratory as soon as possible after collection and certainly within 1 to 2 hours. Ideally, all specimens should be processed immediately; however, this is often not practical or possible. Certain specimens such as urine or sputum may be held overnight in the refrigerator. Many specimens collected on a swab and placed in transport medium can be held several hours at room temperature and at least overnight in the refrigerator. Exceptions are specimens that might contain temperature-sensitive organisms such as *Neisseria* spp. or anaerobic bacteria. These should ideally be processed at once but can be held at room temperature. In fact, in a gassed-out tube with carrier medium, most anaerobic bacteria survive at least 24 hours at room temperature.

Cerebrospinal fluid, other fluids collected by needle aspiration, and specimens obtained in the operating room always should be processed immediately. Essentially, any specimen collected by an invasive procedure should be cultured promptly. They are obtained at considerable cost, discomfort, and possible danger to the patient, and must be handled with care and concern.

Once a specimen arrives in the laboratory, the label and the requisition form are checked to make sure that the same patient information appears on both and that all necessary information is present. The date and time of arrival are noted on the requisition. The following information is needed on the requisition form, specimen label, or both:

> Patient name, sex, age (both)
> Hospital or clinic location, room number (both)
> Provisional diagnosis (requisition form)
> Antimicrobial therapy (requisition form)
> Immune status (requisition form)
> Date and time of collection (requisition form)
> Source (both)
> Examination requested (requisition form)
> Ordering physician (requisition form)

Once the specimen is determined to be properly labeled, the laboratorian has the responsibility then to ascertain its suitability for processing. If the specimen does not fit the guidelines for a suitable specimen, it should be rejected and

Table 39-1 Criteria for rejection of specimens

Criterion	Action
Mislabeled requisition or container	Call nursing station or client; request new specimen, consult clinician if new specimen is unobtainable; do not process until rectified
Unlabeled container	As above; if processed, write "container not labeled" on requisition; do not process until rectified
No source or incorrect source; delay of more than 2 hours in transport	Call nursing station or client; see "Mislabeled requisition" above
Dry swabs	See "Mislabeled requisition"; if processed, write "dry swab unsatisfactory for bacteriologic evaluation" on requisition
Foley catheter tips	Do not process; results unreliable; discuss with clinician
Pooled 24-hour urine, feces, or sputum	Request new specimen; do not process
Improper or unsterile container	See "Mislabeled requisition"; if processed, write "improper container for specimen, may invalidate results"
Nasal secretions for sinusitis	Consult clinician
Sputum with evidence of saliva contamination	See "Mislabeled requisition"
Anaerobic culture request on unacceptable source	Do not process anaerobically; consult clinician

From Rubin SJ: Specimen collection and processing. In Howard BJ and others (editors): Clinical and pathogenic microbiology, St Louis, 1987, Mosby–Year Book, Inc.

the ordering clinician should be notified immediately. Table 39-1 lists some criteria for specimen rejection.

GUIDELINES FOR SPECIMEN PROCESSING

Clinical microbiology requires both solid and liquid (broth) media for growth and isolation. Solid media permit colony isolation, selection or differentiation of potential pathogens from normal flora, and determination of relative numbers of organisms present in a specimen. Broth media allow growth of small numbers of organisms or more fastidious organisms; some are enriched for a particular pathogen.

A nutrient agar base supplemented with 5% blood, most commonly sheep blood, supports growth of most clinical isolates and reveals patterns of bacterial hemolytic activity. More fastidious bacteria, such as *Haemophilus influenzae*, require a chocolatized agar. Blood is heated before being added to the nutrient base to release hemoglobin, or a hemoglobin suspension is added in place of blood. Some pathogenic microorganisms, such as *Legionella pneumophila*, *H. influenzae*, *Neisseria meningitidis*, *Bacteroides* spp. and others, have special growth requirements, and specific media must be inoculated for their isolation.

Clinical microbiologists also include selective and differential media for specimen inoculation. Selective media contain ingredients that inhibit the growth of some organisms but allow others to grow. For example, anaerobic blood agar containing kanamycin and vancomycin inhibits growth of most bacteria except *Bacteroides* spp. Differential media contain compounds such as a sugar and a pH indicator that allow groups of organisms to be separated. Most differential media are also selective. For example, MacConkey agar is selective for many gram-negative rods and differentiates between lactose-fermenting and non–lactose-fermenting bacteria.

Many types of media are commercially available, either completely prepared or in dehydrated form. The number and types used vary from laboratory to laboratory depending on budgets, personnel, and personal preferences. Media selection is governed by the specimen source and the requested tests, which are usually based on a patient's working diagnosis. Media that allow growth of the majority of potential pathogens from a particular source should be included. Some microbiologists advocate using a relatively large number of different selective media, whereas others believe that familiarity with growth patterns on a relatively small number of selective media is better. The choice is made by the microbiology laboratory director and should be properly listed in the procedure manual of each laboratory.

INOCULATION AND ISOLATION TECHNIQUES

Traditional identification methods depend on obtaining isolated colonies. Many clinical specimens contain a mixture of bacteria; therefore, specimens are diluted to produce single colonies of each organism type present. Dilution techniques include streaking with a wire loop, spreading with a glass rod, or inoculating pour plates. The choice depends on the material to be cultured, the result desired, and the laboratory's preference. Everyone in a laboratory should use the same technique.

The streak plate method is practical and fast. All streak plate methods are designed to provide a continuous dilution of the specimen. Either a stainless steel or nickel and chromium (Nichrome) wire, or a plastic bacteriologic loop is acceptable, although Nichrome should not be used for anaerobic bacteria. In the most common method, a portion of the specimen is deposited in one quadrant of an agar plate free of moisture.

Transferring the inoculum to the plate depends on the specimen type. Liquid specimens are usually inoculated by transfer with a sterile pipette or syringe and needle. One or two drops is placed in the first quadrant of the plate. Urine is an exception and must be plated quantitatively.

Specimens received on swabs can be planted directly by rolling the swab over an area about 2 cm in diameter in the first quadrant of the plate. Depending on the nature of the specimen, it may be desirable to then rinse the swab in a tube of suitable broth.

Feces and sputum may be more easily inoculated by dipping a sterile swab into the specimen rather than attempting to use a loop.

After implantation of the inoculum, a wire loop is flamed and cooled, or a sterile plastic disposable loop is selected. The loop is held between the thumb and index finger and passed at a 90° angle several times through the initial inoculum into the second quadrant of the plate. The plate is turned 90°, and the process is repeated, streaking into the third quadrant, and finally, after another 90° turn, into the fourth quadrant. The loop is flamed between quadrants unless the inoculum is light or the medium is selective or inhibitory. When streak plates are used, laboratory personnel can report relative numbers of bacteria present, which may be helpful to the clinician, particularly if different organism types are present.

Several methods of semiquantitation are used. Some laboratories use "very few, few, moderate, or many"; others use "1 + to 4 + ". Sometimes, determining the actual colony count of a specimen is necessary (one colony equals one colony-forming unit, or CFU). For a colony count, the specimen must be in a liquid form. Nonliquid specimens, such as tissue, are weighed, ground, mixed with a known amount of broth, and centrifuged. The supernatant is then treated as a liquid specimen. Three quantitative methods are used: calibrated loop, broth dilution, streak, and pour plates. Precise details may be found in reference texts, and interpretation of quantitative counts will be found in the appropriate chapters of this book.

The choice of media for bacteriology is an individual one and must be carefully thought out in order to be (1) economical, and (2) inclusive of the routinely isolated bacteria. Table 39-2 provides an outline of suggested choices of media for various specimens. It is not dogma nor is it an exhaustive list.

SPECIFIC GUIDELINES FOR SPECIMEN COLLECTION AND PROCESSING
Blood

Because most bacteremias are intermittent (notable exceptions are in endocarditis and endarteritis), blood for culture is collected at various times. After the influx of bacteria into the bloodstream, the patient's temperature may rise, possibly followed by chills. Unfortunately, by the time the temperature is elevated, organisms may already have been cleared from the blood. Generally, blood cultures are collected about an hour apart or at the time of temperature elevation, except when prompt treatment is imperative. Then three sets of blood cultures are collected with a separate needle and syringe for each specimen, alternating arms or other collection sites for venipuncture. The majority of bacteremias is detected with three sets of blood cultures. Rarely are more than five sets needed during a given febrile episode.

Before a blood culture is collected, the skin is decontaminated and blood is obtained by venipuncture. The number of bacteria per milliliter of blood is usually small (1 to 10 CFU/ml), making the volume collected critical. At least 10 ml and preferably 20 ml per culture is collected but no more than 30 ml. Much less blood is required from infants (1 to 5 ml), because the number of organisms per ml is usually $10\times$-$100\times$ more. Blood is inoculated either directly into blood culture broth or into a tube containing the anticoagulant sodium polyanethol sulfonate (SPS) and is rapidly carried to the laboratory for inoculation. Other anticoagulants are inhibitory and should not be used. Conventionally, blood is cultured in a broth or broth-agar combination. Blood-to-medium ratios from 1:5 to 1:30 are acceptable. Lower dilutions may result in bacterial inhibition by serum factors, and higher dilutions prolong detection time.

Table 39-2   Suggested routine culture media*

Source	Microscopic examination	Agar plates	Broth
Blood			EB (CO_2, ANO_2)
Body fluids			
Cerebrospinal	G	BA, CHOC, ABA, THIO (abscess)	EB
Pericardial, peritoneal, pleural	G	BA, CHOC, ABA	EB
Synovial	G	BA, CHOC, ABA, THIO	EB
Catheters (IV)		BA	
Ear			
Otitis media	G	BA, EA, CHOC	EB
Otitis externa	G	BA, EA, CHOC	
Eye			
Conjunctiva	G	BA, EA, CHOC	
Cornea	G	BA, CHOC	
Intraocular	G	BA, EA, CHOC, ABA, AnPEA	EB
Feces or rectal swab	MB	EA, ESAM, ESAH, CSA	EEB
Genital—male			
Urethra	G	MTM/NYC/ML	
Prostatic fluid	G	BA, EA, MTM/NYC/ML	
Aspirates	G	BA, EA, MTM/NYC/ML	EB
Genital—female			
Vagina	G	BA	
Urethra		MTM/NYC/ML	
Cervix		MTM/NYC/ML	
Endometrium	G	BA, EA, MTM/NYC/ML, ABA, PV[a]	EB
Bartholin's gland	G	BA, EA, MTM/NYC/ML, ABA, AnPEA, PV[a]	EB
Upper tract	G	BA, EA, MTM/NYC/ML, ABA, AnPEA, PV[a]	EB
Respiratory tract—upper			
Nose		BA	
Nasopharynx		BA, CHOC	
Throat		BA	
Sinus	G	BA, EA, CHOC, ABA	
Respiratory tract—lower			
Sputum	G	BA, EA, CHOC	
Bronchial aspirate or brushings	G	BA, EA, CHOC	
Tracheal aspirate	G	BA, EA, CHOC	
Transtracheal aspirate	G	BA, EA, CHOC, ABA, AnPEA	EB
Lung aspirate or biopsy	G	BA, EA, CHOC, AnPEA	EB
Urine			
Clean-catch or catheterized	O	BA, EA (0.001 ml/plate)[b]	
Suprapubic bladder tap	G	BA, EA, (0.1 ml/plate)	
Wounds			
Superficial	G	BA, EA	
Burns, ulcers	G	BA, EA	
Abscess	G	BA, EA, ABA, PV,[a] BBE	EB
Tissue	G	BA, EA, ABA, PV,[a] BBE	EB

From Rubin SJ: Specimen collection and processing. In Howard BJ and others (editors): Clinical and pathogenic microbiology, St Louis, 1987, Mosby—Year Book, Inc.

SYMBOLS: CO_2, Incubate with 5% to 10% carbon dioxide   G, Gram's stain   O, Optional
            ANO_2, Incubate under anaerobic conditions   MB, Methylene blue stain   BA, Blood agar[c]
            EA, Enteric agar (MacConkey, eosin—methylene blue, deoxycholate)[d]
       CHOC, Chocolate agar (CO_2)[e]
            ESAM, Enteric selective agar of moderate selectivity (Hektoen enteric, xylose lysine deoxycholate, Salmonella-Shigella, deoxycholate citrate)[c]
            ESAH, Enteric selective agar of high selectivity (bismuth sulfite, brilliant green)[d]
            CSA, *Campylobacter*-selective agar (Skirrow, Butzler, Campy blood agar)[f]
          ML, Martin-Lewis[e]   MTM, Modified Thayer-Martin[e]   NYC, New York City medium[e]
          ABA, Anaerobic blood agar[g] (supplemented with hemin and vitamin K_1)
          EB, Enrichment broth (prereduced brain-heart infusion, enriched thioglycolate, chopped meat glucose)
          EEB, Enteric enrichment broth (GN, selenite F, tetrathionate)
          PV, Paromomycin-vancomycin blood agar
          BBE, *Bacteroides* bile esculin agar (for use in intraabdominal abscesses)

[a]Kanamycin-vancomycin laked blood agar may be used instead of PV agar.
[b]Also 0.01 ml per plate in acute urethral syndrome.
[c]Some laboratories incubate all BA with CO_2, others vary with specimen source.
[d]Incubate in air.
[e]Always CO_2.
[f]Incubate under microaerophilic conditions.
[g]Always ANO_2.

Commercially prepared blood culture media are bottled under vacuum. The atmosphere in the bottle may contain CO_2 in air or an inert gas. The oxidation-reduction potential (E_h) of most unvented bottles is low enough to support the growth of most clinically significant anaerobic bacteria. Because some organisms, such as yeasts or members of the genus *Pseudomonas*, may not grow at this redox potential, two bottles are inoculated. One is left unvented (and may contain a medium that does not support the growth of all aerobic and facultative organisms). The other bottle is transiently vented by inserting a sterile, cotton-plugged needle into the rubber septum of the bottle.

Most commercially prepared blood culture media contain SPS. Not only does SPS prevent clotting, but it neutralizes the bactericidal effect of human serum, inhibits complement activity and phagocytosis, and inactivates aminoglycosides. The SPS concentration used (0.025% to 0.05%) is inhibitory for some species of *Neisseria* and *Peptostreptococcus anaerobius*. This inhibition can be overcome by supplementing the medium with 1.2% gelatin.

In the traditional approach, inoculated bottles are incubated at 35°C to 37°C for 1 week and examined at various intervals. In cases in which slow-growing or more fastidious bacteria are suspected, bottles are incubated an additional week before discarding. Bottles are examined visually (macroscopically), microscopically (by Gram's stain or acridine orange stain), and by subculture to agar medium.

There are automated instruments available for monitoring growth in blood cultures (Bactec, Becton-Dickinson, Cockeyville, Md.; Bact Alert, Organon Teknika, Durham, N.C.) as well as labor-saving devices (Septi-Chek, Roche Diagnostic Systems, Branchburg, N.J.). These methods are reviewed in Chapter 49.

Body fluids

A body fluid specimen is collected by needle aspiration following skin decontamination. The specimen may be delivered in the syringe or in a sterile, screw-capped tube. As much fluid as possible is collected because organism numbers may be small. Bacteria are then concentrated by centrifugation or filtration. For cerebrospinal fluid (CSF), centrifugation at $1500 \times g$ for 15 minutes is sufficient. Cytocentrifugation may also be used on body fluids. There is evidence that differential counts of cellular constituents may be enhanced. Filtration does not seem to offer any advantage and may inhibit bacteria if antimicrobial agents are in the fluid.

Pleural, pericardial, peritoneal, and synovial fluids are processed in the same manner that CSF is. In general, culture of pleural and peritoneal fluid should include anaerobic agar media in addition to blood agar, chocolate agar, and an enriched broth. Cultures of synovial fluid are examined for *Neisseria gonorrhoeae* and other potential pathogens. Pleural and peritoneal fluid may also be cultured for mycobacteria, and pleural fluid for fungi and *Legionella* spp.

Catheters

Foley catheters or tips should not be cultured because they become colonized with urethral flora, and cultures do not correlate with urine culture or urinary tract infection. Vascular cannulas, however, are frequently submitted for culture because they can become colonized, especially with yeasts and staphylococci, and serve as a source of fungemia or bacteremia. Before their removal, the skin is decontaminated. Short catheters (2 to 3 inches) are removed and severed aseptically at a point that was just inside the skin interface. Two segments of about 2 inches each are collected from longer catheters (8 to 24 inches), one from the skin interface and one from a section that was within the blood vessel. Catheter segments are aseptically placed in sterile containers and immediately transported to the laboratory for culture.

Ears

Laboratory diagnosis of otitis media (middle ear infection) is usually attempted only in cases of therapeutic failure or in neonates because specimens must be collected by needle aspiration through the eardrum (tympanocentesis). If the eardrum is ruptured, exudate may be collected by inserting a sterile swab through an auditory speculum. See Chapter 46. Material from otitis externa, which is a bacterial infection of the skin of the auditory meatus, can be collected with a swab.

Eyes

Except in cases of purulent conjunctivitis, swabs are usually inadequate for culture of ocular infections. Specimens should be collected by an ophthalmologist. With corneal infection, the conjunctivae are first swabbed, and then multiple scrapings are collected and inoculated directly onto agar media. Intraocular fluid is collected by needle aspiration and should be processed immediately.

Endophthalmitis is a serious infection caused by a number of organisms including *Staphylococcus aureus*, *Staphylococcus epidermidis*, *Staphylococcus pneumoniae*, *Enterobacteriaceae* spp., *H. influenzae*, *N. meningitidis*, *Bacillus* spp., and *Mycobacterium fortuitum*.

Pus or intraocular fluid is examined by smear and inoculated, as is done for corneal specimens. Media for mycobacteria, fungi, and anaerobic bacteria may be included if such infection is suspected. See Chapter 46.

Gastrointestinal tract

Feces, vomitus, and duodenal contents may be submitted for isolation of bacteria causing diarrhea. Feces are passed directly into a clean, leakproof container or may be collected from a bedpan. Portions containing pus, blood, or mucus are preferred; a 1- or 2-g quantity is sufficient. If passed feces are unobtainable, the specimen can be collected by passing a swab beyond the anal sphincter, rotating carefully, and withdrawing. In acute disease, when large numbers of organisms are shed, a single specimen is probably enough. Most agents responsible for bacterial diarrhea can be isolated in two or three specimens. To rule out the carrier state, three negative specimens in a row are necessary.

Outside the body, stool temperature drops, producing a pH change that particularly affects *Shigella* spp., so ideally, a specimen should be plated directly. If the specimen cannot be plated within an hour or two of collection, it should be mixed with a transport medium and refrigerated. Buffered glycerol/saline is superior to Cary-Blair transport medium for *Shigella*, but is not good for *Vibrio* spp. or *Campylobacter jejuni*. Therefore, whenever culturing will be delayed, use of Cary-Blair transport medium is advisable.

Microscopic examination of feces is useful to determine if leukocytes are present. Feces are mixed on a slide with Löffler methylene blue stain, a coverslip is applied, and the slide is examined on "high dry." A strongly positive smear suggests infection with an invasive organism. See Chapter 47.

Male genital tract

The urethra is the most common male genital site cultured. The laboratory may also receive testicular or epididymal aspirates, or prostatic fluid. Prostatic fluid is obtained by a physician using digital massage through the rectum and is collected in a sterile tube or on a swab. If urethral exudate is present or can be "milked" from the urethra, the usual swab may be used. Otherwise, a thin urethrogenital swab is inserted about 2 cm into the urethra, gently rotated, and removed. Specimens for culture of *N. gonorrhoeae* are planted directly after collection by using one of several culture-transport devices, such as Jembec plates containing either modified Thayer-Martin (MTM), Martin-Lewis (ML), or New York City (NYC) media. A CO_2-generating system can be used to transport inoculated standard laboratory plates containing one of these media. Jembec plates and standard laboratory plates are all incubated in 5% to 10% CO_2 at 35°C to 37°C. In areas where vancomycin-resistant *N. gonorrhoeae* has been isolated or is suspected, MTM (without vancomycin) or chocolate agar should also be inoculated. Plates or bottles are examined after overnight incubation and again after 48 hours of incubation.

Prostatic secretions are sometimes collected to diagnose bacterial prostatitis. Quantitative cultures are performed. Organisms found are the same as those isolated from urinary tract infections, with facultative, gram-negative rods being the most common. The significance of gram-positive isolates is difficult to assess because staphylococci are found in the normal male urethra. See Chapter 50.

Female genital tract

Although anatomic barriers are not well defined, infections of the female genital tract can be described as lower tract (vulva, vagina, cervix) or upper tract (uterus, fallopian tubes, ovaries). With suspected lower tract gonococcal infection, cervical, urethral, or anal specimens may be submitted. A qualified physician is responsible for obtaining specimens from the female genital tract. The cervix is visualized using a speculum moistened with water (no lubricant). The cervical mucous plug is removed, the cervix is compressed gently with the speculum, and exudate is collected on a swab. If no exudate is seen, the swab is inserted into the endocervical canal, rotated, and removed. Urethral exudate may be stimulated by massaging the urethra against the pubic symphysis through the vagina. If no discharge is expressed, a urethrogenital swab is used, as for men. Anal cultures may be collected before and after treatment because the rectum may be the only positive post treatment site. A swab is inserted about 1 inch into the anal canal just inside the anal ring, moved from side to side, and removed. No fecal material should be on the swab.

Pus from Bartholin's or Skene's gland abscesses can sometimes be collected from the respective ducts. Otherwise, material can be carefully aspirated directly by needle and syringe by a physician.

Specimens from the endometrium are best collected by transabdominal aspiration. They should not be collected through the cervix with a swab because they will be contaminated by cervical and vaginal flora—the same bacteria that cause endometritis. Protected swabs may reduce such contamination.

Specimens for the diagnosis of pelvic inflammatory disease (PID) are all collected by invasive techniques. Peritoneal fluid may be collected from the cul-de-sac by aspiration through the posterior vaginal vault (culdocentesis). Material taken directly from the fallopian tubes or ovaries is collected surgically.

Intrauterine devices have been associated with infection and may be submitted for culture. They should be surgically removed to prevent contamination with cervical or vaginal flora, and the entire device, including any pus or secretions, should be placed in a sterile container for transport to the laboratory. See Chapter 50.

Upper respiratory tract

Specimens from the upper respiratory tract include swabs of the anterior nares, nasopharynx, and throat, and aspirates from sinus cavities. Nasal swabs are used for detection of staphylococcal carriers.

Nasopharyngeal secretions are collected by a physician using a small swab on a flexible wire. The swab is gently inserted through the nose into the nasopharynx, carefully rotated, removed, and placed in an appropriate transport medium. If pertussis is suspected, special transport media must be used, or the specimen should be processed within 3 hours.

Throat cultures are obtained by first depressing the tongue with a tongue depressor or swab. A sterile swab is vigorously rubbed over both tonsillar areas, the posterior pharynx, and any inflamed or ulcerated areas. Care should be taken not to touch the cheeks, tongue, uvula, or lips.

The only appropriate specimen for laboratory diagnosis of sinusitis is material directly aspirated from a sinus cavity by a physician. Nasal or nasopharyngeal specimens are not acceptable.

Diagnosis of thrush (oral candidiasis) is dependent on direct visualization of numerous yeast cells and mycelium on a direct KOH preparation or a Gram's stain prepared from a specimen obtained by swabs from suspect areas of the oral cavity. Isolating a few *Candida* organisms from the oral cavity in the absence of suspect lesions and direct visualization is most likely not significant.

Acute epiglottitis is usually a disease of children 2 to 4 years old and is almost always caused by *H. influenzae*. Occasionally, *Streptococcus pyogenes*, *Staph. aureus*, or *S. pneumoniae* is involved. Cultures are not recommended because manipulation of a swollen, inflamed epiglottis can result in serious respiratory obstruction. Diagnosis is essentially clinical, although blood cultures are useful because 50% of the patients are bacteremic. A physician who requests such cultures should obtain the swabs. See Chapter 43.

Lower respiratory tract

Expectorated sputum is the most common specimen submitted from patients with suspected pneumonia, but is the least productive. The patient coughs deeply and expectorates into a sterile container. Sometimes sputum must be induced. If saline nebulization is used, the saline must not contain any bacteriostatic agents. Lower respiratory tract secretions may also be collected by bronchoscopy, suction through tracheostomy or endotracheal tubes, transtracheal aspiration, direct lung aspiration, or biopsy.

Bronchial brushings are preferable to bronchial washings because the washings are more dilute. Specimens collected via bronchoscopy are contaminated with oral microbial flora, which can be greatly reduced by collecting secretions with a triple-lumen bronchoscope.

Transtracheal aspiration is performed by a physician. The trachea below the larynx is normally sterile, except in patients with chronic pulmonary disease or endotracheal or tracheostomy tubes. A needle is inserted through the cricothyroid membrane into the trachea, a catheter is passed through the needle, and the needle is removed. Secretions are then aspirated through the catheter. Because the procedure is invasive, it is usually reserved for critically ill patients who are not producing sputum or who are suspected of having an anaerobic infection and cultures are considered necessary.

Lung aspirates are obtained by direct aspiration through the chest wall (pleural fluid, empyema fluid, thoracentesis fluid). Transtracheal aspirates, lung aspirates, or lung tissue should be transported and processed without delay.

Although sputum is the easiest specimen to collect, expectorated sputum cultures are among the most difficult to interpret. All expectorated sputum is contaminated to some degree by oral flora as it passes through the upper respiratory tract during collection. Virtually all sputum yields anaerobic bacteria from this contamination. Because anaerobic pulmonary infection is caused by normal oral flora, only specimens collected in a way that bypasses the oral cavity are cultured anaerobically.

A Gram-stained smear is made from a purulent portion of the specimen (1) to assess the degree of contamination and therefore the acceptability of the specimen, and (2) to guide the clinician in selection of initial treatment. The smear is first examined under a low power ($100 \times$) for the numbers and types of cells present. An acceptable specimen should contain an abundance of leukocytes and few squamous epithelial cells. Several systems are used. The simplest is to consider the presence of more than 25 squamous epithelial cells per field unacceptable.

Techniques for the isolation of mycobacteria, fungi, or viruses from sputum use decontamination methods and selective media, so the presence of oral flora is less important. If the specimen is unacceptable, the ordering physician must be notified so that a new specimen can be collected.

Specimens obtained by bronchoscopy are contaminated by oral flora during passage of the bronchoscope and therefore should not be cultured for anaerobic bacteria. The smear and culture are performed as for sputum, except that all bronchoscopically collected secretions should be cultured. Their collection entails considerable discomfort and expense for the patient.

Specimens collected through a tracheostomy or endotracheal tube are difficult to evaluate. Patients become colonized with potential pathogens within 24 hours of insertion of the tube and an inflammatory response to it. Thus, the specimen from a patient without lower respiratory disease can contain large numbers of leukocytes and bacteria. Tracheal aspirates are processed like sputum. Transtracheal aspirates, lung aspirates, or lung tissue is processed like sputum. See Chapter 44.

Urinary tract

In patients with symptoms of urinary tract infection (painful urination, urgency, frequency), urine is collected for culture at the onset of symptoms and may be repeated 48 to 72 hours after institution of therapy. If bacteriuria is asymptomatic, two or three specimens may be necessary to confirm an initial positive culture. In suspected renal tuberculosis, three consecutive first-morning urine specimens should be submitted. Pooled 24-hour collection of urine is unacceptable.

Urine is collected by clean-catch, catheterization, or suprapubic aspiration. A midstream clean-catch specimen must be obtained in a manner that prevents contamination by organisms that colonize the distal urethra, vagina, and perineum. The patient is instructed to clean the periurethral area well with a mild detergent, followed by rinsing. The detergent may be bacteriostatic and must be completely rinsed off. The labial folds or glans penis is retracted, the patient begins to void, and then a midstream sample is collected.

To collect a specimen from a catheterized patient, the tubing is cleaned with alcohol and punctured with a 21-gauge needle, and the urine is aspirated with a syringe. Some urinary catheter systems have a special port for culture collection. The catheter is never disconnected from the drainage bag to collect a specimen, nor should urine be collected directly from the bag.

Urine is collected in a sterile container with a screw-cap or other snug-fitting lid. Most bacteria grow well in urine held at room temperature. Therefore, specimens must be processed within 2 hours or refrigerated to prevent overgrowth by small numbers of contaminating bacteria. Alternatively, the urine may be aspirated into commercially available devices that contain a preservative fluid that maintains viable bacteria in the urine for at least 24 hours at room temperature.

Infection of the urinary tract may involve the lower tract (cystitis, acute urethral syndrome) or upper tract (pyelonephritis). Diagnosis is based on demonstrating significant numbers of bacteria in the urine.

Because urine is frequently contaminated with small numbers of organisms during collection, quantitative cultures are mandatory. Broth culture precludes quantitation and thus is never used. Only urine collected by suprapubic bladder tap should be cultured anaerobically, because some anaerobic bacteria are found normally among the urethral colonizing organisms.

Several techniques can be used for quantitating the number of bacteria in urine. Direct streaking with a calibrated loop may be used. A calibrated platinum loop (0.01 ml.) or a 10-μl micropipette is inserted vertically into the urine, and the urine is inoculated onto blood agar and MacConkey agar. Plates are examined after overnight incubation at 35°C.

Urine collected by direct aspiration from the bladder is also cultured quantitatively, but a pipette is used, and 0.1 ml is dropped onto each plate. After drying, the drop is cross-streaked like other urine specimens.

Microscopic examination of unspun urine by Gram-stained smear can provide helpful information. The presence of more than one organism per oil immersion field correlates quite well (75% to 95%) with 10^5 CFU/ml.

Deciding what colony count is significant is related to the clinical situation. In women with asymptomatic bacteriuria or pyelonephritis, $\geq 1 \times 10^5$ CFU/ml correlate with infection, whereas contaminating bacteria (from the distal urethra) are usually present in numbers $<1 \times 10^3$ CFU/ml.

Colony counts between 1×10^3 and 1×10^5 CFU/ml in these people can be difficult to interpret, since significant counts may be decreased because of antimicrobial therapy, frequency of urination, or dilution of the urine from excessive hydration. Counts between 1×10^3 and 1×10^5 CFU/ml are an indication for repeat culture. Most laboratories consider 10^4 CFU/ml or less in a clean-catch specimen to be insignificant.

Low counts (1×10^3 CFU/ml) are probably significant in specimens collected by aspiration from a catheter port. Any number greater than 10/ml of organisms isolated from suprapubic bladder tap specimens is significant.

Women with symptoms of urinary tract infection and pyuria, but with counts of 1×10^3 to 1×10^5 CFU/ml are designated as having acute urethral syndrome.

Three or more different types of bacteria isolated from a clean-catch urine specimen is almost always indicative of contamination. See Chapter 48.

Wounds

Purulent or serosanguinous material from closed wounds or abscesses is best collected by aspiration with sterile needle and syringe after skin decontamination. If collection is done at surgery, a portion of the abscess wall should also be cultured. Specimens from superficial wounds are frequently collected by swab. Certain infections, such as ulcers and burns, are best sampled by biopsy because organisms isolated from surface swabs of these sites usually represent superficial colonization. Tissue and aspirates should be transported to the laboratory and processed without delay. Tissue should be submitted in a sterile container without carrier medium.

Postmortem specimens are often of limited value because of their poor correlation with antemortem cultures; however, they may be useful in selected cases. Ideally, a 6-cm³ specimen with one serosal or capsular surface intact should be collected by a pathologist.

Any material collected from a wound should be initially examined with a Gram-stained smear. The smear may be extremely helpful in selecting initial antimicrobial therapy. For example, gram-positive cocci in chains seen in a specimen from cellulitis are usually *S. pyogenes* (Group A beta hemolytic Streptococci). Early and appropriate therapy may be critical in these infections. The Gram's stain should also be used to correlate the growth of organisms in culture with their clinical significance. See Chapter 51.

SUGGESTED READING

Balows A, et al.: Manual of clinical microbiology, ed. 5, Am Soc Microbiol, 1991, Washington, DC.

Bartlett JG, et al.: Laboratory diagnosis of lower respiratory tract infections, Cumitech 7A, Am Soc Microbiol, 1987, Washington, DC.

Howard BJ, et al.: Clinical and pathogenic microbiology, St. Louis, 1987, Mosby–Year Book, Inc.

Isenberg HD, et al.: Collection and processing of bacteriological specimens, Cumitech 9, Am Soc Microbiol, 1979, Washington, DC.

40

Principles and practices for the laboratory guidance of antimicrobial therapy

Janet A. Hindler
Linda M. Mann

GENERAL CHARACTERISTICS OF ANTIBACTERIAL AGENTS

The drug, the host, and the microorganism all need to be examined when the success or failure of antimicrobial therapy is considered. To be effective, the antimicrobial agent must reach the site of the infection in levels high enough to kill or inhibit the organism causing the infection without harming the host. The agent should not induce or select resistant organisms during therapy. The effect on normal host flora should be minimal. The properties of an ideal therapeutic agent are listed in Box 40-1.

The host immune system is also important in determining treatment outcome. In the presence of a normal host defense, the inhibition of microbial growth by static agents may slow the infectious process so that the immune system can clear the infection. Without a normal host defense, inhibition of growth alone is rarely successful. Bactericidal agents are extremely important in treatment of infections in the immunocompromised host and in sites sequestered from the immune system, such as within a vegetation on a heart valve or deep within an abscess.

Optimal antimicrobial therapy can rarely be achieved without knowledge of the organism causing the infection and the characteristics of the antimicrobial agent. Some organisms have predictable responses to particular drugs, and clinical experience in treating infections caused by such organisms has confirmed the effectiveness of these agents. Antimicrobial susceptibility testing helps predict whether or not treatment with a particular drug will be successful when the organism has a variable antimicrobial susceptibility pattern.

The largest and most widely used antimicrobial agents specifically target bacterial agents of disease and are correctly termed *antibacterial agents;* however, the more general term, *antimicrobial agent,* is normally used. Antibacterial agents are not usually effective against fungi, viruses, or parasites. Antifungal, antiviral, and antiparasitic agents will be discussed in separate sections.

Antibacterial agents and modes of action

Nearly 100 antibacterial agents are now available for clinical use and many more are in development. Many are antibiotics

---

Box 40-1 Properties of an ideal antibacterial agent

Target	Selectively active against the bacterium or bacteria causing the infection; normal flora minimally affected
Toxicity	No side effects for the host
Spectrum of activity	Narrow rather than broad spectrum
Type of activity	Bactericidal rather than bacteriostatic
Resistance	No inherent resistance or acquired resistance seen clinically
Allergenicity	Does not induce an allergic response
Chemical properties	Stable, long acting; water soluble

---

that have been chemically modified to increase effectiveness by increasing stability, resistance to enzymatic attack, spectrum of activity, or other properties. Others are synthesized totally in the laboratory. Agents with the same basic molecular structure have the same modes of actions and general characteristics, and are grouped in families reflecting their structural similarities.

Most antibacterial agents are clinically useful because they preferentially affect the biochemical processes unique to bacteria and, therefore, are least toxic to humans. Antibacterial agents that interfere with bacterial cell wall synthesis are generally very effective and safe since mammalian cells lack cell walls. Agents that target the bacterial ribosome inhibit bacterial protein synthesis without affecting mammalian ribosomes. Other targets of antibacterial activity include the cell membrane, RNA and DNA polymerases, and enzymes of metabolic pathways.

Table 40-1 summarizes the major families of antibacterial agents and describes their modes of action. Several important groups are discussed in detail in this chapter.

Aminoglycosides

Streptomycin, the first aminoglycoside antibiotic, was discovered by Waksman in 1944 in the initial systematic

Table 40-1   Antibacterial agents: modes of action and mechanisms of resistance

Antimicrobial agent	Mode of action	Mechanism of resistance
Aminoglycosides	Interference with protein synthesis at the 30S ribosomal subunit	Inactivation by aminoglycoside-modifying enzymes, decreased permeability
β-lactams	Inhibition of cell wall synthesis	Inactivation by beta-lactamases, alterations in penicillin-binding proteins, decreased permeability
β-lactam + β-lactamase inhibitor combinations	Inactivation of β-lactamases, inhibition of cell wall synthesis	Inactivation by β-lactamases, alteration in penicillin-binding proteins, decreased permeability
Chloramphenicol	Prevents mRNA from attaching to ribosomes	Inactivation by chloramphenicol acetyltransferase, decreased permeability
Clindamycin	Binds to 50S ribosomal subunit blocking initiation of peptide chains	Methylation of 50S ribosomal subunit
Erythromycin	Binds to 50S ribosomal subunit blocking extension of peptide chains	Methylation of 50S ribosomal subunit
Nitrofurantoin	Inhibition of a variety of bacterial enzyme systems	Alternative metabolic pathways
Polymyxins	Disruption of cell membrane	Alterations in cell membranes
Quinolones	Inhibition of DNA gyrase activity	Alteration of DNA gyrase, decreased permeability
Rifampin	Inhibition of DNA-dependent RNA polymerase activity	Alteration in DNA-dependent RNA polymerase
Sulfonamides	Competitive inhibition of folic acid synthesis	Bypass affected metabolic pathway
Tetracyclines	Interference with protein synthesis at the 30S ribosomal subunit	Decreased drug uptake, increased efflux of drug
Vancomycin	Inhibition of cell wall synthesis	Unknown, ? changes in binding sites

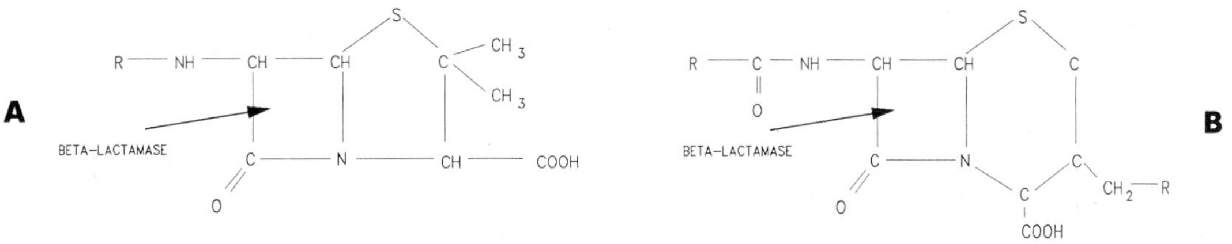

Fig. 40-1   Beta-lactam structure: **A,** Basic structure of penicillin. **B,** Basic structure of cephalosporin. *Arrow* indicates the site of beta-lactamase activity.

effort to isolate antibiotics produced by soil microorganisms. The basic structure of aminoglycosides is composed of an aminocyclitol ring to which various amino-sugars are attached. The more proper name for this family of compounds is aminocyclitols. The family includes streptomycin, kanamycin, gentamicin, tobramycin, amikacin, netilmicin and neomycin. These agents inhibit protein synthesis by binding to the 30S ribosomal subunit, causing misreading of the mRNA. Aminoglycosides are unique among agents that inhibit protein synthesis since they are bactericidal rather than bacteriostatic. They have a broad spectrum of activity but are inactive at low pH and in anaerobic conditions, and are ineffective in treating infections caused by anaerobes or intracellular pathogens. Used in combination with a β-lactam drug, aminoglycosides often show a synergistic killing effect. Aminoglycosides are toxic in high doses and therapy must be carefully monitored.

β-Lactams

By far the largest and most clinically used group of the antimicrobial agents are the β-lactams. The first β-lactam,

penicillin, is an antibiotic produced by the fungus *Penicillium*. Discovered by Fleming in 1924, penicillin was not used clinically until the 1940s when Chain and Florey purified the active compound. Cephalosporin, another β-lactam with a basic structure similar to, but not identical to penicillin was isolated from another fungal species in the genus *Cephalosporium* (now called *Acremonium*). The basic ring structures of penicillin and cephalosporin are shown in Fig. 40-1. Modification of the side chains attached to the rings has improved stability and pharmacokinetic properties as well as increased the activity of the original drugs. An important group of the β-lactam family is the penicillinase-resistant penicillins. Bulky side chains inhibit hydrolysis of the β-lactam ring by β-lactamases increasing the effectiveness of the drugs particularly against β-lactamase producing gram-positive bacteria. β-Lactam inhibitors are compounds that generally have little antibacterial activity but are able to bind to and inhibit β-lactamases. Used in combination with penicillinase susceptible nonpenicillinase-resistant β-lactams, they protect the active agent against hydrolysis by β-lactamases. Table 40-2 lists the classes of β-lactams in more detail.

Table 40-2   The classes of β-lactam agents

β-Lactam	Examples	Comments
PENICILLINS		
Natural penicillins	Penicillin G Penicillin V	Used to treat severe streptococcal, pneumococcal, and meningococcal infections; active against anaerobes other than *Bacteroides fragilis*, effective therapy for treponemal infections
Penicillinase-resistant penicillins	Methicillin Nafcillin Oxacillin Cloxacillin Dicloxacillin	Active against penicillinase-producing staphylococci and, to a lesser extent than natural penicillins, against other gram-positive cocci including pneumococci and group A streptococci
Extended spectrum penicillins Aminopenicillins	Ampicillin Amoxacillin	Slightly less active than penicillin G against pneumococci, streptococci, and meningococci; active against many strains of *Salmonella, Shigella, Proteus mirabilis, Haemophilus influenzae,* and *Neisseria*; inhibitory for enterococci and *Listeria*
Carboxypenicillins	Carbenicillin Ticarcillin	Used to treat serious infections caused by susceptible enterics and *Pseudomonas*; often given in combination with an aminoglycoside
Ureidopenicillins	Azlocillin Mezlocillin Piperacillin	Greater activity than carboxypenicillins against *Enterobacteriaceae* and *Pseudomonas*; active *B. fragilis*; variable activity against *Klebsiella* spp.
Combinations (penicillin + β-lactamase inhibitor)	Ampicillin + sulbactam Amoxicillin + clavulanic acid Ticarcillin + clavulanic acid	Similar to amoxicillin, ampicillin, and ticarcillin with enhanced activity against β-lactamase–producing organisms including staphylococci, *H. influenzae, Bacteroides,* and some *Enterobacteriaceae*
CEPHALOSPORINS		
First generation	Cefaclor Cefadroxil Cefaloridine Cefazolin Cephalexin Cephaloglycin Cephalothin Cephapirin Cephradine	Active against aerobic gram-positive cocci other than methicillin-resistant staphylococci and enterococci; active against some *Enterobacteriaceae* including many strains of *Escherichia coli, Proteus mirabilis, Klebsiella* spp., and most anaerobes other than *B. fragilis*; cefaclor is more active than the others against *H. influenzae*; susceptible to inactivation by many gram-negative β-lactamases
Second generation	Cefamandole Cefixime Cefoxitin Cefuroxime Cefonicid Ceforanide Cefotetan	Slightly more active against enterics; less active than first-generation cephalosporins against staphylococci; increased stability to gram-negative β-lactamases; cefocitin has good activity against *B. fragilis* spp. and *Serratia* spp.; cefuroxime has good cerebrospinal fluid (CSF) penetration; all require parenteral administration
Third generation	Cefmenoxime Cefoperazone Cefotaim Cefotaxime Ceftazidime Ceftizoxime Ceftriaxone Cesulodin Moxalactam	Greatly increased activity against gram-negative bacilli because of increased stability against gram-negative β-lactamases; some have good CSF penetration and/or activity against *Pseudomonas* in contrast to other cephalosporins; less active against gram-positive organisms than other cephalosporins; all have good activity against *H. influenzae*, including β-lactamase–producing strains
MONOBACTAM	Aztreonam	Slightly greater activity than third-generation cephalosporins against *Enterobacteriaceae*; active against gram-positive organisms
CARBAPENEMS	Imipenem	Slightly greater activity than third-generation cephalosporins against *Enterobacteriaceae*; active against many gram-positive cocci including enterococci

The cell walls of bacteria contain peptidoglycan, a macromolecule unique to bacteria that is composed of long chains of alternate N-acetylglucosamine and N-acetylmuramate residues cross-linked by short peptide chains. β-Lactam drugs inhibit bacterial cell wall synthesis by binding to cellular proteins called penicillin-binding proteins (PBP) and interfering in the final step in peptidoglycan synthesis, the cross-linking of the peptides. The effect can be either bacteriostatic or bactericidal. For the β-lactam drug to be effective in killing, the bacterium must be growing and synthesizing peptidoglycan.

Quinolones

The quinolones are compounds synthesized in the laboratory. The basic structure of the quinolones is based on 1,8-napthyrine, and the family includes nalidixic acid, ciprofloxacin, norfloxacin, and ofloxacin. Quinolones inhibit the activity of DNA gyrase, an enzyme required for supercoiling of chromosomal DNA. In the presence of quinolones, DNA gyrase cannot re-ligate DNA strands after supercoiling, which leaves them subject to degradation by nucleases. The quinolones are bactericidal drugs. Nalidixic acid, the first quinolone agent, was used to treat urinary tract infections but is not widely used since resistance is likely to develop during therapy. The newer fluoroquinolones like ciprofloxacin have been modified to produce agents with a broader spectrum of activity. Resistance is still uncommon. However, given the proven adaptability of bacteria and the increasing clinical use of these agents, the appearance of fluoroquinolone-resistant strains is a concern.

Sulfonamides

Dogmagk developed the first sulfa drug, a dye named Prontosil, in 1935. Sulfonamides are similar in structure to para-aminobenzoic acid, a folic acid precursor, and act by competitively inhibiting the synthesis of bacterial dihydrofolate, an essential cofactor in the biosynthesis of purines and pyrimidines. Trimethoprim, an analog of dihydrofolate often used in combination with sulfonamides, interferes with a second step in the metabolic pathway, increasing the effectiveness of therapy and reducing the frequency of development of resistance. Sulfonamides are used most often in the treatment of urinary tract infections and also in the treatment of *Nocardia* infections. The combination of trimethoprim and sulfamethoxazole is an effective antimicrobial agent used in the treatment of *Pneumocystis carinii* pneumonia.

Vancomycin

By the 1950s most hospital strains of *Staphylococcus aureus* were resistant to penicillin and when therapy was changed to tetracycline or erythromycin, resistance to these agents also developed. Vancomycin, a glycopeptide antibiotic isolated from *Streptomyces orientalis* and first approved for use in 1958, was developed as an alternative to penicillin for the treatment of infections due to *S. aureus*. Discovery of the penicillinase-resistant penicillins prevented vancomycin from becoming the drug of choice for *S. aureus* infections in the 1960s, but with the emergence of resistance to the penicillinase-resistant penicillins, vancomycin has become important in the empiric therapy of serious infections and infections in patients allergic to penicillin.

Like the β-lactams, vancomycin interferes with cell wall synthesis by preventing cross-linking of peptidoglycan chains. However, the molecular structure and the actual target of vancomycin differs from that of the β-lactams. With rare exceptions, all gram-positive bacteria are susceptible.

Mechanisms of resistance

Resistance of a microorganism to antimicrobial agents can be either intrinsic or acquired. Intrinsic resistance is common to all or most strains of a given species and results from the normal genetic determinants for that species. The species normally lacks the antimicrobial target or has a modification in the target that prevents antimicrobial activity. For example, penicillin, a cell wall active agent, has no effect on *Mycoplasma* since *Mycoplasma* lack a cell wall. Other examples of intrinsic resistance include: (1) aminoglycosides against anaerobes, (2) vancomycin against gram-negative organisms, and (3) penicillin G against *Enterobacteriaceae*.

Acquired resistance is due to modification of the genetic makeup of the organism. This can result from spontaneous mutations occurring in the chromosomal DNA, which confer a selective advantage when the organism is challenged by an antimicrobial agent. These spontaneous changes may involve a single base or multiple bases and occur at a rate of 10^{-6} to 10^{-13}. If the frequency of change leading to resistance is high, resistance can emerge during therapy and limit the usefulness of an agent clinically. Multiple changes resulting in additive, stepwise increases in resistance are also seen.

Acquired resistance can also result from transfer of genetic material, either chromosomal or extrachromosomal, between bacteria. Mechanisms for gene transfer include transformation, transduction, and conjugation. Currently the most important mechanism of genetic transfer in the development of resistance is conjugation and transfer of plasmids between strains, species, and even genera of bacteria. Plasmids that carry resistance genes are called R factors and may confer resistance to single or multiple agents. Some R factors carry resistance genes called transposons that are able to jump from one plasmid to another or from the plasmid to the chromosome. Once a transposon is established in the chromosome it will be passed on to the progeny of the bacterium.

A microorganism can develop resistance to a single agent and remain susceptible to other antimicrobial agents in the same family. Sometimes, however, changes will result in resistance against several or all agents of the same family or class. For example, acquisition of a particular β-lactamase gene may confer resistance to penicillins as a group but not to the cephalosporins. Changes in permeability often affect the activity of several unrelated agents.

Development of resistance during therapy is related to the particular drug being used, the drug concentration achieved at the site of infection, the bacterial species causing the infection, and the number of bacteria involved. The probability that a microorganism will become resistant to a given agent depends on the species or even strain of organism. For example, *E. coli* appears less likely than *Klebsiella*, *Enterobacter*, or *Pseudomonas* to develop resistance to ciprofloxacin.

One important aspect of detection of resistance in the laboratory is the number of resistant organisms in the population. If the number of organisms tested is small, the probability of detecting resistance is lower than if larger numbers of organisms are tested. The same concept can be applied to the development of resistance during therapy. If the number of organisms in an infection is large, there is a greater chance that resistant organisms are present and that the population will become resistant during therapy.

There are five basic resistance mechanisms: (1) production of enzymes that inactivate the agent, (2) decreased permeability to the agent, (3) modification of receptor or binding sites, (4) development of alternative metabolic pathways, and (5) circumvention of secondary events leading to cell death. Resistance can also result from a combination of mechanisms. Several important examples of resistance mechanisms, discussed in detail, follow.

Aminoglycosides

Resistance to aminoglycosides usually results from the enzymatic inactivation of the agent due to the acquisition of plasmids carrying the genes for modifying enzymes. Several different enzyme activities (acetylases, adenylases, and phosphorylases) are seen and may result in resistance to one or several aminoglycosides. Decreased permeability leading to resistance to aminoglycosides in *Pseudomonas aeruginosa* has also been described. High-level resistance to aminoglycosides due to the production of aminoglycoside-inactivating enzymes is currently of major concern in the treatment of serious *Enterococcus* infections.

β-Lactams

The production of β-lactamases, enzymes that inactivate β-lactam agents, is the major mechanism of resistance to these agents. There are many types of β-lactamases that differ in their specificity and activity against the β-lactams. Penicillinases act preferentially on penicillins, whereas cephalosporinases are more active against the cephalosporins. Resistance due to β-lactamases can result from the acquisition of a plasmid with a β-lactamase gene or deregulation of normal chromosomal β-lactamase genes. β-Lactamases may be inducible and expressed only in response to the presence of the drug, or may result from constitutive expression of β-lactamase genes. A revised Richmond and Sykes classification scheme for β-lactamases based on the spectrum of activity, location, and expression is shown in Table 40-3. Class I and III β-lactamases are currently the subject of much clinical concern. Class I β-lactamases are responsible for much of the resistance against third-generation cephalosporins seen among gram-negative rods. Class III includes the plasmid-mediated transposon TEM responsible for resistance to penicillins in *Haemophilus influenzae* and *Neisseria gonorrhoeae*.

Two other mechanisms of resistance to β-lactams have been observed. Changes occurring in the outer membranes of gram-negative organisms have resulted in resistance by preventing the drug from reaching the site of cell wall synthesis. Changes in the structure of penicillin-binding proteins that prevent or decrease the ability of the drug to bind and block cross-linking reactions will also result in resistance to β-lactams.

Resistance due to the production of β-lactamases is widespread among *S. aureus* strains. Some are also resistant to the penicillinase-resistant agents. Production of β-lactamases is an important factor in the development of resistance to second- and third-generation cephalosporins among the *Enterobacteriaceae*. The susceptibility of pneumococci to penicillin G has been slowly decreasing in recent years. This decrease is due to changes in the penicillin-binding proteins PBP1 and PBP2, resulting in decreased affinity for penicillin G.

Table 40-3   Revised classification scheme for the β-lactamases

Class	Enzyme activity	Location	Expression	Examples
Class I	Cephalosporinase	Chromosomal	Inducible and constitutive	*Enterobacter* *Citrobacter* *Serratia* *Pseudomonas* *Acinetobacter* *Providencia* *Proteus* *Yersinia*
Class II	Penicillinase	Chromosomal	Inducible and constitutive	*Proteus* *Pseudomonas*
Class III	Penicillinase and cephalosporinase	Plasmid	Constitutive	*Enterobacteriaceae* *Haemophilus* *Neisseria* *Pseudomonas*
Class IV	Penicillinase and cephalosporinase	Chromosomal	Constitutive	*Klebsiella* *Enterobacter*
Class V	Penicillinase	Plasmid	Constitutive	*E. coli* *Pseudomonas*
Class VI	Cephalosporinase	Chromosomal	Constitutive	*Bacteroides*

Data from Wong CS:Beta-lactamase inhibitors, *Clin Microbiol Newsletter* 10:177, 1988.

Quinolones

There are two mechanisms by which microorganisms can acquire resistance to the quinolones. The first is to alter the target molecule, DNA gyrase, so that it is less affected by the drug. The second is to prevent the drug from reaching the target by decreasing the permeability of the organism to the drug. Bacteria that become resistant to quinolones because of reduced permeability are usually also resistant to tetracycline, chloramphenicol, and the β-lactams.

Vancomycin

The mechanism of vancomycin resistance is not well understood. Although reports of clinical resistance among *S. aureus* isolates have not been made, vancomycin resistance has been seen among several groups of opportunistic bacteria, including *Leuconostoc, Pediococcus,* and *Lactobacillus.* These bacteria appear to be inherently resistant. Resistance, although uncommon, has also been reported in *Enterococcus* and coagulase-negative staphylococci. Various degrees of resistance have been seen in *Enterococcus.* The high-level resistance (minimum inhibitory concentration [MIC] >256) has caused much concern since it appears to be transferable between *Enterococcus* stains.

APPLICATION OF IN VITRO ANTIMICROBIAL SUSCEPTIBILITY TESTS
Rationale and indications for performing antimicrobial susceptibility tests

The primary functions of a clinical microbiology laboratory are to identify potential pathogens in clinical specimens and to perform antimicrobial susceptibility tests when appropriate. Antimicrobial susceptibility tests are rarely performed on isolates that are probably not contributing to the patient's problem, such as normal flora isolates or isolates that may represent contamination. Reporting antimicrobial susceptibility results in these situations may be misleading and encourage a clinician to treat a patient unnecessarily. Antimicrobial susceptibility tests are not routinely performed on organisms that are predictably susceptible to the drug(s) of choice unless the patient cannot tolerate the drug(s) of choice and alternative agents with less predictable activity are being considered. For example, a patient with a *Streptococcus pyogenes* infection usually requires therapy and these organisms are always susceptible to penicillin, the drug of choice. However, erythromycin is the drug of choice in the penicillin-allergic patient, and in the United States, between 5% to 10% of *S. pyogenes* isolates are resistant to erythromycin. It may be necessary to perform susceptibility tests on isolates from patients who respond poorly to erythromycin. In contrast, a patient with *E. coli* bacteremia obviously requires therapy and the drug(s) of choice include ampicillin with or without gentamicin. The percentage of *E. coli* susceptible to ampicillin may vary considerably from institution to institution, however, in large tertiary care centers 30% to 50% are usually resistant. Whenever *E. coli* is isolated in significant numbers from clinically significant sources, susceptibility studies are performed with ampicillin and other antimicrobial agents that might be useful.

Table 40-4 Factors to consider in determining when antimicrobial susceptibility tests are performed on bacterial isolates from clinical specimens

Factor	Issue	Examples (generally no need to test)	Examples (generally requires testing)
Body site	If normal flora or probable contaminant, no need to test	Viridans streptococci in sputum (normal flora); diphtheroids in a superficial wound probably represents skin contamination	Viridans streptococci in a blood culture; pure culture of >10⁵ CFU/ml diphtheroids in urine (possibly *Corynebacteriuim* D2)
Predictability of susceptibility to drug(s) of choice	If predictably susceptible, no need to test; if variable susceptibility, test	*S. pyogenes* in wound (always susceptible to penicillin); *N. gonorrhoeae* in urethral specimen (always susceptible to ceftriaxone)	*S. aureus* in wound (has variable antibiogram); *E. coli* in blood (has variable antibiogram)
Quantitation (quantitative cultures)	Large numbers, usually test; small numbers, variable	10,000 CFU/ml *E. coli* in urine (asymptomatic female); one colony coagulase-negative staphylococci from IV catheter tip	>10⁵ CFU/ml *E. coli* in urine (clean catch); >15 colonies coagulase-negative staphylococci from IV catheter tip
Presence of other organisms and quantitation	Pure culture, usually test; mixed culture, variable; presence of normal flora and quantitation are important considerations	Many *E. coli, Enterobacter* spp., and *Citrobacter* spp. in wound (probably represents contamination); few *K. pneumoniae* in presence of normal flora in sputum	Pure culture of *E. coli* in wound; pure culture of *K. pneumoniae* in sputum
Patient age	Determine significance of isolate from particular age group	Moderate *H. influenzae* in presence of normal flora in sputum from 22 year old	Moderate *H. influenzae* in presence of normal flora in sputum of 2 year old
Unique host factors	Immunocompetent, follow general rules; immunosuppressed, some isolates otherwise insignificant may require testing in these patients; allergies to drug(s) of choice	Few *Acinetobacter anitratus* in superficial wound from immunocompetent patient; *S. pyogenes* from penicillin-allergic patient who has responded to erythromycin	Many *A. anitratus* in superficial wound from immunocompetent patient; few *A. anitratus* in superficial wound from liver transplant patient; *S. pyogenes* from penicillin-allergic patient who has not responded to erythromycin

A number of factors are considered when deciding which bacteria require complete identification and which require antimicrobial susceptibility testing. Those related to antimicrobial susceptibility testing are listed with examples in Table 40-4.

Because results of antimicrobial susceptibility tests are generally not available until 1½ to 2 days after specimen acquisition, the clinician obviously is not going to wait to initiate therapy. The initial choice of antimicrobial agent is based on the patient's history, clinical condition, symptoms, and site of the infection, and the physician's previous experience treating similar types of infections. Sometimes a Gram stain or other rapid direct test provides additional information. Cumulative antibiogram data from organisms often involved in this type of infection may also be reviewed. Once the etiologic agent is confirmed and susceptibility test results are available, the clinician may alter therapy depending on the patient's clinical response to empiric therapy and the test results. Generally, the trend is to use an agent that is targeted at the etiologic agent (vs. a broad-spectrum agent) that is the least harmful to the patient and can be provided at the lowest cost. Selecting appropriate therapy is becoming more complicated because of the increasing number of antimicrobial agents available, increasing number of immunosuppressed patients, potential interactions with other medications, and introduction of newer medical procedures such as organ transplants.

Supplemental use of antimicrobial susceptibility test information

In addition to guiding therapy, antimicrobial susceptibility test results may be used for other purposes, primarily of an epidemiologic nature. Because most isolates are usually tested against a panel of antimicrobial agents (often 10 or more), the overall susceptibility profile or antibiogram may be useful to establish strain identity and to type bacteria. In a clinical setting, if two or more isolates have different antibiograms, most likely they are not the same strain. In contrast, if two isolates have the same antibiogram, they may be the same strain and even more so if the antibiogram is unusual. For example, *E. coli* are usually susceptible to most of the antimicrobial agents routinely tested. If there were an outbreak of *E. coli* in a neonatal nursery and all of these isolates were ampicillin-, mezlocillin-, tetracycline-, and trimethoprim/sulfamethoxazole-resistant, a common point of origin would be suspected. If the isolates had a variety of antibiograms, it would be unlikely that they were from a common source. If all isolates were susceptible to all agents tested, it would be more difficult to speculate as to whether or not these represented a common strain. Sometimes the biochemical profile can help establish strain identity, however, additional tests that often include molecular analysis (e.g., plasmid profiling) may be needed.

Accrediting agencies require clinical laboratories to compile cumulative antimicrobial susceptibility statistics on bacteria isolated from patients. This involves determining the percentage of each species susceptible to each agent routinely tested. The percent susceptible can vary significantly among species. For example, in most laboratories nearly all (greater than 90%) *Proteus mirabilis* are susceptible to ampicillin, however, less than 5% of *Enterobacter cloacae* are

---

Box 40-2 Important factors to consider when selecting a system to use for routine antimicrobial susceptibility testing

Accuracy
Reliability (instrument, technical support)
Cost
    Capital equipment
    Consumables
    Labor
Availability of results (rapidity)
Workflow-friendly
User-friendly (acceptance by laboratory technologists)
Versatility (testing, data management)
Drug selection flexibility
Interface capabilities
Good backup strategy when system fails
Physical requirements (space, electrical, storage, etc)
Aesthetics (appearance, noise, amount of waste generated)

---

ampicillin-susceptible. By compiling cumulative statistics periodically (usually quarterly, semiannually, or annually), data can be compared to identify any increasing resistance trends. Significant increases would warrant an epidemiologic investigation. Analysis of cumulative statistics might also identify problems with the antimicrobial test system being used. If greater than 5% of *Enterobacter* spp., *Serratia marcescens*, or *Citrobacter freundii* are ampicillin-susceptible, there may be a problem with inoculum preparation since these species are usually resistant and false susceptible results are often due to inadequate inoculum. These types of problems may not be identified by routine testing of the quality control strains. Cumulative statistics from similar agents, such as the third-generation cephalosporins cefotaxime and ceftriaxone, can be compared to see if there is any superiority of one over the other in terms of in vitro activity against the isolates from a particular institution. This information can be taken into consideration when deciding which agent(s) would better serve the hospital formulary.

Selection of a routine test method

It is difficult for microbiologists to decide which antimicrobial susceptibility test system to use for routine testing. There are numerous systems available and each has its unique advantages and disadvantages. The primary factors that should be considered when deciding which system to use are listed in Box 40-2.

The major decision often involves adopting the standard disk diffusion test vs. an alternative system. The simplicity, reliability, and low cost of disk diffusion are attractive features and many laboratories are often unable to justify going beyond this. Box 40-3 lists some advantages and disadvantages to using disk diffusion routinely.

Although qualitative results (susceptible, moderately susceptible, intermediate, or resistant) are usually sufficient, there are some clinical conditions, some bacteria, and some antimicrobial agents for which quantitative results (MICs) are useful. These are listed in Box 40-4. It is recommended that if MICs are reported, a qualitative categoric interpretation should always accompany the MIC result on the pa-

---

Box 40-3 Advantages and disadvantages to using disk diffusion as a routine antimicrobial susceptibility testing method

REASONS FOR ROUTINE USE

Inexpensive
Drug selection flexibility
Easy to perform
Reliable
Much experience with this method
Few consumables needed
Easy to detect mixed test populations

REASONS AGAINST ROUTINE USE

Lacks sophistication?
Not automated; not interfaceable
Rapid results generally unavailable
Subjective interpretation of endpoints
Cannot detect variations of "susceptible" unless zone diameters are monitored (with MICs, can see if isolates are becoming less "susceptible" within "susceptible" range)
Inappropriate for some organisms and clinical situations
Interpretation based on therapeutically achievable blood levels following standard doses
150-mm plate accommodates only 12 disks (12 antimicrobial agents)

Box 40-4 Specific situations in which MICs are useful

CLINICAL CONDITIONS

Endocarditis
Meningitis
Septicemia
Osteomyelitis
Infections in immunosuppressed patients
Infections involving implants or prosthetic devices

BACTERIA

Viridans streptococci
Methicillin-resistant staphylococci (particularly high-level β-lactamase producers)
Enterococcus (for high-level aminoglycoside resistance)
Pseudomonas aeruginosa (particularly aminoglycosides)
Fastidious bacteria for which disk diffusion interpretive criteria is unavailable

ANTIMICROBIAL AGENTS

Agents with low toxic to therapeutic ratio (e.g., aminoglycosides)
"Intermediate" or "moderately susceptible" results
New agents for which disk diffusion interpretive criteria is unavailable
Drugs that diffuse poorly in agar (e.g., polymyxins)

---

tient report. It would not be unusual for a laboratory to perform the disk diffusion test routinely and perform MICs only in select situations. Strategies for accomplishing this would include maintaining a small inventory of commercial microbroth dilution panels or sending the isolate to a reputable reference laboratory.

Although few studies support a significant impact of rapid reporting of antimicrobial susceptibility test results in terms of clinical decision making, with time and continuing education of clinicians, we will probably confirm that rapid results are advantageous. At this time, laboratorians must weigh the advantages of rapid results against the other factors (primarily cost) when deciding whether or not to use a rapid automated antimicrobial susceptibility test system. It must be emphasized that without some mechanism to ensure that results reach the clinician rapidly, rapid testing offers few advantages.

Incorporation of routine and specialized antimicrobial susceptibility tests into the clinical laboratory

Any clinical laboratory that performs routine bacteriology culture and identification tests can also perform routine antimicrobial susceptibility tests. The expertise required for the standard disk diffusion and microbroth dilution MIC test is comparable to that required to perform bacterial identification tests. The specific materials needed are available from a variety of commercial suppliers and instructions for performing these tests are thoroughly described in documents available from the National Committee for Clinical Laboratory Standards (NCCLS). (See NCCLS publications in Suggested Reading list.) Several rapid tests that detect

antimicrobial inactivating enzymes can likewise be performed with minimal effort.

Hospitalized patients who receive antimicrobial agents such as the aminoglycosides, chloramphenicol, vancomycin, and possibly others, may develop toxic side effects if serum levels become excessive. Close monitoring of serum levels and subsequent adjustment of dosages will usually prevent such complications. Several tests for performing serum level assays for these antimicrobial agents have been described, and reagents are commercially available. Because the test method is usually an immunoassay, these tests are often relegated to the chemistry laboratory. Laboratories equipped to perform immunoassays can easily incorporate antimicrobial immunoassays into their system, providing the volume of tests ordered is sufficient for this to be cost effective.

Generally, information provided from routine antimicrobial susceptibility tests is sufficient to guide clinicians in prescribing appropriate therapy. For severe or unusual infections, infections caused by unusual organisms, or infections in immunocompromised patients, specialized antimicrobial susceptibility tests may be useful. These tests, many of which have not been standardized, require considerably more expertise than that for routine disk diffusion and MIC tests. Additionally, they are more labor-intensive and often, special supplies are needed. All of these factors, together with low demand usually results in their performance only in specialized laboratories. A summary of routine and specialized antimicrobial susceptiblity tests is presented in Table 40-5.

A practical strategy for low-volume laboratories is to utilize a reliable reference laboratory for special tests. The

Table 40-5   In vitro antimicrobial susceptibility tests performed in clinical laboratories

Routine tests performed in most clinical laboratories			
Test	**Primarily performed on**	**Description**	**Results reported as**
Disk diffusion (Bauer Kirby)	Aerobic bacteria	Qualitative measure of the ability of an antimicrobial agent to inhibit the growth of a bacteria; interpretation is based on therapeutically achievable blood levels	Susceptible (S), intermediate (I), moderately susceptible (MS), resistant (R)
Minimum inhibitory concentration (MIC)	Aerobic bacteria, anaerobic bacteria	Quantitative measure of the lowest concentration of antimicrobial agent that inhibits the growth of a bacterium; interpretation is based on therapeutically achievable blood levels	μg/ml with S, I, MS, or R interpretation
β-lactamase	*Moraxella catarrhalis*, *Haemophilus* spp., *Neisseria gonorrhoeae*, *Staphylococcus* spp., some anaerobic bacteria	Qualitative measure of the presence or absence of β-lactamase	β-lactamase positive or β-lactamase negative
	Serum (body fluid) from patient receiving aminoglycosides, chloramphenicol, vancomycin	Quantitative measure of antimicrobial agent concentration (μg/ml) in serum or body fluid (usually performed by immunoassay)	μg/ml

Tests performed in specialized laboratories			
Test	**Primarily performed on**	**Description**	**Results reported as**
Chloramphenicol acetyltransferase (CAT)	*Haemophilus* spp.	Qualitative measure of the presence or absence of chloramphenicol acetyltransferase	CAT positive or CAT negative
Antimicrobial level (assay)			
Minimum bactericidal concentration (MBC)	Aerobic bacteria	Quantitative measure of the lowest concentration of antimicrobial agent that kills a bacterium; currently, no standard criteria for interpretation; results must be compared to levels attainable at infection site	μg/ml
Kill curve	Aerobic bacteria	Quantitative measure of the killing capacity of an antimicrobial agent over time; colony counts are performed on suspensions of organisms at various times following exposure to drug to determine rate of killing	Graphic display of number of colonies remaining at various times
Serum bactericidal test (SBT)	Serum from patient receiving antimicrobial agent(s) and the infecting bacterium isolated from the patient	Measure of antimicrobial activity (inhibitory and cidal) of patient's serum against his/her own infecting bacterium	Dilution of patient's serum inhibitory to and dilution cidal to his/her infecting bacterium
Synergism study	Aerobic bacteria	Quantitative measure of the susceptibility of a bacterial isolate to a combination of two antimicrobial agents; both MIC and MBC of each antimicrobial agent alone and in combination can be determined; (kill curves can also be used to test for synergy)	μg/ml
Proportion method (mycobacteria)	Slow-growing mycobacteria	Qualitative measure of the ability of a specific drug concentration to inhibit 99% of the organisms in the test inoculum	Susceptible or resistant
Radiometric method (mycobacteria)	Slow-growing mycobacteria	Qualitative measure of the ability of a specific drug concentration to inhibit growth as determined by production of radiolabeled CO_2	Susceptible or resistant
MIC and minimum fungicidal concentrations (MFC) (fungi)	Yeasts and molds	Quantitative measure of the lowest concentration of antifungal agent that inhibits the growth (MIC) of a yeast/mold; MFC can also be determined	μg/ml
Plaque reduction	Viruses following treatment failure	Quantitative measure of amount of drug required to reduce plaque yield by 50%	μg/ml

primary factors to consider when selecting a reference laboratory would include the laboratory's reputation, consultation services available, and turnaround time.

Selecting antimicrobial agents for routine testing and reporting

It is impractical and unnecessary to test every antimicrobial agent available against each clinically significant isolate. Each laboratory must determine which antimicrobial agents are appropriate for routine testing in their particular setting. Generally, there would be one panel of 10 to 15 drugs for testing *Enterobacteriaceae* and *Pseudomonas*, and another panel for gram-positive bacteria. Sometimes, a special panel containing antimicrobial agents effective against isolates causing lower urinary tract infections is utilized. And with the recent recommendations for testing *Haemophilus* spp. and *Neisseria gonorrhoeae*, separate panels may be formatted for these groups also.

As described previously, some antimicrobial agents are only effective against either gram-negative or gram-positive isolates, and within each of these organism groups there is considerable variability in susceptibility among its members. For example, the first- and second-generation cephalosporins are sometimes active against *Enterobacteriaceae*, but are never active against *Pseudomonas*. Similarly, penicillin is active against most streptococci, but is inactive against most staphylococci. Antimicrobial agents may show activity in vitro but be ineffective clinically; such is the case for the cephalosporins and enterococci. Clearly the first step in the selection process is to obtain guidance on which drugs would be appropriate to test against specific organism groups.

The NCCLS provides a listing in both their disk diffusion and MIC documents of "Suggested Groupings of Antimicrobial Agents that Should be Considered for Routine Testing and Reporting by Clinical Microbiology Laboratories" (Table 40-6). Although a comparable table is not currently included in the NCCLS document for antimicrobial susceptibility testing of anaerobes, general drug selection information is provided in the foreword of this publication. Ad-

Table 40-6 Suggested groupings of antimicrobial agents that should be considered for routine testing and reporting by clinical microbiology laboratories

	Enterobacteriaceae	Pseudomonas aeruginosa and Acinetobacter[a]	Staphylococci	Enterococci[b]	Streptococci (not Enterococci)	Haemophilus
Group A primary test and report	Ampicillin[c]	Mezlocillin Ticarcillin	Penicillin G	Penicillin G[d] or Ampicillin	Penicillin G	Ampicillin[e]
	Cefazolin[c,f] Cephalothin[c,f]	Gentamicin	Oxacillin or Methicillin			Trimethoprim/Sulfamethoxazole[g]
	Gentamicin[c]		Cefazolin[f,h] or Cephalothin[f,h]			
Group B[i] primary test report selectively	Mezlocillin or Piperacillin Ticarcillin	Azlocillin or Piperacillin	Amoxicillin/Clavulanic Acid[h] **or** Ampicillin/Sulbactam[h]	Vancomycin[j]	Cephalothin[f]	Amoxicillin/Clavulanic Acid[g] **or** Ampicillin/Sulbactam
	Amoxicillin/Clavulanic Acid **or** Ampicillin/Subactam Ticarcillin/Clavulanic Acid	Cefoperazone Ceftazidime[k] Aztreonam	Vancomycin		Vancomycin	Cefaclor[g] Cefixime[g]
			Clindamycin[l]			Cefuroxime
	Cefmetazole Cefoperazone Cefotetan Cefoxitin	Imipenem	Erythromycin[l]		Chloramphenicol[l]	Cefotaxime[m] or Ceftazidime[m] or Ceftizoxime[m] or Ceftriaxone[m]
	Cefamandole or Cefonicid or Cefuroxime		Trimethoprim/Sulfamethoxazole			
	Cefotaxime[k] or Ceftizoxime or Ceftriaxone[k]	Amikacin			Clindamycin	Chloramphenicol[m]
	Imipenem	Tobramycin			Erythromycin	Tetracycline[g]
	Amikacin	Ciprofloxacin				
	Ciprofloxacin[c]					
	Trimethoprim/Sulfamethoxazole[c]					

Continued.

Table 40-6 Suggested groupings of antimicrobial agents that should be considered for routine testing and reporting by clinical microbiology laboratories—cont'd

	Enterobacteriaceae	Pseudomonas aeruginosa and Acinetobacter[a]	Staphylococci	Enterococci[b]	Streptococci (not Enterococci)	Haemophilus
Group C[n] supplemental report selectively	**Ceftazidime Aztreonam**	Cefotaxime or Ceftriaxone	**Cefotaxime[h] or Ceftriaxone[h]**		**Cefotaxime[h] or Ceftriaxone**	Cefamandole Cefonicid
		Netilmicin	Imipenem[h]		**Tetracycline**	**Imipenem[o]**
	Kanamycin	Chloramphenicol[p]	**Gentamicin**		Ofloxacin	**Aztreonam**
	Netilmicin	Trimethoprim/ Sulfamethoxazole[p]	Ciprofloxacin **or Ofloxacin**			**Ciprofloxacin[g] or Ofloxacin[g]**
	Tobramycin		Chloramphenicol[i]			Rifampin
	Tetracycline[c]		Rifampin			
	Chloramphenicol[i]		**Tetracycline[q]**			
Group D supplemental for urine only	**Carbenicillin**	**Carbenicillin**	Norfloxacin	Ciprofloxacin Norfloxacin	Norfloxacin	
	Cinoxacin Norfloxacin **or Ofloxacin**	Ceftizoxime	Nitrofurantoin	Nitrofurantoin	Nitrofurantoin	
	Nitrofurantoin	Tetracycline[p,q]	Sulfisoxazole	Tetracycline		
	Sulfisoxazole	Norfloxacin **or Ofloxacin**	Trimethoprim			
	Trimethoprim	Sulfisoxazole				

Permission to use portions of M2-A4 (Performance Standards for Antimicrobial Disk Susceptibility Tests—Fourth Edition; Approved Standard) and M7-A2 (Methods for Dilution Antimicrobial Susceptibility Tests for Bacteria that Grow Aerobically—Second Edition; Approved Standard) has been granted by the National Committee for Clinical Laboratory Standards. NCCLS is not responsible for errors or inaccuracies. The latest M2 and M7 editions and their current supplements may be obtained from NCCLS, 771 E. Lancaster Avenue, Villanova, PA 19085.

NOTE 1: Selection of the most appropriate antimicrobial agents to test is a decision best made by each clinical laboratory in consultation with the infectious disease practitioners, the pharmacy, and the pharmacy and/or infection control committees of the medical staff. The lists comprise agents of proven clinical efficacy for that organism group which show acceptable *in vitro* test performance. **Considerations in the assignment of agents to Groups A, B, C, and D included clinical efficacy, prevalence of resistance, minimizing emergence of resistance, cost, and current consensus recommendations for first choice and alternative drugs, in addition to the specific comments in footnotes i and n.** Tests on selected agents may be useful for infection control purposes.

NOTE 2: The boxes in the table designate clusters of comparable agents that need not be duplicated in testing because interpretive results usually will be similar and clinical efficacy comparable. In addition, an *or* designates a related group of agents which show a nearly identical spectrum of activity and interpretive results and for which cross-resistance and susceptibility is nearly complete. Therefore, usually only one of the agents within each selection box (cluster or related group) need be selected for testing. Agents reported must be tested (**unless reporting based on testing another agent provides a more accurate result, e.g., susceptibility to cefazolin or cephalothin based on oxacillin testing**) and usually should match those included in the hospital formulary, or else the report should include footnotes indicating the agents which usually show comparable interpretive results. **Lastly, unexpected results should be considered for reporting (e.g., resistance of *Enterobacteriaceae* to third-generation cephalosporins or imipenem).**

NOTE 3: Information in boldface type is considered **tentative** for one year.

FOOTNOTES

a. Other non-Enterobacteriaceae should be tested by the dilution method (see M7-A2).

b. Antimicrobial agents not listed in this column such as the cephalosporins, clindamycin, and the aminoglycosides should not be tested and/or reported against the enterococci because the reporting of their results can be dan-

gerously misleading (except for high level aminoglycoside screening for resistance; see text 2.5.3.3 in M7-A2).

c. May be appropriate for inclusion in a panel for testing of urinary tract isolates along with the agents in Group D.

d. Penicillin G susceptibility may be used to predict the susceptibility to ampicillin, amoxicillin, acylampicillins, ampicillin/sulbactam, and amoxicillin/ clavulanic acid to which non-β-lactamase producing enterococci are also "moderately susceptible." However, combination therapy of penicillin G or ampicillin, plus an aminoglycoside, is usually indicated for serious enterococcal infections such as endocarditis. For blood and CSF isolates a β-lactamase test is also recommended.

e. The results of ampicillin susceptibility tests may be used to predict the activity of amoxicillin. The vast majority of clinical isolates of *Haemophilus influenzae* that are resistant to ampicillin and amoxicillin produce a TEM-type β-lactamase. As a result, in most cases, a β-lactamase test alone can be used to predict the activity of these two agents.

f. Cephalothin should be tested to represent cephalothin, cefaclor (except against *Haemophilus*), cephapirin, cephradine, cephalexin, cefadroxil, cefazolin, and loracarbef. Cefazolin can be tested additionally against *Enterobacteriaceae* because strains resistant to cephalothin and other first-generation cephalosporins may be susceptible to cefazolin.

g. The results of tests with agents that are administered only by the oral route should be reported only with isolates of *Haemophilus* spp. from localized, non-life-threatening infections (e.g., uncomplicated cases of otitis media and sinusitis, and selected bronchopulmonary infections).

h. Staphylococci exhibiting resistance to methicillin, oxacillin, or nafcillin should be reported as also resistant to cephalosporins, carbapenems, and β-lactamase inhibitor combinations despite apparent *in vitro* susceptibility of some strains to the latter agents. This is because infections with methicillin-resistant staphylococci have not responded favorably to therapy with β-lactam antibiotics.

i. Group B-**Represents agents which may warrant primary testing but which should be reported only selectively, such as when the organism is resistant to agents of the same family in Group A. Other indications for reporting the**

result might include selected specimen sources (e.g., third generation cephalosporin for isolates of enteric bacteria and **H. influenzae** from cerebrospinal fluid, or trimethoprim/sulfamethoxazole for urinary tract isolates), **stated allergy or intolerance or failure to respond to an agent in Group A, polymicrobial infections, infections involving multiple sites with different microorganisms, or reports to infection control for epidemiologic aid.**

j. Vancomycin is often used for serious enterococcal infections in patients with significant penicillin allergy. It should be reported selectively (or footnoted) as being indicated only in such patients. **Combination therapy with vancomycin plus an aminoglycoside is usually indicated for serious enterococcal infections such as endocarditis.**

k. **Should be reported on isolates from CSF along with agents in Group A.**

l. Not routinely tested against organisms isolated from the urinary tract.

m. The result of testing with one of the extended spectrum cephalosporins and chloramphenicol should be reported routinely with all isolates of *Haemophilus influenzae* recovered from patients with serious, life-threatening infections (e.g., meningitis, bacteremia, epiglottitis, facial cellulitis, etc.)

n. Group C-Represents alternative or supplemental antimicrobial agents that may required testing in those institutions harboring endemic or epidemic strains resistant to one or more of the primary drugs (especially in the same family, e.g., β-lactams or aminoglycosides), or for treatment of unusual organisms (e.g., chloramphenicol for some *Pseudomonas* spp.), or reporting to infection control as an epidemiologic aid.

o. *Haemophilus* **is usually susceptible to imipenem and routine testing may not be necessary.**

p. **May be indicated for primary testing of some *Pseudomonas* spp. other than *P. aeruginosa* and *Acinetobacter* spp. (ampicillin/sulbactam may be tested for strains resistant to other agents).**

q. Doxycycline or minocycline may be tested in place of or in addition to tetracycline for some isolates of *S. aureus* and nonfermentative, gram-negative bacilli (e.g., *Acinetobacter* spp.) but should not be used to predict tetracycline susceptibility.

Table 40-7   Questions that must be addressed when determining which antimicrobial agents to test/report routinely

Question	Comments, examples
What is the age of the patient population?	Some antimicrobials are inappropriate for certain age groups (e.g., quinolones are contraindicated in children because of potential adverse effect on cartilage development)
What is the patient mix in terms of inpatient or outpatients?	It would be inappropriate to test numerous drugs that can only be administered parenterally (IM or IV) in a setting that primarily serves outpatients
Are many patients immunocompromised?	It is often necessary to prescribe broad-spectrum and very "potent" agents to these patients where bactericidal activity is of great importance
What types of infections are encountered?	For more serious infections, include parenteral agents that would get to the site of the infection rapidly (e.g., drugs that cross the blood-brain barrier for meningitis)
	For less serious infections, include oral agents (including urinary tract agents, if appropriate)
	For burn patients who are likely to contract *Pseudomonas aeruginosa* wound infections, include many anti-pseudomonal agents
What drugs are on the hospital formulary?	The hospital formulary includes drugs determined by the medical staff to be appropriate for utilization in the particular institution; efficacy and cost play a major role in formulary decisions
What drugs are actually being used?	If the agent is not being used, there is little reason to test; however, it has been shown that laboratory reporting correlates significantly with antimicrobial agent usage
What are the antibiograms of the isolated bacteria?	It is important to test agents that are likely to have activity against bacteria encountered in a particular setting
What are the most common etiologic agents causing nosocomial infections in your institution?	Often, nosocomial isolates are more resistant and it is important to test agents that are likely to have activity against bacteria encountered in these settings
Are numerous highly resistant bacteria encountered?	It may be appropriate to include a panel containing broad-spectrum agents active against the more resistant bacteria (there may not be room for all of these on the primary panel)

ditional information may be found in the critiques that accompany proficiency testing results coordinated by the College of American Pathologists.

In addition to the NCCLS documents and other reference material, each laboratory must obtain input from pharmacy, infection control, infectious diseases, and other medical services when establishing a policy that would be most beneficial for patient care. In developing this policy, several questions must be asked, which are listed in Table 40-7.

As can be seen, the NCCLS table (Table 40-6) categorizes drugs into four groups: (1) drugs that should be routinely tested and reported, (2) drugs that should be routinely tested but reported selectively, (3) drugs that should be tested only in select situations, and (4) drugs that should only be considered for isolates from the lower urinary tract. There are some drugs that have nearly identical in vitro activity, nearly identical interpretive results, and comparable clinical

efficacy against a particular organism group. An example would be the third-generation cephalosporins cefotaxime, ceftizoxime, and ceftriaxone against the *Enterobacteriacae*. These are identified with "or" connectors in the NCCLS tables and it is usually necessary to routinely test only one of these. If an isolate was susceptible to cefotaxime, it would be susceptible to the others. Despite this ability to extrapolate qualitative results (MIC values may not be identical), exceptions to these rules do exist and the most accurate results are obviously obtained when the specific agent is actually tested. The agent tested is the one that must be reported; however, a footnote indicating the similarities in activities to the other agents might also be included. Because of the similarity in activity, interpretive results, and clinical efficacy among the drugs included in boxed areas in the table, generally, only one is tested. The agent tested is that most commonly used in a particular institution.

In addition to recommending appropriate drugs for testing and reporting, the NCCLS tables convey that certain drugs are inappropriate for testing against particular organisms and that results with these combinations may be misleading. For example, cephalosporins and clindamycin should not be tested against enterococci because these are clinically ineffective despite in vitro activity. As another example, penicillin results should always be used to predict the activity of extended-spectrum penicillinase-labile penicillins (e.g., carbenicillin, mezlocillin, pipercillin, ticarcillin) against staphylococci. The disk diffusion interpretive criteria for the extended-spectrum agents relates primarily to gram-negative bacteria and results may be erroneous if these criteria are applied to staphylococci.

Because the identification of the isolate is usually not known at the time the susceptibility test is performed, it would be impossible to selectively test only those drugs appropriate for reporting on the particular isolate. The most practical and widely used approach is to test a panel of agents and then selectively report those drugs appropriate for the species identified, taking into consideration the overall antibiogram and specimen source.

The panel of drugs tested usually includes several primary and second-line antimicrobial agents. Utilization of a panel that contains primary agents only would result in unnecessary delays in testing and reporting second-line drugs when an isolate is resistant to the primary agent(s). Generally, second-line drugs should only be reported when the isolate is resistant to the primary agent(s). This holds true for antimicrobial agents within a specific class, which can best be illustrated with the aminoglycosides, extended-spectrum penicillins, and cephalosporins. The hierarchy of activities for members of these groups is indicated in Box 40-5. As an example of selective reporting, tobramycin would only be reported on *Pseudomonas aeruginosa* if the isolate is gentamicin-resistant. Similarly, second-generation

cephalosporins would only be reported on *Escherichia coli* if the isolate is resistant to first-generation cephalosporins.

Information is also provided in the NCCLS tables for reporting depending on the body site. For example, drugs that cross the blood-brain barrier such as cefotaxime should be reported on *Enterobacteriaceae* isolated from cerebrospinal fluid even if the isolate is susceptible to cefazolin, which is not effective for meningitis. It is suggested that results for oral agents only be reported from localized, non–life-threatening *Haemophilus* spp. infections. Cinoxacin, norfloxacin, nitrofurantion, trimethoprim, and sulfonamides are only effective against susceptible strains of *Enterobacteriaceae* isolated from urine and it would be misleading to report results for these agents on isolates from other body sites.

The results of all drugs tested should be recorded whether reported or not for statistical and epidemiological purposes and for those select situations when these supplemental results may be clinically useful, such as when the patient cannot tolerate or is not responding to a primary agent.

The goals of selective reporting are to assist the clinician in selecting the most appropriate antimicrobial agent and to prevent indiscriminate use of more costly and toxic agents. Additionally, controlled use of antimicrobial agents will help preserve the spectrum of activity of new agents by

---

Box 40-5 General hierarchy of activity for aminoglycosides, cephalosporins, and extended-spectrum penicillins against *Enterobacteriaceae* and *Pseudomonas aeruginosa*

AMINOGLYCOSIDES

Enterobacteriaceae:	amikacin > tobramycin > gentamicin
Pseudomonas:	amikacin > tobramycin > gentamicin

CEPHALOSPORINS

Enterobacteriaceae:	third generation > second generation > first generation
Pseudomonas:	first- and second-generation agents have no activity against *Pseudomonas aeruginosa*

EXTENDED-SPECTRUM PENICILLINS

Enterobacteriaceae:	piperacillin = mezlocillin > ticarcillin > carbenicillin
Pseudomonas:	piperacillin > azlocillin > mezlocillin = ticarcillin > carbenicillin

---

Table 40-8 Examples of antimicrobial agents reported following a selective reporting* protocol

E. COLI

Source: urine

Primary agents	Result	Second-Line agents
Ampicillin	S	
Cefazolin	S	Not reported
Gentamicin	S	
Norfloxacin	S	
Trimethoprim/sulfa	S	

PSEUDOMONAS AERUGINOSA

Source: blood

Primary agents	Result	Second-Line agents
Mezlocillin	S	
Gentamicin	S	Not reported

E. COLI

Source: wound

Primary agents	Result	Second-Line agents	Result
Ampicillin	R	Ampicillin/sulbactam	R
Cefazolin	R	Cefuroxime	S
Gentamicin	S		

PSEUDOMONAS AERUGINOSA

Source: blood

Primary agents	Result	Second-Line agents	Result
Mezlocillin	R	Amikacin	S
Gentamicin	R	Ceftazidime	S
		Piperacillin	S
		Tobramycin	R

*S, susceptible; R, resistant.

minimizing the potential for development of resistance. Several specific reporting examples following a selective reporting protocol are shown in Table 40-8.

Clinical significance of MIC results

Optimal use of an MIC requires correlation with the antimicrobial level attainable at the site of the infection. Antimicrobial levels vary significantly depending on dosage and body site. Higher drug concentrations are usually attainable in urine compared to blood and the concentration in soft tissue is usually comparable to blood concentrations. This is illustrated for ampicillin and gentamicin in Table 40-9.

The concentration of antimicrobial agent that diffuses into the CSF often depends on inflammation of the meninges. With ampicillin, higher levels result when inflammation is present. Some agents, such as the aminoglycosides, do not adequately cross the blood-brain barrier even if there is inflammation and are usually ineffective in treating meningitis despite in vitro susceptibility.

Generally, it is desirable to obtain a drug concentration at the infection site that is four times the MIC of the infecting isolate. Therefore if an isolate of *E. coli* from blood had an ampicillin MIC of 8 μg/ml, it would be desirable to obtain blood levels of at least 32 μg/ml. Barring unforeseen complications, this could be accomplished with an intravenous 1-g dose. If this same isolate was causing a lower urinary tract infection, an oral dose of 0.25 g would probably be effective since ampicillin is concentrated in urine.

Clinical significance of categoric interpretation of susceptibility test results

It can be misleading to report an MIC result without a qualitative interpretation as it is not uncommon for clinicians to ignore pharmacokinetic factors and select an antimicrobial agent based on the lowest MIC value reported. For example, a clinician may select the more toxic gentamicin over ampicillin for an *E. coli* organism that is susceptible to both agents (ampicillin = 4 μg/ml; gentamicin = 0.5 μg/ml).

Initially, results of antimicrobial susceptibility tests were reported as either "susceptible" or "resistant." However, the NCCLS interpretive tables now include the two additional categories "moderately susceptible" and "intermediate."

The breakpoints used for "susceptible," "moderately susceptible," "intermediate," or "resistant" are based on: (1) therapeutically achievable serum levels, (2) microbiological data that includes population distributions of zone diameters or MICs for the respective agent, and (3) data resulting from extensive clinical treatment trials. The complete NCCLS definitions of the four interpretive categories (which are identical for both disk and MIC procedures) are shown in Box 40-6.

"Intermediate" or "moderately susceptible" results are often misunderstood. For drugs with "moderately susceptible" ranges, increasing the dose beyond standard recommendations may be effective in treating isolates with moderately susceptible zones or MICs. Intermediate results should be considered equivocal and if the isolate is not susceptible to alternative agents that might be used, testing should be repeated. For some drugs (e.g., oxacillin), no "moderately susceptible" or "intermediate" range is defined.

Adequate therapy for "susceptible" organisms may require different dosing regimens (amount, frequency, and route of administration) depending on the severity of the infection, the infection site, and the species causing the infection. For example, therapy for otitis in a child caused by an ampicillin-susceptible *Haemophilus influenzae* organism might be 50 mg/kg/day (orally, four times/day) ampicillin, whereas treatment of the same isolate causing meningitis would be up to 250 mg/kg/day (intravenously every 4 hours). An ampicillin-susceptible *E. coli* organism causing cystitis in an adult might be treated with 250 mg (orally every 6 hours), however, treatment of septicemic pyelonephritis caused by the same isolate would require 2 g (intravenously every 4 hours). When reporting results, the laboratory must make the assumption that the clinician is aware of appropriate therapeutic regimens for the respective situation.

It is important that the laboratory assist clinicians in understanding the meaning of the antimicrobial susceptibility test results. The definitions of "susceptible," "moderately susceptible," "intermediate," and "resistant" can either be included as a footnote or printed on the back of the patient's report. Because of the similarities in "moderately susceptible" and "intermediate" definitions and the difficulties in conveying the differences to clinicians, some have elected to interpret all results that are not susceptible or resistant as

Table 40-9   Levels of ampicillin and gentamicin attainable at various body sites following standard recommended dosages

Antimicrobial agent	Dose (g)	Attainable peak serum levels (μg/ml)	Attainable urine levels (μg/ml)	Bile levels (multiple of serum levels)	CSF inflamed meninges (% of serum levels)	CSF normal meninges (% of serum levels)
Ampicillin	PO 0.25 q6h	1.5-2.5	50-75			
	PO 0.5 q6h	2.5-4.0	250-500			
	PO 1.0 q6h	4.0-6.0	500-1000	100	30%-90%	Nil
	IV 1.0 q4h	40-60	>1000			
	IV 2.0 q4h	80-120	>1000			
Gentamicin	IM or IV q8h (1.5-2.0 mg/kg)	5-7	50-100	0.1-0.2	10%-30%	Nil

either moderately susceptible or intermediate. The definition of the notation selected would obviously require revision. Sometimes it might be helpful to include additional notes on the patient report. For example, a note that suggests the need for combined therapy with a cell wall active agent and an aminoglycoside in the case of serious enterococcal infections would provide a safeguard against misinterpretation.

Correlation of in vitro results with clinical outcome: predictive value of antimicrobial susceptibility test results

Although there is extensive documentation examining the in vitro activity of antimicrobial agents and test methods, there is limited information that addresses the clinical correlation of in vitro results with clinical outcome. In order for an antimicrobial agent to be effective in vivo, an adequate amount of active drug must reach the infecting or-

---

Box 40-6 Summary of NCCLS interpretive categories for antimicrobial susceptibility test results

Susceptible. This category implies that an infection due to the strain may be appropriately treated with the dosage of antimicrobial agent recommended for that type of infection and infecting species, unless contraindicated.

Moderately susceptible. This category includes strains that may be inhibited by attainable concentrations of certain antimicrobial agents (e.g., β-lactams), provided higher dosages are used, or in body sites (e.g., urine) where the drugs are physiologically concentrated.

For enterococci, aerococci, and nonenterococcal streptococci, "moderately susceptible" implies the need for high-dose penicillin or ampicillin, and for serious infections such as endocarditis, combined therapy with ampicillin, penicillin, or vancomycin and an aminoglycoside is indicated to achieve bactericidal activity.

Because all but rare nonenterococcal streptococci are highly susceptible to penicillin or ampicillin, a "moderately susceptible" result warrants retesting and should have an MIC determined in cases of endocarditis. Enterococcal urinary infections may be treated with ampicillin or penicillin alone.

Intermediate. This category provides a "buffer zone" that should prevent small, uncontrolled, technical factors from causing major discrepancies in interpretations (e.g., species that should have few or no end points in this range, or drugs affected by media variation or with narrow pharmacotoxicity margins). For drugs with zones falling within the range defined as intermediate, the results may be considered equivocal and, if the organism is not fully susceptible to alternative clinically feasible drugs, the test should be repeated.

Resistant. Resistant strains are not inhibited by the usually achievable systemic concentrations of the agent with normal dosage schedules and/or a fall in the range where specific microbial resistance mechanisms are likely (e.g., β-lactamases), and clinical efficacy has not been reliable in treatment studies.

From National Committee for Clinical Laboratory Standards. Performance standards for antimicrobial disk susceptibility tests, ed 4, Approved Standard M2-A4, Villanova, PA, 1990, NCCLS.

---

ganisms. This is influenced by a number of factors that include: the degree of protein binding (only unbound drug can diffuse through interstitial spaces and exert an antibacterial effect), dosage and route of administration, antimicrobial level fluctuations, physiologic compartmentalization of the drug (amount distributed in blood, urine, CSF, etc.), and renal and hepatic function of the patient. The suitability of the in vivo environment for antibacterial activity (e.g., pH, oxygenation, antimicrobial inactivating factors that might be present, etc.) plays a major role. The patient's underlying immune status, the virulence of the bacteria causing the infection; and the numbers of organisms present also effect the outcome of therapy.

Therapy with an agent that appears active in vitro may fail in vivo if the organisms develop resistance or tolerance to the agent. Therapy may fail if an infection that requires bactericidal activity such as endocarditis or osteomyelitis, or an infection in immunocompromised patients, is treated with a bacteriostatic agent. If the organism has produced an abscess, drainage is often necessary to enhance exposure of the infecting organisms to the antimicrobial agent.

Sometimes therapy is unsuccessful if the patient's underlying clinical condition worsens or if the patient develops a superinfection. Combination therapy with drugs that are antagonistic may also result in therapeutic failure. Occasionally, the pathogen may be protected by another organism. An example would be a mixed infection with a penicillinase-producing staphylococcus and *Streptococcus pyogenes*. Treatment of the streptococcus with penicillin may be compromised by penicillinase produced by the staphylococcus. Finally, misidentification of the etiologic agent, failure to recover the true etiologic agent in the presence of multiple organisms, or unrecognized polymicrobial infections may result in failure of the prescribed agent to cure the infection.

It has been well documented that for some specific drug/bug combinations, in vitro activity correlates poorly with clinical outcome. Methicillin-resistant staphylococci may appear susceptible to cephalosporins in vitro, but these agents are ineffective in vivo. Similarly, first-generation cephalosporins may appear active against salmonellae and meningococci in vitro, but these agents are of no use clinically. Enterococci often appear susceptible to cephalosporins and clindamycin in vitro, but enterococcal infections cannot be successfully treated with these agents.

Clearly, the predictive value of susceptible results in predicting therapeutic success may vary considerably depending on the host status, the organism causing the infection, and the agent prescribed. The predictive value of a resistant result is much better at predicting therapeutic failure, particularly in serious infections or where there is immunosuppression; however, this correlation is not absolute.

METHODS FOR PERFORMING ANTIMICROBIAL SUSCEPTIBILITY TESTS
Standardized vs. nonstandardized methods

There are a number of in vitro test methods that can be used to assess the effectiveness of antimicrobial agents against specific bacteria. Some of these have been well standardized and generate results that have been shown to be accurate and reproducible. Standardization of a method must take into account many variables of the test, including, but not limited to: concentration of organisms in the test inoculum, media (reagents) used, concentration(s) of antimicrobial agent(s) used, incubation conditions, and measurement of end points.

The standardization methods that are most widely used in clinical laboratories are those described by the National Committee for Clinical Laboratory Standards (NCCLS). In producing their documents, the NCCLS works on a voluntary consensus mechanism. The Subcommittee on Antimicrobial Susceptibility Testing is composed of 13 individuals (representatives from clinical laboratories, laboratory and professional associations, industry, and agencies of the federal and state governments) with significant expertise in antimicrobial susceptibility testing. The NCCLS working

committees continually solicit input from users of the documents and address the concerns of the users in reformulating subsequent editions of each document. The documents currently available from the NCCLS that directly relate to antimicrobial susceptibility testing in clinical laboratories are listed in Table 40-10.

Routine antimicrobial susceptibility testing methods

Disk diffusion testing

The disk diffusion test, often referred to as the Kirby Bauer test, is one of the most widely used antimicrobial susceptibility tests in clinical laboratories. As early as 1940, researchers were immersing pieces of filter paper in solutions of antimicrobial agents and placing these on a freshly inoculated lawn of bacteria on an agar plate. The plate was incubated overnight and examined for the presence of zones of inhibition, which would indicate some antimicrobial activity against the test bacteria. In 1966, the first standardized disk diffusion method was described by Bauer, Kirby, Sherris, and Turck, and this method that incorporates the use of single, high-content antimicrobial disks, is basically the procedure upon which the currently used disk diffusion methods are based.

The standard disk diffusion test is acceptable for testing rapidly growing, nonfastidious aerobic bacteria, including the *Enterobacteriaceae*, *Pseudomonas*, *Acinetobacter*, staphylococci, and enterococci. Slight modifications of the standard method are used for testing *Haemophilus* spp., *Neisseria gonorrhoeae*, and *Streptococcus* spp. (including *Streptococcus pneumoniae*).

The first step in performing the disk diffusion test is inoculum preparation. This is accomplished by either suspending fresh growth taken from an overnight agar plate in saline or broth, or growing organisms in a broth to log phase (2 to 8 hours) to obtain a suspension with turbidity that is equivalent to a 0.5 McFarland turbidity standard (corresponds to approximately 1.5×10^8 CFU/ml). A sterile swab is dipped into this suspension and then used to thor-

Table 40-10 NCCLS documents for antimicrobial susceptibility testing

Document no.	Title
M2-A4	Performance standards for antimicrobial disk susceptibility tests; approved standard
M7-A2	Methods for dilution antimicrobial susceptibility tests for bacteria that grow aerobically; approved standard
M11-A2	Methods for antimicrobial susceptibility testing of anaerobic bacteria; approved standard
M20-CR	Antifungal susceptibility testing; committee report
M23-T	Development of in vitro susceptibility testing criteria and quality control parameters; tentative guideline
M24-P	Antimycobacterial susceptibility testing; proposed standard
M21-P	Methodology for the serum bactericidal test; proposed guideline
M26-P	Methods for determining bactericidal activity of antimicrobial agents; proposed guideline

Obtained from the National Committee for Clinical Laboratory Standards, 771 East Lancaster Avenue, Villanova, PA 19085.

Table 40-11 Zone interpretive standards and equivalent minimum inhibitory concentration (MIC) breakpoints for organisms other than *Haemophilus* and *Neisseria gonorrhoeae*

Antimicrobial agent	Disk content (μg)	Zone Diameter, nearest whole mm				Equivalent MIC breakpoints (μg/ml)	
		Resistant	Intermediate	Moderately susceptible	Susceptible	Resistant	Susceptible
Ampicillin							
When testing gram-negative enteric organisms	10	≤13	—	14-16	≥17	≥32	≤8
When testing staphylococci	10	≤28	—	—	≥29	β-lactamase	≤0.25
When testing enterococci	10	≤16	—	≥17	—	≥16	—
When testing nonenterococcal streptococci	10	≤21	—	22-29	≥30	≥4	≤0.12
When testing *Listeria monocytogenes*	10	≤19	—	—	≥20	≥4	≤2.0
Cephalothin	30	≤14	—	15-17	≥18	≥32	≤8
Gentamicin	10	≤12	13-14	—	≥15	≥8	≤4
Mezlocillin		≤15	—	—	≥16	—	—
When testing *Pseudomonas*	75	≤17	—	—	≥18	≥128	≤64
When testing other gram-negative organisms	75	≤17	—	18-20	≥21	≥128	≤16

From National Committee for Clinical Laboratory Standards: M100-S3: Supplemtal tables for M2-A4, M7-A2, amd M11-A2, Villanova, Pa, 1991, NCCLS.

oughly inoculate the surface of a Mueller-Hinton agar plate. Antimicrobial disks are placed on the inoculated surface. Following overnight incubation at 35° C, the diameters of the zones of inhibition around each disk are measured. Each millimeter value for each drug is compared to a table (see example in Table 40-11) to determine if the isolate is susceptible, of intermediate susceptibility, moderately suscep-

tible, or resistant to the specific antimicrobial agent. For some drugs (e.g., ampicillin), there are separate interpretive criteria to use for testing various species or organism groups.

The disk diffusion test is easy to perform, the materials are reasonably priced and readily available from a variety of commercial sources, no special equipment is required, and by following the standard method as described in the

Table 40-12 Primary variables that must be controlled when performing routine disk diffusion and microbroth dilution MIC tests

Variable	Standard	Comments
Inoculum	Disk diffusion: 1.5×10^8 CFU/ml Microbroth dilution: 5×10^5 CFU/ml (final concentration)	Use "adequate" McFarland turbidity standard (usually 0.5); when preparing direct suspensions (without incubation), do not use growth from plates >1 day old
Media		
Formulation	Mueller-Hinton	Prepare in house or purchase from reliable source; perform media quality control to verify acceptability prior to use for patient tests
Ca^{++} Mg^{++} content	25 mg/L Ca^{++}, 12.5 mg/L Mg^{++}	Excessive concentrations can result in false resistance of *Pseudomonas aeruginosa* to aminoglycosides and decreased activity of tetracyclines (lower concentrations have the opposite effect)
Thymidine content	Minimal or absent	Excessive concentrations can result in false resistance to sulfonamides and trimethoprim
pH	7.2-7.4	Decreased pH can lead to decreased activity of aminoglycosides, erythromycin, clindamycin, and increased activity of tetracyclines (increased pH has the opposite effect)
Agar depth (disk diffusion)	3-5 mm	Possibility for false susceptible results if <3mm; false resistance results if >5 mm
Antimicrobial agents		
Disks	Use disks containing appropriate FDA/NCCLS defined concentration of drug, proper storage, proper placement on agar	Check NCCLS publication or FDA package insert (accompanying disks) for specifications Long-term storage in *non*-frost free freezer at ≤ − 20°C in tightly sealed, desiccated container; short-term storage (≤1 week) at 2°C-8°C in tightly sealed desiccated container; allow to warm to room temperature before opening container ≤12 disks/150-mm plate (no overlapping zones)
Solutions	Prepare from reference standard powders, proper storage	Pharmacy grade antimicrobial solutions are unacceptable, may not show antibacterial activity in vitro; store in *non*-frost free freezer at ≤ − 20°C; ≤ − 70°C needed for some drugs; never refreeze
Incubation		
Atmosphere	Humidified ambient air	CO_2 incubation decreases pH, which can lead to decreased activity of aminoglycosides, erythromycin, clindamycin, and increased activity of tetracyclines
Temperature	34°C - 35°C	Some methicillin-resistant *S. aureus* (MRSA) may go undetected if >35°C
Length	Disk diffusion: 16-18 h Microbroth dilution: 16-20 h (24 h staphylococci with oxacillin*; 24 h sometimes needed for fastidious bacteria)	Some MRSA may go undetected if <24 h
End Point Measurement		
Disk diffusion	Use reflected light and hold plate against black background; measure zones from back of plate (except staphylococci and oxacillin*)	Lawn must be confluent or almost confluent; ignore faint growth of tiny colonies at zone edge; trimethoprim and sulfonamides—end point at ≥80% inhibition; ignore swarm within obvious zone for swarming *Proteus* spp.; retest colonies within zone (except staphylococci and oxacillin*)
	Use transmitted light for staphylococci and oxacillin*	Call resistant if *any* growth within zone (unless possibly artifactual or contaminated)
Microbroth dilution	Use adequate lighting/reading device	MIC = lowest concentration that inhibits growth (turbidity, haze, or pellet); sulfonamides and trimethoprim may trail (ignore trailing <2-mm buttons); justify "skip wells" or repeat; staphylococci and penicillin—perform induced β-lactamase test if MIC is 0.06-0.12 µg/ml; reproducibility within ± 1 twofold dilution

*Includes all penicillinase-resistant penicillins (oxacillin, methicillin, nafcillin, cloxacillin, dicloxacillin, and flucloxacillin).

NCCLS document, accurate and reproducible results are obtained. However, some special precautions must be emphasized regarding controlling the variables when performing this test. These are listed in Table 40-12.

Tests that determine minimum inhibitory concentrations (MIC tests)

A quantitative measure of the inhibitory activity of an antimicrobial agent can be determined by testing a standardized number of bacteria against serial, twofold dilutions of antimicrobial agent in broth or agar. Originally, dilution tests were performed using broth dispensed in test tubes; a separate tube was used for testing each concentration of each drug. This macrobroth dilution method can be reasonably used for testing a few organisms against a few antimicrobial agents, but because of the materials and labor required, it is not practical for use as a routine testing method when it is usually necessary to test a battery of antimicrobial agents against each isolate. Some clinical laboratories may elect to use the macrobroth dilution method as a supplemental method for testing drugs not available in the routine testing system, for testing fastidious organisms where special testing conditions are required, or for performing minimal bactericidal concentration (MBC) tests. However, the macrobroth dilution method has been adapted to multiwell microdilution trays, increasing the number of drugs that can be tested against a single isolate at one time. Many clinical laboratories find it advantageous to utilize this microbroth dilution (MIC) method as their routine testing method.

The standard microdilution tray is constructed of polystyrene and contains 96 wells. Small volumes (generally 0.1 ml) of serial, twofold dilutions of antimicrobial agent in broth are dispensed in each well. The broth most commonly used is Mueller-Hinton that has been adjusted to contain defined concentrations of the divalent cations Ca^{++} and Mg^{++} (cation-adjusted Mueller-Hinton broth). Depending on the number of antimicrobial agents tested, between four and eight concentrations of each are included. The range of concentrations tested for any given drug represents the concentrations attainable in a patient's blood and testing of concentrations that may produce toxic side effects are avoided. Sometimes higher concentrations are tested against bacteria isolated from urine to represent the higher concentrations of antimicrobial agent obtained in urine. Two control wells are included; the positive growth well contains broth plus inoculum and the negative growth well contains broth only. A diagramatic representation of a typical tray format that might be used for testing gram-negative bacteria is shown in Fig. 40-2.

AMK	AMP	AMP/ SUL	CEF	CFUR	CFTX	CFTZ	GENT	MEZ	PIP	TOB	+ CONT
0.25[1]	0.25	0.25	0.25	0.25	0.25	0.25	0.25	2.0	2.0	0.25	- CONT
0.5	0.5	0.5	0.5	0.5	0.5	0.5	0.5	4.0	4.0	0.5	T/S[2] 0.5/ 9.5
1.0	1.0	1.0	1.0	1.0	1.0	1.0	1.0	8.0	8.0	1.0	T/S 1 / 19
2.0	2.0	2.0	2.0	2.0	2.0	2.0	2.0	16.0	16.0	2.0	T/S 2 / 38
4.0	4.0	4.0	4.0	4.0	4.0	4.0	4.0	32.0	32.0	4.0	CIP[2] 0.25
8.0	8.0	8.0	8.0	8.0	8.0	8.0	8.0	64.0	64.0	8.0	CIP 0.5
16.0	16.0	16.0	16.0	16.0	16.0	16.0	16.0	128.0	128.0	16.0	CIP 1.0
32.0	32.0	32.0	32.0	32.0	32.0	32.0	32.0	256.0	256.0	32.0	CIP 2.0

amk=amikacin; amp=ampicillin; amp/sul=ampicillin/sulbactam; cef=cephalothin; cfur=cefuroxime; cftx=cefotaxime; cftz=ceftazidime; cip=ciprofloxacin; gent=gentamicin; mez=mezlocillin; pip=piperacillin; tob=tobramycin; T/S=trimethoprim/sulfamethoxazole

[1] concentrations in μg/ml

[2] fewer dilutions of some drugs may be tested depending on space available

Fig. 40-2 Diagram of microbroth dilution MIC tray layout that might be used for gram-negative bacteria; *amk*, amikacin; *amp*, ampicillin; *amp/sul*, ampicillin/sulbactam; *cef*, cephalothin; *cfur*, cefuroxime; *cftx*, cefotaxime; *cftz*, ceftazidime; *cip*, ciprofloxacin; *gent*, gentamicin; *mez*, mezlocillin; *pip*, piperacillin; *tob*, tobramycin; *T/S*, trimethoprim/sulfamethoxazole.

[1] Concentrations in μg/ml.

[2] Fewer dilutions of some drugs may be tested depending on space available.

In performing the microbroth dilution MIC test, the inoculum suspension is prepared as for the disk diffusion test. The turbidity of the suspension is standardized and subsequently diluted so that the final concentration of organisms tested in each well is approximately 5×10^5 CFU/ml (5×10^4 CFU/0.1-ml well). A multipronged inoculating device is used to simultaneously inoculate all wells. Additionally, it is advisable to subculture the test inoculum to an agar plate to check for purity of the inoculum suspension. Following overnight incubation, the purity plate is checked and if no problems are noted, the tray is visually examined with the aid of a reflecting mirror or light box. The MIC for each drug is determined as the lowest concentration that inhibits growth as demonstrated by the absence of growth or turbidity in the respective well. The NCCLS document contains a table (Table 40-13) for interpreting MIC results as related to therapeutically achievable blood levels. As with the disk test, sometimes different interpretive criteria are used for a single agent, depending on the species or organism group tested.

If an actual MIC value is to be reported, it is suggested that at least five consecutive twofold dilutions are tested. However, fewer dilutions or nonconsecutive concentrations can be tested in order to test more drugs per tray. If two concentrations are tested, these would generally include the concentrations just below the breakpoint for resistance. For example, with ampicillin, 8 μg/ml and 16 μg/ml would be tested. If an isolate did not grow in either well (MIC $\leq$8 μg/ml), it would be considered susceptible. If an isolate grew in 8 μg/ml but not in 16 μg/ml (MIC = 16 μg/ml), it would be interpreted as moderately susceptible, and if it grew in both wells (MIC >16 μg/ml), it would be resistant. Reporting recommendations when testing breakpoint concentrations include reporting categoric interpretations. The corresponding MIC range could be reported, if desired.

An agar dilution method can also be used to determine MICs. Varying volumes of antimicrobial solution are added to cooled, molten agar that is then poured into Petri plates and allowed to solidify. A separate plate is prepared for each test concentration of drug and an abbreviated drug dilution schema (generally three or four) is often used. Thus, for example, when testing ampicillin, separate plates containing 2 μg/ml, 8 μg/ml, and 16 μg/ml are made. The inoculum suspension is prepared as for the other methods described, standardized, and subsequently diluted so the final concentration of organisms tested per "spot" is approximately 10^4 CFU. A replicating device is used to simultaneously inoculate as many as 36 different isolates onto each plate. Following overnight incubation, plates are examined visually and the MIC for each drug is determined as the lowest concentration that allows the growth of no more than two colonies. Although the costs for materials used in agar dilution are low, plate preparation is very time consuming and this method is primarily used in research settings. It is only practical when large numbers of isolates are tested.

Preparation of the dilutions for any of the methods described requires that laboratories first make antimicrobial stock solutions from reference standard antimicrobial powders. Growth media must also be prepared. For the microbroth dilution MIC method, individual panels can be prepared manually by using multichanneled pipettors to first dispense the broth diluent and then dilute the drugs. Alternatively, large volumes of each test dilution in broth can be prepared and dispensed into large numbers of trays using an automated dispensing device. Obviously, this is not something that can be done in the smaller laboratory. However, several commerical companies manufacture prepared microbroth dilution MIC panels containing either dried or frozen antimicrobial agents. The dried panels are reconstituted at the time of inoculation and the frozen panels merely require defrosting prior to inoculation. Utilization of these commercial panels represents a practical solution for MIC testing in many clinical laboratories.

Many of the same test variables important in disk diffusion testing must be considered for MIC methods as well

Table 40-13 MIC interpretive standards (μg/mL) of three categories of susceptibility for organisms other than *Haemophilus* and *Neisseria gonorrhoeae*

Antimicrobial agent	Susceptible	Moderately susceptible	Intermediate	Resistant
Ampicillin				
When testing *Enterobacteriaceae*	$\leq$8	16	—	$\geq$32
When testing staphylococci and *Moraxella catarrhalis*	$\leq$0.25	—	—	$\geq$0.5
When testing *Listeria monocytogenes*	$\leq$2	—	—	$\geq$4
When testing enterococci	—	$\leq$8	—	$\geq$16
When testing nonenterococcal streptococci and other gram-positive organisms	$\leq$0.12	0.25-2.0	—	$\geq$4
Cephalothin	$\leq$8	16	—	$\geq$32
Gentamicin	$\leq$4	—	8	$\geq$16
Mezlocillin				
When testing *Pseudomonas*	$\leq$64	—	—	$\geq$128
When testing other gram-negative organisms	$\leq$16	32-64	—	$\geq$128

From National Committee for Clinical Laboratory Standards: M100-S3: Supplemental tables for M2-A4, M7, 2nd M11-A2, Villanova, Pa, 1991, NCCLS.

(Table 40-12). Additionally, it is important to note that because of the small number of organisms tested (usually 10^4/well), the microdilution MIC method may not always detect penicillin resistance in staphylococci producing small amounts of β-lactamase. Consequently, for those isolates that have penicillin MICs in the susceptible range of 0.06 to 0.12 μg/ml, an induced β-lactamase test must be performed (see text that follows). β-Lactamase positive reactions confirm penicillin resistance and should override the susceptible penicillin MIC result.

Relationship between disk diffusion and MIC tests

There is an inverse linear relationship between the zone of inhibition generated in a disk diffusion test and the $\log_2$ MIC test. As mentioned, there is a specific set of zone-interpretive criteria and MIC-interpretive criteria (breakpoints) for each antimicrobial agent. A defined procedure is followed in establishing breakpoints. For the disk test, the optimum concentration of drug to incorporate into the disk is determined. Then, approximately 100 to 150 clinically significant isolates with comparable growth rates and varying susceptibility to the antimicrobial are tested by both the standard disk diffusion and a standard MIC method. A scattergram is constructed by plotting the zone diameter of inhibition against the $\log_2$ MIC for each isolate. A least squares regression analysis is performed to generate the line of best fit. Based on therapeutically achievable blood levels obtained following standard dosing, MICs representing susceptible, moderately susceptible (or intermediate), or resistant levels are defined. By examining the regression line, these MICs are matched to the corresponding zone diameters, which are subsequently used as the zone diameter breakpoints. A generic representation of the scattergram and regression analysis is shown in Fig. 40-3.

Automated antimicrobial susceptibility test systems

Perhaps the most recent innovation for antimicrobial susceptibility testing in the routine clinical laboratory involves the use of instrumentation. There are several commercial companies that manufacture semiautomated or automated instruments that can be used for organism identification as well as antimicrobial susceptibility testing. For antimicrobial susceptibility testing, organisms are inoculated into one or more concentrations of broth containing antimicrobial agent. Following incubation, various methods are used to detect the growth in the antimicrobial chambers, which is compared to that in a growth control chamber.

The three technologies used to detect growth include (1) turbidimetry, (2) fluorometry, and (3) video image processing. In the turbidimetric systems, a photometric device measures changes in turbidity over time. Fluorometry utilizes substrates conjugated to fluorophores. As organisms grow, enzymes are produced that cleave the substrates, which then release the fluorophore that is detected by a fluorometric sensor. Video image processing involves using a television camera to inspect many points in each well. The camera contains picture elements (pixels) that perceive the density at each point and translates it into digital signals that are analyzed with a computer. One of the advantages of the turbidimetric and fluorometric systems is the rapidity in which results are generated. Since these systems are more sensitive in detecting growth than visual inspection, results can be obtained within 3 to 8 hours for most clinically significant, rapidly growing, nonfastidious organisms. Although growth detection is enhanced with video image processing, at this time, overnight incubation is still required when such a method is used.

There are obvious advantages of using automated antimicrobial susceptibility test systems. Perhaps the most note-

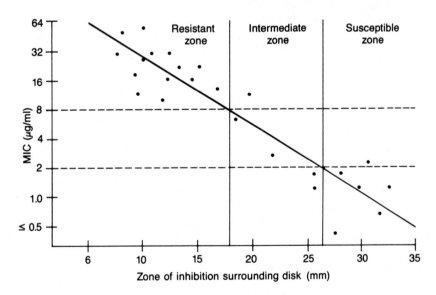

Fig. 40-3 Example of a regression analysis plot used to determine zone sizes that correspond to susceptibility characteristics of the species of bacteria being tested. In this example the maximum achievable serum concentration is 8 μg/ml. Zone sizes ≤18 mm are interpreted as resistant; zone sizes ≥26 are interpreted as susceptible. *From Baron EJ and Finegold SM: Diagnostic microbiology, ed 8, St Louis, 1990, Mosby–Year Book, Inc.*

Box 40-7   Advantages and disadvantages of automated antimicrobial susceptibility test systems

---

POTENTIAL ADVANTAGES (varies among different systems)

Increased standardization of method
Objective interpretation of end points
Rapid results
Reduced labor
Reduced cost/test
Interface capabilities
Tests can be performed by unlicensed personnel (technologist must review reports)
Data management capabilities

POTENTIAL DISADVANTAGES (varies among different systems)

Capital equipment required
Cost
Space and electrical requirements
Backup needed during instrument failure
Inability to test all isolates requiring susceptibility tests (e.g., fastidious, problematic organisms)
Limited flexibility in antibiotic selection
Limited flexibility in methodology

---

worthy include objective interpretation of end points, rapid reporting, and instrument interface capabilities. However, there are some disadvantages and capital equipment cost is a major issue. Box 40-7 summarizes these and other concerns.

A primary concern regarding rapid automated systems is the ability of these systems to detect low-level resistance. If a small subpopulation of resistant organisms is present, it is conceivable that the 3- to 8-hour incubation may not allow sufficient time for these resistant organisms to multiply to the point where they would be detected. To circumvent this and similar problems, some of the systems have incorporated unique media formulations, increased the number of organisms in the test inoculum, and modified algorithms used for interpreting results.

A significant feature of automated systems involves the data management options. Since all of these systems are computerized, the potential exists for entry and storage of culture information (including demographic information on the patient) in addition to organism identification and antimicrobial susceptibility data. The system can thus be used as the primary data management system for the smaller clinical microbiology laboratory. For those laboratories that have a computerized laboratory information system, the automated microbiology system can be interfaced to this for optimal data management. In this situation, susceptibility results can be viewed on the computer screen and verified by the technologist, transmitted across the interface, and reported without any intermediate transcription.

Exceptions to routine testing: methods for antimicrobial susceptibility testing of fastidious and problematic bacteria

Some clinically significant bacteria that may warrant antimicrobial susceptibility testing require special nutrients and sometimes special incubation atmospheres for growth, and cannot be tested using routine testing methods. Although a variety of nonstandardized methods for testing these bacteria have beeen described, the NCCLS has made significant strides in proposing standardized methods that can be used reliably in clinical laboratories. Most of these utilize slight modifications of the routine disk diffusion and dilution procedures.

One of the general recommendations for testing fastidious organisms involves inoculum preparation. Because these organisms grow unpredictably in broth, inocula are usually prepared by suspending growth from colonies on an overnight agar plate into broth and adjusting to the turbidity of a McFarland 0.5 or appropriate standard without incubation of the broth. Additional testing concerns for specific organisms are summarized in Table 40-14.

Haemophilus spp.

A standardized method for testing *Haemopohilus influenzae* and other *Haemophilus* spp. has been described by the NCCLS in their disk diffusion and dilution testing documents. It is suggested that a photometric standardizing device be used to standardize the inoculum to the turbidity of a 0.5 McFarland standard because testing of this genus is particularly sensitive to changes in inoculum concentration. The medium used is *Haemophilus* test medium (HTM) agar for disk diffusion testing and HTM broth for dilution testing. With the disk diffusion test, plates are incubated in CO_2, however, an atmosphere without supplemental CO_2 is satisfactory for broth tests.

There are specific zone diameter and MIC interpretive criteria tables for interpreting results with *Haemophilus* spp. in the NCCLS publications, which include criteria for drugs appropriate for treating infections caused by *Haemophilus* spp. For some agents, such as cefotaxime, there are only susceptible criteria. The reason for this is that there are virtually no cefotaxime-resistant isolates. Consequently, criteria for defining resistance cannot be established at this time. If a clinical laboratory were to encounter an isolate that was not susceptible to cefotaxime or other agents for which there is only susceptible criteria, the isolate should be investigated further.

β-Lactamase testing of *Haemophilus* spp. is useful in identifying ampicillin-resistant isolates. In the United States, approximately 20% of *Haemophilus influenzae* produce a plasmid-mediate β-lactamase and this enzyme is encountered twice as often in type b as compared to non-B isolates. In contrast, only 0.1% of *H. influenzae* are ampicillin-resistant due to altered penicillin-binding proteins. These latter isolates often have higher cephalosporin MICs than either ampicillin-susceptible isolates or β-lactamase–producing isolates, although these MICs still fall in the susceptible range. Approximately 0.5% of *H. influenzae* produce plasmid-mediated chloramphenicol acetyltransferase and this enzyme can be found in β-lactamase–producing or nonproducing isolates.

Because of the predictable susceptibility of *H. influenzae* to many drugs of choice, it is questionable as to whether it is necessary to perform more than a β-lactamase test routinely, particularly if the isolate is not causing an invasive infection.

Table 40-14 Summary of in vitro antimicrobial susceptibility testing concerns for some fastidious and/or problematic bacteria encountered in a clinical microbiology laboratory*

Bacteria	Agar medium for disk diffusion	Medium for MICs	Comments
Haemophilus spp.	*Haemophilus* test medium (HTM)	*Haemophilus* test medium (HTM) broth	Perform β-lactamase test ASAP on blood/CSF isolates
Neisseria gonorrhoeae	GC agar base with defined supplement	GC agar base with defined supplement	Perform β-lactamase test only routinely
Neisseria meningitidis	MHA	MHA	No standard recommendations for testing/reporting
Streptococcus pneumoniae	B-MHA	CAMHB with 2%-5% lysed horse blood	Test oxacillin (1 μg) disk for penicillin results; perform MIC if oxacillin zone <20 mm
Streptococcus spp.	B-MHA	CAMHB with 2%-5% lysed horse blood	Perform penicillin MIC on viridans isolated from endocarditis patients
Staphylococcus spp.	MHA	CAMHB (add 2% NaCl for oxacillin**)	For disk diffusion, examine oxacillin zone using transmitted light; incubate oxacillin tests for 24 h, perform induced β-lactamase test if microbroth dilution penicillin MIC is 0.06-0.12 μg/ml
Enterococcus spp.	MHA	CAMHB	Perform high-level aminoglycoside screen, β-lactamase test, and vancomycin MIC (standard dilution method) on blood/CSF isolates
Anaerobes	Not applicable	Wilkens-Chalgren agar or Wilkens-Chalgren broth	Reference method is agar dilution
Rapidly growing *Mycobacteria* spp.	Not applicable	CAMHB or MHA (disk elution)	Antibacterial (vs. antimycobacterial) agents effective against these

*MHA, Mueller-Hinton agar; B-MHA, Mueller-Hinton agar with 5% sheep blood; CAMHB, cation adjusted Mueller-Hinton broth. For *Moraxella catarrhalis*, perform β-lactamase test only routinely.
**Includes all penicillinase-resistant penicillins.

Neisseria gonorrhoeae

The NCCLS has also recently described a standard method for testing *Neisseria gonorrhoeae* in their disk diffusion and dilution testing documents The medium used is GC agar base containing 1% defined supplement for both disk diffusion and dilution tests. Incubation requires an atmosphere with supplemental CO_2.

As with *Haemophilus* spp., there are specific zone diameter and MIC interpretive criteria tables for interpreting results with *N. gonorrhoeae* and ceftriaxone, penicillin, spectinomycin, tetracycline and several quinolones and other cephalosporins. There are only susceptible criteria for ceftriaxone and a laboratory should investigate any isolate that does not demonstrate ceftriaxone susceptible results.

Prior to 1989, penicillin was considered the drug of choice for treatment of uncomplicated gonococcal infections. However, because of the increased incidence of penicillin resistance, a single intramuscular dose of ceftriaxone combined with 7 days of oral doxycycline (to cover for concomitant chlamydial infection) is now recommended. The incidence of plasmid-mediated penicillinase (β-lactamase) production in *N. gonorrhoeae* (PPNG) is over 5% in the United States and the β-lactamase test is very reliable in detecting this resistance. Chromosomally mediated resistance to penicillin (CMRNG), which can only be detected with the conventional tests, occurs in approximately 6% of gonococcal isolates. Eighteen percent of gonococci are tetracycline-resistant and this resistance may be either plasmid-mediated (TRNG) or chromosomally mediated (see

Schwarcz et al, Suggested Reading). Ceftriaxone resistance has not yet been reported.

Some health departments continue to recommend that clinical laboratories perform the simple β-lactamase test on all *N. gonorrhoeae* isolates, primarily for epidemiologic purposes. Since all gonococci are susceptible to ceftriaxone, there is probably no need for additional routine testing. However, testing should be considered if the patient cannot tolerate ceftriaxone and an alternative agent to which resistance has been described is being considered.

Neisseria meningitidis

Unfortunately, although several nonstandardized methods have been described, there currently are not any standardized methods for antimicrobial susceptibility testing of meningococci. Resistance to penicillin (due to β-lactamase production), the drug of choice, has only been reported in three cases during the past 8 years, and most clinical laboratories are not concerned about routine testing. Because of some recent developments suggesting decreased penicillin susceptibility due to altered penicillin-binding proteins, susceptibility testing may not be considered inconsequential in the future. The varying susceptibility to the sulfonamides and to rifampin, either of which are used as prophylactic therapy for individuals who come in contact with patients with systemic meningococcal infections, suggests that susceptibility testing to these agents may be useful. A disk diffusion method for testing sulfonamides (300-μg disk) where the inoculum is adjusted to minimally visible turbidity was described by Bennett in 1966. (See Suggested Reading.) Isolates with ≥40 mm zones are susceptible. The FDA package inserts that accompany commercially available disks specify a rifampin (5-μg disk) breakpoint of ≥25 mm as susceptible when tests are performed following the standard disk diffusion method.

Streptococcus pneumoniae

For disk diffusion testing of *Streptococcus pneumoniae*, Mueller-Hinton agar supplemented with 5% sheep blood is used. Dilution tests are generally performed in Mueller-Hinton broth supplemented with 2% to 5% lysed horse blood. Incubation is usually in an atmosphere without supplemental CO_2, however, CO_2 may be required to obtain adequate growth of some strains.

Penicillin susceptibility in pneumococci is divided into three categories based on the penicillin MIC: ≤0.06 μg/ml = susceptible; 0.12 to 1.0 μg/ml = relatively resistant; and >1.0 μg/ml = resistant. Penicillin resistance in this species is not due to β-lactamase, but rather to altered penicillin-binding proteins. Consequently, the β-lactamase test should not be performed.

A disk diffusion test to determine penicillin susceptibility has been standardized. Because testing with the standard penicillin disk is unreliable, use of a 1-μg oxacillin disk is recommended. Isolates with oxacillin zones ≥20 mm are considered penicillin-susceptible. MIC tests must be performed when oxacillin zones are <20 mm to determine whether the isolate is resistant or relatively resistant to penicillin. Disk diffusion testing of other antimicrobial agents has not yet been addressed by the NCCLS, however, the standard interpretive criteria for chloramphenicol appears to be acceptable for these organisms.

The importance of differentiating relatively resistant from resistant isolates can be illustrated by the fact that high doses of penicillin may be effective in treating infections other than meningitis (e.g., pneumonia) caused by relatively resistant but not resistant isolates. The incidence of frank penicillin-resistant isolates is very low in the United States and health departments are interested in any isolates that are encountered. Although multiple resistant isolates are seen frequently in Africa and some European countries, these are not common in the United States.

Streptococcus spp.

The media and incubation conditions for testing other *Streptococcus* spp. are the same as those for *Streptococcus pneumoniae*. As for the pneumococci, penicillin resistance in *Streptococcus* spp. is due to altered penicillin-binding proteins and the β-lactamase test has no merit. There are specific disk diffusion zone interpretive criteria for the 10-μg ampicillin and 10-U penicillin disks; the oxacillin disk should not be used. MIC interpretive criteria categorize isolates as penicillin-susceptible (≤0.12 μg/ml), moderately susceptible (0.25 to 2.0 μg/ml), or resistant (>2.0 μg/ml).

Penicillin remains the drug of choice for treating most streptococcal infections caused by penicillin-susceptible isolates. However, in the case of viridans endocarditis, an aminoglycoside is usually added when penicillin MICs are ≥0.25 μg/ml, thus emphasizing the need for clinical laboratories to accurately detect this decreased susceptibility.

Group A β-hemolytic streptococci remain universally susceptible to penicillin. However, occasional isolates may be erythromycin-resistant and erythromycin susceptibility testing may be warranted for the penicillin-allergic patient who is not responding to erythromycin. Groups B, C, and G streptococci likewise remain susceptible to penicillin, however, their MICs may be slightly higher (0.06 to 0.12 μg/ml) than Group A isolates (≤0.06 μg/ml). The number of penicillin-resistent viridans isolates with decreased penicillin susceptibility is increasing particularly in *Streptococcus mitis* and *Streptococcus sanguis II*.

Occasionally, a laboratory may encounter a vancomycin-resistant isolate that morphologically resembles *Streptococcus* spp. Further identification tests will usually reveal that this isolate is either a *Lactobacillus* spp., *Leuconostoc* spp., or *Pediococcus* spp., all of which are intrinsically vancomycin-resistant.

Methicillin-resistant Staphylococcus aureus

One of the penicillinase-resistant penicillins (methicillin, nafcillin, oxacillin, dicloxacillin, or cloxacillin) is often prescribed for treatment of *Staphylococcus aureus* infections. Resistance of *S. aureus* to these agents first appeared in the United States in the 1970s and the incidence of this problematic organism continues to increase.

Staphylococcus aureus isolates that are intrinsically resistant to the penicillinase-resistant penicillins have a unique penicillin-binding protein. Resistance to any one of these agents indicates resistance to the entire group, which can best be detected in vitro by testing oxacillin. Under standard test conditions, there is often phenotypic heterogeneity within a population of cells, and unless test variables are carefully controlled, this clinically significant resistance may go undetected. The standard methods for detecting methicillin-resistant *S. aureus* (MRSA) include disk diffusion and microbroth dilution. A standard agar screen method that utilizes Mueller-Hinton agar supplemented with 4% NaCl and 6 μg/ml oxacillin has also been reliable for detecting MRSA and is often used as a supplemental test with rapid automated systems, which have on occasion failed to detect MRSA. Inocula for all tests with staphylococci and penicillinase-resistant penicillins should be prepared by suspending colonies from an overnight agar plate in broth or saline and adjusting the turbidity accordingly. Oxacillin should be tested as the representative of the group and the broth for microbroth dilution testing should be supplemented with 2% NaCl. Other important variables to control, including incubation and end point determination, are mentioned in Table 40-12. Intrinsically resistant isolates are usually resistant to other agents, including clindamycin, erythromycin, and sometimes chloramphenicol, tetracycline, trimethoprim/sulfamethoxazole, and the aminoglycosides.

Another more subtle type of resistance to the penicillinase-resistant penicillins, sometimes referred to as borderline or acquired resistance, is due to high levels of β-lactamase production. Despite the fact that the penicillinase-resistant penicillins are by definition resistant to inactivation by penicillinase, high concentrations of this enzyme may have an inactivating effect and oxacillin is more vulnerable than the other agents in this group. The MICs for these isolates are often just above the susceptible breakpoint. In contrast to the intrinsically resistant isolates, these isolates are usually not multiply resistant and combinations of β-lactam/β-lactamase inhibitors are active against them.

An isolate that demonstrates resistance to any penicillinase-resistant penicillin should be considered resistant to all β-lactam agents, including penicillins, cephalosporins, β-lactam/β-lactamase inhibitor combinations, and imipenem, even if in vitro results indicate a susceptible isolate. The recommendations for testing *S. aureus* are applicable to coagulase-negative staphylococci also, despite the fact that methicillin-resistant species within this group have not been studied nearly as much as MRSA.

Enterococcus spp.

Several concerns surround the detection of clinically significant resistance in *Enterococcus* spp. Detection of high-level aminoglycoside resistance will be discussed in detail shortly with other methods of detection of enzymatic resistance.

Most enterococci are inhibited but not killed by therapeutically achievable concentrations of cell wall active agents such as ampicillin, penicillin, and vancomycin. Although these agents alone are often effective in treating less serious infections in which the inflammatory response is good, combination therapy with an aminoglycoside is necessary for bactericidal activity for more serious infections, such as endocarditis. This latter condition led the NCCLS to include only moderately susceptible and resistant interpretive criteria for ampicillin, penicillin, and vancomycin. The intent (according to the definition of "moderately susceptible") is to emphasize that these drugs would not be effective alone in treating serious infections, however, either of them as a single agent may be appropriate for less serious infections or for infections in body sites where the drugs concentrate.

Many *Enterococcus faecium* isolates are resistant to ampicillin and penicillin (MIC >16 μg/ml) due to altered penicillin-binding proteins. β-Lactamase production has recently been demonstrated in a few isolates of *Enterococcus faecalis*. Although conventional tests have been able to detect resistance due to altered penicillin-binding proteins, standard disk diffusion, MIC, and automated methods have resulted in susceptible results for β-lactamase–producing isolates. This is due to an inoculum effect and a larger number of organisms than is routinely tested in conventional methods is needed to detect resistance due to β-lactamase production. A practical solution is to use the rapid nitrocefin β-lactamase test, which thus far has been able to reliably detect β-lactamase production in this genus. Interestingly, nearly all β-lactamase–producing isolates have also had high-level gentamicin and often streptomycin resistance, making therapy of these isolates extremely difficult.

Most recently, vancomycin resistance has appeared in enterococci. As with β-lactamase–producing isolates, the incidence is very low. Some isolates have higher vancomycin MICs (≥256 μg/ml) and these are detected by disk diffusion, MIC, and automated systems. However, disk diffusion and automated methods may not always detect resistant isolates that have lower MICs. Undoubtedly, testing methods will be modified to more readily detect the resistance that is appearing in the enterococci.

Anaerobes

Antimicrobial susceptibility testing of anaerobes represents a unique challenge and a single reliable method for testing all clinically significant anaerobic isolates has yet to be described. This is mainly due to the varied results obtained when using different methods, varied growth requirements of the different genera and species of anaerobes, and limited ability to study the clinical correlation of in vitro results because of the complicated clinical situation (e.g., polymicrobial infections, combination antimicrobial therapy, surgical intervention) surrounding the management of anaerobic infections.

The NCCLS reference method for antimicrobial susceptibility testing of anaerobes is an agar dilution method that utilizes Wilkens-Chalgren agar. As mentioned previously, agar dilution testing is usually restricted to research settings. An agar dilution method developed at Wadsworth Veterans Administration hospital (Los Angeles, CA) that utilizes *Brucella* blood agar, a limited agar dilution method, and a macrobroth dilution method have also been described by NCCLS. However, the NCCLS microbroth dilution MIC test is generally used for routine testing of anaerobes in clinical laboratories. The test is performed as for aerobes, however, Wilkens-Chalgren broth is generally used and the number of organisms tested is 1 $\log_{10}$ higher (10^6 CFU/ml). Trays are incubated anaerobically at 35° C for 48 hours before MICs are determined. There is a single breakpoint indicating susceptibility for each drug. The definition of susceptible (MIC ≤ the breakpoint concentration) would include those for susceptible, moderately susceptible, and intermediate as described for routine disk diffusion and dilution tests. A problem with using microbroth dilution routinely is that many anaerobic species will not grow adequately in the base broth, so alternative methods are needed. As for aerobic organisms, commercially manufactured microbroth dilution trays are available for testing anaerobes.

The β-lactamase test may be useful in predicting penicillin resistance in some anaerobes, particularly *Bacteroides* spp. Since virtually all *Bacteroides fragilis* group organisms are β-lactamase producers, it is generally not necessary to test these organisms.

Rapidly growing *Mycobacterium* spp.

The rapidly growing mycobacteria, including *Mycobacterium fortuitum* and *Mycobacterium chelonae*, are resistant to conventional first- and second-line antituberculosis agents, except for the aminoglycosides. However, infections caused by these organisms are often effectively treated with other commonly used antibacterial agents and antimicrobial susceptibility test methods commonly used for aerobic bacteria can be used for testing rapidly growing mycobacteria.

Although antimicrobial susceptibility tests for rapidly growing mycobacteria have not been standardized, there are primarily two methods that are used. The microbroth dilution method is basically the same as that described for aerobic bacteria and cation adjusted Mueller-Hinton broth is used. The inoculum broth is supplemented with 0.02% Tween 80 to help disperse the organisms. Following inoculation and 2 to 3 days of incubation, MICs are determined. Incubation is usually at 35° C in an atmosphere without supplemental CO_2, however, 30° C incubation may be required to obtain adequate growth of some *M. chelonae*. End points may not always be as clear as when testing nonmycobacterial isolates.

An agar disk elution method is sometimes used for testing rapidly growing mycobacteria. Antimicrobial disks are placed in the wells (3.5 × 10 cm) of tissue culture plates. Cooled, molten Mueller-Hinton agar is poured into each well and the agar is allowed to solidify. After the drug has diffused through the agar, plates are inoculated with 10^5 CFU. Plates are examined for growth or absence of growth, indicating susceptible or resistant results following 2 to 3 days of incubation.

Although the rapidly growing mycobacteria can be tested in Mueller-Hinton broth-based microdilution trays, some of the drugs of interest for these organisms, which include amikacin, cefoxitin, ciprofloxacin, doxycycline, imipenem, minocycline, tobramycin, and trimethoprim/sulfamethoxazole, are not available in commercially manufactured trays. To date, no company is manufacturing a tray specific for testing these organisms.

Special tests for detecting enzymatic resistance
β-Lactamase tests

Simple tests to detect β-lactamase production have been useful for testing certain organisms, particularly *Haemophilus influenzae, Neisseria gonorrhoeae, Branhamella catarrhalis,* and *Bacteroides* spp. For these organisms, it has been demonstrated that the production of β-lactamase is the primary mechanism that confers resistance to β-lactam antimicrobial agents (primarily ampicillin and penicillin) that

might be used in treating infections caused by these species. In the case of *B. catarrhalis,* the current NCCLS recommendation is to perform the β-lactamase test only since all isolates to date encountered in the United States are susceptible to the remaining drugs of choice.

More recently, it has been suggested that the nitrocefin β-lactamase test be used to detect β-lactamase production in enterococci. This rare and unique mechanism of ampicillin and penicillin resistance in this genus might not be detected with conventional susceptibility tests because of inoculum effects.

The basic principle behind the β-lactamase tests involves detection of penicilloic acid that is produced following β-lactamase hydrolysis of the substrate β-lactam. The nitrocefin method which utilizes the chromogenic cephalosporin, nitrocefin, is usually used, however, the acidimetric and iodometric methods perform satisfactorily for some organism groups. A description of the three methods and the organisms that can be reliably tested by these are described in Tables 40-15 and 40-16. Several commercial products are available for β-lactamase testing.

For the aforementioned organisms, substantial quantities of β-lactamase are produced constitutively, thus the organisms continuously produce sufficient quantities of the enzyme to be detected. However, β-lactamase production in staphylococci is inducible and some isolates produce low levels of β-lactamase that may not give a positive reaction unless enzyme production is stimulated to detectable levels. This can be practically accomplished by growing the isolate in the presence of subinhibitory concentrations of an inducing β-lactam agent such as cefoxitin. The test is then performed on the cells that have grown in the presence of the inducing agent.

An advantage of the β-lactamase test is that results are often available in a matter of minutes. Consequently, the β-lactamase test can be performed on colonies of probable *H. influenzae* that have grown following 18 hours of cul-

Table 40-15   β-lactamase test methods

Method	Substrate	Reaction	Results
Acidimetric	Citrate buffered penicillin + phenol red	Penicilloic acid produces pH decrease	Positive = yellow, negative = red
Chromogenic cephalosporin	Nitrocefin	Color change when β-lactam ring opened	Positive = red/brown, negative = yellow
Iodometric	Phosphate-buffered penicillin + starch-iodine complex	Penicilloic acid reduces iodine and prevents it from combining with starch	Positive = colorless, negative = purple

Table 40-16   Reliability of various β-lactamase methods for respective bacteria*

Method	Haemophilus	Neisseria gonorrhoeae	Staphylococci	Moraxella catarrhalis	Enterococci	Bacteroides
Acidimetric	X	X	X	—	—	—
Chromogenic cephalosporin (nitrocefin)	X	X	X	X	X	X
Iodometric	—	X	X	—	—	—

*X, reliable results generated.

turing a CSF specimen. In contrast, conventional tests to detect β-lactam resistance may take an additional day. Many of the species for which the β-lactamase test is useful cannot be tested by rapid automated methods because of their fastidious nature.

It must be emphasized that production of β-lactamase may not be the only mechanism of β-lactam resistance in the organisms commonly tested. By definition, an isolate that produces β-lactamase is resistant to ampicillin and penicillin. However, an isolate that gives a negative β-lactamase test reaction must be tested by a conventional method to see if perhaps it is resistant to these β-lactams by an alternative resistance mechanism. In cases where the probability of such resistance is very low (e.g., *B. catarrhalis*), supplemental tests may not be warranted in the clinical laboratory.

Chloramphenicol acetyltransferase test

Like the β-lactamase test, the rapid chloramphenicol acetyltransferase test (CAT) is useful in detecting enzymatic resistance. The CAT test is not used to the extent that the β-lactamase test is used, primarily because chloramphenicol is not a drug of choice for very many infections and the incidence of resistance in organisms causing life-threatening infections where CAT results might be useful is low. Most chloramphenicol-resistant *H. influenzae* organisms produce chloramphenicol acetyltransferase, but again, there may be occasional strains that are chloramphenicol-resistant by another mechanism. Although the extended-spectrum cephalosporins have, for the most part, replaced ampicillin and chloramphenicol for treating severe *H. influenzae* infections, there are some situations when chloramphenicol is indicated. In these cases the rapid CAT test may be useful, particularly if chloramphenicol-resistant isolates have been encountered in the particular geographic area. Although CAT is produced by other organisms (e.g., *Salmonella* spp., *Streptococcus pneumoniae*), it is rarely used for testing these in clinical laboratories. CAT test reagents are commercially available.

Tests for detection of high-level aminoglycoside resistance in *Enterococcus* spp.

There are two types of aminoglycoside resistance in enterococci. Low-level resistance is due to poor drug uptake. MICs are <2000 μg/ml, but are still above achievable serum levels, which precludes use of aminoglycosides such as gentamicin, tobramycin, and streptomycin single agents in treating enterococcal infections. However, when an aminoglycoside is combined with a cell wall active agent such as ampicillin, penicillin, or vancomycin, synergy is possible.

In contrast, some enterococci may have high-level aminoglycoside resistance (HLAR). This resistance is usually due to the production of aminoglycoside-inactivating enzymes and MICs are >2000 μg/ml. When high-level resistance is present, the aminoglycoside does not act synergistically with the cell wall active agent.

Because the incidence of high-level aminoglycoside resistance is increasing, laboratories should test for this on blood and CSF isolates. Although disk diffusion methods that utilize special disks containing 300 μg of streptomycin and 120 μg of gentamicin have been reliable in detecting

HLAR to the respective agent, the high content disks are not yet commercially available. Alternatively, HLAR can be detected using dilution methods. Typically, 2000 μg/ml of streptomycin and either 500 μg/ml or 2000 μg/ml of gentamicin is incorporated in broth or agar, which is then inoculated following standard dilution procedures. The 500-μg/ml concentration for gentamicin has been recommended by some because isolates that produce gentamicin-inactivating enzymes may have MICs near 2000 μg/ml and the higher concentration may not detect these isolates as reliably.

Most enterococci will not have HLAR. For those with HLAR, the most common pattern is HLAR to streptomycin, but not to gentamicin. In these cases, gentamicin would be synergistic with the cell wall active agent. Due to the nature of the enzymes produced, an isolate that shows HLAR to gentamicin would also have HLAR to other aminoglycosides, including amikacin, kanamycin, netilmicin, and tobramycin, but not streptomycin. If the particular isolate lacked HLAR to streptomycin, this agent could be used. However, many isolates with gentamicin HLAR also have streptomycin HLAR. With these, the antibacterial effects of any aminoglycoside is negligible, which presents a significant therapeutic dilemma for the clinician.

Quality control of antimicrobial susceptibility tests

Like any other clinical laboratory test, a good quality control (QC) program is essential to ensure reliability of antimicrobial susceptibility test results. The NCCLS recommends specific reference strains for use with routine disk diffusion and dilution susceptibility tests. These include: *E. coli* ATCC 25922, *S. aureus* ATCC 25923 (for disk diffusion), *S. aureus* ATCC 29213 (for dilution tests), *P. aeruginosa* ATCC 27853, *E. coli* ATCC 35218, and *Enterococcus faecalis* ATCC 29212. Additional strains are recommended for quality control of tests for *Haemophilus* spp, *N. gonorrhoeae*, and anaerobes, which respectively include *H. influenza* ATCC 49247, *N. gonnorhoeae* ATCC 49226, *Bacteroides fragilis* ATCC 25285, *Bacteroides thetaiotaomicron* ATCC 29741, *Clostridium perfringens* ATCC 13124, and *Eubacterium lentum* ATCC 43055. Several investigators have suggested use of *Mycobacterium fortuitum* ATCC 6847 for quality control of tests for rapidly growing mycobacterial species. When disk diffusion inhibition zones or MIC results fall within specific ranges of acceptability for the appropriate QC strain(s), the test system is considered to be in control. Commercial manufacturers of antimicrobial susceptibility test systems often recommend these strains and sometimes additional strains specifically selected for their system.

Testing the recommended reference strains is but one part of an overall quality control program for antimicrobial susceptibility tests. Other components include: satisfactory performance on proficiency surveys, utilization of relevant testing and reporting strategies, assuring technologist proficiency in performing the tests, supervisory review of reported results, utilization of a program for compilation and review of cumulative susceptibility statistics on each species tested over a given time frame, and utilization of antibiogram checks to further verify results on patient isolates. An antibiogram is the antimicrobial susceptibility profile of an

Table 40-17 Various antibiograms that might be obtained with *E. coli**

Antimicrobial agent	Result pattern				
	1	2	3	4	5
Amikacin	S	S	R	**R**	S
Ampicillin	S	R	R	S	R
Cephalothin	S	S	R	S	S
Cefotaxime	S	S	S	S	**R**
Cefuroxime	S	S	S	S	S
Gentamicin	S	S	R	S	S
Ticarcillin	S	S	R	S	S
Tobramycin	S	S	R	S	S
Trimethoprim/ Sulfamethoxazole	S	S	R	S	S

From Hindler JA: Nontraditional approaches to quality control of antimicrobial susceptibility tests, Clinical microbiology newsletter 12:65, 1990.
*1, typical and most common antibiogram; 2, typical, but less common antibiogram; 3, atypical, but possible antibiogram (results of related drugs are reasonable); 4, atypical antibiogram; very unusual to encounter an isolate resistant to amikacin and susceptible to gentamicin and tobramycin; 5, atypical antibiogram; for *Enterobacteriaceae*, unusual to encounter resistance to a third-generation cephalosporin if an isolate is susceptible to first- (cephalothin) and second- (cefuroxime) generation cephalosporins. S, susceptible; R, resistant.

isolate to a battery of antimicrobial agents. Many species have typical antibiograms that can be checked against the organism's identification to verify both the identification and susceptibility results. Additionally, an understanding of the hierarchy of activities of drugs within a specific group can be used to verify susceptibility test results. An example of various antibiograms for *E. coli* is shown in Table 40-17.

Tests to determine minimal bactericidal concentrations

All the tests described thus far examine the inhibitory capacity of an antimicrobial agent. In situations where immune mechanisms contribute little to eradicate infecting organisms, such as in endocarditis, osteomyelitis, or in infections in immunocompromised patients, bactericidal activity of antimicrobial agents is essential. The simplest way to examine bactericidal activity in vitro is with the minimum bactericidal concentration (MBC) test. The NCCLS has provided guidelines for performing MBC tests, although these are not considered standard methods at this time.

A broth dilution (either macro or micro) MIC test can be carried one step further to determine the MBC. Each tube or well showing no growth is subcultured to an agar medium to see if the organisms in the initial inoculum were killed or merely inhibited from multiplying. Any organisms that escaped killing will form colonies on subculture and the end point is the dilution that represents ≥99.9% killing. In order to establish the number of colonies that constitute ≥99.9% killing, it is essential to perform colony counts on the initial inoculum. A diagrammatic representation of an MIC test and subsequent performance of an MBC test is shown in Fig. 40-4. There are numerous additional variables to control in the MBC test as compared to MIC tests. Most importantly, the organisms in the initial inoculum for the MIC/MBC test must be in the log phase of growth; the direct inoculum preparation method cannot be used. This ensures maximum opportunity for the antimicrobial agent

to exert an antibacterial effect, and many antimicrobials, such as β-lactams, will only exert an antibacterial effect on growing bacteria. Other important variables that must be controlled include size of the inoculum, taking precautions to ensure maximum contact of drug with bacteria, minimizing the effect of antimicrobial carryover (which may prevent viable organisms from growing into colonies), and subculturing sufficient volumes of each antimicrobial dilution. Adequate control of all variables will hopefully provide meaningful results, however, some question the reliability of MBC test results even when performed under optimal conditions.

There are several biologic conditions that have been described that have an impact on MBC tests and often complicate interpretation. Sometimes, a small proportion of organisms in the test inoculum escape killing and upon retesting, these organisms are no more resistant than the initial inoculum. These organisms have been described as "persisters." In some cases, more organisms will survive killing at higher concentrations of a drug than at lower concentrations. This paradoxical effect that is most commonly seen with cell wall active agents is believed to be due to higher drug concentrations inhibiting protein synthesis (and consequently growth), which is necessary for some drugs to exert a bactericidal effect. Finally, tolerance is when the MBC is considerably higher than the MIC (sometimes defined as an MBC:MIC ratio of >32). Persistence and the paradoxical effect are two forms of tolerance. Additionally, some isolates may appear tolerant as a result of the in vitro testing conditions and others may actually possess a mechanism, such as a defective autolytic system, that results in high MBCs. Although there are several suggestions that tolerance as determined by MBC tests has significant clinical implications, this remains controversial.

Kill curves: another method to assess bactericidal activity

The kill curve, which is primarily performed in research settings, provides a more dynamic means of assessing bactericidal activity. Bacteria in the log phase of growth are inoculated into one or more concentrations of antimicrobial agent in broth and a broth control tube. Generally ≥10 ml of broth containing drug concentrations at the MIC, one half the MIC, and one fourth the MIC are tested. Samples from each tube are removed for a colony count at 0 hour and the tubes are incubated. Additional colony counts are performed on each tube at specific time intervals such as 4, 8, 12, and 24 hours. Following incubation of the colony count plates, the numbers of colonies are plotted over time on semilog paper with time on the x-axis and colony counts on the y-axis. Bactericidal activity is defined as a 3 $\log_{10}$ decrease in colonies in the drug tubes as compared to the control.

Serum bactericidal tests

The serum bactericidal test (SBT, previously known as the Schlichter test) assesses the inhibitory and bactericidal activity of a patient's serum against the infecting bacteria. The technique used to perform the test is similar to broth dilution tests and procedures for performing the SBT have been described by the NCCLS. Generally, trough and peak serum

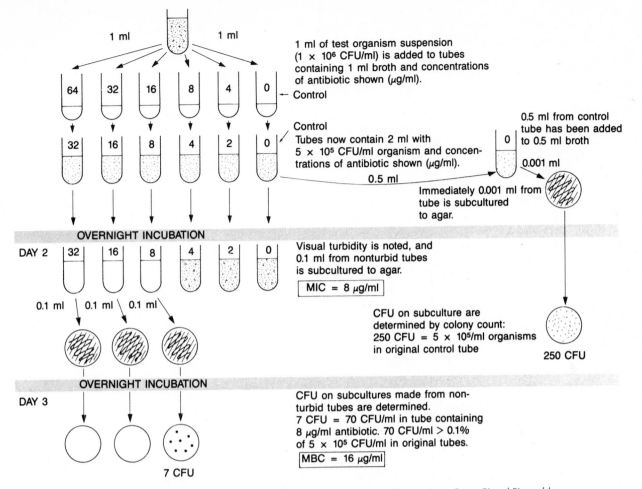

Fig. 40-4 Determining MIC and MBC for one organism and one antibiotic. *From Baron EJ and Finegold SM: Diagnostic microbiology, ed 8, St Louis, 1990, Mosby-Year Book.*

samples are collected from the patient while on antimicrobial therapy: the trough is obtained right before dosing and the peak is obtained 30 to 90 minutes after the antimicrobial agent is administered (30 minutes after completion of an intravenous infusion, 60 minutes after an intramuscular dose, 90 minutes after an oral dose). Serial twofold dilutions of each serum sample are prepared in broth and these are inoculated with a standard inoculum of the patient's organism. Following overnight incubation, the inhibitory dilution is determined as the highest dilution that inhibits visible growth. A sample from each tube demonstrating no growth is subcultured to an agar medium and incubated for 24 to 72 hours as in the MBC test to determine the highest dilution of the patient's serum that results in >99.9% killing. To better stimulate in vivo conditions as related to protein binding of antimicrobial agent, sometimes a diluent containing broth and pooled serum is used, or alternatively, the patient's serum is filtered to remove protein prior to performing the test.

The SBT takes into account pharmacokinetic factors related to the antimicrobial agent and any additional antibacterial factors in the patient's serum (e.g., metabolites of the antimicrobial agent) that may help eradicate the infecting organism. The SBT is sometimes useful when a patient is receiving multiple agents. The primary indications for performing the SBT is to monitor therapy in patients with endocarditis, osteomyelitis, closed space infections such as joint infections, and to assess the effectiveness of switching to oral therapy following parenteral administration.

As with the other tests that assess bactericidal activity, there is controversy as to the reliability of SBT results. Generally, a trough cidal titer of ≥1:8 and a peak cidal titer of ≥1:32 represents adequate therapy, however, most of the studies surrounding these recommendations have been performed on patients with endocarditis, where the outcome was assessed in terms of bacteriologic cure.

Synergism studies

For serious infections and infections in immunocompromised hosts, combination antimicrobial therapy is often prescribed and sometimes it is useful to measure the activity of these combinations in vitro. Advantages of combination therapy include potential for enhanced antibacterial activity through synergistic interactions, a broader spectrum of coverage, particularly when the etiologic agent is unknown, and minimizing the development of resistance. The primary disadvantage is the possibility of antagonistic antimicrobial interactions.

Some antimicrobial agents routinely tested in clinical laboratories are drug combinations that are tested in fixed combinations using either disk diffusion or dilution methods. These include the β-lactam–β-lactamase inhibitor combinations (ampicillin/sulbactam, amoxicillin/clavulanic acid, ticarcillin/clavulanic acid) and trimethoprim/sulfamethoxazole.

Other combinations might be tested if a synergistic action is not predictable or to determine which of several combinations demonstrates the greatest synergism. Usually two drugs are tested, however, some researchers have performed synergism studies with more than two drugs.

The methods most commonly used for synergism studies involve broth dilution (usually microbroth dilution) or kill curves. None of these methods are considered standard for clinical laboratory purposes and results from different methods sometimes produce conflicting results. Consequently, the value of synergism studies remains controversial. In the broth dilution method, each drug alone and a series of combinations of the two agents in a two-dimensional checkerboard format are tested. From this point on, the test is performed identically to that when testing single agents. Synergism occurs when the activity of the combination is greater than that of either drug alone. In contrast, antagonism implies that the activity of the combination is less than that of either drug alone. Indifference is when the activity of the combination is equivalent to that of either drug alone. Results can be inserted into an equation to calculate the type of response that occurred (generally expressed as fractional inhibitory concentration or FIC), or results can also be presented graphically using isobolograms. Generally, if the MIC for each drug in the combination is reduced to one fourth that of the original MIC, synergism has occurred.

Kill curve methods involve testing combinations of the two agents and each drug alone in separate tubes, utilizing the method employed for testing single agents. Synergism occurs when there is a two $\log_{10}$ reduction in the number of colonies with the combination as compared to either drug alone.

Disk diffusion methods can be used to obtain a crude estimation of potential synergistic interactions. The standard disk diffusion method is used and the two different antimicrobial disks are strategically positioned on the bacterial lawn. Synergism is identified by enhanced inhibition in the area where diffusion of the two drugs overlap.

Antimicrobial assays

The amount of antimicrobial agent in serum or body fluid is sometimes measured to ensure that the dosage is sufficient for adequate therapy but does not result in concentrations that may produce toxic side effects. The concentrations attained can vary depending on the patient's clinical condition, particularly renal and hepatic status. Assays are usually performed on drugs that have a low toxic to therapeutic ratio in vivo, in which the toxic concentration is only slightly greater than the therapeutic concentration. Consequently, aminoglycosides, chloramphenicol, and vancomycin are the drugs most frequently monitored. Timing collection of specimens following dosage is critical and generally both trough and peak specimens are assayed. The trough is obtained right before dosing and the peak is obtained 30 to 90 minutes after the antimicrobial agent was administered (30 minutes after completion of an intravenous infusion; 60 minutes after an intramuscular dose; 90 minutes after an oral dose).

There are a number of methods that can be used for antimicrobial assays, which include both microbiological and chemical procedures. The most commonly used microbiological procedure is the bioassay, in which an organism susceptible to the antimicrobial agent is added to molten agar and the agar poured into a Petri plate. The agar is allowed to solidify and standards containing known concentrations of the antimicrobial agent and the patient samples are applied to the agar (wells are cut in the agar and filled with the samples, or the samples are added to filter paper disks that are placed on the agar). Following incubation, the diameters of the zones of inhibition are measured. A graph is constructed from the standards and the amount of drug in the patient sample is determined by extrapolation from the graph.

Several commercial companies have developed kits for aminoglycoside, chloramphenicol, and vancomycin assays. Most of these are based on an immunoassay procedure, such as radioimmunoassay, enzyme immunoassay, fluorescent immunoassay, and fluorescent polarization immunoassay. Similar kits are not available for other antimicrobial agents, primarily because the demand for such is low. Antimicrobial levels can also be determined using chromatographic methods such as gas liquid chromatography and high-pressure liquid chromatography.

Nucleic acid probes for detecting antimicrobial resistance

In this era of molecular diagnostics it is reasonable to speculate that in the clinical laboratory we will some day be using nucleic acid probes to detect resistance to specific antimicrobial agents. These have already found application in the research setting and the remarkable specificity, together with the rapidity in which results can be obtained, makes these probes attractive. There are some concerns related to the use of probes and one of these involves correlation of the presence of the gene with expression of resistance. Nevertheless, breakthroughs in this area are inevitable.

BEYOND TRADITIONAL BACTERIA
Mycobacteria

Mycobacteria can be divided into three groups: 1) *Mycobacterium tuberculosis* and *M. bovis,* 2) slow growing nontuberculous mycobacteria, and 3) rapidly growing mycobacteria. The methods used for antimicrobial susceptibility testing of rapidly growing mycobacteria have been covered previously and will not be discussed here. Tuberculosis is increasing dramatically among both normal and immunocompromised populations. Nontuberculous mycobacterial infections are also increasing in the immunocompromised population, especially among AIDS patients. Treatment of these infections and the clinical usefulness of antimycobacterial susceptibility testing varies between the two groups.

Antituberculous agents

The agents used to treat infections caused by *M. tuberculosis* are listed in Table 40-18 along with their modes of

Table 40-18 Antituberculosis agents recommended for susceptibility testing

	Mode of action/mechanism of resistance/comments
PRIMARY AGENTS	Used in combination for first-line therapy of tuberculosis
Isoniazid	Inhibits synthesis of mycolic acids, also affects NAD metabolism; resistance is probably the result of decreased permeability to the agent; very potent agent with low toxicity; bactericidal against growing mycobacteria
Streptomycin	Inhibits protein synthesis by binding to the bacterial ribosome; resistance can result from alterations in the ribosome or by decreased permeability to the agent
Rifampin	Inhibits DNA-dependent RNA polymerases; resistance results from alterations in the polymerase
Ethambutol	Inhibits cell wall synthesis by interfering with arabinogalactam synthesis
SECONDARY AGENTS	Used for treatment when resistance has developed to primary agents
Ethionamide	Inhibits synthesis of mycolic acids; resistance mechanisms are unknown
Capreomycin	Inhibits protein synthesis by binding to the bacterial ribosome, bacteriostatic
Cycloserine	Analogue of alanine, inhibits cell wall synthesis; resistance is probably the result of decreased permeability to the agent
Kanamycin	Inhibits bacterial protein synthesis by binding to the bacterial ribosome; resistance can result from alterations in the ribosome or by decreased permeability to the agent
Pyrazinamide	Resistance results from loss of the enzyme needed to convert the drug to the active form; converted to active form pyrazinoic acid in vivo, active in killing mycobacteria in the phagolysosome

action and mechanisms of resistance when known. Since treatment of tuberculosis requires long-term drug therapy and the number of organisms involved in an infection is large, it is not unusual for resistance to develop during therapy. Therefore, combinations of two or three agents are generally used to prevent emergence of resistance. Primary agents are normally used to treat newly diagnosed infections caused by susceptible mycobacteria. Secondary agents may be used after treatment failure or when resistance to one or more of the primary agents is detected.

Other antimycobacterial agents

The treatment of infections caused by some nontuberculous mycobacteria like *Mycobacterium kansasii* is similar to the treatment for tuberculosis. However, infections caused by *Mycobacterium avium* and *Mycobacterium intracellulare* in immunocompromised patients do not respond clinically to the primary antituberculous agents. A number of agents, often given in multidrug combinations, are being evaluated. Several of these agents, like amikacin and rifamycin, are

normally used to treat bacterial infections. Others like cycloserine, clofazimine, and ethionamide are also used in the treatment of tuberculosis but as secondary agents.

Antimycobacterial susceptibility testing

There are four purposes for antimycobacterial susceptibility testing: (1) to provide guidance in initial therapy, (2) to determine if development of resistance is responsible for treatment failure, (3) to determine the prevalence of resistant organisms in a particular population, (4) to determine the clinical relevance of current testing methods in predicting clinical response of nontuberculous mycobacteria to particular agents. Most laboratories do not perform antimycobacterial susceptibility testing. Testing is usually available at city, county, or state departments of health and are sometimes performed by reference laboratories as well. The value of antimycobacterial susceptibility testing is well established for *M. tuberculosis* and several standardized methods have been described. Testing of *M. avium* and *M. intracellulare* is of minimal value at this time since in vitro results often do not correlate with in vivo response.

The two methods commonly used in the United States for susceptibility testing of the slowly growing mycobacteria are the proportion and radiometric methods. The NCCLS has published a proposed standard (NCCLS document M24-P) for testing *M. tuberculosis* by the proportion method.

The proportion method is most similar to an agar dilution method since agents are tested in an agar medium, usually Middlebrook and Cohn 7H10 agar. Only one or two critical concentrations of each agent are tested. The agents may be added as solutions to cooled, molten agar or eluted from disks containing agents placed in the plates before the agar is poured. The inoculum can be a standard suspension of organisms from a positive culture (indirect method) or can be prepared by dilution of a smear-positive specimen (direct method). Several inoculum dilutions are plated so that the number of colonies appearing after incubation can be counted and compared to control plates without drug. The isolate is susceptible if 99% of the growth is inhibited by the agent. Testing by the proportion method is only a qualitative measure of susceptibility since the actual concentration of drug needed to inhibit growth is not determined.

The radiometric method is similar to the proportion method in that only one or two concentrations of agents are tested and the results are also qualitative. Both direct and indirect testing may be done. The difference between the methods is the way the response to the drug is measured and the use of broth instead of agar plates. In the radiometric method the amount of CO_2 given off during growth is measured and used to determine the inhibitory effect of the agent compared to a control without drug. The advantage of the radiometric method is the speed at which results are obtained (days vs. weeks for the proportion method). The major disadvantages are the cost of the equipment and the need to use radionuclides.

Fungi
Antifungal agents

Until recently there was only one effective antifungal agent for systemic infections, amphotericin B, a polyene

Table 40-19   Antifungal agents

Agent	Mode of action	Comments
POLYENES		
Amphotericin B	Binds to ergosterol disrupting fungal cell membranes	Broadly active and effective but very toxic; delivery of drug using liposomal carriers may decrease toxic effects; until recently the drug of choice for nearly all serious system fungal infections; has fungicidal properties
Nystatin	Disruption of fungal cell membranes	Topical use only; too toxic for systemic administration
NUCLEOSIDE ANALOGUE		
Flucytosine	Analogue of cytosine; inhibits thymidylate synthetase activity interfering with DNA synthesis and RNA processing	Limited activity, toxicity, and emergence of resistance has limited use; sometimes used in small doses in combination with amphotericin B, fungistatic
AZOLES		All azoles are fungistatic
Clotrimazole	Inhibits ergosterol synthesis and cell membrane function by interfering with carbon metabolism by cytochrome enzymes	Used topically for yeast infections; toxicity and induction of degradation enzymes in the liver limits parental use, fungistatic
Ketoconazole	As above	First oral azole; broad activity with the exception of *Aspergillus* and *Sporothrix*; relatively nontoxic except in high doses; poor penetration into CSF; drug of choice for chronic mucocutaneous candidiasis and less severe infections with *Blastomyces, Histoplasma,* and *Coccidioides; fungistatic*
Miconazole	As above	Toxicity and relapses limit parental use; drug of choice for *Scedosporium* (*Pseudallescheria*) infections; some use against *Candida*; sold over the counter for topical use; fungistatic
Fluconazole	As above	Increased solubility in water allows both oral and parental use; broadly active with good CSF penetration; may be drug of choice for long-term treatment of cryptococcal meningitis; may replace ketoconazole as drug of choice for chronic mucocutaneous candidiasis; fungistatic
Itraconazole	As above	Available in United States for investigational studies; appears more potent than ketoconazole with increased activity against *Aspergillus* and *Sporothrix; fungistatic*

antibiotic that acts by binding to ergosterol, a major structural component of fungal membranes. Amphotericin B, while effective as an antifungal agent, is also a toxic agent and its use is often limited by nephrotoxicity. Several new antifungal agents have been introduced recently (Table 40-19). The fungistatic azole compounds have been clinically useful in therapy of systemic fungal infections. The development of new antifungal agents is currently of major interest because of the increasing importance of fungal agents in causing serious infections in immunocompromised hosts.

Antifungal susceptibility testing

The methods used for antifungal susceptibility testing are similar to the methods used for bacteria and broth dilution, agar dilution, and disk diffusion methods have been described. Both MICs and minimal fungicidal concentrations (MFCs) can be determined. Disk diffusion testing is generally limited to yeasts. The inoculum standardization procedure for yeast is done similarly to the bacterial tests. Inoculum preparation for molds is more problematic because of their filamentous cell structure.

Antifungal susceptibility testing should only be routinely performed in specialized laboratories. There is no general agreement between the methods used by different laboratories and results can vary widely. Factors such as medium, inoculum preparation, and conditions of incubation dramatically affect test results. It is generally agreed that test methods need to be rigorously standardized. In vitro test results may show a poor correlation to clinical outcome. It must be recognized by the clinician that the testing may not accurately predict clinical outcome.

Viruses

Development of chemotherapeutic agents for the treatment of viral infections has presented unique challenges. Since the viruses that cause disease in animals must replicate in animal cells using cellular machinery, development of agents that can selectively inhibit viral processes without significant toxicity for animal cells is difficult. As viral function and structure become understood on a molecular level, more selective and useful antiviral agents can be developed for specific viral targets.

No broad-spectrum antiviral agents are currently available, so selection of antiviral therapy depends upon identification of the specific viral agent causing the infection. Because identification of the virus may take weeks with conventional methods, the increased use of rapid viral identification methods offers obvious advantages.

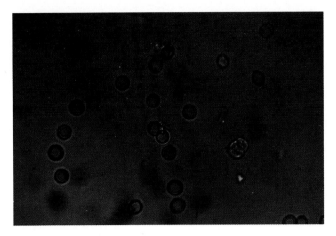

Plate 1. Normal red blood cells, one white blood cells (×400). *From Strasinger SK: Urinalysis and body fluids, ed. 2, Philadelphia, 1989, F. A. Davis.*

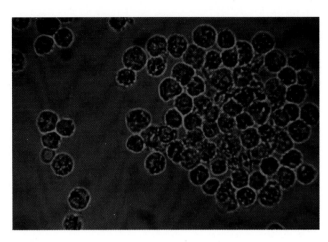

Plate 2. White blood cell clump (×400). *From Strasinger SK: Urinalysis and body fluids, ed. 2, Philadelphia, 1989, F. A. Davis.*

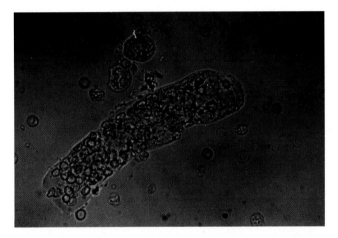

Plate 3. Red blood cell cast. Notice the presence of free red blood cells, including ghost cells (×400). *From Strasinger SK: Urinalysis and body fluids, ed. 2, Philadelphia, 1989, F. A. Davis.*

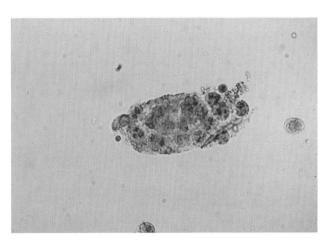

Plate 4. White blood cell cast. Note nuclear detail (×400). *From Strasinger SK: Urinalysis and body fluids, ed. 2, Philadelphia, 1989, F. A. Davis.*

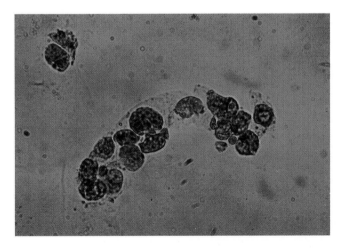

Plate 5. Stained renal tubular epithelial cell cast (×400). *From Strasinger SK: Urinalysis and body fluids, ed. 2, Philadelphia, 1989, F. A. Davis.*

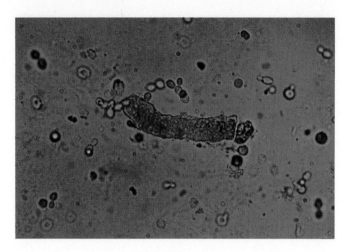

Plate 6. Coarsely granular cast with hemoglobin pigment. A comparison of red blood cells and yeast can also be made from this slide (×400). *From Strasinger SK: Urinalysis and body fluids, ed. 2, Philadelphia, 1989, F. A. Davis.*

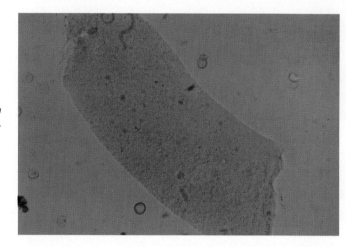

Plate 7. Waxy cast. Notice the irregularly broken ends (×400). *From Strasinger SK: Urinalysis and body fluids, ed. 2, Philadelphia, 1989, F. A. Davis.*

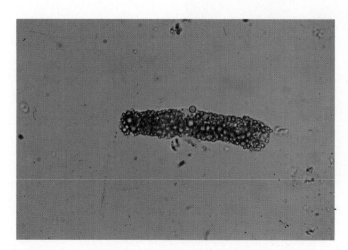

Plate 8. Fatty cast. Observe the refractile fat droplets on the matrix surface (×400). *From Strasinger SK: Urinalysis and body fluids, ed. 2, Philadelphia, 1989, F. A. Davis.*

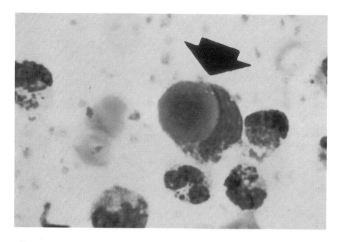

Plate 9. LE (lupus erythematosus) cell; a neutrophil containing a homogenous structureless inclusion body (from lymphocyte nuclei) altered by antinuclear antibody.

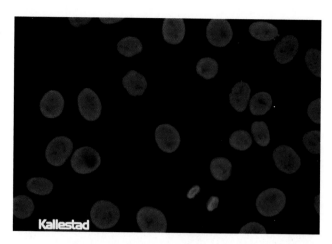

Plate 10. HEp-2 substrate, positive antinuclear antibody, homogeneous pattern, chromosome positive, 400X. *Used with permission of Sanofi Diagnostics Pasteur, Quantafluor immunofluroscence slide series, Chaska, MN.*

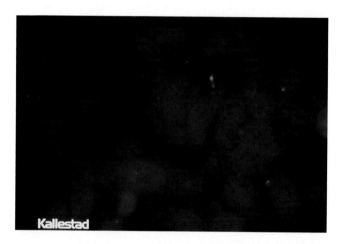

Plate 11. HEp-2 substrate, negative pattern, 400X. *Used with permission of Sanofi Diagnostics Pasteur, Quantafluor immunofluroscence slide series, Chaska, MN.*

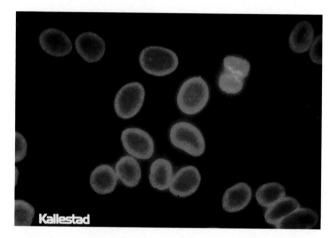

Plate 12. HEp-2 substrate, positive antinuclear antibody, rim pattern, chromosome positive, 400X. *Used with permission of Sanofi Diagnostics Pasteur, Quantafluor immunofluroscence slide series, Chaska, MN.*

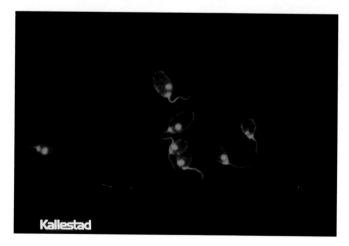

Plate 13. *Crithidia luciliae* substrate, positive kinetoplast, 1000X. *Used with permission of Sanofi Diagnostics Pasteur, Quantafluor immunofluroscence slide series, Chaska, MN.*

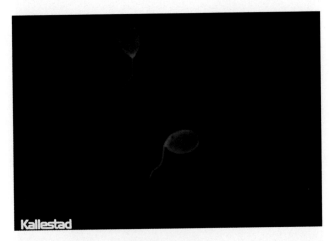

Plate 14. *Crithidia luciliae* substrate, negative reaction, 1000X. *Used with permission of Sanofi Diagnostics Pasteur, Quantafluor immunofluroscence slide series, Chaska, MN.*

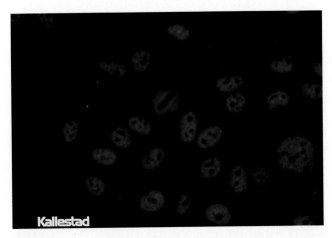

Plate 15. HEp-2 substrate, positive antinuclear antibody, speckled pattern, chromosome negative, 400X. *Used with permission of Sanofi Diagnostics Pasteur, Quantafluor immunofluroscence slide series, Chaska, MN.*

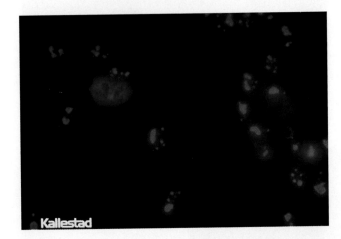

Plate 16. HEp-2 substrate, positive antinuclear antibody, nucleolar pattern, 400X. *Used with permission of Sanofi Diagnostics Pasteur, Quantafluor immunofluroscence slide series, Chaska, MN.*

Plate 17. HEp-2 substrate, positive antinuclear antibody, discrete speckled pattern (centromere), chromosome positive, 400X. *Used with permission of Sanofi Diagnostics Pasteur, Quantafluor immunofluroscence slide series, Chaska, MN.*

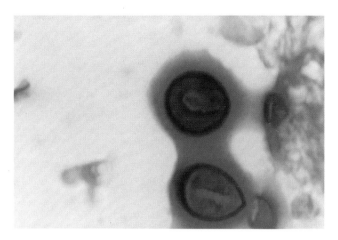

Plate 18. Encapsulated cells of *Cryptococcus neoformans* stained with Southgate's mucicarmine stain (×1000).

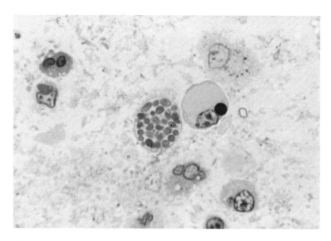

Plate 19. *Toxoplasma gondii* cysts in brain section examined with high resolution light microscopy techniques (×1000).

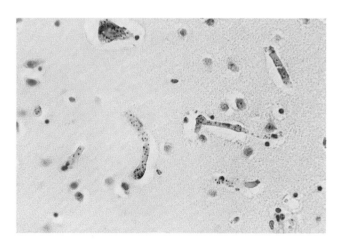

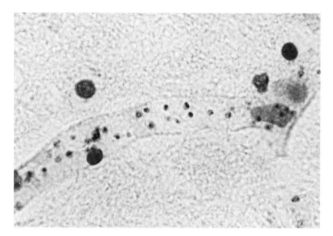

Plate 20. Cerebral malaria: *Plasmodium falciparum* parasitemia in blood vessels of brain (×100 and ×400).

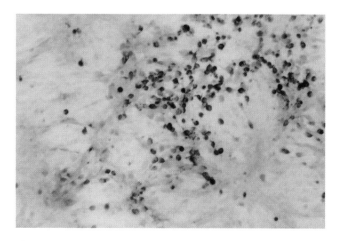

Plate 21. Immunoperoxidase stain of herpes simplex virus-infected rabbit kidney cells (×400).

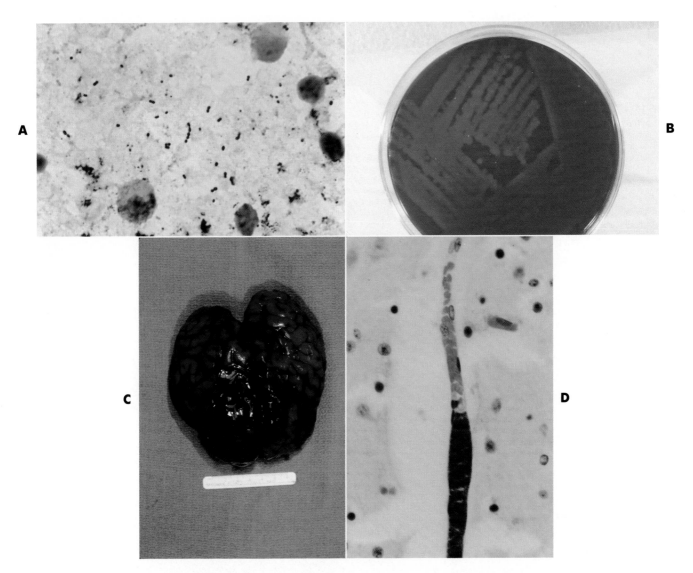

Plate 22. **A,** Direct Gram stain demonstrating *Streptococcus agalactiae* in CSF of infected neonate (×1000). **B,** Blood agar plate demonstrating diffuse β-hemolysis due to Group B streptococci from CSF culture of 3-6a. **C,** Brain at autopsy demonstrating acute hemorrhagic response to *Streptococcus agalactiae* in 3-6a case. **D,** Brain section with blood vessel occluded by Group B streptococci in 3-6a case.

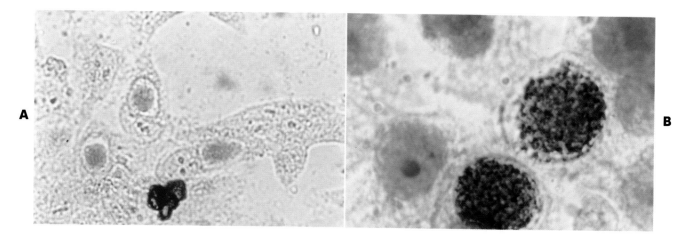

Plate 23. **A,** Iodine-stained glycogen vacuoles in chlamydia-infected McCoy cells (×400). **B,** Immunoperoxidase-stained McCoy cells infected with *Chlamydia trachomatis* (×1000).

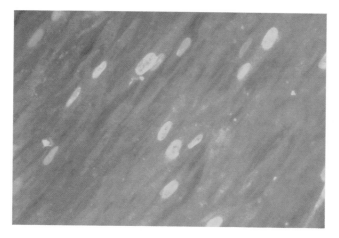

Plate 24. Cytomegalovirus-infected human embryonic fibroblasts stained with fluorescein-labeled monoclonal antibody to early nuclear antigen (×1000).

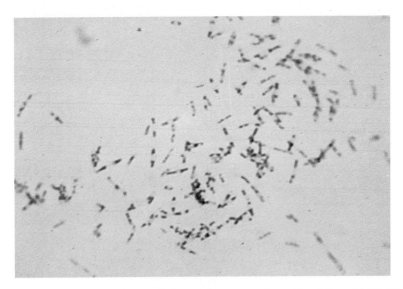

Plate 25. *B. fragilis.* Irregular staining and pleomorphism. *From Baron EJ and Finegold SM: Diagnostic microbiology, ed 8, St. Louis, 1990, Mosby-Year Book, Inc.*

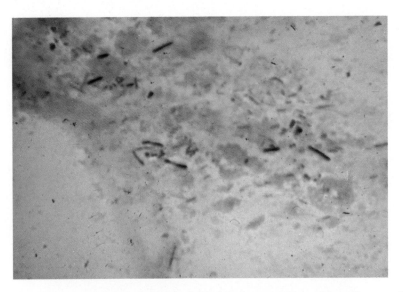

Plate 26. Perineal gas gangrene. *C. perfringens* (large, broad gram-positive rods), coliforms, and white blood cells badly distorted by toxin of *C. perfringens. From Baron EJ and Finegold SM: Diagnostic microbiology, ed 8, St. Louis, 1990, Mosby-Year Book, Inc.*

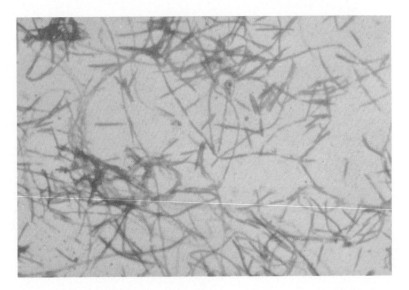

Plate 27. *F. nucleatum.* Thin bacillus with pointed ends. *From Baron EJ and Finegold SM: Diagnostic microbiology, ed 8, St. Louis, 1990, Mosby-Year Book, Inc.*

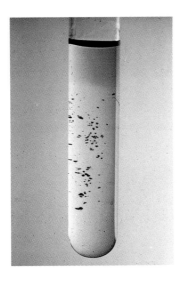

Plate 28. *Actinomyces israelii* in thioglycolate medium. No growth occurs at surface of medium. *From Howard BJ et al: Clinical pathogenic microbiology, St. Louis, 1987, Mosby–Year Book.*

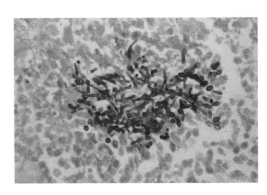

Plate 29. Periodic acid–Schiff stain of kidney tissue showing magenta yeast cells of *Candida albicans.* (×400.) *From Howard BJ et al: Clinical pathogenic microbiology, St. Louis, 1987, Mosby–Year Book.*

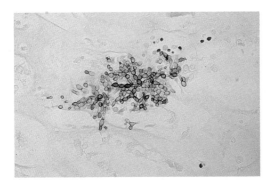

Plate 30. Grocott-Gomori methenamine–silver nitrate stain of *Candida albicans* in kidney. *From Howard BJ et al: Clinical pathogenic microbiology, St. Louis, 1987, Mosby–Year Book.*

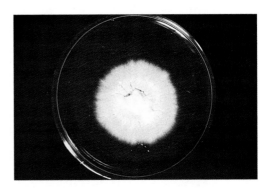

Plate 31. Colony of *Epidermophyton floccosum;* Sabouraud dextrose agar. *From Howard BJ et al: Clinical pathogenic microbiology, St. Louis, 1987, Mosby–Year Book.*

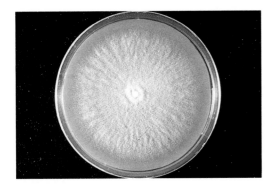

Plate 32. Colony of *Microsporum audouinii,* Sabouraud dextrose agar. *From Howard BJ et al: Clinical pathogenic microbiology, St. Louis, 1987, Mosby–Year Book.*

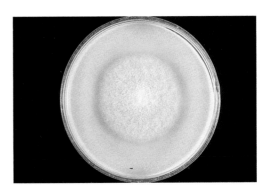

Plate 33. Colony of *Microsporum canis;* Sabouraud dextrose agar. *From Howard BJ et al: Clinical pathogenic microbiology, St. Louis, 1987, Mosby–Year Book.*

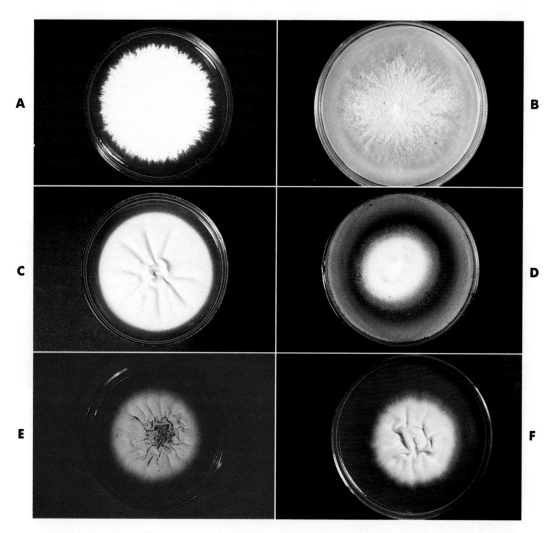

Plate 34. **A,** Colony of *Microsporum gypseum;* Sabouraud dextrose agar. **B,** Colony of *Microsporum nanum;* Sabouraud dextrose agar. **C,** Colony of *Trichophyton mentagrophytes* (var. *quinckeanum*); Sabouraud dextrose agar. **D,** Colony of *Trichophyton rubrum,* Sabouraud dextrose agar. **E,** Colony of *Trichophyton schoenleinii;* Sabouraud dextrose agar. **F,** Colony of *Trichophyton tonsurans;* Sabouraud dextrose agar. **A** to **F** *from Howard, BJ et al: Clinical pathogenic microbiology, St. Louis, 1987, Mosby— Year Book.*

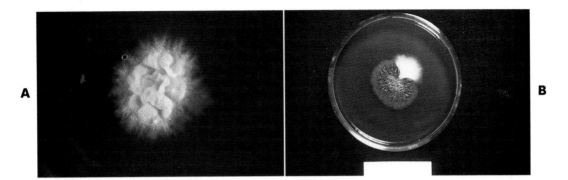

Plate 35. **A,** Colony of *Trichophyton verrucosum;* Sabouraud dextrose agar. **B,** Colony of *Trichophyton violaceum;* Sabouraud dextrose agar. *From Howard, BJ et al: Clinical pathogenic microbiology, St. Louis, 1987, Mosby–Year Book.*

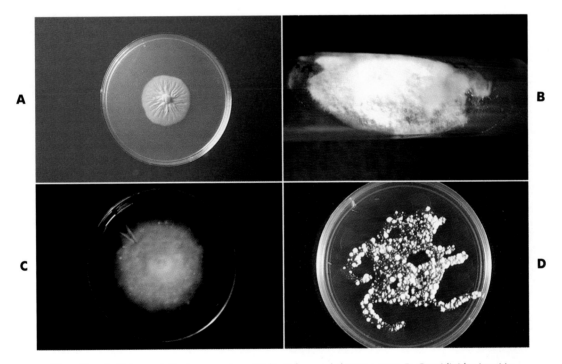

Plate 36. **A,** Colony of *Blastomyces dermatitidis;* Sabouraud dextrose agar. **B,** *Coccidioides immitis;* Sabouraud dextrose agar. **C,** Colony of *Histoplasma capsulatum* (soil isolate); Sabouraud dextrose agar. **D,** *Paracoccidioides brasiliensis* on Sabhi agar. *From Howard BJ et al: Clinical pathogenic microbiology, St. Louis, 1987, Mosby–Year Book.*

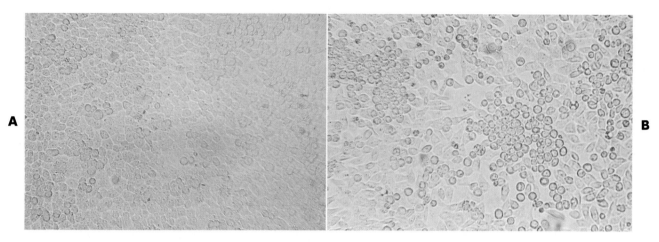

Plate 37. HEp-2 (heteroploid) cell monolayer infected with HSC. **A,** Uninfected monolayer; **B,** 2-3 + due to HSV.

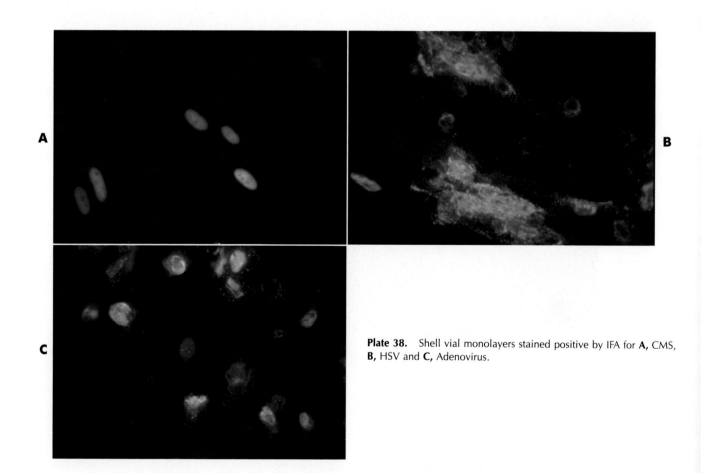

Plate 38. Shell vial monolayers stained positive by IFA for **A,** CMS, **B,** HSV and **C,** Adenovirus.

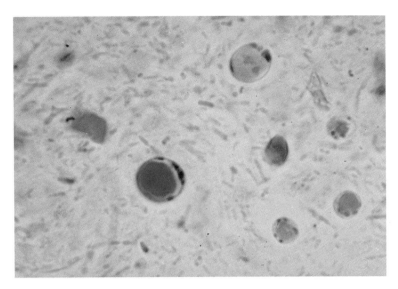

Plate 39. *Blastocystis hominis* (larger objects) and yeast cells (smaller, more homogenous objects). *From Garcia LS: Laboratory methods for diagnosis of parasitic infections. In Baron EJ and Finegold SM: Diagnostic microbiology, ed 8, St. Louis, 1990, Mosby-Year Book.*

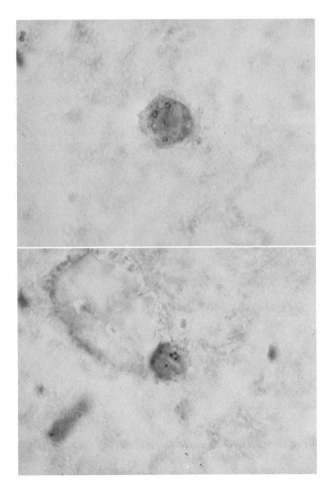

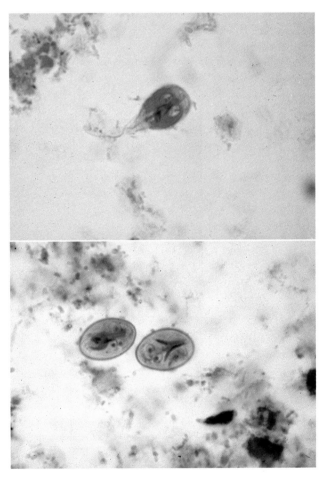

Plate 40. Top, *Dientamoeba fragilis*, two nuclei. Bottom left, *D. fragilis*, one nucleus. *From Garcia LS: Laboratory methods for diagnosis of parasitic infections. In Baron EJ and Finegold SM: Diagnostic microbiology, ed 8, St. Louis, 1990, Mosby-Year Book.*

Plate 41. Top, *Giardia lamblia* trophozoite. Bottom left, *G. lamblia* cyst. *From Garcia LS: Laboratory methods for diagnosis of parasitic infections. In Baron EJ and Finegold SM: Diagnostic microbiology, ed 8, St. Louis, 1990, Mosby-Year Book.*

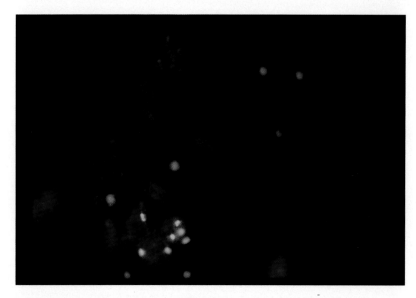

Plate 42. Fluorescein-conjugated monoclonal antibody–stained *T. vaginalis* in vaginal discharge (Courtesy Meridian Diagnostics, Inc. Cincinnati, Ohio.) *From Garcia LS: Laboratory methods for diagnosis of parasitic infections. In Baron EJ and Finegold SM: Diagnostic microbiology, ed 8, St. Louis, 1990, Mosby-Year Book.*

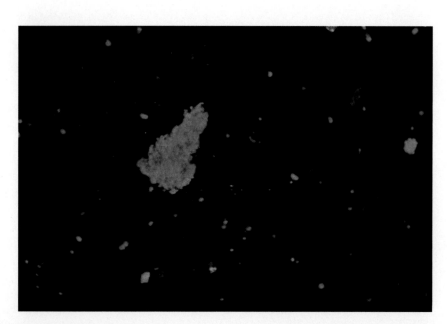

Plate 43. *P. carinii* cysts and trophozoites stained with a monoclonal antibody–fluorescent stain. (Courtesy Meridian Diagnostics, Inc., Cincinnati, Ohio.) *From Garcia LS: Laboratory methods for diagnosis of parasitic infections. In Baron EJ and Finegold SM: Diagnostic microbiology, ed 8, St. Louis, 1990, Mosby-Year Book.*

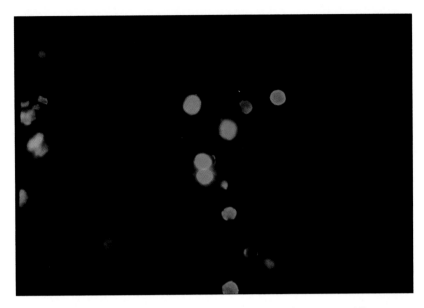

Plate 44. *Cryptosporidium* oocysts stained with monoclonal antibody–conjugated fluorescent reagent. (Merifluor, Meridian Diagnostics, Inc., Cincinnati, Ohio.) *From Garcia LS: Laboratory methods for diagnosis of parasitic infections. In Baron EJ and Finegold SM: Diagnostic microbiology, ed 8, St. Louis, 1990, Mosby-Year Book.*

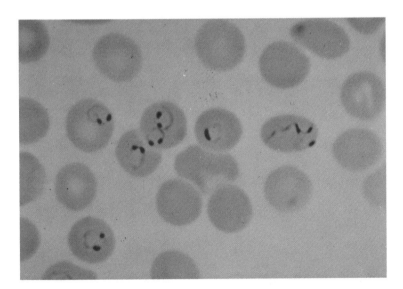

Plate 45. *Plasmodium falciparum* early ring forms. *From Garcia LS: Laboratory methods for diagnosis of parasitic infections. In Baron EJ and Finegold SM: Diagnostic microbiology, ed 8, St. Louis, 1990, Mosby-Year Book.*

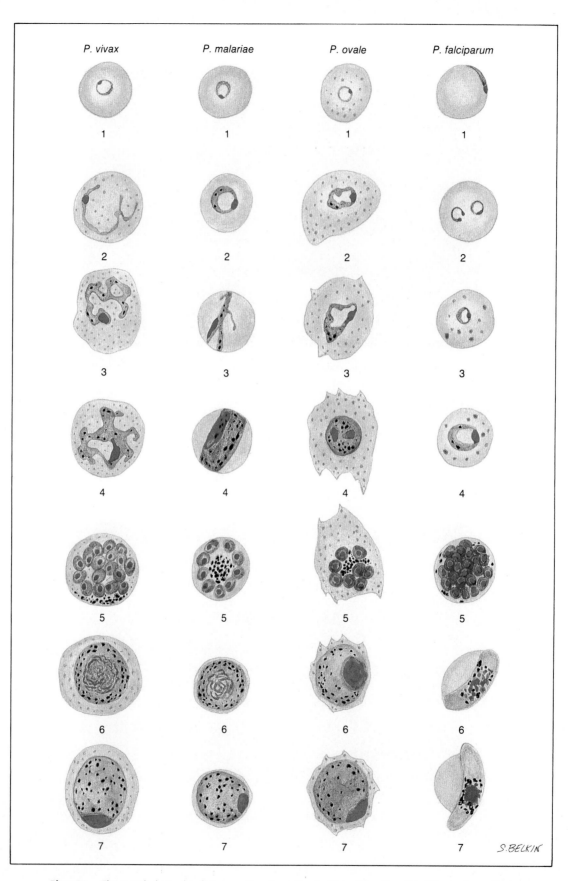

Plate 46. The morphology of malaria parasites. *From Garcia LS, and Bruckner DA, Diagnostic medical parasitology, New York, 1988, Elsevier Science Publishing Co., Inc.*

Table 40-20   Antiviral agents

Agent	Structure	Mode of action	Clinical use
Acyclovir	Analogue of guanine, converted to active phosphorylated form by thymidine kinase	Inhibits herpesvirus DNA polymerase activity and terminates elongation of viral DNA	Active against herpes simplex and varicella-zoster; resistance due to lack or alteration of thymidine kinase, or alteration in the viral DNA polymerase
Amantadine and rimantadine	Tricyclic amines derived from adamantane	Inhibits uncoating of virions, fusion, and assembly; exact target is unknown	Active against influenza A virus when given early in the course of the infection; decreased susceptibility of some strains has been seen recently
Gancyclovir	Analogue of guanine, closely related to acyclovir	Inhibits viral DNA polymerase activity	Active against herpesviruses with enhanced activity against cytomegalovirus; toxicity limits use for serious, life-threatening cytomegalovirus infections
Interferons	Antiviral peptides produced by animal cells	Induces the synthesis of several cellular proteins, increases intracellular resistance to viral infections	α-Interferon may be useful in the treatment of infections due to herpes and respiratory viruses
Ribavirin	Analogue of guanosine	Inhibits capping of viral mRNAs and RNA polymerase activity; decreases cellular GTP pools	Active against both RNA and DNA viruses, used in the treatment of influenza A and B, parainfluenza, and respiratory syncytial virus infections; inactivates the Lassa fever virus
Vidarabine	Analogue of adenosine	Inhibits viral DNA polymerase activity	Active against herpesviruses
Zidovudine (AZT)	Analogue of thymidine	Competitively inhibits reverse transcriptase	Inhibits replication of HIV, host toxicity is a problem, resistance has developed, but clinical importance unknown

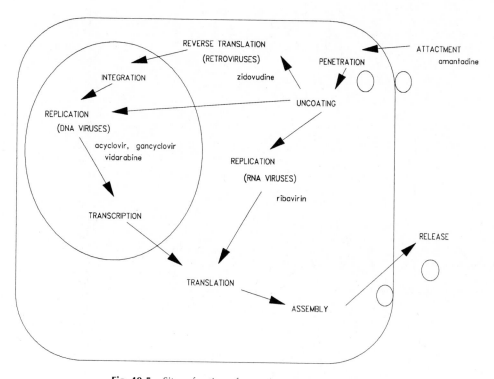

Fig. 40-5   Sites of action of some important antiviral agents.

Antiviral agents

Today, a number of effective antiviral agents are available (described in Table 40-20). Most antiviral agents in clinical use are analogues of purines or pyrimidines and interfere with viral DNA or RNA synthesis. Figure 40-5 illustrates the sites of action for some of these agents. Currently, none of these agents are viricidal nor do they affect latent viruses.

Resistance to antiviral agents has been reported but does not appear, at least at present, to be a significant clinical problem. An exception may be strains of the human immunodeficiency virus (HIV-1), which have developed resistance to zidovudine during long-term therapy is required to suppress the infection.

Antiviral susceptibility testing

Antiviral susceptibility testing is primarily performed in research laboratories. The method commonly used is the 50% plaque reduction assay, which determines the minimal amount of antiviral agent required to reduce by 50% the number of plaques formed in cell culture with a standard inoculum. This method requires careful titration of the virus and can only be used with those viruses that form visible plaques in cell culture. Isolation of the virus is also required and may delay results, so that they are of little clinical use. Methods using DNA probes for the detection of resistance genes or enzyme immunoassays that detect viral replication may make antiviral susceptibility testing quicker and more useful.

Parasites

Numerous antiparasitic agents are available for the treatment of parasitic diseases. Quinine and emetine, used respectively for the treatment of malaria and amebiasis, were among the first antimicrobial agents known. Resistance to antiparasitic agents is rare except among *Plasmodium* spp. Resistance of *Plasmodium falciparum* is of worldwide concern. Susceptibility testing of parasites is not performed except in research laboratories and the effectiveness of antiparasitic agents are determined largely by clinical response.

SUGGESTED READING

American Thoracic Society: Diagnosis and treatment of disease caused by nontuberculous mycobacteria, Am Rev Respir Dis 142:940, 1990.

Baron EJ and Finegold SM (editors): Methods for testing antimicrobial effectiveness. In Bailey and Scott's diagnostic microbiology, ed 8, Philadelphia, 1990, Mosby–Year Book, Inc.

Bauer AW et al: Antibiotic susceptibility testing by a standard single disk method, Am J Clin Pathol 45:493-496, 1966.

Bennett JV, Camp HM, and Eickhoff TC: Rapid sulfonamide disc sensitivity test for meningococci, Appl Microbiol 16:1056-1060, 1968.

Bush K: Beta-lactamase inhibitors from laboratory to clinic, Clin Microbiol Rev 1:109, 1988.

Chambers HF: Methicillin-resistant staphylococci, Clin Microbiol Rev 1:173, 1988.

Conte JE and Barriere SL: Manual of antibiotics and infectious diseases, ed 6, Philadelphia, 1988, Lea & Febiger.

Finegold SM: Anaerobes: problems and controversies in bacteriology, infections, and susceptibility testing, Rev Infect Dis:12(Suppl): S223, 1990.

Fromtling RA: Overview of medically important antifungal azole derivatives, Clin Microbiol Rev 1:187, 1988.

Graybill JR: Antifungal agents of the 1980's, Antimicrobic Newsletter 5:45, 1988.

Hindler JA: Nontraditional approaches to quality control of antimicrobial susceptibility tests, Clin Microbiol Newsletter 12:65-69, 1990.

Hirsh MS and Kaplan JC: Antiviral agents. In Fields BN and others (editors): Virology, ed 2, New York, 1990, Raven Press.

Johnson AP and others: Resistance to vancomycin and teicoplanin: an emerging clinical problem, Clin Microbiol Rev 3:289, 1990.

Klugman K: Pneumococcal resistance to antibiotics, Clin Microbiol Rev 3:171, 1990.

Lorian V: Antibiotics in laboratory medicine, ed 3, Los Angeles, 1991, Williams & Wilkins.

Miller JM, Thornsberry C, and Baker CN: Disk diffusion susceptibility test troubleshooting guide, Lab Med 15:183, 1984.

Murray BE: The life and times of the enterococcus, Clin Microbiol Rev 3:46, 1990.

National Committee for Clinical Laboratory Standards: Antifungal susceptibility testing, Committee report M20-CR. Villanova, PA, 1985, NCCLS.

National Committee for Clinical Laboratory Standards: Methodology for the serum bactericidal test, proposed guideline M21-P. Villanova, Pa, 1987, NCCLS.

National Committee for Clinical Laboratory Standards: Methods for determining bactericidal activity of antimicrobial agents, Proposed Guideline M26-P Villanova, PA, 1987, NCCLS.

National Committee for Clinical Laboratory Standards: Antimycobacterial susceptibility testing, proposed standard M24-P, Villanova, Pa, 1990, NCCLS.

National Committee for Clinical Laboratory Standards: Methods for antimicrobial susceptibility testing of anaerobic bacteria, ed 2, approved standard M11-A2. Villanova, Pa, 1990, NCCLS.

National Committee for Clinical Laboratory Standards: Methods for dilution antimicrobial susceptibility tests for bacteria that grow aerobically, ed 2, approved standard M7-A2. Villanova, Pa, 1990, NCCLS.

National Committee for Clinical Laboratory Standards: Performance standards for antimicrobial disk susceptibility tests, ed 4, approved standard M2-A4. Villanova, Pa, 1990, NCCLS.

National Committee for Clinical Laboratory Standards, M100-S3: Supplemental Tables for M2-A4, M7-A2, and M11-A2, Villanova, PA, 1991, NCCLS.

Sahm DF and others: Current concepts and approaches to antimicrobial agent susceptibility testing, Cumitech 25, Washington, DC, 1988, American Society for Microbiology.

Schwarcz SK et al: National surveillance of antimicrobial resistance in Neisseria gonorrhoeae, JAMA 264:1413-1417, 1990.

Thornsberry C (section editor): Laboratory tests in chemotherapy. In Balows A and others: Manual of clinical microbiology, ed 5, Washington, DC, 1991, American Society for Microbiology.

Washington JA II: Current problems in antimicrobial susceptibility testing, Diagn Microbiol Infect Dis 9:135-138, 1988.

Wolfson JS and Hooper DC: Fluoroquinolone antimicrobial agents, Clin Microbiol Rev 2:378, 1989.

Wong CS: Beta-lactamase inhibitors, Clin Microbiol Newsletter 10:177-184, 1988.

41

Microbial antigen detection

Richard C. Tilton

Timely and appropriate diagnosis and treatment of infectious diseases is, to a large extent, based on rapid and sensitive identification of the etiologic agent as well as determination of the agent's susceptibility to a wide variety of antimicrobial agents. A number of methods exist for rapid detection of microorganisms, including microscopy, detection of organism-specific IgM antibody, microbial antigen detection, molecular probes, and instrumentation methods such as gas chromatography, flow cytometry, and light scattering. With the exception of microscopy, microbial antigen detection is the method most widely used in most clinical microbiology laboratories. A variety of methods are available such as counterimmunoelectrophoresis (CIE), latex agglutination (LA), coagglutination (CA), enzyme immunoassay (EIA), radioimmunoassay (RIA), and immunofluoresence assay (IFA). Antigen detection tests are not limited to bacteria, but include representative fungi, parasites, and viruses.

METHODS

Counterimmuno electrophoresis (CIE) was first used clinically for the detection of "Australia antigen" (HbsAg). Radioimmunoassay soon replaced CIE for HbsAg, but CIE was a valuable immunologic tool for rapid detection of both microbial antibodies and antigens for at least a decade. Latex agglutination and EIA are more sensitive and have replaced CIE in most laboratories. (See Table 41-1.)

Counterimmunoelectrophoresis is a rapid precipitin reaction in which the reactants are driven by an electric current. In 1901 Vincent and Bellot first described the use of the tube precipitin reaction for the detection of meningococcal antigen in cerebrospinal fluid. Dochez and Avery identified the capsular polysaccharide of the pneumococcus in patients' urine. The precipitin reaction is a function of the precipitation of antibody and soluble antigen at the equivalence point. The reaction may take up to 18 hours. CIE combines the advantages of immunodiffusion and electrophoresis. The antigen (Ag) is placed in a well on the cathodic side of a solid support and the antibody is placed on the anodic side. The antigen, if negatively charged, migrates toward the anode, and the antibody, which usually has a weak negative charge, also migrates toward the cathode. This is called endoosmotic flow. If conditions of voltage, current, buffer, pH, antigen/antibody concentration, and quality of antisera are optimal, then a precipitin line appears between the two wells after as little as 30 minutes of electrophoresis.

There are a number of variables that must be standardized if CIE is to be a reliable, reproducible method in the clinical laboratory. These include quality of antisera, buffers, support systems, and electrical parameters.

LATEX AGGLUTINATION

Latex polystyrene beads were first used to detect rheumatoid factor in serum. Either antigen or IgG antibody is nonspecifically absorbed to the surface of the latex polystyrene beads of uniform diameter, usually 0.8 μm. Addition of the specific antibody or antigen visibly agglutinates the milky white latex suspension. Although latex agglutination (LA) tests can be done in test tubes, they are usually performed on slides.

Depending on the system, the procedure for the detection of antigen or antibody by LA may be quite simple. A drop or two of the latex reagent is mixed with a suspension of the colony or the body fluid to be tested. The suspension is incubated at room temperature with occasional rotation of the slide. Agglutination is a positive finding.

Although several commercial reagents are available, preparation of LA reagents in the laboratory is not difficult. One example is the use of an LA test to identify *Legionella pneumophila*. Antiserum, 0.1, is added to a tube containing 1 ml of 10% solution of Dow latex polystyrene and a 1:20

Table 41-1 Sensitivity of antigen detection by counterimmunoelectrophoresis and latex agglutination*

| | Polysaccharide (μg/ml) | | |
| | *Haemophilus influenzae* Type B | *Neisseria meningitidis* | |
Method		Group A	Group C
Counterimmunoelectro-phoresis	20	50	75
Latex agglutination	5	10	25

Modified from Leinonen M and Kayhty H: J Clin Pathol 31:1172, 1978.

solution of glycine-buffered saline containing 0.1% bovine serum albumin. The diluted latex reagent is filtered through a thin layer of absorbent cotton to remove any clumped particles.

A major drawback to LA is nonspecific reactions with specimens such as urine, sputum, serum, and synovial fluid. False-positive agglutination can sometimes be eliminated by heating the specimen to 60°C for 15 minutes or to 100°C for 5 minutes.

COAGGLUTINATION

Kronvall was the first to introduce the coagglutination (CA) technique for the detection of pneumococcal antigens. Certain strains of *Staphylococcus aureus*, in particular Cowan strain I, contain a cell surface protein known as protein A. Antibodies of the IgG class adhere to protein A by their Fc portion, leaving the Fab ends free to bind to complex homologous antigen. The presence of antigen results in the visible agglutination of the staphylococci.

The agglutination of sensitized protein A containing staphylococci may be less distinct than that of latex. The sensitivity of antigen detection by CA is similar to LA. The procedure, like latex agglutination, is subject to nonspecific agglutination in body fluids, such as cerebrospinal fluid, serum, and urine.

The preparation of CA reagents is technically simple, and once prepared, the sensitized staphylococci are more stable than latex reagents. Commercial coagglutination reagents are available.

ENZYME IMMUNOASSAY

The two major types of enzyme immunoassays are homogeneous and heterogeneous. Heterogeneous immunoassays require physical separation of bound and unbound antigen, whereas homogeneous assays do not. Enzyme-multiplied immunoassays (EMIT) are homogeneous assays, and enzyme-linked immunosorbent assays (ELISA) are heterogeneous.

Enzyme-multiplied assay is a competitive assay. The substance to be tested, usually a low molecular weight antigen, is attached to an enzyme. This attachment occurs in such a way that binding of antibody to the antigen sterically blocks substrate binding. In the clinical test, a body fluid that purportedly contains free or unbound antigen is mixed with antibody and the enzyme-labeled or bound antigen. Both free and bound antigen compete for binding sites on the antibody. The more free antigen present, the more enzyme remains unbound and catalytically active on the addition of a specific enzyme substrate. The reaction is read spectrophotometrically; the greater the enzyme activity, the greater the change in absorbance of the substrate. The absorbance change is directly correlated to the concentration of antigen in the patient's specimen.

Figure 41-1 depicts antigen measurement by the enzyme immunoassay (EIA) double sandwich technique. An antibody is bound to a solid support, such as a plastic tube, a tray, or polystyrene beads. The antigen-containing body fluid is layered over the sensitized solid phase. An enzyme-labeled antibody is then added to form an antibody-antigen-antibody "sandwich." After separation of the bound and free enzyme-tagged antibody, a specific chromogenic enzyme substrate is added. The bound enzyme reacts with its substrate to produce a color change, which indicates the presence of antigen. Enzyme substrate combinations commonly used include alkaline phosphatase and nitrophenyl phosphate or horseradish peroxidase and orthophylenediamine.

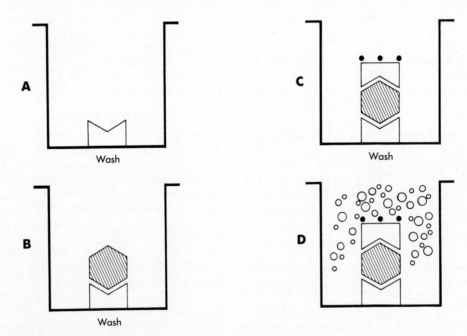

Fig. 41-1 Double antibody sandwich method of EIA for assay of antigen. **A,** Antibody is adsorbed to surface. **B,** Test solution containing antigen is added. **C,** Enzyme-labeled specific antibody is added. **D,** Enzyme substrate is added. Amount of hydrolysis equals amount of antigen present. (**A** to **C** show condition of well after excess, unbound reagents have been washed away.) *From Tilton RC: Immunoserology in the clinical microbiology laboratory. In Howard BJ and others: Clinical and pathogenic microbiology, St Louis, 1987, Mosby-Year Book.*

A competitive ELISA (similar to the competitive RIA) may also be used to detect antigen.

In EIA, the amount of hydrolysis of the substrate is directly related to the amount of antigen or antibody present. The reaction may be read visually or spectrophotometrically. For screening tests, that is, simply determining positive or negative results, manual reading is acceptable. For most applications, however, quantitation of antigen content is desirable.

Antigen/antibody can also be attached to a membrane. Diffusion of the specimen, enzyme conjugate, and substrate through the membrane very rapidly produces a visual signal if positive. The signal can be a dot ● or a + sign.

Although EIA methodology is not conceptually difficult, parameters such as solid phase, the washing process, enzymes, substrates, and reaction termination must be strictly controlled.

RADIOIMMUNOASSAY

Radioimmunoassay (RIA) techniques use a radioisotope, usually iodine-125, to detect antigen-antibody reactions. These techniques combine the specificity of immunology and the sensitivity of radiochemistry. Although the principal use of RIA is in endocrinology for the assay of hormones, all areas of laboratory medicine have found RIA to be a useful tool. Radioimmunoassay has many variations, but in most applications in the clinical setting, a competitive protein binding assay is used to measure antigen. In this assay, a known amount of radiolabeled antigen competes with an unknown quantity of antigen in a patient's serum for available binding sites on a specified amount of homologous antibody. If high concentrations of unlabeled antigen are present in the patient's serum, the amount of labeled antigen bound by antibody is reduced. After equilibrium between the bound and the unbound antigen is reached, the bound fraction is separated from the unbound fraction by precipitation or centrifugation, and the radioactivity in the bound or free phase (or both) is measured in a scintillation counter. The counts are then related to concentration with the use of a standard curve.

FLUORESCENCE IMMUNOASSAYS

The fluorescence immunoassay is similar to the other assays described (RIA, EIA) except that fluorescing compounds are used to tag antigens or antibodies instead of radioisotopes or enzymes. The assays may be competitive or noncompetitive. Plastic beads, disks, tubes, or paddles are coated with an antigen or antibody. If the tests are competitive, fluorescein-labeled compounds compete with nonlabeled compounds for binding sites. As in the other systems, the bound and free components are separated by centrifugation, decanting, and most recently, by the use of magnetic beads.

The Abbott TDX instrument (Abbott Laboratories, Chicago) is based on fluorescence polarization immunoassay (FPIA) and is used in many laboratories. This assay is a nonseparation immunoassay; that is, the bound and free complexes need not be separated before the test is read. Fluorescence polarization immunoassay is also a competitive assay in that bound and free antigen-antibody complexes generate different signals when fluorescent light is polarized in both horizontal and vertical planes. In FPIA, the specificity of an immunoassay is combined with the speed and convenience of a homogeneous method. Methods are currently available for the measurement of aminoglycosides and vancomycin in serum, as well as other low molecular weight substances such as digoxin, cortisol, and illegal drugs. An updated version of the TDX is the Abbott IDX, which detects both high and low molecular weight antigens.

Time-resolved fluoroimmunoassay (TRFIA) reduces background fluorescence by selective detection of long decay fluorescing molecules such as europium and terbium. These molecules, in the form of their lanthanide chelates, have a high quantum yield that enables emission peaks to be discerned from the background. A TRFIA instrument from Wallac (Turku, Finland) is used in Europe for viral antigen detection.

APPLICATION OF MICROBIAL ANTIGEN DETECTION

Bacterial antigens detected by immunologic methods consist primarily of cell envelope molecules ranging from polysaccharide capsular material to major outer membrane proteins (MOMP). Few, if any, internal bacterial structures have been targeted for antigen detection tests. Some constituents, such as capsular polysaccharides, are not tightly cell-associated and are released in substantial quantity to the blood, urine, cerebrospinal fluid, or other body fluids. Capsular antigen can be detected in the absence of whole bacteria. Other components such as MOMP are more tightly cell-associated and cellular components in which bacteria are found, such as *Chlamydia* are necessary for a sensitive antigen detection test. Following is a compilation of some of the available bacterial antigen detection tests applicable to clinical microbiology.

Group A beta hemolytic streptococci (Streptococcus pyogenes)

Rapid tests for group A beta hemolytic streptococci (GABS) were developed and initially marketed during 1984 to 1985. The initial kits were based on detection of antigen by latex agglutination following extraction of the C carbohydrate of the GABS. During the ensuing 7-year period, the number of commercially available test kits increased from 2 to >50. These test kits are based on latex agglutination, coagglutination, or enzyme immunoassay. A wide range of test sensitivity (55% to 95%) has been reported although specificity of most of the products is >95%. Those kits that require extraction of the group antigen appear to be more sensitive. The kits were developed primarily for the physician office market or point-of-use testing. While they can be used in the clinical laboratory, their value is diminished as the time between specimen collection and reporting increases.

Traditional culture for GABS, whether performed in the physician office laboratory, private laboratory, or clinical laboratory is time consuming (48 to 72 hours). Several advantages are readily seen with a test for GABS that requires 10 minutes or less. If the rapid test is positive, then there is >95% assurance that GABS are present. A number of studies now document in children the advantages of rapid treatment, including rapid improvement in clinical condition as well as reduction of the risk of transmission of the bacterium within the family unit. There are also studies that indicate that rapid treatment abrogates antibody formation which results in lack of immunity to the particular M-type. If the rapid test is negative, then the physician may wish to perform a culture depending on the signs and symptoms observed. The recurrence of rheumatic fever in the United States again underscores the necessity of appropriate and prompt treatment of GABS pharyngitis.

Group B streptococcus (Streptococcus agalactiae)

Group B streptococci (GBS) are leading causes of neonatal morbidity and mortality, with an incidence between 1 and 4 per 1000 live births. However, approximately 20% of pregnant women are asymptomatic carriers of GBS. In the newborn, GBS disease may occur as an early onset disease, in which case the bacteria can be isolated from blood and gastric aspirates, or it may occur as a late-onset disease in which the bacteria are usually isolated from the CSF cerebrospinal fluid. A number of studies have indicated that intrapartum chemoprophylaxis reduces the incidence of GBS infection to nearly zero. Hence, the necessity of a rapid test. LA, CA, and EIA tests are available. A number of studies suggest that rapid tests on vaginal secretions can be used to identify women at high risk of delivering infants with GBS disease. Once infected, it is also possible to use the same tests to diagnose GBS in the newborn. A number of reports suggest that the antigen is more readily detected in urine than in blood or cerebrospinal fluid. Consequently, these rapid tests should be used in conjunction with culture on women about to deliver as well as on infected infants. Sensitivity approaching 100% can be realized if urine and one other body fluid from infected infants are tested by LA, CA, or EIA.

Cerebrospinal fluid antigen detection

A number of commercial LA and CA kits for detection of *Neisseria meningitidis, Haemophilus influenzae, Streptococcus pneumoniae,* and group B streptococcal antigens are available. Most kits use polyclonal antibodies with the exception of a monoclonal antibody for group B *N. meningitidis.* The LA and CA tests are rapid and the entire panel can be done in less than 30 minutes. The reagents are approved for cerebrospinal fluid, urine, and serum, although in the author's experience, detection of capsular antigen in serum is rarely useful. All tests include directions for treatment of specimens in the event that nonspecific agglutination occurs. Many reports document the broad range of sensitivity and specificity of these tests. Both of these statistical parameters are a function of the antigen detected and the body fluid analyzed. Unfortunately, none are 100% sensitive and specific.

Two questions are asked when a child presents with signs and symptoms of meningitis. One is, "Does the child have meningitis?" The other, "Is the etiology bacterial, viral, or neither?" Nonmicrobiologic parameters such as cerebrospinal fluid glucose, protein, cellular constituency, and Gram's stain aid in the answers to these questions. Ninety-five percent of cerebrospinal fluid specimens will show no abnormalities. Five percent of the specimens are potential candidates for cerebrospinal fluid antigen detection. However, the sensitivity of antigen detection is approximately the same as the Gram's stain and false-positive agglutinations do occur. Of the 5% of specimens that would suggest bacterial

meningitis, 10% to 15% of these patients will have been partially treated. The cerebrospinal fluid will usually have a negative Gram's stain. It is in these cases that antigen detection is worthwhile. Cerebrospinal fluid antigen detection is costly and should not be performed unless there are a significant number of white blood cells in the cerebrospinal fluid (10 to >100/cu mm) or other chemical constituents that point to bacterial meningitis. Thus, cerebrospinal fluid antigen detection should be reserved for partially treated patients or to confirm positive cerebrospinal fluid Gram's stain results. A number of investigators, however, have indicated that the sensitivity of meningitis diagnosis may be increased by testing concentrated urine specimens.

Chlamydia trachomatis

There are three methods currently available to detect *Chlamydia trachomatis* in human specimens. These include EIA, direct fluorescence antibody microscopy (DFA), and a nucleic acid probe (Gen-Probe, Pace II, San Diego, Calif). The polymerase chain reaction (PCR) is also done experimentally to detect *Chlamydia*-specific DNA.

The detection of *C. trachomatis* antigens has the potential to replace culture for the routine diagnosis of chlamydia cervicitis, urethritis, pneumonitis, and conjunctivitis. Culture is technically difficult, time consuming, and requires a tissue culture facility. To date, however because of sensitivity and specificity problems, antigen detection tests for *C. trachomatis* have not replaced culture but offer an acceptable alternative in populations at high risk for the disease. Enzyme immunoassay detects group antigens that are either genus- or species-specific for a variety of *C. trachomatis* serotypes, depending on the manufacturer. Both polyclonal and monoclonal antibodies directed to either the major outer membrane protein (MOMP) or lipopolysaccharides are used.

Investigators have compared EIA methods to culture. One large study noted that Chlamydiazyme (CZ) (Abbott Laboratories, North Chicago, Ill) was a sensitive and specific test for a high-risk population. However, when tested by CZ, both females at low to moderate risk and asymptomatic males revealed that the kit was less sensitive than for high-risk patients. False-positive results may also occur in both EIA and DFA. There are at least three bacteria that crossreact with monoclonal antibodies against *C. trachomatis* MOMP. It is also possible that false-positive antigen detection tests are, in fact, false-negative culture tests. While this has been suspected in a number of patients, it is likely that neither EIA nor DFA tests are 100% specific. The true sensitivity of culture is not known, but if vials (not microdilution plates), one blind passage, and detection of inclusion bodies by FA are used, it is likely that culture is at least 80% sensitive.

One of the major disadvantages of EIA is that the cellular composition of the specimen, that is specimen quality, cannot be determined. The advantages include time (as little as 1 to 1½ hours), the ability to batch specimens, and the reading of the test by a spectrophotometer, which reduces subjectivity. Enzyme immunoassay tests are more suitable to automated systems and, unlike culture, do not require a viable organism for a positive result. Transportation, then, becomes much less of a problem with the rapid test compared to culture.

A number of solid phase membrane EIAs such as the Abbott Testpak have been introduced. They are rapid (± 30 minutes) and could potentially be performed in a satellite clinic or a physician's office. Recently, however, the Test-Pak was removed from the market.

Because of the nature of culture, it would appear that noncultural methods would be less expensive and much more applicable to the smaller laboratory. In order to be cost beneficial, however, testing should be reserved for groups of patients who might not be routinely treated for chlamydial infection or for those patients in whom the clinical outcome of infection is very serious. Women, because of the consequences of infection, such as salpingitis, and because of their epidemiological importance in transmitting the bacterium, are the best candidates for specific *C. trachomatis* diagnosis. Children who are suspected of being sexually abused must be tested by culture.

Clostridium difficile

Pseudomembranous enterocolitis (PMC) is a life-threatening disease. The primary etiology is *Clostridium difficile*. Most patients are infected following antibiotic therapy, although various studies suggest that *C. difficile* colonization rates range from 2% to 24%, depending on the patient's environment and the administration of antibiotics.

Pathogenic *C. difficile* secretes two toxins, A and B, and a motility factor. There are nontoxigenic strains present, however, that produce neither toxin. Toxin A causes the intestinal pathology observed in animal models and toxin B is primarily responsible for the cytopathology observed in tissue cultures. Recent evidence suggests that toxin A is also cytotoxic. Enzyme immunoassays have been developed for both toxins A and B. Demonstration of *C. difficile* toxin(s) in stool filtrates has relied on the demonstration of characteristic cytopathology in a variety of cell lines, usually human diploid fibroblasts such as WI-38. Some feel that the sensitivity of cytotoxin detection compared to clinical disease may be low, and that toxin B titers do not necessarily correlate with the extent of disease.

In 1986 Marion Scientific Company (Kansas City, Mo) introduced a latex agglutination (LA) test for toxin A. Subsequently, it was shown that the protein detected by LA was not toxin A, but a structural protein of *C. difficile*. The LA reagent cross-reacts with *Clostridium sporogenes* and *Peptostreptococcus anaerobius*. The gene for production of this structural protein has been cloned. The gene product is not toxin A. The LA test, if positive, indicates the presence of *C. difficile* or a cross-reacting bacterium. Both toxigenic and nontoxigenic *C. difficile* will be detected.

A number of studies indicate that LA is an effective screening test for disease. However, if the LA test is positive, it has been suggested that a cytotoxin assay be performed on the stool filtrate. While there have been variations in sensitivity of LA reported, it is generally felt that a negative test correlates with the absence of disease.

Escherichia coli

Escherichia coli K1 antigen has been detected in the cerebrospinal fluid and urine of neonates using *Neisseria meningitidis* group B antiserum. Both antigens are immunologically identical. Commercial LA kits are available. This cross-reactivity must be carefully monitored so as not to confuse meningococcal disease diagnosis with *E. coli* K1 disease. Radioimmunoassay, LA, and ELISA have been used to detect LT and ST toxins of enterotoxic *E. coli*. Kits are not commercially available as demand for such assays has been minimal.

Escherichia coli serotypes, predominantly 0157/H7, which produce Shiga-like toxins (Verotoxin) and have been associated with hemorrhagic diarrhea and hemolytic uremia syndrome, can be detected in stool filtrates using tissue culture. Although EIA for *E. coli* Shiga-toxin detection has been reported, the assays are not commercially available. A latex agglutination test is available for identification of 0157/H7 serotypes of *E. Coli*.

FUNGI
Cryptococcus neoformans

The LA test for the detection of cryptococcal polysaccharide antigen in human serum and cerebrospinal fluid is widely used for the rapid diagnosis of cryptococcosis. Latex agglutination is more sensitive than microscopy and as sensitive as culture. Cross-reactions occur due to rheumatoid factor (RF), so parallel RF testing should be performed on all positive results.

Candida albicans

The diagnosis of disseminated candidiasis is difficult to make by both clinical and laboratory means. Often the diagnosis is made only at autopsy. Isolation of *Candida albicans* from a body site does not indicate infection per se or deep-seated infection specifically. Attempts to more precisely and rapidly diagnose disseminated candidiasis (DC) have been only moderately successful. Mannan is the major component of *Candida* cell walls. Mannan antigenemia is detected at higher rates in immunosuppressed patients, but the sensitivity of the test for DC is between 50% and 70%. *Candida* metabolites such as mannose and arabitol have been detected in serum by gas liquid chromatography. Sensitivity ranges from 64% to 96%. Tests for other *Candida* cell wall antigens have not been successful.

Systemic mycoses

Exoantigen techniques have been reported for *Blastomyces dermatitidis*, *Histoplasma capsulatum*, *Coccidioides immitis*, *Aspergillus*, and *Sporothrix schenckii*. At the present time these antigen detection tests are used to identify fungi on culture and have not been routinely used directly on clinical specimens.

PARASITOLOGY
Pneumocystis carinii

Pneumocystis carinii is a leading cause of pneumonia in patients with HIV-I infection (human immunodeficiency virus). Until recently, laboratory detection was based on detection of the typical cysts and/or trophozoites in a stained sample of respiratory secretions. Although both CIE and EIA have been described for detection of *P. carinii* in clinical specimens, no source is available and has not been corroborated. Both IFA and DFA procedures are available

Table 41-2 Antigen detection methods for viral diagnosis*

Virus	Methods	Comments
Hepatitis B surface antigen (HBsAg)	RIA, EIA, reverse passive LA	HBsAg is the primary screening test for hepatitis B. Appears 1-12 wk after infection.
Hepatitis Be antigen (HBeAg)	RIA, reverse passive hemagglutination, EIA	Within 1 week of HBsAg, e antigen appears and lasts <18 weeks. Indicates highly infectious sera.
Hepatitis delta virus antigen	EIA RIA	Commercial kits are available for the detection of delta virus antigen. The assay should be used for specific diagnosis of delta hepatitis and not for screening, as patients infected with delta virus will also have hepatitis B markers.
Human immunodeficiency virus (HIV-I) p24 antigen	EIA	p24 Antigen detection kits are available commercially. p24 Ag appears early; infection disappears and then reappears. Its reappearance is a poor prognostic sign. p24 Ag may also decrease in response to anti-HIV therapy.
Herpes simplex virus (HSV)	EIA, LA	A variety of EIA and LA products are available for direct detection of HSV in clinical specimens. One EIA claims 96% sensitivity and 100% specificity. Others appear to be much less sensitive, especially in asymptomatic female patients.
Cytomegalovirus (CMV)	In situ microscopy (peroxidase-labeled Ig)	CMV may be detected directly in leukocytes by an indirect monoclonal antibody mediated HRP-stained microscopic evaluation.
Varicella zoster virus (VZV)	IFA, EIA	Fluorescent antibody (FA) microscopy is used to detect VZV in clinical specimens. EIA has been reported, but is not available. FA microscopy may be more sensitive than culture.
Respiratory syncytial virus (RSV)	IFA, DFA, EIA, TRFIA	Since the availability of specific therapy for RSV, rapid methods for detection are essential. EIA appears to be less sensitive than IFA; DFA, is more rapid than IFA. Reports suggest that TRFIA is virtually as sensitive as culture.
Influenza, parainfluenza, adenovirus (respiratory)	TRFIA, DFA, IFA, EIA	With some exceptions, there seems to be no trend to screen all respiratory specimens for the three viruses. Methods that are sensitive and specific are available commercially should a laboratory wish to offer a respiratory virus screening panel.
Norwalk virus	EIA	Research methods are available for direct detection of Norwalk virus in feces.
Rotavirus	LA, EIA, CIE	The routine method for rotavirus detection in feces is either EIA or LA, although EM and CIE have been used. LA is less sensitive than EIA, whereas some EIA products lack specificity.
Adenovirus 40/41	EIA	Cambridge Biotech (Hopkinton, Mass) has available an EIA for direct detection of adenovirus 40/41 in feces.

*RIA, radioimmunoassay; EIA, enzyme immunoassay; LA, latex agglutination; IFA, indirect fluorescent antibody assay; DFA, direct fluorescent antibody; TRFIA, time-resolved fluoroimmunoassay.

for the direct detection of *P. carinii*. The method of choice for most laboratories is DFA.

Giardia lamblia

Giardiasis may be the most prevalent infectious diarrhea in the United States. Diagnosis is based on microscopic detection of the cysts in a series of stool samples. It is often necessary to process multiple stools on successive days to demonstrate the organism. There are commercial EIA kits available for *Giardia* antigen.

The literature substantiates increased sensitivity and specificity of EIA over microscopic examination. There were 30% more cases of giardiasis diagnosed with EIA than with routine methods. In some cases, *Giardia* antigen was present in the absence of cysts.

Toxoplasma gondii

Infection with *Toxoplasma gondii* is widespread and ranges from foodborne toxoplasmosis to intrauterine infections to toxoplasmosis in patients with HIV infection. Diagnosis has

been primarily serological. That is, specific IgG or IgM antibodies have been used to diagnose disease. An antigen detection test might be useful as demonstration of the parasite in infected tissues is not a sensitive procedure. Both CIE and EIA antigen detection procedures have been described, but results have been equivocal.

Trichomonas vaginalis

Trichomoniasis is a widespread and major cause of vaginitis and occasionally, of urethritis in males. Most laboratories detect this parasite microscopically as culture is complicated and time consuming. An EIA has recently been described that detects a GSKD surface polypeptide using a monoclonal antibody. Compared to culture of *T. vaginalis*, sensitivity of the EIA on vaginal specimens was 89% and specificity was 97%.

Virology

Table 41-2 lists viral antigen detection tests commonly used in the clinical microbiology laboratory.

SUGGESTED READING

Balows A, et al: Manual of clinical microbiology, ed 5, Washington, DC, 1991, American Society for Microbiology.

Balows A, Tilton RC, Turano A: Rapid methods and automation in microbiology and immunology, Brescia, Italy, 1989, Brixia Academic Press.

Fung JC and Tilton RC: Detection of bacterial antigens. In Wicher K (editor): Microbial antigenodiagnosis, Boca Raton, Fla, 1988, CRC Press.

Rytel MW: Rapid diagnosis in infectious disease, Boca Raton, Fla, 1979, CRC Press.

Tilton RC: Immunoserology in the clinical microbiology laboratory. In Howard BJ, et al.: Clinical and pathogenic microbiology, St Louis, 1987, Mosby–Year Book.

42 Nucleic acid amplification techniques for the diagnosis of infectious diseases

David H. Persing

The ability of a nucleic acid molecule to specifically recognize and bind complementary sequences to form double-stranded hybrids has been recognized for nearly 30 years. This property, which represents one of the most specific intermolecular interactions in nature, has been largely responsible for bringing about the revolution in molecular genetics that has since occurred. While most of this revolution has occurred in the basic science laboratories, the last decade has witnessed a mounting interest in extending this technology from the basic laboratory to the diagnostic laboratory, particularly in the diagnosis of inherited disorders and infectious diseases.

In principle, if a unique "signature sequence" can be identified in the nucleic acids of an infectious agent and appropriate probes can be generated, the detection of the sequence in a clinical specimen may indicate the presence of the pathogen. Despite the auspicious introduction of such probes for the detection of infectious agents, however, relatively few laboratories employ them on a regular basis. This lack of widespread acceptance is due in large part to three factors. First, despite recent advances, the application of nucleic acid probes is still technically demanding and requires specially trained personnel. Second, most protocols require use of radioactive compounds in order to provide maximum sensitivity. Third, the greatest sensitivity of nucleic acid probes, approximately 10^3 and 10^4 molecules, may not be sufficiently high for them to be used directly on patient specimens. For this reason, probes for infectious agents have been largely confined to culture confirmation and have not yet eliminated the need for primary culture.

This chapter will review in vitro amplification techniques that are under development for enhancing the signal generated by nucleic-acid–based detection systems. The goal of these systems is to improve on the sensitivity of nucleic acid–based tests and to simplify them through the use of automation and the incorporation of nonisotopic detection formats. While these methods are not limited to the diagnosis of infectious diseases, the clinical microbiology laboratory will benefit greatly from their introduction. Amplification techniques will likely revolutionize the detection of pathogens for which in vitro cultivation systems are lengthy, inconvenient, or unavailable, and will thus greatly extend the diagnostic repertoire of the clinical laboratory. Indeed, published reports of new applications for the diagnosis of infectious diseases, in keeping with the technology they exploit, are accumulating at a seemingly exponential rate.

The technology underlying in vitro amplification techniques is complex and in a state of flux. Thus, the ultimate intent of this chapter is to provide a framework for understanding a complex subject matter, so that when improvements and/or innovations are introduced, they can be more easily assimilated. Specifically, we will examine two different approaches to in vitro amplification of nucleic acids: (1) amplification of *target sequences* using the polymerase chain reaction or transcription-based systems, and (2) amplification of the *probe sequences* using Qβ replicase or the recently described ligase amplification reaction. We will provide simple examples of how the various techniques are used. Ancillary technologies will be described that may some day facilitate the transfer of these techniques to the clinical laboratory. Finally, we will review the power and pitfalls of this technology and will speculate on future directions.

TARGET AMPLIFICATION METHODS

Target amplification systems are in vitro methods for replicating portions of a target molecule to levels where it can be readily detected. For our definition of a target amplification technique, the procedure must incorporate target-specific sequence information into the amplification product. Thus, the final product contains sequence information derived from the target that is not present in the reagents at the start of the reaction. Because of this capability, target amplification systems are capable of simultaneously identifying a pathogen and providing useful information that can be used for further characterization. If, for example, a gene specifying serological variants of an organism is amplified using reagents that recognize all of the variants, the intervening amplified sequences might then be used to provide typing information. If, in this case, serological variants are associated with different pathological predilections, analysis of the amplification product may have a direct bearing on patient management.

The polymerase chain reaction

The best studied and most widely used target amplification technique is the polymerase chain reaction (PCR). First described in 1985 by scientists at the Cetus Corporation,

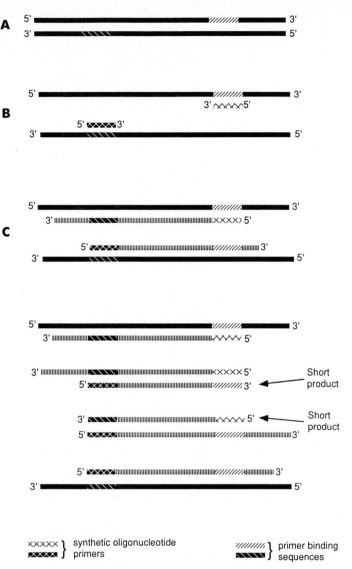

xxxxx }
xxxxx } synthetic oligonucleotide
     primers

//////// }
\\\\\\\\ } primer binding
     sequences

Fig. 42-1 The polymerase chain reaction. First cycle: **A,** A double-stranded DNA target sequence is shown with the primer binding sites indicated by a diagonally hatched line. **B,** These two strands are separated by heat denaturation and two synthetic oligonucleotide primers (cross-hatched lines), anneal to their respective recognition sequences in the 5' to 3' orientation indicated. Note that the 3' ends of each primer are facing each other. **C,** Taq DNA polymerase initiates synthesis at the 3' ends of each primer. Extension of the primer via DNA synthesis *(broken line)* results in new primer binding sites. The net result after one round of synthesis is two copies of the original target DNA molecule.

Second cycle: Each of the four DNA strands shown in **C** anneals to primers (present in excess) to initiate a new round of DNA synthesis. Of the eight single-stranded products, two are of a length defined by the primer annealing sites; this "short product" accumulates exponentially in subsequent cycles. *Reprinted by permission from the American Society for Microbiology. From Persing DH: Polymerase chain reaction: trenches to benches, J Clin Micro 29: 1281–1285, 1991.*

PCR has developed into a mainstay technique in many molecular biology laboratories. This method uses repeated cycles of oligonucleotide-directed deoxribonucleic acid (DNA) synthesis to carry out in vitro replication of target

nucleic acid sequences (Figure 42-1). The oligonucleotides, whose sequence is determined by the target nucleic acid, are synthesized to be complementary to their annealing sites within the two different strands (the sense and nonsense strands) of a target sequence, from approximately 150 to 3000 nucleotide bases apart.

Each cycle of PCR consists of three steps: (1) a denaturing step, in which the target DNA is incubated at a high temperature so that the target strands are melted apart and thus made accessible to specific oligonucleotide primers present in the reaction buffer; (2) an annealing step, in which the reaction mixture is cooled to allow the primers to anneal to their complementary target sequences; and (3) an extension reaction, usually carried out at a moderate temperature, in which the primers are extended on the DNA template by a DNA polymerase. Each time a cycle is completed, there is a theoretical doubling of the target sequence (in practice, however, the method becomes less efficient in the later cycles). Repeating this cycle many times (twenty- to sixtyfold) results in amplification of the target sequence over a millionfold. The target-specific amplification product can be identified by its precisely defined length and the presence of amplified internal target sequences; nonspecific amplification products are only rarely the same size as the target-specific product, and they will not contain internal sequences that are recognized by target-specific hybridization probes.

In a conventional hybridization, imperfect base-pairing of a primer may allow it to anneal in a nonspecific manner, binding to multiple sites in the target or in the co-purifying genomic DNA. Thus, for low-abundance targets, the background of nonspecific binding may be much higher than the true signal. The polymerase chain reaction, however, addresses this problem by requiring *two* specific priming reactions. The two primers are oriented such that they "fire at each other" in initiating DNA synthesis; polymerization proceeds toward the annealing site for the primer on the opposite strand. In order to proceed efficiently, PCR then requires that the second primer anneal to this strand within reasonable proximity to the priming site for the first; the geometric accumulation of the product depends on the primer-directed synthesis of new priming sites. It is this design that gives PCR much of its sensitivity and specificity.

Recent technical innovations have simultaneously simplified and greatly increased the power of PCR. The first is the use of a thermostable DNA polymerase (Taq polymerase) isolated from a thermophilic bacterium, *Thermus aquaticus*, that grows in hot springs at temperatures of 70°C to 75°C. Taq polymerase has a half-life of approximately 40 minutes at 95°C and thus is able to withstand the repeated heating and cooling cycles of PCR. This makes it possible to perform PCR without reopening tubes and adding fresh polymerase to replenish the enzyme that had been denatured in the previous heating step. Taq polymerase is added once at the beginning of the reaction, thus greatly simplifying tube handling. In addition, the ability to perform annealing and extension reactions at a higher temperature significantly reduces nonspecific amplification; the annealing step can be customized for each primer set so that conditions are unfavorable for the formation of imperfectly base-paired complexes between primer and target. A second innovation is the development of the programmable thermal cycler. The thermal cycler, essentially a programmable heating block, is capable of carrying out successive heating and cooling cycles unattended, and eliminates the tedious task of transferring reaction tubes between water baths or heating blocks. Thermal cyclers are now available from many manufacturers and have become standard laboratory equipment.

The polymerase chain reaction has proven to be an extremely powerful technique for finding the nucleic acid equivalent of the proverbial "needle in the haystack"; it can be used to selectively amplify target sequences that are present in small volumes in a background of genomic DNA. This feature makes it potentially very useful for the diagnosis of small numbers of pathogens whose DNA (or RNA ribonucleic acid), co-purifies with human genomic DNA. The best studied example of this is seen in the detection of proviral sequences for human immunodeficiency virus type I (HIV-I). The low prevalence in human mononuclear cells of virus-specific sequences precludes the use of conventional hybridization techniques. The typical PCR-based detection scheme detects sequences located in highly conserved regions of the HIV-I provirus, such as the long terminal repeat (LTR) or the *gag* and *pol* coding regions. The amplification products are then electrophoretically separated and blotted onto nitrocellulose. A labeled oligonucleotide probe is then used to detect sequences flanked by the amplification primers to confirm the presence of the specific amplification products. Several studies of the detection of HIV-I using PCR vs. conventional culture in the peripheral blood of infected individuals have confirmed the sensitivity of the in vitro technique; PCR may become the preferred method for direct HIV detection, if only because it is faster, less costly, and potentially less hazardous than culture.

A good example of the potential advantages of a target amplification technique over other methods is seen in the detection and typing of human papillomavirus (HPV) by PCR. This family of small DNA viruses now includes over 60 types (defined as having less than 50% DNA sequence homology by nucleic acid hybridization); new members are being discovered at regular intervals. As might be expected from the diversity of HPV types, the papillomaviruses are associated with a wide array of human pathology. Some types are found exclusively on the skin (HPV types 1,5), others in the genital tract (HPV types 6,11,16,18,31,33,35). Types 16 and 18 are found almost exclusively in the cervical epithelium and are strongly associated with abnormal cytological findings and neoplasia. Other types are found almost exclusively in benign lesions. Detection of papillomaviruses by conventional techniques such as immunoassay or immunocytochemistry has been elusive because of low sensitivity and limited immunological cross-reactivity between types. Consequently, DNA hybridization is now considered the "gold standard" for HPV detection and typing.

Target amplification methods are ideally suited to the task of detecting diverse types of a given pathogen. Using PCR, over 25 genital HPV strains can be identified (virtually all that have been tested to date) using a "universal" primer set designed to react with a sequence common to most HPV types within the L1 gene. Because the region of DNA bordered by the primers is type-specific, probes can be developed that react only with specific HPV types. This allows the design of a detection system whereby the type-specific

Table 42-1 Application of amplification methods to diagnostic microbiology

Method	Organism
Polymerase chain reaction	Human immunodeficiency virus type I
	Human immunodeficiency virus type II
	Human T-cell lymphotropic virus type I and II
	Human B cell lymphotropic virus
	Human papillomavirus
	Cytomegalovirus
	Rhinovirus
	Hepatitis B virus
	Epstein-Barr virus
	Herpes simplex virus
	Human parvovirus B19
	Enterotoxigenic *E. coli*
	Trypanosoma cruzi
	Toxoplasma gondii
	Borrelia burgdorferi
	Helicobacter pylori
	Legionella pneumophila
	Chlamydia trachomatis
	Leptospira
	Coliform bacteria
Transcript amplification system/3SR*	Human immunodeficiency virus type I

*3SR, self-sustaining sequence replication.

probes are placed on a filter; under conditions of sufficient stringency, the amplified fragments will only bind to the spot on the filter containing the oligonucleotide probe with the type-specific match.

Polymerase chain reaction-based assays are by no means limited to the detection of viruses, although clinical virology stands to benefit greatly from their introduction. Assays for fungal, protozoal, and bacterial pathogens have recently been described. Though only a few of these reports have directly demonstrated the clinical utility of these assays, many laboratories are involved in their development and testing on clinical specimens. Table 42-1 gives a practical list of pathogens detected so far by using PCR.

Transcript amplification systems

An alternative amplification method, based on in vitro transcription, has recently been described (Figure 42-2). Like PCR, the transcript amplification system (TAS) can use DNA or RNA as starting material. Each step of TAS consists of two parts: (1) synthesis of a DNA molecule that is complementary to the target nucleic acid (cDNA), and (2) in vitro transcription using the newly synthesized cDNA as a template. The cDNA synthesis step is primed using a hybrid oligonucleotide primer; one end of the primer consists of a target-specific region, whereas the other end comprises a recognition sequence ("promoter") for phage T7 RNA polymerase. Thus, in the first step, one molecule of DNA is produced for each DNA or RNA target by reverse transcriptase, and a promoter sequence for a DNA-dependent RNA polymerase is incorporated into the newly synthesized strand. T7 RNA polymerase is then added to the cDNA molecules; this results in many molecules of RNA from

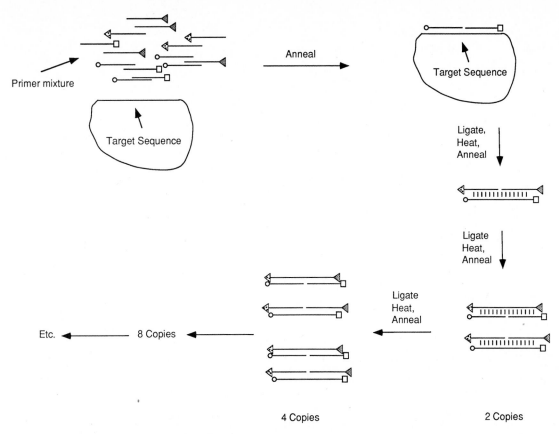

Fig. 42-2   The transcript amplification system. A complementary DNA (cDNA) is synthesized from the RNA target by reverse transcription, followed by an in vitro transcription step using the cDNA as a template. During the cDNA synthesis step, a copy of DNA is produced from each target and a promoter sequence for an RNA polymerase is incorporated into the newly synthesized strand. The 3′ half of the primer consists of a target-specific region, whereas the 5′ end comprises a promoter for the phage T7 RNA polymerase. The newly synthesized cDNA serves as template for the synthesis by T7 polymerase of a large molar excess of RNA, which then serves as the substrate for the next cycle. *Reprinted by permission, Yale University Press.*

each molecule of template, often exceeding a thirty- to fortyfold ratio of RNA product to cDNA template.

The action of T7 polymerase thus provides the amplification step; the newly synthesized cDNA serves as a template for the synthesis by T7 polymerase of a large molar excess of RNA, which then can be used as the substrate for the next cycle. This method has been applied to the detection of the *vif* region of the HIV-I RNA genome, where it was determined that fewer than one HIV-I infected cell could be detected in a population of 10^6 uninfected cells. After completion of four TAS cycles, target sequences were amplified 2 to 5×10^6-fold. The amplified HIV-I-specific RNA was detected after annealing to solid-phase–bound oligonucleotides, an approach facilitated by the single-stranded "sticky" structure of the RNA molecules.

Self-sustaining sequence replication (3SR)

An interesting and potentially powerful modification of the TAS protocol has been recently described, which is based on the enzymology of retrovirus genomic replication. Instead of using heat to denature RNA-cDNA hybrids after reverse transcription (as in the TAS protocol), the enzymatic activity of RNAse H is exploited. RNAse H activity is

present in retroviral reverse transcriptases and as a distinct activity in *E. coli*. RNAse H selectively degrades the RNA strand of RNA-cDNA hybrids, so single-stranded RNA is not affected. The simple addition of this activity results in an isothermal replication and accumulation of sense and/or antisense RNA amplification products of the target sequence, thus eliminating the need for thermal cycling required for TAS.

AMPLIFICATION OF THE PROBE MOLECULE

An alternative strategy for detecting rare target molecules is to amplify the probe molecule itself. Unlike target amplification methods in which target sequences are copied into the molecule that is eventually detected, amplification of the probe molecule does not result in the incorporation of target information. Instead, the end product of the reaction is an amplified version of the original components used to detect the target. Such systems may be useful in settings in which the target-derived sequence information is not necessary, such as in the detection of a "signature sequence" within a pathogen.

The principle underlying probe amplification methods is straightforward; after the probe has specifically annealed to its target and the unbound and/or nonspecifically bound material is washed away, it is enzymatically replicated in vitro to levels that can be readily detected. The problem of reducing the background binding may be formidable; non-specific hybridization of the probe molecule to sequences other than the intended target may result in amplification of background signals, potentially overwhelming the signal generated by a small number of target sequences. However, with the introduction of improvements such as "molecular switches" (described shortly) or target capture (where the target sequence is first processed by nucleic acid capture methods, such as hybridization to oligonucleotide-coated beads), background hybridization can be markedly reduced. If the anticipated problems of nonspecific hybridization can be overcome, probe amplification methods may form the basis for sensitive diagnostic assays.

Qβ replicase amplification of RNA probe molecules

Qβ replicase is an RNA-directed RNA polymerase that replicates the genomic RNA of the bacteriophage Qβ. This unique polymerase specifically recognizes a unique, folded RNA structure ("secondary structure"), formed by intra-molecular base-pairing of the Qβ RNA genome; most other folded forms of RNA are not recognized as substrates. Because one region of a Qβ substrate RNA (mov-1) can tolerate short probe inserts and still be replicated by Qβ replicase, this system can be exploited to provide a means of amplifying hybridization signals by amplifying the probe molecule itself.

Recombinant RNA probes are produced by in vitro transcription of recombinant DNA templates; the probes have a secondary structure that is predicted to be very similar to that of the wild-type origin, except that they harbor extensions in one loop of the folded structure. The size of the inserts must remain short due to the presumed size constraints on the placement of unstructured sequences into the otherwise highly structured replication origin. The molecules are then incubated with purified Qβ replicase; despite the presence of the inserts, the replication of the chimeric molecules can be as efficient as that of the unmodified parent molecule, approaching 10°-fold in a 30-minute incubation.

With this level of amplification, the replicase quickly becomes saturated, and the previously logarithmic reaction kinetics approach linearity. Thus, reactions containing more of the substrate molecules achieve saturation sooner; the further accumulation of replicated RNA is time-dependent. This property may make it possible to greatly extend the range in which such an assay remains quantitative because it allows a direct linear relationship between the number of input probe molecules and the amplified product.

As mentioned, the major obstacle to developing a sensitive assay using probe amplification will be reducing levels of background amplification. One approach to reducing background would be to make the amplifiable probe conformation-dependent; only those probe molecules bound to target would be recognized by the polymerase. Another approach, especially applicable to Qβ replicase, would be to design a "molecular switch" around the properties of site-specific endonucleases (Figure 42-3). The "switch" in this case is a hybridization-dependent RNAse sensitive site in a

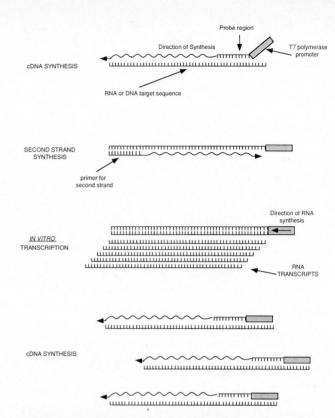

Fig. 42-3 Amplification of the probe by-Qβ replicase. A recombinant RNA molecule contains both a target-specific probe region and an endonuclease cleavage site formed by intramolecular base pairing near the probe region. When the molecule is annealed to the target sequence, it is RNAse resistant. Unbound probe is treated with RNAse and then washed from the reaction mixture. Qβ replicase is added to the probe and the reaction is incubated for a set amount of time, resulting in amplification of the probe.

Qβ substrate molecule. When the probe is hybridized to the target, the molecule is not recognized by RNAse III because the normal duplex substrate for RNAse III cannot form. However, the secondary structure in the absence of target binding (i.e., of the free probe molecule) forms a substrate for RNAse III; sequences unbound to the target are selectively cleaved, thus inactivating them as Qβ substrates. This approach has the potential to markedly reduce background problems.

DNA ligase-dependent amplification

All of the amplification techniques described so far depend on polymerases to copy genetic information in vitro. An alternative method, the ligase amplification reaction (LAR), based on template-dependent ligation of oligonucleotide probes, is now under investigation. This method employs DNA ligase to join two oligonucleotide probes after they have bound to a target sequence in vitro; successful ligation is dependent on both the approximation of the 3′ and 5′ ends of the primers and the presence of perfect base-pairing at the point of ligation. Once the two probes have been ligated together, the ligation product, which now mimics one strand of the original target sequence, can serve as a template for ligation of complementary primers. The com-

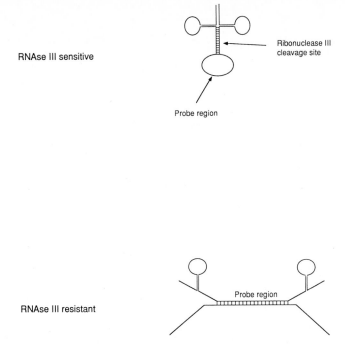

RNAse III sensitive

Ribonuclease III cleavage site

Probe region

RNAse III resistant

Probe region

Fig. 42-4 Ligation amplification reaction. Oligonucleotide primers are annealed to template molecules in a head to tail fashion, with the 3′ end of one probe abutting the 5′ head of the second. When perfect base-pairing is present at the junction, DNA ligase will join the ends to form a duplicate of one strand of the target. A second primer set, complementary to the first, can then use this duplicated strand (as well as the original target) as a template for ligation. Repeating the process results in a logarithmic accumulation of ligation products, which can be detected via the functional groups attached to the oligonucleotides.

ponents are then heated to denature the templates and allowed to anneal at a cooler temperature. Fresh DNA ligase is added at the end of each round, and the reactions are incubated for 30 minutes to 5 hours. Repeating this process theoretically results in a doubling of the ligation products, leading to a geometric accumulation. A diagrammatic summary of this method is shown in Figure 42-4.

Potential problems that may limit the usefulness of ligase-dependent amplification are high levels of background amplification due to blunt-end ligation of primer duplexes, relatively long reaction times (especially in the early cycles of amplification), and relatively nonstringent annealing conditions that may compound the problems of high background. However, many of these criticisms were also valid in the early days of PCR development; the introduction of a thermostable DNA polymerase was largely responsible for the popularity of the present-day technique. Likewise, the introduction of thermostable DNA ligases may lead to similar improvements in ligase-based amplification methods.

Target-directed ligation, either alone or in combination with a target amplification method, are potentially useful for the detection of single nucleotide base mutations. The oligonucleotides can be designed so that their point of ligation straddles the nucleotide position of a known mutation or polymorphism; efficient ligation and the eventual detection of a ligation product will only occur when the probes are perfectly base-paired to the target sequence. Single-base polymorphisms and mutations are now known to be associated with several inherited disorders (β-thalassemia, sickle-cell anemia, phenylketonuria, hemophilia, alpha$_1$-antitrypsin deficiency). Detection of single-base changes in pathogens may also become useful, such as in determining the species of a pathogen by examining ribosomal DNA sequences for characteristic nucleotide differences.

As with target amplification systems, the oligonucleotide probes used in ligation-detection assays can be modified to aid in the detection of the amplification product. For example, if one probe is synthesized with biotin at its 5′ end and the other probe is labeled with a reporter group such as alkaline phosphatase or a fluorescent molecule, only the ligation product will incorporate both moieties. After running the amplification reaction over a streptavivdin matrix and washing to eliminate unligated reporter groups, the bound material is then assayed for enzyme activity or fluorescence. This approach may facilitate automated methods for the detection of target sequences and nucleotide base changes.

POTENTIAL PROBLEMS WITH AMPLIFICATION SYSTEMS

Whereas amplification techniques represent new and powerful additions to the molecular diagnostics laboratory, several technical problems, some created by the technology itself, have recently been identified. One such problem stems from the exquisite sensitivity of these techniques, namely, the issue of how many pathogens constitutes an infection. In some cases relatively small numbers of organisms are tied to the development of disease (such as for infection with HIV), whereas other organisms are ubiquitous, only causing infection when host defenses are attenuated (such as is thought for *Pneumocystis carinii*). The clinician must therefore weigh the results of an extremely sensitive test with the clinical picture, knowing that tiny quantities of a given pathogen may be present in normal individuals.

A second problem arises from the fact that the diagnosis of an organism is based on the presence of DNA and not the intact organism. Most studies to date have treated the "signature fragment" and the organism as synonymous for diagnostic purposes. However, there may be important practical distinctions between the presence of a viable, disease-producing organism and the presence of its nucleic acids. The detection of *Borrelia burgdorferi* sequences in 45-year-old museum specimens of its arthropod vector *Ixodes dammini* is an extreme example of the persistence of pathogen-specific DNA fragments long after the viability of an organism is lost. The issue must be addressed again if the same methods are used in the detection of pathogens after treatment; the persistence of nucleic acid fragments may far outlast the disease-producing capabilities of a pathogen. Likewise, the testing laboratory must be aware that procedures that were once adequate to prevent sample cross-contamination with viable organisms may not be sufficient to prevent the spread of DNA fragments from dessicated, nonviable organisms contaminating the work area.

A third potentially serious problem that has surfaced in laboratories that regularly perform PCR is sample contamination by PCR fragments. Here, the exquisite sensitivity of PCR proves to be its undoing: the transfer of minuscule amounts (and in conventional detection schemes, negligible quantities) of such sequences into a neighboring tube may result in a false-positive. Amplified target sequences are proven substrates for further amplification; they are typically short in length (thus easily replicated and denatured) and contain all the sequence information necessary to be recognized by the oligonucleotides during PCR. This problem rarely surfaces when setting up a new assay because it appears to be related to the accumulation of these fragments in the laboratory over time. Amplification products may potentially contaminate reagents, buffers, laboratory glassware, laboratory garments, racks used to transport specimens, and even the air circulation system.

The issue of contamination of amplification reactions has far-reaching implications for both the basic and clinical laboratories. The magnitude of this problem and the frequency with which it occurs has led to a list of recommendations for avoiding false-positive PCR reactions. Indeed, these recommendations may be valid for any of the amplification methods described in the previous pages:

1. Use of positive-displacement pipettes. This is probably the most important step in reducing fragment contamination. When this is not possible, pipettors should be dedicated for handling unamplified DNA only.
2. Pre-aliquot all reagents used in PCR reactions.
3. Prepare reagents in an area that is physically separated from the area used to amplify and analyze the amplification reactions.
4. Prepare specimens and reactions in an area that is physically separated from the area used for amplification and analysis.
5. Avoid excessive numbers of cycles to reduce the risk of amplifying spurious single-copy fragments. (This recommendation assumes that most pathogens, when associated with disease, will be present in higher numbers.)
6. Include multiple "no template" controls with every diagnostic PCR run. If any of these controls are positive, the validity of the run must be questioned.
7. Run reactions for the detection of other genetically distinct target sequences that are present in the organism. The presence of more than one target sequence in the same sample is generally regarded as confirmation of a positive result.
8. Provide independent verification of the positive specimens in a second laboratory, preferably using non-overlapping primer sets.

Amplicon sterilization techniques

Two amplicon sterilization methods, one enzymatic and one photochemical, have recently been described and are depicted in Figure 42-5. In the enzymatic method, dUTP is substituted for TTP in all amplification reactions, resulting in incorporation of U in place of T in the amplicon. Amplicons can thus be distinguished from authentic target DNA by the presence of an "unnatural" nucleotide base. An *E. coli*-derived DNA repair enzyme, uracil-N-glycosylase (UNG), is then added to the reaction mixes. The normal function of this enzyme is to remove uracil residues from

bacterial DNA. During a brief incubation step prior to amplification, uracil-containing DNA strands that are carried over from previous amplifications are enzymatically and thermally degraded. The UNG protocol therefore allows "live" amplicons to accumulate in the laboratory, but a "pre-PCR" sterilization step selectively eliminates them prior to amplification (Fig. 42-5, left side).

An alternative, "post-PCR" method has recently been described that exploits the photochemical properties of psoralen derivatives. These compounds are added to PCR reaction mixture prior to amplification. After the thermal cycling is complete, the closed tubes are exposed to long-wave ultraviolet light, which penetrates the polypropylene tubes and photochemically activates the isopsoralen, but does not otherwise damage the DNA. The activated psoralen then forms covalent linkages with pyrimidine residues on the amplified DNA that prevent Taq polymerase from completing the process of primer extension.

Both of the aforementioned sterilization techniques are in the early stages of development and refinement, so good laboratory practice is still highly recommended. Nonetheless, sterilization methods are likely to have a major impact on the automation of the technology and on the importation of nucleic acid amplification methods into the clinical laboratory.

PRACTICAL CONSIDERATIONS IN THE USE OF AMPLIFICATION TECHNIQUES
Selection of target sequences

Regardless of the detection scheme that is eventually implemented, target sequences that are specific to the pathogen of interest ("signature sequences") must be carefully selected. The ideal target sequence would be: (1) absolutely unique to an organism or class of organisms, thus conferring specificity to the assay, (2) a sequence present in multiple copies, conferring both sensitivity and some immunity to sequence loss or alteration, and (3) inherently resistant to loss or to mutation that would render the sequence unrecognizable. The chosen target sequences could then be used to generate oligonucleotides to be used as probes or primers in an amplification reaction.

Unfortunately, such sequences rarely exist. Nucleic acid sequences that specify an open reading frame (ORF) for a structural protein may be subject to the effects of "silent mutation," that is, nucleotide substitutions that do not alter the primary protein sequence and thus are not directly selected against. This is possible because of the redundancy in the genetic code, in which several codons, made up of triplets of nucleotides, may code for a single amino acid. A single nucleotide substitution, especially one that is critically located, may be sufficient to markedly reduce hybridization efficiency and/or subsequent amplification. It is possible, however, to design oligonucleotide probes and primers so that their activity is less susceptible to small sequence alterations (see text that follows shortly).

As stable targets for detection or amplification purposes, ribosomal RNA (rRNA) and the genes that specify them (rDNA) have both advantages and disadvantages. Unlike structural protein genes, in which selective pressure occurs at the protein level, the evolutionary pressure to maintain sequence integrity of ribosomal RNA genes occurs at the

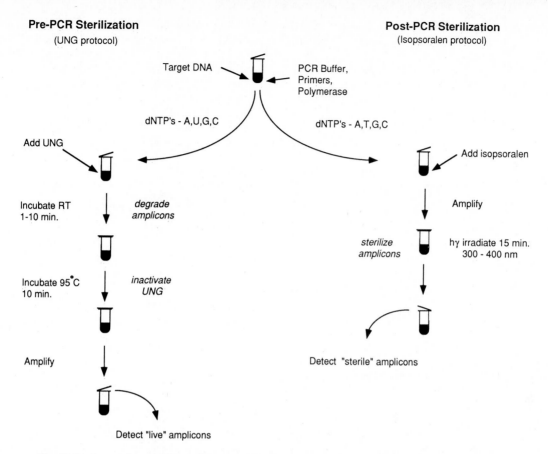

Fig. 42-5   Pre- and post-PCR sterilization methods. In the pre-PCR (enzymatic) method, previously amplified DNA (containing U in place of T) is selectively degraded prior to amplification. In the post-PCR (photochemical) protocol, an isopsoralen compound is included prior to PCR. After amplification, but before the products are removed for analysis, the tubes are exposed to long-wave ultraviolet light, resulting in cross-linking of amplified DNA. *Reprinted by permission, American Society for Microbiology. From Persing DH: Polymerase chain reaction: trenches to benches, J Clin Micro 29:1281–1285, 1991.*

nucleotide level. Because of the direct interactions of rRNA strands with each other and with ribosomal proteins, mutations in the rRNA genes are only rarely tolerated, thus providing us with examples of some of the best conserved genes in nature. Despite the conservation of ribosomal genes, however, there are regions of the coding sequences that can be classified as genus-and even species-specific. This finding has generated interest in using ribosomal DNA or RNA as targets for direct detection using oligonucleotide probes or in amplification schemes. While generally attractive because of the relative immutability of rRNA sequences, methods to detect rDNA sequences or ribosomal RNA within cells will have to be carefully engineered; sequence divergence of only one or a few nucleotides may dictate the differences between known pathogens and normal flora.

Selection and generation of oligonucleotides

The selection and generation of oligonucleotides for use as probes or amplification primers is the second critical step in developing a detection system. Oligonucleotide synthesis has been revolutionized by the introduction of automated nucleic acid synthesizers. The sequence of the desired oligonucleotide is entered on a keyboard; the instrument per-

forms serial coupling reactions between reactive nucleotide derivatives and a growing oligonucleotide bound to a solid substrate. Because the coupling efficiency of each nucleotide addition step is usually greater than 98%, the yield of the full-length, finished product will depend on the length of the oligonucleotide.

Although the actual sequence of the primers used in an amplification technique is probably less important than their placement on the target molecule, there are several specific recommendations for oligonucleotide primer design:

1. Avoid repetitive sequences or long tracts of a single nucleotide.
2. Avoid using sequences with extensive secondary structure potential. This can be determined with any of the popular sequence analysis programs.
3. Use sequences with a relatively even mixture of A-T and G-C base pairs.
4. When using PCR, avoid using sequences that allow oligonucleotides to anneal at their 3′ ends (the end of the primer used to prime DNA synthesis) in order to reduce "primer dimer" artifact.
5. When targeting a conserved coding region with PCR, TAS, or ligase amplification reaction (LAR), the 3′ ends of the oligonucleotides should lie on the first or

second base of a codon to reduce the potential effects of silent mutations (the second position is the least variable).

The exact sequence of the oligonucleotide is best determined by DNA sequence analysis and comparison with corresponding sequences (if available) from related strains; regions that display strain-specific differences will likely be good first choices. The placement of the recognition sequences on the target molecule may also be determined by what type of information is desired. For example, primers may be selected so that the nucleic acid sequence bordered by the primer binding sites contains important information about a pathogenic strain or a virulence factor; this information might then be derived by hybridization with oligonucleotide probes or restriction enzyme analysis.

The selection of target and oligonucleotides sequences should be customized for each infectious agent. If possible, multiple target sequences for each organism should be developed in order to verify negative and rule out false-positive results. The stability and suitability of the targets must then be determined on large numbers of isolates or clinical samples, using currently available techniques for comparison. The consequences of sample transport, storage, and the effects of therapy on the detection of the target sequence must then be determined so that results can be interpreted properly. In addition, proper control, to eliminate the possibility that negative results are due to inadequate specimens or an inhibitory substance, should be included for each specimen. When these issues are evaluated and the many questions answered, amplification techniques may be transformed from clinical research tools into the extremely useful clinical tests that they promise to be.

CONCLUSIONS

What will be the practical implications of the use of in vitro nucleic acid amplification techniques in the clinical laboratory? Several predictions can be made. First, these techniques will greatly facilitate the detection of pathogens whose identification has previously been limited by the lack of a practical culture system. This will add to the litany of organisms that can be detected, increasing both the services and responsibility of the clinical laboratory. Second, the high sensitivity of these methods may alter patient sampling requirements so that they are more convenient and less invasive. For example, buccal epithelial cells derived from a mouthwash have been successfully used to identify carrier status for the cystic fibrosis allele. One can envision the use of urinary sediments in the place of urethral swabs in the diagnosis of urethritis, peripheral blood instead of bone marrow or liver biopsy in the diagnosis of atypical mycobacterial infections, and peripheral blood mononuclear cells instead of bone marrow biopsy specimens in the detection of recurrent leukemias and lymphomas. Third, the emergence of amplification techniques will result in increased automation and a decrease in the dependence on radiolabeled probes; the sensitivity previously attained only with radioactive probes will likely be achieved by combining amplification methods with nonradioactive reporter systems. Fourth, if the potential problems of sample cross-contamination and amplification product carryover can be successfully addressed, amplification methods may form the basis

of a fully automated nucleic acid detection system. Fifth, the technological nature of these methods will create a demand for technologists and laboratory physicians with training in this technology. Continuing medical education programs must be instituted to provide these individuals with updates in this rapidly evolving field. Sixth, quality control testing and standardization of testing methods must be provided by independent agencies such as the College of American Pathologists (CAP) and the National Committee for Clinical Laboratory Standards (NCCLS). Finally, and most importantly, there will be a need to carefully evaluate the data derived from new diagnostic technology in light of the clinical picture. The integration of these data with the clinical impression, patient history, supporting laboratory data, and treatment records will be required to determine the true relevance and importance of these techniques in the establishment of a clinical diagnosis.

SUGGESTED READING

Buchbinder A and others: Polymerase chain reaction amplification and in situ hybridization for the detection of human β-lymphotropic virus, J Virol Methods 21:191, 1988.

Cimino GD and others: Post-PCR sterilization: a method to control carryover contamination for the polymerase chain reaction, Nucleic Acids Res 19:99, 1991.

Demmler GJ and others: Detection of cytomegalovirus in urine from newborns by using polymerase chain reaction DNA amplification, J Infect Dis 158:1177, 1988.

Eisenstein BI: The polymerase chain reaction: a new method of using molecular genetics for medical diagnosis, New Engl J Med 322:178, 1990.

Gama RE and others: Polymerase chain reaction amplification of rhinovirus nucleic acids from clinical material, Nucleic Acids Res 16:9346, 1988.

Guatelli JC and others: Isothermal in vitro amplification of nucleic acids by multienzyme reaction modeled after retroviral replication, Proc Natl Acad Sci 87:1874-1878, 1990.

Isaacs ST and others: Post-PCR sterilization: development and application to an HIV-I diagnostic assay, Nucleic Acids Res 19:109, 1991.

Kwoh DY and others: Transcription-based amplification system and detection of amplified human immunodeficiency virus type I with a bead-based sandwich hybridization format, Proc Natl Acad Sci 86:1173-1177.

Larzul D and others: Detection of hepatitis B virus sequences in serum by using in vitro enzymatic amplification, J Virol Methods 20:227, 1988.

Lench N, Stanier P, and Williamson R: Simple non-invasive method to obtain DNA for gene analysis, Lancet 18;1(8599):1356, 1988.

Lizardi PM and others: Exponential amplification of recombinant RNA hybridization probes. Biotechnology 6:1197, 1988.

Longo MC, Berninger MS, and Hartley JL: Use of uracil DNA glycosylase to control carry-over contamination in polymerase chain reactions, Gene 93:125, 1990.

Mullis KB and Faloona FA: Specific synthesis of DNA in vitro via a polymerase-catalyzed chain reaction, Methods Enzymol 155:335, 1987.

Ou CY and others: DNA amplification for direct detection of HIV-I in DNA of peripheral blood mononuclear cells, Science 239:295, 1988.

Persing DH, and Landry ML: In vitro amplification techniques for the detection of nucleic acids: new tools for the diagnostic laboratory, Yale J Biol Med 62:159, 1989.

Persing DH and others: Detection of Borrelia burgdorferi infection in Ixodes dammini ticks with the polymerase chain reaction, J Clin Microbiol 28:566-572.

Persing DH and others: Detection of Borrelia burgdorferi DNA in museum specimens of Ixodes dammini ticks, Science 249:1420-1423, 1990.

Persing DH: Polymerase chain reaction: trenches to benches, J Clin Micro 29:1281-1285, 1991.

Rayfield M and others: Mixed human immunodeficiency virus (HIV) infection in an individual: demonstration of both HIV type I and type II proviral sequences by using polymerase chain reaction, J Infect Dis 158:1170, 1988.

Saiki RK and others: Enzymatic amplification of β-globin genomic sequences and restriction site analysis for the diagnosis of sickle-cell anemia. Science 230:1350, 1985.

Saiki RK and others: Primer-directed enzymatic amplification of DNA with a thermostable DNA polymerase, Science 239:487, 1988.

Ting YI and Manos M: In Innis M and others (editors): Detection and typing of genital human papilloma-viruses in PCR protocols—a guide to methods and applications, 1990, Academic Press.

White TJ, Arnheim N, and Ehrlich HA: The polymerase chain reaction, Trends Genet 5:185, 1989.

White TJ, Madej R, and Persing DH: The polymerase chain reaction: clinical applications. In Spiegel HE (editor): Advances in clinical chemistry, Vol. 29, San Diego, 1992, Academic Press.

Wu DY and Wallace RB: The ligase amplification reaction (LAR)—amplification of specific DNA sequences using sequential rounds of template-dependent ligation, Genomics 4:560, 1989.

PART SEVEN

MICROBIOLOGICAL ANALYSIS OF CLINICAL SPECIMENS

43 Upper respiratory tract specimens

Michael A. Gerber

THE COMMON COLD

The common cold is a mild, acute, self-limited disease characterized by nasal stuffiness, sneezing, coryza, and throat irritation. It is caused by a large number of different viruses and is the leading cause of acute morbidity as well as visits to a physician in the United States.

The common cold is a frequent illness because of the large number of causative viruses and because reinfection with the same virus type can occur. In the vast majority of cases the primary route of viral inoculation is the inhalation or self-inoculation of virus onto the nasal mucosa. Inoculation can also occur onto the conjunctival surface. Following inoculation, the virus infects the cells of the local respiratory epithelium. This infection spreads locally, producing a large amount of nasal secretions with an increased protein content. The nasal discharge during the second to the seventh day is mucopurulent due to its content of desquamated epithelial cells and polymorphonuclear leukocytes. Initially, there is submucosal edema followed by shedding of the ciliated epithelial cells. Epithelial damage reaches its maximal stage by the fifth day and regeneration occurs over the next 10 days. The nasal mucociliary cleansing mechanism is markedly damaged during an acute illness and slight impairment may persist for as long as a month. Impairment of this mechanism is believed to allow the resident bacterial flora of the upper respiratory tract to invade normally sterile areas such as the sinuses and middle ear. This process is primarily responsible for the secondary bacterial infections that may result from the common cold.

Symptoms of nasal congestion, sneezing, and throat irritation usually begin on the second or third day and are due to both cellular damage and irritation. Viral shedding is usually maximal two to seven days after the onset of illness and may continue, particularly in children, for another two weeks. The common cold is characteristically of short duration and self-limited. The viruses that produce colds are not usually present in asymptomatic people, although subclinical infections can occur. In children, viral carriage may be quite prolonged.

The infection in a cold is restricted to the epithelial surfaces of the upper respiratory tract including the sinuses and eustachian tubes; viremia is unusual. This localization of the infection probably is due to local interferon production.

During the course of the cold, serum and secretory antibodies are produced, although their exact role in the pathologic process has yet to be determined. The role of cell-mediated immunity in the common cold has also yet to be determined. However, high levels of secretory and serum antibodies appear to be protective against reinfection. Unexplained constitutional factors also appear to modulate the clinical manifestations of colds.

Many different groups of viruses are etiologically involved with colds and within each group of viruses there may be many different types. As a group, rhinoviruses are the most common cause of colds in both children and adults. Colds due to reinfections are particularly common with parainfluenza virus and respiratory syncytial virus (Table 43-1).

Identification of the specific virus involved in a cold is usually not possible on the basis of the clinical findings. However, consideration of the typical epidemiologic setting, the characteristic seasonal patterns, and the history of contacts can be helpful in attempting to identify the most likely agent. A specific diagnosis can be made by the isolation of a virus from the nasal secretions, a nasal wash, or a nasopharyngeal culture. Parainfluenza virus, respiratory syncytial virus, and most rhinoviruses and influenza viruses can be isolated in tissue culture relatively easily. However, coronaviruses and some rhinoviruses and influenza viruses can be recovered only with special laboratory techniques.

Serologic diagnosis of influenza, parainfluenza, respiratory syncytial, and adenovirus infections can be made relatively easily. However, serologic diagnosis of rhinovirus infections is not practical because of the many antigenic types. Rapid diagnostic techniques using immunodiagnostic or molecular procedures on respiratory secretions may be available in the future and would be useful if antiviral chemotherapy were also available.

SINUSITIS

Sinusitis is either an acute or chronic suppurative infection of the mucosal lining of one or more of the paranasal sinuses. It probably occurs to some extent with every upper respiratory tract infection associated with rhinitis. However, in the vast majority of these episodes there is spontaneous resolution of the sinus involvement. The signs and symptoms of sinusitis may occur simultaneously with the upper

Table 43-1   Viruses associated with the common cold

	Antigenic types	Estimated % of cases
Rhinoviruses	100 types and 1 subtype	30-35
Coronavirus	3 or more types	≥10
Parainfluenza virus	4 types	
Respiratory syncytial virus	1 type	10-15
Influenza virus	3 types	
Adenovirus	33 types	
Other viruses (Enteroviruses, Reoviruses)		5
Presumed undiscovered viruses		30-35

From Gwaltney JM Jr: The common cold. In Mandell GL, Douglas RG Jr and Bennett JE, eds: Principles and practice of infectious diseases, ed 3, New York, 1990, Churchill Livingstone.

Table 43-2   Bacteriology of acute sinusitis

Bacteriologic agent	Percent of cases	
	Adults	Children
Streptococcus pneumoniae	20-35	25-30
Haemophilus influenzae	6-26	15-20
Moraxella catarrhalis	2	15-20
Streptococcus pyogenes	1-3	2-5
Anaerobes	0-10	2-5
Staphylococcus aureus	0-8	—

Data from Gwaltney JM Jr: Sinusitis. In Mandell GL, Douglas RG Jr and Bennett JE, eds: Principles and practice of infectious diseases, ed 3, New York, 1990, Churchill Livingstone and Wald ER: Pediatr Infect Dis J 7:449, 1988.

respiratory tract infection, but most often they follow. The term "sinusitis" usually refers to infections that persist after the episode of upper respiratory tract infection has resolved. When the signs and symptoms are of relatively short duration (less than three weeks) it is considered acute sinusitis, while a process of longer duration is considered chronic sinusitis. Sinusitis may be complicated by serious intracranial infections such as bacterial meningitis, epidural abscess, subdural abscess, or brain abscess.

The mucosal lining of all of the paranasal sinuses is composed of ciliated columnar epithelium and goblet cells, and is covered in part by a mucous blanket that contains immunoglobulins (IgA, IgG, and IgM) and lysozyme. Under normal conditions the ciliary movement and mucous flow keep the sinuses sterile and clear of pathogens. However, any insult that damages this ciliary epithelium or alters the mucous blanket may allow the inoculation of a large number of pathogens into the sinus which often results in the development of an infection.

The most common insult leading to sinusitis is a viral upper respiratory tract infection. The respiratory viruses involved in these infections can penetrate the mucous blanket of the normal respiratory epithelium and initiate a process that disrupts the normal cleansing mechanism. This opens the way for secondary bacterial invasion. During the acute sinusitis that ensues the mucosal lining becomes inflamed and edematous and an exudate containing a high concentration of both polymorphonuclear leukocytes (>5000 cells/mm³) and bacteria (>10⁵ CFU/ml) is produced. In addition, the sinus ostia become obstructed and spontaneous drainage is no longer possible.

Prolonged and repeated episodes of acute sinus infections in untreated or inadequately treated patients may lead to irreversible damage to the mucosal lining and chronic sinusitis. The normal ciliated epithelium is replaced by stratified squamous epithelium that may eventually fill the entire sinus lumen. Sterility is no longer maintained because of the structural damage to the sinus membrane and acute infectious exacerbations can occur.

Other pathophysiologic mechanisms may be involved. Approximately 5% to 10% of the episodes of maxillary sinusitis result from a dental infection that spreads through the floor of the sinus. Several noninfectious conditions, including defects of ciliary function such as immotile cilia syndrome and Kartagener's syndrome, may cause acute sinusitis. In addition, there may be anatomic abnormalities, such as congenital choanal atresia, septal deviation, foreign bodies, or tumors that predispose to sinusitis. Allergic reactions, nasal polyps, and indwelling nasal tubes are additional conditions that may predispose to sinusitis.

Acute sinusitis is a bacterial infection, with *Streptococcus pneumoniae* and *Haemophilus influenzae* being the most important organisms. In children, *Moraxella catarrhalis* is rapidly increasing in importance as a cause of acute sinusitis. *Streptococcus pyogenes*, viridans streptococci, and occasionally *Staphylococcus aureus* may also be involved. In chronic sinusitis, anaerobic bacteria assume a more important role (see Table 43-2). *Aspergillus* species are the most common cause of fungal sinusitis, but *Zygomycetes*, *Drechslera*, and *Curvalaria lunata* have also been implicated.

Nasal, throat, and nasopharyngeal cultures are of no value in patients with acute sinusitis; the results are not predictive of the bacterial pathogens within the sinus cavity. Even cultures of nasal discharge or of sinus exudate obtained by rinsing through the sinus ostia give unreliable information because of contamination with the normal bacterial flora of the nose. Since the microbial causes of acute sinusitis have been well described, it is not necessary to routinely obtain cultures directly from the infected sinuses of all patients. There are situations where identifying the specific microbial cause is necessary and this can be determined only by culture of the purulent exudate or washings obtained from a sinus by direct needle puncture. The puncture is best performed by the transnasal route through the lateral nasal wall with the needle directed beneath the inferior turbinate. The syringe containing the aspirated specimen should be transported directly to the laboratory for examination by Gram stain as well as for aerobic, anaerobic, and fungal cultures. When available, quantitative cultures of the specimen may be useful in differentiating between accidental bacterial contamination and true sinus infection (>10⁵ CFU/ml).

CROUP

Croup, which is also known as laryngotracheobronchitis, is a viral infection of the upper and lower respiratory tract in young children. It produces inflammation of the subglottic region which results in labored breathing accompanied by a characteristic stridorous noise during inspiration.

Most episodes of croup begin as a viral infection of the nasopharynx which spreads down to involve the larynx and trachea, and in more severe cases, the lower respiratory tract. The virus inhibits the tracheal ciliary function and marked destruction of the epithelium with viral invasion of the lamina propria occurs. As the disease progresses the tracheal lumen becomes obstructed by fibrinous exudate as well as by marked edema and cellular infiltration of the lamina propria, submucosa, and adventitia. The inflammation and obstruction tend to be greatest at the subglottic level. Inflammatory changes may be seen in the epithelium, the mucosa, and the submucosa of the larynx, trachea, and the linings of the bronchi, bronchioles, and even the alveoli.

The most common cause of croup is parainfluenza virus type 1, with parainfluenza virus type 3 also being a common cause. Parainfluenza virus type 1 is the cause of much of the croup that occurs in the fall. Influenza A virus is also a common cause of croup but the croup caused by this agent usually occurs in the winter or early spring, tends to be more severe, and affects a broader age group than parainfluenzal croup. Respiratory syncytial virus and adenovirus are less-common causes of croup.

Croup is usually a clinical diagnosis although A-P and lateral X-rays of the neck may be helpful. Identification of the specific viral agent involved may be accomplished by culturing the throat, trachea, or nasal washings. Identification can also be made by fluorescent antibody staining or one of the other new techniques for rapid viral diagnosis. Serologic diagnosis is unreliable for some of the agents involved and, at best, can only provide a retrospective diagnosis.

EPIGLOTTITIS

Epiglottitis is a rapidly progressive infection of the epiglottis, aryepiglottic folds, and arytenoid soft tissues that has the potential of causing abrupt, complete airway obstruction.

The infection probably arises from direct invasion of the supraglottic region with a subsequent bacteremia. This bacteremia is usually of a relatively short duration and low grade. The supraglottic cellulitis that develops consists of a diffuse infiltrate with polymorphonuclear cells, hemorrhage, and fibrin deposition. It is associated with marked edema. This process progresses to the formation of microabscesses.

Epiglottitis is a bacterial infection with *Haemophilus influenzae* type B as the etiologic agent in almost all cases. Occasionally *S. pneumoniae* or *S. aureus* may be involved and rarely *S. pyogenes* or *H. parainfluenzae*.

Epiglottitis is primarily a clinical diagnosis, with lateral neck X-rays providing supportive evidence and direct visualization of the epiglottis providing the definitive diagnosis. Identification of the etiologic agent can be provided by culturing of the epiglottis, a blood culture, or an antigen-detection test on the serum or urine. Throat cultures are of little value.

OTITIS MEDIA

Acute otitis media is an inflammation of the mucoperiosteal lining of the middle ear cleft including the eustachian tube, tympanic cavity, mastoid antrum, and mastoid air cell system (see Chapter 46). If the inflammation extends beyond

the mucoperiosteal lining, one of the complications of otitis media (e.g., mastoiditis) may develop. Chronic otitis media usually results from recurrent episodes of acute otitis media and is characterized by drainage through a perforated tympanic membrane lasting two to three months or longer.

The middle ear is part of a continuous system that includes the nares, nasopharynx, eustachian tubes, and mastoid air cells. These structures are lined with a respiratory epithelium which contains ciliated cells, mucous-secreting goblet cells, and cells capable of secreting local immunoglobulins. The eustachian tube has at least three physiologic functions with respect to the middle ear—protecting the middle ear from nasopharyngeal secretions, permitting secretions produced in the middle ear to drain into the nasopharynx, and ventilating the middle ear to equilibrate the air pressure with that in the external ear canal. Any anatomic or physiologic dysfunction of the eustachian tube that causes a disruption of these functions can result in otitis media. When the eustachian tube is obstructed, secretions that normally form in the middle ear accumulate. If bacteria from the nasopharynx are then introduced, an infection develops. Purulent exudate accumulates within the middle ear space and exerts pressure against the surrounding bone and tympanic membrane. Viral upper respiratory tract infections are the most common cause of eustachian tube obstruction.

Chronic otitis media may result from an episode of acute otitis media with spontaneous perforation of the tympanic membrane and ongoing infection. Chronic otitis media may also occur as a complication of PE tube insertion for the treatment of serous otitis media. Craniofacial anomalies such as cleft palate are a predisposing factor for chronic otitis media. Allergies may also be a predisposing factor. Chronic otitis media produces edema, fibrosis, and inflammatory cell infiltration of the mucous membranes of the middle ear and mastoid. This in turn may lead to polyps, osteitis, sclerosis, tympanosclerosis, labyrinthitis, and intracranial suppurative complications such as epidural, subdural, or brain abscess.

About one third of the middle ear cultures from patients with acute otitis media will be sterile. The vast majority of the remainder will yield a bacterial pathogen, with *Streptococcus pneumoniae* and *Haemophilus influenzae* being by far the most important (See Table 43-3.). Viral infections are often epidemiologically associated with acute otitis media but viruses are infrequently isolated from the middle ear. Viral agents appear to be an important cause of the upper respiratory tract infections that produce eustachian

Table 43-3 Bacteriology of acute otitis media

Bacteriologic agent	Percent of cases
Streptococcus pneumoniae	33
Haemophilus influenzae	21
Streptococcus pyogenes	8
Moraxella catarrhalis	3
Staphylococcus aureus	2
Miscellaneous bacteria	2
None or nonpathogens	31

From Klein JO: Otitis externa, otitis media, mastoiditis. In Mandell GL, Douglas RG Jr, and Bennett JE, eds: Principles and practice of infectious diseases, ed 3, New York, 1990, Churchill Livingstone.

tube dysfunction. These viral agents are therefore important in setting the stage, rather than actually producing the acute otitis media. However, adenovirus, respiratory syncytial virus, influenza virus, and enteroviruses may occasionally cause acute otitis media. Mycoplasma, chlamydia, and other agents are additional unusual causes of acute otitis media.

The agents that cause chronic otitis media are varied but *Pseudomonas aeroginosa* predominates (See Table 43-4.). Anaerobic bacteria have also been cultured from the middle ear fluid of patients with chronic otitis media. However, the precise role of these organisms in this disease process is still uncertain.

As the microbial causes of acute otitis media have been well established, there is no need to routinely attempt to identify the bacteria involved by culturing either the middle ear effusion or other sites such as the throat or nasopharynx. In selected patients, needle aspiration of the middle ear effusion should be considered in order to identify the bacteria present. These patients would include those who are critically ill, those who do not respond to the initial choice of antibiotic therapy, and those who are immunodeficient. For patients with chronic otitis media, cultures should not be obtained from the drainage in the external canal because of the potential contamination from saprophytes residing in that area. Culture specimens should be obtained from fluid in the middle ear space through the perforation in the tympanic membrane after cleansing of the external ear canal.

OTITIS EXTERNA

Otitis externa is an infection of the external auditory canal and in many ways resembles skin and soft tissue infections elsewhere in the body (see Chapter 46). However, because of the narrow and tortuous nature of the canal, fluid or foreign objects that enter may get trapped, causing irritation and maceration of the superficial tissues. In addition, because of the limited space for expansion of the inflamed tissues, the pain and itching that result may be severe. Malignant otitis externa is a fulminant, necrotizing form of otitis media frequently associated with diabetic microangiopathy and caused by *Pseudomonas aeroginosa.*

The continuous flow of epithelium from the tympanic membrane to the external auditory meatus has three natural mechanisms designed to protect it from infection. First, the rolling motion of the lateral external auditory canal facilitates the removal of debris through the external auditory meatus. In addition, hairs located on the outer one third of the ear canal actively push debris toward the external auditory meatus. Finally, the cerumen in the ear canal provides an acid environment that acts as a chemical barrier to infection. Any factor that disrupts these natural protective

mechanisms may result in otitis externa. Some of the more common predisposing factors include high temperature and humidity, alkaline pH, environmental bacterial contamination, and maceration.

Approximately 30% of all individuals will have sterile external ear canals, while 50% will be colonized with *Staphylococcus epidermidis*, 3% with *Staphylococcus aureus*, and 30% with fungi such as *Aspergillus niger* or *Candida albicans*. In temperate climates *S. aureus* is the most common cause of otitis externa, while in the tropics it is *Pseudomonas aeroginosa*. *Pseudomonas aeroginosa* is the most common cause of malignant otitis externa but anaerobes may also play a role.

MASTOIDITIS

Mastoiditis is a suppurative infection of the mastoid air cells. Mastoiditis that has been present for less than one month is usually considered acute, while mastoiditis that has been present for more than three months is usually considered chronic.

As the mastoid air spaces are contiguous with the middle ear cavity and as both are lined by a continuous mucoperiosteum, all episodes of otitis media are associated with a certain amount of mastoid inflammation. During the early phase of otitis media, there may be merely some hyperemia of the mastoid air cell mucosa. However, as the infection progresses, serum, fibrin, polymorphonuclear leukocytes, and red blood cells begin to accumulate. In time, the pressure builds to the point where the tympanic membrane perforates and allows for drainage of both the middle ear and mastoid air cells. At times there may be so much swelling of the mucoperiosteum that drainage of pus from the mastoid is blocked and mastoiditis develops. If the pressure in the mastoid air cells continues to build, decalcification and resorption of the bony septa may occur as well as osteomyelitis of the adjacent bone.

The most common pathogens in acute mastoiditis are *S. pneumoniae* and *S. pyogenes*. *Staphylococcus aureus* is also a common pathogen, while *Haemophilus influenzae*, coliforms, and *Mycobacterium tuberculosis* are less common. The most common pathogens in chronic mastoiditis are *Pseudomonas aeroginosa* and *Staphylococcus aureus*. Anaerobes are also commonly involved (See Table 43-5.).

Table 43-5 Bacteriology of mastoiditis

Bacteriologic agent	Percent of isolates	
	Acute	Chronic
Streptococcus pyogenes	32	2
Streptococcus pneumoniae	25	1
Staphylococcus aureus	17	9
Haemophilus influenzae	7	—
Pseudomonas species	3	8
Other gram-negative bacilli	3	8
Anaerobes	6	68
Enterococci	3	—
M. tuberculosis	3	—
Miscellaneous others	3	4

From Lewis K and Cherry JD: Mastoiditis. In Feigin RD and Cherry JD, eds: Textbook of pediatric infectious diseases, ed 2, Philadelphia, 1987, WB Saunders Co.

Table 43-4 Bacteriology of chronic otitis media

Bacteriologic agent	Percent of isolates
Pseudomonas aeruginosa	44
Staphylococcus aureus	13
Staphylococcus epidermidis	8
Streptococcus pneumoniae	4
Miscellaneous bacteria	31

From Nelson JD: Pediatr Infect Dis J 7:446, 1988.

As a middle ear culture is an accurate reflection of the organisms in the mastoid air cells, a sterile aspirate through an intact tympanic membrane is the best way to identify the causative agent of the mastoiditis. An aspiration of any postauricular fluctuance is also diagnostic, as would be a surgical specimen. If the tympanic membrane is perforated, one can get an idea of the cause of the mastoiditis by culturing the fluid in the middle ear space through the perforation after cleansing of the external ear canal.

PHARYNGITIS

Pharyngitis is an inflammation of the mucous membranes and underlying structures of the throat characterized by exudate, ulceration, or erythema. Pharyngitis may be either a viral or bacterial infection. Most cases are of viral etiology and occur as part of an upper respiratory tract infection. Group A streptococci is the most important bacterial cause of pharyngitis.

The events that lead to invasion of the pharyngeal mucosa by respiratory viruses are not well understood. Some respiratory viruses (e.g., adenovirus, coxsackie virus) can directly invade the pharyngeal mucosa, but for other respiratory viruses (e.g., rhinovirus) it is not known whether they invade the pharyngeal mucosa directly or if the pharyngeal inflammation is secondary to infection of the respiratory epithelium of the nose. The events that lead to invasion of the pharyngeal mucosa by group A streptococci are also not well understood. Pharyngeal carriage of group A streptococci is commonly observed in asymptomatic people and some of the factors that may influence the balance between colonization and invasive infection include natural and acquired host immunity as well as interference among the bacteria present in the oropharynx.

Multiple factors, including the season of the year, the age of the patient, the status of the host, the environment, potential exposures, and the type of lesions have a bearing on the potential etiology of the pharyngitis. In many cases the etiology is not known. Most cases of pharyngitis, particularly in adults, are due to viruses. Rhinovirus and coronavirus produce a mild pharyngitis often associated with an upper respiratory tract infection. Adenovirus produces a pharyngitis that is often associated with nasal obstruction or discharge and a cough, while herpes simplex virus is associated with ulcerative lesions in the pharynx and in the anterior mouth. Coxsackie and ECHO virus are associated with vesicular or ulcerative lesions, parainfluenza virus is associated with cough and coryza, Epstein-Barr virus is associated with the other signs and symptoms of infectious mononucleosis, and influenzal pharyngitis occurs during outbreaks of influenza in association with the other clinical findings of that illness.

In children, during certain periods of the year, group A streptococci may cause 35% to 40% of the cases of pharyngitis. Non-group A streptococci, particularly group C and group G, have been implicated in primarily food-borne outbreaks of pharyngitis, but their role in endemic pharyngitis is still controversial. Other bacteria that may occasionally cause pharyngitis include *Neisseria gonorrhea, Yersinia enterocolitica, Mycoplasma pneumoniae, Corynebacterium*

hemolyticum, and perhaps, *Chlamydia pneumoniae. H. influenzae* and *S. pneumoniae* may be part of the normal pharyngeal flora and neither has been established as an etiologic agent of pharyngitis. In developing areas of the world *Corynebacterium diphtheriae* is still an important cause of pharyngitis. The role of anaerobic bacteria in pharyngitis remains controversial (See Table 43-6.).

With acute pharyngitis, the primary goal of diagnosis is to distinguish between group A streptococcal pharyngitis and viral pharyngitis, and to recognize unusual causes that are a manifestation of a more serious underlying illness. As one cannot accurately distinguish between streptococcal and viral pharyngitis on clinical findings alone, some form of bacteriologic confirmation is needed to make the diagnosis of group A streptococcal pharyngitis. Either blood agar plate cultures or rapid antigen detection tests can be used to provide that bacteriologic confirmation. However, both suffer from their inability to distinguish between a streptococcal carrier and someone who is truly infected with group A streptococci.

Viral cultures are not usually performed, but when the pharyngeal findings are unique, or when many cases with a similar illness are observed, they may be helpful. Viral serology may also be helpful in these situations. Culture for other pathogens should be reserved for unusual situations suggested by persistent symptomatology, indicative epidemiology, or other pertinent historical data. In cases where anaerobes may be playing a role (e.g., Vincent's angina) Gram stain of the pharynx may be particularly helpful.

ORAL CAVITY

Most oral cavity infections are odontogenic in origin, including dental caries, pulpitis, periapical abscess, gingivitis, and peridontal and deep fascial space infections. These in-

Table 43-6   Microbial causes of acute pharyngitis

Causes	Estimated percentage of cases
Viral	
Rhinovirus	20
Coronavirus	5
Adenovirus	5
Herpes simplex virus	4
Parainfluenza virus	2
Influenza virus	2
Coxsackievirus A, Epstein-Barr virus, Cytomegalovirus	<1
Bacterial	
Streptococcus pyogenes	15-30
Neisseria gonorrheae, Corynebacterium diphtheriae, Corynebacterium hemolyticum, Yersinia enterocolitica, Anaerobes	<1
Chlamydia pneumoniae	unknown
Mycoplasma pneumoniae	<40
Unknown	40

From Gwaltney JM Jr: Pharyngitis. In Mandell GL, Douglas RG Jr, and Bennett JE eds: Principles and practice of infectious diseases, ed 3, New York, 1990, Churchill Livingstone.

fections can spread to adjacent or distal fascial spaces or to the maxilla and mandible, where they may produce serious and potentially life-threatening complications.

One of the potential complications of an oral cavity infection is Ludwig's angina, which is an infection of the sublingual and submandibular spaces, bilaterally. It is characterized by hard, brawny swelling with a minimum of suppuration. It has the potential to progress to the point of causing airway obstruction and death. Another potential complication is that infections of the teeth adjacent to the maxillary antrum may spread into the maxillary sinus and produce acute sinusitis. Finally, orbital and intracranial infections may, on rare occasions, develop. These occur from either direct extension from the oral cavity, from extension through one of the paranasal sinuses, or from hematogenous spread. These infections include orbital cellulitis, cavernous sinus thrombosis, subdural empyema, and brain abscess.

Most severe orofacial infections evolve from a dental infection that is either periapical, peridontal, or pericoronal. These dental infections tend to spread along the anatomic path of least resistance. Therefore, peridontal and pericoronal infections generally drain from the gingival sulcus along the surface of the tooth into the oral cavity and rarely have major sequelae. In contrast, periapical infections can spread to adjacent bone where they produce an osteomyelitis or they can spread to adjacent soft tissue as either a cellulitis or as a soft tissue abscess. Eventually, these soft tissue abscesses may perforate the mucous membrane or the skin and produce a fistulous tract or they may rupture into the maxillary sinus.

The bacteriology associated with odontogenic infections tends to be polymicrobial and complex, generally reflecting the composition of the indigenous oral flora. *Bacteroides, Fusobacterium, Peptostreptococcus, Actinomyces,* and *Streptococci* are the organisms most commonly encountered. But in selected patients with serious underlying conditions, *Staphylococcus aureus* and facultative gram negative rods may play an important role. More serious infections, in which spread to orofacial soft tissues has occurred, tend to present with a mixture of anaerobic and aerobic organisms, with anaerobes predominating in some and aerobes in others. Infections arising solely from the dental periapical tissues are much more likely to be predominantly anaerobic. Those infections that arise from non-odontogenic sources such as facial trauma, surgical manipulation, or tonsillitis are much more likely to be predominantly aerobic.

When collecting appropriate specimens for Gram stain and culture, it is important that they be obtained extraorally or by direct needle aspiration of loculated pus in order to avoid contamination by commensal oral flora. It is also important that all specimens be transported and cultured in a manner appropriate for the isolation of both aerobic and anaerobic organisms.

DEEP NECK ABSCESSES

A deep neck abscess is a collection of pus in a potential space, usually an area of least resistance to the spread of infection, bounded by fascia. These infections may begin as a small area of cellulitis, eventually progress into an abscess, and then extend into the adjacent potential spaces. Deep neck abscesses frequently encompass vital structures found within the neck and it is the compromise or destruction of these structures that represents the major complications of these infections.

Three examples of deep neck abscesses are peritonsillar, pterygomaxillary, and retropharyngeal abscesses. Peritonsillar abscess (quinsy) may follow any severe episode of tonsillitis with extension of the infection through the fibrous tonsillar capsule. Pterygomaxillary abscess may follow an incompletely or inadequately treated episode of bacterial pharyngitis or tonsillitis. It may also follow a peritonsillar abscess, dental infections, bacterial parotitis, mastoiditis, petrositis, cervical adenitis, or a foreign body. Retropharyngeal abscesses are most commonly secondary to suppurative adenitis of the retropharyngeal lymph nodes. In childhood, these nodes are prominent and receive drainage from the nasopharynx, adenoids, and paranasal sinuses. Retropharyngeal abscesses may also follow penetrating foreign bodies, endoscopy, trauma, pharyngitis, vertebral body osteomyelitis, petrositis, and dental procedures.

Group A streptococci and *Staphylococcus aureus* are the organisms most often associated with deep neck abscesses. Recently, oral anaerobic bacteria have also been identified as playing an important role in these infections.

The optimal material for identifying the etiologic agent of a deep neck abscess is pus obtained at the time of surgical drainage. This material should be transported and cultured in a manner appropriate for both aerobic and anaerobic organisms. Gram stains may be helpful. If a Gram stain shows a mixture of organisms, this would suggest a mixed aerobic-anaerobic infection. Throat swabs or swabs of the abscess cavity after drainage are usually not appropriate specimens for culture because of potential contamination with the normal oropharyngeal flora.

CERVICAL LYMPHADENITIS

Cervical lymphadenitis is an inflammation of one or more of the lymph nodes of the neck. This inflammation most often arises from an infection proximal to the involved lymph node that has drained into the node through the connecting lymphatic channels.

Following an acute episode of group A streptococcal pharyngitis or tonsillitis, organisms may spread through the lymphatics to the cervical lymph nodes where suppuration may occur. *Staphylococcus aureus* that is colonizing the anterior nares may also spread through the lymphatics to the cervical lymph nodes and then alone, or in conjunction with group A streptococci, initiate a suppurative process. In addition, peridontal disease may cause local tissue destruction that serves as the portal of entry for normal mouth flora to invade the lymphatics. These organisms, which are predominantly anaerobic, may then drain into the cervical lymph nodes and produce suppuration.

Most cervical adenitis occurs as part of a reticuloendothelial system response to a viral upper respiratory tract infection. Group A streptococci and *Staphylococcus aureus* are the most common bacterial pathogens in cervical lymphadenitis, with anaerobes also playing an important role. Atypical mycobacteria, *Actinomyces israelii,* and *Myco-*

bacterium tuberculosis are less frequently involved as is the gram-negative bacterium of cat scratch disease (*Afipia*).

In the acute stage of cervical lymphadenitis, needle aspiration of the affected node can be helpful in identifying the etiology. This material should be Gram and acid-fast stained as well as cultured for aerobes, anaerobes, fungi, and mycobacteria. If a biopsy is performed, that material can also be stained and cultured in a similar manner.

SUGGESTED READING

Brook I: Pathogenicity and therapy of anaerobic bacteria in upper respiratory tract infections, Pediatr Infect Dis J 6:131-136, 1987.

Feigin RD and Cherry JD: Textbook of pediatric infectious diseases, ed 2, Philadelphia, 1987, W.B. Saunders Company.

Ginsburg CM: Aerobic microbiology of upper respiratory infections in infants and children, Pediatr Infect Dis J 6:843-847, 1987.

Mandell GL, Douglas RG Jr, and Bennett JE: Principles and practice of infectious diseases, ed 3, New York, 1990, Churchill Livingstone.

Moffet HL: Pediatric infectious diseases; a problem-oriented approach, ed 2, Philadelphia, 1981, JB Lippincott Company.

Salit IE: Diagnostic approaches to head and neck infections, Infect Dis Clin NA 2:35-55, 1988.

Van Hare GF and Shurin PA: The increasing importance of *Branhamella catarrhalis* in respiratory infections, Pediatr Infect Dis J 6:92-94, 1987.

44

Lower respiratory tract specimens

Michael A. Saubolle

GENERAL PRINCIPLES

Microorganisms gain access to the lower airways primarily by way of aspiration from the upper respiratory tract or by inhalation of aerosols. Hematologic seeding to the lung from a distant focus occurs infrequently, while direct extension from a contiguous site is also possible but unusual. Outcome of any invasion of the pulmonary tree depends on the balance between the virulence and inoculum size of the potential etiologic agent and the status of the immune mechanism of the host. Thus, diverse settings for pneumonia occur and the number of agents known to cause lower respiratory tract infections continues to increase (Tables 44-1 and 44-2). The etiologies are, however, often predictable, thereby limiting the differential diagnosis to a more manageable size based on epidemiologic, clinical, and preliminary laboratory findings (hematologic, roentgenographic). Although causes of

Table 44-1 More common general bacterial etiologies of pneumonia

Category/organism	General characteristics
AEROBES (OR FACULTATIVE ANAEROBES)	
Gram-positive	
Streptococcus pneumoniae	Most common cause of community-acquired pneumonia (10%—25% overall; 30%—70% of hospitalized cases)
Staphylococcus aureus	Nosocomial (15%—25%); community-acquired (2%—4%)—often associated with tracheostomy, trauma, elderly, or post-viral
Streptococcus pyogenes (Group A)	Rare: often rapidly progressive
Streptococcus agalactiae (Group B)	Associated with neonates and immunocompromised patients
Nocardia spp	Associated with immunocompromised patients, especially those on steroids
Gram-negative	
Haemophilus influenzae	10%—20% community-acquired; associated with pediatrics (serotype b), chronic lung disease (non-typeable), cystic fibrosis, post-viral
Moraxella (Branhamella) catarrhalis	Less than 5% of community-acquired pneumonia; role increases in patients with underlying disease and nosocomially
Neisseria meningitidis	Rare cause of community-acquired pneumonia
Enterobacteriaceae	Up to 50% of nosocomially-acquired pneumonia; especially *Klebsiella*, *Escherichia coli*, *Enterobacter*, and *Serratia*
Pseudomonas aeruginosa	Nosocomial (5%—10%), associated also with cystic fibrosis (mucoid strains)
Acinetobacter	Nosocomially-acquired pneumonia
ANAEROBES	
	Generally, up to 30% of nosocomially-acquired pneumonia, associated with aspiration and necrotizing pneumonias as well as lung abscess
Gram-positive	
Peptostreptococcus	
Actinomyces	
Gram-negative	
Fusobacterium	
Bacteroides	Especially *B. melaninogenicus*, sometimes *B. fragilis*

591

Table 44-2 Etiologies of pneumonia requiring special processing or culture techniques

Category/organism	General characteristics
Legionella	1%—5% of all pneumonias (some areas 15%—25%); at least 17 species associated with human infection, *L. pneumophila* most common, non-pneumophila species associated with the immunocompromised
Mycobacterium	*M. tuberculosis, M. avium* complex, *M. kansasii,* and in some areas *M. xenopi* most common; other nontuberculous mycobacteria less frequent
Chlamydia	*C. psittaci* (ornithosis [psittacosis]-bird exposure), *C. trachomatis* (neonatal pneumonia) and *C. pneumoniae* (TWAR agent; approximately 10% of community acquired pneumonias in certain regions)
Mycoplasma pneumoniae	Commonly associated with young adults
Fungi	May be divided into yeast and moulds categories
Yeasts	*Cryptococcus neoformans* associated with bird droppings; *Candida* spp associated with immunocompromised but rarely cause pneumonia
Moulds	Community-acquired pneumonias caused by regionally common dimorphic fungi *Coccidiodes immitis* (Southwest), *Histoplasma capsulatum* and *Blastomyces dermatitidis* (Midwest, Ohio River Valley regions); infections in immunocompromised patients may be caused by *Aspergillus* and the zygomycetes
Pneumocystis carinii	Pneumonia in immunocompromised patients (especially in AIDS); genetic material resembles that of fungi rather than protozoa
Parasites	
Protozoa	Protozoal infections are rare, pneumonia is not usual primary presentation
Helminths	*Strongyloides stercoralis* is an infrequent cause of hyperinfection and pneumonitis in the immunocompromised; *Paragonimus* may be seen regionally in endemic areas; *Ascaris* and *Trichuris* are encountered with extreme rarity
Viruses	Generally, more commonly involved in pediatric infections (especially when patients hospitalized) or those of immunocompromised host. In adults viral infections may be seasonal or epidemic
Respiratory Syncytial Virus	
Parainfluenza Virus 1, 2, and 3	
Adenovirus	
Influenza Virus A and B	
Cytomegalovirus	
Herpes Simplex Virus	
Varicella-Zoster	
Enterovirus	

pneumonia are frequently derived from the colonizing flora of the upper respiratory tract, it is not possible to identify with any certainty specific etiologies through surveillance cultures of general respiratory flora. Clinical and epidemiologic information, together with suspected organisms, should be provided to the laboratory so that appropriate steps can be taken in processing the specimens.

INDIGENOUS FLORA OF UPPER RESPIRATORY TRACT

The oropharyngeal environment harbors aerobic as well as anaerobic microorganisms. The gingival crevices support large concentrations of the even more fastidious anaerobic bacteria, which may outnumber aerobic bacteria tenfold (Box 44-1). Composition of indigenous flora can be altered by specific changes in a patient's environment or underlying condition. Colonization with potentially pathogenic species may occur during seasonal changes or with increased exposure. Thus, opportunity for colonization with *Streptococcus pneumoniae* and *Haemophilus influenzae* may increase significantly in adults with children recently enrolled in day-care centers. Colonization with Gram-negative bacilli increases in patients hospitalized with acute illnesses, in patients treated with broad spectrum antimicrobics, and in patients suffering from diabetes or chronic alcoholism.

The tracheobronchial tree beyond the larynx is considered to be sterile except for a small number of commonly aspirated microorganisms which are rapidly cleared by the

---

Box 44-1 Predominant organisms indigenous or transient in the upper respiratory tract

NORMALLY COMMENSAL BACTERIA

Anaerobes *(may outnumber aerobes by 5-10:1)*
  Bacteroides (especially *B. melaninogenicus*), *Fusobacterium,* Gram-positive cocci, *Veillonella, Actinomyces,* other Gram-positive rods (including *Eubacterium, Bifidobacterium,* and *Propionibacterium*)
Aerobes *(may be facultative anaerobes)*
  Streptococcus (viridans, non-hemolytic), *Neisseria, Moraxella* (*Branhamella*), *Haemophilus, Staphylococcus* (especially coagulase negative staphylococci), yeasts (especially *Candida*)

POTENTIALLY PATHOGENIC/TRANSIENT COLONIZERS

Streptococcus pneumoniae, beta-hemolytic Streptococcus, Staphylococcus aureus, Haemophilus influenzae b, *Enterobacteriaceae* (especially *Klebsiella, Enterobacter, Serratia, Escherichia coli, Pseudomonas aeruginosa,* other Gram-negative rods (*Acinetobacter, Neisseria meningitidis, Moraxella* [in large numbers], yeasts)

---

mucociliary apparatus. Microbial colonization beyond the larynx, however, increases in patients with bronchial neoplasms, chronic respiratory disease, endotracheal intubation, or in the comatose patient who aspirates. During a pneumonic process, the concentration of organisms in lower respiratory secretions is normally greater than 10^6/ml, unless antimicrobial therapy has been initiated.

INFECTIOUS ETIOLOGIES OF LOWER RESPIRATORY TRACT DISEASE

Practically, the etiologic agents of pneumonia may be divided into two major groups. One group includes organisms harbored as normal commensal flora of the upper respiratory tract whose significance has to be interpreted carefully in light of clinical and laboratory parameters. The second group includes organisms not routinely colonizing the respiratory tract, more frequently recognized as pathogens without interpretational problems, and for whom selective techniques may be used to obviate overgrowth by indigenous flora.

Specimens submitted for routine cultural analysis predominantly yield organisms belonging to the first group (Table 44-1). Of those recovered, *S. pneumoniae* is still the most common overall cause of community-acquired pneumonia, accounting for a quarter of all cases and up to three quarters of those requiring hospitalization. *Staphylococcus aureus* accounts for less than 5% of community-acquired pneumonias, but up to a quarter of nosocomial pneumonias. This organism also has a predilection for patients following viral pneumonia and for those with cystic fibrosis. Other streptococci and staphylococci are far less frequently involved with pneumonia, although *S. agalactiae* (Group B) may predominate in infections of the newborn.

Gram-negative bacteria of respiratory flora which may cause lower tract infections include *H. influenzae* and *B. catarrhalis*. *Haemophilus influenzae* causes up to 20% of community-acquired pneumonias and is associated with pediatric patients (serotype b strains) and adults with chronic lung disease (nontypeable strains). The organism is also recognized in patients recovering from viral illness and in patients with cystic fibrosis. *B. catarrhalis*, a Gram-negative diplococcal bacterium resembling the neisseria, has been documented as a pathogen in patients with underlying respiratory or immunologic problems. *Neisseria meningitidis* is responsible for a small number of community-acquired pneumonias. Anaerobic flora, on the other hand, have a major role in aspiration pneumonia and possibly a larger-than-recognized role in both community as well as nosocomial pneumonias. Frequently, anaerobic infections may be mixed, with both aerobic and anaerobic flora contributing to the process. The role of Gram-negative bacilli of the enteric and *pseudomonas* groups increases dramatically in nosocomial pneumonias. *Klebsiella, Enterobacter, Escherichia, Serratia, Pseudomonas* and *Acinetobacter* genera may all cause disease. In this group, pneumonias caused by *K. pneumoniae* or *P. aeruginosa* are more common, although those caused by *Enterobacter* have recently been gaining prominence. *Pseudomonas aeruginosa* also colonizes and exacerbates those with bronchiectasis, especially in the cystic fibrosis population.

Organisms not routinely colonizing the respiratory tract are frequently searched for by concentration and decontamination techniques, as well as by use of selective media (Table 44-2). Organisms belonging to this group include *Legionella, Mycoplasma, Chlamydia, Nocardia, Mycobacteria,* some moulds, viruses and protozoa, or helminths.

Box 44-2   Specimens commonly used for recovery of organisms causing pneumonia and potential for their being contaminated

POTENTIALLY HEAVILY CONTAMINATED

Expectorated sputum
Induced sputum
Nasotracheal/Endotracheal aspirate
Tracheostomy aspirate

MODERATELY CONTAMINATED

Bronchoscopic washings, brushings
Bronchoalveolar lavage

MINIMALLY CONTAMINATED

Transtracheal aspirate

UNCONTAMINATED (NORMALLY STERILE)

Pleural fluid
Transthoracic needle aspirate
Lung biopsy (open-lung)

OTHER SITE SPECIMENS

Blood (cultures)
Urine (antigen detection for *Haemophilus influenzae* b and *Legionella*)

When these organisms are suspected, specimens are frequently referred to subspecialty areas of the laboratory where specialized techniques are performed. Specific test requests are required for these procedures and appropriate information must be submitted to the laboratory if specific organisms are suspected.

SPECIMEN EVALUATION, CULTURE, AND INTERPRETATION
Routine microbiologic (bacteriologic) examination

Specimens submitted for routine microbiologic evaluation may include 1) those easily collected by noninvasive means, but which may be contaminated with indigenous flora and 2) those collected by more invasive means but which are less likely to be contaminated (Box 44-2). If at all possible, specimens should be collected prior to initiation of antimicrobial therapy. Swabs and 12- to 24-hour collections of sputum are *not* acceptable. Specimens should be processed within two hours of collection or they may be refrigerated up to six to eight hours; longer delays tend to compromise relative numbers of organisms present in secretions or promote overgrowth. Specimens from invasive techniques or from a patient whose condition is rapidly deteriorating should be effectively coordinated and processed as rapidly as possible.

All specimens should be Gram-stained for direct-microscopic evaluation. Potentially contaminated sputum should be screened microscopically for acceptability and rejected if criteria based on oropharyngeal contamination and presence of lower tract secretions (leukocytes: polymorphonuclear cells and/or alveolar macrophages) are not met.

Cultures should be set up for semiquantitative assessment of growth on agar plates based on the numbers of colony-forming units (CFU) seen in consecutive streak areas.

Growth should be recorded as: 1+ (rare; < 10 CFU/1st streak); 2+ (light; > 10 CFU/1st streak, but < 5 CFU/2nd streak); 3+ (moderate; > 5 CFU/2nd streak, but < 5 CFU/3rd streak); 4+ (heavy; > 5 CFU/3rd streak). The relative growth of various organisms can thereby be described and interpreted in conjunction with direct smear evaluation and any discrepancy reviewed.

Potentially contaminated specimens
Sputum

Specimens in this category, including expectorated and induced sputum, as well as nasotracheal, endotracheal and tracheostomy aspirates, may all be heavily contaminated. Experience has shown that induced specimens are usually inferior to expectorated ones for diagnosis of routine bac-

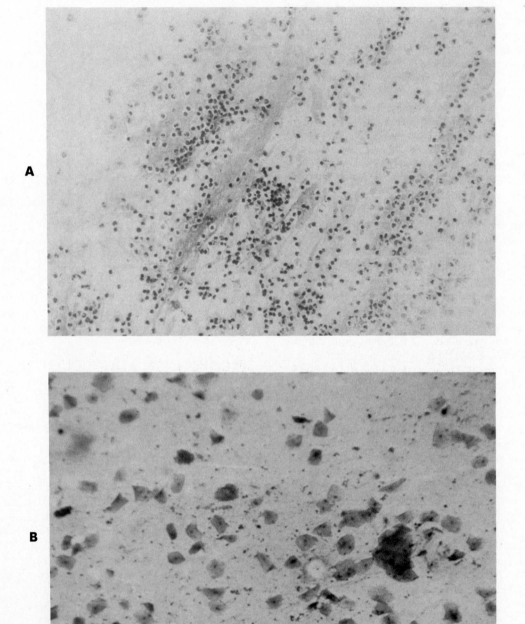

Fig. 44-1   Smears of expectorated sputum for screening (Gram-stain ×100). **A,** ideal sputum, >25 polymorphonuclear cells (PMN), <25 squamous epithelial cells (SEC); **B,** unacceptable specimen, <25 WBC, >25 SEC.

terial pneumonias, but may be useful in other pneumonias. The presence of an endotracheal tube may elicit a leukocyte response and the endotracheal tube may become colonized as well, thus obfuscating the actual disease process in the lung. Results of smears and cultures from the latter specimens are therefore difficult to interpret and may not provide adequate guidance for patient care.

The specimen should be observed carefully for mucopurulent strands and those areas teased out with applicator sticks and applied to a glass slide as a thin, light smear for Gram-stain or wetmount. Initial microscopic screening should be performed at lower magnification ($\times 100$). Several fields should be examined and the most purulent areas selected for grading the specimen.

Criteria for cytologically grading the quality of sputum are based on parallel observation of cytologic and culture results of sputum and transtracheal aspirates. Irrespective of numbers of leukocytes present, culture results of specimens with > 25 squamous epithelial cells (SECs) per low power field correlated poorly with those of transtracheal aspirates. Thus, specimens showing > 25 SECs should normally be rejected (Fig. 44-1). In some instances, specimens having > 25 SECs may also have > 25 leukocytes. Review of these smears may indicate that the contamination is light (ratio of leukocytes to SECs > 10:1) rather than heavy (ratio < 10:1). Observation of one or two bacterial morphologies associated with leukocytes in these specimens may make them appropriate for Gram-stain guided culture (Table 44-3).

Submission of repeat specimens should be recommended only within appropriate time limits and if antimicrobial therapy has not been initiated. If the second specimen fails the screen, the clinician should consider using more invasive diagnostic procedures, if clinically warranted.

Screening techniques may be implemented for routine bacteriologic procedures alone but are not usually necessary when selectively searching for other etiologic agents such as mycobacteria, viruses, or the dimorphic fungi.

Specimens acceptable for routine bacterial study should be microscopically examined under high magnification ($\times 1000$) for evaluation of the organisms around the leukocytes. Normally with bacterial pneumonia, greater than 10 organisms per oil immersion field are present. It has also been suggested that only specimens with greater than 10 organisms per oil immersion field morphologically similar to *Haemophilus* or *Neisseria* need to be cultured to chocolate agar. Gram-stain results should note the predominant organisms and relative content of mixed or otherwise normal indigenous flora. There is usually no value in culturing specimens showing mixed species or presence of organisms resembling anaerobes, irrespective of leukocyte or SEC counts. In these instances, the Gram-stain may remain the best and only guide to diagnosis.

Acceptable specimens should be inoculated to solid agar media to allow semiquantitative grading of growth. The media used should allow isolation of the more common pathogens suspected and may include blood agar for the Gram-positive organisms and MacConkey for Gram-negative organisms. Chocolate agar may also be used or reserved for specimens in which Gram-negative pleomorphic coccobacilli or diplococci are observed in predominant numbers. Enrichment broth media should not be used for sputum specimens. Plates should be incubated at 35 to 37°C in five to 10 percent CO_2, and read after 18 to 24 hours. The cultures may be read again after 48 hours if the patient is on therapy or if there is a discrepancy between the direct smear and culture.

Identification and susceptibility studies should be reserved for those potentially pathogenic organisms showing predominant moderate to heavy growth, and whose presence is recognized in adequate numbers in association with leukocytes in the direct smear. Organisms meeting these criteria should be identified to the extent that pathogens may be recognized. Viridans streptococci should be screened for bile solubility to rule out *S. pneumoniae*. Beta hemolytic streptococci should minimally be typed as being Group A or non-Group A, while staphylococci need only be tested and reported as to coagulase activity. Nonhemolytic streptococci do not routinely require further identification and diphtheroids may be reported as such based on colony and Gram-stain morphology as well as a catalase test. *Nocardia asteroides* should be ruled out if branching Gram-positive or stippled rods are seen.

Table 44-3 Guidelines for grading sputum specimens for routine bacterial culture

Number of squamous epithelial cells/low power field*	Number of WBC/low power field	Grade: quality (comment)
< 25	< 25	Grade 6: acceptable to unsatisfactory (minimal inflammation and contamination; suitability depends on high power Gram-stain evaluation around WBCs; consider leukopenia in immunocompromised)
< 10	> 25	Grade 5: ideal (very suitable for culture)
10-25	> 25	Grade 4: good to acceptable (light contamination, suitable for culture)
> 25	> 25	Grade 3: normally unsatisfactory (suitability depends on extent of contamination, ratio of WBC to squamous epithelial cells [SEC], and ability to find predominant organism involved with WBC. WBC/SEC ratio >10:1—may be acceptable WBC/SEC ratio <10:1—normally unsatisfactory)
> 25	< 25	Grades 1 and 2: not acceptable (minimal inflammation with heavy contamination: "regarded as consisting mostly of saliva")

Data from Geckler, RW, et al: J Clin Microbiol 6:396, 1977.
*Low power field is at 100 to X120 magnification

When indicated by direct smear, *Haemophilus* species should be differentiated to *H. influenzae* and non-influenzae using growth and morphologic characteristics as well as X and V factor growth requirements or porphyrin studies. Serotyping of type b *H. influenzae* is not routinely necessary, but may be helpful in selected instances.

Further identification of oxidase-positive, Gram-negative diplococci may be reserved for those showing etiologic potential in the direct smear. When causing pneumonia, *Neisseria* and *Branhamella catarrhalis* are normally seen in large numbers among the polymorphonuclear cells and may be present intracellularly. Yellow pigmented *Neisseria* species may be reported as indigenous flora; otherwise, biochemical testing is normally required for identification of *N. meningitidis* and *B. catarrhalis*.

Gram-negative bacilli may be identified by conventional means including categorization by lactose fermentation on MacConkey medium, spot tests (indole and oxidase production), motility, short or long biochemical profile sets, and commercial identification kits. Because of the frequency with which Gram-negative bacilli colonize the respiratory tract in the hospital setting, identification should be strictly limited to those isolates that are definitely predominant and in which an association with the leukocytes has been ascertained by direct smear.

The identification and reporting of the pseudomonads is usually limited to *P. aeruginosa* based on oxidase reaction and pyocyanin pigment production. Other pseudomonads may be reported as *Pseudomonas* not-aeruginosa, unless further characterization is epidemiologically or clinically warranted. *Pseudomonas cepacia* should be identified in patients with cystic fibrosis; specimens from such patients may also be cultured on media selective for *P. cepacia*.

Yeasts isolated on routine bacteriologic media are rarely implicated in disease of the lower tract, and their presence does not provide a diagnosis of pneumonia. Therefore, yeast should not be routinely identified from sputum specimens, unless cytologic evidence collected by biopsy indicates its pathogenic role in the tissues. If suspected, *Cryptococcus neoformans* may be ruled out by a negative rapid urease activity test, a positive germ tube test indicating *C. albicans*, or presence of pseudomycelia.

Identification of organisms in cultures showing mixed growth of potential pathogens may be limited to only one or two distinctly predominant isolates (when also supported by direct smear). Otherwise, a statement regarding the morphologic characteristics of the organisms isolated (e.g., lactose-fermenters resembling *Klebsiella/Enterobacter* species, or resembling *E. coli* or *Pseudomonas* species) and a comment such as "mixed culture of potential pathogens— no predominant organism distinguishable; call laboratory if further workup is clinically warranted" is appropriate.

Antibiotic susceptibility studies should be limited to those organisms meeting criteria for identification. In most instances, qualitative susceptibilities provide adequate information for appropriate patient care. Susceptibility reports should only include a limited, selective battery of antimicrobics based on recommendations of the Pharmacy and Therapeutics Committee in conjunction with the clinical microbiologist of each hospital. In the private reference laboratory the choice may be based on careful evaluation of recommendations by the National Committee on Clinical Laboratory Standards and their application to the needs of the specific situation.

Other methods for studying sputum specimens have been described, including antigen detection (counterimmuno-electrophoresis, coagglutination, enzyme-linked-immunoassay) and quellung studies for *S. pneumoniae*, as well as specialized wash and/or liquefaction procedures for routine culturing. Unfortunately, such studies are labor intensive, costly, and are not normally practical for most laboratories. The quellung reaction might be the most useful.

Bronchoscopic specimens

Specimens collected by bronchoscopic aspiration may be heavily contaminated with upper respiratory flora and usually are not better than expectorated sputum specimens for diagnosis of rapidly growing bacterial pathogens. Bronchoscopy should be reserved for patients with infiltrates and a nonproductive cough who pose diagnostic dilemmas or for immunocompromised patients with potentially unusual, opportunistic pathogens. Routine culture results obtained with bronchial washings rarely contribute to patient care and should always be correlated to results of microscopic examination of a direct smear. Anaerobic culture should not be performed. When unusual or opportunistic infections are suspected, additional brushings and biopsies may enhance recovery of causative organisms. The newer modifications of bronchoscopic techniques have attempted to improve both recovery of etiologies and to allow quantitative assessment of bacterial load in the lower respiratory tract.

Bronchoalveolar lavage (BAL) is performed by wedging the fiberoptic bronchoscope into distal affected airways and sampling by serial aliquots of saline. The lavage fluid must be divided to accommodate all the requested studies, including selective isolation of more unusual organisms such as legionellae, fungi, mycobacteria, and viruses. Cytocentrifuge-prepared slides ($\times 500$ g) enhance visualization of organisms by special stains. BAL is useful primarily for recognition of opportunistic pathogens in the immunocompromised host (especially for *Pneumocystis carinii* in the patient with acquired immunodeficiency syndrome [AIDS]).

Collection of lower respiratory secretions using a distally occluded, double-lumen, protected-brush, fiberoptic catheter is considered to be best suited for isolation of routine bacterial pathogens. The brush should be severed into a tube containing 1.0 ml of transport medium (Ringer's lactate without preservative), and transported as quickly as possible to the microbiology laboratory. The brush should be vortexed vigorously; 0.1 ml of the suspension inoculated onto blood, chocolate, MacConkey and anaerobic agars. Additionally, the same agar media should be inoculated with 0.1 ml each of a $1:10^2$ and a $1:10^4$ dilutions of the suspension. After appropriate incubation, the plates are examined for growth and potentially pathogenic organisms having $> 10^3$ CFU/ml (representing $> 10^6$ CFU/ml in the original pulmonary secretions) may be considered possibly significant.

Uncontaminated (normally sterile) specimens

Transtracheal aspirations (TTA) are rarely used although they may provide a relatively safe and sensitive method for diagnosis of many pleuropulmonary infections. These aspirates are considered relatively free of upper respiratory flora, although there may be some minimal contamination due to aspiration. Other normally sterile specimens useful for diagnosis of pneumonia include pleural fluid collected by thoracentesis, transthoracic needle aspirates (TNA), and lung biopsies. These specimens are usually excellent for detection of etiologic agents of pneumonia.

Processing of specimens should include direct studies of either fluid, pus, centrifuged secretions, touch preparations of tissue, or ground tissue, as well as culture for both aerobic and anaerobic bacteria as necessary. Routine aerobic and anaerobic culture media, together with broth media, should be inoculated and incubated according to conventional means.

Isolation of potentially pathogenic organisms should be considered significant and fully worked up. Rare growth of viridans streptococci, coagulase negative staphylococci, or diphtheroids may occur in a few instances and should be considered as contaminating flora.

Microbiologic examination for non-routine organisms

Nocardia

Nocardia asteroides may be isolated from secretions of patients with various underlying immunocompromising conditions and especially from those on steroids. The characteristic Gram-positive or stippled, filamentous, branching rods are often easily recognizable in direct Gram-stained smears. They may be identified presumptively as nocardial bacteria by performing a modified "weak" Kinyoun acid-fast stain using a 0.5 percent decolorizing acid solution; however, only approximately 70% of these in direct smear are discerned as weak acid-fast positive. The Gram-stain seems to be the most sensitive stain for detecting *Nocardia* in most circumstances.

Nocardia may be isolated on routine bacteriologic media (blood and chocolate agar) if incubated for longer than usual intervals. Inoculation of a selective Thayer-Martin medium has been recommended to enhance recovery from contaminated specimens. In general, time to detection averages three to five days, but may require several weeks. If the organisms are not detected in direct smears and routine media is discarded, *Nocardia* may still be isolated on fungal or mycobacterial media, although mycobacterial decontamination techniques may be deleterious.

Identification to species level is based on biochemical studies, while studies of susceptibility to the tetracyclines, sulfas, aminoglycosides, beta-lactams, and imipenem may be performed using a modified disk-diffusion method. Although the significance of isolation of *Nocardia* from some patients sometimes is questioned, the organism should be considered a pathogen if present in direct smears or isolated from a compromised host.

Legionella

Presently, there are more than 25 species and 33 serogroups in the family *Legionellaceae,* with at least 18 species associated with pneumonia. *Legionellae* encompass a broad spectrum of morphotypes ranging from coccobacillary to elongated fusiform types. They have the common traits of being difficult to stain directly in specimens by the Gram method, being Gram-negative on culture, being more easily stained by the Dieterle modification of the silver stain, being fastidious in terms of isolation from clinical specimens, and being ubiquitous in environments containing warm water (e.g., hot water supply pipes and air conditioning water tanks).

Legionellae can be cultured from expectorated sputum if selective and nonselective media and specimen decontamination procedures are used. Tissue or sterile lung fluid provide the best results, while bronchoscopically obtained specimens, endo/nasotracheal aspirates, and expectorated sputum provide a decreasing order of diagnostic efficacy.

Although the risk of working with Legionellae is not high, use of a class II biosafety hood is recommended for procedures creating aerosols. Because *Legionellae* media will support other fastidious potential pathogens (e.g., *Francisella* and *Coccidioides*), use of the hood is also recommended when fungal or unidentified colonies are being examined.

Legionellae cannot be detected directly in specimens by the Gram-stain. They can, however, be detected by either immunofluorescent microscopy, DNA probe studies, or by the Dieterle silver stain. Although the silver stain is not as sensitive or as specific, it may detect a legionella species for which monoclonal fluorescent antibody conjugates are not available.

Specific fluorescent monoclonal antibody reagents for *Legionella pneumophila* (reactive with all serogroups) are available commercially (Genetic Systems Corp., Seattle) as is a DNA probe (Gen-Probe Corp., San Diego). Both reagents have similar sensitivity of approximately 70% for *L. pneumophila* but will not detect other species of *Legionella*. The Genetic Systems' monoclonal antibody is not useful for detecting legionella in formalin-fixed tissues. Detection of legionellae antigens in other body fluids is addressed in Chapter 41.

Normally sterile respiratory tract specimens can be cultured on a nonselective, buffered charcoal yeast extract (BCYE), medium supplemented with alpha-ketoglutarate. Potentially contaminated specimens should additionally be cultured on two selective basal media, one containing cefamandole, polymyxin B, and anisomycin (BMPA) and the second substituting vancomycin for the cefamandole (PAV) since several *Legionella* species may be inhibited by cefamandole.

Heavily contaminated specimens may be decontaminated by pretreatment with acid (pH 2.2 KCl-HCl) prior to plating. To enhance isolation in such specimens, culture of both acid-treated and untreated secretions onto both selective and nonselective plates has been suggested.

Plates should be incubated at 35°C to 37°C in a humidified environment with 3% to 5% carbon dioxide. Incubation should be for at least two weeks, although most isolates are detected within 3 to 5 days. Legionellae may be presumptively identified by its colonial morphology, Gram reaction and growth patterns. The organisms fail to grow on blood or chocolate agar. Further identification to genus and species level requires specific typing sera not available in most laboratories, so submission to referral centers (State Health Department Laboratory or Centers for Disease Control, Atlanta) is commonly necessary.

Susceptibility testing of Legionellae Kolata is unnecessary and not recommended since standard methods for testing rapid-growing bacteria cannot be used. Clinically useful antimicrobials include those that can penetrate intracellularly into the alveolar macrophage (e.g., erythromycin).

Isolation of Legionellae from clinical specimens is always considered significant although mixed infections are possible and may be more frequent in the compromised patient.

Mycoplasma

Mycoplasma pneumoniae causes a wide spectrum of respiratory infections ranging from asymptomatic to frank bronchopneumonia. Overall, the majority of respiratory infections due to mycoplasma are probably diagnosed and treated empirically. Diagnostic studies usually include serologic rather than cultural techniques because of the latter's technical difficulty and delay in detection due to slow growth of the organism. Serologic methods are described in Chapter 34.

Specimens for isolation of *mycoplasma* include swabbings of the pharynx which should be transported to the laboratory in sucrose phosphate (SP-4) medium. If specimens are to be referred to other laboratories and require extended time for transport, they should be frozen at −20°C.

Fresh diphasic and selective agar media are necessary for isolation of *mycoplasma*. Freshly prepared yeast extract may be the critical factor among other serum and peptone components of the medium. Unfortunately, commercially available *mycoplasma* media usually do not perform well and in-house medium preparation is normally recommended. Although growth is usually evident within the first 10 to 14 days, cultures require a minimum of a month-long incubation. The difficulty of media preparation, together with slow growth of the organism, detract from the diagnostic effectiveness of *mycoplasma* cultures.

DNA probes are available for detection of *mycoplasma* directly in respiratory secretions and preliminary studies on these new technical capabilities are promising. Their role in the diagnosis of lower pulmonary tract disease is yet to be ascertained, although may surpass that of culture.

Chlamydia

Three species of *Chlamydia* have been implicated in disease of the lower respiratory tract. Infections caused by *Chlamydia psittaci* (ornithosis), *C. trachomatis* (infant pneumonitis) and *C. pneumoniae* (TWAR strain; pneumonia in young adults and elderly) can be diagnosed by culture, serologies, and, in some instances, by direct detection in specimens. Serologic techniques, which are preferred for the diagnosis of ornithosis and which may be more commonly used for the diagnosis of *C. pneumoniae*, are available only in reference laboratories or state or federal public health laboratories.

Specimens submitted for isolation of chlamydia should be held at 4°C and processed within 24 to 48 hours of collection, or frozen at −70°C if further delay is anticipated. Freezing, however, can lower isolation rates by as much as 20%. Because of low sensitivity of culture and high virulence of *C. psittaci,* routine attempts at isolation of the organism are not recommended. When isolation is at-

tempted, cultures should be performed in an appropriately equipped laboratory and by trained technical staff.

Swabs of secretions which are not to be frozen may be transported in tryptose phosphate or similar broth with vancomycin, gentamicin, and nystatin or amphotericin added to prevent bacterial or fungal overgrowth. Alternatively, 2-sucrose phosphate or sucrose-glutamate-phosphate may be used as a transport medium with addition of 2% to 10% fetal calf serum if storage at −70°C is expected. Viral transport media containing penicillin may be inhibitory to chlamydia and should not be used.

Chlamydia trachomatis and *C. pneumoniae* can be cultivated in monolayers of tissue culture cells. The most consistently effective method for isolation of *C. trachomatis* includes use of McCoy cell monolayers grown on coverslips in shell vials and pretreated with cycloheximide. Centrifugation of specimens (×3000 g for one hour) onto the cell monolayer further enhances isolation. Hela-229 cells are more sensitive than McCoy cells for detection of *C. pneumoniae*. Detection of growth of *C. trachomatis* is accomplished by staining the cell monolayer with either a fluorescein-conjugated monoclonal antibody for intracytoplasmic inclusions, or the Giemsa stain or iodine for accumulations of glycogen produced by the chlamydia after 48 to 72 hours of incubation.

In instances where transportation of specimens is not a problem, culture for *C. trachomatis* remains the most sensitive method for detecting this organism. However, monoclonal immunofluorescent and immunochemical methods, as well as DNA probes, are commercially available for detecting the organisms directly in specimens. Although such methods have been well studied or show great promise for diagnosis of chlamydial infections of other sites, there is a paucity of data regarding their sensitivity, specificity, and efficacy in the detection of these organisms from the lower respiratory tract.

Mycobacteria

Not all laboratories have the facilities or staff expertise to work with mycobacteria within adequate safety or proficiency standards. Specific levels of service dependent on individual laboratory capabilities have been recommended. Services may extend from acid-fast staining and microscopic examination, followed by packaging and submission to referral laboratories, to providing complete studies including isolation, definitive identification, and susceptibility tests of isolated mycobacteria. In intermediate-sized laboratories, extent of service may be limited to specimen inoculation with subsequent referral, to limited isolation and identification of *Mycobacterium tuberculosis*, or to isolation and identification of all mycobacteria but referral of susceptibility studies.

Three to five early-morning expectorated sputum specimens are normally adequate for diagnosis of mycobacteriosis. Sputum collections over a 12- to 24-hour period are not acceptable because of the increased rate of contamination. Procedures involving sputum induction with 3% to 10% sodium chloride or bronchoscopic collection should be limited to patients incapable of providing adequate specimens. Occasionally, post-bronchoscopy expectorated sputum increases the yield of mycobacterial cultures. Cultures of blood and stool are only useful in the immunocompromised patient, especially when *M. avium* is suspected in association with AIDS.

For safety and protection of personnel, manipulation of *any* specimen suspected to contain mycobacteria must be performed within a class II biosafety laminar flow hood at biosafety level 2 in a clean work room that has negative air pressure in relation to surrounding work areas. (See Chapter 2.)

Screening for oropharyngeal contamination is not necessary when processing sputum for mycobacteria. However, recovery of mycobacteria increases significantly when sampling of lower respiratory secretions is adequate. Digestion (liquefaction) and decontamination using strong alkali or other chemicals to which mycobacteria are more resistant because of the high lipid content of their cell walls are used for contaminated specimens. This decontamination also adversely influences the mycobacteria; therefore, a gentle decontamination process should be chosen and the harsher methods reserved for specimens known or expected to be highly contaminated.

More common reagents used in liquefaction and decontamination of sputum include N-acetyl-L-cysteine (mucolytic agent) with 2% sodium hydroxide, dithiothreitol (sputolysin) with 2% sodium hydroxide, or zephiran-trisodium-phosphate. Additionally, survival of mycobacteria in specimens being mailed to referral laboratories for processing is enhanced by treatment with 1% cetylpyridinium and 2% sodium chloride prior to mailing. Specimens suspected of being heavily contaminated with pseudomonads should be decontaminated with 5% oxalic acid.

Following a gentle decontamination, the specimen is neutralized (pH 6.8 buffer), centrifuged at 2000 to $\times 3000$ g in individual centrifuge cups, and the sediment used for inoculation of media after being resuspended in 0.2% bovine albumin. Decontamination is unnecessary for specimens from sterile sites. If specimen sterility is questioned, a portion may be cultured overnight in a nutrient broth to detect contamination.

Smears for staining and microscopic examination may be made before or after specimen concentration. However, the examination of smears prepared directly from unconcentrated specimens are less likely to show acid-fast bacilli than smears prepared from concentrates, since approximately 10^4 to 5×10^4 organisms per milliliter of sputum are necessary for microscopic visualization. Preliminary reports based on microscopic examination of direct smears should be followed by results of the concentrated smear examination.

Several acid-fast stains are available, including the auramine fluorochrome stain, the Ziehl-Neelsen stain, and the Kinyoun cold stain. The fluorochrome method is most sensitive, allowing for rapid screening with lower magnification. However, it may not stain some of the rapid growing mycobacteria. The Ziehl-Neelsen stain is the most difficult to perform, requiring steam heating of the slides and higher magnifications for microscopic screening. It is useful for confirming morphology of mycobacteria detected by auramine stain. Kinyoun's cold stain is comparable to the Ziehl-Neelsen; although it is easier to perform since heating is not necessary.

Table 44-4 Quantitation method for reporting results of direct stained smears for mycobacterial acid-fast bacilli

No. of AFB seen	Report	Interpretation
0	Negative for AFB	Probably negative (Not present in concentrations heavy enough to be directly visible)
1-2/300 fields	Number seen	Not positive (Not considered positive, but additional specimens may be studied if warranted)
1-9/100 fields	Number/100 fields	1+ ; rare
1-9/10 fields	Number/10 fields	2+ ; few
1-9/field	Number/field	3+ ; moderate
> 9/field	> 9/field	4+ ; many

Data from Sommers HM and McClatchy JK: Cumitech 16, Laboratory diagnosis of the mycobacteriosis, Morello JA, coordinating ed, Washington, DC, 1983, American Society for Microbiology.
AFB = acid-fast bacilli
reports based on X800-X1000 magnification of concentrated smears

It has been recommended that quantitation and reports of smears be standardized and based on examination of concentrated material at magnifications of 800 to $\times 1000$ (Table 44-4).

Concentrated specimens are inoculated to nonselective and selective media. Nonselective media may include those that are egg-base (Lowenstein-Jensen and Petragnani); agar-base (Middlebrook and Cohn, 7H10, 7H11); or liquid (7H9 broth, Dubos broth). Selective media contain antimicrobial agents and include modifications of Lowenstein-Jensen (Gruft modification, Mycobactosel) or of 7H10 and 7H11 media. However, selective media may be inhibitory to mycobacteria and should never be used alone.

Recently, a liquid medium with the same characteristics as the selective 7H11 medium was introduced with an added radiolabelled (^{14}C) fatty acid component (7H12 broth). Growth is detected radiometrically by measuring release of CO_2 (BACTEC; Becton Dickinson Diagnostic Instrument Sytems, Towson, Maryland). On the average, the system reduces time to recover mycobacteria by one to two weeks.

All agar or solid media are best incubated at 35°C in air with increased CO_2 (8% to 12%); tubes should have screw caps slightly loosened to allow CO_2 atmosphere penetration. The BACTEC system provides for increased CO_2 in the head space of the bottles. All media should be examined for at least six to eight weeks.

Identification of mycobacteria is important because clinical significance, therapeutic modality, and prognosis may vary according to species. Colonial morphology, chromogenicity (carotenoid pigmentation), and growth rates were used to categorize species differing from *M. tuberculosis* and *M. bovis*. These were placed into divisional units known as Runyon Groups (Table 44-5). Although useful, the groups are not accurate and may be misleading; biochemical profiling identifies the species more accurately. Species resembling each other biochemically and pathogenically may be considered as complexes (e.g., *M. avium* complex).

Table 44-5 Separation of more common mycobacterial species by divisional units (old Runyon Groups), biochemical profiles, and pathogenic potential

Group	Description	Pathogenic or Potentially pathogenic[a]	Rarely pathogenic/most commonly saprophytic[b]
M. tuberculosis Complex	(organisms in this group are always considered pathogens)	*M. tuberculosis* *M. africanum* *M. bovis*	
I.	Photochromogens (slow growth; pigment stimulated by light)	*M. kansasii* *M. simiae* *M. marinum*	
II.	Scotochromogens (slow growth; pigment in presence or absence of light)	*M. scrofulaceum* *M. xenopi*	*M. flavescens* *M. gordonae*
III.	Nonphotochromogens (slow growth)	*M. avium* *M. intracellulare*	*M. gastri* *M. terrae-triviale*
IV.	Rapid growers (growth within seven days)	*M. fortuitum* *M. chelonae*	*M. smegmatis* *M. thermoresistibile*

[a]Other potentially pathogenic species: mycobacterial species—*M. szulgai, M. malmoense, M. ulcerans,* and *M. haemophilum.*
[b]Usually saprophytic species: M. asiaticum, M. phlei, M. vaccae, others.

Identification by biochemical reactions may take one to four weeks or longer to complete. The radiometric BACTEC system has introduced a proprietary chemical reagent capable of differentiating between *M. tuberculosis* complex (*M. tuberculosis, M. bovis, M. africanum*) and nontubercular mycobacteria (NTM) within four to six days of initial isolation if adequate concentrations are available for testing.

Recently, DNA relatedness (DNA/RNA probes) and gasliquid chromatographic studies have facilitated differentiation between mycobacterial species. Technical improvements and cost reduction should make these techniques more readily available.

Susceptibility testing of *M. tuberculosis* is indicated for isolates from treatment failures, for isolates from individuals who acquired their infection outside the United States or Canada, and perhaps for those cultures isolated from individuals who immigrated to the United States or whose families have a history of tuberculosis. Recent reports of resistant isolates of *M. tuberculosis* from various parts of the United States, however, support the practice of routine susceptibility testing of all such isolates. Primary drugs to be tested should include isoniazid, streptomycin, rifampin, ethambutol, and pyrazinamide. A secondary battery of drugs may include ethionamide, capreomycin, cycloserine, kanamycin, and p-aminosalicilate. Historically, susceptibility studies with the nontuberculous mycobacteria have shown poor predictive value for patient outcome. Recent data suggest, however, that use of minimal inhibitory concentrations obtained with the BACTEC system may provide guidance for designing optimal therapy for *M. kansasii, M. fortuitum, M. chelonae,* and members of the *M. avium* complex. All such studies should be performed only by reference laboratories capable of providing the expertise for such procedures.

Isolation of members of the *M. tuberculosis* complex is always significant and should be reported to the attending physician at once. However, the increasing environmental prevalence and low virulence of NTM may cause difficulty for interpretation of positive cultures. Criteria useful for differentiation between clinical disease and colonization include evidence of increased quantity of organisms in the specimen, isolation or visualization from normally sterile sites, and repeated isolations of the same organism from multiple specimens acquired at different times. Additional clues may include progressive roentgenographic changes, an isolate's identity, a chronically ill patient with failure to identify other etiologies, and the presence and extent of host risk factors.

Fungi

Cultural and histologic documentation of fungal infections is more successful than are serologic techniques. As with bacterial isolates, the fungi may be divided into two groups in terms of interpretational ease. Isolation of *Cryptococcus neoformans, Coccidioides immitis, Histoplasma capsulatum,* and *Blastomyces dermatitidis,* should always be considered significant. On the other hand, *Candida albicans* and, less frequently, other members of the genus *Candida* (*C. tropicalis, C. guilliermondi, C. parapsilosis,* etc.) are common colonizers of the oropharynx and their presence in respiratory secretions are not normally predictive of their pathogenicity. The significance of the isolation of aspergilli or the zygomycetes in sputum cultures is also difficult to evaluate, as these (and other fungi) are commonly present as contaminants or colonizers. However, multiple isolations of an *Aspergillus* spp from sputum of immunocompromised patients should raise the index of suspicion for systemic aspergillosis and the attending physician should consider more invasive techniques to obtain specimens for documentation of systemic aspergillosis.

Respiratory specimens are to be processed as quickly as possible or refrigerated. Some pathogens, however, may remain viable for several days at room temperature. Decontamination of sputum using mycobacterial techniques is unnecessary and normally contraindicated. Use of liquefying agents (e.g., dithiothreitol) has been recommended by some workers and although not necessary for culture, may be beneficial for preparation of concentrated smears for wet mount or stain. Addition of potassium hydroxide as a clearing agent may also be useful in preparation of certain tissue specimens for wet-mount observation.

Direct specimen examination is especially useful with bronchoscopically collected material and lung biopsy. Preferentially incorporated into chitin and cellulose components of fungi, the calcofluor white fluorescent stain allows their visualization in wet mounts and may be used in conjunction with KOH.

Histologic studies on tissue biopsies are invaluable and a close liaison should exist between the microbiology and pathology laboratories for obtaining, sharing and processing biopsies. Such studies can clarify the role of potentially pathogenic fungi such as aspergilli, the zygomycetes, and candida by visualizing their invasiveness in lung tissue.

The Gomori methenamine-silver (GMS) stain is the most sensitive for detection of fungi. Other available stains include the periodic acid-Schiff (PAS), the Hematoxylin-Eosin, the Papanicolaou and the Gram stains. The stains have differing sensitivities, and knowledge of their respective capabilities is necessary for their best use in the detection of fungi. Visualization of spherules (Coccidioides), small oval yeasts (Histoplasma), larger broad-based budding yeasts (Blastomyces), fine budding yeasts with mucicarmine staining capsules (Cryptococcus), yeasts with pseudohyphae (Candida), septate hyphae (Aspergillus), and broad, nonseptate hyphae (zygomycetes) can provide early clues as to etiologic agents responsible for an infectious disease process.

Specimens should be inoculated onto nonselective as well as selective media. Enrichment media should be used if Histoplasma is considered. Media for sputum specimens should include a Sabouraud dextrose agar and a brain-heart infusion agar (BHIA) with blood (if Histoplasma is suspected), as well as BHIA containing gentamicin and chloramphenicol. Cycloheximide (inhibitory to Cryptococcus and Aspergillus as well as other normally contaminating molds) should be added to one of two selective media. All media should be incubated at 30°C and held for up to 4 weeks. Most pathogenic fungi may be detected within the first week of incubation, although Histoplasma may require several weeks for detection.

As with mycobacteria, all studies on moulds should be performed in a class II biosafety laminar flow hood. Identification of the moulds is based on morphologic criteria, formation of conidia and growth characteristics, or on conversion from myceliating fungal form to yeast or spherule form at differing temperatures (Histoplasma, Blastomyces) or in specialized media (Coccidioides). Conversion studies are overly difficult with Coccidioides and Histoplasma, so that exoantigen immunodiffusion analyses are usually necessary for timely identification. Recently, genetic probes have become available for rapid identification of the dimorphic fungi.

Candida or yeast-like isolates from respiratory secretions do not routinely need to be identified to species level unless cytologic evaluations indicate their involvement in tissue. Yeasts may therefore only to be routinely screened to rule out Cryptococcus neoformans. Full identification to species level of the more commonly isolated Candida spp can be accomplished, when necessary, using any of several commercially available identification systems.

Serologies may be useful for evaluation of patients suspected of having systemic coccidioidomycosis and histoplasmosis, but play minor roles in the diagnosis of blastomycosis, cryptococcosis, candidosis, and aspergillosis.

Pneumocystis

Prevalence of Pneumocystis carinii in respiratory illness has reached epidemic proportions with the advent of AIDS. Its status as a protozoan is presently challenged by its genetic resemblance to the fungi. Patients presenting with pneumocystis usually have a nonproductive cough requiring either sputum induction or more invasive means of specimen collection. Properly induced sputum has a high enough yield in patients with AIDS to recommend it as an initial diagnostic study (50% to 60% sensitivity) followed by BAL and transbronchial biopsy (approaching 100% sensitivity in patients with AIDS). However, in other non-AIDS immunocompromised patients, the recovery of pneumocystis by induced sputum, BAL, and transbronchial biopsy decreases.

Smears of bronchial washings and lavage may be made either directly by cytocentrifugation ($\times 500$ g for 5 minutes) onto glass slides or by conventional centrifugation ($\times 700$ g for 15 minutes) and smear preparation from the sediment. Alternatively, imprints of lung tissue may be made by touch preparation.

Smears may be stained by either toluidine blue O or Giemsa stains (air-dried stains), or by GMS (methanol or formalin fixed smears). Toluidine blue and GMS both stain pneumocystis cysts, but the latter requires less experience for detection of organisms. Components within cysts as well as trophozoites may be visualized by the Giemsa, but require experience for recognition. Direct staining is now also possible with monoclonal fluorescent antibody reagents and may be the most sensitive method available.

Microscopic evaluations remain the diagnostic methods of choice for Pneumocystis since routine culture techniques are not available. Although susceptibility studies are not available, the organisms are normally responsive to trimethoprim-sulfamethoxazole, pentamidine, and dapsone.

Parasites

Direct visualization of wet-mount preparations or of stained smears of lower respiratory secretions are the diagnostic methods of choice when parasites are suspected. Prevalence of certain helminths may show geographic variation (Paragonimus), whereas symptomatic disease with others may be manifest primarily in the immunocompromised patient (hyperinfection with Strongyloides stercoralis). Strongyloides has been the most frequently encountered nematode and can be identified in sputum outside of endemic areas because of the organism's propensity to autoinfect a patient who may remain asymptomatic for years. Recently, the coccidian Cryptosporidium has been implicated in infections primarily associated with AIDS. In that setting, cryptosporidial oocysts may be visualized by the Giemsa stain, a modified acid-fast stain, or by the newer, direct monoclonal fluorescent antibody reagents.

Occasionally, Entamoeba histolytica or hydatid sand may be present in sputum secondary to a ruptured abscess or cyst, respectively. Migratory larvae of ascarids or hookworm may also be encountered, but rarely.

Table 44-6 Recognition of presence of more common respiratory viruses in tissue culture

	Tissue culture cell line			
Virus	Monkey kidney	Heteroploid (HEp-2)	Human diploid fibroblasts (MRC-5, WI-38)	Average days to recovery
Cytopathic Effect (CPE):				
Adenovirus	+ + +	+ + + +	+	3-7
Respiratory Syncytial Virus	+ +	+ + +	+	3-10
Cytomegalovirus	−	−	+ +	5-21
Herpes Simplex	+ or −	+ + +	+ + + +	1-3
Varicella	−	−	+ + +	5-10
Enterovirus	+ + +	+ or −	+ +	2-8
Rhinovirus	+ or −	+ or −	+ +	4-10
Hemadsorption:				
Influenza Virus	+ + + +	−	+ or −	2-10
Parainfluenza Virus	+ + +	−	−	3-7

+ + + + = strong; + + + = moderate; + + = light; + = weak; − = not evident.

Sputum can be examined either directly or after addition of a mucolytic agent followed by centrifugation and observation of the concentrated sediment. The smears should be examined microscopically at low power so as not to miss the large nematodes. These are often observed while screening sputum specimens for acceptability.

Sputum may be preserved for referral to another laboratory by treating the sediment with an equal volume of 10% buffered Formalin (for nematodes). Alternatively, referral of sputum for observation of amoeba may be accomplished by either preserving a small portion in polyvinyl alcohol fixative or treating smears with Schaudinn fixative.

Viruses

Viruses are not considered normal indigenous flora of the human respiratory tract, although extended shedding can occur after an infection. Therefore, viral isolation in association with appropriate clinical symptoms is often diagnostic. The presence of respiratory syncytial virus (RSV), influenza A and B, and parainfluenza virus 1, 2, and 3 from the respiratory tract is highly suggestive of their etiologic role. However, the presence of herpes, cytomegalovirus, and adenovirus, which may be shed for extensive periods, is suggestive but certainly not conclusive of their participation in a pneumonic process.

Possibility of several etiologies in an infectious process, especially in an immunocompromised patient, should also be considered. In such patients, cytomegalovirus may be present in lung tissue concomitantly with *Legionella,* pneumocystis, and fungal pathogens. Despite these few diagnostic dilemmas, presence or absence of certain viruses in an appropriately processed specimen contributes significantly to a clinical diagnosis.

Specimens for diagnosis of viral respiratory infections include nasopharyngeal and throat swabbings or washings, bronchoscopic aspirates or washes, and lung biopsies. Nasopharyngeal secretions are effective for isolation of RSV and rhinoviruses, while pharyngeal secretions may be more effective for isolation of adenovirus and enterovirus. The two specimen types may be combined if uncertainty as to virus identity exists. Sputum specimens are acceptable for viral isolation, but more likely to be heavily contaminated

by bacterial flora. Potentially contaminated specimens (swabs, washings), as well as small pieces of tissue, should be transported in a medium with high protein content, high buffering capability, and containing antibacterial and antifungal agents. The specimens should be kept cold and processed as quickly as possible.

Processing includes decontamination of contaminated specimens using antimicrobial agents, centrifugation at 4°C, and inoculation into tubes of at least several differing cell culture lines such as monkey kidney, heteroploid (HEp-2), and human diploid fibroblast (MRC-5, WI-38). After overlaying the cell lines at 36°C, the tubes should be re-fed and incubated on roller drums at 36°C for up to 3 weeks.

Additionally, slides may be prepared using the centrifuged sediment or directly using a cytocentrifuge for direct monoclonal fluorescent antibody studies. Reagents for RSV, adenovirus, CMV, herpes virus, influenza virus A and B, and the parainfluenza viruses 1, 2, and 3 are commonly available. Although useful in specific situations, these direct detection studies are usually less sensitive than tissue culture.

Recently, the introduction of shell vial methods have significantly decreased time to viral detection. The methods generally include centrifugation of the specimen onto cell culture monolayers grown on cover slips in shell vial tubes, followed by incubation and early detection of certain viral antigens (CMV, herpes, adenovirus) using monoclonal fluorescent antibody. Using shell vial cultures, detection of CMV can be accomplished within 48 hours instead of the average one to two weeks with conventional systems. (Table 44-6.)

Viral identification is easier than once considered. Observation of the range of cell lines affected by the virus and the type of effect produced, together with clinical data, commonly allows an accurate identification. Viral effect on host cells is detected either directly by observation for areas of characteristic morphologic changes or death (cytopathic effect; CPE), by hemadsorption or hemagglutination, and by specific fluorescent staining for presence of viral inclusions. Characteristic CPE is recognizable with RSV, CMV, and herpes virus and is present with adenovirus, coxsackie B virus, echovirus, rhinovirus and varicella. Influenza virus,

Table 44-7 Summary of recommended evaluations of respiratory secretions for recovery of etiologies of pneumonia

Organisms	Direct exam	Culture
Routine Bacteria		
Contaminated specimens	Gram-stain, screen for acceptibility; quellung?	BAP, Mac, (Choc?)
Bronchoscopy	Gram-stain	Not recommended for routine bact BAP, Mac, (Choc?)
Bronchoalveolar Lavage	Cytocentrifuged smear (Gram-stained)	(Quantitative culture?)
Double-Lumen Occluded Cath Tip	Gram-stain	Quantitative culture: BAP, Choc, Mac, anaerobic
Normally Sterile Specimens	Gram-stain	BAP, Choc, Mac anaerobic
Nocardia	Gram-stain best, confirm with "weak" Kinyoun acid-fast stain	Routine bact media and Thayer-Martin, hold for longer; LJ slants and Sabourauds's agar
Legionella	DFA, Dieterle	Decontaminate; selective and nonselective BCYE
Mycoplasma	DNA probes	Not usually recommended
Chlamydia	DFA (C. trachomatis)	Tissue culture; Serologies usually recommended for C. psittaci and pneumonia
Mycobacteria	acid-fast stain (fluorochrome or Kinyoun)	Decontamination and concentration; 7H12 broth (radio-metric detection), LJ slant, 7H11 agar
Fungi	Calcofluor KOH wet prep, GMS, H&E	Sabouraud's, BHIA, selective agars
Pneumocystis	GMS, Giemsa, Toluidine blue 0, DFA	
Parasites	Wet Prep, Trichrome, Modified acid-fast and Giemsa or DFA for Cryptosporidium	Not normally available
Viruses	DFA, Elisa, DNA Probe?	Tissue culture, conventional and shell vial for selected viruses

BAP: blood agar plate; BCYE: buffered charcoal yeast extract agar; BHIA: brain heart infusion agar; Choc: chocolate agar; DFA: direct fluorescence antigen detection; GMS: Gomori methenamine-silver; H&E: hematoxylin and eosin; LJ: Lowenstein-Jensen; Mac: MacConkey.

parainfluenza virus, and the mumps virus do not usually produce CPE, but are detected by their alteration of the host cells to allow cell adsorption of guinea pig red blood cells. Further elucidation of identity can be accomplished using specific fluorescent antibody techniques in some instances, by neutralization studies (differentiation of polio and other enteroviruses) and acid lability studies (differentiation of acid-stable adenovirus from acid-labile rhinoviruses). Enzyme-linked immunosorbent assays and genetic probe technologies are being improved rapidly and will be more commonly available for both direct studies and identification purposes in the laboratory.

Serologic evaluations are not as commonly used for diagnosis of viral respiratory infections (because of the delay of antibody response) and are reviewed at length in Chapter 34.

A summary of recommendations for recovery of etiologic agents of pneumonia is found in Table 44-7.

SUGGESTED READING

Barnes RC: Laboratory diagnosis of human chlamydial infections, Clin Microbiol Rev 2:119, 1989.

Bartlett JG, O'Keefe P, Tally FP, Louie TJ, and Gorbach SL: Bacteriology of hospital-acquired pneumonia, Arch Intern Med 146:868, 1986.

Bartlett JG, Ryan KJ, Smith TF, and Wilson WR: Cumitech 7A: Laboratory diagnosis of lower respiratory tract infections, Washington JA II, coordinating ed, Washington, DC, 1987, American Society for Microbiology.

Chernesky MA, Ray CG, and Smith TF: Cumitech 15: Laboratory diagnosis of viral infections, Drew WL, coordinating ed, Washington, DC, 1982, American Society for Microbiology.

Clyde WA Jr, Kenny GE, and Schacter J: Cumitech 19: Laboratory diagnosis of chlamydial and mycoplasmal infections, Drew WL, ed, Washington, DC, 1984, American Society for Microbiology.

Heineman HS and DiAntonio RR: Bacteriology of sputum—purpose, significance, problems, and role in diagnosis. In: Lorian V, ed: Significance of medical microbiology in the care of patients, ed 2:169-196, Baltimore, 1982, Williams and Wilkins.

Roberts GD, Goodman NL, Land GA, Larsh HW, and McGinnis MR: Detection and recovery of fungi in clinical specimens. In: Lennette EH, Balows A, Haussler WJ Jr, and Shadomy HJ, eds: Manual of clinical microbiology, ed 4:500-513, Washington, DC, 1985, American Society for Microbiology.

Sommers HM and McClatchy JK: Cumitech 16: Laboratory diagnosis of the mycobacteriosis, Morello JA, coordinating ed, Washington, DC, 1983, American Society for Microbiology.

Washington JA II: Noninvasive diagnostic techniques for lower respiratory infections. In: Respiratory infections: diagnosis and management, ed 2:69-96, Pennington JE, ed, New York, 1988, Raven Press.

45

Central nervous system specimens

Stephen G. Jenkins

CENTRAL NERVOUS SYSTEM INFECTIONS

Infections of the central nervous system (CNS) are among the most serious encountered in clinical medicine and often represent medical emergencies. The pathogenesis and course of such infections are greatly influenced by the anatomy of the brain, spinal cord, and related structures. Most agents causing infection reach the CNS by hematogenous spread from extracranial sites or by retrograde extension within infected thrombi. Organisms producing acute infection, including most bacteria, elicit a polymorphonuclear leukocyte inflammatory response. By comparison, subacute or chronic infections such as those caused by fungi, *Mycobacterium tuberculosis*, or some viruses result in a predominantly mononuclear lymphocytic infiltrate, although significant numbers of neutrophils may be present if there is extensive tissue destruction. Antibody producing plasma cells may also predominate at the site of infection. The inflammatory response within the spinal cord or brain is unique in that it includes microglial cell infiltration and astrocyte proliferation and usually is less intense than in other organs. Unlike abscess formation at other body sites, encapsulation of abscesses within the brain occurs by gliosis, a slower and less complete process than fibrosis. When the brain has suffered an antecedent anoxic event, the inflammatory response may be reduced, and reactive gliosis may not occur.

Recovery from CNS infections involves cell-mediated immunity (CMI), antibody, and complement responses. Extrinsic antibody is normally excluded from the CNS. Detection of immunoglobulin in the CSF therefore suggests antibody diffusion across a damaged blood-brain barrier or local immunoglobulin synthesis by immunocompetent cells that have migrated into the brain parenchyma. Antibody production within the CNS is oligoclonal, indicating that plasma cells responsible for this local antibody synthesis are derived from a limited number of B cells. Systemic humoral antibody serves a major protective role against bacterial CNS infections and is an important determinant in survival in cases of bacterial meningitis. Because the CSF-blood barrier is poorly permeable to immunoglobulins, the serum:CSF antibody ratio is typically above 200. Damage to the blood-brain barrier can lower this ratio nonspecifically whereas intrathecal antibody synthesis directed against a particular infecting agent may selectively alter the ratio for

that agent. Detection of CSF antibody or proof of intrathecal antibody synthesis has sometimes proven useful in diagnosing slow or chronic infections such as Lyme disease, subacute sclerosing panencephalitis, or progressive rubella encephalitis. Since antibody titers increase over time, specific CSF immunoglobulin detection is generally not useful for diagnosis of acute infections such as herpes simplex encephalitis. CMI represents the major defense within the CNS against infections caused by fungi or intracellular parasites such as *M. tuberculosis,* viruses, *Listeria monocytogenes,* and *Toxoplasma gondii.* When CMI is impaired, the CNS is particularly susceptible to infection with such agents and disease can be fatal despite extremely high titers of specific antibody. Complement functions in lysis both of infectious agents and cells expressing viral or other foreign surface antigens. Such action against infected cells, however, may be a major cause of neurologic damage.

In certain infections caused by *Mycoplasma pneumoniae* or certain viruses or after immunization, the host may develop an immune response against both the eliciting agent and also against the basic protein of peripheral or central myelin. Reaction against peripheral myelin results in segmental demyelination and, on occasion, axonal loss within nerve roots and peripheral nerves, causing an ascending motor paralysis, the Guillain-Barre syndrome. Reaction to central myelin results in perivascular inflammation and multifocal demyelination of the optic nerve, spinal cord, and brain. In severe cases necrosis and hemorrhage may occur within the white matter.

Infection and inflammation within the CNS also results in loss of capillary integrity with transudation of intravascular fluid into the brain or spinal cord. The resultant edema is almost invariably noted in cases of CNS infection, occurring around brain abscesses as well as in cases of viral encephalitis and bacterial meningitis.

Clinical specimens

The type of specimen submitted to the laboratory will be a function of the clinical presentation (meningitis, encephalitis, or CNS suppurative process). Cerebrospinal fluid, biopsy tissue, or purulent material from an abscess may be collected for laboratory analysis. Table 45-1 represents a summary of methods a laboratory should consider for the

Table 45-1 Summary of methods suggested for CNS specimen processing

SPECIMEN	TRANSPORT	Microscopic examination					Culture Media† (minimum)			
		BACTERIA	FUNGI	ACID-FAST BACTERIA	PARASITES	VIRUSES	BACTERIA	FUNGI	ACID-FAST BACTERIA	VIRUSES
CSF	sterile screw-capped tube	gram stain, (acridine orange)	India Ink, (PAS, calcofluor white)	acid-fast (rhodamine-auramine)	wet mount	cytospin Giemsa stain	BAP, chocolate, thioglycollate	SAB-DEX	Lowenstein-Jensen	A-549, PMK, HF
Purulent material-Abscess	anaerobic transport vial	gram stain, (acridine orange)	KOH, (PAS, calcofluor white)	acid-fast (rhodamine-auramine)	wet mount	NA*	BAB, ANBAP, thioglycollate	SAB-DEX	Lowenstein-Jensen	NA*
Tissue biopsy	anaerobic transport vial	gram stain, (acridine orange)	KOH, (PAS, methenamine silver, mucicarmine)	acid-fast (rhodamine-auramine)	wet mount	NA*	BAB, ANBAP, thioglycollate	SAB-DEX	Lowenstein-Jensen	A-549, PMK, HF

†BAP, 5% sheep blood agar; ANBAP, prereduced CDC anaerobic blood agar; SAB-DEX, Sabouraud extrose broth; PMK, primary monkey kidney cells; HF, human foreskin fibroblasts.
*NA, not applicable

transport and processing of CNS specimens obtained for general bacteriology, mycobacteriology, mycology, virology and parasitology.

Collection and transport of specimens

Commonly, CSF is collected and divided into three or four sterile tubes for microbiologic, chemical, and hematologic laboratory studies. Scrupulous attention must be given to skin disinfection prior to lumbar puncture; otherwise, contamination of the specimen with normal cutaneous flora (i.e., *Staphylococcus epidermidis* and *Corynebacterium* spp.) can result, sometimes leading to confusion rather than a clinical diagnosis. Tincture of iodine (2%) is rapidly bactericidal and is an example of an effective skin disinfectant. Upon completion of the lumbar puncture, iodine should be removed with 70% alcohol prior to covering the bandage site with a dressing to prevent iodine burns. Iodophors also represent effective skin disinfectants. Since activation of the iodophor occurs through oxidation, it is imperative that the iodophor be allowed to completely dry before lumbar puncture begins. Other disinfectants, including 70% isopropyl alcohol, are also useful topical disinfectants but their effectiveness depends on careful and conscientious use.

Processing of specimens

Like other usually sterile body fluids including blood, the sensitivity of culture methods in detecting infectious agents in CSF is often volume dependent. In early bacterial meningitis it is not uncommon to fail to observe microorganisms on Gram stain, yet isolate small numbers of colonies of the infecting agent by culture. In nonimmunocompromised patients, 5 to 10 ml of CSF are often required to cultivate *Cryptococcus neoformans*. This problem is obviated by use of the cryptococcal antigen latex agglutination test, a technique more sensitive than culture yet requiring less than 1 ml of specimen.

Since a number of laboratory analyses are usually required on such difficult-to-recollect specimens—including hematology, cytology, microbiology, chemistry, and serology tests—decisions often must be made when an insufficient amount of CSF has been obtained as to which analysis is most important. Such priority decisions should always be made in conjunction with the patient's primary physician. Concentration of CSF by centrifugation at $1,500 \times g$ is recommended to increase the sensitivity of culture and staining techniques. When CSF volume is inadequate for all analyses requested, the portions to be used for chemical and serologic tests may be combined and centrifuged; the supernatant can be used for antigen and/or antibody detection and chemical analysis while the sediment can be utilized for cultures and stains.

Purulent material surgically aspirated from brain abscesses should be transported to the microbiology laboratory using sterile techniques that will also ensure anaerobiosis. A syringe and needle capped with a sterile VACUTAINER® top or similar stopper will maintain anaerobic conditions within the aspirate for only a very short period. Alternatively (and preferably), an anaerobic-transport device will maintain anaerobic conditions longer. Such devices are available from a number of commercial sources. Swabs are less desirable than aspirates of abscess material but when the volume of purulent material is small, sterile swabs may be the only option. Swabs used to collect purulent abscess material must also be placed in an anaerobic transport device for rapid delivery to the laboratory. Likewise, tissue obtained by biopsy should be sent to the microbiology laboratory under anaerobic conditions.

Tissue specimens should be carefully homogenized in sterile nonbacteriostatic saline or appropriate microbiologic broth medium in a sterile tissue grinder or with a sterile mortar and pestle. Silica alumina or Carborundum™ sterilized for this purpose should be used to facilitate grinding. To reduce the exposure of potential anaerobes to oxygen, processing time should be kept to a minimum. Homogenized material prepared by this procedure should be used for media inoculation and smear preparation.

In cases of suspected viral CNS infection, efforts should be made to detect the causative agent following an algorithm based on patient age, seasonal prevalence of the agent, and potential for exposure to the virus (Table 45-2). If clinical and/or epidemiological findings imply that less-common agents may be involved, special isolation techniques and serologic tests are often indicated. The diagnosis of viral CNS infection is not always based on isolation of the etiologic agent from CSF or brain tissue. Enteroviral infections (including poliovirus, coxsackievirus, and echovirus) yield positive cultures more frequently from pharyngeal and fecal specimens than from CSF itself. When measles encephalitis occurs, it usually presents concomitantly with other systemic symptoms as evidenced by the classic cutaneous erup-

tion. Mumps virus can also cause encephalitis and can be isolated in most instances from pharyngeal specimens as well as from CSF, whereas stool samples are usually nonproductive. With the advent of acyclovir and other antiviral agents, herpes simplex encephalitis is now considered a treatable disease. Rapid accurate diagnosis is essential for prompt initiation of therapy. The diagnosis is usually based on cultivation of the virus from a brain biopsy, demonstration of viral antigen using a specific fluorescent antibody technique, or detection of viral antigens in clinical materials by a latex agglutination technique. To best accomplish any viral isolation, specimens should be collected during the acute stages of illness (typically within the first four to seven days). When serological methods for diagnosis of viral infection are used, acute (collected during the first seven days of illness) and convalescent (collected two to three weeks after obtaining the acute sample) serum specimens should be run in parallel against viral antigens from suspected agents to detect a fourfold rise in IgG antibody titer. Serum samples tested for acute phase IgM antibodies can sometimes lead to a more rapid serological diagnosis.

One suggested approach is to collect acute serum samples (to be frozen for possible serological analysis), CSF, pharyngeal swabs, and fecal specimens (rectal swab or stool) upon admission when a viral CNS infection is diagnosed. Clinical specimens yield positive viral culture results frequently if appropriate cell lines are challenged prior to freezing.

Table 45-2 Viral CNS infections

Virus(es)	Age group usually affected	Peak season(s)	Environmental/geographic association
Epstein-Barr	Adolescents, children	Year-round	None useful
Cytomegalovirus	Neonates	Year-round	None
Herpes simplex			
Type 1	Adults	Year-round	None useful
Type 2	Neonates, young children	Year-round	None useful
Varicella-zoster	Neonates, young children	Spring	Usually outbreak-associated
Mumps	Children	Winter-spring	None useful
Enteroviruses (coxsackie A, B; polio, echo)	Infants, children	Summer-fall	Commonly outbreak-associated
Rabies	All ages	Summer-fall	Animal bite/scratch
Alphaviridae			Mosquito-borne
Eastern equine encephalitis	Infants, children, elderly	Summer-fall	Eastern U.S. seaboard
Western equine encephalitis	Infants, children	Summer-fall	Several endemic areas in U.S.
Venezuelan equine encephalitis	Infants, children	Summer-fall	South and Central America; southern U.S.
St. Louis encephalitis	Elderly	Summer	Western hemisphere
Bunyaviridae			
California encephalitis	School-aged children	Summer-fall	Upper midwest of U.S.
Measles	Infants, children 10-14 years	Spring	Ubiquitous
Rubella	Neonates, adults (rare)	Spring	Ubiquitous
Lymphocytic-choriomeningitis	Adults	None	Rodent exposure
Human immunodeficiency-type I	Neonates, adults	None	Exposure to contaminated blood, body fluids
Adenovirus	Children	None	Ubiquitous
Progressive multifocal leuk-encephalopathy (JC)	Adults, 40-70 years	None	Immunocompromised status

As CSF is normally a sterile body fluid, cell culture inoculation for viral isolation does not require prior decontamination. Pharyngeal and rectal swabs should be placed in a viral transport medium immediately upon collection. Several formulations are commercially available but most contain a buffered salt solution, sucrose and/or fetal bovine serum as a stabilizer, and antibiotics such as gentamicin (50 micrograms/ml), streptomycin (50 micrograms/ml), and amphotericin B (4 micrograms/ml). Tissue samples and stool specimens should be homogenized to produce an approximate 10% suspension in a balanced salt solution (Hanks) containing antibiotics. With the exception of CSF, all specimens should be clarified by centrifugation at 1,500-2,000 × g for 30 minutes. The supernatant is then used for challenging cell cultures and/or animal inoculation.

Microscopic examination

Bacteria

Following centrifugation, microscopic examination of CSF sediment is an accurate technique for the rapid diagnosis of bacterial meningitis and detects the infectious agent in approximately 75% of cases. Gram-stained smears of CSF sediment often reveal only a very few microorganisms; therefore, meticulous attention must be paid to such samples before reporting them as negative. One should report and semi-quantify the presence (or absence) of leukocytes, erythrocytes, and bacteria. Substituting basic fuchsin for safranin in the Gram-stain procedure will assist in the detection of Gram-negative bacteria that characteristically stain poorly (e.g., anaerobic Gram-negative bacilli including *Fusobacterium* sp.). Acridine orange microscopy may further facilitate the detection of bacteria in samples containing only a small number of microorganisms. Smears stained with acridine orange can be screened with low-power magnification on a fluorescence microscope, thus reducing the time required for microscopic examination and facilitating detection of small numbers of bacteria. Organisms detected under low power should be re-examined for cell morphology under high-dry magnification and verified by Gram stain to assess their Gram reaction. Decolorization of an acridine orange-stained smear is not required prior to performing the Gram stain.

Gram-positive cocci resembling *Streptococcus pneumoniae*, small Gram-negative coccobacilli compatible with *Haemophilus influenzae*, and Gram-negative diplococci looking like *Neisseria meningitidis* may be rapidly identified using capsular swelling techniques with specific antisera, the Quellung reaction.

Fungi

The presence of *Cryptococcus neoformans* in CSF may be detected by negative staining, allowing visualization of the capsule with Nigrosin or India ink. Sufficient ink should be added to the CSF sediment to provide proper contrast yet not so much to prevent detection of yeasts. A mixture of one drop of sedimented CSF from a Pasteur pipet with a bacteriological loopful of India ink consistently yields an appropriate preparation. Convenient dropper dispensers of India ink are now available from commercial sources. The CSF/India-ink mixture should be covered with a cover-slip and examined with a light microscope under high-dry mag-

nification with the substage condenser lowered to provide the best contrast. Before reporting a specimen as positive for "presumptive cryptococci," encapsulated yeasts (Plate 1-1) must be observed. Cryptococcal antigen testing further adds to the sensitivity of microscopic techniques by detecting small amounts of capsular antigens as sometimes occurs with microencapsulated strains of cryptococci and in indolent infections. Although usually detected in a simple wet-mount preparation of CSF sediment, the amoeboflagellates *Naegleria* and *Acanthamoeba* have been observed in India-ink preparations.

Calcofluor white represents an alternative to India ink for examination of CSF sediments. It must be kept in mind, however, that the capsule of *Cryptococcus neoformans* will not stain with this technique and procedures described above are required if cryptococci are considered in the differential diagnosis. After mixing, the calcofluor white/CSF preparation should be covered with a cover-slip and observed under a fluorescence microscope equipped with appropriate filters. Preparations may be examined under low power, changing to high dry for closer scrutiny for potential yeasts. Since calcofluor white only fluoresces when combined with chitin, as seen in cell walls of fungi, white cells are less apt to result in false positives than with contrast techniques such as India ink.

Tissue obtained through biopsy and abscess material submitted for fungal culture should be examined microscopically for budding yeast, hyphae, and other fungal elements following treatment with 10% to 20% KOH. After mixing KOH with the specimen, a coverslip should be gently pressed onto the preparation. Applying gentle heat to the mixture for a brief period results in specimen clarification. The preparation should be examined under a light microscope with lowered condenser to optimize contrast or, alternatively, with a phase-contrast microscope.

Mycobacteria

Stains for acid-fast bacilli (AFB) should be performed on CSF sediment of all specimens submitted for AFB culture. If a fluorescence microscope is available, the rhodamine-auramine stain is preferred over Kinyoun or Ziehl-Neelsen for reasons of increased sensitivity and decreased technical time. Although potentially present, acid-fast bacilli are rarely observed in acid-fast smears of CSF from patients with tuberculous meningitis and meticulous care must be taken in the microscopic examination of stained preparations of CSF sediment.

Parasites

Naegleria and *Acanthamoeba*, free-living amoebae, should be considered in patients with signs of meningeal irritation, headache, vomiting, and a stiff neck who have been recently swimming in warm or stagnant water. CSF examination usually yields elevated protein and depressed glucose levels with a negative Gram stain. Amoebae are best demonstrated by direct microscopic examination of a CSF wet prep with a phase-contrast microscope or light microscope with reduced illumination. Motility differentiates these organisms from macrophages.

Other parasites occasionally causing cerebral infection or resulting in CNS symptoms include *Entamoeba histo-*

Table 45-3 Parasitic infections sometimes resulting in CNS symptoms

Agent	CNS symptom or sign	Geographic foci
Angiostrongylus cantonensis	eosinophilic meningitis	South Pacific, Southeast Asia, Taiwan
Gnathostoma spinigerum	eosinophilic meningitis	Southeast Asia
Baylisascaris procyonis	eosinophilic meningoencephalitis	United States
Trypanasoma sp.	meningoencephalitis	South and Central America, East and West Africa
Plasmodium falciparum	headache, cerebral malaria	Africa, Haiti, New Guinea, Southeast Asia, South America, Oceania
Toxoplasma gondii	encephalitis	Worldwide
Entamoeba histolytica	brain abscess	Worldwide
Acanthamoeba sp.	granulomatous encephalitis	Undefined
Naegleria sp.	meningoencephalitis	Worldwide
Trichinella sp.	encephalitis	Worldwide
Schistosoma japonicum	space-occupying lesion; encephalopathy	Japan, China, Phillipines
Schistosoma mansonii	granulomatous lesions in spinal cord	Arabia, Africa, South America, Caribbean
Schistosoma haematobium	granulomatous lesions in spinal cord	Africa, Middle East
Paragonimus westermanii	space-occupying lesion	West Africa, Far East, Indian subcontinent, Central and South America
Taenia solium	space-occupying lesions, hydrocephalus	Worldwide
Echinococcus granulosus	cerebral hydatid cyst	Worldwide
Multiceps multiceps	cyst; arachnoiditis; posterior fossa syndrome	Worldwide
Strongyloides stercoralis	CNS invasion with secondary gram-negative meningitis	Worldwide

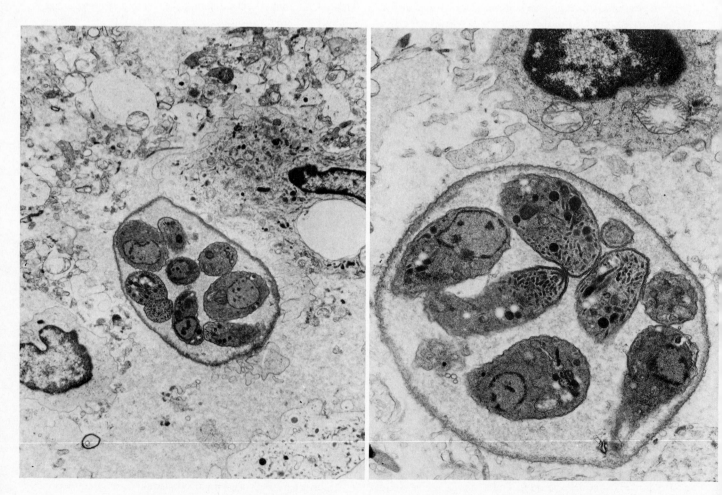

Fig. 45-1 Electron micrographs of *Toxoplasma gondii* cysts in brain section (×13,600 and ×29,600).

lytica, Toxoplasma gondii, and *Taenia solium (Cysticercus cellulosae).* Parasites that may cause CNS infections are listed in Table 45-3. Patients with cerebral amoebic cysts are infrequently assessed because they often are extremely ill due to other manifestations of invasive amoebiasis. Toxoplasma encephalitis has become more common with the advent of the AIDS epidemic. Cerebral toxoplasmosis may present as a singular space occupying lesion or as multicentric disease. Diagnosis is often made based on histologic examination of tissue obtained by brain biopsy. Although cysts can be observed with standard hematoxylin and eosin stains, high resolution microscopic examination of Giemsa-stained sections of tissue embedded in plasticine more readily demonstrates the agent (Plate 1-2). Electron microscopy has also proven useful in some situations in establishing toxoplasmosis (Figure 45-1).

Cerebral malaria represents a late manifestation of *Plasmodium falciparum* infection and is usually diagnosed upon examination of brain sections obtained at autopsy. Usually a large percentage of the erythrocytes are parasitized within the small vessels of the brain (Plate 1-3). Cerebral edema, ring hemorrhages, and central vein necrosis are seen throughout the brain. Most other parasitic CNS infections are diagnosed using serologic techniques rather than through microscopic examination of clinical specimens.

Viruses

Direct detection of viral agents by microscopic techniques can lead to rapid diagnosis and early therapy, critical in diseases such as herpes encephalitis. The most reliable approach to a rapid accurate diagnosis of herpes encephalitis is the brain biopsy. In addition to ruling out other causes of CNS disease through histopathological examination of tissue sections, expeditious detection of viral antigen by immunoperoxidase or direct immunofluorescent staining of impression smears or frozen sections can often lead to diagnosis in less than two hours. Results of such stains should always be confirmed by culture. Epstein-Barr virus encephalitis can also be diagnosed using immunofluorescent staining techniques. In addition, direct immunofluorescent detection of mumps virus antigen in pharyngeal or urinary epithelial cells sometimes provides a rapid diagnosis in cases of suspected mumps encephalitis.

Culture techniques
Bacterial

Cultures of CSF should be performed whenever possible using centrifuged sediment as the inoculum. Using a sterile Pasteur pipet, a 5% sheep blood agar plate and a chocolate agar plate should be inoculated and streaked for isolation. A tube of thioglycollate broth without indicator should be inoculated. Plate media should be incubated at 35°C for 72 hours (before reporting as negative) in an atmosphere of increased CO_2 in a candle jar or in an incubator providing a 5% carbon dioxide environment. The thioglycollate broth should be incubated for five days, also at 35°C, with cap loose to permit air exchange. If patients received penicillin or cephalosporin therapy prior to lumbar puncture, one drop of penicillinase may be added to the thioglycollate tube and to the surface of the plate media prior to inoculation. The sterility of penicil-

linase should be verified for quality-control purposes by concomitantly inoculating a chocolate agar plate and a tube of thioglycollate broth with penicillinase alone and incubating under the same conditions as the media inoculated with the patient specimen. Commercially available penicillinase preparations inactivate most penicillins including the anti-staphylococcal penicillins and some cephalosporins. The drop of CSF sediment should be well mixed with the penicillinase prior to streaking the plates for isolation.

Tissue specimens obtained by biopsy and abscess material should be inoculated onto the same plate media as for CSF and incubated under the same conditions. In addition, a prereduced blood agar plate supplemented with vitamin K and hemin should be inoculated along with an anaerobic broth medium such as thioglycollate enriched with horse serum, peptone-yeast-glucose broth, or chopped-meat-glucose broth. If thioglycollate is chosen it should be prereduced and/or supplemented with sodium bicarbonate to serve as a buffer. The last two media should be incubated under anaerobic conditions. Additional selective media may be inoculated if the Gram stain demonstrates mixed Gram-positive and Gram-negative bacteria. Media incubated in the CO_2 environment should be inspected daily whereas the anaerobic media should be incubated for a minimum of 24 and preferably 48 hours before examination. Media incubated in anaerobe jars may be examined after 24 hours incubation if they are exposed to ambient air for only a short period before reincubation under anaerobiosis.

If the CSF Gram stain revealed microorganisms but the cultures remain negative after 72 hours, plate culture media should be reincubated for an additional four days before issuing a final negative report. Anaerobic broths inoculated with biopsy or abscess aspirate should be incubated for seven days and Gram stained at that point before discarding as negative. If culture for *Nocardia* sp. is requested, incubate all media for seven days before reporting as negative. (See Chapter 53.)

Fungal

It is specifically recommended that specimens submitted for fungal culture be processed in a biological safety cabinet. Since one never knows which specimens contain highly virulent microorganisms, it is probably prudent to process all specimens using such safety precautions. Clinical specimens should be inoculated onto two Sabouraud's dextrose agar plates or slants and incubated at 25°C to 30°C for four weeks. Throughout the incubation period, media should be examined frequently for fungal growth. One of the Sabouraud's dextrose agar tubes or plates may be substituted with alternative media such as brain heart infusion agar or Sabouraud's dextrose agar supplemented with blood. All cultures yielding filamentous molds or yeast-like colonies should be processed in a biologic safety cabinet. Extreme care should be taken when a white filamentous mold is recovered from a CNS specimen, particularly if the patient has a history of living or visiting the southwestern United States. *Coccidioides immitis,* endemic in that area, can result in CNS disease, and infection can take place in laboratory personnel exposed to the agent when a breach of safety technique occurs. (See Chapter 54.)

Mycobacterial

Specimens submitted for mycobacterial culture should always be processed in a biological safety cabinet. Decontamination of abscess material, CSF sediment and biopsy tissue homogenate is not required. The specimen should be inoculated directly onto two Lowenstein-Jensen (L-J) slants or one L-J slant and one Middlebrook 7H11 slant or plate. In addition, a tube of either Dubos or Middlebrook 7H9 broth should be inoculated. Incubation of inoculated media should be at 35°C in an environment of 5% CO_2 for eight weeks. Alternatively, one L-J slant can be replaced with a bottle of C^{14} labeled Middlebrook 7H12 broth especially designed for the BACTEC 460 instrument (Johnston Laboratories, Baltimore, Maryland). Bottles should be run twice a week for eight weeks before discarding as negative. The BACTEC should be the modified version equipped with a laminar flow hood/cover and ultraviolet lights designed for surface decontamination following running of bottles.

Viral

Cell lines used for culture may vary from laboratory to laboratory but usually include human diploid fibroblasts (which will support the replication of mumps, herpes simplex, human cytomegalovirus, and some enteroviruses), primary cynomolgus or Rhesus kidney cells (capable of supporting most enteroviruses), and a heteroploid cell line such as Hela, HEp-2, or A-549. Suckling mice (preferably less than 24 hours old), used almost exclusively in reference and public health laboratories, may be useful in recovering the few strains of Coxsackie A virus associated with CNS infection which fail to replicate in many cell culture systems. Suckling mice are also useful in the isolation of rabies virus and arboviruses. Arbovirus encephalitis is usually diagnosed, however, by serological techniques.

Enteroviral isolation is best accomplished by concomitant culture of CSF (typically unrewarding), fecal material, and a throat swab. Cultures of CSF, throat samples, and sometimes urine yield mumps virus in cases of mumps encephalitis. Arbovirus is only occasionally recovered in CNS infections by culture techniques. Disseminated disease with herpes simplex virus in the neonate may be definitively diagnosed by culture of urine, pharyngeal secretions, vesicles, and other specimens. Aseptic meningitis due to herpes simplex virus type 2 in young adults is usually confirmed by isolation of the agent from CSF and genital lesions. Herpes simplex virus is easily isolated in all of the cell lines listed above. Cytopathic effects observed in infected cell lines can be confirmed as produced by HSV with immunofluorescent or immunoperoxidase techniques (Plate 1-4). Encephalitis due to HSV-1 represents a medical emergency. Rapid diagnosis is essential since specific, effective antiviral therapy with acyclovir is available. However, HSV is infrequently isolated from CSF in such cases; viral isolation from pharyngeal secretions or other peripheral sites may represent stress reactivation of latent HSV virus and should not be interpreted as the probable cause of CNS symptoms. Consultation with the attending physician is in order.

In cases of encephalitis due to human immunodeficiency virus (HIV), the agent can be recovered by culture of tissue obtained by brain biopsy in phytohemagglutinin-stimulated lymphocyte cell lines. HIV cultures should only be performed, however, in facilities with proper containment equipment and by trained, experienced personnel. Cultures are rarely required though, as the diagnosis of HIV infection is usually based on history, clinical findings, and by sensitive and specific serologic techniques. (See Chapter 55.)

Parasitic

Toxoplasma encephalitis can be diagnosed by cultivation of *T. gondii* in cell culture or embryonated eggs, or by recovery of the agent following intraperitoneal inoculation of laboratory mice with biopsy material. Primary amoebic meningo-encephalitis due to *Naegleria fowleri* can be diagnosed by culture of CSF on artificial medium supplied with a living nutrient, such as *Klebsiella pneumoniae*. A heavy suspension of *K. pneumoniae* (approximately equal to a McFarland 3.0 turbidity) should be made in Page's saline and mixed directly on a nutrient agar plate with CSF sediment. After sealing the plate to prevent drying, the system should be incubated at 37°C for up to 14 days. The surface of the agar should be examined daily for motile amoebae under low power ($\times 100$ total magnification). If amoebae are detected, permanently mounted and stained slides can be prepared. (See Chapter 56.)

Nonculture detection techniques

With the development of newer biochemical and serological techniques, clinical specimens can be examined for the presence of microbial products by noncultural methods, even in the absence of viable cells. Although limitations exist when microorganisms are present in small numbers, these procedures supplement microscopic methods for the rapid detection of infectious agents in CSF and other CNS materials.

Antigen detection
Counterimmunoelectrophoresis (CIE)

CIE has been evaluated by many investigators for the detection of bacterial antigens in systemic diseases including meningitis. Specific antisera are used to detect bacterial capsular antigens in CSF of infected patients. Required equipment is relatively inexpensive and takes up little bench space. Commercially available gels make specimen preparation simple, requiring only the addition of CSF and the specific antisera. The test result is usually available within one hour of specimen receipt. This procedure is a rapid, effective method for detecting bacterial antigens in CSF. A drawback to this procedure has been the relative paucity and high expense of quality antisera. Specifics for this technique are published elsewhere. (See Chapter 41.)

Staphylococcal coagglutination

The first practical use for the macroscopic staphylococcal coagglutination technique was reported by Kronvall in 1973 and was for serotyping pneumococci. Reagents are now commercially available for detection of antigens of *Neisseria meningitidis*, groups A, B, C, Y, and W135; pneumococci, group B streptococci; and *Haemophilus influenzae* type b in CSF, urine, and blood. To analyze a CSF specimen for the presence of these antigens, one drop of CSF should be mixed with one drop of each of the specific reagents and observed after 60 seconds for macroscopic agglutination. Extracts of each pathogen for use as positive controls are also commercial available and should be run along with negative controls each time the procedure is performed. Nonspecific agglutination sometimes occurs with staphylococcal coagglutination reagents and can usually be eliminated by heating the specimen to 100°C for 10 minutes prior to performing the test. False-positive and false-negative results occur infrequently and usually are the result of cross-reactions with other bacterial antigens or concentrations of antigen below the detectable sensitivity of the assay. These tests are easy to perform and relatively cost-effective since equipment other than a rotator and boiling water bath are not required.

Latex agglutination

Bacterial antigen detection can be readily accomplished in CSF using latex agglutination techniques. This procedure is more rapid than CIE and can be performed with facility requiring only a rotator and a boiling water bath. Reagents are commercially available for *Streptococcus pneumoniae; Haemophilus influenzae* type b; *Streptococcus agalactiae; Neisseria meningitidis* groups A, B, C, Y, and W135; and *Escherichia coli* K1 (which cross-reacts with *N. meningitidis* group B); as well as for the yeast *Cryptococcus neoformans.* Early identification of these infectious pathogens is important in that it directs the clinician in the choice of appropriate and adequate antimicrobial chemotherapy. Although many bacterial species have been implicated in meningitis, group B streptococci (Plate 1-5) and *E. coli* K1 are the two most common causes of neonatal bacterial meningitis, whereas *H. infuenzae* type b, *S. pneumoniae,* and *N. meningitidis* are the most common agents in older age groups. These bacteria carry specific surface polysaccharide antigens which diffuse into body fluids such as serum and CSF, and are excreted in the urine. These antigens can then be detected by agglutination of polystyrene latex particles coated with specific antibody. The *S. pneumoniae* reagent is sensitized with purified antibodies from an omnivalent serum, whereas the remainder of the reagents are serotype specific.

CSF specimens should be heated for 10 minutes in a boiling water bath or 100°C heat block prior to testing to eliminate potential interference due to rheumatoid factor. Positive and negative controls should be run concomitantly with patient specimens to insure proper reactions. False-positive and false-negative reactions may occur as the result of cross-reacting substances or insufficient antigen concentration in the body fluid.

Enzyme-linked immunoassays

ELISA techniques are sensitive and highly specific methods for bacterial antigen detection in CSF. Sensitive to the picogram range, no false-positive and only rare false-negative results have been reported. The major drawback to this technique is the approximate four-hour turnaround time resulting from relatively long incubation and washing steps. No ELISA kits are currently available commercially for this purpose.

Nucleic acid probes

To date, nucleic acid probes have not proven useful for detection of pathogenic microorganisms directly from clin-ical CNS specimens. Modification of these techniques, however, might result in increased sensitivity and clinical application. Highly specific kits are commercially available for identification of *Mycobacterium tuberculosis* and *Herpes simplex* virus from culture systems and can result in more rapid diagnosis of these disease entities. DNA amplification by polymerase chain reaction is available for detection of HIV-infected lymphocytes in CNS specimens and future applications of this technique should lead to more rapid and specific detection of heretofore difficult to detect pathogens.

Limulus amoebocyte assays

Detection of bacterial endotoxin can be accomplished by coagulation of an amoebocyte extract derived from the horseshoe crab, *Limulus polyphemus.* Although there are several commercial sources for *Limulus* lysate reagents, use of this assay for diagnosis of Gram-negative bacterial meningitis remains, for the most part, a research tool. Gelation of an extractable, clottable protein from *Limulus* blood cells results when the lipid A moiety of bacterial endotoxin activates an enzyme in this system. As little as 0.1 ng of lipid A/ml of body fluid can be detected with this technique. In the procedure for detection of gram-negative meningitis, 0.1 ml of patient CSF should be mixed with 1 ml of *Limulus* lysate reagent, incubated at 37°C, and examined every 30 minutes for signs of turbidity or gelation as compared to appropriate controls. Although the phenomenon is easily visualized when high concentrations of lipopolysaccharide are present, a spectrophotometer facilitates detection of low quantities of endotoxin. Reactions vary from slight flocculation and turbidity to a solid clot and are graded on a 1+ to 4+ basis. Total incubation time is two hours. The assay is one of the most sensitive systems for endotoxin detection, but other substances can lead to false-positive results. As with all diagnostic laboratory techniques, results must be carefully correlated with the patient's clinical symptoms.

Lactic acid determinations

Elevated CSF lactic acid levels are observed in patients with meningitis. Gas-liquid chromatographic techniques have been successfully used to detect and quantitate CSF lactic acid as an indicator of the possible etiology of infectious meningitis. Levels of 35 mg/dl or greater are indicative of bacterial or tuberculous meningitis, whereas lower concentrations suggest viral or other forms of meningitis. GLC is a complex and time-consuming technique requiring lactic acid extraction with organic solvents and relatively expensive gas chromatographic equipment. Commercially available enzymatic assays measured spectrophotometrically are less complex, more rapid (approximately 15 minutes to perform), and equally accurate. With this technique lactic acid concentrations of greater than 20 mg/dl are highly suggestive of bacterial meningitis. This test may be of value in partially treated cases, as increased lactic acid levels in CSF may persist up to 72 hours after initiation of appropriate antibiotic therapy. However, false negative and positive results have been reported. Although elevated CSF lactate does not specifically identify a pathogen, this information may aid clinicians in differentiating viral from bacterial meningitis. Equivocal results, however, have been seen in cases of pediatric meningitis.

Gas-liquid chromatography (GLC)

GLC is capable of detecting metabolic products of various infectious agents in CSF, providing relatively rapid, clinically useful information for slow-growing organisms and microorganisms normally present in only low numbers in CNS infections. Specific chromatographic patterns have been described for *Mycobacterium tuberculosis, Cryptococcus neoformans,* and a few viral pathogens. Information concerning patterns observed with more common bacterial pathogens, however, is generally lacking. In addition, these techniques are complex, time-consuming, and require expensive laboratory instrumentation.

Antimicrobial susceptibility tests

Rapid diagnosis and initiation of appropriate antimicrobial therapy are paramount concerns in the management of acute bacterial meningitis. Since some antibiotics readily cross the blood-brain barrier (e.g., chloramphenicol), and others cross the barrier only to a very limited degree under most circumstances (e.g., gentamicin), the value of antibiotic susceptibility testing is highly drug-dependent. Since bacterial meningitis represents a medical emergency, empiric antibiotic therapy is almost always initiated before culture results are available. Results of Gram stains and other microscopic examinations as well as antigen detection procedures should be communicated to the clinician as soon as available to assist in the selection of appropriate antibiotic agents. Antibiotic therapy is sometimes initiated before obtaining CSF by lumbar puncture, reducing the positive culture rate. Such therapy may also affect smear positivity rates. Knowledge of the sensitivity patterns of common bacterial pathogens is important in the selection of empiric antimicrobial agents. (See Chapter 40.)

Beta-lactamase detection

Many strains of *H. influenzae* type b produce a beta-lactamase capable of hydrolyzing a number of penicillins (e.g., ampicillin) and cephalosporins. This enzyme can be detected by iodometric, acidometric, and chromogenic cephalosporinase techniques often providing valuable information to the clinician within 24 hours of specimen receipt in the laboratory. All isolates of *H. influenzae* from CSF should be tested for beta-lactamase production and results reported to the clinician as soon as possible since ampicillin and chloramphenicol remain useful agents for therapy in cases of pediatric meningitis.

Chloramphenicol acetyltransferase detection

Strains of *H. influenzae* resistant to chloramphenicol, although still relatively rare, have been reported. The mechanism of resistance is through production of an inactivating enzyme, chloramphenicol acetyltransferase. Methods are commercially available for rapid detection of this enzyme in clinical isolates of *H. influenzae*. In settings where chloramphenicol continues to be used as a component of empiric therapy for bacterial meningitis, all *H. influenzae* isolates from CSF should be tested for its production and positive results reported to the physician as soon as available.

Antibiotic susceptibility studies

Strains of *S. pneumoniae* overtly resistant to penicillin have been reported and relatively resistant or moderately susceptible strains (defined as being inhibited by 0.12 to 1 μg/ml of penicillin) are growing in frequency. All such isolates from CSF should be reported as resistant since these levels of penicillin may not be achieved in all cases of CNS infection. Susceptibility testing of *S. pneumoniae* to penicillin can be accomplished with a 1.0 microgram oxacillin disc. Isolates demonstrating zone diameters of inhibition of 19 mm should be further tested for susceptibility to penicillin by a broth or agar dilution technique. Strains inhibited by >1 microgram of penicillin/ml should be considered fully resistant.

Quantitative susceptibility studies on CNS bacterial isolates by broth or agar dilution techniques following guidelines of the National Committee for Clinical Laboratory Standards are recommended over disc diffusion methods. The susceptible, intermediate, and resistant interpretations obtained through disc diffusion methods are based on achievable antibiotic blood concentrations. Typically, CSF antibiotic concentrations are significantly lower than those in blood. It is therefore possible using the disc diffusion test to record as susceptible an isolate which in reality is resistant because the required level of antibiotic is not achievable in CSF by parenteral therapy.

Laboratory result reporting

Since CNS infections are often life-threatening, all positive laboratory results must be communicated to the attending physician as soon as possible. Positive wet-mount, smear, and/or antigen detection results must be telephoned to the primary physician and/or the relevant nursing unit. The name of the person to whom the information was communicated should be recorded along with the time and date of the call. A written report should also be issued. The same course should be followed when a microorganism is cultured from a CNS specimen. To ensure that the laboratory report is accurate and legible, all reports should be reviewed by the supervisor in charge of the microbiology laboratory or designated surrogate before transmission to the nursing unit.

SUGGESTED READING

Balows A, Hausler Jr WJ, and Lennette EH: Laboratory diagnosis of infectious diseases: Principles and practice, Vol 1 and 2, 1988, Springer Verlag, New York.

Braude A, Davis CE, and Fierer JF: Infectious diseases and medical microbiology, ed 2, Philadelphia, 1986, WB Saunders Company.

Feign RD and Cherry JD: Textbook of pediatric infectious diseases, ed 2, Philadelphia, 1987, WB Saunders Company.

Finegold SM and Baron EJ: Bailey and Scott's diagnostic microbiology, ed 7, St. Louis, 1986, Mosby–Year Book, Inc.

Hoeprich PD: Infectious disease, ed 3, Philadelphia, 1983, Harper and Row.

Lennette EH, Balows A, Hausler Jr WJ, Herrmann KL, Isenberg HD, and Shadomy HJ: Manual of clinical microbiology, ed 5, Washington, DC, 1991, American Society for Microbiology.

Mandell GL, Douglas RG, and Bennett JE: Principles and practice of infectious disease, ed 3, New York, 1990, Churchill Livingstone.

National Committee for Clinical Laboratory Standards: Methods for dilution antimicrobial susceptibility tests for bacteria that grow aerobically, M7-A2, Vol 10 No 8, Villanova, Penn, 1990, NCCLS.

National Committee for Clinical Laboratory Standards: Performance standards for antimicrobial disk susceptibility tests, ed 4, M2-A4, Vol 10 No 7, Villanova, Penn, 1990, NCCLS.

Ray CG, Wasilauskas BL, and Zabransky R: Laboratory diagnosis of central nervous system infections, Washington, DC, 1982, American Society for Microbiology.

Reller LB, Murray PR, and MacLowry JD: Blood cultures II, Washington, DC, 1982, American Society for Microbiology.

Rose NR, Friedman H, Fahey JL: Manual of clinical laboratory immunology, ed 3, Washington, DC, 1986, American Society of Microbiology.

Youmans GP, Paterson PY, and Sommers HM: The biologic and clinical basis of infectious diseases, ed 3, Philadelphia, 1985, WB Saunders Company.

46 Eye and ear specimens

Stephen G. Jenkins

OCULAR INFECTIONS

The eye is an organ uniquely predisposed to infection by a variety of microorganisms. Conjunctival hyperemia is the most obvious clinical manifestation of conjunctivitis, the most common ocular infection. Secretions made up of an exudate of inflammatory cells and a fibrin-rich edematous fluid from the blood, combined with denuded epithelial cells and mucus, are almost always a feature of this disease. The exudate may be purulent, mucopurulent, fibrinous, or sero-sanguineous, depending on the severity of illness and its etiology. The eyelids may stick together when the secretions dry. Chemosis (conjunctival edema) may be present in those parts of the conjunctiva that freely move over the lids and globe. The normal transparency of the conjunctiva may be clouded, and it may appear thickened due to leukocytic infiltration of the tissues. The various types of conjunctivitis are rarely differentiated morphologically, since none have pathognomonic features and most have common symptoms and signs.

The inflammation of the cornea (keratitis) can be the result of infection or be caused by noninfectious stimuli such as hypersensitivity, trauma, or other immuno-mediated reactions. As the conjunctival and corneal epithelium are contiguous, forming the ocular surface, agents causing conjunctivitis may also infect the cornea. However, before most infectious agents can invade the stroma of the cornea, an insult to the ocular surface must occur. Defects may result from external trauma, including contact lens irritation, an inverted eyelash, infolding of the margin of the eyelid or abnormal lid margins, or chronic problems including dry eyes, exposure, or neurogenic anesthesia of the cornea. Any inflammatory reaction involving the cornea should be considered sight threatening and should demand prompt medical management. Corneal perforation with resultant eye loss can occur after only 24 hours of infection with microorganisms including *Staphylococcus aureus* and *Pseudomonas aeruginosa*.

An inflammatory reaction involving the ocular cavity and adjacent structures, endophthalmitis, may be classified according to the infecting agent, the route of entry, and location within the eye. Infectious etiologic agents include parasites, viruses, fungi, and bacteria. The infectious agent may be introduced directly into the eye as in cases of surgical contamination and trauma or may reach the eye by hematogenous spread from a distant nidus of infection. Panophthalmitis occurs when the episclera is significantly involved with the inflammatory process.

In infections involving periocular structures, anatomic areas of concern include the eyelids, the lacrimal ducts and associated components, and paranasal and cavernous sinuses, and the orbit.

The techniques used for microbiologic examination are a function of the infection site and severity, as well as the agents most likely responsible for causing a given infectious process. Since the quantity of material which can be collected from anatomical sections of the eye is extremely limited, special collection and processing techniques are often needed. In many cases such procedures must be performed at the patient's bedside, in the examining room, or in the operating room.

Clinical specimens

The type of specimen obtained for culture is a function of the infectious process and presentation of each given patient. Ophthalmologists and clinical microbiologists should jointly formulate methods for specimen collection, transport, and microbiologic examination. In serious eye infections, including suppurative keratitis and endophthalmitis, the ophthalmologist should communicate with the microbiology laboratory to ensure the availability of adequate media and to allow the laboratory sufficient time to prepare for any special procedures which might be required.

Collection and transport of specimens

Cotton, polyester, and calcium-alginate swabs are acceptable for recovery of most bacteria and fungi from clinical specimens. Calcium alginate can be dissolved in sodium salts of organic acids when quantitative cultures are desired. Cotton or polyester swabs are preferred for viral cultures. Several anaerobic transport devices are commercially available for pus or fluid requiring anaerobic culture. Specimens collected on swabs are less satisfactory than syringe aspirates because swabs limit the quantity of specimen available for examination and because anaerobic bacteria are recovered less efficiently.

The preferred topical anesthetic for collecting corneal scrapings for culture is 0.5% proparacaine hydrochloride as it is less antiseptic than tetracaine, cocaine, and others. Glass slides with frosted ends and demarcated circles facilitate labeling and detection of clinical materials when limited quantities are available. Slides should be dipped in methyl alcohol and wiped to remove dust and nonviable bacteria, which can absorb stains, producing false-positive results. Fixation of smears for Giemsa or Gram stain should be accomplished with 95% methanol for 5 to 10 minutes in a Coplin jar.

Conjunctival cultures should be obtained with a cotton-tipped swab by collecting discharge from the inferior tarsal conjunctival fornix. Culture media should be inoculated immediately, otherwise the specimen should be transported to the microbiology laboratory as quickly as possible using a suitable transport system. Swabs without a carrier medium should not be used for transport of the specimen because resulting desiccation can result in a loss of viability for such agents as *Neisseria gonorrhoeae*.

Keratitis

In cases of keratitis the ophthalmologist should use a slit lamp to visualize the affected area of the cornea. Because some infectious agents are inhibited by local anesthetics, conjunctival cultures should be taken before proparacaine topical anesthetic is instilled onto the eye. A sterile Kimura platinum spatula or a sterile scalpel blade should be used to scrape the corneal epithelium and to inoculate appropriate culture media. Smears should be concomitantly prepared for direct microscopic examination.

Preseptal cellulitis

An inflammatory condition of the subcutaneous tissues of the lids, preseptal cellulitis, usually presents with abscess formation and extensive edema. The absence of an open drainage site usually permits aspiration of purulent material containing the causative agent(s) without bacterial contamination from normal skin flora. In cases involving primarily the upper lid, the incision should be made below the brow at the juncture of the lateral 1/3 and medial 2/3 of the lid. In abscesses of the lower lid, the incision should be made at the site of maximum fluctuation, ideally 1 to 2 cm above the rim of the inferior orbit. After cleansing the skin thoroughly with an effective disinfectant, a stab incision can be made with a number 11 Bard-Parker blade. If an open wound or drainage site is present, the adjacent skin should be thoroughly cleansed to reduce bacterial contamination of the specimen. Whenever possible, purulent material should be aspirated with a sterile needle and syringe and inoculated directly to appropriate media. Slides for Gram staining should be prepared by smearing a drop of specimen over the slide surface or by compressing a drop of purulent material between two glass slides and pulling them across each other to spread the specimen. Slides should then be fixed by immersion in 95% methanol for 5 minutes. When direct media inoculation is not practical, all air bubbles should be expelled from the syringe and the needle capped with a sterile rubber stopper. Alternatively, the specimen can be injected into an anaerobic transport vessel and delivered immediately to the microbiology laboratory.

Ocular erysipelis

Swabs of intact skin of involved areas are generally unreliable and conjunctival cultures in such cases only rarely yield *Streptococcus pyogenes*. In cases of ocular erysipelis, a cotton or calcium alginate swab saturated in bacteriologic broth should be rolled across the inferior tarsal conjunctiva and fornix of the ipsilateral and contralateral eyes and inoculated only to a plate of 5% sheep blood agar. Injection and aspiration of sterile saline from subcutaneous tissue is often unrewarding and orbital space needle aspiration is generally contraindicated. Blood cultures should be collected as they sometimes aid in the diagnosis. In culture-negative cases, the diagnosis can often be confirmed by detection of antistreptolysin-O antibodies in acute and convalescent blood specimens.

Orbital cellulitis

When an open wound or drainage site is observed, purulent material should be aspirated in a sterile syringe and immediately inoculated to appropriate media. In cases when this is not feasible, material should be collected and transported to the laboratory as quickly as possible under anaerobic conditions. Identical techniques should be utilized when material is obtained during surgery from a subperiosteal abscess, infected paranasal sinus, or intraorbital abscess. Smears should be prepared for tinctorial studies by smearing the clinical specimen over a clean glass slide. Random orbital needle aspiration is contraindicated. In cases of chronic orbital cellulitis, purulent drainage, when present, should be collected for fungal, bacterial, and mycobacterial examination. The ophthalmologist should biopsy involved orbital tissue when drainage cultures do not lead to identification of the etiologic agent, and the specimen should be submitted for both microbiologic and histopathologic analysis.

Dacroadenitis

Cotton or calcium alginate-tipped applicators should be swabbed in the superotemporal fornix and over the surface of the palpebral lobe and inoculated to media capable of supporting fastidious bacteria, including *Haemophilus influenzae*. The contralateral conjunctiva, even when apparently uninvolved, should be sampled in a similar fashion. Material obtained from swabbing the conjunctival surface and/or exudate, when present, should be spread over an area approximately 1 cm in diameter for Gram staining. Following installation of proparacaine, the conjunctiva in the superotemporal fornix should be scraped with a Kimura spatula and also smeared for Gram staining. Lacrimal gland needle aspiration is contraindicated. Diagnosis of chronic granulomatous dacroadenitis often requires lacrimal gland biopsy. The sample should be submitted for both histopathological and microbiological examination. Cultures should be appropriate for isolation of fungi and mycobacteria. Smears should be prepared for routine Gram stain, acid fast stain, and fungal stain, as well as dark-field examination, when appropriate.

Dacrocystitis

Infection of the lacrimal gland usually involves stasis of the distal drainage structures. Since such infection usually results in obstruction of the distal portion of the canaliculi, thereby interfering with aspiration of purulent material, isolation of the etiologic agents may not be accomplished. Transcutaneous aspiration or incision through the sac wall is usually contraindicated, although spontaneous external fistula formation sometimes occurs providing ready access to clinical material. When present, lacrimal sac drainage material should be aspirated with a sterile syringe and processed appropriately. Microbiological results in cases of chronic dacrocystitis are usually difficult to interpret because a number of microorganisms often contaminate the obstructed sac without causing cellulitis. Dacroliths should be biopsied surgically and submitted for both microbiological and histopathological studies.

Canaliculitis

Acute infections of the canaliculi and lacrimal puncta are uncommon. Chronic canaliculitis, characterized by edema and hyperemia of the lid, punctum dilation, and recurrent epiphora often results in thick, mucopurulent discharge. Although most infections have reportedly been due to *Actinomyces israelii,* the majority are probably caused by *Arachnia propionica.* As skin and conjunctival bacteria often contaminate clinical specimens, cultures reporting mixed aerobic and anaerobic flora are difficult to interpret. Compression of the lid and canaliculus in these cases usually results in expression of pus. A Kimura spatula should be used to collect purulent material, inoculate media, and prepare smears for staining and microscopic examination. These infections often cause formation of large diverticuli containing cheesy to concretious material. A small chalazion curette or sterile spud should be used to scrape the diverticuli to obtain additional culture material. Solid fragments of this material should be crushed between two glass slides to prepare smears for appropriate stains.

Viral blepharitis

Herpes simplex, varicella zoster, and vaccinia viruses can cause a vesicular eyelid and ocular adnexal region eruption without an accompanying diffuse exanthema. Clear vesicles should be selected for study and the vesicular surfaces should be cleaned gently with an alcohol swab. Fluid should be aspirated with a sterile tuberculin needle and syringe and inoculated into viral transport medium. Vesicles should be uncovered, the base scraped with a sterile scalpel blade or Kimura spatula, and cellular material should be smeared on duplicate 1-cm areas of a glass slide. Slides prepared for fluorescent-antibody studies should be fixed in cold acetone ($-20°C$) for 10 to 15 minutes and stored at $-20°C$ to $-70°C$ until staining. Those for Giemsa staining should be immersed for 5 minutes in 95% methyl alcohol.

The fragmented or umbilicated regions of molluscum contagiosum lesions should be scraped with a Kimura spatula or a sterile scalpel blade. Scrapings should be Giemsa stained to demonstrate characteristic eosinophilic molluscum bodies. Biopsy material should be fixed in 10% neutral formalin for standard histopathological microscopic examination. If performed, electron microscopy should reveal dumbbell-shaped elementary bodies making up the molluscum bodies. To date the virus has not been recovered in cell culture.

Bacterial blepharitis

Acute bacterial infection of the lid margin is almost always caused by *Staphylococcus aureus* and *S. epidermidis* and results in uni- or bilateral skin ulceration with eyelid cellulitis. Streptococci and staphylococci can cause superinfections in cases of ulcerative viral blepharitis. Acute Gram-negative bacterial blepharitis is extremely uncommon. A calcium alginate or cotton-tipped applicator saturated with bacteriologic broth should be swabbed across the anterior lid margins and ulcerated areas of both lids of one eye. The procedure should then be repeated with a fresh swab on the contralateral eye.

Chronic staphylococcal blepharitis, or squamous blepharitis, is characterized by thickening and crusting of the anterior lid margin, cilia loss, recurrent hordeola, conjunctival hyperemia, and punctate epithelial corneal erosion. Chronic desquamation, hyperemia, and ulceration of the lateral canthral regions (angular blepharitis) can be caused by *Moraxella* spp., although it may also be a form of eczematoid blepharitis secondary to staphylococcal infection. In cases of chronic blepharitis, eyelid margin cultures should be collected in the same fashion as for acute infections.

Phthiriasis palpebrarum

The crab louse (*Phthirus pubis*) can infect the lashes producing irritation, pruritis, and anterior lid margin hyperemia. Adult lice and ova (nits) can be easily detected using slit lamp biomicroscopy and identified by examination of a simple wet-mount preparation of one or more infected eyelashes.

Bacterial conjunctivitis

Characterized by unilateral or bilateral lid edema and conjunctival hyperemia and edema with a purulent discharge, acute bacterial conjunctivitis is most often caused by *Haemophilus influenzae, Streptococcus pneumoniae, S. pyogenes, S. aureus,* and *Neisseria gonorrhoeae. H. influenzae* often results in serious preseptal cellulitis resembling orbital cellulitis in children less than three years of age. One of the few bacteria capable of penetrating the intact corneal epithelium with resulting suppurative keratitis, *N. gonorrhoeae* must be considered in the differential diagnosis in cases of rapidly progressive infection. Gram-negative enteric bacilli and *Pseudomonas* spp. are almost exclusively associated with nosocomial infection following prolonged hospitalization or in immunocompromised individuals. Even in cases of apparent unilateral conjunctivitis, bilateral bacterial cultures should always be obtained.

As topical anesthetics can interfere with the isolation of certain pathogens, conjunctival cultures should always be collected prior to installation of such agents. Cotton or calcium alginate swabs should be rubbed over the inferior tarsal conjunctiva and fornix of one eye and streaked onto chocolate and blood agar plates. If purulent exudate is present, use of bacterial broth to saturate the swab is not required. The collection procedure should then be repeated on the contralateral eye. One agar plate of each medium is sufficient for culture of both eyes, but inoculation areas should be clearly demarcated. Except in cases of suspected blepharoconjunctivitis with *S. aureus,* lid margin cultures are not required. In immunocompromised hosts and when concomitant infection of the ocular adnexa is evident, media appropriate for the isolation of anaerobic bacteria and fungi should also be inoculated. Gram stains should be prepared from conjunctival exudate and examined in all cases of bacterial conjunctivitis.

Isolation of the etiologic agent(s) is more readily accomplished from conjunctival surface scrapings than from swab cultures of purulent discharge. Following installation of one to two drops of proparacaine hydrochloride, the lower tarsal conjunctiva should be scraped gently with a Kimura spatula by an ophthalmologist. The specimen should be smeared in an approximate 1-cm area on a clean glass slide for tinctorial studies. Scraping the superior tarsal or bulbar conjunctiva is contraindicated. Smears for Gram stain should be prepared from both conjunctivae and slides should be fixed in 95% methanol for 5 minutes.

Viral conjunctivitis

The most common etiologic agents of viral conjunctivitis in the United States are adenovirus and herpes simplex, which are difficult to distinguish from adenovirus infection when skin lesions are absent. Although both can result in lid edema, preauricular lymphadenopathy, serous conjunctival discharge, punctate keratitis, and follicular conjunctivitis, it is important to differentiate the two since effective antiviral therapy (acyclovir) is available for herpes simplex as well as for herpes zoster. Cutaneous lesions, however, are always present in cases of herpes zoster conjunctivitis.

Topical anesthetics should be instilled only after viral culture collection. A dry, cotton-tipped applicator should be swabbed over the tarsal conjunctiva and fornix of the affected eye, immersed in viral transport medium, and rolled with pressure against the side of the collection tube to express virion-containing medium. The swab should then be removed and discarded into a biohazard container as some swab materials can interfere with virus isolation. In cases of bilateral conjunctivitis, the two samples should be combined in one tube of viral transport medium, thereby increasing the probability of viral isolation. Specific indication by the clinican of the suspected etiologic agent assists the laboratory in processing the clinical specimen(s).

Since fluorescent antibody techniques are as sensitive as culture for diagnosing viral conjunctivitis during the acute stages of infection, slides should be prepared for FA staining to expedite specific viral diagnosis. Following installation of a couple of drops of topical anesthetic, the lower and upper tarsal conjunctiva should both be scraped with a Kimura spatula and the specimen smeared in two 1-cm circular areas on each of two clean glass slides for detection of HSV and adenovirus infected cells. The slides should be fixed in cold acetone ($-20°C$) for 10 to 15 minutes and stored at $-20°C$ to $-70°C$ until staining. In cases of unilateral conjunctivitis, material collected from the contralateral eye can serve as a negative control.

Predominantly mononuclear inflammatory cell infiltrates are seen on Giemsa-stained smears of conjunctival scrapings in cases of viral conjunctivitis. This compares to the polymorphonuclear leukocyte response characteristically observed in acute bacterial conjunctivitis. The Giemsa stain,

however, does not differentiate the viral agents responsible for the conjunctivitis nor are multinucleated giant cells or intranuclear inclusions typically detected in conjunctival Giemsa-stained smears.

Serological testing is of limited value in the management of cases of acute viral conjunctivitis since adenovirus infection typically results in antibodies only after a week to 10 days of symptoms and are detectable for years after primary infection. Likewise, seroconversion is not usually noted in cases of recurrent HSV conjunctivitis and a large proportion of the general population is seropositive to the agent as a result of other forms of HSV infection.

Chlamydial conjunctivitis

Two types of conjunctivitis and keratitis result from infection with *Chlamydia trachomatis:* trachoma, which can culminate in blindness, and inclusion conjunctivitis. Caused by serotypes D, E, F, G, H, I, J, and K, inclusion conjunctivitis is seen in children and adults but is most common during the neonatal period. Ubiquitous throughout the world, the agent is usually transmitted to the infant during passage through the birth canal. The reservoir is the genital tract of both males and females. Endemic trachoma is restricted in the United States to a Native American population in the Southwest and is caused by serotypes A, B, BA, and C. Infection is characterized by gradual onset, preauricular lymphadenopathy, conjunctival hyperemia and follicle formation, mucopurulent discharge and pleomorphic punctate keratitis. It may be unilateral or bilateral.

The diagnosis of chlamydial conjunctivitis can be made by Giemsa stain, culture (Plate 1-6), direct fluorescent antibody, and ELISA techniques. Specimens for culture should be collected prior to instillation of topical anesthetic with a calcium alginate swab because cotton swabs are toxic and will inhibit the isolation of chlamydiae. After rubbing the lower and upper tarsal conjunctiva and fornix with a dry swab, the specimen should be agitated in viral transport medium, the fluid expressed into the transport vial, and the vial delivered to the microbiology laboratory as quickly as possible. The specimen can be refrigerated for a short time prior to cell culture inoculation or should be frozen at $-70°C$ if delay is expected.

The Giemsa stain for detection of pathognomonic chlamydial inclusions in conjunctival scrapings from adults with inclusion conjunctivitis is positive in only about 50% of the culture-confirmed cases. The Giemsa stain is as accurate as culture for the diagnosis of neonatal chlamydial conjunctivitis. When typical inclusions are not present, chlamydial conjunctivitis should still be suspected when lymphocytes, neutrophils, stem and blastoid cells, Leber cells, and large epithelial cells are observed in various phases of degeneration. Scrapings should be obtained from the upper and lower conjunctiva of involved eyes, smeared on clean glass slides, and fixed in 95% methanol. Direct fluorescent antibody detection of chlamydia appears to be more sensitive than Giemsa-stain for diagnosis of chlamydial conjunctivitis. Following fixation in 95% methanol, smears prepared for fluorescent antibody examination should be stained and examined for diagnostic elementary bodies. Pools of monoclonal antibodies prepared against the major outer membrane protein present in all 15 described human sources of

C. trachomatis are commercially available and increase both the sensitivity and specificity of the procedure.

Serological tests for diagnosis of chlamydial conjunctivitis are insensitive and nonspecific and are not recommended on a routine basis.

Ophthalmia neonatorum

Neonatal conjunctivitis can occur by three mechanisms: 1) ascending infection from the female genital tract following premature rupture of membranes; 2) infection from contaminated personnel or environmental sources; or 3) genitourinary secretion inoculation during the birthing process. Clinical signs and symptoms do not usually suggest the etiologic agent(s) in the infection. The most common organisms in such infections include *N. gonorrhoeae*, *S. pyogenes*, *S. aureus*, and *C. trachomatis* (serovars D through K). Disseminated or cutaneous infection with HSV-2 can result in herpetic keratitis and/or conjunctivitis. Conjunctivitis due to *P. aeruginosa*, albeit rare, represents a potentially fatal disease in premature infants. Clinical material for smears and culture should be collected as described previously. When HSV infection is suspected, conjunctival specimens should be inoculated into viral transport medium.

Suppurative keratitis

Fungal and bacterial keratitis can result from corneal trauma with contaminated foreign matter or following microbial invasion of a pre-existing epithelial imperfection. Few bacteria (including *Corynebacterium diphtheriae*, *N. gonorrhoeae* and *N. meningitidis*) are capable of penetrating the intact epithelium of the cornea. Clinical symptoms do not provide a clue as to the etiologic agent and often are not indicative of infectious versus noninfectious disease.

The most common agents in bacterial keratitis, *S. aureus*, *S. pneumoniae*, *P. aeruginosa*, and members of the *Enterobacteriaceae*, particularly *Enterobacter*, *Serratia*, *Klebsiella*, *Citrobacter*, and *Proteus*, account for up to 86% of the pathogens in such cases. The most aggressive pathogen is *P. aeruginosa* which can result in perforation of the cornea within 3 days. Anaerobic bacterial infection is uncommon. *Mycobacterium chelonei* and *M. fortuitum* can both cause chronic ulcerative keratitis with a sparse tissue inflammatory response.

Fungal keratitis, usually clinically indistinguishable from bacterial keratitis, most often results from infection with saprophytic, opportunistic molds or yeasts. Keratitis caused by filamentous fungi is more common in the southern United States and generally follows mild trauma to the eye in an outdoor recreational or work-related setting. Species of *Aspergillus*, *Acremonium*, and *Curvularia* and *Fusarium solani* represent the most commonly isolated etiologic fungal agents. Filamentous fungal infection of the cornea can also result during corticosteroid therapy in individuals with a history of epithelial ulceration. Caused primarily by *Candida albicans*, keratitis due to yeasts does not occur with increased frequency in any geographic area and is generally seen in individuals with a prior history of corneal ulceration or in the setting of altered host defense.

Both eyes should be swabbed for culture and inoculated to blood and chocolate agar as well as a broth capable of supporting anaerobic bacteria prior to performing corneal scraping for smear and culture. Corneal scrapings should be inoculated directly to media as outlined in Table 3-3. A minimum of three slides should be smeared for tinctorial studies. Based on results from the routine Giemsa and Gram stains, the third slide may be processed using special stains for fungi or acid-fast organisms as indicated. Potassium hydroxide preparations should not be examined for detection of fungi in corneal smears as they lack sensitivity and are no longer recommended.

An ophthalmologist, using a slit lamp or ocular microscope, should obtain corneal material by scraping diverse areas that demonstrate suppuration or ulceration with a Kimura spatula. Clinical material from the cornea collected on a swab is of no diagnostic value. Specimen from each scraping should be used to inoculate only one piece of medium or prepare one slide for microscopic examination. Both sides of the spatula should be streaked onto the nutrient medium without tearing the agar surface. Enriched thioglycollate broth should be inoculated by collecting clinical material from the spatula with a swab moistened with bacteriologic broth and rotating the swab in the tube of thioglycollate.

Acanthamoeba keratitis

Keratitis caused by the free-living amoeba *Acanthamoeba*, albeit rare, is characterized by chronic multifocal suppuration. When seen, it usually is associated with ophthalmologic corticosteroid therapy and/or previous ocular ulceration. Clinical signs and symptoms are identical to those seen in other types of infectious keratitis. Some *Acanthamoeba* species replicate on routine blood and chocolate agar incubated at 35°C. The recommended isolation technique, however, is inoculation of corneal scraping material onto a nonnutrient agar plate overlayed with heat-killed *Klebsiella pneumoniae* or *Escherichia coli*. In wet preps of corneal scrapings the vegetative stage of *Acanthamoeba* can sometimes be observed. Twenty to 50 μm in length, the slow-moving trophozoite is characteristically covered with spine-like projections called acanthapodia. Typical cysts of *Acanthamoeba* spp. are 10 to 25 μm in length and have double-layered, polygonal walls that give clusters of cysts a honeycomb appearance. Although cysts can be readily demonstrated in Gram- and Giemsa-stained corneal scrapings, trophozoites can be difficult to differentiate from inflammatory cells.

Viral keratitis

Acute viral infection of the corneal epithelium can be caused by herpes simplex, varicella, vaccinia, herpes zoster, and adenoviruses. Since a limited amount of clinical material can be collected from the infected cornea, and since significant pain and discomfort can be associated with such an infection, and since potential risks are associated with sampling the intact epithelium, laboratory diagnosis is usually made by collecting conjunctival exudate and scrapings for viral culture and specific immunofluorescent staining with appropriate antibodies.

Herpes simplex virus can cause recurrent epithelial keratitis with conjunctivitis. Corneal material collected from debridement of infected epithelium should be used for culture and fluorescent antibody staining. Following instillation of a topical anesthetic, the involved epithelium should be scraped with a Kimura spatula and the clinical material should be inoculated into a tube of viral transport medium. Additional specimen should be smeared on a glass slide and fixed in cold acetone for FA staining as described previously for conjunctival infections. Multinucleated giant cells can often be seen in Giemsa- or Papanicolaou-stained smears in cases of herpes simplex epithelial keratitis. Although pathognomonic for herpes group virus infection, this technique fails to differentiate the various herpes family viruses potentially involved in the infectious process. When debridement of the corneal epithelium is not feasible, a cotton-tipped swab should be rolled gently over the surface of the anesthetized cornea and inferior tarsal conjunctiva and placed in a tube of viral transport medium. Collection and culture and/or FA staining of abnormal epithelium may be of value in the diagnosis of late keratitis due to adenovirus, herpes zoster, or varicella.

Endophthalmitis

In microbial endophthalmitis, a serious, sight-threatening eye infection, a high index of suspicion, rapid laboratory examination, and aggressive antibiotic therapy are imperative in order to preserve eyesight. Infection can result from exogenous sources following ophthalmologic surgery, ocular trauma with perforation, corneo-scleral fistula, or corneal penetrating infection. Endophthalmitis can also result from hematogenous spread of microorganisms as a complication of septicemia. Although rare, *Mucor* spp. can directly invade the orbit in cases of mycotic ophthalmic cellulitis.

Exogenous bacterial endophthalmitis

Typically developing within 72 hours of trauma to the orbit, exogenous bacterial endophthalmitis is characterized by blurred vision, pain, lid edema, conjunctival hyperemia, and severe iridocyclitis with hypopyon. Onset of symptoms in cases resulting from infection with nonsporeforming anaerobic bacteria may be delayed for several days. In patients with postsurgical bacterial endophthalmitis, *S. aureus*, coagulase negative staphylococci, *S. pneumoniae*, other streptococcal species, *Proteus mirabilis*, and *Pseudomonas aeruginosa* represent the most commonly incriminated organisms. A variety of organisms have been associated with infection following perforating ocular injury. *Bacillus* spp., often considered skin contaminants in other settings, can result in severe, rapidly progressive intraocular infection. Symptoms in cases of mycotic endophthalmitis are indolent and require weeks to months to develop following surgery or trauma. They include progressively deteriorating vision, iridocyclitis and focal or multifocal vitreous abscesses. Organisms incriminated in these infections include *Aspergillus* spp., *Acremonium* spp., *Paecilomyces lilacinus*, *Volutella* spp., *Neurospora sitophilia*, and others. Epidemic mycotic endophthalmitis has occurred following intraocular lens implantation, and as isolated cases after retinal attachment surgery.

Hematogenous microbial endophthalmitis

Seeding of the orbit with resulting infection via the hematogenous route appears most often in compromised hosts and in intravenous drug abusers. Infection, particularly early *Candida* endophthalmitis, can closely resemble sterile uveitis. Treatment with corticosteroids can severely exacerbate the condition. Bilateral infection is not uncommon. Microorganisms commonly isolated in this condition include *S. aureus*, *S. pneumoniae*, *H. influenzae*, *N. meningitidis*, *Mycobacterium fortuitum-chelonei* complex, and *Bacillus* spp. *Candida albicans* can result in focal or multicentric retinovitritis or diffuse iridocyclitis following intravascular line sepsis and should always be considered as a potential late complication in such cases because it can lead very rapidly to blindness. Other fungi causing infection by the hematogenous route include other *Candida* spp., *Aspergillus fumigatus*, *Coccidioides immitis*, *Cryptococcus neoformans*, *Sporothrix schenckii*, and *Blastomyces dermatitidis*.

Collection and processing of specimens

The specific etiologic agents in cases of endophthalmitis can be determined by examining intraocular fluid in the laboratory collected by an ophthalmologist in an operating room setting. Since vitreous cultures appear to be more specific than aqueous cultures in cases of exogenous bacterial endophthalmitis, specimens should be collected from both sites in patients with post-traumatic or post-surgical infection. Based on disease severity, the ophthalmologist may submit vitreous fluid aspirated with a sterile needle and syringe or material collected with a vitrectomy instrument. Hematogenous endophthalmitis can result in either focal or diffuse vitreous suppuration. Random vitreous aspiration or aqueous fluid aspiration by keratocentesis, therefore, may not be reliable. Intraocular fluid should be collected, when feasible, by vitrectomy under direct microscopic visualization.

To help differentiate contaminants from pathogens in intraocular fluid cultures, specimens from both unanesthetized conjunctivae should be cultured concomitantly. Any potential entry site, such as a wound, abscess or conjunctival bleb, should be swabbed or scraped and processed as would samples in cases of microbial keratitis. In addition to the media indicated in Table 46-1 for intraocular fluid culture, Lowenstein-Jensen agar should be inoculated in cases of suspected mycobacterial endophthalmitis. Slides should routinely be prepared for Gram and Giemsa stain. Additional slides should be prepared, based on specimen volume, for other special stains that might be indicated following initial microscopic examination (PAS, AFB, methenamine silver, calcofluor white, etc.). Papanicolaou- or Giemsa-stained smears of intraocular fluid should be prepared and examined to assist in the diagnosis of conditions that mimic microbial endophthalmitis such as metastatic intraocular neoplasm, leukemia, or lens-induced uveitis.

Ideally, inoculation of aqueous and vitreous fluid to appropriate media should be performed in the operating room by an experienced technologist or ophthalmologist. Otherwise, specimens should be transported to the laboratory in an expeditious manner and processed as soon as possible after receipt. Slides prepared for staining and microscopic examination should be fixed in 95% methanol for 5 minutes. When the specimen is extremely viscous, a small amount of balanced salt solution or saline can be added to a drop of the specimen, mixed, and smeared. The resultant thinner

Table 46-1   Processing recommendations for clinical material from ocular infections

Clinical infection	Specimen source	Stains			Media			
		Gram	Giemsa	Special	Blood agar	Chocolate agar	Enriched[a] thioglycollate	Lowenstein Jensen
Endophthalmitis	Conjunctivae	•			•	•	•	
	Abscess drainage or fistula	•	•		•	•	•	
	Intraocular fluid	•	•	Fungal[b] Acid-fast[c]	•	•	•	•
Viral keratitis	Conjunctivae			Fluorescent[d] antibody				
	Cornea		•	Fluorescent[d] antibody				
Suppurative keratitis	Conjunctivae	•			•	•	•	
	Cornea	•	•	Fungal[b] Acid-fast[c]	•	•	•	•
Acute conjunctivitis	Conjunctivae	•	•	Fluorescent[d] antibody	•	•		
Neonatal conjunctivitis	Conjunctivae	•	•		•	•		
Acute blepharitis	Margin of eyelid				•			
Chronic blepharitis	Margin of eyelid				•			
Viral blepharitis	Vesicular fluid from eyelid		•	Fluorescent[d] antibody				
Acute dacrocystitis	Conjunctivae	•			•	•	•	
	Drainage	•			•	•	•	
Canaliculitis	Purulent material or cheesy concretions	•	•		•	•	•	
Acute orbital cellulitis	Abscess drainage	•	•	Fungal[b]	•	•	•	
Preseptal cellulitis	Abscess drainage	•			•	•	•	

[a]Prereduced thioglycollate without indicator supplemented with 1 ml of horse serum.
[b]Modified Gomori's methenamine silver, periodic acid-Schiff and/or calcofluor white, especially in cases of orbital mucormycosis.
[c]Rhodamine-auramine or Kinyoun. Modified Kinyoun when infection with *Nocardia* spp. is suspected.
[d]In cases of suspected herpes simplex, adenoviral, or herpes zoster conjunctivitis or blepharitis.
[e]For cases of suspected goncoccal conjunctivitis.

smear is more efficiently fixed to the slide for pursuant staining. When large volumes of fluid are collected, filtration should be considered to concentrate pathogens prior to media inoculation.

Corneal and intraocular foreign bodies

Foreign bodies such as wood splinters should be cultured after removal, following corneal trauma, to detect potential causes of secondary microbial keratitis. If only one fragment is available it should be inoculated into a tube of multipurpose broth, such as thioglycollate. If multiple fragments are available they should be inoculated to media appropriate for the isolation of bacterial, fungal, and mycobacterial agents as outlined in Table 46-1.

Toxoplasma retinitis

Caused by intraretinal multiplication and encystment of *Toxoplasma gondii*, toxoplasma retinitis is characterized by unilateral vision loss, focal or multicentric exudative retinitis, vitritis, and/or iridocyclitis. Diagnosis generally is based on clinical features and detection of specific antibodies in serum by one of several available techniques. Although IgM antibodies are indicative of acute infection, the majority of cases of toxoplasma retinitis in patients with acquired immune deficiency syndrome (AIDS) represent recrudescent

infections and specific IgM antibodies are characteristically absent. Toxoplasma IgG antibodies, however, are usually present and titers may be elevated.

Human cytomegalovirus retinitis

Cytomegalovirus (CMV) retinitis in adults is a relatively uncommon complication in patients receiving immunosuppressive therapy, particularly in transplant recipients. It is a fairly common infectious process in AIDS patients, however, often resulting in blindness. CMV can cause unilateral or bilateral vision loss, focal or diffuse necrotizing retinitis, and vitritis. In transplant recipients, isolation of the etiologic agent from urine, bone marrow, or buffy-coat preparations can assist in making the diagnosis. Historically, isolation of CMV in human embryonic fibroblasts often took as long as six weeks. With newer shell vial procedures using monoclonal antibodies directed at early nuclear antigens of CMV (Plate 1-7), laboratory diagnosis can often be made in less than 24 hours. Rapid diagnosis of CMV retinitis is considerably important since gancyclovir is valuable in treating this condition, particularly in patients with AIDS. In cases of acquired adult retinitis, the agent can be isolated from subretinal fluid and from aqueous fluid in neonatal infections. Serological techniques are of limited value since a large proportion of the population has IgG antibodies di-

Sabouraud dextrose agar	BHI broth	Viral transport medium	Chlamydial transport medium	Additional	Supplemental techniques
•					
•	•				
•	•			Anaerobic blood agar	
		•			
					Papanicoulau stain for cytologic exam.
•					
•	•	•		Anaerobic blood agar	Nonnutriant agar precoated with *E. coli* for *Acanthamoeba* spp.
		•	•	Thayer-ᶜMartin	
		•	•	Thayer-ᶜMartin	
•					Eyelid biopsy for a unilateral, atypical inflammatory reaction.
		•			Papanicoulau stain cytologic exam.
•	•			Anaerobic blood agar	
•	•			Anaerobic blood agar	
				Anaerobic blood agar	

rected against human CMV, and production of IgM antibodies is not predictable, even in acute infections.

Toxocara canis endophthalmitis and retinitis

Dissemination of *T. canis* larvae in young children sometimes results in ocular infection characterized by a focal retinal granulomatous reaction, peripheral traction of the retina with detachment, or diffuse retinovitritis. The resultant inflammatory response may be difficult to differentiate from other types of endogenous microbial endophthalmitis and may necessitate collection of intraocular fluid. An eosinophilic response is characteristically seen on examination of Giemsa-stained smears. Detection of antibodies to *T. canis* by an ELISA technique assists in making the diagnosis. In ocular toxocariasis, however, ELISA appears to be somewhat less sensitive than in cases of visceral larva migrans, especially with localized disease and as time passes.

Microscopic examination
Gram stains

In cases of acute bacterial conjunctivitis, microorganisms can be observed both extracellularly and intracellularly within polymorphonuclear leukocytes and are only rarely seen within epithelial cells. Organisms representing the usual conjunctival flora can sometimes be detected in small numbers in conjunctival scrapings (e.g., yeasts, coagulase-negative staphylococci, diphtheroids, etc.). Stains demon-

strating only low numbers of such organisms without the coincident occurrence of PMN's should be interpreted with caution. In true infections, the responsible bacteria are typically present in larger numbers and in areas of the smear with increased numbers of PMN's and necrotic epithelial cells. Similar results are expected in Gram-stained smears of corneal scrapings. Indigenous bacteria of the preocular tear film can sometimes be detected as rare, extracellular organisms distributed randomly throughout the smear.

Gram-stained smears often prove useful for the detection of fungi in cases of mycotic infection. Typically, the cell wall of hyphal elements fails to stain whereas the safranin is inconsistently taken up by the fungal protoplasm, staining the vascular channels pink to red. Yeasts usually retain the crystal violet, staining dark blue. Other fungal elements are not usually observed. The Gram stain is also of value for detecting double-walled *Acanthamoeba* cysts which can stain dark blue or red. Trophozoites are difficult to distinguish from inflammatory cells and epithelial debris in Gram stains of clinical material.

Giemsa stains

The Giemsa stain provides useful information in ocular infections. It helps to characterize the type of inflammatory cell response and the condition of conjunctival epithelial cells, as well as to detect chlamydial intracytoplasmic inclusions. Most bacteria stain deep blue with Giemsa stain, thereby requiring a Gram stain to further delineate microscopic staining characteristics. A predominance of PMN's is seen in bacterial conjunctivitis as well as in non-infectious processes such as allergic, chemical, and irritative conjunctivitis. A PMN predominance can also be seen in early stages of severe adenovirus conjunctivitis. Eosinophils predominate in allergic conjunctivitis and chlamydial conjunctivitis. A predominance of mononuclear cells (monocytes and lymphocytes) characterizes herpes simplex and adenoviral conjunctivitis as well as chronic, drug-induced toxic or allergic conjunctivitis. Plasma cells, large macrophages (Leber cells), and immature blastoid and stem cells can be observed in cases of chlamydial conjunctivitis along with basophilic, intracytoplasmic epithelial inclusions. Chlamydial inclusions are most often seen in areas of the smear demonstrating increased numbers of PMN's and clumps of epithelial cells 10 to 15μm in size (typically larger than leukocytes). Intracytoplasmic inclusions are made up of aggregates of small red-purple staining elementary bodies approximately 300 nm in size, or larger deep-blue staining initial bodies (reticulate particles) approximately 1 μm in diameter.

The Giemsa stain is also useful in revealing *Acanthamoeba* trophozoites with an irregular cell border, vacuolated cytoplasm, and nuclear karyosome. Cyst walls stain deep blue whereas the cytoplasm stains a pale blue. As in the Gram stain, fungal elements incorporate Giemsa stain into the protoplasm appearing blue-purple. Pseudohyphae and yeast cells stain deep-blue. In *Haemophilus* infections, the Giemsa stain will sometimes yield better bacterial morphologic detail than the Gram stain.

Special stains

A modified Gomori's methenamine silver stain (GMS) or periodic acid-Schiff stain (PAS) may be used if Giemsa and Gram stains are unrewarding in cases of suspected mycotic ocular infection. Ideally, corneal scrapings should be smeared on gelatin-coated slides for GMS stain. With this technique, fungal cell walls and septa stain black, contrasting sharply with the relatively transparent background. Fungal elements and yeasts stain a deep pink with the PAS stain. Calcofluor white is valuable in detecting fungal elements in cases of mycotic keratitis.

A rhodamine-auramine or Kinyoun acid-fast stain should be performed in cases of suspected mycobacterial keratitis or if branching Gram positive bacilli, indicative of *Nocardia* spp. and *Actinomyces* spp., are seen on Gram stain.

Culture techniques

In cases of ocular infection, all plate media should be examined daily and broth media should be inspected for the presence of turbidity and/or gas production. Due to the severe nature of keratitis and endophthalmitis, bacterial media should be inspected, if possible, for early microbial growth after 12 to 18 hours of incubation and returned to the incubator immediately if no evidence of growth is present. Isolates should be worked up and identified based on established policies as outlined in the laboratory's procedure manuals drafted in the format outlined by the NCCLS.

Interpretation of the significance of bacterial isolates from eyelid and conjunctival cultures must be accomplished with knowledge of the usual indigenous microflora. Coagulase-negative staphylococci, diphtheroids, *Propionibacterium acnes,* viridans streptococci, *Staphylococcus aureus, Branhamella catarrhalis,* and nonenteric Gram-negative bacilli can be isolated at varying frequencies from normal uninfected conjunctivae. Many of these same organisms can be pathogenic in some circumstances. Microbial growth should be semiquantified by species. Isolates should be identified based on the infectious process diagnosed and, in cases of unilateral infection, on the microbial flora isolated from culture of the contralateral eye.

In corneal cultures, organisms representing usual flora can be isolated from the preocular tear film both in cases of noninfectious and suppurative keratitis. The indigenous microflora, however, are usually present in small numbers in noninfectious processes when compared to quantities observed in cases of true infection and in comparative numbers to the amount seen in ipsilateral conjunctival cultures. Anaerobic cultures should be examined on a daily basis and returned to anaerobiosis immediately if no growth is observed.

The majority of fungi in cases of mycotic keratitis can be observed within five to seven days of media inoculation. All such cultures should be incubated a minimum of 4 weeks before discarding and reporting as negative.

Plates for *Acanthamoeba* detection should be examined under a dissecting microscope using oblique light (45° angle) to espy the thin, serpentine migration lines on the agar surface.

When large volumes of intraocular or irrigation fluid are available for culture, the specimen should be suction-filtered using a sterile 0.45 μm-pore-sized filter. The filter should then be cut into a minimum of six parts with a sterile scalpel, and transferred to media as outlined in Table 46-1. The filter segments should be rubbed gently, filter side down, across the agar surface of individual plate media and positioned, with the filtration side up, in the center of the plates for incubation. Smears can be prepared by scraping filtered specimen from filter segments with a sterile scalpel blade or spatula and transferring the material to clean glass slides for tinctorial studies.

Tissue obtained through biopsy should be homogenized in sterile nonbacteriostatic saline or appropriate microbiologic broth medium in a sterile tissue grinder or with a sterile mortal and pestle. Sterile silica alumina or Carborundum™ should be used to facilitate grinding. Processing time should be kept to a minimum to reduce the exposure of potential anaerobes to oxygen. Homogenized material prepared in this manner should be used to prepare smears for Gram and Giemsa stains and to inoculate media as specified in Table 46-1. Samples of corneal bathing medium should be diluted 1:10 and 1:100 to overcome antimicrobial activity, and aliquots of each dilution should be inoculated into a tube of enriched thioglycollate and incubated as for other specimens. Any unused corneoscleral tissue should be homogenized as above for biopsy tissue and inoculated to appropriate media.

Antimicrobial susceptibility testing

Standard techniques for antimicrobial susceptibility testing should be used for all potentially pathogenic bacterial isolates. The recommended techniques are those outlined by the NCCLS for disk diffusion testing and dilution testing. Since the interpretive results obtained with disk diffusion testing are based on achievable antibiotic blood levels using usual dosing regimens, dilution techniques may give more direction to the ophthalmologist in determining whether a given antibiotic will achieve levels necessary to effectively treat an infection in ocular tissues and in the preocular tear film. Antimicrobials selected for testing should be based on the antibiotic hospital formulary and the organism-specific recommendations outlined by the NCCLS for routine testing and reporting. (See Chapter 40.)

Antifungal susceptibility testing is not routinely performed in most clinical laboratories. Available in some larger hospital and reference laboratories, the value of these studies for directing therapy in mycotic ocular infections has not been determined. The NCCLS is currently in the process of drafting recommendations for standardized techniques for antifungal susceptibility testing. If performed, antimicrobials selected for testing should include agents with proven efficacy in ocular infections. Since several recently discovered antifungals are in various stages of development, such decisions should be based on input from physicians who know the activity of these and more established compounds.

EAR INFECTIONS

Exudative infection of the mucosal lining of the middle ear is one of the most common childhood diseases. The vast majority of children experience at least one episode of otitis media with effusion and approximately ⅓ have repeated bouts during early childhood. The availability of effective antimicrobial agents against the bacteria usually responsible for these infections has significantly decreased the incidence of serious suppurative complications. Such therapy, however, may actually have increased the incidence of persistent recurrent sterile middle ear effusions. Hearing deficits resulting from such effusions may ensue at critical times of language and speech development, potentially leading to learning disabilities with lifelong implications. Otitis externa, infection of the external auditory canal, is similar to other types of skin and soft tissue infection. Because the auditory canal is tortuous and narrow, however, any foreign objects or fluids that gain entry may be trapped, causing irritation and superficial tissue maceration. Pain and itching may become severe due to the limited space available for inflamed tissue expansion. Recent reviews categorize external canal infections into four groups: malignant otitis externa, acute localized otitis externa, acute diffuse otitis externa, and chronic otitis externa. The bacterial flora of the external canal is similar to that on skin elsewhere. *Staphylococcus aureus*, *S. epidermidis*, and diphtheroids predominate and anaerobic bacteria such as *Propionibacterium acnes* are typically present in smaller numbers. When the tympanic membrane is intact, organisms responsible for middle ear infection such as *Morexella catarrhalis*, *Streptococcus pneumoniae*, and *Haemophilus influenzae* are rarely recovered in culture.

Absorbing moisture from the environment, the external otic epithelium desquamates and denudation of superficial epithelial layers may result. The moist, warm microenvironment encourages multiplication of organisms in the canal, which may result in invasion of macerated skin which can be accompanied by inflammation and suppuration. Infecting bacteria include those of the usual skin flora as well as Gram-negative bacilli, especially *Pseudomonas aeruginosa*. In malignant otitis media, a necrotizing infection caused by *P. aeruginosa*, the bacteria invade deeper ear canal tissues causing localized vasculitis, thrombosis, and tissue necrosis. Poor local perfusion of the skin overlying the temporal bone resulting from diabetic microangiopathy may lead to and accentuate the infection. (See Chapter 43.)

Clinical specimens
Collection and transport of specimens

Results of microbiologic examination of middle-ear effusions in patients with otitis media are so consistent that antimicrobial therapy is usually based on knowledge of the bacteriology rather than on results of culture on individual patients. If the patient appears bacteremic or has focal infection at another site, blood cultures and a culture of the infected site should be collected. Tympanocentesis (needle aspiration of middle ear fluid) should be performed following cleansing of the canal and surface of the tympanic membrane with 70% alcohol, in selected circumstances such as: a critically ill patient, a patient failing to respond to 48 to 72 hours of appropriate antimicrobial therapy who appears septic, and the immunodeficient patient (including the neonate). Routine nasopharyngeal cultures are not recommended as they are poorly predictive of the middle ear microflora. If pus is evident in the ear canal, a sample should be obtained for examination. Interpretation of these cultures must appreciate that staphylococci and diphtheroids represent part of the usual indigenous flora of the external auditory canal and often contaminate drainage samples. In cases of mastoiditis, bacterial cultures of ear drainage should be taken carefully to assure collection of fresh drainage as opposed to material from the external auditory canal. The canal should be cleaned prior to obtaining pus as it exudes from the tympanic membrane. Tympanocentesis should be performed to obtain middle ear material in those cases in which the tympanic membrane is intact. If a subperiosteal abscess has developed, pus aspirated from the focus of infection should be cultured. Lumbar puncture to investigate the possibility of a secondary meningitis should be considered.

In cases of otitis externa, an inflammatory condition of any skin section of the external auditory canal, swab specimens of the involved area(s) should be cultured for both bacteria and fungi. Malignant otitis externa, caused by *Pseudomonas aeruginosa*, begins as an infection of the external auditory canal and extends into the temporal bone. The infection can further progress and involve the base of the skull, contiguous soft tissue, and the brain. The disease occurs predominantly in elderly diabetic individuals but has also been reported in patients with hematological malignancies and dyscrasias. The disease should be suspected in cases of otitis externa refractory to therapy, especially if granulomatous tissue is present in the auditory canal concomitantly with a persistent purulent drainage. If the patient has no history of diabetes, a glucose-tolerance test should

Table 46-2 Processing recommendations for clinical material from otic infections

Clinical infection	Specimen source	Stains		Media			
		Gram	Special	Blood agar	Chocolate agar	CNA or PEA[a]	Enriched[b] thioglycollate
Otitis media	tympanocentesis blood (in septic patients)	•		•	•		•
Mastoiditis	pus (if present in ear canal)	•		•	•	•	•
	ear drainage	•		•	•	•	•
	tympanocentesis (if eardrum intact)	•					
	subperiosteal abscess (pus)	•		•	•		•
	lumbar puncture (to rule out meningitis)	•		•	•		•
Otitis externa	swab of involved area	•	•[d]	•	•	•	•
Malignant otitis media	drainage and/or granulomatous tissue	•		•	•	•	•
	lumbar puncture (to rule out meningitis)	•		•	•		•
Tuberculous otitis	middle ear tissue from biopsy	•	•[e]	•	•		•

[a]Columbia CNA agar with 5% sheep blood or phenylethyl alcohol agar with 5% sheep blood.
[b]Prereduced thioglycollate without indicator supplemented with vitamin K_1, hemin, and 16% horse serum.
[c]For infants less than 6 months of age.
[d]KOH or Calcofluor white if *Aspergillus* spp. or *Candida* spp. are suspected.
[e]Rhodamine-auramine and/or Kinyoun's acid fast stain.

be performed. The erythrocyte sedimentation rate is usually elevated. *Pseudomonas* spp. should be isolated from purulent discharge cultures. Lumbar puncture should be considered in serious cases to rule out the possibility of pseudomonal meningitis. In patients without meningeal involvement, the CSF typically demonstrates a mild pleocytosis with normal glucose and negative Gram stain. In patients with meningitis, an increase of PMN's and decreased CSF glucose level are usually observed.

Tuberculous otitis occurs in adults and, more commonly, in children. Neonatal cases have been reported. The usual etiologic agent, *Mycobacterium tuberculosis,* often progresses producing secondary temporal bone infection. Middle-ear tissue biopsies characteristically show caseating epithelioid granulomas. Cultures are infrequently positive. Tuberculin skin tests, however, usually are reactive and may assist in making the diagnosis.

Processing of specimens

Middle-ear effusions collected by tympanocentesis or myringotomy (more traumatic and often contaminated with indigenous microflora obfuscating culture interpretation) should be cultured for bacteria, viruses, and other microorganisms based on clinical findings and the patient's age. Cultures for bacterial pathogens should include media appropriate for the isolation of fastidious bacteria including *Haemophilus influenzae* as well as a broth medium, such as thioglycollate, capable of supporting the growth of anaerobic bacteria.

Epidemiologic investigations have shown a frequent connection between viral infection and acute otitis media. In pediatric studies in a day care setting, viral isolation from the upper respiratory tract was correlated with the clinical diagnosis of acute otitis media. Epidemics of otitis media occurred coincidentally with viral outbreaks due to adenovirus, enteroviruses, and respiratory syncytial virus. By comparison, viruses are only infrequently isolated from middle-ear effusions of children with otitis media.

Chlamydia trachomatis, a relatively common agent in acute respiratory disease in infants less than six months, also causes acute otitis media in this age group and has been isolated from middle-ear fluid collected from infants with acute disease. Rare etiologic agents in otic infections include *Corynebacterium diphtheriae* (diphtheritic otitis); *Clostridium tetani* (otogenic tetanus); and *Ascaris lumbricoides* (otitis). Diagnostic techniques applicable for the specific agent should be used when one of these infections is suspected.

Direct examination and culture techniques

Recommendations for the culture of specimens obtained in otic infections are outlined in Table 46-2. The indigenous microbial flora of the external auditory canal is similar to that found on skin elsewhere. Coagulase-negative staphylococci (especially *S. epidermidis* and *S. auricularis*); diphtheroids; *S. aureus;* and, less often, such anaerobic bacteria as *Propionibacterium acnes* predominate. Pathogens responsible for middle-ear infection are infrequently isolated in cultures of the external auditory canal when the tympanic membrane is intact. Organisms representing usual skin flora of the external ear are listed in Box 46-1.

Bacterial

The bacteriology of otitis media has been well documented by appropriate cultures of middle-ear fluid obtained by tympanocentesis. *Streptococcus pneumoniae* is the most common cause of otitis media. Relatively few serotypes are responsible for the majority of disease and include, in order of decreasing frequency, types 19, 23, 6, 14, 3, and 18.

Lowenstein-Jensen	MacConkey agar	Sabouraud dextrose agar	Viral transport medium	Chlamydia transport medium	Special techniques
			•	•c	Blood culture bottles for aerobic and anaerobic bacteria
	•				
	•				
	•	•			
	•				Glucose tolerance test if no history of diabetes
•		•			Tuberculin skin test may assist in diagnosis

All of these are included in the currently available pneumococcal polysaccharide vaccines.

Otitis media caused by *H. influenzae* is usually due to nontypable strains. Approximately 10%, however, are associated with serotype b and concomitant bacteremia and/or meningitis is seen in approximately 25% of these cases. In the preantibiotic era, otitis media caused by *Streptococcus pyogenes* (group A streptococci) was very common and still represents the third most common cause of this disease. *Streptococcus agalactiae* (group B streptococci) has been isolated from middle-ear effusions in neonates with otitis media frequently in association with bacteremia. Members of the *Enterobacteriaceae* are responsible for approximately 20% of cases of otitis media in neonates but rarely cause disease in older children or adults except in immunocompromised individuals and patients with chronic suppurative otitis with tympanic membrane perforation. Under these circumstances *Proteus mirabilis*, *E. coli*, and the nonfermentative Gram-negative bacilli including *Pseudomonas* spp. have all been associated with disease.

The role of anaerobic bacteria, coagulase negative staphylococci, and *S. aureus* in these infections is unclear. Anaerobic bacteria appear to have a limited role both in chronic and acute otitis media having been found in mixed cultures in up to 50% of specimens collected by tympanocentesis. *Moraxella (Branhamella) catarrhalis* is being recognized increasingly in cases of otitis media having been isolated in 19% of middle-ear effusions in one study of a pediatric population. Seventy percent of these strains were beta-lactamase positive and therefore interpreted as ampicillin resistant. Staphylococci are rarely isolated in pure culture from middle-ear fluid. In cases of chronic otitis externa, by comparison, *P. aeruginosa* (approximately ⅔ of all isolates) and other *Pseudomonas* spp. and *Staphylococcus aureus* (isolated in approximately 30% of cases) represent the predominant bacteria. A single bacterial pathogen is isolated in about ⅔ of all cultures from cases of otitis externa. Other

Box 46-1 Usual microflora of the external auditory canal

ORGANISM	FREQUENCY
Fungi	
Candida spp., not *albicans*	Common
Aspergillus spp., not *fumigatus*	Uncommon
Bacteria	
Gram-positive cocci	
Staphylococcus epidermidis	Very common
Staphylococcus auricularis	Very common
Staphylococcus aureus	Common
Peptococcus spp.	Uncommon
viridans streptococci	Common
Streptococcus pneumoniae	Relatively common
Gram-positive bacilli	
Lactobacillus spp.	Very common
diphtheroids	Very common
Aerobic gram-negative bacilli	
Enterobacteriaceae	Common
Escherichia coli	Uncommon
Enterobacter spp.	Uncommon
Klebsiella spp.	Common
Proteus mirabilis	Relatively common
Pseudomonas aeruginosa	Relatively common

organisms noted in decreasing frequency of isolation are viridans streptococci, *Proteus mirabilis*, *Enterobacter* spp., *Klebsiella* spp., and *E. coli*. As previously underscored, *P. aeruginosa* is the primary pathogen in cases of malignant otitis externa.

Viral

As explained previously, viruses are only infrequently isolated from middle-ear effusions from patients with otitis media even when concomitant acute viral respiratory disease is diagnosed. This may signify that viruses are typically present early in the course of illness but absent by the time inner-ear symptoms develop, that viruses are present in concentrations below the sensitivity of culture systems, or that inhibitory immunomodulators, including antibody and interferons, impede viral isolation efforts. Adenoviruses, influenza and parainfluenza viruses, coxsackie virus, and respiratory syncytial virus (RSV) have, however, all been incriminated in otitis media and isolated from ear aspirates collected by tympanocentesis.

When viral cultures are requested, specimens should be inoculated to cell cultures capable of supporting the replication of the viral agents listed previously. Although each laboratory's choice of cell lines will differ slightly, a Simian kidney cell line (African green monkey kidney or Rhesus monkey kidney); human fibroblasts (MRC-5 or human foreskin fibroblasts); and Hep-2 or A-549 lines should be included. Although RSV can be effectively detected in respiratory specimens by ELISA, data on the sensitivity and specificity of these test systems when applied to middle-ear effusion fluids are not available.

Mycobacterial

When tuberculous otitis is suspected, media appropriate for the isolation of mycobacteria should be inoculated with clinical specimen and acid-fast stains performed. To date, commercially-available genetic probes have not proven sufficiently sensitive for direct detection of mycobacteria in clinical specimens. They are useful, however, in expediting the specific identification of an isolate once detected in a culture system. Radiometric techniques for detection of mycobacteria also decrease the time to positivity and may be useful in these cases.

Mycoplasma

Currently, culture techniques for the isolation of *Mycoplasma pneumoniae* from clinical specimens are not widely offered in most clinical laboratories. As a result, requests for culture of mycoplasmas usually require referral to an outside reference laboratory. Clinical specimens should be sent frozen to the reference lab in transport medium usually made available by the reference center or, as an alternative, in 2 ml of a nutrient broth, such as tryptose phosphate, without antimicrobials. A commercially available culture system for mycoplasmas has facilitated isolation procedures for these microorganisms and might be considered in larger clinical lab settings. Genetic probes, approved for direct detection of *M. pneumoniae* from throat swabs, have not been sufficiently evaluated to recommend their use on middle ear effusions.

SUGGESTED READING

Balows A, Hausler Jr, WJ and Lennette EH: Laboratory diagnosis of infectious diseases: principles and practice, vols 1 and 2, New York, 1988, Springer-Verlag.

Bergstron L: Diseases of the external ear. In: Bluestone CD and Stool SE, eds, Pediatric otolaryngology, Philadelphia, 1983, WB Saunders.

Braude AI, Davis CE, and Fierer JF: Infectious diseases and medical microbiology, ed 2, Philadelphia, 1986, WB Saunders Company.

Finegold SM, Shepherd WE, and Spaulding EH: Practical anaerobic bacteriology, Washington, DC, 1977, American Society for Microbiology.

Harding AL, Anderson P, Howie VM, et al: *Haemophilus influenzae* isolated from children with otitis media. In: Sell SHW and Karzon DT, eds, *Haemophilus influenzae*, Nashville, 1973, Vanderbilt University Press.

Hoeprich PD: Infectious disease, ed 3, Philadelphia, 1983, Harper and Row.

Holt JG, Sneath PH, Mair NS, and Sharpe ME: Bergey's manual of systematic bacteriology, vol 2, Baltimore, 1986, Williams and Wilkins.

Howard BJ, Klaas J, Rubin SJ, Weissfeld AS, and Tilton RC: Clinical and pathogenic microbiology, St. Louis, 1987, CV Mosby Company.

Jones DB, Liesegang TJ, and Robinson NM: Laboratory diagnosis of ocular infections, Washington, DC, 1981, American Society for Microbiology.

National Committee for Clinical Laboratory Standards: Methods for dilution antimicrobial susceptibility tests for bacteria that grow aerobically, M7-T, 3:31, Villanova, Penn, 1983, NCCLS.

National Committee for Clinical Laboratory Standards: Clinical laboratory procedure manuals, GP2-A, vol 4, no 2, Villanova, Penn, 1984, NCCLS.

National Committee for Clinical Laboratory Standards: Performance standards for antimicrobial disk susceptibility tests, ed 3, M2-A3, 4:369, Villanova, Penn, 1984, NCCLS.

National Committee for Clinical Laboratory Standards: Performance standards for antimicrobial susceptibility testing, M100-S2, MZ-A-S2, vol 7, no 10, Villanova, Penn, 1988, NCCLS.

Schachter J: Chlamydiae (psittacosis-lymphogranuloma venereum-trachoma group). In: Lennette EH, Balows A, Hausler Jr WJ, and Truant JP, eds, Manual of clinical microbiology, ed 3, Washington, DC, 1980, American Society for Microbiology.

Schachter J and Dawson CR: Human chlamydial infections, Littleton, Mass, 1978, PSG Publishing Company.

Senturia BH, Marcus MD, Lucente FE: Diseases of the external ear. An otologic-dematologic manual, ed 2, New York, 1980, Grune and Stratton.

47

Gastrointestinal tract specimens

J. Michael Miller

EPIDEMIOLOGY AND PUBLIC HEALTH SIGNIFICANCE

Gastrointestinal illness is a major cause of morbidity and mortality worldwide, particularly in developing countries where sanitation and living conditions offer little to protect those most susceptible to diarrheal disease. Children are especially susceptible in these countries, where it has been estimated that infectious diarrhea is a direct contributor to a death rate of 20 deaths per 1000 children per year. The youngest children, those less than 2-years-old, may experience 2 to 3 episodes of infectious diarrhea per year. Calculating this with the number of children less than 5 years old in Africa, Asia (excluding China), and Latin America, one could expect up to one billion episodes of diarrhea per year, resulting in 4.6 million deaths. The United States as well is not completely protected from experiencing infectious diarrhea in its children or its adults.

The rate of reported salmonella infections has steadily increased since 1955 (Fig. 47-1); the case rate has risen from 13.5 per 100,000 in 1978 to 20.9 cases per 100,000 of the population in 1987. Shigella infection case rates have changed little over the years and stand at 9.8 cases per

100,000 in 1987 (Fig. 47-2). Cholera in the United States has been relatively rare, but appears to present a potential threat along the Gulf Coast where a few cases have occurred since the mid-1970s. Although campylobacterosis and yersiniosis are not reportable to the Centers for Disease Control, these diarrheal illnesses are the subject of frequent case reports and journal articles. Gastrointestinal illness caused by *Campylobacter* spp. is more common in the United States than that caused by *Yersinia* spp. For this reason, most hospitals routinely culture for *Salmonella*, *Shigella*, and *Campylobacter* from stool specimens.

Acute viral gastroenteritis is a common worldwide problem causing high morbidity and mortality. One worldwide study estimated that 40% of the 5 to 18 million deaths attributed to diarrheal illness in one year (1977 to 1978) were related to viral gastroenteritis. Again, most patients were young children. Until the early 1970s, characterizing the cause of nonbacterial or nonparasitic diarrhea was only speculative. Using creative electron microscopic techniques, the 27-nm Norwalk agent was visualized as aggregates in stool samples of volunteers. A 70-nm particle was visualized in the mid-1970s and was later designated as

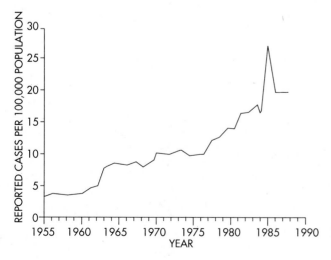

Fig. 47-1 Salmonella (excluding typhoid fever) infections in the United States, 1955 to 1987.

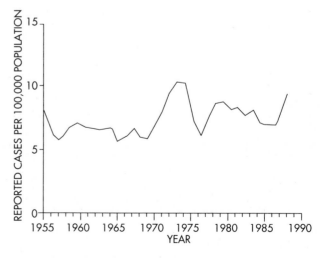

Fig. 47-2 Shigella infections in the United States, 1955 to 1987.

rotavirus. Although effective culture methods are still not available for most agents of viral diarrhea, some viral agents can be detected by a number of commercially available tests.

Diarrhea caused by intestinal parasites may be even more difficult to document because laboratorians and physicians are less able to recognize the etiologic agent microscopically, or to accurately diagnose the illness. In addition, because parasitic illness is not emphasized in their training, physicians may not even know the proper types of specimens to obtain or how they are best submitted to the laboratory.

Clearly, intestinal parasites are a major cause of morbidity and mortality in diarrheal illness worldwide, but there are no accurate figures on the prevalence of such parasites, even in the United States. Complicating the laboratory diagnostic picture is the variety of intestinal protozoa and helminths found in human stool examinations that are not considered pathogens, nor do they all cause diarrhea. The infection rate of amebiasis caused by *Entamoeba histolytica* in the United States is estimated to be 5%, but it is higher among institutionalized persons, male homosexuals, American Indians living on reservations, and in some residents of socioeconomically disadvantaged areas. *Giardia lamblia* is probably the most frequently recognized parasite in American travelers and in campers who drink from natural streams. Since the advent of the acquired immunodeficiency syndrome (AIDS) epidemic in the United States, *Cryptosporidium* spp. have become frequently recognized pathogens in these immunosuppressed individuals and in some day-care center outbreaks. In this country, intestinal helminths cause diarrhea less frequently than do protozoa.

Although yeast and other fungi can be isolated occasionally from stool specimens, these agents rarely are the cause of gastroenteritis in immunocompetent individuals. In AIDS patients and in patients undergoing aggressive antimicrobic therapy, the presence of large numbers of yeast or the isolation of some filamentous fungi suggests a potential etiologic role for these agents. Cessation of antimicrobics allows normal intestinal flora to be reestablished and, in most cases, symptoms will be alleviated.

Patients with AIDS frequently suffer a number of abnormalities in the gastrointestinal system, both infectious and noninfectious. The following list illustrates the potential problems occurring in these individuals:

1. Noninfectious
   a. Kaposi's sarcoma
   b. AIDS enteropathy
   c. Burkitt's lymphoma
   d. Other lymphomas
   e. Squamous cell carcinoma of the tongue
   f. Squamous cell carcinoma of the rectum
   g. Cloacogenic carcinoma of the rectum
2. Infectious
   a. Bacterial: *Salmonella* spp., *Shigella* spp., *Campylobacter* spp., *Mycobacterium fortuitum*, *Neisseria gonorrhoeae*, *Treponema pallidum*, *Clostridium difficile*, *Listeria monocytogenes*
   b. *Chlamydia trachomatis*
   c. Fungal: *Candida* spp.
   d. Viral: Herpes simplex, cytomegalovirus, papillomavirus
   e. Parasitic: *Entamoeba histolytica*, *Giardia lamblia*, *Cryptosporidium* spp., *Isopora belli*, *Sarcocystis* spp., *Enterocytozoon* sp.

NORMAL GASTROINTESTINAL ENVIRONMENT

Because of the ubiquity, diversity, and sheer number of enteric microorganisms, one can appreciate the normal host defenses and the role these defenses play in maintaining an equilibrium and health in most people. Recognizing and understanding these enteric host defenses are important for the clinical microbiologist in order to properly respond to the physician's request for identification of an etiologic agent. The microbiologist should be able to assess the appropriateness of the specimen submitted for examination, as well as interpret the results of the examination. If necessary, the microbiologist must also explain the compromised nature of the results if an error has been recognized in any part of the specimen's total testing process, not just in the analytical portion of processing.

Intestinal host defenses include gastric acidity, immunity, intestinal motility, and commensal flora. One additional factor in host protection is simply personal cleanliness. The inoculum size is critical for most agents of gastrointestinal illness, and routine handwashing may serve to protect individuals by simply reducing the number of organisms on the hands available to be ingested. It has long been known that shigellosis requires only 10 to 100 cells of *Shigella* to initiate infection in susceptible persons, whereas cholera requires the ingestion of up to 100 million *Vibrio*. Shigellosis, therefore, is easily spread by person-to-person contact, and laboratory accidents could easily occur if laboratorians are careless when working with these agents. Cholera and most other enteric infections are spread primarily by the ingestion of large numbers of organisms and less frequently by person-to-person contact.

Gastric acidity offers substantial protection against many agents of diarrheal illness. Neutralizing stomach acidity in experiments with sodium bicarbonate reduced the infective dose of *Vibrio* by 10,000-fold. In patients who are achlorhydric, the frequency and severity of infections with *Salmonella* and *Giardia* are increased. The stomach, however, has little, if any, "normal flora." Transient flora that has been swallowed is usually present but short-lived.

Normal intestinal motility is important in both the elimination of pathogens and in normal absorption of fluid and electrolytes. When intestinal motility is inhibited with diphenoxylate hydrochloride with atropine (Lomotil), treatment for shigellosis is ineffective in reducing symptoms and is associated with prolonged shedding of organisms.

Specific defense mechanisms in the intestines include humoral IgG antibodies and secretory IgA antibodies (coproantibody), which are synthesized locally. In addition, the recent finding of lymphocytes in the lamina propria of the gastrointestinal tract suggested that these lymphocytes can mediate immunologic reactions alone or in conjunction with antibody.

The way normal flora protects against enteric disease has been well documented. The normal flora of the mouth generally arises from the gums and gingival crevices. Upon natural swallowing, this flora, and that from food, enters the stomach. The low pH of the gastric fluid is usually toxic to most organisms. A few, however, can briefly survive in the stomach and enter the small intestine. Generally, only small numbers of commensal flora can be found in the upper portion of the small bowel, and the number increases significantly from the jejunum to the proximal and then the distal bowel, where counts of 100,000 to 10,000,000 are common. The largest number of commensal flora (mostly anaerobes) are found in the colon, where bacterial counts usually reflect those found in feces.

The protective effects of this flora were demonstrated in early studies in mice: when mice were given one dose of streptomycin, the infecting dose of *Salmonella typhimurium* was reduced over 100,000-fold. Reduced resistance correlated with the reduction of commensal colonic flora but was restored by a return of normal flora. In humans, the observation of antibiotic-associated enterocolitis due to *Clostridium difficile* illustrates the protective effect of normal enteric flora.

AGENTS OF GASTROINTESTINAL ILLNESS

There are many etiologic agents of gastrointestinal disease. It must be kept in mind that all parasites found in feces are not pathogenic, nor are all bacteria, yeasts, or viruses. Indeed, one would expect to find a myriad of organisms. To interpret the results of stool cultures to provide accurate, significant, and clinically relevant information to the physician, the laboratorian must have a specimen that has been appropriately selected, collected, and transported to the laboratory. In addition, the physician must communicate the suspected diagnosis to the laboratorian. Knowing which etiologic agent is suspected will guide the laboratorian in the selection of analytic methods that will provide the earliest and most accurate report. The agents commonly considered important in gastrointestinal illness are listed in Box 47-1.

Clinical virology is no longer relegated to retrospective diagnosis. Newer technology has allowed the laboratorian to aggressively look for and detect agents for viral illness, in many cases as quickly as a bacterial diagnosis can be done. Diarrhea of viral etiology is common worldwide and should be ruled out routinely when possible. Most agents of viral gastroenteritis are not routinely cultivated. An excellent review of human viral gastroenteritis has recently been published.

Rotavirus, a double-stranded DNA virus, is the most common cause of viral gastroenteritis in infants and young children and in the elderly. Carriers are frequently asymptomatic, which make its detection more important especially since the virus is spread by the fecal-oral route. Rotavirus infects the small intestine, where it replicates in the epithelial cells on the tips of the villi. Rotavirus is not routinely cultivated. Enzyme immunoassay (EIA) and latex agglutination (LA) tests are available and are frequently used to detect the presence of antigen. Electron microscopy (EM) is also used, employing a negative stain with phosphotungstic acid. Tests available infrequently include counterimmunoelectrophoresis (CIE), complement fixation tests (CFT), immunofluorescence (IF), and radioimmunoassay (RIA). DNA

Box 47-1   Agents of gastrointestinal illness

A. Common cause
1. Viral
   a. Rotavirus
   b. Parvovirus (Norwalk agent)
2. Enterotoxigenic bacterial
   a. Toxigenic *Escherichia coli*
   b. *Clostridium difficile*
   c. *Clostridium perfringens,* food poisoning
   d. *Staphylococcus aureus,* food poisoning
3. Invasive bacterial
   a. *Shigella* spp.
   b. *Salmonella* spp.
   c. Invasive *E. coli*
   d. *Campylobacter jejuni*
   e. *Helicobacter pylori,* gastric ulcers
4. Parasitic
   a. *Entamoeba histolytica*
   b. *Giardia lamblia*
   c. *Cryptosporidium* spp.
B. Rare cases in the United States
1. Bacterial
   a. *Vibrio cholerae*
   b. *Aeromonas* spp.
   c. *Vibrio parahaemolyticus*
   d. *Bacillus cereus*
   e. *Yersinia enterocolitica*
2. Parasitic
   a. *Ascaris* spp.
   b. Hookworm
   c. *Strongyloides* spp.
   d. *Trichuris* spp.
   e. *Schistosoma* spp.
   f. *Taenia* spp.
   g. *Trichinella* spp.
   h. *Blastocystis* spp.*
   i. *Dientamoeba fragilis*
3. Other
   a. *Lymphogranuloma venereum*
   b. Early hepatitis
   c. *Candida* spp.

*May be relatively common causes.

---

probes have been developed, but are not in routine use at this time.

Norwalk and Norwalk-like agents, including the Hawaii agent, the Montgomery County agent, and the Snow Mountain agent, cause outbreaks of gastroenteritis among older children, adolescents, and adults. These agents are often associated with high attack rates. Their incubation period is 24 to 48 hours, with the sudden onset of severe nausea and vomiting, accompanied by low-grade fever and mild diarrhea. These agents are not routinely cultivated in vitro. Since cultivation is difficult, reagents are not available commercially. In addition, routine laboratory diagnosis of these agents is not done since most patients do not require hospitalization, where testing is done. Immune EM using serum specimens from convalescing patients has been used to detect the virus, as has EIA and RIA.

Adenoviruses are double-stranded DNA viruses not uncommonly found in feces by EM. Types 40 and 41 are fastidious adenoviruses often implicated in diarrheal illness. Worldwide, they are the second-most common cause of infantile gastroenteritis after rotavirus. Adenoviruses are usually endemic rather than epidemic and found mostly in children 2 years old and younger. The illness caused by adenovirus is a milder disease with less pronounced vomiting, fever, and diarrhea than rotavirus disease. The CFT test detects the common group antigen and is used in reference laboratories. Electron microscopy, RIA, EIA, and CIE have also been used. Recently developed DNA probes are not yet commercially available.

Other viruses found in children with diarrhea include calciviruses, astroviruses, and coronaviruses. Although astroviruses can be grown in human embryonic kidney cells, the others are not cultivated. Electron microscopy can be used to detect all three.

CLINICAL AND LABORATORY INTERFACE

Because the potential etiologic agents in gastrointestinal illness are so numerous, it is clear that the laboratorian and the clinician must make every effort to communicate. Each must understand the needs, abilities, and limitations of the other. Clearly, the microbiology laboratory will confirm the presence or absence of a potential etiologic agent and will determine, when appropriate, the antimicrobic susceptibility

pattern of the isolate. Tables 47-1 and 47-2 summarize the clinical and laboratory findings in most cases of gastrointestinal illness occurring in the United States.

INITIAL SPECIMEN EXAMINATION AND SCREENING

Once the specimen arrives in the laboratory, it should be logged in and accessioned according to routine laboratory protocol. The request form should be examined to determine whether all pertinent information has been included. The initial processing and plating of the gastrointestinal specimen have been discussed in Chapter 39. In addition to routine plating for growth of bacterial or fungal agents, or the subsequent submission of the specimen to a reference laboratory for testing, some screening procedures can be done to assist the physician.

Although culture remains the preferred method for diagnosis of most bacterial infections of the gastrointestinal tract, some helpful screening activities may assist the physician in the early confirmation and treatment of patients. The advent of DNA probes into the clinical laboratory arena will likely have a positive impact on early diagnosis of infection, but probes are not yet routinely used to detect *Salmonella*, *Shigella*, *Campylobacter*, *Yersinia*, or *Vibrio* spp.

Table 47-1 Clinical and laboratory factors in infectious diarrhea

Case description	Etiologic agent	Therapy	Comments
Child/adult, no travel history, afebrile, no blood or neutrophils in stool	Rotavirus, Norwalk agent, *E. coli*	None or ampicillin	Mild (3 unformed stools/day): replace fluids; moderate (3-5 episodes/day): PeptoBismol®; severe (6 episodes/day): consider ampicillin; antimicrobial therapy clearly indicated in shigellosis, cholera, enterotoxigenic *E. coli*, nontyphoid *Salmonella* (infants less than 12 weeks and immunocompromised); enteroinvasive *E. coli*, campylobacter, protracted *Yersinia*, non-cholera *Vibrio*
Infant	*E. coli* (enteropathogenic)	Neomycin (po)	
Child/adult, febrile, blood or neutrophils in stool, or history of travel	Varies: *Campylobacter*, *E. coli*, *Shigella* spp., *Salmonella* spp., *Aeromonas* spp., *V. cholerae*, *Cryptosporidium* spp.	Ciprofloxacin, norfloxacin, or Trimethoprim-sulfamethoxazole	
Premature infant	Necrotizing enterocolitis: *E. coli*, coag. neg. staph., *P. aeruginosa*, *C. perfringens*	Ampicillin + antipseudomonal aminoglycosidic antibiotic	
Antibiotic-associated colitis	*Clostridium difficile*	Metronidazole (po) or vancomycin (po)	Diagnosis requires toxin detection; avoid Lomotil®
AIDS patients	Same as child/adult + HIV, cytomegalovirus, *Cryptosporidium* sp.		

Table 47-2 Clinical and laboratory factors in nondiarrheal gastrointestinal illness

Case description	Etiologic agent	Therapy	Comments
Duodenal ulcer and type B antral gastritis	*Helicobacter pylori*	Colloidal bismuth subcitrate + tinidazole	Ciprofloxacin is an alternate therapy; cure rate good when organisms are cleared
Perirectal abscess	Enterics, *Bacteroides* spp., enterococci	Cefoxitin/cefotetan, timentin, or augmentin	Surgical drainage critical
Ulcerative colitis (mild to moderate)	Unknown	Sulfasalazine	Consider serology for *Entamoeba histolytica*

The Gram stain has limited use in the early examination of feces. Because of the numbers and morphology of fecal flora, recognizing and reporting specific organisms must be done with caution. Gram's stain is helpful in initial evaluation of cases of pseudomembranous colitis, staphylococcal enterocolitis, and perhaps heavy yeast infection since the etiologic agents are usually present in predominant numbers. Recognizing large numbers of gram-negative, curved bacilli may strengthen the suspicion of *Campylobacter* or *Vibrio* infection. The observation of characteristic gram-negative, intracellular diplococci in specimens from anal lesions suggests *Neisseria gonorrhoeae.*

Observing the cellular content of feces may suggest a mechanism of pathogenicity that could be correlated with a particular etiologic agent. Invasive bacteria usually evoke a polymorphonuclear leukocyte response in the intestine, and the leukocytes can be seen in the Gram stain of feces. Toxigenic organisms usually do not cause a similar response (Table 47-3).

Gastric contents may be submitted for detection of *Mycobacterium tuberculosis*. While culture may take days to weeks, an acid-fast stain or fluorescent stain of the material will quickly reveal the presence of suspicious organisms. A significant contribution in the early laboratory recognition of this organism would be the use of DNA probes for *Mycobacterium* used with direct specimens. The acid-fast stain is also useful for observing suspected *Mycobacterium avium-intracellulare* in the feces of patients with AIDS. Gastric washings are often unproductive for *Helicobacter pylori*. An *H. pylori* screen is discussed below.

Toxin detection in feces is more definitive than culture in the case of certain bacterial diseases and food poisoning. The detection of the toxin of *Clostridium difficile* in feces is necessary in order to implicate *C. difficile* as an etiologic agent. Latex agglutination tests are available commercially that detect proteins in the feces that correlate well to the presence of *C. difficile* toxin in the stool. The test is rapid and convenient to use. Toxin assay in cell cultures remains the reference method of choice.

Toxins of *Staphylococcus* and *Clostridium botulinum* may be detected, even when the organisms are unable to be isolated in the laboratory. The presence of toxins of these foodborne pathogens must be confirmed in order to implicate an etiologic agent. Detection of toxin from *Bacillus* spp. must be correlated with the presence of *Bacillus* spp. in feces and in the implicated food.

When parasites are suspected in gastrointestinal illness, most of the diagnostic work done in the laboratory is done

Table 47-3 Fecal leukocytes in stool specimens from patients with diarrheal disease

Disease	Predominant cell type in feces (acute illness)
Campylobacterosis	Polymorphonuclear
Shigellosis	Polymorphonuclear
Salmonellosis	Polymorphonuclear
Typhoid fever	Mononuclear
Cholera	None
Enterotoxigenic *E. coli*	None
Invasive *E. coli*	Polymorphonuclear

directly on the specimen, and results can be quickly reported. Saline and iodine wet preparations, wet mounts for *Trichomonas,* trichrome stains, acid-fast or fluorescent stains for *Cryptosporidium* or other coccidian parasites such as *Isospora,* and observation of cellophane tape preparation for *Enterobius* (pinworm) are relatively rapid procedures. Whereas the rapidity of the tests and observations may equate them to screening procedures, skilled technologists can actually provide a definitive diagnosis based on careful and complete microscopic study of the specimen.

Direct examination of the bile-stained portion of the string removed from a patient undergoing a "string test" or from aspirated duodenal contents also provides helpful information when fecal examination for *Giardia* and, rarely, *Strongyloides* has been unproductive.

Direct examination of feces for viruses is limited to relatively few procedures. Latex and EIA tests for antigens of rotavirus are available and some larger, better equipped facilities have the capability to perform electron microscopic study on specimens and observe for typical viral morphology. In addition, EIA tests are available for adenovirus types 40 and 41.

A definitive diagnosis of *H. pylori* infection can only be made by culturing antral or duodenal biopsy specimens from patients undergoing upper gastrointestinal tract endoscopy. The organism can be grown on Skirrow's medium as well as on blood and chocolate agar. A prominent feature of *H. pylori* is its unusually high endogenous urease activity, which may protect it from the acidic environment of the stomach by generating large quantities of ammonium and bicarbonate ions from urea. Other *Helicobacter* and campylobacter species pathogenic to humans do not have this property of being able to hydrolyze urea.

Helicobacter pylori is a motile, gram-negative rod with four sheathed flagella. Other similar species have a single flagellum. It grows optimally in a microaerophilic atmosphere when incubated at 35° C but not at 30° C or 42° C. Isolates are oxidase-positive, catalase-positive, indole-negative, nitrate-negative, and do not ferment glucose. *Helicobacter pylori* is highly susceptible to most antibiotics except nalidixic acid, vancomycin, trimethoprim, and sulfonamides.

Helicobacter pylori screen test

The specimen of choice is either an antral or duodenal biopsy specimen. Specimens should be placed in 5 ml of sterile saline and submitted to the laboratory within 30 minutes of collection. Store at 4° C up to 4 hours. Upon its arrival, split the specimen (tissue) into two portions: Mince one portion (or grind with mortar and pestle) in sterile saline or *Brucella* broth and mince or ground the second portion in 0.5 ml of 2% Christensen's urea broth as a direct screen. Colonies selected for testing should be positive for oxidase, catalase, and urease, and appear typical on the Gram stain. Emulsify colonies into urea broth and incubate at 35° C, or dip a swab into urea broth and touch the suspect colony (positive pink will be seen within 30 seconds). The direct screen (minced tissue in urea broth) is read at 1-hour intervals for color change to red or pink. The speed and depth of the color change are proportional to the numbers of organisms present. Some will be positive in an hour, almost half will be positive by 6 hours. The report should read as follows: "*Helicobacter pylori* screen test positive for urease activity in biopsy tissue. While the screen test usually correlates with *H. pylori* infection, a positive culture result will confirm its presence." When *H. pylori* is grown on media, report: "*Helicobacter pylori* isolated from biopsy tissue. Susceptibility tests not routinely performed."

Inoculate one drop of the saline-minced tissue onto a chocolate agar plate and a Skirrow's agar plate. Incubate both plates at 35° C in a microaerophilic atmosphere. If mincing in urea broth was not done, inoculate 1 ml of Christensen's urea broth with 1 to 2 drops of suspension. Incubate at 35° C. A positive color may result in less than 10 minutes if *H. pylori* is present. Incubate for 24 hours. One may also spot-inoculate a urea agar slant, prewarmed to room temperature. Perform a Gram stain on one drop of suspension and look for typical gram-negative helicobacter-like organisms.

At 24 and 48 hours, observe chocolate and Skirrow's agar for typical colonies. Since other organisms may not survive stomach acidity, contamination may be rare, although overgrowth may occur (*Proteus, Pseudomonas, Citrobacter* have been reported). Therefore a positive urease screen must correlate to culture.

Newer technology with molecular or genetically based procedures will potentially facilitate more rapid diagnosis of agents of gastrointestinal illness. The advent of these new procedures should provide for earlier, accurate di-agnosis, leading to shorter morbidity and substantial cost savings to patients and to hospitals. Direct specimen examination is clearly the focus of many modern tests. However, until sensitivity and specificity of newer procedures are improved, current methods, including routine culture, will remain necessary for definitive identification of agents of illness.

SUGGESTED READING

Bellanti JA: Immunologically mediated diseases. In Bellanti JA, editor: Immunology III, Philadelphia, 1985, WB Saunders.

Christensen ML: Human viral gastroenteritis, Clin Microbiol Rev 2:51, 1989.

Dascal A and Blacklow NR: Viral diarrhea. In Gorbach SL, editor: Infectious diarrhea, Boston, 1986, Blackwell Scientific.

Ellner PD: Infectious diarrheal diseases—current concepts and laboratory procedures, New York, 1984, Marcel Dekker.

Hook EW and others, editors: Current concepts of infectious diseases, New York, 1977, John Wiley.

Isenberg HD and others: Cumitech 9—collection and processing of bacteriological specimens, Washington, DC, 1979, American Society for Microbiology.

Miller JM: Handbook of specimen collection and handling in microbiology, ed 2, Atlanta, 1985, Centers for Disease Control.

Sack RB and others: Cumitech 12—laboratory diagnosis of bacterial diarrhea, Washington, DC, 1980, American Society for Microbiology.

Tyrrell DAJ and Kapikian AZ, editors: Virus infections of the gastrointestinal tract, New York, 1982, Marcel Dekker.

Wolfe MS: Parasites. In Gorbach SL, editor: Infectious diarrhea, Boston, 1986, Blackwell Scientific.

48 Urinary tract specimens

Marie Pezzlo

The urinary tract is normally free of microorganisms and, under normal conditions, urine is a sterile fluid. However, any invasive procedure or other disruption of the integrity or disorder of the urinary tract may cause microorganisms to gain access and multiply. Colonization or invasion of the urinary tract tissues by a variety of microorganisms result in urinary tract infections. Infection may occur at one or more sites in the urinary tract, such as in the kidneys, causing pyelonephritis; in the bladder, causing cystitis; in the prostate, causing prostatitis, or in the urethra, causing urethritis.

Urinary tract infections are second in frequency to respiratory tract infections, however, urine specimens represent the majority of samples received in the clinical microbiology laboratory for analyses. The reason for the larger number of urine specimens submitted for microbiologic examinations over respiratory specimens is easily explained. A majority of infections associated with the upper respiratory tract have a viral etiology with symptoms that are not severe, so laboratory tests are usually not required. In contrast, urinary tract infections are usually caused by bacteria and require antimicrobial therapy. Finally, screening of certain patient populations is warranted for detection of asymptomatic infections that may cause serious sequelae if left untreated.

PATHOPHYSIOLOGY OF URINARY TRACT INFECTION
Pathways of infection

Microorganisms invade and spread throughout the urinary tract by three different pathways or routes: ascending, hematogenous, and lymphatic. The ascending route is the usual pathway. Microorganisms from the skin, external genitalia, and feces enter the urethral meatus and ascend into the bladder. Microorganisms also enter the female urinary tract by urethral massage and sexual intercourse. Ascending infection in association with instrumentation is common in both sexes. For most catheter-induced infections, especially in women, bacteria migrate from the rectal area, colonize the urethra, and ascend between the catheter and urethral mucosa. It is presumably the adherence of the microorganisms to the uroepithelial cells of the bladder that initiates the colonization of the urinary tract.

The hematogenous, or descending route, is an important source of infections in the kidneys; however, it occurs less commonly than the ascending route. Large volumes of blood continuously flow through the kidneys and, therefore, any systemic infection can seed the kidneys with blood borne microorganisms. The lymphatic pathway may have very little significance in urinary tract infection, although this route may be associated with prostatitis.

The location of the bladder, anatomy, and short urethra account for the increased numbers of infections in females compared to males. Microorganisms colonize the urethra and may be easily inoculated into the bladder following instrumentation or sexual intercourse, resulting in cystitis or urethritis. Other conditions that predispose the urinary tract to infection include interference with the flushing action of urine outflow and increased pressure on the bladder, forcing urine into the urethra. The latter can occur in normal women during coughing, and as bladder pressure returns to normal, microorganisms are washed into the bladder. Other risk factors incude urinary tract obstruction associated with congenital abnormalities, renal calculi, and urethral occlusion. Patients with a neurogenic bladder, urethral stricture, or prostatic hypertrophy are also predisposed to infection. Also, the increased incidence of pyelonephritis during pregnancy has been associated with loss of urethral peristalsis.

Bladder defense mechanisms

Three defense mechanisms have been described that allow the bladder to defend itself against infection. The primary bladder defense mechanism, or repeated voiding, enables bacteria to be flushed from the bladder. Bacterial counts are greatly reduced with a high fluid intake and frequent voiding. The secondary defense mechanism is the effect of the bladder mucosa on the remaining microorganisms. Lastly, the tertiary bladder defense mechanism includes the antimicrobial properties of urine such as organic acids, low pH, and high concentrations of urea. Additional natural defenses in the urinary tract have been described as anti-adherence mechanisms, the action of phagocytic cells, and immune mechanisms.

CLINICAL MANIFESTATIONS

Infections of the urinary system may involve the upper or the lower urinary tract, with or without symptoms. The infections range from a single episode of acute symptomatic infection, which may result in a spontaneous cure following single-dose antimicrobial therapy, to a more serious recurring infection such as chronic pyelonephritis, caused by a resistant, difficult to treat microorganism.

Upper urinary tract infections

Infections of the upper urinary tract involve the kidneys, renal pelvis, and ureters, and are characterized by flank pain, chills, fever, nausea, and vomiting.

Acute pyelonephritis is an inflammatory disease characterized by upper urinary tract symptoms and the presence of $\geq 10^5$ colony-forming units (CFU) per ml of urine, ≥ 10 white blood cells (WBC)/mm^3, and WBC casts. Acute pyelonephritis may be associated with septicemia, shock, toxemias of pregnancy, diabetes mellitus, pregnancy, hypertension, and kidney stone formation. The disease is usually seen in women of childbearing age and in the elderly.

Chronic pyelonephritis is a term used to describe a prolonged infection associated with the presence of bacteria or the presence of lesions in the absence of active disease. The symptoms range from an acute to a mild infection accompanied by malaise, or the patient may be completely asymptomatic. These patients may also experience nocturia and may produce only dilute urine.

Lower urinary tract infections

Infections of the lower urinary tract involve the bladder (cystitis), the urethra (urethritis), and, in males, the infection of the prostate glands, resulting in prostatitis. The symptoms include painful (dysuria) and frequent urination, with small amounts of urine that may be turbid and bloody but with no systemic involvement. If the infection is in the bladder, large numbers of microorganisms, $\geq 10^5$ CFU/ml, are usually present. However, studies have shown that as few as 10^2 CFU/ml may be found in young women with acute dysuria and lower urinary tract infection.

In contrast, patients with urethritis, also termed the acute urethral syndrome, may have symptoms of dysuria and frequent urination with no recognizable pathogen. One study classified patients with the acute urethral syndrome into four categories: those with $\geq 10^5$ CFU/ml, those with $< 10^5$ CFU/ml, those with unusual urinary pathogens, and those with no recognizable pathogens. Pyuria was a significant finding in the first 3 groups.

It is important for the physician to distinguish between urethritis and vaginitis; in vaginitis, urine cultures are unnecessary. Females with vaginitis have external dysuria compared with the internal dysuria and frequent urination experienced with urethritis. On the other hand, it is not necessary to distinguish between cystitis and the acute urethral syndrome.

Prostatitis may be an acute or a chronic infection. Acute prostatitis may be accompanied by symptoms of tenderness and fever, chills, back pain, dysuria, and pyuria. The prostate gland becomes swollen and prostatic fluid contains many WBC and microorganisms. Pyelonephritis, bacteremia, and prostatic abscesses are some of the complications that may result from infection of the prostate gland. Chronic prostatitis causes relapsing urinary tract infections and is often difficult to cure. Cultures of the urethra, urine, midstream urine, and prostatic secretions, using a quantitative localization technique, are necessary to confirm the diagnosis of chronic prostatitis.

Asymptomatic lower urinary tract infection

Asymptomatic (covert) bacteriuria refers to the presence of significant bacteriuria in the absence of symptoms. The term may be misleading since a majority of these patients have experienced symptoms of a urinary tract infection during the preceding year. Although asymptomatic infections may occur throughout life, they pose a serious threat during pregnancy and to the elderly. Screening of these patient groups for significant bacteriuria may help prevent the increased morbidity and mortality associated with undetected and untreated infections. The diagnosis of an asymptomatic infection may be made by the presence of $\geq 10^5$ CFU/ml of a single organism in at least two consecutive urine cultures collected on separate days.

EPIDEMIOLOGY OF URINARY TRACT INFECTION

All individuals are susceptible to urinary tract infections, however, the prevalence varies with age, sex, and certain predisposing factors. Various studies have demonstrated that infections may begin as early as the first few days of life and continue sporadically throughout life. It has been estimated that 10% to 20% of women experience a urinary tract infection at some time in their lives.

The incidence of infection peaks at various times during life and is associated with both age and sex. Females are more susceptible to urinary tract infections throughout life except as infants and when the infection is catheter-associated. The incidence of infection is four times greater in infant males than in females. This ratio changes to 15:1 among preschool female children and increases to 30:1 for school-age children. It has been estimated that at least 5% of all females will have at least one urinary tract infection prior to completion of high school.

The highest incidence of infection occurs in young adult women with a female-to-male ratio of $> 30:1$. This increased incidence of both acute and recurrent urinary tract infection has been associated with sexual intercourse. Of the approximate 20% of women who have a urinary tract infection during their lifetime, only 3% experience recurrent infection. The explanation may be that the majority of infections in adult women are asymptomatic and resolve spontaneously. However, many women, even those with normal urinary tracts, will experience recurrent symptomatic infections.

Bacteriuria during pregnancy can be very serious to both the mother and the fetus, and infection occurs in 2% to 5% of pregnant women. Asymptomatic infections in this patient population are of great concern because untreated infections can lead to symptomatic pyelonephritis during the third trimester. Pregnant women who have had urinary tract infections during childhood are at greatest risk. These women have 26 times the attack rate of pyelonephritis in pregnancy and are more likely to have low birth weight deliveries and perinatal deaths. The most common cause of hospitalization during pregnancy is pyelonephritis, which is associated with premature deliveries and deficient infant development.

Urinary tract infections in males are uncommon after infancy until the age of 50 years. The major causes of infection among middle-aged men are prostatic obstruction and instrumentation. The cause of persistent and recurrent infection among men results from the inability to completely empty the bladder, causing organisms from the prostate to colonize the urinary tract. Sexual intercourse does not seem to be a common factor for urinary tract infection in men, although an association has been made.

Urinary tract infection in the elderly can be serious and an association has been made between infection and increased mortality. Elderly patients with cardiovascular diseases, dementia, diabetes mellitus, poor bladder emptying capability, urinary obstruction, and stroke are more likely to have urinary tract infections than patients in the same age group without these abnormalities. Boscia and Kaye have suggested that it may be these diseases, rather than the bacteriuria per se, that result in the decreased survival rate.

In contrast to young adults in whom bacteriuria is 30 times more frequent in females than in males, the ratio of infection for patients over the age of 65 dramatically decreases. By the age of 70 years, the incidence of infections in men equals or exceeds that in women. An increased incidence of pyelonephritis has been associated with urinary obstruction in both sexes in the elderly.

Use of urinary catheters is common in acute care hospitals, nursing homes, and chronic care facilities. The urinary catheter, which is a relatively simple tube used to aid in the collection of urine, also allows microorganisms to enter the urinary system; eventually, all catheterized patients become bacteriuric. The risk of acquiring a urinary tract infection associated with catheterization ranges from 1% to 5% after a single brief catheterization, to 100% with an indwelling catheter draining into an open system for longer than 4 days. During the 1960s, closed catheter systems were introduced and they now have become the standard for patients requiring indwelling urethral catheters. Use of a closed system has decreased the risk of infection, however, infection still occurs approximately 20% of the time.

MICROORGANISMS ASSOCIATED WITH URINARY TRACT INFECTIONS

The most frequent causes of urinary tract infections are bacteria, and facultative, aerobic, gram-negative bacilli predominate. Although gram-negative bacilli predominate among all patient populations, gram-positive cocci are responsible for large numbers of infections among hospitalized and institutionalized patients. Table 48-1 lists the various clinical manifestations associated with urinary tract infections and the microorganisms associated with these infections. In an acute care teaching hospital, *Escherichia coli* was the most common isolate. This microorganism is by far the most common isolate among all patient populations, including young adults, pregnant women, the elderly, males with prostatitis, and patients with catheter-associated

Table 48-1   Clinical manifestations and microorganisms associated with various types of urinary tract infections

Infection type	Clinical manifestation	Microorganisms associated with infection	Significant colony count (CFU/ml)
UPPER URINARY TRACT			
Pyelonephritis	Acute: fever, chills, flank pain, nausea, vomiting, WBC casts, tissue invasion		$\geq 10^5$
	Chronic: asymptomatic, mild or acute, presence of lesions, WBC casts		
	Gram-negative bacilli*		
	Staphylococcus aureus		
	Coagulase-negative staphylococci		
	Candida spp.		
	Mycobacterium spp.		
	Mycoplasma hominis		
LOWER URINARY TRACT			
Cystitis	Symptomatic: dysuria, frequent urination	*Escherichia coli** Other gram-negative bacilli*	$\geq 10^5$
	Asymptomatic	*Enterococcus* spp. Coagulase-negative staphylococci	
Urethritis	Dysuria, frequent urination	*Escherichia coli** *Chlamydia trachomatis* *Neisseria gonorrhoeae* *Staphylococcus saprophyticus* *Trichomonas vaginalis* Herpes simplex virus, type 2 *Candida albicans*	$\geq 10^2$
Prostatitis	Acute: fever, chills, back pain Chronic: asymptomatic or acute	≥Gram-negative bacilli* *Ureaplasma urealyticum* *Chlamydia trachomatis*	$\geq 10^3$

*Common isolates.

infections. *Enterococcus* spp., *Pseudomonas aeruginosa,* and *Candida* spp. are present most often in catheter-associated infections. *Enterococcus* spp., an organism commonly found in prostatitis, are common agents of nosocomial urinary infections and are isolated more frequently in males. *Proteus mirabilis* is also more frequently isolated from males at this institution and similar findings have been reported by others.

Streptococcus agalactiae (group B streptococci), an uncommon cause of urinary tract infection, may account for 5% of infections in pregnant females. Although streptococci may be the predominate gram-positive agent of urinary tract infections, the increasing significance of staphylococcal infections has been recognized in recent years. *Staphylococcus aureus* has usually been considered the pathogenic species and coagulase-negative staphylococci have been considered the contaminants or colonizers. However, the pathogenicity of the coagulase-negative staphylococcal species has also been recognized in recent years. *Staphylococcus saprophyticus* is a known urinary tract pathogen, found especially in young women. The incidence of infection may be as high as 30% in young female outpatients between the ages of 16 and 25 years old, and it appears to have a seasonal association, with peaks occurring in late summer and early fall. Other species of coagulase-negative cocci have also been associated with urinary tract infections, and their incidence also has been increasing during recent years. Patients at risk include males undergoing urologic procedures, those with underlying urinary tract pathology, and catheterized patients. During catheterization, the bladder becomes colonized, and if predisposing factors are present, infection with coagulase-negative staphylococci may occur. *Staphylococcus aureus* urinary tract infection is more commonly associated with urinary tract obstruction, neoplasm, and manipulation.

Anaerobic bacteria as agents of urinary tract infection are uncommon. If routine aerobic cultures are negative and there is good clinical reason to suspect anaerobic bacteriuria, urine should be collected by suprapubic aspiration to avoid any chance of contamination. The incidence of anaerobic bacteriuria is less than 2% in patients with significant bacteriuria.

Some microorganisms causing urinary tract infections are not isolated on routine culture media or detected by some of the rapid urine screening methods. Although uncommon, these microorganisms have been implicated in infection of the urinary system. These organisms include *Campylobacter* spp., *Chlamydia trachomatis, Gardnerella vaginalis, Haemophilis influenzae, Legionella pneumophilia, Mycobacterium* spp., *Mycoplasma hominis, Salmonella* spp., *Shigella* app., and *Ureaplasma urealyticum. Chlamydia trachomatis* has been associated with the acute urethral syndrome in young adult women and nongonococcal urethritis in men. This organism has been isolated from a majority of patients with chronic prostatitis as well as from women with cystourethritis. Both *Mycoplasma hominis* and *Ureaplasma urealyticum* have been associated with prostatitis, and *M. hominis* has been described as the causative agent in urinary tract infections of patients with acute pyelonephritis.

Kidney infections caused by *Mycobacterium* spp. can be serious and usually have their primary site in the lung. The organism is spread hematogenously and causes stricture formation, resulting in frequency of urination, hematuria, pain, and, in severe infections, kidney failure and death. Although uncommon, fungi, viruses, and the protozoan *Trichomonas vaginalis* can also cause infection of the urinary tract. The history of a new sex partner may suggest a sexually transmitted infection such as *T. vaginalis, C. trachomatis,* or herpes simplex virus.

Bacteria are definitely the leading cause of urinary tract infections and the most frequently isolated agents in most patient populations. However, the significance of fastidious microorganisms such as anaerobes, chlamydia, fungi, mycobacteria, protozoa, and viruses cannot be ignored. Although unusual, these organisms have been isolated with varying frequency from both symptomatic and asymptomatic individuals.

LABORATORY ANALYSES

Laboratory analysis of a urinary tract infection may involve determination of the presence or absence of the etiologic microorganism and/or the presence or absence of leukocytes (WBCs). A urine specimen is usually submitted for routine urinalysis, including a microscopic examination for bacteria. Although the urinalysis results may suggest infection, they are not confirmatory. When the routine urinalysis procedure includes the microscopic examination of urinary sediment, it should be well defined and standardized. Otherwise, the determination of bacteriuria, and more important, pyuria may be unreliable.

Determination of bacteriuria and pyuria are performed on urine specimens from patients with acute symptoms of infection, as a follow-up to treatment, as part of a septic work-up, to monitor urinary catheters, for prostatitis, and to determine the presence of blood and protein in urine.

In order to establish the etiology of infection, consideration should be given to specimen collection and transport, rapid test methods that can be performed as screening procedures, available culture methods, and the significance of the leukocytes and the microorganism(s) isolated.

SPECIMEN COLLECTION AND TRANSPORT

Urine specimens are collected: for culture from patients with urinary symptoms of urgency, frequency, and dysuria; to rule out sepsis; as a follow-up to antimicrobial therapy; to monitor adverse effects of urinary catheters; and on asymptomatic patients in high-risk groups (e.g., pregnant women and the elderly). The methods of collection include suprapubic bladder aspiration, catheterization, and voided midstream urine specimens.

Suprapubic bladder aspiration yields the most accurate and reliable results, however, this method involves an invasive procedure and should be performed by qualified physicians. Using sterile surgical techniques, urine is aspirated from the bladder using a needle and syringe. The specimens obtained by this method are a true reflection of bladder urine and, therefore, any organism recovered is considered significant. Catheterization is also an invasive procedure for obtaining urine specimens; there is always the possibility of introducing bacteria from the perineum, vagina, and urethra into the bladder when using this collection method and the risk of nosocomial urinary tract infections must be considered. Collection of urine by voiding is the simplest and most commonly employed method. However, if appropriate cleansing techniques of the external genitalia are not employed, especially with females and uncircumcised males, the specimen may be contaminated with the normal microbial flora from the skin, urethra, and external genitalia. To minimize the possibility of contamination, collection instructions should be provided to the patient, especially the female patient. Cleansing is unnecessary for males except if uncircumcised, because cleansing of the external genitalia does not significantly improve specimen quality.

The first voided morning specimen should be collected. If this is not possible, urine should be allowed to remain in the bladder for as long as possible prior to collection. This allows the organisms to increase in number, therefore providing more accurate laboratory results, especially if the urine is to be examined by rapid screening procedures.

A special collection procedure has been described for males with suspected chronic prostatitis. Using this method, three separate samples are collected from the patient: at the beginning of urination (urethral sample), after 10 to 15 ml have been voided (bladder sample), after prostatic massage (semen sample), and, if semen is not expressed, a voided urine is collected following the massage. This collection process aids the physician in establishing the specific type of infection: urethritis, cystitis, or prostatitis.

The collection of urine specimens from infants, pediatric patients, and incontinent patients present special problems. House officers or skilled nurses are best suited to obtain such specimens and initiate their transport to the laboratory.

Once the urine specimen has been collected, it should be transported to the laboratory as quickly as possible for processing. If transport is delayed, urine specimens must be refrigerated. The number of colony forming units per milliliter (CFU/ml) may greatly increase if the specimen is held at room temperature for longer than 2 hours. Use of a urine transport tube containing a preservative has been advocated as an alternative to refrigeration. A basic acid-glycerol-sodium formate preservative may have an inhibiting effect on some microorganisms, especially *E. coli*, and therefore jeopardizes the accuracy of bacteriuria detection. A lyophilized form of the boric acid-glycerol-sodium formate may be less inhibitory to microorganisms than the liquid form.

LABORATORY METHODS FOR DETECTION OF BACTERIURIA AND PYURIA
Culture methods

A variety of methods has been employed for isolation and quantitation of microorganisms in urine specimens (Table 48-2). These include tube dilution pour plate and spread plate methods, the flood plate method, the dipstick and dipslide method, and the semiquantitative calibrated loop method. Calibrated platinum and nickel loops are commercially available that deliver approximately 0.001, 0.01, and 0.003 ml of urine sample. The definitive test for enumeration of bacteriuria was the tube dilution pour plate method; in 1960 the calibrated loop method was proposed for plating urine specimens from asymptomatic patients. However, because of its simplicity and despite its varied accuracy, the calibrated loop method has become the most widely used method for quantitating CFU/ml in urine specimens. Users of this method should be aware of its variability associated with the sample volume, the container size, and the angle of sampling.

For the culture method, selection of media should include agar plates that allow for the growth of commonly isolated facultative, gram-positive cocci and gram-negative bacilli (Table 48-1). Use of a broth medium is not recommended since it does not allow for quantitation of microorganisms and, in most cases, low count bacteriuria ($<10^3$ CFU/ml) is not considered significant. However, when detection of low count bacteriuria (10^2 CFU/ml) is required, lower di-

Table 48-2 Microbiologic approach to urine bacteriology

Parameter	Method/interpretation	Comment
Microscopic exam		
Gram stain	≥1 organism/OIF* = ≥10^5 CFU/ml	Uncentrifuged urine
Hemacytometer count	≥8 WBC/mm³ (μl)	Equivalent to leukocyte excretion rate (≥4 × 10^5 WBC/hour)
Selection of media	5% Sheep blood agar	
	MacConkey or eosin-methylene blue (EMB) agar	
	Optional: colistin-nalidixic blood agar (CNA)	For isolation of streptococci or yeast
Quantitation of cultures		
Pour plate	1. 9.9 ml saline + 0.1 ml urine (mix) (10^{-2})	Classical standard method; rarely used; cumbersome to perform
	2. 9.9 ml saline + 0.1 ml of 1st dilution (10^{-4})	
	3. Add 1 ml of each of above dilution to 150-mm Petri dish	
	4. Pour melted agar, mix, incubate overnight at 35°C	
Surface streak	Calibrated loop; 0.001 ml or 0.01 ml; 95% platinum and 5% rhodium	Easiest, most widely used
Incubation	Overnight at 35°C to 37°C aerobically	Prolonged incubation only if clinical condition and Gram's stain do not correlate with culture

*Oil immersion field.

lutions of urine should be plated rather than using a broth medium for isolation. The majority of microorganisms causing urinary tract infections are isolated from cultures incubated aerobically overnight. However, an additional 24 hours of incubation may be required to isolate some microorganisms that may be partially inhibited by antimicrobials.

Although the culture method allows for the isolation and enumeration of the etiologic agents of urinary tract infections, it does not provide for the same-day reporting of negative specimens. For this reason, rapid urine screening tests have been introduced. Many factors have influenced the development of these tests, including the number of samples tested, the need for rapid turnaround time for test results, and the need for cost-effective testing. Rapid reporting of negative specimens eliminates the need for culture and, therefore, allows the microbiologist to spend more time on the positive specimens. Some of the rapid screening methods also enable the detection of pyuria, an important finding in the presence of low-count or negative bacteriuria. The presence of pyuria also helps differentiate colonization from infection.

A number of rapid methods for detection of urinary tract infections are available and have been reviewed in detail elsewhere. These include microscopic, enzymatic, colorimetric filtration, and photometric methods. A brief description of some of the more widely used methods follows and they are summarized in Table 48-3.

Microscopic methods

The Gram's stain is a rapid and reliable microscopic method for estimating bacteriuria at $\geq 10^5$ CFU/ml; the presence of at least one organism per oil immersion field from an uncentrifuged specimen correlates with significant bacteriuria. The method is also simple to perform. Despite these advantages, it does not have widespread use as a urine screen. Its decreased sensitivity at colony counts of $<10^5$ CFU/ml may be one reason for its limited use. Another problem is that it is a subjective test and it can be a tedious and time-consuming procedure because there may be very little dif-

ference between a positive and negative test. Also, it has no cost advantage over other screens that require more objective interpretation, and it is less sensitive than the colorimetric filtration methods for detecting clinically significant bacteriuria. Although this method may not be practical for routine use, it should be available upon request of the physician. Positive findings of bacteria and WBCs may guide the physician in initiating antimicrobial therapy.

The most widely used method for detection of pyuria is the microscopic examination of urinary sediment; however, this procedure is not reliable unless it is standardized. The method variables include the volume of urine centrifuged, suspended, and examined; the speed and time of centrifugation; and observer bias. The method lacks precision and does not correlate with the leukocyte excretion rate. Simpler and more reliable methods have been described for measuring pyuria from uncentrifuged urine. The presence of ≥ 8 WBC/mm^3 correlates with significant pyuria.

In recent years, microscopic examination of urine has been automated. The Yellow IRIS (International Remote Imaging Systems, Inc, Chatsworth, Calif) incorporates a flow microscope, in which an uncentrifuged urine specimen is presented to a video camera. Aliquots of the following specimens are taken as stop-motion pictures by the video camera. The resulting pictures are digitized and delivered to the image processing computer, which recognizes the individual particle images by size.

Enzymatic methods

Enzymatic tests have been used as bacteriuria and pyuria screens primarily as part of the urinalysis screen rather than the microbial evaluation. These tests are based on the detection of specific enzymes associated with bacteria and WBCs and usually are available in dipsticks. The most widely used tests include detection of catalase, glucose oxidase, leukocyte esterase, and nitrate reductase. Although these tests are rapid and inexpensive screening methods, a high number of false-negative and false-positive results can occur. Some of the factors that contribute to low sensitivity

Table 48-3 Rapid urine screening methods*

Method	Detection time (min)	Sensitivity (%) CFU/ml			Detects pyuria	Cost per test ($)†	Automated
		10⁵	10⁴	10³			
Microscopic							
Gram stain	2	96	90	73	Yes	1.17	No
Enzymatic							
Chemstrip LN	2	85	—	70	Yes	0.44	No
Uriscreen	2			95**	Yes	0.80	No
UTIscreen	15	96	86	72	No	0.97	Yes
Filtration							
Bac-T-Screen	2	96	85	76	Yes	1.08	Yes
FiltraCheck-UTI	2	95	89	84	Yes	1.25	No
Photometry							
Autobac	≤6h	97	90		No	0.60	Yes
Vitek	≤13h	96	91		No	1.00	Yes

*Data from cited literature.
†Includes technical time.
**Includes pyuria

and specificity are low concentration of enzyme in the specimen, the presence of interfering substances, and misinterpretation of borderline results by the observer. For these reasons, a single test method should not be used alone for bacteriuria and pyuria screens. Combination testing of two or more enzymes has been shown to improve the overall sensitivity of these methods. Overall sensitivity of bacteria and WBC may be improved when these tests are used in combination with another urine screen. The Chemstrip LN (Bio-Dynamics, Division of Boehringer Mannheim Diagnostics, Indianapolis, Ind) and Uriscreen (API, Analytab Products, Inc.) are two tests that detect two or more enzymes.

Use of bioluminescence as a urine screen was described as early as 1944. Since that time, the technology and methodology have developed into practical, easy-to-use urine screens. The method is based on the enzymatic bioluminescent reaction of adenosine 5'-triphosphate (ATP) with luciferin and luciferase, that is measured by a luminometer. One such method, the UTIscreen (Los Alamos Diagnostics, Los Alamos, NM), compares favorably with other screening methods with respect to sensitivity, predictive value of a negative test, ease of performance, and cost. Additionally, it is possible to perform batch tests, the interpretation is objective, and this method has a higher specificity than the enzyme dipstick and colorimetric filtration methods.

Colorimetric filtration

Use of filtration and staining has been described for the rapid detection of bacteriuria. A sample of urine is passed through a filter, and if cells are present, they are trapped on the surface of the filter. Safranin O dye is used to stain the trapped cells. Acetic acid is used as both the urine diluent and the decolorizer to remove the dye from the filter fibers. This procedure has been adapted for use with a semiautomated instrument, the Bac-T-Screen (Vitek Systems, Inc, Hazelwood, Mo) and a manual filtration device, the FiltraCheck-UTI (Applied Polytechnology, Inc, Houston, Tex). Both urine screening methods have the ability to rapidly detect clinically significant bacteriuria with a high degree of accuracy. Initial evaluation of these methods reported high false-positive findings; however, modification of the decolorizing reagent has improved specificity.

Photometric methods

The first generation of bacteriuria screens utilized changes in light transmission for detection of growth. This method differs from those previously described, in that growth is required prior to detection and, as a result, detection times are delayed from 30 minutes up to 13 hours. Three commonly available instruments, the Autobac System (Organon Teknika Corp, Durham, NC), the Vitek System (Vitek Systems, Inc), and the ARx Avantage (Abbott Laboratories, Irving, Tex) employ this principle of detection. These methods compare favorably to culture. The need for incubation may limit their use as urine screens in some laboratories, although each instrument has other applications, including identification and antimicrobial susceptibility testing. Also, interfacing these instruments with laboratory and hospital information systems may provide results automatically without technical intervention.

Endotoxin tests

The *Limulus* amoebocyte lysate endotoxin test has been described for detection of gram-negative bacteriuria. The major disadvantage of this test is that gram-positive pathogens are not detected. Although the method has a high sensitivity for detection of gram-negative bacilli, it cannot be used alone as a urine screen. Combination testing, to include a parameter for detecting gram-positive organisms, would make this an excellent rapid screen.

INTERPRETATION OF TEST RESULTS

The clinical microbiology laboratory must carefully consider the demographics of patient population served to determine the best interpretive approach in the evaluation of urine specimens being analyzed for evidence of UTI. Numerous studies have established certain criteria that should be applied to this decision-making process. Existing data strongly support the criteria listed in Table 48-1 for pyelonephritis, cystitis, urethritis, and prostatitis. Additionally, selection of an accurate and effective criterion must be based on the prevalence of disease. It may be necessary to select more than one criterion to evaluate these specimens.

Cumitech 2A and Table 48-4 present guidelines for interpretation of urine culture results. The Cumitech guidelines are based on the principle that four factors (number

Table 48-4   Interpretive guidelines for urine cultures

Colony count (CFU/ml)	Clinical condition collection method	Organism(s) present	Work-up required
0	—	None	None
10^2	Symptomatic female*	Pure culture of gram-negative rods	Organism identification
10^3	Catheter urine; symptomatic male	Pure culture of probable pathogens	Organism identification
10^4	Catheter urine	Two species of probable pathogens	Organism identification
		≥3 Species	None; report multiple species present
10^5	Voided urine	Pure culture of probable pathogens if ≥2 species are present	Organism identification
			None; report multiple species present
≥1	Suprapubic bladder aspirates	All species at any concentration	Organism identification

*Inoculation of media is usually performed using 0.001 ml of urine, therefore, 10^3 is the lowest achievable colony count. Inoculation of 0.01 ml of urine is performed following physician's request.

of isolates, density of isolates, type of specimen, and clinical information) must be considered to assess the significance of an isolate(s) and to determine the amount of time and effort, and the cost that should be expended to characterize the isolate. These guidelines suggest that when three or more different colony types are evident, as many as two organisms should be identified, especially if the specimen was collected by instrumentation. These guidelines can be used to develop flow diagrams (algorithms) to assist with specimen identification.

Keeping in mind that quantitative urine cultures alone cannot be used to detect infection in some patient populations unless lower colony counts are considered, a rapid screen may be a more practical approach than the culture method. Although 10^5 CFU/ml may be used as the standard interpretive breakpoint for most patient populations, it may be necessary to lower that breakpoint to 10^2 CFU/ml when evaluating cultures from young, symptomatic females. Also, incorporating the detection of pyuria may be important in making the diagnosis of a urinary tract infection. The interpretive protocol should be practical, efficient, and cost effective, and most important, it should be compatible with the patient population. Clearly, it is of utmost importance for the medical and laboratory staff to work together in establishing how urine specimens should be collected, transported to the laboratory, processed, and reported.

SUGGESTED READING

Boscia JA and Kaye D: Asymptomatic bacteriuria in the elderly. In Andriole VT, editor: Urinary tract infections, Infect Dis Clin N Amer 1:893, 1987.

Clarridge JE, Pezzlo MT, and Vosti KL: Cumitech 2A, Laboratory diagnosis of urinary tract infections, Weissfeld AL (coordinating editor) Washington, DC, 1987, American Society of Microbiology.

Johnson JR and Stamm WE: Diagnosis and treatment of acute urinary tract infections. In Andriole VT, editor: Urinary tract infections, Infect Dis Clin N Amer 1:773, 1987.

Kass EH: Horatio at the orifice: the significance of bacteriuria, J Infect Dis 138:546, 1978.

Kaye D and Santoro J: Urinary tract infection. In Mandell GL, Douglas RG, and Bennett JE, editors: Principles and practice of infectious disease, New York, 1979, John Wiley & Sons.

Kunin CM: Detection, prevention and management of urinary tract infections, Philadelphia, 1987, Lea & Febiger.

Meares EM: Prostatitis: a review, Urol Clin N Amer 2:3, 1975.

Pazin GJ and Braude A: Pyelonephritis. In Hoeprich PD, editor: Infectious diseases: a modern treatise of infectious processes, Hagerstown, Md, 1977, Harper & Row.

Pezzlo MT: Detection of urinary tract infections by rapid methods, Clin Microbiol Rev 1:268, 1988.

Sobel JD: Pathogenesis of urinary tract infections; Host defenses. In Andriole VT, editor: Urinary tract infections, Infect Dis Clin N Amer 1:751, 1987.

Stamm WE and others: Causes of acute urethral syndrome in women, N Engl J Med 303:409, 1980.

49 Blood specimens

Melvin P. Weinstein

Infections of the cardiovascular system are among the most serious encountered in clinical medicine. Many such infections are characterized by the presence of bacteremia. Indeed, bacteremia is the common denominator in infective endocarditis and other endovascular infections, and no discussion of endocarditis should be undertaken without an understanding of the pathogenesis and diagnosis of bacteremia.

BACTEREMIA

Invasion of the bloodstream by living microorganisms occurs either as a consequence of direct entry via needles and various other intravascular devices, or from extravascular primary foci of infection via the lymphatic system. The latter circumstance is an indication that the patient's host defenses have failed to contain the infection at its primary site, or that the physician has failed to remove, drain, or otherwise adequately treat the primary infection. Ordinarily, a sudden influx of microorganisms into the blood is cleared in minutes to hours, due in large measure to efficient phagocytosis by macrophages in the liver and spleen. However, prompt clearance of microorganisms does not occur when overwhelming infection or an intravascular focus of infection is present.

Conceptually, it is useful to think of bacteremia as either transient, intermittent, or continuous. Transient bacteremia is most common and occurs after manipulation of infected tissue such as abscesses and furuncles, during certain surgical procedures, after instrumentation of contaminated mucosal surfaces (e.g., dental procedures, cystoscopy, and gastrointestinal endoscopies), and at the onset of infections such as bacterial pneumonia, acute osteomyelitis, septic arthritis, and bacterial meningitis. Intermittent bacteremia—that is, bacteremia that occurs, clears, and recurs in the same patient due to the same microorganism(s)—is associated characteristically with the presence of an undrained abscess. Continuous bacteremia is a key clinical and laboratory feature of infective endocarditis and other endovascular infections (e.g., suppurative thrombophlebitis, mycotic aneurysm), and continuous bacteremia also is present in the early weeks of typhoid fever and brucellosis.

The sources of bacteremia are diverse. Most commonly, the primary foci for bacteremia are infections in the respiratory tract, the genitourinary tract, or the abdomen (e.g, biliary infection, bowel disease, intraabdominal abscess). Other primary foci for bacteremia are the skin and soft tissues, including surgical and traumatic wounds or burns, and indwelling intravascular or genitourinary catheters. Difficult to explain but nonetheless true, even after intense clinical evaluations, is the inability to determine the source for bacteremia in one quarter to one third of all episodes.

Not unexpectedly, the etiologic agents causing bloodstream infections reflect the microbial flora associated with the common primary foci of infection. The most common microorganism causing bacteremia in most studies has been *Escherichia coli,* which generally resides in the gastrointestinal and female genitourinary tracts. Other enteric gram-negative rods also frequently cause bacteremia. The most common gram-positive blood pathogen is *Staphylococcus aureus,* and streptococci also are common isolates. The coagulase-negative staphylococci such as *Staphylococcus epidermidis,* which are normal flora of the skin and frequent contaminants when grown from blood cultures, have become more important as pathogens in association with the increased use of long-term, indwelling, intravascular catheters and the presence or implantation of prosthetic materials and devices (e.g., dialysis shunts, joint and vascular prostheses, and artificial heart valves). Decisions regarding the clinical significance of coagulase-negative staphylococcal isolates from blood cultures may be very difficult.

Ultimately, the epidemiology of bacteremia in any laboratory or institution depends upon the types of patients being cultured. For example, in pediatric medical centers, *Haemophilus influenzae* and *Streptococcus pneumoniae* are frequent isolates, whereas gram-negative bacteria are less common. By contrast, microbiology laboratories in institutions with many adult surgical and gynecologic patients are more likely to isolate enteric gram-negative rods and anaerobic bacteria, the common microflora of the bowel and female genitourinary tract.

BLOOD CULTURES

The means by which bacteremia is detected is the blood culture. Quite simply, a blood culture is obtained by venipuncture in a sterile fashion and, in most commercially available blood culture systems, blood is inoculated to two culture bottles containing broth media and atmospheric conditions that can support the growth of aerobic, facultative, and anaerobic pathogens. Many variables influence the sensitivity of blood cultures, and alternatives to broth-based culture systems, such as lysis centrifugation, are commercially available. The interested reader is referred to the reports of Aronson and Bor, Reller and others, Tilton, and Washington and Ilstrup for more detailed discussion of issues and controversies in blood culturing, all of which cannot be reviewed here.

One of the most important, if not the most important, factors in the detection of bacteremia is the volume of blood that is cultured (Box 49-1). Studies at the University of Colorado Medical School and the Mayo Clinic have shown a direct relationship between the volume of blood cultured in adults and the yield of positive culture results. For example, the results reported by Ilstrup and Washington demonstrated a 61% increase in yield when the volume of blood cultured was increased from 10 to 30 ml. Based on these data, the recommended volume of blood per culture from adults now is 20 to 30 ml; in no case should less than 10 ml per culture be obtained since too many bacteremias will be missed. Fewer data are available from children. However, it has been shown that cultures of <1 ml of blood result in a lower yield than cultures of 1 ml or more, and volumes of 1 to 5 ml per culture usually are recommended.

The number of blood cultures needed to detect bacteremia depends in part upon the volume of blood obtained per culture. When 10 ml of blood were obtained per culture at the Mayo Clinic, the first culture detected 80% of bacteremias, the first two cultures detected 88%, and the first three cultures detected 99%. When 15 ml of blood were obtained per culture at the University of Colorado Health Science Center, the first culture detected 91% of bacteremias, and the first two blood cultures detected more than 99% of bacteremias. Thus, fewer blood cultures are necessary to detect bacteremia when larger volumes of blood are obtained with each culture. An important corollary is that more than three blood cultures from a patient during an episode of suspected bacteremia seldom are necessary.

As a general rule, single blood cultures are discouraged since the volume of blood obtained often will be suboptimal for detecting bacteremia and interpretation of a positive result may be more difficult for the clinician. Indeed, one of the most reliable means used to distinguish between contaminated cultures and true infection is to evaluate the results of two or more blood cultures obtained in sequence by separate venipunctures. For example, the significance of a single positive blood culture growing *S. epidermidis*, a viridans streptococcus, or a diphtheroid is unknown. However, if other blood cultures obtained in sequence are negative, the isolates almost certainly represent contamination (Fig. 49-1). Alternatively, if subsequent blood cultures are all positive, there is strong evidence of true bacteremia and, in appropriate clinical circumstances, endocarditis or other intravascular infection (Fig. 49-1).

The interval between sequential blood cultures depends in large measure on the urgency of the clinical situation. When patients are seriously ill and need antimicrobial therapy promptly, blood cultures may be obtained minutes apart, whereas in less urgent situations, blood cultures may be obtained at intervals of 1 hour or more. Recommendations for obtaining blood cultures in specific clinical situations are as follows:

1. Acute infection (for example, bacterial pneumonia or meningitis, or suspected septicemia from an unknown focus): Obtain two separate blood cultures (separate venipunctures) before starting empiric antimicrobial therapy.
2. Fever of uncertain etiology in an otherwise stable patient: Obtain two blood cultures over several hours. If, after 1 to 2 days of incubation, these cultures are negative and the patient's clinical status continues to suggest an infectious cause, obtain two more blood cultures. If these remain negative, bacteremia is exceedingly unlikely, and further blood cultures will have little or no incremental yield. Diagnostic studies in addition to blood cultures should, of course, be undertaken.

Box 49-1 Blood cultures: selected clinical issues

Volume of blood: Adults: 10-30 ml per culture
Infants and small children: 1-5 ml per culture
Number of blood cultures: Adults: volume-dependent; 10-ml culture, minimum of 3; 15-30–ml culture, minimum of 2
Children: Two sets recommended

Timing:

Acute infection in which therapy is urgent: two cultures 5 to 15 minutes apart

Fever in an otherwise stable patient: two cultures several hours apart

Acute infective endocarditis: three cultures during first 1 to 2 hours of evaluation

Subacute infective endocarditis: three cultures during first 24 hours of evaluation

---

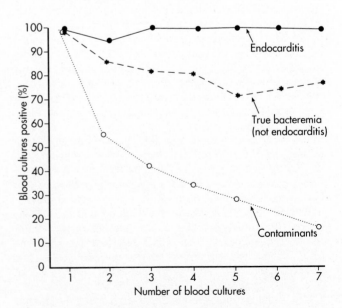

Fig. 49-1 Patterns of positivity in successive blood cultures: evidence of the diagnostic importance of separate cultures.

3. Acute infective endocarditis: Obtain three blood cultures during the first hour or two of evaluation and begin empiric antimicrobial therapy.

4. Subacute infective endocarditis: Obtain three blood cultures during the first 24 hours of evaluation. If these remain negative after 2 days of incubation, obtain two or three more blood cultures.

5. Suspected infective endocarditis in patients who have received prior antimicrobial therapy during the weeks immediately preceding evaluation: Obtain two blood cultures on the first day of evaluation. If cultures remain negative, obtain two additional cultures daily on the second and third days of evaluation. Although prior antibiotic therapy may cause blood cultures to be negative, more often growth is just delayed, and longer incubation times are necessary.

The technique for obtaining blood cultures centers on careful aseptic preparation of the culture site to minimize the chance that microorganisms that inhabit the skin will contaminate the blood culture (Box 49-2). Usually, contaminants should be present in fewer than 3% of blood cultures obtained in any given laboratory or institution. The venipuncture site should be cleansed with 70% isopropyl or ethyl alcohol, followed by 10% povidone-iodine (1% available iodine) that should be allowed to dry for 1 to 2 minutes before the actual venipuncture. The stoppers or rubber diaphragms of the blood culture bottles also should be cleansed with alcohol prior to inoculation. Blood may be obtained with needle and syringe or a Vacutainer-type device (Becton-Dickinson Vacutainer Systems, Rutherford, NJ). If the Vacutainer-type device has been used, blood is drawn directly into a transport tube or, alternatively, to a culture bottle designed to fit the device. Because of the increased probability of contamination and the difficulty in interpreting the significance of a positive result, blood cultures never should be obtained from indwelling venous or arterial catheters. Finally, there is no evidence that arterial blood cultures have any clinical advantage over venous blood cultures.

Box 49-2 Blood cultures: selected technical issues

Media: Many enriched broths are satisfactory (e.g., Trypticase soy®, brain-heart infusion, Brucella, supplemented peptone, Columbia)

Anticoagulant: Sodium polyanetholsulfonate (SPS) used in all commercial media in United States

Blood-to-broth dilution: 1:5 to 1:10 is generally recommended

Agitation: Recommended for aerobic bottle during first 24 to 48 hours of incubation

Subcultures: Recommended for macroscopically negative aerobic bottle, after first overnight incubation, to chocolate agar. Not needed for instrumented detection systems. Routine terminal subcultures are not necessary.

Mycobacterial blood cultures: Lysis centrifugation (ISO-LATOR, Wampole Laboratories) or radiometric (BACTEC) most sensitive systems

Fungal blood cultures: Lysis centrifugation (ISOLATOR) most sensitive system

---

Most microbiology laboratories incubate blood cultures for 7 days, based on data suggesting little value in longer incubation times for routine blood cultures. However, under special circumstances such as suspected fungemia or endocarditis, longer incubation periods may be desirable. Indeed, some authorities recommend a minimum incubation period of 2 weeks when endocarditis or fungemia is suspected.

INFECTIVE ENDOCARDITIS

Infection of the heart valves or endocardium, the latter usually occurring in areas of turbulent blood flow related to congenital or acquired cardiac defects, is termed infective endocarditis. Bacteria cause the great majority of these infections, but fungi, chlamydiae, rickettsiae, and possibly viruses also may be pathogenic agents of endocarditis. Endocarditis has fascinated and challenged generations of clinicians, in part because of its extraordinarily varied presentations and also because of the difficulties in managing patients with this infection.

Although there is great interest in endocarditis among physicians and clinical microbiologists, the disease actually is relatively uncommon. Most cases of endocarditis occur in adults, and the disease is quite rare in children. In recent years, the age of patients with endocarditis has increased, and hospital-acquired endocarditis associated with devices such as central intravascular catheters and pacemaker wires has become more frequent. Still, the most important clinical problems that predispose to infective endocarditis are rheumatic and congenital heart disease, intravenous drug abuse, age-related calcification of valves, and other lesions such as mural thrombi or, as more recently recognized, mitral valve prolapse.

The primary event in the pathogenesis of infective endocarditis is usually a transient and asymptomatic bacteremia. Typical examples include the transient bacteremias associated with dental, bowel, or genitourinary manipulations. In all probability, infection first occurs in an area of endothelial damage where there is a high pressure gradient across a narrow orifice, for example, the atrial side of a calcified regurgitant mitral valve. Although the actual sequence of events is not completely known, a reasonable hypothesis would suggest that microthrombi consisting of platelets and fibrin implant at an area of endocardial irregularity, resulting in a small, sterile vegetation that provides a focus for seeding during a transient bacteremia. Once microorganisms are established in the vegetation, bacteremia becomes continuous, and the lesion enlarges as more platelets, fibrin, and microorganisms adhere to it.

The terms *acute* and *subacute* have been used for many years to describe the clinical syndromes of endocarditis. In the pre-antibiotic era, these terms referred to the speed with which patients with endocarditis died. The terms remain useful clinically in the current era, but for different reasons; patients with subacute endocarditis often have insidiously progressive symptoms over weeks to months, whereas patients with acute endocarditis have an abrupt onset of symptoms and are toxic at the time of presentation. Although the characteristic syndromes of acute and subacute endocarditis will be described, it is important to realize that these syndromes are not mutually exclusive and that overlap occurs.

Acute infective endocarditis is characterized by sudden onset and a rapid course. High, spiking fever almost always is present and often is associated with shaking chills. Most patients with acute endocarditis do not have a history of underlying heart disease, and any valve may be involved. Intravenous drug abusers frequently get this form of endocarditis, and there is an increased frequency of right-sided valvular infection, especially the tricuspid valve, in these patients. Septic emboli from the infected vegetation are common, and patients may have multiple sites other than blood from which cultures are obtained and sent to the laboratory. *Staphylococcus aureus* is the most common etiologic agent of acute endocarditis.

In contrast to acute endocarditis, subacute endocarditis is characterized by an insidious onset and slow progression of symptoms. Fever is almost always present, but it is low grade and not associated with shaking chills. Most, but not all, patients have a history of some form of underlying heart disease, and the mitral and aortic valves most often are involved. Patients usually are not toxic, and septic emboli are less common than in acute endocarditis. However, other extracardiac manifestations of endocarditis such as enlargement of the spleen and the presence of petechiae on the distal extremities and in the conjunctivae or retina are more frequent than in acute endocarditis. Although many microorganisms have been reported to cause subacute endocarditis, the viridans group of streptococci continue to be the most common etiologic agents.

Endocarditis occurs not only on native heart valves. Patients with prosthetic heart valves have an increased risk of this infection, either shortly after implantation of the valve prosthesis or many months or years later. Prosthetic valve endocarditis that occurs within 2 months of implantation may be due to fungi, gram-negative bacilli, or other bacteria resistant to antimicrobial agents administered during the earlier hospitalization, and is associated with high mortality. Prosthetic valve endocarditis that occurs more than 2 months after implantation usually is caused by gram-positive cocci and diphtheroids, and is associated with lower mortality, although the infection still may be difficult to cure with antimicrobial agents alone.

An extraordinary number of different microorganisms have been implicated as the etiologic agents of infective endocarditis, but the great majority of infections, perhaps more than 75% to 80%, are due to streptococci and staphylococci. Historically, streptococci have been the most common causative agents, but staphylococci have become more common and now exceed streptococci in frequency in some institutions.

The viridans group of streptococci (note that viridans is not a species designation but rather a designation for a group of streptococci, all of which produce alpha [green] hemolysis on sheep blood agar) are the prototypic agents of subacute endocarditis. These microorganisms are normal flora of the oropharynx and the skin, and a history of dental manipulation within the prior 4 to 6 months often is obtained from a patient with viridans streptococcal endocarditis. Speciation of the viridans streptococci may be difficult and usually is not necessary. However, for the reasons outlined shortly, these microorganisms should be differentiated from the enterococci and nonenterococcal group D streptococci that may produce alpha hemolysis.

The nonenterococcal Lancefield group D streptococci, such as *Streptococcus bovis,* and the enterococci, most commonly *Enterococcus faecalis* (formerly *Streptococcus faecalis*) also are important causes of endocarditis, and differentiation of these group D strains is important both prognostically and therapeutically.

The normal habitats for the enterococci and nonenterococcal streptococci are the bowel and genitourinary tracts, and a history of disease of these regions or trauma to the bowel or genitourinary mucosa may be elicited. *Streptococcus bovis* has been demonstrated to be a marker for gastrointestinal malignancies, and all patients with *S. bovis* bacteremia should be evaluated for such lesions. Enterococcal endocarditis occurs with greater frequency in older males and women of childbearing age, perhaps related to the increased frequency of genitourinary procedures or disease in these patients. The enterococci, in contrast to most streptococci, are not killed by penicillins alone and require combination therapy with aminoglycosides for cure of endocarditis. The differentiation of these microorganisms should not be difficult. Although both *S. bovis* and the enterococci hydrolyze bile esculin, only the enterococci will grow in 6.5% sodium chloride. Since some viridans streptococcal strains also hydrolyze bile esculin and fail to grow in 6.5% sodium chloride, further testing is necessary to definitively identify *S. bovis.*

Some streptococcal strains causing endocarditis have special nutritional requirements and have proved difficult to isolate on solid culture media. These nutritionally variant strains require pyridoxal (vitamin B_6) and usually grow in the broth blood culture media but not on sheep blood agar or some lots of chocolate agar. Supplementation of agar with 0.001% pyridoxal will permit growth but may inhibit other microorganisms. As a useful alternative for isolation of these microorganisms, blood agar can be cross-streaked with *Staphylococcus aureus,* which will permit satelliting growth of the nutritionally variant streptococcus around the staphylococcal streak.

Although other streptococci can cause endocarditis, they are uncommon. In the pre-antibiotic era, *S. pneumoniae* was a frequent cause of endocarditis and produced a fulminant syndrome with valve destruction. Fortunately, pneumococcal endocarditis now is rare.

Both *Staphylococcus aureus* and the coagulase-negative staphylococci cause endocarditis, but the clinical manifestations of disease and underlying factors predisposing to infection usually are quite different. As mentioned earlier, *S. aureus* endocarditis represents the prototype of the "acute" syndrome and occurs with increased frequency in individuals who use illicit drugs intravenously. When *S. aureus* infects the mitral or aortic valves, a fulminant course with systemic emboli, metastatic foci of infection, and high mortality may be the result. In intravenous drug users, there is an increased incidence of right-sided valvular infection, more often involving the tricuspid valve. Patients with this syndrome have lower mortality and often a less severe course compared to patients with mitral or aortic valve (left-sided) endocarditis.

Endocarditis caused by coagulase-negative staphylococci, most commonly *S. epidermidis,* differs from *S. aureus* endocarditis in that its clinical syndrome is most often subacute and the valves infected more often are prosthetic than native. Indeed, *S. epidermidis* is a rare cause of native valve endocarditis but the most common cause of prosthetic valve endocarditis. These infections may be more problematic therapeutically because of the greater frequency of methicillin-resistance among coagulase-negative staphylococci and because infections involving foreign bodies often are more difficult to cure medically (i.e., without surgical removal of the device).

Despite the frequency with which gram-negative bacteria invade the bloodstream, they are relatively uncommon causes of endocarditis. The reasons for this paradox are not known completely but relate at least in part to the fact that gram-negative microorganisms do not adhere as well as gram-positive cocci to the fibrin-platelet microthrombi on the endocardium. Endocarditis due to gram-negative bacteria occurs primarily in addicts and in the early post-operative period after prosthetic valve implantation. The enteric gram-negative rods such as *Escherichia coli* are distinctly uncommon etiologic agents of endocarditis. Both *Pseudomonas aeruginosa* and *Serratia marcescens* have been reported with some frequency in drug addicts, although these infections have been reported most often from specific geographic areas (Detroit and San Francisco, respectively). Fastidious gram-negative bacteria that usually reside in the oropharynx such as *Haemophilus parainfluenzae, Haemophilus paraphrophilus, Haemophilis aphrophilus, Actinobacillus actinomycetemcomitans,* and *Cardiobacterium hominis,* as well as the nonpathogenic *Neisseria* spp. all may cause subacute endocarditis. The fastidious nature of some of these species is such that growth may be slow and the organisms undetectable unless blood cultures are incubated for more than the usual 7 days (see discussion that follows). *Neisseria gonorrhoeae,* an important etiologic agent of endocarditis in the pre-antibiotic era, still is seen occasionally and may cause a fulminant syndrome with valve destruction and high mortality.

Other bacteria are uncommon causes of endocarditis. Although a few cases of endocarditis due to *Bacillus* species, *Listeria monocytogenes,* and *Erysipelothrix rhusiopathiae* have been reported, the most important gram-positive rods are diphtheroid bacteria of the genus *Corynebacterium,* which may be important causes of prosthetic valve endocarditis. Anaerobic bacteria, particularly species of *Bacteroides* and *Fusobacterium,* also are rare causes of endocarditis.

The known nonbacterial etiologic agents of endocarditis include fungi, rickettsiae, and chlamydiae. Fungal endocarditis occurs in drug addicts, patients with prosthetic heart valves, and patients who have received long-term intravenous or antibiotic therapy. The most common agents are *Candida* and *Aspergillus* spp., but many other fungi can cause this infection. Diagnosis of fungal endocarditis may be made more difficult by the inability of some blood culture systems to detect these microorganisms. The rickettsia, *Coxiella burnetii,* causes Q fever endocarditis. This infection is more common in Australia, Great Britain, and Ireland, but has occurred in the United States. Endocarditis due to *Chlamydia psittaci,* the etiologic agent of psittacosis, also has been reported. Most recently, *Legionella pneumophila* has been reported to cause prosthetic valve endocarditis.

Some patients have a syndrome compatible with infective endocarditis, but the diagnosis cannot be confirmed micro-biologically. These patients sometimes are diagnosed as having "culture-negative" endocarditis, and the reasons for culture negativity have been the subject of much speculation and investigation. Certainly, many culture-negative endocarditis cases from the past would be detected in the current era using modern blood culture media, increased volumes of blood for culture, and incubation periods of at least 2 weeks. Nevertheless, culture-negative endocarditis will continue to occur rarely. Possible explanations for negative cultures include improper methods or processing, as already alluded to, the presence of microorganisms (e.g., *C. psittaci, C. burnetii, L. pneumophila,* and some fungi) that will not grow in conventional blood culture broth or on subculture media, prior antimicrobial therapy, noninfective endocarditis, or an incorrect diagnosis. In the author's personal experience, unequivocal culture-negative endocarditis has occurred in only 2 of more than 200 episodes of endocarditis seen during the past 14 years.

Although blood cultures clearly are the most important modality in the laboratory diagnosis of endocarditis, other microbiologic studies may be useful. For example, when blood cultures are negative, bone marrow cultures may provide the means by which an etiologic agent is identified. Endocarditis caused by *Histoplasma capsulatum* and other fungi, *Brucella* spp., *Salmonella* spp., and *Mycobacterium tuberculosis* (in an exceedingly rare case of miliary tuberculosis) may be diagnosed only by culture of the bone marrow. Serologic tests for antibodies to *C. burnetii, C. psittaci,* and *Legionella* spp. are critical to the diagnosis of these culture-negative endocarditides.

Other laboratory abnormalities may be seen in patients with endocarditis, but these will not be diagnostic. Hematologic studies often show a normochromic normocytic anemia, leukocytosis, and an elevated erythrocyte sedimentation rate. Urinalysis may reveal microscopic or gross hematuria, casts, and proteinuria. The presence in serum of rheumatoid factor, circulating immune complexes, and reduced levels of complement all have been noted. The presence of high levels of antibodies to staphylococcal teichoic acids have been suggested to be helpful in differentiating staphylococcal endocarditis from bacteremia without endocarditis; at present, the clinical utility of this test is not known. Finally, imaging studies such as the echocardiogram, although not in the domain of the clinical laboratory, may be of great help in confirming the presence of valvular vegetations.

Once the diagnosis of endocarditis has been made, the role of the laboratory is to assist in assuring optimal therapy. The usual tests of antimicrobial susceptibility measure inhibitory rather than bactericidal activity. However, since the cure of endocarditis requires bactericidal therapy, the routine tests can provide only an initial therapeutic guide. Standardized methodology for tests of bactericidal activity (minimum bactericidal concentration [MBC] and serum bactericidal test [SBT]) recently have been proposed, and the interested reader is referred to these documents for a detailed description of the methods (see both references to National Committee for Clinical Laboratory Standards).

The SBT has the potential advantage of measuring not only the activity of the antimicrobial agent against the infecting microorganism, but also the combined effect of absorption and elimination of drug in the patient's serum, the binding of drug to serum proteins (only free drug is active), and the effect of drug interactions (synergy or antagonism) during combination antibiotic therapy. The test is a modification of the broth dilution susceptibility test. Serum obtained from the patient being treated is diluted serially, and the bactericidal activity is measured against that patient's infecting microorganism. The prognostic value of proposed standardized tests was studied by Weinstein and others in 129 patients with endocarditis. Peak serum bactericidal titers of 1:64 or greater and trough titers of 1:32 or greater by the microdilution method were associated with 100% bacteriologic cure. However, many patients with lower titers also were cured bacteriologically; thus, the test was not a good predictor of bacteriologic failure. The study also showed that ultimate clinical outcome could not be predicted by the SBT, which is not surprising since multiple other factors (e.g., underlying disease, embolic phenomena, cardiac function) affect outcome as well. In sum, the SBT appeared to be able to predict bacteriologic cure but not bacteriologic failure or ultimate clinical outcome. Additional studies of the standardized SBT are needed.

Some microorganisms, such as the enterococci, cannot be killed by single antimicrobial agents. Usually, penicillin or ampicillin (or vancomycin in penicillin-allergic patients) is combined with an aminoglycoside such as gentamicin in order to achieve bactericidal antimicrobial activity. Recent reports have described enterococci that have high-level resistance to aminoglycosides and are, thereby, resistant to the synergistic effects of aminoglycosides in combination therapy. Methods to screen for such resistance have been published, and all enterococcal isolates from patients with endocarditis should be screened for high-level aminoglycoside resistance.

Other methods are available for determining whether or not synergy is present in vitro. Used most frequently have been: (1) the checkerboard technique, in which varying concentrations of two drugs are tested against the infecting microorganism, and (2) the time-kill curve, in which the speed of killing the infecting microorganism by specified concentrations of antimicrobials is measured over time. These techniques are not widely available and generally are not practical for monitoring therapeutic efficacy.

MYOCARDITIS

Myocarditis is an inflammatory disorder of the heart muscle that has been associated with many infectious agents and with noninfectious etiologies such as hypersensitivity reactions, radiation, chemicals, physical agents, and drugs. Discussion of the noninfectious myocarditides will not be undertaken here.

The syndrome of myocarditis may be either acute or chronic. Many patients never become symptomatic; those that develop symptoms usually have arrythmias (disturbances of heart rhythm), other electrocardiogram abnormalities, and congestive heart failure that sometimes may be fatal. Although viral etiologies are much more common, bacterial myocarditis is more likely to be associated with signs and symptoms. These include fever, chest discomfort, a weakened pulse, poor quality heart tones, and associated murmurs or gallops (extra heart sounds).

By far, the most common etiology for myocarditis is viral infection, especially due to the enteroviruses. Patients with

enteroviral myocarditis frequently have pericarditis as well, and some authorities prefer the term *myopericarditis*. Most likely, infection occurs in association with gastrointestinal viral replication and subsequent viremia. Coxsackievirus B strains are the most frequent pathogens, but coxsackievirus A, poliovirus, and the echoviruses also cause myocarditis. Other viruses that cause myocarditis include influenza, adenovirus, rubella, and rubeola.

Direct bacterial invasion of the myocardium is uncommon but sometimes occurs as a complication of endocarditis, especially due to *S. aureus* and the enterococci, or during disseminated sepsis as in gonococcemia or meningococcemia. Direct invasion of the myocardium by *Borrelia burgdorferi* has been reported in Lyme disease. Lyme carditis usually is a mild disease of relatively short duration. Other bacterial pathogens may be associated with myocarditis but not necessarily as a result of direct invasion of the myocardium. For example, the myocarditis of diphtheria is caused by an exotoxin produced by *Corynebacterium diphtheriae*, and the myocarditis of acute rheumatic fever is part of an immune response to recent group A streptococcal infection.

Rickettsial infections that have been associated with myocarditis include Rocky Mountain Spotted Fever (RMSF) and scrub typhus. Untreated or severe RMSF may be complicated by cardiovascular collapse with myocarditis and pulmonary edema. The myocarditis of scrub typhus usually is not severe, consisting of electrocardiographic changes and first-degree heart block.

Many fungi have been implicated as etiologic agents of myocarditis. In nonimmunocompromised hosts, both histoplasmosis and, rarely, coccidiodomycosis have been complicated by myocarditis. In immunocompromised patients, other fungi (e.g., *Aspergillus* spp.) and yeasts (e.g., *Candida* spp.) occasionally have invaded the heart as part of disseminated infection.

At least two parasitic agents, *Toxoplasma gondii* and *Trypanosoma cruzi*, are capable of invading the myocardium. Toxoplasma myocarditis occurs in immunocompromised adults. In Chagas' disease, caused by *T. cruzi* and endemic in parts of South and Central America, myocarditis is predictable and may be extensive. Clinical illness usually develops many years after initial infection and may result in severe congestive heart failure and death.

The diagnosis of myocarditis usually is based on clinical criteria; the contribution of the clinical laboratory depends on the etiologic agent. In viral myocarditis, laboratory identification of the etiologic agent may be difficult. The best means of making an etiologic diagnosis includes both viral isolation from the pharynx and stool, and demonstration of a fourfold rise in type-specific neutralizing, hemagglutinating, or complement-fixing antibodies between acute and convalescent serum specimens. The presence of a fourfold rise in antibody titer only, or positive viral cultures from pharynx and stool only, is weaker evidence for an etiologic diagnosis. Sensitive and specific IgM antibody assays for the various viral agents that cause myocarditis are not yet widely available but may be useful in the future.

In the case of pyogenic bacterial myocarditis and many cases of fungal myocarditis, identification of the etiologic agent is not difficult since disseminated infection often is present and blood cultures are positive. Fungi often are more difficult to isolate from blood cultures than are bacteria, and prolonged incubation or special methods (e.g., biphasic blood culture systems or lysis-centrifugation methodology) may be needed. Alternatively, serologic tests for fungal antibodies may be helpful, at least for the diagnosis of *Histoplasma* and *Coccidioides* myocarditis. The diagnosis of Lyme carditis (and Lyme disease in general) cannot be made by routine culture methods; at this time, presence of antibodies to *B. burgdorferi* in an appropriate clinical setting provides support for the diagnosis.

The laboratory diagnosis of rickettsial or parasitic myocarditis rests primarily on detection of antibodies in serum to *Rickettsia rickettsii* (RMSF), *Rickettsia tsutsugamushi* (scrub typhus), *T. gondii*, or *T. cruzi*. In general, a fourfold rise in species-specific antibody titer between acute and convalescent specimens now is preferred to the Weil-Felix test for the diagnosis of rickettsial infections. For early diagnosis of RMSF, skin can be biopsied and examined by immunofluorescence microscopy. However, this promising diagnostic technique is not yet widely available. In Chagas' disease, since myocarditis is a manifestation of chronic rather than acute infection, a rise in *T. cruzi* antibody titer would not be expected. Rather, the etiologic diagnosis in this disease depends on the presence of antibody in a patient with an appropriate history of exposure and consistent clinical findings. In toxoplasma myocarditis, most patients are immunocompromised, and the antibody response may be blunted (i.e., a fourfold rise in titer may be absent). Consistent clinical findings and the presence of toxoplasma IgG antibodies (determined by the Sabin-Feldman dye test, indirect fluorescent antibody test, enzyme-linked immunosorbent assay or other methods) may be the only data available for laboratory confirmation of the diagnosis.

PERICARDITIS

The pericardium consists of two thin tissue layers that form a sac around the heart; the two layers normally are separated by a small amount of serous fluid. Pericarditis is an inflammation of the pericardium that may be either acute or chronic, and, like myocarditis, has both infectious and noninfectious causes. The latter, which will not be discussed here, are quite diverse and include direct injury (trauma, surgery, irradiation), connective tissue diseases (e.g., systemic lupus erythematosus, rheumatoid arthritis) and hypersensitivity reactions (serum sickness), neoplasia, metabolic diseases (myxedema, uremia), and drugs (e.g., procainamide, hydralazine, minoxidil).

The most common clinical syndrome is acute pericarditis characterized by sharp, stabbing, pleuritic chest pain (i.e., exacerbated by inspiration) and worse when the patient is recumbent. Fever is almost always present. At auscultation, the physician often hears a pericardial friction rub (due to the rubbing together of the inflamed pericardial layers that occurs with each myocardial contraction). The inflammatory process may result in a marked increase in the amount of fluid present between the two pericardial layers—a pericardial effusion). The presence of an effusion is important for several reasons: (1) for the clinician, the physical examination may be altered with the rub no longer heard and the heart sounds muffled by the increased fluid around the heart; (2) detection of an effusion using echocardiography helps confirm the clinical diagnosis; (3) the fluid provides

a focus from which cultures may be obtained and an etiologic agent identified.

The infectious agents that cause pericarditis usually reach the pericardium either via the bloodstream or by direct extension from contiguous foci of infection. In acute pericarditis, a viral etiology is usually assumed but seldom proven. The most common viruses identified as causes of pericarditis are coxsackievirus B and echovirus, but many other viruses have been implicated as etiologic agents, including adenovirus, influenza, herpes simplex, herpes varicella-zoster, and mumps.

Both pyogenic bacteria and mycobacteria cause pericarditis. Disease due to pyogenic bacteria is relatively rare and usually occurs as a complication of bacteremia or endocarditis, or less commonly, as a direct extension from a pulmonary, pleural, or mediastinal infection. The major bacterial pathogens are *Staphylococcus aureus*, *Streptococcus pneumoniae* and other streptococci, *Neisseria meningitidis*, and *Haemophilus influenzae*. Patients with purulent pericarditis due to these microorganisms usually are very ill as a result of disseminated bacterial infection, and blood cultures often are positive. Pericarditis due to *Mycobacterium tuberculosis* complicates fewer than 5% of tuberculous infections and the syndrome may be an acute, subacute constrictive, or chronic constrictive pericarditis. Tuberculous pericarditis is the most common cause of chronic pericardial effusion. Constitutional symptoms characteristic of tuberculosis, such as fever, anorexia, and weight loss, often are present.

Fungal etiologies for pericarditis include *Histoplasma capsulatum*, *Coccidioides immitis*, *Blastomyces dermatiditis*, *Candida* spp, and *Aspergillus* spp. These agents tend to cause a chronic, granulomatous infection, sometimes with constriction. The higher bacteria such as *Nocardia* and *Actinomyces* are capable of causing pericarditis and clinically behave in a fashion similar to the fungi.

A few parasitic organisms cause pericarditis, although parasitic etiologies are quite rare in the United States. Most notable are *Toxoplasma gondii*, which is occasionally seen in compromised hosts, and *Entamoeba histolytica*, which causes pericardial disease usually by direct extension of infection through the diaphragm from a preexisting amebic liver abscess.

As in myocarditis, the diagnosis of pericarditis is based largely on clinical criteria. Most often, an etiologic diagnosis is not made, nor is one considered necessary because the course of the patient's illness is self-limited. For definitive microbiologic diagnosis, pericardial fluid usually must be obtained either by needle aspiration (pericardiocentesis) or by an open surgical procedure. The fluid is examined by Gram's stain or other stains (e.g., acridine orange) and cultured for viruses, pyogenic bacteria, fungi, and mycobacteria as appropriate.

If pericardial fluid is not obtained, microbiologic diagnosis rests on other studies that may be both less sensitive and less specific. In suspected viral pericarditis, isolation of virus from pharynx or stool specimens, and demonstration of a fourfold rise in antibody titer to that virus, is suggestive of an etiologic association. In suspected pyogenic bacterial pericarditis, blood cultures may be positive before pericardiocentesis or open drainage is undertaken. Positive blood cultures and clinical evidence of purulent pericarditis represent strong evidence for an etiologic diagnosis. Although drainage may not be necessary for diagnosis, it is often needed therapeutically. Tuberculous pericarditis is best diagnosed by obtaining pericardial tissue itself for mycobacterial culture and histologic examination. Culture of the pericardium is more likely to yield *M. tuberculosis* than is culture of pericardial fluid. In suspected fungal pericarditis, blood cultures are less likely to be positive; acute and convalescent sera showing a fourfold rise of specific fungal antibodies support the diagnosis.

SUGGESTED READING

Aronson MD and Bor DH: Blood cultures, Ann Intern Med 106:246, 1987.

Ilstrup DM and Washington JA II: The importance of volume of blood cultured in the detection of bacteremia and fungemia, Diagn Microbiol Infect Dis 1:107, 1983.

Murray PR: Determination of the optimum incubation period of blood culture broths for the detection of clinically significant septicemia, J Clin Microbiol 21:481, 1985.

National Committee for Clinical Laboratory Standards: Methodology for the serum bactericidal test; proposed guideline, Doc 21-P, Villanova, Pa, 1987, NCCLS.

National Committee for Clinical Laboratory Standards: Methods for determining bactericidal activity of antimicrobial agents; proposed guideline, Doc M26–P, Villanova, Pa, 1987, NCCLS.

Reller LB, Murray PR, and MacLowry JD: Cumitech 1A, blood cultures II. Coordinating editor, Washington JA II, American Society for Microbiology, Washington, DC, 1982.

Tilton RC: The laboratory approach to the detection of bacteremia, Ann Rev Microbiol 36:467, 1982.

Washington JA II: Blood cultures: principles and techniques, Mayo Clin Proc 50:91, 1975.

Washington JA II and Ilstrup DM: Blood cultures: issues and concepts, Rev Infect Dis 8:792, 1986.

Weinstein MP and others: Multicenter collaborative evaluation of a standardized serum bactericidal test as a prognostic indicator in infective endocarditis, Am J Med 78:262, 1985.

50 Genital specimens

Sandra A. Larsen

The microorganisms causing infections in the genitals and reproductive system are numerous and varied, and include viral, bacterial, fungal, and protozoal diseases. Most are sexually transmitted, but some are commensal and patients only become symptomatic when their hormonal, chemical, or immune system deviates from normal. The clinical manifestations range from none, to open lesions, to infertility. Some infections are localized to the reproductive organs, whereas others become systemic or may be transmitted to the neonate. Mixed infections are not infrequent, and the diagnosis of all infectious agents involved is essential to provide quality health care to the patient.

Safety of the clinician and laboratory worker must be of primary concern in handling specimens from the genital-reproductive system. Patients who are at risk for the sexually transmitted diseases covered in this chapter are also at risk for human immunodeficiency virus (HIV) and hepatitis B virus (HBV), which are not addressed in this section. Universal precautions, discussed in Chapter 2, must be followed for specimen collection and all laboratory procedures.

CHANCROID

Although chancroid is less common in the United States than other sexually transmitted diseases, the global incidence of the disease exceeds that of syphilis. Outbreaks of chancroid periodically occur in the United States; the most recent cases occurred in Florida, Texas, New York City, and California. Like other genital ulcer diseases, chancroid plays a role in the transmission of HIV.

The organism

The causative organism of chancroid, *Haemophilus ducreyi*, was first described by Ducrey in 1889. The appropriateness of the *Haemophilus* classification has been questioned, based on results of DNA studies showing only limited relatedness to several other members of the genus. On Gram's stain, *H. ducreyi* appears as gram-negative, small, pleomorphic rods, 0.5 to 0.5 μm in width and 1.6 to 2 μm in length, in short chains arranged in "schools of fish" or "railroad track" patterns.

Clinical diagnosis

The lesion that guides the clinical diagnosis initially appears as a tender papule after a 3- to 10-day incubation period. Within 12 to 24 hours the papule ulcerates to form a deep, painful, necrotic, and purulent lesion with ragged edges. The lesions of chancroid can be confused with those of syphilis, herpes simplex, and granuloma inguinale; subsequently, these infections should be ruled out. Darkfield or direct fluorescent antibody and serologic tests for syphilis should be performed, as well as a viral culture for herpes simplex.

Laboratory diagnosis

Although isolation rates are only 60% to 85%, isolating *H. ducreyi* is the only means for definitive diagnosis of chancroid. For specimen collection, if the lesion is crusted over with pus, gently soften the crust with saline and remove the crust or other superficial debris with a swab. Using either a cotton or calcium alginate swab, collect exudate from the ulcer's base or margins for a Gram's stain. Roll the swab over the microscope slide to preserve cellular morphology and arrangement. For culture, use a second swab or bacteriologic loop to collect material from the base or margins of the lesion, and transfer it directly to a primary isolation medium. The ability to use transport media for *H. ducreyi* has not been thoroughly evaluated.

Because *H. ducreyi* is extremely fastidious, the culture medium used is critical to isolating the organism. More than one culture medium may be needed to increase isolation rates. The following culture media yield the highest isolation rates: (1) Hammond's medium composed of gonococcal agar base plus 1% or 2% hemoglobin, 5% fetal bovine serum, 1% cofactors-vitamins-amino acids (CVA enrichment), or 1% IsoVitaleX with 3 mg of vancomycin/liter of medium; (2) heart infusion agar with 10% fetal bovine serum; and (3) Mueller-Hinton agar plus 5% chocolatized horse blood and 1% CVA or 1% IsoVitaleX with 3 mg of vancomycin/liter. Mueller-Hinton agar with horse blood has the lowest isolation rate, but some isolates that will not grow on Hammond's medium will grow on Mueller-Hinton agar with horse blood.

Inoculate the specimen onto plates, streak for isolation and incubate the plates in 5% CO_2 in a water-saturated environment at 33°C to 35°C for at least 48 hours prior to initial reading. *Haemophilus ducreyi* does not grow well at 37°C, and temperatures above 37°C are lethal to the organism. Hold plates for at least 5 days before reporting as culture-negative.

Identify *H. ducreyi* by colony morphology and Gram's

stain. The colonies of *H. ducreyi* are characteristic of the organism. Colonies are small, yellow to gray, smooth, and dome-shaped. The waxy colonies can be moved intact across the agar with the edge of a loop without pitting the agar. Confirm identification with a positive oxidase test using N-N-N-N-tetramethyl-p-phenylenediamine dihydrochloride, a positive nitrate reductase reaction, and a negative porphyrin test, demonstrating a requirement of *H. ducreyi* strains for exogenous hemin (X factor). The reagent for the porphyrin test is a test fluid consisting of 2 mM δ-aminolevulinic acid and 0.8 mM $MgSO_4$ in 0.1 M phosphate buffer, pH 6.9. Mix a heavy suspension of organisms from a 48-hour culture in the test reagent, and incubate for 18 or 24 hours at 37°C. Detect production of porphyrins with a Wood's ultraviolet lamp. If porphyrin is produced, the reagent in the test tube will emit a red fluorescence. An alternate method is to detect the production of porphobilinogen or porphyrin by adding an equal volume of Kovac's reagent to the test tube. A red color in the aqueous phase indicates a positive test and the lack of a requirement for hemin. The test reaction of *H. ducreyi* is thus negative.

Antigen detection

Techniques such as DNA probes and polymerase chain reaction (PCR) methods for the detection of *H. ducreyi* are in the early stages of evaluation and development. When these techniques are refined, probes should facilitate the laboratory diagnosis of chancroid.

CHLAMYDIA

Chlamydial infections are probably the most frequently occurring sexually transmitted disease in developed countries. Infections of the genitalia are most common, followed by infections of the conjunctivae, mucosal surfaces of the pharynx, urethra, and rectum. Lymphogranuloma venereum (LGV) was the first form of veneral disease recognized as a chlamydial infection. Although LGV is rare in the United States, LGV is common in central Africa. Also present in developing countries are infections involving *Chlamydia trachomatis,* which is one of the most frequent causes of preventable blindness.

The organism

Chlamydia trachomatis belongs to the order Chlamydiales and, until recently, shared the genus with only *Chlamydia psittaci*. Recently, *Chlamydia pneumoniae,* previously known as TWAR, was recognized as a separate species and as the causative agent of human respiratory disease. The chlamydiae are bacteria that are also obligate intracellular parasites because of their incomplete metabolic capabilities. Chlamydiae have a complex life cycle. The infectious form, the elementary body (EB), is approximately 350 nm in diameter and undergoes endocytosis by susceptible host cells. The EB is metabolically inactive, but once ingested, the EB converts to a metabolically active, vegetative form, the reticulate body (RB). The RB competes with the host cell for metabolic precursors and replicates by binary fission. Following replication of the reticulate bodies, the RBs condense to the EB form and are subsequently released from the infected host cell to begin the cycle again in vivo.

Serotyping using monoclonal antibodies is a method of classifying *C. trachomatis* strains into 15 types. Serotypes L1, L2, and L3 are associated with LGV, whereas trachoma is usually associated with serotypes A, B, Ba, and C. Genital infections may be caused by multiple serotypes.

Clinical diagnosis

In men, chlamydial infections result in urethritis. The majority of the cases of urethritis are characterized by urethral discharge, dysuria, or pruritus. However, approximately one fourth of men with urethral *C. trachomatis* infection are asymptomatic. Rarely do chlamydiae cause acute epididymitis. In women the most serious complication is acute salpingitis. Symptoms may be nonspecific but severe, resulting in scarring of the fallopian tubes and subsequent infertility. However, up to 70% of chlamydial genital infections in women are asymptomatic. In neonates, chlamydial infection may be present as a self-limited conjunctivitis, and some 10% of neonates born to mothers with chlamydial infection will develop pneumonitis.

Laboratory diagnosis

With the exception of trachoma, the clinical signs and symptoms in chlamydial infections are nonspecific. Thus laboratory assistance is necessary, and cell culture is still the preferred method for identification of chlamydial infection. Collect specimens before the patient is treated with antimicrobial agents. The sample should include epithelial cells and not urethral or cervical exudate, semen, or blood alone. Recovery rates of *C. trachomatis* depend on the training of the individual collecting the specimens, the materials used to collect the specimens, the transport media, and the timeliness of the culture after specimen collection. Use swabs made of rayon, Dacron, or cotton on plastic or flexible metal shafts or a cytobrush. Some lots of swabs may be toxic and should be checked for toxicity or inhibition of chlamydial growth with a laboratory strain, or request quality control performance from manufacturer.

Once the specimen has been collected, swirl the swab in transport media and express liquid from the swab by pressing it against the side of the test tube. Use transport medium (2 SP) composed of 0.2 M sucrose and 0.02 M phosphate, final pH 7.2, with gentamicin at 10 μg/ml, vancomycin at 100 μg/ml, and nystatin at 25 units/ml or amphotericin B at 2.5 to 4.0 μg/ml. Sterile glass beads may be added to facilitate vortexing at the time of culture. If the transport medium containing the specimen must be stored prior to culturing, store at −70°C and add 2% to 10% fetal bovine serum to the transport medium. For best recovery, process specimens within 24 to 48 hours after collection. Rates of recovery decrease by 20% when specimens are frozen at −70°C. Keep specimens to be processed within 24 hours at 4°C.

To culture specimens, vortex or sonicate transport medium containing the specimen, and inoculate tissue culture monolayers. McCoy cells of mouse fibroblast origin in 1-dram shell vials containing 12-mm coverslips are commonly used monolayers. However, other cell lines, such as HeLa 229, treated with diethylamino-ethyl dextran (DEAE-D) or BHK-21 cells, can be used. Inoculate 0.1 to 0.3 ml of the vortexed sample onto 24-hour confluent McCoy cell monolayers (approximately 1×10^5 to 2×10^5 cell concentration). Centrifuge inoculated shell vials for 1 hour at 2000 to 3000 × g at 30°C to 35°C. After centrifugation, hold the vials for 2 hours at 35°C. Aspirate the inoculum; rinse the cell layers once with Eagle's minimum essential medium, containing 0.5 to 2 μg per ml of cycloheximide, and incubate for 48 to 72 hours at 35°C. To detect chlamydial infection of the monolayer, stain with either immunofluorescent antibody or iodine and examine microscopically for cytoplasmic inclusion bodies containing granular-appearing RBs. To improve culture sensitivity, pass cultures in which inclusion bodies are not found to fresh monolayers at least once. To ensure that monolayers, culture media, and staining methods are working properly, run positive and negative controls with each set of cultures. Use a previous genital isolate as the positive control and an uninoculated monolayer as the negative control.

Antigen detection

Although culturing is the most sensitive method of detecting chlamydial infection, other methods have been developed that are less labor-intensive. Of the direct antigen detection methods, the fluorescent antibody staining method is the most sensitive. To perform the test, roll the specimen-containing swab or cytobrush onto a slide. Air dry the slide, fix with acetone, and apply fluorescein isothiocyanate (FITC)-conjugated antichlamydial monoclonal antibody. Incubate the slide for 30 minutes at room temperature and rinse with distilled water to remove unbound antibody. (Incubation times and temperatures vary among commercial kits.) Mount slides with coverslips and read them using an incident light fluorescent microscope. Elementary bodies and RBs appear as apple-green dots against a red-brown background. As with other fluorescent microscopic techniques, the microscopist should be well trained. Commercial kits are available from a number of manufacturers. Some investigators prefer monoclonal antibody conjugates prepared against the surface-exposed major outer membrane proteins of chlamydiae to those monoclonal antibody conjugates prepared against the genus-specific lipopolysaccharides (LPS).

A number of enzyme immunoassays (EIA) have been developed for the detection of chlamydial infections and appear to be useful when a large number of specimens are screened. The sensitivities of the EIA techniques appear to be comparable to those of fluorescent antibody techniques; however, the EIA methods may be less specific. Currently, nucleic acid probe and PCR technologies are being evaluated for antigen detection.

Under no circumstances should rapid methods be used for *Chlamydia* in the laboratory investigation of sexually abused children. Culture of proper specimens for *Chlamydia* is necessary.

Antibody detection

Serologic tests for chlamydial infections have only limited applicability and are not recommended for diagnosing lower genital tract infections or for diagnosing conjunctivitis. Complement fixation tests are used for the diagnosis of LGV and psittacosis, whereas the microimmunofluorescence test is clinically useful in identifying chlamydial pneumonitis in infants.

GONORRHEA

Although rates of gonorrhea have decreased in the past years, gonorrhea is still the most frequently reported sexually transmitted disease in the United States. Gonorrhea is generally a disease of persons under the age of 30 who have had multiple sexual partners and reside in socioeconomically disadvantaged areas. Most men with gonococcal urethritis are symptomatic, whereas the majority of women with cervical infections are asymptomatic and serve as a reservoir for heterosexual transmission. The rapid development, typically within 5 years, of the organism's resistance to new therapeutic agents presents a challenge to the control of gonorrhea.

The organism

Neisseria gonorrhoeae was first described in 1879 as the etiologic agent of venereal discharges and ophthalmia neonatorum by A. Neisser. The organism belongs to the family Neisseriaceae, which also includes *Branhamella, Kingella, Moraxella,* and *Acinetobacter* spp. These other members of the *Neisseriaceae* family may be incorrectly identified as *N. gonorrhoeae,* a fact to be particularly alert for in suspected child abuse cases. Strains of *N. gonorrhoeae* can be classified by auxotype, serotype, or colony type. Classification is important epidemiologically in identifying antimicrobial-resistant strains in a population.

Clinical diagnosis

Most gonococcal infections are uncomplicated and occur within the mucosal surfaces of the female endocervix, male urethra, rectum, or pharynx. The eyes of newborns may be infected at birth, and the infection can result in blindness if not treated. Complications in adults can occur if treatment is not properly administered. Disseminated gonococcal infections are characterized by skin lesions and arthralgias, and occasionally will progress to endocarditis or meningitis. Pelvic inflammatory disease (PID) may develop in as many as 8% of women with cervical gonorrhea. This disease is the most devastating complication of gonorrhea, in the female, resulting in infertility or ectopic pregnancies.

Laboratory diagnosis

Initial diagnosis of gonococcal infection can be made by performing a Gram's stain of male urethral, female cervical, and rectal specimens. On Gram's stain, *N. gonorrhoeae* appears as gram-negative, kidney-bean–shaped diplococci with adjacent sides flattened and usually within polymorphonuclear leukocytes. Collect specimens for Gram's staining on a swab. Sterile cotton swabs may be used to obtain specimens from the endocervical canal, rectum, and vagina. If urethral exudate is not readily expressed in the male, use a sterile calcium alginate swab on an aluminum wire. A speculum must be used to obtain endocervical and vaginal samples. Gram's staining is not recommended as a presumptive diagnosis for specimens collected from the rectum of women or from the oropharynx of either sex. The sensitivity of the Gram's stain depends on the anatomical site from which the specimen was collected. The sensitivity and specificity of urethral Gram's stain is greater than 95% in symptomatic males and 50% to 70% sensitive in female endocervical smears.

Gram's stain procedure

To perform the Gram's stain, prepare a thin smear by rolling the swab across the slide. Air dry the smear. Heat fixing is not necessary because genital specimens usually contain enough albumin to adhere to the slide. Flood the slide with crystal violet solution for 30 seconds, rinse with tap water, and drain. Flood the slide with Gram's iodine for 30 seconds, rinse, and drain. Next, decolorize with acetone alcohol until the blue color is no longer detectable in the drops falling from the slide. Immediately rinse the slide and drain. Finally, flood the slide with safranin for 15 to 30 seconds, rinse, drain, and pat or air dry. Examine the slide using a light microscope with a $\times 100$ objective. Although demonstrating gram-negative intracellular diplococci in exudate from a symptomatic male is an acceptable basis for diagnosis, a culture should be obtained for antimicrobial susceptibility testing.

Culture procedure

Collect specimens for culture (before the patient is treated) in a manner identical to collection for Gram's staining. The specimens can be transported if direct plating is impossible. Do not refrigerate specimens, but inoculate onto transport or isolation medium (such as Jembec or Transgrow) and incubate overnight, as described shortly, before shipping by courier or an express mail service. If direct plating is possible, inoculate specimens onto selective media such as modified Thayer-Martin, Martin-Lewis, or New York City. These media are commercially available and are composed of GC agar base or the equivalent medium supplemented with growth factors. Antimicrobials and antifungals are added to the selective media: vancomycin to inhibit gram-positive bacteria; colistin to inhibit gram-negative bacteria; trimethoprim lactate to prevent swarming of *Proteus* spp., and nystatin or anisomysin to inhibit yeast. In geographic areas where vancomycin has been reported to inhibit gonococcal growth, use nonselective media such as chocolate agar composed of GC agar base, hemoglobin, and a supplement such as IsoVitaleX in addition to selective medium.

Inoculate the plate by rolling the swab across it in a Z pattern, using a loop cross-streak through the Z pattern to ensure separation of colonies. Incubate plates immediately at $35°C$ to $36°C$ in an atmosphere of 5% to 8% CO_2 and 70% humidity for at least 24 to 48 hours. The proper CO_2 atmosphere can be provided by use of a CO_2-generating tablet, a CO_2 incubator, or a candle extinction jar.

Colonies of *N. gonorrhoeae* grown on selective media appear as translucent white to gray to brownish colonies, measuring 0.5 to 1.0 mm in diameter, after 24 hours incubation. After 48 hours, the colonies may reach 3 mm in diameter. The edges of the colonies may be smooth or rough. Frequently, a mixture of colony types will occur. Pick representative colonies, perform a Gram's stain, and examine for oxidase production. Oxidase production may be determined either by placing a drop of 0.5% tetramethylparaphenylenediamine hydrochloride directly on a few colonies, or by rubbing a few representative colonies on filter paper moistened with a 1% solution of the oxidase reagent. A platinum loop must be used to transfer the colonies. Oxi-

dase-positive colonies will rapidly turn dark blue. Colonies rubbed on the oxidase strips will turn the paper purple within 10 seconds. Commercial oxidase strips are also available. As an adjunct to the oxidase test and Gram's stain, a superoxol test to measure catalase production is a useful, presumptive test. Using 30% hydrogen peroxide, drop the peroxide on typical colonies and look for instant vigorous bubbling.

If the Gram's stain of colonies is typical and colonies are oxidase-and superoxol-positive, then perform additional confirmatory tests. A variety of confirmatory test methods are available commercially. Traditional confirmatory biochemical tests for *Neisseria* include acid production from glucose, lactose, maltose, and sucrose, and reduction of nitrate. For carbohydrate degradation tests, use cystine trypticase agar in tubes containing phenol red and 1% to 2% concentrations of glucose, lactose, maltose, or sucrose. Use a pure, 18-hour subculture from growth on a nonselective medium as the inoculum. Stab the agar tubes in the upper third of the medium. Incubate them at $35°C$ without CO_2 for 24 hours. In positive tests, the area of the inoculum should be pale yellow. *Neisseria gonorrhoeae* is positive only in glucose. Most other species of *Neisseria* produce positive results with maltose or other sugars, whereas a few (*Neisseria cinerea*) do not utilize these sugars at all.

Rapid detection methods

In addition to the traditional techniques, a number of rapid biochemical tests and antigen detection methods are available commercially. Most require a pure culture. Species of *Neisseria* produce enzymes that may be used to identify them. For example, *Neisseria lactamica* produces beta-D-galactosides, *Neisseria meningitidis* produces gamma-glutamylaminopeptidase, *N. gonorrhoeae* produces hydroxypropyl aminopeptidase, whereas *Branhamella catarrhalis*, often confused with gonococcus, produces none of these enzymes. The fluorescent antibody test has been used for many years for antigen detection. Newer versions now employ monoclonal antibodies. The Gonozyme test (Abbott Laboratories, North Chicago, Ill) is an antigen detection test that is useful to screen high-risk populations. A positive Gonozyme test result should be confirmed by culture if results have medicolegal implications. Also commercially available are coagglutination tests made up of a pool of a number of monoclonal antibodies directed toward gonococcal protein 1, which have been absorbed to *Staphylococcus aureus* cells that produce protein A. Cross-reactions with nongonococcal *Neisseria* and missed *N. gonorrhoeae* strains have been reported with this method. The commercially available reagents should be used according to the manufacturers' directions. A prototype nucleic acid probe test (PACE-II, GenProbe, San Diego, CA) has yielded high sensitivity and specificity in preliminary evaluations.

Antimicrobial susceptibility testing

Once *N. gonorrhoeae* has been isolated, antimicrobial susceptibility testing should be performed as an integral part of a routine evaluation at a sexually transmitted disease clinic. Methods for performing susceptibility tests are described elsewhere.

HERPES SIMPLEX VIRUS

The most common cause of genital ulcerations in the developed world is herpes simplex virus (HSV). Two distinct types of HSV exist. The etiologic agent for more than 90% of orolabial infections and herpetic keratitis is HSV-1, whereas HSV-2 accounts for 90% of genital infections. Herpes simplex virus is spread primarily by intimate oral or sexual contact, with the virus entering through mucous membranes or microscopic cracks in the skin. Unlike most other sexually transmitted diseases, symptomatic genital HSV infections are more prevalent in middle to upper-income white populations than in disadvantaged populations. However, HSV-2 antibody prevalence rates are higher in nonwhite populations, suggesting that the HSV-2 infection may be asymptomatic.

The organism

Herpes simplex virus is a member of the Herpesviridae family. Other members of the family that cause human infection are varicella-zoster, Epstein-Barr, cytomegalovirus (CMV), and human herpesvirus-6. All members of the family are similar in structure, consisting of one molecule of double-stranded viral DNA wrapped around a proteinaceous spool and surrounded by a capsid composed of viral proteins. The space between the capsid and outer envelope, the tegument, consists of an amorphous material. The outer envelope is composed of lipoprotein with spikelike projections occurring at regular intervals. The diameter of the virus is approximately 140 to 200 nm. Herpes simplex virus is an obligate intracellular parasite.

Clinical diagnosis

Herpes simplex virus infections can be subdivided into four categories. The primary episode or initial infection with genital HSV is usually the most painful, with a greater tendency for the infection to become generalized than in subsequent recurrences. Clinical manifestations of the primary infection occur approximately 1 week after contact with an infected individual. At that time discrete vesicles appear, which evolve into pustules that eventually coalesce to form ulcers. Pain associated with the lesions as well as with urination can be severe. The virus is shed for at least 10 days, and the lesions heal in appproximately 20 days. Virus isolation from lesions is related to the length of time the lesion has been present and the stage of the infection. Virus titers are highest early in the infection when vesicles or pustules are present; thus isolation is easier. The second category is a nonprimary first episode, or the first infection with HSV-2 in an individual with antibodies to HSV-1. This infection is usually less severe, both in the numbers of lesions and the pain associated with the infection, than the primary episode. As with the primary episode, virus isolation is easier when done early in the infection process. The third category includes recurrent episodes of genital herpes. Recurrences may be triggered by a variety of factors both internally and externally. The episodes are usually mild and isolation of the virus is more difficult because viral shedding usually lasts only 4 days and the lesion lasts 10 days. The final category of genital herpes is asymptomatic shedding. Individuals in this category shed the virus without noticeable lesions present. These individuals are infectious, however, and the virus can be isolated. During the period between episodes, HSV-2 lies dormant in the sensory or autonomic root ganglia and the individual is not infectious.

Extragenital complications of HSV-2 are rare with the exception of the development of a stiff neck, headache, and photophobia. A major concern is possible neonatal infection as the result of asymptomatic herpes infection in the maternal genital tract at the time of delivery. Since neonatal herpes is serious, any neonatal cutaneous vesicle, bulla, or erosion should be cultured.

Laboratory diagnosis
Cytologic stains

Perhaps the most commonly used methods for the initial diagnosis of HSV are cytologic stains. With stains such as Papanicolaou's, Giemsa, and Wright-Giemsa (Tzanck), changes in host cell architecture can be detected by light microscopy. The most characteristic feature of infection with members of the Herpesviridae family is the formation of multinucleated cells. Samples may be collected from cervical or mucocutaneous lesions. To collect specimens from the female genital tract, use a wooden vaginal spatula. Take scrapings from the endocervical surface, the external os, vagina, and labia. Smear each sample on a separate microscope slide and fix immediately. Either spray the slide with a commercial fixative or fix slides by placing in 95% ethanol for 1 hour. Stain with a modified Papanicolaou's stain. Scan slides for cells that show nuclear and cytoplasmic enlargement with nucleolar lysis and cytoplasmic hyalinization, which imparts a "ground glass" appearance to the nucleus. These changes are consistent with early changes. Later changes include the development of multinucleated giant cells with marginated chromatin and molding of individual nuclei against one another but without overlapping. The specificity of cervical cytology approaches 95%, however, sensitivity is only 50% to 60%.

To collect samples from mucosal or cutaneous lesions, gently scrape fresh lesions with a flat applicator, scalpel, or curet. Remove the top from vesicles and scrape the base. For Giemsa and Wright-Giemsa stains, spread the specimen on a clean glass slide. Air dry smears without additional fixation and stain. Scan slides for cell architecture described earlier.

Antigen detection

Large quantities of HSV antigens are produced during infection, thus conjugated antibodies can be used in direct and indirect staining procedures. Sensitivities of these techniques are greater than 80%, and the procedures are relatively uncomplicated. Fluorescein-isothiocyanate-conjugated monoclonal antibodies are available that distinguish HSV-1 from HSV-2 infections. Generally the direct fluorescent antibody (DFA) tests are performed as follows. Collect scrapings from mucocutaneous lesions as described earlier. Make two smears on each slide. Fix air-dried smears in acetone or methanol. Once the slide has again dried, dip the slide in phosphate-buffered saline (PBS), pH 7.2, and add appropriately diluted conjugates to the slide: anti-HSV-1 to one smear and anti-HSV-2 to the other. Place the slide within a moist chamber and incubate for 30 minutes at 37°C. Rinse the slide in PBS three times for 10 minutes each time. Then rinse the slide in running distilled water, drain, air dry, mount a coverslip with glycerol in PBS or elvanol and examine the slide using a fluorescent microscope. Look for apple-green intracellular fluorescence.

Antigen detection with immunoperoxidase (IP) staining is an alternative to the immunofluorescent (IF) method. The test is performed in a manner similar to that for indirect fluorescent antibody technique. As an example, add unlabeled anti-HSV monoclonal antibody to the fixed smear and incubate, then rinse. Next add anti-mouse globulin conjugated with horseradish peroxidase, incubate and rinse. Then, treat the sample with diaminobenzidine (DAB). The DAB reacts with the horseradish peroxidase, and the area where the antibody has bound appears as reddish brown granules when examined under a light microscope. Still another rapid detection method is the HSV enzyme-linked immunosorbent assay (ELISA), an antigen-capture technique. An abbreviated procedure is described here.

Collect a specimen on a swab from vesicular fluid or genital tract lesion and extract into serum-free medium by swirling the swab and expressing it against the side of the test tube. Place the clinical sample in a micro-well strip coated with HSV antibody. Incubate for 1 hour and wash three times. Next add horseradish peroxidase-conjugated herpes simplex antibody, incubate for 1 hour and wash five times. Then add enzyme substrate, orthophenylenediamine. Stop the reaction after 30 minutes with a 2 N HCl and read at 490 nm.

Several rapid detection methods for HSV based on DNA probe technology are currently commercially available. The tests, which use biotinylated probes, are comparable in sensitivity and specificity to IF methods. To perform the in situ DNA hybridization, place the specimen, which was collected on a Dacron swab moistened with saline or curet, on a glass slide. Air dry the slide and fix in acetone. Next add biotinylated HSV DNA probe and apply a coverslip. On a heating block, heat the slide at 92°C for 2 to 3 minutes. Remove the slide from the block and leave at room temperature for 10 to 20 minutes. Remove the coverslip and wash with a probe solution containing formamide and PBS, pH 7.0, for 5 to 10 minutes. Rinse with PBS containing ethylenediamine tetraacetic acid (EDTA) for 5 to 10 seconds and drain slide. Add avidin-biotinylated horseradish peroxidase complex and incubate for 10 to 20 minutes. Wash the slide and add the chromogen substrate solution. Incubate at room temperature for 20 minutes; rinse, and apply fast green counterstain. Wash slide and apply the mounting medium and coverslip. Scan slides under a light microscope with ×100 magnification and confirm at ×400 magnification. Read for red nuclear staining in intact nonsuperficial epithelial cells.

Culture method

Although the sensitivity of DNA probe techniques approaches that of viral isolation in early genital lesions, the sensitivity of the probe method appears to be decreased in specimens from asymptomatic individuals. The preferred specimen for culture is vesicle fluid aspirated with a needle and syringe, but collection on Dacron, rayon, or cotton swabs is also an acceptable method. Immediately place the swab or vesicle fluid in a transport medium such as Hanks balanced salt solution with antibiotics or veal infusion broth with antibiotics. Vigorously swirl swab in medium and express fluid against the side of the tube. Herpes simplex virus is stable at 4°C for up to 72 hours; however, the virus is rapidly inactivated at room temperature or -20°C.

A number of cell lines will support the growth of HSV. Some investigators prefer to use cell lines in which cytomegalovirus will not grow, such as rabbit kidney, Vero, HeLa, and baby hamster kidney, because the cytopathic effect of the two organisms is similar. Inoculate cell culture tubes containing a confluent monolayer with 0.25 ml of culture extract. Place on a roller drum at 36°C and examine daily at a magnification of ×125 for cytopathic effect. The earliest change observed in the monolayer is rounding of the cells, followed by swelling of the cells and a glassy appearance. Finally the cells detach from the culture tube and die. To confirm HSV as the cause of the cytopathic effect, use an immunologic method such as direct fluorescent antibody test. For DFA, scrape cells exhibiting cytopathic effect from the culture tube and place into glass well slides. Fix in acetone and add anti-HSV conjugate; incubate and wash. Read slides for intracellular fluorescence.

Even though the cytopathic effect of HSV is observed within 2 to 3 days on the average in the standard culture technique, several investigators have devised methods of using shell vials and low-speed centrifugation to decrease culture time to approximately 16 hours. For this technique, inoculate 0.2 ml of specimen extract onto confluent monolayer growing on a 12-mm round coverslip in 3.7-ml shell vials, and centrifuge at 700 × g for 40 minutes at 30°C. After viral absorption, add 1.0 ml of Eagle's minimal essential medium and incubate at 36°C for 16 hours. Wash coverslips two times with PBS and fix in acetone for 20 minutes. Stain as outlined earlier and read for intracellular fluorescence at ×200 magnification.

Antibody detection

Numerous serologic tests for HSV have been developed. Currently the main function of these tests is to delineate primary from nonprimary infection in individuals experiencing genital herpes for the first time. Serologic tests that will distinguish HSV-1 from HSV-2 antibodies are currently being developed based on the use of cloned antigens.

HUMAN PAPILLOMA VIRUS

The recent rise in infections with human papillomavirus (HPV), now estimated to be approximately one million new cases per year, has focused public attention on this agent, and the relationship of the infection with cervical cancer and to a lesser degree with penile cancer has received some scrutiny. At present, 60 genotypes of HPV have been identified based on DNA cross-hybridization; at least 17 types (types 6, 11, 16, 18, 31, 33, 35, 39, 40, 42, 43, 44, 48, 53, 54, 55, 56) have been described in lesions of the genital tract.

The organism

Human papilloma virus belongs to the Papovaviridae family, based on its form and capsid structure. The human papilloma viruses are small (approximately 55 nm in diameter), nonenveloped icosahedral virons. Their DNA genomes are 7.9 kilobases $\pm 10\%$ in length, double-stranded, convalently closed, and circular. Their capsids are composed only of proteins, which form 72 capsomers. Human papilloma virus infects the skin and mucous membranes, probably through small abrasions, and replicates in the nuclei of infected epithelial cells. Basal cells are nonpermissive for viral replication, but HPV induces basal cell proliferation, and basal cells appear to serve as a reservoir for viral infection.

Clinical diagnosis

The clinical presentation of genital HPV infection is varied. Condylomata acuminata, or the classic warts, are flesh-colored, soft, bulky, pedunculated growths, usually associated with HPV types 6 and 11. Condylomata acuminata may become so large that normal physical structures become deformed. Condylomata plana, or flat warts, are flesh-colored or nearly invisible flat papules. When 3% to 5% acetic acid is applied, a whitened area of slightly raised epithelium may be observed with a hand lens or colposcope. Most genital HPV types have been identified in these lesions; however, types 16 and 18 occur more commonly when condylomata plana and cervical intraepithelial neoplasia occur together. A third form of HPV infection is termed *bowenoid papulosis*. This type of lesion is a flat, small, pink or reddish brown, multicentric papule. Bowenoid papulosis typically resolves itself spontaneously and is rarely associated with the development of advanced neoplasia. Because the lesions of HPV and syphilis may be similar, direct microscopic examination of lesion material by darkfield microscopy or fluorescent staining should be performed, as well as serologic tests for syphilis, to ensure the correct diagnosis.

Laboratory diagnosis

Human papilloma virus cannot be grown in tissue culture or transmitted to laboratory animals because of the extreme species specificity of the virus. Thus laboratory diagnosis is limited to the recognition of specific histopathologic changes in tissue samples and identification is based on various DNA probe techniques.

Nucleic acid hybridization

Southern blot and dot blot (modified Southern blot) are widely used techniques. A Southern blot kit is available from Oncor, Inc., Gaithersburg, Md., and two dot blot kits, one for screening and one for diagnosis are available from Digene Co., Silver Springs, Md. The dot blot methods are only slightly less sensitive than Southern blot techniques, and when RNA-DNA hybrids are used, the nonspecific reactivity associated with the dot blot techniques is reduced.

For Southern and dot blot methods, punch biopsies and cervical scrapings serve as specimen sources. Collect scrapings on a wooden spatula or a swab. Transfer the collected cells to buffered saline. For extraction of viral DNA, the samples must be kept frozen at $-20°C$. Details of Southern blot and dot blue techniques are found in references by Schneider and Mifflin. Briefly, extract DNA from the tissue sample, denature, and then mix with a radioactive-labeled HPV-DNA probe. In the Southern blot method, cut the DNA extracted from the specimen into fragments by restriction endonuclease digestion, separate by molecular weight through agarose gel electrophoresis, denature, and then transfer to a nitrocellulose or nylon membrane. The target DNA on the membrane and the radioactive-labeled HPV probe then hybridize. Detect the reaction by autoradiography. In the dot blot method, "dot" extract DNA from the patient's specimen in an area of 0.5 to 1.0 cm in diameter directly onto the membrane, then react with the HPV probe.

The simplest form of viral nucleic acid detection is the filter in situ hybridization (FISH) technique. Place a cell suspension from the patient on a nitrocellulose filter, lyse the cells with alkali to denature the DNA, neutralize the filters and bake; then hybridize with the human papillomavirus DNA probe. This method is not applicable to biopsy material. For tissue samples, tissue in situ hybridization (TISH) methods are available. TISH methods are carried out on microscope slides. Treat cytologic smears or paraffin-embedded specimens to expose and denature the DNA, then react with a biotinylated probe to yield a colorimetric reaction. Several kits are commercially available for TISH. Whereas TISH is less sensitive than the membrane techniques, its advantage lies in the rapidity of the test and the use of nonradioactive probes.

Polymerase chain reaction (PCR) techniques represent a new approach to the diagnosis of HPV. Specimen sources may vary from cervical scrapes to urine. The PCR technique is based on selective in vitro amplification of a specific region of DNA. A pair of oligonucleotide primers that flank a 200 to 300 base-pair region direct the synthesis of the fragment with DNA polymerase in opposite and overlapping directions. Extracted DNA from the patient's sample and the newly synthesized DNA fragments, after heat denaturation, bind again to the primer molecules and serve as templates for further DNA synthesis. Amplification through heating and cooling cycles can feasibly be 10^6-fold or more. Final identification of amplified DNA is usually by Southern or dot blot methods. The utility of the PCR method in the clinical laboratory has not been established as of this writing.

Histopathology

For specimen collection, perform a biopsy either by punch or by surgical excision. Spread the tissue out to dry on paper for 1 to 2 minutes, then place in 10% neutral buffered formalin. Note the lesion site and previous treatment, if any, on the laboratory request form. Stain sections of the tissue with hematoxylin and eosin.

According to Lever, all warts share certain histologic features; however, each of the three forms of HPV has characteristic features. In condylomata acuminata, look for the presence of koilocytes in the stratum spinosum and stratum granulosum epidermides. Koilocytes are large epithelial cells in which the cytoplasmic organelles congregate at the cell's periphery, creating the appearance of clear vacuoles of cytoplasm. The nuclei of these cells are dense, irregular, and may be slightly enlarged. In addition, the mitotic index may be increased and multinucleated, and dyskeratotic cells may be present. Changes in the submucosa include moderate to mild inflammation and occasionally, edema and vascular dilation. The characteristics to look for in flat condylomata of the cervix are the lack of conspicuous papillations and the presence of koilocytes. For bowenoid papulosis of the external genitalia, look for full-thickness intraepithelial neoplasia. Keratinocytes with hyperchromatic and pleomorphic nuclei are characteristically present, producing a pattern of squamous cell carcinoma in situ. Koilocytosis is rare. (More detailed histopathology is beyond the scope of this chapter.)

MYCOPLASMAS

At least seven species of mycoplasmas have been isolated from the urogenital tract of sexually active individuals. Three species, *Ureaplasma urealyticum, Mycoplasma hominis,* and *Mycoplasma genitalium* are known or believed to cause disease. *Ureaplasma urealyticum* and *M. hominis* do not cause disease in the lower female genital tract, but are suspected to cause disease in the upper female genitourinary tract, e.g., pelvic inflammatory disease, as a result of *M. hominis* infection. In the male, urethritis may be the result of infection with *U. urealyticum.* Two reports have linked *M. genitalium* with nongonococcal urethritis (NGU). A definite association between *M. hominis* and postabortion and postpartum fever has been established, as has the association of *U. urealyticum* isolation from the placenta with chorioamnionitis, funisitis, stillbirth, and perinatal morbidity and mortality. In addition, *U. urealyticum* and *M. hominis* cause respiratory disease, particularly in very low birth weight infants, and may be among the most common causes of central nervous system infections in preterm infants. Evidence indicates that these respiratory infections are acquired in utero.

The organism

Mycoplasma spp. and *Ureaplasma* spp. belong to the family *Mycoplasmataceae.* Mycoplasmas, which range in size from 0.42 to 0.5 μm, are the smallest known free-living microorganisms and are not visible on a Gram's stain. Mycoplasmas are unique because they lack a cell wall and thus are included in a separate class, Mollicutes. The small size of the mycoplasmal genome (5×10^8 daltons) limits their biosynthetic abilities and to some extent explains the fastidiousness of these organisms in vitro. However, in vivo, the mycoplasmas are extracellular pathogens.

Laboratory diagnosis

Mycoplasma cultivation is demanding and attempts to perform cultures should be limited to those clinical conditions in which mycoplasmas have been proven as the etiologic agent. Specimens suitable for culture are blood (collected without anticoagulant), synovial fluid, urine, prostatic fluid, amniotic fluid, tissues, cervical swabs, male urethral swabs, tracheal secretions, tissues, sputum, and placenta. If swabs are taken, the swab tips should be made of Dacron, calcium alginate, or polyester. Place swabs immediately in mycoplasma media. Do not break the swab stick off in the medium, but rather agitate the swab in the medium and press against the side of the culture tube to express most of the fluid. Other types of samples should be inoculated into the medium within an hour after collection. Keep the inoculated tube at 2°C to 8°C until it is transported, and transport it refrigerated. Dilute body fluids at a 1:10 concentration in transport media. Mince tissues and suspend in transport medium at a concentration of approximately 10%. Prepare additional dilutions to at least 1:1000 of the minced tissue

in transport medium. If the specimen cannot be transported within 72 hours, freeze the medium containing the specimen at −70°C or store in liquid nitrogen and transport it in its frozen state. Media used for transport are 2SP composed of 0.2 M sucrose in 0.02 M phosphate buffer, pH 7.2, with 10% heat-activated fetal calf serum and trypticase soy broth, with either 0.5% bovine serum albumin or 10% to 20% horse serum.

In the laboratory, process specimens immediately. Thaw previously frozen specimens in a 37°C water bath. Recovery rates are improved if the specimen is first inoculated into liquid medium, serially diluted, then subcultured to liquid and agar media. Several liquid culture media have been successfully used; Shepard's 10B broth prepared from PPLO broth, supplemented with yeast extract and horse serum; A8 agar and SP-4 medium, prepared from beef infusion broth supplemented with yeast extract; and heat-treated fetal bovine serum and glucose. Glucose, arginine, or urea and the pH indicator phenol red are added in order to detect growth. Various batches of media may or may not support the growth of mycoplasmas; therefore, monitoring quality control by using stock strains and fresh isolates is critical to isolation. No single medium will support the optimal growth of *M. hominis, U. urealyticum,* and *M. genitalium;* however, all three grow on SP-4 broth and agar with the appropriate pH and additives. Transfer 0.2 ml of clinical material or transport medium with clinical sample into three tubes containing 1.8 ml of medium; one tube supplemented with 0.002% phenol red and 0.1% arginine, the second tube supplemented with 0.022% phenol red and 0.1% glucose, and the third tube supplemented with 0.002% phenol red and 0.1% urea. Prepare tenfold dilutions of each in like media. Incubate broth cultures for *M. hominis* and *U. urealyticum* at 37°C under atmospheric conditions. Incubate broth culture for *M. genitalium* in 95% N_2 and 5% CO_2 at 37°C. The length of incubation depends on the number of organisms in the original specimen. Color changes may be noted for ureaplasmas within 48 hours. *Mycoplasma hominis* usually grows more slowly, with color change occurring within a week. *Mycoplasma genitalium* may take up to 50 days to produce a color change. In SP-4 broth with an initial pH of 7.4, *M. hominis* converts arginine to ammonia, which is indicated by a color change from red to deep fuchsia. This color change is due to the presence of the enzyme urease in ureaplasmas, which breaks down urea to ammonia. *Mycoplasma genitalium* and *Mycoplasma fermentans* convert glucose to lactic acid, indicated by a color change from red to yellow. Subculture any culture showing a color change into fresh broth and onto agar plates. Incubate agar plates in 95% N_2 and 5% CO_2 at 37°C. On A8 agar, *M. hominis* produces a colony 200 to 300 μm in diameter with a fried egg appearance, whereas ureaplasmas produce tiny colonies, 15 to 30 μm in diameter, with a granular, brown appearance. *Mycoplasma genitalium* colonies have no distinct appearance on agar. Further specific species identification is based on serologic methods, either through inhibition of colony development around a disk containing specific antiserum, or epi-immunofluorescence or immunoperoxidase techniques. These techniques are more frequently found in reference and research laboratories than in clinical laboratories.

Antibody detection

Antibody detection tests have little significance if both acute and convalescent serum samples are not available because of the ubiquity of mycoplasmas. Thus, serodiagnosis is not recommended for routine diagnostic purposes.

Antigen detection

Antigen detection test methods, including DNA probes, have not been evaluated extensively. Limited evaluation has shown the probes to be less sensitive than cultures.

SYPHILIS

Currently, rates of syphilis are approaching levels not seen since the late 1940s. Recent surveys indicate that syphilis is most prevalent in heterosexual, lower socioeconomic, recreational drug users. Persons with syphilis are infectious to their sexual partners when skin lesions are present, as in the primary and secondary stages. Infected women may transmit the infection to their infants during any stage of syphilis, but are less likely to transmit the disease during the latent stage. Many individuals with syphilis are also coinfected with human immunodeficiency virus type 1 (HIV-1). Studies are underway to define the influence of HIV-1 infection on syphilis test outcome.

The organism

The causative agent of syphilis is *Treponema pallidum* subspecies *pallidum,* a member of the order Spirochaetales. Unlike the other pathogenic spirochetes, *Borrelia* and *Leptospira,* pathogenic species and subspecies of *Treponema* cannot be cultivated on artificial media. *Treponema* do not take up Gram's stain, but can be visualized through darkfield microscopy or direct fluorescent antibody staining for *T. pallidum* (DFA-TP).

Clinical diagnosis

Syphilis is a disease with multiple characteristics or stages. Although the treponemes disseminate throughout the body within hours after initial contact with the organism, preferential multiplication occurs at the site of entry. Usually within 3 to 4 weeks after infection, the primary lesion or chancre appears as a single, painless lesion. In the secondary stage, which occurs 6 weeks to 6 months after infection, nonspecific symptoms develop, including fever, headache, sore throat, arthralgias, and anorexia. A generalized rash appears, with diverse manifestations often resembling other dermatoses. After a year or two, syphilis becomes latent and no clinical symptoms are present. Late manifestations are rare and usually occur many years after the initial infection (but may appear within a year); they include cardiovascular syphilis, neurosyphilis, or late benign syphilis.

Laboratory diagnosis
Microscopic

The most specific and immediate means of diagnosing syphilis is to visually identify *T. pallidum* using direct microscopic examination of specimens collected from an infected person. To collect specimens from external lesions for direct microscopic examination, if necessary, clean the lesion with 0.9% saline, then dry and squeeze the lesion to provoke exudate. The exudate should be collected directly on the microscope slide or transferred with a bacteriologic loop to the slide. Transporting specimens for darkfield examination is impossible. Perform the darkfield examination immediately after specimens are collected, because identification is based on the characteristic motility of *T. pallidum.* With darkfield microscopy, treponemes appear as delicate, corkscrew-shaped organisms with rigid, uniform, tightly wound, deep spirals and unique motility. The length of the organism is 6 to 14 μm, the width is 0.25 to 0.30 μm, length of the spiral wave is 1.0 to 1.15 μm, and the spiral depth is 0.5 to 1.0 μm.

The characteristic motion of *T. pallidum* is a deliberate forward and backward movement with rotation about the longitudinal axis. Rotation may be accompanied by a soft bending, twisting, or undulation of the organism from side to side. When attached to or obstructed by heavier particles, the organism may contort, convolute, or bend and thereby distort the coils, but the organism will snap back to its original form in a coil-like manner. Organisms easily confused with *T. pallidum* are *Treponema refringens* and *Treponema denticola.*

Collect specimens for DFA-TP either on the microscope slide or in capillary tubes sealed with a plastic closure or putty, and store at 2°C to 8°C until they are tested or shipped. Air dry smears prepared on microscope slides. Reagents for the test include phosphate-buffered saline (PBS) with pH 7.2; PBS (pH 7.2) with 2% Tween 80; reagent grade acetone or reagent grade methanol; mounting medium (1 part PBS, pH 7.2, plus 9 parts glycerine); fluorescein isothiocyanate (FITC)-labeled, anti-*T. pallidum* globulin conjugate, and controls. The conjugate should have been absorbed with the nonpathogenic *Treponema phagedenis* biotype *Reiter* treponeme or should be a monoclonal antibody to *T. pallidum.* Include appropriate controls in each test run. Place material from the capillary tube on a clean slide and air dry. Fix slides in acetone or methanol. Dilute the conjugate to a working dilution and place on slides, then stain, rinse, drain, and blot slides. If present, *Treponema pallidum* appears as a corkscrew-shaped, brightly fluorescing organism.

Serologic tests

Because lesions may not always be accessible or present, serologic tests for syphilis are performed. Initially, screen serum specimens in a nontreponemal test, then confirm reactivity with a treponemal test. Collect specimens for serologic tests by venipuncture without using anticoagulant and follow universal precautions. Aseptically separate the serum from the clot and mail or take specimens to the laboratory in leakproof tubes.

Nontreponemal tests

Five nontreponemal tests are currently considered standard tests for syphilis. They are divided into microscopic and macroscopic tests. The microscopic tests include the Venereal Disease Research Laboratory (VDRL) slide test and the unheated serum reagin (USR) test. The macroscopic tests include the rapid plasma reagin (RPR) 18-mm circle-card test, the reagin screen test (RST), and the toluidine-red unheated serum test (TRUST). The tests, other than the VDRL test, are modifications of the VDRL antigen made by stabilizing the suspension and by adding various visualization agents. All the nontreponemal tests (1) measure IgG and IgM antibodies, (2) can be used as qualitative tests for initial screening, (3) can be used as the quantitative tests to follow treatment of the patient, (4) are similar in sensitivity and specificity, and (5) are performed in a similar manner.

Macroscopic card tests, the most commonly used tests, are available in kit form to use for both qualitative and quantitative test procedures. The card tests are performed on disposable, plastic-coated cards imprinted with circles. Samples may be heated or unheated serum specimens or unheated plasma. Additional reagents for the quantitative test not provided in the kits are 0.9% saline and a 1:50 dilution of serum that is nonreactive for syphilis prepared in 0.9% saline. This diluent is used for making dilutions of a patient's serum with titers of 1:32 or greater. The antigen must be tested daily with control serum specimens, which are graded reactive, minimally reactive, and nonreactive. Reagents and serum specimens should be at room temperature, 23°C to 29°C (73°F to 85°F). To perform the test, place 50 µl of serum into one of the circles on the test card, using a dispensing or automatic pipetting device. Spread the specimen to fill the entire circle and add a drop of antigen suspension to each test area that contains serum. Rotate the card for the specified amount of time with the specified number of revolutions per minute under a humidity cover. Read the test reactions in the wet state under a high-intensity light immediately after the card is removed from the rotator. Results are reported as reactive or nonreactive. Specimens that show any degree of reactivity as well as rough nonreactive samples should be quantitated to an endpoint titer. To quantitate, use 50 µl of 0.9% saline as the diluent for 50 µl of serum and prepare twofold dilutions. Continue the dilution until it reaches 1:16. Starting at the highest dilution, spread the specimen within each circle. Add one drop of antigen to each circle, then rotate and read the card as previously described.

Quantitative results are reported as the highest titer that produces a reactive (R,Rm) result. If the endpoint titer is not reached at the highest dilution (1:16), then prepare a 1:16 dilution of test serum in 0.9% saline. Place 100 µl of the 1:16 dilution on the card and continue twofold dilutions in the 1:50 dilution of the nonreactive serum. Perform the test as previously described. Reactive nontreponemal tests may indicate past or present infection with pathogenic treponemes that may or may not have been adequately treated. Likewise, a reactive test may also be false-positive. A nonreactive test may be interpreted as no current infection or as an effectively treated infection. A nonreactive test does not rule out incubating-stage syphilis, however. Generally, a fourfold increase in titer (e.g., 1:16 to 1:64) indicates infection, reinfection, or treatment failure, whereas a fourfold decrease in titer indicates adequate therapy in the early stages of syphilis.

Although the overall sensitivity of the nontreponemal tests is approximately 90%, the results will be nonreactive in up to 28% of patients with early primary syphilis during their initial visits. In addition, in approximately 30% of the cases of late, untreated syphilis, patients' nontreponemal tests will be nonreactive. Specificity for the nontreponemal tests is 98%. However, the specificity of the test is greatly influenced by the population tested. The nontreponemal tests

are reactive in patients with secondary syphilis; almost without exception, titers will be 1:16 or greater, regardless of the test method used. Less than 2% of these patients will have serum specimens that exhibit a prozone. Nontreponemal test titers in early latent syphilis are similar to those titers obtained in secondary syphilis. However, as the length of the latent stage increases, the titer decreases.

Treponemal tests

The treponemal tests are reserved for confirmatory testing when the clinical signs or patient history disagrees with the reactive nontreponemal test results. Three treponemal tests are currently considered standard tests for syphilis: the fluorescent treponemal antibody absorption (FTA-ABS) test, the FTA-ABS double staining (DS) test, and the microhemagglutination assay for antibodies to *T. pallidum* (MHA-TP). All treponemal tests use *T. pallidum* subspecies *pallidum* as the antigen, and all are based on the detection of antibodies directed against treponemal cellular components. The treponemal tests are qualitative procedures and cannot be used to monitor the efficacy of treatment.

The FTA-ABS and FTA-ABS DS tests are the most popular of the treponemal tests and therefore will be described here. For the FTA-ABS tests, a microscope with transmitted illumination is used, and for the FTA-ABS DS test, a microscope with incident illumination is used. Reagents may be purchased in kit form from a variety of commercial manufacturers and include *T. pallidum* subspecies *pallidum* antigen, sorbent, conjugates, and control serum samples. The fluorescein isothiocyanate (FITC)-labeled antihuman conjugate used in the FTA-ABS tests principally recognizes heavy-chain IgG. The FTA-ABS DS test's tetramethyl-rhodamine isothiocyanate (TMRITC)-labeled antihuman conjugate should recognize heavy-chain IgG only. The FITC-labeled antitreponemal conjugate (counterstain) of the FTA-ABS DS test should stain the treponemes at a 3+ to 4+ intensity. For both tests, the control serum samples consist of a reactive 4+ control, a minimally reactive 1+ control (which may be a dilution of the 4+ control), and a nonspecific serum control. Other reagents are PBS, pH 7.2 ± 0.1; 2.0% Tween 80 (polysorbate 80); mounting medium; and acetone.

To prepare antigen slides, resuspend and mix treponemes until they are adequately dispersed, as seen by darkfield examination before slides are prepared. On thoroughly cleaned slides, make a very thin antigen smear within each circle using a standard platinum wire loop. Air dry slides for at least 15 minutes, then fix smears in acetone for 10 minutes and thoroughly air dry. Slides fixed in this manner may be stored frozen indefinitely.

There are seven controls for the FTA-ABS tests. Prepare two reactive 4+ controls. Place 30 µl of each of the following dilutions on separate antigen circles. The reactive 4+ control should demonstrate 4+ staining when diluted 1:5 in PBS and 3+ to 4+ staining when diluted 1:5 in sorbent. The minimally reactive (1+) control is a dilution of a reactive serum in PBS to point where the minimal degree of fluorescence that is reported as reactive is observed. Do *not* dilute this control further in sorbent. Place the 1+ control on an antigen circle. Use this control as the reading standard for the day's test run. Prepare the two nonspecific serum controls from a serum specimen of a person without syphilis. The serum should give 2 + staining when diluted 1:5 in PBS and essentially no staining when diluted 1:5 in sorbent. Place 30 μl of each of the two 1:5 dilutions on separate antigen circles. Prepare the two reagent specificity controls by simply adding PBS to one antigen smear and sorbent to another antigen smear.

Heat the serum samples to be tested for 30 minutes at 56°C. Then prepare a 1:5 dilution of the heated serum in sorbent. Place the diluted serum on the antigen smear and incubate the slide, along with the control slides, within a moist chamber at 35°C to 37°C for 30 minutes. After incubation, rinse slides with running PBS for approximately 5 seconds, then place them in a staining dish containing PBS. While the slides are in the PBS, agitate them by dipping them in and out at least 30 times. Change the PBS after 5 minutes and again agitate the slides. Next, rinse the slides in running distilled water for approximately 5 seconds and then gently blot to remove excess water droplets.

If the FTA-ABS DS test is being performed, at this point place TMRITC-labeled antihuman IgG globulin, which has been diluted in PBS containing 2% Tween 80 to its working titer, on each smear. Incubate, rinse, and blot the slides as already described. Then place FITC-labeled anti-treponemal globulin, which has been diluted in PBS containing 2% Tween 80 to the working titer on each smear, and incubate the slides for 20 minutes, then rinse and blot as previously described.

For the FTA-ABS test, after the initial serum incubation and rinsing and blotting of slides, place FITC-labeled antihuman immunoglobulin properly diluted in PBS containing 2% Tween 80 on each antigen smear. Then incubate, rinse, and blot the slides as after the initial serum incubation.

In both FTA-ABS tests, mount the slides by placing a small drop of mounting medium on each smear and apply coverslips. The slides should be examined as soon as possible. However, if a delay in reading is necessary, place slides in a darkened room and read within 4 hours.

For the FTA-ABS test, use the darkfield condenser and the tungsten light to verify the presence of treponemes on nonreactive slides. For the FTA-ABS DS test, locate treponemes and focus the microscope using the FITC filter system, then switch to the TMRITC filters to read specific fluorescence.

Read both tests in the same manner. Record the intensity of staining as follows: ± or <1 + when there is visible staining but it is less than the 1 + reading standard, 1 + when the intensity is equivalent to the minimally reactive 1 + control, and 2 + to 4 + when the intensity is moderate to strong. If there is no staining or if treponemes are vaguely visible but without distinct fluorescence, record the reading as −. Repeat the test with any specimen staining 1 +. Specimens reading 2 + to 4 + are reported as reactive (R). Specimens staining 1 + on repeat tests are reported as reactive minimal (RM) with a notation that in the absence of historical or clinical evidence of treponemal infection, this test result should be considered equivocal. A second specimen should be submitted for serologic testing. Specimens read initially as negative or repeating as negative should be reported as nonreactive.

A reactive treponemal test usually indicates past or present infection with pathogenic treponemes. Usually, once the treponemal tests are reactive, they remain reactive for a lifetime. In fact, in some patients with late syphilis, a reactive treponemal test may be the only means of confirming the suspected diagnosis. Generally, a nonreactive test indicates no past or present infection. However, when treatment is begun in early syphilis, for example, in the primary or secondary stage, about 14% of these patients will test nonreactive within 2 years after treatment. The treponemal test also may be nonreactive for incubating-stage syphilis.

The overall sensitivity of the FTA-ABS test, approximately 98%, is greater than that of the other three treponemal tests, which have sensitivities of approximately 95%. The major difference in sensitivities is found in the primary stage. The specificities of the four treponemal tests are 98% for the FTA-ABS test and 99% for the other three treponemal tests.

Antigen detection

Specific tests are needed for the diagnosis of congenital syphilis and neurosyphilis. Antigen detection tests are in the early stages of evaluation.

VAGINOSIS/VAGINITIS

Although complaints of vaginal discharge, odor, pruritus (itching), and irritation account for numerous physician office visits yearly, the diagnosis of vaginitis/vaginosis may also be an incidental finding during a routine pelvic examination. Infections of the vagina are usually bacterial, fungal (yeast), or protozoan in origin, and may or may not be associated with sexual transmission. Male partners of women with vaginosis may have inapparent, transient infections, or overt manifestations of urethritis, prostatitis, or epididymitis.

Bacterial causes

Bacteria are the most common cause of vaginosis and the infection may be the result of an alteration in the natural flora or change in the pH of the vagina. Because the organisms associated with infection may also be a part of the normal flora, disease may be a result of a break in the complex symbiotic relationship between lactobacilli, other aerobic, facultative anaerobic, and anaerobic bacteria that normally colonize the vagina. Clinical diagnosis of bacterial vaginosis is based on finding at least three of the following signs: (1) a thin, homogeneous, gray discharge clinging to the vaginal walls; (2) a foul odor (amine or fishlike) associated with vaginal secretions intensified by the addition of 10% potassium hydroxide (KOH); (3) a vaginal pH of greater than 4.5; and (4) the presence of epithelial cells (clue cells) on wet mount.

Gardnerella vaginalis (Haemophilus vaginalis, Corynebacterium vaginale)

First, collect two specimens of vaginal fluids on two cotton-tipped or calcium alginate swabs, one for culture and one for microscopy. For culture, immediately press the swab onto a plate containing primary isolation medium such as Columbia agar with colistin and nalidixic acid, supplemented with 1% proteose-peptone No. 3 and 5% whole human or rabbit blood, or human bilayer agar. Incubate the plate in an atmosphere of 5% to 10% CO_2 (in a candle jar) or in an anaerobic chamber at 35°C to 37°C and examine for 2 to 3 days. At 48 hours the colonies of *G. vaginalis* are 0.3 to 0.5 mm in diameter, smooth, opaque, gray-white, and have sharp outlines, surrounded by diffuse beta hemolysis. A Gram's stain revealing pleomorphic, gram-variable rods gives a presumptive identification of *G. vaginalis.* If specimens must be transported, place the swab in 0.5 ml of an enriched medium such as Columbia, trypticase soy, Amies transport, or Stuart and plate within a few hours or freeze at −50°C or below.

From a second swab prepare a wet mount or a Gram's stain smear. (The Gram's stain smear is preferable.) On Gram's stain, *G. vaginalis* organisms are gram-negative or gram-variable, pleomorphic coccobacilli or rods, 0.4 × 1.5 µm in size, and often are attached to vaginal epithelial cells (clue cells). The presence of clue cells and the absence or a low number of *Lactobacillus* spp. on Gram's stain correlate with a diagnosis of bacterial vaginosis.

For definitive identification of *G. vaginalis,* several biochemical tests are used (Table 50-1). More than 85% of the *G. vaginalis* strains are positive for hippurate, starch hydrolysis, and α-glucosidase, and are negative for catalase.

To detect hippurate hydrolysis, suspend colonies from growth medium such as heart infusion agar supplemented with 5% defibrinated rabbit blood or chocolate agar or Columbia agar in 0.5 ml of a 1% solution of sodium hippurate in 0.067 M Sorensen phosphate buffer (pH 6.4). After the tubes have been incubated for 2 hours at 35°C, add 0.2 ml of a solution of 3.5% ninhydrin in equal parts of acetone and butanol. The development of a deep purple color within 5 minutes indicates a positive test.

To demonstrate α-glucosidase, add a loopful of bacteria from an overnight culture to 0.5 ml of a substrate solution containing 0.1% 4-nitrophenyl-alpha-D-glycopyranoside in 0.67 M Sorensen phosphate buffer (pH 8.0). For β-glucosidase, inoculate the culture into 0.067 M Sorensen phosphate buffer (pH 8.0) containing 0.1% 4-nitrophenyl-beta-D-glycopyranoside. Incubate the tubes for 4 hours in a 35°C water bath. The development of a yellow color indicates a positive test. *Gardnerella vaginalis* is positive for α-glucosidase and negative for β-glucosidase.

To detect starch hydrolysis, flood colonies on a Mueller-Hinton agar plate containing 5% horse serum with Lugol iodine. Clearing is characteristic of hydrolysis. On purple agar base plus 1% cornstarch, the growth area is yellow with a clear area surrounding it.

Although acid production from various sugars is not necessarily recommended for the identification of genital isolates, if degradation of glucose and maltose is to be determined, use a proteose-peptone medium. Another method of

Table 50-1 Biochemical identification of Gardnerella vaginalis

Positive tests	Negative tests
Acid phosphatase	Catalase
Hippurate hydrolysis	Oxidase
Starch hydrolysis	β-Glucosidase
α-Glucosidase	Mannitol
Acid from glucose, maltose, sucrose (85%)	Nitrate reduction
	Urease
	Indole

identification is the API 20 Strep system (API System La Balme Les Grottes, Montalieu-Vercieu, France) consisting of 20 biochemical tests. The inoculum for the strip must be equivalent to a McFarland standard of 4.

Mobiluncus spp

Although *Gardnerella* and *Mobiluncus* spp. are not the sole bacterial etiologic agents of vaginosis, the association of *Peptostreptococcus, Peptococcus,* and *Bacteroides* spp. is even less clear. Members of the genus *Mobiluncus* ("mobile hooks") are anaerobic, curved rods made motile by subpolar flagella. The species within the genus differ in their Gram's stain reaction, length, and ability to migrate through soft agar. *Mobiluncus curtisii* subspecies *curtisii* and *holmesii* are small (±1.7 µm), gram-variable rods. Nitrate reduction or the lack thereof is the basic difference between the two subspecies. *Mobiluncus mulieris* spp. are larger (±2.9 µm) gram-negative rods.

For preliminary identification, plate a cotton-tipped or calcium alginate swab of vaginal fluid on enriched medium such as Columbia agar with 5% rabbit blood supplemented with colistin and nalidixic acid to inhibit other bacteria, or on a semiselective bilayer agar. Incubate the plates anaerobically at 35°C to 37°C for at least 5 days. Colonies of *Mobiluncus* spp. are minute, translucent, gray, and convex. On medium containing rabbit blood, *M. mulieris* produces spotty or weak hemolysis, and *M. curtisii* produces little or no hemolysis.

Perform Gram's stain on suspect colonies and transfer to translucent GC Base agar supplemented with IsoVitaleX and 0.1% cornstarch to demonstrate starch hydrolysis. Oxidase and catalase tests are negative. *Mobiluncus curtisii* strains produce ornithine, citrulline, and ammonia from arginine; *M. mulieris* strains do not. *Mobiluncus mulieris* strains produce acid from glycogen and do not hydrolyze hippurate.

Because culture techniques for *Mobiluncus* spp. and other vaginal bacteria are laborious, and because simply isolating a specific organism from vaginal secretions does not necessarily confirm that particular bacterium as the cause of the vaginosis, other methods such as Gram's stain, DNA probes, and gas-liquid chromatography (GLC) may be more sensitive and as specific as culture techniques. A detailed method for GLC has been described by Spiegel.

Fungal causes

The yeast causing vaginitis (as the bacteria causing vaginosis) also may be part of the endogenous vaginal flora; most women have at least one symptomatic infection during their lifetime. Predisposing risk factors to symptomatic infection include pregnancy, diabetes, use of birth control pills, corticosteroids, and systemic antimicrobials and immunosuppression.

Clinically, pruritus (with or without vaginal discharge) is the most common symptom. When a discharge does occur, it is usually white, thick, and curdlike (cottage-cheese–like). There is no offensive odor.

Candida albicans

Candida spp. are the most frequent cause of infection, with *Candida albicans* the most common species. *Candida albicans* occurs in both yeast and mycelial forms. In the vagina, the yeasts multiply by forming buds that elongate and do not detach from one another. Such forms are called pseudohyphae, because, unlike true hyphae, no mycelium is formed. Preliminary diagnosis may be made by wet mount or Gram's stain. Initially, for a wet mount use a cotton-tipped applicator to transfer a small amount of discharge to a drop or two (50 to 100 μl) of 10% KOH on a glass slide. Place a coverslip on top and gently heat the slide. Examine the slide with a microscope equipped with a brightfield condenser under low power ($\times 100$) magnification for the presence of yeasts. Examination of the slide at high power ($\times 400$) will permit detailed observation of the organism. The yeasts are oval cells about 2.5×4 μm in diameter. The Gram's stain is as sensitive as a wet mount for the detection of *Candida* spp. On Gram's stain, the yeast are stained an intense purple.

The most sensitive method for the detection of *Candida* is culture. The most frequently recommended medium is Sabouraud dextrose agar with chloramphenicol. Streak the specimen swab on one plate of Sabouraud medium with antibiotic and on a second plate without the antibiotic. Incubate plates at 30°C for 48 to 72 hours. Examine colonies for germ tube and chlamydospore formation.

Protozoan causes

Symptomatic trichomoniasis, *Trichomonas vaginalis* vaginitis, is clinically characterized by vaginal itching, usually with an accompanying discharge. Commonly, the discharge is purulent and often described as yellow-green and foamy. As in bacterial vaginosis, an odor may occasionally be noticed, probably indicating an overgrowth of anaerobic microorganisms.

Trichomonas vaginalis

Current practice is to initially collect vaginal secretions for wet mount. Use a Dacron-tipped swab for collection. After collection, either place the swab in a tube containing a small amount of normal saline and swirl or gently vortex and then place 50 μl on a microscope slide, or mix the swab with 50 to 100 μl of saline directly on a microscope slide. Place a coverslip over the specimen and examine the slide by light (brightfield) or phase-contrast (darkfield) microscopy. Under low power, the trichomonads are ovoid in shape, approximately the size of lymphocytes (10 to 20 μm), and move with a characteristic jerky motion. Under high power, confirm the presence of four anterior flagella with a trailing fifth flagellum attached to an undulating membrane. The wet mount is a rather insensitive technique. Sensitivity is optimal when the specimen is examined within 15 to 20 minutes after collection, the concentration of the parasite is high ($\geq 10^5$/ml), and the miscroscopist is experienced. When the specimen must be transported, a variety of staining methods for use with vaginal smears are available. Acridine orange and immunofluorescent techniques appear to be more sensitive than other staining methods. Specimens that test positive by wet mount or direct staining techniques do not need to be confirmed by culture.

Culture methods are estimated to detect twice the number of infections as wet mounts alone. *Trichomonas vaginalis* is an aerotolerant anaerobe with a fermentative metabolism. Many liquid media are available for the growth of these organisms. In a recent study, Schmid and others found Diamond's medium to be superior to others evaluated. Inoculate culture medium at room temperature with a portion (0.2 ml) of the saline in which the vaginal swab was placed for wet mount examination. Incubate the culture tube either aerobically or anaerobically at 33°C to 35°C for up to 7 days. Each day examine a drop of fluid from the bottom of the culture tube by wet mount for the presence of trichomonads. If daily examination is impossible, then examine cultures at day 3 or 4 and again at day 7.

SUGGESTED READING

Ahearn DG and Schlitzer RL: Yeast infections. In Balows A (editor): Diagnostic procedures in bacterial, mycotic and parasitic infections, ed 6, Washington, DC, 1981, American Public Health Association.

Ashley RL: Genital herpes infections. In Judson FN (editor): Clinics in laboratory medicine, vol 9, Philadelphia, 1989, WB Saunders.

Barnes RC: Infections caused by Chlamydia trachomatis. In Morse SA, Moreland AA, and Thompson SE (editors): Atlas of sexually transmitted diseases, New York, 1989, Gower Medical Publishing.

Barnes RC: Laboratory diagnosis of human chlamydial infections, Clin Microbiol Rev 2:119, 1989.

Cassell GH, Waites KB, and Taylor-Robinson D: Genital mycoplasmas. In Morse SA, Moreland AA, Thompson SE (editors): Atlas of sexually transmitted diseases, New York, 1989, Gower Medical Publishing.

Corey L: Genital herpes. In Holmes KK and others (editors): Sexually transmitted diseases, ed 2, New York, 1989, McGraw Hill.

Douglas JM and Werness BA: Genital human papillomavirus infections. In Judson FN (editor): Clinics in laboratory medicine, vol 9, Philadelphia, 1989, WB Saunders.

Fiumara NJ: Herpes simplex. In Clinics in dermatology, vol 7, Philadelphia, 1989, JB Lippincott.

Gissmann L and Schneider A: The role of human papillomavirus in genital cancer. In de Palo G, Rike F, and zur Hausen H (editors): Herpes and papillomavirus, vol 31, New York, 1986, Raven Press.

Glatt AE, McCormack WM, and Taylor-Robinson D: Genital mycoplasmas. In Holmes KK and others (editors): Sexually transmitted diseases, ed 2, New York, 1989, McGraw Hill.

Grayston JT and others: Chlamydia pneumoniae sp. nov. for Chlamydia sp. strain TWAR, Int J Syst Bacteriol 39:88, 1989.

Kenney GE: Genital mycoplasmata. In Wentworth BB and Judson FN (editors): Laboratory methods for the diagnosis of sexually transmitted diseases, Washington, DC, 1984, American Public Health Association.

Lever WF: Histopathology of the skin, ed 4, London, 1967, Pitman.

Mathews HM: Trichomoniasis. In Balows A and others (editors): Laboratory diagnosis of infectious diseases: principles and practice, vol 1, New York, 1988, Springer-Verlag.

Mifflin TE, Bruns DE, and Savory J: Detection of papillomavirus DNA, Clin Chem 34:1359, 1988.

Schachter J: Chlamydiaceae: the Chlamydiae. In Balows A and others (editors): Laboratory diagnosis of infectious diseases: principles and practice, vol 1, New York, 1988, Springer-Verlag.

Schmid GP and others: Evaluation of six media for the growth of Trichomonas vaginalis from vaginal secretions. J Clin Microbiol 27:1230, 1989.

Schmid GP, Schalla WO, and DeWitt WE: Chancroid. In Morse SA, Moreland AA, and Thompson SE (editors): Atlas of sexually transmitted diseases, New York, 1989, Gower Medical Publishing.

Schneider A: Methods of identification of human papillomavirus. In Syrjanen K, Gissmann L, and Koss LG (editors): Papillomavirus and human disease, Berlin, 1987, Springer-Verlag.

Secor RMC: Bacterial vaginosis: a comprehensive review, Nurs Clin N Am 23:865, 1988.

Spiegel CA: Vaginitis. In Wentworth BB and Judson FN (editors): Laboratory methods for the diagnosis of sexually transmitted diseases, Washington DC, 1984, American Public Health Association.

51

Wound, body fluid, and surgical specimens

Robert C. Jerris

Wound cultures, surgical specimens, and sterile body fluids other than cerebrospinal fluid represent a significant proportion of the total specimen load in the clinical microbiology laboratory. Infections at these sites may be caused by bacteria, fungi, viruses, and occasionally by parasites. Each specimen type poses a unique set of challenges both to the physician and to the microbiologist. Agents responsible for significant morbidity range from relatively common organisms to agents that are difficult for the laboratory to isolate and identify. Due to this fact and the ever increasing patient population who are immunocompromised, the optimum recovery of pathogens requires ardent communication between clinician and laboratorian.

WOUND CULTURES
Skin and soft tissue

Infection of the skin may occur from direct invasion of microorganisms or may be a secondary complication of surgery or trauma, or may result from a disseminated systemic infection. Lesions observed on the skin often give significant clues as to the type of etiologic agent responsible for infection. These cutaneous surface lesions can be simplistically categorized using the following definitions.

Macules are non-elevated, non-depressed, circumscribed regions of discolored skin resulting from extravasation of blood or pigment. Special forms of maculae include purpura, petechia, and ecchymosis. Endocarditis and meningococcemia are examples of embolic infection that can present this way.

Papules are solid lesions less than 1 cm in diameter elevated above the skin. Although primarily due to dermal hyperplasia, a number of infectious agents, primarily viruses, present with maculopapular lesions. A *verrucous lesion* is a type of papule consisting of multiple, closely packed elevations. Warts, orf, tuberculosis, leprosy, nocardiosis, and the cutaneous fungi may demonstrate verrucous lesions.

Elevated, circumscribed lesions containing serum, lymph, or blood are defined as *vesicles* (if less than or equal to 0.5 cm in diameter) or *bullae* (if greater than 0.5 cm in diameter). Although most commonly caused by viral agents, significant bacteria may demonstrate these skin

manifestations. Noteworthy among the bacteria are *Staphylococcus aureus* and *Streptococcus pyogenes* in cases of impetigo, *Pseudomonas aeruginosa* in cases of ecthyma gangrenosum, *Clostridium perfringens* with a concomitant bronze discoloration of the skin, *Vibrio vulnificus*, and miscellaneous enteric gram negative bacilli. *Pustules* are vesicles filled with pus and are commonly associated with pyogenic bacteria.

Ulcerative lesions result from loss of the epidermal and dermal layers of the skin. Agents responsible for these types of lesions include *Corynebacterium diphtheria, Bacillus anthracis, Francisella tularensis, Nocardia* species, *Mycobacterium marinum, Sporothrix schenkii*, the systemic fungal pathogen *Blastomyces dermatitidis*, and agents of sexually transmissable diseases (Chapter 50). Table 51-1 details some of the skin lesions associated with specific agents. Fungal infections including superficial dermatophytic and yeast infections are dealt with in Chapter 52.

Many infectious diseases involving skin manifestations may be directly related to occupational, environmental, or animal exposure. Table 51-2 lists some of the more common associations.

In addition to the previously described agents, several other noteworthy infectious diseases demonstrate skin lesions. *Scarlet fever*, caused by an erythrogenic toxin as a result of the beta-phage being inserted in certain strains of *S. pyogenes*, is manifest on the skin as a diffuse erythematous (red) eruption. *Scalded skin* and *toxic-shock syndromes* are caused by toxins from *S. aureus*. Both syndromes manifest as a rash with subsequent desquamation of the affected skin. In both cases the organism producing the toxin is located at an infection site remote from the lesions. *Erythrasma*, a superficial infection caused by *Corynebacterium minutissimum* is often confused with fungal dermatophytic infections. This infection shows dry, scaly, pink to brown lesions of the skin and is most often located in the groin, pubis, axillary, intergluteal, or intermammary folds. *Erysipelas* is a common infection caused primarily by *S. pyogenes* and other beta hemolytic streptococci, notably Groups C and G. A marked, fiery-red inflammatory lesion with raised edematous borders is apparent.

When microorganisms gain access to the dermis and sub-

Table 51-1 Skin involvement in selected infectious diseases

Manifestation	Agent(s)/syndrome	REF
Viruses/rickettsia		
Vesiculopustules	Herpes simplex, Variola, Vaccinia, Varicella, Rickettsiapox, Coxsackievirus A and B, Reovirus 2, *Mycoplasma pneumonia, ECHO 4, Orf	4
Maculopapules	*Secondary syphilis, *Scarlet fever, ECHO 9 and 16 Erythema infectiosum, Rubella, Rubeola, Hepatitis Coxsackie A5, A9, A16, B5, Reovirus 2, Arbovirus Rickettsioses	
Petechia	*Bacterial endocarditis, ECHO 9, Mononucleosis Rubella, Coxsackie A5, A9	
Bacteria		
Primary pyoderma impetigo	*Staphylococcus aureus*, group A streptococci	37
Folliculitis, carbuncle, furuncle	*S. aureus*	
Paronychia	*S. aureus*, group A streptococci, *Pseudomonas aeruginosa*	
Ecthyma	*P. aeruginosa*, group A streptococci	
Erysipelas	Group A streptococci	
Cellulitis	Group A streptococci, *S. aureus*, others (see text)	
Erythrasma	*Corynebacterium minutissimum*	

*Although not virus/rickettsia class, these agent(s)/syndromes are included in these categories because of their similar skin manifestations.

cutaneous tissues, an abscess may develop. This localized accumulation of pus, not visible through the intact skin, is the most common response to pyogenic bacteria. *S. aureus* and *S. pyogenes* account for the vast majority of these types of infections including folliculitis, furunculosis, and carbuncles. These agents, in particular *S. aureus*, are occasionally present with mixed flora in cases of botryomycosis,

a skin lesion often containing a granule consisting of dense clumps of the organisms. Deep-seated abscesses may spontaneously rupture and erode to the skin surface, resulting in draining sinus tracts. The causative organisms vary dramatically depending on the underlying disorder. The laboratory must be prepared to culture slow-growing anaerobic organisms including *Actinomyces* species, bacteroides, fu-

Table 51-2 Select skin and soft tissue infections related to reservoir, occupation, and environmental factors*

Disease	Organism(s)	Predisposing factor/reservoir
Bacteria		
Anthrax	*Bacillus anthracis*	Sheep, goats, animal products—wool, ivory
Brucellosis	*Brucella* species	Meatpacking, livestock grazers veterinarians, cattle, swine
Erysipeloid	*Erysipelothrix rhusiopathae*	Swine, fish, shellfish, poultry
Glanders	*Pseudomonas mallei*	Horses
Leptospirosis	*Leptospira icterrohemorrhagiae*	Farmers, hunters, wild animals
Pet bite infections	*Pasteurella multocida DF-2*	Dogs, cats, others
Rat bite fever	*Streptobacillus moniliformis*	Rodents, prairie dogs
Tularemia	*Fransicella tularensis*	Hunters, trappers, furriers rodents, rabbits, foxes
Plague	*Yersinia pestis*	Rodents, prairie dogs
Trachoma	*Chlamydia trachomatis*	Towel sharing
Syphilis	*Treponema pallidum*	Glassblowing
Miscellaneous	*Aeromonas* species, *Vibrio vulnificus*, other *Vibrio* species, *Mycobacterium marinum*	Fisherman, divers, shellfish
Protozoa		
African trypanosomiasis	*Trypanosoma gambiensis*	Tsetse fly
American trypanosomiasis	*T. cruzi*	Triatomid bugs, dogs, cats, monkeys, rodents
Leishmaniasis	*Leishmania donavani, L. braziliensis, L. tropica*	Mosquitoes (*Phlebotomus* species)
Helminths		
Schistosomiasis	*Schistosoma hematobium, S. mansoni, S. japonicum*	Snails
Cutaneous larva Migrans	*Ancylostoma braziliensis* *A. caninum*	Dogs, cattle
Trichinosis	*Trichinella spiralis*	Swine
Sparganosis	*Spirometra mansoides*	Snakes, birds, pigs, frogs, cats, dogs
Cutaneous loiasis	*Loa loa*	Biting fly (*Chrysops* species)

*From Simmons RL and Arhenholz DH: Infection of the skin and soft tissue. In Howard RJ, and Simmons RL, eds: Surgical infectious diseases, ed 2, Appleton & Lange, 1988.

sobacteria, and mycobacteria, as well as the more commonly seen agents of *S. aureus* and various members of the *Enterobacteriaceae*.

The expanding diffuse infection of the skin and subcutaneous tissue known as cellulitis, is typified by pain, tenderness, erythema, and edema and may be associated with fever and regional lymphadenopathy. Classically, *S. aureus* and *S. pyogenes* are involved; however, *S. pneumoniae, S. agalactiae* and the viridans streptococci may be isolated. Note that cellulitis differs from erysipelas in that there is no distinct demarcation of the border of the lesion with cellulitis. The clinical history is particularly important, as cellulitis is often a complication of infections with unusual pathogens like *Erysipelothrix rhusiopathiae*, from environmental soil exposure; *Aeromonas hydrophila*, from exposure to natural fresh and saltwater; and *Haemophilus influenzae* in the upper extremities, especially the face and neck in young children. In addition, fulminant rapidly spreading lesions may be due to *Clostridium perfringens*. Typically, cellulitis involves all layers of the skin and subcutaneous tissue without suppuration or necrosis.

Lymphadenopathy is frequently observed in Cat Scratch Disease. The etiological agent of Cat Scratch Disease has recently been described. It is a pleomorphic gram negative bacillus named *Afipia Felis* and is isolated with difficulty from infected lymph nodes. The medium of choice is buffered charcoal-yeast extract agar.

Certain groups of organisms infect the subcutaneous tissue and spread in the fascial cleft's overlying muscle. As the blood supply to the skin is interrupted, skin gangrene results. These syndromes can be collectively termed necrotizing fasciitis and include: clostridial anaerobic cellulitis caused primarily by *C. perfringens* and *C. septicum;* nonclostridial anaerobic cellulitis caused by a mixed anaerobic flora excluding clostridia species; and mixed synergistic necrotizing cellulitis caused by a mixture of aerobic and anaerobic species.

Muscle involvement may be a prominent manifestation in many infections as organisms gain entry into the deeper tissues. Although the pathologic processes and predisposing factors may be quite variable, wound specimens are required for diagnosis. Gangrenous infections involving muscle include clostridial myonecrosis and classic gas gangrene, and may be a rapidly progressive, life threatening, toxemic infection. Although *C. perfringens* is most commonly involved, other species, including *C. novyi, C. septicum,* and less frequently *C. bifermentans, C. histolyticum,* and *C. fallax,* have been isolated. Non-clostridial myonecrosis may be caused by anaerobic streptococci alone or in a mixed synergistic infection with different species of anaerobes. Discrete primary involvement of muscle tissue has been described with *S. aureus* and more rarely with *S. pneumoniae* and *Escherichia coli.*

The sources of the majority of the previously described organisms are endogenous, that is, part of the normal microbial flora of the host. The clinical syndromes associated with traumatic and punctative wound infections may involve organisms from exogenous sources in the environment. Two significant wound infections of serious consequence are botulism and tetanus. *C. botulinum* secretes a neurotoxin responsible for an acute descending flaccid paralysis. Of the seven antigenically distinct toxins, designated A-F, the ma-

jority of human wound infections are caused by Groups A and B. Clinically, wound botulism differs from foodborne botulism in that wound botulism usually does *not* involve fever, nausea, or vomiting. Additionally, the incubation period of wound botulism is generally longer (4-14 d versus 18-36 h). The specific diagnosis depends on microbiological culture, with identification of the organism and demonstration of the toxin.

The exotoxin tetanospasmin, produced by *C. tetani,* is responsible for the disease tetanus (lockjaw). Two basic forms of the syndrome have been described. Local tetanus is confined to the site of the wound and is characterized by spasms of the affected muscles. Systemic involvement is characterized by tonic spasms of the involuntary muscles and may eventually result in respiratory arrest. The diagnosis is made primarily on clinical grounds and may be prevented by immunization with tetanal toxoid.

Many types of organisms may be responsible for infections secondary to trauma and often represent the ubiquitous flora inhabiting the specific environment at the site of the accident. The laboratorian is guarded against the casual dismissal of these potential pathogens as simple "environmental" organisms.

BODY FLUIDS

Excessive fluid accumulation in various body sites is the primary reason for collecting specimens for examination in the laboratory. The stimuli for excessive production may be due to toxic influences, trauma, hemodynamic derangements, immunologic and infectious causes. The composition of the fluid differs dramatically depending on the stimuli. Fluid, usually devoid of cellular material, with a specific gravity of less than 1.102 is known as a transudate and generally results secondarily to causes other than infection. Exudates are inflammatory extravascular fluids with high specific gravity (greater than 1.012) and contain a prominent white blood cell component. Exudates are most commonly associated with infection.

Body fluids to be covered in this chapter include synovial, pericardial, pleural, and peritoneal including peritoneal dialysate fluid, and bile.

Synovial fluid

Synovial, or joint, fluid is secreted by the membrane cells lining joints and is responsible for lubrication and decreasing friction. Infections most commonly arise from the hematogenous route. Characteristically, the infections are monoarticular involving one of the large joints, most commonly the knees or hips, followed by the ankles, elbows, wrists, or shoulders. The affected joint usually demonstrates a typical inflammatory response with swelling, pain, redness, increased temperature, and limitation of motion. The most common etiologic agent of all cases of septic arthritis is *S. aureus*. In children less than two years old, *H. influenzae* predominates, while in adults under 30 years, *Neisseria gonorrhoeae* is most common. Less commonly involved in joint infections are members of the *Enterobacteriaceae*, Group A and B streptococci, *S. pneumoniae, Enterococcus* species, and, rarely, anaerobes including the bacteroides and fusobacteria. Mycobacteria and *Nocardia* species may also be isolated.

Infection of prosthetic joints occurs rarely (in less than 1% of operations). However, the types of organisms differ dramatically from those previously described. Most commonly involved are coagulase negative staphylococci and anaerobic non-sporeforming rods of the *Propionibacterium* species. These organisms are presumably inoculated into the wounds at the time of surgery and at some later time demonstrate infections.

Noninfectious arthritic manifestations accompany a large number of infectious diseases including Lyme disease, meningococcal diseases, and others and are presumed to be the result of the cascade of events following antigen-antibody complexes.

Pericardial fluid

Approximately 20 ml of clear, serous pericardial fluid bathe the heart. This fluid is contained by the pericardium, the protective covering of the heart and its major vessels. Hemodynamic involvement secondary to congestive heart failure or systemic edema associated with liver or renal disease may lead to an increase in the volume of this fluid. Inflammation of the pericardium (pericarditis) may have the same effect. The most common agents infecting the pericardium are viruses. Coxsackie A and B predominate as infectious agents, while echoviruses, adenoviruses, influenza viruses and others have a lesser role.

Bacteria play a smaller role in pericarditis and usually manifest with a purulent reaction. *S. aureus*, *S. pneumoniae*, *Enterobacteriaceae*, and other gram-negative rods, as well as anaerobes, have all been recovered from pericardial fluid. *M. tuberculosis*, *Nocardia*, and *Actinomyces* species may also be found. Parasites very infrequently detected include *Entamoeba histolytica* and *Toxoplasma gondii*. The rapidly growing mycobacterium, *M. chelonei* has been isolated from pericardial fluid secondary to infected porcine aortic valves. Most non-viral infections of the pericardium occur in patients with severe underlying disorders.

Pleural fluid

Found between the lungs and the pleura, pleural fluid is frequently referred to as thoracentesis fluid. Like pericardial fluid, increases in the normal volume of pleural fluid occur in many systemic diseases where hemodynamic derangements occur. Infections generally create an exudative effusion. Frank purulent exudates of the pleural cavity are termed empyema.

Microorganisms found in the pleural fluid most frequently gain access through contiguous spread from an intrapulmonary source, secondary to pneumonia. As such, the common agents of infection include *S. pneumoniae*, *S. aureus*, *H. influenzae*, *Enterobacteriaceae*, pseudomonads, and mixed aerobic and anaerobic flora from aspiration pneumonia. Agents recovered less frequently from pleural fluid include *M. tuberculosis*, nontuberculous mycobacteria, *Nocardia* species (particularly in immunocompromised hosts), and *Actinomyces* species. Smaller volumes of pleural effusions seen with bacteria may be evident with mycoplasma and viruses.

Alternative routes to seeding of the pleural cavity include spread from subdiaphragmatic or hepatic abscesses. The agents subsequently isolated will more closely reflect the endogenous flora of the colon.

Peritoneal fluid

Peritoneal fluid bathes the liver, pancreas, kidneys, spleen, stomach, bladder, intestinal tract, Fallopian tubes, and ovaries and is contained by the peritoneal cavity. The fluid is generally serous in nature. The collection of edema fluid in the peritoneal cavity, secondary to serious systemic disease (primarily portal hypertension) yielding a transudative effusion, is known as ascites. As with other body fluids, infectious agents stimulate an exudative response. Microbes that infect the peritoneal fluid may gain access to the peritoneum by many different routes, including: direct extension through perforation of the bowel, contiguous spread from infected organs, implantation secondary to trauma or surgery, and hematogenous dissemination. These infections are sometimes referred to as secondary peritonitis, as opposed to primary peritonitis, a less common infectious process in which there is no apparent source of contaminating organism. Agents recovered in primary peritonitis are usually monomicrobic and include *S. pneumoniae*, *S. pyogenes*, and *Enterobacteriaceae*.

The diverse groups of specific microorganisms involved in secondary peritonitis reflect the underlying process from which they were derived. For example, peritonitis arising from a perforated appendix or diverticulitis will yield organisms indigenous to the gastrointestinal tract. As such, cultures routinely yield mixed aerobic and anaerobic isolates. Infection secondary to female genital tract infections may involve *N. gonorrhoeae* and *Chlamydia trachomatis*. Traumatic wound infections may yield microorganisms introduced from outside the body. Less commonly, *Mycobacteria* species, *Nocardia* species, and *Actinomyces* species may be involved.

Continuous ambulatory peritoneal dialysate

Continuous ambulatory peritoneal dialysis (CAPD) is currently used for thousands of patients with end-stage renal disease. In CAPD, dialysis fluid in a sterile plastic bag is instilled directly into the peritoneal cavity through a permanent catheter. Following five to six h, the dialysis fluid is drained back into the bag. Current practices have reduced the risk of peritonitis in CAPD from one episode every six months to one every 17 months. Gram positive cocci including coagulase negative staphylococci and *S. aureus* account for up to 65% of isolates with incidences of 30% to 40% and 10% to 25% respectively.

Bile

Bile is continually produced by liver cells and secreted into the hepatic duct. It may then either enter the common bile duct and pass into the duodenum or be diverted through the cystic duct for concentration and storage in the gallbladder. Bacterial infection is almost always secondary to a primary biliary complication like cholecystitis or cholangitis. Obstruction of the cystic duct leads to an increased concentration of bile, which may be infected by organisms from the gut through the portal system directly into the bile, by direct ascent from duodenum through the bile duct, or by hematogenous spread. By 72 h post obstruction, as many as 80%

of patients develop infections. The organisms commonly involved in infection are bile-resistant aerobic and anaerobic species found in the normal intestine, including bacteroides, enterobacteriaceae, *Enterococcus* species, and clostridia.

SURGICAL SPECIMENS

Although operative tissue specimens may be submitted from any site, those most frequently received for microbiological evaluation include intra-abdominal, obstetrical and gynecological, thoracic and pleuropulmonary, and central nervous system specimens. Surgical specimens pose a unique set of challenges to the microbiologist. First, unlike many other specimen types, surgical specimens are not easily amenable to obtaining a repeat specimen. Once the surgeon has made final closure, additional specimens from the original site cannot be collected. Second, due to the high likelihood that infecting organisms will include anaerobes, optimal techniques must be in place for collection, transport, and processing of these specimens.

Over the past two decades, intensive interest in the role of anaerobes in infection has yielded important information regarding the pathogenesis of infections and laboratory aspects for culture of these organisms. Simplistically, anaerobes may be defined as bacteria that fail to grow on solid media of nutritive nature, such as sheep blood agar or chocolate agar incubated in ambient air, or in a CO_2-enriched (5% to 10%) atmosphere. From a practical standpoint, an organism can be identified as an anaerobe in the clinical laboratory following tests for aerotolerance, where growth is recognized on nutritively rich anaerobic media but no growth is detected on plates incubated in CO_2.

Organisms can be divided based on the atmospheric conditions required for growth: anaerobes, as previously defined; aerobes, demonstrating good growth in room atmosphere; microaerophiles, demonstrating best growth in an atmosphere of reduced oxygen tension; and capnophiles, growing best in a CO_2 environment (usually 5% to 10% more CO_2 than in room air). Facultative anaerobes grow under either aerobic or anaerobic environments.

Anaerobic bacteria are ubiquitous in the environment and in food, as well as in and on animals. In humans, anaerobic bacteria are found as indigenous flora on the skin and on all mucous membranes including the oral cavity, gastrointestinal tract, and the genitourinary tract. The anaerobic species outnumber their aerobic counterparts in both the oral cavity and the colon, where the ratio of anaerobes to aerobes may be as great as 1000:1. The ecological factors that favor anaerobes in these sites include a warm, moist environment with a reduced oxidation-reduction potential (Eh) that is created from the normal metabolism of organisms utilizing available oxygen for respiration. The presence of anaerobes as normal flora renders the following sites unsuitable for anaerobic culture: throats, nasopharyngeal, and gingival specimens; sputum, tracheostomy suctions, and routine bronchoscopic washings; clean-catch and catheterized urine samples; routine vaginal and cervical swabs; gastric and bowel contents (exept in "blind loop" and similar syndromes); and feces (except for *C. difficile* in pseudomembranous actitis and *C. perfringens* and *C. botulinum* in foodborne outbreaks).

In infection, anaerobes may be found in any organ of the body when environmental conditions are suitable. In the pathogenesis of most anaerobic infections, a predisposing event such as malignancy, surgery, trauma, vascular stasis, or tissue necrosis provides a favorable environment for anaerobes to infect. The vast majority of these types of infections are polymicrobic, involving facultatively anaerobic and anaerobic organisms most commonly from endogenous sources. As the organisms multiply, they maintain an environment suitable for growth. Factors responsible for the pathogenicity and synergism among these organisms include: production of leucocidins, hemolysins, and cytotoxins; maintenance of a low redox potential, initially by the facultative organism; secretion of growth factors (such as vitamin K by the facultative species required by *Bacteroides [Porphyromonas] melaninogenicus* for growth); production of antiphagocytic capsules (by certain bacteroides species); and elaboration of penicillinases, cephalosporinases, lipases, and heparinases (by certain bacteroides and fusobacterium species).

Numerous studies detail the survival of anaerobic bacteria following exposure to different concentrations of oxygen and following exposure to ambient air for different time durations. Such studies indicate that the anaerobic species that normally colonize mucosal surfaces are extremely sensitive to oxygen. These organisms rarely represent species found in infections. For anaerobes commonly involved in infections—including *B. fragilis* and the *B. fragilis* group, *B. (P.) melaninogenicus* and the other black pigmenting *Bacteroides* species, *Fusobacterium nucleatum*, *Peptostreptococcus* species and most *Clostridium* species—surface growth occurred in oxygen concentrations of 2-8% and there was minimal loss in viability after exposure to ambient air for 80 minutes. Additionally, studies utilizing large-volume purulent specimens obtained by syringe aspiration yielded minimal decrease in both qualitative and quantitative recovery of common anaerobic clinical isolates on exposure to air for up to 24 h.

Intraabdominal processes

Abscesses may be found throughout the abdomen with the many reflections and recesses of the intra- and retro-peritoneal spaces. The processes that give rise to these infections include: diseases of the gastrointestinal tract such as appendicitis, diverticulitis, neoplasms, gangrene of the bowel or perforation of an ulcer; and traumatic injury with perforation of the uterus, bladder, stomach, or bowel. In addition, infection may be found in any abdominal organ, including the liver, pancreas, spleen, kidneys, and genital system. Perirectal abscesses are a common problem in immunocompromised individuals. In the rectum, only a single layer of columnar epithelium separates viable tissue from fecal microorganisms and any breach in the integrity of the wall may cause infection. Organisms may also gain entrance through the anal ducts and glands.

Most infections involve mixtures of facultatively anaerobic and aerobic organisms. Anaerobic species tend to outnumber aerobic species. Isolated organisms frequently include *E. coli* and other facultatively anaerobic gram-negative rods, *B. fragilis* and other *Bacteroides* species, *Enterococcus* species, *Fusobacterium* species, *C. perfringens*, *Actinomyces* species, and anaerobic cocci. A primary infection extending to the abdominal cavity may be associated with less common organisms like *M. tuberculosis*, *Salmonella typhi*, and the protozoan amoeba, *Entamoeba histolytica*.

Obstetric and gynecologic

The lower female genital tract represents a unique ecosystem characterized by dynamic changes in the species and concentrations of organisms at different times of the menstrual cycle, during pregnancy, hormonal therapy, and menopause. The normal facultative flora includes large amounts of *Lactobacillus* species as well as *Corynebacterium* species, coagulase negative staphylococci, and *Streptococcus* species. Gram-negative facultative flora is less frequently seen, with *E. coli* being the most common. The anaerobic species include the anaerobic gram-positive cocci, *Bacteroides bivius*, *B. (P.) melaninogenicus*, *B. disiens*, and *Fusobacterium* species. *B. fragilis* is an infrequent isolate as normal flora.

Conditions predisposing to infection in the female genital tract include pregnancy, puerperium, abortion, malignancy irradiation, surgery, cervical cauterization, fibroids, the use of intrauterine contraceptive devices, and preexisting intraabdominal infections.

Infections of the upper female genital tract are preferably referred to by the nature and site of infection, such as salpingitis (Fallopian tubes), oophoritis (ovary), or postpartum endometritis. Although the term "pelvic-inflammatory disease" is commonly used, this imprecise description most often refers to acute infection of the Fallopian tubes or acute salpingitis. Common infections of the female genital tract include: endometritis, myometritis, parametritis, and abscesses of the Bartholin's and Skene's glands, vulva, vaginal wall, ovaries, and Fallopian tubes.

Organisms involved in infection may include not only agents of sexually transmitted disease (see Chapter 50) but also more common mixtures of the facultative and anaerobic organisms that comprise the usual flora. Many of the anaerobic species, including *Actinomyces* species, *B. bivius*, *B. disiens*, and *B. melaninogenicus*, are slow growing, fastidious microorganisms that may require prolonged incubation for isolation.

Although less commonly seen, *B. fragilis* and *C. perfringens* are associated with more serious infections and complications.

Thoracic and pleuropulmonary

Chest infections may be located in the chest wall, pleural spaces, lungs and airways, and mediastinum. Infection here may be predisposed by: aspiration of oral secretions; periodontal disease and gingivitis; otitis and mastoiditis; preexisting pulmonary conditions such as obstructive foreign body, carcinoma, bronchiectasis and pulmonary tuberculosis; endocarditis; and intraabdominal infectious processes. The primary routes of infection are from contiguous site of infection and bacteremic spread. Common infections from contiguous pulmonary conditions that may require surgical intervention for diagnosis and/or therapy include aspiration pneumonia, abscesses (lung and chestwall), necrotizing pneumonia, and empyema.

The organisms recovered in these infections reflect the underlying conditions of the host and the predisposing fac-

tors. When inappropriately treated, the common agents of pneumonia (Chapter 44) may be seen in these infections with some frequency. Most commonly, a mixture of facultative and anaerobic organisms predominates with organisms representative of the usual oral flora. The anaerobic organisms that may be recovered include *F. nucleatum* and other *Fusobacterium* species; black pigmenting bacteroides; anaerobic gram-positive cocci; bile-sensitive *Bacteroides* species; non-sporeforming gram-positive rods (*Eubacterium* species, *Lactobacillus* species, *Bifidobacterium* species); *Veillonella* species; *C. perfringens* and other *Clostridium* species; and, more rarely, *B. fragilis* and the *B. fragilis* group.

Chronic pulmonary disease may be associated with very different groups of etiologic agents. Fungi (Chapters 52, 54); mycobacteria (*M. tuberculosis*, *M. avium-intracellulare*, *M. zenopi*, *M. fortuitum-chelonei*, *M. scrofulaceum*); *Actinomyces* species; *Nocardia* species; and the parasite *E. histolytica* may all be recovered. The cyst of the tapeworm *Echinococcus* species may also be seen in lung parenchyma in locations where sheep and cattle are raised.

Central nervous system

Operative specimens from the central nervous system most commonly are brain abscesses. These arise secondary to direct penetration from surgery or trauma, from adjacent infections such as otitis media, osteomyelitis of the skull, or sinus/mastoid infections, or from hematogenous spread (commonly from infection of the lungs or pleural space). During the first decade of life, a high incidence of abscesses has been related to cyanotic congenital heart disease. With traumatic, penetrating injuries, the etiology depends on environmental factors, but *S. aureus* and *C. perfringens* are frequently seen. With endogenous infection, the organisms recovered correlate closely with the species involved in the infection at another body site from which they spread. Anaerobes are a major component in these abscesses; anaerobic and microaerophilic streptococci are particularly common. In cases of otogenic temporal abscesses, the organisms recovered include anaerobic and microaerophilic streptococci, *B. fragilis*, and *Enterobacteriaceae*. Abscesses secondary to chronic sinusitis may contain anaerobic streptococci, *S. pneumoniae*, *H. influenzae*, non-fragilis *Bacteroides* species, veillonella, black pigmenting bacteroides, and fusobacteria species. In abscesses secondary to pulmonary infection, *Fusobacterium* species, anaerobic, microaerophilic and viridans streptococci, as well as *Bacteroides* species, *Actinomyces* species, and *Nocardia* species may be recovered. Less frequently, the fastidious pathogens *Haemophilus aphrophilus* and *Actinomyces actinomycetemcomitans* may be isolated. Brain abscesses secondary to abdominal or genitourinary tract infection often contain *Enterobacteriaceae* and anaerobes. Subdural empyemas and epidural abscesses that may require surgical intervention often yield the same groups of organisms, since the pathogenesis of infection is similar.

Infrequent organisms that may be involved include: *M. tuberculosis*; *E. histolytica* from disseminated infection; the free living amoeba, *Naegleria fowleri*; and even less frequently, the hydatid cyst of *Echinococcus* species, the cysticercus of *Taenia solium*, and granulomas secondary to schistome infection. In immunocompromised hosts *Toxoplasma gondii* may also be seen.

Infections secondary to shunting procedures are usually caused by organisms of low virulence including coagulase negative staphylococci and *Propionibacterium* species.

Laboratory aspects
Collection and transport

Surface wounds. Specimens must be collected from the active site of infection, and enough material must be obtained for optimal laboratory work up. In general, tissue, aspirates, and fluid specimens are superior to swab specimens. Surface wounds must be carefully sampled because a large number of colonizing microorganisms may be present. The eschar, if present, should be soaked with a sterile saline-soaked gauze and gently removed. The advancing erythematous edge of the lesion must be sampled by separating the wound margins with the thumb and forefinger of one hand (wearing a sterile glove), while placing the swab deep into the bordering edge of the lesion. A minimum of two swabs must be used. For superficial closed abscesses and vesicles, the skin surface should be disinfected with 70% alcohol or povidone iodine and sampled by aspiration with a needle and syringe. Alternatively, pus may be expressed onto two swabs. When viral isolation is required, a portion of vesicular fluid must be transferred to a protein-rich transport (2-SP, etc.) and immediately refrigerated. If swabs are used where Herpes virus is suspected, it is important to avoid the use of calcium alginate, which may inhibit viral replication. Surface abscess specimens can be delivered to the lab in the capped syringe. Plating of specimens onto appropriate media must be done as soon as feasible. Due to the fastidious nature of organisms that may be recovered in petechial lesions, it is imperative to make stains and to plate these specimens immediately.

Although controversial, surface-wound specimens are occasionally submitted to quantitatively determine the bacterial counts to aid in medical or surgical management. The method for dilution and plating of Lyman may be used.

The significance of microbiological data from processing of decubitus ulcers is dubious. These superficial wound infections most commonly contain mixtures of aerobic and anaerobic organisms. The flora of these lesions change with different stages of healing and, in addition, samples obtained from different sites of the same lesion show marked variability in the organisms isolated. The clinical management of the lesion focuses on debridement, topical cleansing agents, and reducing the factors that inhibit wound healing. These are compelling reasons to reject these specimens from analysis or to do minimal analysis, such as detailing only the morphotypes of organisms present.

Deep wounds. Deep wounds, spreading lesions of the skin and subcutaneous tissue (gangrene), fistulas, and sinus tracts should be processed for facultative and anaerobic bacteria. A properly collected specimen from these sites requires surface decontamination and aspiration of at least 1 ml of pus or sampling the advancing margin of the lesion with at least two swabs as previously described. Excessive air should be expelled from the syringe. One of the approved anaerobic transport devices must be used for prompt delivery to the laboratory. (See Chapter 39.)

Body fluids. These specimens are invariably obtained by trained personnel using aseptic methods, often under the guidance of fluoroscopic techniques. It is essential to receive in a sterile container an adequate amount of fluid—3-5 ml if possible—because the microbial burden may be low. These specimens must be delivered immediately to the laboratory for processing. For CAPD, the entire dialysis bag should be delivered promptly to the laboratory. Although procedures vary widely, a volume of 50-100 ml aseptically obtained from the bag usually is sufficient for processing.

Surgical specimens. Tissue or aspirated pus should be required for all surgical specimens submitted for microbiological evaluation. If swabs are collected, at least two should be submitted in an anaerobic transport device. These specimens should be delivered promptly to the laboratory. The importance of using appropriate procedures in collecting and processing clinical specimens for anaerobes has been documented by Spaulding and co-workers. In their work, nearly three times more anaerobes were recovered using appropriate anaerobic techniques compared to suboptimal methods with aerobic transport and routine processing.

Specimen processing

Once received in the laboratory, processing is required for most body fluids and tissue specimens prior to inoculation of media. Body fluids greater than 1 ml should be centrifuged at 1,500 g for 15 minutes to concentrate microorganisms. The sediment is used for stains and plating. Alternatively, the Cytocentrifuge (Shandon Corp., Pittsburgh) may be used for preparation of slides. Tissue specimens should be gently homogenized in sterile saline using a sterile tissue grinder and silica. A 10%-20% suspension should be made. Stains should be made from the homogenate and plates should be inoculated immediately to avoid undue exposure to oxygen. Often a proteinaceous clot will develop, particularly with synovial fluid. To solubilize, it is essential not to add substances that will enhance precipitation. A small volume of sterile saline can be added with gentle vortexing to aid in breaking the clots.

Stains

All specimens submitted for microbiologic evaluation discussed in this chapter require immediate stains to aid in patient management and microbiological work up. A small sample from the aspirate, fluid, or tissue is placed on the center of the slide. Care must be taken not to prepare too thick a slide. This may be accomplished by gently spreading the specimen over the slide with a sterile applicator stick. Occasionally, specimens of high-protein content peel off the slide. A small drop of sterile albumin may be applied as a precoating to affix the specimen. Swabs should be gently rolled on the slide to ensure optimal transfer of the specimen.

Gram stain. The Gram stain remains the stat procedure in clinical microbiology. Data from the Gram stain provides: the differential staining characteristics of organisms, immediate clues as to the general group of organisms responsible for infection, the host cellular response, direction for the types of plating media to be used, indications for the length of time to hold inoculated media, and quality control for culture adequacy.

Acridine orange (AO) stain. This stain has gained widespread use with body fluids and exudates where bacterial counts are low or where proteinaceous debris on the slide may confuse gram-stain interpretation. The AO stain detects microbial DNA and fluoresces orange-red when viewed under a long-wave ultraviolet light source. Slides may be rapidly screened under low power, with confirmation at high or oil power. Once organisms are demonstrated with AO, a Gram stain must be performed to establish the organism's differential staining properties.

Acid-fast (AF) stains. When mycobacteria or nocardia are suspected in clinical specimens, the appropriate AF stains should be performed. The fluorochrome stain for mycobacteria is recommended for a sensitive-screening procedure. Positives should be confirmed by Kinyoun's or Ziehl-Neelson stains. It is critical to use optimal techniques for detection of these organisms in clinical specimens as detection of growth on plates may require 4 to 6 weeks of incubation. The modified Kinyoun's stain may be used to detect *Nocardia* species. It should be noted that frequently acid-fast stains for nocardia on direct specimens are negative. However, the branching, beaded gram-positive morphology on Gram stain is often apparent. Culture on glyc-

erol-containing media enhances the acid-fast characteristics of these organisms.

Other stains. Fluorescent antibody stains to detect the *B. fragilis* group and certain members of the black-pigmenting bacteroides are commercially available (Rapid Detect *Bacteroides fragilis*, Rapid Detect *B. (p.) melaninogenicus*, Organon-Technica, Durham, N.C.).

Media

Media must be carefully selected to provide optimal nutrients for growth, selection, and differentiation of the most likely pathogens encountered in a particular specimen. With the majority of these infections containing mixed flora of both aerobes and anaerobes, a variety of differential and selective media may be required to expeditiously isolate and presumptively identify the organisms. Table 51-3 details the guidelines for media selection.

Routine nutritive media

Five percent sheep blood agar added to trypticase soy (BA), Columbia base, or beef-heart infusion agar is routinely employed for cultivation of fastidious organisms and

Table 51-3 Suggested primary plating media for bacteriology*

Specimen type	Direct smear	Plated media† Aerobic BA	CHOC	GNS/D	GPS	Anaerobic ANABA	LKV	Liquid media‡ Enriched thioglycollate (without indicator)	Comments‡
Abscesses	+	+	+	+	+	+	+	+	1, 2
Fistulas	+	+	+	+	+	+	+	+	1, 2
Draining sinus tract	+	+	+	+	+	+	+	+	1, 2
Body fluids									3
Bile	+	+	+	+	+	+	+	+	4
Joint	+	+	+					+	12
Pericardial	+	+	+					+	12
Peritoneal	+	+	+	+	+	+	+	+	1,2
Pleural	+	+	+	+	+	+	+	+	5
CAPD	+	+	+					+	6, 12
Skin deep wound	+	+	+	+	+	+	+	+	1, 2, 10
Punctative traumatic surface lesion	+	+	+	+	+			+	1, 2, 7
Rashes	+	+	+	+	+			+	11
Tissue operative/biopsy	+	+	+	+	+	+	+	+	8, 1, 2
Intraabdominal	+	+	+	+	+	+	+	+	
OB/GYN	+	+	+	+	+	+	+	+	9, 10
Thoracic/pleuropulmonary	+	+	+	+	+	+	+	+	5
Central nervous system	+	+	+	+	+	+	+	+	

*Abbreviations: BA = 5% sheep blood agar; CHOC = Chocolate agar; GNS/D = Gram negative selective/differential; GPS = Gram positive selective; ANABA = Anaerobic blood agar; LKV = laked kanamycin-vancomycin agar; CAPD = chronic ambulatory peritoneal dialysate.
†Incubate: BA, CHOC in 5-10% CO_2; GNS/D, GPS in air; ANABA, LKV anaerobically; Liquid Media in air; all at 35°C.
‡Comments:
1. Additional media as indicated by the direct smear.
2. Additional length of incubation if *Actinomyces* species are suspected.
3. Centrifuge for 15 min. at 1,500 × g. Use sediment for processing.
4. No anaerobic culture if collected by oral route.
5. May include media for *Legionella* and *Chlamydia* species as needed.
6. Filtration technique or BACTEC is also acceptable.
7. If crepitant (gas) or foul-smelling, process also for anaerobes.
8. Grind tissue, make @ 10% suspension.
9. Include additional selection media for *N. gonorrheae*.
10. It is emphasized that these specimens require stringent techniques in collection to avoid the normal flora.
11. Process immediately if *N. meningitidis* is suspected.
12. Routinely are monomicrobic infections with aerobic organisms.

determination of hemolytic reactions. Chocolate agar (CHOC), which contains 2% hemoglobin or Isovitalex (BBL, Cockeysville, Md.), is routinely employed for isolation of *Haemophilus* species and *N. gonorrhoeae* and other fastidious gram-negative rods.

Anaerobic blood agar (ANABA) of CDC formulation is recommended for routine culture of anaerobic organisms. Enriched with L-cystine, hemin, and vitamin K, this media supports the growth of the most nutritively demanding and fastidious organisms, including thiol-dependent streptococci, *Fusobacterium necrophorum,* and the strict anaerobe *C. novyi* type B. The media may be prereduced in an anaerobic environment for several hours prior to plating, which may allow more rapid detection of organisms. Optimal recovery of anaerobes is achieved with freshly prepared media.

Selective and differential media

Two commonly used Gram-positive selective (GPS) media for aerobes are phenylethyl alcohol agar and colistin-nalidixic acid agar. Both media permit isolation of streptococci and staphylococci with inhibition of most gram-negative rods. A wide variety of selective and differential media are available for facultatively anaerobic gram-negative rods. Of these, MacConkey agar (MAC) or eosin methylene blue agar (EMB) are routinely used. These media select for gram-negative rods, inhibit gram positive cocci and permit differentiation of lactose-fermenting and non-lactose-fermenting organisms.

Selective and differential anaerobic media have been developed for many different species. For routine use, however, selective media for the *B. fragilis* group is recommended due to the frequent incidence of these organisms in mixed infections and the impact of their presence on therapy. Laked kanamycin vancomycin medium selects for *Bacteroides* species and inhibits most facultatively anaerobic gram-negative rods and aerobic and anaerobic gram positive cocci. Bacteroides bile esculin agar may also be used to select these organisms and to differentiate them on the basis of esculin hydrolysis. When the gram stain from the clinical specimen demonstrates gram-positive rods suggestive of *Clostridium* species, an egg yolk agar plate may be included to detect lipase and/or lecithinase production.

Liquid media

Thioglycollate medium, enriched with hemin and vitamin K, is a general purpose enrichment broth recommended as a supplement to plated media. This permits growth of a wide variety of aerobic or anaerobic organisms, and is a useful backup when there is a small volume of specimen containing few organisms.

Anaerobic systems

Comparative studies have demonstrated at least three general systems as being satisfactory for recovery of anaerobes. These include the anaerobic jar, the anaerobic glove box, and the less commonly used roll-tube and roll-streak method; the latter is not further reviewed.

In the anaerobic jar, a gas-generating kit is generally employed to create an anaerobic environment. This is achieved by complexing hydrogen with oxygen in the presence of a catalyst (palladium) to yield water. The catalyst may be contained within the gas-generating kit (GasPak Plus, BBL, Cockeysville, Md.) or may be affixed to the jar lid. The volatile metabolic end products of metabolism, including hydrogen sulfide, may render the catalyst inactive. As such, the palladium-coated silica pellets attached to the jar lid must be reactivated after each use by heating at 160°-170° C for two h and then stored in a dry, clean container, preferably a desiccator. An alternative method to achieve an anaerobic environment in the jar is the evacuation-replacement technique. In this technique, a vacuum removes the air from the jar. The air is replaced with a mixture of 85% N, 10% H, and 5% CO. This cycle is repeated three times.

A unique modification of the jar technique is a transparent bag that contains its own gas-generating system and palladium catalyst (Bio-Bag Environmental Chamber [Type A], BBL, Cockeysville, Md.). A further modification of the transparent bag system is available (Anaerobe Pouch System Catalyst Free, Difco Laboratories, Detroit, Mich.). This system lacks a catalyst, and an anaerobic environment is created when water is added to a sachet containing iron powder, which reduces molecular oxygen to iron oxides. Designed to hold individual petri dishes, this system allows examination of plates without breaching the integrity of the anaerobic environment. In all of these systems, an anaerobic indicator such as methylene blue or resazurin must be used as quality control of the anaerobic environment. Both are colorless under anaerobic conditions.

The anaerobic glove box is an air-tight, self-contained anaerobic system that allows manipulation of specimens and observation of media in a completely anaerobic environment. Specimens, media, and supplies are introduced and removed through an airtight chamber. Manipulations are performed through neoprene gloves affixed to a clear plastic front which permits direct visualization of media. Incubators may be installed within the chamber. Anaerobiosis is maintained by palladium catalysts and gas mixtures. Current modifications on the design of anaerobe chambers include molded plexiglas units with gloves, as well as a gloveless system (Sheldon Manufacturing, Cornelius, Oregon).

Inoculation of media

Using a sterile pipette, one drop from the sediment from centrifuged body fluids or tissue homogenates is placed on each agar plate and on a slide for direct smear. For thioglycollate broth inoculation, 1 ml of sample (or as much as possible) is added to the bottom of the fluid. Alternative procedures for processing CAPD include the inoculation of Bactec (Johnston Laboratories, Cockeysville, Md.) bottles or passage of the fluid through filters, with subsequent placement of the filters directly on media. Each procedure seems adequate to concentrate organisms from a large volume of fluid. For swab specimens, one of the swabs is removed from the transport tube and gently rolled over a quarter of the agar surface. The swab is then placed in thioglycollate broth taking care to break off the applicator stick below the site where the gloved finger touched the stick. The second swab is used to make a slide for direct smears. One drop from aspirated specimens can be directly applied to plated media and 1 ml, or as much as possible, should be inoculated into thioglycollate broth. One drop should be placed on a slide for direct smear. The residual specimen not used for inoculation should be stored for at least two weeks at 4° C.

Incubation

All plates are incubated at 35°-37° C.

The BA and CHOC plates are incubated in a CO_2-enhanced atmosphere. The gram-positive selective and gram-negative selective/differential media and thioglycollate broth are incubated in the ambient air, while the anaerobe plates are incubated in an anaerobic environment.

The duration of primary incubation for anaerobically isolated plates prior to examination is critical. For laboratories using the jar technique, a full two days of incubation is recommended to reduce the loss of O_2-sensitive strains. Additional rationale for this procedure is owed to the fact that strains of *B. melaninogenicus,* certain anaerobic cocci, *Actinomyces* species, *Eubacterium* species, and *F. nucleatum* may be retarded in their growth rate on frequent exposure to oxygen. *B. fragilis* and *C. perfringens* may frequently grow after overnight incubation. To permit efficient screening for these pathogens, a second jar may be set up on initial plating to be opened at 24 h. Alternatively, the BioBag system or anaerobic glove box may be used to permit daily observation without breaching the anaerobic environment. While the majority of clinically significant anaerobic isolates will be detected by 72 h of incubation, it is generally recommended to incubate anaerobic plates 7 d.

Examination of primary culture

Plates incubated aerobically and in CO_2 should be examined daily. Identification and susceptibility testing (when warranted) should be done as soon as possible using pure isolates.

ANABA plates incubated in BioBags or in an anaerobic glove box may be examined at 24 h for evidence of growth not detected on aerobic plates. Likewise, selective plates incubated in these systems can be examined for growth and, if detected at 24 h, the isolates can be screened for aerotolerance. (See Fig. 51-1.) Anaerobic plates incubated by the jar technique should be removed from the jar and examined at 48 h. Upon removal from the primary anaerobic system, anaerobic plates should be stored in a holding jar while awaiting observation and colony selection for aerotolerance testing. The holding jar should contain either the anaerobic gas mixture as previously described or O_2 free N_2 gas.

The test for aerotolerance distinguishes anaerobes from facultative organisms. Anaerobic plates should be screened carefully for colonial morphology with the assistance of a stereomicroscope. Using $\times 10$ to $\times 25$ magnification, one colony of an isolate suspected of being an anaerobe should be picked with a sterile needle and incubated to a BA plate, to an ANABA plate, and to a slide for a Gram stain. The BA plate should be incubated in a CO_2 environment, while the ANABA should be incubated anaerobically. Following overnight incubation, both plates should be examined for growth and purity. If growth occurs on the plate incubated

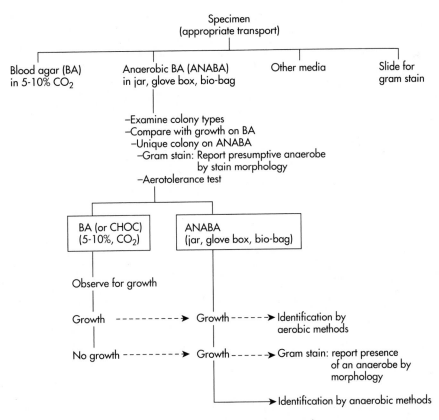

Fig. 51-1 Flow chart for processing anaerobes.

Table 51-4 Common features of frequently isolated anaerobes

Organism	Gram stain	Aerotolerance	Key feature(s)
B. fragilis group	GNR, rounded ends	—	Opalescent colonies, growth on LKV, colonies > 1mm in diameter
Pigmented Bacteroides species (Porphyromonas sp.)	GNR, GN coccobacillus	—	Dark pigmenting (brown to black, colony fluoresces brick red under long wave ultraviolet light
B. ureolyticus group	GNR	—	Colonies pit the agar
F. nucleatum	GNR, pointed ends	—	Breadcrumb or speckled colonies
C. perfringens	GPB, uniform boxcar shape	—	Double zone beta hemolysis
Other Clostridium species	GPB	— (+)	Spores frequently seen on Gram stain
Non-sporeforming Gram positive rods	GPB	— (+)	

*Abbreviations: GNR = gram negative rod; GN = gram negative; GPB = gram positive bacillus.

in CO_2, the organism should be identified by aerobic means. If growth occurs only on the anaerobic plate, it should be identified by anaerobic techniques. Both plates should be held at least 48 h. This duration may be required to detect the slower growing anaerobes. Fig. 51-1 details the work flow for processing and isolating anaerobes. Table 51-4 gives common characteristics of some of the frequently isolated anaerobic organisms.

Certain *Clostridium* species including *C. tertium* and *C. hemolyticum* (Sutter) may grow luxuriantly on anaerobic plates but poorly on plates incubated in CO_2. These aerotolerant strains should be identified by anaerobic methods. Occasionally, *Haemophilus* species may grow on initial isolation only on the ANABA. Therefore, when small gram-negative rods are detected on gram stain of the ANABA, it is recommended to pick these isolates to CHOC for incubation in CO_2. Thioglycollate broth should be examined daily. Subculture of the media is recommended if growth is detected in the broth and no growth is detected on the aerobic or anaerobic plates or if the direct gram stain indicated morphotypes of organisms not isolated from the primary plates. Subculture should be made to a BA plate and to an ANABA plate with subsequent incubation in a CO_2 environment and in an anaerobic environment, respectively. Selective and differential media may also be inoculated base on the Gram stain morphology of the broth. These media should be observed as previously noted.

Special considerations

Adjunctive procedures should be used for specimens suspected of containing *Actinomyces* species to ensure optimal recovery. These procedures should be employed when granules are submitted as part of the specimen, when direct gram stain or histopathology slides demonstrate elongated gram-positive rods, or when specifically requested for isolation.

A separate ANABA should be inoculated for *Actinomyces* species. These plates should be incubated for at least three to five days prior to initial observation and should be held at least 14 days prior to discarding.

Identification of all isolates may proceed as directed in subsequent chapters.

SUGGESTED READING

Altemeir WA, Culbertson WR, et al: Intra-abdominal abscesses, Am J Surg 125:70, 1973.

Balows A, Hausler WJ, et al: Manual of Clinical Microbiology, ed 5, American Society for Microbiology, 1991.

Barron EJ and Finegold SM: Diagnostic microbiology, ed 7, Mosby-Year Book, Inc., 1986.

Dowell VR, Lombard GL, et al: Media for isolation, characterization, and identification of obligate anaerobic bacteria, US Dept of HHS, Centers for Disease Control, 1981.

Finegold SM: Anaerobic bacteria in human diseases, Academic Press, 1977.

Finegold SM, Shepherd EW et al: Practical anaerobic bacteriology, Cumitech 5, American Society for Microbiology, 1977.

Gorbach SL, Thadepalli H, et al: Anaerobic organisms in intraabdominal infections. In Balows A, DeHaan RM, et al, eds: Anaerobic bacteria: Role in disease, Charles C. Thomas, 1974.

Hill GB, Eschenbach DA, et al: Bacteriology of the vagina. In Mardh PA, Taylor-Robinson D, eds: Bacterial vaginosis, Almquist and Wiskell International, 1984.

Howard RJ and Simmons RL: Surgical Infectious Diseases, ed 2, Appleton and Lange, 1988.

Koneman EW, Allen SD, et al: Color atlas and textbook of diagnostic microbiology, ed 3, JB Lippincott, 1988.

Lorber B and Swenson RM: The bacteriology of intraabdominal infections, Surg Clin N Amer 55:1349, 1975.

Rosenblatt JE, Fallon AM, et al: Comparison of methods for isolation of anaerobic bacteria from clinical specimens, Appl Microbiol 25:77, 1973.

Sutter VL, Citron DM, et al: Wadsworth anaerobic bacteriology manual, ed 4, Star Publishing Co, 1985.

52

Hair, skin, and nail specimens

Nancy L. Anderson

The potential spectrum of infections diagnosed from hair, skin, and nail specimens is vast. This is due in part to the number and variety of microorganisms existing as transient or resident flora at these sites, becoming pathogenic when conditions are altered. It is also affected by differences in the cellular composition of the layers of skin. Fungal organisms known as dermatophytes are able to invade and utilize keratinized tissues down to the layer of the dermis. The viable dermal tissue, containing blood vessels and lymphatics, is able to support the growth of bacteria, viruses, and other fungi, but dermatophytes are inhibited at this level.

The diagnoses of bacterial, viral, and parasitic infections of the cutaneous tissue and identification of their etiologic agents are described elsewhere in this book. The focus of this chapter is the evaluation of hair, skin, and nail specimens for the diagnosis and differentiation of fungal disease in these tissues.

FUNGAL DISEASE OF HAIR, SKIN, AND NAILS
Superficial infections

The mycoses that infect only the outermost epidermal layer, the stratum corneum, and the suprafollicular portion of the hair are known as superficial infections. Because these infections do not invade living tissue, they often go unnoticed or are diagnosed as a result of cosmetic effects. Although the agents of these infections can be cultured, the diseases are usually diagnosed clinically, or by the detection of fungal elements in a skin or hair specimen on direct exam.

Piedra. There are two types of piedra, a nodular infection of the external hair shaft: black piedra, whose etiologic agent is the darkly pigmented *Piedraia hortae,* and the rarer white piedra, caused by the filamentous yeast, *Trichosporon beigelii.* Although both are found on man and animals in tropical climates, especially in South America and the Far East, white piedra has been sporadically reported elsewhere, including the United States and Europe.

Both black and white piedra present as adherent nodules along the hair shaft, but there are differences between the two. *P. hortae* mainly infects scalp hair, forming hard, crusty, brown to black (dematiaceous) masses which are difficult to remove. *T. beigelii* infects hair on other areas of the body, commonly the axilla, the beard, and the groin. The white to tan nodular fungal masses which form

this infection are softer and less adherent than those of black piedra. They can be confused with attached nits, and white piedra must be differentiated from the more commonly seen ectoparasites causing pediculosis.

The agents of piedra can be identified on direct microscopic examination of the nodules. Masses formed by *P. hortae* consist of septate, dematiaceous mycelium, 4-8 μm diameter, aligned surrounding oval asci, each containing eight curved ascospores. *T. beigelii* produces nodules made up of hyaline hyphae, 2-4 μm diameter, oval to rectangular arthroconidia, and budding blastoconidia.

Tinea nigra (palmaris). Tinea nigra is a cosmetic problem, an asymptomatic infection of the stratum corneum, which manifests as brown to black, patchy lesions on the palms of the hands or soles of the feet. The dark, smooth macules resemble silver nitrate stains and can be confused with serious conditions including malignant melanoma. The infection is rarely seen outside of tropical areas such as Central and South America.

Exophiala werneckii (syn. *Phaeoannellomyces werneckii*), a dematiaceous mold, is the major etiologic agent of tinea nigra, with a second species, *Stenella araguata,* isolated rarely. In direct mounts of skin scrapings, *E. werneckii* is seen as light brown to olive green septate hyphae, 1.5-3 μm diameter, mixed with swollen and yeast-like cells.

Tinea versicolor. This superficial mycosis is caused by *Malassezia furfur* (syn. *Pityrosporum orbiculare*), a yeast that is part of man's normal skin flora. The disease, common worldwide and also known as pityriasis versicolor, presents as slightly raised, scaling lesions on the skin, which enlarge and coalesce as the infection spreads. These lesions are found on areas of the body with high numbers of sebaceous glands, such as the scalp and upper torso. The lesions tend to appear hyperpigmented on light skin and hypopigmented on dark skin, resulting in a variety of colors, even on the same individual. The disease is often noticed when the infected areas fail to tan as deeply as surrounding skin.

M. furfur can cause several other cutaneous infections including folliculitis and seborrheic dermatitis, but most significant is its association with systemic disease. This lipophilic yeast has been isolated in cases of fungemia in patients receiving parenteral fat emulsions through intravascular catheters or hyperalimentation. Organisms from the

673

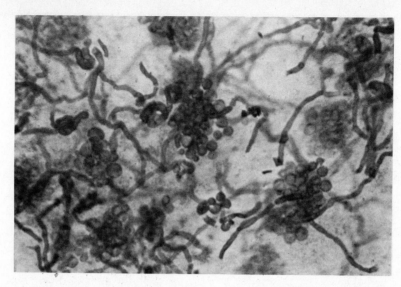

Fig. 52-1 Hyphae and yeast cells of *Malassezia furfur,* as seen on direct smear. *Courtesy of MG Rinaldi, San Antonio, TX.*

skin around the catheter insertion enter the bloodstream and proliferate due to the high lipid concentration. The catheter-related sepsis has been seen most often in infants with predisposing conditions, and *M. furfur* has recently been implicated in an outbreak in a neonatal intensive-care unit.

Tinea versicolor is easily diagnosed on direct exam of scrapings from its lesions. The pathognomonic feature of the disease, seen microscopically, is a mixture of hyphal fragments of varying lengths and clusters of round yeast cells, which have been termed "spaghetti and meatballs" (Figure 52-1). Due to the nutritional requirement for lipid by *M. furfur,* successful growth in culture depends on an oil-enriched medium. Sabouraud dextrose agar overlaid with sterile olive oil, or glucose yeast extract-peptone agar with sterile lipid supplements can be used. The organism has been isolated from commercial blood culture media when a source of lipid has been added to it.

Malassezia pachydermatis, a second species in this genus, is recovered from skin, but is not known to cause disease in humans. It grows on media used to isolate *M. furfur* but does not have the requirement for lipid. This characteristic can be used to differentiate the two.

Infections of skin and cutaneous tissue

The molds known as dermatophytes are one group of fungi isolated from lesions on the hair, skin, and nails. Yeast are also detected quite often in cutaneous specimens, and other filamentous fungi infect this keratinized tissue rarely. The correct diagnosis of mycotic infection, and its differentiation from other cutaneous diseases, is critical in proper management of any of these conditions.

Dermatophytoses. The closely-related fungi termed dermatophytes are classified in the anamorph (asexual) genera *Epidermophyton, Microsporum,* and *Trichophyton. Microsporum* and *Trichophyton* also exist in sexual states, in the teleomorph genera *Nannizzia* and *Arthroderma,* respectively. These molds cause a variety of syndromes referred to as "tineas" or "ringworm," because of the circular nature

of the lesions produced. The clinical manifestations range from mild to severe, depending on the etiologic agent and area of the body. Common dermatophytoses are described and categorized according to affected body site in Table 52-1.

Table 52-2 summarizes the most frequently isolated dermatophytes. Overall, these fungi have a cosmopolitan distribution, with some geographic variation among the species. Each agent can produce several diseases and, conversely, the same clinical syndrome can result from infection by one of several organisms.

The tissue forms of the dermatophytes, as seen on exam of clinical material, are different from their microscopic morphology in culture. Skin and nail specimens infected with these fungi contain hyaline, septate hyphae, 2-4 μm diameter, that occasionally branch; and thick-walled, barrel-shaped arthroconidia (Figure 52-2). The appearance of *Microsporum* or *Trichophyton* in hair specimens depends on the type of hair invasion, that differs according to the infecting species. Some of the *Trichophyton* species invade the hair shaft and produce hyphae that break up into arthroconidia on the interior only (endothrix) (Figure 52-3). The *Microsporum* and other *Trichophyton* species invade the hair shaft and form a sheath around the exterior, which results in an arrangement of arthroconida and hyphae externally as well (ectothrix) (Figure 52-4). *Trichophyton schoenleinii* has a unique form of hair invasion (favic) in which long hyphal fragments are seen within the hair shaft, but no arthroconidia are produced.

Although the dermatophytes cannot be speciated based on their appearance in a direct exam, a preliminary diagnosis can often be made, and the presence of a mycotic infection confirmed. Culture characteristics, as well as physiologic and nutritional tests, are used to differentiate the species.

Cutaneous Yeast Infections. Unlike the filamentous fungi, yeast are found as normal flora in many areas of the body, including the skin, without signs of disease. Organisms which are frequently part of the resident skin flora

Table 52-1   Manifestations of common dermatophytoses

Disease	Site of infection	Clinical presentation
Tinea capitis	Scalp, eyebrows, eyelashes	Variable, depending on agent; mild, scaling erythema to severe inflammation with abscesses, leading to scarring and alopecia.
Tinea corporis	Glabrous skin	Circular, scaling, erythematous lesions with central healing and advancing vesicular borders.
Tinea cruris	Groin, upper thighs	Dry, scaling lesions with raised, vesicular, well-demarcated borders.
Tinea pedis	Feet, mainly toe webs and soles	Chronic—noninflammatory, mild, scaling lesions. Acute—severe inflammation, vesicle and bullae formation.
Tinea ungium	Nail plates	Discoloration and dystrophy of nail with buildup of subungual debris.

Table 52-2   Characteristics of human dermatophytes

Species	Natural habitat	Geographic distribution	Disease in man
Trichophyton rubrum	Anthropophilic*	Worldwide	Dry scaling on feet, glabrous skin, nails; occasionally beard infected.
Trichophyton mentagrophytes	Anthropophilic	Worldwide	Infects all body sites: Ectothrix hair invasion; vesicular inflammation in other areas.
Epidermophyton flocossum	Anthropophilic	Worldwide	Inflammatory lesions of groin, feet.
Trichophyton tonsurans	Anthropophilic	North, Central America, Europe, Caribbean	Endothrix hair invasion with hair breakage at the scalp; smooth skin also infected.
Microsporum canis	Zoophilic†	Worldwide	Ectothrix hair invasion with inflammation, suppuration; smooth skin also infected.
Microsporum audouinii	Anthropophilic	Africa, USA	Ectothrix hair invasion with scaling, little inflammation; smooth skin also infected.
Trichophyton verrucosum	Zoophilic	Worldwide	Ectothrix hair invasion with suppurative folliculitis; kerion formation.

*Preferred host is man.
†Preferred hosts are animals.

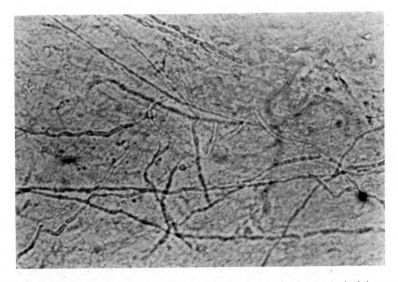

Fig. 52-2   KOH preparation of nail scrapings containing branching hyphae typical of dermatophytes. *Courtesy of MG Rinaldi, San Antonio, TX.*

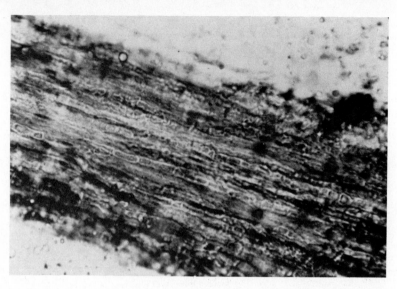

Fig. 52-3 Endothrix invasion of hair demonstrating hyphae and arthroconidia within the shaft. *Courtesy of MG Rinaldi, San Antonio, TX.*

Fig. 52-4 Ectothrix invasion of hair with numerous arthroconidia surrounding exterior of shaft. *Courtesy of MG Rinaldi, San Antonio, TX.*

include species of *Candida, Torulopsis, Trichosporon, Geotrichum,* and *Rhodotorula*. Cutaneous yeast infections are common but usually occur as a result of a change in the metabolism or defenses of the host. Examples of these changes include diabetes, pregnancy, AIDS or other immunodeficiencies, treatment with cytotoxic or immunosuppressive drugs, physical factors such as severe burns, or continual moisture on the skin surface.

Candida albicans, an endogenous organism in the alimentary tract and the mucocutaneous surfaces of man, is not part of the normal skin flora. It is, however, the agent isolated most frequently in cutaneous yeast infections. The clinical manifestations of cutaneous candidiasis are varied and are summarized in Table 52-3. The most common conditions are those of paronychia, onychomycosis, and infection of the intertriginous areas of glabrous skin. Other than *Candida* species, yeast which are occasionally isolated in onychomycosis and cutaneous disease include *Geotrichum candidum, Trichosporon beigelii,* and, rarely *Hendersonula toruloidea.*

Prompt microscopic examination of freshly collected clinical material is beneficial in the diagnosis of a cutaneous yeast infection. Because these organisms can be present on skin surfaces, the detection of yeast cells on a direct smear does not necessarily indicate infection. However, the presence of budding yeast, with mycelial forms and pseudohyphae (Figure 52-5), suggests invasion rather than mere colonization of tissue. Because *Candida* multiplies rapidly and can produce pseudohyphae in stored specimens, it is important to perform direct exams as quickly as possible. If biopsies are examined using histopathology stains, invasion of tissue by mycelial forms of the infecting agent can also be detected.

Some yeast, including *Geotrichum,* do not produce hyphal forms, but are seen only as arthroconida on direct smears and in tissue. For this reason, and because the portion of material examined may not contain fungal elements, cul-

Table 52-3   Cutaneous manifestations of candidiasis

Disease	Clinical presentation	Predisposing conditions
Paronychia/onychomycosis	Erythematous swelling of folds surrounding nail; invasion of nail plate causing thickening, discoloration, brittleness, ridges.	Frequent or prolonged immersion of hands in water.
Intertrigo	Papules or vesicopustules in folds of glabrous skin, which rupture and coalesce; result is erythematous, weeping base bordered by ragged, white membrane.	Physiologic disorders (diabetes, malignancy), obesity, environmental factors (heat, humidity, friction).
Diaper dermatitis	Red, scaly patches in diaper area; satellite lesions appear, rarely spread.	Prolonged contact with unclean diaper; often seen with oral infection.
Congenital candidal dermatitis	Generalized maculopapular rash on many body surfaces with post-inflammatory desquamation.	Intrauterine candidal infection due to maternal candidiasis.
Disseminated systemic infection	Widespread erythematous papules, nodules, or abscesses.	Broad spectrum antibiotics, immunosuppressive therapy, malignancy, burns.

ture and identification of a yeast isolate is important in the determination of its significance to disease. Growth of a pure culture of an organism or repeated positive cultures from the same source indicate infection in the presence of clinical disease.

The degree to which yeast isolates are identified varies among laboratories. Because *C. albicans* is the most common agent of candidiasis and can be easily identified, laboratories should speciate this organism. This is done by testing for germ tubes and chlamydoconidia (chlamydospores), both of which are produced by *C. albicans*. Other yeasts are speciated by morphology combined with carbohydrate assimilation patterns. A number of commercial products are available for yeast identification.

Other Cutaneous Mycoses. Primary infections of the skin or nails by other filamentous or yeast-like fungi occur sporadically, especially in patients with predisposing conditions. These are often caused by opportunistic organisms generally considered nonpathogenic. Species of *Aspergillus*, *Alternaria*, *Fusarium*, and *Pseudallescheria* have been reported in cases of cutaneous infection in cancer patients or individuals undergoing chemotherapy, or in those with burn or puncture wounds. Primary cutaneous zygomycosis (mucormycosis) is a severe, fulminating disease produced by members of the genus *Rhizopus*, the common bread mold. This rare infection, documented in diabetics, immunocompromised patients, burn victims, and trauma patients, must be rapidly diagnosed and treated because these organisms can disseminate and cause necrotizing lesions. Nosocomial cutaneous infections have also resulted from the use of surgical tape or wrapping contaminated with *Aspergillus* and *Rhizopus* species.

Onychomycosis, as discussed with manifestations of candidiasis, is a nail infection produced by yeast, or filamentous fungi. The organism isolated most often in this disease is *Scopulariopsis brevicaulis*, which is sometimes mixed with a dermatophyte infection. Molds rarely isolated include species of *Aspergillus*, *Fusarium*, *Acremonium*, *Chaetophoma*,

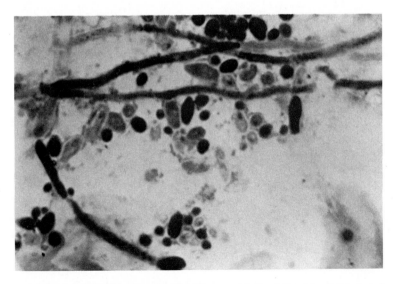

Fig. 52-5   True hyphae, pseudohyphae, and budding yeast cells of *Candida albicans* on direct smear from skin. *Courtesy of MG Rinaldi, San Antonio, TX.*

and *Microascus*. Although onychomycosis occurs in both healthy and diseased individuals, it is usually preceded by trauma or dystrophy of the nail, resulting in a physical abnormality. The infection most commonly affects the nail of the big toe, many times in elderly patients.

The etiologic agents of these cutaneous infections can be demonstrated in microscopic exams of scrapings from the lesions, or nail shavings, where each agent has its characteristic tissue form. Identification is made after isolation in culture. Since many of these opportunistic pathogens are ubiquitous in nature, and frequently found as culture contaminants, detection of tissue invasion by fungal elements in a direct exam is often more significant than growth of the organism.

Subcutaneous mycoses

The subcutaneous mycoses are infections which result from traumatic implantation of organisms through the skin to the deeper subdermal tissue, producing local lesions that slowly spread, sometimes over a period of years. When the fungi disseminate into surrounding tissue or through the lymphatics, lesions often appear on the skin or cutaneous tissue. These infections must be differentiated from primary cutaneous disease. The major clinical conditions which result from subcutaneous fungal infections include sporotrichosis, chromoblastomycosis, phaeohyphomycosis, and mycetoma. Rhinosporidiosis and lobomycosis are very rare subcutaneous mycoses not included in this chapter.

Sporotrichosis. The infectious disease caused by the fungus *Sporothrix schenckii* has several manifestations, most commonly involving the lymphocutaneous tissue. The organism is ubiquitous in soil and on decaying plants, and causes infection when there is contact with the contaminated vegetation through a break in the skin. The usual clinical presentation is the development of a small, hard, painless nodule at the site of inoculation, sometimes months after the organism was implanted. This nodule enlarges and ul-

cerates, and, simultaneously, secondary lesions frequently develop along local lymphatics.

In areas such as Mexico or South America, where *S. schenckii* is endemic, much of the population is sensitized to the organism without having clinical signs of disease. When these people are infected, the lesions tend to remain restricted to the cutaneous tissue at the inoculation site with no lymphatic involvement. These infections are termed "fixed cutaneous sporotrichosis."

Although *S. schenckii* infects healthy individuals, sporotrichosis is seen as an opportunistic disease in patients with underlying conditions such as malnutrition, alcoholism, or AIDS. In these cases, the infections are generally more severe, disseminating from the cutaneous site, most commonly to the bone and joints. The other manifestation of sporotrichosis, rarely reported, is primarily pulmonary infection, which results after inhalation of *S. schenckii*.

The diagnosis of sporotrichosis depends on its differentiation from similar clinical conditions, examples being atypical mycobacteriosis, other fungal infections, anthrax, tularemia, cutaneous malignancy, and nocardiosis. Culture of *S. schenckii* from an aspirate or swab of a lesion, or from a tissue biopsy, is the usual method of definitive diagnosis.

S. schenckii is a dimorphic fungus, existing in a yeast form both in tissue and in culture at 37°C, but growth is mycelial at 25°C. Demonstration of conversion of this organism from mold to yeast form in the laboratory is used in its identification. The yeast forms are tiny (2-6 μm), stain poorly, and are difficult to detect in direct smears of clinical material, biopsy, or tissue section (Figure 52-6). They are oval or cigar-shaped and when seen on a gram stain are gram positive or irregularly stained. Fluorescent antibody staining techniques can be used to specifically stain these organisms in clinical specimens or in culture.

The characteristic tissue reaction to *S. schenckii* produces what is called an asteroid body, seen on tissue sections stained with hematoxylin and eosin. Asteroid bodies consist

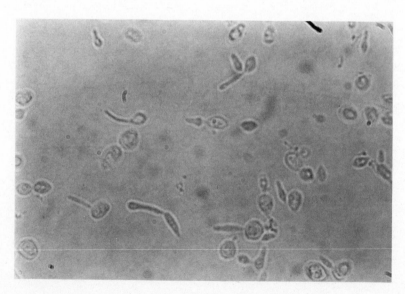

Fig. 52-6 Cigar-shaped yeast cells typical of tissue form of *Sporothrix schenckii Courtesy of MG Rinaldi, San Antonio, TX.*

Table 52-4 Agents of chromoblastomycosis and subcutaneous phaeohyphomycosis

Chromoblastomycosis	Subcutaneous phaeohyphomycosis
Fonsecaea pedrosoi	Exophiala jeanselmei
Fonsecaea compacta	Exophiala spinifera
Phialophora verrucosa	Phialophora richardsiae
Cladosporium carionii	Phialophora parasitica
Rhinocladiella aquaspersa	Phialophora verrucosa
	Wangiella dermatitidis
	Xylohypha bantiana (Cladosporium bantianum)
	*

*Other species rarely isolated.

Table 52-5 Agents of human mycetoma

Species	Granule characteristics	Size range (mm)
Eumycotic Mycetoma		
Madurella mycetomatis	Hard, black	0.5-5.0
Madurella grisea	Soft, black	0.3-0.6
Pseudallescheria boydii	Soft, white	0.5-1.0
Leptosphaeria senegalensis	Hard, black	0.5-2.0
Acremonium species	Soft, white	0.2-0.5
*		
Actinomycotic Mycetoma		
Nocardia brasiliensis	Soft, white	.025-.15
Nocardia asteroides	Soft, white†	.025-.15
Actinomadura madurae	Soft, white-yellow-red	1.0-5.0
Actinomadura pelletieri	Soft, deep red	0.3-0.5
Streptomyces somaliensis	Hard, yellow-brown	1.0-2.0
*		

*Other species rarely isolated.
†Granules rarely found in clinical material.

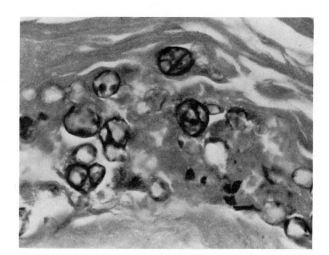

Fig. 52-7 Pigmented sclerotic bodies of chromoblastomycosis within keratin layer of skin. *From Chandler FW and Watts JC: Pathologic diagnosis of fungal infections, Chicago, 1987, American Society of Clinical Pathologists.*

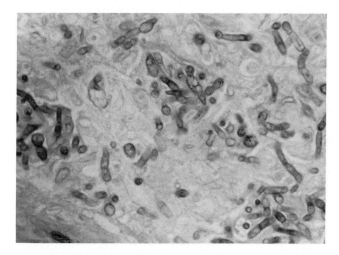

Fig. 52-8 Pigmented hyphae and yeast cells in subcutaneous phaeo-hyphomycosis caused by *Alternaria alternata. From Chandler FW and Watts JC: Pathologic diagnosis of fungal infections, Chicago, 1987, American Society of Clinical Pathologists.*

of a central, degenerated yeast cell, surrounded by radiating, eosinophilic material composed of precipitated antigen-antibody complexes. Because this reaction occurs with other mycoses, it is not diagnostic for sporotrichosis.

Chromoblastomycosis, Phaeohyphomycosis, and Mycetoma. These three subcutaneous mycoses are caused by a number of organisms (Tables 52-4 and 52-5) with a diversity of clinical presentations. They are seen most often in tropical and subtropical climates and are very rare in temperate regions. The infections are commonly found on the extremities, which have the highest degree of exposure to the environment.

The term "chromoblastomycosis" is used to describe infections in which warty, verrucose lesions slowly develop in the skin and subcutaneous tissue at the site of traumatic inoculation. The infections begin as small, scaly, raised, erythematous papules which enlarge and coalesce with satellite lesions that develop. This process sometimes continues for years, resulting in large, tumorous masses resembling cauliflower heads. The characteristic tissue form of any of the etiologic agents is the same and can be demonstrated on microscopic exam of material from the lesions or biopsy. The organisms appear as thick-walled, round, sclerotic bodies, which are brown-pigmented with muriform (vertical and horizontal) septations (Figure 52-7). Septate, branched, dematiaceous hyphae are also seen. When isolated in culture, the agents are speciated by their microscopic morphology and method of conidia production.

Phaeohyphomycosis is a group of mycotic diseases characterized by the presence of dematiaceous hyphal elements in tissue. The most common clinical manifestation is either a subcutaneous abscess similar to those of chromoblastomycosis, or a subcutaneous nodular cyst. Other forms of infection include the superficial diseases black piedra and tinea nigra, cutaneous invasion, and cerebral and systemic disease. The morphology of these fungi in tissue is varied. Hyphae, pseudohyphae, yeast cells, and distorted fragments are seen (Figure 52-8), but no round, sclerotic bodies are present. After isolation in culture, microscopic examination of the organisms is used in speciation.

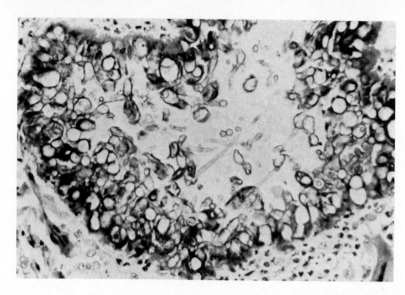

Fig. 52-9 Dematiaceous hyphae and chlamydoconidia embedded in cement-like substance, from granule produced by *Curvularia geniculata. From Chandler FW and Watts JC: Pathologic diagnosis of fungal infections, Chicago, 1987, American Society of Clinical Pathologists.*

Mycetoma is another infection that results after traumatic inoculation of microorganisms into subcutaneous tissue. There are two categories of this disease, eumycotic and actinomycotic, based on the etiologic agent of infection (See Table 52-5). Eumycotic mycetoma develops as a result of infection by a number of filamentous fungi, and actinomycotic mycetoma is caused by members of the family of aerobic, branching, filamentous bacteria, the *Actinomyce-taceae*. The lesions produced in these infections remain localized, but the organisms invade cutaneous tissue, and sometimes bone, at the site of inoculation. Painful swelling, draining sinus tracts, and the presence of granules within the infected tissue and discharged material are the hallmarks of a mycetoma. The color and consistency of the granules, as seen on direct exam (Figure 52-9), are helpful in determining the infectious agent, and final identification is established after culture of the organism. Because bacterial infection can mimic mycetoma and different therapy is appropriate for each form of the disease, it is critical that the correct etiologic agent be identified.

Cutaneous manifestations of systemic mycoses

Dimorphic pathogens. Although many opportunistic fungi can cause systemic mycoses, the "true pathogens" associated with these infections include *Blastomyces dermatitidis, Coccidioides immitis, Histoplasma capsulatum,* and *Paracoccidioides brasiliensis.* These organisms can produce disease in a healthy host if a heavy dose of inoculum is present. Clinical symptoms of infection are similar, and accurate diagnosis of disease depends on the recovery of the etiologic agent.

Systemic fungal disease usually begins by inhalation of the infectious stage of these organisms into the lungs, resulting in a respiratory infection that may be asymptomatic. From this point, the fungi disseminate, particularly in patients that are debilitated or immunocompromised. With some of these pathogens, the skin is a frequent site for secondary lesions to develop.

The agents of systemic mycoses, as described in Table 52-6, are dimorphic fungi, which, like *S. schenckii*, are mycelial at 25°C and convert to a yeast form at 37°C. Their natural geographic distribution is restricted, but travel to endemic areas and transport of contaminated material has resulted in isolation of these fungi in other locales. *B. dermatitidis* and *C. immitis* are most likely to present with cutaneous dissemination. *B. dermatitidis* is also isolated in primary cutaneous disease. *H. capsulatum* rarely disseminates to cutaneous tissue but has been isolated from these lesions, especially in AIDS patients, where it must be differentiated from a number of possible skin diseases.

The tissue forms of the dimorphic pathogens can be seen on exam of lesional material or histopathologic stain of tissue biopsy (Figures 52-10 to 52-13). Because the yeast of *H. capsulatum* is small and difficult to differentiate on routine fungal stains, either Giemsa or Wright stain is used to aid in visualizing budding cells. Fluorescent antibody stains also are available for the specific detection of each of these fungi in tissue.

After isolation in culture, these systemic fungal agents can be identified by demonstration of conversion from mold to yeast form at 37°C. This method, however, takes a minimum of 48 hours for *B. dermatitidis* and does not always work for the other pathogens. A faster, more sensitive, and more specific method of identifying *B. dermatitidis, C. immitis,* and *H. capsulatum,* is the exoantigen test, an immunodiffusion technique which identifies specific antigens present in extracts of these organisms. Molecular probe assays are also being developed for rapid culture confirmation of the systemic pathogens.

Cryptococcosis. This opportunistic yeast infection, caused by *Cryptococcus neoformans,* also produces cutaneous lesions as a result of disseminated disease. As these

Table 52-6   Dimorphic agents of systemic mycoses

Species Disease synonyms	Endemic areas	Appearance in clinical material

Blastomyces dermatitidis
  Blastomycosis
  North American Blastomycosis
  Gilchrist's Disease
	North-central, Southeastern U.S.; parts of
	Latin America, Africa, Middle East
		Thick-walled, spherical yeast, 8-15 μm; single
		buds attached by broad base.

Coccidioides immitis
  Coccidioidomycosis
  San Joaquin Valley Fever
  Desert Rheumatism
	Southwestern U.S.; Northern Mexico; parts of
	Central, South America
		Thick-walled, nonbudding spherules, 20-60 μm,
		containing endospores, 2-4 μm.

Histoplasma capsulatum
  Histoplasmosis
  Darling's Disease
  Reticuloendotheliosis
	Mississippi, Ohio River Valleys; Mexico; parts
	of Central, South America
		Small, oval yeast cells, 2-4 μm; single buds,
		narrowly attached; may be intracellular.

Paracoccidioides brasiliensis
  Paracoccidioidomycosis
  South American Blastomycosis
  Paracoccidioidal Granuloma
	Brazil; parts of Columbia, Venezuela; north-
	ern Argentina; Paraguay
		Thick-walled yeast cells, 10-60 μm; multiple
		buds, narrowly attached.

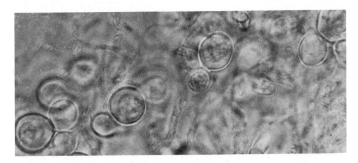

Fig. 52-10   Budding yeast cells of *Blastomyces dermatitidis*.

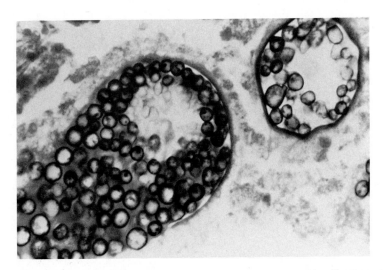

Fig. 52-11   Spherules of *Coccidioides immitis* containing endospores. *From Chandler FW and Watts JC:*
Pathologic diagnosis of fungal infections, Chicago, 1987, American Society of Clinical Pathologists.

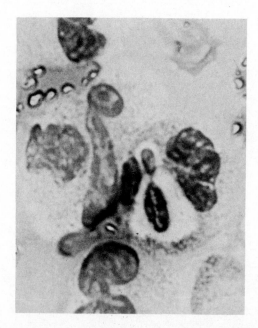

Fig. 52-12   Single budding yeast cell of *Histoplasma capsulatum* within a macrophage. *Courtesy of L Ajello, Centers for Disease Control.*

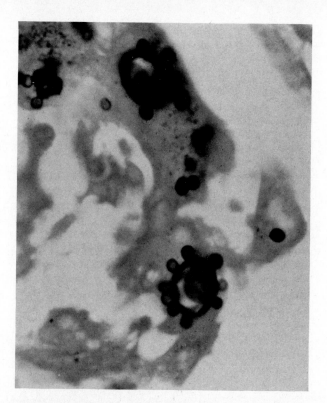

Fig. 52-13   Yeast cells of *Paracoccidioides brasiliensis* covered with uniform, oval blastoconidia. *From Chandler FW and Watts JC: Pathologic diagnosis of fungal infections, Chicago, 1987, American Society of Clinical Pathologists.*

organisms spread from the primary pulmonary infection, there is a predilection for the central nervous system, with rare cutaneous involvement. Among the immunosuppressed, cryptococcosis often presents as a primary cutaneous disease. The lesions that result from infection by *C. neoformans* are variable, presenting as papules, pustules, or abscesses, most commonly seen on the face or scalp. Secondary cryptococcal lesions resembling molluscum contagiosum have been reported in AIDS patients with systemic disease. Primary infections caused by this organism often heal spontaneously, but secondary lesions in the compromised patient tend to be more severe.

The preliminary diagnosis of cutaneous cryptococcosis is made by observing oval, budding, encapsulated yeast on a stained tissue biopsy or in clinical material (Figure 52-14). Methods used for direct exam when *Cryptococcus* is suspected are the India ink technique or the Mayer's mucicarmine stain on tissue smears. The identification of *C. neoformans* is made by isolation of the organism in culture, followed by carbohydrate and nitrate assimilation tests. This yeast can also be identified by many commercial yeast identification reagents.

LABORATORY EXAMINATION OF CUTANEOUS SPECIMENS
Specimen collection and transport

Proper collection and transport of any specimen in the microbiology laboratory is essential for the efficient recovery and identification of pathogens. Cutaneous specimens sub-

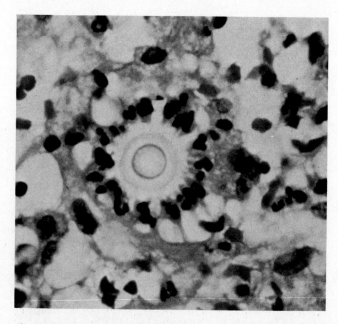

Fig. 52-14   Encapsulated yeast cell of *Cryptococcus neoformans* bordered by polymorphonuclear leukocytes. *From Chandler FW and Watts JC: Pathologic diagnosis of fungal infections, Chicago, 1987, American Society of Clinical pathologists.*

mitted for fungal examination and recovery of dermatophytes generally include hair, skin scrapings, and nail shavings. Aspirates and biopsies are occasionally submitted when other fungi are suspected. Infected hair should be plucked, rather than clipped, and skin and nail scrapings or shavings should be collected after cleaning the diseased area with 70% alcohol. When obtaining any specimen for culture of dermatophytes, care should be taken to avoid bleeding because blood inhibits the growth of these organisms. Aspirates of vesicular or pustular lesions should be collected in a syringe, using sterile technique, and biopsies should be taken from the advancing edge of lesions, where viable organisms are most likely found. Swab specimens submitted for mycological evaluation are unacceptable for cutaneous lesions because tissue invaded by fungi cannot be adequately collected in this manner. In addition, fibers in the tip of the swab may be displaced and can be confused with hyphae when viewed microscopically.

Skin, hair, and nail specimens should be transported in a sterile, dry petri dish or a clean envelope. Dry conditions help suppress overgrowth of bacteria and saprophytic fungi, without injuring dermatophyte species. Biopsies, on the other hand, should be kept moist. They should be transported either in gauze soaked in sterile, distilled water or in a small tube of sterile water. Syringes containing aspirated material and biopsies should be processed and cultured immediately upon receipt in the laboratory as the organisms likely to be isolated from these specimens are fragile and sensitive to drying or prolonged storage. Specimens for dermatophytes should be processed as soon as possible in the laboratory. However, organisms have been recovered from these specimens even after delays of up to 48 hours.

Direct Microscopic Examination

Direct microscopic examination of clinical specimens for fungi is a rapid method of obtaining useful diagnostic information. The visual observation of characteristic fungal elements quickly provides a physician with information about an organism that could take weeks to culture or may not grow at all. It also allows the differentiation of mycotic disease from other infections, or conditions such as malignancies, with which mycotic infections are frequently confused. Several techniques are routinely used in the laboratory for direct examination of hair, skin, or nails, and special stains are performed when specific organisms are suspected.

The use of 10% (or 20%) potassium hydroxide (KOH) for processing cutaneous specimens is common because it is easy to perform and requires no special equipment. Specimens are mixed with a drop of KOH on a microscope slide and gently heated. This clears proteinaceous material without altering fungal elements. The correct examination of slides prepared using this method is difficult, as it requires experience and patience to accurately interpret results. The slides must be viewed under low-intensity light in order to visualize the clinical material. When the tissue cells in the specimen are detected, it is often difficult to discern fungal elements from background debris. Many artifacts may be seen using this procedure, and upon standing, KOH distorts even fungi.

There are alternative methods to the KOH technique which can increase the sensitivity and specificity of the direct exam. A number of these are available to laboratories with a fluorescent microscope. One is the use of a fabric brightener, calcofluor white, along with KOH, to detect fungi in clinical specimens. This nonspecific fluorochrome has an affinity for chitin and cellulose in fungal cell walls, and produces a bright apple-green fluorescence when viewed with ultraviolet, violet, or blue light. Another fluorochrome reportedly used is Congo red. This reagent, with an affinity for cellulose, stains fungal elements in clinical material a bright fluorescent red, as observed using a green-band filter. Acridine orange, a fluorescent stain which binds to DNA in living cells, is also used to stain fungi in skin, hair, and nails, producing a bright fluorescence against a dark background under blue-violet light. Although these dyes simplify reading and increase the detection of fungi in the microscopic preparation, the slides which result are, again, only temporary.

The permanent method of staining used routinely in mycology for clinical material is the periodic-acid Schiff stain (PAS). Use of this technique increases the sensitivity of the direct exam and has been recommended as a follow-up to a negative KOH result. However, PAS is more time consuming than the other methods described, as more steps are involved in fixing and staining the specimen. After staining with PAS, the fungi are a magenta color against a light pink

Table 52-7   Special fungal or histopathology stains used in mycology

Technique	Features
Fluorescent antibody	Monoclonal antibodies to fungal antigens, conjugated to fluorescent dyes, detect specific organisms in clinical material or culture when viewed with fluorescent microscope.
Giemsa or Wright stain	Method of detecting intracellular *H. capsulatum,* particularly in blood films; yeast cells are dark blue with pale blue halo.
Gomori methenamine silver stain	Tissue stain; brown to black precipitate on cell walls delineates fungal elements.
Gridley fungus stain	Tissue stain; fungal cell walls colored red to purple.
Hematoxylin and eosin	Stain used to study tissue response to disease; fungi are visualized but sometimes stain poorly.
India ink	Negative stain used to demonstrate encapsulated yeast, especially *C. neoformans;* background is black with clear capsule surrounding yeast cell.
Mayer's mucicarmine	Method of staining polysaccharide capsule of *C. neoformans;* some *B. dermatitidis* also positive, staining bright red.
Modified acid-fast stain	Method of detecting and differentiating *Nocardia* species, which are acid-fast, from fungi, which are not.

background. Histopathology stains are also used in the detection of fungi in clinical material, biopsies, and tissue sections. Table 52-7 lists a number of special stains that are routinely used, with a brief description of their characteristic features.

Culture techniques

Material from cutaneous lesions can be directly inoculated to culture media in the mycology laboratory, for isolation of either yeast or moulds. In most cases, Sabouraud dextrose agar is used, often with the addition of antibiotics to prevent bacterial overgrowth. Chloramphenicol and cycloheximide are frequently added and are available commercially in the media sold as Mycosel (BBL Microbiology Systems, Cockeysville, Md.) or Mycobiotic (Difco Laboratories, Detroit). Because cycloheximide inhibits the growth of saprophytic fungi, some of which may be pathogenic, a second medium should be included in all cultures set up. Penicillin and streptomycin is an antibacterial combination that can be added to a medium without suppressing the growth of fungi.

A medium often used in physician office laboratories is Dermatophyte Test Medium (available commercially from various suppliers), which is made selective for these fungi by including cycloheximide, gentamicin, and chlortetracycline. It is also differential due to the pH indicator, phenol red, which changes the medium from yellow to red as the dermatophytes grow and metabolize.

All cultures from hair, skin, and nail specimens should be incubated at 25-30°C and held for four to six weeks before being discarded as negative. Colonies of yeast generally appear in the first 24 to 48 hours, but some molds require a longer incubation period. Following initial isolation, fungi should be subcultured to obtain pure growth. A variety of techniques are routinely employed for identification.

SUGGESTED READING

Balows A et al: Manual of clinical microbiology, ed 5, Washington, DC, 1991, American Society for Microbiology.

Koneman EW and Roberts GD: Practical laboratory mycology, ed 3, Baltimore, 1985, Williams and Wilkins.

Rippon JW: Medical mycology, ed 3, Philadelphia, 1988, W.B. Saunders Co.

Sindrup JH, et al: Skin manifestations in AIDS, HIV infection, and AIDS-related complex, Int J Dermatol 26:267, 1987.

Standard PG, et al: Exoantigen test—rapid identification of pathogenic mould isolates by immunodiffusion, Atlanta, 1985, U.S. Department of Health and Human Services, Public Health Service.

PART EIGHT

THE SYSTEMATIC IDENTIFICATION OF CLINICALLY SIGNIFICANT MICROORGANISMS

53 Bacteriology

David L. Sewell

The laboratory diagnosis of an infectious disease depends on communication between the medical staff and the clinical microbiology laboratory staff. The patient's history, physical examination, and clinical findings determine the appropriate specimens and other pertinent information that are submitted to the laboratory. The laboratory's responsibility is to select procedures that will most likely lead to the isolation and identification of the infectious agent. These tests include inoculation of appropriate media, microscopic examination of smears prepared from the specimen, immunologic methods, and direct detection of microbial antigens or products.

The extent of microbiological services a laboratory provides depends on multiple factors such as needs of the patient population and clinical staff, the expertise of the laboratory staff, the availability of the test at a reference laboratory, the cost-effectiveness of performing the test in-house, and the proficiency of the laboratory performing the test.

This chapter is organized to conform to the flow of work in a clinical microbiology laboratory, regardless of size. The emphasis is placed on how the laboratory proceeds in a general way to identify clinically significant bacteria through direct microscopic examination of specimens, morphology of organisms, culture results (including special growth requirements), and laboratory tests required for a presumptive or definitive identification of the isolate. Detailed descriptions of stains, media, tests, and methods of identification are not included in this text but are available in the excellent general references at the end of the chapter.

DIRECT EXAMINATION OF SPECIMENS

The direct examination of clinical specimens by microscopy is a rapid and cost-effective technique that provides much information for the initiation of appropriate therapy, assists in the evaluation of the quality of a specimen, and serves as a guide to interpretation and quality control of culture results. However, the accurate interpretation of microscopic results requires a certain degree of technical expertise. The sensitivity of the procedure is related to the number of organisms that must be present (usually 10^4-10^5/ml) in the specimen for detection. Smears are less valuable when low

numbers ($< 10^4$/ml) are present or the site is colonized with normal flora.

Methods and application

Specimens submitted for bacteriologic culture can be examined by a number of microscopic methods. Unstained preparations can be viewed by phase-contrast or darkfield microscopy while stained specimens are usually observed by light or fluorescent methods. Staining techniques include Gram, acridine orange, and acid-fast, or specific antibodies labeled with a fluorescent dye or enyzme. Cytocentrifugation of normally sterile body fluids increases the sensitivity of the microscopic examination.

The Gram stain is used for the direct examination of specimens submitted from patients with suspected bacterial pneumonia and meningitis, bacteriuria, genital infections, and pyogenic infections of tissue or normally sterile body fluids. The sensitivity of the Gram- or acridine orange-stained smear of cerebrospinal fluid (CSF) ranges from 60 to 80% and is directly related to the number of organisms present in CSF. The concentration of bacteria in CSF varies with early versus late meningitis and prior antimicrobial therapy.

Microscopic examination of expectorated sputum is widely accepted as a tool for assessing the quality of the specimen and acceptability for culture. The presence of numerous squamous epithelial cells (> 25/LPF) indicates that the specimen is heavily contaminated with oropharyngeal secretions and should not be processed. The presence of polymorphonuclear leukocytes or alveolar macrophages indicates that lower respiratory tract secretions were collected.

The Gram stain is very useful for ruling out urinary tract infections of 10^5 or more CFU/ml (sensitivity equals 80 to 90%) and providing rapid diagnostic information based on observed microbial morphology. However, the technique is not helpful for infections with fewer than 5×10^4 CFU/ml (which may occur in obstructive uropathies, over-hydration, chronic pyelonephritis, women with acute dysuria, during antimicrobial therapy, or following urinary tract surgery).

The sensitivity of a Gram-stained smear of urethral ex-

Table 53-1   Gram-stain morphology of frequently encountered aerobic bacteria

Organism	Morphology	
GRAM-POSITIVE COCCI		
Staphylococcus	Occur in "grape-like" clusters, may appear singly, in pairs, short chains, or tetrads.	
Streptococcus	Occur in short or long chains, occasionally pairs.	
S. pneumoniae	Occur in pairs; oval, distal ends pointed; usually encapsulated.	
GRAM-NEGATIVE COCCI OR COCCOBACILLI		
Neisseria and *Branhamella*	Occur in pairs with adjacent sides flattened giving a "kidney-bean" appearance, longer in width than length.	
Acinetobacter and *Moraxella*	Occur in pairs or singly, may be pleomorphic, longer in length than width.	
Haemophilus	Small coccobacillus, occurs singly or in pairs, short chains, may be pleomorphic.	
GRAM-NEGATIVE BACILLI		
Enterobacteriaceae	Occur singly or in pairs, occasionally short chains, barrel-shaped, pleomorphic, stain darker at ends of cell.	
Pseudomonas	Occur singly, in pairs, occasionally short chains, cells are straight, more slender, and less pleomorphic than enterics, stain evenly.	
GRAM-POSITIVE BACILLI		
Bacillus	Large, occurs singly, pairs, short chains.	
Coryneforms	Small, occur singly, pairs, short chains, or clumps, rounded or club-shaped ends, may be pleomorphic.	

Modified from Belsey RE, Baer DM, Statland BE and Sewel DL: The physician's office laboratory, Oradell, NJ, 1986, Medical Economics Books.

udate from men with symptomatic urethritis is over 90% but only 50 to 70% in asymptomatic males. The sensitivity of Gram-stained smears of endocervical secretions collected from women with uncomplicated gonorrhea is also low (50 to 70%). The presence of "clue cells" in vaginal secretions is an indication of vaginosis due to *Gardnerella vaginalis* and other anaerobic microorganisms.

The Gram and acridine-orange stains are also useful for detecting pyogenic infections of tissue or normally sterile body fluids. The identification of a mixed anaerobic, staphylococcal, streptococcal, or gonococcal infection plays an important role in the decision of empiric therapy.

The examination of respiratory specimens by carbol-fuchsin or fluorochrome stains for detection of mycobacterial species has a sensitivity of approximately 40 to 60%. The fluorochrome stain is somewhat more sensitive because the smear can be examined with a lower-power objective and therefore more fields can be viewed in less time. The quality of the specimen, centrifugal force used for concentration, therapy, and type of disease (cavitary versus noncavitary) influence the sensitivity of the method. Laboratories that use acid-fast smears for detecting mycobacteria should have fewer than 1% false positive smears.

All aspirates of normally sterile body fluids, tissues collected during surgery or by biopsy, abscesses, bone marrow, urethral discharges, bronchial washings or lavages, and sputum should be routinely examined microscopically. Specimens that may be examined microscopically by request include external ear, conjunctiva, superficial wounds, endocervical secretions, vaginal discharge, urine, feces, and tissue from autopsy or burn specimens.

PRELIMINARY/PRESUMPTIVE IDENTIFICATION OF BACTERIA

Clinical microbiology is concerned with developing the most practical, rapid, and clinically relevant approach to detect and identify organisms in specimens. This has produced a variety of culture methods, stains, and identification schemes based on biochemical reactions, immunology, and, more recently, nucleic-acid probes. The ideal approach to the detection, isolation, and identification of an infectious agent depends on the needs of the clinical staff and expertise of the specific laboratory (i.e., office, community, or academic). The extent of identification of the organism is based primarily on the clinical significance of the particular isolate. Seldom is it clinically relevant or cost-effective to identify organisms without clinical significance from specimens which are contaminated with normal flora (i.e., throat, sputum, gastrointestinal specimens). It is more important to provide clinicians with preliminary information which can be used to initiate antimicrobial therapy.

The identification of bacteria usually begins with examination and interpretation of a stained smear of the specimen (Table 53-1). Based on knowledge of the morphology of bacteria and the most likely agents causing the infection, the appropriate media are inoculated and incubated at the optimal temperature and atmosphere. Bacteria are then categorized according to: 1) growth characteristics on the primary isolation media (i.e., colony morphology, odor, hemolysis, etc.); 2) type of media that supports growth; 3) Gram-stained smear of the colony; 4) atmosphere of incu-

Table 53-2 General growth characteristics of bacteria on initial isolation

Characteristic	Organism	
	Gram-positive	Gram-negative
Growth in air ± CO_2		
Blood agar	Staphylococcus	Neisseria
	Streptococcus	Branhamella
	Corynebacterium	Pasteurella
	Bacillus	Gardnerella
	Listeria	Capnocytophaga
	Erysipelothrix	Kingella
	Other GPB	Brucella
		Bordetella
		Eikenella
		Moraxella
		Cardiobacterium
Blood and MacConkey agars		Enterobacteriaceae
		Aeromonas
		Pleisiomonas
		Vibrio
		Acinetobacter
		Flavobacterium
		Chromobacterium
		Achromobacter
		Alcaligenes
		Moraxella
Chocolate agar only		Haemophilus
Special media		Legionella
		Francisella
		Leptospira
Growth in 5% oxygen		Campylobacter
Growth anaerobically only		
Blood agar		Veillonella
		Fusobacterium
Laked blood agar		Bacteroides

Modified from Washington JA, ed: Laboratory procedures in clinical microbiology, ed 2, New York, 1985, Springer-Verlag.

bation (i.e., room air, increased CO_2, decreased oxygen, anaerobic conditions); and 5) results of spot tests performed directly on the colony (Table 53-2). The resultant information is used to presumptively identify the organism or to narrow the possibilities so that a definitive identification can be made based on additional biochemical reactions, immunologic tests, or presence of specific nucleic-acid sequences (Figures 53-1 and 53-2). The specimen may also be examined directly by a variety of tests for the presence of a specific organism.

AEROBIC GRAM-POSITIVE COCCI
Micrococcaceae

The family *Micrococcaceae* contains three genera: *Staphylococcus*, *Micrococcus*, and *Planococcus*. Members of the genus *Planococcus* are not isolated from clinical specimens, and members of the genus *Micrococcus*, although part of the normal skin flora, are rarely implicated in significant infections and when isolated are misidentified and are usually reported as coagulase negative staphylococci (CNS). The genus *Staphylococcus* contains over 20 species of the

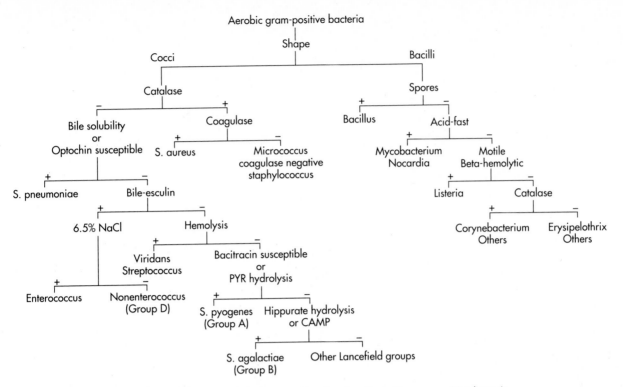

Fig. 53-1 Flow chart for the preliminary identification of aerobic gram-positive bacteria.
*Definitively identifed by latex agglutination tests.

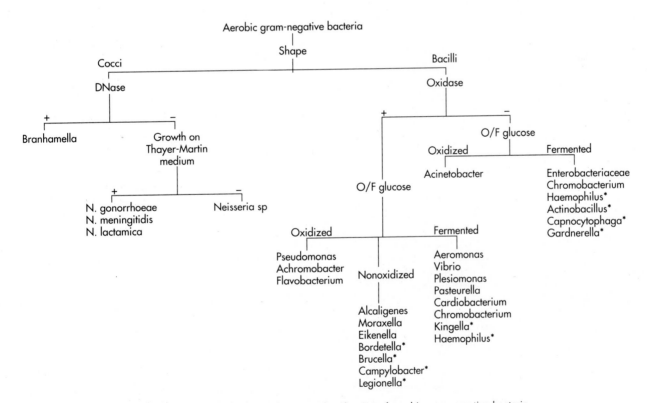

Fig. 53-2 Flow-chart for the preliminary identification of aerobic gram-negative bacteria.
*Requires special media for growth, incubation conditions, or is slow-growing.

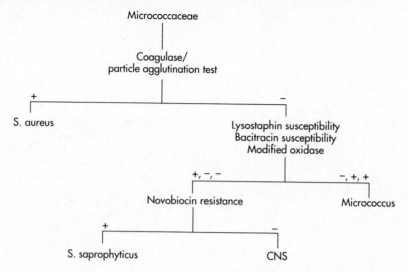

Fig. 53-3   Flow-chart for presumptive identification of gram-positive cocci.

normal flora of skin and mucous membranes in humans and animals. *S. aureus* is the major pathogen of the genus, producing infections ranging from localized boils to life-threatening systemic infections. The CNS are common inhabitants of the skin and are frequently isolated from clinical specimens as contaminants. However, with the increased numbers of immunocompromised patients and implantation of foreign material into patients, the CNS are becoming increasingly important as pathogens, especially *S. epidermidis*. *S. saprophyticus* is a common uropathogen in young, sexually active women. Species less commonly implicated as pathogens include *S. haemolyticus*, *S. hominis*, *S. warnari*, *S. sarcharolyticus*, *S. cohnii*, and *S. simulans*. *S. lugdunensis* is a newly described coagulase negative species that may cause soft tissue infection. Staphylococcal species rarely isolated as pathogens include *S. capitis*, *S. auricularis*, and *S. xylosus*.

Morphology and general characteristics

Staphylococci are gram-positive cocci, 0.5 to 1.5 um in diameter, occurring singly, in pairs, and in tetrads. They characteristically divide in more than one plane to produce irregular grape-like clusters. Aged cells or cells exposed to cell-wall active compounds may lose their ability to retain crystal violet and appear gram-negative. Staphylococci are nonmotile, oxidase-negative, usually strongly catalase-positive, and unencapsulated. Staphylococci grow well on any peptone-containing medium under aerobic or anaerobic conditions. Most strains grow in the presence of up to 10% NaCl and between the temperatures of 18 and 40°C. Some stains exhibit beta-hemolysis on bovine blood agar.

Figure 53-3 shows an abbreviated scheme for presumptively identifying staphylococci. When clinically important to differentiate between CNS and micrococci, seven tests are useful. Three relatively simple methods recommended for routine clinical laboratories include susceptibility to bacitracin, susceptibility to lysostaphin, and the modified oxidase test. Staphylococci are resistant to bacitracin, susceptible to lysostaphin, and are oxidase negative.

Staphylococcus aureus

S. aureus grows well on most nonselective agar and broth media (i.e., blood agar, trypic-soy, brain-heart infusion) producing 1-2 mm colonies in 18 to 24 hours of incubation. The colonies range from non-pigmented to yellow or orange. Many strains are beta-hemolytic. Rare isolates have increased nutritional requirements for hemin, menadione, thiamine, or pantothenate and can be grown on chocolate agar containing IsoVitaleX and menadione.

The coagulase test is used to identify *S. aureus*. In those rare instances when the coagulase test is equivocal, the thermostable deoxyribonuclease test, a commercial identification system, or conventional biochemicals tests can be used. The standard tube and slide coagulase test have been replaced in large part by rapid particle agglutination tests which measure the bound coagulase and protein A content of the cell wall. Although these systems are quite accurate, they may miss a small percentage of methicillin resistant *S. aureus*.

Coagulase negative staphylococcus

CNS are negative for tube coagulase (except *S. intermedius* and *S. hyicus*) and protein A. Colonies are usually gray to gray-white (non-pigmented) on nonselective media. Table 53-3 shows selected biochemical reactions useful for the identification of clinically significant CNS. More extensive tables, commercial identification kits, and instrument systems are available for the definitive identification of the CNS.

Streptococcus, Enterococcus and Aerococcus
Classification

Medically important streptococci are broadly classified according to three different classification schemes, each of which is partly useful in the clinical laboratory. Classification of organisms based on their hemolytic action on blood agar, as described by Brown in 1919, is used by most laboratories for the preliminary differentiation of streptococci into beta-, alpha-, and non-hemolytic (or gamma) groups.

Table 53-3 Abridged identification of coagulase negative *Staphylococcus* species

| Species | Arginine utilization | Urease | Acid from | | | Novobiocin resistance |
			Mannitol	Sucrose	Trehalose	
S. epidermidis	+	+	−	+	−	−
S. saprophyticus	−	+	+ / −	+	+	+
S. haemolyticus	+	−	+ / −	+	+	−
S. hominis	− / +	+	−	+	+ / −	−
S. warneri	− / +	+	+ / −	+	+	−
S. cohnii	−	−	+ / −	−	+	+
S. simulans	+	+	+	+	+ / −	−
S. saccharolyticus	+	NT	−	−	−	−

Finegold SM and Baron EJ: Bailey and Scott's diagnostic microbiology, ed 7, St. Louis, 1986, Mosby-Year Book.
+ = > 90% of strains positive.
− = > 90% of strains negative.
+ / − = Variable results; results more often positive.
− / + = Variable results; results more often negative.
NT = Not tested.

In the 1930s, Lancefield developed a serologic classification system based on the presence of group-specific antigens. More recently, the availability of commercial particle agglutination kits has made the serologic identification of some streptococci a simple and accurate procedure.

With the exception of the group D streptococci, the majority of alpha- (viridans strep) and non-hemolytic streptococci can only be classified by physiologic tests as proposed by Sherman. Historically, the group D streptococci

have been divided into enterococcal and nonenterococcal groups based on salt tolerance. Based on genetic relatedness, enterococci have been placed in a separate genus *Enterococcus*. The genus is composed of *E. fecalis*, *E. faecium*, *E. durans*, *E. avium*, etc. The non-enterococcal group D isolates, *S. bovis* and *S. equinus* would remain as streptococci.

In addition, a group of streptococci, which have been referred to as *S. milleri* by European and British authors

Table 53-4 Classification of streptococci

Species	Group antigen (Lancefield classification)	Sherman classification	Hemolysis (Brown classification)	Main habitat
S. pyogenes	A	Pyogenic	β, γ	Humans
S. agalactiae	B	Pyogenic	β, γ	Cattle; humans
S. equisimilis	C	Pyogenic	β	Many animals; humans
S. zooepidemicus	C	Pyogenic	β	Many animals
S. equi	C	Pyogenic	β	Horses
S. anginosus	F, None (A, C, G)[a]	Pyogenic	β	Humans
E. faecalis	D	Enterococci	α, β, γ	Feces of mammals
E. faecium	D	Enterococci	α, γ	Feces of mammals
E. durans	D	Enterococci	α, β, γ	Feces of mammals
S. avium	D	Enterococci	α, γ	Feces of birds
S. bovis	D	Nonenterococci	γ	Feces of mammals
S. bovis variant	D	Nonenterococci	α, γ	Feces of mammals
S. equinus	D	Nonenterococci	α	Feces of horses
S. mutans	None[b]	Viridans	γ	Humans, other animals
S. uberis	None[b]	Viridans	α	Cattle, soil
S. intermedius	None[b]	Viridans	α, γ	Humans
S. constellatus	None[b]	Viridans	α, γ	Humans
S. sangius I	None[b]	Viridans	α	Humans
S. sangius II	None[b]	Viridans	α	Humans
S. salivarius	None[b]	Viridans	γ	Humans
S. mitis	None[b]	Viridans	α	Humans
S. morbillorum	None[b]	Viridans	α	Humans
S. acidominimus	None[b]	Viridans	γ	Cattle

Modified from Facklam RR: Clin Microbiol Newsletter 7:91, 1985; and Parker MT: Streptococci and lactobacillus. In Wilson G and Miles A, ed: Topley and Wilson's principles of bacteriology, virology, and immunity, vol 2, ed 7, London, 1983, Edward Arnold.
[a]Approximately 75% of *S. anginosus* have group F antigen, approximately 15% are nongroupable, and approximately 10% possess group C, G, or A antigen (RR Facklam, personal communication).
[b]Approximately 75% of viridans streptococci do not have group antigens. Remaining 25% may have any streptococcal group antigen (A-O) with the exception of B and D (RR Facklam, personal communication).

and as three separate species *(S. intermedius, S. constellatus and S. anginosus)* by American authors, have been shown to be genetically related at the species level. It has been proposed by Coykendall, et al that their official name be *S. anginosus.* The interrelationship of the three classification schemes is depicted in Table 53-4.

Initial characterization

Catalase-negative, gram-positive cocci are considered to be streptococci (includes *Enterococcus* and *Aerococcus*). It is important to keep in mind that rare isolates of staphylococci may be catalase negative and that the colonial morphology of *Listeria* (a genus of gram positive bacilli and catalase positive) resembles beta-hemolytic streptococci. Microscopically, streptococci are typically round, ovoid, or lancet shaped but may elongate to resemble gram-positive rods. Most often they occur in pairs or chains. *S. pneumoniae* typically appear lancet-shaped, encapsulated, and in pairs but may form short chains. Streptococci grow on standard blood containing infusion media. Nutritionally variant streptococci (pyridoxal-dependent) can be cultured by use of a "Staph" streak, by adding pyridoxal HCl to the growth medium, or by placing sterile disks containing pyridoxal on blood agar plates. Streptococci are facultative anaerobes, often requiring increased CO_2 for best growth. Recovery of beta-hemolytic streptococci is definitely enhanced by anaerobic incubation.

Hemolysis is a key feature for determining which additional tests are required for the differentiation of streptococci. After the hemolytic pattern is established, clinically significant isolates of beta-hemolytic streptococci are definitively identified by serological tests that place the organism in Group A, B, C, D, F, or G. Non- or alpha-hemolytic strains are tested only with Group D and B antisera. Nongroup B, D, and other streptococci are identified by physiologic tests.

Identification of beta-hemolytic streptococci

Beta-hemolytic streptococci are definitively identified by the detection of group-specific cell wall carbohydrate antigen by the classical Lancefield precipitin reaction, immunofluorescent staining, or particle agglutination reagents.

In addition to serogrouping, the beta-hemolytic streptococci can be presumptively identified by a few, easy-to-perform tests such as the determination of susceptibility to bacitracin and trimethoprim-sulfamethoxazole; hydrolysis of L-pyrrolidonyl-beta-naphthylamide (PYR test) and hippurate; and production of the CAMP factor (Table 53-5). Smaller laboratories may choose to presumptively identify all streptococci entirely by physiologic tests. Group A streptococci are susceptible to bacitracin and yield a positive PYR test. The PYR test is more sensitive and specific than the bacitracin test. Group B streptococci are hippurate and CAMP positive but PYR negative. The other beta hemolytic-streptococci are susceptible to trimethoprim-sulfamethoxazole but are negative in the other tests.

Identification of Enterococcus, Aerococcus, and alpha- and non-hemolytic streptococci

Alpha-hemolytic colonies are tested for bile solubility or optochin susceptibility. *S. pneumoniae* is positive for both tests while other streptococci are negative. Enterococci and Group D nonenterococci can be identified by testing for the ability to hydrolyse esculin in the presence of bile. Group D isolates are bile esculin positive. *Enterococcus* spp. can be separated from non-enterococci by growth in 6.5% NaCl and hydrolysis of PYR. If serologic testing is not performed, some isolates of *S. bovis* may be misidentified as viridans streptococci and some aerococci may be confused with enterococci. Aerococci are alpha-hemolytic, grow in 6.5% NaCl and may be bile esculin positive. However, they lack the Group D antigen and microscopically appear as gram-positive cocci in tetrads. Other physiologic reactions for aerococci and group D organisms are seen in Table 53-6.

Most viridans streptococci do not possess group antigens and must be identified, when clinically indicated, by physiologic tests (Table 53-6). If the proposal to combine the different species of streptococci into a single species named *S. anginosus* is accepted, it can be presumptively identified by the characteristics listed in Table 53-7. Commercially

---

Table 53-5 Presumptive identification of streptococci and enterococci

Category	Hemolysis	Susceptibility to Bactracin	Susceptibility to SXT	Hydrolysis of Hippurate	Hydrolysis of PYR	CAMP	Bile esculin	Growth in 6.5% NaCl	Optochin and Bile[a]
Group A	Beta	+	−	−	+	−	−	−	−
Group B	Beta[b]	−[b]	−	+	−	+	−	+[b]	−
Beta-hemolytic streptococci (not group A, B, or D)	Beta	−[b]	+	−	−	−	−	−	−
Group D, enterococcus	Alpha, beta, none	−	−	−[b]	+	−	+	+	−
Group D, nonenterococcus	Alpha, none	−	+[b]	−	−	−	+	−	−
Viridans group	Alpha, none	−[b]	+	−[b]	−	−	−[b]	−	−
Pneumococcus	Alpha	±	?	−	−	−	−	−	+

From Facklam RR and Carey RB: Streptococci and aerococci. In Lennette EH, et al, eds: Manual of clinical microbiology, ed 4, Washington, DC, 1985, American Society for Microbiology.
SXT = Trimethoprim-sulfamethoxazole
PYR = L-Pyrrolidonyl-β-naphthylamide
+ = Positive reaction or susceptible
− = Negative reaction or resistant
[a] Optochin susceptibility and bile solubility.
[b] Exceptions occasionally occur.

Table 53-6 Differentiation of group D streptococci, *Enterococcus* spp., viridans streptococci, and aerococci found in human infections

Test	E. faecalis	E. faecium	E. avium	E. durans	Aerococci	S. bovis	S. mutans	S. uberis	S. intermedius	S. bovis (var.)	S. constellatus	S. equinus	S. sanguis I	S. salivarius	S. mitis	S. sanguis II	S. morbillorum	S. acidominimus
HEMOLYSIS																		
Alpha	+	+	+	+	+	−a	−a	+	−a	−a	+	+	+	−a	+	+	−a	+
Beta	+	−	−	+	−	−	+	−	−	−	−	−	−	−	−	−	−	−
None	+	+	+	+	−a	+	+	+	+	+	−a	−	−a	+	−a	−a	+	−a
PHYSIOLOGIC																		
Bile esculin	+	+	+	+	v	+	−a	−	−a	+	−a	+	−a	−a	−	−	−	−
Growth in 6.5% NaCl	+	+	+	+	+	−	−	−a	−	−	−	−	−	−	−	−	−	−
Growth at 10° C	+	+	−	+	−	−	−	−	−	−	−	−	−	−	−	−	−	−
Pyruvate	+	−	+	−	−	−	−	−	−	−	−	−	−a	−	−	−	−	−
Arginine	+a	+	−	+	−	−	−a	−	+a	−	+a	−	+	−	−	−a	−	−
Esculin	+	+	+	+	v	+	+a	+	+	+	+a	+	+a	+a	−	−	−	−
Starch	−	−	−	−	−	+	−	−	−a	−a	−	−	+a	−a	−	−a	−	−
Hippurate	v	v	−	v	+a	−	−	+a	−	−	−	−	−	−	−	−	−	+a
Sucrose	+a	+	+	−a	+	+	+	+	+	+	+	+	+	+	+	+	+	+
Lactose	+a	+	+	+	+a	+	+	+	+	+	−	+	+a	+	+	−	−	−
Mannitol	+	+	+	v	+	+	+	+	−	−	−	−	−	−	−	−	−	−
Sorbitol	+a	−	+	−	−	+	+	+	−	−	−	−	−a	−	−	−	−	−
Arabinose	−a	+a	+	−	−	−	−	−a	−	−	−	−a	−	−	−	−	−	−
Sorbose	−	−	+	−	−	−	−	−	−	−	−	−	−	−	−	−	−	−
Inulin	−	−a	+a	−	−a	+a	+a	+a	−	−	−	−	+	+	−	−	−	−
Raffinose	−a	+a	+	−a	v	+a	+a	+a	v	v	−a	−a	−a	+a	−	+	−	−
Glucan	N	N	N	N	N	L	D	N	Na	Na	N	N	Da	La	N	Da	N	N

Modified from Facklam RR, and Carey RB: Streptococci and aerococci. In Lennette EH, et al, editors: Manual of clinical microbiology, ed 4, Washington, DC, 1985, American Society for Microbiology.
+ = Positive reactions   N = No glucans
− = Negative reactions   L = Levans
v = Variable reactions   D = Dextran
aOccasional exceptions occur.

available rapid systems are also available for the identification of many of the streptococci.

AEROBIC GRAM-NEGATIVE COCCI (NEISSERIA AND BRANHAMELLA)
Classification

The family *Neisseriaceae* consists of four general genera: *Neisseria*, *Moraxella*, *Acinetobacter*, and *Kingella*. Based on genetic relatedness studies, the genus *Branhamella* has been reclassified as a subgenus of *Moraxella*. Because of a common usage, similar morphology, and common biochemical identification systems, *Moraxella (Branhamella) catarrhalis* will be referred to as *B. catarrhalis*.

Morphology and general characteristics

Neisseria and *B. catarrhalis* are gram-negative, kidney bean-shaped cocci that appear most often in pairs with their adjacent sides flattened. In general, the plane of division between adjacent cells is longer than the width of the cell. Intracellular overdecolorized *S. aureus* or gram-negative

Table 53-7 Presumptive identification of the proposed species *S. anginosus*

Streptococcus	Characteristics
Nonhemolytic or alpha-hemolytic	Positive VP, arginine hydrolysis; negative sorbitol fermentation, growth in 0.5% NaCl and PYR hydrolysis.
Beta-hemolytic, Group A	Positive VP, resistant to bacitracin; negative PYR hydrolysis.
Beta-hemolytic, Group C or G	Positive VP.
Beta-hemolytic, Group F	All isolates are *S. anginosus*.
Other beta-hemolytic organisms	Do complete identification; most isolates are *S. anginosus*.

Modified from Ruoff KL: *Streptococcus anginosus* ("Streptococcus milleri"), Clin Microbiol Newsl. 10:65-68, 1987.

coccobacilli (e.g., *Moraxella* and *Acinetobacter*) may be confused with these organisms. *Neisseria* and *B. catarrhalis* are oxidase- and catalase-positive aerobic organisms that grow best on enriched media containing serum or blood in a humid atmosphere of 2-8% CO_2. *N. gonorrhoeae* requires chocolate agar for growth whereas *N. meningitidis* will grow on blood agar. *B. catarrhalis* and other *Neisseria* spp. can grow on medium devoid of blood. A selective medium (e.g., modified Thayer-Martin, Martin-Lewis, or New York City agar) is a requirement for isolation of pathogenic *Neisseria* (*N. gonorrhoeae* and *N. meningitidis*) from specimens that are contaminated with other bacterial flora. The plates should be incubated 72 hours before reporting as negative.

Preliminary identification

All suspicious colonies (i.e., 0.5 to 1 mm in diameter, gray-white, glistening) growing on selective agar that are oxidase-positive, gram-negative diplococci with adjacent sides flattened can be reported as pathogenic *Neisseria* and then definitively identified. *N. lactamica* and *N. cinerea* may grow on selective media and morphologically resemble pathogenic *Neisseria*. The indoxyl butyrate strip test has recently been recommended as a rapid method for the presumptive identification of *B. catarrhalis*.

Definitive identification

Carbohydrate utilization tests (e.g., cystine-tryptic agar, rapid-fermentation tests, and other physiological parameters) have historically been used to identify the *Neisseria* species and *B. catarrhalis* (Table 53-8). *N. gonorrhoeae* grows on selective medium and produces acid from glucose while *N. meningitidis* produces acid from both glucose and maltose. *B. catarrhalis* can be differentiated from other *Neisseria* sp by growth on blood agar at 22°C, growth on

Table 53-8 Characteristics of *Neisseria* spp. and *Branhamella catarrhalis*

Species	Colony morphology	Growth on			Acid production from					Reduction of		Polysaccharide Synthesis	DNAse
		MTM, ML, or NYC medium	Chocolate or blood agar at 22°C	Nutrient agar at 35°C	Glucose	Maltose	Lactose	Sucrose	Fructose	NO₃	NO₂		
N. gonorrhoeae	Gray to white, smooth, five colony types on subculture from primary	+	0	0	+	0	0	0	0	0	0	0	0
N. meningitidis	Nonpigmented or gray to white, some yellowish, smooth, transparent, encapsulated strains mucoid	+	0	0	+	+	0	0	0	0	V	0	0
N. lactamica	Nonpigmented or yellowish, smooth, transparent	+	V	+	+	+	+	0	0	0	+	0	0
N. sicca	Nonpigmented, wrinkled, coarse and dry, adherent	0	V	+	+	+	0	+	+	0	+	+	0
N. subflava	Greenish yellow, smooth, often adherent	0	V	V	+	+	0	V	V	0	+	V	0
N. mucosa	Sometimes yellowish, mucoid appearance due to capsule production	0	+	+	+	+	0	+	+	+	+	+	0
N. flavescens	Yellow, opaque, smooth	0	+	+	0	0	0	0	0	0	+	+	0
N. cinerea	Grayish white, slightly granular	V	V	+	0	0	0	0	0	0	+	0	0
N. elongata[a]	Grayish white, slight yellowish tinge, flat, glistening, dry, clay-like consistency	0	+	+	0	0	0	0	0	0	+	0	0
B. catarrhalis	Nonpigmented or gray, opaque, smooth	0	+	+	0	0	0	0	0	+	+	0	+

From Morello JA, Janda WM and Bohnhoff M: *Neisseria* and *Branhamella*. In Lennette EH, et al, eds: Manual of clinical microbiology, ed 4, Washington, DC, 1985, American Society for Microbiology.
+ = Strains typically positive, but genetic mutants that lack the requisite enzyme activity are occasionally encountered
0 = Most strains negative
V = Variable characteristic
[a]Weakly positive or negative catalase test, in contrast to other *Neisseria* spp.

Table 53-9 Abbreviated scheme for identification of gram-positive bacilli

Genus or species	Microscopic morphology[a]	Catalase	Grows better anaerobically	Motility	Esculin	H₂S (TSI)	TSI acid slant/butt[b]	Nitrate reduction	Urease	Hemolysis	Comments
Bacillus	Medium-large regular rods, spores	+	–	v	+	–	v/v	v	v	B, A, N	
Kurthia	Chains, plump rods	+	–	+	–	–	–/–	–	+/–	N	Strict aerobe; feathery growth; grow best at 20 to 30°C
Listeria monocytogenes	Small rods, coccobacilli	+	–	+	+	–	+/+	–	–	B	Umbrella motility
Oerskovia	Coccoid, branching filaments	+	–	+	+	–	+/+	v	v	N, A	Yellow pigment
Brevibacterium	Coccoid, short rods	+	–	+	+	–	+/+	v	–	v	Golden yellow
Rothia dentocariosa	Coccoid, diphtheriod, branching filaments	+	–	–	+	–	+/+	+	–	N	Coccoid in broth
Mycobacterium fortuitum	Slender rods	+	–	–	–	–	–/–	+	v	N	Acid-fast
Rhodococcus equi	Coccoid, branching filaments	+	–	–	v	–	–/–	v	v	N	Pink, coral pigment, acid fast
Corynbacterium	Diphtheroid, curved, pleomorphic	+	–	–[c]	–	–	v/v	v	v	v	
Arcanobacterium	Diphtheroid curved, pleomorphic, slender	–	+/–[d]	–	v	–	+/+	–	–	B	
Arachnia	Diphtheroid, pleomorphic	–	+	–	–	–	+/+	–	–	N	
Actinomyces	Diphtheroid, branching filaments	–[e]	+	–	+	–	+/+	+/–[d]	–	N	
Lactobacillus	Thin rods, thick rods, chains	–	+/–[d]	–	v	–	+/+	–	–	N, A	Some grow on tomato juice agar
Erysipelothrix	Pleomorphic, chains, small rods	–	–	–	–	+	+/+	–	–	N, A	
Propionibacterium	Diphtheroid	+	+	–	v	–	+/+	–	–	B, A, N	

Modified from Clarridge JE, and Weissfeld AS: Clin Microbiol Newsletter, vol 6:115, Elsevier Science Publishing Co, Inc, 1984.

+ = > 90% of strains positive   A = Alpha-hemolytic   N = Nonhemolytic
– = < 10% of strains positive   B = Beta-hemolytic
v = variable reaction

[a]Small is < 0.5 μm in diameter; medium is 0.5 to 0.9 μm; large is > 0.9 μm.
[b]+ reaction indicates acid production.
[c]Some species are positive.
[d]There is discrepancy in literature as to whether reaction is positive or negative.
[e]*A. viscosus* is positive.

nutrient agar at 35°C, lack of carbohydrate fermentation, reduction of nitrate and nitrite, and production of DNase. In addition to physiologic parameters, rapid commercial systems which utilize a heavy inoculum to measure the presence of preformed enzymes are available for the identification of *Neisseria* and *B. catarrhalis*. Nonbiochemical tests (e.g., fluorescent antibody, nucleic-acid probes, en-zyme-linked immunoassays) are also available for the identification of *N. gonorrhoeae* and *N. meningitidis*.

AEROBIC GRAM-POSITIVE BACILLI

The gram-positive aerobic to facultatively anaerobic rods comprise a heterogeneous group of organisms which are difficult to identify based on a few simple laboratory tests

Table 53-10 Identification of *corynebacterium* and other coryneform organisms

Genus and species	Tinsdale halo	Glucose utilization	Nitrate reduction	Urease production	Glucose	Maltose	Sucrose	Beta-hemolysis	Motility	Comments
C. diphtheriae	100[a]	F	91[b]	0	99	94	1	67	—	Respiratory pathogen
C. ulcerans	100	F	0	100	100	94	19	50	—	Respiratory pathogen
C. pseudotuberculosis (ovis)	100	F	77	96	100	100	79	62	—	Associated with horses
C. xerosis		F	100	0	100	100	100	ND	—	
C. striatum		F	100	0	100	0	100	58	—	
C. matruchotii		F	83	6	83	67	88	0	—	
C. kutscheri		F	100	100	100	93	100	20	—	Associated with rats
C. renale		F	100	90	90	0	0	36	—	Associated with cattle
C. pseudodiphtheriticum (hofmannii)		O	100	100	0	0	0	29	—	
C. minutissimum		F	0	0	100	100	100/0[c]	—	—	
CORYNEFORM GROUPS										
A3[e]		F	100	0	100	100	100	33	100	
A4[e]		F	13	0	100	100	100	28	58	Yellow
A5[e]		F	29	4	100	100	100	32	48	Yellow
ANF-1		O	0	0	0	0	0	20	—	
ANF-3		O	100	0	0	0	0	13	—	
B-1		O	16	0	100	33	42	25	—	
B-3		O	0	8	0	0	0	19	—	
D-2 (C. urealyticum)		O	0	100	0	0	0	16	—	
F-1		F	48	100	100	82	100	ND	—	Isolated from humans, especially genitourinary tract
F-2		F	39	88	100	100	0	ND	—	
G-1		F[d]	100	0	100	25	100	25	—	
G-2		F[d]	0	0	100	49	100	14	—	
I-1		F	100	0	100	0	0	44	—	
I-2		F	100	0	100	100	0	ND	—	
C. jeikeium (group JK)		F	2	0	100	43	0	—	—	May need serum; antibiotic resistant
C. bovis[e] (unassigned)		F	—	—	+	v	—	—	—	May need serum
C. aquaticum[e] (unassigned)		O	16	6	94	92	90		66	Yellow
Actinomyces pyogenes		F	0	0	100	87	68	100	—	Catalase negative
Arcanobacterium haemolyticum		F	7	0	71	100	31	100	—	Catalase negative
Rhodococcus equi		O	43	76	28	13	2	—	—	Pink, acid fast

Modified from Hollis DG and Weaver RE: Identification of gram positive bacilli, Atlanta, 1981, Centers for Disease Control.

+ = > 90% positive
− = < 10% positive
v = 10% - 90% positive
ND = No data available
[a]Numbers throughout table represent percent positive reactions. Reactions may be delayed up to seven days.
[b]C. diphtheriae, ssp. mitis var. belfanti is nitrate negative.
[c]One biotype is positive, and the other biotype is negative.
[d]May require added serum.
[e]Does not conform to definition of genus.

(Table 53-9). Fifteen different genera fit this description, some of which will be discussed in other sections (i.e., *Mycobacterium, Nocardia,* organisms which grow better anaerobically). More extensive identification schemes for these organisms are available in the general reference at the end of this chapter.

Most of the gram-positive bacilli are ubiquitous inhabitants of the environment or are found on skin and mucous membranes of humans and animals. Although most are opportunistic pathogens, some species (*C. diphtheriae, Listeria, B. anthracis,* etc.) are highly pathogenic.

Corynebacterium
Morphology and general characteristics

Corynebacterium are gram-positive, catalase positive, aerobic or facultatively anaerobic, nonmotile, club-shaped rods that frequently appear in palisades or form *L*s and *V*s. Some *Corynebacterium* species are common inhabitants of the skin and mucous membranes, and are often isolated in the laboratory but dismissed as contaminants. However, many species are capable of producing disease in the compromised host (e.g., *Corynebacterium* jeikeium [group JK]) or in patients with implants. When corynebacteria are the predominant or only isolate, they should be identified at least to the genus level.

Corynebacterium grow well on most routine enriched media (e.g., blood agar) and produce colonies that are opaque, white or gray. In cases of suspected diphtheria, selective agar (e.g., cystine-tellurite agar, modified Tinsdale agar) and Loeffler coagulated serum medium should be inoculated in addition to routine media.

Identification

The identification of *Corynebacterium* species begins with the direct Gram-stain examination of the specimen, looking for a predominance of coryneform organisms. The absence of organisms, however, doesn't rule out their involvement. In cases of suspected diphtheria, growth from the Loeffler's slant is stained with alkaline methylene blue, looking for typical coryneform morphology and metachromatic granules which suggest *C. diphtheriae.* On cystine-tellurite medium, colonies of *C. diphtheriae* appear grayish-black and the colonial morphology has been used to identify three subspecies: *gravis, mitis,* and *intermedius.* All suspected isolates of *C. diphtheriae* must be definitively identified (Table 53-10) and shown to be toxogenic by in vivo

or in vitro tests. Only *C. diphtheriae, C. ulcerans,* and *C. pseudotuberculosis* lack pyrazinamidase.

The biochemical test reactions for *Corynebacterium* sp are listed in Table 53-10. Many species require the addition of serum to the tests. Due to the difficulty of definitive identification of these organisms, only identification of clinically relevant isolates should be attempted.

Listeria

The genus *Listeria* consists of five species, of which only *L. monocytogenes* and, rarely, *L. ivanovii,* are pathogenic for man. Because species other than *L. monocytogenes* are very infrequently isolated from clinical specimens, their identification will not be discussed here but can be found in the general references.

Morphology and general characteristics

L. monocytogenes is a gram-positive (gram-variable with age or in clinical material) pleomorphic rod that may appear coccoid (resembling streptococci) to rod-shaped (resembling "diphtheroids"). The organism grows on most ordinary laboratory media and is a facultative anaerobe. Selective media and cold enrichment is useful for isolation from a contaminated specimen. Colonies of *L. monocytogenes* on sheep-blood agar are small (less than 1 mm), translucent, whitish-gray, and produce a narrow zone of beta-hemolysis which sometimes is best seen after removal of the colony from the medium.

Identification

As shown in Tables 53-9 and 53-11, *Listeria* can be separated from most other gram-positive bacilli and cocci by positive tests for catalase, tumbling motility at room temperature, esculin hydrolysis, and beta-hemolysis on sheep-blood agar. L. monocytogenes may be differentiated from other *Listeria* species by fermentation of carbohydrates and the CAMP test.

Erysipelothrix
Morphology and general characteristics

Erysipelothrix rhusiopathiae is a facultatively anaerobic, gram-positive, pleomorphic rod which may decolorize easily. The organism grows on blood containing medium but growth can be enhanced by culturing in infusion broth containing 1% glucose.

Table 53-11 Differentiation of *L. monocytogenes* from other bacteria it resembles*

Organism	Catalase	Esculin hydrolysis	Motility	Beta hemolysis	Growth in 6.5% NaCl
L. monocytogenes	+	+	+	+	+
Corynebacterium sp.	+	−	− / +	− / +	+ / −
Propionibacterium sp.	+	+ / −	−	+ / −	+
Arcanobacterium	−	+ / −	−	+	−
S. agalactiae (group B streptococci)	−	−	−	+	−
Enterococci	−	+	−	− / +	+

From Baron EJ and Finegold SM: Diagnostic microbiology, ed 8, St. Louis, 1990, Mosby-Year Book, Inc.
*+ = > 90% of strains positive; − = > 90% of strains negative; + / − = variable (most strains positive); − / + = variable (most strains negative).

Table 53-12 Identification of *Bacillus* spp.[a]

	Usual cell diameter (µm)	Penicillin (10 units)	Motility	Wide zone lecithinase	Beta-hemolysis	Spores swell cells	Voges-Proskauer	Nitrate reduction	Starch	Distinguishing characteristics
GROUP I										
B. anthracis	≥0.9	S	0	27	−	−	85	100		Produces capsule
B. cereus	≥0.9	R	99	100	+	−	84	89		
B. mycoides	≥0.9	R	63	100	−	−	50	100		Rhizoid colony
B. megaterium	≥0.9	V	42	0	−	−	0	10		
B. thuringiensis	≥0.9	R	+	+	+	−	V	+		Insect pathogen that produces toxin crystals
GROUP II										
B. subtilis	<0.9	S	84	−	V	−	71	89	80	
B. pumilus	<0.9	S	100	−	V	−	78	0	6	
B. licheniformis	<0.9	S	80	−	+	−	83	100	100	
B. firmus	<0.9	S	90	−	V	−	0	70	50	
B. coagulans	<0.9	S	+	−	V	−	V	0		Grows at 55° and 35° C
GROUP III										
B. circulans	<0.9		+	−	−	+	6	76		Colonies may migrate on agar
B. sphaericus	<0.9		+	−	−	+	0	26		Produces spherical spores
B. laterosporus	<0.9		+	V	−	+	0	90		Produces canoe-shaped spores
B. brevis	<0.9		+	−	−	+	−	26		
B. polymyxa	<0.9		+	−	−	+	100	0		
B. alvei (H$_2$S + *Bacillus*)	<0.9		+	−	V	+	V	+		
B. stearothermophilus	<0.9		+	−	−	+	V	0		Grows at 65° C, no growth at 35° C

From Clarridge JE: Miscellaneous gram-negative coccobacilli. In Howard BJ, et al: Clinical and pathogenic microbiology, St. Louis, 1987, Mosby-Year Book, Inc.
+ = > 90% positive
− = < 10% positive
V = 10-90% positive
[a]Percentages are given when available.

Identification

The biochemical characteristics of *E. rhusiopathiae* are presented in Table 53-9. It is the only catalase-negative gram-positive bacillus that produces H$_2$S in a triple sugar iron or Kligler's iron agar slant.

Bacillus

The genus *Bacillus* contains over 40 species that are normal inhabitants of the soil and environment and are frequent contaminants in the laboratory. With the exception of *B. anthracis* and *B. cereus,* most species are not clinically significant. Strict safety precautions must be used for specimens and cultures suspected of containing *B. anthracis*. All work must be done in a biologic safety cabinet, personnel should wear gloves, and all equipment and bench areas disinfected.

Morphology and general characteristics

Bacillus species are aerobic or facultatively anaerobic, catalase-positive spore-forming rods of variable size. They grow well on ordinary media and produce a wide range of colonial morphology and pigment. Because some strains stain gram-variable or negative and are oxidase-positive, they are often confused with gram-negative bacilli.

Identification

Three tests are helpful to differentiate overdecolorized *Bacillus* species from gram-negative bacilli. *Bacillus* species are spore-formers (sporulation may be stimulated on esculin or TSI agar), are usually vancomycin susceptible, and are resistant to KOH.

Tests to differentiate some of the *Bacillus* species are shown in Table 53-12. Anthrax in humans is extremely rare in the United States and *B. anthracis* is seldom encountered in clinical laboratories. Colonial morphology, hemolytic activity, motility, penicillin susceptibility, and reduction of nitrate are useful screening tests for the presumptive identification of *B. anthracis*. *Bacillus* species that produce medusa-head colonies, are nonmotile, nonhemolytic, penicillin susceptible, and nitrate positive need confirmatory identification as possible *B. anthracis*.

NONFASTIDIOUS, FACULTATIVELY ANAEROBIC BACILLI

Gram-negative rods are initially grouped based on their growth characteristics and oxidase reaction. Nonfastidious organisms grow rapidly (24 hours) on nonselective routine media while fastidious organisms require specialized media or nutrients, special atmosphere of incubation or are slow growing (48 hours or longer).

Table 53-13 Appearance of commonly isolated *Enterobacteriaceae* on various enteric media

	MacConkey (MAC) agar	Eosin–methylene blue (EMB) agar	Hektoen enteric (HE) agar	Xylose–lysine deoxycholate (XLD) agar	Salmonella-Shigella (SS) agar	Deoxycholate citrate (DC) agar	Bismuth sulfite (BS) agar	Brilliant green (BG) agar
Escherichia coli Lac +	Flat; red or dark pink; surrounded by zone of precipitated bile	Red black with metallic sheen[a]	Yellow-orange	Yellow	Pink	Deep red-pink	Usually do not grow	Usually do not grow
Lac –	Colorless	Colorless	Yellow-orange or green	Yellow	Colorless	Colorless	Usually do not grow	Usually do not grow
Klebsiella	Pink; mucoid	Purple	Yellow-orange	Yellow	Pink	Pink	Usually do not grow	Usually do not grow
Enterobacter	Pink; not usually as mucoid as *Klebsiella*	Purple	Yellow-orange	Yellow	Pink	Pink	Usually do not grow	Usually do not grow
Citrobacter, Serratia, Hafnia, Providencia	May appear colorless after 24 hr or slightly pink in 24 to 48 hr	Lavender or colorless	Colorless	Red, yellow, or colorless with or without black centers	Colorless	Colorless	Usually do not grow	Usually do not grow
Proteus, Morganella, Edwardsiella	Colorless[b]	Colorless	Colorless	Red, yellow, or colorless with or without black centers	Colorless	Colorless	Usually do not grow	Usually do not grow
Salmonella	Colorless	Colorless	Green or blue-green	Pink to red with black center	Colorless with black center	Colorless	Green-black	Pink-white opaque; surrounded by brilliant red medium
Shigella	Colorless	Colorless	Green or blue-green	Colorless	Colorless	Colorless	Usually do not grow	Usually do not grow
Yersinia	Colorless to peach	Colorless or purple[c]	Salmon	Yellow	Colorless	Colorless	Usually do not grow	Usually do not grow

From Farmer JJ III, Howard BJ, and Weissfeld AS: Enterobacteriaceae. In Howard BJ, et al: Clinical and pathogenic microbiology, St. Louis, 1987, Mosby-Year Book, Inc.

[a]Not all strains produce a metallic sheen; on the other hand, other species of enteric bacilli (for instance, *Yersinia enterocolitica*) may produce a sheen.

[b]*Proteus mirabilis, Proteus vulgaris,* and *Proteus penneri* may swarm.

[c]*Yersinia enterocolitica,* a non-lactose-fermenter that ferments sucrose, produces colorless colonies on Levine EMB agar and purple colonies on the modified Holt-Harris Teague formula, which contains sucrose.

Table 53-14 Typical reaction patterns of *Enterobacteriaceae* on triple sugar iron agar and lysine iron agar

LYSINE IRON AGAR	Triple sugar iron agar					
	K/Ⓐ H₂S+	K/Ⓐ	A/Ⓐ H₂S+	K/A	A/Ⓐ	A/A
R/A	*Proteus vulgaris*, *Proteus mirabilis*	*Morganella morganii*, *Providencia* spp.	*P. vulgaris*, *P. mirabilis* (rare), *Proteus penneri*	*M. morganii* (rare), *Providencia* spp.	*P. penneri*	*Providencia* spp., *P. penneri*
K/K or K/NC H₂S+	*Salmonella typhi*, *Salmonella* spp.	*Salmonella* spp., *Edwardsiella* spp.	*Salmonella* spp. (rare)	*S. typhi*		
K/K or K/NC	*Salmonella* spp. (rare)	*Escherichia coli*, *Hafnia alvei*, *Klebsiella* spp. (rare), *Serratia* spp. (rare), *Enterobacter gergoviae*		*S. typhi*, *Serratia* spp. (rare), *Klebsiella* spp. (rare), *E. coli*	*Klebsiella* spp., *E. coli*, *Serratia* spp., *Enterobacter aerogenes*, *E. gergoviae*	*Serratia* spp.
K/A H₂S+ K/A	*Citrobacter freundii*	*Salmonella paratyphi A*, *Escherichia agglomerans* (occ), *Enterobacter cloacae*, *Enterobacter taylorae*, *E. coli* (occ), *M. morganii*, *S. paratyphi A*, *Shigella flexneri*, *Citrobacter diversus*, *Citrobacter amalonaticus*	*C. freundii*	*E. coli*, *Shigella* spp., *M. morganii*, *E. agglomerans*, *Yersinia* spp., *Serratia* spp. (rare)	*E. coli* (occ), *C. diversus*, *C. amalonaticus*, *Serratia* spp., *E. cloacae*, *Enterobacter sakazakii*, *E. gergoviae*, *E. taylorae*	*E. coli*, *Enterobacter* spp., *Citrobacter* spp., *Yersinia* spp., *E. agglomerans*, *Serratia* spp.

Modified from Hall CT: Bacteriology I; January 1973 summary analysis – proficiency survey, Atlanta, 1973, Centers for Disease Control.
R = Red, oxidative deamination of lysine
K = Alkaline slant
A = Acid slant
/K = Alkaline butt
/A = Acid butt
/Ⓐ = Acid + gas in butt
/NC = No change in butt
H₂S+ = Hydrogen sulfide production

The extent to which members of the *Enterobacteriaceae* and other gram-negative rods are identified depends on the technical expertise of the personnel, the clinical significance of the isolate, the clinical need for the information, and cost considerations. Many laboratories identify "enterics" by a multisystem approach depending on the above considerations. Nonsignificant isolates may simply be reported as gram-negative rods (lactose-positive or negative). Significant isolates from non life-threatening infections may be identified by colonial morphology and a few spot tests or by a commercial identification system. Lastly, isolates not identified by the other systems can be identified by a full set of biochemicals or sent to a reference laboratory.

Oxidase-negative organisms: Enterobacteriaceae
General characteristics

The family *Enterobacteriaceae* is composed of more than 25 genera of gram-negative rods which, in general, are oxidase-negative, ferment glucose, reduce nitrate to nitrite, are catalase-positive, are peritrichously flagellated if motile, grow luxuriantly on routine media, and, within 24 hours, produce colonies that are 1 to 3 mm in diameter. Colonies on blood agar are usually dull gray, entire, opaque, and may be mucoid (e.g., *Klebsiella*). Some strains (especially *E. coli*) are hemolytic. Some *Proteus* species exhibit swarming on blood agar. Many species produce characteristic colonial morphology on certain selective media (Table 53-13). *E. coli* 0:157 produces a colorless colony (sorbitol-negative) on sorbitol-MacConkey agar.

Screening tests for stool pathogens

Three media (urea, triple sugar iron, and lysine iron agar) are used to screen stool cultures for potential pathogens within the Enterobacteriaceae. (Table 53-14). Urea is used to screen out urea-positive *Proteus* and *Providencia* species. Latex agglutination tests are commercially available to iden-

tify colonies of *Shigella, Salmonella,* or *E. coli* 0:157 and can be used as a screening test. A number of screening tests are being evaluated for the detection of verocytotoxin-producing *E. coli*.

Presumptive identification

Significant isolates from non life-threatening infections can be presumptively identified by colonial morphology and a few rapid tests as depicted in Figure 53-4. The identification is based on lactose fermentation on MacConkey agar, colonial morphology on MacConkey and blood agars, spot indole reaction, motility and ornithine decarboxylase. The typical susceptibility pattern is also used as an aid to identification (Table 53-15).

Definitive identification

Definitive identification of members of the *Enterobacteriaceae* is accomplished by inoculation of up to 25 conventional biochemicals (Table 53-16) or one of the many commercial systems. The identification of *Salmonella, Shigella,* and *E. coli* 0:157 needs to be confirmed by serologic agglutination.

Table 53-15 Typical antimicrobial resistance of selected members of the Enterobacteriaceae

Organism	Antimicrobial agent
E. coli.	None
Enterobacter	Ampicillin, cephalothin
Klebsiella	Ampicillin, carbenicillin
P. mirabilis	Tetracycline
P. vulgaris	Ampicillin, cephalothin

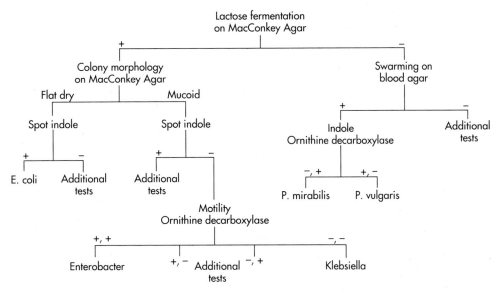

Fig. 53-4 Presumptive identification of common members of the *Enterobacteriaceae From Hicks MI and Ryan KJ: Simplified scheme for identification of prompt lactose-fermenting members of the Enterobacteriaceae, 1976, J Clin Microbiol, 4:511-514.*

Table 53-16 Biochemical reactions of the named species, biogroups, and enteric groups of the family *Enterobacteriaceae*

Species	Adonitol fermentation	l-Arabinose fermentation	Arginine dihydrolase	Citrate (Simmons')	Dulcitol fermentation	Gelatin hydrolysis (22°C)	d-Glucose – acid	d-Glucose – gas	Hydrogen sulfide (TSI)	Indole production	KCN (growth in)	Lactose fermentation	Lysine decarboxylase	Malonate utilization	d-Mannitol fermentation	Methyl red	Motility (36°C)	myo-Inositol fermentation	Ornithine decarboxylase	Phenylalanine deaminase	Salicin fermentation	d-Sorbitol fermentation	Sucrose fermentation	Urea hydrolysis	Voges-Proskauer
BUTTIAUXELLA																									
B. agrestis	0[a]	100	0	100	0	0	100	100	0	0	80	100	0	60	100	100	100	0	100	0	100	0	0	0	0
CEDECEA																									
C. davisae[b]	0	0	50	95	0	0	100	70	0	0	86	19	0	91	100	100	95	0	95	0	99	0	100	0	50
C. lapagei[b]	0	0	80	99	0	0	100	100	0	0	100	60	0	99	100	100	80	0	0	0	100	0	0	0	80
C. neteri[b]	0	0	100	100	0	0	100	100	0	0	65	35	0	100	100	100	100	0	0	0	100	100	100	0	50
C. species 3[b]	0	0	100	100	0	0	100	100	0	0	100	0	0	0	100	100	100	0	0	0	100	0	50	0	50
C. species 5[b]	0	0	50	100	0	0	100	100	0	0	100	0	0	0	100	100	100	0	50	0	100	100	100	0	50
CITROBACTER																									
C. freundii[b]	0	100	65	95	55	0	100	95	80	5	96	50	0	15	99	100	95	3	20	0	5	98	30	70	0
C. diversus[b]	98	100	65	99	50	0	100	98	0	99	0	35	0	90	100	100	95	0	99	0	20	99	45	75	0
C. amalonaticus[b]	0	100	85	85	0	0	100	97	0	100	95	50	0	0	100	100	98	0	95	0	40	100	15	80	0
C. amalonaticus biogroup 1[b]	0	100	85	1	4	0	100	93	0	100	96	19	0	0	100	100	99	0	65	0	0	100	100	45	0
EDWARDSIELLA																									
E. tarda[b]	0	9	0	0	0	0	100	100	100	99	0	0	100	0	0	100	98	0	100	0	0	0	0	0	0
E. tarda biogroup[b]	0	100	0	0	0	0	100	50	100	100	0	0	100	0	100	100	100	0	100	0	0	0	0	0	0
E. hoshinae	0	13	0	0	0	0	100	35	0	13	0	0	100	100	100	100	100	0	95	0	50	0	100	0	0
E. ictaluri	0	0	0	0	0	0	100	50	0	0	0	0	100	0	100	100	0	0	65	0	0	0	0	0	0
ENTEROBACTER																									
E. aerogenes[b]	98	100	0	95	5	0	100	100	0	0	98	95	98	95	100	5	97	95	98	0	100	100	100	2	98
E. cloacae[b]	25	100	97	100	15	0	100	100	0	0	98	93	0	75	100	5	95	15	96	0	75	95	97	65	100
E. agglomerans[b]	7	95	0	50	15	2	100	20	0	20	35	40	0	65	100	50	85	15	0	20	65	30	75	20	70
E. gergoviae[b]	0	99	0	99	5	0	100	98	0	0	0	55	90	96	99	5	90	0	100	0	99	0	98	93	100
E. sakazakii[b]	0	100	99	99	0	0	100	98	0	11	99	99	0	18	100	5	96	75	91	50	99	1	100	1	100
E. taylorae[b]	0	100	94	70	0	0	100	100	0	0	98	5	0	100	100	5	99	1	99	0	92	9	0	1	100
E. amnigenus biogroup 1[b]	0	100	9	100	0	0	100	100	0	0	100	70	0	91	100	7	92	9	55	0	91	100	100	0	100
E. amnigenus biogroup 2	0	100	35	100	0	0	100	100	0	0	100	35	0	100	100	65	100	100	100	0	100	100	0	0	100
E. intermedium	0	100	0	65	100	0	100	100	0	0	65	100	0	100	100	100	89	100	89	0	100	100	65	0	100
ESCHERICHIA-SHIGELLA																									
E. coli[b]	5	99	17	1	60	0	100	95	1	98	3	95	90	0	98	99	95	1	65	0	40	94	50	1	0
E. coli – inactive[b]	3	85	3	1	40	0	100	5	0	80	1	25	40	0	93	95	5	1	20	0	10	75	15	1	0
Shigella – serogroups A, B, and C[b]	0	60	5	0	2	0	100	2	0	50	0	0	0	0	93	100	0	0	1	0	0	30	0	0	0

	S. sonnei[b]	E. fergusonii[b]	E. hermannii[b]	E. vulneris[b]	E. blattae	E. americana[b]	H. alvei[b]	H. alvei biogroup 1	K. pneumoniae[b]	K. oxytoca[b]	K. Group 47 (indole and ornithine positive)	K. planticola	K. ozaenae[b]	K. rhinoscleromatis[b]	K. terrigena	K. ascorbata[b]	K. cryocrescens[b]	M. wisconsensis	M. morganii[b]	M. morganii biogroup 1[b]	O. proteus biogroup 2	P. mirabilis[b]	P. vulgaris[b]	P. penneri[b]	P. myxofaciens	P. rettgeri[b]	P. stuartii[b]	P. alcalifaciens[b]	P. rustigianii[b]	R. aquatilis[b]
	0	0	0	0	0	95	85	70	98	95	70	98	0	0	100	0	0	0	0	0	0	50	0	0	0	0	0	0	0	100
	0	0	45	8	0	0	4	0	95	90	100	98	10	0	0	0	0	0	98	100	0	0	98	95	0	98	30	0	0	0
	1	0	45	8	0	0	10	0	99	100	100	100	20	75	100	98	81	100	0	0	0	15	97	100	100	15	50	15	35	100
	2	0	1	0	0	0	0	0	99	99	100	92	65	100	100	40	45	0	0	0	0	0	0	0	0	1	1	1	0	94
	65	40	30	0	0	80	13	55	99	100	100	100	97	98	100	100	100	0	0	0	0	0	50	0	0	50	2	1	0	100
	0	0	0	0	0	0	0	0	0	1	0	0	0	0	0	0	0	0	95	100	0	98	99	99	100	98	95	98	100	95
	98	100	0	0	0	0	98	45	0	0	100	0	3	0	20	100	100	0	98	95	100	99	0	0	0	0	0	1	0	0
	0	0	0	0	0	0	0	0	95	98	95	100	55	95	80	0	0	0	0	0	0	90	95	1	0	90	95	1	0	0
	100	93	99	100	0	60	85	0	0	0	0	100	0	0	80	98	90	0	95	0	0	95	95	85	100	94		96	30	6
	100	100	100	100	0	84	40	85	10	20	96	100	98	100	60	100	100	100	97	95	15	97	95	100	100	93	100	99	65	88
	99	98	100	100	0	100	99	55	99	99	100	100	100	100	100	100	95	60	0	0	0	0	10	0	0	100	10	2	0	100
	0	35	85	100	0	0	50	45	93	98	100	100	3	95	100	96	86	0	1	5	0	2	0	0	0	0	0	0	0	100
	2	95	6	85	100	0	5	0	98	99	100	100	40	0	100	98	23	0	0	100	100	0	0	0	0	0	0	0	0	0
	2	0	45	15	0	70	5	0	98	100	100	100	30	0	100	98	95	100	1	0	0	2	2	1	0	5	2	0	0	100
	0	0	94	15	0	5	95	0	98	97	100	100	88	80	100	92	86	70	98	91	0	98	99	99	100	97	100	100	100	0
	0	98	99	0	0	0	0	0	0	99	100	20	0	0	0	92	90	0	98	100	0	2	98	0	0	99	98	99	98	0
	0	0	0	0	0	0	0	0	0	0	0	0	0	0	0	0	0	0	5	41	0	98	95	30	0	0	0	0	0	0
	0	95	97	97	100	0	98	0	97	97	100	100	50	0	80	93	95	0	90	91	0	96	85	45	100	10	0	85	35	98
	100	100	100	100	100	100	100	100	100	100	100	100	100	100	100	100	100	100	100	100	100	100	100	100	100	100	100	100	100	100
	0	0	0	0	0	0	0	0	0	0	0	0	0	0	0	0	0	0	0	0	0	90	91	50	100	0	0	0	0	0
	0	95	97	97	100	0	98	0	97	97	100	100	50	0	80	93	95	0	90	91	0	96	85	45	100	10	0	85	35	98
	0	0	60	19	0	0	0	0	30	55	10	15	2	0	20	25	0	0	0	0	0	0	0	0	0	0	0	0	0	88
	2	17	1	0	50	95	10	0	98	95	100	100	30	0	40	96	80	80	0	0	0	65	15	0	50	95	93	98	15	94
	2	5	0	30	0	0	6	0	0	6	0	0	6	0	0	0	0	0	0	0	0	0	0	0	0	0	0	0	0	0
	95	98	100	100	100	0	95	0	99	98	100	100	98	100	100	100	100	0	0	0	0	0	0	0	0	0	1	1	98	0
	0	0	0	0	0	0	0	0	90	99	100	100	97	100	100	0	0	100	0	0	0	0	0	0	0	0	5	0	0	0

Continued.

Table 53-16 Biochemical reactions of the named species, biogroups, and enteric groups of the family *Enterobacteriaceae* — cont'd

	Voges-Proskauer	Urea hydrolysis	Sucrose fermentation	D-Sorbitol fermentation	Salicin fermentation	Phenylalanine deaminase	Ornithine decarboxylase	myo-Inositol fermentation	Motility (36° C)	Methyl red	D-Mannitol fermentation	Malonate utilization	Lysine decarboxylase	Lactose fermentation	KCN (growth in)	Indole production	Hydrogen sulfide (TSI)	D-Glucose — gas	D-Glucose — acid	Gelatin hydrolysis (22° C)	Dulcitol fermentation	Citrate (Simmons')	Arginine dihydrolase	L-Arabinose fermentation	Adonitol fermentation
SALMONELLA																									
Subgroup 1 serotypes[b] — most	0	1	1	95	0	0	97	35	95	100	100	0	98	1	0	1	95	96	100	0	96	95	70	99	0
S. typhi[b]	0	1	0	99	0	0	0	0	97	100	100	0	98	1	0	0	97	0	100	0	0	0	3	2	0
S. choleraesuis[b]	0	0	0	90	0	0	100	0	95	100	98	0	95	0	0	0	50	95	100	0	5	25	55	0	0
S. paratyphi A[b]	0	0	0	95	0	0	95	0	95	100	100	0	0	0	0	0	10	99	100	0	90	0	15	100	0
S. gallinarum[b]	0	0	0	1	0	0	1	0	0	100	100	0	90	0	0	0	100	0	100	0	90	0	10	80	0
S. pullorum[b]	0	0	0	10	0	0	95	5	0	90	100	0	100	0	0	0	90	90	100	0	0	0	10	100	0
Subgroup 2 strains[b]	0	1	1	100	5	0	100	5	98	100	100	95	100	1	1	2	100	100	100	2	90	100	90	100	0
Subgroup 3a strains[b] (*Arizona*)	0	0	1	99	0	0	99	0	99	100	100	95	99	15	1	1	99	99	100	0	1	99	70	99	0
Subgroup 3b strains[b] (*Arizona*)	0	0	5	99	0	0	99	0	99	100	100	95	99	85	1	2	99	99	100	0	1	98	70	99	0
Subgroup 4 strains[b]	0	2	0	100	60	0	100	0	98	100	98	0	100	0	95	0	100	100	100	0	90	98	70	100	5
Subgroup 5 strains[b]	0	0	0	100	0	0	100	0	100	100	100	0	100	0	100	0	100	80	100	0	100	100	100	100	0
SERRATIA																									
S. marcescens[b]	98	15	99	99	95	0	99	75	97	20	99	3	99	2	95	1	0	55	100	90	0	98	0	0	40
S. marcescens biogroup 1[b]	60	0	99	92	92	0	65	30	17	100	96	0	55	4	70	0	0	0	100	30	0	30	4	0	30
S. liquefaciens group[b]	93	3	100	95	97	0	95	60	95	93	100	2	95	10	90	1	0	75	100	90	0	90	0	98	5
S. rubidaea[b]	100	2	98	1	99	0	0	20	85	20	100	94	55	100	25	0	0	30	100	90	0	95	0	100	99
S. odorifera biogroup 1[b]	50	5	99	100	98	0	100	100	100	100	100	0	100	70	60	60	0	0	100	95	0	100	0	100	50
S. odorifera biogroup 2[b]	100	0	100	100	45	0	94	100	100	60	97	0	94	97	19	50	0	13	100	94	0	97	0	100	55
S. plymuthica[b]	80	0	100	65	94	0	0	50	50	94	100	0	0	80	30	0	0	40	100	60	0	75	0	100	0
S. ficaria[b]	75	0	100	100	100	0	0	55	100	75	100	0	0	15	55	0	0	0	100	100	100	100	0	100	0
Serratia fonticola[b]	9	13	21	100	100	0	97	30	91	100	100	88	100	97	70	0	0	79	100	100	91	91	0	100	100
TATUMELLA																									
T. ptyseos[b]	5	0	0	0	55	90	0	0	0	0	0	0	0	0	0	0	0	0	100	0	0	0	0	0	0

YERSINIA

Organism																		
Y. enterocolitica[b]	0	98	0	0	0	100	5	0	98	97	2	30	95	0	20	99	95	75	2
Y. frederiksenii[b]	0	100	0	15	0	100	40	0	100	100	5	20	95	0	92	100	100	70	0
Y. intermedia[b]	0	100	0	5	0	100	18	5	100	100	5	15	100	0	100	100	100	80	5
Y. kristensenii[b]	0	77	0	0	0	100	23	0	100	92	5	15	92	0	15	100	0	77	0
Y. pestis[b]	0	100	0	0	0	100	0	0	97	80	0	0	0	0	70	50	0	5	0
Y. pseudotuberculosis[b]	0	50	0	0	0	100	0	0	100	100	0	0	0	0	25	0	0	95	0
Yersinia ruckeri	0	5	0	0	30	100	5	50	100	97	0	0	100	0	0	50	0	0	10

XENORHABDUS

Organism																		
X. luminescens (25° C)	0	0	0	50	50	75	0	0	0	0	100	0	0	0	0	0	0	25	0
X. nematophilus (25° C)	0	0	0	0	80	80	0	0	0	0	100	0	0	0	0	0	0	0	0

Organism																		
Enteric Group 17[b]	0	100	21	100	0	100	95	3	100	100	0	0	95	0	100	100	100	60	2
Enteric Group 41[b]	100	100	0	0	0	100	100	50	100	100	100	0	0	0	100	0	100	50	0
Enteric Group 45[b]	0	100	22	100	0	100	89	0	100	100	100	0	100	0	11	0	0	0	0
Enteric Group 57[b]	0	90	0	40	50	100	60	0	0	70	0	0	0	0	0	0	0	0	0
Enteric Group 58[b]	0	100	0	85	0	100	85	85	100	100	100	0	85	0	100	100	0	70	0
Enteric Group 59[b]	0	100	60	100	0	100	100	90	100	100	100	0	0	30	100	0	0	0	0
Enteric Group 60[b]	0	25	0	0	0	100	100	100	100	50	75	0	100	0	0	0	0	50	0
Enteric Group 63	0	100	0	0	0	100	50	0	100	100	65	0	100	0	100	100	0	0	0
Enteric Group 64	100	100	50	50	0	100	100	100	100	100	100	0	0	0	100	0	0	0	0
Enteric Group 68[b]	0	0	0	0	0	100	100	100	100	100	0	0	0	0	50	100	100	0	50
Enteric Group 69	0	100	100	100	100	100	100	100	0	100	100	100	100	0	100	100	25	0	100

From Farmer JJ, III, et al: J. Clin. Microbiol. 21:46, 1985.

[a]Each number gives the percentage of positive reactions after two days of incubation at 36° C (except *Xenorhabdus* organisms, which were incubated at 25° C). The vast majority of these positive reactions occur within 24 hours. Reactions that become positive after two days are not considered in the table.

[b]Organism is known to occur in clinical specimens.

Table 53-17 Differential characteristics of *Aeromonas* and *Plesiomonas*

Organism	DNase	Esculin hydrolysis	Voges-Proskauer	Lysine decarboxylase
A. hydrophilia	+	+	+	+
A. caviae	+	+	−	−
A. sobria	+	−	+	+
P. shigelloides	−	−	−	+

Oxidase-positive organisms
Aeromonas and Plesiomonas

Aeromonas and *Plesiomonas* are facultatively anaerobic gram-negative, oxidase- and catalase-positive, motile rods. Both organisms grow well on blood and MacConkey agars and variably on other enteric screening agar. *Yersinia*-selective agar (CIN) supports the growth of *Aeromonas* species and may be used to screen stool specimens. Many strains of *A. hydrophilia* and *A. sobria* are beta-hemolytic on blood agar.

The presumptive identification of *Aeromonas* and *Plesiomonas* is based on the reactions of a limited number of tests (Figure 53-5). Commercial identification systems will generally identify *Aeromonas* and *Plesiomonas* to the genus level. Table 53-17 lists key differential characteristics of *Aeromonas* species and *P. shigelloides*. Definitive identification to the species level can be performed with a battery of conventional biochemical tests.

Vibrio

Vibrio species are oxidase positive (except *V. metschnikovii*), motile, catalase positive, gram-negative straight or curved rods that are facultative anaerobes. *Vibrio* spp. will grow on most laboratory media. Thiosulfate-citrate-bile salts - sucrose (TCBS) agar is useful for the recovery of *V. cholerae* and other diarrheogenic vibrios from feces al-though not all *Vibrio* species grow on TCBS. Many halophilic vibrios require the addition of 1% or more of NaCl to biochemical testing media to insure growth.

The sucrose-fermenting vibrios *(V. cholerae, V. alginolyticus, V. fluvialis, V. metschnikovii and V. furnissii)* appear as yellow colonies on TCBS after 24 hours incubation while the other species appear green. Most of the commercially available identification systems will identify *Vibrio* species if a saline suspension is used as the inoculum. Otherwise, routine biochemicals supplemented with 1 to 3% NaCl can be used (Table 53-18).

Pasteurella

The genus *Pasteurella* has undergone proposed reclassification leading to new species associated with animal bites. These are *P. canis* (formerly *Pasteurella* new species 1 or "gas" and some *P. pneumotropica*) and *P. stomatis* (formerly *P. multocida* biotype 6). In addition, it has been proposed that *P. pneumotropica, P. ureae,* and *P. hemolyticum* be transferred to the genus *Actinobacillus*.

Pasteurella species are catalase- and oxidase-positive, nonmotile, facultatively anaerobic, gram-negative bacteria that range morphologically from small coccobacilli to filamentous rods. All species reduce nitrates to nitrites. The organisms grow well on blood and chocolate agars but with the exception of *P. aerogenes* and *P. haemolytica* don't grow on MacConkey agar. Colonies are usually smooth and gray although rough and mucoid variants can occur. Many strains produce a brownish discoloration on blood agar. The *Pasteurella* species are associated with animal bites and *P. multocida* is the species most frequently isolated.

The isolation of a gram-negative rod from an animal bite that grows on blood agar and not MacConkey agar and is oxidase-, indole- and ornithine-positive is strong presumptive evidence of *P. multocida*. Differential characteristics of *Pasteurella* species are shown in Table 53-19 and most commercial identification systems will identify *Pasteurella* to the species level. *Pasteurella* species are susceptible to pencillin G.

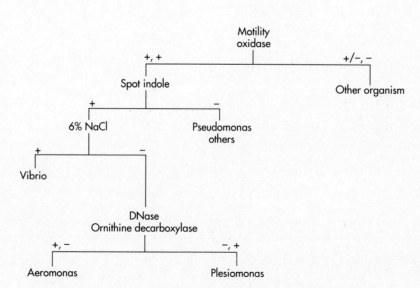

Fig. 53-5 Presumptive identification of *Aeromonas* and *Plesiomonas*.

Table 53-18 Tests for differentiation of members of the *Vibrionaceae* from humans[a]

Test	V. cholerae 01 and non-01	V. mimicus	V. parahaemolyticus	V. vulnificus	V. alginolyticus	V. cincinnatiensis	V. fluvialis	V. furnissii	V. damsela	V. hollisae	V. metschnikovii	Aeromonas spp.	Plesiomonas spp.
Oxidase	+	+	+	+	+	+	+	+	+	+	−	+	+
NO$_3$-NO$_2$ + 1% NaCl	+	+	+	+	+	+	+	+	+	+	−	+	+
Indole + 1% NaCl	+	+	+	+	+	−	−	−	−	+/−	−/+	+/−	+
Voges-Proskauer + 1% NaCl	+/−	−	−	−	+/−	+	−	−	+	−	+/−	+/−	−
Urease	−	−	−/+	−	−	−	−	−	+	−	−	−	−
Lysine decarboxylase + 1% NaCl	+	+	+	+	+	+	−	−	+/−	+/−	+/−	−/+	+
Ornithine decarboxylase + 1% NaCl	+	+	+	+/−	+/−	−	−	−	−	−	−	−	+
Arginine dihydrolase + 1% NaCl	−	−	−	−	−	−	+	+	+	−	+/−	+/−	+
Fermentation of													
Sucrose	+	−	−	−/+	+	+	+	+	−	−	+	+/−	−
Lactose	(+)/−	+/−	−	+	−	−	−	−	−	−	+/−	−/+	+/−
L-Arabinose	−	−	+	−	−	+	+	+	−	+	−	+/−	−
Gas from glucose	−	−	−	−	−	−	−	+	−/+	−	−	−/+	−
Growth in nutrient broth													
0% NaCl	+	+	−	−	−	−	−	−	−	−	−	+	+
3% NaCl	+	+	+	+	+	+	+	+/−	+	+	+	+	+
6% NaCl	+/−	+/−	+	+/−	+	+	+/−	+/−	+	+/−	+	−	−
8% NaCl	−	−	+	−	+	−	−	−	−	−	+/−	−	−
10% NaCl	−	−	−	−	+/−	−	−	−	−	−	−	−	−
Susceptibility to O/129													
10 µg	S	S	R	S	R	R	R	R	S	R	S	R	R/S
150 µg	S	S	S	S	S	S	S	S	S	S	S	R	S
Growth on TCBS	Y	G	G	G/Y	Y	Y	Y	Y	G	G/−	Y	−	−

From Janda JM, Powers C, Bryant RG, and Abbott SL: Current perspectives on the epidemiology and pathogenesis of clinically significant *Vibrio* spp, Clin Microbiol Rev. 1:245-267, 1988.
[a] + = Most strains positive; − = most strains negative; +/− or −/+ = variable reaction (predominant reaction shown as the numerator); ( ) = delayed reaction; S = susceptible; R = resistant; Y = yellow colonies; G = green colonies.

Table 53-19 Characteristics of *Pasteurella* spp.

Species	Hemolysis	Ornithine decarboxylase	Arginine decarboxylase	Urease	Indole	Glucose fermentation	Gas from glucose	Acid from maltose	Growth on MacConkey agar	Comments
P. multocida	Alpha (60)[a]	+	−	−	+	+	−	−	−	Many animals, cats and dogs especially
Pasteurella new species 1	Alpha (33)	−	−	v	+	+	v	+	−	Associated with dogs and cats
P. pneumotropica	Alpha (33)	+	−	+	+	+	−	+	v	Usually isolated from rodents
P. gallinarum	Nonhemolytic	−	+	−	−	+	−	+	v	Associated with poultry; usually commensal
P. hemolytica	Beta (72)	−	−	−	−	+	−	+	v	Infections in sheep and cattle
P. ureae	Alpha (16)	−	−	+	−	+	−	+	−	Human respiratory tract, usually commensal
P. aerogenes	Alpha (56)	v	−	+	−	+	+	+	+	Associated with swine, usually commensal

From Clarridge JE: Miscellaneous gram-negative coccobacilli. In Howard BJ, et al: Clinical and pathogenic microbiology, St. Louis, 1987, Mosby-Year Book, Inc.
+ = 90% positive
− = < 10% positive
v = 10-95% positive
[a] Number in parentheses: percent positive.

Table 53-20 Key characteristics for the identification of Chromobacterium violaceum

Character	C. violaceum	Aeromonas	Plesiomonas	Pseudomonas	Vibrio	Enterobacteriaceae
Oxidase	+	+	+	+	+	−
Indole	−	+	+	−	+	v
Lysine decarboxylase	−	v	+	v	+	v
Ornithine decarboxylase	−	−	+	v	+	v
Acid from:						
Glucose	+	+	+	−	+	+
Mannitol	−	+	−	−	+	v
Maltose	−	+	+	−	+	v

Chromobacterium

C. violaceum is a motile, oxidase- and catalase-positive, facultatively anaerobic, gram-negative rod that grows on blood and MacConkey agars.

Most colonies exhibit a characteristic violet pigment (produced optimally at 22°C) after 24 hours. Colonies may appear black on blood agar and often produce an odor of cyanide (almond odor). Nonpigmented strains need to be differentiated from *Aeromonas, Plesiomonas, Vibrio, Pseudomonas,* and *Enterobacteriaceae.* (Table 53-20).

NONFASTIDIOUS, AEROBIC, NONFERMENTATIVE GRAM-NEGATIVE BACILLI

The nonfermentative gram-negative bacilli (NFB) are ubiquitous in nature and can be found on the mucous membranes of humans and animals. They comprise approximately 15% of the gram-negative rods isolated in the clinical laboratory with *P. aeruginosa* accounting for 70% of these isolates. The next most frequently isolated species include *Acinetobacter calcoaceticus, P. cepacia,* and *X. maltophilia.* Definitive identification of the other NFB is often difficult, requiring specialized tests. The extent to which these isolates are identified and the degree of accuracy depends on the underlying condition of the patient (high risk for an opportunistic infection), the source of the specimen (colonized or sterile body site), the sole or predominant isolate from the specimen, the need for epidemiologic surveillance, and the available resources and technical expertise of the laboratory. The definitive identification of the NFB is beyond the scope of this text and the reader is referred to other excellent reviews in the general references.

Classification

The classification of the NFB is constantly undergoing change. The reader is referred to general references for a discussion of the nomenclature of these organisms. In this chapter, the organisms will be referred to by their former names and not their reclassified names. The genus *Kingella* and EF-4 group are listed in the tables here because they are sometimes mistaken for nonfermentive bacteria.

General characteristics

The isolation methods used for members of the *Enterobacteriaceae* will generally suffice for the recovery of the NFB

from clinical specimens, since most genera grow on unsupplemented blood agar. With the exception of *Eikenella, Moraxella,* and some *Flavobacterium* species, the NFB will also grow on MacConkey agar. The NFB are obligate aerobes and do not grow well under anaerobic conditions. Although most strains grow at 35°C, some require incubation at 25 to 30°C for optimal growth on plates or in biochemical tests. The Gram-stain morphology can help group these organisms. In general, *Pseudomonas* is a thin rod with parallel sides, *Acinetobacter* and *Moraxella* are fat coccobacilli (may resemble *Neisseria*) and *Eikenella* is a small coccobacillus. Growth conditions may affect the morphology. The description of colonial morphology of the NFB on primary isolation media is included in Table 53-21).

Initial characterization of nonfermentative bacilli

The initial characterization of NFB is based on the oxidase test, growth on MacConkey agar, motility, and whether the organisms oxidize carbohydrates fermentatively or oxidatively (Table 53-22). (*Enterobacteriaceae* are oxidase-negative, grow on MacConkey agar, and ferment glucose as detected by a yellow butt in TSIA, KIA or in O-F medium.) Motile organisms can be further classified by the arrangement of their flagella. Commercial identification systems may be used for some of the more easily identified species.

Presumptive identification of nonfermentative bacilli

Pseudomonas

P. aeruginosa is the most frequently isolated NFB. On blood agar, colonies are flat with a feathered edge or rough. They may be beta-hemolytic and produce a grape-like odor. Most strains produce a pyocyanin pigment (blue-green to green) pyoverdin (fluorescein), pyorubin (red), or pyomelanin (brown). If pyocyanin is present, the isolate can be identified as *P. aeruginosa* without any additional tests. Pigment production can be enhanced by growth on Pseudomonas agar (Difco) or TECH agar (BBL). Fluorescein pigment is enhanced by Pseudomonas F agar (Difco), FLO agar (BBL), or GNF agar (Flow Laboratories).

The differential characteristics of *P. aeruginosa* and other pseudomonads are listed in Table 53-23. The minimal characteristics for identification of strains as *Pseudomonas* species are gram-negative rod, asporogenous, polar monotrichous or tuft of flagella, motile, glucose-oxidizer or non-

Table 53-21 Colonial morphology of the nonfermentative bacteria

Organism	Description
Pseudomonas aeruginosa	Several colonial forms; usually large (2 mm in diameter), irregularly round, effuse colonies with matte surface and floccular internal structure; colonies have ground-glass appearance with raised butyrous centers and usually produce metallic sheen on blood agar and distinct grapelike odor; mucoid forms commonly seen in patients with cystic fibrosis
Pseudomonas fluorescens	Tiny colonies (less than 1 mm); increase in size after extended incubation
Pseudomonas cepacia	May appear as sulfur-yellow colonies or as colorless colonies
Pseudomonas diminuta	Colonies brown
Pseudomonas putida	Circular, smooth, raised, amorphous with entire edge
Pseudomonas stutzeri	Usually buff colored to yellow, wrinkled, and coherent, although smooth stains not uncommon
Xanthomonas maltophilia	Young colonies lavender colored but become gray-green with age (yellow colonies seen on peptone medium); colonies produce odor of ammonia
Pseudomonas putrefaciens	Colonies slightly mucoid and initially tan in color; color becomes reddish brown or pink after 48 hours
Pseudomonas pseudomallei	Young colonies white but become buff to brown after few days; colonies may produce earthy smell
CDC Ve	Form wrinkled yellow colonies after 48 hours of incubation wrinkles may be lost after numerous sub-cultures
Achromobacter xylosoxidans	Small, convex, circular, smooth, glistening, and butyrous with an entire margin; may or may not exhibit indeterminate lysis of blood cells
Alcaligenes faecalis	Nonpigmented, glistening, convex, almost clear colonies surrounded by greenish brown discoloration
Alcaligenes odorans	Feather-edged colonies usually surrounded by zone of green discoloration; produce highly characteristic fruity odor
Acinetobacter	Raised, creamy, circular, smooth, opaque, grayish, white; resembles *Enterobacteriaceae*; *A. alcaligenes* and *A. haemolyticus* beta-hemolytic
Flavobacterium meningosepticum	Circular with entire edge, convex, smooth or slightly mottled, glistening, butyrous, and pale yellow (cream) in color
Flavobacterium breve	Same as for *F. meningosepticum*, except yellow-orange in color
Flavobacterium (Sphingobacterium) multivorum	Small, circular, convex, smooth, opaque with pale yellow pigment; pigmentation develops after overnight incubation at room temperature
Flavobacterium indologenes	Same as for *F. breve*
Flavobacterium sp. group IIf	Small colonies at 24 hours but increasing in size and developing a distinctive, tan, mucoid appearance with continued incubation
Moraxella	Form tiny (less than 1 mm), translucent to semiopaque colonies after overnight incubation; *M. osloensis* and *M. nonliquefaciens* may form slightly larger colonies; *M. lacunata, M. nonliquefaciens,* and *M. atlantae* may show pitting; pitting colonies of *M. atlantae* and *M. nonliquefaciens* may also show surface spreading; all colonies are white except for *M. atlantae* and *M. phenylpyruvica,* which may appear slightly pink
Eikenella corrodens	*Forms characteristic grayish, dry, flat, radially spreading colony with irregular periphery and moist central core; when colonies are examined with stereoscopic microscope, three distinct zones of growth may be noted: (1) innermost clear, moist center, apparently devoid of growth, (2) highly refractile, speckled, pearl-like zone resembling mercury droplets, and (3) outer refractile spreading perimeter; when colonies are scraped from agar surface, pitting or corroding may be observed*
Kingella	May appear as smooth, entire, convex colonies or as colonies that pit the agar and have thin, spreading zone of growth around outer edge

From Oberhofer TR and Howard BJ: Nonfermentative gram-negative bacteria. In Howard BJ: Clinical and pathogenic microbiology, St. Louis, 1987, Mosby-Year Book, Inc.

Table 53-22 Characteristics of genera of nonfermentative bacteria

Genus	Oxidase	Growth on MacConkey agar	Motility	Utilization of glucose
Pseudomonas	+[a]	Good	Motile by means of polar flagella	Oxidative
Achromobacter	+	Good	Motile by means of peritrichous flagella	Oxidative
Alcaligenes	+	Good	Motile by means of peritrichous flagella	Inactive
Acinetobacter	−	Good, except for few strains of var. *lwoffi*	Nonmotile	Oxidative or inactive
Flavobacterium	+	Variable according to species	Nonmotile	Oxidative
Moraxella	+	Variable according to species	Nonmotile	Inactive
Eikenella	+	Negative	Nonmotile	Inactive
Kingella	+	Variable according to species	Nonmotile	Delayed fermentative

From Oberhofer TR and Howard BJ: Nonfermentative gram-negative bacteria. In Howard BJ: Clinical and pathogenic microbiology, St. Louis, 1987, Mosby-Year Book, Inc.
+ = Positive
− = Negative
[a] *X. maltophilia* is usually oxidase negative. *P. cepacia* may be negative.

Table 53-23   Differential characteristics of *Pseudomonas*

Characteristics†	*P. aeruginosa*	*P. putida*	*P. cepacia*	*P. maltophilia*	*P. fluorescens*	*P. pseudomallei*	*P. stutzeri*	*P. putrefaciens*
O-F Glucose	+	+	+	+	+	+	+	+
O-F Maltose	− / +	− / +	− / +	+	+	+	+	+ / −
O-F Xylose	+ / −	+ / −	+ / −	+ / −	+	+	+ / −	−
O-F Lactose	−	− / +	− / +	+	+	−	+ / −	−
Oxidase	+	+	+	+ / w	+ / w	+	−	+
Motility	+	+	+	+	+	+	+	+
Polar flagella	1	>1	>1	>1	>1	1	>1	1
Gas from nitrate	+ / −	−	−	+	−	+	−	−
Pyocyanin	+ / −	−	−	−	−	−	−	−
Pyoverdin	+ / −	+	+ / −	−	−	−	−	−
Growth at 42°C	+	−	−	+	+ / −	+ / −	− / +	+ / −
H₂S	−	−	−	−	−	−	−	+
Arginine dihydrolase	+	+	+	+	−	−	−	−
Lysine decarboxylase	−	−	−	+	−	+	−	−
Extracellular DNase	− / +	−	−	−	+	−	+	−
Polymyxin susceptibility	+	+	+	−	−	+	+	+
Gelatin hydrolysis	+ / −	+	−	+	+ / −	−	+	+ / −

From Sewell DL: In Wentworth BB, ed, Procedures for bacterial infections, ed 7, American Public Health Association, Inc., Washington, DC, 1987.
†Signs: + = 90% or more positive; − = 90% or more negative; + / − = most strains positive; − / + = most strains negative; w = weakly reactive

oxidizer, oxidase-positive or negative, and catalase-positive. *P. maltophilia* is oxidase negative and has been moved to the genus *Xanthomonas*. The majority of pseudomonads produce an alkaline slant and no change in the butt of TSIA or KIA.

Acinetobacter

The taxonomy of the genus *Acinetobacter* is confusing. Bouvet and Grimont lists six species of *Acinetobacter*, Gilardi recognizes four biotypes and Rubin, et al uses the widely accepted nomenclature of *A. calcoaceticus* var *anitratus* or var *lwoffi* (see general references). All species of *Acinetobacter* are nonmotile, oxidase-negative, nitrate-negative, catalase-positive, gram-negative rods that grow well on MacConkey agar and can initially be confused with the *Enterobacteriaceae* (Table 53-24). Morphologically, cells of *Acinetobacter* are plump coccobacilli (resemble *Neisseria*) but may also form filaments.

Eikenella

E. corrodens is a small, coccobacillus that is oxidase-positive, catalase-negative, indole-negative, reduces nitrate to nitrite, is unable to utilize carbohydrates and fails to grow on MacConkey agar. On initial isolation, the organism requires hemin for growth. *Eikenella* is usually recognized by its ability to "pit or corrode" the agar and its ability to produce small (0.2 to 0.5 mm), yellowish colonies that have a bleachlike odor. Strains that do not corrode the agar produce dome-shaped translucent colonies. Ornithine and lysine are decarboxylated when a heavy inoculum is used and help differentiate *Eikenella* from other NFB (Tables 53-22 and 53-25). *Eikenella* is susceptible to penicillin but resistant to clindamycin.

Moraxella

The genus *Moraxella* is composed of six species that are gram-negative coccobacillary rods that grow on blood agar and variably on MacConkey agar and may be confused with *Neisseria*. The species are catalase- and oxidase-positive, nonmotile, penicillin-susceptible, and unable to utilize carbohydrates. Other key characteristics are shown in Table 53-26.

Alcaligenes and Achromobacter

The genera *Alcaligenes* and *Achromobacter* include gram-negative, peritrichously flagellated, oxidase- and catalase-positive short rods. *B. bronchiseptica* and some CDC IVC species can be separated based on a positive-urea hydrolysis test. It has been proposed that the *Achromobacter* species be included in the genus *Alcaligenes*. All species of both genera are biochemically relatively inactive. Key characteristics are listed in Table 53-27.

Flavobacterium

The genus *Flavobacterium* is undergoing taxonomic changes with the addition of some CDC groups and the proposed transfer of *F. multivorum* and *F. spiritivorum* to the genus *Sphingobacterium*. The members of the genus *Flavobacterium* are recognized by their typical yellow pigment and formation of indole (xylene extraction required). The genus may be divided into oxidative and nonoxidative species. The species show variable growth on MacConkey agar, are nonmotile and catalase- and oxidase-positive. Blood agar colonies are usually surrounded by a lavender-green discoloration. *F. odoratum* (indole negative) and *F. indologenes* produce a fruity odor. Other characteristics are listed in Table 53-28. The cell morphology is a long thin rod with slightly bulbous ends.

Table 53-24 Biochemical characteristics of oxidase-negative, nonmotile *Acinetobacter* spp.

Test or substrate[a]	*A. anitratus*[b] (265)[c]	*A. lwoffii* (137)	*A. haemolyticus* (25)	*A. alcaligenes* (7)
Motility[d]	0[c]	0	0	0
Oxidase[d]	0	0	0	0
Urease	53	4	11	0
Phenylalanine deaminase	0	0	15	29
Nitrite production	0	0	6	0
Gelatinase[d]	1	64	1	57
Litmus milk peptonized[d]	5	88	3	86
Lecithinase	3[f]	56	9	100
Growth at 42° C	99	54	59	42
Growth on SS agar[d]	5	52	7	43
Growth on MacConkey agar	100	100	94	100
Hemolysis[d]	0	100	0	100
Oxidative-fermentative				
Glucose[d]	100	100	0	0
Lactose	95	88	0	0
Sucrose	0	0	0	0
Maltose	13[f]	16[f]	0	0
Mannitol	0	0	0	0
Xylose[d]	100	100	0	0
Fructose	0	0	0	0
Amides/salts				
Acetamide	2	0	12[f]	0
Allantoin	3	4	1	0
Citrate	98	88	47	100
Malonate	83	48	30	71
Tartrate	49	16	3	0
Colistin susceptible	100	100	100	100

From Oberhofer TR and Howard BJ: Nonfermentative gram-negative bacteria. In Howard BJ, et al: Clinical and pathogenic microbiology, St. Louis, 1987, Mosby–Year Book, Inc.
[a]All strains tested were negative for pyocyanin, fluorescein, gluconate oxidation, lysine and ornithine decarboxylase, arginine dihydrolase, denitrification, DNAse, starch hydrolysis, esculin hydrolysis, cetrimide tolerance, pigment, and beta-D-galactosidase.
[b]All organisms are biotypes of *A. calcoaceticus.*
[c]Figures in parentheses indicate number of strains tested.
[d]Key characteristics.
[e]Results expressed as percent positive after 7 days' incubation.
[f]Weak reaction.

Table 53-25 Biochemical and morphologic characteristics of fastidious, nonoxidative, gram-negative bacteria

Test or substrate[a]	*Kingella denitrificans* (15)[b]	*Kingella indologenes* (2)	*EF-4* (10)	*Kingella kingae* (3)	*Eikenella corrodens* (18)
Motility[c]	0[d]	0	0	0	0
Oxidase[c]	100	100	100	94	100
Indole[c]	0	0	100	0	0
Urease	0	0	0	0	0
Phenylalanine	0	0	0	0	20
Nitrite production[c]	80	0	0	100	100
Denitrification[c]	100	0	0	0	60
Lysine decarboxylase	0	0	0	50	0
Arginine dihydrolase	0	0	0	0	50
Ornithine decarboxylase[c]	0	0	0	94	0
Gelatinase	0	0	0	0	10
Litmus milk peptonized[c]	0	100	100	0	0
Growth on TSI agar[c]	Poor	100	100	Poor	100
Growth on MacConkey agar	0	0	0	0	0
Growth on Martin-Lewis agar	93	0	0	0	0
Growth at 42° C	NT[c]	0	0	NT[c]	100
Hemolysis[c]	0	100	0	0	0
Pitting					
Blood agar	38	67	50	78	0
Chocolate agar	46	67	50	61	0
TSA plate					
Growth[c]	0	100	100	0	100
X factor[c]	0	0	0	94	0
CO₂ enhanced[c]	100	0	0	100	0
Odor (bleach)	0	0	0	78	0
Glucose-fermentation[c]	13	100	100	0	100

From Oberhofer TR and Howard BJ: Nonfermentative gram-negative bacteria. In Howard BJ, et al: Clinical and pathogenic microbiology, St. Louis, 1987, Mosby–Year Book, Inc.
[a]All strains were negative in tests for pyocyanin, fluorescein, gluconate, cetrimide, starch hydrolysis, esculin hydrolysis, H₂S, alkalinization of amides and salts, beta-D-galactosidase, lecithinase, and deoxyribonuclease.
[b]Figures in parentheses indicate number of strains tested.
[c]Key characteristics.
[d]Results expressed as percent positive after 7 days' incubation.
[e]Not tested.

Table 53-26 Characteristics of *Moraxella* species

	Growth on MacConkey agar	Urease	Phenylalanine deaminase	Nitrate→ nitrite	Nitrite→ gas	Sodium acetate utilization
M. atlantae	+/−	−	−	−	+/−	+/−
M. lacunata	−	−	+/−	+	ND	−
M. nonliquefaciens	−	−	−	+	ND	−
M. osloensis	+/−	−	+/−	+/−	−	−
M. phenylpyruvica	+/−	+	+	+/−	−	+/−
M. urethralis	+	−	+	−	+	+/−

Finegold SM and Baron EJ: Bailey and Scott's diagnostic microbiology, ed 7, 1986, Mosby–Year Book, Inc.
+, ≥90% positive; −, ≥90% negative; +/−, variable results; ND, not done.

Table 53-27   Key characteristics of *Alcaligenes* and *Achromobacter*

Character*	A. faecalis	A. denitrificans	A. odorans	Achromobacter
Motility	+	+	+	+
Oxidase	+	+	+	+
Urease	−	−	−	−
Decarboxylases	−	−	−	−
Nitrate reduction	− / +	+	−	+ / −
Nitrate to gas	−	+	−	+ / −
Fruity odor	−	−	+	−
O/F Glucose	−	−	−	+ / −
O/F Xylose	−	−	−	+
Colistin susceptibility	+	−	+	+ / −

Modified from Oberhofer TR and Howard BJ: Nonfermentative gram-negative bacteria. In Howard BJ, Klaas II J, Rubin SJ, Weissfeld AS, and Tilton, RC, eds: Clinical and pathogenic microbiology, St. Louis, 1987, Mosby—Year Book, Inc.
* + = 90% or more strains positive; − = 90% or more strains negative; +/− = most strains positive; −/+ = most strains negative

Table 53-28   Characteristics of *Flavobacterium*

Character*	F. meningosepticum	F. indologenes	F. breve	F. multivorum	F. sp. II F	F. odoratum
Motility	0	0	0	0	0	0
Oxidase	100	100	100	100	100	100
Indole	100	72	100	0	97	0
Urease	0	10	0	100	0	100
Pigment	30	100	100	100	100	100
Nitrate reduction	10	25	0	11	0	0
O/F Glucose	100	100	100	100	0	0
DNase	100	34	100	9	72	29
ONPG	100	36	0	91	0	0
Colistin susceptibility	0	0	0	0	+	−

Modified from Oberhofer TR and Howard BJ: Nonfermentative gram-negative bacteria. In Howard BJ, Klass II J, Rubin SJ, Weissfeld AS, and Tilton RC, eds: Clinical and pathogenic microbiology. St. Louis, 1987, Mosby—Year Book, Inc.
*Results are expressed as percent positive after seven days; + = majority of strains positive; − = majority of strains negative.

FASTIDIOUS OR SLOW-GROWING AEROBIC OR FACULTATIVELY ANAEROBIC GRAM-NEGATIVE BACILLI

The microorganisms discussed in this section are not usually isolated on routine laboratory media (i.e., blood and MacConkey agar) after 24-hour incubation. They may be slow-growing (require at least 48 hours of incubation); require special growth conditions (i.e., specialized medium or atmospheric conditions); and may be unusual organisms not easily classified or associated with a specific clinical syndrome. In general, the organism must be considered by the health-care team before the specimen is inoculated so that special laboratory procedures are performed. Many of these organisms pose a considerable challenge regarding their diagnosis, isolation, identification, and characterization.

Campylobacter

Morphology and general characteristics

Campylobacter species are slender, curved, gram-negative rods (0.5 to 5 μm long) that may be comma, *S*, gull-winged, or spiral in shape. They are oxidase-positive, motile, microaerophilic and capnophilic (5% O_2, 10% CO_2, and 85% N_2), and inactive toward carbohydrates. *Campylobacter* species grow well at 35°C on blood agar but *C. jejuni*, *C. laridis*, and *C. coli* grow best at 42°C. Selective media and 42°C incubation temperature are necessary for the optimal isolation of enteric *Campylobacters* from stool specimens. Colonies are 1 to 2 mm in diameter, smooth, convex and translucent. With enteric *Campylobacters*, two colony types are observed: round and raised or flat and watery with irregular edges.

Direct microscopic examination

A presumptive diagnosis of *Campylobacter* enteritis can be made by a wet-mount or Gram-stain examination of the stool specimen. A wet mount of stool in broth is observed by darkfield or phase-contrast microscopy. *Campylobacter* will appear comma-shaped with a darting motility. A Gram-stain of the stool specimen demonstrating organisms with the typical cellular morphology of *Campylobacter* can also be diagnostic. Since the organisms stain faintly, the safranin should remain on the smear for two to three minutes.

Presumptive identification

The presumptive identification of *Campylobacter* from stool specimens can be made if the isolate has the typical cellular morphology, is oxidase- and catalase-positive and exhibits a darting motility, or suspect colonies can be tested by a commercially available latex agglutination test. *Helicobacter pylori* can be presumptively identified by inoculation of Christensen's urea broth with a portion of a gastric biopsy. The test will usually turn positive within one to two hours if *H. pylori* is present.

Table 53-29   Differential characteristics of *Campylobacter* species related to human disease

	Growth			Nitrate reduction	TSI	H₂S in lead acetate paper	Hippurate hydrolysis	Susceptibility to 30 μg disk		C-19 fatty acid production
	25°C	**37°C**	**42°C**					**Celphalothin**	**Nalidixic acid**	
C. jejuni	−	+	+	+	−	+	+	R*	S*	+
C. coli	−	+	+	+	−	+	−	R	S	+
C. laridis	−	+	+	+	−	+	−	R	R	−
C. fetus subsp. fetus	+	+	d*	+	−	d	−	S	R	−
C. hyointestinalis	d	+	d	+	+	+	−	S	R	−
C. cineadi	−	+	−	+	−	+	−	S	S	−
C. fennelliae	−	+	−	−	−	+	−	S	S	−
C. pylori	−	+	−	−	−	+	−	R	R	+
C. upsaliensis†	−	+	+	+	−	+	−	S	S	−

From Blaser MJ and Wang WL: Campylobacter infections. In Wentworth BB, ed: Diagnostic procedures for bacterial infections, ed 7, American Public Health Association, Inc, Washington, DC.
*R = resistant; S = susceptible; d = variable; † = catalase negative or weak

Definitive identification

Table 53-29 shows the results of confirmatory tests for the identification of *Campylobacter* species. The following text should be consulted for setting up the biochemical tests.

Legionella
Morphology and general characteristics

Legionella species are nutritionally fastidious (require L-cysteine), slow-growing (two to five days), aerobic, motile, gram-negative rods that vary in length from short to filamentous. They stain faintly with a routine Gram stain. Visualization is enhanced by staining with safranin for two to three minutes, replacing safranin with carbol-fuchsin, or staining only with crystal-violet and Grams iodine without decolorization. *Legionella* do not grow on ordinary laboratory media. The preferred medium is buffered charcoal yeast extract supplement with alpha-ketoglutaric acid (BCYE). Colonies are initially pinpoint but reach three to four mm in five to seven days, are gray, convex, and glistening with a ground-glass appearance when viewed with a dissecting microscope. *Legionella* are biochemically inactive.

Direct detection of antigen

A presumptive diagnosis of legionellosis can be made by direct detection of antigen in clinical specimens with commercially available immunofluorescent reagents, nucleic acid probes, or EIA/RIA. Since the immunologic reagents may not detect all species or serotypes of *Legionella*, the preferred means of diagnosis is by isolation in culture.

Presumptive identification

Suspect colonies on BCYE agar are subcultured to blood and CBYE agar. Organisms that grow only on BCYE agar are presumptively identified as *Legionella* species.

Definitive identification

Identification of the isolate to the genus level can be made with commercially available immunologic reagents or nucleic-acid probes. Legionella can be separated into groups by using the tests depicted in Table 53-30. The isolate should be submitted to a reference laboratory with the necessary expertise for definitive identification. Since the therapy for infections caused by all *Legionella* spp. is the same, the clinical laboratory initially needs to identify the isolate to the genus level; in the event of an outbreak, complete identification is needed. Assistance is available from the Centers for Disease Control or the state health department laboratory.

Haemophilus
Morphology and general characteristics

Members of the genus *Haemophilus* are facultatively anaerobic, nonmotile, pleomorphic, coccoid to coccobacillary, gram-negative bacilli that require hemin (Factor X) or nicotinamide adenine dinucleotide (Factor V) or both for growth. They are usually oxidase- and catalase-positive and growth of some species is enhanced by 5-10% CO_2. Optimum incubation temperature is 35 to 37°C. The colonial and cellular morphology of *Haemophilus* species is depicted in Table 53-31. Enriched chocolate agar is the preferred medium for culture except for *H. ducreyi* which requires a selective agar for optimum recovery. Body fluids (e.g., cerebrospinal fluid) can be directly examined by Gram stain or particle agglutination tests for a rapid diagnosis of *Haemophilus* infection.

Identification

Many laboratories identify *Haemophilus* species on the basis of X and V factor requirements (Table 53-32); more definitive identification of species and biotypes requires additional biochemical tests. Commercial systems are available for the rapid identification of *Haemophilus* species including *H. ducreyi*.

Actinobacillus
Morphology and general characteristics

Members of the genus *Actinobacillus* are fastidious, slow-growing, small, nonmotile, gram-negative, coccoid to

Table 53-30 Phenotypic properties of the Legionellae

Species	Oxidase	Catalase	Motility	Beta-lactamase	Fluorescence	Hippurate	Brown pigment	Gelatin	Number of serotypes
L. pneumophila	v	+	+	+	Y	+	+	+	10
L. feeleii	−	+	+	−	Y	v	+w	−	2
L. spiritensis	+	+	+	+	Y	+w	+	+	1
L. longbeachae	+	+	+	V	Y	−	+	+	2
L. jordanis	+	+	+	+	Y	−	+	+	1
L. oakridgensis	−	+	−	+w	Y	−	+	+	1
L. wadsworthii	−	+	+	+	Y	−	+	+	1
L. sainthelensi	+	+	+	+	Y	−	+	+	1
L. hackeliae	+	+w	+	+	Y	−	+	+	1
L. maceachernii	+	+	+	−	Y	−	+	+	2
L. jamestowniensis	−	+	+	+	Y	−	+	+	1
L. santicrucis	+	+	+	+	Y	+	+	+	1
L. micdadei	+	+	+	−	Y	−	−	−	1
L. bozemanii	V	+	+	V	BW	−	+	+	2
L. dumoffii	−	+	+	+	BW	−	v	+	1
L. gormanii	−	+	+	+	BW	−	+	+	1
L. anisa	+	+	+	+	Va	−	+	+	1
L. cherrii	+	+	+	+	BW	−	+	+	1
L. steigerwaltii	−	+	+	+	BW	−	+	+	1
L. parisiensis	+	+	+	+	BW	−	+	+	1
L. rubrilucens	−	+	+	+	R	−	+	+	1
L. erythra	+	+	+	+	R	−	+	+	1

Modified from Brenner DJ, et al: Int J Syst Bacteriol 35:50, 1985.
*Most strains of *L. anisa* fluoresce blue-white.
+ = Positive
− = Negative
+w = Some strains may be only weakly positive
V = Variable
Y = Yellow
BW = Blue-White
R = Red

coccobacillary rods. They ferment carbohydrates and grow best on blood and chocolate agar with increased CO_2. After 24 hours at 35°C, colonies of *A. actinomycetemcomitans* on blood agar are punctate to 0.5 mm and adherent. On continued incubation, a figure resembling a four- to six-pointed star may be seen in the center of the colony.

Identification

Actinobacillus needs to be differentiated from other similar genera (Table 53-33). Because of the variability of the biochemical tests, confirmation of an isolate as an *Actinobacillus* species requires a comprehensive test battery. The biochemical characteristics of the *Actinobacillus* species are listed in Table 53-34.

Cardiobacterium
Morphology and general characteristics

The genus *Cardiobacterium* contains one species, *C. hominis*. The organism is a fastidious, facultatively anaerobic, nonmotile, pleomorphic gram-negative rod with one rounded and one tapered end (resembling a teardrop). It may occur in clusters resembling rosettes. It does not grow on MacConkey agar and growth is enhanced by high humidity and 5-10% CO_2. Colonies on blood agar after 48 to 72 hours are 1 to 2 mm in diameter, circular, and glistening. A slight green to brown color may develop around the colony and some strains pit the agar.

Identification

Differentiation of *C. hominis* from biochemically similar genera may be done by indole production (requires xylene extraction), catalase, and fermentation of carbohydrates (see Table 53-33). The biochemical characteristics of *C. hominis* are shown in Table 53-35.

Capnocytophaga
Morphology and general characteristics

Capnocytophaga species are fastidious, facultatively anaerobic, capnophilic, gram-negative, fusiform bacilli that exhibit gliding motility. Optimal recovery occurs under anaerobic conditions. The organisms are slow-growing, requiring two to three days of incubation at 35°C and do not grow on MacConkey agar. Colonies are yellow, nonhemolytic, and spreading with finger-like projections.

Table 53-31   Morphologic characteristics of *Haemophilus*

Organism	Microscopic morphology	Colonial morphology[a]
H. influenzae	Coccobacilli or small, regular rods, 0.3 to 0.5 × 0.3 to 0.5 μm	Small (0.5 to 1 mm), smooth, translucent, grayish, convex with entire edge and a "mousy" odor; encapsulated strains larger (1 to 3 mm) and more mucoid, with tendency to coalesce
H. aegyptius	Long slender rods, 0.2 to 0.3 × 2 to 3 μm	After 48 hours appear small (0.5 mm), smooth, low, convex, grayish, and translucent
H. haemolyticus	Small coccobacilli or short rods with occasional filamentous forms	Resemble *H. influenzae* but are beta-hemolytic on blood agar
H. ducreyi	Slender rods in pairs or chains, 0.5 × 1.5 to 2.0 μm; "schools of fish" arrangement may be observed	After 48 to 72 hours on selective media, most appear small (~0.5 mm in diameter), flat, smooth, yellow-gray, and translucent to opaque; colonies may be pushed intact across agar surface
H. parainfluenzae	Small pleomorphic rods usually with long filamentous forms	Resemble *H. influenzae* except for their slightly larger size (up to 3 mm in diameter)
H. parahaemolyticus	Small pleomorphic rods usually with long filamentous forms	Similar to *H. parainfluenzae* but is beta-hemolytic on blood agar
H. paraphrohaemolyticus	Short- to medium-length rods, 0.75 to 2.5 μm and 0.4 to 0.5 μm in width with occasional short filaments when incubated in 10% CO_2; without extra CO_2 short to long coarse rods with twisted filaments	Resembles *H. aphrophilus* but is beta-hemolytic on blood agar
H. aphrophilus	Short regular rods, 0.45 to 0.55 × 1.5 to 1.7 μm; occasional filamentous forms	Highly convex, opaque, granular, yellowish, ranging in diameter from 1 to 1.5 mm; growth in broth is granular with heavy sediment on bottom of tube, and colonies adhere to walls of tube
H. paraphrophilus	Short regular rods with occasional filamentous forms	Identical to *H. aphrophilus*
H. segnis	Pleomorphic rods; irregular filamentous forms predominate	After 48 hours convex, grayish white, smooth or granular, and 0.5 mm in diameter

From Howard BJ: Haemophilus. In Howard BJ, et al: Clinical and pathogenic microbiology, St. Louis, 1987, Mosby–Year Book, Inc.
[a]On chocolate agar after 24 hours' incubation unless otherwise indicated.

Table 53-32   Principal differential characteristics of *Haemophilus* spp.

Species	Factor requirement X[a]	V	Hemolysis	Fermentation of Glucose	Sucrose	Lactose	Presence of catalase	CO_2 enhances growth
H. influenzae (*H. aegyptius*)	+	+	−	+	−	−	+	−
H. haemolyticus	+	+	+	+	−	−	+	−
H. ducreyi	+	−	−[b]	−[c]	−	−	−	−
H. parainfluenzae	−	+	−	+	+	−	D	−
H. parahaemolyticus[d]	−	+	+	+	+	−	D	D
H. segnis	−	+	−	W	W	−	D	−
H. paraphrophilus	−	+	−	+	+	+	−	+
H. aphrophilus	−	−	−	+	+	+	−	+

From Kilian M: Haemophilus. In Lennette EH, et al, ed: Manual of clinical microbiology, ed 4, Washington, DC, 1985, American Society for Microbiology.
+ = 90% or more of strains positive
− = 10% or less of strains positive
D = 11%-89% of strains positive
W = Weak fermentation reaction
[a]As determined by porphyrin test.
[b]Some strains may show delayed, weak beta-hemolysis.
[c]Clinical isolates usually appear to be asaccharolytic. However, under favorable growth conditions some strains show a late positive reaction for glucose fermentation.
[d]*H. parahaemolyticus* and *H. paraphrohaemolyticus* differ only in their requirement for CO_2. *H. paraphrohaemolyticus* requires CO_2, whereas *H. parahaemolyticus* does not.

Table 53-33   Differentiation of *Capnocytophaga* spp. and phenotypically similar genera and species

Genus and species	Catalase	Oxidase	Indole	Urease	Fermentation of glucose	Nitrate reduction	Motility
Capnocytophaga spp.	−	−	−	−	+	v	+
Cardiobacterium hominis	−	+	+	−	+	−	−
Chromobacterium spp.	+	v	v	v	+	+	+
Actinobacillus actinomy-cetemcomitans	+	v	−	−	+	+	−
Pasteurella spp.	+	+	v	v	+	+	−
Eikenella corrodens	−	+	−	−	−	+	−
Kingella spp.	−	+	v	−	+	v	−
Haemophilus aphrophilus	−	v	−	−	+	+	−

From Weissfeld AS, et al: Miscellaneous pathogenic organisms. In Howard BJ, et al: Clinical and pathogenic microbiology, St. Louis, 1987, Mosby−Year Book, Inc.
+ = ≥90%
− = ≤10%
v = Variable reactions

Table 53-34   Biochemical characteristics of *Actinobacillus* spp.

	Reaction			
Characteristic	*A. lignieresii*	*A. equuli*	*A. suis*	*A. actinomycetemcomitans*
Triple sugar iron agar (TSI)	Acid/acid	Acid/acid	Acid/acid	Acid/acid
H₂S (butt/paper)	− / −	− / −	− / −	− / −
Kligler iron agar (KIA)	Acid/acid	Acid/acid	Acid/acid	Acid/acid
Catalase	v	v	v	+
Oxidase	+	+	+	v
Motility	−	−	−	−
Growth on MacConkey agar	v	v	+	−
Growth on Salmonella-Shigella agar	−	−	−	−
Simmons citrate	−	−	−	−
Urea hydrolysis	+	+	+	
Gelatin liquefaction	−	v	−	−
Indole	−	−	−	−
Nitrate reduction	+	+	+	+
Lysine decarboxylase	−	−	−	−
Ornithine decarboxylase	−	−	−	−
Arginine dihydrolase	−	−	−	−
Esculin hydrolysis	−	−	+	−
ONPG (production of beta-galactosidase)	+	+		−
Gas from glucose	−	−	−	v
Acid from:				
Arabinose	+	v		−
Dulcitol	v	−		−
Fructose	+	+		+
Galactose	+	+		v
Glucose	+	+	+	+
Lactose	v	+	+	−
Maltose	+	+	+	+
Mannitol	+	+	v	v
Melibiose	−	+	+	−
Raffinose	v	+	+	−
Rhamnose	−	v		−
Salicin	−	v		−
Sucrose	+	+	+	−
Trehalose	−	+	+	−
Xylose	+	+	+	v

From Weissfeld AS, et al: Miscellaneous pathogenic organisms. In Howard BJ, et al: Clinical and pathogenic microbiology, St. Louis, 1987, Mosby−Year Book, Inc.
v = Variable; >10% but <90% positive; reaction may be delayed
+ = 90% or more strains positive
− = 90% or more strains negative

Table 53-35 Biochemical characteristics of *Cardiobacterium hominis*

Characteristic	Reaction
Triple sugar iron (TSI) agar	Acid/acid
H_2S (butt/paper)	−/+ weak
Kligler iron agar (KIA)	Alkaline/acid
Catalase	−
Oxidase	+
Motility	−
Growth on MacConkey agar	−
Growth on Salmonella-Shigella agar	−
Simmons citrate	−
Urea hydrolysis	−
Gelatin liquefaction	−
Indole	+ weak
Nitrate reduction	−
Lysine decarboxylase	−
Ornithine decarboxylase	−
Arginine dihydrolase	−
Esculin hydrolysis	−
ONPG (production of beta-galactosidase)	−
Hippurate hydrolysis	−
Gas from glucose	−
Acid from:	
Adonitol	−
Arabinose	−
Dulcitol	−
Fructose	+
Galactose	−
Glucose	+
Inositol	−
Lactose	−
Maltose	+
Mannitol	+
Raffinose	−
Rhamnose	−
Salicin	−
Sorbitol	+
Sucrose	+
Trehalose	−
Xylose	−

From Weissfeld AS, et al: Miscellaneous pathogenic organisms. In Howard BJ, et al: Clinical and pathogenic microbiology, St. Louis, 1987, Mosby−Year Book, Inc.
+ = 90% or more strains positive
− = 90% or more strains negative

Table 53-36 Key biochemical characteristics of *Capnocytophaga* spp.

Characteristic	C. ochracea	C. sputigena	C. gingivalis	C. canimorsus
Anaerobic growth	+	+	+	+
Aerobic growth in 5% to 10% CO_2	+	+	+	+
Growth in air	−	−	−	−
Starch hydrolysis	v	−	−	
Nitrate reduction	−	+	−	−
Oxidase production	−	−	−	+
Catalase production	−	−	−	+
Indole production	−	−	−	−
Urease production	−	−	−	−
Acid production from:				
Glucose	+	+	+	+
Lactose	v	v	v	+
Maltose	+	+	+	+
Mannitol	−	−	−	−
Sucrose	+	+	+	
Xylose	−	−	−	−

From Weissfeld AS, et al: Miscellaneous pathogenic organisms. In Howard BJ, et al: Clinical and pathogenic microbiology, St. Louis, 1987, Mosby−Year Book, Inc.
+ = ≥90%
− = ≤10%
v = Variable reactions

nocytophaga from similar genera is shown in Table 53-33. Other characteristics are listed in Table 53-36.

Kingella

Members of the genus *Kingella* are facultatively anaerobic, nonmotile, oxidase-positive, catalase-negative, straight, gram-negative rods that don't grow on MacConkey agar. CO_2 enhances growth on blood agar and the organisms may pit the agar.

Pertinent characteristics for differentiation of *Kingella* from other genera are shown in Table 53-33. Key characteristics for the identification of *Kingella* species are listed in Table 53-25.

Gardnerella

Gardnerella vaginalis is a small, pleomorphic, fastidious, facultatively anaerobic, nonmotile gram-negative to gram-variable bacillus. The organism grows on semi-selective human blood bilayer agar with Tween 80 (HBT), on non-selective vaginalis agar (V-agar) and on Columbia-colistin-nalidixic agar (CNA). It is beta-hemolytic on medium containing human blood (HBT or V-agar). It does not grow on MacConkey agar. After 48 hours in 5-10% CO_2, colonies on HBT agar are beta-hemolytic, gray, and approximately 0.5 mm in diameter.

G. vaginalis can be identified presumptively on the basis of catalase- and oxidase-negative, beta-hemolytic colonies on HBT agar. Confirmatory tests include starch and hippurate hydrolysis and alpha- and beta-glucosidase tests as well as a commercially available identification system.

Capnocytophaga canimorsus (DF-2)

C. canimorsus is a filamentous, sometimes curved, gram-negative rod associated with dog bites. The organism does not grow on MacConkey and requires approximately four days incubation at 35°C in 5-10% CO_2 for growth on chocolate agar. It is oxidase- and catalase-positive, indole, urease, and nitrate negative. It is susceptible to most beta-lactam antibiotics but resistant to gentamicin and kanamycin.

Identification

A yellow fusiform gram-negative bacillus that exhibits gliding motility and grows only anaerobically or in 5-10% CO_2 is presumptive identification. Differentiation of *Cap-*

Table 53-37   Characteristics of *Bordetella* spp.

Characteristic	B. pertussis Phase 1	B. pertussis Phase 4	B. bronchiseptica	B. parapertussis
Time to grow on Bordet-Gengou plates	3-4 days	1-2 days	1-2 days	1-2 days
Appearance on Bordet-Gengou plates at 3-4 days	Half pearl, entire, <1 mm	Larger than phase 1, rougher	Pitted; larger than phase 1 of *B. pertussis*	Larger and duller than phase 1 of *B. pertussis*
Growth on blood agar	−	+	+	+
Inhibited by fatty acids and sulfides	+	−	−	−
Urease	−	−	+ (4 hours)	+ (24 hours)
Nitrate	−	−	+	−
Pigment, brown soluble	−	−	−	+
Exotoxin	+	−	−	−
Pili	+	−	−	−
Filamentous hemagglutinins	+	−	−	−
Occurrence	Human respiratory tract	Laboratory	Animals (respiratory and wound); rarely from humans	Humans

From Clarridge JE: Miscellaneous gram-negative coccobacilli. In Howard BJ, et al: Clinical and pathogenic microbiology, St. Louis, 1987, Mosby−Year Book, Inc.
+ = 90% positive
− = <10% positive

Bordetella

The genus *Bordetella* consists of aerobic, small, coccoid, bipolar, pale-staining gram-negative bacilli. Staining can be enhanced by prolonged staining with safranin (two to three minutes) or using a carbol-fuchsin counterstain. On initial isolation, *B. pertussis* requires special media (e.g., Bordet-Gengou or Regan-Lowe) and appears as a small (less than 1 mm) gray, translucent colony with a pearl-like luster after three to four days incubation at 35°C in 5-10% CO_2. The appearance, growth characteristics, and biochemical tests useful for differentiating *Bordetella* species are listed in Table 53-37. Because of the difficulty in isolation of *B. pertussis*, direct smears of the clinical specimen should be sent to a reference laboratory for staining by direct fluorescent antibody stains. This reagent can also be used for a rapid presumptive identification of a suspicious colony. Methods to directly detect *B. pertussis* antigens or nucleic acid in nasopharyngeal secretions are currently being evaluated.

Brucella

The genus *Brucella* is characterized as gram-negative, non-motile, usually oxidase-positive, catalase-positive, glucose-oxidizing or non-oxidizing bacillus that reduces nitrate to nitrite and may produce H_2S or urease. *Brucella* are slow-growing, requiring three to four days incubation in 5-10% CO_2 to produce pinpoint, gray colonies on blood agar. Blood cultures should be held at least three weeks. Increased CO_2 is necessary for the isolation of some biotypes of *B. abortus*. Differential characteristics separating *Brucella* from other similar genera are shown in Table 53-38. Presumptive identification of *Brucella* species is based on urease, H_2S production, and requirement for CO_2 (Table 53-39). Definitive identification should be performed by a reference laboratory.

Francisella

F. tularensis is an obligately aerobic, small (0.2 by 0.3 to 0.5 μm), nonmotile, gram-negative rod that requires enriched media with added cystine or cysteine for isolation. In addition to the specialized media, BCYE agar (used for *Legionella*) will support growth of *Francisella*. On recommended media, colonies are pinpoint, gray, and smooth after 24 hours incubation at 35°C. *F. tularensis* can be separated from other similar genera in that it is oxidase-negative, is obligately aerobic, requires cystine or cysteine for growth, is nonmotile, and does not require CO_2 (Table 53-38). Specimens can be examined for organisms by a direct fluorescent antibody test. The definitive identification of *F. tularensis* should be performed by a reference laboratory since this organism is highly infective and special biosafety precautions are required.

Calymmatobacterium

C. granulomatis is usually visualized as clusters of safety pin-shaped rods in the cytoplasm of histocytes in scrapings of lesions by Wright or Giemsa stain. The organism can be cultured but it is difficult and the diagnosis is usually based on smear results.

Bartonella

These organisms can be isolated from blood cultures and on media containing blood, are motile, and stain gram-negative. The diagnosis of bartonellosis is most often made by demonstrating pleomorphic, rod or ring-shaped bacteria on or within the red blood cells in thick and thin blood films stained with Wright or Giemsa stain. In cutaneous nodules, the organisms appear within endothelial cells. The patient's history is critical if the laboratory is requested to look for

Table 53-38   Characteristics of some small gram-negative bacilli

Genus	Fermentation of glucose	Oxidase	Motility	Growth on MacConkey agar	Urease	Needed growth factors	Mol % G+C of DNA
Francisella	−	−	−	−	−	Cysteine or cystine	33-36
Bordetella	−	v	v	+[a]	v	Nicotinamide	66-70
Brucella	−	+	−	v	+	Thiamine	55-58
Pasteurella	+	+	+	v	v	—	40-45
Actinobacillus	+	+[b]	−	+[b]	v	—	40-43
Haemophilus	+	+/−	−	−	v	X and/or V	38-44
Yersinia	+	−	+	+	v	—	46-50

From Clarridge JE: Miscellaneous gram-negative coccobacilli. In Howard BJ, et al: Clinical and pathogenic microbiology, St. Louis, 1987, Mosby—Year Book, Inc.
+ = ≥90% positive
− = ≤10% positive
v = 10-90% positive
[a]*B. pertussis* does not grow on MacConkey agar.
[b]*A. actinomycetemcomitans* is usually negative.

Bartonella, because the bacterium is transmitted by sandflies (*Lutzomyia* sp) found only in South America.

Streptobacillus

Streptobacillus moniliformis is an etiologic agent of rat-bite fever that is seen in the western part of the world. The organism may be isolated from clinical specimens but requires the presence of blood, ascitic fluid or serum. A second rarely reputed agent of rat-bite fever is reputed to be a spiral organism that has not been cultivated. The disease has been reported only in Japan. For a discussion of isolation and identification of *S. moniliformis*, refer to the Suggested Reading.

MYCOBACTERIUM

Most mycobacteria are characterized by slow growth, acid-fastness, and high lipid content in their cell walls. Although the incidence of mycobacterial disease is high in developing nations, it is declining in industrialized nations with the exception of individuals suffering from severe immune deficiency disorders. Many laboratories receive only a small number of specimens making it difficult to sustain technical proficiency in all areas of mycobacteriology. Based on workload, facilities, and need, it has been suggested that laboratories limit their work to a) examination of smears only; b) smear, culture, identification, and susceptibility testing of *M. tuberculosis;* or c) performance of all aspects of mycobacteriology. Approximately 1000 specimens per year are usually necessary to maintain acceptable proficiency at the highest level (i.e. a, b & c). Procedures and required laboratory facilities relating to the safe collection, processing, and culturing of specimens for the isolation of mycobacteria, as well as test procedures are discussed in the texts listed in the Suggested Reading. See Chapter 2 on biosafety.

Table 53-39   Characteristics of *Brucella* spp.

Species	Urease[a]	H2S produced[b]	CO2 required
B. abortus	1-2 hr	+	v
B. melitensis	v	−	−
B. suis	<30 min	−	−
B. canis	<30 min	−	−

From Clarridge JE: Miscellaneous gram-negative coccobacilli. In Howard BJ, et al: Clinical and pathogenic microbiology, St. Louis, 1987, Mosby—Year Book, Inc.
+ = 90% positive
− = < 10% positive
v = 10-90% positive
[a]Warm the urea slant and inoculate heavily.
[b]Detected by a lead acetate strip above a slant, such as brain heart infusion, inoculated with *Brucella* organisms.

Table 53-40   Suggested method for reporting acid-fast bacilli in fuchsin-stained smears

Number of bacilli[a]	Report
0	No acid-fast bacilli found
1-2/300 fields	±
1-9/100 fields	1+
1-9/10 fields	2+
1-9/field	3+
> 9/field	4+

From Kent PT and Kubica GP: Public health mycobacteriology: a guide for the level III laboratory, Atlanta, 1985, Centers for Disease Control.
[a]All observations are made using ×800 to ×1000. All reports should state staining method used and actual number of organisms observed.

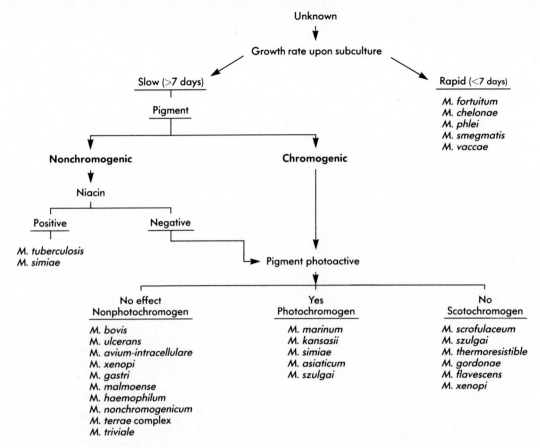

Fig. 53-6 Preliminary subdivision of the mycobacteria. *From Kubica GP and David HL: The mycobacteria. In Sonnenwirth AC and Jarett L, eds: Gradwohl's clinical laboratory methods and diagnosis, ed 8, vol 2, St. Louis, 1980, Mosby-Year Book, Inc.*

Direct examination of clinical specimens

Smears prepared from clinical specimens can be examined for mycobacteria by either a standard carbol-fuchsin acid-fast or fluorochrome procedure. The sensitivity of a smear for detecting acid-fast bacilli in unconcentrated sputum is approximately 30-40% but increases to 60-80% when the specimen is concentrated. At least 10^5 organisms per ml of sputum must be present to be assured of observation microscopically. When mycobacteria are observed they should be enumerated and reported according to the scheme in Table 53-40. Since acid-fast artifact may be present, it is important to look critically at the morphology of the organism. *M. tuberculosis* usually appears as a relatively thin, slightly curved bacillus with tapered ends whereas other mycobacteria are usually thicker and may appear beaded.

Preliminary identification

All growth from mycobacterial media should be stained by a carbol-fuchsin stain to confirm that it is acid-fast and is not contaminated with other bacteria. Colonial morphology, texture, and pigmentation are noted. The colonial morphology, niacin production, rate of growth, pigment production, and photoreactivity tests can be used to initially group the isolate (Figure 53-6). If the Bactec instrument is being used, susceptibility of the isolate to o-nitro-l-acetyl-amino-beta-hydroxy-proprophene (NAP) identifies the iso-

late as belonging to the *M. tuberculosis* complex (*M. tuberculosis, M. bovis, M. africanum*). With conventional tests, isolates that are nonchromogenic, slow-growing (more than seven days), and produce niacin can be tentatively reported as *M. tuberculosis*.

Definitive identification

After an isolate has been placed in a subgroup based on the results of growth rate and pigment production, additional biochemical tests depicted in Table 53-41 can be used to identify the species or complex. All the tests listed in the table should be performed and used for identification of the isolate.

ANAEROBES
Extent of identification of anaerobes

The extent to which anaerobes are identified will depend primarily on the available facilities, the technical competence of the laboratory personnel, and the clinical need for the information. In addition, the availability of rapid tests and the length of time required to identify an isolate are important.

The type and quality of the specimen submitted for anaerobic culture must be considered. Wounds and abscesses (especially perirectal abscesses) often contain multiple anaerobic and facultatively anaerobic organisms. Assessment

Table 53-41 Distinctive properties of mycobacteria encountered in clinical specimens

Runyon group	Complex name[a]	Species name	Growth rate 45° C	37° C	31° C	24° C	Usual colony morphology	Pigmentation	Niacin	Susceptibility to TZH (5 µg/ml)	Nitrate reduction	Semiquantitative catalase (>45 mm)	68° C catalase	Tween hydrolysis (5 days)	Tellurite reduction (3 days)	Tolerance to 5% NaCl	Iron uptake	Arylsulfatase (3 days)	MacConkey agar	Urease	Pyrazinamidase (4 days)	Agglutination tests available
I	TB	M. ulcerans	-	-	S	-	r	N	-	-	-	-	+	-		-			+	+	-	
		M. tuberculosis	-	S	S	-	r	N	+	-	+	-	-	-		-				+	+	+
		M. bovis	-	S	S	-	r, t	N	-	+	-	-	-	-		-	-		-	+	-	+
		M. marinum	-	I	M	M	s/sr	P	±	-	-	+	+	+		-	-	-[b]		+	-	+
		M. kansasii	-	S	S	S	sr/s	P	-	-	+	+	+	+		-		+		+	-	+
		M. simiae	-	S	S	S	s	P	+	-	-	+	+	-		-				+	+	+
		M. asiaticum	S	S	S	S	s/r	P	-	-	-	+	+	+		-				-	+	-
II	Scrofulaceum	M. scrofulaceum	S	S	S	S	s	Sc	-	-	-	+	+	-		-		-[b]	-	+	±	+
		M. szulgai	-	S	S	S	s/r	Sc/P[c]	-	-	+	+	+	-[d]/+		-		±[b]/+		+	±	-
III		M. gordonae	-	S	S	S	s	Sc	-	-	-	+	+	+	-	-		-		+	±	+
		M. flavescens	-	M	M	M	s	Sc	-	-	+	+	+	+	-	+		-[b]		+	±	-
		M. xenopi	S	S		-	s, f	Sc[e]	-	-	-	+	+	-	-	-		-		-	+	+
		M. avium	±	S		±	s, t/r	N	-		-	-	+	-	+	-		-		-	+	+
		M. intracellulare	±	S		±	s, t/r	N	-		-	-	+	-	+	-		-		-	+	+
		M. gastri	-	S		S	s/sr/r	N	-		-	-	-	+	-	-		-		-	+	-
		M. malmoense	-	S	S	S	s	N	-		-	-	+	+	>	-		-		-	+	+
		M. haemophilum	-	-	S[i]	-	r	N	-		-	-	-	+		-				-	>	
		M. nonchromogenicum		S		S	sr	N	-		-	+	+	+	-	-		-		-	+	
IV	Terrae	M. terrae	-	S	S	S	sr	N	-		+	+	+	+	-	+		-		+	-	
		M. triviale	-	S	S	S	r	N	-		+	+	+	+	-	+		-		+	±	
	Fortuitum	M. fortuitum	-	R	R	R	s, f/r, f	N	-		+	+	+	±	>	+	+	+	+	+	+	+
		M. chelonae	-	R	R	R	s/r	N	v		-	+	+	-	>	v[g]		+	+	+	+	+
		M. phlei	R	R	R	R	r	Sc	-		+	+	+	+	+	+		-	-	+		
		M. smegmatis	R	R	R	R	r/s	N	-		+	+	+	+	+	+	+	-	-	+		
		M. vaccae	-	R		R	s	Sc	-		-	+	+	+	+	v	+	-		+		

From McClatchy JK and Tsang AY: Nontuberculous mycobacteria: laboratory and clinical aspects, workshop sponsored by the American Society for Microbiology. Reference cultures for these organisms are available from the Mycobacterial Culture Collection.[76]

+ = Present
– = Absent
v = Variable
Blank = Information unavailable or property unimportant

[a] For most clinical laboratories, designation to "complex" is usually sufficient.
[b] Positive after 14 days.
[c] Scotochromogenic at 37° C, photochromogenic at 25° C.
[d] Positive after 10 days.
[e] Young cultures may be nonchromogenic or possess only pale pigment that may intensify with age.
[f] Requires hemin as growth factor.
[g] Absent in M. chelonae ssp. chelonae; present in M. chelonae ssp. abscessus.

S = Slow, ≥21 days
M = Moderate ~12 days
R = Rapid, < 7 days
I = Intermediate
r = Rough

s = Smooth
sr = Intermediate in roughness
t = Thin or transparent
f = Filamentous extensions
P = Photochromogenic

Sc = Scotochromogenic
N = Nonphotochromogenic

of the quality of the specimen (quantity of WBC and squamous epithelial cells present) and discussion of the preliminary culture and Gram-stain information with the clinician can limit the extent of workup of the culture. However, in serious infections or infections which don't respond to therapy, the anaerobes need to be identified.

Not all laboratories have the resources or expertise to definitively identify anaerobic isolates but all laboratories should be able to presumptively identify isolates based on cellular and colonial morphology and a few key characteristics. In serious cases the isolates can be submitted to a reference laboratory for definitive identification.

Collection, processing, and inoculation of specimens

Procedures for the collection, processing, and incubation of specimens are discussed in Chapter 39. Specimens for anaerobic culture should be inoculated to nonselective anaerobic blood agar, selective agar, and an enriched liquid medium. The types of selective media will depend on the specimen and the results of the direct microscopic examination of the clinical material.

Direct examination of specimens

The presence of the anaerobes in a specimen is suggested when the material has a foul odor or large amounts of gas, has a black discoloration that fluoresces red under ultraviolet light, or contains sulfur granules.

The direct Gram stain of the specimen may provide early presumptive information on the presence of anaerobes for use in starting empiric therapy and suggest additional media to set up. Cellular morphology, characteristic of some genera or species, may be observed on the direct smear. *Bacteroides* (Plate 1-8) appear as pale, pleomorphic gram-negative rods with bipolar or irregular staining. A smear of material from possible gas gangrene which demonstrates few leukocytes and large gram-positive rods with blunted ends suggests *C. perfringens* (Plate 1-9). *Fusobacterium nucleatum* (Plate 1-10) appears as a pale, slender, long gram-negative rod with tapered ends, while other *Fusobacterium* species may appear as pale, filamentous, irregular stained, pleomorphic, gram-negative rods with swollen areas. Clusters and chains

of irregularly stained gram-positive cocci are suggestive of *Peptostreptococcus* but would also include the aerobic gram-positive cocci. *Actinomyces* may appear as thin, branching, gram-positive bacilli with beaded staining.

Other direct analysis methods of specimens include commercially available fluorescent antibody reagents for detection of the *B. fragilis* group and *B. melaninogenicus* group; and analysis of pus or body fluids for short-chain fatty acids by gas-liquid chromatography (GLC) as presumptive evidence of *Bacteroides* or *Fusobacterium* species.

Examination of primary plates

It is generally recommended that primary plates in anaerobic jars be incubated at 35°C for 48 hours before examination, although Rosenblatt found that examination of the plates after 24 hours (if kept in a holding jar for under 40 minutes) did not diminish recovery. The use of a holding jar is recommended during examination and subculture of all anaerobes. Growth on the blood agar plate incubated in 5-10% CO_2 is compared to that on the anaerobic plates. Bacteria with the same colonial and cellular morphology are considered facultative anaerobes. The primary anaerobic plates should be examined with long-wave ultraviolet light to detect fluorescent colonies. Colonial morphology should be observed with a dissecting microscope or at least a hand-held lens. Each distinctive colony type should be noted and Gram stained. The cellular and colonial morphology of anaerobes can be helpful in a rapid presumptive identification of certain species or groups (Table 53-42). Fluid backup media should be Gram stained and subcultured if any morphologic types appear on smear that aren't seen on the primary plates. All primary plates are incubated for five to seven days.

Initial subculture of isolates

Probable anaerobes are subcultured to anaerobic blood agar plates which are incubated anaerobically and in 5-10% CO_2. After a minimum 24 hours incubation (or longer for slow growers), the plates are examined and those isolates which are anaerobes are identified. Gram-positive cocci which are capnophiles, may not grow in CO_2 on initial subculture and require a second subculture to demonstrate growth.

Table 53-42   Level I identification*

Organism	Cell shape	Gram reaction	Aerotolerance	Distinguishing characteristics
B. fragilis group	B	−	−	Growth on BBE with colony size >1 mm in diameter
Pigmented *Bacteroides* sp.	CB	−	−	Dark pigmenting or brick red fluorescing colony
B. ureolyticus-like group	B	−	−	Pitting colonies
F. nucleatum (presumptive)	B	−	−	Slender bacillus with pointed ends; breadcrumb, speckled colony
Anaerobic gram-negative bacillus	B CB	−	−	
Anaerobic gram-negative coccus	C	−	−	
Anaerobic gram-positive coccus	C	+	−	
C. perfringens (presumptive)	B	+	−	Double zone of beta hemolysis; boxcar shaped cells
Other *Clostridium* sp.	B	+	−⁺	Spores seen on Gram stain
Anaerobic gram-positive bacillus	B	+	−⁺	No boxcar shaped cells; no spores

From Sutter VL, Citron DM, Edelstein MAC, and Finegold SM: Wadsworth anaerobic bacteriology manual, ed 4, Belmont, Calif, 1985, Star Publishing Co.
*B = bacilli; CB = coccobacilli; C = cocci; + = most strains positive; − = most strains negative; superscripts indicate reactions of some strains.

PURE COLONY ISOLATES

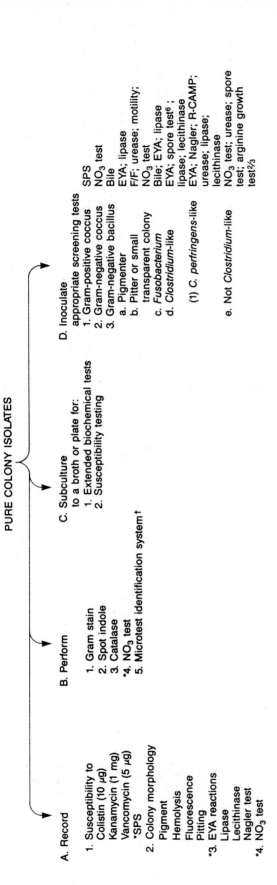

A. Record

1. Susceptibility to
   Colistin (10 µg)
   Kanamycin (1 mg)
   Vancomycin (5 µg)
   *SPS
2. Colony morphology
   Pigment
   Hemolysis
   Fluorescence
   Pitting
*3. EYA reactions
   Lipase
   Lecithinase
   Nagler test
*4. NO₃ test

B. Perform

1. Gram stain
2. Spot indole
3. Catalase
*4. NO₃ test
5. Microtest identification system†

C. Subculture
   to a broth or plate for:
1. Extended biochemical tests
2. Susceptibility testing

D. Inoculate
   appropriate screening tests
1. Gram-positive coccus   SPS
2. Gram-negative coccus   NO₃ test
3. Gram-negative bacillus   Bile
   a. Pigmenter   EYA; lipase
   b. Pitter or small   F/F; urease; motility;
      transparent colony   NO₃ test
   c. *Fusobacterium*   Bile; EYA; lipase
   d. *Clostridium*-like   EYA; spore test§ ;
                                 lipase; lecithinase
      (1) *C. perfringens*-like EYA; Nagler; R-CAMP;
                                 urease; lipase;
                                 lecithinase
   e. Not *Clostridium*-like   NO₃ test; urease; spore
                                 test; arginine growth
                                 test‡/§

Key: * =if available at this time; SPS=sodium polyanethol
sulfonate; EYA=egg yolk agar; F/F=formate-fumarate growth test;
R-CAMP=reverse CAMP test
† Use test systems selectively and with appropriate
  organisms. See Section 34.5g for guidance.
‡ Perform when spores are not detected on Gram stain.
§ Perform on tiny gram-positive rod.

Fig. 53-7 Pure culture isolate processing scheme. *From Sutter VL, Citron DM, Edelstein MAC, and Finegold SM: Wadsworth anaerobic bacteriology manual, ed 4, 1985, Belmont, Calif, Star Publishing Co.*

Table 53-43   Level II group and species identification of anaerobic gram-negative organisms*

	Cell shape	Slender cells with pointed ends	Kanamycin (1 mg)	Vancomycin (5 µg)	Colistin (10 µg)	Growth in 20% bile	Catalase	Indole production	Lipase	Growth stimulated by formate-fumarate	Nitrate reduction	Urease	Motility	Pitting	Pigment	Brick-red fluorescence
B. fragilis group	B		R	R	R	+	V	V	−							−
Other *Bacteroides* sp.	B		R	R	V	−	−	V	−		−⁺					−
Pigmented *Bacteroides* sp.	CB/B		R	V	V	−	−	V	V						+	+⁻
B. intermedius			R	R	S	−	−	+	+⁻							
B. loescheii			R	R	V	−	−	−	−⁺							
B. ureolyticus-like group	B		S	R	S	−		−		+	+	V	V	V		
B. ureolyticus			S	R	S	−		−		+	+	+	−	V		
B. gracilis			S	R	S	−		−		+	+	−	−	V		
Wolinella sp.			S	R	S	−		−		+	+	−	+	V		
Fusobacterium sp.	B	V	S	R	S	V	−	V	V							−
F. nucleatum		+	S	R	S	−		+	−							
F. necrophorum		−	S	R	S	−⁺		+	+⁻							
F. mortiferum-varium		−	S	R	S	+		V	−							
Gram-negative coccus	C		S	R	S						V					
Veillonella sp.	C		S	R	S						+					−⁺

From Sutter VL, Citron DM, Edelstein MAC, and Finegold SM: Wadsworth anaerobic bacteriology manual, ed 4, Belmont, Calif, 1985, Star Publishing Co.
*B = bacilli; C = cocci; CB = coccobacilli; R = resistant; S = sensitive; V = variable; + = most strains positive; − = most strains negative; superscripts indicate reactions of occasional strains.

Table 53-44   Level II group and species identification of anaerobic gram-positive organisms*

	Cellular morphology	Survives ethanol spore test	Kanamycin (1 mg)	Colistin (10 µg)	Vancomycin (5 µg)	Sodium polyanethol sulfonate (SPS)	Indole production	Nitrate production	Catalase	Arginine stimulation	Lecithinase	Nagler test	Reverse CAMP test	Boxcar-shaped cells	Double zone beta hemolysis	Urease	Ground glass yellow colonies on CCFA medium
Anaerobic gram-positive coccus	C	−	V	R	S	V	V		−⁺	V							
Peptostreptococcus anaerobius	C/CB	−	R	R	S	S	−										
Peptostreptococcus asaccharolyticus	C	−	S	R	S	R	+										
Clostridium species	B	+	V	R	S					V							
Nagler positive *Clostridium* sp.	B	+	S	R	S						+	+					
C. perfringens	B	+	S	R	S		−				+	+	+	+	+		
C. bifermentans	B	+	S	R	S		+				+	+	−	−	−		
C. sordellii	B	+	S	R	S		+				+	+	−	−	−	+⁻	
Nagler negative *Clostridium* sp.	B	+	S	R	S					V	−						
C. difficile	B	+	S	R	S								−	−	−		+
Non-spore-forming bacilli	CB/B	−	S	R	S												
Propionibacterium acnes	B	−	S	R	S		+⁻	+⁻	+⁻								
Eubacterium lentum	CB/B	−	S	R	S		−	+	−	+							

From Sutter VL, Citron DM, Edelstein MAC, and Finegold SM: Wadsworth anaerobic bacteriology manual, ed 4, Belmont, Calif, 1985, Star Publishing Co.
*B = bacilli; C = cocci; CB = coccobacilli; S = sensitive; R = resistant; V = variable; + = most strains positive; − = most strains negative; superscripts indicate reactions of occasional strains.

Presumptive identification

Do not inoculate or read tests unless adequate growth of a pure culture is present. The pure-culture isolate of sufficient growth is further processed as shown in Figure 53-7. The presumptive grouping and identification of many frequently encountered gram-negative and positive organisms can be made based on the reactions shown in Tables 53-43 and 53-44. The taxonomy and classification of anaerobes are continuously updated based on new data. Table 53–45 shows many of the recent changes in gram-negative anaerobes.

Definitive identification

The definitive identification of anaerobes by conventional methodologies requires a battery of biochemical tests, GLC analysis, serologic tests, etc., and is beyond the scope of this chapter. For detailed discussions refer to the texts in the suggested reading.

For the non-reference laboratory, commercial microsystems that detect preformed enzymes aerobically a few hours after inoculation provide rapid, accurate alternatives to the more costly, labor-intensive conventional methods for identification of anaerobes.

SPIROCHETES
Morphology

Spirochetes of medical importance are in the genera *Leptospira, Borrelia,* and *Treponema.* The pathogenic spirochetes are restricted to a living host, are not free-living in the environment, and are heterogeneous in regard to physiology and habitat. Common features include morphology and unique flexous motility related to the presence of axial filaments located in the periplasmic space between the outer membrane and protoplasmic cylinder. The organisms are motile by a corkscrew-like motion. The spirochetes can be loosely grouped into genera by their morphology. In general, the spirochetes are slender, flexible, helical-shaped bacteria. Treponemes are 7-15 μm long and 0.1-0.2 μm wide with regular spaced coils and exhibit a rotational back and forth motility with some bending and snapping. The *Leptospira* are normally 6-20 μm long and 0.1-0.2 μm wide with very tightly wound coils that may be hooked at one or both ends. They exhibit a rapid darting back and forth motion. The borreliae are 10-20 μm long and 0.2-0.5 μm wide with fewer and more loose coils than the other two genera.

Leptospira general characteristics

The genus *Leptospira* consists of two species, *L. biflexa* which is a nonpathogenic free-living spirochete composed of over 60 serovars and *L. interrogans* which causes leptospirosis in humans and animals and consists of over 180 serovars. Leptospires are aerobic, require certain nutrients (e.g., long-chain fatty acid) for growth at 28-30°C, and prefer a neutral to slightly alkaline pH (7.2-7.4).

Identification

The diagnosis of leptospirosis requires the demonstration of *L. interrogans* in clinical specimens (by culture or direct examination) or by serology (see Chapter 34.). Anticoagulated blood, spinal fluid, or urine may be concentrated by differential high-speed centrifugation and examined by darkfield microscopy. Although direct microscopy is rapid, it is rarely positive because so few organisms are present. *L. interrogans* is readily cultivated in two types of media: those supplemented with bovine serum albumin and polysorbate 80 (EMJH) or those enriched with rabbit serum (Fletcher or Stuart). Approximately two to three drops of blood or CSF collected during the first week of illness is added to each of three to five tubes of medium. One to two drops of undiluted and a 1:10 dilution of urine collected after one week of illness is added to each of three to five tubes of medium with and without 200 mg/ml of 5-fluorouracil (prevents bacterial overgrowth). All cultures are

Table 53-45 Recent taxonomic changes

New nomenclature	Previous nomenclature
Anaerorhabdus furcosus	*Bacteroides furcosus*
Bacteroides caccae	*Bacteroides sp. "3452A"*
B. forsythus	New species
B. galacturonicus	New species
B. merdae	New species
B. pectinophilus	New species
B. salivosus	New species
B. stercoris	New species
B. tectum	New species
Bilophila wadsworthia	New genus and species
Centipeda periodontii	New genus and species
Fibrobacter succinogenes	*Bacteroides succinogenes*
F. intestinalis	New species
Fusobacterium alocis	New species
F. sulci	New species
F. ulcerans	New species
Megamonas hypermegas	*B. hypermegas*
Misuokella multiacida	*B. multiacidus*
M. dentalis	New species
Selenomonas artemidis	New species
S. dianae	New species
S. flueggei	New species
S. infelix	New species
S. noxia	New species
Porphyromonas asaccharolytica	*B. asaccharolyticus*
P. endodontalis	*B. endodontalis*
P. ginigivalis	*B. ginigivalis*
Prevotella bivia	*B. bivius*
P. buccae	*B. buccae*
P. buccalis	*B. buccalis*
P. corporis	*B. corporis*
P. denticola	*B. denticola*
P. disiens	*B. disiens*
P. heparinolytica	*B. heparinolyticus*
P. intermedia	*B. intermedius*
P. loescheii	*B. loescheii*
P. melaninogenica	*B. melaninogenicus*
P. oralis	*B. oralis*
P. oris	*B. oris*
P. oulora	*B. oulorum*
P. ruminicola	*B. ruminicola*
P. veroralis	*B. veroralis*
P. zoogleoformans	*B. zoogleoformans*
Rikenella microfusus	*B. microfusus*
Ruminobacter amylophilus	*B. amylophilus*
Sebaldella termitidis	*B. termitidis*
Tissierella praecuta	*B. praecutus*
Wolinella curva	New species

From Jousimies-Somer, HR and Finegold, SM: Manual of Clincal Microbiology, ed 5, Washington D.C., 1991, American Society for Microbiology.

incubated in the dark at 30° C for up to six weeks. Tubes are examined weekly for macroscopic growth in the form of a ring 1-3 cm below the surface and by darkfield microscopy. *L. biflexa* and *L. interrogans* can be differentiated by growth at 13°C, growth in the presence of purine analogues or conversion to spheroplasts in the presence of 1M NaCl. Radiometric methods for culture may reduce the time for recovery of organisms.

Borrelia

Borrelia recurrentis is the etiologic agent for louseborne (epidemic) relapsing fever transmitted by the human louse, *Pediculus humanus*. Species of *Borrelia* responsible for tick-borne (endemic) relapsing fever are named after the species of *Ornithodoros* tick that transmits the organisms. The *Ixodes* ticks transmit *B. burgdorferi* which causes Lyme disease.

Relapsing fever

Borreliae are present in blood during the febrile period of the illness and can be visualized by darkfield microscopy (after 1:2 dilution of the blood) or in Giemsa- or Wright-stained thick and thin smears of blood. Although the organism can be cultured in Kelly medium, it is a low-yield procedure and not generally recommended. Serology is generally useful for making the diagnosis during the acute stage of the illness.

Lyme disease

Isolation of *B. burgdorferi* is difficult; direct microscopy of the organism in clinical specimens is rarely positive. Standardized serologic tests are used to make the laboratory diagnosis (see Chapter 34).

Treponema

The pathogenic treponemes can be continuously cultured only by animal passage and consist of two species, *T. carateum* (the causative agent of pinta) and *T. pallidum*, which consist of three subspecies: *pallidum* (causes syphilis), *pertenue* (causes yaws), and *endemicum* (causes endemic syphilis or bejel). These organisms are serologically and morphologically indistinguishable and the diseases are separated based on clinical manifestations and geographic area.

Identification of T. pallidum ssp. pallidum

The diagnosis of syphilis is based on clinical signs and symptoms, demonstration of the organism in specimens by darkfield microscopy and serological testing (see Chapter 34). The microscopic demonstration of the treponeme in moist lesion material provides rapid diagnosis of the disease in patients who present with primary or secondary syphilis. The darkfield microscopic examinations of material from oral or anal lesions must be interpreted with great caution because of the presence of morphologically similar saprophytic treponemes. The darkfield microscopic examination of any suspect lesion must be done with care and by a qualified individual. The direct fluorescent polyclonal antibody test on lesion material is commercially available but is not widely used. Newer methods for direct detection of *T. pallidum* in lesion material include radio- or fluorescein-labeled monoclonal antibodies and a DNA probe.

SUGGESTED READING

Appelbaum PC: Advances in rapid preliminary and definitive identification of anaerobes. Clin Microbiol Newsl, 11:89-93, 1989.

Balows A, et al: Manual of clinical microbiology, ed 5, Washington, DC, 1991, American Society for Microbiology.

Balows A, Hausler Jr WJ, Ohashi M, and Turano A: Laboratory diagnosis of infectious diseases: principles and practice, vol 1, New York, 1988, Springer-Verlag.

Coykendall AL, Wesbecher PM, and Gustafson KB: "*Streptococcus milleri*," *Streptococcus constellatus*, and *Streptococcus intermedius* are later synonyms of *Streptococcus anginosus*, Int J Syst Bacteriol, 37:222-228, 1987.

Dealler SF, Abbott M, Croughan MJ, and Hawkey PM: Identification of *Branhamella catarrhalis* in 2.5 minutes with indoxyl butyrate strip test, J Clin Microbiol, 27:1390-1391, 1989.

Dowell VR and Hawkins TM: Laboratory methods in anaerobic bacteriology, Atlanta, 1977, Centers for Disease Control.

Edmonds P, Kassman N, Judd RL, and Rudert CS: Clinical and microbiological features of *Campylobacter pylori*—associated gastric ulcers in humans, Clin Microbiol Newsl, 10:97-100, 1988.

Finegold SM and Baron EJ: Bailey and Scott's diagnostic microbiology, ed 7, St. Louis, 1986, Mosby-Year Book, Inc.

Fournier JM, Boutonnier A, and Bouvet A: *Staphylococcus aureus* strains which are not identified by rapid agglutination methods are of capsular serotype 5, J Clin Microbiol, 27:1372-1374, 1989.

Freney J, Brun Y, Bes M, Meugnier H, Grimont F, Grimont PAD, Nervi C, and Fleurette J: *Staphylococcus lugdunensis* sp nov and *Staphylococcus schleiferi* sp nov, two species from human clinical specimens, Int J Syst Bacteriol, 38:168-172, 1988.

Friedman RL: Pertussis: the disease and new diagnostic methods, Clin Microbiol Rev, 1:365-376, 1988.

Holdeman LV, Cato EP, and Moore WEC: Anaerobe laboratory manual, ed 4, Blacksburg, Va, 1977, Virginia Polytechnic Institute and State University Anaerobe Laboratory.

Howard BJ and Ducate MJ: Streptococci. In Howard BJ, Klaas II J, Rubin SJ, Weissfeld AS, and Tilton RC: Clinical and pathogenic microbiology, St. Louis, 1987, Mosby-Year Book, Inc.

Howard BJ, Klass II J, Rubin SJ, Weissfeld AS, and Tilton RC: Clinical and pathogenic microbiology, St. Louis, 1987, Mosby-Year Book, Inc.

Jenkins SG: Rat-bite fever, Clin Microbiol Newsl, 10:57-59, 1988.

Karmoli MA: Infection by verocytotoxin-producing *Escherichia coli*, Clin Microbiol Rev, 2:15-38, 1989.

Manca N, Verardi R, Colombrita D, Ravizzola G, Savoldi E, and Turano A: Radiometric method for the rapid detection of *Leptospira* organisms, J Clin Microbiol, 23:401-403, 1986.

Murray PR: Microscopy. In Wentworth BB, ed: Diagnostic procedures for bacterial infections, ed 7, Washington, DC, 1987, American Public Health Association, Inc.

Penner JL: The genus *Campylobacter*: a decade of progress, Clin Microbiol Rev, 1:157-172, 1988.

Pfaller MA and Herwaldt LA: Laboratory, clinical, and epidemiological aspects of coagulase-negative staphylococci, Clin Microbiol Rev, 1:281-299, 1988.

Saubolle MA: Leptospirosis. In Wentworth BB ed: Diagnostic procedures for bacterial infections, ed 7, Washington, DC, 1987, American Public Health Association, Inc.

Sulea IT, Pollice MC, and Barksdale L: Pyrazine carboxylamidase activity in *Corynebacterium*, J Clin Microbiol, 30:466, 1980.

Sutter VL, Citron DM, Edelstein MAC, and Finegold SM: Wadsworth anaerobic bacteriology manual, ed 4, Belmont, Calif, 1985, Star Publishing Co.

Washington II JA: Rapid diagnosis by microscopy, Clin Microbiol Newsl, 8:135-138, 1986.

Washington JA: Laboratory procedures in clinical microbiology, ed 2, New York, 1985, Springer-Verlag.

Weaver RE and Hollis DG: Gram-positive organisms: a guide to presumptive identification, Atlanta, 1983, Centers for Disease Control.

Wentworth BB: Diagnostic procedures for bacterial infections, ed 7, Washington, DC, 1987, American Public Health Association, Inc.

54 Fungi

Richard C. Tilton

There are approximately 50,000 to 100,000 accepted species of fungi. About 180 species have been shown to be pathogenic under some circumstances. Because concepts of pathogenicity for all microorganisms have become more clearly defined in the past decade, we are beginning to understand why only a very small portion of the fungi that humans encounter may cause disease. Notwithstanding advances in cancer chemotherapy, which often lower the normal host defenses, several factors are necessary for fungi to invade human tissue. Typically, these factors include the ability to grow at temperatures of 35° to 37°C, the ability to bridge the specific and nonspecific defense barriers of the host, and the ability to use available in vivo substrates as sources of nutrients and energy for growth.

Like animals, fungi are heterotrophic and must obtain preformed organic substances from the environment. However, fungi have an absorptive type of nutrition, whereas animals have an ingestive type. Fungi release hydrolytic enzymes into their immediate surroundings. These enzymes degrade substrates into smaller subunits, which the fungus then absorbs. Human pathogenic fungi possess the enzymes necessary to obtain nutrients directly from the living host.

For years mycologists have recognized that fungi are very different from plants. All fungi possess a cell wall composed of cellulose. Furthermore, as previously mentioned, fungi synthesize lysine by the L-alpha-adipic acid biosynthetic pathway, whereas plants synthesize lysine by the meso-alpha-diaminopimelic acid pathway. Unlike plants, fungi do not have chloroplasts and thus are not photosynthetic.

STRUCTURAL ORGANIZATION OF FUNGI

Fungi are identified in the laboratory according to the vegetative or growth structures they produce and according to their reproductive structures. The fungi most commonly seen in the laboratory exist in one or both of two vegetative forms, yeasts or molds.

Credit for much of the information in the chapter is given to Dr. Michael R. McGinnis, a coauthor with Richard C. Tilton of a series of chapters in mycology in Howard BJ, et al: Clinical and pathogenic microbiology, St. Louis, 1987, Mosby-Year Book.

Molds

Molds form dry, fluffy, filamentous colonies consisting of branching hyphae. Hyphae, the primary element of the vegetative form of a mold, are cylindric, tubelike structures that elongate by growth at the tip or apical end. The aerial hyphae are responsible for the fluffy, filamentous nature of the mold. They range in diameter from approximately 3 to 20 μm, depending on the species.

Hyphae usually have cross-walls called septa that divide the hyphae into numerous cells. Septa have tiny pores, so the cytoplasm is continuous throughout the hypha. Hyphae that contain septa are referred to as septate. Hyphae lacking septa have in the past been called aseptate or nonseptate. Because all hyphae may have some septa, the term "sparsely septate" is more accurate.

A mass of hyphae is called mycelium, (because the term "mycelium" may be singular or collective, "mycelia" is inappropriate). There are three basic types of mycelium: vegetative mycelium, which penetrates the surface of the medium and absorbs nutrients; the aerial mycelium that grows above the agar surface; and the fertile mycelium that bears conidia or spores for reproduction and may be located anywhere in the colony. The mycelium composing the colony gives the colony its texture, tenacity, topography, and color. To subculture a fungus, it is necessary to remove a portion of the colony and transfer it to a new nutrient agar.

The vegetative mycelium of a fungus may also produce several unique structures that aid in identification.

Yeasts

Yeasts form discrete, smooth, moist colonies consisting of spherical to ellipsoidal cells 3 to 15 μm in diameter, which reproduce by budding. Unlike molds, which are identified on the basis of morphology alone, yeasts are identified by morphology and physiologic testing. Some yeasts are very small *(Torulopsis glabrata)*, whereas others are large *(Cryptococcus neoformans)*. *C. neoformans* produces a polysaccharide envelope or capsule. If yeast cells do not separate, a chain of blastoconidia may be found. These blastoconidia may elongate to form a pseudohypha. Table 54-1 compares true hyphae and pseudo hyphae.

When a yeast cell of *C. albicans* produces a filament by

Table 54-1 Differentiation between hyphae and pseudohyphae

Characteristic	Hyphae	Pseudohyphae
Growth	Occurs at hyphal apex by linear elongation with subsequent formation of septa	Results from blowing-out process and subsequently appearing basal constriction of each new blastoconidium, without separation of each blastoconidium from its parent cell
Terminal cell	Typically longer than preceding cell just behind first septum; usually cylindric	Typically shorter than or equal to preceding cell just behind first septum; usually rounded
Walls	Typically parallel with no invagination at septa	Typically contain marked constrictions at septa
Septa	Refractive and straight	Often difficult to discern and usually curved
Side branches	Not constricted at their point of origin; first septum typically some distance from main hypha	Constricted at their point of origin; septum at origin of branch

From McGinnis MR: Laboratory handbook of medical mycology, New York, 1980, Academic Press, Inc.

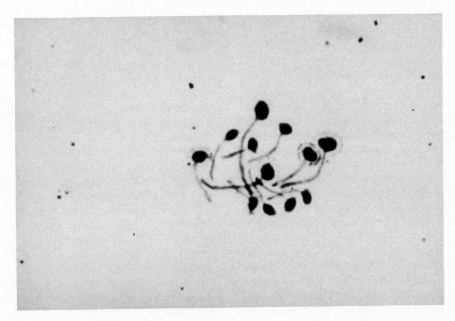

Fig. 54-1 Germ tubes of *Candida albicans*. Courtesy L. Ajello.

apical elongation without a constriction at the origin of the filament from the parent cell, the filament is called a germ tube (Figure 54-1). The germ tube is the beginning of the formation of a hypha. Most mycologists consider a germ tube to be a hypha once the first septum is laid down. This typically occurs some distance from the origin of the germ tube from the parent cell. Germ tube formation is a useful method of recognizing *C. albicans* in the clinical laboratory.

Dimorphic fungi

Fungi that are able to grow in two different forms are considered dimorphic. This ability is usually temperature dependent, e.g., the fungus that causes blastomycosis, *Blastomyces dermatitidis*, grows as a yeast at 37°C and in tissue but as a mold at room temperature (23 to 25°C). Another dimorphic fungus, *Coccidiodes immitis*, forms spherules in tissue and produces hyphae at room temperature.

REPRODUCTIVE STRUCTURES OF FUNGI

Fungi reproduce by asexual, sexual, and parasexual means. For the clinical microbiologist, asexual reproduction is the most important because most pathogenic fungi do not reproduce sexually in the laboratory.

Asexual reproduction

Asexual reproduction may involve the formation of spores or, more frequently, conidia. (Only the zygomycetes typically reproduce asexually by forming spores). Spores may be produced sexually as well as asexually. Sexual spores are produced following meiosis, whereas asexual spores are produced following mitosis.

Conidia are nonmotile, reproductive structures, and like spores, are produced after mitosis. Conidia usually are produced on aerial hyphae by a process called conidiogenesis. There are a number of classification schemes based on the ways conidia are formed. However, rapid and precise identification of fungi requires an understanding of conidiogenesis, which includes

1. conidium ontogeny (thallic or blastic),
2. conidiogenous cell development,
3. conidial septation, color, and arrangement,
4. conidiophores, and
5. site of conidial development.

During the past several years, a number of medically important fungi have been either reclassified or better defined because of a clearer understanding of conidiogenesis.

Sexual reproduction

Sexual reproduction in the fungi involves meiosis. Before meiosis can occur, two compatible nuclei must unite. In the first step, plasmogamy, or fusion, of two protoplasts—but not their nuclei—must occur. Occurring next is karyogamy, which is the actual fusion of the two haploid (n) nuclei to produce a diploid (Zn) or zygote nucleus. Meiosis now takes place, resulting in four haploid (n) nuclei. There may be a long period between plasmogamy, karyogamy, and meiosis. Sometimes the two haploid nuclei do not fuse but behave as if they were a single nucleus. Such a condition is called dikaryotic (n + n).

Most fungi are heterothallic, that is, sexually self-sterile. For sexual reproduction to occur, two compatible isolates are required. In some instances, only a specific isolate of one mating type crosses with a specific isolate of the second mating type. Sexual compatibility systems help explain why sexual spores are not typically seen in clinical isolates. These isolates usually represent only one mating type. The presence of sexual spores typically means that the isolate is homothallic, or sexually self-fertile. Each isolate of a homothallic species is able to reproduce sexually under appropriate conditions.

The zygomycetes are characterized by the production of sexual spores called zygospores. (Zygomycetes may form sexual and asexual spores). These spores are round, thick-walled reproductive structures that result from the union of

Table 54-2 A clinical classification of fungal infections

Nature of infection	Body sites	Mycosis	Representative etiologic agents
Superficial	Hair	Black piedra	*Piedraia hortae*
	Hair	White piedra	*Trichosporon beigelii*
	Skin	Pityriasis versicolor	*Malassezia furfur*
	Skin (thick) or palms, feet	Tinea nigra	*Phaeoannellomyces*[a] *werneckii*
Cutaneous	Keratinized tissue (hair, nail, skin)	Dermatophytosis	*Epidermophyton floccosum, Microsporum canis, Trichophyton rubrum*
	Skin, nails	Candidiasis	*Candida albicans*
	Nails	Onychomycosis	*Aspergillus fumigatus, C. albicans, Scopulariopsis brevicaulis*
	Eye	Keratomycosis	*Aspergillus flavus, Bipolaris spicifera, C. albicans, Fusarium solani*
	Ear	Otomycosis	*Aspergillus niger, C. albicans*
Subcutaneous	Skin and lymph nodes	Sporotrichosis	*Sporothrix schenckii*
	Skin and subcutaneous tissue and bone (often feet and hands)	Mycetoma	*Madurella mycetomatis, Pseudallescheria boydii*
	Skin and subcutaneous tissue (often legs)	Chromoblastomycosis	*Cladosporium carrionii, Fonsecaea pedrosoi, Phialophora verrucosa*
	Skin and subcutaneous tissue	Zygomycosis	*Basidiobolus ranarum, Conidiobolus coronatus*
	Mucosa of nose	Rhinosporidiosis	*Rhinosporidium seeberi*
	Skin and subcutaneous tissue	Lobomycosis	*Loboa loboi*
	Skin and subcutaneous tissue	Phaeohyphomycosis	*Exophiala jeanselmei, Wangiella dermatitidis*
Systemic	Any organ system may be affected	Blastomycosis	*Blastomyces dermatitidis*
		Coccidioidomycosis	*Coccidioides immitis*
		Cryptococcosis	*Cryptococcus neoformans*
		Histoplasmosis	*Histoplasma capsulatum*
		Paracoccidioidomycosis	*Paracoccidioides brasiliensis*
Opportunistic mycoses	All organs	Disseminated candidiasis	*C. albicans*
	Lung	Aspergillosis	*A. fumigatus*
	Nasal sinuses, lungs, gastrointestinal tract	Zygomycosis	*Rhizopus arrhizus*
	Brain	Phaeohyphomycosis	*Xylohypha*[b] *bantiana*
	Any organ, deep tissue, blood	Systemic fungal disease	*Bipolaris hawaiiensis, Penicillium marneffei, Pseudallescheria boydii, Torulopsis glabrata, Trichosporon beigelii,* virtually any other fungus

[a]Previously classified as *Exophiala werneckii.*
[b]Previously classified as *Cladosporium bantianum.*

two gametangia, which are cells containing nuclei involved in sexual reproduction.

Ascomycetes produce sexual spores called ascospores in a special saclike structure known as an ascus. Clinically important ascomycetes usually form antheridia (cells that will fuse with ascogonia to provide them with nuclei for sexual reproduction) and ascogonia (cells that will receive nuclei for sexual reproduction from antheridia). A nucleus (n) is passed from the antheridium into the ascogonium. Ascogneous hyphae having a dikaryotic (n + n) nuclear condition develop from the ascogonium.

Basidiomycetes are unique because their vegetative cells are typically dikaryotic (n + n). Theoretically, only one of these cells could give rise to sexual spores. To maintain the dikaryotic hyphal condition, many basidiomycetes have clamp connections (hyphal bridges) that permit the simultaneous mitosis of the two nuclei to occur in such a manner that the n + n nuclei are duplicated. Usually the terminal cell of a dikaryotic hypha becomes a basidium. The basidium enlarges and karyogamy occurs, resulting in a diploid (2n) nucleus. Meiosis then occurs, resulting in four haploid (n) nuclei. Each of the haploid nuclei migrate through one of the sterigmata (tubelike extensions from the basidium) into a basidiospore. The uninucleate basidiospore is then forcibly discharged from the sterigma.

Taxonomy

Fungal taxonomy is confusing. It is complicated by the fact that several schemes have been proposed to classify fungi. The reader is referred to Howard, et al (1987) for a comprehensive discussion of taxonomy. It is clear, however, that fungi represent an advanced level of taxonomic organization and should be included in their own kingdom. Fungi are multicellular, multinuclear eukaryotes, as are plants and animals. Distinguishing features such as an absorptive nutrition readily separate the kingdom Fungi.

The average clinical microbiology laboratory encounters only the most common zygomycetes, ascomycetes, and the fungi imperfectii. Reference will be made to each of these major groups. Perhaps of even more use to the laboratory-oriented person is the clinical classification proposed in Table 54-2.

ULTRASTRUCTURE

Fungi have a characteristic nuclear membrane that comprises two parallel membranes with many nuclear pores where the membranes join. The endoplasmic reticulum, also a complex membrane system, is closely associated with the nucleus. On the endoplasmic reticulum, the ribosomes and the Golgi apparatus can be seen. The mitochondria in fungi are about 1 to 1.5 μm in diameter. This is the approximate size of some bacteria. These are the respiratory and metabolic energy organelles of the fungus.

Fungi also contain vacuoles, which are membrane bound. These vacuoles contain hydrolytic or digestive enzymes for the breakdown of substrates. Lipid and glycogen granules may also be present in the fungal cell.

The cytoplasmic membrane is a typical eukaryotic bilayered membrane. This membrane controls the diffusion of solutes and nutrients, as well as the energy-dependent and energy-independent transport of amino acids and sugars.

The cytoplasmic membrane is composed of phospholipids, proteins, glycoproteins, and sterols. The most prevalent lipids are phospholipids and sphingolipids. The major sterol is ergosterol, in contrast to cholesterol in mammalian cells. The greater affinity of amphotericin B for ergosterol rather than cholesterol is at least partially responsible for its effectiveness as an antifungal antibiotic. Amphotericin B binds to the membrane sterols and causes a rapid leakage of potassium, which inhibits metabolic processes such as glycolysis and respiration.

The amount of DNA present in a single fungal cell is approximately four to 10 times that of a bacterium, but only 1/1000 to 1/10,000 of that in a plant or animal cell.

Cell wall

Fungal walls are complex structures that serve multiple purposes for the cell. The wall imparts rigidity, acts as an osmotic barrier, determines the shape of the organism, and is a primary factor in fungal morphogenesis. The fungal cell wall also mediates the contact of the organism with its environment. Fungi can exist as spheroplasts without cell walls after the wall is removed by lytic enzymes. As in bacterial cells, these fungal protoplasts are osmotically unstable. No free-living fungi devoid of cell walls exist.

The cell wall constitutes 90% of the dry weight of the fungus. Generally, yeast cell walls are thicker than mold walls. Walls of old cells appear thicker and more resistant to hydrolytic enzymes. Under light microscopy, the cell wall appears as a thick, refractile covering. Electron photomicrographs reveal a structure that is smooth on the outside but fibrillar on the inside. These fibrils may be linear or crosshatched. Polysaccharides make up 80% to 90% of the dry weight of isolated cell walls. These polysaccharides include chitin, glucans, chitosan, galactans, and mannans. The remaining 10% to 20% is protein and glycoprotein. The wall polysaccharides are specific for particular fungal groups.

METABOLISM

Fungi require carbon, nitrogen, and many other elements. Carbon is used for the synthesis of compounds such as carbohydrates, proteins, lipids, and nucleic acids. Their oxidation provides energy required by the fungus. Fungi secrete extracellular enzymes such as amylase, protease, and lipase, which degrade organic macromolecules into smaller subunits that can be transported into the fungus. Various systems move these subunits across the membrane. Some transport systems are always present, and some are inducible. Simple diffusion may occur with certain lipids. Most carbon sources are taken up by either diffusion or active transport. Environmental factors such as temperature, pH, and inhibitors are important in these processes.

Nitrogen is required for the synthesis of cellular constituents including amino acids, proteins, purines, pyrimidines, nucleic acids, glucosamine, chitin, and various vitamins. Either inorganic nitrogen sources or organic sources such as amino acids can be used by most fungi. Most sources (protein is an exception) enter the cell directly by diffusion. Their utilization is governed by metabolism other than transport.

Most fungi are aerobic but some—yeasts and molds such

as *Mucor*—are facultative; that is, they can grow in a reduced oxygen environment. None are strict anaerobes.

Fungi are able to tolerate a wide variation in pH values (2 to 10). However, they grow best at a pH of approximately 7. Fungi prefer a moist environment. However, the conidia and spores can survive in a dry atmosphere. Although the optimal growth temperature for many fungi is 25° to 37°C, even the casual observer will note that some fungi grow in the refrigerator and others, such as *Aspergillus fumigatus*, which is associated with piles of decomposing leaves, grow at 45°C.

THE DETECTION, ISOLATION, AND IDENTIFICATION OF FUNGI AND ACTINOMYCETES IN THE CLINICAL MICROBIOLOGY LABORATORY

The pathophysiology and clinical aspects of fungal diseases are reviewed in Chapters 44, 45, and 52. This section will present practical but not exhaustive information on the detection, isolation, and identification of fungi and actinomycetes from human specimens. While not specifically mentioned in this section, the awareness of laboratory safety guidelines in mycology cannot be overstressed. Fungal colonies typically release spores and conidia when exposed to air currents. Simply opening a plate with fungi growing on it may pose a significant risk to the technologist.

Because fungi tend to grow slower than other microorganisms (e.g., bacteria), a great deal of emphasis is placed on direct examination of clinical specimens. Direct examination may provide important information regarding diagnosis, appropriate therapy, and the use of special media or conditions for recovery of the suspected pathogen. Since mycology is a morphology-based science, important decisions can be made by detecting the presence of pathogenic fungi.

Many media and techniques have proved useful for the isolation of pathogenic fungi. However, no universal agreement exists on how fungi should be recovered.

DIRECT MICROSCOPIC EXAMINATION OF CLINICAL SPECIMENS

Direct microscopic examination of clinical specimens submitted for mycologic analysis is performed for several reasons. Because of the long period of time it takes to recover some pathogenic fungi, it is important to provide the physician with rapid information that can assist the diagnosis and choice of therapy. A clinical specimen can be examined in minutes by direct microscopy, and sometimes the observed morphology of the fungus can provide valuable clinical information. The second purpose of direct examination is to provide the laboratory technologist with information that can effectively isolate the suspected etiologic agent.

Several methods of direct microscopic analysis of specimens are available. They include potassium hydroxide (KOH) preparations, periodic acid-Schiff stain, acid fast stain, India ink preparation, Giemsa stain, calcifluor white stain, and fluorescent antibody stains. Table 54-3 summarizes the essential characteristics of these stains.

Once stained, fungal elements may be identified by characteristic morphology. Table 54-4 lists fungal elements most commonly seen in direct specimen smears.

Guidelines for initial processing of specimens for isolation of fungi may be found in Chapter 39. While microscopic examination of patient specimens yields important information, attempts to culture the fungi are essential. Most clinical microbiologists base their choice of media on per-

Text continued on p. 54-12.

Table 54-3   Essential characteristics of stains for direct examination of fungi

Stain	Biological basis	Limitations	Utility
Potassium hydroxide (KOH) preparation	Digests protein; clears keratinized tissue.	May be insensitive, nonspecific, poor contrast; may dissolve hyphae.	Good general stain for fungal elements in tissue; improves clarity.
Periodic acid-Schiff stain (PAS)	C-C bonds in carbohydrates oxidized by periodic acid to aldehydes; aldehydes combine with basic fuchsin to form magenta colored complex.	Must be strictly controlled because of deterioration of periodic acid; may be heavy background staining if reagents are old.	Differentiation of fungi is easier if counterstain (fast green) is used; yeast and hyphae will be magenta against green background.
Acid fast stain	Mycobacteria and Nocardia resist decolorization with acid alcohol after staining with basic fuchsin.	Some yeast and *Streptomyces* spores are acid fast; decolorization must be strictly controlled.	Specific for *Mycobacterium* variable results with *Nocardia*.
India ink	A negative stain which highlights the capsular polysaccharide of *Cryptococcus neoformans*.	May be false positives with yeasts, other cryptococci, RBC, and WBC.	Specific if capsules and cryptococcal morphology are apparent.
Giemsa/Wright's stain			Used to stain bone marrow for *Histoplasma*.
Fluorescent antibody stains	Specific antigen/antibody reaction made visible by fluorescein labelling of antibody.	Lack of antibody specificity; Nonspecific fluorescence.	Used to detect *Actinomyces*, *Coccidiodes*, *Histoplasma*, *Blastomyces*, *Sporothrix Candida*.
Calcifluor White (celluflor)	Calcifluor non-specifically binds to chitin in fungal cell wall; acts as a "brightener" when added to KOH.		Enables better visualization of fungal elements in clinical specimens.

Table 54-4   Actinomycete and fungal elements observed in clinical specimens

Element	Specimen	Suggested infection or organism	Diagram
Gram-positive, branched, filaments 1 to 1.5 μm; tangled elements typically acid fast.	Respiratory secretions, pus, tissue	Nocardiosis	Plate 11
Hyphae organized into granules; some cells often swollen.	Pus, tissue biopsy	Mycetoma; suspect *Pseudallescheria boydii* in United States	Figure 54-2
Large (5 to 20 μm), sparsely septate, irregularly branching, hyaline hyphae.	Lesion drainage, pus, tissue, respiratory secretions	Zygomycosis	Figure 54-3
Septate, dichotomous branching, hyaline, 2 to 3 μm, septate hyphae.	Lesion drainage, pus, tissue, ear debris, respiratory secretions	Aspergillosis; possibly *P. boydii*	Figure 54-4
Oval hyaline yeast cells, pseudohyphae, hyphae, or any combination; cells 5 to 7 μm.	Urine, respiratory secretions, blood, skin, mucocutaneous lesions	Candidiasis; may represent invasion or colonization	Plates 12 and 13
Round, hyaline yeasts; capsules typically present; blastoconidia attached by narrow neck; cells 8 to 10 μm.	Cerebrospinal fluid, blood, lung biopsy, bone marrow, pus, respiratory secretions, urine	Cryptococcosis	Figure 54-5
Round, hyaline, thick-walled yeast cells; broad-based budding cells 8 to 15 μm.	Tissue, draining pus, respiratory secretions	Blastomycosis	Figure 54-6
Spherules (20 to 60 μm), containing endospores.	Respiratory secretions, tissues, pus	Coccidioidomycosis	Figure 54-7
Oval, hyaline, intracellular yeast (3 to 5 μm).	Respiratory secretions, bone marrow	Histoplasmosis	Figure 54-8
Thick-walled, brown cells with cross-walls in two planes (10 to 12 μm); hyphae may be present.	Subcutaneous tissue, skin	Chromoblastomycosis	Figure 54-9
Arthroconidia in and around hair shaft; cuticle destroyed (ectothrix).	Hair	Tinea capitis	Figure 54-10
Arthroconidia only inside hair shaft; cuticle intact (endothrix).	Hair	Tinea capitis	Figure 54-11
Hyphae, occasionally arthroconidia in keratinized tissue.	Skin, nails	Dermatophytosis	Figure 54-12
Carbonaceous, black, hard, hyphal nodules.	Hair	Black piedra	Figure 54-13
Short, hyaline hyphae and clusters of bottle-shaped unicellular yeast cells (3 to 7 μm).	Skin	Pityriasis versicolor	Figure 54-14
White to tan nodular masses composed of hyphae and arthroconidia.	Hair	White piedra	Figure 54-15

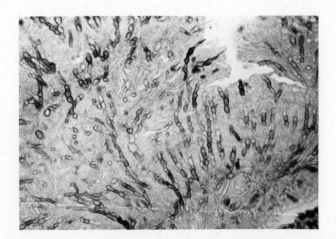

Fig. 54-2   Gomori methenamine-silver stain of biopsy specimen from foot of patient with mycetoma. Some of the mycelial strands of *Madurella mycetomatis,* the etiologic agent, contain vesicles.

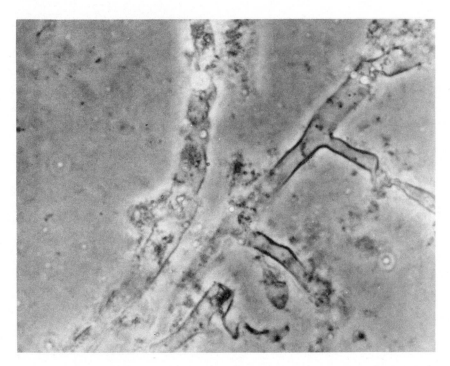

Fig. 54-3   Large branching hyphae of *Cunninghamella* (a zygomycete) in sputum of patient with zygomycosis. (Potassium hydroxide preparation.)

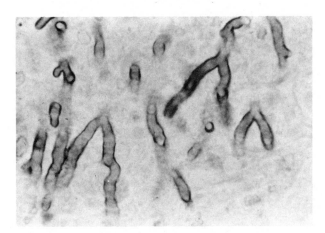

Fig. 54-4   Septate, dichotomous branching hyphae of *Aspergillus* in lung tissue.

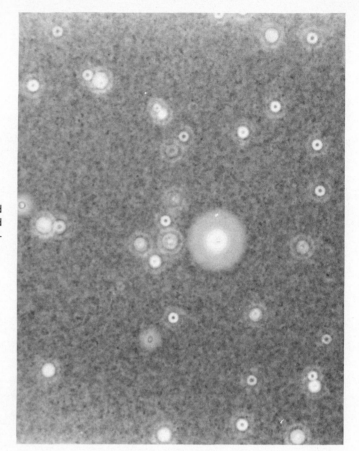

Fig. 54-5   India ink preparation showing capsule surrounding round yeast cells of *Cryptococcus neoformans*. Note how ink has created dark background that highlights colorless (hyaline) polysaccharide capsule.

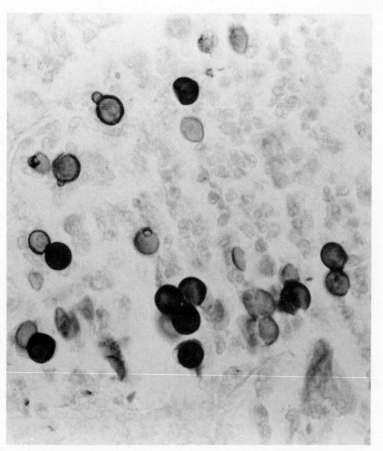

Fig. 54-6   Gomori methenamine-silver stain of lung tissue of patient with blastomycosis. Note broad base of attachment of blastoconidia of *Blastomyces dermatitidis*.

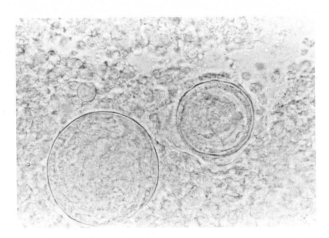

Fig. 54-7   Thick-walled spherules of *Coccidioides immitis* in sputum. *From CDC Mycology Collection C-73780.*

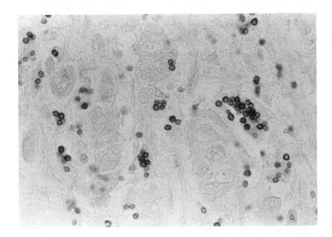

Fig. 54-8   Small intracellular oval yeast cells of *Histoplasma capsulatum* in Gomori methenamine-silver-stained tissue.

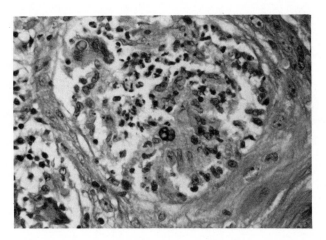

Fig. 54-9   Hematoxylin and eosin stain of subcutaneous microabscess showing thick-walled chestnut brown spherical cells and sclerotic bodies of *Fonsecaea pedrosoi.*

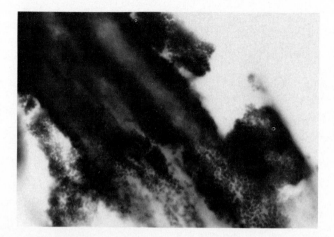

Fig. 54-10   Periodic acid-Schiff (PAS) stain of ectothrix hair invasion by *Microsporum canis.* Note that arthroconidia are within and outside hair shaft. Cuticle of hair is damaged.

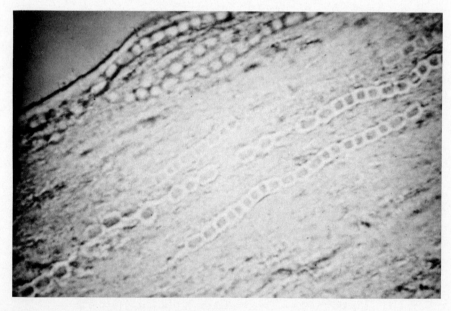

Fig. 54-11   Endothrix hair invasion of *Trichophyton tonsurans.* Note arthroconidia within hair shaft. *Courtesy L. Ajello.*

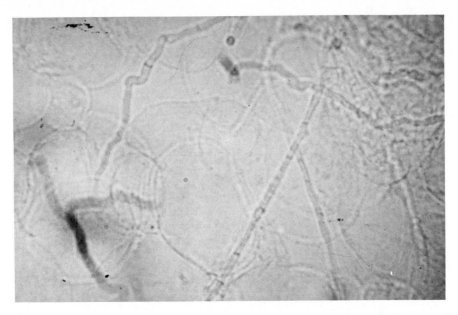

Fig. 54-12   Hyaline hyphae of *Epidermophyton floccosum* in skin scrapings mounted in 15% potassium hydroxide.

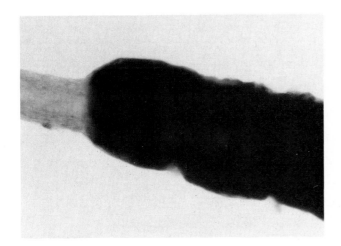

Fig. 54-13   Hard carbonaceous nodule of *Piedraia hortae* surrounding hair shaft.

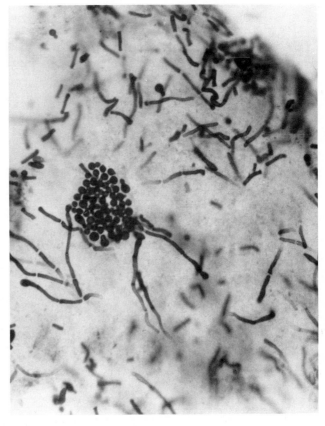

Fig. 54-14   Periodic acid-Schiff (PAS) stain of skin showing bottle-shaped yeast cells of *Malassezia furfur,* indicative of pityriasis versicolor.

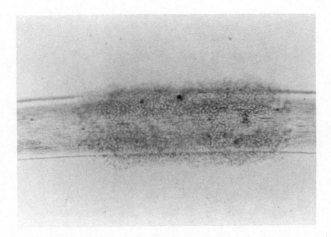

Fig. 54-15   White piedra. Note white to tan nodular masses produced by *Trichosporon beigelii. Courtesy L. Ajello.*

Table 54-5   Guidelines for media selection for primary isolation of fungi from clinical specimens[a]

Clinical specimens	Brain heart infusion agar			Inhibitory mold agar	Mycosel or mycobiotic	Sabhi agar	Yeast extract–phosphate agar[27]
	Plain	Blood	Antimicrobics				
Blood[b]	+	+		+			
Bone marrow[c]	+	+		+			
Cerebrospinal fluid	+			+			
Ear	+			+			
Eye	+		+	+			
Hair, nail, skin				+	+		
Oral cavity scrapings	+			+			
Respiratory secretions (sputum, aspirates, and washings)	+			+		+	+
Sterile fluids (peritoneal, pleural, and synovial)	+	+		+			
Tissue	+			+			
Urine	+			+			
Vaginal	+			+			

+ = Appropriate choice
[a]These are general guidelines only. Specific choice of medium is based on types of fungi recovered, which varies depending on geographic area, types of patients, and so on.
[b]Blood processed with DuPont Isolator.
[c]Nutrient broth for small specimen.

sonal experience, geographic location, and endemicity of specific fungal diseases. However, suggestions that any microbiologist may follow are presented in Table 54-5.

Many other media may be used to isolate or identify fungi. Specific types are discussed in this section when the identification of specific fungi is presented.

ENVIRONMENTAL REQUIREMENTS

Cultures for fungi are incubated at either 30°C or at room temperature (22° to 25°C). Thirty degrees Celsius is recommended because most pathogenic fungi grow better and faster at this temperature. Incubating primary isolation media at 35° to 36°C may actually inhibit or greatly retard the growth of some pathogenic fungi and thus should be avoided. However, incubation of supplemental media at even higher temperatures may be useful in some situations. *Aspergillus fumigatus*, for example, is thermotolerant and may be distinguished from other *Aspergillus* spp. by growth at 45°C.

Dimorphic fungi may grow as yeasts or as spherules at 37°C or in tissue and as molds at 25°C. This ability to grow in two forms and at two temperatures distinguishes dimorphic fungi from morphologically similar fungi. Although these organisms grow at 37°C, they grow faster at 30°C. Initial isolation, incubated at 35° to 36°C, is not cost effective because it does not provide an isolation advantage over media incubated only at 30°C.

Even when isolation plates are sealed and tubes capped, they can dry out after extended incubation if humidity is low. To prevent this, either the incubators should be humidity controlled or water should be placed in a pan in the incubator.

GENERAL SUGGESTIONS FOR THE IDENTIFICATION OF FUNGI

- Fungal cultures should be incubated at least four weeks.
- Yeast colonies should be transferred when they appear (two to three days) and the original plates reincubated.
- When examining colonies, note colony size, shape, color, and texture.
- When observations of colonies have been completed, microscopic examination is necessary. It can be done in one of several ways:

Teased preparation

Portions of colonies may be "teased" apart with a bent dissecting needle or small insect-mounting pins in a needle holder. A safety cabinet should *always* be used. Usually a sample is taken midway between the colony's center and edge. If no structures are seen, additional samples are collected closer to the center. The material is transferred to a drop of lactophenol cotton blue (LPCB) on a clean slide and teased apart with two needles. With a phase contrast microscope, lactophenol without cotton blue is used. A coverslip is applied, and the preparation is observed microscopically under both low and high power. Fungal elements that have taken up the cotton blue are readily visible. Although LPCB kills the fungi, the slides still should be autoclaved before disposal. The slides may be preserved, however, by sealing the edges of the coverslip with clear finger nail polish.

Slide culture

The slide culture is used when it is necessary to see how the conidia or spores are produced. Because a tease mount involves teasing the hyphae apart, conidiogenesis is often difficult to study. The slide culture permits the microbiologist to see how and where the conidia and spores are produced. All procedures involving slide cultures should be performed in a biologic safety cabinet. Either LPCB or lactophenol without cotton blue is used as the mounting medium. Potato dextrose agar, cornmeal agar, or V-8 juice agar should be used as the growth medium. The following steps should be followed:

1. Cover the bottom of a Petri dish with a piece of filter paper.
2. Place a bent V-shaped glass rod or bent V-shaped wooden applicator sticks on the filter paper.
3. Place a clean glass microscopic slide on the V-shaped rod.
4. Sterilize this setup by autoclaving at 121°C for 15 minutes (if disposable plastic Petri dishes are used, sterilize the components separately and then add to the Petri dish).
5. Cut a sterile agar square (1 cm) out of the growth medium and place on a sterile glass slide on the side opposite the frosted edge (more than one kind of medium can be placed on a single sterile glass slide).
6. Inoculate the four sides of agar square with isolate.
7. Using a sterile forceps, place a sterile coverslip on top of the agar square. Sterilize the forceps by passing through a flame.
8. Moisten the filter paper with 2 to 3 ml of sterile distilled water.
9. Incubate the slide culture in the dark at 22° to 25°C for approximately two weeks. It may be helpful to expose the setup to light for a day or so.
10. Add sterile water to the Petri dish if the culture begins to dry out.
11. When the slide culture has matured, remove the coverslip and quickly pass it through a flame to fix the structures. Add a drop of mounting medium to a clean microscope slide and place the coverslip at the edge of the drop of mounting fluid. Carefully lower the coverslip.
12. Discard the agar block from the microscope slide used in the slide culture setup. The microscope slide may be used as a second mount.
13. Gently heat the microscope slide, add a drop of mounting medium, and cover with a clean coverslip.
14. Seal both slide preparations by placing clear fingernail polish around the edge of the coverslips. Label the slides.

Transparent-tape preparation (Scotch® tape preparation)

The transparent-tape preparation should never be used for suspected dimorphic fungi. For other isolates, however, it is a rapid method for observing the undisturbed arrangement of conidia. Because the tape is not sterile, the isolate may become contaminated. The tape preparation should be made using a duplicate culture. The procedure follows:

1. Place a drop of LPCB on a slide.
2. Press transparent tape, sticky side down, on the surface of the mold colony and then onto the slide containing the LPCB.
3. Observe the slide microscopically and then discard it. This is a temporary preparation, and great care must be taken to avoid contamination of the fingers.

IDENTIFICATION OF FUNGI AND AEROBIC ACTINOMYCETES
Aerobic actinomycetes

Actinomycetes are bacteria, not fungi. They are susceptible to antibacterial agents but not to antifungal agents. They are included in the mycology section of this book because their morphology superficially resembles that of fungi, and they cause similar diseases. Actinomycetes are either aerobic or anaerobic. Anaerobic actinomycetes are discussed in Chapter 51. The most recent classification (1984) of the aerobic actinomycetes can be seen in Table 54-6. The genus *Mycobacterium* is discussed in Chapter 53; the other genera are discussed in this chapter.

Aerobic actinomycetes form gram-positive, filamentous elements that tend to branch. These filaments are 0.5 to 1 μm in diameter, smaller in diameter than fungal hyphae. Multiplication is by binary fission, sporulation, or fragmentation. The primary constituents of the cell wall are LL-diaminopimelic acid (DAP) and glycine; meso-DAP, arabinose, and galactose; and lysine, aspartic acid, and galactose. Because the composition of the actinomycete cell wall is extremely stable, analysis of the cell wall is a reliable means of identification.

Some of the aerobic actinomycetes may be acid fast (*Nocardia* spp.), whereas others (*Streptomyces* spp.) may only have spores that are acid fast. Not all clinical isolates of *Nocardia* are acid fast. Testing acid fastness is a useful way to identify organisms in clinical specimens but is variable in work with cultures.

Micropolyspora, Micromonospora, and *Saccharopolyspora* spp. are thermophilic actinomycetes; that is, their optimal growth temperature is approximately 50° to 55°C. Members of these genera are rarely isolated in the clinical laboratory—they can be isolated only with special procedures and media. Diagnosis is most often made by detecting specific antibodies (IgE) of these organisms in patients' serum specimens. (Lacey)

Aerobic actinomycetes normally occur in soil and are associated with plant material. They can be found in the dust of the hospital environment. These organisms cause a variety of diseases, including mycetoma and nocardiosis.

Laboratory diagnosis

The laboratory is aided in isolating and identifying aerobic actinomycetes if clinical information suggests a diagnosis of either nocardiosis or actinomycotic mycetoma. Whether or not such information is available, the tissue or biopsy specimens must be thoroughly searched for granules. The presence of granules indicates a mycetoma. If granules are found, they are teased and crushed for microscopic examination. If granules are not found, the tissue should be teased apart and macerated in sterile saline before direct examination and culture. Tissue specimens examined for *Nocardia* organisms may be very small, especially if collected by needle biopsy. Sterile saline, 0.25 to 0.5 ml, should also be added to these specimens before maceration.

Actinomycetes have been recovered from both concentrated and unconcentrated specimens. The decision to concentrate should be based on the volume of the specimen. If sufficient volume is present, then concentration by centrifugation should improve recovery.

Morphology of actinomycetes observed microscopically in direct smears can be noted in Table 54-7.

Specimens should be inoculated onto 7H10 agar, Lowenstein-Jensen agar, and brain heart infusion (BHI) agar. Agar containing chloramphenicol should *not* be used because it inhibits actinomycetes. The plates should be well sealed with parafilm. One 7H10 plate and a BHI plate without antibiotics are incubated at 35°C. The other plates and slants are incubated at room temperature (22° to 25°C). The cultures are held for four weeks before discarding.

The colonial morphology of the aerobic actinomycetes is summarized in Table 54-8. An acid-fast stain should be performed on all isolates suspected to belong to the genus *Nocardia*. It should be noted, however, that acid fastness is variable among *Nocardia* isolates, and although the presence of acid fastness is highly suggestive of this organism, a negative result from an isolated colony has little value.

Table 54-6 Classification of aerobic actinomycetes

Family	Genus	Representative species
Dermatophilaceae	*Dermatophilus*	*D. congolensis*
Mycobacteriaceae	*Mycobacterium*	*M. tuberculosis*
Nocardiaceae	*Nocardia*	*N. asteroides, N. brasiliensis, N. caviae*
	Rhodococcus	*R. rhodochrous*
Streptomycetaceae	*Streptomyces*	*S. somaliensis*
Thermomonosporaceae	*Actinomadura*[a]	*A. madurae, A. pelletieri*
	Nocardiopsis[a]	*N. dassonvillei*[b]
	Micropolyspora	*M. faeni*
	Micromonospora	*M. chalcea*
	Saccharopolyspora	*S. viridis*

[a]Mishra, Gordon, and Barnett have included *Actinomadura* and *Nocardiopsis* as members of the genus *Nocardia*. However, *Actinomadura* and *Nocardiopsis* are listed in the "Approved Lists of Bacterial Names" as separate taxa.
[b]Previously classified as *Actinomadura dassonvillei.*

Table 54-7   Direct microscopic appearance of specimens in which aerobic actinomycetes may be present

Specimen	Appearance	Possible cause
Pus and respiratory secretions (suspected nocardiosis)	Granules absent; variably acid-fast, gram-positive, irregularly stained, beaded, branched filaments (0.5-1 μm in diameter); filaments may be clumped or scattered	*Nocardia asteroides, Nocardia brasiliensis, Nocardia caviae*
Tissue (suspected mycetoma)	Granules present; when crushed, reveal clumped, intertwined, branching, variably acid-fast, gram-positive filaments; description of granules:	
	0.5-5 mm, white, soft	*Actinomadura madurae*
	0.3-0.5 mm, red, soft to hard	*Actinomadura pelletieri*
	0.5-2 mm, yellow, hard	*Streptomyces somaliensis*
	15-200 mm, white, soft	*N. brasiliensis, N. caviae, Nocardiopsis dassonvillei*

Table 54-8   Colonial appearance of aerobic actinomycetes[a]

Genus and species	Macroscopic appearance[b]	Microscopic appearance[c]
Actinomadura		Fine, intertwining, branched filaments with delicate aerial hyphae; nonfragmenting and may form short chains of spores
A. madurae	Waxy, heaped, folded, membranous, and tough; white, tan, pale orange, pink, or red	
A. pelletieri	Heaped, irregular, waxy, and granular; areas of bright and dark red; sparse aerial hyphae	
Mycobacterium		Do not show aerial filaments
Nocardia (*N. asteroides, N. brasiliensis, N. caviae*)	Orange colonies, glabrous, heaped, and folded; may also be white to pink with aerial hyphae; dry, crumbly, and adherent (Figure 54-16)	Fine, intertwining, branched filaments with delicate aerial hyphae; may have hyphal fragmentation to produce spores from aerial hyphae
Nocardiopsis dassonvillei	Orange colonies, glabrous, heaped, and folded; may also be white to pink with aerial hyphae; dry, crumbly, and adherent	
Rhodococcus		Do not show aerial filaments
Streptomyces somaliensis	Leathery, heaped, and folded; wide range of pigmentation from cream to brown-black; white aerial hyphae	Fine, intertwining, branched filaments with delicate aerial hyphae; nonfragmenting and often forms chains of spores

[a]On Sabouraud dextrose agar at 25° to 37° C.
[b]A dissecting microscope is best for macroscopic observation.
[c]Slide cultures must be set up if the original culture shows no aerial hyphae.

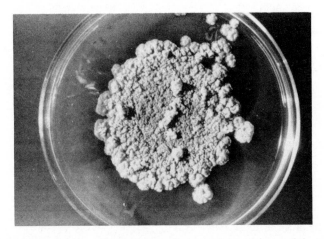

Fig. 54-16   Dry, crumbly colonies of *Nocardia asteroides* on Sabouraud dextrose agar.

Table 54-9 Physiologic characteristics of the aerobic actinomycetes

Test	Actinomadura madurae	Nocardiopsis dassonvillei	Actinomadura pelletieri	Streptomyces griseus	Nocardia asteroides	Streptomyces somaliensis	Nocardia brasiliensis	Streptomyces spp.[a]	Nocardia caviae
Acid from:									
Arabinose	+	–	–	–	–	v	+[b]	–	v
Cellobiose	+	–	–	–	–	+	+	–	v
Inositol	v	–	–	+	+	–	v	–	v
Mannitol	+	–	–	+	+[c]	+	+	–	v
Xylose	+	–	–	–	–	v	+	–	v
Hydrolysis of:									
Casein	+	+	–	+	–	+	+	+	+
Gelatin	+	+	–	+	–	+	+	+	+
Hypoxanthine	+	+[b]	–	+	+	+	+	+	+
Tyrosine	+	+	–	+	v	+	+	+	+
Urea	–	–	+	+	+	v	+	–	v
Xanthine	–	–	–	–	+	+	+	–	+[d]
Lysozyme resistance	–	–	+	+	+	–	–	–	v
Cell wall type	IIIB	IIIB	IV	IV	IV	IIIC	I	I	I

From Mishra SK, Gordon RE, and Barnett DA: J Clin Microbiol 11:728, 1980.
+ = ≥90% of strains positive except where indicated
– = ≥90% of strains negative
v = Variable
I = LL-diaminopimelic acid (DAP) plus glycine
III = Meso-DAP
IIIB = Meso-DAP plus 3-O-methyl-D-galactose (madurose)
IIIC = Same as IIIB, except madurose is absent
IV = Meso-DAP plus arabinose and galactose
[a]Includes *S. albus*, *S. lavendulae*, and *S. rimosus*.
[b]≥75% of strains positive.
[c]81% of strains positive.
[d]≥90% of *S. lavendulae* and *S. rimosus* positive; 86% of *S. albus* positive.

Acid fastness may be enhanced if the organism is grown in litmus milk or on Lowenstein-Jensen agar. A colony of *Nocardia* can be observed in Figure 54-16.

When morphology cannot distinguish genera of the actinomycetes, physiological testing must be done. Most tests are within the capability of the average laboratory, while others (e.g., cell wall analysis) should be left to reference or research laboratories. Table 54-9 summarizes the physiological characteristics of aerobic actinomycetes.

IDENTIFICATION OF FUNGI THAT INFECT HAIR, SKIN, AND NAILS

Many species of fungi infect hair, skin, and nails. They include:

1. fungi (e.g., *Malassezia furfur*, *Phaeoannillomyces werneckii*, *Tridiosporon beigelii*, and *Piedraia hortae*) that attack the outer keratinized tissues of the skin and hair;
2. dermatophytes (e.g., *Epidermophyton*, *Trichophyton*, and *Microsporum*) that attack hair, skin, and nails; and
3. a variety of fungi that infect the subcutaneous layers of skin as well as other organ systems.

The pathology and clinical significance of these infections are reviewed in Chapter 52.

Laboratory diagnosis

The specimens most commonly submitted for examination are hair, skin, and nails. A short clinical summary accompanying the specimen greatly assists the laboratory. The laboratory then can begin to narrow the broad range of fungi potentially infecting the patient. If superficial mycotic infection is suspected, then direct examination of specimens is usually adequate to a diagnosis. In some cases, culture may be indicated.

Skin scrapings

A potassium hydroxide (KOH) preparation should be made from skin scrapings. If *M. furfur* is present, short, truncated, unbranched hyphae and clusters of round to bottle-shaped yeast cells will be present (see Figure 54-14). *P. werneckii* appears as pale brown- to olive-colored hyphae and budding yeast cells. The hyphae are septate and branched and often have thickened cell walls.

Culture is not required and generally not recommended for *M. furfur* because of the lipophilic nature of this organism. For situations in which a culture is necessary, however, the organisms can be isolated on a medium such as Mycosel or Mycobiotic agar. The scrapings are mixed in a very small drop of sterile olive oil and then spread on the agar surface; the oil serves as a lipid source. The inoculated medium is incubated at 35° to 37°C. Immature colonies are cream colored, glossy, and raised. They later become dull, dry, and beige.

Skin scrapings suspected to contain *P. werneckii* are inoculated onto the surface of Mycosel or Mycobiotic agar and then incubated at 30°C. *P. werneckii* is not sensitive to 0.5 g/L of cycloheximide. The colonies are initially moist, flat, pasty, black, and yeastlike. With age, they become black to gray or olive colored with some aerial hyphae. The predominant and distinctive form of this yeast consists of cylindric to spindle-shaped cells having a septum. The former name of this fungus is *Exophiala werneckii*.

Hair

The hard carbonaceous nodules of *P. hortae* are tightly attached to the hair shaft, and if the hair is pulled through two tightly pressed fingers, the nodules do not separate from the hair. The nodules of *T. beigelii*, however, are easily stripped off the hair.

Infected hairs should be examined using a KOH preparation. Microscopic examination of the crushed nodules of *T. beigelii* hair reveal hyphae and many arthroconidia.

Hairs infected with *T. beigelii* should be cultured on Sabouraud dextrose agar (SDA) with chloramphenicol but without cycloheximide (to which *T. beigelii* is sensitive). Although direct microscopic examination of *P. hortae* is definitive, this organism may also be recovered on SDA with chloramphenicol.

T. beigelii grows in three or four days and produces a raised, heaped, creamy, yeastlike colony. In one to two weeks, it becomes yellowish gray.

The colonies of *P. hortae* grow slowly and are black to dark brown with a velvety appearance.

Some of the most common microscopic and cultural procedures in a clinical microbiology laboratory are the processing of hair, skin, and nail specimens for dermatophytes.

As in the case with superficial mycotic infections, clinical information is very helpful. Isolation can be easily accomplished without specialized media and identification of dermatophytes is usually morphologic.

Direct examination

The Wood's lamp (UV light) may be useful for clinical differentiation of the dermatophytoses. Hair that is infected with a dermatophyte may fluoresce under UV light. Fluorescing hairs should be selectively examined and cultured because they contain the fungi. The UV light is also useful for differentiating ringworm of the skin from erythrasma, an infection caused by *Corynebacterium minutissimum;* dermatophyte lesions do not fluoresce, whereas *Corynebacterium* infections do.

In addition to culture, a portion of the clinical specimen consisting of skin, nail, or hair is placed into a drop of 20% potassium hydroxide (KOH) preparation on a clean microscope slide. The slide is gently warmed and then examined with both the low- and high-power objectives of the microscope. If the result is negative, the specimen should be reexamined after the tissue has been cleared for some additional time. Skin and pulverized nail scrapings typically contain septate, branched, hyaline hyphae. Occasionally, chains of arthroconidia are present. If the hair is invaded, the invasion may be favic, endothrix, or ectothrix.

Favic hair invasion is caused by *T. schoenleinii.* Invasion of the hair by the fungus produces hyphae parallel to the long axis of the hair shaft (Figure 54-17). The hyphae degenerate, leaving tunnels within the hair shaft. These tunnels are best observed by examination immediately after placing the hair in the KOH solution. The fluid fills the tunnels, and in the process air bubbles can be seen rushing down the hair shaft. This is characteristic of *T. schoenleinii.*

Endothrix hair invasion is caused by *T. tonsurans, T. soudanense,* and *T. violaceum.* The hyphae grow down the

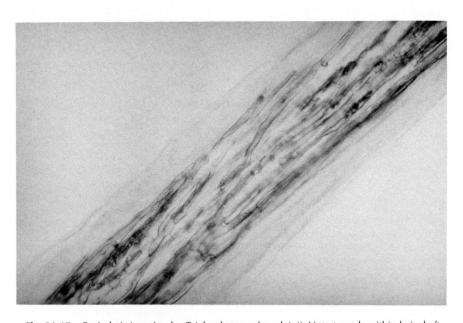

Fig. 54-17   Favic hair invasion by *Trichophyton schoenleinii.* Note tunnels within hair shaft.

Table 54-10 Colonial and microscopic morphology of commonly isolated dermatophytes

Organism	Colonial appearance[a]	Microscopic appearance
Epidermophyton floccosum	Mature colonies become yellow or mustard yellow to tan; surface is flat with radial folding; reverse colony is deep orange; white, cotton tufts of sterile mutants may appear on surface of colony	Numerous, club-shaped, two- to four-septate conidia (6 to 12 μm × 20 to 40 μm) that occur singly or in groups of two to three (Figure 54-18); cell walls are smooth and thick; microconidia are absent
Microsporum audouinii[b]	Colony is cream or tan to light brown; reverse colony is orange-tan to salmon pink; colony is flat, velvety, and slightly raised in center	Terminal, swollen cells occasionally present; hyphae usually sterile; microconidia may be formed; macroconidia infrequent, but when present, they are large, irregularly spindle shaped, and thick walled with roughened surface (Figure 54-19)
Microsporum canis	Colony initially white, becoming bright yellow at edge; reverse colony is yellow, becoming orange to brown; colonies silky, becoming cottony with irregular tufts or concentric rings	Macroconidia are spindle shaped, large (35 to 110 μm × 12 to 25 μm); thick outer wall; thin inner cell wall; microconidia one celled, clavate, and smooth walled (Figure 54-20)
Microsporum fulvum	Colony is flat, light tan to medium brown or cinnamon brown, powdery to velvety; reverse colony is rosy buff to cinnamon	Macroconidia and microconidia similar to *M. gypseum*
Microsporum gypseum	Same as *M. fulvum*	Macroconidia numerous (25 to 60 μm × 8 to 15 μm); thick walled with four to six septa of similar thickness to outer cell wall; microconidia one celled, clavate, smooth walled (Figure 54-21)
Microsporum nanum	Flat colonies, powdery, cream to buff to medium brown; reverse colony is orange at first, becoming dark red to brown; similar to *M. gypseum*	Numerous small (12 to 18 μm × 5 to 7 μm) macroconidia, oval to elliptic, rough walled with one to three septa; microconidia one celled, clavate, smooth walled (Figure 54-22)
Trichophyton mentagrophytes	Colony is flat and may be velvety or powdery *(T. mentagrophytes* var. *interdigitale)* and even granular *(T. mentagrophytes* var. *mentagrophytes);* white to creamy tan; reverse of colony is white to reddish brown	Microconidia are round to subglobose, one celled, and hyaline (Figure 54-23); they occur in clusters, along the hyphae, or both; macroconidia typically absent, but may be produced on Sabouraud dextrose agar containing 5% NaCl; when present, they have one to four septa, are cylindric to clavate, and are smooth walled; spirals and nodular bodies may be present
T. rubrum	Mature colonies grown in 1 to 2 weeks and are white and granular to cottony; reverse of colony is white, light brown, or dark red; bright red reverse may be produced when isolate is grown on cornmeal agar	Microconidia similar to *T. mentagrophytes,* except they are clavate; in cottony isolates, microconidia rare or absent; macroconidia typically absent, but when present, are cylindric, have two to seven septa, and are smooth walled
T. schoenleinii	Colony is white and becomes tan with age; colony is raised and folded, leathery, glabrous, waxy, granular to velvety, agar tends to crack; reverse of colony is buff to light brown	Conidia typically absent; favic chandeliers common (Figure 54-24); mycelium have irregular diameter; numerous chlamydoconidia typically present
T. tonsurans	Colony is flat, compact, and glabrous to granular, becoming heaped and folded with maturity; may be cream or yellow to rose, buff, or brown; reverse colony yellow to mahogany red; growth enhanced by thiamine	Numerous microconidia, varying in size; globose, elongate to bulging, borne at right angle to hyphae; macroconidia are rare, but when produced they are cylindric and smooth walled and have one to six septa; fertile hyphae are broader than vegetative hyphae (Figure 54-25)
T. verrucosum	Surface of colony is dull white or gray to yellowish tan; glabrous to waxy, becoming powdery; aerial hyphae may develop in old colonies; growth more rapid at 37° C	Characteristic chains of chlamydoconidia (Figure 54-26) seen at 37° C; on thiamine rich media, microconidia are present sides of hyphae; macroconidia are seen
T. violaceum	Heaped and folded colonies with smooth, waxy, or velvety surface; buff to lavender but with a deep purple, diffusible, reverse pigment	Microconidia and macroconidia very rare; thiamine often stimulates conidial production

[a]Colonial characteristics based on growth at 25° to 30° C on Sabouraud dextrose agar with 4% sugar and two weeks' incubation.
[b]Rarely seen in North America.

hair follicle and then penetrate the hair shaft. The fungus grows within the hair, and the cuticle of the hair remains intact. The hyphae within the hair are converted into arthroconidia (see Figure 54-11).

Ectothrix hair invasion is usually associated with *M. audouinii, M. canis, M. gypseum, M. nanum,* and *T. verrucosum* infections. The arthroconidia can be seen both inside and outside the hair shaft. The arthroconidia surrounding the hair look like a sheath. Ectothrix hair infection develops like endothrix, except that the hyphae destroy the hair cuticle and grow around the hair shaft (See Figure 54-10.). The hyphae then converted into arthroconidia are virulent infective propagules.

A KOH preparation that does not contain fungal elements does not rule out a dermatophyte infection. On the other hand, a positive result for the KOH preparation only confirms that an infection exists. Because the hyphae of different dermatophytes are morphologically similar in keratinized tissues, identifying the particular species involved requires isolating the fungus.

Culture and isolation

Clinical specimens—including skin, hair, and nails—suspected of containing dermatophytes are inoculated onto media with and without 0.5 g/ml of cycloheximide. All media are incubated at 30°C. All cultures are held for three weeks before being discarded as negative.

When colonies appear on primary media, they should immediately be transferred to Sabouraud dextrose agar (SDA), incubated at 25° to 30°C and checked to ensure purity.

Molds, yeasts, and bacteria may contaminate dermatophyte cultures. In some instances, a dermatophyte culture may contain two different dermatophytes. The original isolation plates should be reincubated while purification is being formed.

Pure colonies of suspicious dermatophytes are examined grossly and then microscopically in either slide culture or teased preparations. Table 54-10 contains information regarding the colonial and microscopic features of the dermatophytes most commonly isolated. The descriptions for fungi are based on isolates grown on SDA.

The genus *Trichophyton* contains morphologically similar species, i.e., *T. verrucosum* and *T. schoenleinii.* Physiologic tests may be necessary to identify these fungi. Table 54-11 summarizes these tests.

The laboratory diagnosis of fungal infections of the subcutaneous skin layer is complicated by the fact that these fungi may be difficult to identify. Therefore the cost and clinical effectiveness of the laboratory is a direct function of access to clinical information and communication with the ordering clinician. The mycology of these organisms is difficult, and precise identification may be better obtained by reference laboratories. By astute observation, however, the routine clinical microbiology laboratory should be able to provide preliminary information regarding the presence of fungi in clinical specimens.

Specimens like skin scrapings, exudates, biopsy material, lesion crusts, pus, and aspirated debris are examined in 10% potassium hydroxide (KOH) after gentle heating of the slide to dissolve the clinical material. Tissue specimens should be homogenized or macerated but only after a search for purulent or necrotic areas that can be examined directly. Since demonstrating *Sporothrix schenckii* in a clinical spec-

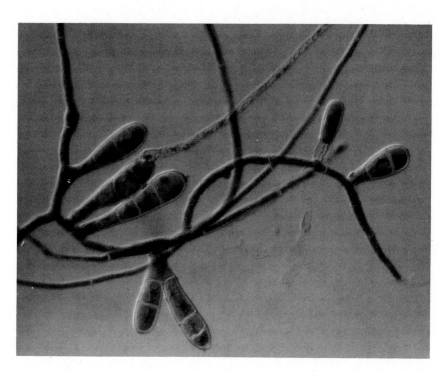

Fig. 54-18 *Epidermophyton floccosum.* Club-shaped conidia with two to four septa produced singly or in groups.

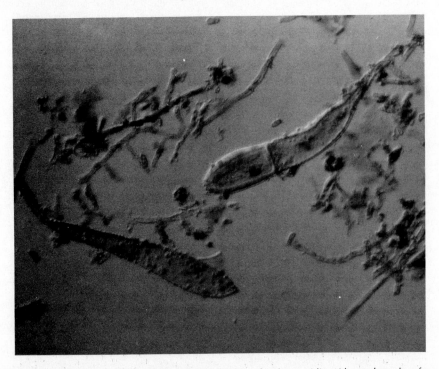

Fig. 54-19   *Microsporum audouinii.* Large spindle-shaped macroconidia with roughened surface.

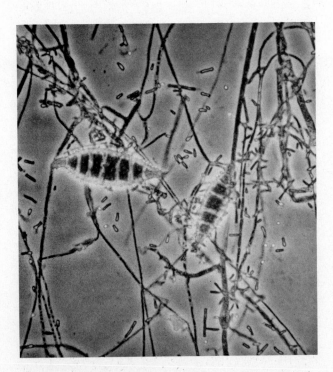

Fig. 54-20   *Microsporum canis.* Spindle-shaped macroconidia typically have septa that are thinner than outer conidial wall. Note extremely roughened texture of outer cell wall.

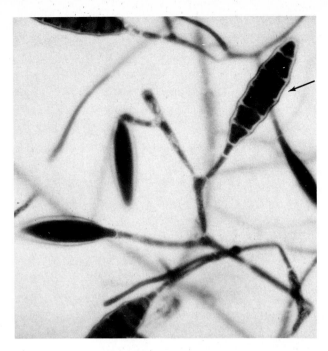

Fig. 54-21   *Microsporum gypseum*. Various developmental stages of thallic macroconidia are present. In mature macroconidium *(arrow)* outer cell wall tends to collapse slightly.

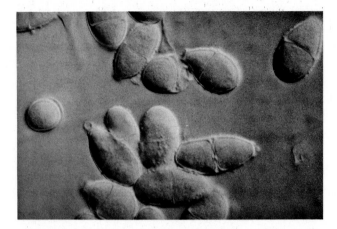

Fig. 54-22   *Microsporum nanum*. Most clinical isolates produce two-celled roughened macroconidia with flattened bases (truncate).

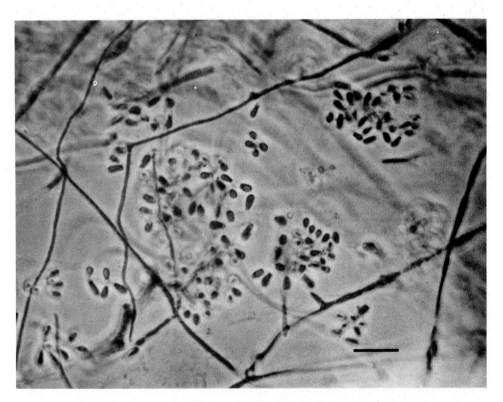

Fig. 54-23   *Trichophyton mentagrophytes*. Microconidia are one celled and round (globose) to nearly round (subglobose). *From McGinnis, M.R., et al.: Pictorial handbook of medically important fungi and aerobic actinomycetes, New York, 1982, Praeger Publishers.*

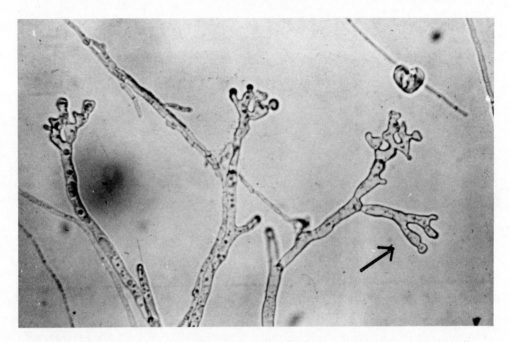

Fig. 54-24   Characteristic favic chandeliers *(arrow)* of *Trichophyton schoenleinii. Courtesy L. Ajello.*

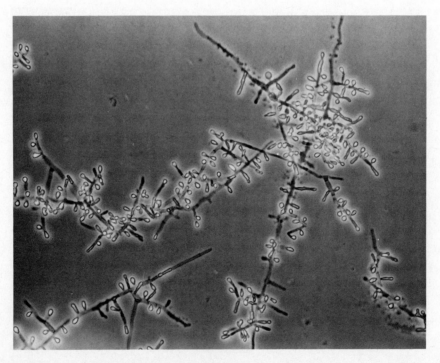

Fig. 54-25   *Trichophyton tonsurans.* Conidia that vary from round (globose) to elongate resembling matchsticks characterize this dermatophyte. *From McGinnis, M.R.: Laboratory handbook of medical mycology, New York, 1980, Academic Press, Inc.*

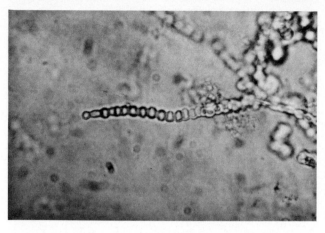

Fig. 54-26 Typical chains of chlamydoconidia of *Trichophyton verrucosum. Courtesy J. Kane.*

Table 54-11 Physiologic tests available for the differentiation of some members of the genus *Trichophyton*

Test	Differential characteristics
Urease Production	*T. mentagrophytes* hydrolyzes urea in 3-7 days. *T. rubrum* rarely is urease positive.
Pigment production	*T. rubrum* produces a deep red pigment on cornmeal agar with 1% dextrose in 2-4 weeks. *T. mentagrophytes* does not.
In vitro hair perforation	*T. mentagrophytes* perforates hair in a wedge shape. *T. rubrum* does not. May be the most reliable differential test.
Growth temperature	*T. verrucosum* and *T. mentagrophytes* grow at 37°C. *T. terrestre* does not.
Growth on rice grains	*Microsporum audouinii* does not grow but produces brown discoloration on polished, unfortified rice grains. *M. canis* and other fungi grow on rice grains.

Table 54-12 Direct microscopic appearance of some clinical specimens containing agents of subcutaneous mycoses

Disease	Representative fungi	Direct microscopic appearance
Chromoblastomycosis	*Fonsecaea pedrosoi, Phialophora verrucosa, Cladosporium carrionii*	Pigmented hyphal elements at skin surface; sclerotic bodies thick walled, muriform, chestnut brown structures, approximately 10 μm in diameter, and often are covered with crusty layer of refractile material; in crusts, dematiaceous, septate, branched hyphae often present
Lobomycosis	*Loboa loboi*	Large, hyaline, thick walled, spherical to oval yeasts (10 μm), occurring in short chains with tubular connections between each cell of the chain
Mycetoma	*Pseudallescheria boydii, Exophiala jeanselmei, Madurella mycetomatis*	Examine specimen for granules; composed of hyphae
Phaeohyphomycosis	*Bipolaris spicifera, E. jeanselmei, Xylohypha bantiana*	Pale brown to brown yeastlike cells, hyphae, or both; hyphae regular to irregular, often with swollen cells
Sporotrichosis	*Sporothrix schenckii*	Direct microscopic examination not recommended
Subcutaneous zygomycosis	*Basidiobolus ranarum, Conidiobolus coronatus*	Broad, irregularly branching hyphae (5 to 18 μm), sparsely septate; surrounded by eosinophilic material

imen by a KOH preparation is difficult, stained tissue sections or fluorescent-stained material should be examined. The differential microscopic appearance of clinical specimens is described in Table 54-12.

Specimens examined for the recovery of fungal agents of subcutaneous infections should be cultured on media with and without antimicrobial agents. Some dermatiaceous fungi are sensitive to 0.5 mg/ml of cycloheximide. All grow well at 30°C, and viable colonies are present in one to two weeks. Some do not grow at 37°C. Plates should not be discarded for at least four weeks. In cases of mycetoma, the granules should be cultured on media with and without antimicrobial agents. When actinomycetes are involved, they are sensitive to antibacterial agents like chloramphenicol.

When colonies appear on the isolation media, they must be purified before identification. Dermatiaceous fungi should be subcultured to potato dextrose agar or cornmeal agar because these stimulate conidial formation. McGinnis suggests that an isolate resembling *Sporothrix schenckii* be subcultured to a blood agar plate (BAP), incubated at 36°C to confirm its dimorphic nature. One BAP is incubated at 22° to 25°C, the other at 35°C in a candle jar. Yeast forms should be present at 35°C. It is not necessary for the entire colony to be converted to a yeast to show dimorphism.

Table 54-13 describes the macroscopic and microscopic morphology of commonly isolated fungi. As with other fungi, all cultural and microscopic preparation should be performed in a biologic safety cabinet.

Table 54-13 Microscopic and macroscopic morphology of some fungi causing subcutaneous infections

Organism	Microscopic morphology	Macroscopic morphology
Bipolaris spicifera	Erect, pale brown, sympodial conidiophores giving rise to ellipsoidal conidia with three septa and slightly protruding hila (Figure 54-27) (hila [sing. *hilum*] are scars at base of conidium)	Rapid growing; first white, rapidly becoming olive green to black; texture velvety to woolly
Cladosporium carrionii	Erect, dematiaceous conidiophores giving rise to acro-, petally branched chains of one-celled, pale brown blastoconidia (Figure 54-28); chains are fragile; conidia close to conidiophore apex, often resembling shields; termed "shield cells" (*Cladosporium carrionii* resembles *Xylohypha bantiana* but is differentiated as discussed under *X. bantiana*)	Rapidly growing, dark-olive to black colony; black submerged hyphae; woolly to cottony; slightly raised
Exophiala jeanselmei	Conidiophores are pale brown, giving rise to cylindric to flask-shaped annellides; conidia are one celled, hyaline to pale brown, and accumulate in a cluster at the apex of the annellide (Figure 54-29)	Moderately fast growing, moist, glistening, gray to black colony, becoming woolly as colony matures
Fonsecaea pedrosoi	Form primary one-celled conidia arising from sympodial conidiophores; primary conidia function as sympodial conidiogenous cells to form secondary one-celled conidia; some conidia occur as branched chains of blastoconidia; may also produce phialides with collarettes and clusters of one-celled conidia; *Fonsecaea* organisms produce three types of anamorphs: (1) those similar to that seen in *Rhinocladiella* spp. (incorrectly called *Acrotheca*-like), (2) those similar to that found in *Cladosporium* spp., and (3) those similar to that found in *Phialophora* spp.	Slow growing, black-brown, gray-black, olive-gray, or black colony; texture velvety to cottony; *F. pedrosoi* and *P. verrucosa* indistinguishable macroscopically
Madurella mycetomatis	Isolates typically sterile, but some fresh isolates on potato dextrose agar (PDA) may produce phialides with collarettes having conidia in balls at their apices; better growth observed at 35° than 30° C	Most isolates form slow-growing, raised to heaped, woolly, olive to gray, yellow, or brown colonies
Phialophora verrucosa	Conidiophores short when present; conidiogenous cells dematiaceous, cylindric to flask-shaped phialides having collarettes; conidia ovoid to cylindric, one celled, hyaline, and occur in balls at the apices of the phialides (Figure 54-30)	Moderately fast growing, dark olive-gray to black colony; initially dome-shaped but becomes woolly to cottony
Pseudallescheria boydii	Cleistothecia are black, spherical (140 to 200 μm in diameter) structures that occur in medium below colony surface and its junction with agar (Figure 54-31); ascospores one celled, ovoid to ellipsoidal, pale brown to copper, with eight ascospores per ascus; anamorphs *Scedosporium apiospermum*, *Graphium* spp.; produce one-celled, hyaline to pale brown, subglobose to elongate conidia; borne on synnemata	Colony initially white, becoming gray; rapid growing, cottony
Sporothrix schenckii	Dimorphic fungus; at 25° C, two kinds of conidia present: (1) hyaline, globose to clavate, one-celled conidia on denticles that develop along hyphae or laterally from sympodial conidiophores, and (2) dark, one-celled, thick-walled conidia along hyphae; identity confirmed by conversion of mold form to yeast form at 37° C (Figure 54-32)	Fast growing; young colonies may be white, glabrous, yeastlike, becoming cream to dark brown; at first moist, becoming wrinkled; leathery to velvety in texture
Wangiella dermatitidis	Conidiophores hypha like; conidiogenous cells are phialides without collarettes; phialoconidia are one celled, smooth, hyaline to pale brown, forming in clusters at apices of phialides; isolates also commonly produce yeast forms; *W. dermatitidis* readily grows at 40° C, which helps to distinguish it from most other dematiaceous fungi	Rapidly growing; on initial isolation, moist, glistening, olive to black, becoming velvety and olive gray
Xylohypha bantiana	Previously known as *Cladosporium bantianum* or *C. trichoides*, fungus was reclassified as *X. bantiana* because its conidiophores are hypha like and extremely long chains of blastoconidia are sparsely branched; it is differentiated from *C. carrionii* by lacking erect, distinct conidiophores, having longer conidia, and ability to grow at 42° to 43° C; *C. carrionii* does not grow at the latter temperature	Moderately fast growing, like *C. carrionii*

From McGinnis MR, et al: Pictorial handbook of medically important fungi and aerobic actinomycetes, New York, 1982, Praeger Publishers.

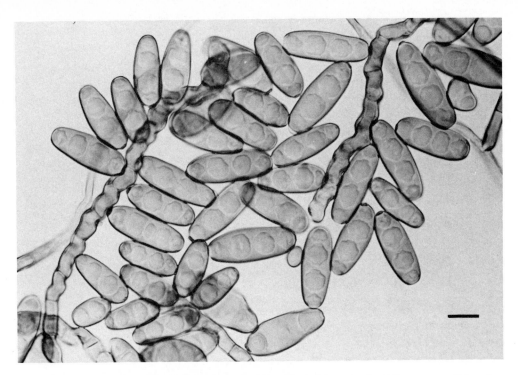

Fig. 54-27   *Bipolaris spicifera.* Note septate conidia with slightly protruding hila on sympodial coni-diophores. (Bar = 10 μm.)

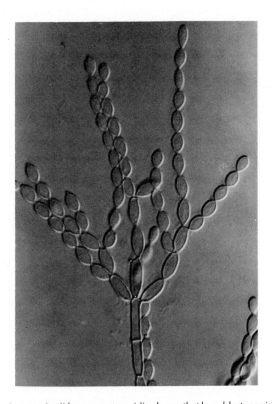

Fig. 54-28   *Cladosporium carrionii* forms erect conidiophores that bear blastoconidia in branched chains.

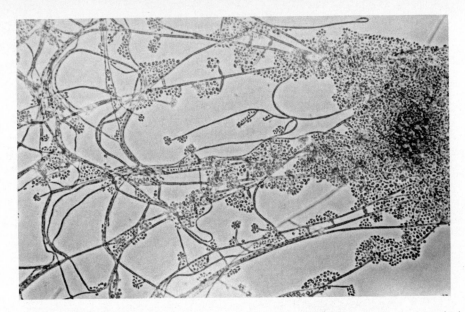

Fig. 54-29   One-celled annelloconidia accumulating at tips of annellides is characteristic of *Exophiala jeanselmei*.

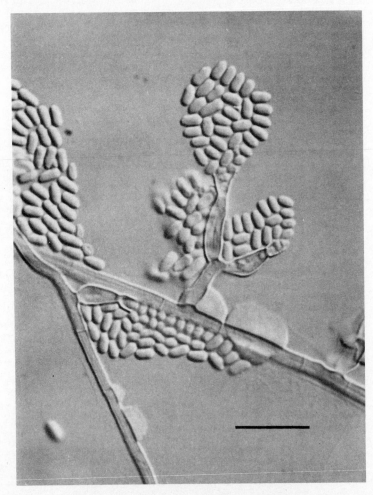

Fig. 54-30   *Phialophora verrucosa*. Flask-shaped phialides with collarettes give rise to cylinderic one-celled conidia that occur in balls. (Bar = 10 μm.) *From McGinnis, M.R., D'Amato, R.F., and Land, G.A.: Pictorial handbook of fungi and aerobic actinomycetes, New York, 1982, Praeger Publishers.*

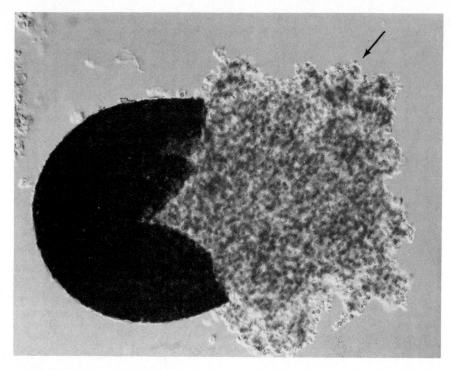

Fig. 54-31 Ascospores *(arrow)* have been released from mature cleistothecium of *Pseudallescheria boydii*. Many asci, which cannot be seen because their walls have dissolved within cleistothecium as it matured, are randomly dispersed within structure.

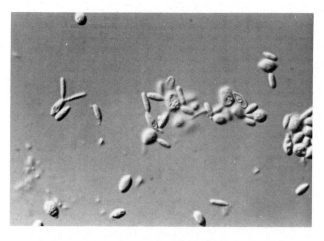

Fig. 54-32 Yeast form of *Sporothrix schenckii* at 37° C.

ISOLATION AND IDENTIFICATION OF FUNGI THAT CAUSE SYSTEMIC MYCOSIS

The four fungi traditionally thought to cause systemic disease are *Histoplasma capsulatum*, *Blastomyces dermatitidis*, *Coccidioides immitis*, and *Paracoccidioides brasieliensis*. They are usually grouped together because they 1) have similar epidemiology, 2) are dimorphic, and 3) require similar techniques for specimen processing, isolation, and identification. It must be recognized that other fungi such as *Rhizopus, Mucor, Candida, Cryptococcus,* and others cause

systemic disease as well. Relatively few fungi, however, are thermally dimorphic, that is, they grow as yeasts at 37°C and as molds at room temperature (25°C). *Sporothrix schenckii* and *Penicillium marheffei* are also dimorphic.

Laboratory diagnosis

While Chapter 2 discusses biosafety in the clinical laboratory, it must be stressed that the fungi described in this section are dangerous and must be handled with utmost care. Manipulations of specimens must be done in a biological safety cabinet, plates should be sealed with parafilm, technologists should *never* smell plates, and all materials should be autoclaved. Specimen collection and transport in microbiology is reviewed in Chapter 3. Specimens for mycologic examination should be delivered to the laboratory and processed without delay. *H. capsulatum,* for example, is very sensitive to environmental conditions or to contaminated overgrowth. Unlike most fungi, it does not survive for extended periods of time in the refrigerator.

All specimens for systemic fungi should be examined at the time of their receipt. In some instances, a specific diagnosis can be made rapidly; this may influence the therapeutic regimen or alert the laboratory worker to use additional media or techniques for isolation. If specimens must be concentrated, microscopy should be subsequently performed as soon as possible. The sediment can be examined directly. It is sometimes necessary to clear the specimen with potassium hydroxide (KOH) before evaluation. KOH preparations, use of calcifluor, Gram stains, periodic acid-Schiff (PAS) stain, phase-contrast microscopy, and fluores-

Table 54-14 Microscopic appearance in clinical and tissue specimens

Organism	Microscopic appearance
Blastomyces dermatitidis	Large spherical yeast cells 8 to 12 μm, with thick walls; blastoconidia attached to parent cell by broad base (Figure 54-33)
Coccidioides immitis	Spherules round, hyaline, large, 30 to 60 μm, thick-walled structures filled with one-celled, hyaline, small, 2 to 5 μm endospores (Figure 54-34)
Histoplasma capsulatum	Rarely seen in sputum; may be evident in touch preparations of lymph nodes, bone marrow, and blood smears of patients with AIDS; small (2 to 5 μm) oval yeasts resembling *Torulopsis glabrata* (Figure 54-35); oil immersion is recommended; in tissue sections the small yeasts are intracellular in polymorphonuclear leukocytes, giant cells, or macrophages
Paracoccidioides brasiliensis	Multiple budding blastoconidia around large one-celled, hyaline, thick-walled cells; blastoconidia are variable in size and arranged radially around the parent cells, attached by narrow tubular denticles; they are often described as a "pilot's wheel" (Figure 54-36)

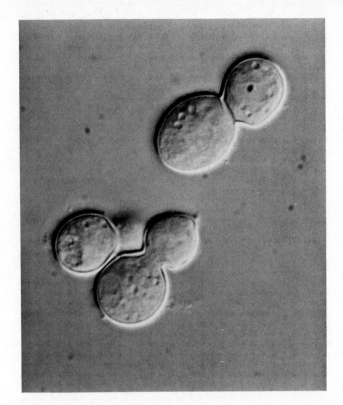

Fig. 54-33 *Blastomyces dermatitidis* in its yeast form. Note broad base of attachment of blastoconidium to parent cell.

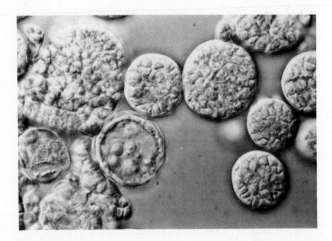

Fig. 54-34 Thick-walled spherules of *Coccidioides immitis*.

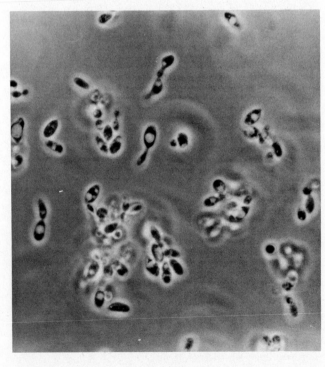

Fig. 54-35 *Histoplasma capsulatum*. Small oval yeast cells producing blastoconidia.

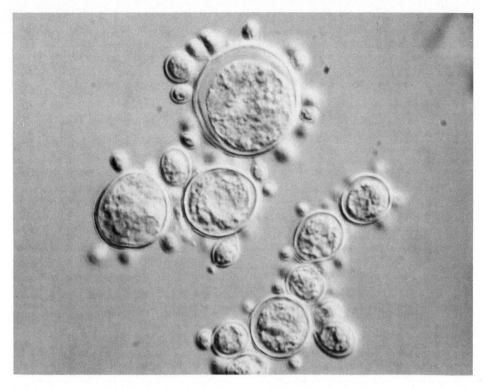

Fig. 54-36 *Paracoccidioides brasiliensis.* Yeast cells are round with multiple blastoconidia attached to parent cell by narrow necks.

cent antibody (FA) stains can provide useful and important data.

Table 54-14 describes structures seen on direct smears of specimens for systemic fungi.

Culture and isolation

Media with and without antimicrobial agents must be used when culturing systemic fungi. *Cryptococcus neoformans, Pseudallescheria boydii, Aspergillus* spp., and some zygomycetes are sensitive to cycloheximide. *H. capsulatum* is inhibited by high concentrations of gentamicin and chloramphenicol, especially when incubated at 37°C. *Actinomyces* spp. and the aerobic actinomycetes, such as *Nocardia asteroides,* are susceptible to chloramphenicol and other antimicrobics, such as penicillin.

Yeast extract-phosphate medium should be used to recover *H. capsulatum* from contaminated respiratory specimens, such as sputum. In HIV-infected patients, the Isolator blood culture system (Wampole) is useful for the detection of *Histoplasma* fungemia.

Isolation plates or slants are incubated at 30°C and inspected every two to four days for evidence of growth. Plates should be sealed entirely around their edges with oxygen-permeable tape. The lids of the Petri dishes should not be removed during inspection—this prevents accidental contamination of workers and the environment. Plates are inspected within a BSC. When oxygen-permeable tape is used to seal the entire dish, the unopened dish can be examined under a good light source.

Of the four dimorphic fungi described in this chapter,

Coccidioides immitis grows fastest (four to five days), and *H. capsulatum* and *Paracoccidioides brasiliensis* grow slowest (two to three weeks). The microbiologist cannot assume that a saprophytic fungus is present simply because colonial growth appears in a few days.

Lactophenol cotton blue preparations should be made on all colonies to evaluate the nature of conidiogenesis. Contaminated cultures must be purified before their identification.

Morphology

At 30°C *H. capsulatum* grows as a white to brownish mold. Other morphologic characteristics are summarized in Table 54-15. At 37°C on special media the colony is slow growing and consists of yeastlike cells. At room temperature, both one-celled microconidia and macroconidia are typically produced on short, hyphalike condidiophores. The macroconidia are round (7 to 12 μm in diameter) with thickened cell walls that are typically tuberculate. The microconidia are 2 to 5 μm, round, and smooth walled. The conidia of some *Chrysoporium* and *Sepedonium* spp. are similar to those of *Histoplasma,* but neither genus contains species that are dimorphic. However, because of the morphologic similarity of these two genera to *H. capsulatum,* suspected isolates of *H. capsulatum* must be confirmed as such by exoantigen testing.

There are actually two varieties of *H. capsulatum.* The variety isolated in the United States is *H. capsulatum* var. *capsulatum. H. capsulatum* var. *duboisii* is the cause of African histoplasmosis. These two varieties are morpho-

Table 54-15   Colonial appearance and microscopic morphology of the systemic fungi at room temperature

Organism	Colonial appearance	Microscopic morphology
Blastomyces dermatitidis	Young colonies may be thin and membranous; older colonies may be glabrous to woolly; color varies from dirty white to tan; slow to moderate growing	Small, oval, smooth-walled conidia borne on short, lateral, hyphalike conidiophores (Figure 54-37)
Coccidioides immitis	Young colonies glabrous and grayish, becoming white and cottony; with age, becoming white to brown to dark gray; rapid growing	Alternating one-celled, thin-walled, barrel-shaped arthroconidia and disjunctor cells (Figure 54-38)
Histoplasma capsulatum	Colonies woolly, cottony, or granular; initially white, becoming brown in color; slow growing	Macroconidia one celled, round (7-12 μm), and tuberculated; microconidia small, one celled (2-5 μm), round, smooth walled (Figure 54-39); hypha-like conidiophores
Paracoccidioides brasiliensis	Colonial forms vary and may be glabrous, leathery, flat to wrinkled, folded, or velvety; color of colony white to beige; slow growing	Hyphae are typically sterile; fresh isolates may produce one-celled, hyaline conidia similar to those produced by *B. dermatitidis*

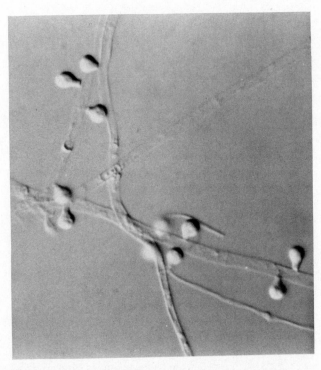

Fig. 54-37   *Blastomyces dermatitidis* in its mold form. Hyphalike conidiophores give rise to small, one-celled conidia.

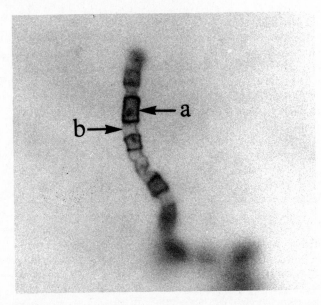

Fig. 54-38   Arthroconidium *(a)* and disjunctor cell *(b)* of *Coccidioides immitis. From Mycopathol. Mycol. Appl. 45:269, 1971.*

logically indistinguishable in culture. When their isolates are crossed with each other, *Ajellomyces capsulatus*, the teleomorph, is produced. Clinically, the infections are different, and in tissue *H. capsulatum* var. *duboisii* is much larger.

The colonial and microscopic morphology of *C. immitis* is described in Table 54-15. The arthroconidia of *C. immitis* must be confirmed. The exoantigen test is recommended.

Colonies of *B. dermatitidis* growing at room temperature may be membranous, smooth, and cream colored with no aerial hyphae, or they may be woolly with a white to tan

color. This mold form of *B. dermatitidis* produces oval, smooth-walled, one-celled conidia (3 to 5 μm) borne on short lateral hyphal branches. Some isolates of *B. dermatitidis* produce echinulate conidia. At 35°C, the colonies are yeastlike in appearance. The yeast are thick walled, spherical, one celled, and hyaline and produce a single blastoconidium attached to the parent cell by a wide base. The yeast cells are 10 to 15 μm in diameter. The conidia of *B. dermatitidis* resemble conidia produced by some species of *Chrysoporium* and must be confirmed. *Blastomyces der-*

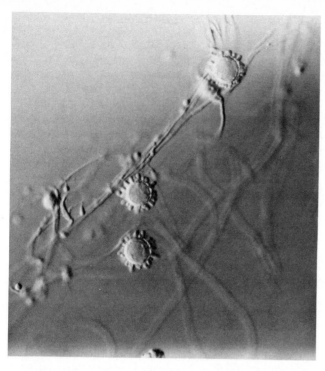

Fig. 54-39 *Histoplasma capsulatum.* Large, single, thick-walled macroconidia with robust projections from the cell wall develop on hyphalike conidiophores.

As already discussed, identification of the systemic fungi must be confirmed by converting the mold form to either the corresponding yeast form (*H. capsulatum, B. dermatitidis, P. brasiliensis*) or the spherule form *(C. immitis)* on conversion media or by using specific antigens obtained from culture filtrates in the exoantigen test. With the advent of good conversion media and the exoantigen tests, animal inoculation is unnecessary. The use of exoantigens is recommended. Specific procedures for mold to yeast or spherule form may be found in a number of reference sources including *Clinical and Pathogenic Microbiology,* Howard, et al, 1987. Table 54-16 summarizes media use and morphology of dimorphic fungi.

The five systemic fungi can also be identified immunologically through detection of cell-free antigens from culture filtrates. A 10-day-old (or older) Sabouraud dextrose agar slant culture is extracted with an aqueous merthiolate solution for 24 to 48 hours at 25°C. The extract is concentrated by ultracentrifugation or a disposable microconcentrator (Minicon, Amicon, Inc., Danvers, Mass.) and tested by immunodiffusion with a homologous antibody for each fungi.

ISOLATION AND IDENTIFICATION OF YEASTS

In the past, *Candida albicans* and *Cryptococcus neoformans* were considered the only true pathogenic yeasts. Indeed, in many laboratories these are still the only yeasts identified to the species level. The advent of cancer chemotherapy, radiotherapy, steroids, and antimicrobial agents has contributed to a milieu in which not only are cellular and humoral immune functions compromised, but the normal microbial flora is altered or destroyed. One result of this complex change in the human biosphere is an environment where opportunistic microorganisms thrive without competition. *C. albicans* and *C. neoformans* are still major yeast pathogens, but the so-called non-pathogenic yeasts are being implicated with greater frequency as opportunistic pathogens in the compromised host.

Yeasts can be friends and enemies to humans. They have numerous applications in food preparation. Yet yeast infections of the mucous membranes, such as thrush and *Candida* vaginitis, afflict millions worldwide. Although localized yeast infections may be merely a nuisance, other yeast infections can be deadly. Yeasts in the bloodstream (fungemia) are often a result of intravenous catheterization or parenteral

matitidis readily converts from mold to yeast form at 37°C on enriched media. The exoantigen procedure is also an excellent method to confirm its identification.

Isolates of *P. brasiliensis* are slow growing, and its hyphae are typically sterile. Some fresh isolates produce one-celled, hyaline, smooth-walled, small conidia laterally from the hyphae on short hyphae-like conidiophores. When grown at 37°C, the fungus produces large, one-celled, thick-walled yeast cells that have multiple blastoconidia attached by narrow tubular necks. This is often referred to as "multiple budding." Some of the yeast cells may be as large as 30 μm in diameter. Because isolates may either be sterile or resemble isolates of *Chrysoporium*, their identification must be confirmed. The exoantigen is recommended procedure because of its accuracy and speed.

Table 54-16   Mold-to-tissue conversion of the dimorphic fungi

Fungus	Media and conditions	Morphologic form obtained	Some similar fungi at 25° C
Blastomyces dermatitidis	KT medium, Kelley agar, or blood agar, 37° C	Yeast	*Chrysosporium* spp.
Coccidioides immitis	Modified Converse medium, 40° C, 5% to 10% CO_2	Spherules containing endospores	*Malbranchea* spp.
Histoplasma capsulatum	Pines medium or glucose-cysteine-blood (GCB) agar,[a] 37° C	Yeast	*Sepedonium* spp., *Chrysosporium* spp.
Paracoccidioides brasiliensis	BHI agar, 37° C	Yeast	*Chrysosporium* spp., Mycelia Sterilia
Sporothrix schenckii	BHI agar, 37° C, 5% to 10% CO_2	Yeast	*Acrodontium* spp., *Sporothrix* spp.

[a]GCB agar is 1% glucose, 0.1% cysteine, and 10% rabbit or sheep blood.

nutrition (hyperalimentation). Invasion of the heart valves by yeasts can follow the installation of artificial valves, resulting in endocarditis. Overwhelming disseminated yeast infections can contribute to the death of cancer patients and, more recently, patients with acquired immunodeficiency syndrome (AIDS).

Because yeasts are part of the normal human microflora, their isolation from clinical specimens that originate from nonsterile sites may create misunderstanding about their significance. Yeasts in mixed culture and in small numbers from a site contiguous to mucous membranes (sputum, urine, feces, and vagina) are not usually treated as pathogens without additional clinical information. Yet their isolation from a sterile body fluid or tissue specimen is cause for concern. The presence of yeasts in pure culture and in large numbers from any body site is highly suspect. Effective and rapid communication with the physician should be used to determine the significance of an isolate.

Laboratory identification

Yeasts are frequently recovered from sputum and urine; less frequently from blood, and cerebrospinal fluid. No special techniques are necessary for isolating yeasts from clinical specimens. For direct specimen examination, material from the vagina, mouth, or other sites contiguous to mucous membranes may be Gram stained. KOH, which unlike Gram stains does not distort the yeast, can also be used. Figure 54-40 shows budding yeast and pseudohyphae of *C. albicans* in sputum.

Culture and isolation

A variety of media are available for the initial isolation of yeasts. In practice, yeasts are most commonly isolated on either mycology media without antimicrobial agents or enriched bacteriologic media, such as brain heart infusion agar, trypticase soy agar, or Columbia agar. Media with cyclohex-

imide (0.5 mg/ml) are never used alone because yeasts such as *C. neoformans* are inhibited by cycloheximide. Caffeic acid agar is a good isolation medium for *C. neoformans*. This yeast produces a characteristic brown-black pigmented colony because of the enzymatic deposition of melanin in the cell wall.

Most pathogenic yeasts grow well at both 25° and 35°C. The inability of some yeasts to grow at 35°C typically denotes a saprophytic nature.

Reference texts provide sophisticated schemes for identifying yeasts. Because of the expanding role of yeasts in human disease, simple approaches like the germ-tube test may need supplements. A number of commercial yeast identification kits that markedly increase the proficiency of laboratories are available. When a yeast is isolated, the following procedure should be performed: microscopic morphology, germ-tube test, chlamydospore production, physiological tests.

Microscopic morphology

The microscopic morphologic structure of yeast is evaluated by using a wet mount. The presence of capsules and ascospores and the purity of the culture can be determined in a wet mount. Capsule formation can be confirmed with an India ink preparation. If capsules are seen, a rapid swab urease test may be performed to presumptively confirm the identity of *C. neoformans*. The presence of ascospores suggests ascosporogenous yeasts such as *Saccharomyces* and *Pichia*. Because special media and physiologic tests are required to identify these organisms, ascomycetous yeasts are usually sent to a mycology reference laboratory.

Germ-tube test

A rapid screening for *C. albicans* is the germ-tube test (see Figure 54-1). A light suspension of yeast is added to 0.5 ml of bovine, sheep, or human serum. (If human serum is

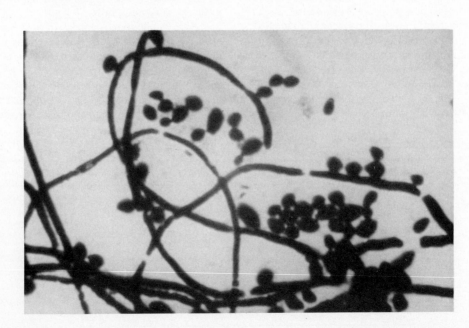

Fig. 54-40   Gram stain of sputum showing budding yeast cells and pseudohyphae of *Candida albicans*.

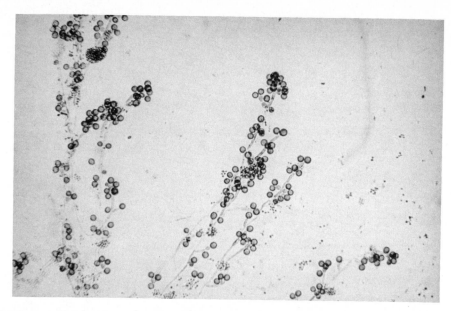

Fig. 54-41 Typical thick-walled chlamydospores produced by *Candida albicans* on cornmeal agar. *Courtesy L. Ajello.*

used, it must be hepatitis B surface antigen [Hb$_s$Ag] and HIV antibody free). The inoculated serum is incubated in a water bath at 35°C for two to three hours. If germ tubes are present, they can be seen readily with the ×40 high-dry objective. A germ tube has parallel walls at its origin from the yeast cell. Because germ tubes are the beginning of the formation of hyphae, they grow by linear elongation from the yeast cell. Hence their walls at the union of the cell are parallel and not constricted, as in elongated blastoconidia. Virtually all *C. albicans,* as well as rare isolates of *C. stellatoidea,* produce germ tubes. *C. tropicalis* may rarely produce germ tubes.

Chlamydospore production

If the germ-tube test is negative, more extensive morphologic analysis, such as chlamydospore production, is required. The culture is inoculated to either cornmeal agar with 0.3% Tween-80, rice extract agar, or yeast morphology agar. The yeast inoculum is diluted on the medium in the form of streak lines on the surface. A cover glass through which the fungus can be microscopically observed is placed on the agar surface. The agar plates are incubated at 22° to 25°C for one to two days. *C. albicans* and *C. stellatoidea* produce thick-walled chlamydospores (Figure 54-41.) *Cryptococcus, Rhodoturula,* and *Torulopsis* organisms are unicellular, nonfilamentous yeasts. Their differential morphology is outlined in Figure 54-42.

Physiologic tests

Precise identification of yeasts to the species level cannot be made on the basis of morphology alone. Tests for carbohydrate assimilation, alcohol assimilation, nitrate utilization, urease production, and, occasionally, carbohydrate fermentation must be performed.

Assimilation is the aerobic utilization of a carbon source

by a yeast. Glucose, for example, is oxidized to carbon dioxide and water. Assimilation can be measured by observing growth in the presence of the assimilable carbon substrate.

It is recommended that one of the commercial assimilation systems, such as the API 20C yeast identification kit or the Uni-Yeast-Tek identification system be used.

Fermentation is the anaerobic utilization of a carbohydrate, resulting in the production of CO_2 and ethanol. Detection of fermentation, therefore, occurs by gas production (CO_2) and not by pH change. Sugars used for yeast fermentation differ from sugars used for testing bacterial fermentation. Some of the kits for rapid yeast identification also incorporate fermentable substrates. Fermentation tests are rarely necessary for identifying yeasts. The physiologic patterns of yeasts can be seen in Table 54-17.

ISOLATION AND IDENTIFICATION OF OPPORTUNISTIC FUNGI

The most common opportunistic fungi are zygomycetes, *Aspergillus, Candida,* and *Cryptococcus.* This section summarizes the mycologic basis for their identification. The other fungi are discussed in previous sections. In addition, other saprophytic fungi that are usually contaminants but that may be pathogenic are presented both in tabular form and in photomicrographs. Under the appropriate conditions, most of the so-called saprophytic fungi are probably capable of causing opportunistic infection in a compromised host.

Direct examination

Sputum, other pulmonary specimens, and tissue should be placed on a microscope slide containing a drop of 10% to 20% potassium hydroxide (KOH) and then examined. Tissue is minced in sterile saline. Body fluids, which are usually sterile, should be centrifuged. Caseous tissue should be

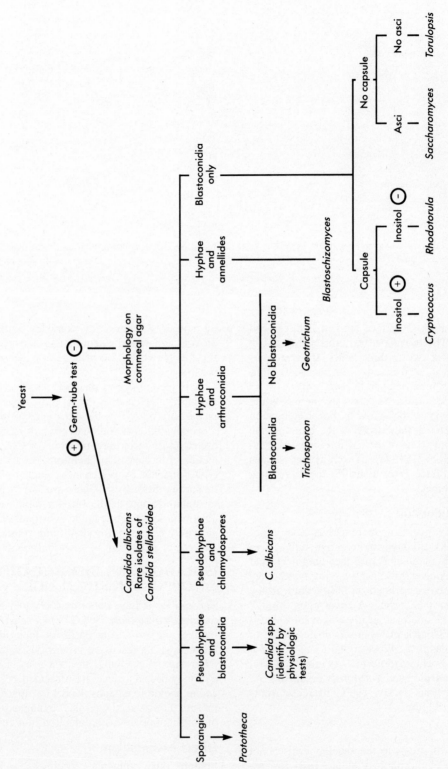

Fig. 54-42   Practical approach to initial identification of yeasts and yeastlike fungi.

Table 54-17 Physiologic patterns of the various yeasts

Genus and species	Celliobiose	Inositol	Melibiose	Trehalose	Germ-tube production	Growth at 37°C	KNO₃ utilization	Urease production	Galactose	Lactose	Raffinose	Xylose	Glucose	Maltose	Sucrose
Blastoschizomyces capitatus	−	+/v	+	−	−	−	−	−	−	−	−	−	+	−	−
Candida albicans	−	+	+	−	−	+	−	−	−	−	−	+	+	−	−
Candida guilliermondii	+	+	+	−	−	+	+	+	+	+	+	−	+	−	−
Candida krusei	−	−	+	−	−	−	−	−	−	−	−	−	+	−	+/v
Candida parapsilosis	−	+	+	−	−	+	−	−	+	+	+	−	+	−	−
Candida pseudotropicalis	+	+	+	−	+	−	−	+	+	−	+/v	−	+		
Candida rugosa	−	−	+	−	−	+	−	−	−	−	−	−	−	−	−
Candida stellatoidea	−	+	+	−	−	+	−	−	−	+/v	+	+	+	−	−
Candida tropicalis	+/v	+	+	−	−	+	−	−	+	+	+	−	+	−	−
Cryptococcus albidus var. *albidus*	+	−/v	+	+	+/v	+	−/v	+	+	+	+	−	+	+	+
Cryptococcus albidus var. *diffluens*	+	−/v	+	+	−	+	+/v	+	+	+	+	−	+	+	+
Cryptococcus gastricus	+	+	+	+	−	+	−	−	−/v	+	+	−	−	−	+
Cryptococcus laurentii	+	+	+	+	+	+	+/v	+/v	+	+	+	−	+	−	+
Cryptococcus luteolus	+	+	+	+	−	+	+	−/v	+	+	+	−	+	−	+
Cryptococcus neoformans	+	+/v	+	+	−	+	−	+/v	+	+	+	−	+	−	+
Cryptococcus terreus	+	+/v	+	+	−/v	+/v	+	−	−/v	+	+	−	+	+	+
Cryptococcus unguttulatus	−/v	−/v	+	+	−	+	−/v	+/v	+	+/v	+	−	+	−	+
Geotrichum candidum (not a yeast but may be confused with yeasts)	−	+	+	−	−	−	−	−	−	−	+	−	−	−	−
Rhodotorula glutinis	+/v	+	+	−	−	+	−	+/v	+	+	+/v	+/v	+	+	+
Saccharomyces cerevisiae	−	+	+	−	−	+	−	+	+	−	+	−	+/v	−	−
Trichosporon beigelii	+	+	+	+/v	+	+/v	+/v	+/v	+/v	+/v	+/v	−	+/v	−	+
Torulopsis candida	+	+	+	−	+/v	+	+/v	+	+	+	+	−	+	−	−
Torulopsis glabrata	−	−	+	−	−	−	−	−	+	−	−	−	+	−	−

Symbols: + = Positive
            − = Negative
            v = Variable reaction

Table 54-18 Colonial and microscopic morphology of some clinically significant zygomycete genera

Genus	Colonial morphology	Microscopic appearance
Absidia	Rapid growing; woolly to cottony; olive gray	Sporangiophores branching, rising from stolons between rhizoids; sporangia pear shaped and contain one-celled, globose to ovoid sporangiospores; columella round, merging with apophysis
Cunninghamella	Rapid growing; cottony; white to dark gray	Elongate branched sporangiophores with terminal vesicle on which one-celled, globose spores form on denticles
Mucor	Rapid growing; woolly to cottony; white to gray brown	No rhizoids; branching or simple sporangiophores arising from hyphae; sporangia round, containing one-celled sporangiospores; columella variable
Rhizomucor	Rapid growing; cottony; white; becoming smoke-gray to brown	Sporangiophores develop from simple or branched aerial hyphae or stolons; rhizoids poorly developed; sporangia round, containing one-celled, round sporangiospores; columella round; thermotolerant; growth at 50° to 55° C
Rhizopus	Rapid growing; cottony; white to brownish gray; colonies tenacious	Sporangiophores long, dark, unbranched, solitary or in clusters; rhizoids at base of sporangiophores; sporangia black, round, containing one-celled, globose sporangiospores; columella hemispheric
Saksenaea	Rapid growing; woolly; white	Flask-shaped sporangia with long necks and rhizoids at base of sporangiophore

From McGinnis MR, D'Amato RF, and Land GA: Pictorial handbook of medically important fungi and aerobic actinomycetes, New York, 1982, Praeger Publishers.

Table 54-19 Colonial and microscopic morphology of some genera of fungi

Organism	Colonial morphology	Habitat	Microscopic appearance	Clinical aspects
Acremonium	Rapid growing; flat, membranelike; white-yellow-rose; older colonies with aerial hyphae	Soil; decaying organic matter	Conidiophores thin, erect, with tapering phialides; phialoconidia one celled and globose to cylindric, accumulating in balls at tip of phialides	Mycotic keratitis; mycetoma; opportunistic infections; occasional contaminant
Alternaria	Rapid growing; cottony to woolly; gray-white to olive	Soil; plants; decaying vegetable matter	Conidiophores sympodial, giving rise to branching chains of conidia; conidia acropetal and muriform, having swollen basal portion and terminal beak; walls darkly pigmented, olive brown to black, and smooth or rough	Implicated in allergy; occasional contaminant
Arthrographis	Moderately rapid growing; downy to powdery; cream-white to buff	Soil	Chains of one-celled, hyaline, cylindric arthroconidia on short hypha-like conidiophores	Occasional contaminant
Aureobasidium	Moderately rapid growing; moist and mucoid to pasty; white to pink; occasionally black; colonies become wrinkled	Soil; wood; fruit	One-celled oval to cylindric hyaline conidia developing from hyphae; conidia often bud to produce blastoconidia; thick-walled, dematiaceous arthroconidia often present	Unusual contaminant
Bipolaris	Rapid growing; woolly to cottony; olive green to black	Soil; plants; vegetable matter	Conidiophores sympodial, geniculate, brown; conidia multicelled, fusoid to cylindric, light brown, with slightly protruding dark hila	Mycotic keratitis and other forms of phaeohyphomycosis, especially sinusitis; unusual contaminant
Chrysosporium	Moderately rapid growing; granular; woolly to cottony; white to pale brown	Soil	Conidia one celled, broader than vegetative hyphae, terminal or along sides of hyphae; annular frill at base of conidium; random arthroconidia that are larger than parent hyphae typically present	Sensitive to cycloheximide; unusual contaminant; morphologically similar to *Blastomyces dermatitidis* and *Histoplasma capsulatum*
Cladosporium	Moderately rapid growing; velvety to woolly; grayish green to olive green	Soil; plants; vegetable matter	Erect conidiophores; septate, pigmented conidia one to four celled, pale brown with dark hila, in branching acropetal chains; conidia near conidiophore often shield shaped	Allergin but rare pathogen; occasional contaminant

Table 54-19   Colonial and microscopic morphology of some genera of fungi—cont'd

Organism	Colonial morphology	Habitat	Microscopic appearance	Clinical aspects
Curvularia	Rapid growing; woolly; olive green to black	Soil; vegetable matter	Conidiophores sympodial, geniculate, brown; conidia several celled, curved, with enlarged central cell and end cells lighter in color than other cells	Mycotic keratitis; endocarditis; other forms of phaeohyphomycosis; unusual contaminant
Exophiala	Slow to rapid growing; often yeastlike; becoming woolly; gray to black	Soil; wood; vegetable matter	Conidiophores hyphalike; annellides cylindric to flask shaped; conidia one celled, hyaline to pale brown, accumulating in balls; *Phaeoannellomyces* yeast anamorph often present	Occasional agent of phaeohyphomycosis; occasional contaminant
Exserohilum	Rapid growing; woolly to cottony; olive green to black	Soil; plants; vegetable matter	Conidiophores sympodial, geniculate, brown; conidia cylindric, multicelled, light brown, with strongly protruding dark hila	Phaeohyphomycosis, especially sinusitis; unusual contaminant
Fusarium	Rapid growing; woolly to cottony; white to purple	Grain; soil; decaying plant matter	Conidia of two types: macroconidia, multicelled, curved or sickle shaped, with foot cell, smooth walled; microconidia typically one celled, in balls or occasionally chains, similar to *Acremonium*; microconidia and macroconidia produced by phialides	Mycotic keratitis; mycetoma; burn infections; other opportunistic mycoses; occasional contaminant
Geotrichum	Rapid growing; cottony; white	Milk; fruit; soil; vegetable matter	Hyaline hyphae; arthroconidia cylindric to globose, one celled, in chains; conidiophores absent; blastoconidia absent	Rare opportunistic pathogen; occasional contaminant
Paecilomyces	Rapid growing; cottony to ropy; white to olive brown	Soil; vegetable matter	Erect, branching, septate conidiophores; phialides with tapering apices, in pairs, groups, or verticils; chains of one-celled, ovoid to fusoid conidia forming entangled chains; conidia may be pigmented	Endocarditis; other opportunistic mycoses; occasional contaminant
Penicillium	Rapid growing; velvety; usually in some shade of green	Soil; decaying organic matter	Conidiophores unbranched or branched; conidiogenous cells flask-shaped phialides produced directly on metulae; phialoconidia one celled, in basipetal, unbranched chains	Common contaminant
Scedosporium	Rapid growing; cottony; white becoming smoky-brown	Soil; vegetable matter	Conidiophores short, hyphalike, giving rise to cylindric annellides that often have swollen area just below apex; conidia one celled, nearly round to elongate, pale brown, accumulating in balls; some conidia solitary along hyphae	Pulmonary infections; mycetoma; other mycoses; occasional contaminant
Scopulariopsis	Moderately rapid growing; granular to powdery white, becoming tan	Soil; organic matter	Branched or unbranched conidiophores; conidiogenous cells annellides; conidia one-celled basipetals in chains, round, rough walled and flattened at basal portion	Nail infection; occasional contaminant
Sepedonium	Rapid growing; woolly to cottony; white to tan	Soil	Large, one-celled, hyaline to golden conidia on slender hyphalike conidiophores; phialides occasionally present	Sensitive to cycloheximide; rare contaminant, morphologically similar to *Histoplasma capsulatum*
Syncephalastrum	Rapid growing; cottony; white or gray to black	Soil	Sporangiospores formed in row within long cylindric sporangia (merosporangia); tip of sporangiophore swollen; rhizoids present	Rare contaminant
Verticillium	Rapid growing; velvety to cottony; white to pinkish brown	Soil; plants; vegetable matter	Conidiophores erect, hyaline to pigmented, often branched; phialides long, hyaline, arising in whorls; branches also in whorls; conidia one celled, ovoid to allantoid, accumulating in balls	Rare pathogen; rare contaminant

digested with pepsin before microscopic observation. This procedure breaks down the tissue and allows the microbiologist to see the characteristic structures of the aspergilli, that is, hyaline, dichotomously branched, septate hyphae. In the fungus ball, the hyphae may already be dead, and no growth occurs. If debris from the ears or material from the nose is examined directly, conidiophores may be seen. In acute aspergillosis, swollen, empty, enlarged hyphae also may be seen.

The zygomycetes are characterized by large (6 to 25 μm) hyphae, (see Figure 54-3). Tissue sections may be stained with periodic acid-Schiff (PAS), methenamine-silver, or eosin (H and I) hematoxylin stain to see the hyphae of both *Aspergillus* organisms and the zygomycetes. H and E-stained sections are often the best.

Culture and isolation

Specimens should be cultured on primary isolation media. Sterile bread without preservatives is also an excellent culture medium for zygomycetes. Cycloheximide should be excluded from the medium because many of the saprophytic fungi are susceptible to it at 0.5 mg/ml. Since the specimens received for mycologic examination are often heavily contaminated with bacteria, gentamicin or streptomycin and polymyxin B can be added to the isolation media. The sealed plates are incubated at 30°C.

Both aspergilli and the zygomycetes form colonies within a few days. The identification of both groups is based on morphologic examination; therefore, lactophenol cotton blue preparations of the isolated colonies and slide cultures should be initiated as soon as colonies are evident.

Reference mycology tests should be consulted for precise identification of both the zygomycetes and aspergilli. Table 54-18 summarizes the colonial and microscopic morphology of some zygomycetes.

Saprophytic fungi

Many normally saprophytic fungi can become opportunistic pathogens in compromised hosts. A few of these fungi may be confused with primary fungal pathogens because they have a similar morphologic structure. Table 54-19 summarizes the colonial and microscopic morphology of some of these saprophytes that are isolated from various clinical specimens.

SUGGESTED READING

Balows A, Hausler WJ Jr, Herrmann KL, et al.: Manual of Clinical Microbiology, ed 5, Am Soc Microbiol, 1991, Washington, DC.

Howard BJ, Klass J, Rubin SJ, et al.: Fungi and actinomycetes, part 3 in clinical and pathogenic microbiology, St Louis, 1987, Mosby-Year Book.

Kaufman L, Standard PG: Specific and rapid identification of medically important fungi by exoantigen detection, Annu Rev Microbiol 41:209-225, 1987; Annu Rev Inc, Palo Alto.

McGinnis MR: Laboratory handbook of medical mycology, New York, 1980, Academic Press.

Mishra SK, Gordon RE, and Barnett DA: Identification of nocardiae and streptomycetes of medical importance, J Clin Microbiol 11:728, 1980.

Rippon JW: Medical mycology, the pathogenic fungi and the pathogenic actinomycetes, ed 3, Philadelphia, 1988, WB Saunders Co.

Salkin IF and Robinson BE: Section 1 Mycology. In Wentworth BB, ed, Diagnostic procedures for mycotic and parasitic infections, Washington DC, 1988, Am Pub Health Assoc, Inc.

55 Viruses

Mark A. Neumann

Viruses are obligate intracellular microorganisms that range in size from under 30 nm to 300 nm. As a group, viruses are the most common cause of infectious illness in humans and, in the case of deoxyribonucleic acid (DNA) tumor viruses, are now known to contribute to the development of 20% of world cancers. Several characteristics—including size, simple organization, mode of replication, and nucleic acid content—distinguish viruses from other microorganisms. Viruses do not multiply by binary fission and contain only a single type of nucleic acid as genetic material rather than both ribonucleic acid (RNA) and deoxyribonucleic acid (DNA). Viruses may be specific for humans, animals, plants, or bacteria (bacteriophage). Within each group, viruses may infect only certain cell types or species.

The International Committee on Nomenclature of Viruses (ICNV) has assigned approximately 1400 viruses to approved taxa. About 500 more have been designated as "probable" or "possible" members of these taxa. Of the more than 61 families of viruses recognized by the ICNV, 21 contain viruses that infect humans and animals: seven contain DNA and 14 contain RNA. Although a wide range of these viruses may cause disease in humans, a much smaller number are frequent causes of disease. Thus, medical laboratories must be able to detect at least the viruses most frequently associated with disease. Detection of all potentially pathogenic viruses, however, is not yet possible nor practical because of limited knowledge of their pathogenesis or clinical role and because of the lack of technical methods and immunoreagents available to identify all potentially clinically relevant viruses.

DIAGNOSTIC CLINICAL VIROLOGY

Over the past decade exponential progress has occurred in diagnostic clinical virology. The impetus for this evolution of diagnostic clinical virology in part is due to:

1. explosive growth in understanding specific viral pathogens and their role in human disease, particularly in the neonate and immunocompromised patient;
2. newly discovered viruses such as human immunodeficiency virus (HIV) have posed a major public health threat;
3. recent evolution of antiviral chemotherapeutic agents—including adenosine arabinoside (Ara-A) and acyclovir (Zovirax) for treating herpes simplex virus (HSV) infections; ganciclovir for treating cytomegalovirus (CMV) and HSV infections; amantadine (Symmetrel) and rimantandine for treating influenza A virus infections; zidovudine (Retrovir) for managing infection with HIV; and Ribavirin for treating moderately severe infection with respiratory syncytial virus (RSV) in the very young—along with an ever expanding pharmacopeia of antiviral agents under development;
4. commercial availability of reliable, diverse mammalian cell cultures for ready isolation of many common, clinically important viruses and;
5. commercial availability of reliable immunologic reagents for a) identifying specific viruses in clinical specimens, b) confirmatory identification of viruses in cell culture, and c) acute-phase serologic diagnosis of specific viral infection.

With these clinical, epidemiological, and technical developments, diagnostic clinical virology has evolved at a time when increased economic pressures make it imperative to provide rapid, clinically useful, and cost-effective laboratory results.

In this chapter, the basic fundamentals of clinical virology are described. A methods approach for the laboratory diagnosis of viral infection is presented, including cell culture techniques, direct detection and identification of viruses in clinical specimens and culture, and rapid immunoserological diagnosis of viral infection using patient serum. Basic laboratory format and procedures are outlined as they pertain to the routine clinical virology laboratory. It is beyond the scope of this chapter, however, to present a detailed review of all methods and procedures of the clinical laboratory. However, a number of excellent references are available for this purpose at the end of the chapter.

VIRUS STRUCTURE AND COMPOSITION

Much of our current knowledge about viral structure has come from examining electron micrographs of negatively stained particles (virions). Each virus, or virion, consists of a nucleic acid core and a protein coat termed a capsid (Figure 55-1). The capsid of some viruses may be surrounded by another membrane called an envelope.

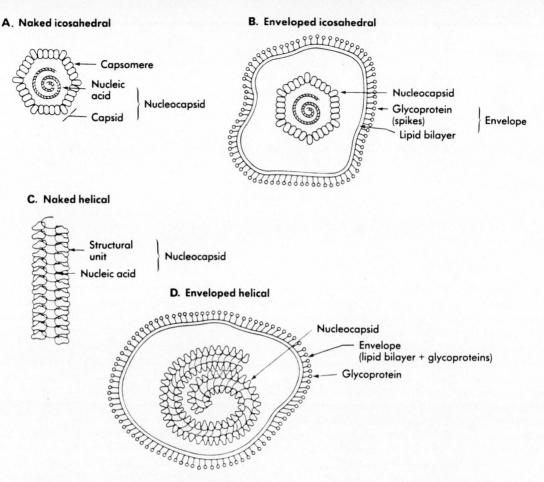

A. Naked icosahedral

Capsomere
Nucleic acid
Capsid
Nucleocapsid

B. Enveloped icosahedral

Nucleocapsid
Glycoprotein (spikes)
Lipid bilayer
Envelope

C. Naked helical

Structural unit
Nucleic acid
Nucleocapsid

D. Enveloped helical

Nucleocapsid
Envelope (lipid bilayer + glycoproteins)
Glycoprotein

Fig. 55-1   Schematic representation of morphologic groups of viruses. *From Freeman BA: Burrows textbook of microbiology, ed 22, Philadelphia, 1984, WB Saunders Co.*

The nucleic acid core of the virion is either DNA or RNA and encodes from three to four genes in small viruses to several hundred genes in large viruses. The capsid surrounding the nucleic acid core serves as a protective protein coat and is necessary for the virion to attach to the host cell. The nucleic acid core and capsid complex comprise the nucleocapsid (Figure 54-1). Nucleocapsids may have an icosahedral or helical symmetrical structure (Figure 55-1).

In some viruses, such as members of the herpes family, the nucleocapsid is surrounded by a loose membrane envelope (Figure 55-1). The envelope is composed of a lipid bilayer, glycoprotein, and matrix proteins. The envelope proteins are predetermined by the viral genome. However, the lipid and carbohydrate moieties of the same virus may differ in the presence of different host cells. The glycoproteins on the outer surface of the envelope appear as spike-like structures (Figure 55-1). The matrix proteins layer the inner surface of the envelope and may serve to connect the envelope and capsid. The presence of a lipid envelope causes a virus to be susceptible to inactivation by lipid solvents such as chloroform or ether. This property has served a great value in the effort to identify and classify certain virus groups.

The morphology of viruses is determined to a large extent by the size, shape, and symmetry of the virion and by the presence or absence of an envelope. Non-enveloped, or "naked," helical viruses appear as long rods; whereas naked icosahedral viruses are spherical in shape (Figure 54-1). Enveloped viruses, on the other hand, are pleomorphic since their outer membrane is not rigid.

The use of high-resolution X-ray crystallographic techniques has recently provided atomic-level views of viral structure. Identifying key microstructures, such as receptor sites or immunodominant domains, will likely provide the framework for a better understanding of structural features in virus-cell interactions.

VIRUS CLASSIFICATION AND TAXONOMY

The present universal system of virus taxonomy is set arbitrarily at hierarchical levels of family and in some cases subfamily, genus, and species. Viruses are classified by families on the basis of their morphologic structure and composition. Some of the characteristics used to classify viruses include: type and form of nucleic acid genome, size, shape, substructure, mode of replication of the virion, and the presence or absence of an envelope. Virus families are designated by the suffix *viridae* (Table 55-1).

Classification of virus families into genera and species

Table 55-1 Practical guide to laboratory diagnosis of common virus infections

Laboratory diagnosis of viral infections depends on appropriate selection and collection of clinical specimens early in the course of the patient's illness. Optimally, specimens should be obtained with the first three to five days of onset. Following collection, all specimens should be kept cold and transported immediately to the virology laboratory. For optimal specimen handling and processing, a brief clinical history specifying the date of onset, type of infection (or virus) suspected, and the major clinical findings should be included on the test request form.

Disease category	Associated virus(es)	Specimens that should be collected routinely	Special comments
RESPIRATORY TRACT			
Upper respiratory infection (including pharyngitis and common cold)	Rhinoviruses, Parainfluenza 1-3, Influenza A&B, Adenoviruses, Enteroviruses, Herpes simplex virus (HSV), Respiratory syncytial virus (RSV), Epstein Barr virus (EBV) and Coronaviruses	For children 2 yrs of age or less: Nasopharyngeal secretions or aspirate or nasopharyngeal swab, or throat swab; place specimen in Chlamydia/Viral Transport Medium tube.	1) If Cytomegalovirus (CVM) is suspected submit urine and blood (EDTA tube); submit serum/blood for acute-phase serology; store all specimens cold.
Croup	Parainfluenza 1-3, Respiratory syncytial virus (RSV), Adenovirus, Influenza A&B	For adults & children over 2 yrs of age: Throat washings or throat swabs or nasopharyngeal secretions or sputum or bronchial washings; place specimen in chlamydia/viral transport medium tube.	2) If Respiratory syncytial virus (RSV) is suspected, nasopharyngeal aspirates submitted in viral transport media for direct antigen detection using IFA or ELISA generally superior to culture.
Bronchiolitis	Parainfluenza 1-3, Respiratory syncytial virus (RSV), Adenovirus, Influenza A&B		
Pneumonia (children)	Respiratory syncytial virus (RSV), Parainfluenza 1-3, A, adenovirus, Varicella-Zoster virus (VZV), measles, (*Chlamydia trachomatic* in infants less than 6 months of age)		3) If *Chlamydia trachomatis* is suspected, collect a nasopharyngeal swab specimen and prepare a smear on glass slide and/or place in Chlamydia/Viral Transport Medium; be certain ample cellular material has been collected.
Pneumonia (adults)	Influenza A&B viruses, Adenovirus (rarely), (Herpes simplex virus, Varicella-Zoster virus, Cytomegalovirus, Respiratory syncytial virus)		4) If rotavirus is suspected, collect sputum in sterile tightly sealed screw-cap container.
EXANTHEM			
Vesicular rash	Herpes simplex virus (HSV), Varicella-Zoster virus (VZV), enteroviruses (coxsackievirus, echovirus)	Vesical fluid and scrapings and/or throat swab or throat washings and/or stool; place specimen in chlamydia/viral transport medium tube.	1) If cytomegalovirus (CMV) is suspected submit urine and blood (EDTA tube); submit serum/blood if acute-phase serology is desired
Maculopapular rash	Measles, Rubella, Enteroviruses, Adenoviruses, Cytomegaloviruses (CMV), Epstein-Barr virus (EBV), Parvovirus B-19, Human Herpes virus-6 (HHV-6)		2) If Varicella-Zoster virus (VZV) is suspected, collect scrapings of vesicle, prepare a smear on a clean glass slide and submit for direct IFA examination.
			3) If Epstein-Barr virus (EBV) rubella, or measles is suspected, submit 1.0-2.0 ml of serum for serologic testing; acute and convalescent sera (two weeks apart) will be required.
GENITOURINARY TRACT			
Vulvovaginitis, cervicitis (Female) penile lesions, (urethritis male)	Herpes simplex virus (HSV), *Chlamydia trachomatis*, Varicella-Zoster virus (VZV) (rarely)	HSV, VZV: Vesicle fluid (aspirate or swab; be certain to collect cellular material from base of lesion) and/or endocervical swab (female); place swab in chlamydia/viral transport medium tube. Chlamydia: Endourethral swab (male) or endocervical swab (female); use male/female chlamydia specimen collection packet.	1) A smear for direct immunofluorescent microscopy for Chlamydia is preferred at this time; a chlamydia specimen collection packet for males and females is available; if Chlamydia culture is desired, collect specimen as described; place swab in chlamydia viral transport medium tube.

Continued.

Table 55-1 Practical guide to laboratory diagnosis of common virus infections—cont'd

Disease category	Associated virus(es)	Specimens that should be collected routinely	Special comments
Acute hemorrhagic	Adenovirus	Urine: Collect 10 ml of urine in a clean or sterile screw-cap cup or vial.	
CENTRAL NERVOUS SYSTEM			
Aseptic meningitis	Enteroviruses (coxsackieviruses) echoviruses, herpes simplex virus type 2, Varicella-Zoster virus (VZV), mumps virus, lymphocytic choriomeningitis virus (LCM)	CSF, throat swab and/or stool blood (optional); submit CSF in sterile screw-cap tube; place throat swab or stool in chlamydia/viral transport medium tube; collect blood in a Lavender-top tube for culture.	1) If mumps virus is suspected submit urine. 2) In addition to culture, serology for HSV, VZV, mumps, and LCM is suggested as a diagnostic supplement to culture if these agents are clinically suspected. 3) If Togavirus (Arbovirus) (i.e. SLE, EEE, WEE, Dengue) is clinically suspected, submit serum for Togavirus (Arbovirus) serology; acute serum is acceptable for testing.
Encephalitis	Herpes simplex virus type I, Varicella-Zoster virus (VZV), arboviruses (togaviruses) (i.e., SLE, EEE, WEE, Dengue)	Brain biopsy and blood; submit brain biopsy in sterile screw-cap container (keep tissue moist); submit 2.0 ml of serum or serum separator tube, spin and refrigerate.	
GASTROENTERITIS	Rotavirus, norwalk-like agent, adenovirus types 40 & 41, caliciviruses, astroviruses	Stool: Collect 1-5 ml or 1-5 gm of stool in a clean screw-cap container.	1) Direct antigen detection (ELISA) is performed for rotavirus and adenovirus types 40 & 41. 2) Norwalk agent, caliciviruses, and astroviruses are detected using electron microscopy.
OPHTHALMIC			
Conjunctivitis, Keratitis	Herpes simplex virus (HSV), adenovirus, Varicella-Zoster virus (VZV), Enterovirus (Type 70-rarely), *Chlamydia trachomatis*	Conjunctival swab, corneal or conjunctival scraping, place swab (specimen) in chlamydia/viral transport medium tube.	1) Direct smear of clinical material for HSV, adenovirus and chlamydia may also be performed if requested; submit scrapings in chlamydia/viral transport medium tube.
CONGENITAL & NEONATAL			
Teratogenic	Rubella, Cytomegalovirus (CMV)	CMV: Urine, throat, (Blood is also suggested but not essential); collect 5-10 ml of urine in a clean or sterile screw-cap cup or vial; place throat swab in chlamydia/viral transport Medium tube: Collect and submit blood in a lavender-top tube for cultures. Rubella: Throat swab; place swab in chlamydia/viral transport medium tube.	1) Acute phase serology for CMV rubella, and/or toxoplasma may also be performed. Submit 1.5 ml of serum (or serum separator tube, spin and refrigerate).

Table 55-1 Practical guide to laboratory diagnosis of common virus infections—cont'd

Disease category	Associated virus(es)	Specimens that should be collected routinely	Special comments
Disseminated disease	Enteroviruses (Coxsackieviruses, Echoviruses), Cytomegalovirus, Herpes simplex virus, Varicella-Zoster virus, Hepatitis B	Throat or nasal swab, eye swab, urine, blood, swab and/or scrapings of skin lesions. Place swab(s) or scrapings in chlamydia/viral transport medium tubes; collect 5-10 ml of urine in a clean or sterile screw-cap cup or vial; collect and submit blood in a lavender-top tube.	1) Suspected hepatitis B must be diagnosed by serologic methods alone. 2) Acute phase serology for HSV, VZV, CMV, Toxoplasma and/or hepatitis B may also be performed.
HERPANGITIS, STOMATITIS	Enteroviruses (Coxsackieviruses, Echoviruses), Herpes simplex virus	Throat swab or swab of oral lesion; place in chlamydia viral transport medium tube.	
LYMPHADENOPATHY	Epstein-Barr virus, Cytomegalovirus, Human immunodeficiency virus (HIV)	CMV: Urine, or throat swab, tissue (blood is also suggested but not essential); collect 5-10 ml of urine in a clean or sterile screw-cap cup or vial; place throat swab or tissue in chlamydia/viral transport medium tube; collect and submit blood in a lavender-top tube for CMV culture.	1) Evaluation for infection with EBV and HIV must be made by serologic testing; acute-phase serology may also be performed for CMV and toxoplasma.
HEPATITIS	Hepatitis A, B, C, D (Delta virus), Cytomegalovirus, Epstein-Barr virus, Adenovirus, Herpes simplex virus	Hepatitis A&B: Submit serum with request for acute hepatitis profile. Delta virus: Submit serum. Hepatitis C (non-A-non-B Hepatitis): submit serum. HSV: Submit serum for acute-phase serology; collect blood in EDTA tube for HSV culture. Adenovirus & Enterovirus: Throat and/or stool; place specimen in chlamydia/viral medium tube; collect and submit blood in EDTA tube for viral culture Label all specimens "blood precautions."	1) Evaluation for delta virus should only be done if patient is positive for HBsAg with compatible clinical history. 2) Positive screen test for HVC should be confirmed with bead neutralization test or RIBA
NON-SPECIFIC FEBRILE ILLNESS	Cytomegalovirus (CMV), Epstein-Barr virus (EBV), Human immunodeficiency virus (HIV), Human T-lymphotropic virus I (HTLV-1), Hepatitis viruses (see under Hepatitis).	Serum	
MISCELLANEOUS			
Carditis	Enteroviruses (particularly Coxsackie B)	Enteroviruses: Throat swab, and/or stool, pericardial fluid, and blood; place throat swab or stool in chlamydia/viral transport Medium tube; collect and submit blood in tube for culture; place pericardial fluid in sterile tube; submit for Coxsackie B serology.	
Myositis	Togaviruses (formally called Arboviruses), enteroviruses (Coxsackie A&B, and echoviruses), Influenza virus (particularly Influenza B).		
Parotitis, pancreatitis, orchitis	Mumps, Enterovirus, (particularly Coxsackieviruses)		
Arthritis	Rubella, Hepatitis B, Influenza viruses (rarely)	Mumps: Collect 5-10 ml of urine in a sterile container; submit serum for serology.	

Continued.

Table 55-1 Practical guide to laboratory diagnosis of common virus infections—cont'd

Disease category	Associated virus(es)	Specimens that should be collected routinely	Special comments
		Rubella: Submit serum for serology. Influenza: Throat swab or throat washings; place specimens in chlamydia/viral transport medium tube. Hepatitis B: Submit serum/blood for hepatitis B serology. Togavirus (Arbovirus): Submit serum/blood for Togavirus serology. Label specimen tubes "blood precautions."	
Acquired Immunodeficiency	Human Immunodeficiency virus (HIV1/2)	Serum	1) For screening or diagnosis for HIV1/2 submit serum for testing by ELISA and, if repeatably reactive, confirmation by IFA or Western blot. 2) PCR currently is the most sensitive technique for early antigen detection (submit ACD yellow top tube). PCR testing may be preferred for detection of HIV antigen before seroconversion. 3) Serum or plasma for HIV P24 antigen testing ELISA provides early definitive diagnosis in the newborn, detection of HIV in spinal fluid, and is useful in following therapeutic response. 4) Serum by HIV-IgA immunoblot assay provides early diagnosis of perinatal HIV infection.
Malignancy	HTLV-I (adult T-cell leukemia/lymphoma, tropical spastic parapesis): submit serum HTLV-II (adult hairy-cell leukemia?): submit serum Human papilloma virus (HPV): submit cervical scrapings or biopsy for nucleic acid in situ hybridization.		

is based on antigenicity and other physiochemical and biological properties. Virus genera are designated by the suffix *virus* (Table 55-1). The term "virus" generally represents groups of species that share certain characteristics and are distinct from other groups of species. The taxonomic application of virus species has yet, to be fully defined. Nor have associated nomenclature problems been resolved by virology taxonomists. The ominous task of virus classification and nomenclature has been largely undertaken and published by the ICTV, entitled *The Classification and Nomenclature of Viruses,* in the journal Intervirology.

Table 55-2 lists the characteristics, classification, and nomenclature of the major viruses that infect humans. Figure 55-2 illustrates the morphology of many of these viruses.

VIRUS REPLICATION

Unlike bacteria, viruses have few or no enzymes and can produce only in susceptible host cells, where they utilize the host cell's replicative "machinery" for synthesis of their progeny. The virion's separate components are synthesized and then assembled. Viral nucleic acid must then enter the host cell nucleus and specify the synthesis. This process takes place in a number of ways, depending on the virus and the type and configuration of its nucleic acid. Regardless

Table 55-2   Classification of important DNA viruses infecting humans

Capsid symmetry	Envelope	Site of capsid assembly	Size (diameter in nm)	Family	Genus	Common name
Icosahedral	No	Nucleus	45-55	Papovaviridae	Papovavirus A Papovavirus B	Wart virus BK and JC viruses
Icosahedral	No	Nucleus	18-26	Papovaviridae	Papovavirus	Possibly Norwalk agent
Icosahedral	No	Nucleus	45-55	Adenoviridae	Mastadenovirus	Adenovirus
Icosahedral	Yes	Nucleus	100	Herpesviridae	Alphaherpesvirinae Betaherpesvirinae Gammaherpesvirinae	Herpes simplex virus, Varicella-Zoster virus Cytomegalovirus Epstein-Barr virus
Complex	Complex coats	Cytoplasm	230 × 300	Poxviridae	Orthopoxvirus	Smallpox virus (variola), Vaccinia virus
Complex	Yes	Unknown	42	Hepadnaviridae	Not classified	Hepatitis B virus

Classification of important RNA viruses infecting humans

Capsid symmetry	Envelope	Site of capsid assembly	Size (nm)	Configuration of RNA	Family	Genus	Common Name
Icosahedral	No	Cytoplasm	24-30	SS(+)	Picornaviridae	Enterovirus	Poliovirus, Coxsackie Echovirus, Hepatitis A virus
						Rhinovirus	Rhinovirus (cold virus)
			70	DS(segmental)	Reoviridae	Rotavirus	Rotavirus
	Yes	Cytoplasm	60	SS(+)	Togaviridae	Alphavirus	Arbovirus (Group A)
			40			Flavivirus	Arbovirus (Group B)
			60			Rubivirus	Rubella virus
Helical	Yes	Cytoplasm	80-120	SS(−) segmental	Orthomyxoviridae	Influenzavirus	Influenza virus
			150-300	SS(−)	Paramyxoviridae	Pneumovirus Paramyxovirus Morbillivirus	Respiratory syncytial virus Parainfluenza virus, Mumps virus Measles virus
			60 × 180	SS(−)	Rhabdoviridae	Lyssavirus	Rabies virus
Unknown/ unsymmetric	Yes	Cytoplasm	50-300	SS	Arenaviridae	Arenavirus	Lymphocytic choriomeningitis meningitis virus, Lassa fever virus
			80-100	SS(+)	Coronaviridae	Coronavirus	Human coronavirus
			100	SS	Bunyaviridae	Bunyavirus	Bunyamwera, California encephalitis virus
Icosahedral capsid with probable helical nucleocapsid	Yes	Cytoplasm	100	SS(+)	Retroviridae Subfamily Oncoviridae Subfamily Lentiviridae	Oncovirus Lentivirus	Leukosis, Sarcoma, Mammary tumor viruses Slow-acting viruses

SS = Single stranded
DS = Double stranded
+ = Positive strand; strand that functions as mRNA
− = Negative strand; strand that must first be transcribed

of nucleic acid type, however, the classic cycle of viral replication involves the following steps:

1. Attachment and adsorption. The first step in replication is when virus attaches to specific host cell receptor sites.
2. Penetration. Penetration rapidly follows adsorption. Viruses may penetrate host cells in one of two ways, fusion or phagocytosis, depending on whether or not the virus is enveloped.
3. Uncoating. The viral capsid is shed, probably as a result of host cell enzymes, exposing nucleic acid.
4. Eclipse. During the eclipse phase, viral nucleic acid

functions as a template for the production of "messenger" RNA (mRNA), which codes and directs the synthesis of viral proteins. Viral nucleic acid is duplicated and viral structural proteins are then synthesized, followed by random assembly. Protein synthesis occurs in the host cell cytoplasm, but capsid formation may occur in the cytoplasm or nucleus.
5. Maturation. Assembly of intact virions proceeds in the host cell cytoplasm.
6. Release. During the final replicative step, mature assembled virions are extruded from the host cell. The nucleocapsid of enveloped viruses migrate to the host

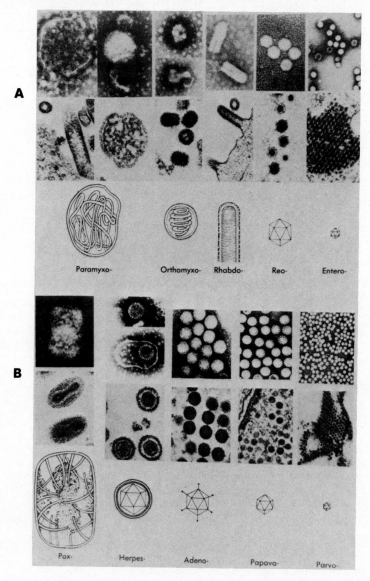

Fig. 55-2 Electron micrographs. **A,** RNA viruses and **B,** DNA viruses in negatively stained preparations (top row) and in thin sectioned cells (middle row) as compared with schematic drawings (bottom row). *From Hsiung G, Fong CKY, and August MJ: Prog Med Virol 25:133, 1979.*

cell nuclear or cytoplasmic membrane, depending on the virus. The membrane then surrounds the nucleocapsid to form the envelope. Enveloped viruses are released by a process that is the reverse of penetration.

VIRUS INFECTION

How viruses interact with an intact living host to produce the signs and symptoms of disease remains a fundamental challenge to clinical virologists and, at this time, can only be conceptualized from lessons learned from the study of virus-cell interactions in in vitro tissue cultures. The process by which a virus produces disease in a living host is referred to as pathogenesis. The capacity of a viral infection to produce disease or death in a susceptible host is referred to as virulence.

In general terms the process of viral infection may be pictured as follows:

1. The process of virus-host interaction starts with a susceptible host's exposure to infectious virus under conditions that are conducive for transmission. Effective transmission of viral infection often is virus and host specific and depends on the presence of sufficient inoculum of virus particles in respiratory aerosols or droplets, in focally contaminated food or water, or in a body fluid or tissue (e.g., blood, saliva, urine, semen, or transplanted organ) to which the susceptible host is exposed. Transmission may also occur through direct inoculation of the host by an insect or animal bite (i.e., togaviruses and rabies virus). Certain viral infections can also be transmitted

vertically from mother to fetus or newborn child through virus in the mother's blood (e.g., hepatitis B virus [HBV], and human immunodeficiency virus [HIV]); birth canal (e.g., herpes simplex virus HSV, cytomegalovirus CMV); or breast milk (e.g., HBV, CMV). In some cases virus infection may result from the reactivation of endogenous latent virus, as may occur with varicella-zoster virus (VZV), CMV, HSV, HIV, and Epstein-Barr virus (EBV), rather than from de novo exposure to exogenous virus.

2. Following exposure, effective transmission, and initial infection, viral replication occurs within susceptible target cells, tissues, or organs, leading to local spread or viremia.
3. Primary viremia may result in parasitism of reticuloendothelial cells.
4. Following viral replication within reticuloendothelial cells, secondary viremia can occur with spread of the infection to distal visceral cells.

The onset of symptoms of viral infection vary depending on the type of virus and the infected host cell type. The onset of symptoms generally occurs with the initial invasion of susceptible host cells during the early course of infection, as with rhinovirus and coronaviruses. In other instances, symptoms may not appear until after secondary viremia and the invasion of target tissue or organs, as seen in poliomyelitis. In latent or dormant virus infections (e.g., HIV 1/2, HTLVI/II) or "slow" virus infections (e.g., progressive multifocal leukoencephalopathy [PML]), symptoms of disease may not develop for many months or years.

LABORATORY DIAGNOSIS OF VIRUS INFECTIONS

The spectrum of disease potential for any virus can be quite broad. A corollary to this is that certain infectious clinical syndromes may be caused by a number of different viruses (Table 55-1). However, careful clinicoepidemiologic and symptomatologic assessment frequently narrows the spectrum of possible viruses. Via-à-vis the patient's clinical symptoms and history are the most important factors in deciding which virus(es) may be the etiologic agent, and which diagnostic approaches will be most helpful to establish a definitive diagnosis. The most critical steps to establish the viral etiology are the determination of the most appropriate laboratory test(s) together with proper and optimal specimen collection, specimen transport, and performance of the laboratory tests by trained personnel (Table 54-1). Despite the broad range of viruses responsible for human disease, relatively few are detected in the diagnostic clinical virology laboratory with any frequency (Tables 55-1 and 55-2).

Approach to laboratory diagnosis

To accurately detect viruses in clinical specimens, clinicians must know which virus(es) are associated with diseases, which body site(s) need to be sampled to detect the infecting virus(es), and which diagnostic test method(s) are most proficient for virus detection for any given infection or body site. Table 55-1 is a practical guide to laboratory diagnosis of common virus infections. Table 55-3 assesses the three

basic laboratory approaches to detecting viruses of clinical relevance:
1. culturing of viruses in cell culture,
2. direct detection of virus antigen in clinical specimens and,
3. serodiagnosis.

The remainder of this chapter reviews these basic approaches to diagnosing viral diseases and describes the levels of services different categories of clinical microbiology laboratories should be able to provide.

LEVELS OF LABORATORY TEST SERVICES

The clinical microbiologist or virologist must carefully plan clinical virology test services that best meet local or regional needs and are consistent with the laboratory's philosophy and capability. The demands of physicians who utilize the laboratory also figure in these decisions. Laboratories should be classified according to level of service provided:

Level 1: Collecting and transmitting specimens to a reference laboratory.

Level 2: Limited isolation or detection of antigen for specific agents for which reagents are commercially available (e.g., herpes simplex virus or *Chlamydia trachomatis*). Other specimens are sent to a reference laboratory.

Level 3: Recovery of all viral groups that grow in commonly used cell cultures. Definitive identification of agents for which simple immunologic procedures suffice (e.g., immunofluorescence or hemagglutination inhibition).

Level 4: Level 3 plus definitive serotypic identification of all commonly isolated viruses including use of neutralization tests and typing of strains of influenza virus A and B.

Level 5: Isolation and complete identification of all viruses, including inoculation of animals where appropriate (see Chapter 2).

Levels 1 and 2 are most appropriate for small to mid-sized community hospitals. Levels 3 and 4 might be appropriate for large community hospitals and university medical centers. Level 5 is generally unwarranted and impractical for laboratories other than national reference laboratories that have proper containment facilities and well-trained personnel.

CELL CULTURE

The primary ("gold standard") diagnostic technique for most viral infections is isolation of viruses in cell culture. Other culture methods for isolating viruses, including animal inoculation and inoculation of embryonated hens eggs, are not practical for routine diagnostic virology laboratories and are used only by large public health and reference laboratories.

The term "cell culture" is used to describe animal or human derived cells growing in vitro that have lost their differentiation. Cells in culture may be grown as a single layer of cells on an internal surface of a glass or plastic container referred to as a cell monolayer. Cell cultures are of three types:
1. primary

Table 55-3 Modes of detection for common viral pathogens

Virus	Direct antigen detection	Cell culture	Serology	Comments
Adenovirus	+ +	+ + +	+	a) Culture and direct antigen detection using IFA or ELISA are preferred methods of diagnosis. b) For enteric (gastroenteritis-producing) adenoviruses types 40 & 41 direct antigen detection using a monoclonal antibody-based ELISA is the diagnostic method of choice. c) Clinical significance of isolate must be interpreted in relationship to serotype, clinical findings, and history.
Coronaviruses	0	0	+ +	a) Diagnostic testing not routinely available.
Cytomegalovirus	+ +	+ + +	+ +	a) Culture and direct antigen detection using IFA are preferred methods of diagnosis. b) Combination of conventional cell culture tubes and shell vial culture amplification greatly enhances detection of CMV and shortens time of detection. c) Acute-phase (IgM and IgG) serologic test kits are commercially available, allowing for rapid detection of CMV infection, particularly in primary infection.
Delta agent (Hepatitis D)	0	0	+ + +	a) Acute-phase (IgM and IgG) Serologic testing is preferred method of diagnosis.
Enteroviruses	+ /0	+ + +	+	a) Cell culture is preferred for diagnosis, particularly for Coxsackie B, Echoviruses, and Polioviruses. Cell culture is insufficient for some Coxsackie A viruses and inferior to culture-neutralization in suckling mice. b) Serologic testing is of greatest benefit in determining Coxsackievirus B 1-6 as a causative etiology in cases of myopericarditis. c) Direct antigen detection of enterovirus using nucleic acid hybridization holds promise for future. d) Clinical significance of isolate must be interpreted in relation to site infected, serotype, clinical findings, and history.
Epstein-Barr virus	+ /0	+ /0	+ + +	a) Serology for EBV-specific antigens using IFA or ELISA is the most sensitive and specific means of diagnosis and assessing stage of illness. b) Nonspecific heterophile antibodies (e.g., Monospot) are most readily available, but not reliable in children <4 years old. False-negative results in 10%-15% of cases during the first two weeks of illness.
Hepatitis virus A & B	+ /0	0	+ + +	a) Serology for Hepatitis A and B-specific antigens using RIA or ELISA are readily available.
Human immuno-deficiency (HIV-1/2)	+ +	+ /0	+ + +	a) Serologic testing using ELISA with confirmation of positive test results using IFA or western blot is preferred method of virus detection. b) Direct antigen detection of HIV in peripheral blood is generally useful for determining presence of HIV infection in infants using ELISA or PCR.
Human papilloma virus	+ + +	0	0	a) Direct antigen detection of HPV using in situ nucleic acid hybridization or southern blot analysis is currently available.
HTLV-1	0	+ /0	+ + +	a) Serologic testing using ELISA with confirmation of positive test results using western blot is preferred method of virus detection. b) PCR technology is now available for detection of peripheral leukocytes and spinal fluid.
Human herpes virus-6 (HHV-6)	+ +	+ +	+ + +	a) Serology for IgM and IgG antibody by IFA is commercially available. b) PCR is preferred for direct antigen testing from peripheral leukocytes.
Influenza virus A & B	+ +	+ + +	+ + +	a) Culture and direct antigen detection using IFA are preferred methods of diagnosis. b) Combination of conventional cell culture tubes and shell vial culture amplification may enhance detection of influenza virus and decreases positive culture detection by 50% in most cases.
Measles	0	+ +	+ + +	a) Acute-phase (IgM and IgG) serologic testing is preferred method of diagnosis.
Mumps	0	+	+ + +	a) Acute-phase (IgM and IgG) or acute and convalescent sera collected 10-14 days apart are the most widely available methods for diagnosis.
Norwalk agent	+ + +	0	+ / −	a) Diagnostic testing not routinely available. b) Direct detection of viral antigen using EM or IEM remains the "gold standard" for diagnostic testing.
Parainfluenza viruses	+ +	+ + +	+ + +	a) Culture and direct antigen detection using IFA are preferred methods for early diagnosis.

+ + + = Preferred and most available (commercial reagents) mode of detection
+ + = Secondary or less efficient or available mode of detection
+ = Not routinely available or consistently reliable
IFA = Immunofluorescent antibody assay
ELISA = Enzyme-linked immunosorbent assay
IEM = Immune electron microscopy
FAMA = Fluorescent antibody to membrane antigen

Table 55-3 Modes of detection for common viral pathogens—cont'd

Virus	Direct antigen detection	Cell culture	Serology	Comments
Respiratory syncytial virus	+++	++	++	a) Direct detection of RSV in nasopharyngeal secretions using IFA or ELISA is the preferred method of diagnosis. b) Shell vial culture amplification is rapid and more sensitive for isolation of RSV compared to conventional cell culture tube technique.
Rhinovirus	0	+++	−	a) Cell culture is the only routinely available method for rhinovirus detection.
Rotavirus	+++	0	+	a) Direct detection of rotavirus in the stool samples using EM, IEM, or ELISA is the most sensitive and efficient means of diagnosis.
Togaviridae and flaviviridae (alphavirus and flavivirus)	+	++	+++	a) Acute-phase serology using IgM antibody capture ELISA is the most rapid and promising means of diagnosis. b) Culture is not routinely available.
Varicella-Zoster virus	+++	+	+++	a) Direct detection of VZV in clinical samples using IFA or ELISA is often superior to culture in speed and sensitivity. b) FAMA is regarded as the most sensitive and preferred method for serodiagnosis; ELISA and anticomplement IFA are also acceptable for serodiagnosis.
Parvovirus B-19	+	0	+++	a) Serodiagnosis by IFA or ELISA for IgM and IgG specific antibodies is preferred for early diagnosis.

2. diploid
3. heteroploid

Primary cell cultures consist of a mixture of cells (e.g., kidney or lung) obtained by dissociation of cells from the minced organ. Generally, these cells can be maintained in culture for a limited time. Once subcultured ("passage") in vitro, a primary cell culture becomes a "cell line." The most commonly used cell lines are composed of fibroblasts obtained from kidney or embryonic lung. A cell line is diploid if at least 75% of the cells have the same karyotype as the normal cells of the tissue type from which they were derived. Such cell lines can undergo only a limited number (ca., <50-70) of passages in vitro. A cell line is heteroploid if more than 25% of the cells have an abnormal karyotype compared to the normal cells of the tissue type from which they were derived. Such cell lines can undergo unlimited or "continuous" passages in vitro. Cell cultures commonly employed by clinical virology laboratories include the following:

1. *Primary*
   a. RMK (from rhesus monkey kidney)
   b. CMK (from cynomolgus monkey kidney)
   c. RK (from rabbit kidney)
   d. AGMK (from African green monkey kidney)
   e. HEK (from human embryonic kidney)
2. *Diploid*
   a. WI-38 (from human embryonic lung)
   b. MRC-5 (from human embryonic lung)
   c. HEK (from human embryonic kidney)
3. *Heteroploid*
   a. HeLa (from carcinoma, human cervix)
   b. HEp-2 (from carcinoma, human larynx)
   c. Vero (from African green monkey kidney)
   d. A-549 (from carcinoma, human lung)

Since specific cell lines are susceptible only to certain viruses, most clinical virology laboratories employ one of each major cell type to provide a broad host range. The majority of clinically significant viruses can be recovered in at least one of the three cell culture types. Specimens submitted for isolation of viruses requiring less commonly used cell culture lines (i.e., coxsackie A, togaviruses) are forwarded to large reference laboratories. However, areas where coxsackie A and B viruses are highly endemic may require additional cell culture lines such as RD (rhabdomyosarcoma) or BGM (Buffalo green monkey). All of the cell culture lines discussed are available from a number of reliable commercial sources (Whittaker Bioproducts, Walkersville, Md.; Viromed, Minnetonka, Minn.; and Bartels Immunodiagnostic, Supplies, Bellevue, Wash.).

Cell cultures require two types of media, growth and maintenance, for their sustenance. Cell culture media require essential vitamins, amino acids, and serum factors for optimal cell viability. Growth media contain these essential nutrients along with a high (ca. 10%) serum concentration to produce active cell growth (replication); and are employed to produce cell monolayers. Maintenance media consist of the same nutrients but only a 2% to 5% serum concentration to keep cells in a steady state of metabolism. The latter is employed during virus isolation in cell culture. Most virologists do not use serum in media formulations for maintenance of primary monkey kidney cell cultures. In practice, once a confluent cell monolayer is produced, growth medium should be replaced with a maintenance medium prior to and during inoculation with clinical specimens for virus isolation. Eagle's Minimum Essential Medium (MEM) is commonly used both for growth and maintenance of cells, and is available through commercial suppliers. The vitamin and amino acid supplements in MEM remain stable when stored at 4°C, except for l-glutamine, which may need to be replenished on a weekly basis. It is critically important that the serum supplement used in preparation of these media be free of any infectious agents, including the mycoplasmas, and not contain antibodies to any viruses that may be present in clinical specimens. For this reason, either fetal, newborn, or agammaglobulinemic calf serum, available from commercial suppliers, should be used.

To reduce the risk of bacterial or fungal contamination, which may be harmful to cell cultures and/or obviate virus isolation, MEM may be supplemented with antibiotics such as penicillin (200 μg/ml), streptomycin (200 μg/ml) or gentamicin (50 μg/ml), and amphotericin B (1.25 μg/ml). Certain cell cultures may be contaminated with viruses indigenous to the tissue from which they were derived. This occurs with monkey kidney cells containing simian viruses (SV40, SV5, Foamy agent) that can destroy cell monolayers. In an attempt to control this problem, simian virus antiserum can be added to monkey kidney cell lines. Unfortunately, these antisera may inhibit some strains of parainfluenza virus types 2 and 3.

Virus isolation

To facilitate proper virus isolation in cell culture, the clinical virology laboratory must be appropriately equipped and staffed. In turn the staff must ensure the appropriate selection of clinical specimens and the optimal transport of specimens to the laboratory.

Laboratory equipment

Equipment for the routine diagnostic clinical virology laboratory includes the following:

1. Appropriate grade (generally Class II A) laminar flow hood(s) to conduct specimen and cell culture manipulations.
2. One or more aerobic incubator(s) set at 35°C and equipped to hold the required number of roller drums (based on test volume) and sufficient shelf space to store one week's supply of cell cultures.
3. Roller drums to hold inoculated cell culture tubes and a sufficient number of motor-driven bases to rotate the drums.
4. Inverted light (phase-contrast optional) microscopes with ×4 and ×10 objectives to examine cell culture tubes (or flasks).

5. Temperature controlled horizontal head centrifuge(s).
6. Refrigerator(s) with −20°C freezer (non self-defrosting) for reagent and media storage.
7. Ultra low (−70°C or below) freezer to store reagents, virus isolates, and other materials.
8. Ultra-violet microscope for reading immunofluorescent antibody test procedures.
9. Other miscellaneous equipment items: vortex mixer, a 35°C and 56°C waterbath, a vibrating platform, electric pipetters, and sonicator (optional).

Specimen selection and transport

Table 55-1 details specimens that should be collected routinely for specific virus infections/syndromes. Generally, specimens collected three to five days after the onset of illness have a poorer yield in virus isolation. Aspirates, fluids, and tissues should be transported to the laboratory in a sterile leak-proof container. Swabs should be placed into a transport medium that includes antibiotics (penicillin, streptomycin or gentamicin, and amphotericin B). A number of transport media (e.g., Hank's, Leibovitz-Emory, Richard's, veal infusion broth) are available from reliable commercial vendors. Common collection devices include Virocult (Medical Wire and Equipment Co., Cleveland) and Viral Culturettes (Becton Dickinson, Cockeysville, MD). Standard bacterial culturettes that contain Stuart's medium may be used if necessary and if processed within four to 24 hours of collection. All specimens should be refrigerated (4°C) or kept on wet ice until they are inoculated into cell cultures because certain viruses (e.g., cytomegalovirus, respiratory syncytial virus) are labile to freezing. If specimen inoculation to cell culture must be delayed beyond four days, storage at −70°C or below is appropriate. Viruses such as RSV should be cultured within three hours post collection, or preferably at the patient's bedside, for optimal yield.

Inoculation and incubation of cell cultures

The basic procedural cycle for processing specimens for viral culture is detailed in Figure 55-3. In brief, transport

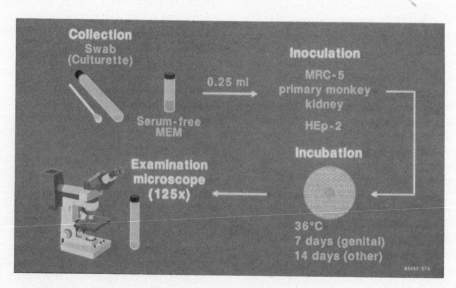

Fig. 55-3 Steps in processing specimens for viral culture. *Courtesy of TM Smith.*

tubes or vials that contain swabs should be vortexed and material from the swab expressed into the antibiotic containing medium. Alternatively, if Culturettes are received, they should be placed in a sterile 15 ml conical centrifuge tube containing 2 ml of serum-free MEM plus antibiotics. The tube should be vortexed and the excess fluid should be expressed on the swab and then discarded. Tissue samples should be minced and homogenized in a small volume of serum-free MEM plus antibiotics. Tissue or respiratory specimens that contain excessive debris or mucus may be clarified by low-speed centrifugation.

Fecal specimens should be centrifuged at 1000 xg for 15 to 20 minutes, followed by harvesting the supernate, filtering it through a 0.4 μm membrane filter and diluted 1:10 in serum-free MEM plus antibiotics to obviate potential cell culture toxicity.

Urine specimens should be centrifuged if visibly cloudy and treated with antibiotics as previously described. The pH of the urine sample should be between 6.9 and 7.2 to obviate potential pH-related toxicity to cell monolayers. Urine pH can generally be equilibrated by adding a few drops of sodium bicarbonate. Other normally sterile fluids such as CSF may be directly inoculated to cell cultures. Blood samples collected in EDTA (Vacutainer "lavender top") tube may be processed using the Sepracell-MN method (Sepratech Corp., Oklahoma City, Okla.) to harvest leukocytes. The Sepracell-MN method is quicker, more sensitive, less tedious, and less expensive than the conventional Ficoll-Paque procedure. Any specimen that is potentially contaminated with other flora should be treated with serum-free MEM plus antibiotics for 30 minutes at 4°C before further processing or cell culture inoculation.

Properly treated and processed specimens should be inoculated to appropriately selected cell culture tubes containing confluent monolayers. Maintenance medium from the cell culture tubes should be decanted using aseptic technique. Each cell culture tube should be inoculated in the following order: "diploid" cell culture tube(s), "heteroploid" cell culture tube(s), "primary" cell culture tube(s) with 0.25 ml of specimen. The order of cell culture tube inoculation will obviate the risk of cross contamination with viruses indigenous to primary cell lines. Inoculated cell culture tubes should be placed in a roller drum or horizontal test tube rack and incubated at 36°C for 30 to 60 minutes to achieve viral adsorption. Following adsorption, the inoculum medium in each cell culture tube should be replaced with 1.5 ml of fresh MEM plus antibiotics. MEM plus 2% fetal calf serum is recommended for diploid and heteroploid cell culture monolayers. MEM without fetal calf serum is preferred for primary cell monolayers. Any remaining specimen should be stored at 4°C for 24 hours in case reinoculation of cell culture tubes is necessary if toxicity has occurred in the initial culture tubes. Specimens should then be stored at −70°C or below for future studies.

Inoculated cell monolayers should be incubated at 35-37°C for recovery of most viruses. The optimal temperature of incubation for respiratory viruses is 33°C, but recovery of other viruses may be reduced at that temperature. Therefore, two incubators, one set at 35-37°C and a second at 33°C, are often used. Generally, two weeks of incubation is adequate for the recovery of most viruses. Viruses such as cytomegalovirus (CMV) may require 21 days for optimal recovery. If the recovery of only herpes simplex virus (HSV) is sought, the period of incubation may be shortened to five to seven days. More rapid recovery (72 hours or less) of viruses may be accomplished with specialized techniques such as shell vial procedures.

Identification of viruses for cell cultures

Most viruses produce certain types of cellular changes or cellular damage referred to as cytopathic effect (CPE). CPE can be observed by viewing the inoculated cell culture tubes on an inverted light or phase-contrast microscope at ×4 and ×10 magnification. CPE may occur as discrete foci or involve the entire cell monolayer. The type of CPE produced is often characteristic of the infecting virus in specific cell culture monolayers (Table 55-4). Thus, observing the time interval in which CPE is produced, and the cell culture type in which CPE occurs, generally helps to focus on a provisional diagnosis of a specific virus or virus group. Plate 1-11 is a photomicrographic representation of a HEp-2 cell monolayer infected with HSV. The cell monolayer reveals typical rounded swollen cells that become detached from the glass, a finding typical of HSV infection in this type of cell monolayer. CPE may be quantitatively assessed as follows:

- $+/- = <25\%$ of cell monolayer exhibits CPE
- $1+ = 25\%$ of cell monolayer exhibits CPE
- $2+ = 50\%$ of cell monolayer exhibits CPE
- $3+ = 75\%$ of cell monolayer exhibits CPE
- $4+ = 100\%$ of cell monolayer exhibits CPE

Cell cultures demonstrating $2+$ CPE or greater may be processed for definitive virus identification. Cell cultures that demonstrate only suspicious or low-grade CPE are subcultured to fresh cell culture tubes with fresh maintenance medium to stimulate enhanced viral replication. Blind subpassages (no CPE present) are not performed in most clinical virology laboratories due to the extremely low yield of such passages.

Some viruses, including the myxovirus and paramyxovirus groups (e.g., influenza, parainfluenza and mumps viruses), often produce little or no detectable CPE. As a result, certain procedures that capitalize on the hemadsorbing characteristics of these viruses are employed to determine the presence of these viruses. A hemadsorption (HAD) test (Box 55-1) should be performed on all primary monkey kidney cell cultures, particularly for specimens from respiratory sites, on day three, five, and 10 of incubation.

Once CPE reaches $2+$ and a provisional virus or virus group identification is made, more definitive identification of the virus can be made using an immunological technique. The mainstay of identifying viruses in cell culture is the direct or indirect immunofluorescence antibody (IFA) test (Box 55-2). A wealth of high-quality monoclonal (and polyclonal) antibody pools are available from a number of reliable commercial sources. Immunoperoxidase (IP) staining is a common alternative to IFA for virus identification. Like IFA, IP staining may be performed as a direct or indirect technique and has been applied in a modified peroxidase-antiperoxidase (PAP) stain. IP staining is identical to IFA staining except for the labeling method. In IP staining, the label is a peroxidase enzyme rather than fluorescein.

Table 55-4 Laboratory identification of common viral pathogens by cell culture

Virus	Primary PMK	Cell culture line[a] diploid HDF	Continous HEp-2	A549	No. of days isolation: mean (range)	Descriptive evidence of viral replication by CPE[c]
Adenovirus	+ +[b]	+	+ +	+ + +	5 (4-10)	Enlarged, rounded, grape-like clusters or lattice formation most predominant in A549 cell line.
Cytomegalovirus	0	+ + +	0	0	9 (3-21)	Compact or elongated small foci of enlarged rounded cells with slow contiguous progression.
Enteroviruses (polio-, echo-, coxsackie-)	+ + +	+	+	0	3 (2-5)	Focal swollen or shrunken refractile which may detach from glass of cell culture tube. Buffalo green monkey kidney cells enhance speed and recovery of a broad range of enteroviruses. MRC-5 cells provide the best overall isolation rate. Some coxsackie A strains are best isolated in suckling mice.
Herpes simplex virus	+	+ + +	+ +	+ + +	2 (1-5)	Enlarged-ballooned granular cells with occasional multinucleate giant cell formation. CPE often begins at the edge of the cell monolayer with rapid progression.
Influenza virus	+ + +	0	0	0	2.5 (1-6)	CPE may not occur at all or may appear as focal enlarged granular or vacuolated cells followed by sloughing and rapid progression. HAD[d] with guinea pig or human erythrocytes is generally necessary to demonstrate presence of viral infectivity.
Measles	+	0	+	0	8 (6-14)	If CPE occurs at all it appears as vacuolated syncytial giant cells. HAD with guinea pig erythrocytes may be necessary to demonstrate presence of viral infectivity.
Mumps	+ + +	+	0	0	7 (6-11)	Enlarged syncytial giant cells.
Parainfluenza virus	+ + +	0	0	0	7 (5-11)	CPE may not occur at all or may appear as focal rounding and multinucleated giant cells (type 2 & 3). HAD with guinea pig or human erythrocytes is generally necessary to demonstrate presence of viral infectivity.
Respiratory syncytial	+ +	0	+ + +	0	5 (4-10)	Enlarged refractile or ground-glass appearing cells with some syncytial formation.
Rhinovirus	+	+ +	0	+ + +	6 (2-9)	Compact or elongated foci of enlarged or shrunken rounded cells. Slow contiguous progression of CPE is enhanced by use of growth medium.

[a]PMK = primary monkey kidney cells; HDF = human diploid fibroblasts (e.g., WI38 and MRC-5)
WI38 = Wistar Institute human lung fibroblasts; MCR-5 = medical reserach human lung fibroblasts
HEp-2 = human laryngeal carcinoma cells; A549 = human lung carcinoma cells
[b]+ + + = Optimal cell line for virus isolation and detection of CPE
  + + = good (acceptable) cell line for virus isolation and detection of CPE
    + = generally insensitive cell line for virus isolation (CPE may occasionally be observed)
    0 = insensitive cell line for virus replication (CPE does not usually occur)
[c]CPE = cytopathic effect; may vary depending on the strain and concentration of virus and type, condition and age of cell culture
[d]HAD = Hemadsorption

IP techniques depend on the action of the active peroxidase enzyme on a suitable substrate to produce a color change. This change or indicator can be detected macroscopically using a standard light microscope.

Viruses that do not produce CPE (e.g., myxoviruses and paramyxoviruses) but are HAD positive can be identified using an antibody-antigen-specific hemagglutination inhibition (HAI) test (Box 55-3). The enterovirus group is comprised of 71 antigenically distinct serotypes. Thus they are not amenable to identification by IFA or IP procedures. Identification of enteroviruses is generally performed using a cell culture neutralization assay.

Alternative cell culture techniques

HSV isolation and identification systems

Because HSV accounts for approximately 80% of clinical virology isolates, considerable attention has been devoted to isolating these agents. Several commercially produced isolation systems have been designed specifically for rapid detection and identification of HSV. These packaged systems contain a cell culture isolation system specific for HSV and HSV-specific antibody labeled stain (usually immunoperoxidase) for detection of HSV antigen in cell culture following the established incubation period (usually 48 hours). Some of the more commonly used packaged systems include: Selecticult-HSV kit (Adams Scientific, West Worwick, RI), Cultureset (Ortho Diagnostics Systems, Inc., Raritan, NJ), and Cellmatics kit (Difco Laboratories, Detroit, MI).

The sensitivity of these systems compared to conventional cell culture varies. However, their specificity is good. These commercially packaged systems generally provide confirmation of HSV infection more rapidly than do conventional cell cultures. This is not unexpected because these

Box 55-1   Hemadsorption (HAD) test, for detection of orthomyxovirus and paramyxoviruses

PRINCIPLE

Members of the orthomyxovirus and paramyxovirus groups (e.g., influenza, parainfluenza, and mumps viruses) often fail to produce visible cytopathic effect (CPE) in infected cell cultures. However, as these viruses mature in the plasma membrane of cells within a susceptible cell monolayer, they insert virus-specific hemagglutinins into the membrane. These hemagglutinins combine with erythrocytes (hemadsorption) of certain animal species, permitting visual detection of virus infected cell monolayers by the HAD test. Viruses that both hemadsorb and hemagglutinate guinea pig RBCs are usually influenza A or B. The parainfluenza viruses and mumps virus generally produce only hemadsorption.

The HAD test should be performed on cultures of respiratory specimens (or urine in the case of suspected mumps) at three days postinoculation during influenza and parainfluenza season, and at five and 10 days postinoculation.

MATERIALS AND REAGENTS

1. Guinea pig (or human O or chicken) erythrocytes (RBCs) washed three times in dextrose-gelatin-veronal (DGV) buffer (commercially available). Use low-speed centrifugation between each wash step to prevent hemolysis. Prepare a 10% RBC stock suspension by adding 3.6 ml DGV and 0.4 mL of packed erythrocytes. The RBC stock suspension should not be kept for more than one week at 4°C. On the day of testing, prepare a 0.4% suspension of the RBCs by diluting the 10% suspension (0.4 ml) with MEM (9.6 ml).
2. Two uninoculated (negative control) primary monkey kidney cell culture tubes.
3. Two primary monkey kidney cell culture tubes; one inoculated with influenza virus and one inoculated with parainfluenza virus 2 (positive control).
4. Primary monkey kidney cell culture tube(s) inoculated with patient samples.

PROCEDURE

1. Transfer fluid medium from the control and patient cell cultures to sterile tubes using aseptic technique. A portion of the MEM may be used in the hemagglutination inhibition test if the hemadsorption test is positive.
2. Pipet 0.8 ml of fresh serum-free MEM and 0.2 ml of the 0.4% RBC suspension to each cell culture tube. Be careful not to cross-contaminate tubes; positive controls should be handled last.
3. Place cell culture tubes in a horizontal rack so that the RBC suspension covers the monolayer. Incubate at 4°C or room temperature for 30 minutes.
   NOTE: Cell cultures determined ↓ to be HAD positive following incubation at 4°C for 30 minutes may be reincubated at 20°C for one hour. If repeat microscopic examination reveals elution of RBCs, then the hemadsorbing virus is likely to be parainfluenza virus.
4. Rock the tubes gently and observe them microscopically for presence of hemadsorption. Hemadsorption must be evident in the positive control tube(s) and absent in the negative control tubes for the test to be considered valid.

INTERPRETATION

Hemadsorption is characterized by the presence of foci or plaques of RBCs adhering to the cell monolayer and microscopic agglutination of RBCs in the fluid phase. Hemadsorbing viruses may be definitively identified by detecting virus specific antigen in infected cell monolayers by immunofluorescence or immunoperoxidase staining or by performing a hemadsorption inhibition test or hemagglutination inhibition test.

MEM = Eagles's minimal essential medium

HSV isolation systems rely on immunologic identification of HSV antigen in the cell monolayer, whereas conventional HSV culture depends on CPE production by the virus. However, the commercially packaged HSV culture-identification systems lack the ultimate sensitivity of conventional culture and suffer somewhat with false-positive results. These systems are suboptimal in a reference clinical laboratory, but they may serve a useful purpose in smaller laboratories where HSV testing is desired and a quality reference laboratory is not immediately available or for laboratories only performing HSV testing.

Rapid shell vial culture technique

In 1984, Gleaves, et al reported their findings for rapid culture detection of CMV using a spin-amplification technique employing cell monolayers on 12-mm round coverslips contained in 1-Dram (3.7 ml) shell vials, and staining for early CMV antigen, "pre-CPE," at 36 hours postinoculation. The use of this culture technique compared to conventional culture demonstrated a promising rate of sensitivity and specificity of 100% and 94.7%, respectively. Since CMV CPE may not be detected in conventional cell culture for five to 21 days (average nine days) postinoculation, this culture concept revolutionized cell culture technology for clinical virology laboratories. To date, the rapid shell vial culture technique has been applied to early detection of a broad range of viruses (Table 55-5). The general incubation period for pre-CPE detection of these viruses ranges from 16 to 72 hours, thus allowing the clinical virology laboratory to report test results much sooner than with conventional culture. An added advantage of the shell vial culture technique is that it is amenable to batch testing. At this time, however, it may not be wise to totally replace conventional culture with the shell vial culture technique.

Box 55-2   Immunofluorescence microscopy

PRINCIPLE

Immunofluorescence microscopy provides a useful means of detecting viral antigen directly in clinical specimens and of providing specific immunologic identification of isolates from cell culture. If the viral antigen is known, the presence of specific antibodies in a test serum may also be determined. Immunofluorescence microscopy employs virus-specific antibody (monoclonal or polyclonal) conjugated to fluorescein isothiocyanate (FITC). After incubation and FITC-conjugated antibody and viral antigen, the presence of a reaction is detected by observing fluorescence viewed through a microscope equipped with a source of ultraviolet light. Either a direct (FITC-labeled antibody plus antigen) or an indirect (antibody 1 plus antigen followed by FITC-labeled anti-antibody x antibody) is used when performing immunofluorescence testing. Generally, the indirect method offers greater test sensitivity.

MATERIALS AND REAGENTS

1. FITC-conjugated specific antibody (direct method)
2. Unconjugated specific antibody and FITC-conjugated anti-species immunoglobulin. Note: Reagents from 1 and 2 are diluted to the optimal dilution (two- to fourfold below the last dilution that shows 3-4+ fluorescence intensity with a known positive specimen).
3. Phosphate-buffered saline (PBS)
4. Phosphate-buffered glycerol
5. High-quality fluorescence microscope, preferably epifluorescence with interference filters.

PROCEDURE

1. Apply specimen to a scrupulously clear glass slide, allow to dry, and fix in cold acetone for 10 minutes. For testing isolates from cell culture, decant cell culture fluid, scrape cell monolayer with a rubber policeman or typsinize cell monolayer, rinse the cell culture tube with PBS, and harvest cells, then proceed as if testing a clinical specimen.
2. a. In the direct test for viral antigen, the FITC-conjugated virus specific antibody is added over the fixed antigen substrate on the glass slide in a single step.
   b. In the indirect test for virus antigens, a two-step procedure is employed:
      i) Nonconjugated virus specific antibody is added to the portion of the glass slide containing specimen.
      ii) Following incubation (see step 3), the slide is rinsed to remove unrelated antibody. Then, add a FITC-conjugated anti-species immunoglobulin as in step 2a.
3. Incubation for step 2a and b is performed in a moist chamber for 30 to 60 minutes at either room temperature or 37°C.
4. Rinse slides three times in PBS, blot carefully and mount with buffered glycerol and add a glass coverslip.
5. Examine under an ultraviolet microscope.

INTERPRETATION

1. Specific fluorescence (usually >1+, preferably 3-4+) that has the pattern expected of the virus antigen sought and is not present in negative controls is a positive result.
   A positive and negative control antigen should be included with each rung or on each day of testing.

A good idea is to use this technology as an adjunct to conventional culture. In this fashion, clinical virology laboratories will enhance their overall, culture sensitivity resulting in a high yield of virus isolation. Some laboratories have conducted their own studies, however, and found that the shell vial technique in some instances may be used alone. Laboratory directors and supervisors are cautioned against this practice unless carefully designed in-house studies support their decision. Box 55-4 details the general methodology employed in the shell vial culture technique. Plate 1-12 shows representative photomicrographs of shell vials stained for CMV, HSV, and adenovirus using a monoclonal IFA.

Interpretation of viral culture results

Interpreting viral culture results with regard to the clinical significance of a specific virus isolate must be carefully based on a number of important factors. Clinicians and clinical microbiologists must be knowledgeable of the normal viral flora in the site sampled, the epidemiologic behavior of viruses and the clinical findings of the patient. A number of publications are available to assist with inter-

pretation of virus culture results. The following is a brief review of viral culture interpretation.

Viruses in tissue and body fluids

A virus isolate from CSF, blood, the eye, vesicular fluid, or tissue is almost always clinically significant. Viruses other than CMV recovered from urine are also almost always clinically significant of infection. Examples include adenovirus associated with hemorrhagic cystitis and mumps. The recovery of CMV from urine and tissue merits more careful consideration for assessing clinical significance. Briefly, CMV recovered from urine of newborns within the first three weeks of life essentially is diagnostic for congenital CMV, whereas the onset of viral excretion after four weeks of life reflects intrapartum or postpartum infection. CMV recovered from urine or tissue of adult patients is more difficult to interpret since CMV may be excreted in urine for a prolonged period of time after initial infection. Or it may be present in urine or tissue as a result of reactivated latent infection and therefore may not reflect the primary cause of the patient's symptoms. However, if CMV is isolated from multiple sites (e.g., urine, blood, tissue)

Box 55-3   Hemagglutination inhibition (HAI) test for detection of orthomyxoviruses and paramyxoviruses

PRINCIPLE

A number of viruses encode virus specific surface proteins that agglutinate erythrocytes of a variety of species. The viral hemagglutinating antigen (hemagglutinin) serves as a bridge between the receptor sites of erythrocytes, thus causing hemagglutination. The principle of hemagglutination can be used to detect certain viruses in infected cell cultures (or egg fluids for influenza virus). The identity of the virus or of antibodies in a patient's serum can be determined by specific inhibition of that hemagglutination using a hemagglutination inhibition (HAI) test. The HAI test is commonly employed for diagnosis of infections caused by the orthomyxovirus and paramyxovirus groups (influenza A & B, parainfluenza 1-3, mumps virus). The HAI test may also be used for diagnosing infection caused by "arboviruses" (togaviruses including rubella, flaviviruses and bunyaviruses) and adenovirus.

MATERIALS AND REAGENTS

1. Clinical isolate which produced a positive HAD test.
2. Influenza A specific immune serum.
3. Influenza B specific immune serum.
4. Parainfluenza type 1 specific immune serum.
5. Parainfluenza type 2 specific immune serum.
6. Parainfluenza type 3 specific immune serum.
7. Mumps specific immune serum.
8. Phosphate buffered saline (PBS) pH 7.2.
9. Guinea pig erythrocytes, 0.4%, in PBS, pH 7.2.

PROCEDURE

1. Treatment of sera.
   a. Removal of nonspecific inhibitors in sera is necessary for most viruses. Removal may be accomplished by physical means, such as kaolin, by enzymes such as neuraminidase or the receptor destroying enzyme (RDE) of *Vibrio cholerae,* or by a combination. The choice varies with the virus to be tested.
2. Prepare a dilution of the test fluids that contain 4 HA units per 0.025 ml. To determine the correct dilution of virus containing 4 HA units per 0.025 ml, divide by 8 the titer determined in preliminary titrations of 0.05 ml volumes. For example, if cell culture fluid was titrated in microtiter wells with an equal volume of 0.4% guinea pig erythrocytes (total volume 0.05 ml) and incubated for 4 hours at room temperature with a resulting maximum hemagglutination titer of 1:160, then a 1:20 dilution would contain 8 HA units per 0.05 ml or 4 HA units per 0.025 ml. Two milliliters of each antigen is required for the test. Standardize the diluted antigen with a back titration according to the following procedures:
   a. Carefully mark and label a microtitration plate.
   b. Using a 0.05 ml microdiluter, prepare serial twofold dilutions of each standardized specimen (undiluted to 1:32) in 0.05 ml volumes of PBS.
   c. After completing the dilution, place the loop in 0.5% sodium hypoclorite for 1 minute. Remove, blot, rinse in distilled water, and blot.
   d. Add 0.05 ml of a 0.4% guinea pig erythrocyte suspension to each well after completing procedure 6.
3. Prepare serial twofold dilutions of each serum, 1:10-1:5, 120 in 0.025 ml volumes of PBS and add 0.025 ml of a 1:10 dilution of each serum to the serum control well.
4. Add 0.025 ml of the standardized virus (4 HA units) to the wells containing sera.
5. Prepare a cell control by adding 0.05 ml PBS to a well.
6. Shake the plate on a mechanical shaker to mix. Allow the plate to stand at room temperature for 30 minutes.
7. After incubation, add 0.05 ml of 0.4% guinea pig erythrocytes suspension to all of the wells. Mix on a mechanical shaker, seal with tape, and allow the cells to settle at room temperature. Read and record the results.

INTERPRETATION

1. The endpoint is the last well at which partial or complete agglutination of the red cells occurs. A smooth or jagged shield of cells or an irregular button indicates agglutination. Observation of the movement of the button of red cells when the plate is tilted may help to clarify the end point.

with clinical findings suggestive of disease, it is generally viewed as clinically significant. Other test parameters, including histologic and serologic findings, may support or refute the significance of CMV from these sites.

Viruses in respiratory specimen

Isolation of respiratory syncytial virus (RSV), influenza virus, parainfluenza virus, measles, or mumps from respiratory sites is almost always significant because these viruses are rarely shed for long periods and asymptomatic carriage

is rare. Isolation of other viruses from the respiratory tract is more difficult to interpret. Enteroviruses can be shed for weeks, and adenoviruses, HSV and CMV, can be shed intermittently for months.

Viruses isolated from skin

The most common viruses isolated from skin lesions (usually vesicular lesions) are HSV, varicella-zoster virus (VSV), and some enteroviruses. When recovered from skin lesions, these viruses are always clinically significant.

Table 55-5 Performance characteristics of virus isolation using shell vials for low-speed centrifugation culture amplification

Virus	Shell vial cell line	Duration of incubation	Antigen detection confirmation method	Comparison to conventional cell culture tube		Special comment
				Sensitivity	**Specificity**	
Adenovirus	HEp-2	(24) 48h	IFA-Mab (CBC)	(52%) 97%	100%	
	Human foreskin fibroblasts	72h	IFA-Mab (Cambridge Bio.)	86.7%	100%	
Cytomegalovirus	MRC-5	36h	IFA-Mab (Biotech)	100%	94.7%	
	MRC-5	16-48h	IFA-Mab (Syva)	91%	96%	
	MRC-5	36h	IFA-Mab (DuPont)	86.4%	100%	Significantly more CMV positive specimens were detected by shell vial culture (n = 154; 84.6%) than in conventional cell culture (n = 126; 69.2%)
	MRC-5	16h	IFA-Mab (Biotech)	—	100%	Shell vial culture demonstrated greater sensitivity than conventional cell culture
	Human foreskin fibroblasts	16-18h	IFA-Mab (DuPont)	100%	92%	Less optimal for diagnosis of CMV pneumonia; 71% sensitivity and 50% specificity
Herpes simplex virus	MRC-5	16h	IFA-Mab (Syva)	97%	99%	
	MRC-5	16h	DNA probe (Pathogene, Enzo Biochem)	98%	99%	
	MRC-5	16h	IFA-MAb (Syva)	100%	95.6%	
	MRC-5 (24-well plate)	16h	IFA-Mab	70%	99.8%	
	Primary rabbit kidney	(8h) 20h	IFA-Mab (Syva)	(63%) 91%	(99%) 97%	Use of an 8h incubation for HSV shell vials is unacceptable for diagnostic use
	MRC-5	36h	ELISA (Ortho)	93.1-96.1%	99.9-100%	Pretreatment of shell vial cell monolayers with 10^{-5}M dexamethasone enhanced the detection of HSV and shortened the time of incubation
Influenza virus A & B	Medin-Darby canine kidney	40h	IFA-Mab (CDC)	84%	100%	
	Primary monkey kidney	(24h) 48h	IFA-Mab (CDC)	(56%) 60%	100%	
	Rhesus monkey kidney	16-18h	IFA-Mab (Wellcome Diagnostics)	90.9%	97.6%	Sensitivity and specificity for frozen samples was 87.5% and 100% respectively
Respiratory syncytial virus	MRC-5	72h	IFA-Mab (Whittaker Bio)	100%	91%	
Varicella Zoster virus	MRC-5	48h	IFA-Mab (Ortho)	100%	100%	The combination of direct IFA on clinical specimens and culture using the shell vial low-speed centrifugation method enhanced detection of VZV by 30%

IFA-Mab = Immunofluorescent monoclonal antibody; ELISA = enzyme linked immunosorbent antibody.

Viruses in fecal specimens

The most common fecal isolates are enteroviruses and adenoviruses. Their significance is often questionable because both can be shed in feces for many weeks (enteroviruses) or months (adenoviruses). Clinical significance is more likely if both respiratory and fecal specimens contain the same virus, less likely if only the respiratory specimen is positive, and least likely if virus is isolated only from feces. In these cases, serologic tesing for a rise in antibodies to the virus isolate can help determine clinical significance.

DIRECT DETECTION OF VIRUSES IN CLINICAL SPECIMENS

Direct detection of virus particles, their antigens, or their nucleic acids in clinical specimens is the most direct and generally the most rapid means for obtaining a specific viral diagnosis. Detection of virus particles requires electron microscopy, and detection of nucleic acids requires hybridization methods. Antigen detection, on the other hand, is done by immunologic methods using specific hyperimmune sera or monoclonal antibodies.

Box 55-4   General methodology for shell vial culture amplification

1. Culture system: 3.7 ml (l-dram) shell vials, each containing a 12-mm round coverslip seeded with a cell line monolayer (ca. 50,000 cells per ml) capable of supporting growth of the viral pathogen(s) of interest.
2. Remove maintenance medium from shell vial cell monolayer.
3. Inoculate not less than two shell vials with 0.2 ml each of treated specimen.
   a. Contamination of cell cultures can be prevented by treating clinical specimen suspensions with antibiotic; penicillin (200 µg/ml), gentamicin (50 mg/ml) and amphotericin B (1.25 µg/ml).
4. Close vials with a sterile rubber stopper, then centrifuge at 700 × g for 45 minutes at 30°C.
5. Add 1 ml of Eagles's minimal essential medium (MEM) containing 0%-2% heat inactivated fetal calf serum.
6. Incubate at 35°C. Duration of incubation must be based on the replication rate of the viral pathogen of interest and the antigen or epitope target of the immunoglobulin used for virus detection.
7. Following incubation remove cell culture medium and wash the coverslip cell monolayer twice with calcium and magnesium free phosphate buffered saline (PBS).
8. Fix coverslip cell monolayers in cold acetone for 20 minutes.
9. Stain with specific monoclonal or polyclonal reagent.

Direct detection of viruses in clinical specimens is the only primary means of diagnosing a number of viruses including enteric adenovirus 40/41, rotavirus, other gastroenteritis viruses, human papilloma viruses, and rabies virus (See Table 55-3). Direct detection of viruses in clinical specimens serves as a useful complement to culture or serodiagnosis for a number of other viruses including respiratory syncytial virus (RSV), other respiratory viruses (influenza A,B, adenovirus and parainfluenza virus 1-3), varicella-zoster virus (VZV), herpes simplex virus (HSV), hepatitis B, cytomegalovirus (CMV), and human immunodeficiency virus (HIV) (See Table 55-3). Following is a brief review of the primary methodologies used for detecting viruses in clinical specimens.

Light microscopic detection of viral inclusions

The detection of viral inclusions in smears or tissues by light microscopy has been the traditional means of directly demonstrating viral infections. In general, viruses that are assembled in the nucleus (usually DNA viruses) produce intranuclear inclusions, whereas cytoplasmic assembly (predominantly RNA containing viruses) yields cytoplasmic inclusions. This approach is generally used for detecting the presence of viral CPE in cells contained in the specimen and is most commonly applied to examining PAP smears (for HSV), eye scrapings (for HSV, adenovirus enterovirus), scrapings of cutaneous vesicles (HSV, VZV), urine cell sediment (CMV), and tissues suspected of viral infection. Diagnostic CPE of these viruses in clinical specimens can be reviewed elsewhere. Although this method of viral diagnosis is crude and insensitive (ca. 50%) compared to immunologic or hybridization methods, it serves a useful function in providing a rapid and inexpensive presumptive viral diagnosis.

Electron microscopy for detecting virus particles

Electron microscopy (EM) remains the "gold standard" to which other virus antigen detection methods are compared. Two basic techniques are used: negative staining and thin sectioning. Negative staining is simple and rapid. Clinical material is placed on a Formvar-carbon-coated copper grid, stained with potassium phosphotungstate, or uranyl-acetate and examined. Stain surrounds the virus particle, and the electron beam cannot pass through this metalic background but can pass through the low electron density of the virus. Therefore, a light virus is seen against a dark background. Virus particles are evaluated for size, shape, and symmetry, thus yielding likely identification. If necessary, immune electron microscopy (IEM) can be employed for definitive virus identification or typing. Specimens of vesicular fluid, serum, urine, respiratory samples, and feces are most suited for negative staining. It is the method of choice for tissue. EM is the only current means of detecting Norwalk agent as well as other gastroenteritis viruses (astroviruses, caliciviruses, coronaviruses). Unfortunately EM scopes are generally only available to those laboratories located in medical centers, research institutes, and some large commercial laboratories.

Latex agglutination

This method incorporates tiny polystyrene beads coated with virus-specific antibody (polyclonal or monoclonal) in a liquid suspension. A drop of clinical specimen in liquid form is added to a drop of virus-specific, antibody-coated polystyrene beads on a glass surface with a dark background. The presence of virus antigen will cause an antibody-antigen reaction with the virus-specific, antibody-coated polystyrene beads resulting in lattice formation producing visible agglutination. The latex agglutination test is most notably used in diagnostic clinical virology laboratories for detecting rotavirus in fecal specimens. This method offers good sensitivity and specificity for detecting rotavirus and compares favorably with ELISA tests. Latex agglutination has also been favorably used for detecting HSV in cell culture fluids but has not performed well in detecting HSV in vesicular fluids. Latex agglutination tests are generally inexpensive, rapid, require no special equipment or special technical skills, and are useful for laboratories with low test volumes. Further virus antigen test applications of latex agglutination will depend on achievable test sensitivities and specificities.

Immunofluorescence microscopy

With the surge in commercially available fluorescein isothiocyanate (FITC) conjugated polyclonal and monoclonal antibody reagent kits, immunofluorescence microscopy has become the accepted standard for detecting viral antigens. This procedure can be used for either direct viral antigen detection in clinical specimens or for the identification of virus isolates from cell culture. In addition, immunofluorescence antibody (IFA) microscopy is useful for detecting and quantitating patient antibody to known antigens. Flouresant antibody testing can be performed with a direct immunofluorescence (DFA) technique or an indirect immunofluorescence (IFA) technique. With the DFA technique, virus-specific FITC-conjugated antibody is reacted with antigen. In the IIFA test, virus-specific antibody is reacted with antigen and then reacted with FITC-conjugated antiimmunoglobulin antibody. Generally the IIFA test offers greater sensitivity. Overall, this technique is simple and quick (30 to 90 minutes). IIFA offers a high degree of sensitivity and specificity and gives virologists an opportunity to visualize the viral antigen-antibody reaction and pattern with an ultraviolet microscope. Because of its popularity in clinical virology, a brief review of the procedure is detailed in Box 55-2.

The IFA test is most commonly used to detect respiratory viruses (influenza A & B, respiratory syncytial virus [RSV], adenovirus, and parainfluenza virus 1-3) and the herpes virus group (herpes simplex virus [HSV], varicella-zoster virus [VZV], and cytomegalovirus [CMV]). The IFA test is crucial for detecting RSV and VZV since these viruses are extremely labile and either grow slowly in cell culture or they do not grow at all. Indirect IFA testing, which employs monoclonal pooled antibody, provides a sensitivity of 80% to 95% for RSV and VZV with excellent specificity. These reagents are available from a number of commercial vendors. Rapid detection of RSV with IFA (or ELISA) is crucial for early treatment of infants and young children with Ribavin. In addition, rapid detection of VZV in hospitalized patients helps prompt infection control intervention.

One commercial source (Bartels Immunodiagnostic Supplies, Bellevue, Wash.) has produced an IFA monoclonal pool and individual stains for detecting the seven most common respiratory viruses (influenza A & B, RSV, adenovirus, parainfluenza 1-3) in clinical specimens. These methods also identify isolates from cell culture. The overall sensitivity and specificity reported by Stout, et al was 69% and 97%, respectively.

IFA has been particularly useful in detecting CMV antigenemia by examining CMV "early" antigens in harvested leukocytes from peripheral blood, providing diagnostic results much sooner than cell culture. The usefulness of DFA for direct detection of HSV in clinical specimens has also been well established.

Solid phase immunoassays

The most commonly used solid phase immunoassay for detecting virus antigen in clinical specimens is the enzyme-linked immunosorbent assay (ELISA or EIA). The principle of ELISA is simple. The capture antibody is bound to a solid phase, which is usually a polystyrene microtitration well, bead, or tube. The specimen is incubated with solid-phase antibody, the nonbound material is washed away, and biotin-labeled or nonlabeled antibody, followed by labeled anti-immunoglobulin or enzyme-labeled avidin is added. After another wash, the bound label is measured in optical density units based on the degree of indicator color change.

ELISA commercial assays have been designed for a number of viruses including rotavirus, enteric adenoviruses, RSV, HSV, VZV, and HIV. Overall, ELISA has the advantage of being amenable to testing large batches of specimens and generally is as sensitive as IFA. ELISA testing is a great diagnostic benefit in detecting HIV infection in infants and CSF of HIV patients with abnormal CNS findings. ELISA also allows clinicians to stage and monitor HIV infection in patients.

Molecular diagnostic techniques

Nucleic acid hybridization, commonly referred to as DNA and RNA probe technology, offers promise for detecting viral nucleic acids in clinical samples. DNA probes, small fragments of complementary DNA labeled with enzymes (e.g., biotin) or radioactive substances, are now commercially available. These probes are prepared from areas of each viral genome that contain unique sequences. The labeled probe is capable of hybridizing (attaching to) complementary nucleic acid strands of DNA or RNA to form stable double strands. To perform a DNA probe assay, clinical samples or infected cells from cell cultures are heat treated to produce disruption of cells and separation of double-stranded DNA. The unknown target nucleic acid is immobilized by fixation to a microscope slide or in a semisolid medium such as polyacrylamide gel or electrophoresed in agarose and transferred to a membrane (e.g., nylon), (i.e., Southern blot). The DNA probe is applied and hybridizes over time to complementary viral DNA or RNA segments in the sample. Following the hybridization period, unattached probe DNA is removed by rinsing, or alternatively, the nucleic acid hybrids are harvested with hydroxyapatite and centrifugation. The hybridized probe is measured. Enzyme-labeled probes are detected by the action of the enzyme on a specific substrate solution; radiolabeled probes are measured by a scintillation counter or by autoradiography.

DNA probe technology can be use to detect essentially any virus. Clinical virology laboratories especially like DNA probe technology for detecting enteroviruses and human papilloma viruses. Beyond testing these two virus groups, DNA probe technology continues to improve with regard to sensitivity and specificity when compared to other diagnostic methods such as cell culture. In time, however, these problems may be resolved.

Probably the most powerful diagnostic tools in clinical virology are the molecular amplification techniques such as the polymerase chain reaction (PCR). Briefly, PCR is a molecular technique in which target nucleic acid sequences are amplified 3 million times within 3 hours. Thus, minute amounts of viral nucleic acid that may go undetected by other methods can be targeted, amplified, and then more easily detected by a DNA probe. This technique is being applied to a number of viruses and, to date, is probably the best method for detecting HIV in patient specimens.

SEROLOGIC DIAGNOSIS OF VIRAL INFECTIONS

Prior to the 1980s serologic methods for testing acute and convalescent serum (collected two to four weeks apart) were the primary methods for diagnosing viral infections. More recently, conventional serologic testing has been overshadowed by technical advances in cell culture techniques (shell vial assay) and newer methods for direct detection of virus antigen in clinical specimens. Both allow for more rapid viral diagnosis. However, a number of common viruses—including Epstein-Barr virus (EBV); cytomegalovirus (CMV); varicella-zoster virus (VZV); measles; mumps; rubella (and other togaviruses); human immunodeficiency virus (HIV); other retroviruses (HTLV-I, HTLV-II); and the hepatitis viruses (A,B,C,D,E), parvovirus B-19 and HHV-6 to name a few—are difficult, impractical, or not yet possible to grow in cell culture or detect with current direct antigen detection methods. Therefore serologic procedures must be used to effectively diagnose infections caused by these viruses. The relative frequency and proficiency for serodiagnosis of a number of common viruses are illustrated in Tables 55-3 and 55-6.

Viral serology serves a number of useful purposes in evaluating and managing patients. Its primary purposes are to detect and/or quantitate virus-specific antibody (or antigen) to diagnose current or recent infection, and to assess a patient's previous exposure (immune status) to a virus or response to a vaccination. Serology can also play an important role in diagnosing certain viral syndromes (e.g., myopericarditis) that result from immune-related tissue/organ damage secondary to a previous virus (e.g., coxsackie B 1-6) infection.

General considerations

Although antibody response depends on the virus and the immunologic status of the infected host, the following antibody pattern generally occurs: After exposure to viral antigen, IgM antibody appears in one or two weeks followed one or two days later by IgG. IgM antibody titers generally peak in three to six weeks and then drop to undetectable levels in two to three months. IgG titers generally peak in four to twelve weeks, remain elevated for many months

Table 55-6 Frequency and distribution of virus serology yielding diagnostic results[a] at a virus diagnostic laboratory Services, Inc., over a one-year period (1988-1989)

Virus	Number	% of total
Human immunodeficiency virus	182	39.7
Epstein-Barr virus	78	16.9
Hepatitis B virus	70	15.3
Cytomegalovirus	64	13.9
Hepatitis A virus	62	13.5
Varicella-Zoster virus	2	0.4
Measles	1	0.2
Rubella	0	0
Total	459	100%

[a]Overall viral serology diagnostic yield (459/7,038) 6.5%

and, with some virus infections or immunizations, may persist for life.

A definitive serologic diagnosis is generally made by testing and evaluating patient serum collected in the acute phase of illness and serum collected two to four weeks later. The "paired" serum samples must be tested in tandem to generate reliable results. The presence of IgM antibody (when tested on carefully controlled conditions) and/or a fourfold or greater rise in IgG antibody titer is considered indicative of recent or active infection. The absence of IgM antibody and a stable IgG titer implies infection (or in some cases immunization) with the virus at some undetermined time in the past.

Although the detection of virus-specific IgM antibody is a useful diagnostic indicator of probable acute infection, a number of factors must be carefully considered and controlled during testing of patient serum, and testing must be performed in the correct clinical settings for results to be reliable. Problems related to testing for virus specific IgM antibody include:

1. Rheumatoid factor (RF) anti-IgG IgM antibody found in serum of adults with rheumatoid conditions, some normal adults, and a fairly high percentage of normal infants. The fetus can produce IgM antibody against maternally transferred virus-specific IgG. When serologic tests using labeled anti-human IgM are performed, false-positive results may occur.
2. If patient serum contains high levels of IgG in the presence of IgM, the IgG competes with IgM for the antigen binding sites. Thus the IgG blocks the IgM, resulting in false-negative results.
3. Detection and quantitation of virus-specific antibody is generally not useful for viruses (HSV, CMV) that produce chronic or recurrent infection because IgM antibody levels can increase with asymptomatic viral shedding. In addition, with some viruses, IgM levels may persist longer than two or three months.

The problems mentioned above for IgM antibody detection can be essentially alleviated by pretreatment. A number of physicochemical methods for separation or fractionation of IgM from serum have been employed with a good degree of success. These include sucrose density gradient ultracentrifugation, chromatographic gel filtration, ion-exchange chromatography, affinity chromatography, and protein A absorption. Recent technical advances in immunoassays (reverse "capture" solid-phase IgM assays) avoid the problems of competitive interference and nonspecific reactivity inherent in other types of immunoassays by employing a reverse IgM antibody capture method. This method of detecting antiviral IgM antibodies employs a solid phase coated with anti-IgM antibody to "capture" and bind the IgM antibodies in a serum specimen, after which IgG and any immune complexes in the specimen are washed away. Exposure of the bound IgM antibody to specific viral antigen, followed by the addition of a second, labeled antiviral antibody, completes the test. Reverse "capture" solid-phase IgM enzyme immunoassays have proved to be very sensitive and specific. This method has been successfully applied to detect IgM antibodies to a growing number of viruses.

Other solid-phase indirect immunoassays in common use—including indirect immunofluorescence (IFA), the enzyme-linked immunosorbent assay (ELISA), and radioimmunoassay for detecting virus-specific IgM antibodies—use anti-human IgM antibody in a "sandwich" assay system. In these methods, the test serum is incubated with viral antigens bound to a solid phase surface, and specific IgM antibodies bound to the antigen are subsequently detected with anti-human IgM antibody labeled with a suitable marker. Because of the technical simplicity of these methods, indirect immunoassay IgM kits for several viruses—including CMV, HSV, VZV, EBV, hepatitis viruses (A,B,C,D), rubella, and measles—have become commercially available. However, this method of serologic testing is prone to problems mentioned previously for IgM antibody testing. Therefore, patient serum samples must be pretreated to remove interference and competitive factors such as RF and aggregated IgG.

Approach to serologic testing

Serologic tests include complement fixation (CF), neutralization (Neut), hemagglutination inhibition (HI), passive hemagglutination (PHA), indirect immunofluorescence antibody (IFA), anticomplement immunofluorescence (ACIF), enzyme-linked immunosorbent assay (ELISA), radioimmunoassay (RIA), immune-electron microscopy (IEM), immune adherence hemagglutination (IAGA), counter immunoelectrophoresis (CIE), and immunoblotting (IB). Of these, IFA, RIA, ELISA and IB are most commonly employed by routine clinical virology laboratories because of their simplicity, reliability, and commercial availability in kit form for most viruses of clinical concern. See Chapter 34 for additional information on the diagnosis of infectious diseases using immunological tests.

Serodiagnosis of viruses of special concern

Viral hepatitis

A rapid, specific diagnosis of hepatitis A, B, C, delta or D, is considerably important in determining patient prognosis and long-term management. In addition, a rapid diagnosis of acute hepatitis B infection is imperative for early infection preventive measures (e.g., administration of hepatitis B immune globulin [H-BIG] and hepatitis B vaccine) for individual intimate contacts at risk of acquiring infection. This is most imperative with a newborn whose mother has active hepatitis B infection. Such newborns must be treated with H-BIG and hepatitis vaccine within the first two to 12 hours of life to obviate the risk of disease. In the case of hepatitis A infection, early serodiagnosis of a patient will allow close contacts to receive immunoprophylaxis with immune serum globulin.

Serodiagnosis of viral hepatitis is somewhat complex because of the number of serologic markers employed to determine the stage of illness (Table 55-7). In most instances patients suspected of having acute hepatitis require rapid testing to assess whether infection is caused by hepatitis A or B. Some laboratories offer an acute-hepatitis serologic profile that detects the three primary serologic markers for acute hepatitis A and B virus (Table 55-8). In this era it is important to evaluate patients with evidence of hepatitis B surface antigen (HBsAg) for concomitant infection with

Table 55-7 Serologic markers for viral hepatitis

Hepatitis marker	Description	Significance
HBsAg	Hepatitis B surface antigen.	Present in acute, active, chronic or carrier state of hepatitis B infection.
anti-HBc IgM	IgM = specific antibody to hepatitis B core antigen.	Present in acute hepatitis B infection.
anti-HBc	Total antibody to hepatitis B core antigen.	Present in acute stage of hepatitis B infection between the disappearance of HBsAg and the appearance of anti-HBs (associated with anti-HBc IgM and negative anti-HBs). Generally remains detectable following resolution of infection.
anti-HBs	Total antibody to hepatitis B surface antigen.	Appears during convalescent phase of hepatitis B infection and generally persists for life.
HBeAg	Hepatitis B "e" antigen.	Present in early acute and chronic hepatitis B. Persistence suggests poor prognosis.
anti-HBe	Total antibody to hepatitis B "e" antigen.	Present in the nonreplicative phase of hepatitis B infection. May be detectable in active disease or convalescence. Associated with a favorable prognosis.
anti-HAV IgM	IgM-specific antibody to hepatitis A.	Present in acute hepatitis A infection.
anti-HAV	Total antibody to hepatitis A.	When present in the absence of anti-HAV IgM indicates past infection with hepatitis A.
anti-Delta IgM	IgM-specific antibody to hepatitis D (Delta agent).	Present, coexisting with HBsAg indicates acute or active infection with hepatitis D.
anti-Delta	Total antibody to hepatitis D.	Present in acute, active or recovery phase of hepatitis D infection.
anti-HCV	Total antibody to recombinant protein (c100-3)	Present in most individuals with current or past infection. Reactive serology by ELISA or RIA must be confirmed by immunoblot containing recombined proteins (e.g., 5-1-1, c100-3, c33c, and c22-3). A reactive immunoblot is based on 1+ or greater reactivity of any two recombinent bands.

Table 55-8 Differential diagnosis of acute viral hepapatitis

Acute viral hepatitis panel (viral markers)			
HBsAg	Anti-HBc IgM	Anti-HAV IgM	Interpretation and recommendations
+	0	0	The patient has early acute or chronic hepatitis B infection and should be considered infectious. Retest patient for HBsAg and anti-HBc IgM in two weeks. Further testing will most likely reveal one of the following: 1. HBsAg (+), anti-HBc IgM (+) indicates acute hepatitis B. Test for anti-HBs in 3-6 months to confirm resolution (convalescence) of infection. 2. HBsAg (+), anti-HBc IgM (−) most likely reflects a chronic carrier state or chronic hepatitis B. Anti-HBc, HBeAg, and anti-HBe may be indicated for further clinical and prognostic evaluation of the patient. Consider patient history and risk factors to determine need for testing (anti-HD IgM and total anti-HD) for co-infection with hepatitis D (Delta agent).
+	+	0	The patient has acute hepatitis B infection. Test for anti-HBs in 3-6 months to confirm resolution (convalescence) of infection. Consider patient history and risk factors to determine need for testing (anti-HD IgM and total anti-HD) for co-infection with hepatitis D (Delta agent).
0	0	+	The patient has acute or recent hepatitis A infection. Test for total anti-HAV in 4-6 weeks to confirm resolution (convalescence) of hepatitis A infection.
0	0	0	There is no serologic evidence of infection with hepatitis A or B. If hepatitis of infectious etiology remains clinically suspected, testing or monitoring for hepatitis C, Cytomegalovirus or Epstein-Barr virus is suggested.

HBsAg = Hepatitis B surface antigen.
anti-HBc IgM = IgM specific antibody to hepatitis B core antigen
anti-HBs = Antibody to hepatitis B surface antigen
HBeAg = Hepatitis B e-antigen
anti-HBe = Antibody to hepatitis B e-antigen
anti-HD IgM = IgM specific antibody to hepatitis D (Delta Agent) antigen
anti-HD IgG = antibody to hepatitis D (Delta Agent) antigen
anti-HAV IgM = IgM specific antibody to hepatitis A virus

hepatitis D (Delta virus) or HIV. The primary methodologies employed for hepatitis serology include commercially available ELISA and RIA kits.

Previously designated "Non A, Non B" hepatitis has been found to be due to two distinct viruses, Hepatitic C virus (HCV) and Hepatitis E virus (HEV). HCV is parenterally transmitted and is the major cause of post blood transfusion hepatitis. Requests for screening and confirmatory tests are in demand and ELISA and western blot reagents are commercially available. HEV is enterically transmitted, and is a major concern in developing countries; cases have not been diagnosed in the United States and testing is not indicated. Tests for HEV are available at CDC, Altanta, GA.

Epstein-Barr Virus (EBV)

Because of its role in infectious mononucleosis, interstitial pneumonia in pediatric patients with AIDS, Burkitt's lymphoma, nasopharyngeal carcinoma, and other lymphoproliferative disorders, serologic testing for EBV remains in great demand. A number of serologic markers are used in testing for EBV to determine the presence and stage of illness (Table 55-9). Additional markers for assessing antibody to EBV nuclear antigens (EBNA 1-5) are available only in a few large reference facilities. Tests with sera from the "chronic mononucleosis or EBV syndrome" have revealed absence of antibody to that component encoded by EBNA-1 in some patients. The primary test methods used for EBV serology include commercially available IFA and ELISA kits.

Human immunodeficiency virus (HIV)

Infection with HIV is most commonly documented by detection of antibody using ELISA for initial screening and employing more specific procedures (Western Blot, IFA) for confirmation. The ELISA test measures antibody to one or more HIV envelope proteins (glycoprotein-120). The Western Blot assay determines the presence of antibody to each of several viral antigens including core protein (p24) and glycoprotein-41 (gp41). The IFA test detects antibody directed at antigens expressed on the surface of infected cells. Because current ELISA screening tests are designed with such a high degree of sensitivity, some degree of specificity has been sacrificed. As a result, false-positive screening tests sometimes occur. Because of this and the serious consequences of HIV infection, appropriate confirmatory testing using IFA or Western Blot must always be performed. Interpretation and reflex test measures for HIV serology are outlined in Figure 55-4. Clinicians and clinical microbiologists must remember that not all patients infected with HIV test positive for the antibody. HIV antibody response is generally slow to develop, often requiring four to 12 weeks, and sometimes six to 18 months or more in up to 5% of individuals infected. As a result, repeat antibody testing may be necessary or testing for HIV antigen using ELISA for detecting HIV p-24 antigen in serum, HIV-specific polymerase chain reaction using heparinized whole blood or HIV culture.

The most complex setting for HIV testing is the newborn of a mother known to be HIV positive. These infants nat-

Table 55-9   Serologic reaction patterns of Epstein-Barr virus (EBV) infection

VCA-IgM	VCA-IgG	EBNA	EA-D/R	Interpretation
	EBV serologic markers			
+	+	0	+	Acute primary infection
0	+	+	+	Infection at some undetermined time in the past. Elevated EA-D/R titers (≥1:160) may reflect possible reactivated or chronic EBV infection. Serologic findings must be carefully correlated with clinical findings and patient history for accurate diagnostic assessment.
0	+	0	+/0	EBV infection of uncertain status. Such serologic patterns occur in the following clinical settings: 1) EBV infection within the past 1 to 6 months where VCA-IgM has fallen below detectable levels prior to the appearance of EBNA antibody. EA-D/R antibody will often be present in this setting. 2) Past infection with EBV where EBNA antibody has fallen below detectable levels as occurs with immunosuppression or advancing age. 3) Possible chronic EBV infection in a patient unable to produce EBNA. Diagnosis may be confirmed if serologic pattern persists beyond 6-8 months. EA-D/R antibody titers will often be elevated. Serologic findings must be carefully correlated with clinical findings and patient history for accurate diagnostic assessment.
0	+	+	0/+	Past infection.
0	0	0	0	No serologic evidence of infection with EBV.

VCA-IgM = IgM specific antibody to EBV viral capsid antigen
VCA-IgG = antibody to EBV viral capsid antigen
EBNA = Epstein-Barr nuclear antigen antibody
EA-D/R = EBV early antigen (diffuse/restricted) antibody

urally acquire HIV IgG maternal antibody, which may remain present for 15 months or longer, thus possibly producing false-positive test results. In this setting, testing for HIV p-24 antigen in infant's serum, using ELISA or the HIV-specific polymerase reaction to detect HIV in heparinized whole blood or HIV culture, should be performed. See chapter 36 for a more complete discussion of HIV tests.

Human T-lymphotropic viruses I/II (HTLV-I/II)

Like HIV, HTLV-I and II are human retroviruses known to infect human lymphocytes following transmission modes similar to those observed with HIV. Unlike HIV, however, HTLV-I/II cause lymphoproliferation of lymphocytes resulting in adult leukemia, lymphoma or tropical spastic parapesis. Since transmission of these viruses parallels that of HIV with regard to the route of transmission and risk groups, the American Association of Blood Banks and the Food and Drug Administration require that all donated blood products be screened for HTLV-I and II antibodies using ELISA testing, with repeatably reactive blood samples confirmed for the presence of HTLV-I/II specific antibodies using a Western blot assay.

Parvovirus B-19

Parvovirus B-19 has been known for some time to be the etiologic cause of erythema infectiosum (fifth disease) in young children. Typically, infected children are presented with a self-limiting mild illness with a low-grade fever, a malar rash, and occasionally arthralgias. Symptoms generally resolve uneventfully over a 4 to 7 day period. In recent years, however, Parvovirus B-19 has been strongly associated as a cause of a number of other clinical problems

including: Flu-like illness in association with joint inflammation, rash and occasionally purpura in young adults; hydrops fetalis and fetal loss in up to 10% of cases in pregnant women with primary infection; transparent aplastic crisis in patients with underlying chronic hemolytic anemias and; chronic severe anemia in patients with AIDS. In view of the recently discovered spectrum of disease caused by Parvovirus B-19, laboratory diagnosis has come into great demand. Serologic testing for Parvovirus B-19 specific IgM and IgG antibodies can now be performed by IFA or ELISA through several commercial sources.

Human herpes virus-6 (HHV-6)

HHV-6 formally called human B-lymphotropic virus (HTLB) when first described and characterized in the mid-1980s, is the etiologic agent of roseola *(exanthem subitum)*. Roseola usually occurs in infants 6 months to 3 years of age, and is characterized by an abrupt onset of high fever (40° C), followed in 2 to 4 days by a rapid drop in temperature that coincides with the appearance of an erythematous maculopapular rash, listlessness, and irritability lasting from 2 to 7 days. Leukopenia may also be present but is transient in nature. HHV-6 infection is also speculated to occur in adults. Illness in adults is characterized as mild, afebrile, with dull headache, slight fatigue, and cervical lymphademopathy which may persist up to 3 months. Serologic diagnosis can be performed using commercially available IFA or ELISA kits that measure HHV-6 IgM and IgG specific antibodies.

Serologic testing for TORCH agents

One of the most controversial uses of serology is the TORCH testing. TORCH stands for *t*oxoplasma (not a virus

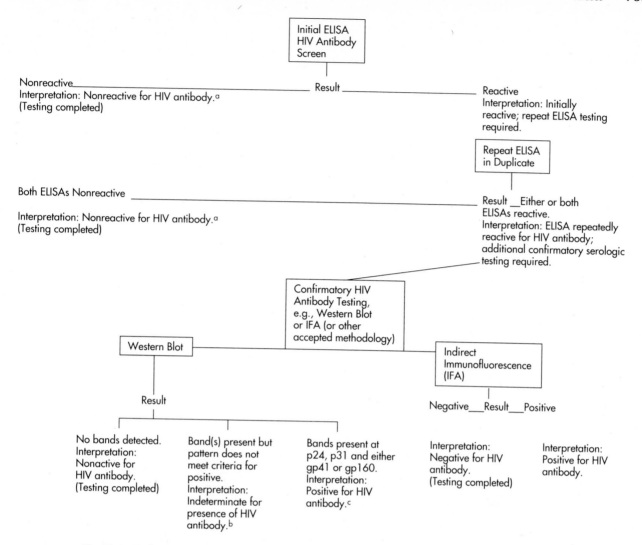

Fig. 55-4 Performing and interpreting HIV antibody testing.

a A negative test in an individual with a high likelihood of HIV infection may indicate that the sample was obtained prior to seroconversion, and testing of a second sample obtained 2 to 6 weeks later should be seriously considered.

b Indeterminate results may reflect false-positive results due to nonspecific serum interference factors or possibly early-stage HIV seroconversion. Indeterminate results characterized by presence of env-encoded glycoprotein bands (e.g., gp41, gp120 and/or gp160) but absence of core-gag protein (p24) may occur in 50% of AIDS patients. Therefore, test findings must be carefully evaluated against clinical findings and patient history. Repeat testing at monthly intervals or testing using an alternative confirmatory method such as the indirect immunofluorescence test may be indicated for further diagnostic assessment.

c These criteria are proposed to apply to interpretation of test results for blood donors and other individuals without a corroborating history or risk for HIV infection. Less stringent criteria (i.e., presence of bands at gp41 and p24) may be applied as "diagnostic" for situations where the serologic diagnosis is carefully corroborated by clinical findings and patient history.

infection), *r*ubella virus, *c*ytomegalovirus and *h*erpes simplex virus. TORCH is most commonly employed in suspect congenital infection, or perinatally to assess infection or immune status (toxoplasma, rubella) and used arbitrarily in cases of fever of undetermined origin. There are a number of pitfalls and concerns regarding TORCH testing. First, serology for HSV is generally unrewarding and unreliable since most adults acquire antibody to HSV early in life and, due to the latency of this virus, demonstrate frequent fluc-

tuations in HSV IgG antibody titers. In addition, persons previously infected with either HSV or CMV may have transient appearance of virus-specific IgM antibody in the absence of disease. Because of this, viral cultures for HSV and CMV, when clinically suspected, are generally more rewarding. Serologic testing for these viruses is best done when "primary" infection with one of these viruses or toxoplasma is suspected.

Deciding whether or not to use serologic testing for rubella virus or toxoplasma follows careful assessment of the patients' clinical findings and history including immunization history. Infection with rubella or toxoplasma can be ruled in or out on these grounds alone, since infections with these agents are associated with rather characteristic findings. However, in the setting of suspect illness, testing for both IgM and IgG antibody may be of diagnostic benefit. For pregnant females, the presence of specific IgG antibody in the absence of IgM implies previous infection (or immunization) and lasting immunity (rubella) and immune protection of her fetus (toxoplasma).

Most congenital or perinatal infections are best diagnosed by virus isolation (HSV, CMV), even though a serologic approach is often attempted. *In utero,* the fetus does not produce IgG. The fetus does produce IgM after the first trimester, but IgM is at low levels at birth. Maternal IgG antibody crosses the placenta into fetal circulation, whereas IgM does not. Thus at birth the newborn has IgG of the same specificity as its mother's. If the fetus is infected *in utero,* virus-specific IgM is synthesized and is present at birth. After birth the infant begins to produce virus-specific IgG. If infection with one of the TORCH agents is suspected at the time of delivery, the infant and maternal serum must be tested together. Repeat parallel serologic testing of infant and maternal serum may need to be repeated at one, three, and six months of age. If both titers are negative or if the mother's titer is greater, congenital infection caused by the agents being tested is unlikely. If the infant's titer is significantly higher (fourfold or greater) than the mother's, a presumptive diagnosis can be made. In the presence of infant virus-specific IgM, when detected using the appropriate methods previously described, a more reliable diagnosis may be made. In the infected infant the IgG titer remains elevated; in the uninfected infant maternal IgG drops to undetectable levels in about two to four months.

Diagnosis of other viral infections

Diagnosis of some viral infections is beyond the scope of most hospital clinical microbiology laboratories because the infections are rare or exotic, the etiologic agents are hazardous, or special diagnostic facilities are necessary. Tests for rabies, togavirus infections, and hemorrhagic fevers are generally performed in state or local public health laboratories or at the Centers for Disease Control.

SUMMARY

Figure 55-5 summarizes the means and impetus for rapid diagnosis of viral diseases. Over the past fifteen years a number of treatments for viral diseases have developed. These include: a better understanding of the role of viruses in human disease, the epidemiology of viruses, introduction of newer technologies and methods for rapid diagnosis of viral diseases, and an ever-expanding pharmacopeia of antiviral agents. The clinical microbiology laboratory plays a pivotal role in the process of patient management by providing rapid detection of viruses in patient specimens. Any

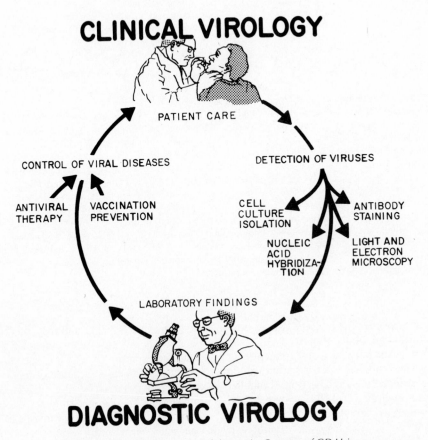

Fig. 55-5 The scope of rapid viral diagnosis. *Courtesy of GD Hsiung.*

well-staffed and well-equipped microbiology laboratory can provide some level of diagnostic services because technology can detect a wide range of viruses.

SUGGESTED READING

Balows A, and others: Manual of clinical microbiology, ed 5, Washington, DC, 1991, American Society for Microbiology.

Baron EJ and Finegold SM: Diagnostic microbiology, ed 8, St. Louis, 1990, Mosby–Year Book, Inc.

Belshe RB: Textbook of human virology, Littleton, Mass, 1984, PSG Publishing Company, Inc.

de la Maza LM and Peterson EM, eds: Medical virology 8: Shell vial centrifugation culture method (SVCCM) for early detection of respiratory syncytial virus, New York, 1989, Plenum Press.

Evans AS: Viral infections of humans: epidemiology and control, ed 3, New York, 1989, Plenum Medical Book Co.

Forbes B. Acquisition of cytomegalovirus infection: an update, Clin Microbiol Rev, 2:204, 1989.

Gleaves CA, Smith TF, Shuster EA, and Pearson GR: Rapid detection of cytomegalovirus in MRC-5 cells inoculated with urine specimens by using low-speed centrifugation and monoclonal antibody to an early antigen, J Clin Microbiol, 19:917, 1984.

Howard BJ, Klaas J, Rubin SJ, Weissfeld AS, and Tilton RC: Clinical and pathogenic microbiology, St. Louis, 1987, Mosby–Year Book, Inc.

Hsiung GD: Diagnostic virology, ed 3, New Haven, 1982, Yale University Press.

Koneman EW, Allen SD, Dowell VR, Janda WM, Sommers HM, and Winn WC: Color atlas and textbook of diagnostic microbiology, ed 3, Philadelphia, 1988, JB Lippincott Co.

Lafferty WE, Krofft S, Remington M, Giddings R, Winter C, Cent A, and Corey L: Diagnosis of herpes simplex virus by direct immunofluorescence and viral isolation from samples of external genital lesions in a high-prevalence population, J Clin Microbiol 25:323, 1987.

Lennette EH, Halonen P, and Murphy FA: Laboratory diagnosis of infectious diseases; principles and practice: viral, rickettsial and chlamydial diseases, vol II, New York, 1988, Springer-Verlag.

Mandell GL, Douglas RG Jr, and Bennett JE: Principles and practice of infectious diseases, ed 3, New York, 1990, Churchill Livingstone Inc.

Marx JL: How DNA viruses may cause cancer, Science 243:1012, 1989.

Mims CA and White DO. Viral pathogenis and immunology, Oxford, Blackwell Scientific Publications, 1984.

Minnich LL, Smith TF, Ray CG, and Spector S, eds: Cumitech 24: rapid detection of viruses by immunofluorescence, Washington, DC, 1988, American Society for Microbiology.

Pouletty P, Chomel JJ, Thouvenot D, Catalan F, Rabillon V, and Kadouche J: Detection of herpes simplex virus in direct specimens by immunofluorescence assay using a monoclonal antibody, J Clin Microbiol, 25:958, 1987.

Rossier E, Miller HR, and Phipps PH: Rapid viral diagnosis by immunofluorescence, Ottawa, Canada, 1989, University of Ottawa Press.

Specter S and Lancz GJ: Clinical virology manual, New York, 1986, Elsevier Science Publishing Company, Inc.

Stout C, Murphy MD, Lawrence S, and Julian S: Evaluation of a monoclonal antibody pool for rapid diagnosis of respiratory viral infections, J Clin Microbiol, 27:448, 1989.

Tenover FC: Diagnostic deoxyribonucleic acid probes for infectious diseases, Clin Microbiol Rev, 1:82, 1988.

56 Parasites

Lynne S. Garcia

The basic approach to diagnostic clinical parasitology should be no different from that used in other areas of microbiology. Specific recommended procedures for this field have been published. If these procedures are not followed, then the clinician must be informed of the limitations of the substitute or modified methods. Patient care becomes particularly important when the number and types of compromised patients seen in most facilities are considered. Increased information concerning patients with the acquired immune deficiency syndrome (AIDS) has led to a greater awareness of parasitic infections in the compromised patient.

The main emphasis should be on recognizing potential parasitic infections, knowing what procedures may provide confirmation of the diagnosis, and recognizing the implications and limitations of information provided to the physician. If there is a lack of understanding of requirements for quality diagnostic testing, then incomplete or inaccurate information will be transmitted to the clinician. The laboratory and the clinician must develop a greater awareness of the importance of this discipline within microbiology.

The majority of this chapter will be presented in tabular form, both for quick reference and to maximize the amount of relevant material. General information regarding body sites and proper specimen collection can be found in Table 56-1, and parasites that can be recovered from specific body sites are seen in Table 56-2. These tables provide a concise review of the clinically relevant information necessary to collect and submit specimens to the laboratory for proper diagnostic workups. This chapter does not include every parasite known to infect humans. The reader is referred to the end of the chapter for a number of excellent publications that provide additional information.

COLLECTION, PRESERVATION, PROCESSING, EXAMINATION, AND REPORTING: HUMAN SPECIMENS SUBMITTED FOR RECOVERY AND IDENTIFICATION OF PARASITES
Fecal specimens
Collection, processing, and examination of specimens

Specimens should be collected every other day (within no more than 10 days). A series of three specimens is the recommended number/series. Less than three will probably result in missed organisms, with the exception of *Giardia lamblia,* which is often very difficult to recover even with a series of three stools.

Fecal specimens should be collected in one of the following manners:
1. Two Vial Collection Kit: Polyvinyl alcohol (PVA with mercuric chloride base), 10% formalin
2. One Vial Collection Kit: PVA
3. One Vial Collection Kit: Sodium acetate, acetic acid, formalin (SAF)
4. Two Vial Collection Kit: PVA with non-mercuric chloride base, 10% formalin
5. One Vial Collection Kit: PVA with non-mercuric chloride base
6. One Vial Collection Kit: Merthiolate-iodine-formalin (MIF)
7. Submission of fresh fecal specimen (not recommended due to potential problems with lag time between passage of the specimen and preservation). This approach is still used for in-house specimens, but the problem of lag time still remains. Fresh stool can be placed into 10% formalin for concentration, and a smear can be placed in Schaudinn's fixative (mercuric chloride base for PVA) for a permanent stained smear.

The "gold standard" is one option. The formalin-ethyl acetate sedimentation concentration can be performed from the 10% formalin vial and a permanent stained smear (trichrome or iron hematoxylin) can be prepared using the PVA-fixed fecal specimen. For safety reasons, ethyl acetate has been substituted for ether.

Other options are less desirable for the following reasons:
1. SAF may not produce optimal results when coupled with the trichrome stain; however, when used with iron hematoxylin, the results are much better.
2. PVA prepared with any non-mercuric chloride base does not provide fixation as good as mercuric chloride. However, with current changes in waste disposal regulations, all laboratories may have to switch to non-mercury based fixatives.
3. MIF is normally not used for permanent stained smears using either trichrome or iron hematoxylin. However, some laboratories do use this fixative.

Table 56-1   Body sites and specimen collection

Site	Specimen options	Collection method
Blood	Smears of whole blood	Thick and thin films
		Fresh (1st Choice)
	Anticoagulated blood	Anticoagulant (2nd Choice)
		EDTA (1st Choice)
		Heparin (2nd Choice)
Bone marrow	Aspirate	Sterile
CNS	Spinal fluid	Sterile
Cutaneous ulcers	Aspirates from below surface	Sterile plus air-dried smears
	Biopsy	Sterile, non-sterile-histopathology
Eye	Biopsy	Sterile (in saline)
	Scrapings	Sterile (in saline)
	Contact lens	Sterile (in saline)
	Lens solution	Sterile
Intestinal tract	Fresh stool	½-pint waxed container
	Preserved stool	5% or 10% Formalin, MIF, SAF, Schaudinn's, PVA
	Sigmoidoscopy material	Fresh, PVA or Schaudinn's smears
	Duodenal contents	Entero-Test™ or aspirates
	Anal impression smear	Cellulose tape (pinworm exam)
	Adult worm/worm segments	Saline, 70% alcohol
Liver, spleen	Aspirates	Sterile, collected in 4 separate aliquots (liver)
	Biopsy	Sterile, non-sterile-histopathology
Lung	Sputum	True sputum (not saliva)
	Induced sputum	No preservative (10% Formalin if time delay)
	Bronchoalveolar lavage (BAL)	Sterile
	Transbronchial aspirate	Air-dried smears
	Tracheobronchial aspirate	Same as above
	Brush biopsy	Same as above
	Open lung biopsy	Same as above
	Aspirate	Sterile
Muscle	Biopsy	Fresh-squash preparation
		Non-sterile-histopathology
Skin	Scrapings	Aseptic, smear or vial
	Skin Snip	No preservative
	Biopsy	Sterile (in saline)
		Non-sterile-histopathology
Urogenital system	Vaginal discharge	Saline swab, Culturette (no charcoal), culture medium air-dried smear for FA
	Urethral discharge	Same as above
	Prostatic secretions	Same as above
	Urine	Unpreserved spot specimen or 24-hr unpreserved specimen
		Midday urine

The traditional Ova and Parasite Examination (O&P) is composed of three parts:

1. The *direct smear* detects protozoan motility in fresh stool material with physiological saline. D'Antoni's or Lugol's iodine can also be added to provide some color, although this will kill the organisms. The benefits of fixation immediately after stool passage, far outweighs the unlikely benefits of seeing motile organisms; as a result, many laboratories have deleted the direct stool examination. The 22 × 22 mm coverslip preparation should be examined under × 100 (entire coverslip) and × 400 (1/3-1/2 coverslip).

2. The *concentration* is for protozoan cysts and helminth eggs and larvae. Although zinc sulfate flotation is available, most laboratories use the formalin-ethyl acetate sedimentation method. The coverslip preparation should be examined for the direct smear.

3. The *permanent stained smear* is the most important method used for the identification and confirmation of the intestinal protozoa. The trichrome stain is most widely used, although iron hematoxylin also produces excellent results and is specifically recommended when using SAF fixative. A minimum of 300 oil immersion (× 1000) fields should be examined before calling the slide negative.

The recommended approach for an O & P examination is as follows:

1. Every specimen submitted should have at least the following:
   A. Concentration (sedimentation recommended). Note: Reagents (FA, ELISA) are now available and being used routinely for the direct detection of *Giardia lamblia* and *Cryptosporidium parvum* in fecal specimens. Fecal material should be submitted in 5% or 10% formalin, SAF, or as fresh specimens. The concentrate sediment is used for

Table 56-2 Body sites and possible parasites recovered (diagnostic stage) (trophozoites, cysts, oocysts, spores, adults, larvae, eggs, amastigotes, trypomastigotes)

Site	Parasites	Site	Parasites
Blood		Intestinal tract (continued)	Hookworm
Red cells	Plasmodium spp.		Strongyloides stercoralis
	Babesia spp.		Trichuris trichiura
White cells	Leishmania donovani		Hymenolepis nana
	Toxoplasma gondii		Hymenolepis diminuta
Whole blood, plasma	Trypanosoma spp.		Taenia saginata
	Microfilariae		Taenia solium
Bone marrow	Leishmania donovani		Diphyllobothrium latum
CNS	Taenia solium (Cysticercosis)		Opisthorchis sinensis (Clonorchis)
	Echinococcus spp.		Paragonimus westermani
	Naegleria fowleri		Schistosoma spp.
	Acanthamoeba-Hartmanella spp.		Heterophyes sp.
	Toxoplasma gondii		Metagonimus sp.
	Trypanosoma spp.	Liver, spleen	Echinococcus spp.
Cutaneous ulcers	Leishmania spp.		Entamoeba histolytica
Eye	Acanthamoeba spp.		Leishmania donovani
	Naegleria spp.		Opisthorchis sinensis (Clonorchis)
	Taenia solium (Cysticerci)		Fasciola hepatica
	Loa loa	Lung	Pneumocystis carinii
	Microsporidia		Echinococcus spp.
Intestinal tract	Entamoeba histolytica		Paragonimus westermani
	Entamoeba coli		Cryprosporidium parvum
	Entamoeba hartmanni		Ascaris lumbricoides
	Endolimax nana		Larvae
	Iodamoeba bütschlii		Hookworm larvae
	Blastocystis hominis	Muscle	Taenia solium (Cysticerci)
	Giardia lamblia		Trichinella spiralis
	Chilomastix mesnili		Onchocerca volvulus (Nodules)
	Dientamoeba fragilis		Trypanosoma cruzi
	Trichomonas hominis		Microsporidia
	Balantidium coli	Skin	Leishmania spp.
	Cryptosporidium parvum		Onchocerca volvulus
	Isospora belli		Microfilariae
	Microsporidia	Urogenital system	Trichomonas vaginalis
	Blue-green algae (cyanobacteria)		Schistosoma spp.
	Ascaris lumbricoides		
	Enterobius vermicularis		

Note: This table does not include every possible parasite found in a particular body site. However, the most likely organisms have been listed.

testing. New reagents for the detection of *Entamoeba histolytica* and *Dientamoeba fragilis* are also under development.

B. Permanent stained smear (trichrome recommended unless using SAF)

Note: The direct smear can be done if fresh specimens are submitted to the laboratory. However, if the stool is formed, there is very little chance that motile organisms would be present, thus there is no need to perform the direct mount. Motile protozoan trophozoites tend to be seen in liquid or soft stools (diarrhea or dysentery). When the intestinal motility is more normal (formed stools), the trophozoites generally tend to encyst (cysts are non-motile).

2. If either the concentration or permanent stained smear is not performed, there is a high probability that some organisms may be missed and/or misidentified.

Reporting of intestinal parasites

Genus name, species name, and stage (trophozoite, cyst) should be reported for intestinal protozoa. *Blastocystis hominis* (Plate 1-13) which may cause symptoms when present in large numbers, is the only intestinal protozoan that needs to be quantitated. Therefore it should be reported as rare, few, moderate, many, or packed. Some laboratories report *B. hominis* when only moderate or greater numbers are seen. However, recent reports suggest that smaller numbers of the protozoan can cause symptoms. Ultimately, the decision to initiate therapy must be based on a patient's clinical condition.

Other findings should also be quantitated such as Charcot-Leyden crystals, polymorphonuclear leukocytes (PMNs), macrophages, and red blood cells. Yeast (budding or the presence of pseudohyphae) should only be reported if the stool was examined within 30 to 60 minutes after passage or was submitted in preservative. Otherwise, the report may be misleading for the clinician, particularly if the specimen has been standing at room temperature for some time prior to fixation (yeast will continue to grow, bud, and produce pseudohyphae).

Typical laboratory reports are as follows:

1. *Giardia lamblia* cysts
   Moderate *Blastocystis hominis*
   Entamoeba histolytica trophozoites and cysts
   Moderate macrophages
   Few Charcot-Leyden crystals
   Few PMNS
2. *Entamoeba coli* cysts
   Dientamoeba fragilis trophozoites (Plate 1-14)
   Endolimax nana cysts

Note that non-pathogens are reported as well as pathogens. The presence of any of these protozoa indicates that the patient has ingested something contaminated with fecal material.

Helminths are generally not quantitated in the report. Exceptions would be *Trichuris trichiura* (light infections may not be treated) and *Schistosoma* spp. (monitoring egg production).

Typical laboratory reports are as follows:

1. *Ascaris lumbricoides* eggs (some laboratories choose to report fertilized or unfertilized eggs, which is not really relevant for therapy)
   Trichuris trichiura eggs
2. *Strongyloides stercoralis* larvae
   Hookworm eggs (the eggs of both species look alike)

A typical mixed infection report is as follows:

1. *Strongyloides stercoralis* larvae
   Entamoeba histolytica trophozoites
   Entamoeba hartmanni trophozoites and cysts
   Entamoeba coli trophozoites and cysts
   Endolimax nana cysts
   Moderate macrophages and PMNs
   Few Charcot-Leyden crystals

Note that the pathogens (*Strongyloides* and *E. histolytica*) are listed first.

Shipping fecal specimens for subsequent examination

Preserved fecal specimens can be shipped via U.S. mail, provided double mailing containers are used. The recommended collection vials are PVA and 10% formalin. The kit should contain specific directions for collecting the specimen and mixing it with the appropriate fixatives. Once the stool specimen is preserved, shipment via regular mail does not present a time-lag problem other than problems encountered in turn-around time.

Other specimens from the intestinal tract and urogenital system

Examination for pinworms

Enterobius vermicularis is distributed worldwide. Infections are often treated symptomatically because six consecutive negative tape preparations are required to rule out the infection. There are sampling paddles and tapes available commercially for physicians who want to submit preparations to the laboratory. Plain cellulose tape can also be used (do not use opaque tape).

Examination for tapeworms

Unless the patient receives a purge after therapy (niclosamide recommended) for a tapeworm infection, the worm will not be passed in any condition to be identified. It will also be impossible to recover the scolex using normal screening techniques. Gravid proglottids that are passed prior to therapy can be identified using the India-ink injection method or clearing compounds.

Sigmoidoscopy material

Material obtained from sigmoidoscopy can be helpful in diagnosing amebiasis. However, these samples are not a substitute for stool specimens submitted for routine ova and parasite examination. Material from six different areas of the mucosal surface should be aspirated or scraped but should not be obtained with a cotton swab. The specimens should be immediately fixed in Schaudinn's fixative. Alternatively the mucus can be simultaneously spread and fixed onto a slide at the same time using three drops of PVA to one drop of specimen. After air drying, the slide can be stained with either trichrome or hematoxylin. If sufficient material is available, direct wet examinations can be performed, looking for motile amebae. Permanent stains are very important, not only as confirmation for suspicious organisms, but to differentiate human cells which can be confused with protozoa.

Duodenal contents

In suspected cases of giardiasis or strongyloidiasis where routine stool examinations have been negative, sampling of duodenal contents can help confirm the diagnosis. These two organisms, particularly *G. lamblia* (Plate 1-15) can be difficult to recover in stool. Fluid submitted for examination should be centrifuged and the sediment examined as wet preparations and permanent stained smears (trichrome or hematoxylin). Often the organisms may be trapped in the mucus, and motility may be very difficult to see. Typical "falling leaf" motility, as described for *Giardia,* is rarely seen in clinical specimens. The duodenal capsule technique (Entero-Test™) can also be very effective. The device consists of a length of nylon yarn coiled inside a gelatin capsule. Yarn protrudes through one end of the capsule. This end of the yarn is taped to the side of the patient's face. The capsule is then swallowed, the gelatin dissolves in the stomach, and the weighted yarn is carried by peristalsis into the duodenum. After four hours the line is retrieved. Bile-stained mucus clinging to the yarn is removed by pulling the yarn between gloved thumb and finger. The mucus is collected in a small Petri dish (usually four to five drops are obtained and can be examined as wet preparations and/or permanent stained smears [trichrome or hematoxylin]). Very specific directions accompany the capsules.

Urogenital specimens

The identification of *Trichomonas vaginalis* (Plate 1-16) is often based on the examination of wet preparations of vaginal and urethral discharges and prostatic secretions or urine sediments. Multiple specimens may need to be examined to confirm the diagnosis. Monoclonal antibody (fluorescent detection) kits are now available and can be used with dry smears submitted to the laboratory from an out-

Table 56-3   Examination of tissue/body fluids

Suspect causative agent	Disease	Appropriate test	Positive result
PROTOZOA			
Naegleria fowleri	Primary amebic meningoencephalitis (PAM)	1. Wet exam of CSF (Not in counting chamber) 2. Stained preparation of CSF sediment	Trophozoites present and identified
Acanthamoeba spp.	Amebic keratitis Chronic meningoencephalitis	1. Culture/stained smears 2. Biopsy/routine histology	Trophozoites and/or cysts present and identified
Entamoeba histolytica	Amebiasis	Biopsy/routine histology	Trophozoites present and identified
Giardia lamblia	Giardiasis	1. Duodenal aspirate 2. Duodenal biopsy/routine histology 3. Entero-Test™ Capsule	Trophozoites and/or cysts

Leishmania spp. (Cutaneous lesions)	Cutaneous leishmaniasis	1. Material from under bed of ulcer
		  a. smear
		  b. culture
		  c. animal inoculation
		2. Punch biopsy
		  a. routine histology
		  b. squash preparation
		  c. culture
		  d. animal inoculation
			Amastigotes recovered in macrophages of skin, or from animal inoculation; other stages recovered in culture

Leishmania spp. (Mucocutaneous lesions)	Mucocutaneous leishmaniasis	As cutaneous leishmaniasis	Amastigotes recovered in macrophages of skin and mucous membranes, or from animal inoculation; other stages recovered in culture

Leishmania spp. (Visceral)	Visceral leishmaniasis (Kala-Azar)	1. Buffy coat
		  a. stain
		  b. culture
		  c. animal inoculation
		2. Bone Marrow
		  As above
		3. Liver/spleen biopsy
		  a. routine histology
		  b. As above
			Amastigotes recovered in cells of reticuloendothelial system

Pneumocystis carinii	Pneumocystosis	1. Open lung biopsy/histology 2. Lung needle aspirate 3. Bronchial brush 4. Transtracheal aspirate (TTA) 5. Bronchoalveolar lavage (BAL) 6. Induced sputum (AIDS patients) 7. Calcofluor	Trophozoites or cysts present and identified Trophozoite- and cyst-specific stains available Monoclonal antibody reagents (fluorescent detection of cysts and trophs)

Toxoplasma gondii	Toxoplasmosis	1. Lymph node biopsy
		  a. routine histology
		  b. tissue culture isolation
		  c. animal inoculation
		2. Serology
			Identification of organisms *plus* appropriate serologic test results

Cryptosporidium parvum	Cryptosporidiosis	1. Duodenal scraping
		2. Duodenal biopsy
		  a. stain
		  b. routine histology
		3. Punch biopsy
		  a. routine histology
		  b. squash preparation
		4. Sputum
			Identification of organisms in microvillus border or in other tissues (lung and gall bladder have also been involved); routine stains plus monoclonal antibody reagents to identify oocysts in stool (fluorescent detection)

Microsporidia
  Nosema spp.
  Pleistophora spp.
  Encephalitozoon spp.
  Enterocytozoon spp.
  Microsporidium spp.
	Microsporidiosis	Routine histology (fair); acid fast, PAS stains recommended (spores); animal inoculation not recommended/latent infections; electron microscopy helpful	These organisms have been found as insect or other animal parasites; route of infection probably ingestion; detection of spores in tissues (GI tract, muscle, CSF, eye, etc.)

Table 56-3   Examination of tissue/body fluids—cont'd

Suspect causative agent	Disease	Appropriate test	Positive result
HELMINTHS			
Larvae (Ascaris, Strongyloides)	"Pneumonia"	1. Sputum	This is an incidental finding, but has been reported in severe infections; Rarely adult worms in lung (eggs in sputum)
Eggs (Paragonimus)	Paragonimiasis	1. Sputum	Eggs will be coughed up and will appear as "iron filings"; eggs could also be found in stool
Hooklets (Echinococcus)	Hydatid Disease	1. Sputum	Rare finding, but hooklets can be found when the hydatid cyst is in the lung
Onchocerca volvulus Mansonella streptocerca	Onchocerciasis	1. Skin	Skin snips examined in saline; microfilariae may be present
Schistosoma spp.	Schistosomiasis	1. Rectal valve biopsy 2. Bladder biopsy	Eggs present and identified

patient clinic situation. Although culture is considered an excellent method for organism recovery and identification, it is not widely used.

The examination of urinary sediment may be indicated in certain filarial infections and in suspect cases of schistosomiasis (particularly with *Schistosoma haematobium*). Various concentration techniques are available for handling the urine, and filtration methods are also applicable.

Tissue and body fluids: sputum, aspirates, CSF, and biopsy material

Although these specimens are not frequently submitted to the laboratory, correct processing and examination can yield or confirm the diagnosis. Protozoa tend to be the most frequent organisms recovered from these types of specimens. Some examples can be seen in Table 56-3.

Sputum

Organisms found in sputum include: migrating larvae of *Ascaris lumbricoides*, *Strongyloides stercoralis*, and hookworm; the eggs of *Paragonimus* spp.; *Echinococcus granulosus* hooklets; *Pneumocystis carinii*; and the protozoa, *Entamoeba histolytica*, *Entamoeba gingivalis*, *Trichomonas tenax*, and *Cryptosporidium parvum*. Sputum is usually examined microscopically as a wet mount (saline or iodine) using low and high dry lenses. If the sputum is thick, the specimen can be digested as performed for acid-fast bacteriology study but digestion should not take place if looking for protozoa. Unless the collection is induced, sputum is not recommended for the recovery of *P. carinii*, and may not be acceptable from a non-AIDS patient; more invasive procedures often are recommended. Monoclonal reagents (FA) for the direct detection of both *Cryptosporidium parvum* oocysts and *Pneumocystis carinii* trophozoites and cysts are now commercially available and being used routinely.

Aspirates

The examination of aspirates can be very helpful in recovering parasitic organisms, particularly when more rou-

tine methods have failed to confirm the clinical diagnosis. It is important that these specimens be transported to the laboratory immediately after collection.

Lung and liver. *Pneumocystis* (Plate 1-17) infection is often the primary suspect in cases of pneumonia, particularly in compromised patients. In non-AIDS patients, invasive procedures are often recommended for specimen collection. Other methods of tissue collection may not yield the same high percentage of positives as the open lung biopsy. AIDS patients often are not able to undergo an invasive procedure. Consequently bronchoalveolar lavage (BAL) is more widely used, as is the induced sputum. A number of stains are available, some of which stain the cyst wall (silver methenamine) and some of which stain the trophozoites (Giemsa). Monoclonal antibody reagents are also available for direct organism detection. Liver aspirate specimens can be examined for the confirmation of extraintestinal amebiasis (amebic abscess). This procedure is rarely performed. Extraintestinal amebiasis is often confirmed serologically (after visualizing an abscess formation on scan).

Lymph nodes, spleen, bone marrow, spinal fluid, and eye specimens. Aspirates from these body sites can be examined for parasites as wet preparations and/or permanent stained smears (trichrome or hematoxylin; Giemsa). Depending on the suspect organism, some of the material can also be cultured or used for animal inoculation.

CSF

A counting chamber is routinely used to examine spinal fluid. For the detection and identification of parasites, the CSF should be placed on a glass slide with a coverslip and examined as a wet preparation. When placed in a counting chamber, amebae will round up and mimic white blood cells. This could lead to a critical error in diagnosis if *Naegleria fowleri* were missed in a case of primary amebic meningoencephalitis (rare, but fatal if misdiagnosed and incorrect therapy given). Since the CSF can be purulent and mimic that seen in bacterial meningitis (containing WBCs), it is critical to differentiate amebae from these human cells.

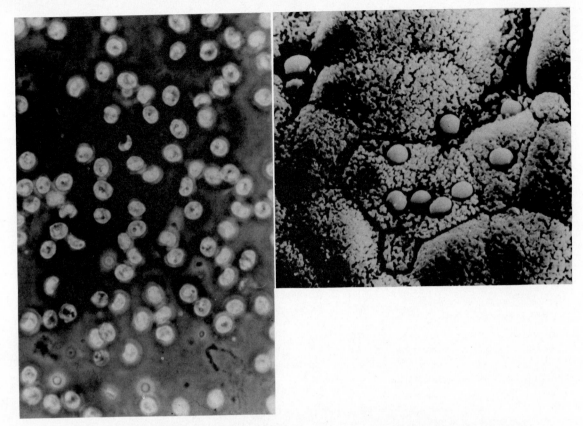

Fig. 56-1 *Cryptosporidium.* **A,** Oocysts recovered from a Sheather's sugar flotation; organisms measure 4-6 μm. **B,** Scanning electron microscopy view of organisms at brush border of epithelial cells. *In Baron EJ and Finegold SM: Diagnostic microbiology, ed 8, St Louis, 1990, Mosby-Year Book, Inc.*

Biopsy material

In certain cases a biopsy may be recommended to confirm a parasitic infection. If the specimens are also intended to be examined as fresh, wet mounts or cultured, they should be submitted in sterile saline. Other samples should be submitted to histopathology. Particular tissues and the corresponding parasites are seen as follows: skin (*Onchocerca volvulus, Mansonella streptocerca, Entamoeba histolytica, Leishmania* spp., ectoparasites); lymph nodes (*Trypanosoma gambiense, T. rhodesiense, Leishmania* spp., *Trypanosoma cruzi, Toxoplasma gondii*); muscle (*Trichinella spiralis, Trypanosoma cruzi,* cestode larval stages, microsporidia); rectal or bladder *(Schistosoma mansoni, S. japonicum, S. haematobium);* colon *(Entamoeba histolytica);* and any part of the intestine (*Cryptosporidium parvum* [Plate 1-18 and Fig. 56-1], microsporidia [Figs. 56-2 to 56-5]).

Blood parasites

Some parasites can be detected in fresh blood by their characteristic morphology and motility. However, most organisms must be confirmed on a permanent stained smear. Giemsa stain is best for blood parasites, although most organisms could be identified using Wright's stain or a Wright-Giemsa combination. Most of the original malarial drawings and descriptions were based on Giemsa-stained smears.

Thick and thin blood films and various concentration and culture techniques are available for organism recovery and identification.

Blood should be drawn when the patient is first seen. This is very important in suspected cases of malaria where the patient may not exhibit the typical fever pattern (Fig. 56-6). If the patient has a *Plasmodium falciparum* infection (Plate 1-19), the symptoms may not correlate with the severity of the infection (patient may be very ill without the typical fever pattern). If fresh blood is used to prepare thick and thin films, the blood on the thick film must be thoroughly stirred to prevent fibrin strand formation. If blood is collected with an anticoagulant, EDTA is recommended over heparin to maintain good parasite morphology. Both thick and thin films should be prepared; the thick film (after laking the red cells, white cells, platelets, and parasites are visible) allows examination of a larger quantity of blood and the thin film (less blood but parasite can be seen within the red cell) provides information regarding the relationship between the infected and uninfected red cells (Plate 1-20). These smears should be prepared on separate glass slides.

Blood films should be carefully examined under low power (×100) for microfilariae and under oil immersion (×900 to ×1000) for trypanosomes, leishmaniae, *Babesia,* (Fig. 56-7) and malaria. A minimum of 300 fields per film

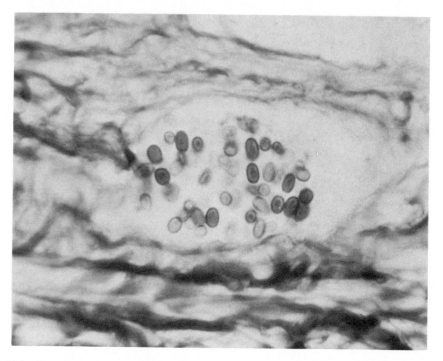

Fig. 56-2 Nosema spores in muscularis of jejunum (GMS ×1260). (Armed Forces Institute of Pathology photograph 71-5887.) *From Garcia LS and Bruckner DA: Diagnostic medical parasitology, New York, 1988, Elsevier Science Publishing Co., Inc.*

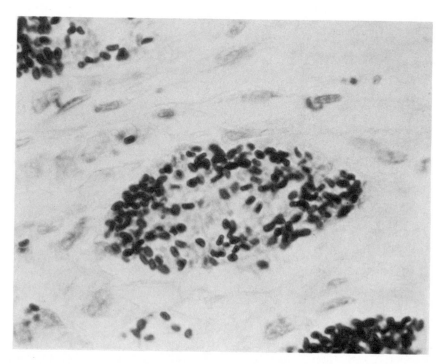

Fig. 56-3 Heart. Some *Nosema* spores are acid fast (photographed with green filter, Ziehl-Neelsen, ×1080). (Armed Forces Institute of Pathology photograph 71-864.) *From Garcia LS and Bruckner DA: Diagnostic medical parasitology, New York, 1988, Elsevier Science Publishing Co., Inc.*

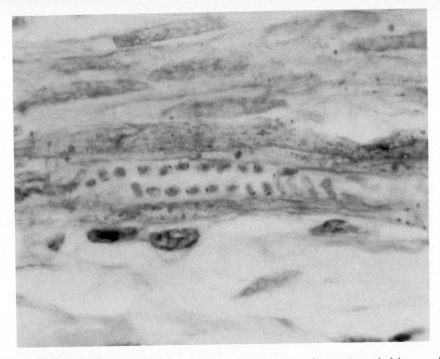

Fig. 56-4 Section of appendix showing *Nosema* spores in muscularis. The anterior end of the spore has a PAS-positive granule (arrows) (PAS × 1260). (Armed Forces Institute of Pathology photograph 71-5883.) *From Garcia LS and Bruckner DA: Diagnostic medical parasitology, New York, 1988, Elsevier Science Publishing Co., Inc.*

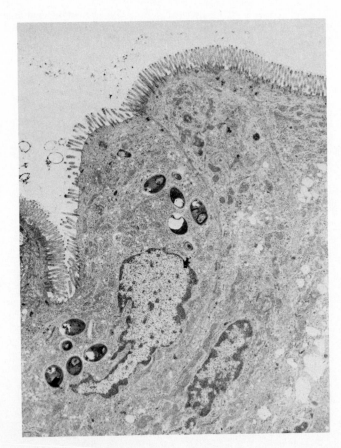

Fig. 56-5 Microsporidia spores in cytoplasm of intact jejunal enterocyte of a man with intractable diarrhea and malabsorption. Transmission electron micrograph of a jejunal suction biopsy. *Courtesy of RL Owen. From Farthing MJG, Keusch GI, eds: Enteric infection: mechanisms, manifestations and management, London, 1987, Chapman and Hall.*

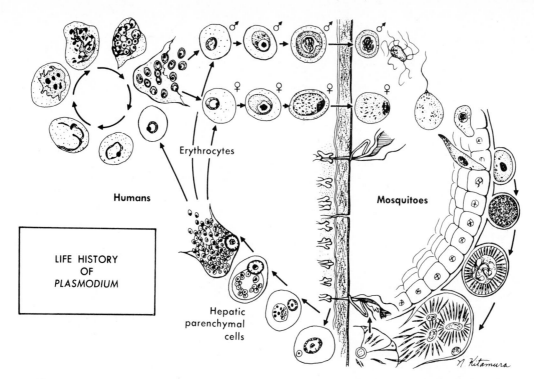

Fig. 56-6 Life cycle of *Plasmodium. Adapted from Wilcox A: Manual for the microscopical diagnosis of malaria in man. Washington, D.C., 1960, U.S. Public Health Service. Illustration by Nobuko Kitamura.*

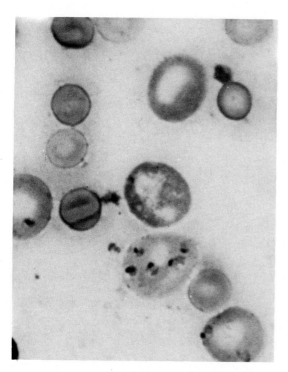

Fig. 56-7 *Babesia* in red blood cells. *Photomicrograph by Zane Price. From Markell EK, Voge M, and John DT: Medical parasitology, ed 6, Philadelphia, 1986, W.B. Saunders Co.*

should be examined under oil immersion. Various concentration techniques are also available for the recovery of other parasites: buffy coat films (leishmaniae); Knott concentration; membrane filtration technique; gradient centrifugation (microfilariae); triple centrifugation method; microhematocrit tube concentration (trypanosomes). The buffy coat preparations can be cultured for the recovery of leishmaniae, and the buffy coat layer from the hematocrit tube can also be used to culture for trypanosomes and/or leishmaniae.

Culture, animal inoculation, and serological diagnosis of parasitic infections

Culture

Although various culture media have been developed for recovering parasites, their use is not widespread. It is mandatory that a positive control be set up with every specimen submitted for culture. Thus the procedures are neither very practical nor cost-efficient. This is particularly true because of the necessity to maintain positive cultures of all the organisms that are needed to provide for controls. Of all the organisms, only three have been routinely cultured in a diagnostic laboratory setting (*Entamoeba histolytica, Trichomonas vaginalis,* and *Leishmania* spp.).

Animal inoculation

As with culture, these methods are not routinely available for several reasons: the cost of maintaining animals, the length of time for many animals to "turn positive," and the time and expertise needed to maintain and offer such services. In the past, the mouse has been used for the recovery

Table 56-4   Intestinal tract/urogenital system protozoa: key characteristics

Amebae	Trophozoite	Cyst	Comments
Entamoeba histolytica Pathogenic	Cytoplasm clean, presence of RBCs is diagnostic, but may also contain some ingested bacteria; peripheral nuclear chromatin is evenly distributed with central, compact karyosome.	Mature cyst contains 4 nuclei; chromatoidal bars will have smooth, rounded ends.	Considered pathogenic; should be reported to Public Health; trophs can be confused with macrophages, cysts with WBCs in the stool.
Entamoeba hartmanni Non-pathogenic	Looks identical to *E. histolytica*, but size is smaller (<12 μm); RBCs will not be ingested.	Mature cyst contains 4 nuclei, but often stops at 2; chromatoidal bars often present and will look like those found in *E. histolytica*; size <10 μm.	Shrinkage occurs on the permanent stain (especially in the cyst form); *E. histolytica* may actually be below the 12 and 10 μm cutoff limits; could be as much as 1.5 μm below the limits quoted for wet preparation measurements.
Entamoeba coli Non-pathogenic	Cytoplasm dirty, may contain ingested bacteria/debris; peripheral nuclear chromatin is unevenly distributed with a large, eccentric karyosome.	Mature cyst contains 8 nuclei, may see more; chromatoidal bars (if present) tend to have sharp, pointed ends.	If a smear is too thick or thin and if stain is too dark or light, then *E. histolytica* and *E. coli* can often be confused; much overlap in morphology.
Endolimax nana Non-pathogenic	Cytoplasm clean, not diagnostic; great deal of nuclear variation; may even be some peripheral nuclear chromatin; normally only karyosomes are visible.	Cyst is round to oval with the 4 nuclear karyosomes visible.	There is more nuclear variation in this amebae than any other; can be confused with *Dientamoeba fragilis* and/or *E. hartmanni*.
Iodamoeba bütschlii Non-pathogenic	Cytoplasm contains much debris; organisms usually larger than *E. nana*, but may look similar; large karyosome.	Cyst contains single nucleus (may be "basket nucleus") with bits of nuclear chromatin arranged on the nuclear membrane (karyosome is the basket, bits of chromatin are the handle); large glycogen vacuole.	Glycogen vacuole will stain brown with the addition of iodine in the wet preparation; "basket nucleus" more common in cyst, but can be seen in troph; vacuole may be so large the cyst collapses on itself.

Flagellates	Trophozoite	Cyst	Comments
Giardia lamblia Pathogenic	Trophozoites are teardrop shaped from the front, like a curved spoon from the side; contain nuclei, linear axonemes, and curved median bodies.	Cysts are round to oval, containing multiple nuclei, axonemes, and median bodies.	Organisms live in the duodenum and multiple stools may be negative; may have to use additional sampling techniques (aspiration, Entero-Test®).
Chilomastix mesnili Non-pathogenic	Trophozoites are teardrop shaped; cytostome must be visible for ID.	Cyst is lemon-shaped with 1 nucleus and curved fibril called "Shepherds Crook."	Cyst can be identified much easier than the troph form; troph will look like other small flagellates.
Dientamoeba fragilis Pathogenic	Cytoplasm contains debris; may contain 1 or 2 nuclei (chromatin often fragmented into 4 dots).	No known cyst form.	Tremendous size/shape range on a single smear; trophs with 1 nucleus can resemble *E. nana*.
Trichomonas vaginalis Pathogenic	Supporting rod (axostyle) is present; undulating membrane comes half-way down the organism; small dots may be seen in the cytoplasm along the axostyle.	No known cyst form	Recovered from genito-urinary system; often diagnosed in clinic with wet preparation (motility)
Trichomonas hominis Non-pathogenic	Supporting rod (axostyle) is present; undulating membrane comes all the way down the organism; small dots may be seen in the cytoplasm along the axostyle.	No known cyst form	Recovered in stool; trophs may resemble other small flagellate trophs.

Ciliates

Table 56-4   Intestinal tract/urogenital system protozoa: key characteristics—cont'd

Coccidia and microsporidia	Tissue stages	Stages in specimen	Comments
Balantidium coli Pathogenic	Very large trophozoites (50-100 μm long) covered with cilia; large bean-shaped nucleus present.	Morphology not significant with exception of large, bean-shaped nucleus.	Rarely seen in U.S.; causes severe diarrhea with large fluid loss; seen in proficiency testing specimens.
Cryptosporidium parvum Pathogenic	Seen in intestinal mucosa (edge of brush border), gall bladder, and lung; seen in biopsy specimens.	Oocysts seen in stool and/or sputum; organisms acid fast, measure 4-6 μm; hard to find if few in numbers.	Chronic infection in the compromised host (internal autoinfective cycle), self-cure in the immunocompetent host; numbers of oocysts correlate with stool consistency (watery diarrhea—more oocysts); can cause severe, watery diarrhea; oocysts are immediately infective when passed (implicated in nosocomial transmission)
Isospora belli Pathogenic	Seen in intestinal mucosal cells; seen in biopsy specimens; does not seem to be as common as *Cryptosporidium parvum*.	Oocysts seen in stool; organisms are acid fast; best technique is concentration from 10% formalin, not permanent stained smear.	Thought to be the only *Isospora* that infects humans; oocysts are not immediately infective when passed. Poorly seen when concentrated from PVA.
Microsporidia Pathogenic *Nosema* spp. *Pleistophora* spp. *Encephalitozoon* spp. *Enterocytozoon* spp. *Microsporidium* spp.	*Enterocytozoon* spp. usually associated with intestinal tract disease; developing stages small (may require EM for diagnosis).	Spores found in stool; however, size (1-2 μm) makes them very difficult to identify.	High index of suspicion necessary for diagnosis by routine histology; EM usually required; development of monoclonal reagents may lead to methods for identification of spores in stool and/or urine.

of *Toxoplasma gondii*, the hamster for *Leishmania* spp, and the steroid treated rat for *Pneumocystis*.

Serologic methods

Serologic methods have been available for a number of years, both for protozoa and helminths. Results from this type of testing have been helpful but often difficult to interpret: Little standardization exists from method to method, many reagents are "home grown," cross reactions occur among the different but closely-related organisms, and testing may not be widely available. The two most common infections where serologic results can be very helpful are toxoplasmosis and amebiasis. The serology is most important in the diagnosis and/or confirmation of toxoplasmosis. The reader is referred to the Centers for Disease Control in Atlanta or a qualified microbiology reference laboratory for expert advice when considering parasitic serologies. Often the clinical relevance of the result is difficult to interpret, and the Centers for Disease Control can provide valuable information.

IDENTIFICATION OF HUMAN PARASITES (PROTOZOA, HELMINTHS, BLOOD PARASITES)
Protozoa (sites other than blood)

Although the key morphologic characteristics of protozoa can be placed in table form, it takes practice at the microscope to find and identify these small organisms. A number of variables influence the final preparation, not the least of which is specimen collection and preservation. If specimen collection and processing are not handled properly, then even the most experienced parasitologist will miss or misidentify organisms. For these reasons, the reader is referred to clinical parasitology texts with more detailed information, line drawings, and photographs. Some texts are listed at the end of this chapter. Again, even photos will be of limited help unless actual positive clinical specimens have been examined. Information on protozoa that can be recovered from the intestinal tract and the urogenital system are presented in Table 56-4. Those recovered in tissue are listed in Table 56-5.

Helminths (sites other than blood)

Helminth eggs, larvae, and adult worms are most often recovered from the intestinal tract. However, other body sites can contain these organisms. The information in Table 56-6 includes the Nematodes (roundworms), Cestodes (tapeworms), and the Trematodes (flukes). Roundworm and tapeworm infections occur frequently in the United States. With the influx of refugees in the last few years and the expansion of proficiency testing programs, laboratories have identified trematode eggs as well. Some helminth eggs may not always appear typical, and if too much iodine is used in the wet preparations, the eggs can be misidentified as debris. The sedimentation concentration method (part of the ova and parasite examination) is the most effective method for egg/larvae recovery.

Table 56-5   Tissue protozoa

Species	Shape and size	Other features
Toxoplasma gondii[1] Trophozoites (Tachyzoites)	Crescent shaped 4-6 μm long by 2-3 μm wide	Found in peritoneal fluid of experimentally infected mice; intracellular forms somewhat smaller and not usually seen in humans; may be isolated in tissue culture, particularly from CSF; diagnosis is most frequently based on clinical history and serological evidence (acute and convalescent sera).
Cysts (Bradyzoites)	Generally spherical 200 μm to 1 mm in diameter	Cysts occur in many tissues of the body (approximately 30% to 50% of the U.S. population have these organisms in the tissues, indicating past infection); many infections are asymptomatic; infections in the compromised host are very serious and involve the CNS; in these patients, particularly those with AIDS, diagnostic serologic titers may be very difficult to demonstrate.
Pneumocystis carinii Trophozoites	Ameboid in shape; measure about 5 μm; nucleus is visible with Giemsa or hematoxylin stain	Patients with AIDS may have a longer incubation period with an average of about 40 days, but up to 1 year; reports indicate that in as many as 28% of these patients, chest X-rays are normal and physical signs in the chest are absent or ill defined; rales may or may not be detected; serologic studies indicate that by age 4, approximately 80% of those tested are positive; diagnosis is based on actual demonstration of the organism.
Cysts	Usually round; when mature, contain 8 trophozoites; often measure 5 μm and contain very small trophozoites (1 μm)	Before AIDS, the recommended procedure was open lung biopsy; currently, bronchoalveolar lavage (BAL), transbronchial biopsy, and collection of induced sputum specimens are more widely used; No commercial reagents presently available for serologic diagnosis; monoclonal reagents for direct organism detection commercially available.
Cryptosporidium parvum[2]	Oocyst usually round, 4-5 μm, each mature oocyst containing sporozoites (infective on passage)	Oocyst usually diagnostic stage in stool, sputum, and possibly other body-site specimens; Various other stages in life cycle can be seen in biopsy specimens taken from the GI tract (brush border of epithelial cell/intestinal tract) and other tissues (lung, gall bladder); a number of modified acid fast stains have been used successfully; direct detection methods available using monoclonal reagents.
Isospora belli	Ellipsoidal oocyst; usual range 20-30 μm long, 10-19 μm wide; sporocysts rarely seen broken out of oocysts, but measure 9-11 μm	Mature oocyst contains 2 sporocysts with 4 sporozoites each; usual diagnostic stage in feces is immature oocyst containing spherical mass of protoplasm (diarrhetic stool); developing stages can be recovered from intestinal biopsy specimens; oocysts are also acid fast and could be detected during acid fast staining of stool for *Cryptosporidium*; oocysts are often detected in the concentration sediment from 10% formalin (wet preparation).
Microsporidia *Nosema* spp. *Pleistophora* spp. *Encephalitozoon* spp. *Enterocytozoon* spp. *Microsporidium* spp.	Spores are extremely small, have been recovered in all body organs, including the eye	Have been found as insect or other animal parasites; route of infection probably ingestion; histology results vary (acid-fast); PAS stains recommended (spores); animal inoculation not recommended—lab animals may carry occult infection; electron microscopy may be necessary for identification; although rare (may just be difficulty in identification), infections found in several AIDS patients (*Enterocytozoon*, *Pleistophora*) in the intestinal tract and in muscle respectively; very difficult to diagnose this infection by examining stool specimens; development of monoclonal antibody reagents should be very helpful (detection of spores in stool).
Sarcocystis hominis *S. suihominis* *S. bovihominis*	Oocyst thin-walled, contains 2 mature sporocysts, each containing 4 sporozoites; frequently thin oocyst wall ruptures; ovoidal sporocysts measure 9-16 μm long and 7.5-12 μm wide	Thin-walled oocyst or ovoidal sporocysts occur in stool; in the compromised host, may be reports of fever, severe diarrhea, abdominal pain and weight loss, although number of patients has been small; infections occur from the ingestion of uncooked pork or beef; life cycle occurs within the intestinal cells with eventual production of sporocysts in stool.
S. "lindemanni"	Shapes and sizes of skeletal and cardiac muscle sarcocysts vary considerably	When humans accidentally ingest oocysts from other animal stool sources, sarcocysts that develop in human muscle apparently do little, if any harm; can be identified with routine histologic methods.

[1] Note: Organisms identified in histologic preparations or isolated in animals/tissue culture systems may or may not be the causative agent of the symptoms.
[2] The infection in the immunocompetent host is self-limiting. However, in the immunodeficient patient (AIDS), the infection is chronic due to an autoinfective capability in the life cycle. The number of oocysts usually correlate with the symptoms (watery diarrhea—many oocysts in the specimen). The more normal the stool, the more difficult it is to find the oocysts. Clinicians should be aware that risk groups include: animal handlers, travelers, immunocompromised individuals, children in daycare centers, and anyone who comes in contact with these individuals. Since the oocysts are immediately infective, nosocomial transmission has been documented.

Table 56-6   Helminths: key characteristics

Helminths		
Nematodes (roundworms)	**Diagnostic stage**	**Comments**
Ascaris lumbricoides Pathogenic	Egg: both fertilized (oval to round with thick, mamillated/tuberculate shell) and unfertilized (tend to be more oval/elongate with bumpy shell exaggerated) eggs can be found in stool; Adult worms: 10-12″ found in stool; rarely (in severe infections) migrating larvae can be found in sputum.	Unfertilized eggs will not float with the flotation concentration method; adult worms have tendency to migrate when irritated (anesthesia, high fever); thus patients from endemic areas should be checked for infection prior to elective surgery.
Trichuris trichiura (whipworm) Pathogenic	Egg: barrel-shaped with two clear, polar plugs; Adult worm: rarely seen; eggs should be quantitated (rare, few, etc.) since light infections may not be treated.	Dual infections with *Ascaris* may be seen (both infections acquired from egg ingestion in contaminated soil); in severe infections, rectal prolapse may occur in children or bloody diarrhea can be mistaken for amebiasis (usually not seen in the U.S.)
Enterobius vermicularis (pinworm) May cause symptoms in some patients (itching)	Egg: football-shaped with one flattened side; Adult worm: about ⅜″ long, white with pointed tail; female migrates from the anus and deposits eggs on the perianal skin.	Test of choice is Scotch tape preparation; 6 consecutive tapes necessary to "rule out" infection; symptomatic patient often treated without actual confirmation of infection; eggs become infective within a few hours.
Ancylostoma duodenale (Old world hookworm) *Necator americanus* (New world hookworm) May cause symptoms in some patients (blood-loss anemia on the differential smear in heavy infections) Pathogenic	Eggs: identical; oval with broadly rounded ends, thin shell, clear space between shell and developing embryo (8-16 ball stage); Adult worms: rarely seen in clinical specimens.	If stool remains unpreserved for several hours or days, the eggs may continue to develop and hatch; rhabditiform larvae may resemble those of *Strongyloides stercoralis*.
Strongyloides stercoralis Pathogenic May see unexplained eosinophilia, abdominal pain, unexplained episodes of sepsis and/or meningitis, pneumonia (migrating larvae) in the compromised patient.	Rhabditiform larvae (non-infective) usually found in the stool (short buccal cavity or capsule with large/genital primordial packet of cells ("short and sexy"); in very heavy infections, larvae can occasionally be found in sputum, and/or filariform (infective) larvae can be found in stool (slit in the tail).	Potential for internal autoinfection can maintain low-level infections for many years (patient will be asymptomatic/elevated eosinophilia); hyperinfection can occur in the compromised patient (leading to disseminated strongyloidiasis and death).
Ancylostoma braziliensis (dog/cat hookworm) Cause of Cutaneous Larva Migrans (CLM) Pathogenic	Human: accidental host; skin penetration of infective larvae from the soil; larvae will wander through the outer layer of skin creating tracks (severe itching, eosinophilia); no practical microbiological diagnostic tests.	Typical setting for infection: dogs and cats defecate in sand boxes, hookworm eggs hatch and penetrate human skin when in contact with infected sand/soil.
Toxocara cati or *caninum* (dog/cat ascarid) Cause of Visceral Larva Migrans (VLM) Cause of Ocular Larva Migrans (OLM) Pathogenic	Human: accidental host; ingestion of dog/cat ascarid eggs in contaminated soil; larvae wander through deep tissues (including the eye); can be mistaken for cancer of the eye; serologies helpful for confirmation; eosinophilia.	Often, requests for laboratory services will originate in the ophthalmology clinic.
Cestodes (tapeworms) *Taenia saginata* (Beef tapeworm) Can cause symptoms in some individuals (adult worm)	Scolex (4 suckers, no hooklets), gravid proglottid (>12 branches on a single side) are diagnostic; eggs indicate *Taenia* spp. only (thick, striated shell, containing a six-hooked embryo or oncosphere); worm usually about 12′ long.	Ingestion of raw/poorly cooked beef; usually only a single worm per patient; individual proglottids may crawl from the anus; proglottids can be injected with India ink in order to see the uterine branches for identification.

Continued

Table 56-6   Helminths: key characteristics—cont'd

Helminths		
Cestodes (tapeworms)	**Diagnostic stage**	**Comments**
Taenia solium (Pork tapeworm) Can cause GI complaints in some individuals (adult worm) Cysticercosis (accidental ingestion of eggs can cause severe symptoms in the CNS)	Scolex (4 suckers with hooklets), gravid proglottid (<12 branches on a single side) are diagnostic; eggs indicate *Taenia* spp. only (thick, striated shell, containing a six-hooked embryo or oncosphere); worm usually about 12′ long.	Ingestion of raw/poorly cooked pork; usually only a single worm per patient; occasionally 2-3 proglottids may be passed (hooked together); proglottids can be injected with India ink in order to see the uterine branches for identification; cysticerci are normally small and contained within an enclosing membrane; occasionally they may develop as the "racemose" type where the worm tissue grows in the body like a metastatic cancer.
Diphyllobothrium latum (Broad fish tapeworm) Can cause GI complaints in some individuals	Scolex (lateral sucking grooves), gravid proglottid (wider than long, reproductive structures in the center "rosette"), eggs are operculated.	Ingestion of raw or poorly cooked freshwater fish; life cycle has 2 intermediate hosts (copepod, fish); worm may reach 30′ in length; associated with vitamin B$_{12}$ deficiency in genetically susceptible groups
Hymenolepis nana (Dwarf tapeworm) Can cause GI complaints in some individuals	Adult worm not normally seen; egg round to oval, thin shell, containing a six-hooked embryo or oncosphere with polar filaments lying between the embryo and egg shell.	Ingestion of eggs (only life cycle where intermediate host/grain beetle can be bypassed); life cycle of egg to larval to adult can be completed in the human; most common tapeworm in the world.
Hymenolepis diminuta (Rat tapeworm) Uncommon Egg can be confused with *H. nana*	Adult worm not normally seen; egg round to oval, thin shell, containing a six-hooked embryo or oncosphere with no polar filaments lying between the embryo and egg shell.	Eggs will be submitted in proficiency testing specimens and must be differentiated from those of *H. nana*.
Echinococcus granulosus Pathogenic Human accidental intermediate host.	Adult worm found only in the carnivore (dog); hydatid cysts develop (primarily in the liver) when humans accidentally ingest eggs from the dog tapeworms; cyst contains daughter cysts and many scolices; laboratory should examine fluid aspirated from cyst at surgery.	Normal life cycle is sheep/dog, with the hydatid cysts developing in the liver, lung, etc. of the sheep. Humans may be asymptomatic unless fluid leaks from the cyst (can trigger an anaphylactic reaction) or pain is felt from the cyst location.
Echinococcus multilocularis Pathogenic Human accidental intermediate host	Adult worm found only in the carnivore (fox, wolf); hydatid cysts develop (primarily in the liver) when humans accidentally ingest eggs from the carnivore tapeworms; cyst grows like a metastatic cancer with no limiting membrane.	Prognosis in this infection is poor; surgical removal of the tapeworm tissue is very difficult; found in Canada, Alaska, and less frequently in the northern U.S.
Trematodes (flukes)		
Fasciolopsis buski (Giant intestinal fluke) Symptoms depend on worm burden	Eggs are found in stool; very large and operculated (morphology like that of *Fasciola hepatica* eggs).	Acquired from ingestion of plant material on which metacercariae have encysted (water chestnuts); worms hermaphroditic.
Fasciola hepatica (Sheep liver fluke) Symptoms depend on worm burden	Eggs are found in stool; can't be differentiated from those of *F. buski*.	Acquired from ingestion of plant material on which metacercariae have encysted (watercress); worms hermaphroditic.
Opisthorchis sinensis (Chinese liver fluke) (Clonorchis) Symptoms depend on worm burden	Eggs are found in stool; very small, <35 μm; are operculated with shoulders into which the operculum fits.	Acquired from ingestion of raw fish; eggs can be missed unless ×400 power is used for examination; eggs can resemble those of *Metagonimus yokogawai* and *Heterophyes heterophyes* (small intestinal flukes); worms hermaphroditic.
Paragonimus westermani (Lung fluke) Symptoms depend on worm burden and egg deposition	Eggs are coughed up in sputum (brownish "iron filings'—egg packets); can be recovered in sputum or stool (if swallowed); are operculated with shoulders into which operculum fits.	Acquired from ingestion of raw crabs; eggs can be confused with those of *D. latum*; infections seen in the Orient; infections with *P. mexicanus* found in Central and South America; worms hermaphroditic but often cross-fertilize with another worm if present.

Table 56-6 Helminths: key characteristics—cont'd

Helminths		
Trematodes (flukes)	**Diagnostic stage**	**Comments**
Schistosoma mansoni (Blood fluke) Pathogenic	Eggs recovered in stool (large lateral spine); specimens should be collected with no preservatives (to determine egg viability); worms in veins of large intestine.	Acquired from skin penetration of single cercariae from the freshwater snail; pathology caused by body's immune response to the presence of eggs in tissues; adult worms in veins cause no problems; adult worms are separate sexes.
Schistosoma haematobium (Blood fluke) Pathogenic	Eggs recovered in urine (large terminal spine); specimens should be collected with no preservatives (to determine egg viability); worms in veins of bladder.	Acquired from skin penetration of single cercariae from the freshwater snail; pathology as with *S. mansoni;* 24-hour and spot unless should be collected; chronic infection has association with bladder cancer; adult worms are separate sexes.
Schistosoma japonicum (Blood fluke) Pathogenic	Eggs recovered in stool (very small lateral spine); specimens should be collected with no preservatives (to determine egg viability); worms in veins of small intestine.	Acquired from skin penetration of multiple cercariae from the freshwater snail; pathology as with *S. mansoni;* infection usually most severe of the three due to original loading infective dose of cercariae from the freshwater snail (multiple cercariae stick together); pathology associated with egg production, which is greatest in *S. japonicum* infections.

Blood parasites

Of all the parasites found in blood, malaria is the most important in terms of clinical relevance. THE PREPARATION AND EXAMINATION OF BLOOD FILMS IS CONSIDERED A TRUE STAT IN THE MICROBIOLOGY DIVISION OF THE LABORATORY AND COVERAGE MUST BE PROVIDED 24 HOURS A DAY, SEVEN DAYS A WEEK. Some of the key points to remember are as follows:

1. Patients may come into the emergency room with a steady low grade fever (NOTHING to indicate that malaria may be the problem).
2. Blood specimens should be drawn ON ADMISSION. Do NOT wait for periodicity to develop (patient may be severely ill by that time).
3. One of the MOST IMPORTANT QUESTIONS TO HAVE ANSWERED: Has the patient received any malarial medication within the last 24 hours? If so,

Table 56-7 Parasites found in blood

Protozoa		
Malaria	**Diagnostic stage**	**Comments**
Plasmodium vivax (Benign tertian malaria)	Rings are ameboid; presence of Schüffner's dots; all stages seen in peripheral blood; mature schizont contains 16-18 merozoites.	Infects young cells; 48-hour cycle; large geographic range; tends to have "true relapse" from the residual liver stages.
Plasmodium ovale (Ovale malaria)	Rings are non-ameboid; presence of Schüffner's dots; all stages seen in peripheral blood; mature schizont contains 8-10 merozoites; red cells may be oval and have fimbriated edges.	Infects young cells; 48-hour cycle; narrow geographic range; tends to have "true relapse" from residual liver stages.
Plasmodium malariae (Quartan malaria)	Rings are thick; no stippling; all stages seen in peripheral blood; presence of "band forms" and "rosette"-shaped mature schizont; lots of malarial pigment.	Infects old cells; 72-hour cycle; narrow geographic range; associated with recrudescence and "nephrotic syndrome"; no true relapse.
Plasmodium falciparum (Malignant tertian malaria)	Multiple rings; appliqué/accolé forms; no stippling (rare Mauer's clefts); rings and crescent-shaped gametocytes seen in peripheral blood (no other developing stages—rare exception/mature schizont).	Infects all cells, 36- to 48-hour cycle; large geographic range; no true relapse; most pathogenic of four species; plugged capillaries can cause severe symptoms/sequelae (cerebral malaria, lysis of rbcs, etc.).

Continued

Table 56-7 Parasites found in blood—cont'd

Protozoa	Diagnostic stage	Comments
Babesia		
Babesia spp.	Ring forms only (resemble *P. falciparum* rings); seen in splenectomized patients; endemic in the U.S. (no travel history necessary); if present, "Maltese Cross" configuration diagnostic.	Tick-borne infection; associated with Nantucket Island; infection mimics malaria; ring forms more pleomorphic than malaria; more rings/cell (usually) than in malaria.
Trypanosomes and leishmania		
Trypanosoma brucei gambiense (West African Sleeping Sickness)	Trypomastigotes long, slender, with typical undulating membrane; lymph nodes/blood can be sampled; microhematocrit tube concentration helpful; examine spinal fluid in later stages of the infection.	Tsetse fly vector; tends to be chronic infection, exhibiting the real symptoms of sleeping sickness.
Trypanosoma brucei rhodesiense (East African Sleeping Sickness)	Trypomastigotes long, slender, with typical undulating membrane; lymph nodes/blood can be sampled; microhematocrit tube concentration helpful; examine spinal fluid in later stages of the infection.	Tsetse fly vector; tends to be more severe, short-lived infection (particularly in children); patient may expire before progressive symptoms of sleeping sickness appear.
Trypanosoma cruzi (Chagas' Disease) (South American Trypanosomiasis)	Trypomastigotes short, stumpy, often curved in "C" shape; blood sampled early in infection; trypomastigotes enter striated muscle (heart, GI tract) and transform into the amastigote form.	Reduviid bug vector ("Kissing bug"); chronic in adults; severe in young children; great morbidity associated with cardiac failure and loss of muscle contractility in heart and GI tract.
Leishmania spp. (Cutaneous) Not actually blood parasite, but presented as comparison with *L. donovani*	Amastigotes found in macrophages of skin; presence of intracellular forms containing nucleus and kinetoplast diagnostic.	Sand fly vector; organisms recovered from site of lesion only; specimens can be stained or cultured in NNN and/or Schneider's medium; animal inoculation rarely used (hamster).
Leishmania braziliensis (Mucocutaneous) Not actually blood parasite, but presented as comparison with *L. donovani*	Amastigotes found in macrophages of skin and mucous membranes; presence of intracellular forms containing nucleus and kinetoplast diagnostic.	Sand fly vector; organisms recovered from site of lesion only; specimens can be stained or cultured in NNN and/or Schneider's medium; animal inoculation rarely used (hamster).
Leishmania donovani (Visceral)	Amastigotes found throughout the reticuloendothelial system; spleen, liver, bone marrow, etc; presence of intracellular forms containing nucleus and kinetoplast diagnostic.	Sand fly vector; organisms recovered from buffy coat (rarely found), bone marrow aspirate, spleen or liver puncture (rarely performed); specimens can be stained or cultured in NNN and/or Schneider's medium; animal inoculation rarely used (hamster); cause of Kala-Azar.

the parasitemia on the smear may be extremely low (difficult to diagnosis).

4. Remember, if you see developing stages on the smear (older trophozoites/rings, developing schizonts, round gametocytes), then it is one of the three species other than *P. falciparum*, although one always has to consider the rare possibility of a mixed infection (combination of *P. vivax* and *P. falciparum* most likely).

5. If you can not rule out *P. falciparum* from the patient history, then it is important to make sure that the physician realizes that ONE NEGATIVE SET OF BLOOD FILMS DOES NOT RULE OUT MALARIA INFECTION. The use of the QBC™ tube (QBC™ capillary blood tubes, Becton Dickinson, Franklin Lakes, N.J.) may also be helpful, but does not take the place of thick and thin blood films.

6. A typical patient within the U.S. may come in with non-specific symptoms. If you see ring forms only and can't speciate, IT MUST BE A PHYSICIAN DECISION TO WAIT FOR ANOTHER BLOOD DRAW SIX HOURS LATER. If another blood sample is drawn, and you again see only young rings—THIS IS EXTREMELY STRONG EVIDENCE THAT *P. FALCIPARUM* IS PRESENT. In the early phases of the infection, THE TYPICAL CRESCENT-SHAPED GAMETOCYTES WILL NOT BE PRESENT.

The presence of other blood parasites tends to be rare, but proficiency testing samples may contain some of the other organisms, often microfilariae. Information on the blood parasites can be found in Table 56-7. Automated differential instruments are not recommended for the diagnosis of blood parasites.

Table 56-7 Parasites found in blood—cont'd

Helminths		
Filariae	**Diagnostic stage**	**Comments**
Wuchereria bancrofti Pathogenicity due to presence of adult worms	Microfilaria sheathed, clear space at end of tail; nocturnal periodicity seen; elephantiasis seen in chronic infections.	Mosquito vector; microfilariae recovered in blood (membrane filtration, Knott concentrate, thick films); hematoxylin will stain sheath.
Brugia malayi Pathogenicity due to presence of adult worms	Microfilaria sheathed, subterminal and terminal nuclei at end of tail; nocturnal periodicity seen; elephantiasis seen in chronic infections.	Mosquito vector; microfilariae recovered in blood (membrane filtration, Knott concentrate, thick films); hematoxylin will stain sheath.
Loa loa (African eye worm) Pathogenicity due to presence of adult worms	Microfilaria sheathed, nuclei continuous to tip of tail; diurnal periodicity; adult worm may cross the conjunctiva of the eye.	Mango fly vector; history of Calabar swellings, worms in the eye; microfilariae difficult to recover from blood; hematoxylin will stain sheath.
Mansonella spp. Pathogenicity mild and due to presence of adult worms	Microfilaria unsheathed, nuclei may or may not extend to tip of tail (depending on species); nonperiodic; symptoms usually absent or mild.	Midge or Black fly vector; microfilariae recovered in blood (membrane filtration, Knott concentrate, thick films).
Mansonella streptocerca Pathogenicity mild and due to presence of adult worms and/or microfilariae	Microfilaria unsheathed, nuclei extend to tip of tail; when immobile, tail curved like "shepherd's crook"; adults in dermal tissues.	Midge vector; microfilariae found in skin snips; microfilarial tails are split rather than blunt.
Onchocerca volvulus Pathogenicity due to presence of microfilariae	Microfilaria unsheathed, nuclei do not extend to tip of tail; adults in nodules.	Black fly vector; microfilariae found in skin snips; microfilariae migrate to optic nerve, cause of "river blindness."

SUGGESTED READING

Ash LR and Orihel TC: Atlas of human parasitology, ed 2, Chicago, 1984, Am Soc Clin Pathol.

Ash LR and Orihel TC: Parasites: a guide to laboratory procedures and identification, Chicago, 1987, Amer Soc Clin Pathol.

Beaver CP, Jung RC, and Cupp EW: Clinical parasitology, ed 9, Philadelphia, 1984, Lea & Febiger.

Binford CH and Connor DH, eds: Color atlas of tropical and extraordinary diseases, Vols I and II, Washington DC, 1976, Armed Forces Institute of Pathology.

Committee on Education, American Society of Parasitologists: Procedures suggested for use in examination of clinical specimens for parasitic infection, J Parasitol 63:959-960, 1977.

Garcia LS and Bruckner DA: Diagnostic medical parasitology, New York, 1988, Elsevier.

Garcia LS, Shimizu RY, and Bruckner DA: Blood parasites: problems in diagnosis using automated differential instrumentation, Diagn Microbiol Infect Dis 4:173-176, 1986.

Garcia LS and Turner JA: Malaria, Am J Med Tech 46:17-20, 1980.

Garcia LS and Voge M: Diagnostic clinical parasitology: Proper specimen collection and processing, Am J Med Tech 46:459-467, 1980.

Kagan IG: Serodiagnosis of parasitic diseases. In Rose NR and Friedman H, eds: Manual of clinical immunology, Washington, DC, 1980 American Society of Microbiologists.

Markell EK, Voge M, and John DT: Medical parasitology, ed 6, Philadelphia, 1986, W.B. Saunders Co.

Melvin DM and Brooke MM: Laboratory procedures for the diagnosis of intestinal parasites, ed 3, Dept Health, Education, and Welfare publication No. (CDC) 82-8282, Washington DC, 1982, U.S. Government Printing Office.

Parasitology Subcommittee, Microbiology Section of Scientific Assembly, American Society of Medical Technology: Recommended procedures for the examination of clinical specimens submitted for the diagnosis of parasitic infections, Am J Med Tech 44:1101-1106, 1978.

Sapero JJ and Lawless DK: The MIF stain-preservation technique for the identification of intestinal protozoa, Am J Trop Med Hyg 2:613-619, 1953.

Spencer FM and Monroe LS: The color atlas of intestinal parasites, ed 2, Springfield, Ill, 1976, Charles C. Thomas.

Taylor AER and Baker JR, eds: Methods of cultivating parasites in vitro, London, 1978, Academic Press.

Yamaguchi T, ed: A colour atlas of clinical parasitology, Philadelphia, 1981, Lea & Febiger.

Yang J and Scholten T: A fixative for intestinal parasites permitting the use of concentration and permanent staining procedures, Am J Clin Pathol 67:300-304, 1977.

PART NINE

HEMATOLOGY

57 Hemopoiesis and cell kinetics

Jay E. Valinsky

In adult humans, the blood is the most massive and wide-spread tissue in the body. It is estimated that 3×10^9 red blood cells/kg, 1×10^9 myeloid cells/kg, and 6×10^9 platelets/kg of body weight are produced each day. The suggestion that the bone marrow is the tissue principally responsible for the production of this enormous number of cells was probably first stated between 1868 to 1869 almost concurrently by Ernst Neumann and by Guido Bizzozero. In a series of papers, these investigators, working independently, suggested that both red cells and white cells were produced in the bone marrow. Although it is clear that the anatomical distribution of blood-forming elements in the marrow described by these authors was incorrect, the basic principle was sound.

During the last 40 years, it has been convincingly demonstrated that the mammalian blood-forming, or hemopoietic system is composed of a hierarchy of cells that descend from a bone marrow-derived precursor, the pluripotent hemopoietic stem cell. The hemopoietic stem cell not only gives rise to all of the recognizable elements of the blood through a complex sequence of proliferation and differentiation steps, but also is responsible for homeostasis in the system. As in all stem cell systems, homeostasis is maintained because of the capacity of the pluri- or multipotent cells for self-renewal and because of the reciprocal relationship between proliferation and cell differentiation (Fig. 57-1). This model for homeostasis in the hemopoietic system implies an extraordinary level of regulation, and this occurs at both the cellular and the humoral levels. Indeed, perturbations from equilibrium caused by inappropriate regulation of the system may lead to disease.

In this chapter, structural, functional, and regulatory elements of hemopoiesis will be discussed. Emphasis will be placed on the interactions of hemopoietic cells with recently isolated protein modulators of the hemopoietic system, the hemopoietic growth factors, which influence all aspects of proliferation and differentiation.

DEVELOPMENT OF THE HEMOPOIETIC SYSTEM
Hemopoiesis in the embryo

Hemopoiesis begins in the early stages of embryogenesis in virtually all species. In mammals, hemopoietic activity pro-gresses from one organ to the next until it is established in the bone marrow at the end of gestation and into early postnatal life (Fig. 57-2). Hemopoietic stem cells presumably arise from mesenchymal precursors, migrate through the developing embryo at precisely defined times, and establish colonies of blood-forming cells in specific organs. This migration occurs both passively in the circulation and actively through developing tissues through the intermediacy of extracellular matrix receptors and enzymatic digestion of the substratum. In each of the organs involved, yolk sac, liver, spleen, and bone marrow, microenvironments suitable for the seeding of hemopoietic stem cells and subsequent differentiation must be established prior to colonization of the tissue by the hemopoietic precursors.

In mammals, the earliest signs of hemopoietic activity appear in the yolk sac. This is an extraembryonic tissue of mesenchymal origin. In all cases, yolk sac hemopoiesis is restricted to red cell differentiation. Erythropoiesis is first observed in regions of the yolk sac referred to as blood islands. These consist primarily of centrally located, mesenchymally derived cells that are surrounded by a capillary endothelium. This morphologically identifiable unit lies directly adjacent to the embryonic endoderm, which provides nutrients and possibly growth factors for continued erythropoiesis. The cells that give rise to the red cells in the yolk sac appear in the center of the blood islands and are derived from pools of hemopoietic stem cells that may either be of embryonic or extraembryonic origin.

Studies in avian and in some mammalian systems suggest that red cell maturation in the blood islands occurs in two waves. A series of red cells called "primitive red cells" appears first. These cells are nucleated, do not proceed to terminal differentiation, and contain embryonic hemoglobins. The second wave of cells, the "definitive" red cells, enucleates, proceeds to terminal differentiation, and undergoes hemoglobin switching to more mature forms.

The factors responsible for the regulation of hemopoiesis in the yolk sac are poorly defined. For example, red cell differentiation in the yolk sac is essentially unresponsive to erythropoietin, the principal regulator of erythropoiesis in the adult. Further, it has been demonstrated in avian systems that yolk sac erythropoiesis continues after the embryo has been removed or destroyed, suggesting that red cell pro-

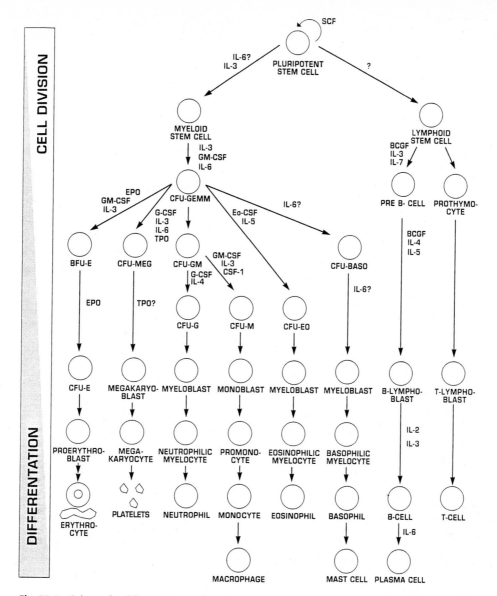

Fig. 57-1 Scheme for differentiation and proliferation in the hemopoietic system. Lineages are denoted by arrows. Growth factors acting at specific stages of differentiation are noted. The curved arrow associated with the pluripotent stem cell denotes "self-renewal." ?, implies the existence of growth factors as yet uncharacterized.

duction does not require factors produced by the embryo itself. These observations suggest that the stem cells that are active in the yolk sac are either maximally stimulated, are subject to autocrine regulation, or are responsive to factors produced locally in the yolk sac.

Hemopoiesis in the yolk sac is a transient process. In the human embryo, yolk sac hemopoiesis begins in the first 6 weeks of gestation and is no longer detectable by the tenth week. The blood islands soon become contiguous with the rapidly developing circulation. Once this occurs, a certain amount of differentiation occurs intravascularly. It is not clear, however, whether the hemopoietic precursors in the yolk sac migrate through the circulation and home to other sites that are receptive to hemopoiesis, or whether stem cells

that subsequently populate the various hemopoietic organs are derived from intraembryonic pools.

The liver is typically the next organ in the sequence (Fig. 57-2). Once the liver has differentiated sufficiently, it is receptive to colonization by hemopoietic stem cells. In humans, hemopoiesis in the liver has been observed as early as 6 weeks of gestation. By week 12, the liver is the principal hemopoietic center. In contrast to hemopoiesis in the yolk sac, liver hemopoiesis is not restricted to erythropoiesis. Myelopoiesis and megakaryocytopoiesis follow the appearance of red cells. Lymphoid differentiation is also observed. This unrestricted hemopoietic activity is clearly due to the presence in the liver of precursor cells that give rise to these lineages and implies that regulatory factors that lead to the

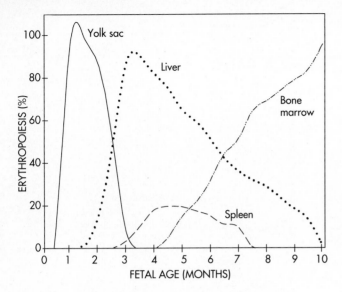

Fig. 57-2 Hemopoiesis in the human embryo.

commitment of multipotential stem cells to specific lineages are also present. The population of hepatic hemopoietic precursors is a stable population of cells that remain in the liver during the entire hemopoietic period. There do not appear to be waves of migration of new stem cells into the liver, as is the case for the yolk sac and thymus. The mechanisms for regulation of liver hemopoiesis in the embryo are unclear. As in the yolk sac, the precursors are relatively insensitive to growth factors such as erythropoietin.

Hemopoiesis begins in the human fetal spleen when yolk sac hemopoiesis is at an end (12 weeks) and peaks between 16 to 20 weeks. It occurs concurrently with liver hemopoiesis. The spleen appears to be colonized by hemopoietic cells in two phases. The first phase consists of the migration of precursor cells from the circulation into the so-called red pulp of the spleen to form hemopoietic foci. These precursors are probably derived from the liver. In the second phase, lymphoid precursors migrate from the circulation into reticular sheaths that surround arterioles to form the so-called white pulp. The lymphoid elements remain in clearly defined zones in the spleen. Splenic hemopoiesis generally does not account for more than 20% of the total hemopoietic activity of the fetus.

By 16 to 18 weeks, the human fetal bone marrow begins to develop into a hemopoietically active tissue. At the end of gestation, the bone marrow is essentially the sole hemopoietic tissue. Bone marrow is formed following the migration of mesenchymal cells that invade calcified cartilaginous tissue during the development of tubular bones. These mesenchymal cells presumably have hemopoietic potential and, in fact, may include stem cells derived from other hemopoietic tissue. There is contrasting evidence that suggests, however, that the marrow stem cells are derived from an independent pool. The mesenchymal cells and associated blood vessels form a reticular network that supports subsequent hemopoiesis, a so-called inductive microenvironment. In the human embryo, this microenvironment is apparently not restrictive; both myelopoietic and erythropoietic

activities are evident from the early stages of marrow development, and lymphoid and megakaryocyte differentiation soon follow. In addition, hemopoietic activity in the fetal bone marrow is compartmentalized, namely, red cell production occurs intravascularly and myeloid cell production appears to occur extravascularly. Following birth erythropoiesis becomes extravascular as well.

Cell types, distribution and structure of the bone marrow

In an adult human, the bone marrow accounts for approximately 3% to 4% of the total body mass. Though precise figures for human bone marrow are not readily available, as in most animals, about 50% of the marrow is found in the limbs, 30% in the trunk, and 20% in the skull. The bone marrow is distributed diffusely in the body in virtually all bones and its composition varies with location and age. Marrow in the peripheral skeleton (yellow marrow) contains a preponderance of adipose tissue, which is not directly involved in hemopoiesis. Adipose tissue may be important, however, in establishing an effective hemopoietic microenvironment. In the axial skeleton where hemopoiesis is most intense (red marrow), there is less adipose tissue. With advancing age, red marrow changes to a more adipose-rich marrow, especially in the long bones. The reappearance of hemopoietically active marrow at sites of deposition of fatty marrow has also been postulated. This, in theory, would raise the possibility of mobilizing a marrow reserve. However, there is no strong evidence to suggest that this conversion actually occurs, even under stress on the hemopoietic system.

The bone marrow itself is a reticulum that is highly vascularized and rich in cells. Table 57-1 shows the approximate differential count of nucleated cells in the normal human bone marrow. The counts are approximate because it is very difficult to distinguish between blastic cells of different lineages on the basis of morphology alone. While all hemopoietic cell lineages are represented; erythroid and myeloid cells predominate. The human fetal marrow contains a relatively high percentage of mononuclear cells (30% as compared to about 10% to 12% in the adult), including lymphocytes, monocyte precursors, and transitional cells, that is, cells that look like small lymphocytes, but which include, in all probability, populations of lineage-specific or multipotential stem cells.

There are two principal compartments in the bone marrow, the hemopoietic cells and the supporting stromal cells. The hemopoietic cells constitute the vast majority of the cells in the marrow. With the probable exception of some precursor cells, the blood cells are present in the marrow only transiently. Following maturation, the cells migrate from the bone marrow to enter the circulation and/or to colonize various organs (e.g., lymph nodes, thymus, spleen, lungs, liver). The stromal elements of the marrow do not migrate. The stroma has two principal functions: to provide a structural meshwork in which hemopoiesis can take place and to provide an appropriate milieu for the proliferation and differentiation of hemopoietic cells. As will be discussed in sections that follow, the stromal cells of the marrow not only produce humoral factors that are active in the regulation of hemopoietic activity, but modulate the activity

Table 57-1 Normal values and kinetic properties of human bone marrow cells*

Cell type	Range (%)	Compartment	Transit time† (hr)
MYELOID CELLS			
Stem cells, progenitors	<0.1	P	
Myeloblasts	0.3-5.0	D	12
Promyelocytes	1.0-8.0	D	12
Myelocytes	7.0-20.0	M	24
Metamyelocytes, early bands	10.0-30.0	M	24
Neutrophils (late bands)	15.0-35.0	S	36
Neutrophilis (segmented)			48
Eosinophils	0.5-3.0	S	
Basophils	0-1.0	S	
ERYTHROID CELLS			
Stem cells, progenitors	<0.1	P	
Proerythroblasts	0.2-4.0	D	16
Basophilic normoblasts	1.0-6.0	D	16
Polychromatophilic normoblasts	5.0-25.0	D	48
Orthochromic normoblasts	2.0-20.0	M	48
Reticulocytes‡	25.0-35.0	S	43
Erythrocytes§		S	~120 days
MONONUCLEAR CELLS/MEGAKARYOCYTES‖			
Lymphocytes	2.0-12.0	S	
Plasmacytes	0-2.0	S	
Monocytes (all stages)	0.5-5.0	S	
Megakaryocytes	<0.01	S	

*P, proliferative compartment; D, differentiation compartments; M, maturation compartment; S, storage compartment.
†Transit time refers to the amount of time a cell remains associated with a particular compartment. Intermitotic intervals for the myeloid series is about 12 hours and 16 hours for erythroid cells.
‡Reticulocytes are found both in the bone morrow and in the peripheral blood. Approximately 2% of the total erythroid cells are reticulocytes.
§Erythrocytes are found primarily in the peripheral blood. The half-life of these cells is approximately 120 days. This is noted as their transit time through the storage compartment.
‖Limited data are available regarding the transit times through the various compartments for lymphocytes, monocytes, and megakaryocytes. These cells are predominantly found in storage pools. For lymphoid cells, transit time in the thymus and other primary lymphoid tissues is about 3 days. Transit times in other sites may exceed 30 days.

of precursor cells through a complex set of cell-cell interactions.

Hemopoietic foci and organization of blood vessels

Figure 57-3, a schematic cross-sectional view through a tubular bone, shows the major organizational features of the bone marrow. Arteries that penetrate the bone ramify and form specialized structures called marrow sinuses or sinusoids. The individual sinuses do not contact the venous system directly, but rather, several combine and lead to the central vein. Blood flows toward the periphery of the bone and then back centrally.

The vessels of the bone marrow are highly specialized structures that permit the constant traffic of very large numbers of cells from the marrow into the blood. The principal morphological modification of the veins, arteries, and sinusoids in the marrow is the relative thinness of the vessel walls. Cells exit the bone marrow by extravasation through the vessel walls. It is astonishing that the structure of the thin vessel walls can remain intact in light of the constant flux of maturing blood cells through the endothelial layer of these vessels.

Hemopoietic activity is most intense at the periphery of the marrow cavity. It is not surprising, then, that morpho-

logical evidence suggests that the highest concentration of hemopoietic precursor cells is in these peripheral regions as well. As noted earlier, hemopoiesis occurs in different compartments in the marrow. In adult mammals all hemopoietic activity occurs extravascularly. At a particular terminal stage in differentiation, cells migrate from the marrow by traversing the vascular endothelium and entering the circulation. The mechanisms involved in this migratory behavior are not clear, but may involve the selective loss, from the cell surface, of antigens that interact with extracellular matrix components in the marrow. These interactions presumably hold the cells in place. Once the antigens are lost, migration to the circulation is enhanced.

The various hemopoietic cell lineages proliferate and differentiate in distinct compartments in the marrow. Erythroid cells differentiate in erythroblastic islands in close association with specialized macrophages called nurse cells. These cells appear to be required for successful erythropoiesis and may be involved in the enucleation process. Granulocyte differentiation occurs in foci, which are anatomically less distinct. Megakaryocytes appear to differentiate in regions in close approximation to the sinusoidal endothelium. Electron microscopy suggests that cytoplasmic extension from the megakaryocytes invaginate the endothelium, thus anchoring the cells to the vessel wall.

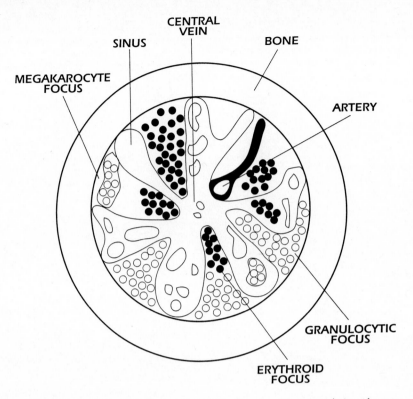

Fig. 57-3 Sites of hemopoiesis in the bone marrow. The drawing shows a rendering of a cross section through an actively hemopoietic bone.

Stromal elements and their role in hemopoiesis

The second principal component of the marrow is the stroma. As noted earlier, the stroma creates a microenvironment in which hemopoiesis can take place. This microenvironment consists of cellular elements, extracellular matrix molecules (e.g. Saminin, fibronectin, collagen), and humoral factors that define and regulate hemopoietic activity. The population of stromal cells is heterogeneous in nature. It consists primarily of endothelial cells, fibroblasts, adipocytes, macrophages, and adventitial reticular cells. These cells produce growth factors necessary to sustain hemopoiesis and are also involved in cell-cell interactions that regulate the activity of hemopoietic precursors.

In addition to the cellular interactions in the stroma, growth factor production is affected by the interactions of stromal cells with a variety of cytokines and lymphokines. For example, factors produced by monocytes (e.g., IL-1 [Interleukin-1] and tumor necrosis factor) can stimulate the production of several hemopoietic growth factors (e.g., G-CSF, M-CSF, and GM-CSF [granulocyte-colony stimulating factor, macrophage-colony stimulating factor, and granulocyte-macrophage colony stimulating factor]) by several different cell types (e.g., endothelial cells, fibroblasts). This illustrates the intimate relationships that are emerging between cell and humoral factors in the stromal regulation of hemopoiesis.

Kinetic and quantitative considerations

As noted at the outset, hemopoiesis in the bone marrow accounts for the vast majority of daily blood cell production. Cell proliferation and differentiation in the marrow must be coordinated so that sufficient numbers of functional cells are produced and the marrow stem cell pools are maintained.

The recognizable precursors and terminally differentiated cells in the hemopoietic system can be classified both with regard to their mitotic activity and the degree to which they have differentiated. This classification defines the aforementioned pools or compartments. There have been several attempts to define these compartments. We can define four pools: (1) the proliferative compartment contains stem cells capable of self-renewal, multipotent progenitors capable of extensive cell division, and lineage-restricted progenitors and recognizable precursors capable of clonal expansion; (2) the differentiation compartment contains lineage-restricted cells with limited capacity for mitosis (perhaps 1 to 3 cell divisions); (3) the maturation compartment contains recognizable precursors that have essentially lost the capacity for cell division and that are programmed toward terminal differentiation; (4) the storage compartment contains the terminally differentiated recognizable cells of the hemopoietic organs and the peripheral blood. These cells are functionally active or can be activated in response to humoral or cellular stimuli.

Calculation of the flux of cells through the various hemopoietic compartments and in the various lineages must take into account the total marrow volume, the proliferative potential of particular precursors, the circulatory half-lives of some types of cells, the rate and extent of cell death, and the extent to which cells marginate or migrate into sites in the tissue. These calculations have been hampered somewhat by imprecise measurements. Nonetheless, estimates of cell transit times have been made for erythroid, myeloid, and lymphoid elements. Table 57-1 illustrates the distribution and transit times for selected cell types in the bone marrow.

Red cell traffic

Transit of erythroid cells through the circulation has been measured precisely using chromium-51–labeled cells. In the adult human, the half-life for a circulating red cell is 120 days. Calculations based on the mitotic indices of red cell precursors in the marrow, the total red cells, and the life span, indicate that there are about 5×10^9 red cell precursors/kg of body weight, or in a 70-kg human, 3.5×10^{11}. From the total number of red cells and the circulatory half-life, it can be estimated that the marrow is required to produce 2.1×10^{11} red cells per day. Given the number of precursors available per day, one can see that there is a minimal reserve of red cells available under normal conditions; that is to say, the daily output of the marrow barely matches the need for red cells. It has been suggested that there is a small reserve of reticulocytes, which can be mobilized upon demand, that may take up the short fall in nucleated erythroid precursor.

Myeloid cell traffic

Granulocytes have very short half-lives in the circulation. The flux of precursor cells into the pool of myeloblasts has been estimated to be 0.4×10^7 cells/kg/hour. This rate suggests that, unlike erythroid precursors, there is a considerable reserve of granulocyte precursors in the bone marrow and in humans, may be ten- to twentyfold. After several mitotic divisions, mature granulocytes appear in the peripheral blood. It is estimated that the average turnover time for a bone marrow granulocyte is about 72 hours. Granulocytes remain in the circulation for only a few hours (<8 hours) before they marginate. Further, the precursor cells can undergo rapid proliferative bursts and cells can be mobilized into the circulation upon demand. This has been shown in pulse radiolabeling experiments. Under normal conditions, it takes approximately 100 hours for mature granulocytes to emerge from the bone marrow. Stimulated by infection, this rate may increase twofold, to about 48 hours.

Lymphocyte traffic

The bone marrow is only one site for the proliferation and differentiation of lymphocytes, and as such, a description of the kinetics of lymphocyte traffic is difficult. In humans, as in most mammals, consideration of lymphocyte traffic must include the lymphoid populations in lymph nodes, thymus, lymphoid nodules, spleen, and lymphoid tissue in the gastrointestinal tract. Lymphocytes in the peripheral blood presumably recirculate through the lymphatic system, using the lymph nodes as way stations in their transit back to the blood. Lymphoid cells in the marrow and more than 80% of the cells in the thymus have very short life spans, probably just a few days. In contrast, splenic lymphocytes and lymphocytes in the lymph nodes may have life spans of months to years.

THEORETICAL CONSIDERATIONS OF HEMOPOIESIS

The scheme in Fig. 57-1, which depicts the hierarchical structure of the hemopoietic system, has several salient features: (1) as noted several times previously, all cells in all lineages derive from a pluripotent stem cell that is capable of self-renewal and that has limited proliferative capacity; (2) progenitor cells arising from the differentiation of the pluripotent stem cell have increased proliferative capacity relative to the pluripotent stem cell and are committed increasingly to specific cell lineages; (3) proliferation and differentiation are regulated by proteins, the hemopoietic growth factors, which have lineage specificity; (4) these factors work singly and/or in combination to direct the flux of cells through the hemopoietic pathways; (5) as differentiation proceeds to the terminal stages, the proliferative capacity of the cells diminishes; and (6) as differentiation proceeds, the capacity for self-renewal in all but the pluripotent stem is lost.

This depiction of the hemopoietic system appears straightforward and suggests that differentiation proceeds in a number of discrete steps that relate parent to progeny. However, there is not necessarily a simple linear time course relating the events as described. It has been suggested, for example, that several programs of cell division/differentiation in any lineage may occur concurrently, making the system very heterogeneous and complex. Further, it has been suggested that there is considerable plasticity in the hemopoietic system, namely, that the movement of cells through branch points in the system is highly fluid, that some steps in the system may not be irreversible, and that interconversions between pathways may not be uncommon.

The maintenance of homeostasis in the hemopoietic system results from the aforementioned properties of the hemopoietic stem cell. As in all stem cell systems, for example, seminiferous epithelium, small intestine, and epidermis, a small population of multipotential cells gives rise, through regulated processes of proliferation and differentiation, to a set of functional, mature cells. The most intriguing aspect of stem cell biology, however, is the capacity of the pluri- or multipotent stem cell for self-renewal. This concept, first advanced over 30 years ago for the hemopoietic stem cell, suggests that during cell division, a progenitor cell may produce daughter cells that are identical to the parent (self-renewal) or may differentiate to more mature progeny. This is believed to be a random or stochastic process. Maintenance of the proportional relationships among hemopoietic cells in the steady state levels of hemopoiesis requires that the population of stem cells is renewed throughout the life of the individual and that the number of stem cells ultimately capable of proliferation and differentiation essentially remains constant.

The validation of the notion of stem cells in the hemopoietic system was given in a set of observations concerning the frequency distribution of hemopoietic colony forming cells in the spleens of lethally irradiated mice following intravenous injection of bone marrow. Cells from these spleens were passaged serially into a second set of mice and the frequency of colonies was obtained. The appearance of colonies was consistent with mathematical models that reinforced the notion of a random process. While it is now clear that these colonies did not derive from the most primitive stem cells, the mathematical model still holds. Recent data suggest, however, that hemopoiesis may not be as dominated by stochastic processes as previously believed, but rather, the system is set up to proceed in a more predetermined manner. In this view there may be the orderly and progressive loss of lineage potential until complete lineage restriction is achieved. While conclusive evidence is not yet available to settle this dispute, it is clear that self-renewal must occur at a frequency great enough to maintain the pool of progenitor cells.

Properties of the hemopoietic stem cell

At the top of the hierarchy of cells in the hemopoietic system (Fig. 57-1) are the pluripotent stem cells, which give rise to all cell lineages. These cells are defined operationally as those capable of long-term reconstitution of the bone marrow following marrow transplantation. The number of pluripotent stem cells in the human bone marrow has been estimated statistically by fluctuation analysis to be perhaps 1000 or less. This number is consistent with the general stem cell hypothesis and numbers of stem cells found in other systems. These estimates, and the distribution of chromosomal, DNA sequence or retroviral markers in the progeny of hemopoietic precursors identified during the repopulation of the bone marrow following transplants into lethally irradiated mice, indicated that hemopoiesis is clonal. This is to say that all cells in the hemopoietic systems of these irradiated mice derive from the expansion of a single progenitor. This clonality is believed to be reflected not only in normal hemopoiesis, but also in clonal hemopathies such as acute myeloid leukemia and polycythemia rubra vera. Two corollaries of the clonal dominance view are that (1) one or, at most, a very small number of pluripotent stem cells are active at any given time and (2), that hemopoietic clones are recruited sequentially throughout the life of the individual. Contrasting opinion holds that this is not the case, but rather, hemopoiesis may take place within the framework of multiple progenitors that are in an active, proliferative state.

Pluripotent stem cells have not been isolated or described morphologically. Their presence in hemopoietic tissue, notably in bone marrow, has been pointed to by functional assays in which progeny of the stem cells can be detected in a variety of in vivo and in vitro clonogenic assays (see text that follows). Recent attempts to purify the pluripotent stem cell from murine or human marrow have yielded enriched populations of cells that, at least in the case of mice, give rise to multiple cell lineages and are capable of long-term repopulation of the marrow in lethally irradiated animals.

The two principal kinetic properties of the stem cell are its capacity for self-renewal and its limited proliferative potential. It has been suggested that the pluripotent stem cell is a quiescent cell that resides in G_o. This is a phase of the cell cycle in which cells are non-dividing and in a maintenance mode. The limited proliferative potential of the stem cell has been pointed to first in tritiated-thymidine suicide experiments, which indicated that only a small portion of cells that gave rise to multiple lineages were active in the cell cycle. Later, it was determined that the quiescent cells

were indeed the ones capable of long-term repopulation of the bone marrow in lethally irradiated mice. Self-renewal, an essential property of all stem cells, was demonstrated by serial transplantation of colony forming cells in the spleen in vivo and also by serial passage of progenitors in cell culture. For the system to work properly, the rate of self-renewal must be consistent with the daily requirements of the program or the stem cell pool will be rapidly depleted. Even though stem cells are for the most part in G_o, they do not appear to respond, in a kinetic sense, only to emergency situations or stresses on the system. Rather, they appear to be continuously responsive to external stimuli.

Recent evidence suggests that the pluripotent stem cells may be in close association with the stromal cells in the bone marrow. The intimate cell-cell interactions that this association implies are believed to play important regulatory roles in hemopoiesis. One school of thought contends that the hemopoietic microenvironment in the bone marrow not only stimulates hemopoiesis, but also provides a milieu that inhibits the proliferation of progenitors, or at least one that prohibits uncontrolled expansion of the hemopoietic clones. Loss of the inhibitory aspect of the microenvironment, either by abnormal production of inhibitory factors, loss of important receptors, or improper responses to inhibitory stimuli, could result in uncontrolled growth and disease.

The ability to stimulate the pluripotent stem cell from G_o in vitro has enormous consequences for bone marrow transplantation and for our understanding of the regulation of hemopoiesis. From the point of view of understanding the regulation of hemopoiesis, the interactions of combinations of purified growth factors on purified stem cells could provide valuable information about the mechanism of self-renewal and commitment to particular differentiation programs at the molecular level. In very recent studies, for example, a glycoprotein, stem cell factor (SCF) has been isolated from rat liver. Initially identified as a mast cell growth factor, SCF appears to act in synergy with other growth factors to stimulate quiescent stem cells into the cell cycle and to differentiate into cells capable of colony formation in vitro. Further, it has been found that this protein is a product of the steel (S1) locus, which is required for maintenance of hemopoiesis. This protein appears to act through the c-kit receptor (i.e., SCF is the c-kit ligand) and is now thought to be a more general stimulator of pluripotent stem cells in the hemopoietic as well as in other systems. The synergy observed between SCF and other hemopoietic growth factors (e.g. Interleukin-3) is typical of growth factor interactions in the hemopoietic system (v. infra).

Hemopoietic progenitor cells: general considerations

Progenitor cells are defined operationally in this context as multipotential or lineage-restricted cells that give rise to differentiated progeny (Table 57-2). Progenitors of the various hemopoietic lineages, like the pluripotent stem cell, have never been purified to homogeneity. Evidence for their existence comes primarily from the observation of their functional activities in vitro and in vivo. Proliferation of progenitor cells and subsequent differentiation into the various recognizable elements of the bone marrow and peripheral blood are modulated by lineage-specific growth factors

Table 57-2   Hemopoietic progenitor cells*

Progenitor cell	Differentiated cell	Growth factor
CFU-GEMM	Multilineage (G, mega, mac, E, T-cells[?])	IL-3, GM-CSF
Blast colony	Blasts, multilineage, self-renewal	IL-3, G-CSF, IL-6
HPP-CFC	Mac, G, mega	CSF-1 plus IL-3, IL-1; or other combinations of factors
BFU-E	Erythroid	EPO plus IL-3, GM-CSF, IL-4
CFU-E	Erythroid	EPO
GM-CFU	G, Mac	GM-CSF, G-CSF, CSF-1?
G-CFC	G	CSF-1
M-CFC	Mac	CSF-1, GM-CSF?, IL-3?
BFU-M	Mega	IL-3, GM-CSF, TPO
CFU-M	Mega	IL-3, GM-CSF, G-CSF, IL-6, TPO
CFU-S (mouse)	E, mega, G, mac, self-renewal	IL-3
Thy-1^{10}Lin$^-$Sca-1$^+$ (mouse)	T, B, myeloid	Multifactors

*G, granulocyte; Mac, macrophage; E, erythroid; mega, megakaryocyte; T, T-lymphocytes; B, B-lymphocytes; CFU, colony forming unit; CFC, colony forming cell; HPP, high proliferative potential; IL-3, interleukin-3; IL-6, interleukin-6; EPO, erythropoietin; TPO, thrombopoietin-like activity; CSF, colony stimulating factor; ?, indicates some doubt as to the precise effects of this factor on the system in question. Thy-1^{10}Lin$^-$Sca-1$^+$ (mouse) refers to a multipotential stem cell isolated from mouse bone marrow.

which will be described later. They act selectively on responsive cells that possess specific cell surface receptors for these factors. The following sections describe cellular and biological aspects of the interactions of growth factors with hemopoietic progenitors.

Functional assays for progenitor cells

Progenitor cells differ from pluripotent hemopoietic stem cells in two respects, they have an enhanced capacity for proliferation and, as differentiation proceeds, they become increasingly lineage-restricted. The existence of these progenitor cells was first suggested in vivo following the transplantation of bone marrow into mice that had been lethally irradiated. Following the transplant (10 to 14 days), hemopoietic foci developed in the spleens of these mice. These foci contained erythroid and myeloid elements, but typically no lymphoid elements. Serial transplantation of the cells from the hemopoietic foci suggested that they arose from single progenitor cells that were at least multipotent. Approximately 20 colonies could be formed in the spleen from 10^5 nucleated bone marrow cells that were transplanted. This suggested that approximately 0.02% to 0.1% of the nucleated cells in the bone marrow were capable of giving rise to these foci. Colonies can be found in the spleen after 8 to 10 days which are slightly different from those observed after 10 to 14 days. The 8 to 10 day colonies are derived presumably from more mature precursors with higher proliferative capacity. Both types of colonies are stimulated by interleukin-3 and probably other growth factors. The colony forming cells were called CFU-S, for colony forming unit-spleen, and were, for a considerable period, considered to be candidate pluripotent stem cells. The ability of candidate stem cells to successfully repopulate the bone marrow of lethally irradiated, or congenitally stem-cell–deficient mice, remains, after more than 30 years, the most convincing evidence for the presence of pluripotential cells in the bone marrow.

It was soon found, however, that lineage-restricted hemopoietic colonies derived from precursors in the bone marrow could be identified and studied in cell culture. Bone marrow, or in fact other hemopoietic tissue (e.g., spleen cells), can

be cultured in a semisolid medium (e.g., agar, methyl cellulose). The addition of serum and a source of hemopoietic growth factor(s) resulted in colony formation. After a certain time (e.g., 7 to 14 days) in culture, foci of cells could be seen in the semisolid media. The number of colonies and the size of the colonies are dependent upon the concentration of growth factor and the number of hemopoietic cells added. Initially, these growth factors, called colony stimulating factors, were derived from biological fluids (e.g., erythropoietin derived from human urine), cell culture medium conditioned by a variety of cell lines, or lectin-stimulated peripheral blood leukocytes. The disadvantage of these preparations was that the colony stimulating factors were typically impure mixtures of proteins and, in many cases, contained inhibitory activities. In more recent years, purified or recombinant growth factors have replaced the cruder preparations. Morphological examination revealed that, depending on the mix of growth factors used, the colonies could be homogeneous or mixed.

Experiments of this type permitted the establishment of lineage relationships commonly accepted in the hemopoietic system and, by counting the colonies produced, one could determine the approximate frequency of a particular progenitor cell in the hemopoietic cell population under study. As a variation of this technique, liquid culture of progenitors in the presence of serum and growth factors, or under serum-free conditions, has also been achieved. The activity of the progenitors cultured in this way can be assessed by subsequent culture in semisolid media as described earlier or by transplantation into mice to analyze bone marrow reconstitution.

Other functional assays for the presence of progenitor cells have also been developed. Diffusion chambers, made of 0.2 μm nitrocellulose filters suspended in Lucite rings have been transplanted to the peritoneal cavity of rodents or other animals. Several experiments have also been conducted in human volunteers. The chamber created by the filters is seeded with hemopoietic, or other (e.g., tumor cells) cells prior to transplant. The filters are impermeable to cells, but are permeable to proteins. Thus, humoral hemopoietic growth factors present in the host animal will induce the proliferation and differentiation of the cells suspended in the chamber, and the effects of specific pharmacologic manipulations of the host on hemopoiesis can be monitored.

Colony formation in the diffusion chamber is measured following removal of the chamber and culturing the cells in plasma clot formed inside the chamber. Colony forming cells of the types seen in semisolid media can then be enumerated and evaluated morphologically. The advantage of the diffusion chamber technique is that the cells inoculated into the chamber can be of a defined type (e.g., bone marrow, tumor cells). The principal disadvantage of the diffusion chamber is that, while it is implanted in vivo, it provides an artificial environment in which the progenitors can grow. The stromal elements of the marrow in vivo are not present. While there are considerable kinetic and quantitative differences in the behavior of progenitors in the bone marrow and in diffusion chambers, the latter technique is often considered the best in vivo system for studying the effects of humoral regulators on hemopoiesis.

Long-term bone marrow cultures (LTC) are systems that support the prolonged self-renewal, proliferation and differentiation of hemopoietic precursors in vitro. These cultures are prepared by seeding tissue culture flasks with bone marrow. After several days in culture under proper conditions of temperature, CO_2, and medium, a monolayer of cells forms in the flask that, with additional time in culture, becomes confluent. This layer contains bone marrow stromal cells (e.g., fibroblasts, endodermal cells, macrophage, adipocytes). The composition of this adherent layer of cells may vary depending on the source of the marrow and on the precise culture conditions. The continuous proliferation of progenitors in these cultures can be demonstrated by removing 50% of the original marrow and replacing it with a fresh inoculum weekly (or by removing all of the adherent cells and replacing the medium) and monitoring the colony forming capabilities of cells from the nonadherent layer in semisolid media. The results indicated that if, for example, 50% of the nonadherent cells were removed, the number of CFU would be decreased proportionately. However, during the ensuing 7 to 10 days, the number of progenitors would come back to the original starting point. In the murine system, this process could be repeated essentially indefinitely. In the human system, even with careful control of the incubation conditions, the system tends to run down, implying that there were missing stimulatory elements. It has subsequently been shown that the stromal layer in long-term cultures produces a variety of growth factors (e.g., GM-CSF, M-CSF, G-CSF, TNF-α, TGF-β, and perhaps interferons). The hemopoietic microenvironment created in these long-term cultures mimics to some degree the microenvironment in the bone marrow. To the extent that this is true, long-term bone marrow cultures will continue to have a significant place in studies of regulation of hemopoiesis, cell kinetics, and the nature of stromal-progenitor interactions.

Hemopoietic growth factors

Hemopoiesis in vitro or in vivo requires the obligatory action of factors that modulate proliferation and differentiation. Regulation of hemopoiesis by growth factors assumes two aspects: (1) the regulation of normal, baseline hemopoiesis; (2) the response of the hemopoietic system to stress (e.g., infection, anoxia). In the former case, maintenance of homeostasis is the goal. In the second case, enhanced production of growth factors occurs, with consequences for amplification of the system (e.g., increased production of erythropoietin at high altitude stimulates increases in the size of the erythron). Hemopoietic growth factors are typically glycoproteins. Many have now been purified, cloned, sequenced, and expressed in yeast or *Escherichia coli*. The hemopoietic growth factors are a subset of cytokines, some of which are unique to the hemopoietic system. A listing of several of these factors and a summary of their biological activities is provided in Table 57-3. Considerations of the regulatory mechanisms involved in the synthesis and activity of these factors must include regulation of cytokine gene expression at both the transcriptional and translational levels, posttranslational modification of the growth factors, and modulation of growth factor receptor activity.

Hemopoietic growth factors were, for the most part, identified initially in media conditioned by tumor cell lines, B- and T-cell lines, fibroblasts, stromal fibroblasts, endothelial cells, dendritic cells, peripheral blood mononuclear cells, spleen cells, placenta, biological fluids (e.g., serum, urine), and a variety of other tissues. Production of factors by these cells have been shown to be constitutive in some cases and inducible in others. The induction may be autocrine or regulated by other growth factors, lymphokines or cytokines. Two classes of factors were initially identified, namely, factors that stimulated myeloid and or erythroid differentiation and factors that stimulated lymphoid differentiation. In the latter category, many of these factors were found to be the same ones that have such profound effects on the modulation of the cellular and humoral immune systems, namely, the interleukins. In general, factors that stimulate myeloid/erythroid colony formation in vitro (e.g., erythropoietin, colony stimulating factors) appear to be specific to the hemopoietic system, although the interleukin family of cytokines, which are potent modulators of the hemopoietic system, are also strongly bioactive in the immune system.

The myeloid and erythroid colony stimulating factors were defined primarily through the use of colony formation assays in semisolid media as already described. Initial investigations using conditioned media and partially purified materials as a source of factors suggested that many of the myeloid factors acted on specific cell lineages. As the purity of the preparations increased and recombinant factors became available in large quantities, it became clear that: (1) colony stimulating factors may have multiple biological activities; (2) some hemopoietic growth factors stimulate across lineages (e.g., GM-CSF, IL-3). These factors tend to act on more immature precursor cells (CFU-GEMM, BFU-E, CFU-Meg, CFU-GM) and do not drive the cells to terminal differentiation; (3) Some hemopoietic growth factors are more lineage restricted (e.g., erythropoietin, G-CSF, M-CSF, IL-5). These factors tend to act on more mature progenitors (e.g., CFU-E) and stimulate the final mitotic divisions through terminal differentiation; (4) Cells that respond to colony stimulating factors and interleukins and other factors (e.g. TGF.B) generally do so through cell surface receptors. The responses to these receptor-mediated

Table 57-3   Summary of biological activities of hemopoietic growth factors

Growth factor	Biological activity
GM-CSF	Stimulates granulocyte-macrophage colony growth in vitro
	Induces proliferation of myeloid cells in vivo
	Erythroid burst promoting activity in presence of EPO
	Stimulates proliferation of multipotent progenitors
	Has stimulatory effects on cytotoxicity, cell adhesion, phagocytosis, and cell viability in the myeloid and macrophage lineages
G-CSF	Stimulates granulocyte colony formation in vitro
	Stimulates blast and megakaryocyte colonies in synergy with IL-3
	Enhances cellular immune responses and chemotaxis of myeloid cells
Erythropoietin	Stimulates erythroid colony formation (CFU-E, BFU-E) in vitro
	Stimulates erythroid proliferation and differentiation in vivo
	Potentiates CFU-M production in vitro in the presence of other factors
Stem cell factor	Stimulates primitive progenitors capable of long-term marrow repopulation into cell cycle, in synergy with other factors
	May stimulate self-renewal and proliferation in nonhemopoietic lineages
	Stimulates mast cell proliferation
Interleukin-1	Acts synergistically with GM-CSF, G-CSF, CSF-1, IL-3 to potentiate the formation of many types of colonies in vitro
	Induces production of cytokines and growth factors from hemopoietic and other cells (e.g., fibroblasts, bone marrow stromal cells)
	Induces a library of cellular immune and proliferative responses in myeloid cells and monocytes/macrophages and cell lines
	Modulates B-cell maturation
Interleukin-3	Stimulates CFUs of multiple lineages and multilineage progenitors in vitro
	Acts in conjunction with EPO to produce primitive erythroid colonies in vitro
	Stimulates formation of blast cell colonies in vitro
	Stimulates HPP-CFC in vitro in conjunction with CSF-1
	Initiates cell cycle in CFU-S
	Induces proliferation of myeloid and erythroid elements in vivo in combination with GM-CSF and/or CSF-1
	Induces a library of cellular immune and proliferative responses in myeloid cells and monocytes/macrophages and cell lines
Interleukin-4	Activates and induces gene expression in B-cell lineage
	Promotes G- or GM-CFC formation in vitro in combination with G-CSF
	Enhances CFU-E, BFU-E, and CFU-GEMM production in vitro
Interleukin-5	Induces differentiation of B cells
	Stimulates CFU-Eo in vitro
Interleukin-6	Acts synergistically with IL-3 to stimulate multipotent hemopoietic progenitors (mouse)
	Potentiates growth of CFU (neutrophil, mac, eos, mast cells, mega) in vitro
Interleukin-7	B-cell maturation
Interleukin-8	Neutrophil-activating protein
	Stimulates neutrophil chemotaxis and degranulation
Interleukin-9	Enhances erythroid BFU-E production in vitro

processes are pleiotropic and include proliferation, differentiation, and cell survival; enhanced rates of DNA synthesis and protein synthesis; decreased rates of protein degradation; and increases in membrane receptor phosphorylation; (5) The concentration of factors necessary to induce optimal effects is generally very low (Dissociation constant $Kd <10^{-9}$ M); (6) combinations of factors may be required to achieve maximum stimulation (inhibition) of cell proliferation and/or differentiation in a particular cell lineage; (7) combinations of factors may show additive or synergistic effects; (8) some factors (e.g., stem cell factor IL-6) may have no intrinsic hemopoietic growth factor activity, but act only in synergy with other factors. These synergistic effects appear to be a general mechanism throughout hemopoiesis. It is the appropriate combination of stimulatory and inhibitory factors that regulates the responses of given cells in the hemopoietic scheme.

Multipotential progenitor cells

The first multipotential hemopoietic precursor identified was the murine CFU-S. This cell gave rise to myeloid/erythroid colonies in the spleen of lethally irradiated or congenitally stem-cell deficient mice. There is no human equivalent for the murine CFU-S. However, a number of in vitro assays have been developed that have revealed the presence of multipotential cells in the human bone marrow. These progenitors, variously called CFU-GEMM or CFU-MIX, give rise to several cell lineages when cultured in the presence of specific growth factors. Initially, these colony forming cells were identified in cultures of bone marrow prepared in the presence of serum, erythropoietin, to stimulate erythropoiesis, and medium conditioned by phytohemagglutinin-stimulated human leukocytes or by tumor cell lines. Conditioned media have now been replaced in these cultures by purified recombinant growth factors.

Table 57-4 Numbers of human colony forming cells in vitro and in vivo

Colony type	No. per 2 × 10⁵ nucleated bone marrow cells
CFU-S (mouse spleen)	30-40
CFU-GEMM	10-30
CFU-GM	200-400
CFU-Meg	50-100
BFU-E	50-200
CFU-E	100-500

Table 57-4 indicates that there are relatively few CFU-GEMM colony forming cells in the normal marrow. CFU-GEMM colonies contain granulocytes, macrophages, erythroid cells, and megakaryocytes. Not all colonies contain cells of all of the lineages. The clonal origin of the cells found in CFU-GEMM colonies is most strongly supported by analysis of G6PD isozyme patterns. All cells in the colonies shared the same G6PD isozyme. While lymphoid cells are not typically found in CFU-GEMM colonies. However, in the few instances in which they have been observed, the G6PD studies identified T lymphocytes that shared the same isozyme pattern as the myeloid and erythroid cells. These results suggest that some of the CFU-GEMM precursors might give rise to both myeloid and lymphoid cells. Serial subculture of cells found in the CFU-GEMM colonies suggest that these colonies have a limited capacity for self-renewal.

Myeloid progenitors and myelopoiesis

Myeloid cells develop in the bone marrow, presumably from the CFU-GEMM pool of precursors. The myeloid progenitor cells ultimately give rise to the recognizable precursors in the bone marrow and the terminally differentiated granulocytes and monocytes of the peripheral blood. The morphological features of many of these recognizable precursors is clear. However, distinctions among the stages of differentiation in the myeloblast population has been difficult. Monoclonal antibody immunophenotyping in the myeloid series has defined a set of antigens associated with some stages of myeloid differentiation. The CD classifications of these antibodies and the cellular immunophenotypes obtained, for the most part, by multiparametric, flow cytometric analysis, are detailed in Chapter 60 and in detailed compilations of immunophenotypes. The immunophenotypes of the myelomonocytic lineages are given in Table 57-5.

Myeloid cells lead a transient existence in the circulation and, as noted earlier, extravasate and enter the tissue, especially into areas where acute infections occur. The principal cellular immune function of these cells, namely the destruction of bacterial and other infectious agents, occurs in the tissue. Thus, the myeloid pool must be in constant readiness to proliferate and differentiate into functional cells.

Granulocyte/macrophage precursor cells were essentially the first hemopoietic precursors identified in vitro through the use of the semisolid colony assay techniques

Table 57-5 Immunophenotypes of human myeloid cells and precursors

Cell type	Immunophenotype
MYELOID STEM CELL (CFU-GEMM)	HLA-DR, CD34, (TdT), (CD13), (CD33), (CD7)
MYELOMONOCYTIC STEM CELL	HLA-DR, CD34, CD13, CD33, (CD4), (CD15), (MPO)
Myeloblast	(HLA-DR), CD34, CD13, CD33, CD15, MPO
Promyelocyte	CD13, CD33, (CD15), MPO, (CD11b)
Myelocyte	CD13, CD33, CD15, MPO, CD11b
Granulocyte	CD13, CD15, MPO, CD11b, CD16, CD67
Monoblast	HLA-DR, CD13, CD33, CD14, (CD11b), (MPO)
Promonocyte	HLA-DR, CD13, CD33, CD14, CD11b, MPO
Monocyte	HLA-DR, CD13, CD33, CD14, CD11b, MPO
Macrophage	HLA-DR, (CD13), (CD33), (CD14), CD11b, CD1, CD68, RFD9
ERYTHROID SERIES	
Proerythroblast	H-antigen, (glycophorin a), TRF-R
Erythroblast	H-antigen, glycophorin a, TRF-R
Reticulocyte	H-antigen, glycophorin a, (TRF-R)
Erythrocyte	H-antigen, glycophorin a
MEGAKARYOCYTE SERIES	
Immature Megakaryoblast	HLA-DR, CD34, CD33, (CD41/CD61), (CD42)
Megakaryoblast	CD41/CD61, CD42, (CD9)
Megakaryocyte	CD41/CD61, CD42, CD9
Platelets	CD41/CD61, CD42, CD9

*HLA-DR, major histocompatibility class II antigen with DR specificity; CD (followed by number), cluster designation assigned by the Fourth International Workshop of Leucocyte Typing (The assignments and information about the antigens involved are found in Chapter 60); TdT, terminal deoxynucleotidyl transferase mpo, myeloperoxidase; TRF-R, transferrin receptor. Parentheses indicates that only a fraction of the cells in a particular subset are positive for the marker.

described earlier. In the mouse, these cells were called CFU-C (colony forming unit, culture) and were distinguishable from the CFU-S foci in the spleen in that they contained only granulocytes and/or macrophages, but not erythroid cells. From this finding, it was presumed that these colonies were formed by the progeny of a more lineage-restricted precursor than CFU-S. CFU-C colonies could be induced by a variety of agents obtained from conditioned media as already described. Morphological examination of the colonies revealed that some were composed either of neutrophils or macrophages, and some were mixed and, accordingly, this colony type was reclassified GM-CFU. This early data in the mouse suggested that multiple factors might be at work in these cultures, which stimulated the proliferation and differentiation of a common precursor to macrophages and granulocytes and that several branch points might exist in the differentiation scheme. Similar results were obtained in cultures of human marrow. Subsequently, at least four factors that affect myeloid differentiation have been isolated, purified, cloned, sequenced, and expressed, namely, GM-CSF, G-CSF, M-CSF, and IL-3.

GM-CSF is a glycoprotein of molecular weight 22,000 daltons. The protein has been cloned and sequenced, and is available through recombinant DNA technology in amounts large enough for therapeutic use. This factor has been shown to elicit a number of activities in the hemopoietic system. Some of these activities are summarized in Table 57-3. The table illustrates that GM-CSF not only stimulates the proliferation and differentiation of progenitors that give rise to a series of myeloid elements, but also has effects on cellular immune functions, chemotaxis, biosynthetic activity, and antigen expression in mature myeloid cells (e.g., macrophage, eosinophils, basophils, neutrophils). In addition, GM-CSF can stimulate the proliferation of erythroid burst-forming units (see text that follows) and perhaps T-cell lines. Thus, GM-CSF could be considered a multilineage factor. As is the case for most growth factors, GM-CSF elicits its effects through high and low affinity receptors. The mechanism of signal transduction in the case of the GM-CSF receptor is still unclear, though it may involve the intermediacy of G proteins.

GM-CSF elicits responses in vivo that mimic the activities observed in colony assays in vitro. Recent studies in animal models and clinical trials in humans have demonstrated the pleiotropic effects of this growth factor. The proliferation of neutrophils, eosinophils, and monocytes has been observed along with immune activation of monocytes and the production of cytokines (e.g., interleukin-1). The stimulation of myeloid differentiation in vivo results in a decrease in the time necessary for the recovery from neutropenia. In the future, GM-CSF has already become a critical component in the supportive therapy following chemotherapy and bone marrow transplantation. Additional studies are underway to assess the effects of GM-CSF on other lineages in vivo.

G-CSF is a lineage-restricted growth factor whose principal activities are in the stimulation of myeloid progenitors. As such, this factor presumably acts at a stage of myeloid differentiation beyond the CFU-GEMM. A significant difference between GM-CSF and G-CSF is that G-CSF does not appear to induce the expression of other hemopoietic growth factors or cytokines. In addition, G-CSF activity is detected in vitro by its stimulation of colonies composed purely of granulocytes. In addition to its activities in vitro, G-CSF enhances the production of neutrophils in vivo and of chemotactic and other cellular immune responses of neutrophils and monocytes. Clinical trials of this agent, in settings similar to those described for GM-CSF, have revealed its potential as an agent for the amelioration of leukocytosis following chemotherapy and marrow transplantation.

Macrophage/monocyte differentiation is coordinately regulated by several different growth factors. Macrophage colonies are found in semisolid medium cultures of bone marrow following stimulation with GM-CSF. These colonies arise several days following the appearance of granulocyte colonies. Colony formation is also stimulated by IL-

3. Lineage-specific monocyte growth factors like CSF-1 (M-CSF) also stimulate the formation of colonies in vitro. CSF-1 is another glycoprotein factor composed of a single polypeptide chain (molecular weight ~40,000 daltons). CSF-1 also ensures the survival of macrophages and monocytes, and stimulates mature macrophages to carry out differentiated functions, such as cytotoxicity, oxidative metabolic activity, release of proteases, and cell adhesions/migration. CSF-1 mediates its effects through a high-affinity receptor. This protein is expressed on monocytes, macrophages, and their committed progenitors.

It has been shown that the CSF-1 receptor is probably identical to a protein encoded by the cellular proto-oncogene, c-fms. The CSF-1 receptor is a member of a family of growth factor receptors that are related to proto-oncogenes and that have intrinsic tyrosine kinase activities. Because these receptors, and the corresponding cellular proto-oncogenes, are likely to be involved in the regulation of hemopoiesis, the possibility exists that mutations in the proto-oncogenes may modify cellular responses to growth factors, induce latent transforming potentials associated with these oncogenes, and therefore contribute to the development of hemopoietic malignancies.

The preceding sections have noted the positive effectors of myeloid differentiation. However, it is clear that myelopoiesis, and indeed all of hemopoiesis, is regulated by both stimulatory and inhibitory factors. It is the balance between these two effects that is crucial for the maintenance of the system. Considerable investigation has been made into the effects of a number of molecules on the inhibition of myelopoiesis. For example, lactoferrin, an 80 kd iron-binding protein, has been shown to inhibit myelopoiesis significantly. Treatment of animals with very low concentrations of lactoferrin results in a decrease in the absolute number of GM-CFU in the bone marrow and in the spleen, and a profound inhibition of GM-CFU colonies in vitro. In addition to effects on myeloid cells, lactoferrin inhibits CFU-GEMM and BFU-E colonies in vitro. Other potent inhibitors of myelopoiesis include transforming growth factor β and (TGF-β), acidic isoferritins, interferons, and prostaglandins.

Megakaryocyte differentiation

Megakaryocytes are the precursors of platelets. Megakaryocytes are generally found in the bone marrow, although extramedullary sites (e.g., lungs) have been suggested in the adult. In the embryo, megakaryocytes can be found in all of the hemopoietically active tissues (e.g., yolk sac, liver, spleen, bone marrow). Platelets are derived as cytoplasmic fragments of megakaryocytes containing multiple granules that contain enzymes, prostaglandins and precursors, nucleotides, and a variety of bioactive agents. The mechanism by which platelets form from megakaryocytes is poorly understood. However, the lineage relationship between platelets and megakaryocytes has been demonstrated on the basis of antigenic similarities (see Table 57-5), microcinematography, and radiolabeling experiments. Megakaryocytes are multinucleated, polyploid cells; the ploidy of these cells varies. Maturation of megakaryocytes, and the subsequent production of platelets occurs only after all of the DNA destined to be found in any given megakaryocyte has been synthesized. During the synthetic phase, the nuclei do not undergo mitotic division and the megakaryocytes increase in size. Megakaryocytes can have degrees of polyploidy exceeding 32 N. Platelets can be produced from megakaryocytes of any degree of ploidy. The number of platelets produced is roughly proportional to the ploidy, but this is an indirect relationship, since the number of platelets produced is really linked to the size of the megakaryocyte. Platelets do not contain nuclei and are intimately involved in hemostasis and growth factor and hormone production and release.

Megakaryocytes presumably arise as progeny of CFU-GEMM. Megakaryocytes or megakaryocyte precursors are found in CFU-GEMM colonies in vitro and have been found in CFU-S colonies in vivo. The precursors of megakaryocytes have been classified recently into three subgroups. The distinctions among these groups are difficult to sort out, and for that reason, definitive placement in the cell lineage diagram of Fig. 57-1 has been avoided. The three groups are burst-forming, unit-megakaryocyte (BFU-MK), colony forming, unit-megakaryocyte (CFU-MK), and the low density precursor (LD-CFU-MK). Each of these colony forming cells have been identified in semisolid medium assays; they are distinguished primarily on the basis of colony size and rate of formation in culture and, more recently, on the basis of antigenic differences. An additional cell type, the transitional immature megakaryocyte, has also been identified. Such cells are presumably further along in differentiation in that they have lost their colony forming capacity. These are small cells with characteristic nuclei. Most are 6 N or 8 N and are therefore undergoing mitosis.

By analogy to other hemopoietic lineages, the existence of a specific growth factor that regulates megakaryocytopoiesis has been postulated for some time. This postulate is based upon observation of increases in the number and DNA content of bone marrow megakaryocytes following induction of thrombocytopenia in experimental animals. Several groups of investigators have claimed the existence of a so-called thrombopoietin that could account for the response to thrombocytopenia in these animals, however this factor has never been isolated or characterized. A megakaryocyte colony stimulating factor, which stimulates CFU-MK formation in culture, has been found in serum and other biological fluids, but has not been purified. Other well-characterized growth factors, namely GM-CSF, IL-3, and IL-6, have MK-CSF activity. The effects of GM-CSF and IL-3 on megakaryocyte colony formation are additive. In vivo studies in animals and in humans indicate that GM-CSF can increase the platelet count, but the results have been inconsistent in a number of clinical trials. Inconsistent results have also been obtained on the effects of erythropoietin on megakaryocyte production. TGF-β, platelet factor 4, and other platelet-derived factors appear to have inhibitory effects on megakaryocyte colony formation.

Erythropoiesis

Red cell differentiation is among the most extensively studied in the hemopoietic system, both in terms of the regulatory factors and cellular morphology. Enucleated red cells probably arise from the CFU-GEMM through a set of nucleated and enucleated bone marrow precursors. Morphol-

ogical identity of erythroblasts and other precursors in the red cell series has been well established. These cells are identifiable on the basis of the amount of hemoglobin present, nuclear morphology, and, in later stages of differentiation, by the absence of the nucleus. Recently, cell surface phenotyping using monoclonal antibodies and flow cytometry has indicated that blasts in the red cell series can be distinguished from other blastic cells on the basis of the presence or absence of particular cell surface antigens. Thus, antibodies directed against the transferrin receptor can label red cells at all stages up to the late reticulocyte stage; mature cells lose this receptor. In a similar manner, loss of the fibronectin receptor has been observed at the time red cells are released from the bone marrow, suggesting that association of immature cells with the extracellular matrix might be involved in keeping the developing cells in the bone marrow. On the other hand, antibodies that react with glycophorin detect cells only later in the red cell maturation sequence; this antigen persists throughout the circulatory lifetime of the mature erythrocyte. Recent studies of the appearance and distribution of blood group antigens on red cell precursors might provide a means of distinguishing among the early precursors.

The composite of the total erythropoietic capacity of an organism has been referred to as the erythron. This term takes into consideration both the production and the destruction of red cells. Several calculations have been made that estimate the content of the erythron under normal conditions. The cell numbers, given in Table 57-6, are based upon radioiron (Fe-59) labeling studies.

Erythropoietin (EPO) is the principal regulator of erythropoiesis and was among the first growth factors purified and studied at the molecular level. This growth factor is extremely lineage-specific in that its activities are confined exclusively to the red cell series. As isolated from human urine, EPO is a 34,000 dalton glycoprotein. Recombinant EPO (hrEPO), expressed in CHO cells, has an apparent molecular weight of 30,400 daltons. The differences may be due to carbohydrate content. Erythropoietin is synthesized primarily in the kidney and to some extent in the liver. The cells in the kidney that produce EPO are not well-described morphologically but appear to be peritubular interstitial cells. Both Kupfer cells and hepatocytes have been implicated in the liver, but evidence is sparse. Erythropoietin is unique among the hemopoietic growth factors in that there is a well-defined bioassay as well as radioimmunoassay or enzyme-linked immunosorbent assay (ELISA).

The principal function of red cells is oxygen carriage and transport to the tissues and as might be imagined, eryth-

Table 57-6 Principal components of the human erythron

Cell type	Total cell number
Nucleated red cells	3.5×10^{11}
Pronormoblasts plus basophilic normoblasts	1.5×10^{11}
Polychromic/orthochromic normoblasts	4.5×10^{11}
Reticulocytes	4.5×10^{11}
Mature red cells	2.6×10^{13}

ropoiesis is highly reactive to environmental conditions. A feedback control system typical of many biological processes is operational. Hypoxic conditions demand an increased number of red cells to deliver adequate supplies of oxygen. Accordingly, hypoxia leads to an increased synthesis of erythropoietin and a concomitant increase in the number of red cells. Recent studies have indicated that the level of EPO mRNA in EPO-producing cell lines is responsive to oxygen tension. At least thirtyfold increases in the amount of EPO mRNA have been observed under hypoxic conditions. This essentially validates the hypothesis that EPO is newly synthesized under stress conditions rather than mobilized from intracellular pools. Similar studies must be performed on EPO-producing kidney cells in vivo. The mechanism by which the kidney responds to hypoxic conditions to initiate the production of EPO is not well understood. It has been suggested on the basis of a series of in vivo experiments, that EPO-release may be dependent upon prostaglandins and cyclic AMP (cAMP). Thus, under hypoxic conditions in the kidney, release of prostaglandin E_1 increases the levels of cAMP, which in turn may increase EPO levels. This hypothesis remains to be proven, however.

Erythropoietin acts on specific colony forming cells in the bone marrow that are committed to erythroid differentiation. These progenitors, burst-forming units-erythroid (BFU-E) and colony forming units-erythroid (CFU-E), are identified as erythroid by the presence of hemoglobin in the differentiated cells present in the colonies and by morphological features of the progeny. BFU-E cells are immature cells and appear to have limited proliferative capacity. They require EPO to differentiate and proliferate but also require other factors (e.g., IL-3, GM-CSF) to enhance in vitro colony formation. In the presence of these factors, colonies of 500 or more erythroid cells develop in vitro in about 2 weeks of culture. This combination of IL-3 and GM-CSF constitute what was previously referred to as burst-promoting activity (BPA), a factor that enhanced erythroid bursts in vitro. BFU-E cells are present in bone marrow at frequencies of 0.01% to 0.1% of nucleated cells. Recently, enriched populations of BFU-E have been obtained using a combination of monoclonal antibody reactivity and flow sorting. In these enriched populations, it was shown that IL-3 was required for initial proliferation in vitro and independently of EPO. Erythropoietin sensitivity appears later and is maintained throughout subsequent differentiation stages. These changes in dependency upon growth factors constitute the basis for classification of BFU-E into several stages of differentiation.

CFU-E are much more highly proliferative cells than BFU-E cells and are generally considered to be more differentiated. They are present in bone marrow at frequencies comparable to BFU-E. The CFU-E cells are responsive to very low concentrations of EPO and give rise to small colonies (<50 cells) in about 7 days of culture. While CFU-E cells do not appear to require the intermediacy of factors other than EPO to support erythroid differentiation, recent studies on enriched populations of CFU-E suggest that insulin-like growth factor may be an accessory factor in their differentiation.

Erythropoietin appears to mediate its effects through the intermediacy of specific cell surface receptors. In several animal and human systems, high- and low-affinity EPO receptors have been identified. The EPO receptor protein is rapidly internalized and degraded following binding of EPO to CFU-E. This receptor has structural features common to a number of growth factor receptors, including those for IL-2, IL-3, GM-CSF, and G-CSF.

Several clinical trials of human recombinant-EPO therapy in end-stage chronic renal disease have led to the conclusion that EPO is effective in increasing and maintaining the hematocrit for extended periods. Additional clinical trials in anemic patients with rheumatoid arthritis and in patients with Acquired Immune Deficiency Syndrome receiving azidothymidine (AZT) therapy have both indicated the efficacy of EPO treatment in sustained improvements in the hematocrit with a minimum of side effects.

Lymphocyte differentiation

Hemopoiesis in the lymphoid series has been extensively studied. Lymphocytes are cells principally involved in cellular and humoral immune responses. The detailed immunology of lymphocytes will be covered in other chapters. In this discussion, an attempt will be made to summarize current information regarding the initial phases of lymphocyte maturation, what is known about the factors that regulate lymphoid differentiation, and the immunophenotypes of cells in this series.

Lymphoid maturation occurs both in the bone marrow and at extramedullary sites. The primary lymphoid organs in mammals are the bone marrow and thymus. At these sites, lymphocytes derived from a stem cell pool proliferate and differentiate into mature effector cells. In humans, T cells mature in the thymus and B cells in the bone marrow. In birds, B-lymphocyte differentiation occurs in a specific organ, the bursa of Fabricius. Lymphocytes develop their repertoire of antigenic responses in the primary lymphoid organs. Lymphoid precursors from the primary organs migrate and colonize secondary lymphoid tissues, namely, the spleen, lymph nodes, tonsils, and Peyer's patches. The microenvironment of the secondary lymphoid organs provides a milieu of cellular and humoral interactions that condition the immune responsiveness of the lymphocytes through their responses to antigen-presenting cells, phagocytes, and other accessory cells.

It has been suggested that the pluripotent hemopoietic stem cells give rise to a lymphoid stem cell, which in turn subsets and differentiates into the principal lymphoid subsets, namely T and B lymphocytes (Figure 57-1). The most recent evidence for this contention has come from studies on very highly enriched pluripotent cells from the mouse bone marrow (Thy-1^{lo}Lin$^-$Sca-1$^+$ cells), which give rise to both myeloid and lymphoid elements under a variety of culture conditions. The identity and purity of these populations remains in question, however. This lymphoid precursor has not been identified either morphologically or functionally. In part, this is because of the paucity of colony assays for lymphoid precursor cells, which parallel those found in the myeloid and erythroid series. Tables 57-7 and 57-8 indicate that certain cell surface markers (TdT, HLA-DR, CD34) may be associated with the putative lymphoid stem cell, but these markers are not exclusive to this cell type.

Table 57-7 Immunophenotypes of human T cells and precursors*

Cell type	Immunophenotype
Lymphoid stem cell	TdT, HLA-DR, CD34
Prothymocyte	TdT, HLA-DR, CD34, CD7, CD2, CD3
Immature thymocyte	TdT, CD7, CD2, CD3, CD5
Common thymocyte	TdT, CD7, CD2, CD3, CD5, CD1, CD4/CD8, (TCR-CD3), (CD10)
Mature thymocyte-H	(TdT), CD7, (CD3), CD4, CD5, TCR-CD3
T-helper/inducer	(CD7), CD2, CD5, CD4, TCR-CD3
Activated T-helper/inducer	(CD7), CD2, CD5, TCR-CD3, HLA-DR, CD25
Mature thymocyte-S	(TdT), CD7, (CD3), CD4, CD5, TCR-CD3
T-suppressor/Cytotoxic	CD7, CD2, CD5, CD8, TCR-CD3, (CD16)
Activated T-suppressor/Cytotoxic	CD7, CD2, CD5, CD8, TCR-CD3, HLA-DR, CD25
Natural killer (NK) cells	CD7, (CD2), (CD8), CD16, CD56, (CD57)

*HLA-DR, major histocompatibility class II antigen with DR specificity; CD (followed by number), cluster designation assigned by the Fourth International Workshop of Leucocyte Typing. The assignments and information about the antigens involved are found in Chapter 60. TdT, terminal deoxynucleotidyl transferase; TCR, T-cell receptor. Parentheses indicate only a fraction of the cells in a particular subset are positive for the marker.

Table 57-8 Immunophenotypes of human B cells and precursors*

Cell type	Immunophenotype
Lymphoid stem cell	TdT, HLA-DR, CD34
Pro-B cell	TdT, HLA-DR, CD34, CD19, CD22, (CD9)
Pre-pre-B cell	TdT, HLA-DR, CD34, CD19, CD22, (CD9), CD10, (CD20)
Pre-B cell	TdT, HLA-DR, (CD34), CD19, CD22, (CD9), CD10, (CD20), weak Ig
Early B cell	HLA-DR, CD19, CD22, (CD9), (CD10), CD20, (CD21), CD37, SmIg
Intermediate B cell	HLA-DR, CD19, CD22, (CD9), CD20, CD21, CD37, SmIg, (CD5), (CD11c), (CD25)
Mature B cell	HLA-DR, CD19, CD22, CD20, (CD21), CD37, SmIg, FMC7
Immunoblast	HLA-DR, CD19, CD22, CD20, CD37, SmIg, FMC7
Immunocyte	HLA-DR, CD19, CD22, (CD20), (CD37), SmIg, CytoIg
Plasma cell	(HLA-DR), CD38, CytoIg

*HLA-DR, major histocompatibility class II antigen with DR specificity; CD (followed by number), cluster designation assigned by the Fourth International Workshop of Leucocyte Typing. The assignments and information about the antigens involved are found in Chapter 60. SmIg, surface immunoglobulin; CytoIg, cytoplasmic immunoglobulin; TdT, terminal deoxynucleotidyl transferase. Parentheses indicate that only a fraction of the cell in a particular subset are positive for the marker.

T-Cell differentiation

Stem cells, or at least very early precursors in the lymphoid series, colonize the thymus in both mammals and birds during early embryogenesis. The migration of stem cells to the thymus occurs in discrete stages when the thymus is receptive for colonization. The signals that induce migration are poorly defined. It is also not clear whether the lymphoid stem cells that migrate to the thymus are committed to the T-cell lineage prior to migration, or whether the local microenvironment conditions their subsequent differentiation. It should be stressed that despite the apparent wealth of information available about the ontogeny of the lymphoid system, very little is known about the distribution of T-cell precursors. There are well-demarcated microenvironments in the thymus that condition the differentiation of lymphoid precursors following their colonization of this organ. The vast majority of the lymphocytes in the thymus are found in the cortex; about 15% to 20% of the thymocytes are found in the medulla. Both cortical and medullary thymocytes come in contact with an array of accessory cells and humoral factors (e.g., thymosin, thymopoietins). Recent studies in human and animal models indicate that freshly isolated T-cell precursors from the bone marrow contain receptors for IL-3 and IL-4, and that fetal thymocytes contain receptors for IL-2 and IL-4, but not IL-3 receptors. These findings suggest a distinct role for these growth factors at specific stages in the differentiation of lymphoid precursors.

It has been suggested that the normal rate of stem cell seeding into the thymus is low. However, once the precursors are in place in the thymic microenvironment, there is an extensive and rapid expansion of lymphoid cells. In the mouse, at least 30% of the cortical thymocytes turn over each day. Medullary thymocytes turn over at a much slower rate. What is more striking is the estimate that only about 1% of thymocytes escape to the circulation and that the 30% noted earlier that die, do so before their maturation is complete. Thus, most cortical cells do not become medullary cells; these lymphocytes are at a maturational dead end and die intrathymically.

The antigenic differences noted in Table 57-7 indicate that the cortical T cells are probably more immature than the medullary cells and that there appears to be traffic between the two compartments. This implies, but does not prove, a parent-progeny relationship between the cells in these areas of the thymus. The immunophenotypes of T cells change considerably during maturation and differentiation. Table 57-7 describes the complement of antigens typically associated with various T-cell subsets. It should be noted that: (1) maturation is accompanied by the retention of some cardinal T-cell markers (e.g., CD7, CD2), progressive loss of others (e.g., TdT), and the acquisition of yet a third set (e.g., TCR-CD3); (2) there is a branch point in differentiation when a bipotential cell (CD4+/CD8+) gives rise to functionally differentiated cells, the CD4+ T-helper/inducer cells and the CD8+ T-supressor/inducer cells; and (3) immune activation of mature lymphocytes is associated with the reappearance of markers lost during the maturation process (e.g., HLA-DR) and the appearance of new activation markers (e.g., CD25).

In addition to the expression of specific antigens during the maturation of T cells, gene rearrangements and activation or inactivation of specific genes are hallmarks. This is illustrated graphically in the case of the T-cell receptor (TCR). This receptor is composed of two disulfide-linked polypeptide chains, α and β. The TCR is associated with the CD3 antigen on the cell surface. The CD3 antigen itself is a heterodimeric protein. By analogy to the immunoglobulins, the TCR is encoded by variable (V), diversity (D), and joining (J) segments that are specifically rearranged throughout T-cell ontogeny. The association of TCR with CD3 is obligatory for TCR expression. The TCR functions in antigen recognition, whereas the CD3 component of the complex may be involved in signal transduction during T-cell activation.

The T-cell receptor/CD3 complex genes undergo rearrangement during maturation from early pre-T cells through mature thymocytes. It is possible that the earliest progenitors can be identified by the presence of the T-cell receptor (TCR) gene in the germline configuration, that is, the gene has not yet rearranged. At this stage there is no transcription of the CD3 genes. As differentiation proceeds, the TCR gene undergoes a series of complex rearrangements and CD3 genes are transcribed. The rearrangement of these genes and the differential expression of classes of CD3 antigens defines functional subsets of antigen-responsive cells.

Speculation exists over the precise parent-progeny relationships in the T-cell lineage. One possible scheme for differentiation of T-lymphocytes might be summarized as follows:

1. A population of $CD4^-CD8^-$ cells is a common precursor in T-lymphocyte development. In the mouse, these cells are typically large, perhaps granular lymphocytes, and are localized in the thymic cortex. Repopulation of mouse bone marrow with these cells gives rise to both cortical and medullary thymocytes. The $CD4^-/CD8^-$ cells clearly constitute a heterogeneous population. These cells express both TCR and CD3. Two lineages of cells appear to co-exist, one that expresses $TCR_{\gamma,\delta}$ and one that expresses $TCR_{\alpha,\beta}$, the predominant form among circulating lymphocytes.

2. Subsequently, α-gene and β-gene rearrangements occur in this transitional cell population with the concomitant conversion of the cells to the $CD4^+/CD8^+$ phenotype. Populations of these cells also become $CD3^+$, whereas others remain $CD3^-$. All of the $CD3^-$ cells appear to die intrathymically.

3. Positive selection of $CD4^+/CD8^+$ cells occurs by virtue of their interactions, through the TCR, with MHC class I and class II antigens in the thymic epithelium. In principal, these interactions result not only in the survival of selected cells biased toward reactivity with foreign antigens, but also result by default in the intrathymic death of those that do not react. This is another case of stromal cell-hemopoietic cell interactions that regulate differentiation.

4. Binding of precursor cells to class I or class II antigens in the thymic microenvironment determines whether or not there is a phenotypic and functional change to $CD4^+/CD8^-$ or $CD4^-/CD8^+$ cells. Those cells that

possess a sufficiently high affinity for "self" antigens are eliminated and the remainder, with presumed biases toward foreign antigens, are selected for the final steps of maturation.

B-Cell maturation

In the fetus, B-cell differentiation is observed first in the liver and then progressively in the bone marrow. In birds, a specialized organ, the bursa of Fabricius, is the site of B-cell maturation. B cells presumably arise in a series of differentiation steps from the same lymphoid precursor as the T-cell lineage. As in the case with T cells, B-cell differentiation requires both cell-cell interactions in the primary lymphoid organs and humoral factors. The exact nature of these interactions at the earliest stages of B-cell differentiation is not well understood.

Studies in chimeric avian embryos have shown unequivocally that hemopoietic stem cells from the circulation traverse blood vessels and colonize the bursa of Fabricius at about 8 to 9 days of incubation. In the ensuing 4 to 5 days they establish themselves in the bursal epithelium and differentiate into B cells capable of antibody production. This differentiation process is enhanced and supported by factors derived from the subjacent bursal mesenchyme. The latter portion of the organ is a site of myelopoiesis during this same period, and it is likely that myeloid elements in the mesenchyme are the source of growth factors for B-cell differentiation. It is presumed, but not definitely established, that epithelial-mesenchymal interactions of this type are at work in mammalian embryos as well. At about 16 to 17 days of incubation, the maturing B cells emigrate from the bursa and colonize the circulation and secondary lymphoid tissues.

Recent studies using long-term bone marrow culture have indicated that stromal interactions are important in B-cell differentiation, at least in vitro. Stromal cells in these cultures appear to be sources of factors that are both stimulatory and inhibitory for B-cell maturation. What is evident from studies of these cultures is that cells that produce growth factors for myelopoiesis and lymphopoiesis are present simultaneously and that a variety of factors may work additively or synergistically in paracrine networks to affect the differentiation of all cell types in the cultures. Messenger RNA associated with GM-CSF, M-CSF, IL-3, IL-6, IL-7, and others have been identified in these cultures, but it must be determined whether these regulators, and others, are involved in the maintenance of the normal steady state of B-cell production or whether they are responsive only as a consequence of the stress of cell culture. Interleukin-7, a 25-kd protein, (see Table 57-3) has been shown to be a potent stimulator of B-cell production in these cultures. Interleukin-1, IL-3, IL-4, and IL-6 have also been shown to be potentiators of B-cell maturation under certain proscribed sets of conditions. Inhibition of lymphopoiesis has also been observed by factors that are present in stromal cell preparations. The most potent of these is perhaps TGF-β; this factor has been shown to block B-cell maturation at several stages. It is not clear whether TGF-β blocks lymphopoiesis through direct action on the B-cell progenitors, on the stroma, or both.

As in the case of T cells, B-cell maturation is signaled

Table 57-9 Proposed growth factor responses during the maturation of human B cells*

Cell type	L-BCGF	H-BCGF	IL-1	IL-2	IL-3	IL-4	IL-5	IL-6	IL-7
Pro-B	+	−	−	−	+	−	−	−	+
Pre-pre-B	+	(+)	(+)	−	+	−	−	−	+/−
Pre-B	+	(+)	(+)	−	+	−	−	−	−
Immature B	+	(+)	−	−	−	+	−	−	−
Mature B	+	−	−	−	−	+	−	−	−
Activated B	+	+	+	+	−	+	+	+	−
Blast B	+	+	+	+	+	−	+	+	−
Memory B	−	+	−	−	−	−	−	−	−
Plasma cells	−	−	−	−	−	−	−	+	−

*L-BCGF, low molecular weight B-cell growth factor; H-BCGF, high molecular weight B-cell growth factor; IL, interleukin. Symbols in parentheses denote reactivity with leukemic cells; +, denotes presence of growth factor receptor; −, denotes absence of growth factor receptor; +/−, denotes expression of receptor at some stages of maturation of the particular cell type or that not all cells with the particular phenotype express the receptor.

by the appearance or disappearance of specific cell surface antigens. Detailed immunophenotypes obtained by monoclonal antibody reactivity and flow cytometry are provided in Table 57-8. In addition, immunoglobulin gene rearrangements, analogous to those observed for the T-cell receptor, are seen in the early stages of differentiation. These rearrangements result in the generation of antibody diversity. The details and implications of immunoglobulin gene rearrangements are found in selected readings and in other chapters of this text.

The functional roles of many of the cell surface antigens described in the pathways of B-cell maturation are unknown. However, the differentiation of B-cell precursors to mature, functional cells can be described by the complement of cell surface antigens found on B-cell precursors. One of many schemes proposed for B-cell maturation is described in Table 57-9. The scheme is based on multiparametric fluorescent flow cytometric analyses of lymphocytes derived from a variety of normal tissues (e.g., bone marrow, fetal liver) and from cells from patients with B-lineage acute lymphocytic leukemias.

While the details of the several proposals vary, some general principals about B-cell differentiation have emerged from these analyses: (1) there is a progressive change in the cell surface immunophenotype of B-cell precursors that parallels the expression of immunoglobulin in these cells; (2) differences in expression of antigens on lymphocytes derived from different organs may reflect local differences in the response of cells to microenvironmental stimuli; (3) leukemic and normal cell phenotypes do not necessarily match, even in cells that are functionally similar; (4) biphenotypic lymphoid precursors that give rise to both B- and T-lymphocytes can be identified in the bone marrow in very small numbers. These cells have the immunophenotype, HLA-DR$^+$TdT$^+$CD2$^+$CD19$^+$. It has been proposed that the selection of the T- or B-cell differentiation programs is conditioned by interactions of these precursor cells with the stroma.

SUMMARY AND PERSPECTIVES

The preceding discussions illustrate, in broad overview, the complexities involved in understanding how the hemo-poietic system manages to generate daily, and with fidelity, the tremendous number of blood cells required to sustain life. While well studied in vitro, the pluripotent hemopoietic stem cell has not been unequivocally identified, and has not been studied in depth in vivo. The availability in recent years of recombinant hemopoietic growth factors has permitted the beginnings of investigations into the detailed nature of interactions of these factors with hemopoietic precursors. As yet, the precise combination of factors required to induce differentiation of cells in a given hemopoietic lineage in vivo has not been established.

Despite all of the work that needs to be accomplished, a considerable number of advances have been made. The availability of recombinant human growth factors (e.g., EPO, GM-CSF) have pointed to new modalities of therapy for several classes of patients who have received marrow suppressive treatments. This would have the potential salutary effect of reducing the utilization of blood and blood components as supportive therapy in these cases. In addition, combinations of growth factors may be found that can stimulate quiescent hemopoietic stem cells in vitro, making it possible to expand these cells in culture. A final outcome of this work will be a more thorough understanding of the development of the normal hemopoietic system and those points at which inappropriate responses to regulatory factors lead to disease.

SUGGESTED READING

Bizzozero G: Zentralbl. Med. Wissensch, 10:149, 1869.

Cairnie AB, Lala PK, and Osmond DG (editors): Stem cells of renewing cell populations, New York, 1976, Academic Press.

Dexter TM, Garland JM, and Testa NG: Colony stimulating factors, New York, 1990, Marcel Dekker.

Fathman CG and Metzger H (editors): Annual reviews of immunology, vol 9, Palo Alto, 1991, Annual Reviews, Inc.

Golde DW (editor): Hematopoiesis, In Methods in hematology, vol 11, New York, 1984, Churchill Livingston.

Hoffman R: Regulation of megakaryocytopoiesis, Blood 74:1196, 1989.

Knapp W and others (editors): *Leucocyte typing IV:* white cell differentiation antigens, Oxford, 1989, Oxford University Press; also see Leucocyte typing database IV, compiled by WR Gilks, Oxford University Press, 1989.

Krantz SB: Erythropoietin, Blood 77:419, 1991.

Moore MAS: The clinical use of colony stimulating factors. In Paul WE.

Neumann E: Zentrabl. Med. Wissensch, 6:689, 1868.

Tavassoli M and Yoffey JM: Bone marrow: structure and function, New York, 1983, Alan R. Liss.

Torok-Storb B: Cellular interactions, Blood 72:373, 1988.

Uckun FM: Regulation of human B-cell ontogeny, Blood 76:1908, 1990.

van Ewikj W: T-cell differentiation is influenced by thymic microenvironments. In Paul WE, Fathman CG, and Metzger H (editors): Annual reviews of immunology, vol 9, Palo Alto, 1991, Annual Reviews, Inc.

58 Morphology of the hematopoietic system

Robert F. Reiss

The hematopoietic system is comprised of tissues normally involved in the production of blood cells and the mature cells circulating in the peripheral blood. As previously described, after the fifth or sixth month of fetal life, the marrow is populated with hematopoietic tissue, and after birth, the marrow becomes the principle site of proliferation, differentiation, and maturation of the myeloid cell lines (erythrocytic, granulocytic, and megakaryocytic). Hematopoiesis in the marrow is termed *medullary hematopoiesis*. The spleen, lymph nodes, and thymus, as well as lymphoid follicles in the marrow, remain as lymphopoietic tissues after birth and, with the exception of the thymus, are capable of again becoming sites of extramedullary hematopoiesis.

At birth all marrow spaces are filled with active red marrow. In the normal adult some of the marrow space is occupied by fatty tissue. By 20 years of age, the shafts of the long bones normally contain only fatty (yellow) marrow, red marrow being found only in the proximal epiphyseal end. The marrow-containing bones in the adult are skull, clavicles, scapulae, sternum, ribs, vertebrae, pelvis, and the proximal end of long bones. With advancing age, even the marrow in these bones changes in the amount of fatty tissue they contain; whereas the bone marrow in a normal young adult is half fatty and half red, that of men and women of advanced age (late sixties, seventies, and eighties) is normally two-thirds fatty and one-third red.

When there is stimulation of hemopoiesis, for whatever reason, fatty marrow is replaced by red marrow to various degrees. When hemopoiesis is very active, as in pernicious anemia or leukemia, not only is all marrow red but, even within this, very little fatty tissue can be seen. In infants and children, the marrow spaces being already filled with red marrow, increased hemopoietic activity, as in hemolytic anemia, is accommodated by an enlargement of the marrow space that produces typical roentgenographic findings (Fig. 58-1).

Lymph nodes are discrete nodules of lymphoid tissue located at anatomically constant points along the course of lymphatic vessels (Fig. 58-2). They have a fibrous capsule from which connective tissue trabeculae extend into the node

in a roughly radial arrangement. The connective tissue framework between the trabeculae consists of a network of reticulum fibers, and this stroma supports primitive reticuloendothelial cells, scattered phagocytic histiocytes, and the predominant lymphocytes. In the medullary (central) portion of the lymph node the small lymphocytes are packed tightly in sheets and cords. In the peripheral or cortical portion the lymphocytes are condensed into roughly spherical lymphoid follicles. These may consist entirely of small lymphocytes when the lymph node is in a completely resting or nonreactive state. When stimulated, the primary lymphoid nodules develop germinal or reactive centers that consist of medium and large lymphocytes (some in mitosis), and some plasma cells. The proliferating germinal center is usually pale-staining and sharply circumscribed by the crowded dark-staining small lymphocytes at the periphery that form a corona around the reactive center. The deeper paracortical areas of the node are populated by T lymphocytes, whereas the lymphoid follicles are composed of B lymphocytes and their progeny is active in the synthesis of immunoglobulin.

Lymph enters the node through afferent vessels and empties into a distinct subcapsular sinus that is continuous with sinuses running along the trabeculae. These ultimately form efferent lymphatics that leave the node at the hilus. The sinuses are lined by flat littoral or lining cells, called endothelial cells; and by cells that are phagocytic, and as such they are active in performing a house-cleaning function in the lymph.

The cells of the peripheral blood are normally comprised of functional and fully differentiated and mature hematopoietic cells. Their numbers and structure are routinely examined by the performance of the complete blood count (see Chapter 59) and examination of the peripheral blood smear.

EVALUATION OF THE PERIPHERAL BLOOD SMEAR

The peripheral blood smear is prepared from either ethylenediaminetetraacetic acid (EDTA) anticoagulated blood or non-anticoagulated blood taken from a finger stick (see Chapter 3). Smears may be prepared on glass slides or coverslips, which are then mounted on glass slides. These

Much of this material has been taken from Miale JB: *Laboratory medicine: hematology*, ed 6, St Louis, 1982, Mosby–Year Book.

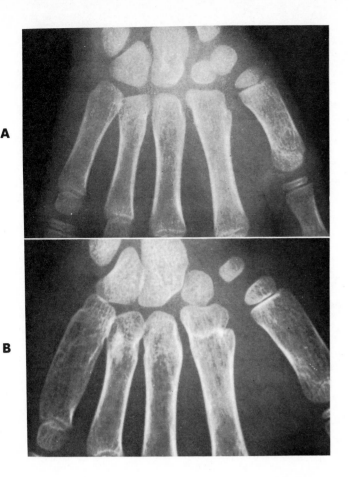

Fig. 58-1 Typical roentgenographic findings in severe erythroid hyperplasia. Enlargement of marrow space due to increased hemopoietic activity. **A,** Hand of normal 9-year-old child. **B,** Hand of 9-year-old child having marked erythroid hyperplasia (sickle-cell anemia). *Courtesy of Dr. Catherine Poole. From Miale JB: Laboratory medicine: hematology, ed 6, St Louis, 1982, Mosby–Year Book.*

Fig. 58-2 Lymph node, normal structure. The capsule, subcapsular sinus, cortex with follicles, paracortical region, and medulla are shown. *Redrawn from Weisz-Carrington: Principles of clinical immunohematology, Chicago, 1986, Year Book Medical.*

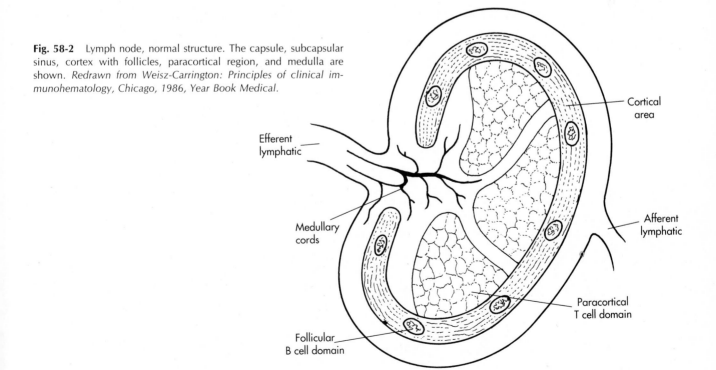

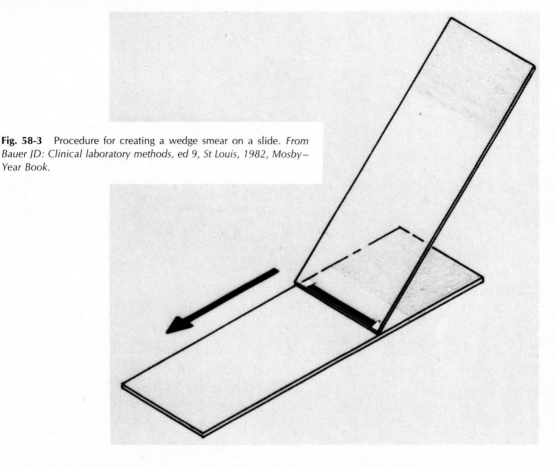

Fig. 58-3   Procedure for creating a wedge smear on a slide. *From Bauer JD: Clinical laboratory methods, ed 9, St Louis, 1982, Mosby—Year Book.*

smears are stained with a Romanovsky type stain and examined microscopically.

Although manually made coverslip preparations can yield excellent smears when prepared by expert technologists, most workers find that an even distribution of cells is difficult to obtain. For this reason smears prepared on glass slides by either manual or automated methods are more generally used.

After placing a drop of blood one third from the end of a clean slide, manual smears are made by placing a second slide (spreader slide) ahead of the blood drop at an angle of 45%, pulling this slide to the drop allowing the blood to spread between the two surfaces, then lowering the slide to 30° and pushing the slide away, thereby creating a smear (Fig. 58-3). A well-made smear should occupy the middle one third to one half of the slide, should not extend to the lateral edges of the slide, and should have a typical wedge shape (Fig. 58-4). Such smears will show progressive thinning from the origin to the terminal, slightly arched and stretched "feather" edge. The quality of the smear is documented by microscopic examination, which shows a large area in from the feathered edge where the red cells form a monolayer, with the cells touching but not overlapping each other. In proper smears, leukocytes will be evenly distributed throughout.

Automated slide preparers are available as either stand-alone instruments or are integrated into some automated differential counting instruments (see Chapter 59). Different models prepare either push or spin smears. Spun smears are

usually superior because the distribution of the white cells is more even.

Romanovsky stains

The peripheral smear, as well as smears of bone marrow aspirates, are examined routinely after staining with one of the Romanovsky type stains. The stain may either be applied manually on the slide, by immersion of the slide into Coplin jars containing the stain, or by semiautomated and automated stainers which are available either as stand alone instruments or are integrated into some automated differential cell counters (see Chapter 59). Romanovsky stains are those that belong to the family that use methylene blue and eosin or their derivatives. These stains include the Wright-Giemsa, and May-Grünwald stains. Among these, the Wright-Giemsa stain is very widely utilized.

With the Wright-Giemsa stain, the alkaline methylene blue stains acidic cellular structures including nuclear DNA and cytoplasmic RNA; the acidic eosin stains hemoglobin and the granules of eosinophils; whereas the other cytoplasmic structures stain neutrally. Classically, air-dried smears are stained with freshly made Wright-Giemsa stain after fixation in absolute methanol. Currently, numerous types of commercial stains are available as prepared stable solutions having very short staining periods and requiring no alcohol fixation of the smear. When bone marrow smears are stained with Wright-Giemsa stains, longer fixation times and slightly longer staining times are used.

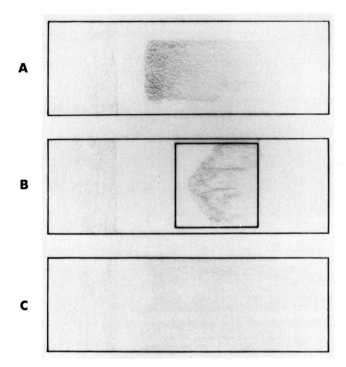

A

B

C

Fig. 58-4 Peripheral blood smears made by **(A)** Wedge technique; **(B)** coverslip technique; **(C)** automated spin technique. *From Bauer JD: Clinical laboratory methods, ed 9, St Louis, 1982, Mosby—Year Book.*

EVALUATION OF THE BONE MARROW

Examination of the peripheral blood reveals its cellular content at the time of sampling and yields data necessary for qualitative and quantitative classification of abnormalities, but it gives limited information about the pathogenesis of an abnormal state. Hematologic diagnosis depends on knowing as much as possible about three processes: cell production, cell release, and cell survival. Since the mechanisms of cell release are least understood, diagnosis is usually based on a determination of the balance between rate and quality of hemopoietic activity on the one hand and rate of cell survival on the other. Qualitative and quantitative data on medullary hemopoiesis are obtained by examination of marrow tissue.

Properly handled marrow tissue can give a wealth of information. Wright-stained or Wright-Giemsa–stained smears give excellent cytologic details, and duplicate smears may be stained for other cytochemical reactions. Paraffin sections of isolated marrow particles and trephine biopsy samples of the marrow stained with hematoxylin and eosin not only give an accurate measure of the relative cellular and fat content, but also are essential for diagnosis of granulomatous diseases such as tuberculosis, in which the his-

tologic pattern is more reliable than the structure of individual cells. Marrow tissue may also be cultured to isolate and identify bacteria and other pathogenic agents.

Techniques for obtaining marrow tissue

The techniques for obtaining marrow consist of aspiration, trephination, and surgical excision.

Aspiration is the most common technique and will usually yield an adequate specimen. Occasionally, a dry tap occurs when aspiration fails to yield marrow tissue. Dry taps sometimes occur when the marrow is involved with metastatic tumors, lymphomas, sarcoidosis, histoplasmosis, or miliary tuberculosis. Occasionally, they will be experienced in pernicious anemia or leukemia because of the difficulty of aspirating a thick, hypercellular, or gelatinous marrow. In other cases, failure to obtain a specimen by aspiration is later explained when acellular, fibrotic, or sclerotic marrow is demonstrated by different techniques. In no case should a diagnosis of aplastic or fibrous marrow be based only on a failure to obtain marrow by aspiration. If repeated aspirations fail, trephination or surgical excision must be performed if trephine biopsy had not been routinely performed at the time of aspiration.

Needles of various designs are available, some of which can be used for both aspiration and biopsy. Others can be used only for aspiration.

Local analgesia is achieved by infiltrating the area with a 1% solution of procaine hydrochloride or other local anesthetic. Two potentially painful areas must be carefully infiltrated. They are the skin and the periosteum. Effective subperiosteal infiltration is accomplished by firmly fixing the point of the hypodermic needle in the bone and injecting the analgesic agent under pressure.

The ilium, sternum, and other sites usually yield comparable samples, but at times aspiration will be unsuccessful at one site and successful at another. The choice of site for aspiration is usually a matter of personal preference but may be based on specific indications, for example, the very thin cartilaginous sternum of infants makes sternal puncture difficult and dangerous.

Posterior ilium aspiration technique (Fig. 58-5)

The posterior ilium is in many ways an ideal site for bone marrow puncture. The marrow cavity here is quite large. Furthermore, the direction of the aspirating needle can be parallel to the inner and outer cortex, thus avoiding the risk of perforating the deep bony table. One can take advantage of this to obtain marrow tissue by biopsy at this site by using a Jamshidi-Swaim, Vim-Silverman, or other biopsy needle.

Aspiration is carried out with the subject prone or positioned as for a lumbar puncture, lying on his or her side with knees drawn up and the back comfortably flexed. After the usual infiltration of skin and periosteum with procaine, a 3 mm skin incision is made with a scalpel blade at a point 1 cm cephalad to the posterosuperior iliac spine. The needle is placed through the incision. The posterior iliac crest is penetrated with the usual clockwise and counterclockwise boring motion, the needle being directed toward the anterosuperior iliac spine. After the marrow cavity has been entered, the stylet is unlocked and removed, a tightly fitting

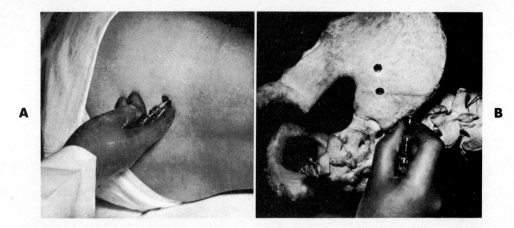

Fig. 58-5 **A,** Aspiration of bone marrow from posterior ilium. **B,** Anatomic relationships. *From Miale JB: Laboratory medicine: hematology, ed 6, St Louis, 1982, Mosby—Year Book.*

10-ml syringe is inserted in its place, and forceful aspiration is effected. No more than 0.2 ml of marrow should be aspirated, thus minimizing dilution of the marrow with sinusoidal blood. This first material obtained is used to prepare thin smears. A second syringe may be then applied and about 1 ml of marrow is aspirated, from which additional marrow particles for particle smears and permanent paraffin sections can be obtained.

Trephine biopsy technique

The Jamshidi-Swaim needle is recommended to perform a biopsy of bone marrow from the posterior iliac crest (Fig. 58-6). The technique is basically the same as that used for marrow aspiration. Biopsy should be performed after aspiration and follow repositioning of the needle. After the point of the needle has entered the marrow cavity, the stylet is removed. The needle is then advanced with continued clockwise-counterclockwise motions for approximately 2-3 cm. The marrow core is then separated by rotating the needle several times. The needle is removed slowly with a rotating motion. The core is removed through the needle base by inserting the probe through the tapered tip. It is placed in Zenkers fixative after making imprints on glass slides.

Sternal marrow aspiration technique (Fig. 58-7)

The preferred point of aspiration is the body of the sternum opposite the second interspace. At this level in the adult, the outer lamina averages 1.35 mm and the inner lamina 1.42 mm, with an average marrow cavity of 7.5 mm (Fig. 58-8).

After adequate analgesia is achieved, the second interspace is located by using the index finger and thumb of the left hand to outline the lateral borders of the sternum. The

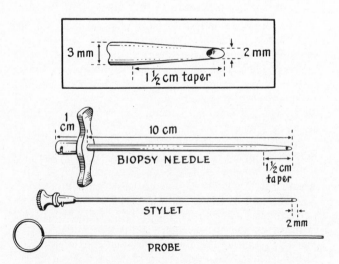

Fig. 58-6 Components of the Jamshidi-Swaim biopsy needle. *From Jamshidi K and Swaim WR: J Lab Clin Med 77:335, 1971.*

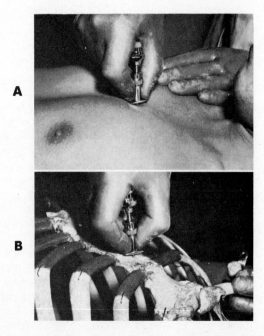

Fig. 58-7 Aspiration of sternal marrow. **A,** Photograph of actual aspiration. **B,** Anatomic relationships. *From Miale JB: Laboratory medicine: hematology, ed 6, St Louis, 1982, Mosby—Year Book.*

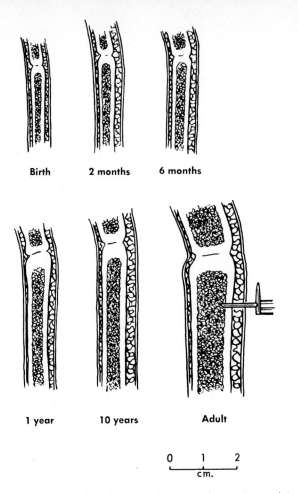

Birth   **2 months**   **6 months**

1 year   **10 years**   **Adult**

0   1   2
cm.

Fig. 58-8 Midsagittal sections through sternum showing in actual size the average thickness of the laminae and the depth of the marrow cavity at different ages. *From Miale JB: Laboratory medicine: hematology, ed 6, St Louis, 1982, Mosby—Year Book.*

needle point is then centered exactly midway between the borders of the sternum. The needle is inserted with a bording motion and steady but not excessive pressure. The pressure should be so gauged as to avoid any sudden penetration when resistance is lessened. Once the marrow cavity is entered, aspiration is performed as previously described.

Preparation of marrow tissue for study

The first material aspirated, about 0.2 ml of marrow, is used for the preparation of several thin smears. A 24-gauge needle is attached to the syringe, and small drops are individually placed on clean glass slides or coverslips. These are smeared out as for a peripheral blood smear (Fig. 58-9). If particle smears are desired as well, the remaining material from the first aspiration is expressed on a slide, and the small particles are identified, transferred to another slide, crushed gently, and then smeared.

Material from a second aspiration of approximately 1 ml is expressed into a small test tube containing one drop of standard full-strength heparin solution, then mixed thoroughly with the anticoagulant and used to make paraffin sections of marrow particles. There are various ways of collecting these particles, one of the simplest being that of straining material through lens paper or some similar type of fine, hard filter paper. After straining, the particles remaining on the paper are pushed together with an applicator stick and immediately fixed in Bouin's or other fixing fluid.

If marrow aspiration is carried out chiefly for bacteriologic diagnosis, the second aspiration is expressed into a sterile tube containing 1 ml of 1% sodium citrate and mixed thoroughly. From this, routine and special bacteriologic studies can be made.

Smears are stained with Wright-Giemsa stain for routine studies, and a minimum of 500 nucleated cells is enumerated

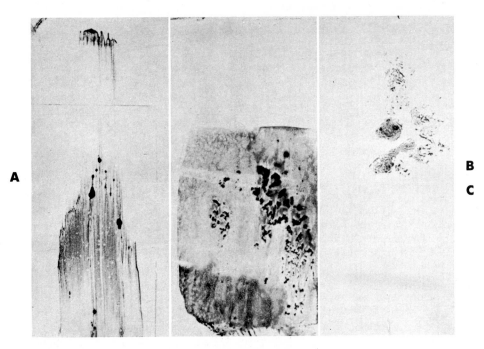

A   **B**   **C**

Fig. 58-9 Bone marrow preparations. **A,** Thin smear. **B,** Particle smear. **C,** Paraffin section. *From Miale JB: Laboratory medicine: hematology, ed 6, St Louis, 1982, Mosby—Year Book.*

BONE MARROW STUDY

Name_____ Age_____ Date_____

Doctor_____ Ward_____ Chart No._____

			Normal	Range	Observed
		Blasts, unclassified			
		Myeloblasts	1.2	0.3- 5.0	
		Progranulocytes	3.0	1.0- 8.0	
		Myelocytes	8.7	0.9-20.3	
		Neutrophilic	7.0	5.0-19.0	
		Eosinophilic	1.4	0.5- 3.0	
		Basophilic	0.3	0 - 0.5	
		Metamyelocytes	11.0	13.0-32.0	
	57.4%	Neutrophilic	9.0	5.6-22.0	
		Eosinophilic	1.5	0.3- 3.7	
		Basophilic	0.3	0 - 0.3	
70%		Band cells	17.9	6.1-36.0	
		Neutrophilic	16.0	15.0-30.0	
		Eosinophilic	1.6	0.2- 2.0	
		Basophilic	0.2	0 - 0.3	
		Segmented	15.6	8.7-27.0	
		Neutrophils	13.4	7.0-30.0	
		Eosinophils	2.0	0.5- 4.0	
		Basophils	0.2	0 - 0.7	
		Lymphoblasts			
		Prolymphocytes	9.8	2.7-24.0	
		Lymphocytes			
		Monoblasts			
	12.6%	Promonocytes	1.4	0.7- 2.8	
		Monocytes			
		Plasmoblasts			
		Proplasmocytes	0.6	0.1- 1.5	
		Plasmocytes			
		Megakaryoblasts			
		Promegakaryocytes	0.2	0.03-0.4	
		Megakaryocytes			
		Promegaloblasts			
		Basophilic megaloblasts			
		Polychromatophilic megaloblasts	0	0	
		Orthochromic megaloblasts			
19.1%	19.1%	Pronormoblasts	0.5	0.2- 4.0	
		Basophilic normoblasts	2.4	1.5- 5.8	
		Polychromatophilic normoblasts	11.7	5.0-26.4	
		Orthochromic normoblasts	4.5	1.6-21.0	
10.9%	10.9%	Unidentified	1.7	0.02-3.3	
		Disintegrated cells	9.2	1.1-20.8	
		Reticulum cells	0.2	0.2- 2.0	

Fig. 58-10   Useful form for reporting results of bone marrow examination. Figure 58-11 shows reverse side of this form. *From Miale JB: Laboratory medicine: hematology, ed 6, St Louis, 1982, Mosby—Year Book.*

for a differential count. A form such as that shown in Figs. 58-10 and 58-11 is useful for reporting the results. Interpretation is made in conjunction with a study of the peripheral blood and other laboratory investigations.

EXAMINATION OF LYMPH NODE CYTOLOGY

Study of the morphology of individual cells, as seen in imprints from the freshly cut surface of a lymph node or from smears of aspirated material, is a useful adjunct to the histopathologic appearance. Histologic sections are essential for determining the relationship of cells to each other and to the architecture of the tissue, but cellular details are partially obscured by fixation and by the thickness of the section.

Imprints are made by gently touching (not smearing) the freshly cut surface of the node to a glass slide. The imprints are then stained with Wright's stain and also cytochemical

stains (oil red O, α-naphthyl acetate esterase, acid phosphatase, tartrate-resistant acid phosphatase, and methyl green-pyronine).

THE CELL MATURATION-STRUCTURE RELATIONSHIP

Before outlining the characteristics of individual cells, it is advisable to discuss the general features of cell differentiation and maturation. In any cell series an almost infinite gradation of cells exists between the most immature blast form and the mature definitive cell.

One other basic consideration is that since a cell is composed of several component parts, each must undergo transformation. Normally, the changes are simultaneous and parallel, a developmental synchronism that simplifies description and analysis. However, abnormal hemopoiesis may be characterized by different rates of maturation for the nucleus

Description:

Diagnosis:

NORMAL VALUES FOR CHILDREN	Control Figures for Various Age Groups									
	1-2 Mo.	3-12 Mo.	1-2 Yr.	3-4 Yr.	5-6 Yr.	7-8 Yr.	9-10 Yr.	11-12 Yr.	13-14 Yr.	15-16 Yr.
Myeloblasts	1.6	1.9	0.7	1.4	1.8	1.0	1.4	1.1	1.2	1.3
Progranulocytes	5.6	1.8	3.4	3.2	3.2	1.8	2.0	1.7	1.1	1.9
Myelocytes	18.1	16.7	13.3	15.9	17.2	17.4	16.5	15.31	16.4	16.8
Metamyelocytes	25.6	23.9	21.8	22.0	22.9	23.4	26.1	22.2	21.6	23.2
Bands and segs	9.3	7.2	14.1	16.4	12.6	12.3	10.9	12.2	12.2	13.3
Pronormoblasts	0.8	0.6	0.8	0.4	0.5	0.4	0.3	0.2	0.4	0.5
Basophilic normoblasts	1.9	2.1	1.2	1.0	1.2	1.7	1.6	1.8	1.3	2.2
Polychromatophilic normoblasts	12.6	14.5	19.5	16.4	17.3	19.4	19.1	21.8	18.3	15.1
Orthochromic normoblasts	1.6	2.5	2.1	1.2	3.6	3.4	2.4	2.7	3.1	2.5
Lymphocytes	19.7	25.4	19.3	18.6	17.5	13.6	13.6	16.0	18.0	17.4
Myeloid: erythroid ratio	5.5	3.5	2.5	3.4	2.8	2.6	2.9	2.3	2.7	3.3

Fig. 58-11 Reverse side of form shown in Fig. 58-10. These normal values were obtained years ago in our laboratory. Rosse and others have tabulated the normal values for 88 infants and children as they matured from birth to 18 months of age. Forty-five children were followed up for the entire 18 months. Their values differ significantly from the above, primarily showing a change in the percentage of lymphocytes after the first month from 14.42% ± 5.54% to values of more than 40%. *From Miale JB: Laboratory medicine: hematology, ed 6, St Louis, 1982, Mosby–Year Book.*

and cytoplasm, called asynchronism, producing cells often called atypical or bizarre but whose structure is just as easily analyzed as that of normal cells.

The transformation from an immature to a mature cell always involves the cytoplasm and nucleus and is generally accompanied by reduction in cell size. It is only for convenience that each is described and diagrammed separately (Fig. 58-12).

Cytoplasmic differentiation
Loss of basophilia

The cytoplasm of immature cells is generally deeply basophilic, basophilia referring to the affinity for a basic dye such as the methylene blue present in Wright's and other polychrome stains. Basophilia is proportional to the cytoplasmic content of ribonucleic acid (RNA). As the cell matures, there is a gradual loss of cytoplasmic RNA and cytoplasmic basophilia.

Cytoplasmic granules

In myeloid cells cytoplasmic differentiation is characterized by the appearance of granules. Some common properties such as lipid content or the presence of peroxidase and other enzymes exist and may be useful in distinguishing myeloid granules from all others.

When cytoplasmic granules first appear, they are few, coarse, and wine red, the nonspecific granules. As the granulocyte differentiates and matures, three types of specific granules appear. The number gradually increases, and the granules differentiate into three types. Each type has an affinity either for acid or for basic dyes. Those that are acidophilic or eosinophilic stain orange-red and are characteristic of the eosinophil leukocyte. The basophilic granules are blue-black and identify the basophil leukocyte, whereas those that stain with both the basic and the acid dyes of a compound stain, called neutrophilic, characterize the neutrophilic leukocyte and are purplish.

Elaboration of hemoglobin

A different type of cytoplasmic differentiation is seen in the synthesis of a characteristic cytoplasmic constituent such as hemoglobin. This is a special feature of the maturation of erythroid cells. At first the immature cell contains no visible hemoglobin, though the greatest rate of hemoglobin synthesis occurs in the pronormoblast and basophilic normoblast. However, this is obscured by the basophilia cy-

Cytoplasmic differentiation

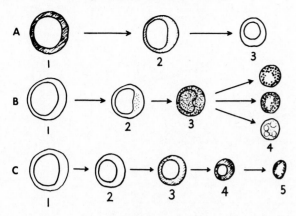

Nuclear maturation 1

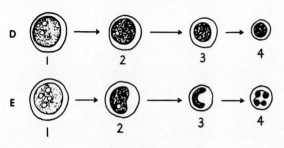

Reduction in cell size

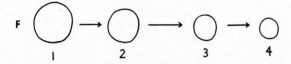

Fig. 58-12 Principles of cell differentiation and maturation. **A,** Loss of cytoplasmic basophilia. **B,** Elaboration and differentiation of cytoplasmic granules. **C,** Elaboration of specific cytoplasmic constituent (hemoglobin). **D,** Reduction in nuclear size, condensation of chromatin, and reduction of nucleoli. **E,** Alteration of nuclear shape. **F,** Reduction in cell size. *From Miale JB: Laboratory medicine: hematology, ed 6, St Louis, 1982, Mosby–Year Book.*

toplasmic RNA in stained smears, and it is only when the RNA content is reduced that hemoglobin becomes visible. Gradually a little appears and then a great deal, the most mature normal cell containing a standard and maximal amount of this respiratory pigment.

Nuclear maturation

Nuclear maturation is concerned with changes in the structure and chemical composition of the nuclear chromatin and nuclei, reduction in size of the nucleus with condensation of chromatin, and in some cases, with striking changes in nuclear shape.

Structure and cytochemistry

The immature nucleus is round or oval. The nucleus-to-cytoplasm (N/C) ratio is high, and the netlike or spongelike nuclear chromatin is very delicate. As the cell matures, the chromatin strands become increasingly coarse and clumped,

Table 58-1 Nomenclature used in this text compared with that proposed by American Society of Clinical Pathologists, Committee for Clarification of the Nomenclature of Cells and Diseases of the Blood and Blood-Forming Organs

Nomenclature used in this text	Nomenclature proposed by ASCP
Myeloblast	Myeloblast
Progranulocyte	Progranulocyte
Myelocyte	Myelocyte
Metamyelocyte	Metamyelocyte
Band granulocyte	Band granulocyte
Segmented granulocyte	Segmented granulocyte
Lymphoblast	Lymphoblast
Prolymphoctye	Prolymphoctye
Lymphocyte	Lymphocyte
Monoblast	Monoblast
Promonocyte	Promonocyte
Monocyte	Monocyte
Plasmablast	Plasmoblast
Proplasmacyte	Proplasmocyte
Plasmacyte	Plasmocyte
Megakaryoblast	Megakaryoblast
Promegakaryocyte	Promegakaryocyte
Megakaryocyte	Megakaryocyte
Platelet	Thrombocyte
Pronormoblast	Rubriblast
Basophilic normoblast	Prorubricyte
Polychromatophilic normoblast	Rubricyte
Orthochromic normoblast	Metarubricyte

whereas their staining properties change from purplish to blue. Simultaneously, a reduction in the number of nucleoli is noted. At the same time, there are striking changes in the distribution of nucleic acids. The nucleus of the young cell is characterized by nuclear chromatin that is rich in deoxyribonucleic acid (DNA). The nucleoli contain RNA and are therefore Feulgen-negative. As the cell matures, the RNA-positive nucleoli disappear, and in their place is found DNA-positive, nucleolus-associated heterochromatin.

Changes in shape

Nuclear maturation of some cell types produces striking changes in shape. This is particularly true of the granulocytes in which the end result is a nucleus containing two or more lobulations connected by filaments of nuclear membrane. The more mature the cell, the more polymorphous the nuclear structure.

Reduction in cell size

Reduction in cell size is a feature of maturity in all cells except those of the megakaryocytic series, in which the youngest cell (diploid) is smaller than the fully developed megakaryocyte (polyploid). In most cells nuclear consideration is greater than the reduction in total cell volume. The nucleus-to-cytoplasm ratio is therefore high in the young cells and low in mature cells.

Nomenclature

A revision and clarification of existing hematologic nomenclature was undertaken in 1949 by a special committee of

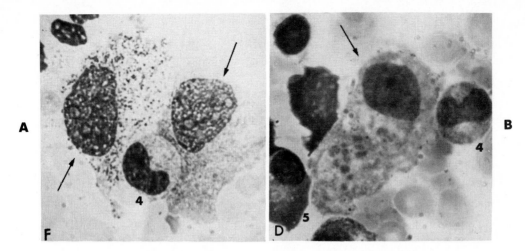

Fig. 58-13 **A,** Reticulum cell of the "Ferrata" type *(arrow)* (Wright's stain; ×950). **B,** Reticulum cell in chronic hemolytic anemia *(arrow)* (Wright's stain; ×950). *From Miale JB: Laboratory medicine: hematology, ed 6, St Louis, 1982, Mosby–Year Book.*

the American Society of Clinical Pathologists. A real contribution was made in proposing a standard and acceptable nomenclature for most cell types. The nomenclature proposed for cells of the erythrocytic series, however, seems awkward and artificial. We use instead the terminology outlined in Table 58-1.

DESCRIPTION OF WRIGHT-STAINED BLOOD AND BONE MARROW CELLS

See summary in Table 58-2.

Reticulum cell (Fig. 58-13)

The use of the term *reticulum cell* is not easy to defend. In a differential count on bone marrow the name *reticulum cell* can be used for two cells, one having a rather abundant frayed cytoplasm, a nucleus with ropy chromatin and prominent parachromatin, and large blue nucleolus, "reticulum cells of Ferrata"; the other being obviously phagocytic.

Size: 15 to 25 μm; usually irregular in outline.
Nucleus: Usually oval; delicate nuclear membrane. Nuclear chromatin forms an irregular network of light violet strands and small irregular clumps. The parachromatin is light blue or pink and sharply demarcated from the chromatin. Nodular thickenings are common where chromatin strands cross.
Nucleoli: one to three, irregular in shape, somewhat hazy in outline, and usually light blue.
Cytoplasm: Abundant; nucleus-to-cytoplasm ratio 1:1 or less; pale blue and mottled. It usually is not granular but may contain a few large azurophilic granules or a large number of red granules or strands (Ferrata reticulum cell). The cytoplasm of the phagocytic reticulum cell contains cellular debris, iron granules, and sometimes parasites.

Myeloblast (Fig. 58-14)

Size: 10 to 20 μm; round.
Nucleus: Round or oval; thin nuclear membrane. The chromatin is abundant, stippled, finely reticulated, and light

purple. The parachromatin is sparse, pale blue or pink, and sharply demarcated.
Nucleoli: Two to five; rather well outlined; round or oval; pale blue. The chromatin tends to be clearer next to the nucleoli.
Cytoplasm: Sparse to moderately abundant; nucleus-to-cytoplasm ratio 5:1 to 7:1; variously basophilic and usually not lighter in the perinuclear zone. It contains no granules.

Progranulocyte (Fig. 58-15)

The chief identifying feature of this cell is that it contains peroxidase-positive azurophilic granules.
Size: 14 to 20 μm; round or oval.
Nucleus: Large, round, or oval; thin nuclear membrane. The chromatin is in the form of a network, slightly coarse and with some slight clumping, especially near the nucleoli.

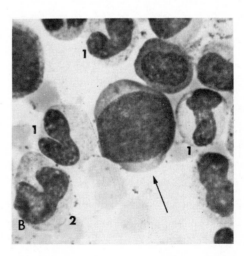

Fig. 58-14 Myeloblast *(arrow)* (Wright's stain; ×950). *From Miale JB: Laboratory medicine: hematology, ed 6, St Louis, 1982, Mosby–Year Book.*

Table 58-2 Summary of characteristics of blood and bone marrow cells (Wright's stain)

Cell	Size (µm)	Nucleus	Nucleoli	Cytoplasm	N/C ratio	Comments
Reticulum cell	15–25	Irregularly oval; delicate membrane; sharply demarcated parachromatin	1–3, irregular and faint	Abundant, pale blue, mottled, usually no granules but may have a few azurophilic granules	1:1	In marrow smears, cell outlines usually indistinct; cytoplasm usually mottled and may appear vacuolated; nucleus often shows thickenings at intersections of chromatin strands
Myeloblast	10–20	Large, oval or round; thin membrane; stippled or finely reticulated chromatin; sparse, sharply demarcated parachromatin	2–5, distinct	Sparse, no granules, deeply basophilic	5:1–7:1	Usually does not show clear perinuclear halo as in lymphoblast, nor is chromatin as coarse as in lymphoblast nucleus; in pathologic proliferation these cells may be very large (macromyeloblasts) or about the size of young lymphocytes (micromyeloblasts); latter easily mistaken for lymphocytes, but micromyeloblast contains finer chromatin
Progranulocyte	14–20	Large, round or oval; thin membrane; chromatin netlike with some clumping next to nucleoli; parachromatin sparse	1–3, not as prominent	Sparse, basophilic, but not as intense as in myeloblast	5:1	Distinguished from myeloblast chiefly by presence of granules and from later cells by small number of granules; at times granules large and round, but usually fine and irregular
Myelocyte Neutrophilic Eosinophilic Basophilic	10–18	Indistinct when cell heavily granulated; chromatin fairly coarse; parachromatin sparse	0–1, indistinct	Moderate, heavily granulated (granules may obscure nucleus)	2:1	Most heavily granulated of blood cells; granules may be purplish at early stage of development, later differentiate into basophilic, eosinophilic, or neutrophilic
Metamyelocyte Neutrophilic Eosinophilic Basophilic	10–18	Kidney shaped; heavy nuclear membrane; chromatin coarse; parachromatin sparse	0	Fairly abundant, pinkish, contains specific granules	1.5:1	Indentation of nucleus indicates greater maturity; granules of neutrophilic metamyelocytes vary in size; in eosinophilic or basophilic cells, granules remain large and usually obscure nuclear outline
Band granulocyte Neutrophilic Eosinophilic Basophilic	10–15	Sausage or band shaped; coarse, deeply staining purple chromatin; parachromatin very scanty	0	Abundant, pinkish, contains specific granules (fine when neutrophilic)	1:2	Nucleus may be constricted at one or more points, but as long as there is visible chromatin between nuclear membranes, cell called band form; when nucleus folded but constriction not visible, should be classified as a band form; nuclear outline in basophilic and eosinophilic cells usually obscured by granules
Segmented granulocyte Neutrophilic Eosinophilic Basophilic	10–15	Lobules of dense chromatin connected by one or more thin filaments	0	Abundant, pinkish, contains specific granules	1:3	Presence of one or more thin filaments identifies cell as segmented granulocyte; neutrophilic granules very fine; eosinophilic and basophilic granules large and round, obscuring the nucleus
Lymphoblast	10–18	Round or oval; definite nuclear membrane; chromatin in thin strands or stippled, light red-purple	1–2	Homogeneous and moderately basophilic, often shows lighter perinuclear zone	7:1–5:1	Not easily distinguished from other blast cells; lighter perinuclear zone may be helpful; also relatively few nucleoli
Prolymphocyte	10–18	Oval or slightly indented; chromatin varies from fine to slightly coarse; parachromatin indistinct	1	Sparse, moderately basophilic, homogeneous	5:1	At times difficult to distinguish prolymphocytes from lymphoblasts, particularly in lymphocytic leukemia; may contain a very few azurophilic granules
Lymphocyte	6–18	Round or oval, slightly or deeply indented; chromatin in coarse clumps; indistinct sparse parachromatin	0	Sky blue or medium blue, clear and glassy	5:1–2:1	Vary in size, chiefly because of variation in amount of cytoplasm; may contain a number of large azurophilic granules; sky blue, clear cytoplasm characteristic

Cell	Diameter (μm)	Nucleus	Nucleoli	Cytoplasm	N:C ratio	Remarks
Monoblast	14–18	Round or oval; thin membrane; chromatin fine and delicate; parachromatin abundant	1–2	Basophilic, homogeneous, nongranulated	6:1	Differentiated with difficulty from other blast cells; is said to have more basophilic cytoplasm than myeloblast and less basophilic cytoplasm than lymphoblast; actually all gradations seen in monocytic leukemias
Promonocyte	14–18	Moderately indented; thin membrane; chromatin in coarse clumps; indistinct sparse parachromatin	0–1	Moderately abundant, gray-blue and opaque, few extremely fine pink granules	5:1	Characterized by presence of very fine pink granules, "azurophilic dust"; however, demonstration of such granules requires most critical staining technique
Monocyte	12–18	Indented or folded, delicate, pale staining; fine chromatin with much parachromatin	0	Gray or gray-blue, opaque, very fine pink granules	4:1	Adult monocyte easily identified in thin well-stained smear, but in thick or overstained smears characteristics lost; one helpful feature is that monocytic nucleus stains much lighter than similar cells
Pronormoblast	14–19	Round or very slightly oval, central or slightly eccentric; fine reticular chromatin; sparse indistinct parachromatin	1–2, very faint	Scanty, deeply basophilic, homogeneous, opaque	8:1	Superficially similar to other blast cells, but characteristically has rounder, more centrally placed nucleus
Basophilic normoblast	10–15	Round, slightly eccentric; chromatin coarse and dark staining; parachromatin sparse but distinct	0–1	More abundant, intensely to moderately basophilic, opaque, royal blue	6:1	Distinguished from pronormoblast by coarse chromatin of nucleus, from lymphocytes by opaque basophilic cytoplasm; cytoplasmic basophilia characteristically vivid royal blue
Polychromatophilic normoblast	8–12	Round, eccentric; chromatin coarse and dark staining; parachromatin distinct	0	More abundant, pink to orange hemoglobin localized in patches or diffused throughout orange-tinged cytoplasm	4:1	Distinguished from earlier cell of erythrocytic series by appearance of hemoglobin, from lymphocytes by distinct parachromatin and opaqueness of cytoplasm
Orthochromic normoblast	7–10	Small and shrunken, dense; may be round or bizarre; no parachromatin visible	0	Orange-red as in adult cell	1:2	Gradations between polychromatophilic normoblasts and orthochromic normoblasts commonly seen
Promegakaryocyte	25–50	Irregular and polylobulated, quite large; darker staining than younger cell	0–2	Moderately to faintly basophilic, few to many fine azurophilic granules near nucleus	6:1	Nucleus usually more irregular than megakaryoblast, larger and more delicate than megakaryocyte
Megakaryocyte	40–100	Multilobular and bizarre; chromatin irregularly clumped	0–many	Abundant, pale, with granular pink aggregates	1:1–1:2	Cell appearance so varied that typical cell is not easily described; may seem to be multinucleated; but must be distinguished from osteoclasts, which are truly multinucleated and in which each nucleus contains a sharply defined nucleolus
Plasmablast	15–25	Round or oval, eccentric; chromatin reticulated; parachromatin distinct	2–4	Moderately to deeply basophilic, granules absent	1:1–2:1	Cell has same nuclear structure as reticulum cell except for less parachromatin and somewhat coarser chromatin strands
Proplasmacyte	15–25	Oval or round, eccentric; chromatin moderately coarse	1–2	Azure blue, with lighter perinuclear zone	1:1–2:1	Characteristic brilliant basophilia of plasmacyte appears in this precursor and is usually typical; may resemble basophilic normoblast (and vice versa) but in normoblast blue is darker
Plasmacyte	10–20	Round or oval, eccentric; very coarse clumped chromatin; sharp but sparse parachromatin	0	Azure blue, with lighter perinuclear zone	1:2	Nucleus quite eccentrically located; color of cytoplasm typical

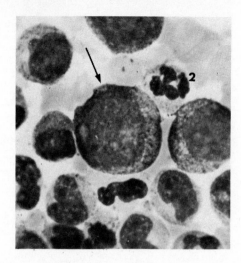

Fig. 58-15 Progranulocyte *(arrow)* (Wright's stain; ×950); *2,* segmental neutrophil. *From Miale JB: Laboratory medicine: hematology, ed 6, St Louis, 1982, Mosby–Year Book.*

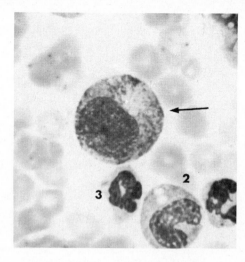

Fig. 58-16 Myelocyte *(arrow)* (Wright's stain; ×950); *2,* metamyelocytes; *3,* band neutrophils. *From Miale JB: Laboratory medicine: hematology, ed 6, St Louis, 1982, Mosby–Year Book.*

Nucleoli: One to three less prominent than in the myeloblast; pale blue; round or oval.

Cytoplasm: Sparse; nucleus-to-cytoplasm ratio about 5:1; basophilic but lighter than myeloblast. It contains a few purplish granules that may be either large and round or fine and irregular.

Myelocyte (Fig. 58-16)

Specific granules (neutrophilic, eosinophilic, or basophilic) appear first in late myelocytes and characterize the later metamyelocytes, bands, and segmented forms. On Wright-stained smears the numerous nonspecific granules in myelocytes disappear as the specific granules develop, and specific granules are peroxidase-negative and alkaline phosphatase-positive.

Size: 10 to 18 μm; round or oval.

Nucleus: Indistinct, thin nuclear membrane, particularly if the cell is heavily granulated. The chromatin network is coarse with irregular patches of blue- or pink-staining parachromatin.

Nucleoli: Usually absent or invisible.

Cytoplasm: Moderate in amount; nucleus-to-cytoplasm ratio about 2:1. In more mature cells the specific granules appear as definitely eosinophilic (brick red), basophilic (deep blue), or neutrophilic (lilac). When present in large numbers, the cytoplasmic granules usually obscure the nuclear outline.

Metamyelocyte (Fig. 58-17)

At this stage the nucleus first shows a definite alteration from a round to a kidney shape. Nuclear condensation coarsens the chromatin and the nucleolus is not visible. As in the myelocyte, different types of granules will be found in the neutrophilic metamyelocyte, the eosinophilic metamyelocyte, and the basophilic metamyelocyte.

Size: 10 to 18 μm.

Nucleus: Kidney shaped; nuclear membrane heavy. The chromatin is coarse or in thick strands, staining deep

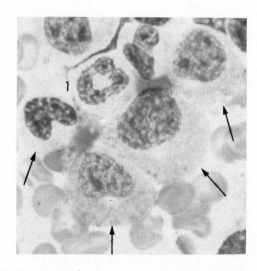

Fig. 58-17 Metamyelocytes *(arrows)*. Various stages of maturity (Wright's stain; ×950); *1,* stab neutrophils. *From Miale JB: Laboratory medicine: hematology, ed 6, St Louis, 1982, Mosby–Year Book.*

purple, and much darker than in younger cells. The parachromatin is scanty but distinct. The nucleolus is not usually visible.

Cytoplasm: Fairly abundant; nucleus-to-cytoplasm ratio about 1.5:1. The cytoplasm is pink. The specific granules are either eosinophilic, basophilic, or neutrophilic and are smaller than in the myelocyte and less uniform in size.

Band granulocyte (Fig. 58-18)

Here the nucleus undergoes further condensation, forming a sausage-shaped band or stab form.

Size: 10 to 15 μm.

Nucleus: Sausage or band shaped. It may be constricted at one or more points, but a significant amount of chromatin

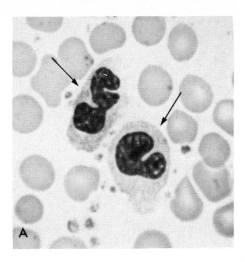

Fig. 58-18   Band granulocytes *(arrows)* (Wright's stain; ×950). *From Miale JB: Laboratory medicine: hematology, ed 6, St Louis, 1982, Mosby–Year Book.*

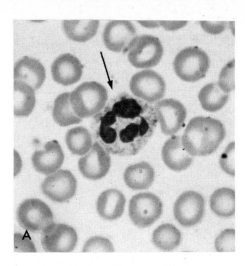

Fig. 58-19   Segmented neutrophilic granulocyte *(arrow)* (Wright's stain; ×950). *From Miale JB: Laboratory medicine: hematology, ed 6, St Louis, 1982, Mosby–Year Book.*

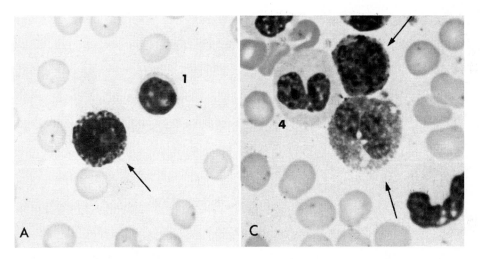

Fig. 58-20   **A,** Basophilic granulocyte *(arrow)* (Wright's stain; ×950). **B,** Eosinophilic granulocyte *(arrow)* (Wright's stain; ×950). *From Miale JB: Laboratory medicine: hematology, ed 6, St Louis, 1982, Mosby–Year Book.*

is seen in the constriction. The chromatin is coarse and deep purple-blue. The parachromatin is scanty; the nucleolus is not visible.

Cytoplasm: Abundant; pale blue or pink; nucleus-to-cytoplasm ratio about 1:2.

Segmented granulocyte (Figs. 58-19 and 58-20)

Mature granulocytes are characterized by segmentation of the nucleus into lobes connected by fine filaments of nuclear membrane, within which no chromatin can be seen.

Size: 10 to 15 μm.

Nucleus: Chromatin coarse and dense; staining deep purple-blue, with scant parachromatin. Two or more lobes of nuclear chromatin are connected by thin filaments.

Cytoplasm: Abundant; nucleus-to-cytoplasm ratio about 1:3; light pink or blue. Specific granules are fine and

pink or lilac (neutrophilic), large and brick red (eosinophilic), or large and blue-black (basophilic).

Lymphoblast (Fig. 58-21)

This cell is either absent in normal bone marrow or present in extremely small numbers.

Size: 10 to 18 μm.

Nucleus: Fairly centrally located; definite nuclear membrane. The chromatin is in thin strands or stippled light red-purple. The parachromatin is moderately abundant, sharply demarcated, and light blue. The nucleus is generally round or oval.

Nucleoli: One to two; small; pale blue.

Cytoplasm: Homogeneous and moderately to heavily basophilic; sparse, with nucleus-to-cytoplasm ratio 5:1 to 7:1. There are no granules.

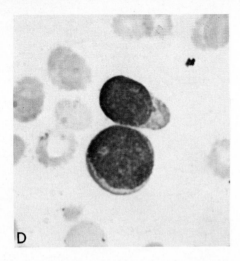

Fig. 58-21   Lymphoblast (Wright's stain; ×950). *From Miale JB: Laboratory medicine: hematology, ed 6, St Louis, 1982, Mosby–Year Book.*

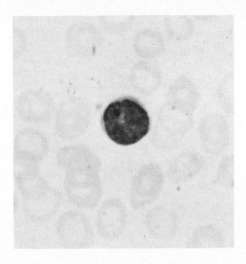

Fig. 58-23   Lymphocyte (Wright's stain; ×950). *From Miale JB: Laboratory medicine: hematology, ed 6, St Louis, 1982, Mosby–Year Book.*

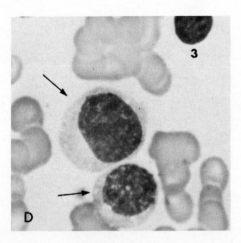

Fig. 58-22   Prolymphocyte *(arrows)* (Wright's stain; ×950). *From Miale JB: Laboratory medicine: hematology, ed 6, St Louis, 1982, Mosby–Year Book.*

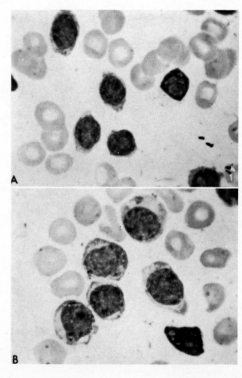

Fig. 58-24   Size of lymphocytes in a smear is markedly affected by the thinness of the smear. These cells are the same but have been photographed from thick, **A,** and thin, **B,** portions of the same peripheral blood smear (chronic lymphocytic leukemia). (Wright's stain; ×750). *From Miale JB: Laboratory medicine: hematology, ed 6, St Louis, 1982, Mosby–Year Book.*

Prolymphocyte (Fig. 58-22)

Whereas the lymphoblast and the adult lymphocyte vary but little from their fellows, the prolymphocyte includes a large spectrum of intermediates.

Size: 10 to 18 μm; average smaller than lymphoblast.

Nucleus: Round or oval; may be slightly indented. The chromatin is more clumped than in the lymphoblast but is still relatively fine and dark red-purple. The parachromatin is generally not as well defined as in the lymphoblast or as smudged as in the adult lymphocyte.

Nucleoli: Usually one; round, blue, and sharply outlined.

Cytoplasm: Tends to be more abundant than in the lymphoblast; nucleus-to-cytoplasm ratio closer to 5:1; light blue to medium dark blue. Occasionally it has azurophilic granules.

Lymphocyte (Fig. 58-23)

The presence of small, medium, and large lymphocytes in the blood of the adult and the predominance of medium and large lymphocytes in the blood of infants are common observations. The size can be easily changed by the thickness of the smear (Fig. 58-24), so that the classification of lymphocytes into large, medium, and small is technically untrustworthy and of doubtful significance.

Size: Small, 6 to 8 μm; medium, 8 to 14 μm; large, 8 to 18 μm.

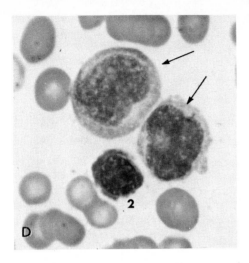

Fig. 58-25   Monoblasts *(arrows)* (Wright's stain; ×950). *From Miale JB: Laboratory medicine: hematology, ed 6, St Louis, 1982, Mosby—Year Book.*

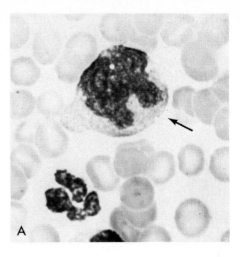

Fig. 58-26   Promonocyte *(arrow)* (Wright's stain; ×950). *From Miale JB: Laboratory medicine: hematology, ed 6, St Louis, 1982, Mosby—Year Book.*

Nucleus: Round or oval; may be slightly or deeply indented; usually somewhat eccentric. The nuclear membrane is heavy. The chromatin is in the form of large, coarse clumps blending into sparse, pale blue to pink parachromatin, so that the differentiation between chromatin and parachromatin is not sharp.

Nucleoli: One may occasionally be seen in the larger cells; generally none.

Cytoplasm: Typically sky blue, but may be medium blue; clear and homogeneous. There are occasional azurophilic granules.

Monoblast (Fig. 58-25)

Size: 14 to 18 μm.

Nucleus: Round or oval; thin nuclear membrane. The chromatin structure is similar to the myeloblast, but appears to stain lighter. The parachromatin is abundant, sharply demarcated, and pale pink or blue.

Nucleoli: One to two.

Cytoplasm: Moderate; basophilic; no granulation in the blast stage. The presence of fine lilac granules indicates maturation to the promonocyte or monocyte stage.

Promonocyte (Fig. 58-26)

Size: 14 to 18 μm.

Nucleus: Moderately indented; thin nuclear membrane. The chromatin is fine and threadlike, giving the nucleus a pale appearance in comparison to other cells. The parachromatin is abundant.

Nucleoli: None to one.

Cytoplasm: Gray-blue; opaque, with very fine lilac granules.

Monocyte (Fig. 58-27)

Size: 12 to 18 μm.

Nucleus: Indented or folded over; delicate; pale staining. The chromatin is in fine strands; the parachromatin is abundant and distinct.

Nucleoli: Usually none; occasionally one.

Cytoplasm: Light gray or gray-blue; opaque; characteristically numerous, fine, dustlike lilac granules.

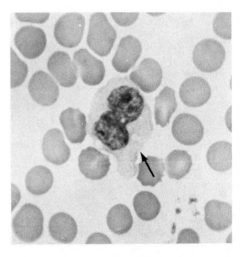

Fig. 58-27   Monocyte *(arrow)* (Wright's stain; ×950). *From Miale JB: Laboratory medicine: hematology, ed 6, St Louis, 1982, Mosby—Year Book.*

Pronormoblast (Fig. 58-28)

This is the most immature cell in the normoblast series.

Size: 14 to 19 μm.

Nucleus: Round or slightly oval; thin nuclear membrane; may be central or slightly eccentric. The chromatin varies from finely reticular, as in the myeloblast, to coarsely reticular with a tendency to clump. The parachromatin is indistinct and scant.

Nucleoli: One to two; usually very faint and pale blue.

Cytoplasm: Small in amount; nucleus-to-cytoplasm ratio usually greater than in myeloblast; moderately basophilic, homogeneous, and opaque.

Basophilic normoblast (Fig. 58-29)

This cell is similar to the pronormoblast, but obviously is more adult, since nucleoli are generally absent and the nuclear chromatin is coarser. The degree of basophilia varies

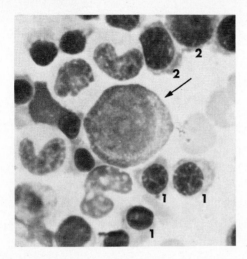

Fig. 58-28 Pronormoblast *(arrow)* (Wright's stain; ×950). *From Miale JB: Laboratory medicine: hematology, ed 6, St Louis, 1982, Mosby—Year Book.*

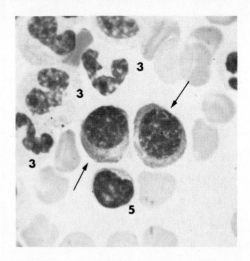

Fig. 58-30 Polychromatophilic normoblast *(arrow)* (Wright's stain; ×950). *From Miale JB: Laboratory medicine: hematology, ed 6, St Louis, 1982, Mosby—Year Book.*

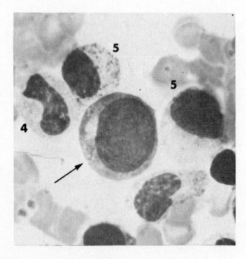

Fig. 58-29 Basophilic normoblast *(arrow)* (Wright's stain; ×950). *From Miale JB: Laboratory medicine: hematology, ed 6, St Louis, 1982, Mosby—Year Book.*

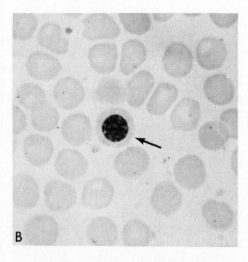

Fig. 58-31 Orthochromic normoblast *(arrow)* (Wright's stain; ×950). *From Miale JB: Laboratory medicine: hematology, ed 6, St Louis, 1982, Mosby—Year Book.*

from intense to moderate and is greater than in the pronormoblast.

Size: 10 to 15 μm.

Nucleus: Smaller than in the pronormoblast; generally round and slightly eccentric; nuclear membrane thin. The chromatin is coarse and irregular, so that the nucleus stains dark. The parachromatin is sparse but distinct.

Nucleoli: None to one.

Cytoplasm: Appears more abundant than in the pronormoblast because of the smaller nucleus. It varies from intense to moderately basophilic and is royal blue and opaque.

Polychromatophilic normoblast (Fig. 58-30)

This cell is characterized by the first appearance of visible hemoglobin, usually perinuclear, so that the cytoplasm stains pink to basophilic, either irregularly if the hemoglobin

is localized or diffusely blue-orange when the hemoglobin is distributed throughout the cytoplasm.

Size: 8 to 12 μm.

Nucleus: Round and smaller than in precursors; usually eccentric; thick nuclear membrane. The chromatin is very coarse and clumped so that the nucleus stains very dark. The parachromatin is distinct in contrast to lymphocyte, with which it may be confused if the hemoglobin content is not recognized.

Nucleoli: None.

Cytoplasm: Relatively more abundant than in precursors; varies from basophilic, with perinuclear areas of pink-staining or orange-staining hemoglobin, to diffusely lilac (polychrome).

Orthochromic normoblast (Fig. 58-31)

This term applies to the fully hemoglobinated form of the

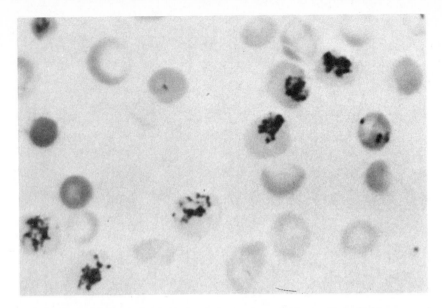

Fig. 58-32 Reticulocytes stained with a supravital stain. *From Bauer JD: Clinical laboratory methods, ed 9, St Louis, 1982, Mosby—Year Book.*

normoblast. When found in the peripheral blood (e.g., hemolytic disease), the cytoplasm is truly orthochromic, in other words, the normal color of the adult nonnucleated erythrocyte. There is usually no trace of basophilia. In bone marrow smears, however, it is unusual to find orthochromic normoblasts with a pure orange cytoplasm, most showing various degrees of basophilia. The bizarre shape sometimes seen in the nucleus is pyknosis preceding extrusion of the nucleus to form the nonnucleated erythrocyte.

Size: 7 to 10 μm.

Nucleus: Small and shrunken; dense and dark staining because of marked condensation of chromatin. Little structure is recognizable, with the parachromatin no longer distinguishable. It may be round, oval, or have various bizarre forms and is usually eccentric.

Nucleoli: None.

Cytoplasm: Orange-red, as in adult erythrocyte.

Polychromatophilic macrocyte or reticulocyte (Fig. 58-32)

After the orthochromic normoblast loses its nucleus, a small amount of the basophilic substance characteristic of immature forms remains in the cytoplasm. The vestige of cellular immaturity is composed of RNA and protoporphyrin. In Wright-stained smears, the basophilic substance may be evenly distributed throughout the erythrocyte (diffuse basophilia), or it may have a patchy distribution, giving the cell a mottled appearance, with orange (hemoglobin) and blush areas (polychromasia). Because these cells are larger than mature red cells, some have termed them polychromatophilic macrocytes. Most characteristically, after staining with supravital stains (e.g., new methylene blue and brilliant cresyl blue), the basophilic substance aggregates into granules and filaments that stain darkly with the dye. The cells are then known as reticulocytes.

Size: 8 to 10 μm.

Nucleus: Anucleate.

Cytoplasm: Uniformly grayish orange (diffuse basophilia) or mottled with basophilic and orange areas (polychromasia). No central pallor. Basophilic reticulum formation when stained with supravital stains.

Erythrocyte (Fig. 58-33)

Size: 7 to 8.5 μm.

Nucleus: Anucleate.

Cytoplasm: Biconcave disc, with central pallor occupying approximately one third to two thirds of the cell diameter, cytoplasm stains orange-pink.

Megakaryoblast (Fig. 58-34)

The megakaryocytic series is characterized by several unusual features: (1) the youngest cell type is generally much smaller than the adult; (2) repeated nuclear division without cellular division takes place, so that instead of the usual diploid nucleus present in other cells, the megakaryocytic nucleus is polyploid; (3) the functional end product, the blood platelet, is a cytoplasmic fragment.

Size: 25 to 35 μm.

Nucleus: Round or oval; large; with delicate purple-staining chromatin and sparse parachromatin.

Nucleoli: Two to six; small and indistinct.

Cytoplasm: Scanty; nucleus-to-cytoplasm ratio about 10:1; irregularly basophilic; occasionally shows blunt extrusions.

Promegakaryocyte (Fig. 58-35)

Size: 25 to 50 μm.

Nucleus: Irregular and large; coarser than in the megakaryoblast. It may appear to be lobulated, and sometimes two or more distinct nuclei are seen.

Nucleoli: None to two; difficult to see.

Cytoplasm: Moderately basophilic with some polychro-

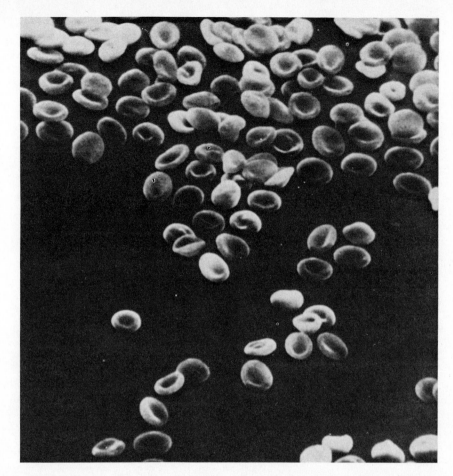

Fig. 58-33 Normal red cells, scanning electron microscopy. *From Salsbury AJ and Clarke JA: Triangle 8(7):261, 1968.*

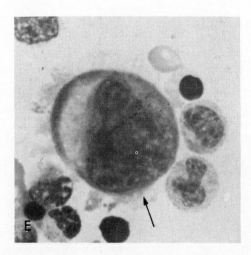

Fig. 58-34 Megakaryoblast *(arrow)* (Wright's stain; ×950). *From Miale JB: Laboratory medicine: hematology, ed 6, St Louis, 1982, Mosby–Year Book.*

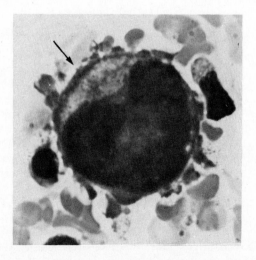

Fig. 58-35 Promegakaryocyte *(arrow)*, (Wright's stain; ×950). *From Miale JB: Laboratory medicine: hematology, ed 6, St Louis, 1982, Mosby–Year Book.*

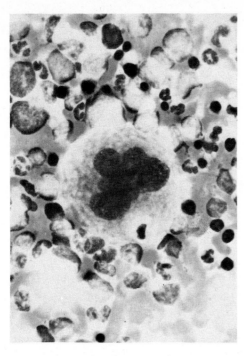

Fig. 58-36 Megakaryocyte (Wright's stain; ×400). *From Miale JB: Laboratory medicine: hematology, ed 6, St Louis, 1982, Mosby–Year Book.*

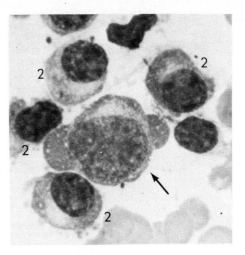

Fig. 58-37 Plasmablast (Wright's stain; ×950). *From Miale JB: Laboratory medicine: hematology, ed 6, St Louis, 1982, Mosby–Year Book.*

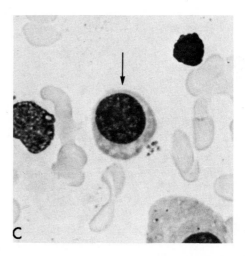

Fig. 58-38 Proplasmacyte (Wright's stain; ×950). *From Miale JB: Laboratory medicine: hematology, ed 6, St Louis, 1982, Mosby–Year Book.*

masia. It contains a few fine azurophilic granules in the perinuclear area. Sometimes there is early platelet formation at the periphery.

Megakaryocyte (Fig. 58-36)

It is the largest of the blood cells and varies so much in appearance that it is difficult to describe a single typical form. It usually has a single nucleus showing extreme pleomorphism.

Size: 40 to 100 μm.

Nucleus: Multiform; usually resembles a staghorn calculus. The chromatin is coarse and irregularly clumped.

Nucleoli: None to many; usually not visible, but in a thinned-out cell, many small nucleoli may be seen, reflecting polypoid endomitotic divisions of the nucleus.

Cytoplasm: Abundant, pale, with azurophilic granules either evenly dispersed or clumped. It may show pseudopod-like projections and shedding of the cytoplasm to form platelets.

Plasmablast (Fig. 58-37)

Size: 15 to 25 μm.

Nucleus: Round or oval; eccentric. The chromatin is reticulated and slightly coarse, and the parachromatin is distinct and moderate in amount.

Nucleoli: two to four.

Cytoplasm: Moderately to deeply basophilic fairly abundant; nucleus-to-cytoplasm ratio about 1:1 or 2:1. It may be mottled; granules are absent.

Proplasmacyte (Fig. 58-38)

Size: 15 to 25 μm.

Nucleus: Oval or round; eccentric; moderately coarse. It may be as large as that of the plasmablast.

Nucleoli: One to two; may be very large in abnormal forms.

Cytoplasm: Brilliant blue or azure, with lighter perinuclear zone common; appears opaque; nucleus-to-cytoplasm ration 1:1 or 2:1.

Plasmacyte (Fig. 58-39)

Size: 10 to 20 μm.

Nucleus: Round or oval; eccentrically placed. It has coarse, clumped chromatin, with sparse but sharp parachromatin. The wheelspoke pattern is seldom seen in bone marrow smears, since this appearance in tissue sections is probably due to fixation.

Nucleoli: None in normal cells. One giant nucleolus is usually present in abnormal forms.

Cytoplasm: Brilliant azure, with a pale perinuclear zone in

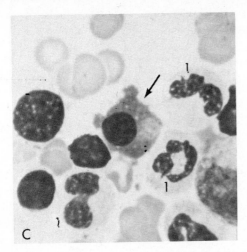

Fig. 58-39 Plasmacyte *(arrow)* (Wright's stain; ×950). *From Miale JB: Laboratory medicine: hematology, ed 6, St Louis, 1982, Mosby—Year Book.*

normal cell; may contain clear distinct values; nucleus-to-cytoplasm ratio 1:2.

CHARACTERISTICS OF NORMAL MARROW

The values for a normal differential count shown in Fig. 58-10 are derived from counts on marrows from 500 supposedly normal adults. The results are similar to other published normal values. In some categories the range is wide as may be expected when one realizes that aspiration samples a very small volume of marrow tissue. Further, the usual differential count done on 500 cells is not based on a sufficiently large number of cells to provide a critically narrow range of normal values. Since it is customary in many laboratories to count 500 marrow cells, the control values are based on 500-cell differential counts of normal marrows. Fig. 58-11 shows control values for children (see legend).

We consider a marrow specimen normal if it is appropriately cellular for the age of the patient as determined by a paraffin section, if the differential cell count falls within the normal range (myeloid:erythroid ratio of 2 to 3:1), if one or two megakaryocytes are seen per high-powered field, and if no foreign or abnormal cells are present.

Normal constituents such as osteoclasts and osteoblasts (Fig. 58-40) should not be confused with metastatic tumor cells or atypical megakaryocytes. They are found most frequently in specimens from infants and children, but may also be seen in adult specimens. Osteoblasts have a deeply basophilic cytoplasm and an eccentric nucleus. These two features give the osteoblast an appearance superficially similar to a plasma cell. Differential features are as follows: (1) an osteoblast is about twice the size of a plasma cell, (2) an osteoblast almost always shows an irregularly round, pale-staining area of the plasma cell that surrounds the nucleus, and (3) the nucleolus of the osteoblast usually shows one or more distinct nucleoli. Osteoclasts may be confused with megakarocytes since both are large, but they can usually be distinguished from megakaryocytes by the presence

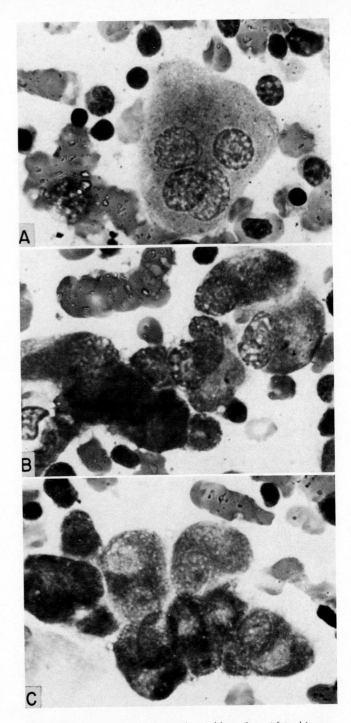

Fig. 58-40 Osteoclasts *(upper)* and osteoblasts *(lower)* found in normal marrow (Wright's stain; ×950). *From Miale JB: Laboratory medicine: hematology, ed 6, St Louis, 1982, Mosby—Year Book.*

of an even number of distinct round or oval nuclei, all of which are identical in appearance. Another normal finding is illustrated in Fig. 58-41, which shows a lymphoid nodule. These areas are usually sharply defined and consist of small lymphocytes.

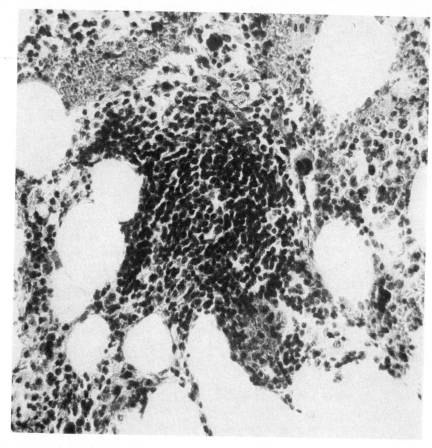

Fig. 58-41   Lymphoid nodule found in normal marrow, paraffin section. (Hematoxylin-eosin stain; ×450). *From Miale JB: Laboratory medicine: hematology, ed 6, St Louis, 1982, Mosby–Year Book.*

QUALITATIVE ABNORMALITIES OF THE MARROW

Qualitative abnormalities are identified by a careful microscopic study of the smears and sections. It is strongly recommended that these be studied first under low magnification to avoid overlooking clumps of abnormal cells. In multiple myeloma the characteristic cells are often present in large numbers and may be identified easily under low power magnification.

Megaloblastic cells may also be easily identified under low power, but other features of megaloblastic dyspoiesis require oil-immersion magnification and attention to minute details. Tumor cells are usually present in clumps (Fig. 58-42) that are visible under low magnification.

The lipid storage diseases such as Gaucher's, Neimann-Pick, and Hand-Schüller-Christian disease usually show such a strikingly abnormal picture that the diagnosis is obvious at first glance. Tuberculosis of the bone marrow shows typical tubercles (Fig. 58-43). Acid-fast organisms of various kinds can be demonstrated by the acid-fast stain. Necrosis of bone marrow tissue may be found in a variety of diseases: neoplastic, infectious, or nutritional. There is no common etiology, with the possible exception of vascular occlusion caused by sickle-cell disease or sickle cell-he-

moglobin C hemoglobinopathy, or disseminated intravascular coagulation.

QUANTITATIVE ABNORMALITIES OF THE MARROW

Quantitative abnormalities may be relative or absolute. Aplasia, hypoplasia, or hyperplasia may affect the marrow as a whole or may be selective for only one cell type. If all cell types are affected, the differential count may be normal, and the quantitative abnormality becomes apparent only on study of the paraffin sections. If one cell type is predominantly affected, the differential count will reveal the relative disproportion among cell types, and the paraffin section will determine whether or not the increase of disease is relative or absolute.

One of the common indications for examination of the bone marrow is to estimate storage iron after staining with Prussian blue stain, which stains hemosiderin iron in macrophages as large confluent blue granules and ferritin deposits in developing red cells as fine blue cytoplasmic deposits (sideroblasts and siderocytes). Iron stores are reported as decreased, normal, or increased. Note that the estimation of storage iron should be done on smears rather than on histologic sections of tissue obtained by core biopsy (Fig.

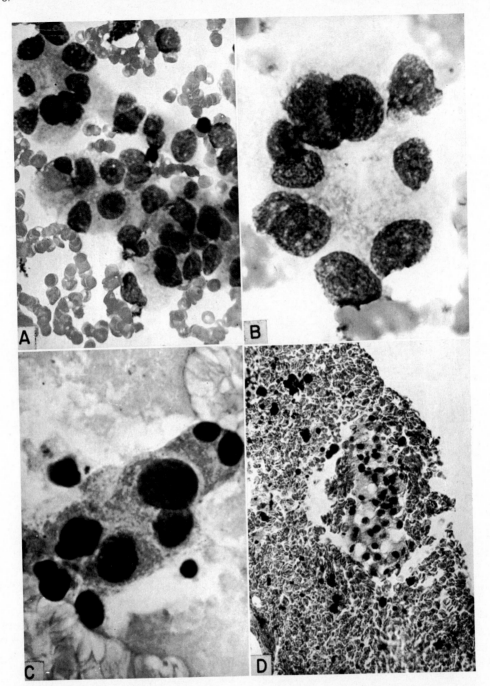

Fig. 58-42 Metastatic tumor cells in marrow aspirates. **A,** Metastatic adenocarcinoma of prostate (Wright's stain; ×450). **B,** The same (×950). **C,** Carcinoma of prostate, undifferentiated (Wright's stain; ×950). **D,** Carcinoma of breast, paraffin section (Hematoxylin-eosin stain; ×450). *From Miale JB: Laboratory medicine: Hematology, ed 6, St Louis, 1982, Mosby–Year Book.*

58-44). It is probable that the loss of stainable iron is caused by decalcification procedures, because histologic sections prepared from formalin-fixed particles compare favorably with the smear preparations.

Normal bone marrow has a supporting lattice of lacy connective tissue, referred to generally as reticulin. It consists of two types of fibers, those that stain by silver im-

pregnation but not with the trichrome stain (true reticulin) and those that stain with the trichrome stain (collagenous reticulin). Reticulin is increased in most pathologic marrow, such as is present in agnogenic myeloid metaplasia, lipid granulomas, chronic lymphocytic leukemia, monoclonal macroglobulinemia, myeloma, polycythemia vera, and myelofibrosis.

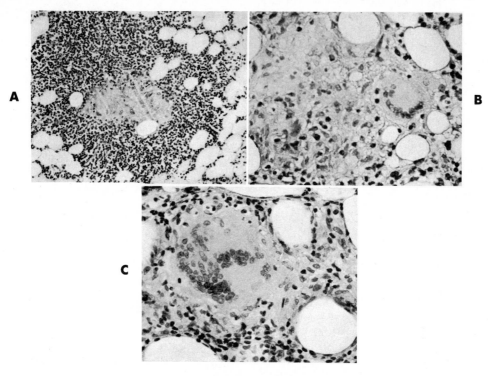

Fig. 58-43 Tubercle (*Mycobacterium tuberculosis* infection), bone marrow (hematoxylin-eosin stain; **A,** ×120; **B** and **C,** ×400). *From Miale JB: Laboratory medicine: hematology, ed 6, St Louis, 1982, Mosby–Year Book.*

SPECIAL TECHNIQUES USED FOR STUDYING BLOOD AND BONE MARROW CELLS

Although diagnosis in hematology has been and will continue to be based primarily on the standard techniques of Romanovsky staining of films and hematoxylin-eosin staining of paraffin-embedded tissue, the special techniques of phase-contrast microscopy, electron microscopy, and cytochemistry have each contributed to the understanding of the structure and function of blood cells.

Phase-contrast microscopy

Phase-contrast microscopy intensifies relatively minute differences in optical density and allows one to see the intimate details of cells and cytoplasmic structures. The chromatin of the nucleus, the mitochondria, the centrosome, and specific granules of the cytoplasm are all clearly visible in the living, unstained, and undamaged cell. Platelets are seen so distinctly with this illumination that they can be counted directly in special counting chambers.

Phase-contrast microscopy depends on two optical principles: (1) light waves out of phase cancel each other entirely or partially, depending on whether they are of the same or of different amplitudes, and (2) the speed of light passing through a substance varies with the refractive index of the substance. The chief features of a phase-contrast microscope (Fig. 58-45) are the following: Instead of the usual Abbe condenser used in standard microscopes, there is a special phase condenser that contains an annular diaphragm below the lower-most lens, which transmits light only around the

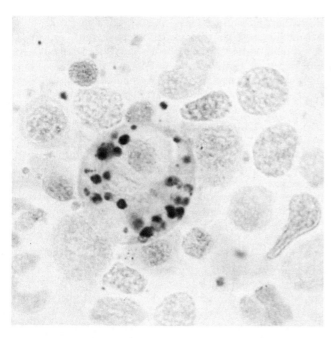

Fig. 58-44 Hemosiderin deposits in marrow macrophages (Prussian blue stain). *From Bauer JD: Clinical laboratory methods, ed 9, St Louis, 1982, Mosby–Year Book.*

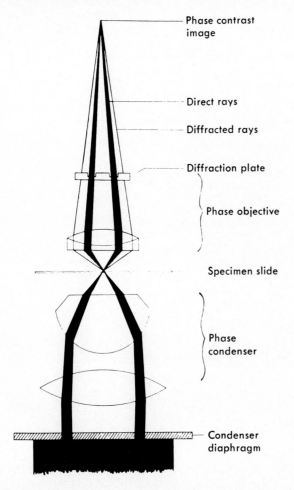

Phase contrast image

Direct rays

Diffracted rays

Diffraction plate

Phase objective

Specimen slide

Phase condenser

Condenser diaphragm

Fig. 58-45   Optics of phase microscopy (schematic). The phase contrast image is produced by two superimposed light wave systems, not in phase with each other, so that minute differences in optical density are intensified. The objective in a phase system acts essentially as a diffraction grating, whereas the position of the phase condenser determines the degree of phase contrast. *From Miale JB: Laboratory medicine: hematology, ed 6, St Louis, 1982, Mosby–Year Book.*

cause they differ little from adjacent areas in refraction thus become clearly delineated. In standard microscopy, differential staining is used to bring out such structures, at the expense of killing the cell and subjecting its components to harsh chemical insults. With phase-contrast microscopy, on the other hand, the living and undistorted cell can be examined.

Electron microscopy

Whereas images obtained by phase-contrast microscopy are due to different optical densities of the cell structures with respect to the passage of light out of phase, those images obtained with the electron microscope are caused by differences in density to the passage of electrons. When ultrathin (0.02 to 0.03 μm) sections are studied by electron microscopy, a very high degree of resolution is made possible—2 to 3 nm as compared to the optimum resolving power of the standard microscope, 0.2 μm. Thus the resolving power of the electron microscope approaches that needed to visualize monolayers of macromolecules. The ultrastructural composite features of blood cells are shown in Fig. 58-46.

The nucleus appears very much the same as in phase-contrast images. It is denser and darker than the remainder of the cell, the density increasing in older cells as the chromatin condenses. The internal structure is a confused network of chromatin strands with no obvious organization. The nucleus is surrounded by a dense nuclear membrane, enveloped in turn by an extremely delicate external membrane. The space between the two membranes, the perinuclear space, connects with the cytoplasmic matrix and contains cytoplasmic rather than nuclear material. The nucleolus presents as a dark granular or netlike structure.

The matrix of the cytoplasm is a reticular network of flattened bags of canals, and this network is called the endoplasmic reticulum. This structure is found in all cells except the mature erythrocyte. It is abundant in young cells, where it takes the form of flattened, parallel lamellae. In older cells, the endoplasmic reticulum is sparse and is presented as isolated bags. The endoplasmic reticulum has been likened to a network of canals, defined at one end by the cytoplasmic membrane and at the other end by the perinuclear space. The granules of Palade are minute (10 to 20 nm) granules adhering to the external surface between the canals. They are electron-dense and therefore appear dark in photographs and may represent units of riboprotein.

In electron microscopy the mitochondria are seen to have a complex structure. Each mitochondrion is limited by a membrane, 10- to 25-nm thick, which then extends toward the interior in the form of cristae that appear sometimes villous, sometime lamellar. When greatly magnified, the outer membrane and the cristae are seen to consist of two layers each about 8-nm thick and separated by a space about 5-nm wide. In the matrix of the mitochondrion one sees small (2 to 3 nm) granules.

The granules of leukocytes are striking and characteristic for each type of granulocyte. The nonspecific (undifferentiated) granules of early myeloid cells, staining deeply azurophilic with Romanovsky stains, are round, rather homogeneous, and usually larger and paler than the specific gran-

annulus at the circumference, the center being blacked out. Phase objectives are also different; a ring of fine film is applied at the rear focal plane, either on a separate disk or directly on the surface of the rear lens. This film acts as a diffraction grating, with the light passing through it being thrown out of phase. When the phase optical system is viewed through the special centering eyepiece, the phase-shifting annular film of the objective appears black, whereas the image of the condenser annulus is bright. When the two rings are exactly concentric and superimposed, the optical system is such that light rays, diffracted only a little while passing through a specimen, are out of phase by one fourth of a wavelength with rays that are diffracted more and that pass chiefly through the center of the objective. That portion of the specimen that is a greater impediment to light waves because of greater thickness or diffraction is seen as a dark structure against the lighter background made by areas that diffract light waves less. Differences are thus markedly accentuated. Structures invisible by standard microscopy be-

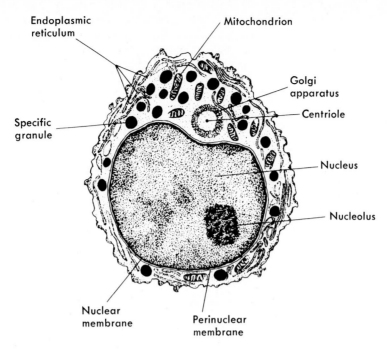

Endoplasmic reticulum

Mitochondrion

Golgi apparatus

Centriole

Specific granule

Nucleus

Nucleolus

Nuclear membrane

Perinuclear membrane

Fig. 58-46 Diagram of the ultrastructure of a blood cell, in this case a neutrophilic myelocyte. *From Miale JB: Laboratory medicine: hematology, ed 6, St Louis, 1982, Mosby–Year Book.*

ules. Neutrophilic granules are smaller, denser, and slightly elongated. Basophilic granules are large, very dense, and homogenous. Eosinophilic granules differ from the others in that they contain dense crystalloid inclusions. They vary in size and shape but are generally rectangular or trapezoidal.

Cytochemistry of blood cells

Cytochemical reactions should be used as an adjunct to standard morphology. They are most useful in (1) distinguishing among some of the leukemias, (2) distinguishing between granulocytic leukemia and a granulocytic leukemoid reaction, (3) distinguishing between classic Auer rods and other crystalline inclusions, (4) identifying the lymphocyte of leukemic reticuloendotheliosis, and (5) identifying the ringed sideroblasts in the sideroblastic anemias. Tables 58-3 and 58-4 summarize the major cytochemical reactions.

Peroxidase (myeloperoxidase)

The peroxidase reaction has been used for many years as a specific marker for the granules of cells of the myeloid series. Myeloperoxidase is present exclusively in azurophilic (nonspecific) granules. Synthesis of myeloperoxidase has begun by the progranulocyte state, so that progranulocytes, myelocytes, metamyelocytes, and band and segmented neutrophils are strongly peroxidase-positive. Eosinophils are strongly peroxidase-positive; the peroxidase is located within the matrix of specific granules. Lymphocytes are peroxidase-negative. Basophils are peroxidase-negative by the classic benzidine technique, but when 3,3'-diaminobenzidine tetrahydrochloride is used, the granules are per-

oxidase-positive. Monocytes show only a few peroxidase-positive granules.

By definition, the myeloblast contains no azurophilic granules; however, some peroxidase activity may be present that is associated with the rough endoplasmic reticulum and Golgi apparatus from which the azurophilic granules are derived.

The peroxidase reaction depends on the oxidation by hydrogen peroxide of a suitable substrate to form a chromogenic oxidized product. The substrate may be benzidine, benzidine dihydrochloride, diaminobenzidine, 3,3',5,5'-tetramethylbenzidine dihydrochloride, ortho-tolidine, or 4-chloro-1-naphthol. Peroxidase is unstable, and the reaction must be performed on freshly made smears.

Lipids

Sudan black B reacts with a variety of lipids, including neutral fats, phospholipids, and steroids. With this stain the granules of neutrophils and basophils stain intensely black or gray. In contrast, the granules of eosinophils stain only on the surface, giving the impression that they have an external lipid envelope. Myeloblasts contain minute, sudanophilic mitochondria.

Lymphocytes usually show only a few variable sudanophilic mitochondria. Monocytes have a few, very small, sudanophilic granules that are usually concentrated near the region of the nucleus. Megakaryocytes show fine punctate staining of the cytoplasm and platelets are faintly sudanophilic.

Peroxidase activity is unstable, demonstrated only in fresh smears, whereas sudanophilia is not affected by storage of smears.

Table 58-3   Cytochemical reactions in normal and abnormal blood cells

Cell	Peroxidase	Sudan	PAS	Alkaline phosphatase
NORMAL				
Myeloblast	Neg to ±	Neg	Neg	Neg
Progranulocyte	+ + + +	+ + + +	+ +	±
Myelocyte	+ + + +	+ + + +	+ + +	±
Metamyelocyte	+ + + +	+ + + +	+ + +	+
Adult neutrophil	+ + + +	+ + + +	+ + + +	+ to + + + +
Eosinophil	+ + + +	+ + + +	Neg to +	Neg
Basophil	Neg	+ + + +	Neg to +	Neg
Lymphocyte	Neg	Neg	Neg*	Neg
Monocyte	± to + +	± to +	± to +	Neg
Megakaryocyte	Neg	±	+ + + +	Neg
Platelet	Neg	±	+ + + +	Neg
Normoblast	Neg	Neg	Neg	Neg
ABNORMAL				
Leukemic lymphoblast	Neg	Neg	+ to + + + + †	Neg
Myelomonocytic cell	Neg to + + + ‡	Neg to + + + ‡	Neg to + + + ‡	Neg
Monocytic (histiocytic) leukemic cell	Neg to ±	Neg to ± ‡	Neg to +	Neg
Leukemic myeloblast	Neg to ±	Neg§	±	Neg
Erythroleukemic cell	Neg	Neg	+ +	Neg
Lymphocyte in chronic lymphocytic leuke- mia	Neg	Neg	+ to + +	Neg
Auer bodies	+ + + +	+ + + +	Neg	Neg

*A few normal lymphocytes may show fine to medium-sized PAS-positive inclusions.
†PAS-positive inclusions are coarse.
‡Varies with maturity; blasts are negative, whereas more mature cells are positive.
§Mitochondria may stain faintly.

Table 58-4   Cytochemical reactions: esterase

Cell	NAS-DC*	NAS-DA†	NAS-DAF‡	α-NB§
Myeloblast, (normal)	Neg	Neg	Neg	+
Myeloblast, leukemic	+ + + +	+ + + +	+ +	Neg
Auer bodies	+ + + +	+ + + +	+ +	+
Progranulocyte	+ + + +	+ + + +	+ + + +	+
Neutrophil, adult	+ + +	+ + +	+ + +	+
Basophil	+	+	+	Neg
Eosinophil	Neg	+	+	+
Monocyte	+	+ + +	0 to +	+ + +
Lymphocyte	Neg	Neg	Neg	Neg
Plasma cell	Neg	+	Neg	+ +
Myelomonocytic leukemia	+ to + +	+ to + +	+ to + +	+
Monocytic leukemia	+ to + + +	+ to + + +	Neg	+ + +
Erythroleukemia	+ + +	+ + +	+ + +	+ +
Acute lymphocytic leukemia	Neg	Neg	Neg	Neg

*NAS-DC, Naphthol ASD chloroacetate.
†NAS-DA, Naphthol ASD acetate.
‡NAS-DAF, NAS-DA reaction after inhibition by fluoride.
§α-NB, α-naphthyl butyrate.

Glycogen

Glycogen is stained by the periodic acid-Schiff (PAS) reaction. Periodic acid splits C-C bonds of glycogen at CHOH-CHOH groups, producing aldehydes (CHO). The Schiff reagent then reacts with the aldehydes to form a colored product, magenta when basic fuchsin is used. The reaction must be timed carefully because prolonged exposure to periodic acid can oxidize the aldehydes and cause a false-negative reaction. Glycogen is the only diastase-sensitive, PAS-positive substance, so that saliva or malt diastase is used to check the specificity of the reaction. Cytochemical studies using this reaction have yielded the following interesting data: Normal lymphocytes occasionally show PAS-positive granules but generally are PAS-negative; normal lymphoblasts are PAS-negative, but leukemic lymphoblasts and the small lymphocytes of chronic lymphocytic leukemia may have fine to coarse PAS-positive granules.

In the granulocytic series, PAS positivity increases in the maturation sequence: the myeloblasts are PAS-negative, the adult polymorphonuclear cells are strongly PAS-positive, and cells of intermediate maturity show intermediate PAS positivity. The granules of eosinophils are PAS-negative, but the cytoplasm shows diffuse staining. The same is true of basophils. Monocytes often show fine or moderately coarse PAS-positive granules. Megakaryocytes and platelets are strongly PAS-positive. Megakaryoblasts are PAS-negative, and promegakaryocytes are intermediate. Normal normoblasts are PAS-negative, but the abnormal normoblast or megaloblasts in erythroleukemia show strong PAS positivity. Plasma cells and Russell's bodies are PAS-negative on smears but PAS-positive in tissue sections.

Esterases

Leukocytes contain esterases, a group of lysosomal enzymes that hydrolyze both aliphatic and aromatic esters. Esterases are associated with the azurophilic (nonspecific) granules.

The substrates commonly employed for the demonstration of esterases are naphthol ASD chloroacetate, naphthol ASD acetate, o-naphthyl acetate, and o-naphthyl butyrate. The latter is considered more specific for monocytic esterase than is o-naphthyl acetate. As shown in Table 58-4, the reactions with naphthol ASD chloroacetate are seen chiefly in granulocytes. Monocytes react more strongly with naphthol ASD acetate, and this reaction, as well as a similar one in the cells of pure monocytic leukemia, is inhibited by fluoride. Positivity in granulocytes is not inhibited by fluoride. Naphthol ADS acetate also shows strong reactions with megakaryocytes, whereas o-naphthyl acetate reacts strongly only with monocytes and plasma cells.

Data on esterase reactions in various leukemias are contradictory. It is agreed that the cells of acute lymphocytic leukemia are esterase-negative. In myelomonocytic leukemia the blasts are usually negative or weakly positive, whereas the more mature cells with cytoplasmic granulation are esterase-positive with no inhibition by fluoride. In pure monocytic (histiocytic) leukemia the cells are variably esterase-positive, and when positive, the reaction is inhibited by fluoride. Auer rods are esterase-positive. The abnormal erythroid cells in erythroleukemia are strongly positive; naphthol ASD chloroacetate is considered to be a specific substrate for granulocytic esterase, whereas o-naphthyl butyrate is monocyte-specific.

Alkaline phosphatase

Phosphatases, more specifically phosphomonoesterases, are enzymes that liberate orthophosphoric acid from alcohol or phenolic monoesters. Based on pH requirements, two types are commonly distinguished, acid phosphatase and alkaline phosphatase. Fluorides inhibit the acid, but not the alkaline enzyme.

At least two alkaline phosphatases are present in leukocytes, one being activated by magnesium ions and the other by zinc ions. The zinc-activated enzyme is involved in the elevated phosphatase activity seen in infection and leukemoid reactions.

In leukemic leukocytes, zinc is low, particularly when the count is high and the disease is in relapse. This may explain why the cells in chronic granulocytic leukemia seem to have little alkaline phosphatase. In contrast to peroxidase activity, alkaline phosphatase activity is a property of specific granules. Young neutrophils have a lower alkaline phosphatase activity than the older neutrophils.

Except in one special situation (hypophosphatasia), there is little or no correlation between serum and leukocyte alkaline phosphatase. The enzyme in leukocytes is not absorbed from the serum, because it cannot be increased by incubating leukocytes in serum having a high alkaline phosphatase activity. In hypophosphatasia the leukocytes have no alkaline phosphate activity and neither does the serum, but here there is an inborn error of metabolism affecting all tissues.

The cytochemical demonstration of alkaline phosphatase depends on the formation of a colored precipitate at the site of hydrolysis of substrate. The Gomori method, modified slightly by several investigators, depends on incubating smears with glycerophosphate at pH 9 in the presence of calcium and magnesium ions. Insoluble calcium phosphate is formed at the site of reaction and is then visualized by being converted to black cobalt sulfide. Kaplow's modification of earlier techniques uses fixation in 10% formalin in absolute methanol at 0° C, sodium o-naphthyl phosphate in the substrate, and fast blue RR as the diazonium salt.

Kaplow described a further modification of the original method that gives very good results. The new method uses naphthol AS-BI phosphate and fast red violet LB buffered with propanediol at pH 9.7. The final coupled product is brilliant ruby red, and the smears are somewhat easier to score according to the degree of alkaline phosphatase activity.

Kaplow proposed rating the degree of positivity of phosphatase staining in each neutrophil on a 0 to 4 scale, the score for a given smear being the sum of ratings for 100 neutrophilic leukocytes. The criteria for rating a given cell are as follows:

0 = Colorless
1 = Diffuse but slight positivity, with occasional granules
2 = Diffusely positive, with a moderate number of granules
3 = Strongly positive, with numerous granules
4 = Very strongly positive, with very dark confluent granules

The reference range for normal individuals is 15 to 70.

Increased phosphatase activity is noted in the leukocytosis caused by various infections. Very striking increases are noted in leukemoid reactions and most myeloproliferative disorders, but not in chronic myelocytic leukemia. Thus the alkaline phosphatase reaction is often useful in differentiating both leukemoid states from leukemia and polycythemia vera from erythrocytosis.

Leukocyte alkaline phosphatase is high in the newborn and in a variety of stressful situations. Administration of adrenocorticotropic hormone (ACTH) produces high values;

cortisone does not. Elevated values are often encountered in normal pregnancy, as early as the fifth week after the last menstrual period. Activity is high in Down syndrome. Low values have been reported in idiopathic thrombocytopenic purpura, in paroxysmal nocturnal hemoglobinuria, and in collagen diseases.

Acid phosphatase

Acid phosphatase is found in almost all cells and therefore has little application in the identification of blood cells. An important exception is in leukemic reticuloendotheliosis. Whereas the acid phosphatase reaction in most blood cells is inhibited by tartrate, it is not inhibited in the "hairy" cells of this disease. Tartrate resistance (no inhibition by tartrate) is a feature also of Sézary cells and prolymphocytic leukemia.

Iron

Hemosiderin storage iron deposits in bone marrow macrophages are stained deep blue with the Prussian blue stain comprised of a 2% potassium ferrocyanide solution acidified with hydrochloric acid. Stains can be performed on marrow smears fixed in methyl alcohol or paraffin-embedded biopsy sections. A modification of the Prussian blue stain can demonstrate ferritin granules in sideroblasts and siderocytes.

SUGGESTED READING

Batjer JD: Preparation of optimal bone marrow samples, Lab Med 10:101, 1979.

Beckstead JH: The bone marrow biopsy: a diagnostic strategy, Arch Pathol Lab Med 110:175, 1986.

Hyun BH, Gulatti GL, and Ashton JK: Bone marrow examination: techniques and interpretation, Haemato Oncol Clin N Amer 2:513, 1988.

Kass L and Elias JM: Cytochemistry and immunocytochemistry in bone marrow examination: contemporary techniques for the diagnosis of acute leukemia and myelodysplastic syndromes, Haematol Oncol Clin N Amer 2:537, 1988.

Sun T: The selective use of cytochemistry and surface markers for the diagnosis of leukemias and lymphomas: a practical approach, Lab Med 12:424, 1981.

59 Quantitative evaluation of the hematopoietic system

Edward R. Burns
Barry Wenz

PRINCIPLES OF QUANTITATIVE HEMATOLOGY

Hematology is a science whose roots are based in the morphological description of the hematopoietic system. Microscopy was the primary tool of the hematologists of the early twentieth century, and with it they defined hundreds of diseases of varied etiologies. The use of the microscope, together with carefully chosen histochemical and cytochemical stains, allowed for the detailed delineation of the morphological features of normal and diseased tissue. The subsequent recognition of the dynamic nature of these diseases led to an understanding that quantitative shifts of the various blood cell populations accompanied the unique morphologic changes, and that these alterations required accurate enumeration for correct diagnosis and management.

Until recently, the practice of quantifying and classifying these changes was also the domain of the microscopist. Special counting chambers and diluting pipettes were devised to allow the trained technician to visually count a small sample of a total cell population and, using mathematical algorithms, to calculate a presumed cell count. The data derived from these procedures are known to be imprecise. Several well-defined aspects of the analytic procedure contribute to this imprecision. These include inadequate mixing, improper or inconsistent dilution, and nonrandom distribution of the sample or cell population in the counting chamber or on the glass slide. In addition, inconsistency in the identification of cells and observer bias yield data that do not precisely reproduce and are frequently inaccurate.

Automated cell counters developed in the early 1960s provide consistency in the quantitative measurement of blood cells. The instruments use measurements of electrical conductivity or light scatter, mechanically mix and dilute samples uniformly, and provide analysis independent of observer bias. These methods improve analytic accuracy and precision. The sophistication of automated hematology cell counters has evolved to become far superior to that of the manual methods they have replaced. However, traditional morphology still remains the primary means of identifying discrete cell populations associated with disease.

MANUAL CELL COUNTS IN HEMATOLOGY
General principles

The cellular elements of blood, red cells, white cells, and platelets can all be enumerated by examining a dilute suspension of cells under a microscope and counting a representative sample. The number of cells counted is then multiplied by the dilution factor and the actual volume of suspension is counted to calculate the concentration of cells in the original sample of whole blood. Until the early to mid-1960s all hematologic cell counts were performed with this methodology. The development of automated cell counters quickly made inroads so that red cell and white cell counts were routinely performed with these instruments by most clinical laboratories. In the 1970s, automated platelet counts became available, but many laboratories continued to perform manual counts because they had invested in equipment that did not have this capability. Today, most new instruments provide full cell counting capabilities of whole blood. Nevertheless, manual methodology remains important to clinical laboratory personnel for several reasons. First, manual methods can be used as reference methods for the calibration of automated instruments. In practice, though, this technique is being supplanted by the use of commercial calibrating reagents that are used directly with the automated instrument.

The most important current use of the manual methodology is for performing cell counts on body fluids such as spinal, pleural, abdominal, and joint fluids. Most current automated instruments are designed to analyze whole blood and cannot adequately provide accurate counts on body fluids. As such, the technique of chamber counting remains important for the modern clinical laboratory.

Most laboratories utilize the improved Neubauer hemocytometer as the counting chamber of choice. This device is a thick glass slide with precisely ruled lines etched into the glass, forming a grid. The grid is 9 mm² and 0.1 mm deep. The four corner squares, measuring 1×1 mm, are subdivided into 16 smaller squares and are used for white cell counts. The center 1 mm² box is used for platelet counting and is also subdivided into 25 smaller boxes used for red cell counting. Blood is usually taken up into a specialized pipette designed either for red cells with a final dilution of 1:200 or for white cells with a final dilution of 1:20. Alternatively, the Unopette system (Becton Dickinson, Rutherford, NJ) may be used. This consists of a plastic reservoir prefilled with a calibrated volume of diluent. A capillary tube extends into the reservoir and is used to collect blood directly from a fingerstick or heelstick. The blood is drawn into the reservoir and mixed, accomplishing the desired dilution. Mixed diluted blood is dispensed either from the diluting pipette or from the Unopette onto the counting chamber.

A number of common potential problems tend to make manual cell counting inherently inaccurate. These include poorly calibrated diluting pipettes, inadequate mixing of the cell suspension in the diluting pipette, and uneven filling of the counting chamber. To partially compensate for this, the counts are always done in duplicate, utilizing both sides of the counting chamber and averaging the results.

Red blood cell counting

The reference method for red blood cell enumeration involves the use of a diluting red cell pipette and the microscopic enumeration of erythrocytes in a hemocytometer loaded with a 1:200 dilution of blood in an isotonic diluting fluid. The number of cells counted within designated red cell areas of the hemocytometer (five center boxes each consisting of 16 small squares) is multiplied by the dilution factor as well as a constant that reflects the volume of the chamber and the percentage of that volume actually counted (0.02 mm^3). The result is expressed in numbers per μl. Thus, if 500 cells were counted, then the number of red cells per μl would be:

$$500/0.02 \times 200 = 5,000,000/\text{mm}^3$$

The method has two major limitations, namely, variation in the dilution between specimens and the relatively small number of cells actually counted. Both serve to magnify errors because of the large multiplication factors used in the final arithmetic conversions. A coefficient of variation (CV) of ±5% to 10% is common in routine clinical practice.

White blood cell counting

The principles of white blood cell counting are similar to those for red cells with two exceptions. First, the diluting fluid used lyses red cells so that they do not obscure the leukocytes. A 2% solution of acetic acid is frequently used. Second, the dilution factor of the white cell pipette is 1:20. The four large outer boxes of the hemocytometer are used for a total volume counted of 4 × 1 mm^2 × 0.1 mm = 0.4 mm^3. Thus, if 100 cells are counted, then the total white blood cell (WBC) count would be:

$$100/0.4 \times 20 = 5,000/\text{mm}^3 \text{ or number counted} \times 50 = \text{cells}/\text{mm}^3$$

When counting body fluids that appear relatively clear, it is customary not to use a diluting pipette. In that case the fluid is loaded directly onto the hemocytometer and the dilution factor is not used in the calculations.

Platelet counting

Anticoagulated whole blood is diluted 1:200 in a 1% solution of ammonium oxalate, using a calibrated red cell pipette. Following a prescribed period of rotation, during which the platelets are evenly suspended, clumps are dispersed and red blood cells (RBCs) are lysed, the counting chamber of an improved Neubauer hemocytometer is filled with the suspension. The hemocytometer is divided into two mirror images; each half is filled using suspensions created with individual pipettes. Parallel counting of these chambers improves precision. The platelets are allowed to sediment for 15 minutes in a humidified chamber. Both debris and platelets may be refractile under phase microscopy, but only the latter have an internal granular structure. Platelets are counted in the large central square of the hemocytometer, which is composed of 25 subdivisions and 400 still smaller total squares. Generally, a minimum of 100 platelets are counted. Each counted square contains 1/250 μl. By averaging the number of platelets counted per small square and multiplying this figure to adjust for dilution ($\times 200$) and sampling volume counted ($\times 250$), the platelet count per μl is obtained. As an example, if 300 platelets were counted in the two central squares (each 1 mm × 1 mm) of both sides of the hemocytometer, then the count would be:

$$300/0.2 \times 200 = 300,000/\text{mm}^3 \text{ or number counted} \times 1000 = \text{cells}/\text{mm}^3$$

The CV of this technique exceeds 10% at physiological levels and is greater in the thrombocytopenic patient. Structural features such as platelet size and clumping are assessed by examining a Wright-stained blood film.

A numerical platelet estimate can be determined by examining ten oil immersion ($\times 1000$) fields of a Wright-stained peripheral blood smear and averaging the number of platelets per field. This number is then multiplied by 20,000 to give the estimated platelet count. Care should be taken to ensure that the platelets are evenly distributed on the smear, which is best accomplished by using freshly drawn anticoagulated blood.

AUTOMATION IN HEMATOLOGY

The ability to count, size, and classify cells is common to all state-of-the-art hematology analyzers. Available instruments use different analytical technologies to perform complete blood counts (CBC) and leukocyte differentials. The basic complete blood count is performed either by measurement of electrical impedance or by measurement of light scatter (Table 59-1). These methods provide the conventional RBC, WBC and platelet count, RBC indices, and new parameters such as the platelet distribution width (PDW) and hemoglobin distribution width (HDW), which are just beginning to find acceptance in clinical management.

Leukocyte differentials are performed by a variety of procedures, including selective cell lysis and sizing by impedance measurement, and flow cytometry employing histochemical, light scatter, depolarization and/or absorption technologies.

Table 59-1   Major automated hematology instruments

Manufacturer model	Analytical principles	Parameters					
		No.	DIFF	IM WBC	Flags	Hist/Cyt	Miscellaneous
COULTER							
T540	EI/CyM	7	2	–	+	– / –	Platelet count
T660	EI/CyM	8	2	–	+	– / –	
T890	EI/CyM	10	2	–	+	– / –	
JT(2)	EI/CyM	16	3	–	+	+ / –	QC program
JT3	EI/CyM	18	3	–	+	+ / –	
JS	EI/CyM	18	3	–	+	+ / –	5PT elec. diff
ST	EI/CyM	18	3	–	+	+ / –	Expanded DP
STKR	EI/CyM	18	3	–	+	+ / –	
STKS	EI/CyM/VCS	20	5	+	+	+ / +	Full featured
SERONO-BAKER							
130 SERIES	EI/CyM	3	–	–	–	– / –	
150 SERIES	EI/CyM	5	–	–	–	– / –	
170 SERIES	EI/CyM	7	–	–	–	– / –	
SYSTEM 8000	EI/CyM	8	–	–	+	+ / –	Platelet count
SYSTEM 9000	EI/CyM	8	–	–	+	+ / –	QC program
SYSTEM 9000Rx	EI/CyM	10	1	–	+	– / –	Expanded DP
SYST 9000Diff	EI/CyM	18	3	–	+	+ / –	
SYSTEM 9000Ax	EI/CyM	18	3	–	+	+ / –	
ABBOTT DIAGNOSTICS							
CELL-DYN400	EI/CyM	4	–	–	–	– / –	Hematocrit
CELL-DYN500	EI/CyM	5	–	–	–	– / –	Mean corpuscular volume
CELL-DYN610	EI/CyM	10	2	–	+	+ / –	Platelet count
CELL-DYN700	EI/CyM	7	–	–	+	– / –	
CELL-DYN900	EI/CyM	9	–	–	+	– / –	
CELL-DYN1500	EI/CyM	16	3	–	+	+ / –	QC, CRT
CELL-DYN1600	EI/CyM	16	3	–	+	+ / –	5PT elec. diff
CELL-DYN2000	EI/CyM	16	3	–	+	+ / –	
CELL-DYN3000	EI/CyM/MAPS	22	5	+	+	+ / +	Full featured
TOA (SYSMEX)							
F-300	EI/CyM	3	–	–	–	– / –	WBC, RBC, HGB
F-500	EI/CyM	5	–	–	–	– / –	
F-800	EI/CyM	15	3	–	+	+ / –	Platelet count
K-1000	EI/CyM	18	3	–	+	+ / –	
M-2000	EI/CyM	18	3	–	+	+ / –	QC program
E-2500	EI/CyM	18	3	–	+	+ / –	Data terminal
E-5000	EI/CyM/HF	18	3	–	+	+ / –	Expanded DP
NE-5500	RF-DC/CyM/HF	23	5	+	+	+ / +	
NE-8000	RF-DC/CyM/HF	23	5	+	+	+ / +	Full featured
TECHNICON							
H*1	CyM/HF/HS/S	23	5	+	+	+ / +	Full featured

*Manufacturer's instruments are ranked in ascending order of complexity. Each machine incorporates all of the features of the one above it.

No., parameters reported; Diff, variety WBC detected; IM WBC, detects blasts or immature WBC; Flags, abnormal cells; Hist/Cyt, histograms/cytograms; EI, electronic impedance; CyM, cyanmethemoglobin; QC, quality control; VCS, volume, conductivity, scatter; DP, data package; MAPS, multiple angle polarized scatter; HF, hydrodynamic focusing; RF-DC, radio frequency-direct current; HS, histochemical staining; S, laser light scatter.

Electronic aperture-impedance instruments

The Coulter principle patented by Wallace Coulter in 1956 uses low frequency electrical impedance measurements to count and size RBCs, and WBCs, and platelets. Cells that are conceptualized as packets of electrical insulating material are passed through an aperture immersed in a conducting solution (Fig. 59-1). The cell is a poor conductor compared to the diluent that it displaces and causes a measurable change in resistance passing through the aperture.

Each cell passage momentarily increases the impedance, causing a change in the voltage across the electrodes of the aperture. Each impulse is recorded as a single event (Fig. 59-2A). The number of impulses recorded is equal to the cell count per volume of blood analyzed. Computer editing of the pulses corrects for coincidence counting, that is, counting more than one cell at a time that simultaneously pass the aperture. The magnitude of the change in impedance (pulse height) is proportional to the volume of the cell,

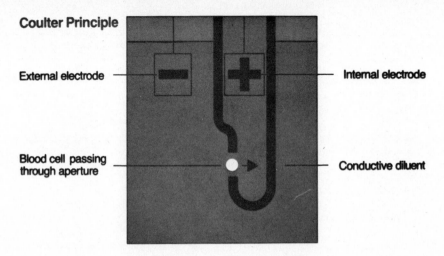

Coulter Principle

External electrode

Internal electrode

Blood cell passing through aperture

Conductive diluent

Fig. 59-1 Schematic illustration of the aperture-impedance principle of Coulter. *Courtesy of Coulter Electronics, Hialeah, Fla.*

namely, a given volume displaces an equal volume of conducting diluent, which allows for the measurement of cell size as well as number. As for coincidence counting, algorithmic compensations are made for those cells that pass near the electrically dense edge of the aperture, causing distorted volume measurements. Onboard computers tally the number of cells processed in separate RBC/platelet and WBC channels. The size and frequency data are combined to construct histograms for these elements (Fig. 59-2B), and from these, RBC and platelet indices are derived. In those instruments capable of performing platelet counts on whole blood samples, the red cell/platelet aperture which is 50 μm in diameter, recognizes pulses greater than 36 μm^3 as RBCs and smaller pulses as platelets. In the leukocyte channel, which is 100 μm in diameter, any pulse greater than 45 μm^3 is tallied as a WBC.

Recently, high frequency electromagnetic energy (RF) has been used to measure the conductivity of cells. The cell walls act as conductors, passing it into and through the cell. Specific alterations in the RF pattern relate the unique chemical, nuclear, and cytoplasmic composition of different cell types. This technology has been combined with those of low frequency impedance and/or light scatter to enable the newest analyzers to better define white cell populations. The clinical utility of this approach will be discussed in the section on white cell analysis.

Light scatter instruments

Modern flow cytometers, typified by the Technicon H*1 system and its predecessors the D90 and H6000, utilize conventional tungsten-halogen light sources as well as laser optics to measure light scatter and absorbance of RBCs, WBCs, and platelets (Fig. 59-3). Blood is hydrodynamically focused by sheathing rapidly moving columns of cells in a manner that causes them to pass in single-file fashion through optical detectors. The individual cell interrupts the

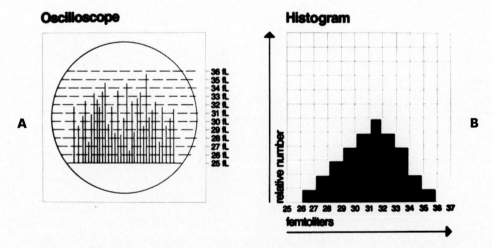

Oscilloscope

Histogram

A

36 fL
35 fL
34 fL
33 fL
32 fL
31 fL
30 fL
29 fL
28 fL
27 fL
26 fL
25 fL

relative number

25 26 27 28 29 30 31 32 33 34 35 36 37
femtoliters

B

Fig. 59-2 **A,** Representation of oscilloscope display (Coulter Instrument) demonstrating cell size measured by multichannel pulse height analysis. **B,** Cell size-frequency histogram derived from data displayed in Fig. 59-2A. *Courtesy of Coulter Electronics, Hialeah, Fla.*

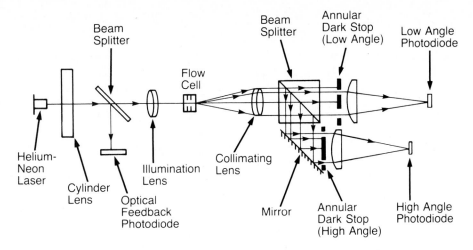

Fig. 59-3 Schematic diagram of optics bench of the Technicon H*1 analyzer. The low and high angle scatter detectors are emphasized. *Published with the permission of Technicon Instruments Corporation, Tarrytown, NY.*

light path and each interruption is noted and accumulated by sensors coupled to a computer system. The detectors enumerate the passing cells and simultaneously record the degree of light scatter and absorbance caused by the cell. These latter measurements are used for size and structure determinations. According to the Mei theory, the degree or angle of light scatter is proportional to the size of the disruptive particle or cell. This information is linked by onboard computers with the cell enumeration data to produce cell size frequency histograms similar to those of the impedance instruments, and similar parameters are derived from these histograms. In this system RBCs and platelets are simultaneously analyzed in one channel by careful selection of size thresholds for each cell type. Unlike manual methods, however, the presence of large platelets or microcytic RBCs causes spurious results. Figure 59-4 illustrates these principles for red cells.

The use of histochemical reagents to stain WBCs allows the flow cytometer to analyze the differential light absorbance of various subpopulations and produce a histochemical leukocyte differential. The machinations of the light-based instruments, as well as the laser technology employed to further define red cell populations, is addressed in the specific sections dealing with the various cell types. Table 59-1 lists the currently available automated instruments along with their predominate technology (aperture-impedance or light scatter) and specific features.

Advantages of automation

Analytic superiority and efficiency are the major benefits afforded by automated blood cell analyzers. Accuracy is improved by elimination of observer subjectivity, and precision is enhanced because of the large number of cells analyzed. Rumke's axiom defines precision as being inversely related to the number of cells analyzed. When few cells are counted, as is the case with manual methods, the chance of not locating cells present in low incidence is very great. This creates a large margin of error in duplicate tests performed by a single observer and even greater imprecision

between analyses performed by different observers. Automated cell analyzers process thousands of cells for each specimen, an impossible task for a human observer. Therefore, even low-incidence populations of cells are well represented in the total survey, greatly increasing precision and accuracy.

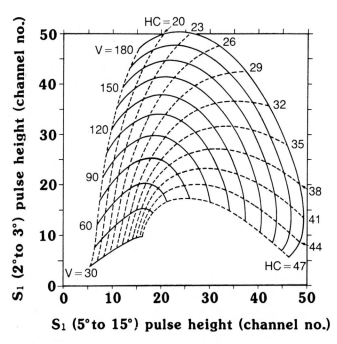

Fig. 59-4 Illustration of the Mei principle, whereby low angle scatter is plotted against high angle scatter to provide information concerning a cell's volume and refractive index or hemoglobin concentration. The solid lines represent constant volume, whereas the dashed lines reflect constant hemoglobin concentration. The precise location of a single cell on this cytogram defines its volume and hemoglobin concentration. *Published with the permission of Technicon Instruments Corporation, Tarrytown, NY.*

There are important clinical benefits to these increased analytical capabilities. For example, when following patients whose hematologic parameters are expected to change as a result of treatment or disease, it is important to be able to distinguish between physiologic changes and those caused by analytic imprecision. If one follows the course of eosinophilia in a patient in whom the coefficient of variation (CV) of the microscopic eosinophil count is 25%, any number between 15% and 25% represents a true eosinophil count of 20%. A change from 25% to 15% over the course of several days might indicate improvement or merely analytic variation. If the CV of the measurement is reduced to 5%, then the true eosinophil count of 20% varies between 19 to 21, and a change from 25% to 15% is definitely ascribed to a change in clinical status rather than analytical variation. Similar examples can be advanced for platelet counts, total leukocyte counts, and hemoglobin determinations. In summary, the high degree of precision made possible by automated methods allows more accurate serial tracking of patients.

An additional advantage of automation not to be overlooked is the ability to perform multiple analyses on very small aliquots of blood. The newer hematology analyzers use only 0.1 ml of blood for complete CBC and leukocyte differential analysis, minimizing the iatrogenic blood loss so common in hospitalized patients. The positive impact this has on the care of critically ill neonates is particularly important.

Disadvantages of automation

Because the operator of an automated instrument doesn't actually see what is being measured, the results generated occasionally represent artifact rather than truth. Examples include the spuriously high mean corpuscular volume (MCV) and low hematocrit generated on specimens with cold agglutinins, or the spurious thrombocytopenia seen in conjunction with ethylenediaminetetraacetic acid (EDTA)-mediated platelet clumping. For this reason, all data generated on automated instruments must be checked for internal consistency. For example, the hemoglobin should be three times the RBC count and the hematocrit should be three times the hemoglobin. Exceptions to internal consistencies must be validated by independent means. Other checks to be made include peripheral smear validation of low platelet counts generated automatically. Careful examination of the cell histograms displayed by advanced modern instruments can alert the operator to artifacts leading to spurious results. Finally, one must be aware that the methods used in automation do not mimic those employed in manual techniques. As the tools of measurement are entirely different, the results rarely are too. For this reason, despite the known correlation of automated methods with reference techniques, a periodic correlation of results is appropriate, especially when new results appear strange.

RED BLOOD CELL COUNTING AND MEASUREMENTS
Hemoglobin concentration

The RBC count, hemoglobin, hematocrit, and indices are most commonly evaluated to screen for anemia, polycythemic states, and to follow the course of patients who are bleeding, hemolyzing, or who require RBC transfusions. The most accurate of these measures, hemoglobin concentration, involves red cell lysis and conversion of the liberated hemoglobin to cyanmethemoglobin, which is spectrophotometerically measured at 540 nm. Conversion of hemoglobin requires a primary reaction with ferricyanide to form methemoglobin, and a subsequent reaction with cyanide to produce cyanmethemoglobin. The manual method has been modified and adapted for use as a dedicated channel in all automated hematology analyzers as well as stand alone hemoglobinometers.

Hematocrit determination

The packed cell volume (PCV) or hematocrit is determined by measuring the percentage of a whole blood column occupied by its red cell mass after the latter has been packed by centrifuging the blood. Centrifugation can be performed in either a long tube (Wintrobe method) or a small capillary tube (microhematocrit method). The determination is easily performed without expensive instrumentation. It is suitable for clinical areas that are remotely located from the hospital laboratory, such as surgical operating suites, emergency rooms, and intensive care units. The microhematocrit measurement is made by filling the small-bore capillary tube with blood and centrifuging at 8000 g for 5 minutes. Inaccuracies result from either careless reading of the RBC: whole blood column ratio or from inconsistent plasma trapping among oddly shaped red cells (e.g., sickle-cell anemia). The plasma trapping may cause the microhematocrit reading to vary from that obtained by automated analyzers by 2% to 3% in normal individuals to as much as 6% in patients with sickle-cell anemia. Newer microhematocrit centrifuges can process microhematocrit tubes in only 1 minute and employ built-in digital readers to maximize reading accuracy.

Most hematocrits are obtained from automated hematology analyzers. These are derived, not measured values, obtained as the product of the directly measured red cell count and the RBC mean corpuscular volume. Although highly reproducible for a given sample, inaccuracies are common because of possible incorrect measurement of the MCV and/or RBC count, which frequently occurs in the presence of RBC cold agglutinins.

Red blood cell count

Most RBC counts are performed using automated analyzers that enumerate the RBC count using light scatter or aperture impedance technology. The replicate error is less than 3%, but is also subject to artifacts. Three distinct phenomena cause spurious red cell counts:

1. Red cell agglutination in the sample tube, most commonly as a result of cold agglutinins, cause many red cells to be counted as doublets, thus spuriously lowering the actual red cell count.
2. Lymphocytosis can artifactually raise the RBC count when present in sufficient numbers to comprise a significant percentage of the total red cell count (e.g., >5%). This may occur in chronic lymphocytic leukemia, a condition frequently typified by marked elevations of small lymphocytes and a corresponding anemia, with its attendant reduction of the RBC

count. In this case the small lymphocytes are counted in the red cell channel and are added to the total red cell count.

3. Red cell fragmentation can occur in microangiopathic hemolytic anemia, sickle-cell anemia, and in association with malfunctioning cardiac prosthetic valves. The small fragments fall below the threshold for the red cell channel and are therefore excluded from the automated RBC count.

Red blood cell indices

In the late 1800s morphologists described the relationship between red cell size and various clinical syndromes. Smaller than normal cells (microcytes) were reported to be seen in chlorosis (iron deficiency), and larger than normal cells (macrocytes) were described in association with pernicious anemia. The first detailed delineations of red cell diameters in health and disease were made by Price-Jones and were reported in a monograph in 1933. His meticulous method involved projecting cells from a stained blood film onto paper and measuring the maximum and minimum diameters of 500 or 1000 cells that had been outlined with pencil. A cell diameter frequency histogram could be constructed, termed a Price-Jones curve, that was somewhat specific for various disease states of erythrocytes. Although judged highly accurate, the method was too laborious for routine use. Price-Jones curves enjoyed a brief period of popularity when dedicated pattern recognition-based hematology instruments, which analyzed individual blood cells microscopically and categorized them using computer-aided artificial intelligence, were sold in the United States. Accurate measurements of red cell diameters and Price-Jones curve generation was readily provided by these now no longer manufactured instruments which are no longer manufactured.

In 1929 Wintrobe introduced the terms mean corpuscular volume (MCV), mean corpuscular hemoglobin (MCH), and mean corpuscular hemoglobin concentration (MCHC), and described their method of calculation. Table 59-2 defines these parameters, called the red cell indices. These indices have found widespread clinical utility as adjuncts in the diagnosis of various red cell disorders.

The classical Wintrobe indices address cell size by calculating mean volume and hemoglobin content. Variations in cell size have also been found to correlate with specific hematologic syndromes. Although variation in cell size, anisocytosis, can be appreciated by examination of the stained blood film, quantitation of cell size variability by this method is imprecise because of the subjectivity of the observer and the nonrandom distribution of cells that occur on a blood film. Price-Jones attempted to quantitate anisocytosis by calculating the coefficient of variation (CV) of the Price-Jones cell diameter curve. Although reproducible, this determination is subject to the same difficulties inherent in generating the curve. In the 1960s and 1970s different groups led by Brecher, England, and Bessman described the measurement of anisocytosis by defining the CV of red cell volume distribution curves. The term *RDW* (red cell distribution width) was popularized by Bessman, who conducted clinical studies that defined the utility of this new parameter. The RDW is now generated by all state-of-the-art hematology analyzers, albeit using different technologies. It can be used as a substitute for peripheral blood smear assessment of anisocytosis when available.

The use of laser optics to measure high angle and low angle light scatter of red cells led to the development of techniques for measuring the hemoglobin content of individual cells. In the H*1, manufactured by Technicon Instruments, a hemoglobin concentration distribution curve can be developed that serves as the source for the newest red cell parameter, the hemoglobin distribution width (HDW). Technical and clinical details of all of these parameters will now be discussed.

Mean corpuscular volume

The delineation of average RBC size provides clinical information regarding differential diagnosis. Armed with this knowledge, the physician can limit his or her deliberations to diagnoses categorized by small, normal, or large red cell populations.

The original measurement of mean corpuscular volume (MCV) was derived using the formula devised by Wintrobe (Table 59-2). Wide scale use of automated analyzers now makes direct measurement of the MCV routine. In the electrical impedance method, each cell is subjected to a shear force as it is projected through the aperture. The shear elongates RBCs into an ellipsoid shape. The almost uniform shape change response of fresh red cells minimizes the potential variation in electrical effects due to differences in their initial shapes, whereas diluting the blood with an isotonic medium eliminates variations in the conductivity of the individual's plasma. These two critical components of the sizing method allow consistent measurements of different specimens.

Table 59-2   Calculation of red cell indices*

Parameter	Definition	Calculation	Example
MCV (fl)	Average volume of a red cell in a given sample	$\dfrac{\text{PCV (Hct)} \times 1000}{\text{RBC count} \times 10^{12}/\text{L}}$	$\dfrac{0.45 \times 1000}{5.0} = 90$
MCH (pg)	Average weight of Hgb per red cell in a sample	$\dfrac{\text{Hgb (g/dL)} \times 10}{\text{RBC} \times 10^{12}/\text{L}}$	$\dfrac{15 \text{ g/dL} \times 10}{5.0} = 33$
MCHC (g/dl)	Average Hgb concentration of all red cells in a sample	$\dfrac{\text{Hgb (g/dL)}}{\text{PCV (Hct)}}$	$\dfrac{15 \text{ g/dL}}{0.45} = 33$

*MCV, mean corpuscular volume; PCV, packed cell volume; RBC, red blood cell, MCH, mean corpuscular hemoglobin; hgb, hemoglobin; MCHC, mean corpuscular hemoglobin concentration.

As previously discussed, Coulter predicted that particle volume was proportional to impulse size in volts as derived from the following equation:

$$\text{Particle volume} = \frac{(\text{aperture area})^2 \times \text{particle impulse}}{\text{medium resistivity} \times \text{applied current}}$$

Several caveats pertain to this formula. First, because changes in the cross-sectional area of the orifice exert such a large effect on the result of the equation, it is crucial to ensure that the aperture orifice remain free of blockages. Even small obstructions become magnified as increases in impulse size with subsequent spurious increases in particle volume. Current instruments deal with this problem by employing three separate apertures that can be monitored independently by the operator. Should one orifice become blocked, the results generated by that subsystem will differ markedly from those generated by the other two. Careful monitoring of the congruity of these results can be utilized as a prime aspect of quality control of these instruments.

The second caveat relates to cell shape. Although most deformable cells assume the shear stream-induced ellipsoid shape, some do not. This can lead to disparities in size since the impulse generated by the cell passing though the orifice is measured along its diameter. If the expected shape change does not take place, the diameter measured will not be directly related to actual cell volume. Accordingly, in disorders such as sickle-cell anemia, in which substantial numbers of nondeformable, irreversible, sickled cells exist, the measured MCV may be inaccurate.

Despite these caveats, it is apparent that the MCV measurement produced by the aperture impedance instruments is generally quite accurate and certainly more precise than the calculated MCV derived from spun hematocrits and red cell counts. Spuriously high microhematocrit results occur when red cells are unable to properly sediment. Abnormalities in red cell shape cause this phenomenon, which results in increased trapping of plasma within the matrix of poorly packed red cells. The measured column of packed red cells is greater and the resulting hematocrit is falsely elevated. Sickle-cell anemia and various echinocytic disorders exemplify conditions associated with increased plasma trapping. For the most part, the electronically measured MCV is more reliable in these conditions.

The MCV is measured differently by the most modern light scattering instruments. The Technicon H*1 measures the low angle (forward) light scatter from a helium-neon laser source to assess cell volume. The amount of light scattered by a cell illuminated by the laser at low angle (0° to 5°) is related to its volume. In addition, the H*1 employs the measurement of high angle (5° to 15°) to measure the refractive index of each cell (Fig. 59-4). The refractive index of a red cell is a function of its hemoglobin concentration, therefore, the accumulated measurements of refractive index on 5000 to 10,000 red cells allows the direct computation of the cellular hemoglobin concentration mean (CHCM).

The property of light scattering by a particle at low and high angles was described by Mei. It can be appreciated that both cell volume and hemoglobin concentration can be plotted for each red cell on this scattergram, and that com-

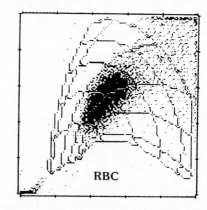

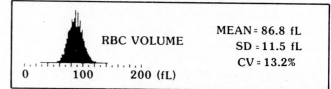

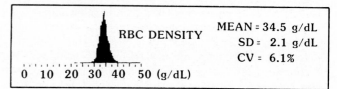

Fig. 59-5 Normal red cell cytogram displayed by the H*1 system. Red cell volume and hemoglobin concentration histograms are derived from the cytogram. *Published with the permission of Technicon Instruments Corporation, Tarrytown, NY.*

puter-generated histograms for both cell volume and hemoglobin concentration can be drawn (Fig. 59-5).

The Mei light scattering theory just referred to predicts cell size and refractive index for geometric spheres. Accordingly, in the Technicon system, the red cells are all isovolumetrically sphered by a reagent containing sodium dodecylsulfate in phosphate buffered saline (PBS). The cells are then fixed with 0.1% glutaraldehyde. The fixation ensures that the spherical shape of the red cell is not altered by the shear forces applied to the stream of red cells being shot through the analytic flow cell.

The clinical advantage of this system is that it minimizes the previously mentioned effect of red cell shape and deformability on cell size determination because all cells presented to the laser are spheres. In addition, because cell deformability is primarily determined by the cytoplasmic viscosity, which, in turn, is a function of hemoglobin concentration, these variables are essentially eliminated by the isovolumetric nature of the cell-sphering process. This adds to improved accuracy of the MCV determination.

This system is also not foolproof. Experimental evidence indicates that irreversibly sickled cells are resistant to sphering, rendering the MCV measurements less than optimal with samples of sickle-cell blood. More critical is the effect of hydration on the cell. As red cells incubate over time in the collection tube, they are prone to changes in water content. This effects the hemoglobin concentration and indirectly affects the MCV. Using the current generation H*1, one can obtain different MCV values for the same specimen over time. Since samples may be analyzed anywhere from minutes to days following collection, widely disparate MCV measurements may be obtained for individual patients, which reflect neither physiologic nor pathophysiologic variation. This problem is being addressed by the manufacturer.

Red blood cell volume distribution width

Red blood cell volume distribution width (RDW) as measured by aperture-impedance or light scattering instruments are approximately symmetrical in normals. Anisocytosis or heterogeneity of red cell size is reflected by the width of the red cell volume distribution curve. The wider the curve, the greater the degree of anisocytosis. The width of the curve is expressed mathematically as the standard deviation (SD) of the mean. However, use of the SD alone may give a false impression of the degree of red cell heterogeneity because a given SD may be normal or abnormal depending upon the MCV. As an example, in a normal subject with an MCV of 80, the SD may be 10. In a subject with severe iron deficiency, the MCV might be 65, yet the SD might also be 10. To best describe anisocytosis mathematically, then, the SD must be normalized for the MCV. The SD is normalized as the coefficient of variation (CV) of red cell size, termed RDW for red cell distribution width. The formula for RDW is:

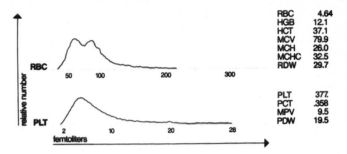

Fig. 59-6   Red cell and platelet histograms from a Coulter Instrument demonstrating a dual red cell population in a patient being successfully treated for iron deficiency. Note the low MCV, high RDW, and double-peaked histogram. *Courtesy of Coulter Electronics, Hialeah, Fla.*

$$RDW(CV)\% = \frac{SD}{MCV} \times 100$$

In the previous example, the normal individual's RDW is 12.5, whereas the patient with iron deficiency has an RDW of 15.4, an abnormal value. In practice, there is no such thing as a low RDW. Increasingly high values for the RDW reflect greater degrees of anisocytosis.

Elevations of the RDW may reflect either a general increase in cell size heterogeneity, as found in iron deficiency, or the presence of two or more discrete cell populations. Examples of the latter are patients recovering from iron

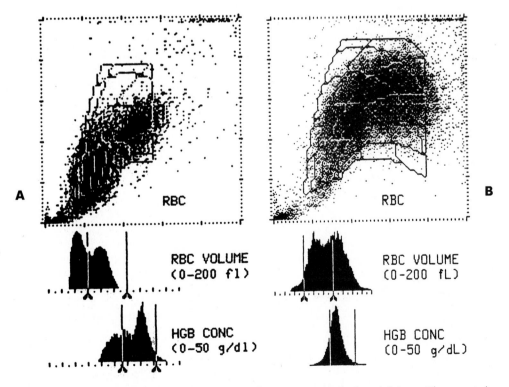

Fig. 59-7   **A,** H*1 display of a patient receiving adequate treatment for iron deficiency. The expected dual cell population is easily appreciated. **B,** H*1 display of a patient being successfully treated for pernicious anemia. Again, a dual cell population is displayed, but is shifted to the right, consistent with an increased MCV. *Published with the permission of Technicon Instruments Corporation, Tarrytown, NY.*

Table 59-3 Classification of anemias using automated indices

MCV Low		MCV High	
Normal RDW	High RDW	Normal RDW	High RDW
Heterozygous thalassemia	Iron deficiency	Aplastic anemia	Folate or B_{12} deficiency
Chronic disease	Sickle cell-thalassemia	Hypothyroidism	Autoimmune hemolysis
	Hemoglobin H		Sickle-cell disease
			Cold agglutinin
			Preleukemia

deficiency or pernicious anemia (Figs. 59-6 and 59-7). Actual examination of the red cell volume histogram is necessary to distinguish between these.

The clinical utility of the RDW becomes apparent when it is combined with the MCV. In general, nutritional anemias due to deficiency of iron, vitamin B_{12}, or folic acid have elevated RDW values. The hypoproliferative anemias not due to vitamin or mineral deficiencies tend to have normal RDW values.

Finally, the hemolytic anemias are inclined to show elevation of the RDW in proportion to the severity of the anemia. Narrowing of the diagnostic possibilities becomes possible when the MCV is either low or high because normal MCV anemias are too numerous to allow adequate discrimination with the RDW. A convenient classification of anemias can be adapted from the publications of Bessman and co-workers using the MCV and RDW (Table 59-3).

Mean corpuscular hemoglobin concentration

The mean corpuscular hemoglobin concentration (MCHC) is an index of the average density of the red cell population. It may be calculated using manual techniques and Wintrobe's formula, but it is most often automatically derived from the directly measured hemoglobin and calculated hematocrit. The clinical utility of the MCHC is somewhat limited inasmuch as there are few disorders in which the value is abnormal. However, high MCHC values should alert the clinician to the possibility of spherocytosis.

Cellular hemoglobin concentration mean

In the Technicon H*1, the cellular hemoglobin concentration mean (CHCM) is calculated from the directly measured cellular hemoglobin distribution curve. This curve is analogous to the red cell volume distribution curve and is derived from the high angle scatter measurements of individual red cell refractive indices.

Hemoglobin distribution width

This new parameter, the hemoglobin distribution width (HDW), is analogous to the RDW but represents the CV of the hemoglobin concentration distribution curve generated by the Technicon H*1. Although not as widely studied as the RDW, elevated HDW values have been documented in sickle-cell anemia, thalassemia major, and spherocytosis.

Changes in the HDW have been seen in individual patients with sickle-cell anemia during vaso-occlusive crises.

Mean corpuscular hemoglobin

The mean corpuscular hemoglobin (MCH) has little value in the diagnosis of anemia. Its major importance is its utility in quality control programs. The MCH is the most stable red cell index for the RBCs of a given individual. Although the hemoglobin, leukocyte count, and platelet count may vary from day to day in sick patients, the MCH tends to stay constant. As such, the longitudinal tracking (delta check) of a constant MCH in a patient assures that one is dealing with the correct patient's laboratory results even if major changes in the other CBC parameters are evident.

Reticulocyte count

Reticulocytes are red cells that have been recently released from the bone marrow. They are identified structurally by their characteristic filamentous inclusions when stained with methylene blue or brilliant cresyl blue. The inclusions are precipitated ribosomal ribonucleic acid (RNA), which persists in red cells for up to 3 days following bone marrow release.

The conventional reticulocyte count is performed by examining 500 to 2000 supravitally stained red cells microscopically and calculating the percentage containing bluish-black filaments or dots. Since the normal lifespan of a red cell is approximately 120 days, and the normal lifespan of a reticulocyte in the peripheral circulation is 1 day in the absence of stress on erythropoiesis, it follows that the normal reticulocyte count should range between 0.8% and 1.2%.

A major problem is the high level of imprecision with the conventional reticulocyte count. Imprecision results because of the following: only a minute cohort of the total red cell population is counted, there is nonrandom distribution of reticulocytes in the blood film, and there is marked interobserver bias in identifying reticulocytes. This imprecision accounts for major discrepancies in the reticulocyte count performed on identical samples when performed by different observers and makes serial tracking of this parameter quite difficult.

Imprecision can be minimized by the use of automated techniques. Staining of red cells with fluorescent dyes such as acridine orange, auramine O, or pyronin Y allows precise enumeration of positively stained reticulocytes when fluorescent flow cytometers are used. Another new technique utilizes a routine hematology analyzer to calculate the ratio of the MCV of the neocyte fraction of blood, separated by density gradient techniques, and the whole blood sample. This MCV ratio is linearly correlated to the reticulocyte count and has a CV of less than 1%. Refinement of this or of the stained techniques on new generation hematology analyzers may eventually lead to a reticulocyte channel as part of the routine CBC.

As will be discussed, the reticulocyte count when calculated as a percentage of red cells must be corrected for anemia. A simple formula is:

$$\text{Corrected reticulocyte count} = \frac{\text{Patient hematocrit}}{\text{Normal hematocrit (45)}} \times \text{Reticulocytes \%}$$

Thus, a 2% observed reticulocyte count in a patient with a hematocrit of 25% translates to a corrected reticulocyte count of only 1.1%, a low value for such a degree of anemia.

PLATELET COUNTING AND SIZING

Historically, platelet counting was performed by phase microscopy. The technique is still used as a reference method, but has been supplanted in most routine laboratories by automated methods.

Instruments using electronic impedance employ measurements identical to those used in RBC analysis to count and size platelets. Early instruments manufactured by Coulter Electronics (Thrombocounter) used platelet-rich plasma (PRP) prepared from anticoagulated whole blood spun in a capillary tube using a dedicated centrifuge (Thrombofuge). The PRP was analyzed and a hematocrit conversion factor was employed to determine the final platelet count. Modern instruments enumerate platelets using whole blood with the same reagent channels and electronics used for red cells. Particles that are equal to or greater than 36 fl in volume are accepted as RBCs, whereas those measuring 2 to 20 fl are counted as platelets. Data are collected, digitized, and grouped into a 64-channel size distribution histogram. If the derived count equals or exceeds 2×10^4 platelets/μl, two minimum and one maximum data points are identified and a log normal curve is fitted to these data by least squares analysis. This curve is next analyzed for an acceptable distribution, namely, the curve is positive, the mode falls between 3 to 15 fl, and the platelet distribution width (described shortly) does not exceed 20. If the curve is found to fulfill these criteria, the counts from all three (and minimally, two apertures) are averaged, corrected to reflect concentration per microliter and reported (Fig. 59-8). If any of the criteria in the described algorithm are not met, the reported data are appropriately flagged.

Platelet counts are usually linear between 10,000 and one million/mm^3 so that confirmation of counts using the manual chamber method is rarely necessary. However, the initial evaluation of a low platelet count must include examination of a stained peripheral blood film to rule out platelet clumping and confirm that the platelet estimate agrees with the automated count. The reason for this precaution is that EDTA-induced platelet clumping within the CBC tube may cause a spuriously low count on the automated instruments. If platelet clumping is found on the smear, a fresh sample of blood may be obtained using sodium citrate as the anticoagulant and the sample is reanalyzed. The resulting platelet count is usually higher and reflects the true status of the patient. If no clumping is found on the smear, the machine count should be considered accurate and further numerical confirmation is unnecessary.

The mean platelet volume (MPV), a measure analogous to the RBC MCV, normally varies inversely with the total platelet count in an inverse curvilinear fashion (Fig. 59-9). As such, it is useful in the differential diagnosis of thrombocytopenia and in assessing bone marrow activity vis-á-vis platelet production. In the face of a falling platelet count, the MPV will rise as the bone marrow produces younger, and consequently, larger platelets. When the bone marrow is incapable of responding to the challenge of thrombocytopenia, platelets released by the megakaryocyte are small. This is reflected in an MPV that is inappropriately low for the given platelet count (Fig. 59-10A). In disorders of peripheral platelet destruction, such as idiopathic thrombocytopenic purpura (ITP), in which the bone marrow's capacity to produce new platelets is normal, the MPV will rise as the platelet count falls (Fig. 59-10B). The utility of the MPV in the diagnosis of thrombocytopenic disorders, based on the published clinical studies of Bessman, is illustrated (Table 59-4).

Because the MPV measurement is derived from the analysis of large numbers of platelets, it should be more accurate in assessing average platelet size than microscopic analysis based on examination of a few platelets. Unfortunately, MPV may vary by as much as $\pm25\%$ within the first 3 hours of venipuncture as a result of K_3EDTA-induced artifact. Since the artifact equally affects both small and large platelets, it remains valid to assume that an elevated MPV in the face of thrombocytopenia and otherwise normal CBC parameters strongly suggests active megakaryocytopoiesis. In the appropriate clinical setting, this information is sufficient to manage isolated thrombocytopenic disorders without the necessity of performing a bone marrow examination to document megakaryocyte activity.

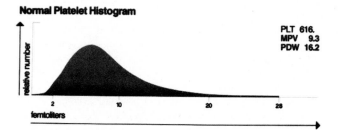

Fig. 59-8   The normal platelet histogram: A frequency analysis of 64 channels, grouping particles from 2 to 20 fl, is performed; the curve is smoothed and analyzed for confidence, as described. The MPV and PDW are derived from the curve. *Courtesy of Coulter Electronics, Hialeah, Fla.*

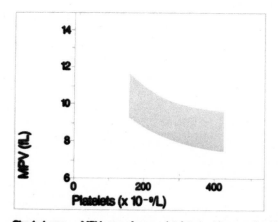

Fig. 59-9   The normal MPV nomogram: There is a predictable reciprocal relationship between an individual's physiological platelet count and the MPV. *Courtesy of Coulter Electronics, Hialeah, Fla.*

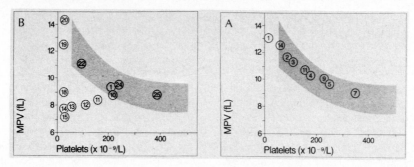

Fig. 59-10   A, The MPV in thrombocytopenia due to bone marrow suppression: Failure of the marrow to repopulate the peripheral circulation with platelets in a manner similar to immune thrombocytopenia creates a population of disproportionately small platelets and disturbs the normal reciprocal relationship between MPV and platelet count. Numbers within the shaded curve represent days of hospitalization. *Courtesy of Coulter Electronics, Hialeah, Fla.* **B,** The MPV in megakaryocytic thrombocytopenia: In the presence of normal bone marrow activity and thrombocytopenia such as immune thrombocytopenia, the predictable relationship between platelet count and MPV persists. *Courtesy of Coulter Electronics, Hialeah, Fla.*

The platelet distribution width (PDW), which is a measure comparable to the RBC RDW and reflects the coefficient of variation (%) of the platelet distribution, together with the MPV, are mathematically derived from the measured parameters as described for the RBC. There is insufficient clinical data to recommend specific use of the PDW.

Principles employed in the TOA Sysmex and the Unipath Cell-Dyn 3000 instruments to enumerate and size platelets are identical. TOA claims that their use of hydrodynamic focusing to maintain particles (RBC/platelets) in the middle of the detection aperture improves the accuracy of the sizing process. This point remains debatable.

The Technicon hematology analyzers assess platelets on the basis of the light scatter phenomenon. As is the case for the impedance system, a single detector is used to measure RBCs and platelets. The sensor employed in the hydrodynamically focused flow stream is a darkfield optical detector that monitors light from a red laser (632.8 nm) at low (2° to 3°) and high (5° to 15°) angle scatter. It is only the data derived from monitoring high angle scatter at low gain that relate to platelet size and counts, and in turn, that relate to the distribution histogram produced. The histogram is analyzed for confidence parameters (fit) similar to those described earlier, and is used to provide an MPV; a PDW is not produced. Precision, linearity, and accuracy of platelet analysis by this method compare favorably to all other systems.

Table 59-4   Use of the MPV in the diagnosis of thrombocytopenia

Low	Appropriate to count*	High
Aplastic anemia	ITP†	Bernard-Soulier
Chemotherapy	Eclampsia	May-Heglin
Megaloblastic anemia		
Hypersplenism		
Wiskott-Aldrich		

*MPV rises as platelet count falls.
†ITP, immune thrombocytopenia.

WHITE BLOOD CELL ANALYSIS AND THE LEUKOCYTE DIFFERENTIAL

White blood cells were historically quantified by light microscopy in a hemocytometer. This remains the reference method for total white cell enumeration. Using a calibrated WBC pipette, a 1:20 dilution of anticoagulated whole blood in 3% acetic acid is placed in both sides of the counting chamber. Following a brief period to allow for RBC lysis and WBC sedimentation, all of the cells in the four large corner squares of the chambers are counted and averaged. One large square represents a total volume of 0.1 μl, therefore, multiplying the average cell count per square by 10 to correct for number per microliter and 20 to adjust for initial dilution, the WBC count per microliter is obtained. The prevision (CV) of this technique varies between 6% and 9% within physiologic range.

The traditional qualitative evaluation of leukocytes in blood films is aided by use of panoptic stains that enhance and characterize diverse structural features of the formed elements. Giemsa stain, Wright's stain, or a combination of both are the most commonly used dyes. Based on clinical suspicion and the information provided by the initial stains, secondary special staining techniques may be used to accentuate certain structural features or to support a diagnosis. For example, the peroxidase stain reaction is used to stain eosinophils, neutrophils, basophils, monocytes, and Auer's rods.

Normal WBC counts are influenced by factors such as physical activity, stress, age, race, and sex. The normal WBC count in children varies from 5000 to 15,000 cells/μl, and in adults from 5000 to 10,000 cells/μl. The leukocyte differential also differs in different groups of individuals. Children's blood normally contains 0% to 2% basophils, 0% to 5% eosinophils, 25% to 75% neutrophils, 30% to 70% lymphocytes, and 0% to 8% monocytes. The percentage of neutrophils in the adult varies from 45% to 75% and lymphocytes range from 20% to 45%. Detection of subtle shifts in this type of distribution is therefore neither possible nor meaningful. It is rather the confirmation of a gross change, the establishment of a trend, or the detection of an abnormal population of cells that provides significant clinical data.

In addition to the physiological and disease influences that control the microscopic leukocyte differential, the precision and accuracy of the analysis is also subject to observer bias, the number of cells examined, the homogeneity of the preparation, and the fields examined. In multiple surveys the coefficient of variation obtained by quantifying different cell cohorts by the microscopic technique can exceed 100%. Furthermore, the ability to detect an abnormal population of cells in a random sampling of leukocytes approaches the 95% confidence level only when the population exceeds 3% of the total. The majority of these limitations are dispelled by use of automated differential WBC counting. In general, automated techniques survey ten times as many leukocytes as the microscopic procedure, making the precision of the automated technique more than three times that of the conventional procedure. The objectivity established by the various machine algorithms, the use of dynamic flow cytometry, and cross-checks such as the use of confidence curve analysis greatly improve the accuracy of most data generated by machine counts. Nevertheless, the use of special stains and structural verification of the data derived remain an essential element of the technologist's function.

Three different technologies for the performance of routine leukocyte differentials have been found to be clinically acceptable. The first of these, pattern recognition, is now of historical interest only because equipment is no longer commercially available, reflecting an inability to compete with the current technologies. The pattern recognition system most closely simulates the microscopic differential. A uniform thin blood film, created by centrifugal or mechanized smear technique, was stained with Wright's reagents and placed on a robotic stage, on which WBCs were individually examined using an oil immersion objective lens.

The derived information was digitized on the basis of individual and adjacent pixels and analyzed by a computer algorithm based on a Golay-type binary image processor. The resultant data relate to color, density, shape, and proportionality of components analogous to human vision. The system's advantages included the ability to count a greater number of WBCs per unit time, an objective analytical data base that increased precision and the potential to recognize cells with unique shape characteristics rather than individual cytochemical properties, such as the band neutrophil, blasts, nucleated red cells, and atypical lymphocytes. Unfortunately, the instrument lacked the minimal throughput volume required by most laboratories.

The Technicon Corporation (Tarrytown, NY) has pioneered the performance of leukocyte differentials by flow cytometry technique through several generations of analyzers. The principles employed in their current equipment, the H*1, will be discussed, but are largely applicable to their previous machines. This analyzer capitalizes on the differential staining of various WBCs with peroxidase reagents and an ability to maintain the cellular integrity of basophils, while stripping cytoplasm from other WBCs. By use of hydrodynamic focusing and detergent-mediated red cell lysis, WBCs are presented to various detectors on an individual basis and are so analyzed.

Peroxidase, an intracellular enzyme present in different concentrations in granulocytes and monocytes, together with hydrogen peroxide and an electron receptor chromogen and formaldehyde, will cause the formation and subsequent precipitation of a dark pigment within the cell.

The use of discriminatory electronic thresholds allows the optical distinction between eosinophils, other granulocytes, monocytes, and unstained cells such as lymphocytes, on the basis of their forward light scatter characteristics, which relate to relative cell size and their respective pattern of decreasing absorbance (Fig. 59-11A).

The cells are characterized and counted by channeling the information collected on each through photodiodes to computer logic circuits. Although these channels do not

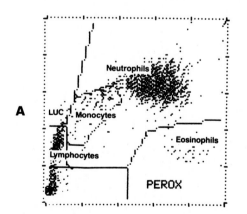
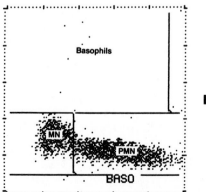

Fig. 59-11　**A,** The H*1 peroxidase channel: Particles are displayed in a scattergram depicting peroxidase content *(OD)* as a function of cell size *(scatter)*. Note, eosinophils appear to be smaller than neutrophils because of their intense absorbance characteristic. **B,** The H*1 basophil/lobularity index: Selective cell lysis, followed by two angle light scatter measurements allows for a scattergram display that quantifies basophils, determines a WBC nuclear lobularity index, and detects shifts in the latter distribution. Atypical lymphocytes, blast cells, are flagged by contrasting the data from the peroxidase channel with that from the basophil channel. *Published with the permission of Technicon Instruments Corporation, Tarrytown, NY.*

directly recognize atypical lymphocytes, nucleated red cells, and blast cells, the operator is alerted to the possibility of the presence of these abnormal elements by flags generated via analysis of the shape and spatial properties of cytograms, unusual features in histograms, or the relationship of data derived from both the peroxidase and basophil/lobularity channels to one another (Fig. 59-11B).

Under controlled conditions a mixture of phthalic acid and surfactant will induce the rupture and subsequent loss of cytoplasm by all WBCs except basophils. The H*1 system capitalizes on this observation by subjecting blood to both hemolysis and differential WBC lysis and analyzing the residual population of intact cells and naked nuclei by two-angle laser scatter. This provides signals that clearly quantify basophils, mononuclear leukocytes, and polymorphonuclear WBCs. In addition, a WBC lobularity index is produced that is used to produce flagging criteria for the possibility of a left-shifted differential, blast cells, atypical lymphocytes, and nucleated RBCs.

Preliminary studies suggest that the accuracy of this system compares favorably with that of the leukocyte differential obtained by the conventional microscopic and automated pattern recognition methods. Blast cells are detected and identified more consistently than with microscopy alone; however, this is accomplished at the expense of a higher rate of false-positive flags. It has also been observed that the degree of flagging and the subsequent review make the system less efficient for the analysis of samples from neonates.

The use of a flow cytometer in the Technicon system provides the laboratory with the capability of performing off-line analysis of lymphocyte subsets. Using peroxidase-conjugated monoclonal antibodies against specific surface markers, the H*1 can quantitate lymphocyte subtypes and produce histograms analogous to those provided by fluorescent activated cell analyzers.

The three-cell leukocyte differential count generated by electronic impedance principles has been widely popularized by Coulter Electronics (Hialeah, Fla), although other manufacturers' versions are available, such as the TOA E-5000 (Kobe, Japan). The relationship of signal height (amplitude) to cell volume derived from the changes in conductivity across an electrically charged orifice has been addressed. When these principles are applied to a blood specimen rendered free of RBCs by lysis, population histograms for various WBCs can be generated.

To enhance precision, total WBC counts are performed by three separate apertures for a period of 4 seconds. All particles generating an electronic pulse equal to or greater than 35 femtoliters (fl) are accepted as WBCs. After reconciling for agreement between the three apertures and data editing according to mathematical smoothing formulas that adjust for coincidence counting and abnormal path trajectories across the orifices, an absolute WBC count is calculated. The volume distribution of each cell is digitized into 256 size channels, from which a corresponding histogram is produced. The histogram is subsequently divided into three size categories: particles between 35 and 90 fl corresponding to lymphocytes, particles between 90 and 160 fl corresponding to mononuclear cells, and particles between 160 and 450 fl, representing granulocytes (Fig. 59-12). The volume distributions do not reflect the native volumes of these elements because of the use of proprietary lysing reagents prior to analysis, which collapse the cytoplasm around the cell nucleus and granules. By use of the relative percentage of these WBCs and the absolute count, their total numbers are derived.

Quantified within the lymphocyte area can be atypical lymphocytes and small variant WBCs; within the mononuclear area can be blast cells, other immature WBCs, and plasma cells; and within the granulocyte area can be band cells and metamyelocytes. A series of flags derived from abnormalities in the shape of the histogram alert the operator to the possibility of nucleated red cells, cell fragments, clumped platelets, atypical lymphocytes, blast cells, plasma cells, immature granulocytes, and relative abnormalities in the number of eosinophils and basophils present. The leukocyte differential based on volumetric distinction and interpretive reporting does not provide the traditional five-cell discrimination, but rather a three-cell differential with flagging capability for eosinophilia and basophilia.

The system has many proponents who have published data that underscore the contention that this degree of differentiation suffices for the vast majority of clinical needs. Evaluation of the system, ranging from tertiary care facilities and oncology services to community hospitals and emergency rooms, concludes that the three-part leukocyte differential combined with flagging criteria is an adequate substitute for the conventional microscopic analysis. When used in such settings, 60% to 85% of the manual leukocyte differentials can be eliminated without adverse clinical impact. However, competitive technology and the desire to remain

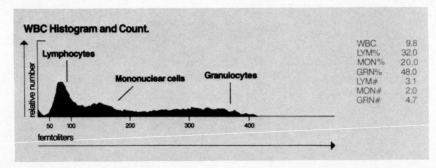

Fig. 59-12 The impedance three-cell leukocyte differential: Cell lysis and electronic sizing enumerates lymphocytes, monocytes, and granulocytes. Curve analysis allows increased numbers of eosinophils and basophils to be flagged. *Courtesy of Coulter Electronics, Hialeah, Fla.*

in the forefront of an emerging automation have provided additional methods for performing routine complete five-cell leukocyte differentials.

The Coulter VCS method (volume, conductivity, and light scatter) routinely analyzes 8000 WBCs per machine cycle. Unlike the method used in the systems based solely on impedance monitoring, the reagent systems employed with the VCS maintain the native integrity of the leukocyte throughout the analysis. Particles are simultaneously analyzed by: (1) the previously described electrical impedance technology, which provides cell volume data and readily discerns lymphocytes from mononuclear cells and granulocytes; (2) by high frequency electromagnetic probes that provide information about the internal composition of the cell, specifically the structure of its nucleus, granule content, and cytochemistry, thereby separating lymphocytes, monocytes, and granulocytes; and (3) by light scatter, whose pattern furnishes a profile of the surface and shape characteristics unique to all five subclasses of WBCs. The result is an integrated three-dimensional plot that effectively separates the five major WBC cohorts and many of their variants.

The system provides the operator with a variety of individual display screens in the form of scattergrams and histograms. It allows the isolation of distinct populations and presentation of data derived from one or all three of its analytical systems, and permits rotation of some screens, simulating the three-dimensional character of the data (Figs. 59-13A to D). Qualitative irregularities in the cell distribution will trigger one or more of seven flags that call attention to the possibility of abnormal cell types or artifacts such as blast cells, immature granulocytes, band neutrophils, atypical lymphocytes, and nucleated RBCs and platelet clumps. Preliminary studies suggest that the VCS's accuracy is equal to or exceeds that of the microscopic differential; its precision rivals that of the Technicon flow cytometry system, as does its ability to detect low incidence populations of abnormal cells. The VCS differential technology has been incorporated into the latest generation Coulter CBC analyzer, the STKS.

Baxter Healthcare Corporation (McGraw Park, Il) distributes the Sysmex NE-8000, manufactured by TOA Medical Electronics (Kobe, Japan), which shares features and technologies described for the Coulter VCS system. The major differences between the systems are as follows: TOA employs three specific WBC lysing reagents that selectively work on all WBCs, eosinophils, and basophils, respectively; only two detection methods are used to discriminate between

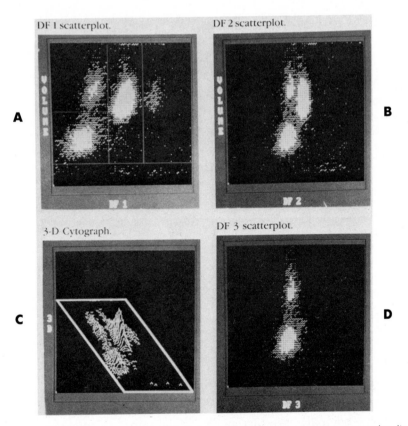

Fig. 59-13   **A,** The discriminant function (DF 1) of the VCS: Light scatter properties are used to distinguish and quantify lymphocytes, monocytes, eosinophils, and neutrophils. *Courtesy of Coulter Electronics, Hialeah, Fla.* **B,** The DF 2: Conductivity measurements distinguish lymphocytes, monocytes, and neutrophils. **C,** The three-dimensional cytograph: This image, which can be rotated, depicts all cell populations. **D,** The DF 3: This scattergram is identical to the DF 2 except for the absence of the neutrophil population; it displays lymphocytes, basophils, and monocytes.

the subsets of leukocytes, radiofrequency (conductivity), and impedance; cell scattergrams are generated in two dimensions rather than three. The initial two-dimensional scattergram (size/conductivity) provides for the division of leukocytes into lymphocytes, monocytes, and granulocytes. Eosinophils and basophils are quantified separately in individual detector blocks.

The unique abilities of the lyse reagents used in the eosinophil and basophil measurements to shrink all WBCs to a greater degree than the corresponding cell allow these cells to be discriminated on the basis of size alone. The neutrophil population is quantified by subtracting the eosinophils and basophils from the directly measured granulocyte number. The interpretive messages regarding abnormal WBC parameters are similar for all systems. We have evaluated the precision and accuracy of the leukocyte differentials of the H*1, STKS, and NE-8000 instruments as compared to 200 cell manual differentials. The instruments tend to be quite similar in their ability to correctly identify the various leukocyte cell types and flag abnormal white cell structure.

A recent entrant into the automated five-cell leukocyte differential arena is the Cell-Dyn 3000, distributed by Abbott Diagnostics (Mountain View, CA). The equipment differentiates among the various classes of leukocytes by the use of fixed angle measurements of polarized light scatter; a process that is referred to as multiple angle polarized (laser) scatter (MAPS). Prior to WBC analysis, the whole anticoagulated blood is mixed with a proprietary diluent that virtually renders the red cells transparent to the optical detectors at the angles employed. As in all flow cytometers, the WBCs are placed in a laminar flow stream and hydrodynamically focused to enable their analysis on a one at a time, single flow basis. A highly coherent polarized source of laser light is focused on the core of the sample stream. As WBCs enter the flow cell, the light is disrupted in all directions. The size and internal composition of each leukocyte determines the characteristic pattern of this disruption.

Four detectors are employed to measure the scattered light at critical angles, while direct laser light is gated from the system. Forward polarized light scatter measured between 1° to 3° varies with the size of the cell, whereas high angle light scatter measured at 3° to 10° correlates with the structure of the WBCs. When these parameters obtained from the photodiodes are plotted on the x and y axis of a scattergram, the various populations of leukocytes are readily discerned. In addition, it has been proven that the granules of eosinophils uniquely cause polarized orthogonal (90°) light to depolarize. Polarized light is measured by a photomultiplier that receives signals from a coverglass angled at 45°, whereas the 90° depolarized light is detected by an independent photomultiplier. These data are also presented in the form of a scattergram that clearly segregates the eosinophil from the rest of the leukocyte populations that appear as individual clusters in a fusiform continuum. By precise volumetric metering to the flow cell, an accurate total WBC count is derived, which allows the subpopulations of leukocytes to be reported as absolute and percentage figures. Flags, monitoring, and interpretive reports are similar in scope and capability to those described for the other automated five-cell leukocyte differential systems.

These superb technologies notwithstanding, it should be acknowledged that recent investigators have concluded that in the majority of clinical settings, the total leukocyte count without the differential provides as much clinical data regarding diagnosis, prognosis, therapeutic intervention, and disposition as the most accurate leukocyte differential. This lack of correlation is not believed to be a measure of poor analytical performance, but rather a reflection of the leukocyte differential's inherent limitations. Leukocyte differentials are best used in populations unable to mount a leukocytosis, such as in the neonate and geriatric patient; to detect specific hematological disease such as leukemia; and for the serial assessment of patients with known leukocyte abnormalities.

QUALITY CONTROL OF AUTOMATED HEMATOLOGY ANALYZERS

As with all methods in clinical laboratory medicine, the accuracy and precision of laboratory data generated by automated hematology analyzers must be verified periodically. We can define accuracy as the ability of an instrument to generate a correct answer (e.g., a correct platelet count or leukocyte differential). Accuracy is ensured by maintaining a properly calibrated instrument. Precision may be defined as the ability of the instrument to repeatedly provide an essentially identical result on a single sample or a single lot of a stable control media. Precision is best monitored by repetitive analysis of single samples or lots to determine stability of results. The two terms are intimately related as imprecision can clearly effect accuracy.

A comprehensive quality control program ensures that every result generated on patient samples is accurate. It begins by proper calibration of an instrument so that each parameter measured is done so accurately. A calibrant is measured repeatedly and the instrument is adjusted so that each parameter registers a reading identical to the known assay value of the commercial calibrant. Alternatively, fresh whole blood may be assayed repeatedly by reference methods to obtain a mean assay value and that same sample is used as a calibrant.

Once an instrument is properly calibrated, the goal is to ensure that it remains so. This is accomplished by repeat analysis of stable control material to ensure that the control values measured by the instrument remain stable. In practice, a broad range of control material is employed (low, normal, and high), reflecting the range of values one would encounter in patients in clinical practice. When a new lot of commercial reagent arrives at the laboratory, it is assayed 10 to 20 times to obtain the laboratory mean and standard deviation. An acceptable range, which usually is defined as two standard deviations around the mean, is then established for each level of control. The necessity for multiple analysis of the control material initially relates to the need to incorporate into the acceptable range the expected analytic variation that always occurs with automated instruments. Following this, the controls are assayed periodically, the minimum being once each shift of use. If the control values fall within the acceptable range, then the system (instruments and reagents) is considered to be functioning properly and patient samples may be run. If the control value is out of range, then some remedial action must be taken (e.g., check integrity of control or reagents, check operation or calibration of instrument). Patient samples should not be analyzed until a repeat analysis of the quality control reagent, following remedial action, falls within the acceptable range.

In order to conserve costs of commercial controls while still performing quality control (QC) often during the day (e.g., every hour), it is acceptable to perform replicate testing on a single patient sample or pooled ABO compatible sample throughout a given day. To utilize this method, the sample is analyzed ten times in the morning and an acceptable range is determined (mean ± 2 SD). This sample is then reanalyzed throughout that day as a QC sample, looking for drift.

This simplified scheme of quality control has many variations. It is recommended that QC data be plotted on a graph that includes the laboratory mean, ± 3 SD, of the hematologic parameter studied plotted on the y-axis and days of the month (1 to 31) plotted on the x-axis. The daily plotting of data on this Levy-Jennings chart gives clues as to trends toward imprecision. One may, for example, notice a daily progressive rise in the QC data despite the fact that each point falls within the acceptable range. This may be an early warning of instrument failure, reagent spoilage, or miscalibration.

An additional method of QC is available on some automated instruments. This employs the moving average method of Bull. A mean of a specific parameter from the previous 20 samples is displayed on a CRT as a point on a Levy-Jennings plot. Since patient means are relatively stable, one should not see drift during the day. Significant drift is a sign of problems. When a batch of known abnormal patient specimens are run, such as from an oncology ward, one or two points from the moving average table may have to be deleted.

The quality control of automated leukocyte differentials presents another problem vis-á-vis accuracy. As adequate calibrating and control materials are not available, it is necessary to correlate the automated differential with a reference method daily. One approach would be to prepare two or three peripheral blood smears from fresh samples each morning and perform a 200-cell manual differential on each slide in duplicate (preferably by two different observers). The averaged values of the manual differential should then be compared to the automated differential. If they agree within 10%, then the automated differential is deemed acceptable.

Another method of detecting a poorly functioning instrument employs the concept of delta checking. In this system, current patient results are compared to previous recent results from the same patient. Hematologically stable parameters such as the MCH should not change in a patient from day to day. If major changes are detected, this could signify either a problem with the system, or more commonly, a mislabeled specimen from a different patient. As long as one or more of these methods are employed constantly during the operation of automated systems, the accuracy of patient data can be ensured.

THE ERYTHROCYTE SEDIMENTATION RATE

The erythrocyte sedimentation rate (ESR) occupies a time-honored role in hematologic analysis as a screening test for various nonhematologic disease states. The test measures the rate of descent in millimeters/hour of a vertical column of blood within a tube of defined length. The Westergren tube, which is 30 cm long, is most commonly used. The rate of fall of red cells suspended in plasma depends primarily on their mass, in other words, the greater the red cell mass, the faster the rate of fall. When individual cells stack together to form rouleaux, the mass of the aggregate per unit of surface area is greater than that of each individual cell. This causes an increase in the rate of sedimentation. Anything that promotes rouleaux formation can thus be predicted to increase the ESR.

Red cells in suspension are kept apart by a dielectric cloud that surrounds each erythrocyte, termed the zeta potential. Negatively charged sialic acid residues on the cell membrane account for this cloud. Elevated levels of fibrinogen and/or plasma globulins can attenuate the zeta potential, leading to increased rouleaux formation and a subsequent elevation of the ESR.

Predictably, the ESR is elevated in those conditions typified by increases in plasma fibrinogen or gamma globulins. Since fibrinogen is an acute phase reactant, it and the ESR are elevated in most infectious, inflammatory, and generalized neoplastic diseases. In addition, the ESR is elevated in multiple myeloma and Waldenström's macroglobulinemia because of the increase in plasma globulins associated with these conditions.

The zeta sedimentation ratio (ZSR) is a modification of the ESR. It utilizes a specially designed centrifuge that subjects a column of blood in a capillary tube to four 45-second cycles of alternating compression and dispersion. The ultimate degree of red cell packing depends on the attenuation of the zeta potential of the red cells by fibrinogen and/or gamma globulin and is linearly related to these plasma proteins. A ratio is calculated relating the patient's hematocrit to the controlled red cell packing (zetacrit). The normal range is 40% to 51%, with levels over 60% considered significantly elevated. Although the technique is much faster than the ESR, has a similar range for men and women, and is not affected by anemia, it has not achieved widespread popularity because of the need for specialized equipment and the requirement for a simultaneous hematocrit determination on each specimen.

Because of its nonspecificity, the ESR is rarely used today as a diagnostic tool. It can, however, be useful as a tracking parameter for the serial observation of defined disease entities. Thus, changes in the ESR reflect disease activity in lupus erythematosus, rheumatoid arthritis, and multiple myeloma. Some physicians use the test as an objective means to assess the efficacy of therapeutic maneuvers or to screen for disease recurrence in patients thought to be in clinical remission. The sensitivity and specificity of the test, when used in this manner, has not been critically evaluated.

USE OF RADIOISOTOPES IN QUANTITATIVE HEMATOLOGY

Blood cells can be labeled with various radionuclides to allow measurement of their lifespan, distribution within the body, and total mass. A wide variety of tests can be performed that can measure hematopoiesis, ferrokinetics, granulocyte and platelet imaging, and bone marrow function. In practice, though, these tests are rarely performed because of their complexity and/or interpretive difficulties. We will focus the discussion on those nuclear medicine tests in common usage in diagnostic hematology.

Red blood cell survival test

In certain instances, the mechanism of anemia, in other words, decreased erythropoiesis, increased erythrocyte destruction, sequestration, or loss cannot be adequately determined from conventional hematologic studies. In such cases, the demonstration of a normal or reduced survival of autologous red cells within the circulation can differentiate among the potential mechanisms. By tagging red cells with a radioactive label that does not elute during the lifespan of the red cell, and by injecting an aliquet of these cells, one can calculate, based upon sequential studies of the fall off in radioactivity, the mean lifespan. One important caveat that allows accurate measurement of red cell survival is that no hemorrhage occur during the study. Should the patient be bleeding, then radioactivity will be lost from the circulation because of external loss, and inference regarding decreased survival can have no validity.

Chromium-51 (Cr-51) sodium chromate is most often used to tag the cells. This isotopic label binds to the beta chain of hemoglobin and is considered a random label inasmuch as cells of all ages are labeled. This is in contradistinction to a cohort or pulse label, which is taken up primarily by marrow precursor cells.

A 10-ml sample of the patient's blood is collected into acid-citrate-dextrose anticoagulant and is centrifuged to remove all plasma. The remaining cells are mixed with 0.5 μCi/kg of Cr-51 sodium chromate for 15 minutes, then washed twice to remove unbound isotope. Alternatively, in another method, ascorbic acid is added to reduce incubation time and ensure proper removal of unbound label. The labeled cells are then resuspended to the original 10-ml volume using isotonic saline. A carefully measured portion of the cells is then injected into the patient and allowed to equilibrate. A 5-ml sample is then drawn at the following times for gamma counting: 10 minutes, 60 minutes, 24 hours, and every other day for 3 weeks. Each sample is subjected to a hematocrit check to ensure a steady state (i.e., no blood loss), and 2-ml aliquots are saved at 4° C until the end of the study for counting. The count for each sample is divided by its own hematocrit and the resulting corrected counts in counts per minute (cpm) are plotted on semi-logarithmic paper (or calculated for the first exponential by least squares fitting) against days. The normal half-time survival (T ½) is 25 to 35 days (Fig. 59-14).

Because normal red cell survival is about 120 days, one would expect a T ½ of about 60 days. One reason for the observed discrepancy is that approximately 10% of the chromium label is lost during the first 24 hours, possibly as a result of RBC damage by the labeling technique. Furthermore, approximately 1% of the chromium label elutes off of the red cell each day, thereby reducing the T ½ to about 30 days. Patients with hemolytic anemias may evidence markedly shortened survivals in the range of 2 to 5 days (Fig. 59-14).

The accuracy of the described technique is also dependent on normal leukocyte and platelet counts. Random labels such as chromium are nonselective as to the cells they tag. Although Chromium-51 binding efficiency to RBCs averages 90%, it also binds to white blood cells and platelets.

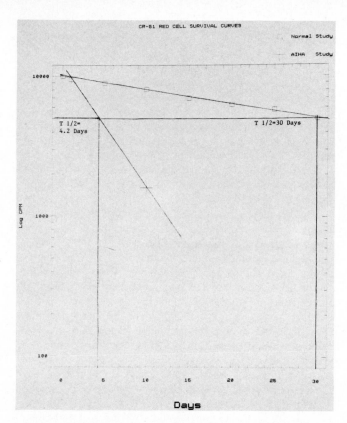

Fig. 59-14   Red cell survival curves for a normal patient and a patient with autoimmune hemolytic anemia (AIHA).

Since these cells have totally different survival rates from RBCs, when present in excessively large proportions, they bias the survival results.

In addition to T ½, external localization of RBC sequestration can be determined by monitoring radiation over the precordium, liver, and spleen. In normal individuals, the spleen-to-liver counts are equal, however, with splenic sequestration or excessive splenic destruction of red cells, the ratio markedly increases. A normal red cell survival in the face of a rising spleen-to-liver ratio suggests hypersplenism, rather than hemolysis. An increased spleen-to-liver ratio accompanying reduced red cell survival confirms the diagnosis of hemolysis. In autoimmune hemolytic anemia, which is refractory to medical therapy, the finding of an increased spleen-to-liver ratio implies that splenectomy may be of therapeutic benefit. However, the predictive value of the test for success is inadequate.

Red blood cell volume

The differential diagnosis of erythrocytosis or an elevated hematocrit includes three major possibilities, primary erythrocytosis (polycythemia vera, a myeloproliferative disorder), secondary erythrocytosis (due to physiologically increased erythropoietin production or tumor-related increases in erythropoietin), or relative erythrocytosis. The last condition reflects a decrease in plasma volume secondary to hemoconcentration, which causes a spurious erythrocytosis in the presence of a normal total red cell mass. Before embarking on a diagnostic work-up for the etiology of erythrocytosis, it is necessary to confirm whether or not the red cell volume is increased.

The test involves measuring the in vivo dilution of a labeled volume of Cr-51. A standard volume of Cr-51–labeled red cells is compared to that of a blood sample taken from the patient 10 or 40 minutes following injection of a similarly labeled sample. It thus employs the principle of hemodilution, which equates blood volume with the quotient of the quantity of the tracer divided by the concentration of the diluted tracer at equilibrium.

In practice, red cells are labeled in a manner similar to that employed for red cell survival studies using 35μCi of Cr-51. One aliquot is diluted into 1000 ml of distilled water for a standard and a 5-ml sample of labeled red cells in saline is injected into the patient. Samples are drawn from the patient after 10 and 40 minutes. Following the determination of the hematocrit of each of the samples, 2.0 ml are counted in a gamma counter. Red cell volume is calculated as follows:

$$RCV = \frac{CPM/ml\ standard \times hematocrit \times 0.98 \times 1000 \times 5}{CPM/ml\ blood\ sample\ (10\ or\ 40\ min)}$$

The results using the 10-minute sample are used if they are similar to those of the 40-minute sample. If the 40-minute sample results are greater, then those values are preferable inasmuch as they probably better reflect the equilibrium state. The normal red cell volume for males is 30 ml/kg (25 to 35), whereas that of females is 25 ml/kg (20 to 30). Values greater than these suggest true erythrocytosis due either to polycythemia vera or increased erythropoietin. When spurious erythrocytosis is suspected based on a normal or decreased red cell volume, a concomitant determination of the plasma volume using radiolabeled albumin is indicated.

Plasma volume

Although theoretically plasma volume could be calculated if the red cell volume and venous hematocrit are known, this is not always the case. The ratio of whole body to venous hematocrit is 0.9 in normal patients. However, in patients with splenomegaly, common in polycythemia vera, this ratio may be increased to 1.0 or greater. In such cases plasma volume must be measured directly. The test involves injecting a bolus of 5 μCi of iodine-125–labeled human serum albumin after first obtaining a 2-ml plasma background counting sample. At 10, 20, 30, and 60 minutes following injection, 5-ml aliquots of blood are withdrawn from the patient and the plasma is separated by centrifugation. The plasma is counted with a gamma counter and the zero time patient count is determined by extrapolation from the timed samples plotted on semi-logarithmic graph paper. An additional 5 μCi of radiolabeled albumin is added to a 1000-ml volumetric flask filled with saline; a 2-ml aliquot of this mixture is removed for gamma counting. Plasma volume is then calculated:

$$PV(ml) = \frac{(net\ cpm \times 1000\ standard)}{(net\ cpm\ plasma\ sample)}$$

Normal values for red cell volume and plasma volume in milliliters/kilogram are presented shortly. It should be noted that the diagnosis of true erythrocytosis as manifested in polycythemia vera requires an elevated red cell volume in the face of a normal plasma volume. If plasma volume is reduced, then an elevated hematocrit is due to volume contraction and is termed spurious polycythemia.

	MALES	**FEMALES**
Total blood volume	55-80	50-75
Red cell volume	25-35	20-30
Plasma volume	30-45	30-45

In vivo crossmatch

Occasionally, the hospital blood bank is unable to provide compatible units of donor blood for transfusion because of recipient antibodies that cause a panagglutination reaction with all donor cells. In such cases an incompatible unit is selected and may be tested using in vitro crossmatching.

A 0.5-ml aliquot of donor cells is labeled with Cr-51 as described for the red cell volume. A red cell volume is performed using Tc-99 labeled cells, or the red cell volume is estimated from tables according to the patient's total body surface area. Blood samples are obtained at 3-, 10-, and 60-minute intervals following injection of Cr-51 radiolabeled cells into the patient. If there is no significant difference in the radioactivity of the three samples and if no significant radioactive activity is present in the plasma of the samples (i.e., no hemolysis), then one can assume no major incompatibility exists. Alternatively, the red cell volume of the 10-minute sample can be calculated and compared to the Tc-99 or predicted RCV. If the values do not differ by more than ±10%, then no major incompatibility exists. Although one can slowly and safely transfuse the donor blood, it is still possible that delayed hemolysis can occur. Careful analysis of a curve that plots the percentage of labeled cells in the circulation vs. time, with additional samples being obtained at 18 and 24 hours, can provide clues as to the likelihood of delayed reactions. Nevertheless, in emergent situations, a negative 60-minute test can provide adequate assurance of the safety of the transfusion.

Platelet survival

Although the study of platelet kinetics have provided a bountiful degree of information about platelet function in health and disease, there are relatively few indications for performing platelet survival tests for the clinical management of patients. In the evaluation of thrombocytopenic disorders, low platelet count is usually due either to inadequate bone marrow production or increased peripheral destruction. The distinction is usually made by evaluating the bone marrow for the presence of megakaryocytes, the precursor cells of peripheral platelets. Adequate megakaryocytes in the face of a low platelet count suggests peripheral platelet destruction. In many cases, the finding of an elevated mean platelet volume (MPV) in the face of an isolated thrombocytopenia can provide similar discriminating information.

In immune thrombocytopenia (ITP), antiplatelet antibodies mediate the splenic sequestration and destruction of platelets. The disorder is diagnosed by the finding of thrombocytopenia, elevated MPV, and elevated levels of platelet-associated IgG (PAIgG) or IgM. Bone marrow confirmation of megakaryocytic hyperplasia may be obtained, but is usually not necessary. Treatment consists of corticosteroids or intravenous gamma globulin. Those patients who are refractory to, or cannot be weaned off of, pharmacologic therapy become candidates for splenectomy.

In certain rare instances, the diagnosis of ITP may not be clear-cut. Platelet antibodies may not be present or megakaryocyte mass may be diminished. In these situations, before a splenectomy is performed it is reasonable to document decreased platelet survival. If found to be shortened, then the supposition that the patient has a peripheral destructive disorder is supported and a splenectomy can be performed. If the survival is normal, then the patient might be suffering from ineffective megakaryocytopoiesis. In such a case, a splenectomy would hardly be expected to be beneficial and should not be performed.

Autologous platelet-rich plasma may be labeled with either Cr-51 or Indium-111 oxine. The T ½ of Cr-51–labeled platelets is 4.5 to 5.5 days and platelet lifespan has been calculated to average 9.5 days. In ITP, the T ½ may be as short as 30 minutes. Indium-111 is the preferred platelet label since it lends itself to external imaging. It should be noted, though, that the response to splenectomy in ITP correlates poorly with splenic localization of radioisotope so that imaging adds little to the data obtained from the kinetic studies. The procedure for platelet survival is analogous to that of the red cell survival test, but blood is obtained from the patient at the following intervals: 15, 30, 60, and 120 minutes as well as 1, 2, 3, and 4 days. The blood sample counts are plotted against time on semi-logarithmic paper. Normal disappearance half-time for Indium-111–labeled platelets is greater than 100 hours (4 days).

The Schilling test

Patients suspected of having megaloblastic anemias are usually evaluated with tests for serum vitamin B_{12} and serum or red cell folic acid. Low levels of serum vitamin B_{12} may be due to pernicious anemia (deficiency of intrinsic factor), malabsorbtion of vitamin B_{12} (due to bacterial overgrowth), or secondary malabsorbtion due to atrophic changes in the intestine because of vitamin B_{12} deficiency. The distinction can be made by the Schilling test. Occasionally, the Schilling test may be performed even when the serum vitamin B_{12} level is normal when the patient is suspected of having recently received parenteral vitamin B_{12}. The test is done in this case to positively rule out pernicious anemia. The importance of this relates to the fact that untreated vitamin B_{12} deficiency can lead to severe neurologic disease.

First described by Robert Schilling in 1953, the classic Schilling test involves the oral administration of 0.5 μCi cobalt-57–labeled vitamin B_{12} to the patient, who is then given a 1-mg injection of nonlabeled vitamin B_{12} parenterally. This flushing dose of nonlabeled vitamin B_{12} saturates the circulating vitamin B_{12}-binding proteins so that any labeled vitamin B_{12} absorbed via the intestine will be excreted by glomerular filtration. A complete 48-hour urine collection is obtained and aliquots are counted in a gamma counter. Normal individuals excrete greater than 10% of the labeled vitamin B_{12}. Less than 6% excretion usually signifies intrinsic factor deficiency. If the test is abnormal, then a repeat dose of labeled vitamin B_{12} is administered orally, together with exogenous intrinsic factor several days later, and the test is repeated.

An improvement in vitamin B_{12} excretion to greater than 10% suggests that the original abnormality was due to in-

trinsic factor deficiency. The patient may then be given the diagnosis of pernicious anemia. If part two of the Schilling test does not improve, then the patient may be suffering from malabsorbtion due either to the blind loop-bacterial overgrowth syndrome or malabsorption secondary to long-standing pernicious anemia. The patient may then be treated with broad-spectrum antibiotics to kill the bacteria and be subjected to a repeat Schilling test. If this part does not improve, then the patient should be treated with vitamin B_{12} for several months to overcome the atrophic intestinal mucosa and have the test repeated.

Recently, the modified Schilling test has come into widespread use. In this version, the patient is simultaneously given two capsules of radiolabeled vitamin B_{12}, each with a different isotope of cobalt. The vitamin B_{12} in one of the capsules contains intrinsic factor, whereas the other does not. Urine is collected as usual and is counted on two gamma counter channels. Normal individuals excrete similar amounts of the two isotopes. Patients with pernicious anemia will only excrete the isotope bound to intrinsic factor, whereas patients with malabsorbtion excrete only small amounts of both isotopes. A third modification of the test, using a serum sample obtained 8 hours following ingestion of the radiolabeled vitamin B_{12} has been tried but is not generally accepted because of reports of false-negative tests.

The Schilling test has been used less frequently in recent years because of the availability of serum levels of anti-intrinsic factor antibodies. The finding of high levels of these specific immunoglobulins is a highly sensitive and fairly specific test for pernicious anemia. Nevertheless, the Schilling test, in one of its several forms, continues to be the gold standard for the specific diagnosis of this disease.

SUGGESTED READING

Alavi JB and Hansell J: Labelled cells in the investigation of hematologic disorders, Semin Nucl Med 14:208, 1984.

Bessman JD, Gilmer PR, and Gardner FH: Improved classification of anemia by MCV and RDW, Am J Clin Pathol 80:332, 1983.

Bessman JD: Use of mean platelet volume improves detection of platelet disorders, Blood Cells 11:127, 1985.

Burns ER and others: Performance characteristics of state of the art hematology analyzers, Clin Lab Sci 5(No 2), 1992.

Burns ER, Goldberg SN, and Wenz B: A new assay for quantifying human reticulocytes, Am J Clin Pathol 88:338, 1987.

Charache S and others: A clinical trial of three-part electronic differential white blood cell counts: Arch Intern Med 145:1852, 1985.

Dutcher TF: Automated differentials; a strategy, Blood Cells 11:49, 1985.

Koepke JA (editor): The white blood cell differential, I, Blood Cells 11:1, 1985.

Krause JR, Costello RT, and Penchasky L: Use of the Technicon H*1 in the characterization of leukemias, Arch Pathol Lab Med 112:889, 1988.

McIntyre PA: The blood and blood forming organs. In Wagner HW (editor): Nuclear medicine, New York, 1975, HP Publishing.

Mohandas N and others: Accurate and independent measurement of volume and hemoglobin concentration of individual red cells by laser light scattering, Blood 68:506, 1986.

d'Onofrio GS and others: Identification of blast cells in the peripheral blood through automatic assessment of nuclear density, Br J Haematol 66:473, 1987.

Schoentag RA: Hematology analyzers, Clin Lab Med 8:653, 1988.

Wenz B and others: The clinical utility of the leukocyte differential in emergency medicine, Am J Clin Pathol 30, 1986.

Wenz B, Ramirez MA, and Burns ER: The H*1 hematology analyzer: its performance characteristics and value in the diagnosis of infectious disease, Arch Pathol Lab Med 111:521, 1987.

60 Flow cytometry and phenotyping of hemopoietic cells

Jay E. Valinsky

HISTORICAL PERSPECTIVES

Flow cytometry is a technique of identifying, characterizing, and isolating single cells through the analysis of physical, chemical, or immunological properties, which can be measured by optical means. These properties include, but are not limited to, cell size, cell shape, DNA content, antigen distribution, and enzymatic activities. Table 60-1 illustrates various attempts to purify specific subpopulations from heterogeneous mixtures of cells for study of their specific biological and molecular properties. While all of these methods have advantages and disadvantages, flow cytometry clearly has emerged as the method of choice for obtaining significant numbers of highly purified cells.

The development of flow cytometry over the past 30 years has been driven by the following:

1. the need for rapid quantitative techniques to analyze the properties of cells;
2. the need to distinguish normal from abnormal cells on the basis of biochemical, functional, and antigenic properties; and
3. the need to use this information in relevant clinical settings.

Specific examples of clinical applications which have prompted these technological advances are illustrated most strikingly in the characterization of normal and abnormal blood cells; the classification of cells from patients with leukemias, lymphomas, and immunodeficiency syndromes with a view towards therapy; and the analysis of cellular DNA content and cell cycle kinetics in applications related to cancer prognosis and treatment.

Flow cytometry has roots in instruments developed as early as the 1930s for particle counting. Flow technology was stimulated in the 1950s and early 1960s by the development of instrumentation for automated differential blood counting, and the concurrent development of fluorescence microscopy, fluorescence staining methods, and techniques for automating the examination of cytological preparations (e.g., PAP smears). Before these innovations, virtually all cytological and morphological measurements of clinical importance were made by light microscopy. This technique employs a variety of vital or supravital dyes or probes that enhance the visibility of particular subcellular structures. While extremely valuable in many clinical settings, light microscopy techniques are slow and very labor-intensive. In addition, the observations and interpretations in many respects are subjective and give rise to semi-quantitative data at best. The great value of microscopic observation is that the distinctive properties of individual cells can be noted, recorded, and classified by trained observers. The visual impact of a cell with abnormal morphology is often quite striking and revealing. Thus microscopy techniques remain critical components of clinical diagnosis and practice.

At the other end of the analytical spectrum are biochemical measurements of, for example, enzymatic activities or metabolite levels on preparations of cells, tissues, or body fluids. Cellular preparations are often very heterogeneous in composition, and, because the measurements typically require homogenization of the cells or tissue, information about identifiable subpopulations of cells is lost.

By the 1950s, the limitations of light microscopy and biochemical measurements underscored the need for methods that could provide quantitative information about single cells or subpopulations of cells in a rapid, automated manner. Though work on automated cell analysis has continued for nearly 60 years, the breakthrough in clinical flow analysis came with the issuance of a series of patents in the 1940s and 1950s. One set of patents was issued for electronic particle sizing instruments, which were immediately employed in automated blood cell counting. Patents were also issued for the development of techniques for the hydrodynamic focusing of cells or particles in a liquid stream, which were required for accurate single particle counting.

Ten to 15 years later instruments designed to make automated measurements not only of cell or particle size but also of the DNA content of single cells became available, both flow systems and microscope-based image analyzers. In the case of flow systems, particle size was measured by electronic volume and later by light scattering. Estimates of DNA or protein content were made by chemical, spec-

Table 60-1   Cell separation methods

Method	Basis for separation	Comment

Sedimentation
    Unit gravity
    Isopycnic
    Elutriation
	Cell size, buoyant density	Rapid, large number of cells, high yields, low to moderate purity

Affinity chromatography "Panning"	Cell surface antigens, lectins	Difficult to recover cells from supports; moderate yields; variable purity
Counter current distribution	Affinity partitioning between two phases	Low yield, poor viability
Electrophoresis	Surface charge	Small numbers of cells; low yield
Flow cytometry/flow sorting	Light scattering and/or fluorescence	Expensive; complex; high purity; small numbers of cells; variable yield

trophotometric, or fluorescence means. Eventually, fluorescence techniques took center stage. A series of fluorescent molecules that interacted specifically and quantitatively with DNA or nucleic acids was developed, and microscope techniques that could detect cells labeled with specific, fluorescently labeled antibodies were adapted for flow cytometry. At about the same time, flow-based blood cell analyzers, which used light scattering and spectrophotometric measurements to distinguish among peripheral blood cells, began to make their appearance.

Like their earlier counterparts, modern flow cytometers incorporate laser-based optical systems and the capability to physically separate cells of choice. However, data analysis with pulse-height analyzers has been rapidly supplanted by sophisticated computer systems which are used for instrument operation as well as data reduction. Thus, modern flow cytometers solve some of the problems posed by conventional light microscopy. For example, they permit high rates of analysis, reduce labor intensity, and improve quantitation, especially with regard to cell sizing and measurements of intrinsic and extrinsic fluorescence.

Enormous strides have also been made in the field of image analysis in the last five years. Computerized, digitizing microscopes capable of providing quantitative, structural information on cytological preparations are now readily available. These instruments can analyze cells and tissues processed by routine histological procedures or by fluorescence techniques. Image analysis works better than flow cytometry in specific applications (e.g., analysis of tissue specimens). Like flow systems, the analytical rates of image analyzers can be very high. However, unlike flow systems, the operator can actually visualize cells and can perform repeated analysis on any given cell. From a quantitative point of view, image analyzers can generate data on a large number of morphometric parameters, which are difficult to assess in flow systems. Thus, cells can be classified not only by their dye-staining intensity, but also by their size and shape and numbers of subcellular organelles. Image analysis bridges the gap between personal observation of cells by microscope and electronic analyses of the same preparations.

THEORY, INSTRUMENTATION, AND DATA ANALYSIS

Despite the apparent complexity of design, flow cytometers are simply optical microscopes that 1) make measurements on single cells 2) process data obtained from these cells electronically. Most commercial flow cytometers consist of three integrated components: a fluidics (i.e., fluid handling) system; an optical system, which includes an illumination source, optical filters, and light collectors; and an electronics module, which may include photomultipliers to amplify light signals and a computer capable of multiparametric data acquisition and analysis. The merging of these components into a working flow cytometer is described below.

The primary objective of flow cytometry is to generate information about subpopulations of cells that can be identified on the basis of one or several characteristic biological properties. These properties may be revealed by extrinsic fluorescent probes (e.g., DNA stains, fluorescently labeled antibodies, fluorogenic substrates for enzymes) or by evaluating intrinsic properties of the cells (e.g., size, light scattering, intrinsic fluorescence).

In flow cytometry, appropriately labeled cells suspended in an electrolyte (e.g., buffered saline or similar media) are caused to flow single file in a fluid stream. Individual cells in the stream are "interrogated" by a beam of light, thereby initiating the analysis. Measurements of cell size, cell volume, fluorescence, or other optical properties ensue, followed by computerized analysis of the data. Data is finally presented in the often complex frequency distributions (histograms), which display the measured property(ies) as a function of cell number. These frequency distributions can then be analyzed in quantitative terms in light of the specific biological property under investigation.

Elements of the system:

Fluidics and hydrodynamic focusing

The success of flow cytometric analysis depends to a large extent on the stability and uniformity of the system's liquid flow and the way cells or particles are integrated into the flow. Uniformity and stability are required since the illumination system and the optical and electronic sensors and detectors all are precisely aligned such that measurements can be made on the cells as they flow by (Figure 60-1). Single-cell suspensions are required for flow analysis. The cells are typically prepared in a solution of an electrolyte that is compatible with cell viability, structural integrity, and functional activities. In most flow cytometers, the suspension of cells is forced under pressure or pumped through plastic tubing into a flow chamber. The exit port of this flow chamber is an orifice typically 50 to 200 μm in diameter.

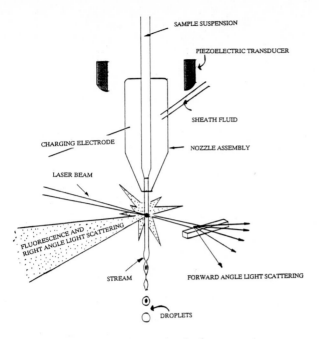

Fig. 60-1 Schematic diagram of a flow cytometer.

Ideally, cells passing through the orifice will follow a uniform laminar trajectory in the fluid stream and will therefore align with the elements of the optical system. However, as in most systems, the real situation is far from ideal. In the stream of a simple flow system, a large percentage of cells emerging from the orifice do not follow the ideal trajectory and thus are off line. This affects the efficacy of the analysis, the coefficients of variation of the frequency distributions, the flow rate, and may even result in clogging the orifice. These problems have largely been solved by the use of an additional fluid stream, the so-called sheath solution, which consists of a cell-free electrolyte that is compatible with the cells under study. The hydrodynamic properties of the system are such that the cells are injected and "hydrodynamically focused" to the center of the sheath fluid stream. This creates what can be envisioned as two concentric streams with the sheath on the outside and the cells on the inside. This process keeps the cells flowing laminarly throughout the analysis, thereby reducing the number of cells off trajectory. It also reduces clogging of the orifice and tightens the coefficients of variation of the data distributions.

Optical and electronic measurements of cellular properties

In some flow cytometers, cells in the fluid stream are ejected from the orifice and analyzed in a jet of liquid in air. In other configurations, the cells enter a quartz flow cell and the subsequent analysis takes place within its confines. Optical measurements of cells occur after cells 1) pass through the orifice or 2) enter the flow cell.

The optical system of a flow cytometer is composed of an incident light source, optics for collecting emitted or scattered light, optical filters, a detector, and devices (e.g., photomultipliers) that amplify weak signals for further electronic processing. As seen in Figure 60-1, the cells in the liquid stream pass one at a time through the incident light

source, which is focused at a precise position on the fluid stream. This focal point is called the *"point of intersection"* or "point of interrogation." The light source in most modern flow cytometers is a laser. The choice of laser depends on the requirements of the measurement. Some lasers produce excitation at a single wavelength (e.g., He-Ne laser, 633 nm); others can be optically adjusted or "tuned" to produce a number of useful lines in the UV and visible regions of the electromagnetic spectrum. For example, argon-ion lasers, commonly used in commercial flow cytometers, produce 450 to 530 nm of incident light and with quartz optics, spectral lines in the ultraviolet. Argon-ion lasers are commonly tuned to 488.8 nm, a wavelength compatible with the absorption spectra of some of the most widely used fluorochromes (Table 60-2). The optical configurations of many flow cytometers can accommodate more than one laser. Multiple lasers can be combined to provide a wide range of excitation wavelengths for the simultaneous analysis of several fluorescent probes. While past multiple-laser systems were quite expensive, low-cost, air-cooled, low-wattage lasers are now common.

Why are these expensive illumination sources required? First, lasers deliver monochromatic light to the sample, thereby taking best advantage of the absorptive properties of the fluorophore without using complex sets of excitation filters. Second, a laser beam can be focused very precisely (a spot <1 mm in diameter) on the fluid stream and thus on the cells that flow through. Most importantly, high-intensity illumination is required since the amount of light emitted or scattered from a cell is typically of very low intensity. High-intensity incident light assures that the amount of fluorescent or scattered light generated by the interaction of the cells with the light beam is adequate for consistent, reproducible measurements. At the point of intersection, where light energy is most concentrated, lasers produce light intensities much higher than those obtained in a light microscope. The cells are thus exposed to high fluences (>10 μwatts/μ^2) during their short transit time (a few microseconds) through the light beam. Since for most stable fluorophores, there is a proportionality between the incident light intensity and the intensity of the emitted light, the output signal is maximized through the use of lasers.

As an alternative to the laser, a highly focused beam from a mercury or xenon arc lamp has been employed in some systems. This type of illumination source has several advantages, notably access to wavelengths (250 to 280 nm) in the ultraviolet region of the spectrum and low cost. However, these advantages are offset by the relative instability of arc lamps, the need for more elaborate optical systems for focusing the beam and for optical filtration of the exciting light.

Measurable parameters

Several parameters can be measured simultaneously during flow cytometric analysis. In addition to light scattering and fluorescence, which are the most common, flow cytometers can perform electronic particle sizing, fluorescence polarization, and absorbance measurements, to name a few.

Light scattering

As particles pass through a beam of light, some of the light is deflected from the forward path, or scattered. A

Table 60-2 Spectral properties of fluorescent probes commonly used in flow cytometry

Application	Fluorophore	Excitation maximum (nm)	Emission maximum (nm)
Antibody labeling	Fluorescein (FITC)	490	520
	TRITC	554	573
	XRITC	580	602
	Phycoerythrin-R	480-565	578
	Texas Red	596	620
	Allophycocyanine	650	660
	"Duo-Chrome"*	480-565 (PE)	550-595 (PE)
			597-640 (TR)
DNA/RNA Stains	Hoechst 33342	340	450
	DAPI	350	470
	Ethidium Bromide	510	595
	Propidium Iodide	536	623
	Acridine Orange (DNA)	480	520
	Acridine Orange (RNA)	440-470	650
	Thiazole Orange	453	480
Intracellular pH	6-carboxyfluorescein	450, 495	520
Calcium Flux	Fura-2 (High Calcium)	335	512-518
	Fura-2 (Low Calcium)	360	505-510
	Indo-1 (High Calcium)	360	390-410
	Indo-1 (Low Calcium)	360	482-485
Membrane Potential	DiO-Cn-(3)	485	505
	Rhodamine 123	511	
Enzyme Substrates	di-arg-CBZ-Rhodamine	495	523
	Coumarin-glucosides	316-370	395-419

*Duo-Chrome is a conjugate of phycoerythrin (PE) and Texas Red (TR). Excitation of the PE component leads to a fluorescence emission at 550-595 nm which, in turn, is absorbed by the Texas Red component. The process of energy transfer results in final emission at about 620 nm. Using this probe, one can perform three-color fluorescence analyses (FITC, PC, Duo-Chrome) with the excitation at one wavelength (488.8 nm).

common example is the reflection of light often observed on dust particles suspended in a sunbeam. In the ideal case, an opaque, spherical particle that passes through a beam of light will scatter the light homogeneously (i.e., at 360°). The scattered light can then be measured by placing a detector at any angle relative to the incident light source. The intensity of light scattered from a particle depends on the angle at which the detector is placed. It follows that information obtained from light scattering data also depends on the angle of measurement. In most commercial flow cytometers, light scattering is measured at two angles. Forward angle light scattering (FALS) is measured at low angles (0° to 10°) from the incident light beam. Orthogonal, or right-angle, light scattering is measured at 90° from the incident light beam. The light-scattering detectors are placed at these particular angles not only because the locations are convenient with regard to the physical configuration of most commercial instruments, but because of the structural information that can be obtained from measurements at these angles.

Light scattered at low angles to the incident beam is collected with a lens that focuses the light on the detector, typically a photodiode. The incident laser light is effectively prevented from falling on the detector by placing a metal bar ("obstruction" or "obscuration" bar) in the light path (Figure 60-1). This blocks the light at approximately 0 to 2°. Failure to block the incident laser light results in saturation of the detector and the loss of all information about the cells. Scattered light that passes the obscuration bar at 2 to 10° angles from the incident beam is collected and

analyzed. A similar system permits the collection of light scattered at 90° from the incident light beam. In this case, however, the scattered light is generally collected with a high numerical aperture microscope objective or with a fiber optic.

A comprehensive discussion of information derived from light scattering measurements is beyond the scope of this review. However, for present purposes it is sufficient to say that forward-angle light scattering provides an estimate of the *relative size* of cells. Thus, the greater the forward angle light scattering intensity, the "larger" the particle appears. However, it must be emphasized that the "size" of a particle determined by light scattering is *not* the absolute size of the particle. This is because the measured forward angle light scattering intensity depends on the wavelength of light employed, the precise angle at which it is measured, the refractive index and absorptive properties of the cells, the viability of the cells, and the nature of the medium in which the cells are suspended.

Right-angle light scattering provides less information about the size of the cells than about their internal, shape, and surface topography. Thus, in complex mixtures of cells, the effects of cytoplasmic granules, nuclear morphology, nuclear/cytoplasmic ratios, among other parameters, on light scattering intensity are valuable in distinguishing among all types in the cell population. The simultaneous analysis of forward- and right-angle light scattering has proven to be a useful procedure. For example, it is possible to obtain a respectable three-part differential count (lymphocytes, monocytes, polymorphonuclear leukocytes) on peripheral blood leukocytes on the basis of combined FALS and right-angle light scattering measurements alone. In addition, combining the two measurements often permits the discrimination of live cells from dead cells.

Electronic particle sizing

While forward-angle light scattering provides estimates of relative cell size, it does not provide an accurate measure of cell volume. Electronic particle sizing, which has been widely used in automated blood cell counters for many years, is the better technique for measuring cell volume. While electronic particle sizing has been applied to flow cytometers, light scattering is still the most widely used flow cytometric technique for cell sizing.

In making these electronic volume measurements, an electrolyte is induced to flow through an orifice of defined size (usually <100 μm). A voltage is applied across the orifice and the system is allowed to come to equilibrium at a constant impedance. Because of its small size, the orifice contributes significantly to the impedance of the entire system. Thus, if a cell or particle enters the orifice, there is a change in the impedance. A voltage change corresponds to the change in impedance and is directly proportional to the volume of the particle. Particles can then be ranked by size according to the voltage change and the results displayed as a histogram. Cell volume can then be combined and analyzed.

Fluorescence measurements

In addition to light scattering, excitation of cell-bound fluorescent probes at the point of laser intersection results in the emission of fluorescent light, which can be collected and quantified. The optical element used to collect the emitted light is, in most cases, a high numerical aperture microscope objective set orthogonally to the incident beam and to the stream (Figure 60-1). In most cases, it is the same objective used to collect light scattered at 90°. Following collection of light by the microscope objective, the incident laser light is removed by optical filters, which transmit only the emitted fluorescent light and the scattered light. The fluorescence and right-angle light scattering signals are separated by a series of dichroic mirrors and optical filters. A small portion of the light (<10%) is diverted for measurement of right-angle light scattering. The remainder of the light is used to measure emitted fluorescence.

Fluorescence emission is measured after extensive optical filtration of the collected light. Beam splitters and dichroic mirrors direct the emitted light to different optical filter sets and subsequently to the detectors. The primary optical filters are chosen to be compatible with the emission wavelengths of the fluorochromes, which are used to label the cells. These are typically glass filters that transmit light at selected ranges of wavelengths. Combinations of filters are used to restrict wavelengths of light analyzed to those emitted by specific fluorochromes.

Flow cytometers may have several sets of dichroics and optical filters, which direct the emitted light along different optical paths. This affords the opportunity to analyze the light emitted from several fluorophores simultaneously. For example, emitted light may be directed along two optical paths, one of which permits green light to pass through the filters, the other red light.

In these so-called multiparametric fluorescence analyses, the choice of optical filters is critical. If a cell is labeled with two or more fluorochromes, accurate analysis depends on the ability to distinguish the two probes optically. This is accomplished first by choosing probes with emission spectra that are significantly different and secondly by choosing optical filters that effectively isolate these spectral lines. For example, both fluorescein isothiocyanate and R-phycoerythrin can be excited by an argon-ion laser at 488.8 nm. However, the emission spectra of the two probes are different enough that they can be conveniently separated optically. On the other hand, fluorescein and some rhodamine derivatives are not easily separated optically and thus are not typically employed together in flow cytometric analyses. Because the absorption and emission spectra of several commonly used fluorophores overlap significantly, optical separation may be incomplete. Electronic "compensation" circuits are often used to correct this optical insufficiency.

Electronic analysis

After the laser beam "interrogates" the cells, scattered and optically filtered light from the cells is directed to the detectors (e.g., photomultiplier tubes, photodiodes) for further electronic processing. When a light signal falls on the detector, a current pulse is generated, and information about pulse height, shape, width, and so forth is obtained. These data are displayed in histograms, which are derived by ranking the intensities complitudes of the voltage signals from the amplifiers and relating the pulse heights to the number of events in each voltage range. Events falling into preset voltage ranges (typically 0 to 10 volts) are expressed as digital signals and are typically displayed on a linear scale. This linear voltage scale is suitable for many measurements. But the signals derived from some cells may not fit into the linear scale. For example, a heterogeneous population of cells may exhibit very large differences (e.g., orders of magnitude) in fluorescence intensities. This problem can be solved by passing the signals through a logarithmic amplifier, which is capable of ranking the signals over several (three to five) decades of fluorescence intensity. In this case, all of the signals will be on scale, and signals with intensities which fall over a wide range of intensities can be analyzed. In early flow cytometers, data from the various detectors were processed by multichannel analyzers. More recently, multichannel analyzers have been replaced by mini- or microcomputers, which allow the analysis, computation, and display of multiparameter data in a variety of ways.

Instruments currently available from commercial sources, can analyze cells at rates of up to 10,000 per second. Some noncommercial instruments are capable of analyzing cells at nearly 10 times this rate. These high-speed rates are necessary for many applications involving rare-event analysis in which cells present in populations at frequencies less than 1/100,000 must be detected and analyzed.

Data presentation and analysis

The preceding discussions implied that with the appropriate optical systems and detectors, several pieces of data can be obtained simultaneously from a given cell. For example, the data available for analysis may include two or more light-scattering signals, cell volume, several fluorescence signals, or other parameters (e.g., polarization, absorbance, etc.). Some flow cytometers are capable of simultaneous acquisition of more than eight parameters. While accumulating so much data on a given cell may seem desirable at first, the ability to interpret multiparametric data on heterogeneous cell populations decreases exponentially as the complexity of the analysis increases.

How data are acquired by a flow cytometer dictates the way data are ultimately displayed and analyzed. Most flow cytometers acquire data with computers and store data in computer files. Data may be stored and processed in two ways. In the first, the so-called list mode format, raw data from each detector (photomultiplier or photodiode) are stored in files that can be manipulated following data acquisition. This is the most flexible way of storing data and is best suited to analyze multiparametric data, since pairwise comparisons of the measured parameters, taken in different combinations, is often required. Alternatively, data

from the photodetectors can be processed immediately in a multichannel analyzer or a computer and the resulting calculated data stored and/or displayed. This mode of data reduction is perhaps best suited to single parameter data analysis. Data processed in this manner can no longer be extensively re-analyzed.

Statistical and graphical analysis of the vast amount of data acquired during a typical flow cytometric analysis has been possible only since the incorporation of computers into the operating systems. As noted previously, flow cytometric data is typically expressed in frequency distributions. These distributions represent relative intensities of fluorescence, light scattering, or any other measurable parameter. The relative intensity scale is divided into "channels," a term left over from the time when flow data were analyzed on multichannel analyzers. Each channel represents a particular voltage level derived from the output of the photomultipliers or photodiodes; each channel can be expressed either linearly or logarithmically.

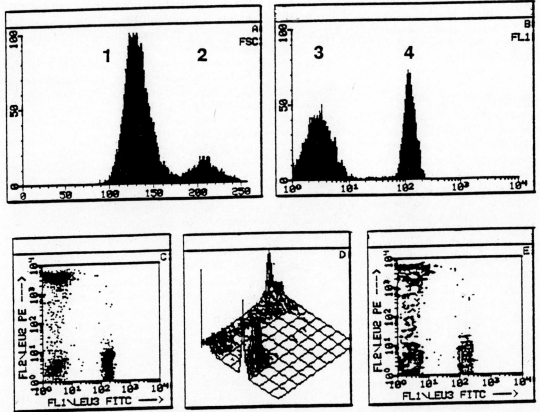

Fig. 60-2 Flow cytometric data displays.
Panel A—Single parameter forward angle light scattering intensity histogram. Region 1, "small" cells; Region 2, "large" cells. Horizontal axis, light scattering intensity; vertical axis, cell number.
Panel B—Single parameter fluorescence intensity histogram. Region 3, "dim" cells; Region 4, "bright" cells. Horizontal axis, log fluorescence intensity; vertical axis, cell number.
Panel C—Dual parameter forward angle light scattering and fluorescence intensity histogram—"Dot Plot." Horizontal axis, light scattering intensity; vertical axis, log fluorescence intensity.
Panel D—Dual parameter forward angle light scattering and fluorescence intensity histogram—Isocontour Plot. X-axis, light scattering intensity; Y-axis, log fluorescence intensity; Z-axis, cell number.
Panel E—Dual parameter forward angle light scattering and fluorescence intensity histogram—Contour Plot. Horizontal axis, light scattering intensity; vertical axis, log fluorescence intensity; Contour levels denote cross sections through the Iso-contour Plot of Panel D.

Frequency distributions may be presented in several formats. The more common representations are illustrated in Figure 60-2. These are single-parameter displays and correlated, multiparameter displays. In the single-parameter representations (Figure 60-2A, B), data are displayed for only one measured parameter (e.g., light scattering, fluorescence) at a time. This presentation is most useful if the cell population is homogeneous.

If there are subpopulations of cells in the preparation, correlated data analysis is more useful (Figure 60-2C-E). Closer examination of the single-parameter histograms of Figure 60-2 A and B reveals the problem with single-parameter displays. These figures show fluorescence and light scattering data obtained from a particular cell preparation. Figure 60-2A shows both "small" cells (Peak 1) and "large" cells (Peak 2), as measured by forward-angle light scattering. Some of these cells are weakly fluorescent or autofluorescent (Figure 60-2B, Peak 3), and some are brightly fluorescent (Figure 60-2B, Peak 4). Upon inspection, one can not predict which subpopulation in the fluorescence-intensity distribution (i.e., Peak 3 or 4) is associated with which different-sized cell population displayed in Peaks 1 and 2.

This problem can be resolved by using correlated data analysis obtained from list mode files. In this case, two or more parameters associated with a given cell are compared and displayed coordinately. Figures 60-2C-E illustrate the various dual-parameter, correlated data displays commonly employed. Figure 60-2C shows a "dot display." Each dot represents correlated, dual-parameter data for an individual cell. In other words, a cell with the coordinates, or properties, (X,Y) is represented by a dot displayed on the grid. Thus, as dots accumulate in a particular region of the grid, a cluster appears. The cluster represents cells with the same

or similar properties. Eventually, as data accumulate, the regions of highest frequency overwhelm the distribution, making the patterns hard to quantitate visually. However, the numerical frequencies can still be obtained from the complete data set stored in the computer.

Figure 60-2D shows an alternative graphic representation, the iso-contour plot. In this case, the frequency distribution of the correlated data is displayed in three dimensions. Two of the axes represent relative intensity; the third represents cell number. The final type of display is the contour plot. The contour plot (Figure 60-2E) is derived by taking cross sections at different levels of the three-dimensional iso-contour plot and then displaying the cross sections in two dimensions. Thus, only selected sections of the frequency distribution are displayed. The contour levels can be adjusted by the operator to accentuate or attenuate particular regions of the distribution. Contour diagrams are extremely useful in defining small populations or the degree to which populations are skewed, provided that the cross sections through the iso-contour plots are taken at the appropriate levels.

Given the ability to acquire and display flow cytometric data, how does one analyze the data in terms of the biological properties of the cells in question? Generally, the analysis consists of calculating the frequency at which a particular marker, or set of markers, appear in the test cell population. To illustrate the procedure, flow cytometric analyses of several preparations of blood leukocytes are presented in Figure 60-3. Figure 60-3A shows a single-parameter fluorescence distribution of peripheral lymphocytes incubated with a fluorescently labeled, nonreactive control antibody. Figure 60-3B shows a single-parameter fluorescence distribution of the same cells following treatment with an antibody that reacts only with T-lymphocytes. In order to determine the

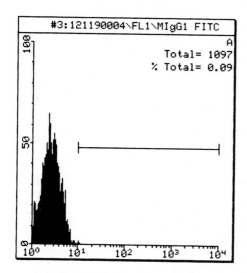
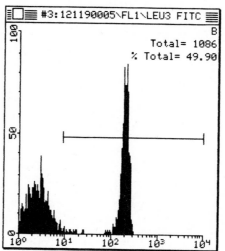

Fig. 60-3 Computation of percentage of antibody positive cells by flow cytometry.
Panel A—Fluorescence intensity histogram of human peripheral blood lymphocytes incubated with a T-helper cell specific antibody control antibody. The horizontal bar indicates the threshold level described in the text. Approximately 0.09% of the cells are "positive" with the control antibody.
Panel B—Fluorescence intensity histogram of human peripheral blood lymphocytes incubated with a T-helper cell specific antibody control antibody. The horizontal bar indicates the threshold level described in the text. Approximately 50% of the cells are "positive" with this antibody.

percentage of "antibody positive" cells, in this case, T-lymphocytes, in the total population, one establishes an electronic limit (threshold) on the control sample. This threshold indicates the amount of detectable fluorescence which is attributable to cellular autofluorescence and/or nonspecific binding of the fluorescent antibody. The marker that appears as the horizontal bar in the figures indicates the threshold. This marker is arbitrarily set at a point such that, in the control sample, fewer than 2% of the fluorescent signals have relative fluorescence intensities greater than the threshold. By definition, any cell with a relative fluorescence intensity greater than the threshold is considered reactive or "positive." The percentage of cells with intensities greater than that of the marker can be easily calculated by summing the number of events exceeding the threshold and dividing by the total number of cells analyzed. In the present example, 50% of the cells are "positive" for this antibody. A similar scenario could be applied to any parameter measured in the experiment.

The analysis of correlated, multiparametric data is somewhat more complex. The example in Figure 60-4 illustrates

procedure. In this case, peripheral blood leukocytes were incubated with two antibodies that recognize different subpopulations of lymphocytes. The antibodies were covalently conjugated to two different fluorophores (FL1 and FL2), which can be distinguished on the basis of their characteristic emission spectra.

In the data-acquisition phase of the experiment, four parameters (forward- and right-angle light scattering, FL1 and FL2) were collected simultaneously and stored in list mode data files for subsequent analysis. Once the data has been collected, how can one determine the percentage of lymphocytes labeled by antibody FL1, labeled by antibody FL2, labeled by both or labeled by neither?

First, one must identify the lymphocytes in the complex mixture of peripheral blood cells. This can be accomplished in several ways. For example, one can exploit the characteristic light scattering properties of lymphocytes. Using dual-parameter, right-angle and forward-angle light scattering distributions (Figure 60-4A), the lymphocytes can be identified and marked electronically (R1 in Figure 60-4A). The fluorescence properties of the cells in this electronic

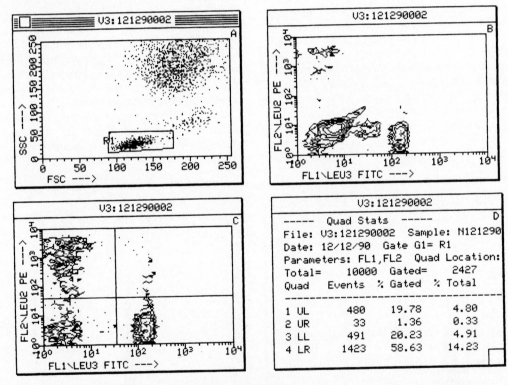

Fig. 60-4   Analysis of multiparametric flow cytometry data.
Panel A—Dual parameter forward and right angle light scattering distribution of peripheral blood leukocytes prepared by the whole blood lysis technique. Box indicates electronic "gate" set on lymphocytes.
Panel B—Ungated dual parameter fluorescence intensity distribution of peripheral blood leukocytes, treated with anti-CD4 (Leu-3) and anti-CD8 (Leu 2) antibodies.
Panel C—Dual parameter fluorescence intensity distribution of peripheral blood leukocytes, treated with anti-CD4 (Leu-3) and anti-CD8 (Leu 2) antibodies gated on lymphocytes. The gate in this panel is the one defined in Panel A.
Panel D—Calculation of percentages of positive cells using multiparametric fluorescence analysis. Cells in each of the quadrants are counted and the percentage of antibody positive cells in the gated population are counted. The absolute number of cells in a particular region can be computed from the WBC and the differential count as described in the text. UL, upper left quadrant; UR, upper right quadrant; LL, lower left quadrant; LR, lower right quadrant.

"gate" can then be analyzed in a dual-parameter fluorescence analysis in which FL1 is compared to FL2. The effects of this gating procedure can be seen in the fluorescence distributions in Figures 60-4B and C. Figure 60-4B shows an "ungated" fluorescence distribution in which FL1 and FL2 staining in all of the leukocyte populations (e.g., lymphocytes, monocytes, polymorphonuclear leukocytes) are displayed simultaneously. As seen in Figure 60-4C, the pattern is simplified considerably when one adds the lymphocyte gate outlined by the box in the light-scattering distributions of Figure 60-4A. In addition, the antibody positive lymphocyte populations are accentuated (Figure 60-4C, upper-left and lower-right boxes). As noted, the grid has been divided into four sectors, or quadrants, which can be used to count the cells. In the four regions one finds:

1. cells that have not reacted with either the FL1 or FL2 antibodies (bottom left);
2. cells that have reacted only with FL2 (upper left);
3. cells that have reacted with both FL1 and FL2 (upper right); and
4. cells that have reacted only with FL1 (lower right).

One can then enumerate the cells in each population and relate the numbers to the total population to obtain the population frequencies. The results of such an analysis are tabulated in Figure 60-4.

Instead of using quadrants, electronic windows can be drawn by pixel mapping around discrete populations and the cells counting. An extension of this procedure involves calculation of the absolute number cells in a population rather than the percentage. One only need know the concentration of cells in the starting population. In the previous example, one would need to know the total white cell count, from the CBC, and the percentage of lymphocytes from the differential white count. By applying the equation:

(WBC) × (% lymphocytes) × (% positive cells by flow cytometry) = Total number of lymphocytes in the subset

While the illustrations in the preceding section involved lymphocytes, this same method can be applied to any population of cells in a complex mixture.

One important caveat concerns the practice of using forward- and/or right-angle light scattering as the sole identifiers of particular cell populations. The light-scattering properties of cells are extremely complex, and disparate cells types may display similar patterns (e.g., lymphocytes and some nucleated red cell precursors). Therefore, additional information about the cell populations must be obtained before unequivocal identification can be made. This data may be obtained by fluorescence-activated cell sorting and biochemical or immunological analysis of the separated cells or by fluorescence gating using antibodies that unequivocally identify the cell population in question.

Sensitivity of flow cytometric methods

Fluorescence measurements on stained cells typically are exquisitely sensitive. There are, however, subtle qualitative differences between fluorescence microscopic analyses and flow cytometric measurements, as well as quantitative ones. First, in microscopy, punctate fluorescence (e.g., "capping" of antigens) is much easier to visualize than diffuse cell surface staining. The reverse appears to be true for the optical systems of a flow cytometer. Secondly, the ability of the human eye to detect low-intensity staining is very great, but is also very wavelength dependent. For example, the yellow-green fluorescence of fluorescein isothiocyanate is easier to visualize than R-phycoerythrin, which emits in the red region of the electromagnetic spectrum. For a flow cytometer, optical filtration and wavelength-specific photomultipliers compensate for these spectral effects.

The sensitivity of most commercial flow cytometers extends downward to fewer than 500 molecules of fluorophore per cell. That is to say, 500 antigenic or other types of binding sites can be detected with ease. Fortuitously, these numbers typically are in the lower end of the range of many antigens present on human blood cells. Modified flow cytometers and specialized fluorescence staining procedures (e.g., the use of fluorescent microbeads) can extend the effective range of detection to fewer than 100 sites per cell. In some instances, it has even been possible to detect a single molecule of a fluorophore in a flow experiment.

A second sensitivity issue concerns the fraction of cells in a population that can be conveniently detected in a flow cytometry experiment. One fact of flow cytometric analysis, mentioned at the outset, is that large numbers of cells may be processed over a short period of time (e.g., up to 10,000 cells per second). Thus, a statistically significant number of events can be counted in a short time. For example, if a subpopulation of 0.1% (1 per 1000) of the total were to be analyzed effectively, and at least 100 cells should be analyzed to give a statistically significant result, a minimum of 100,000 cells should be analyzed. Given the analytical rates commonly attained in flow cytometers (1000 to 5000 per second) this analysis would take less than two minutes.

However, as events become more infrequent, that is, in the range of fewer than 1 per 10,000 (rare-event analysis) statistical considerations become more important and the analytical times become more extended. When the expected frequencies are extremely low ($<1/10^6$), it is often impossible to have enough cells to analyze, and a procedure that enriches the cells of interest prior to flow analysis might be required.

The problem of rare-event analysis is one of effectively identifying two cell populations when one is a very minor proportion of the total. The ability to distinguish the two populations is a function of mean intensities (e.g., fluorescence) of the two peaks and their coefficients of variation (CV) (in this context, the CV effectively describes the peak width). Thus, the greater the CVs and the closer the mean intensities of the two peaks, the less likely it is that the minor peak contains only cells of one population, since there may be considerable statistical overlap of the two populations. Computer algorithms have been designed to approximate the degree to which the distributions overlap and to resolve the distributions mathematically. These algorithms may be applied in worst-case situations but are not generally needed.

Rare-event analysis has recently been applied to:

1. detection of somatic mutations, which occur at very low frequencies (<1 per million);
2. detection of fetal cells in the maternal circulation;
3. estimation of the extent of fetal-maternal hemorrhage;

4. estimation of minimal residual disease in cancer patients;
5. estimation of in vivo survival of transfused red cells;
6. detection of chimeras and mosaics; and
7. identification of hemopoietic progenitor cells.

FLOW SORTING

The analytical mode of operation of flow cytometers described in the preceding sections represents one of two ways in which these instruments can be used. The other is flow sorting. In this mode, cell populations can be physically separated and collected according to specific criteria. Any parameter available in the analytical mode of operation can be used as the basis for flow sorting. The details of the separation techniques vary, but the principle is to: 1) identify the cells of choice; 2) isolate them as single cells from others in the population; and 3) collect the isolated cells for further analysis. This must be done with speed and fidelity and the resulting population of cells must be of high (>95%) purity. A schematic representation of a flow-sorting system is shown in Figure 60-5.

In the first step, cells are selected on the basis of combinations of fluorescence, light scattering, or other properties using the analytical procedures described in preceding sections. Once the cell populations have been chosen, they are defined by electronic "gates," which can be created on single or dual-parameter frequency distributions. Two populations may be chosen for sorting at one time.

Once specified, the two populations are separated. This task is accomplished by isolating the cells in microdroplets

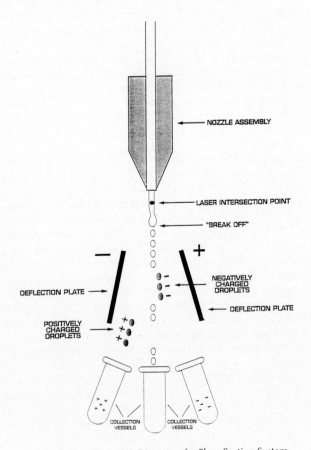

Fig. 60-5 Schematic Diagram of a Flow Sorting System.

of an electrolyte (e.g. sheath fluid), which are not much larger than the cells. These droplets are then induced to move in a defined trajectory to the waiting collection vessels. The first problem is to produce droplets of uniform size. Consider a fluid stream that forms a liquid jet in air as it flows through an orifice of defined size. An observer of this stream would note that at some considerable distance from the orifice, the stream becomes disorganized and finally, under the influence of gravity, disintegrates into droplets that are rather nonuniform in size. However, it was discovered that if the liquid stream is vibrated at high frequency, droplets that are quite uniform in size detach from the stream very close to the orifice, and the cells are entrapped in the droplets at this "break-off" point. Operationally droplets are formed by the activation of an acoustic transducer (i.e., a piezoelectric crystal), which vibrates typically at 25 to 40 kHz (Figures 60-1 and 60-5). Vibration of the nozzle assembly produces droplets of the desired size and at the desired rate.

In most flow cytometers, it takes 25 to 100 μsec. for a cell to travel from the intersection point to the point where it breaks off from the stream in an independent droplet. During this brief time the cells must be analyzed and the populations of choice selected for sorting. An electronic circuit tracks the flight of the selected cell from the intersection point to the break off point. If the cell meets the pre-selected criteria, an instantaneous voltage pulse (e.g., ±5 volts) is applied to the entire nozzle assembly and ultimately to the stream. The timing circuit assures that the charge is applied to the selected cell just as it breaks off of the stream. One of the selected populations is given a positive charge, the other a negative charge. Cells that do not meet the pre-selected criteria are not charged. To increase the probability of the desired cell being collected, it is common practice to charge several drops at a time: for example, the one before the cell of choice, the one containing the cell of choice, and the one after. The applied charge is retained by the droplets containing the cells, first because they are composed of an electrolyte (the sheath fluid) and secondly because the droplets are separated in space. The relatively high electrical resistance of the air inhibits dissipation of the charge, at least during the time of the experiment. Separation of the positively and negatively charged droplets is accomplished as they pass between two deflection plates, set at an angle to the stream. The potential difference across the plates is 200 to 600 volts. Positively charged droplets are deflected slightly toward the negative plate and negatively charged droplets to the positive plate. Uncharged (i.e., unselected) droplets are not deflected and the cells are discarded. The sorted cells are collected in tubes or other vessels placed appropriately in the path of the deflected droplets. Thus, as noted previously, two cell populations can be sorted at once (Figure 60-5). In most cases, sorted cells are collected in test tubes or similar containers and recovered by centrifugation. Other devices permit the deposition of single cells in wells of a microtiter plate for subsequent expansion in cell culture for biochemical or functional analysis.

Cell sorting can be carried out at rates between 1000-10,000 cells per second. The sorting rate depends on the concentration of the cell suspension, the stability of the fluidics system, the rate of droplet generation, the number of droplets charged, the reset time of the analytical circuitry, and proper function of the sort logic. Performed correctly, cell sorting can yield populations more than 95% pure, highly viable and, if desired, sterile.

Ultimately the *rate* at which cells can be sorted may dictate the success of the sort. For example, suppose the cells of choice represent 1% of the total population, and biochemical or other analyses requires 1 million cells (not an uncommon set of circumstances). If one assumes 90% recovery (often a best case result) and 95% purity, it would be necessary to sort about 1.2×10^8 cells to achieve the desired result. At a sort rate of, for example, 2000 cells per second, it would take approximately 16.7 hours to complete the task; at 5000 cells per second, it would take 6.7 hours. This is certainly feasible, but cell viability, instrument stability, operator fatigue, and maintenance of sterility can affect the outcome.

Thus, flow sorting is not always the best first approach to collecting pure populations of cells, especially in cases where large numbers of cells are required. In some cases, enrichment of the desired cells by alternative means (e.g., panning, differential centrifugation, etc.) should be considered.

Good recoveries of sorted cells absolutely depend on the proper adjustment of all flow and electronic parameters, especially droplet generation, charging, and the way cells are handled during and after the sort. Collection medium, collection vessels (e.g., glass or specific plastics), temperature and, viability of the cells over time are important factors. In most cases, only relatively small numbers of cells (perhaps $<10^7$) can be collected efficiently. Cell sorting may be most useful in studies where the sorted cells can be expanded in cell culture for subsequent investigation or to provide the final increment of purification of minor subpopulations that have been enriched by pre-sorting procedures.

APPLICATIONS OF FLOW CYTOMETRY

The number of applications of flow cytometry has multiplied enormously since the technique was introduced in the mid-1960s. Describing all of them in detail is beyond the scope of this discussion. References to appropriate methodologies are in the list of selected readings. Table 60-3 summarizes some of the primary applications of flow cytometry and lists the fluorescent probe(s) typically employed.

Immunophenotyping of human blood cells

One of the principal applications of flow cytometry is the analysis of antigens expressed by human blood cells. This type of analysis has proven tremendously useful in identifying hemopoietic precursor cells, characterizing the stages of differentiation in the hemopoietic system; differentiating normal and abnormal (e.g., leukemic) cells, and classifying and staging hemopoietic disorders.

Leukocyte phenotyping by flow cytometry: definition of normal and abnormal phenotypes in the hemopoietic system

The mammalian hemopoietic system is characterized by a hierarchy of cells that descend from precursor cells in the bone marrow, the hemopoietic stem. All recognizable precursors and terminally differentiated blood cells found in the bone marrow, lymphatic system, and peripheral blood derive from these precursors. A scheme of this hierarchy of cells is illustrated in Figure 60-6. The salient features of this scheme will be described in Chapter 57. However, certain points pertinent to this discussion can be made:

1) Each type of cell in the hemopoietic system can be classified by antigens expressed at different stages of cell differentiation. These antigens may be associated with specific cell lineages (i.e., lymphocytes, granulocytes, monocytes, platelets, red cells, etc.), or they may be expressed on multiple cell lineages.

2) Many antigens that define the various hemopoietic lineages and stages of differentiation have been identified by studies of the interactions of blood cells with specific antibodies. The spectrum of antibody reactivities defines the immunophenotype of the cell. Immunophenotypes have been obtained by immunocytochemistry, immunofluorescence microscopy, and more recently by flow cytometry. In addition, the biochemical properties (e.g., apparent molecular weight, sugar content, etc.) of many differentiation-related antigens have been described. However, quantitating cells with particular antigens or combinations of antigens has been made feasible primarily by flow cytometric techniques. Flow studies have also afforded estimates of the relative number of antigenic sites per cell.

3) Phenotyping of hemopoietic cells became possible during the last 15 years, when methods to produce specific immunological probes were developed. At one point, polyclonal sera derived from immunized humans or animals were the only immunological reagents available for cell surface phenotyping. While many of these antisera displayed remarkable specificity for cellular antigens, several problems became apparent:

1. the immunoglobulins were non-homogeneous in terms of binding affinity;
2. antibody subtypes varied considerably. Many potent antibodies were IgMs and were therefore difficult to use in experimental settings;
3. specific antibodies reactive against single epitopes were difficult to purify from serum, even with the use of affinity chromatographic techniques;
4. sera varied considerably from animal to animal, making it difficult to produce large supplies of consistent, well-characterized reagents; and
5. because the antibodies were difficult to purify, it was generally necessary to use indirect immunofluorescence methods (v. infra), which involved additional procedural steps and which often led to increased levels of nonspecific binding.

4) The production of monoclonal antibodies in vitro by somatic cell hybrids ("hybridomas")—derived from the fusion of splenic B cells from immunized mice or rats and tumor-derived B-lymphoid cell lines—provided the way to prepare a virtually unlimited supply of specific immunological reagents. With diligence it is now possible to prepare immunological reagents reactive with virtually any antigen. Monoclonal antibodies can also be produced on a commercial scale with standardized preparations. After the antibodies are purified, it is possible to prepare directly labeled fluorescent or biotin conjugates for immunophenotyping probes. These reagents resolve most problems associated with polyclonal sera noted previously.

Table 60-3 Applications of flow cytometry

Cellular property	Probe	Application
Cell surface and intracellular antigens	Fluorescent antibody conjugates —FITC, PE, APC, TR1 tandem2, cyanine-labeled antibodies, lectins, ligands —Biotin/avidin system	—Immunophenotyping —Lymphocyte subsets —Leukemia/lymphoma/tumor immunology —Cell differentiation —Hybridoma selection —Oncogene products
DNA/RNA	Propidium iodide Ethidium bromide Acridine orange Hoechst dyes Chromomycin A3 Mithramycin Olivomycin DAPI BrdU/anti-BrdU Oxazines, thiazines Thiazole orange	—Cell cycle analysis —DNA content/ploidy —Tumor biology —Analysis of archived materials —Flow karyotypes —Chromosome isolation —Chromatin structure —Reticulocyte counts
Cell structure and function —Membrane properties	Oxycarbocyanines Merocyanines DPH Propidium iodide Ethidium bromide Fluorescein diacetate Calcifluor white	—Membrane potential —Ion fluxes —Membrane fluidity —Cell viability
—Metabolism	NBT DCFH-DA 4-methyl umbelliferyl, -naphthol, resorufin derivatives o-phthaldialdehyde Anthracyclines Methotrexate derivatives FITC-dextrans Fluorescent microspheres FITC labeled ligands Quin-2 Fura-2 Indo-1 ADB, DCH, BCECF Rhodamine 123	—Enzyme activity —Glutathione metabolism —Drug metabolism —Endocytosis/phagocytosis —Calcium flux —Cell activation —Intracellular pH —Mitochondria, ATP content, general metabolic activity
—Cell Structure	Fluorescein diacetate NBD-phallicidin Nile red Filipin	—Cytoplasmic structure, polarization —Cytoskeleton —Neutral lipids —Cholesterol

(1) Abbreviations used: ABD = 1,4,diacetoxy-2,3-dicyanobenzene; APC = allophycocyanine; BCECF = bis(carboxyethyl)-5,6-carboxyfluorescein; BrdU = bromodeoxy uridine; DAPI = 4'-6-diamino-2-phenylindole; DCH = 2,3-dicyanohydroquinone; DCFH-DA = 2,7-dichlorofluorescein diacetate; DPH = 1,6-diphenyl-1,3,5-hexatriene; NBT = nitro blue tetrazolium; PE = phycoerythrin; TR = Texas Red;
(2) "tandem," refers to chemical conjugates of dyes (e.g. R-phycoerythrin-Texas Red), which are used in three-color fluorescence analyses and work by energy transfer mechanisms.

5) Because monoclonal antibodies are relatively easy to produce, a large number of reagents are available for immunophenotyping applications. Although many of the useful reagents have identical or similar specificities for cells and antigens, they were nonetheless prepared in different ways and generally bear different names. Consequently, it became necessary to classify these regents by specificity and to develop a universal system for naming them. Table 60-4 summarizes the latest attempts of the International Workshop and Conference on Human Leukocyte Differentiation Antigens to classify panels of monoclonal reagents according to cellular and antigenic reactivities. The basis for this classification is the CD (cluster of differentiation) designation. All antibodies that react with cells in standard panels

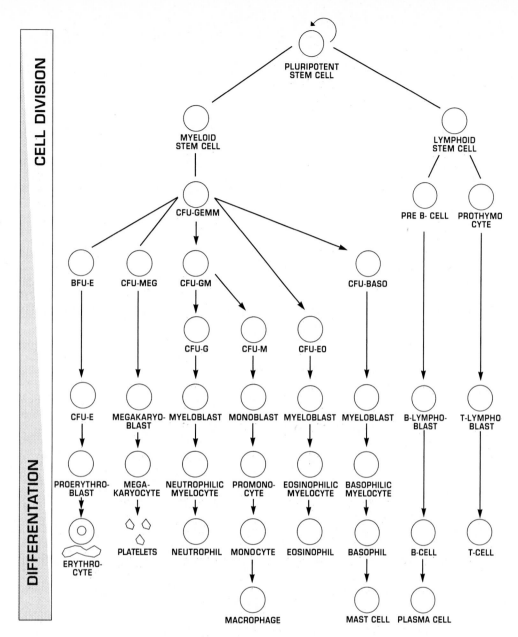

Fig. 60-6   A Model of the Human Hemopoietic System.
Abbreviations used: CFU, colony forming unit; BFU, burst colony forming unit; GEMM, granulocyte erythroid, megakaryocyte. monocyte; Eo, eosinophil; Baso, basophil; Mega, megakaryocyte. As noted in the side panel, as cell division rates decrease, the number of cells in terminally differentiated states increases. The curved arrow associated with the pluripotent stem cell denotes self renewal.

and that identify identical antigens are assigned the same CD number. Monoclonal antibodies, defined by CD designations, are available for the phenotyping of nearly all types of leukocytes. These antibodies are useful in defining cell lineage, the extent of differentiation, and in some cases functional activities.

6) In most cases, abnormal immunophenotypes in the hemopoietic system are defined not by the expression of specific disease-associated antigens, but by the *quantitatively abnormal expression of normal antigens* on a particular cell type or by the appearance of cells bearing specific

markers in compartments in which they are not normally found (e.g., bone marrow precursor cells in the peripheral blood). Immunophenotyping by flow cytometry is proving increasingly useful in diagnostic and prognostic settings. However, flow cytometric data used in clinical contexts should clearly be correlated with all available clinical data, including morphological analysis of the cells. Differing methods of cell preparation, monoclonal antibody specificity, and lack of universally accepted instrumentation standards and controls all contribute to difficulties in the clinical interpretation of flow data.

Table 60-4 Cluster designations for human leukocyte antigens

CD No.	Cell type	Antibodies	Antigen (Mr, KDa)	Comments
CD1a	Thy	Leu-6, OKT6, NA1/34, T6	gp45/12	Langerhans Cells
CD1b	Thy	T6	gp49	Assoc. with B-2 microglobulin
CD1c	Thy	L161, M241, 7C6	gp43	Antigen presentation
CD2	T	Leu-5b, OKT11, 9.6, T11	gp50	E rosette positive
CD2R	Act. T	T11.3, VIT13, D66	gp50	Activated T-cells
CD3	T	Leu4, OKT3, UCHT1, T3	gp19-29	CD3-complex
CD4	T	Leu3, OKT4, OKT4a, T4	gp56	T helper/inducer
CD5	T	Leu1, T1, T101, JML-H5	gp67	Co-mitogen for T-cells
CD6	T	MB06, 12.1, T12	gp100	Unknown function
CD7	T	Leu9, 3A1, WT1	gp41	Immature
CD8	T	Leu2, OKT8, T8	gp32-33	T suppressor/cytotoxic
CD9	M, pre-B, P	BA-2, DU, A11-1	gp24	Many reactive cells
CD10	Pre-B, cALL	J5, BA-3	gp100	Neural endopeptidase
CD11a	Leuk.	LFA-1	p180/95	α-chain
CD11b	M, G	Mac-1, Mo1, OKM1	p160/95	C3Bi receptor
CD11c	M, G	LeuM5, Ki-M1	p150/95	C3Bi receptor(?)
CDw12	M, G	M67	90-120?	Unknown function
CD13	M, G	LeuM7, My7, DU-HL60-4	p130/150	Aminopeptidase N
CD14	M, FDC	LeuM3, MY4, Mo2,	gp55	Induces oxidative burst
CD15	M, G	LeuM1, MCS1, MY1	n/a	X-hapten
CD16	G, NK	Leu11a-c, 3G8, Vep13, L23	p50-60	FcR (low)
CDw17	G	T5A7, GO35, Huylum-13	n/a	Lactosylceramide
CD18	Leuk.	LFA-1	p180/95	B-chain LFA-1; ICAM-1 receptor
CD19	B	B4, HD37, HD237	p90	Inhibits B-cell activation
CD20	B	Leu16, B1	p37/355	B-cell activation; ion transport
CD21	B	HB-5, B2	p140	C3d receptor
CD22	B	Leu14, T015, B3	P135	B-cell activation
CD23	B	BLAST-2, B6	p45	Fc e receptor
CD24	B	BA-1, VIB-E3	p41/38	Some leukemias
CD25	T	2A3, Tac, B1, IL2, 2R1	p55	Activated T cells, IL2-R
CD26	T	TS-145	P120/200	Activated T cells
CD27	T	OKT18a, Ta1	p120	Activated T cells
CD28	T	9.3, Kolt-2	p44	T cell subset
CD29	T	4B4, K20	p135	T cell subset
CD30	T, B	Ki-1, BERH4	gp105	Activated, T and B cells, infectious mononucleosis
CD31	M, G, P	SG134,,TM3	gp130/140	gpIIa
CD32	M, G, P, B	2E1, C1KM5, 1V3	gp40	FcRII
CD33	Myeloid	LeuM9, MY9	gp67	early myeloid, AML, MAP
CD34	Progenitors	HPCA-1, 12-8, B1-C35	gp115	AML, ALL, precursors
CD35	M, G, B, E	CR1, TO5, C3bR	p220	CR1
CD36	M, P	5F1, C1Meg	p85	gpIV
CD37	B	G28-1	gp40-45	Unknown function
CD38	T, PC	Leu17, OKT10, T10	gp45	Activated T
CD39	B, mac	G28-8	p80	Unknown function
CD40	B	G28-5	p50	B cell subset
CD41	P	J15, CLB-thromb-7	gpIIb:120/23 gpIIIa:110	gpIIb/IIIa
CD42a	P	FMC25, BL-H6	gp23	gpIX
CD42b	P	PHN89, AN51	135/25	gpIb
CD43	T, G, E, Br.	Leu22, G10-2	p95	Activation of T, B, M, NK
CD44	T, G, Pre-B	1-173	p65-85	In(a), (b) blood group
CD45	Leuk.	HLE-1, T29/33, LCA	p220-180	T200 family
CD45RA	T	Leu18, 2H4, HB10	p220, 205	T cell subset, T220
CD45RB	B, T, M	PD-7/26/16	220, 205, 190	T200 family

From the Fourth International Workshop and Conference on Human Leucocyte Differentiation Antigens, Leucocyte Typing IV: White Cell Differentiation Antigens, W. Knapp, et al, eds, Oxford University Press, 1989.

B = B cells; T = T cells; G = granulocytes; M = monocytes; Mac = macrophage; P = platelets; E = erythroid cells; NL = reactivity is not lineage specific; NK = natural killer cells; Thy = thymocytes; Leuk = all leukocytes; p(nnn) = protein of apparent molecular weight NNN (reduced); gpNNN = glycoprotein with apparent molecular weight NNN (reduced); n/a = not applicable; Mr + apparent molecular weight; KDa, Kilodaltons.

Table 60-4   Cluster designations for human leukocyte antigens—cont'd

CD No.	Cell type	Antibodies	Antigen (Mr, KDa)	Comments
CD45RO	B, T, M	UCHL1	180	T200 restricted
CD46	Leuk, P	HuLym5, 122-2, J48	p66/56	MCP, fibroblasts
CD47	All cells	BRIC126, BRIC125, CIKM1	p47/52	Rh associated
CD48	Leuk.	WM68, LO-MN25	p41?	PI associated antigens
CDw49b	NL	CLB-thromb/4, Gi14	p167	VLA α-2 (collagen R)
CDw49d	M, T, B	B5G10, HP2/1	p132/25	VLA α-4 (Homing R)
CDw49f	P, Mega	GoH3	p120/30	VLA α-6 (Laminin R)
CDw50	Leuk.	101-1D1, 140-11	p140/108	Unknown function
CD51	NL	13C2, 23C6, NKI-M7	p120/24	VNR α-chain
CDw52	NL	CAMPath-1	p25-30	Cell adhesion molecule
CD53	NL	MEM-1	p32-40	Stim. oxidative burst
CD54	NL	ICAM-1	p85	Cell adhesion molecule
CD55	All hemop. cells	134-30, BRIC110	p70	Decay accelerating factor
CD56	NK, M, NE	MY31, NKH-1	p220/135	Neural cell adhesion
CD57	NK, NL	HNK-1	p110	Unknown function
CD58	Leuk.	LFA-3	p45-46	LFA-3
CD59	Leuk.	MEM-3	p18-20	Inhibits complement membrane attack complex
CDw60	Leuk.	M-T32, M-T41	p120	Ceramide
CD61	Leuk.	Y2/51, VI-PL2	p114	GPIIIa/VNR β-chain
CD62	P (activated)	CLB-thromb/6, RUU.SP1	p150	GMP-140 (PADGEM)
CD63	Leuk.	CLB-gran/12, RUU-SP2.28	p53	Activation
CD64	M	mAb32.3, mAb22	p75	FcIgG Receptor I
CDw65	G, M	VIM2, HE10, CF4, VIM8	n/a	Fucoganglioside
CD66	G	CLBgran/10, YTH71.3	p180-200	Activation
CD67	G	B1 3.9, G10F5	p100	PI linked activation
CD68	Mac	EMB11, Y2/131	p110	Unknown function
CD69	Act, T, B, M, NK	Leu23	p78	Activation marker
CDw70	B, T	Ki-24	unknown	B, T activation, Reed-Sternberg cells
CD71	L-blasts, M, E	OKT9, B3/25	p90	Transferrin receptor
CD72	B	S-HCL-2	p43/39	Increases B-cell proliferation
CD73	B, T subset	1E9.28.1, 7G2.2.11	p69	ecto 5'NT
CD74	B, Mac	LN2, BU43, BU-45	p41, 35, 33	MHC Class II invariant chain
CDw75	B, T subset	LN-1	p53	Mature B
CD76	B, T subset, G	Cris-4	p85/67	Mature B
CD77	B	Gb3	n/a	Globotriaosylganglioside p^k blood group
CDw78	B, Mac	Leu-21	p67	Unknown function

Methodology for immunophenotyping of human leukocytes

Collection and storage of hemopoietic cells for flow cytometry. Phenotyping of human blood cells for flow cytometric analysis requires the preparation of uniform, single-cell suspensions of peripheral blood cells, bone marrow cells, or cells from lymphatic or other tissue.

Blood collected by venipuncture is the primary source of material for leukocyte phenotyping. Blood can be collected in EDTA, heparin, or in acid-citrate-dextrose (ACD solution A). EDTA is the anticoagulant of choice if CBC and differential blood counts are used in conjunction with the flow cytometric measurements. It has been recommended that CBC and differential counts be obtained within six hours of collection if these numbers are used in calculating absolute numbers of cells (v. supra). For most clinically relevant procedures (e.g., lymphocyte subset analysis), blood should be processed as soon after collection as possible. Unseparated blood should be stored at 18 to 22°C for no more than 24 hours. Storage at lower temperatures (e.g., 4°C) could result in selective cell or antigen loss. However, each laboratory must define conditions appropriate to its specific analytical needs.

Preparing leukocytes from peripheral blood for immunophenotyping is straightforward in that the cells are already in suspension in the blood. The most significant problem is the removal of red blood cells which could interfere with the flow cytometric analysis. Because only 0.01% of peripheral blood cells are leukocytes, it is often difficult to resolve leukocytes from red cells by light scattering alone, since the leukocyte population is effectively obscured in such an analysis.

Two techniques, density gradient centrifugation and "whole blood lysis" are typically employed to remove red cells and to prepare cells for flow analysis. In the first method, diluted, anticoagulated whole blood is first carefully layered over a separation medium (e.g., Ficoll-Hypaque) with density adjusted to 1.077 g/ml. The two layers are centrifuged. Cells with buoyant densities greater than 1.077 g/ml sediment to the bottom of the tube. Cells with buoyant densities less than 1.077 g/ml typically collect at the liquid/liquid interface between the separation medium and the plasma. Cells that collect at the bottom of the tube include red blood cells and polymorphonuclear leukocytes. Mononuclear cells (e.g., lymphocytes, monocytes), blasts and precursor cells and nucleated red cells are found in the layer at the interface. Platelets are found in suspension in the plasma layer. The cells at the interface are collected, washed, and re-suspended in appropriate buffers for fluorescence staining. Relatively large volumes (>5 ml) of whole blood are required in this procedure and recoveries of 80%-90% of the peripheral blood mononuclear cells can be obtained.

Other density centrifugation procedures (e.g., Percoll), which employ continuous or discontinuous gradients with precisely adjusted buoyant density levels, are used to prepare highly enriched (>90%) populations of granulocytes, monocytes, and low-density precursor cells for further study. Density centrifugation procedures work most effectively on freshly isolated cells or on cells stored for less than 12 hours at ambient temperatures. Changes in cell density on prolonged storage, or upon refrigeration, alter the distribution of subpopulations of cells within the gradient and may compromise the recovery and viability of the product.

The second procedure, "whole blood lysis," was developed not only to eliminate red cell contamination, but also to provide a rapid means of preparing peripheral blood cells for flow cytometric analysis. This procedure takes advantage of differences in osmotic fragility between red cells and leukocytes. Red cells can be hemolysed under a variety of conditions that leave leukocytes essentially undamaged. In most cases, fluorescent antibody staining is carried out prior to lysis of the red cells. Fluorescently-conjugated antibodies are incubated with a small volume of blood (0.05 to 0.1 ml). The lysing agent (e.g., 0.17 M buffered ammonium chloride, detergents, hypotonic buffers) is added, and after a short incubation, red cell membrane debris and hemoglobin are removed by successive washing by centrifugation. The leukocytes are recovered in the final centrifugation pellet. The success of the whole blood lysis method depends on precise timing and temperature control since, left long enough, all cells in the preparation will be destroyed. The advantages of this method are that all classes of leukocytes are retained in the cell pellet, aged specimens (<24 hours after collection) can be analyzed effectively, small volumes of blood are required, and manipulation of the blood cells is kept to a minimum. One disadvantage of the lysis method is that it requires a chemical step, which might result in the depletion of sensitive cell populations or to the destruction of sensitive antigens.

Preparing hemopoietic cells from bone marrow or lymphatic tissue presents a separate set of problems. Cells from bone marrow aspirates can be prepared for flow cytometry in a manner similar to that described for peripheral blood.

Cellular fractionation on density gradients is often used to selectively enrich for particular subpopulations (e.g., hemopoietic precursors). However, because of the way they are collected, bone marrow aspirates may be significantly "hemo-diluted," i.e., contaminated by peripheral blood. It is important, for purposes of quantitative analyses, to estimate the extent of this contamination. This is less of a problem in the analysis of marrow samples obtained by curettage of marrow directly from samples of bone.

Preparing cells from lymphatic tissue (e.g., lymph nodes), or for that matter, any tissue, tumors, etc., requires dissociation of that tissue to obtain single cell suspensions. To assess the validity of these preparations: a) it must be ascertained, by independent means, that the cells obtained after dissociation of the tissue are representative and that extensive, selective cell loss has not occurred; b) care must be taken to use dissociation conditions that minimize clumping of the cells. Cell aggregates can not pass through the flow cell of the flow cytometer and will clog the system. While it is possible to remove clumps prior to flow analysis by filtration of the preparation through a 50 micron nylon mesh, one must be sure that the filtration does not remove cells of interest; and c) during the dissociation one must be careful to avoid the use of proteolytic or other enzymes that could degrade sensitive cell surface antigens.

Two other aspects of cell preparation must be considered. First, the viability of the cells must be carefully monitored during all phases of the preparation. A disproportionate number (>10%) of dead cells indicates a poor preparation. Dead cells are often nonspecifically, and sometimes rather intensely, stained by fluorescent antibodies and therefore contribute to high rates of false positive results. Some of the most common reasons for excessive cell death are poor laboratory practice (e.g., improperly prepared reagents), adverse storage or handling conditions, and cryopreservation procedures. Estimating the number of dead cells can be done microscopically at several stages during the preparation by trypan blue exclusion or similar methods. Alternatively, estimates may be made by fluorescence techniques and flow cytometry. For example, dead cells are stained by dyes such as ethidium bromide and propidium iodide whereas the dyes are excluded from live cells. Thus dead cells can be excluded from the analysis by gating techniques. The percentage of dead cells can be calculated from the number of ethidium bromide or propidium iodide positive cells, and appropriate arithmetic corrections made. It is good practice to monitor the viability of the cells just prior to analysis.

The second consideration concerns fixation of stained cells. This issue has become more significant since the analysis of retrovirus (e.g., HIV-1) infected lymphocytes has become a routine clinical flow cytometric procedure. It has therefore, become good practice to fix all potentially biohazardous cells prior to analysis. Aerosols produced in the flow cytometer can disperse potentially infectious cells rapidly into the laboratory environment. Fixation must be rapid, irreversible, and must not degrade either cellular antigens or the fluorophors bound to the cell. In general, it is advisable to fix cells only after staining with fluorescent antibodies is complete. Finally, the fixative must not produce fluorescent products that could interfere with the cell analysis (e.g., glutaraldehyde). In most cases, the fixative of choice is formaldehyde or paraformaldehyde.

Fluorescent antibody staining procedures. As noted, immunophenotyping techniques are based on the interaction of specific antibodies with cellular antigens. The application of multiparametric fluorescence analysis has demonstrated clearly that *the immunophenotypes of blood cells can not be assigned on the basis of the reactivity of single antibodies*. This is primarily because antigens/epitopes may be common to several subpopulations of cells or because the specificities of the antibodies used in immunophenotyping are not absolute. Rather, the combination of antigens/epitopes, which are coordinately expressed on the cells, is the critical factor. Multiple antigens may be analyzed through the simultaneous use of at least two antibodies conjugated to different fluorophores.

Two procedures are commonly employed in immunophenotyping, namely, direct and indirect immunofluorescence. The methodologies applied to flow cytometry are essentially the same as those used in microscopy. However, because of the quantitative nature of flow cytometric measurements, careful attention must be paid to:

1. the choice of primary and secondary antibodies;
2. the choice of fluorescent conjugate(s);
3. methods to eliminate nonspecific binding of primary and secondary reagents;
4. appropriate antibody titers; and
5. appropriate control reagents.

Direct immunofluorescence involves a single incubation of the cells with primary antibodies that are directly, chemically conjugated to the fluorophore. This incubation is followed by a series of washes with protein containing buffers to remove nonspecifically bound antibodies. The tightly bound antigen-fluorescent antibody complex marks the cells for subsequent analysis by flow cytometry. Fluorescent conjugates routinely used in these direct-staining procedures are described in Table 60-2. Indirect staining involves at least two steps. The cells are first incubated with a non-fluorescent primary antibody and then with a fluorescently labeled antibody. The second antibody should be species and subtype/isotype specific for the primary antibody. The formation of an antigen-primary antibody-fluorescent secondary antibody "sandwich" marks the cells for subsequent flow cytometric analysis. In both direct and indirect fluorescence techniques, all antibodies must be titrated to assure that they are present at saturating concentrations. *The optimal concentration must be determined by flow cytometry,* since the antibody concentration at which saturation is achieved may be different for the flow measurements than for other procedures (e.g., immunocytochemistry, fluorescent microscopy). For indirect methods, an arbitrary, but relatively high dose of the secondary reagent is chosen and the primary reagent concentration is varied until saturation is reached. A second titration is then performed, in which a saturating dose of the primary reagent is chosen and the secondary antibody is varied until saturation is reached. Thus the optimal dose for each reagent can then be found.

In a variant of the indirect antibody staining procedure, cells are first incubated with primary antibodies that have been chemically conjugated with biotin rather than to a fluorescent probe. In the second step, an incubation is carried out with a fluorescently labeled derivative of avidin or streptavidin. Avidins bind to biotin with extremely high affinity ($K_d \sim 10^{-15}$ M). The binding of the fluorescent avidin derivative marks the cells for subsequent flow cytometric analysis. Because of the very high affinity of avidins for biotinylated molecules, and the high degree to which avidins can be labeled by fluorescent probes, the sensitivity of the method may be enhanced three- to tenfold over the corresponding reactions of fluorescently labeled secondary antibodies.

Cells can also be labeled with fluorescent latex beads (<1 micron diameter) that have been clinically conjugated with specific antibodies. Beads prepared in this way have been shown to bind with relatively high affinity to cells. The advantage of this technique is that the beads can be infused with extremely high concentrations of the fluorophore, thereby enhancing the sensitivity of the measurement. Thus if even a few beads (<10 in some cases) are bound, the cells can be detected. The disadvantage of the method is that only a limited number (perhaps <200) of these relatively large beads can be bound to the surface, making quantitation of the actual number of antigenic sites difficult.

Both direct and indirect immunofluorescence assays can be employed in multiparametric fluorescence analysis, but direct staining is the method of choice. Indirect staining methods can be used if the two (or more) primary antibodies can be distinguished either by subclass (e.g., IgG vs. IgM), isotype (e.g., IgG1 vs. IgG2a), or species in which the antibody was prepared (e.g., mouse vs. goat). If these criteria are met, the primary antibodies may be added simultaneously to the test cells. In the next step, secondary antibodies, specific for the primary reagents, can also be added simultaneously.

Appropriate control samples must be included in the experimental protocol to complement the analyses of the test samples. These should provide quality-control checks for instrument performance, for the staining methodology, and for the quality of the reagents. The controls should also compensate for cellular autofluorescence and for the nonspecific binding of primary or secondary antibodies.

At the time of this writing, there are no universally accepted standards for the performance of immunophenotyping by flow cytometry. This is true for instrumentation, antibodies, controls or quality control procedures. Guidelines have been suggested by the National Committee for Clinical Laboratory Standards (NCCLS) and several regulatory bodies (e.g., ASTPHLD, College of American Pathologists, local departments of health).

While universally acceptable panels of instrumentation quality control standards have not been clearly defined for flow cytometers, instrument performance should be monitored daily using an internally consistent quality-control regime. Quality-control procedures should assure that the instrument is optically aligned and electronic calibrations are optimized. These checks on the system operation are most effectively done with a non-biological preparation, typically plastic microbeads, which have specific, stable fluorescence and light-scattering properties.

A biological control (usually a sample of "normal" blood cells) should also be analyzed to ensure the integrity of the staining method and the reagents. A cell with known antibody reactivities should be tested daily against the panel of reagents usually employed in the laboratory and "normal" ranges established. In effect, this procedure provides a positive control value that can be monitored daily. This protocol is most valuable in clinical settings where standard analyses are carried out, it has less value in research settings where new reagents or unknown cell types are being evaluated. Considerable controversy exists over the nature of this positive control specimen. Guidelines noted earlier may provide the basis for more uniformity in clinical laboratory practice.

In terms of test-result interpretation the most important experimental controls are the negative controls. For these, a nonreactive antibody is incubated with the test cells, and the amount of residual, nonspecific fluorescence is measured in the flow cytometer. The fluorescence intensity of the control specimen can then be compared to the reactivity of the test antibody and the number of antibody positive cells can be calculated. In addition, the mean fluorescence intensity of the negative control is a scalar for the fluorescence intensity of the test sample and can thus provide a semi-quantitative estimate of the relative—but not the absolute—number of antibody binding sites.

In direct fluorescence methods, the nonreactive, control antibody may be a fluorescent conjugate of an immunoglobulin known not to react with the cells under study. In some cases, this may be a myeloma protein obtained from cultured hybridoma cells. In the best case, the control reagent should be of the same isotype as the test reagent. In indirect immunofluorescence assays, the control reagent should be a nonreactive antibody that is species, subclass, or isotype matched with the primary reagent. After incubation of the control antibody with the cells, a titrated dose of the secondary, fluorescent antibody is added. Flow analysis can then take place. In multiparameter fluorescence analyses, control antibodies which match each of the test antibodies are required. For direct multiparameter fluorescence analysis, a separate control antibody is required for each fluorophore. In experiments in which the biotin-avidin system is used, the non-biotinylated derivative of the first antibody should be employed as the control. In all of the cases cited, the concentration of the control antibody should match that of the optimal dose of the test antibody as determined by titration.

Fluorescent antibody staining procedures—intracellular staining. In addition to the cell surface phenotyping discussed in the preceding sections, it is often possible to use flow cytometry to classify cells by the presence or absence of cytoplasmic or nuclear antigens. It is necessary to render the cells permeable to antibodies so that they can react with the intra-cellular antigens. This can be accomplished by treating the cells with alcohols, acetone, or low concentrations ($<0.1\%$ w/v) of non-ionic detergents (e.g., Nonidet P-40). The treatment used to permeabilize the cells must not significantly destroy the antigen(s) of interest. Fluorescent antibody staining protocols similar to those described previously can then be employed.

The analysis of red cells by flow cytometry

It is ironic, perhaps, that the red cell—the most extensively studied cell of biochemistry and immunology, and the most widely analyzed and utilized cell of medical practice—has been largely overlooked in applications of flow cytometry. In routine practice, red cells are generally analyzed by differential hemagglutination reactions. These tests are based on Landsteiner's work in the early part of the century and on the work of Ashby and Coombs. Despite the sensitivity of hemagglutination tests, they are semi-quantitative and somewhat subjective. More quantitative approaches to red cell analysis, such as enzyme-linked immunoassays, are effective, but generate a new set of problems (e.g., lower sensitivity, nonspecific reactions). While serological techniques are still the methods of choice in most clinical applications involving analysis of red blood cells, flow cytometry brings a new quantitative dimension to the characterization and enumeration of red cell populations. Flow cytometric methods have several advantages over conventional serological procedures:

1. flow techniques are less subject to error than are manual, labor-intensive analyses of mixed-field agglutination, especially when the enumeration of small populations is required;
2. in flow techniques, red cell populations can be phenotyped definitively and the number of antigenic sites estimated by monitoring the binding of antibodies to single cells; and
3. flow analysis affords the opportunity to study two or more phenotypes simultaneously by means of multiparameter fluorescence analysis.

Analytical methods for red cells

The same serological reagents used in traditional immunohematology can be used in flow cytometry. These reagents include polyclonal human antisera derived from immunized individuals as well as murine and human monoclonal antibodies. The activity of these reagents in direct or indirect agglutination tests is not necessarily the best index of potency in immunofluorescence assays. Frequently, the agglutination titer of a particular serum or monoclonal antibody is ten- to 100-fold higher than the "fluorescence" titer of the same reagent determined in flow experiments. The

---

Box 60-1 Clinical applications of flow cytometric analysis of red blood cells

INDUCED MOSAICISM

Fetal-maternal hemorrhage
Quantitation of immunoglobulin bound to red cells
Estimation of red cells survival in vivo

GENETIC MOSAICISM AND CHIMERISM

Identification of mosaic blood types in female carriers of X-linked disorders
Analysis of red cell somatic variants; calculation of mutation frequencies
Measurement of gene dosage effects

HEMATOLOGY

Reticulocyte counts
Measurement of levels of parasitemia

discrepancy between hemagglutination and fluorescence results can be accounted for, in part, by cell surface phenomena. Most blood group antigens are present in fairly high copy number per cell (e.g., ABO, ~10^6 per cell). Agglutination induced by anti-blood group IgMs, for example, may require as few as 50 to 500 binding sites per cell; IgGs may require more sites. Since most commercial flow cytometers detect 2000 to 5000 fluorescein molecules per cell, flow measurements should, in principle, be nearly as sensitive as agglutination reactions. However, agglutination is cooperative and is potentiated by processes that have minimal effects on the equilibrium binding constant of fluorescent antibody conjugates. Consequently, at concentrations of fluorescent antibody that permit the detection of red cell antigens, agglutination may have already occurred, making flow determinations impossible. This problem may be bypassed by fixation procedures that reduce agglutinability of the red cells. Fluorescent antibody staining of red cells can then be performed by standard direct or indirect immunofluorescence techniques.

Clinical applications of red cell analysis

Flow cytometry has been used increasingly in the analysis of red cells in particular clinical settings and especially in rare-event analysis. The analysis of red cells by flow cytometry is concerned primarily with identifying and enumerating two or more phenotypically distinct red cell populations that coexist in the circulation. In classical serological tests, multiple populations of red cells of different phenotypes are often revealed as mixtures of agglutinated and non-agglutinated cells—so-called mixed field agglutination. In flow measurements, multiple phenotypes are detected as distinct antibody positive and negative populations in fluorescence-intensity histograms. The use of flow cytometry is indicated especially in those instances where the population of interest is minute (e.g. < 1/100) and where

analysis of these rare events is difficult by conventional tests. A summary of these applications is provided in Box 60-1.

Flow cytometric techniques applied to analysis of red cells are not only useful adjuncts to classical serological methods, but they provide unique, quantitative information unobtainable by antiglobulin tests. This is most apparent in measurements of red cell blood group antigen density, the quantitation of antibody bound to red cells, the characterization of phenotypic heterogeneities in normal and pathological red cell populations, and in analysis of rare events. It is clear that the development of more automated, clinically-oriented instruments and software, new probes of cellular structure and function, and new quantitative tests will not only accelerate acceptance of flow techniques as valid methods for the analysis of red cells but will also broaden the scope of clinical and basic investigations.

SUGGESTED READING

Darzynkiewicz Z and Crissman HA, ed: Flow Cytometry, methods in cell biology vol 33, New York, 1991, American Press.

Harlow E and Lane D: Antibodies: a laboratory manual, Cold Spring Harbor, NY, 1988, Cold Spring Harbor Laboratory.

Knapp W, Dorken B, Gilks, et al, eds: Leucocyte typing IV: white cell differentiation antigens, Oxford, 1989, Oxford University Press. Also see, Leucocyte typing database IV, compiled by WR Gilks.

Landay A, Auer R, Duque R, et al: Clinical applications of flow cytometry: quality assurance and immunophenotyping of peripheral blood lymphocytes, document H42-P, vol 9, Number 13, Villanova, Penn, 1989, National Committee for Clinical Laboratory Standards.

Lillie RD, ed: HJ Conn's biological stains, ed 9, Baltimore, 1977, Williams and Wilkins.

Shapiro HM: Practical flow cytometry, ed 2, New York, 1988, Alan R Liss.

Van Dilla MA, Dean PM, Laerum OD, Melamed MR: Flow cytometry: instrumentation and data analysis, Orlando, Fla, 1985, Academic Press.

61

Laboratory diagnosis of erythroid disorders

Robert F. Reiss

CLASSIFICATION AND EVALUATION OF ANEMIAS

The basic parameters for measuring the adequacy of erythroid cell content in the peripheral blood are the red cell count, the concentration of hemoglobin in the blood, and the hematocrit. The reference mean values for these parameters vary with age and sex and are listed in Table 61-1. Anemia is the condition that exists when the hemoglobin concentration and/or hematocrit falls below 2SD of these mean values, assuming that the plasma volume is not increased as in some physiological conditions (e.g., pregnancy).

Approach to laboratory evaluation of anemia

Evaluating a patient for anemia begins with determining the red cell count, hematocrit, and hemoglobin determination, together with the preparation and examination of a peripheral smear. The mechanism by which the hemoglobin concentration or hematocrit can fall may be related to a decrease in the red cell count, the presence of poorly hemoglobinized red cells, the production of small red cells, or a combination of these factors. As previously discussed, calculation of the red cell indices permits the investigator to define the interrelationships of these factors, and therefore the mechanism by which the hemoglobin concentration or hematocrit has decreased (Table 61-1). Since the red cell indices are mean values, the smear is examined to see if there is one population of cells or if the values obtained reflect the mean of different sizes (anisocytosis) and degrees of hemoglobinization. (Similar information regarding variation in size is furnished by the histogram calculated and displayed by the current generation cell counters). Examining the peripheral smear is required to show marked variations in red cell morphology (poikilocytosis), diagnostically characteristic red cells (e.g., sickle cells, spherocytes, etc.), types of white cells, and platelet quantity, which are suggestive or diagnostic of a given disease. Finally, although the presence of polychromasia suggests the early release of reticulocytes from the bone marrow, a reticulocyte count should always be determined in order to adequately estimate effective marrow erythropoietic activity, as will be discussed.

The quantification of total erythroid activity in the marrow is established by examining a bone marrow biopsy and smear. Such examination, however, does not reflect the quantity of erythroid cells developing into normal mature red cells (effective erythropoiesis) as opposed to the production of increased ($>10\%$) numbers of cells that die within the marrow (ineffective erythropoiesis). The reticulocyte production index is the calculation that allows the determination of effective erythroid activity by quantifying the number of reticulocytes delivered to the periphery. As previously discussed, under stable situations, and at normal hematocrit levels, the life span of a reticulocyte in the peripheral blood is one day and the life span of the red cell 120 days; therefore the reticulocyte count in the peripheral blood is about 1%. An increased percent of reticulocytes would be expected to reflect increased erythropoiesis, but the reticulocyte count alone tends to overestimate the effective erythropoiesis because: 1) as a percentage it is also raised if the number of red cells are reduced and 2) as the number of red cells or hemoglobin concentration falls, the life span of the reticulocytes in the peripheral blood increases due to the earlier release of these cells from the marrow. Calculation of the corrected reticulocyte count (multiplying the observed count by the observed hematocrit, divided by 45) is therefore considered by some to still overestimate the true rate of reticulocytes production and release. As a rule, the peripheral life span increases by a half-day for every 10% decrease in the hematocrit from a normal of 45 (e.g., at a hematocrit of 25, the life span is two days). To adjust for the prolonged peripheral maturation time, the corrected reticulocyte count is divided by the maturation time, which is measured in days. The resultant value is known as the reticulocyte production index: Corrected reticulocyte count $\div$ maturation time in days = reticulocyte index.

In the presence of a reticulocyte index less than three, the bone marrow does not usually need to be examined since it would be anticipated that erythroid hyperplasia would be found. In such cases, anemia is due to the premature peripheral destruction of red cells and the next diagnostic measures would be directed toward eliciting an exact cause of such destruction. If the reticulocyte index is less than two, and often, if it is between two and three, a bone marrow biopsy and aspirate smear may be performed to assess marrow cellularity, M:E ratio, cytologic characteristics of the hemopoietic cells, iron stores, and presence or absence of

Table 61-1 Normal values for the red blood cell compartment of "apparently healthy" subjects, White and Black*

Subjects	HGB (Gm/dl)	RBC (millions/mm³†)	HCT (%)	MCV (fl‡)	MCH (pg§)	MCHC (%)
Adult men	15.1 (13.9-16.3)	5.1 (4.3-5.9)	47 (39-55)	90 (80-100)	30 (25.4-34.6)	34 (31-37)
Adult women	13.5 (12.0-15.0)	4.5 (3.5-5.5)	42 (36-48)	88 (79-98)	30 (25.4-34.6)	33 (30-36)
Boys						
Birth	20.0 (18.5-21.5)	5.6 (5.0-6.3)	59 (53-65)	105 (95-115)	36 (30-42)	33 (32-34)
1 month	17.0 (15.5-18.5)	5.2 (4.7-5.9)	50 (44-56)	101 (92-110)	36 (30-42)	32 (31-33)
3 months	15.0 (13.5-16.5)	4.5 (3.8-5.2)	45 (39-52)	100 (92-110)	33 (28-38)	33 (32-34)
6 months	14.0 (13.0-16.0)	4.6 (3.8-5.1)	46 (39-51)	100 (92-109)	30 (27-34)	30 (29-31)
9 months	13.0 (12.0-14.0)	4.6 (3.7-5.2)	45 (39-52)	97 (90-104)	28 (24-32)	28 (27-30)
1 year	12.1 (10.0-14.0)	4.2 (3.5-4.9)	41 (37-45)	95 (87-98)	27 (24-32)	29 (28-30)
2 years	12.3 (10.5-14.2)	4.2 (3.5-5.9)	40 (36-47)	88 (80-95)	28 (24-32)	30 (28-31)
4 years	12.6 (11.2-14.3)	4.2 (3.7-5.0)	37 (30-44)	89 (80-96)	28 (24-32)	28 (27-29)
8 years	13.4 (12.0-14.8)	4.6 (4.0-5.1)	41 (37-45)	87 (80-94)	29 (23-34)	29 (28-30)
14 years	14.0 (12.5-15.0)	4.7 (3.9-5.3)	41 (36-46)	88 (80-95)	29 (23-34)	30 (29-31)
Girls						
Birth	19.5 (18.0-21.0)	5.6 (5.0-6.3)	58 (51-65)	103 (94-114)	34 (28-40)	34 (33-35)
1 month	17.0 (15.8-18.9)	5.2 (4.7-6.0)	49 (42-56)	102 (92-112)	36 (30-42)	32 (31-33)
3 months	14.8 (13.3-16.4)	4.4 (3.8-5.2)	44 (39-51)	104 (92-112)	33 (27-39)	33 (32-34)
6 months	13.8 (12.8-14.8)	4.2 (3.5-4.9)	44 (39-50)	100 (91-109)	30 (25-35)	32 (31-33)
9 months	12.8 (11.7-13.9)	4.2 (3.5-4.9)	43 (37-50)	98 (90-105)	28 (23-34)	30 (29-31)
1 year	12.2 (10.0-14.0)	4.2 (3.4-5.0)	43 (37-49)	95 (87-100)	27 (22-30)	30 (29-31)
2 years	12.2 (10.5-14.2)	4.2 (3.5-5.0)	43 (36-50)	94 (86-101)	27 (22-30)	30 (29-31)
4 years	12.7 (11.3-14.2)	4.4 (3.8-5.2)	43 (36-51)	88 (80-95)	28 (23-31)	28 (27-29)
8 years	13.0 (11.5-14.5)	4.5 (3.9-5.1)	40 (36-46)	89 (80-96)	29 (23-33)	28 (27-29)
14 years	13.2 (11.6-14.8)	4.5 (3.8-5.2)	40 (36-47)	87 (80-94)	29 (23-33)	29 (28-30)

From Miale JB: Laboratory medicine: hematology, ed 6, St. Louis, 1982, Mosby-Year Book, Inc.
*Values represent the mean and 95% range. Data from Coulter S or Hemac cell counters.
†To convert to SI units: millions × $10^{12}/1$.
‡fl is new symbol for cubic microns (μ^3).
§pg is new symbol for micromicrograms ($\mu\mu$g). To convert to SI units (fmol): pg × 0.0155.

extrinsic cellular infiltrates. This examination, along with specific laboratory tests, is usually able to separate anemias due to decreased erythropoesis from those due to ineffective erythropoiesis.

The quantification of peripheral red cell life span and subsequent destruction (hemolysis) is most commonly determined by a red cell survival study. Usually, this test is performed on a mixed population of autologous cells from the peripheral blood by isotopic techniques (Chapter 59). The normal T ½ of ^{51}Cr tagged red cells is approximately 25 to 35 days. The survival of a mixed aliquot of homologous cells can be measured by similar isotopic methods. Of historical interest are methods for measuring homologous cell survival by the Ashby technique, in which the persistence of red cells bearing antigens not possessed by the propositus can be directly measured by classical red cell agglutination techniques.

Increased hemolysis of red cells is accompanied by the accumulation and excretion of large quantities of the products of hemoglobin catabolism as well as a fall in the serum levels of various hemoglobin binding proteins, as will be extensively discussed later in this chapter.

Classification of anemia

Classification may be based on either the morphological characteristics of the red cells or the pathogenesis of the anemia.

Morphological classification

According to this classification, the red cell indices classify the anemias into general groups and distinctive morphologic characteristics (e.g., sickle cells) further assist in classification (Box 61-1). The major groupings are as follows:

a) Normocytic, Normochromic Anemias (normal MCV and normal MCHC)
b) Microcytic, Hypochromic Anemias (decreased MCV and decreased MCHC)
c) Macrocytic, Normochromic Anemias (increased MCV and normal MCHC)

Classification by pathogenic mechanism

According to this system, the presence or absence of effective hematopoiesis is assessed and, on this basis, the anemias are divided into hypoproliferative anemias and hemolytic anemias (Box 61-2). This assessment is primarily done by the determination of the reticulocyte index (<2 or >3) and when this determination is inconclusive by bone marrow examination or other laboratory studies. The hypoproliferative anemias are further divided by the cytological characteristics of maturation as determined by examination of the peripheral smear and bone marrow smear into those with synchronous maturation and those with asynchronous maturation. The anemia of acute blood loss is not appropriately classified under this system and is listed separately.

Box 61-1   Morphologic classification of anemia

I. NORMOCYTIC-NORMOCHROMIC ANEMIAS

A. Acute bleeding
B. Hemolytic anemias
   Extracorpuscular
      Immune
      Non-immune
   Intracorpuscular
      Membrane
      Metabolic
      Hemoglobinopathies
C. Marrow Failure
   Aplastic anemia
   Pure red cell aplasia
   Anemia of chronic disease
   Anemia of renal failure
   Anemia of endocrine disorder
   Myelophthisic anemia

II. MICROCYTIC HYPOCHROMIC ANEMIAS

A. Iron deficiency
B. Sideroblastic anemias
   Refractory
   Reversible
   Pyridoxine responsive
C. Thalassemias

III. MACROCYTIC-NORMOCHROMIC ANEMIAS

A. Megaloblastic anemia
   Vitamin B_{12} deficiency
   Folate deficiency
   Others
B. Non-megaloblastic macrocytic anemias

Box 61-2   Pathogenic classification of anemias

I. HYPOPROLIFERATIVE ANEMIAS (RI <2)

A. Synchronous maturation
   1. Decreased erythropoetin production or demand
      a) Anemia of renal disease
      b) Anemia of endocrine disorders
      c) Anemia due to Hb with decreased O_2 affinity
   2. Marrow failure
      a) Aplastic anemia
      b) Pure red cell aplasia
      c) Myelophthisic anemia
B. Asynchronous maturation
   1. Decreased hemoglobin synthesis
      a) Decreased iron incorporation
         Iron deficiency anemia
         Anemia of chronic disease
      b) Decreased globin synthesis
         α Thalassemia
         β Thalassemia
         Other thalassemias
      c) Decreased porphyrin synthesis
         (Sideroblastic anemias)
   2. Abnormal nuclear development
      a) Megaloblastic anemias
         Vitamin B_{12} deficiency
         Folate deficiency
         Others

II. HYPERPROLIFERATIVE (HEMOLYTIC) ANEMIAS (RI >3)

A. Extracorpuscular
   1. Immune
   2. Non-immune
B. Intracorpuscular
   1. Membrane abnormalities
   2. Metabolic abnormalities
   3. Hemoglobinopathic abnormalities

III. ACUTE BLOOD LOSS

ANEMIA OF ACUTE BLOOD LOSS

With modest hemorrhage, cardio-circulatory changes compensate for the slightly reduced blood volume and maintain adequate perfusion and oxygen transport to the peripheral organs. With more severe hemorrhage, the body is threatened by loss of blood volume resulting in shock. In such cases the hematocrit may be normal for several hours. The subsequent fall in hematocrit is evident as hemodilution from mobilized extravascular fluids occurs. The full extent of red cell deficit may not be evident for one to two days. The resultant anemia is normochromic and normocytic. After hemorrhage the rate of recovery of red cell mass depends on the iron stores available. In individuals with available iron stores, a reticulocytosis is noted after six to 10 days. Continued bleeding results in a depletion of iron stores leading to a hypoproliferative anemia.

THE HYPOPROLIFERATIVE ANEMIAS

As previously discussed, the hypoproliferative anemias are defined for our purposes as those characterized by deficient effective erythropoiesis (reticulocyte index <2). Some may be characterized by marrow erythroid hypoplasia, while others are associated with erythroid hyperplasia. Peripherally, some may also have shortened red cell survival, but the anemias are classified with the hypoproliferative rather than the hemolytic anemias because the primary defect, as judged by the reticulocyte index, is deficient effective erythropoiesis.

Aplastic anemia

Aplastic anemia is characterized by the loss of all hemopoietic elements from the marrow, resulting in a normocytic, normochromic anemia and pancytopenia, which in severe cases presents with a markedly decreased corrected reticulocyte count (<1%), as well as neutropenia (<500/mm^3) and thrombocytopenia (usually <20,000/mm^3), resulting in susceptibility to infection and hemorrhage.

Congenital aplasias as an isolated defect or associated with other developmental anomalies (Fanconi's Anemia and Dyskeratosis Congenita), arise within the first ten years of life. Acquired cases may arise after infections (miliary tuberculosis and more commonly, hepatitis B and C), following radiation, or after drug ingestion (Box 61-3). Patients who are treated with chloramphenicol undergo a reversible myelosuppression, the severity of which is dose related. Rare patients (1:30,000) undergo a nonreversible severe hypoplasia, which is not dose related ("hypersensitivity").

Several mechanisms may be operative in the pathogenesis

Box 61-3   Some drugs implicated in hemopoietic suppression*

Acetophenetidin (1, 3)	Cycloheximide (3)	Para-aminosalicylic acid (3, 4)
Acetylsalicylic acid (aspirin)	Dextromethorphan HBr (2)	Penicillin (1, 2, 3, 4)
(1, 2, 3)	Diethylstilbestrol (2)	Phenobarbital (1, 2, 3, 4)
Acetyl sulfisoxazole (3)	Phenytoin (Dilantin) (4)	Phenylbutazone (Butazolidin)
Aminosalicylic acid (3, 4)	Dipyrrone (3)	(1, 2, 3)
Ammonium thioglycolate (3)	Ethinamate (2)	Primidone (1)
Amodiaquin HCl (3)	Fumagillin (3)	Prochlorperazine (Compazine) (2, 3)
Arsenicals (1, 2, 3, 4)	γ-Benzene hexachloride (1, 3)	Pyrimethamine (Daraprim) (1, 2, 3)
Arsphenamine (1, 2)	Hair lacquer (3)	Quinidine (2)
Atabrine (1, 2)	Imipramine HCl (3)	Quinine (2, 3)
β-Naphthoxyacetic acid (2)	Iproniazid (1)	Reserpine (2)
Benzene (1, 2, 3, 4)	Isoniazid (1, 3, 4)	Stibophen (2)
Bishydroxycoumarin (3, 4)	Lead (1)	Streptomycin (1, 2, 3)
Carbamide (2)	Lithium carbonate (1)	Sulfamethoxypyridazine (Kynex)
Carbon tetrachloride (1)	Mephenytoin (Mesantoin) (1, 2)	(2, 3, 4)
Carbutamide (Orabetic) (2)	Meprobamate (1, 2, 3)	Tetracycline (3)
Chloramphenicol (1, 2, 3, 4)	Methaminodiazepoxide (Librium)	Thenalidine tartrate (3)
Chlordane (1)	(3)	Thioridazine HCl (3)
Chlorophenothane (DDT) (1, 2)	Methapyrilene HCl (4)	Tolazoline HCl (1, 2)
Chlorothiazide (3)	Methylpromazine (3)	Tolbutamide (1, 2, 3)
Chlorpheniramine maleate (3)	Mezapine (2)	Tolbutamide (Orinase) (2)
Chlopromazine (Thorazine) (3)	Nitrofurantoin (4)	Trifluoperazine (1, 3)
Chlorpropamide (2)	Novobiocin (4)	Trifluoperazine (Stelazine) (3)
Chlortetracycline (1, 3)	Nystatin (2)	Trimethadione (Tridione) (1, 2)
Cinophen (3)	Oxyphenabutazone (2)	
Coldricine (2, 3)		

From Miale JB: Laboratory medicine: hematology, ed 6, St. Louis, 1982, Mosby-Year Book, Inc.
*More than 500 are listed in the last report of the American Medical Association Subcommittee on Blood Dyscrasias. The drugs listed in this table are those which when given alone have been implicated in the production of dyscrasias. Most reports are of isolated cases with no firm evidence other than clinical experience. 1 = pancytopenia; 2 = thrombocytopenia; 3 = leukopenia; 4 = anemia.

of the acquired forms of aplastic anemia. Those which appear secondary to the action of defined myelotoxins commonly are caused by defective stem cell proliferation resulting in absent production of differentiating elements. Less frequently, a disturbance in the marrow microenvironment or immunologic suppression of stem cell differentiation is responsible for the aplasia.

The diagnosis is made by examining the bone marrow biopsy, which shows replacement of the marrow by fat (Figure 61-1). In cases of rapid loss of hematopoetic tissue, the void is not as quickly filled with fat, but contains a gelatinous material. Patients with early Fanconi's Anemia may show pancytopenia and reticulocytopenia with mild erythroid hyperplasia and dyserythropoesis of the bone marrow. With progression, however, they too develop an empty marrow. In addition, patients with chloramphenicol induced aplasia may show vacuolization of the residual hematopoietic precursors (Figure 61-2).

The serum iron levels are elevated, and, as will be discussed, ferrokinetic studies reveal prolonged clearance of ^{59}Fe from the plasma and markedly decreased uptake into the red cells. In patients with Fanconi's Anemia and others with congenital pancytopenia, increased chromosome breaks can be detected. Most patients with aplastic anemia have a marked increase in hemoglobin F levels. Some patients show associated paroxysmal nocturnal hemoglobinuria (PNH) defects, while others develop acute myelogenous leukemia.

The prognosis of congenital and acquired idiopathic and post infectious cases of aplastic anemia is poor—only 25%

surviving five years. Many patients develop transfusion hemosiderosis during the course of their disease. Death is usually related to infection or hemorrhage.

Pure red cell aplasia

Selective hypoplasia of red cell precursors may be seen on a congenital basis (Diamond-Blackfan syndrome) or after exposure to the various etiologic agents described under aplastic anemia. Idiopathic cases in women are often associated with thymomas, while most men with red cell aplasia do not have these tumors. A special type of red cell aplasia is the transitory aplastic crisis that sometimes occurs in the course of congenital hemolytic anemias. These crises often occur after intercurrent viral infections (most commonly parvovirus). The most common form of acquired red cell aplasia in children is known as Transient Erythroblastopenia of Childhood. It occurs in early childhood, lasts several weeks, spontaneously resolves, and is associated with IgG suppression of CFU-E and BFU-E activity. As with aplastic anemias, the red cells are normochromic and normocytic. The diagnosis is confirmed by the bone marrow examination, which shows a selective loss of erythroid precursors. The congenital cases may have elevated levels of fetal hemoglobin and increased expression of the "i" antigen, while acquired cases lack these features.

Congenital dyserythropoietic anemias

The congenital dyserythropoietic anemias (CDA) are a rare group of hereditary hypoplastic anemias characterized by

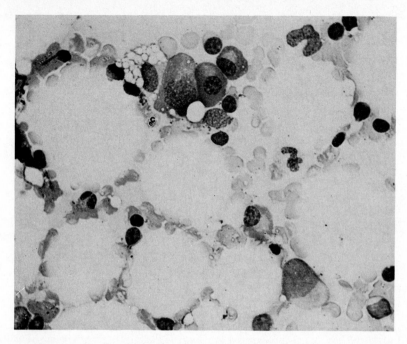

Fig. 61-1   Bone marrow aspirate, aplastic anemia. Residual cells consist mainly of lymphocytes, plasma cells, and histiocytes. *From Sonnenwirth AC and Jarett L: Gradwohl's clinical laboratory methods and diagnosis, vol 1, ed 8, St. Louis, 1980, Mosby–Year Book, Inc.*

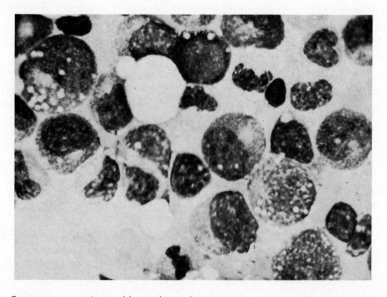

Fig. 61-2   Bone marrow aspirate, chloramphenicol toxicity. Hemopoetic cells are heavily vaculated. *From Sonnenwirth AC and Jarett L: Gradwohl's clinical laboratory methods and diagnosis, vol 1, ed 8, St. Louis, 1980, Mosby–Year Book, Inc.*

ineffective erythropoiesis and morphologically abnormal red cell differentiation (dyserythropoiesis). They are characterized by variable anemia, a low reticulocyte index, erythroid hyperplasia of the marrow, and splenomegaly. Peripheral cell survival is variably decreased and laboratory studies reflect this hemolysis. Iron stores are increased. If performed, ferrokinetic studies indicate increased PITR and decreased red cell iron reutilization.

This group of anemias has been classified on the basis of their morphological, serological, and clinical characteristics into three principle types.

Type I CDA is characterized by moderate macrocytic anemia occuring in infancy or adolescence and is inherited as an autosomal recessive trait. The red cell precursors are very large, many are binucleate, and show the stigmata of megaloblastic maturation, which will be described later in this chapter.

The most common type of anemia is Type II CDA, which in some patients arises in infancy and may be severe. It is inherited as an autosomal recessive trait. The anemia is generally normochromic and is characterized by marked aniso- and poikilocytosis. Numerous erythroid precursors are multinucleate. The red cells continue to express increased quantities of "i" antigen and increased amounts of fetal hemoglobin (HbF). They also demonstrate increased complement-mediated hemolysis when exposed to acidified serum, similar to cells from patients with paroxysmal nocturnal hemoglobinuria (PNH). Importantly, however, in this connection, the hemolysis follows the fixation of complement by the classical pathway resulting from the sensitization of red cells by antibodies directed against antigenic sites on the cells while fixation to PNH cells occurs via the alternate pathway, as will be discussed later in this chapter. Because of these features, cells belonging to type II PDA are also known as HEMPAS cells. (Hereditary Erythroid Multinuclearity with a Positive Acidified Serum test).

Type III CDA is the rarest syndrome and is characterized by the presence of giant multinucleated erythroblasts in the marrow, giant erythrocytes in the peripheral blood and prominent basophilic stippling. The few cases described have had negative acidified serum tests. Transmission seems to be as an autosomal-dominant trait.

Myelophthisic anemias

These anemias result from marrow replacement or infiltration by nonhemopoietic tissue or hemopoietic tumor. A normocytic, normochromic anemia results with neutropenia and thrombocytopenia. Examination of the peripheral blood smear reveals polychromasia and poikilocytosis with typical teardrop-shaped cells. Nucleated red cells and immature granulocytes are present (leukoerythroblastic picture). Many of the platelets seen are very large ("giant platelets") (Figure 61-3).

Anemias associated with decreased erythropoietin production

These anemias are commonly normocytic and normochromic and are associated with reticulocytopenia and a mild decrease in the quantity of erythroid precursors in the marrow. The decreased production may result from renal pa-

renchymal disease; decreased O_2 consumption by tissues in cases of endocrine dysfunction (hypopituitarism or hypothyroidism); or lastly, the maintenance of constant O_2 delivery in the face of decreased hemoglobin levels when the abnormal hemoglobin involved has decreased oxygen affinity.

The most frequent is the anemia of renal failure, a complex disorder. Besides its predominant cause (decreased erythropoietic production), decreased cell survival, decreased iron utilization, and microscopic blood loss through the gastrointestinal tract may also play roles in the pathogenesis of the anemia of renal failure.

Anemias associated with abnormal heme synthesis

Hemoglobin is synthesized in the cytoplasm of the developing red cells from two basic units: heme moieties and globin chains. Synthesis of the globin chains will be discussed later in this chapter. The heme moiety is a tetrapyrole containing Fe^{+2} (Figure 61-4). Heme synthesis occurs in both the mitochondria and in the cytoplasm (Figure 61-5). In the mitochondria, succinate and glycine are converted into Δ-aminolevulinic acid, which in turn is transformed into porphobilinogen. These monopyrole molecules leave the mitochondria and in the cytoplasm condense via methane bridges to form uroporphyrinogen III which, in turn, forms coproporphyrinogen III. This product reenters the mitochondria, where it is transformed into protoporphyrin III (9), which then combines with the Fe^{+2} to form heme.

Hemoglobin can be oxygenated only when the iron is in the $+2$ state. If the iron is oxidized to the $+3$ state, the resultant "methemoglobin" cannot bind oxygen. Small amounts are continuously produced but then reduced through a NADH diaphorase enzyme system. Patients deficient in the NADH diaphorase system, or with an abnormal hemoglobin M, have congenital methemoglobinemia. The production of methemoglobin is increased in patients exposed to oxident drugs or toxins. Detection of methemoglobins was described in a previous chapter.

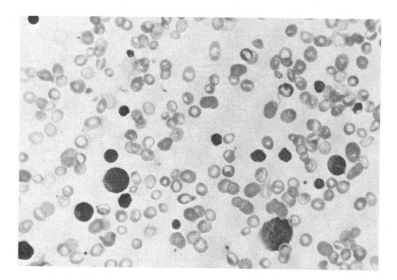

Fig. 61-3 Peripheral blood smear, leukoerythroblastosis. Appearance of immature granulocytic elements, nucleated red cells, and "tear drop" cells in the peripheral blood in patients with extensive replacement of normal marrow architecture. *From Nathan DG and Oski FA: Hematology of infancy and childhood, ed 2, Philadelphia, 1981, WB Saunders Co.*

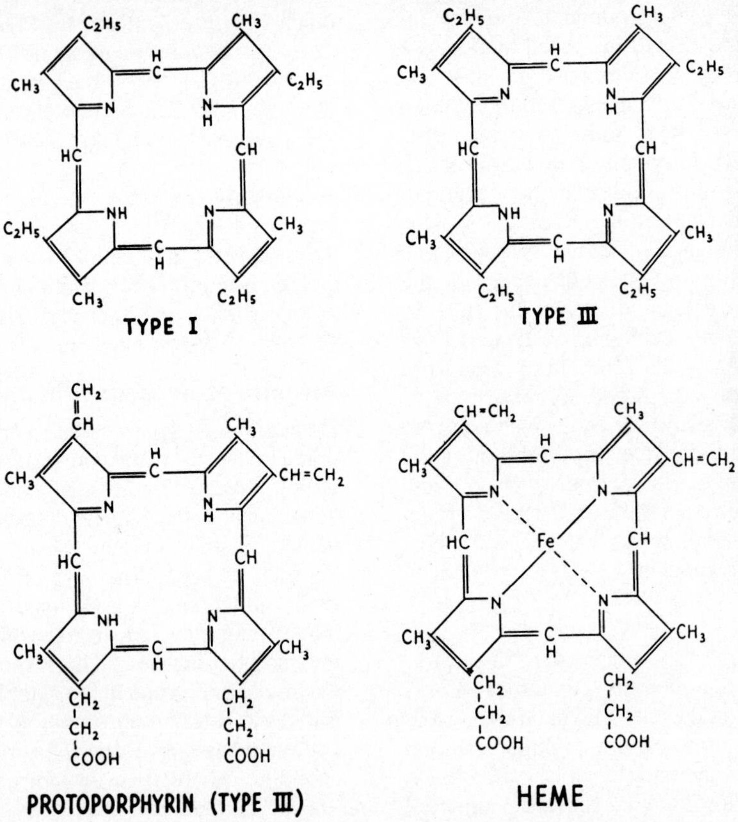

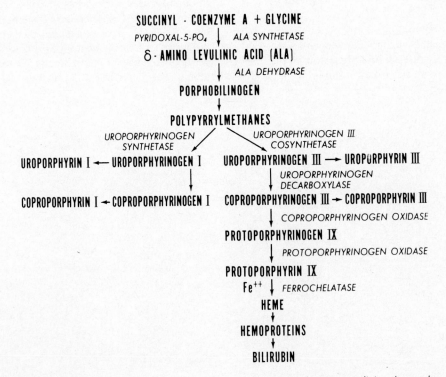

TYPE I

TYPE III

PROTOPORPHYRIN (TYPE III)

HEME

Fig. 61-4 Structure of porphyrin compounds. Type I and Type III isomers, protoporphyrin (Type III) and heme. *From Miale JB: Laboratory medicine: hematology, ed 6, St. Louis, 1982, Mosby–Year Book, Inc.*

SUCCINYL · COENZYME A + GLYCINE

PYRIDOXAL-5-PO₄ ↓ *ALA SYNTHETASE*

δ · AMINO LEVULINIC ACID (ALA)

↓ *ALA DEHYDRASE*

PORPHOBILINOGEN

↓

POLYPYRRYLMETHANES

UROPORPHYRINOGEN SYNTHETASE ↙   ↘ *UROPORPHYRINOGEN III COSYNTHETASE*

UROPORPHYRIN I ← UROPORPHYRINOGEN I   UROPORPHYRINOGEN III → UROPORPHYRIN III

↓ *UROPORPHYRINOGEN DECARBOXYLASE*

COPROPORPHYRIN I ← COPROPORPHYRINOGEN I   COPROPORPHYRINOGEN III → COPROPORPHYRIN III

↓ *COPROPORPHYRINOGEN OXIDASE*

PROTOPORPHYRINOGEN IX

↓ *PROTOPORPHYRINOGEN OXIDASE*

PROTOPORPHYRIN IX

Fe⁺⁺ ↓ *FERROCHELATASE*

HEME

↓

HEMOPROTEINS

↓

BILIRUBIN

Fig. 61-5 Biosynthesis of porphyrins and heme. *From Miale JB: Laboratory medicine: hematology, ed 6, St. Louis, 1982, Mosby–Year Book, Inc.*

Iron deficiency (sideropenic) anemia

Review of normal iron metabolism. The total body iron content in a 70 kg man varies from 3 to 4 gm., (65% to 70% in hemoglobin, 10% to 20% in storage iron and 10% to 15% in myoglobin, enzymes and bound to transport proteins in the plasma). Red cells contain about 1 mg/ml of cells. Iron is stored in one of two forms: 1) Ferritin, composed of a core of Fe^{+3} chelate surrounded by a water-soluble shell of protein molecules (apoferritin). Ferritin is present in most body tissues, developing normoblasts, and in the serum in small quantities; 2) Hemosiderin is comprised of non-ferritin micellar iron and other proteins. It is found in reticulo-endothelial system cells appearing as gray-green granules in hematoxylin and eosin-stained marrow sections and deep blue when stained with Prussian blue stain.

A typical diet contains about 6 mg of elemental iron per 1000 calories. The absorption of 1 mg of elemental Fe per day balances normal losses in the adult male, about 1 mg. This loss occurs from sloughing of ferritin-laden mucosal cells through the G.I. tract and microscopic bleeding from the gut (<1 ml/day). The remainder of daily iron need is met by the iron returned to the storage pool from red cell senescence. The daily iron requirements may be in excess of 1 mg/day when blood loss or iron utilization increases. Physiologic losses occur in females through menstruation, pregnancy, and lactation. Pathologic bleeding may be occult.

Iron in the diet is largely in the Fe^{+3} inorganic form or bound in hemoglobin. Medicinal iron is in the Fe^{+2} inorganic form. The best absorbed form is heme form, followed by Fe^{+2}. Fe^{+3} is poorly absorbed. In the stomach, HCl solubilizes Fe^{+3} and allows it to be chelated to amino acids, sugars, or the ascorbate secreted in gastric juice. These chelates remain soluble in the alkaline environment of the duodenum (instead of precipitating as $Fe(OH)_3$), where bile substances reduce Fe^{+3} to Fe^{+2}, which can be absorbed into the mucosal cells. Hemoglobin is split into heme and globin by proteolytic enzymes in the duodenum. Heme is soluble in alkaline pH and thus is absorbed in the mucosal cells as intact metalloporphyrin.

Under normal conditions, 5% to 10% of dietary iron is absorbed into the mucosal cells of the duodenum (approximately 1 mg/day), while in iron deficiency, 20% to 30% may be absorbed. Likewise, a high percentage of medicinal iron in the Fe^{+2} form is absorbed. Once absorbed, the Fe^{+2} ion, as well as the Fe^{+2} freed from porphyrin in the cell, combines with apoferritin to form ferritin (Fe^{+3}). This ferritin is a local mucosal storage form which releases Fe^{+2} for transport across the mucosal cell membrane to bind with an iron-binding protein (transferrin) in the serum. One mole of transferrin binds one or two atoms of Fe^{+3}.

The quantity of transferrin (Tf) in the serum is measured as the total iron-binding capacity of serum, which is normally 250 to 450 μgm/dl. The normal level of serum iron is 50 to 150 μgm/dl. Therefore, transferrin serum is normally 20% to 40%. Methods of measuring serum Fe and TIBC were discussed previously (Chapter 11). Most of the iron bound does not derive immediately from dietary input, but from senescent red cells broken down in the RES. When serum iron levels are low, transferrin is produced and the TIBC rises.

The transfer of Fe^{+3} to a developing normoblast depends on association of the Tf Fe^{+3} complex to a Tf receptor on the cell. Following this, the transferrin molecule enters the cell by surface endocytosis and Fe dissociates from Tf. Fe enters cytoplasmic ferritin deposits, which release iron as needed into the mitochondria to form heme. Developing red cells with cytoplastic ferritin deposits are called "sideroblasts." This extraction to the developing red cell is possible at low transferrin saturation. At high saturation, iron is also unloaded into other tissues, especially the liver, where it is stored as ferritin and hemosiderin.

The availability of iron in the cell cytoplasm regulates the rate of hemoglobin synthesis. In turn, it appears that the rate of hemoglobin synthesis regulates the number and timing of cell divisions. A lack of iron, therefore, decreases hemoglobin synthesis and increases the number of cell divisions in the differentiation compartment, giving rise to smaller cells.

Etio-pathogenesis of iron deficiency anemia. The cause of iron deficiency in infants is usually nutritional, given their large growth demand. Premature infants are most vulnerable. Pure milk diets lead to iron deficiency. The onset of menstruation, associated with the growth demand of adolescence, contributes to iron deficiency in young women. Pregnancy usually totally depletes the iron reserves. Iron deficiency in adult men implies abnormal bleeding unless proven otherwise. Malabsorption is an uncommon cause of iron deficiency (50% of patients with a subtotal gastrectomy eventually develop iron deficiency). Iron deficiency is the most common cause of anemia: 10% of women in the United States may be affected (Box 61-4).

Anemia arises as the last manifestation of the following series of events:

1. Iron depletion: loss of iron stores and decreased serum ferritin levels.
2. Iron deficiency without anemia: absent storage iron, low serum iron concentration, and later increased TIBC and decreased saturation (<12% is diagnostic).
3. Iron deficiency anemia: characterized first by a decreased reticulocyte count, then by microcytosis, and, lastly, hypochromia.

Clinical picture. The clinical manifestation of iron deficiency anemia are nonspecific. Severe anemia (below a hemoglobin of 7 gm/dl) may be associated with pallor, fatigue, decreased exercise tolerance, mild tachycardia, etc. In addition, loss of iron-containing enzymes may cause epithelial atrophy (smooth tongue, atrophic gastritis, and in some populations, esophageal webbing associated with dysphagia, which is known as the Plummer-Vinson syndrome).

Laboratory findings. The peripheral blood picture is variable, and, as previously discussed, depends on the severity of iron deficiency. In the full-blown case, the patient may be significantly anemic (Hg <7 gm/dl) and have microcytic hypochromic indices. The reticulocyte index is low. Mild to moderate thrombocytosis is frequently observed. Examination of the peripheral smear shows moderate aniso-poikilocytosis with hypochromia and numerous microcytes.

Box 61-4   Etiologic factors in iron deficiency

Increased physiologic requirements
    Rapid growth: infancy, preadolescence
    Menstruation
    Pregnancy
Decreased iron assimilation
    Iron-poor diet
    Iron malabsorption
        Sprue, nontropical sprue
        Gastric resection
        Pica
Blood loss
    Gastrointestinal bleeding
        Milk-induced enteropathy
        Peptic ulcer disease
        Inflammatory bowel disease
        Meckel's diverticulum
        Drugs: salicylates
        Hookworm infestation
    Fetal-maternal transfusion
    Hemoglobinuria: prosthetic heart valve
    Iatrogenic
    Idiopathic pulmonary hemosiderosis
    Intense exercise

From Miller DR and Baehner RL: Blood diseases of infancy and childhood, ed 6, St. Louis, 1990, Mosby–Year Book, Inc.

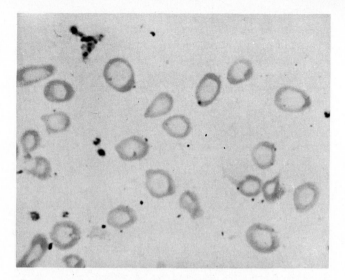

Fig. 61-6   Peripheral blood smear, iron deficiency anemia. Note hypochromia, microcytosis, anisocytosis, and poikilocytosis. (Wright's stain, ×950.) *From Miale JB: Laboratory medicine: hematology, ed 6, St. Louis, 1982, Mosby–Year Book, Inc.*

(Figure 61-6). Some target cells are often visible.

Although often not performed in the presence of usual serum iron study results, the bone marrow shows mild erythroid hyperplasia with under-hemoglobinized normoblasts and absent identifiable sideroblasts and iron stores.

The diagnosis is confirmed by the serum iron studies. In cases of fully developed iron deficiency anemia, they show decreased serum iron levels and increased total iron-binding capacity due to the increased synthesis of transferrin. A resultant saturation of less than 12% is considered diagnostic. Alternatively, decreased serum ferritin levels indicate iron deficiency. Because of the decreased synthesis of heme due to the unavailability of iron in these patients, increased "free" erythrocyte porphyrin levels are present. Although nonspecific for iron deficiency, since it is also elevated in cases of lead poisoning and other sideroblastic anemias, the determination of these levels has been proposed as an effective method for mass screening.

Studies of the kinetics of iron utilization (ferrokinetic studies) are not widely used but are valuable research tools and may be helpful in evaluating select anemias. To perform these studies, ^{59}Fe in the form of ferric citrate or chloride is injected intravenously. Following infusion, the level of radioactivity in the blood is measured periodically and external scanning over the sternum, sacrum, liver, and spleen is performed. The rate of decrease of radioactivity represents the *Plasma Iron Disappearance Time* (PIDT), the T-½ of which is normally 60 to 120 minutes. By deriving the quantity of iron removed from the plasma per minute from the PIDT, one can calculate the mg of iron leaving the plasma per dl of whole blood per day, which is termed the *Plasma Iron Turnover Rate* (PITR) and is normally found to be 25 to 40 mg/day. The PITR reflects total erythropoetic activity.

Simultaneous external scanning can either confirm that most of the iron is taken up by the bone marrow during the first 24 hours or identify alternate significant sites of uptake. Effective erythropoesis is reflected in *Red Cell Iron Reutilization Rate* (RCIRR). As samples are collected periodically over a two-week period, radioactivity reappears in the peripheral blood as newly formed red cells appear in the circulation. Normally, an excess of 80% is incorporated into the red cells at 14 days. Increased effective erythropoesis may not only increase the reutilization rate modestly but may dramatically shorten the time required to peak (Table 61-2).

Patients with iron deficiency anemia demonstrate a decreased PIDT, increased PITR, localization in the bone marrow, and increased RCIRR.

Following treatment with oral iron replacement, the earliest sign of therapeutic response is the reticulocyte count which begins to rise after five to 10 days. Generally, normalization of the hemoglobin concentration requires one to two months. Replenishment of tissue iron stores requires two to six months of iron administration after correction of anemia.

Anemia of chronic disease

The term "anemia of chronic disease" refers to a heterogeneous group of anemias characterized by normochromic or slightly hypochromic and normocytic or slightly microcytic indices noted during the course of chronic infections, other inflammatory or neoplastic diseases. The reticulocyte index is decreased, while the bone marrow is normocellular. Both the serum iron and the total iron-bonding capacity are decreased. Serum ferritin levels and marrow iron stores are increased. The apparent decreased reutilization of iron from storage sites also results in increased "free" erythrocyte porphyrin levels.

The cause of this decreased reutilization is obscure but

Table 61-2 Ferrokinetic studies in normal and anemic individuals

Condition	Retic index (x basal)	Plasma iron (μg/dl)	Tf sat (%)	T-½ (min)	RCU (%)	PIT (mg/dl/d)	ETU (μmol/L/d)
Normal subjects	1	112 ±43	35 ±11	80 ±15	85 ±4	0.71 ±0.17	60 ±12
Pure red cell aplasia	0.1 ±0.1	253 ±56	94 ±5	363 ±94	3 ±3	0.57 ±0.15	12 ±11
Renal failure	1.2 ±0.6	206 ±38	80 ±15	232 ±55	26 ±10	0.73 ±0.16	35 ±11
Renal failure (no transfusions)	1.5 ±0.7	79 ±24	28 ±6	81 ±22	71 ±13	0.77 ±0.18	73 ±21
Hemolytic anemia	5.7 ±1.9	126 ±70	44 ±24	27 ±9	72 ±19	3.86 ±1.45	400 ±130
Ineffective erythropoiesis	0.8 ±0.5	156 ±68	66 ±25	28 ±11	30 ±11	5.11 ±1.85	474 ±147

From Cazzola M et al: Blood 69:296, 1987.
Tf = transferrin; RCU = red cell utilization; PIT = plasma iron turnover; ETU = erythron transferrin uptake.
Values are mean ± 1 S.D.

may be related to increased macrophage activity in these disorders. It has been proposed that such increased activity may be mediated by increased levels to IL-1 released at the site of inflammation. In addition to this defect in iron re-utilization, some patients demonstrate lowered levels of serum erythropoetin, while others have modestly shortened red cell survivals, which do not appear due to intrinsic cell defects.

Refractory (sideroachrestic) anemias

A mixed group of idiopathic acquired anemias characterized by a hypercellular marrow, defective utilization of iron in developing red cells, and increased iron stores which are refractory to treatment, are termed "refractory (Sideroachrestic) anemias." Some are characterized by the development of ringed sideroblasts (acquired idiopathic sideroblastic anemia) or are associated with abnormalities in maturation of other marrow elements (e.g., refractory anemia with excess of blasts). Most authorities now refer to these entities as myelodysplastic syndromes and feel that some cases may evolve into acute leukemia over a period of time ("preleukemic syndromes"). These will be more fully discussed later in this section (Chapter 62).

Sideroblastic anemias

Sideroblastic anemias are characterized by a defect in porphyrin synthesis and a secondary accumulation of iron as non-micellar complexes within the mitochondria of the normoblasts, which leads to a typical appearing cell termed a "ringed sideroblast" in which the nucleus is encircled with iron deposits (Figure 61-7). This iron collection leads to eventual destruction of the mitochondria and premature death of the normoblast (intramedullary hemolysis).

Etiologic classification

Refractory sideroblastic anemias

Hereditary. A sex-linked recessive state characterized by a deficiency of ALA synthetase and/or heme synthetase.

Acquired forms. Found in pernicious anemia, porphyria, diGiugliamo's syndrome, or as an idiopathic state.

Reversible sideroblastic anemias

Toxic. Related to toxic inhibition of ALA synthetase and heme synthetase (INH, cycloserine, chloramphenicol, alcohol, and lead poisoning).

Nutritional. Nutritional lack of pyridoxine leads to decreased activity of ALA synthetase due to loss of the coenzyme activity of pyridoxal phosphate.

Pyridoxine responsive. A few patients without nutritional deficiency respond to very high doses of pyridoxine.

Diagnosis. These anemias are hypochromic and often slightly microcytic. The smear is usually dimorphic with considerable anisocytosis. The reticulocyte index is decreased. Serum iron levels and iron saturation are both increased, as is the serum ferritin level. The bone marrow shows erythroid hyperplasia with increased iron stores and numerous ringed sideroblasts. If performed, ferrokinetic studies reveal an increased PITR and decreased red cell iron reutilization, which further substantiate the ineffective erythropoesis characteristic of these conditions. Free erythrocyte porphyrin is also increased.

The thalassemia syndromes

As previously discussed, the hemoglobin molecule exists as a tetramer of four globin chains, each associated with a heme moiety. The globin polypeptide chains are synthesized on the cytoplasmic ribosomes. Four chains are produced in the adult: α chains are present in all hemoglobin molecules, and synthesis is begun in fetal life; β chains are present in the predominate hemoglobin of the adult, HbA >95%; δ chains are present in a minor adult hemoglobin, HbA$_2$ <2% to 3%; and γ chains are present in the fetal hemoglobin which persists in small quantity in adulthood, HbF <1% to 2%. ζ and ξ chains are embryonic chains produced only in early fetal life and are present in the embryonic Gower I, Gower II, and Portland hemoglobins (Figure 61-8).

The α chains contain 141 amino acids, while the β, δ and γ chains contain 146 amino acids. The primary structure of the protein is simply delineated by its amino acid sequence, each chain being distinctive. Two types of γ chains exist as a mixture in the HbF; one, G-gamma, has a glycine residue located at position 136; the other, A-gamma, has alanine at that position. The N terminus of this polypeptide chain is defined by amino acid residue one, while the C

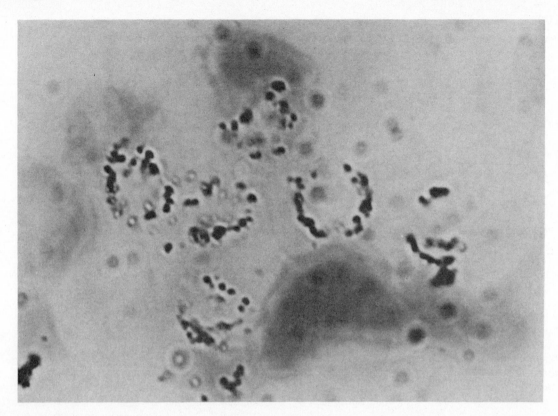

Fig. 61-7 Bone marrow aspirate, sideroblastic anemia. Ringed sideroblasts. Note the perinuclear arrangement of coarse iron laden mitochondria. (Iron stain, ×1000.) *From Miale JB: Laboratory medicine: hematology, ed 6, St. Louis, 1982, Mosby–Year Book, Inc.*

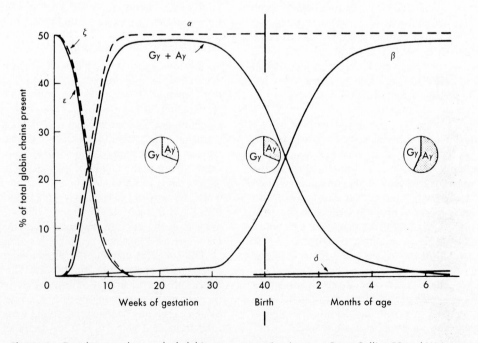

Fig. 61-8 Developmental control of globin gene expression in man. *From Collins FS and Weismann SM: Progress in Nucleic Acid Research and Molecular Biology 31:312, 1984.*

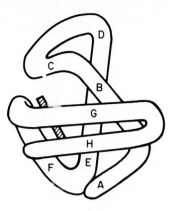

Fig. 61-9 β-Chain of human hemoglobin with the helices lettered A to H. *Modified from Schroeder WA and Jones RT: Fortschr Chem Org Nautrst 23:113, 1965.*

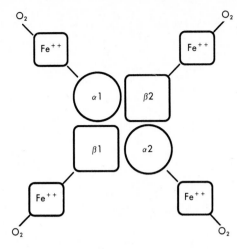

Fig. 61-10 Schematic drawing of human hemoglobin. Hemoglobin is composed of two α- and two β-chains, with each of the subunits having a heme prosthetic group. Oxygen combines with the ferrous heme iron. *From Miller DR and Baehner RL: Blood diseases of infancy and childhood, ed 6, St. Louis, 1990, Mosby–Year Book, Inc.*

terminus is either residue 141 or 146. Eighty percent of this chain is coiled into an α helix, thereby defining its secondary structure. The helices are separated by straight interhelical segments. Each helical segment is assigned a letter. β chains have eight helices (A through H), while α chains have seven (D is absent). The tertiary convoluted structure depends on bending in the non-helical portions of the chains. Proline residues are usually located in these bends (Figure 61-9). A heme moiety is inserted into hydrophobic niches formed between helical segments E and F of each chain in HbA. The iron atom of each heme is attached to the proximal F histidine (β92 or α87) and distal E histidine (β63 or α58) residues. The individual monomeric chains form αβ dimers that in turn form tetramers, which represent the quaternary structure of hemoglobin (Figure 61-10). The tetramer therefore contains two α chains with 2 β chains in HbA ($\alpha_2\beta_2$); two γ chains in HbF ($\alpha_2\gamma_2$); or two δ in HbA$_2$ ($\alpha_2\delta_2$). The embryonic hemoglobin tetramers are formed as follows: Gower I ($\zeta_2\xi_2$); Gower II ($\alpha_2\xi_2$; and Portland ($\zeta_2\gamma_2$). The HbA tetramer has an asymetrical configuration with a shorter distance between the iron of the α chain of one dimer and the β chain of the other ($\alpha_1\beta_2$ contact) than between the α and β chain of the same dimer ($\alpha_1\beta_1$ contact). The distances between O$_2$ binding sites are therefore unequal and not constant.

The structural characteristics of the hemoglobin tetramer are of critical importance to the reversible binding of O$_2$ to the hemoglobin because of the configurational change between the dimers, which occurs during oxygen binding and release. At high oxygen tension, oxygenation of one heme iron of deoxygenated hemoglobin occurs and causes rotation of the chains thereby creating a 7Å decrease in distance between the β chains. This in turn makes the other heme pockets more available so that two more oxygen molecules can be attached with only a slight increase in O$_2$ tension. The reverse movement of chains occurs as hemoglobin tends to unlock oxygen at low O$_2$ tension. This allosteric effect (heme-heme) interaction is largely reponsible for the sigmoidal shape of the oxygen dissociation curve (Figure 61-11). The Bohr effect also regulates the oxygen affinity of hemoglobin in that increasing pH causes a decreased affinity with a shift of the O$_2$ dissociation curve to

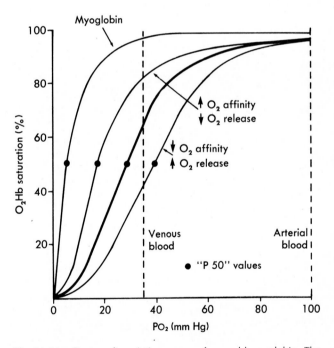

Fig. 61-11 Oxygen dissociation curves of normal hemoglobin. The heavy middle tracing shows the dissociation curve of normal adult hemoglobin at pH 7.4 and temperature 37°C, which has a P^{50} value of 27 mm Hg. The curve shifts to the right with increased temperature or decreased pH (Bohr effect) and increased 2,3 DPG levels. The opposite effects are noted with decreased temperature, increased pH and decreased 2,3 DPG levels. *From Sonnenwirth AC and Jarett L: Gradwohl's clinical laboratory methods and diagnosis, vol 1, ed 8, St. Louis, 1980, Mosby–Year Book, Inc.*

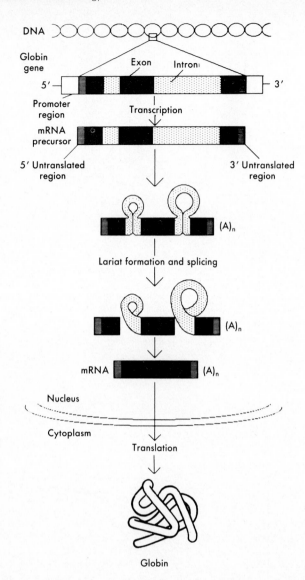

Fig. 61-12 Globin chain synthesis. DNA information is transcribed from the globin gene to mRNA precursor in the nucleus. After the removal of intervening sequences (introns) by splicing, the exons fuse to form mature mRNA. The mature mRNA leaves the nucleus to enter the cytoplasm, where globin chains are synthesized. *From Miller DR and Baehner RL: Blood diseases of infancy and childhood, ed 6, St. Louis, 1990, Mosby–Year Book, Inc.*

the right (i.e., in an acidic environment, oxyhemoglobin, which is more acidic than deoxyhemoglobin, will tend to deoxygenate). Aside from heme-heme interaction and the Bohr effect, the availability of 2,3 DPG, a product of the Embden-Meyerhoff glycolytic pathway, is also important in modulating the O_2 affinity of hemoglobin. During periods of oxygen lack, 2,3 DPG synthesis is increased. 2,3 DPG binds with hemoglobin undergoing deoxygenation on a mole-for-mole basis by establishing a bond from one β chain to the opposite β chain. It stabilizes the deoxyhemoglobin conformation and thereby lowers O_2 affinity and permits O_2 release. Inversely, DPG synthesis is decreased with increased O_2 availability, and the deoxygenated hemoglobin is able to be readily oxygenated.

The synthesis of these globin chains is controlled by their

respective genes. The β, γ, δ and ξ genes are located closely together on chromosome 11 while pairs of genes for α and ζ chains are on chromosome 16. Their production depends on appropriate initiation and termination of transcription from DNA to complementary RNA nucleotide bases; excision of introns, which separate the coding or structural exons at determined splice junctions; and transport of finished mRNA to cytoplasmic microsomes for translation. The rate of transcription is controlled by promotor regions upstream from the 5'terminus of the genes and by certain base sequences within their intron regions (Figure 61-12). Transcription termination is related to polyadenylation of the 3'terminus of the mRNA.

While mutations and deletions occuring in the structural exon regions give rise to production of abnormal globin molecules (hemoglobinopathies), such changes in the promotor, initiator, terminator, intron, and splice junction regions may give rise to decreased chain production.

Thalassemias are a group of hereditary anemias characterized by defective hemoglobin formation due to decreased globin chain synthesis. Depending on the deficient chain(s), thalassemia is classified as β, α, δ, βδ, etc. (Box 61-5).

Beta thalassemias

These syndromes result from the presence of an abnormal β-chain gene expression leading to reduced β-chain production. The β^{thal+} genes allow the production of decreased amount of β-chain, while $\beta^{thal\,0}$ genes allow no detectable β-chain to be formed. The molecular defects underlying these decreased gene expressions can be correlated to specific defects in the β globin chain region. Most of the β^+ defects result from single base changes in the promotor region upstream from the 5'end of the β gene or in the mid intron regions, while deletions or mutations in the structural exons or at the 5' or 3'splice junctions of the introns account for β^0 defects (Box 61-6). Patients homozygous for an aberrant β^0 or doubly heterozygous for β^0 and β^+ gene activity are said to have Thalassemia Major or Cooley's anemia. Some homozygous patients with milder disease may be those with β^+ genes and have Thalassemia Intermedia. Heterozygotes for β^0 or β^+ have Thalassemia Trait or Thalassemia Minor. Beta thalassemias disorders arise in and are most prevalent among populations of the Mediterranean basin.

Beta thalassemia minor

These patients have only slight anemia, with marked microcytosis and moderate hypochromia (resulting in a normal or near normal MCHC), elliptocytosis, leptocytosis, and basophilic stippling of their red cells. The reticulocyte index is normal. Fe and TIBC are normal. Characteristically, erythrocytic porphyrin levels are also normal, and this test has been proposed as a quick screening tool to differentiate iron deficiency and lead poisoning from thalassemia minor. The diagnosis is confirmed by finding an elevated level of hemoglobin A_2 in the range of 4-5-6.0%. In addition, some patients have a slight elevation of HbF.

While quantification of the major normal hemoglobins and hemoglobin variants can be performed most easily by cellulose acetate hemoglobin electrophoresis and densitometry, as will be discussed later in this chapter, these tech-

---

Box 61-5   Classification of the thalassemias

I. β-Thalassemia
  A. Homozygous $β^+$-thalassemia: $α_2β_2{}^{thal\ +}$
  B. Homozygous $β^0$-thalassemia: $α_2β_2{}^{thal\ O}$
  C. Heterozygous $β^+$-thalassemia: $α_2ββ^{thal\ +}$
  D. Heterozygous $β^0$-thalassemia: $α_2ββ^{thal\ O}$
II. δβ-Thalassemia
  A. Homozygous δβ-thalassemia: $α(δβ)^{thal}α(δβ)^{thal}$
  B. Heterozygous δβ-thalassemia: $αβα(δβ)^{thal}$
  C. Doubly heterozygous δβ-β-thalassemia: $αβ^{thal}(δβ)^{thal}$
III. α-Thalassemia
  A. Homozygous α-thalassemia: $α^{thal\ 1}βα^{thal\ 1}β$
  B. Heterozygous α-thalassemia: $αβα^{thal\ 1}β$
  C. Homozygous mild α-thalassemia (H disease): $α^{thal\ 1}βα^{thal\ 2}β$

  D. Heterozygous mild α-thalassemia: $αβα^{thal\ 2}β$
  E. Heterozygous α-Q-Thalassemia: $α^{thal\ 1}βα^Qβ$
  F. Heterozygous α-Constant Spring thalassemia: $α^{thal\ 1}βα^{Constant\ Spring}β$
IV. δ-Thalassemia
  A. Homozygous δ-thalassemia: $α_2β_2(δ_2{}^{thal})$
  B. Heterozygous δ-thalassemia: $α_2β_2(δ^{thal})$
V. The Lepore syndromes: $α_2(δβ)_2$
VI. Hereditary persistence of fetal hemoglobin (HPFH)
  A. Negro type
  B. Greek type
  C. Swiss type
VII. Double heterozygosity of above categories with each other or structural variants

From Miale JB: Laboratory medicine: hematology, ed 6, St. Louis, 1982, Mosby–Year Book, Inc.

niques are generally inadequate in quantifying the minor hemoglobins. Prior attempts to measure HbA_2 by this methodology were unable to be standardized sufficiently to eliminate considerable interlaboratory variation. Densitometric quantification of hemoglobin F was never considered possible because of the low level measured and the difficulty in achieving good separation from other hemoglobins by electrophoresis.

Although some success has been reported in the quantification of HbA_2 after separation by electrophoresis if the HbA_2 and other hemoglobins were eluted into buffer and measured spectrophotometrically, the most widely adopted techniques for HbA_2 quantification are now those based on separation of hemoglobins by column chromatography and their measurement spectrophotometrically. Application of a hemolysate over a DEAE-Sephadex or cellulose column, followed by addition of an alkaline buffer (e.g., Tris/HCL, pH 8.4) permits the differential elution of HbA_2. The remainder of the bound hemoglobin A is eluted by a less alkaline buffer (e.g., Tris/HCL, pH 6.5-7.0). The optical density (O.D.) of the eluted HbA_2, measured at 415 nm, divided by the sum of the O.D.'s of the HbA_2 and other hemoglobins eluted, equals the percentage of HbA_2. Samples containing hemoglobin variants that have an intermediate charge between the negative HbA and relatively positive HbA_2 (e.g., HbS), may be eluted separately by sequential use of a buffer at pH 8.1-8.2 after elution of the HbA_2 fraction. Because hemoglobin C has a similar charge, HbA_2 cannot be quantified in the presence of HbC by most such techniques. Chromatography is readily performed in routine clinical laboratories since good-quality, small-volume prepared columns are now commercially available. Other methods of hemoglobin A_2 quantification include starch block electrophoresis, which was considered the classical reference method prior to the development of chromatographic techniques and which, although highly precise and accurate, was tedious and time-consuming; and bulk hemoglobin absorption in which all hemoglobins except hemoglobin A_2 are absorbed onto a suspension of DEAE-Cellulose and the optical densities of the hemolysate prior to and after absorption are compared.

Hemoglobin F quantification is based on the resistance of this hemoglobin to alkali denaturation. In this test, 1.2

Box 61-6   β-thalassemia mutations

	Principle Categories
$β^0$	5′ or 3′ Exon Deletions (rare)
$β^0$	5′ or 3′ Splice Junction Point Mutations
$β^0$	Exon Nonsense or Frame Shift Mutations
$β^+$	5′ Promotor Region Point Mutations
$β^+$	3′ Polyadenylation Site Point Mutations
$β^+$	Intron Point Mutations

N sodium hydroxide is added to a diluted hemolysate and the denatured hemoglobin is then precipitated by a saturated ammonium sulfate solution. Both the post-precipitation supernatant and the original diluted hemolysate are then added to Drabkins solution (potassium cyanide and potassium ferricyanide), and the O.D. of each solution is measured at 415 nm.

The amount of HbF in red cells is not distributed equally in blood from adults; less than one percent of the cells contain detectable levels. In cord blood samples almost all cells have high levels while only half the red cells from infants at three months have HbF. The identification of cells with HbF by the acid elution technique (Kleinhauer-Betke) depends on the insolubility of HbF in a citric acid-Na_2HPO_4 buffer (pH 3.3). This test is performed by immersing ethanol fixed blood smears into the buffer and subsequently staining the slide with eosin. Cells containing HbF stain red while all other red cells appear as unstained ghosts. In thalassemia minor, HbF levels may be increased to 3% to 5%, and the distribution of HbF in the red cells is shown to be heterogeneous among the red cells (Figure 61-13).

Beta thalassemia major

Patients with thalassemia major have a grave disease and, until recently, rarely reached adulthood. Patients with thalassemia intermedia have a somewhat milder disease. In these disorders the lack of production of β chains leads to the compensatory production of HbF and the relative excess of intracellular α chains which tend to form tetramers. These α tetramers spontaneously denature and form intracellular precipitates in the red cells, which are subsequently pitted

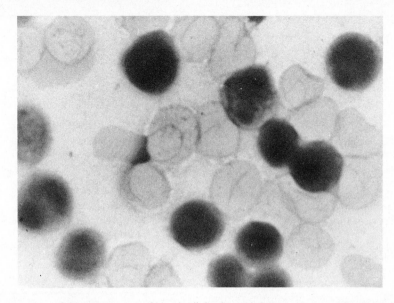

Fig. 61-13 Hemoglobin F demonstrated in red cells by the acid elution technique. The dark cells contain HbF. *From Miale JB: Laboratory medicine: hematology, ed 6, St. Louis, 1982, Mosby—Year Book, Inc.*

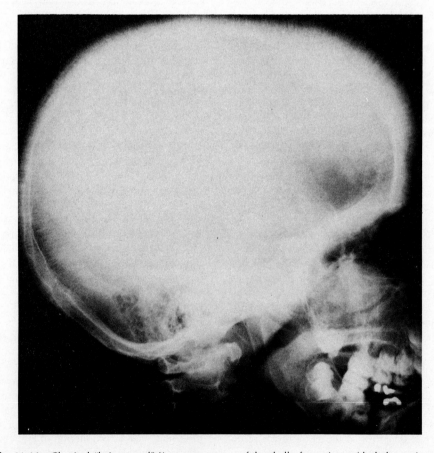

Fig. 61-14 Classical "hair on end" X-ray appearance of the skull of a patient with thalassemia major, resulting from the widening of the diploic spaces. *From Miller DR and Baehner RL: Blood diseases of infancy and childhood, ed 6, St. Louis, 1990, Mosby—Year Book, Inc.*

and culled by macrophages in the bone marrow and the peripheral reticulo-endothelial system.

Severe anemia therefore results from decreased hemoglobin synthesis and from intra-medullary destruction (ineffective erythropoiesis) and extra-medullary hemolysis. In addition, the compensatory synthesis of HbF, a hemoglobin with high O_2 affinity, further increases tissue hypoxia. All of this leads to marked erythropoietin production, extreme erythroid hyperplasia of the marrow, and retarded growth and deformities of flat bones (Figure 61-14). Extra-medullary hematopoiesis leads to striking hepatosplenomegaly. Iron retention results from recycled iron derived from hemolysed cells, increased iron absorption in the duodenum, and tranfused red cells. This iron results in eventual hemosiderosis and development of myocardial fibrosis and heart failure.

The severe anemia is characterized by a markedly lowered reticulocyte index. Severe microcytosis and hypochromia of the peripheral red cells is accompanied by extreme poikilocytosis with target cells, leptocytes, and elliptocytes (Figure 61-15). Basophilic stippling may be striking. Numerous nucleated red cells and marked polychromasia may be present. Hemoglobin A_2 is usually normal, but HbF is markedly elevated, often >90%. The distribution of the HbF as determined by the Kleinhauer-Betke stain is heterogenous. As previously stated, the bone marrow is hypercellular with a markedly inverted M:E ratio (Figure 61-16). The iron stores are markedly increased, as are the serum ferritin and iron levels.

Alpha thalassemias

The genetic background of the α thalassemia syndrome is considerably different from the β thalassemias. Since the α globin gene is duplicated with two genes per chromosome, there is normally a total of four α genes per diploid cell. The globin chain synthetic defect in α thalassemia usually results from deletions in α genes, and the severity of the disorder is related to the number of genes deficient. α Thalassemias are disorders that arise in and are most prevalent among Far Eastern populations and American blacks.

α Thal 2 (carrier state): One of four α-genes is deficient. There is no anemia, but the red cells may be slightly microcytic and hypochromic.

α Thal 1 (α thal trait): Two of four α genes are deficient. There may be mild anemia. The disorder resembles β thal trait, but HbA_2 and HbF are not increased. Diagnosis rests on the cell indices, normal iron studies, morphology, and dominant inheritance.

HbH disease: Three of four α genes are deficient, resulting in a mild to moderately severe thalassemia syndrome. The hemolysis is due to the presence of an unstable hemoglobin HbH (β tetramer) associated with the cell membrane.

HbBart's syndrome (Hydrops Fetalis): All four genes are deficient. Infants are prematurely stillborn or die shortly after birth. The cells contain only HbBarts (γ tetramer). The hemoglobin has such a high O_2 affinity that the condition is incompatible with life.

Other thalassemia syndromes

Extended deletions in the γ or δ region may result in depressed synthesis of HbF or HbA_2 respectively, conditions

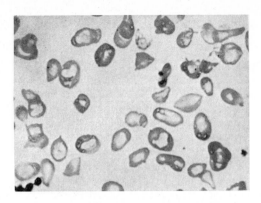

Fig. 61-15   Peripheral blood smear, thalassemia major. Note extreme poikilocytosis and microcytosis. Target cells and normoblasts are also usual findings. *From Bauer JD: Clinical laboratory methods, ed 9, St. Louis, 1982, Mosby–Year Book, Inc.*

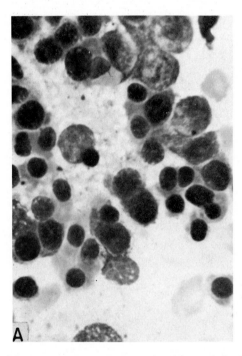

Fig. 61-16   Bone marrow aspirate, erythroid hyperplasia. Note inversion of M:E ratio due to marked hyperplasia of erythroid precursors such as seen in thalassemia major. (Wright's stain, × 950.) *From Miale JB: Laboratory medicine: hematology, ed 6, St. Louis, 1982, Mosby–Year Book, Inc.*

not associated with clinical disease. Deletions involving both the β and δ gene regions, βδ or F thalassemia, lead to an anemia of varying severity, depending on whether the condition is homozygous. HbF makes up to 20% of the total hemoglobin in heterozygotes, where it is heterogeneously distributed between cells, while no HbA or HbA_2 is made by homozygous patients. A variant form of βδ thalassemia in which all cells persist in making high levels of HbF is termed Hereditary resistence of fetal hemoglobin (HPFH). Heterozygous patients are differentiated from those with βδ thalassemia trait by the uniform distribution of HbF among the cells when stained by the Kleinauer-Betke technique. Homozygous patients possess 100% HbF and have polycythemia related to the increased oxygen affinity of fetal hemoglobin.

Patients in whom the non-α chain is a hybrid of the N terminal portion of the δ chain and the C terminus of the β chain resulting from a cross-over between adjacent β and δ chain gene loci possess Hemoglobin Lepore. These patients have a decreased production of this abnormal chain and a relative excess of α chains. Homozygous patients will therefore have a syndrome similar to β thalassemia major, while heterozygous patients present as β thalassemia minor. This abnormal hemoglobin is easily detected by cellulose acetate hemoglobin electrophoresis at pH 8.4 as it migrates to a position identical to HbS. Solubility tests for sickling hemoglobins are negative. Homozygous patients have from 70% to 80% HbF and 20% to 30% Hb Lepore, while heterozygotes possess up to 10% to 15% Hb Lepore.

An α thalassemia-like syndrome can be seen when Hemoglobin Constant Spring is produced. The alpha chain of this hemoglobin is elongated because of a mutation in the terminator position of the gene and is produced in reduced quantity. The severity of the resulting thalassemia syndrome depends on the zygosity of the patient and the number of chains affected. Hb Constant Spring is identified on cellulose acetate hemoglobin electrophoresis by its limited migration to a position between the origin and HbA$_2$.

Antenatal diagnosis of thalassemia

The antenatal diagnosis of the thalassemia syndromes was previously based on tests of globin chain synthetic rates in fetal blood samples. These tests, which were associated with occasional fetal deaths due to blood sampling, have been largely replaced by analysis of restriction enzyme fragments of amniotic cell DNA by oligonucleotide probes specific for known thalassemia point mutations.

Megaloblastic anemias

These anemias are characterized by asynchronous development of red cells with nuclear development lagging behind cytoplasmic development. The morphological characteristics of megaloblastic anemias are due to defective DNA synthesis and prolonged cell cycle time with continued protein synthesis. These cells have increased volumes with large nuclei containing a looser nuclear chromatin than would be expected from the degree of hemoglobinization (Figure 61-17). Such megaloblastic features are also seen in granulocytic cells and in most epithelial cells (e.g., gut).

The red cells have a shortened life span both in the marrow (ineffective erythropoiesis) and in the periphery (hemolysis). Ineffective granulocytopoiesis and thrombopoiesis are also present.

Usually, they are related to inadequate availability or utilization of tissue folate necessary for DNA synthesis, resulting either from folate deficiency or the lack of vitamin B$_{12}$ necessary for normal folate metabolism. About 5%, however, are secondary to drugs, associated with hematologic neoplasias and refractory anemias, or found in other rare congenital and acquired metabolic abnormalities (Box 61-6).

Folate and B$_{12}$ metabolism

Folic acid (pteroyglutamic acid, Figure 61-18) is present in a variety of foods in a polyglutamate form. It is absorbed

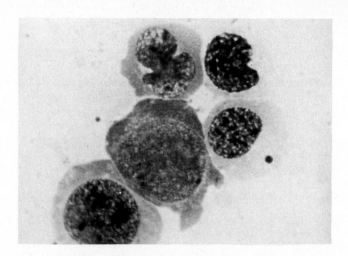

Fig. 61-17 Bone marrow aspirate, megaloblastic anemia. Note the marked nuclear-cytoplasmic asynchrony of these erythroid precursors. Also note the prominent parachromatin spaces and the fineness of the chromatin strands, which give rise to the distinctive "salt and pepper" appearance of the nucleus. (Wright's stain, ×950.) *From Miale JB: Laboratory medicine: hematology, ed 6, St. Louis, 1982, Mosby–Year Book, Inc.*

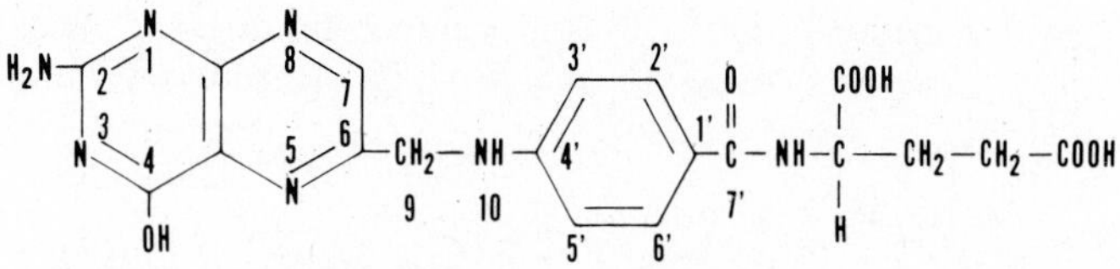

Fig. 61-18 Pteroylmonoglutamic acid (folic acid) showing the convention for numbering the atoms where some substitutions occur. Additional glutamic acid residues are added by linking the amino group to the terminal carboxyl group. *From Miale JB: Laboratory medicine: hematology, ed 6, St. Louis, 1982, Mosby–Year Book, Inc.*

in the jejunum as mono- to triglutamate forms after splitting of the polyglutamate by the enzyme "intestinal conjugase." The absorbed folate is reduced in many parenchymal cells, especially the liver, to dihydro- and then tetrahydrofolate acid (THFA) by dihydrofolate reductase:

EQ 61-1

$$FA + NADPH + H^+ \rightarrow DHFA + NADP^+$$
$$DHFA + NADPH + H^+ \rightarrow THFA + NADP^+$$

THFA (FH4) functions as a one-carbon carrier in numerous metabolic pathways and therefore multiple C substitution forms are described (e.g., 5CH$_3$ [methyl], 5,10 CH$_2$ [methylene], 5 CHNH$_2$ [foramino], etc.). The folate function of interest in the pathogenesis of the megaloblastosis is related to the synthesis of thymidylate, the pyrimidine necessary for DNA synthesis, from deoxyuridylate:

EQ 61-2

$$dUMP + N5,10\text{—}CH_2THFA \rightarrow dTMP + DHFA$$

The DHFA formed regenerates more N5,10-CH$_2$THFA by the following reactions:

EQ 61-3

DHFA + NADPH + H⁺ → THFA + NADP⁺

THFA + Serine → Glycine + N5,10—CH₂THFA

The predominate circulating form is N5-CH₃THFA. THFA is stored in cells conjugated to polyglutamate. Stores are sufficient to last three to six months.

Vitamin B₁₂ (cyanocobalamine) is present as the methyl and deoxyadenosyl analogues in the body (Figures 61-19). The methyl analogue is essential for the continued availability of THFA necessary for the synthesis of the various active one-carbon derivatives of folate needed. As stated, the principle circulating form of folate is N5-CH₃THFA. It is thought that folate present in the cells in this form is not available for most reactions. According to one theory (the methyltrap hypothesis), it can only be made available by its transformation into THFA during the conversion of homocysteine into methionine, a reaction which requires the methylcobalamine as an essential co-enzyme for the action of the appropriate methyltransferase. Furthermore, N5-CH₃THFA rapidly leaks out of the cell.

EQ 61-4

Homocysteine + N5—CH₃THFA $\xrightarrow{B_{12}}$ methionine + THFA

The transformation of methylmalonic acid (a metabolite of proprionic acid) to succinic acid, which can enter the TCA cycle, is dependent on the adenosyl analogue of B₁₂ as it is a co-factor for the activity of methylmalonyl CoA mutase.

Vitamin B₁₂ is present only in animal foods and is ultimately derived from bacterial synthesis. Physiologic absorption requires peptic separation of B₁₂ from animal protein. B₁₂ (extrinsic factor) then combines with a glycoprotein (intrinsic factor) produced by gastric parietal cells. The B₁₂-IF complex is absorbed on specific receptors in the terminal ileum. B₁₂ is then actively transported to the plasma, which contains three binding proteins. Transcobalamin I and III are storage binders released from the white blood cells, which bind and release vitamin B₁₂ slowly. Transcobalamin II is produced in the liver and other cells and is the principal transport protein with a rapid turnover of bound B₁₂. The B₁₂-TCII complex binds to receptors on tissue cells. Vitamin B₁₂ is released into and stored in the liver (Figure 61-20). Adequate stores last for years.

Etiopathogenesis of the megaloblastic anemias

Folate deficiency may occur from decreased intake in patients with poor diets (e.g., in alcoholics). Decreased absorption may occur in malabsorption syndromes (e.g., sprue) or from ingestion of drugs that inhibit intestinal conjugase (diphenylidantoin and oral contraceptives). Increased utilization occurs in infancy, during pregnancy, and in cases of hemolytic anemia. Finally, folate deficiency can occur from inhibited utilization after administration of the antifolate drug, methotrexate, which inhibits the activity of dihydrofolate reductase (Box 61-7).

B₁₂ deficiency only rarely results from a decreased intake in patients who are strict vegetarians. It usually results from malabsorption due to a gastric abnormality resulting in a lack of intrinsic factor, to an ileal abnormality, or to a hereditary deficiency of TC II (Box 61-7). The most important

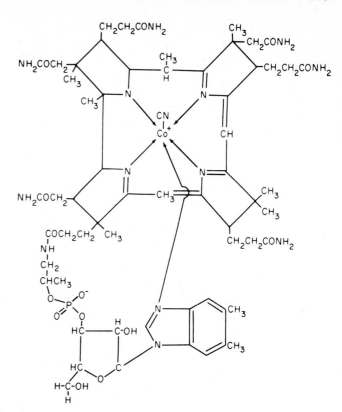

Fig. 61-19 Formula of cyanocobalamin (vitamin B₁₂). *From Miale JB: Laboratory medicine: hematology, ed 6, St. Louis, 1982, Mosby—Year Book, Inc.*

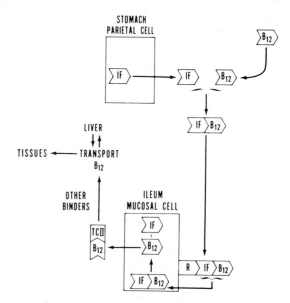

Fig. 61-20 Absorption, transport, and storage of vitamin B₁₂. IF = intrinsic factor; R = ileal receptors; TC II = transcobalamine II. *From Miale JB: Laboratory medicine: hematology, ed 6, St. Louis, 1982, Mosby—Year Book, Inc.*

Box 61-7   Classification of anemia caused by deficiency of vitamin B$_{12}$ or folate

I. Vitamin B$_{12}$ deficiency
   A. Caused by deficient intake (vegans)
   B. Resulting from lack of intrinsic factor
      1. Classic pernicious anemia
         a. In adults
         b. In children
      2. After gastrectomy
      3. After destruction of gastric mucosa
      4. Because of biologically inert intrinsic factor
   C. Due to disease of small intestine
      1. Blind loop syndrome
      2. Diseased or resected ileum
      3. In *Dibothriocephalus latus* infection
      4. Pancreatic dysfunction
   D. Familial selective vitamin B$_{12}$ malabsorption (Imerslund's syndrome)
   E. Deficiency of transcobalamin II
   F. Drug-induced malabsorption

   G. Zollinger-Ellison syndrome with steatorrhea
   H. Increased requirements
II. Folate deficiency
   A. Dietary deficiency
   B. Increased folate requirements
      1. Pregnancy (megaloblastic anemia of pregnancy)
      2. Infancy (megaloblastic anemia of infancy)
      3. Increased cellular proliferation (leukemia, hemolytic anemia)
   C. Due to malabsorption of folate
      1. Congenital folate malabsorption
      2. Drug-induced folate malabsorption
      3. Steatorrheas
   D. Due to defective folate interconversion
III. Megaloblastic anemia of uncertain etiology
   A. In hemochromatosis
   B. In Di Guglielmo's syndrome (erythroleukemia)
   C. Pyridoxine-responsive megaloblastic anemia

From Miale JB: Laboratory medicine: hematology, ed 6, St. Louis, 1982, Mosby–Year Book, Inc.

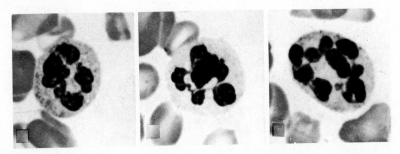

Fig. 61-21   Peripheral blood smear, megaloblastic anemia. Hypersegmented neutrophils. (Wright's stain, ×950.) *From Miale JB: Laboratory medicine: hematology, ed 6, St. Louis, 1982, Mosby–Year Book, Inc.*

gastric etiology of B$_{12}$ is the so-called Classical Pernicious Anemia (PA). This is a familial trait (dominant with variable penetrance) characterized by the adult onset of atrophic gastritis with absent IF, achylia, anacidity, anti-parietal cell, and anti-intrinsic factor antibodies (of both the blocking and binding types) and an increased incidence of gastric carcinoma. Juvenile P.A. is identical to the classic form, but develops in children. Congenital P.A. is transmitted as a recessive trait and manifests itself prior to three years of age. In this condition the sole defect is the lack of production of IF. Gastric atrophy and anti-IF antibodies are not features. Rarely, adult patients may suffer from an acquired P.A. without a familial history. Many post-gastrectomy patients develop P.A. Ileal causes of malabsorption include hereditary defect in B$_{12}$-IF binding sites (Inserslund's Syndrome), sprue, ileal resection, bacterial overgrowth in diverticulae and blind loops, and Diphyllobothrium latum infestation.

Clinical manifestations

Aside from the nonspecific signs and symptoms of anemia, many patients demonstrate slight scleral icterus and jaundice from the release of bilirubin from cells undergoing intramedullary and extramedullary destruction. In addition, patients may develop anemia severe enough to cause conges-

tive heart failure. In patients with pernicious anemia, the megaloblastic changes occuring in the gastrointestinal mucosa can be associated with the finding of a beefy red tongue and development of a malabsorption syndrome.

In addition to these manifestations, B$_{12}$ deficiency gives rise to demyelination and degeneration of the dorsal and lateral columns of the spinal cord known as "subacute combined system disease." The pathogenesis of the neurologic changes is poorly understood. There is some evidence that the defect in methionine synthesis from homocysteine results in a decrease in availability of adenosyl methionine, which may be required for the synthesis of a myelin protein.

Laboratory features

The anemia is macrocytic and normochromic and may be severe and accompanied by granulocytopenia and thrombocytopenia. Reticulocyte index is low. Examination of the peripheral smear shows numerous macroovalocytes. When the hematocrit is very low (<20%), megaloblastic normoblasts may be seen. The neutrophils are large and have hypersegmented nuclei (typically, more than 5% have five or more lobes). (See Figure 61-21.) The bone marrow shows erythroid hyperplasia with nuclear-cytoplasmic asynchrony, giant bands, and increased iron stores (Figure 61-22). Serum iron levels may be increased. A mild increase of indirect bilirubin is commonly found. A marked elevation of serum LDH resulting from the ineffective erythropoesis is found. Notably, LDH 1 is more elevated than LDH 2 and reflects the increased content of the former isoenzyme in megaloblastic red cell precursors.

The diagnostic findings of folate deficiency are decreased serum and red cell folate levels with a normal serum B_{12} level. Assays for these vitamins are discussed elsewhere (Chapter 20). Patients with folate deficiency also demonstrate increased urinary excretion of formimino-L-glutamic acid (Figlu) after an oral loading dose of histidine because tetrahydrofolate is required to transform Figlu, an intermediary metabolic product of histidine into glutamic acid. This test has now been replaced by the direct assay of folate because the vitamin level falls before the Figlu excretion test becomes abnormal.

In patients with B_{12} deficiency, the serum B_{12} level is decreased and the serum folate level may be normal or elevated while the red cell folate level may be decreased or normal. These patients also demonstrate increased urinary excretion of methylmalonic acid following an oral loading dose of valine because B_{12} is required as a co-factor to transform methylmalonic acid, a metabolic product of valine, into succinic acid. This test has now been replaced by the direct assay of B_{12} because the vitamin level falls before the excretion test becomes abnormal. It is also abnormal in the rare case of congenital methylmalonic aciduria.

The usual test used to differentially diagnose the causes of B_{12} deficiency is Schilling's test. As previously discussed (Chapter 59), this test depends on the excretion of orally administered isotope labeled B_{12} in the urine, following an IM "flushing dose" of nonlabeled B_{12}. If more than 7% of the small orally administered radioactive dose is excreted in the urine over the following 24 hours, the cause of the B_{12} is nutritional. If less is excreted, the test is repeated, along with oral administration of intrinsic factor. If this regimen corrects the excretion pattern, the diagnosis of P.A. is made. If it does not correct the excretion pattern, then the B_{12} deficiency is due to either an ileal defect or lack of TC II (Box 61-8).

Because of its diagnostic specificity, many investigators believe that the workup of an adult patient with known B_{12} deficiency can be initiated with a test for anti-intrinsic factor antibodies, and that the Schilling's test be performed only if the serum is not found to contain antibodies. The immunoassays for antibodies to intrinsic factor measure the presence of both blocking and binding types. The test for blocking antibodies is based on the ability of test serum to inhibit complex formation between reagent intrinsic factor and subsequently added ^{57}Co-B_{12} while binding antibody assays detect the formation of immune complexes formed between ^{57}Co-B_{12}-IF and antibody contained in the test serum. Although the assays are highly specific for pernicious anemia, approximately 25% of patients with proven disease do not possess such antibodies. Although in excess of 90% of adult patients with pernicious anemia have anti-parietal antibodies, the poor specificity of this finding precludes its use as a routine diagnostic procedure.

Recommendations to perform routine gastric aspirate analysis of pH following stimulation with a histamine analog

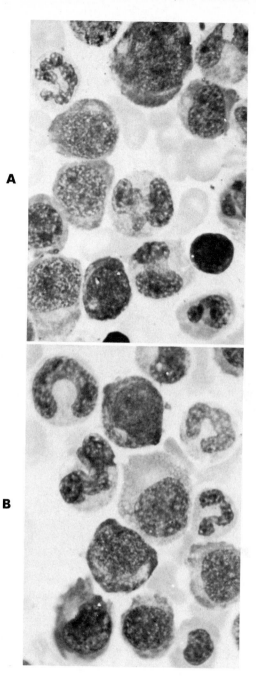

Fig. 61-22 A & B. Bone marrow aspirate, megaloblastic anemia. Hypercellular marrow with marked erythroid hyperplasia **(A)** cells show marked megaloblastic features **(A)**. Note the giant band **(B)**. (Wright's stain, ×950.) *From Miale JB: Laboratory medicine: hematology, ed 6, St. Louis, 1982, Mosby–Year Book, Inc.*

in order to detect achlorhydria and achylia in cases of classical pernicious anemia have now been replaced by the tests described previously. Similarly, the performance of therapeutic trials with small amounts of each vitamin (1-2μg B_{12} IM or 100-200 μgm of folic acid p.o.), to establish differential diagnoses between the two causes of megaloblastic anemia is unnecessary, unless it is impossible to obtain serum vitamin levels. These trials are based on the

---

Box 61-8 Pattern of results of Schilling test when there is a vitamin B_{12} deficiency state

I. Normal Schilling test
  A. Dietary deficiency of vitamin B_{12}
II. Malabsorption pattern (abnormal with no change after intrinsic factor is given)
  A. Malabsorption syndrome (tropical sprue, celiac disease, idiopathic steatorrhea)
  B. Malabsorption secondary to intestinal abnormalities
    1. Regional enteritis
    2. Stricture of small intestine
    3. Shunting anastomoses of small intestine
    4. Multiple diverticula of small intestine
    5. Resection of ileum
    6. Pancreatic dysfunction
    7. *Dibothriocephalus* infection
    8. Deficiency of transcobalamin II
III. Pernicious anemia pattern (abnormal standard test, normal excretion after intrinsic factor is given)
  A. Pernicious anemia (adult and juvenile)
  B. Gastrectomy
  C. Hypothyroidism
  D. Intrinsic factor inhibitor in gastric juice

From Miale JB: Laboratory medicine: hematology, ed 6, St. Louis, 1982, Mosby–Year Book, Inc.

---

fact that if such small physiologic doses are administered, the patient responds with a reticulocyte elevation after five to seven days only to the vitamin that is deficient.

With progressive deficiency, manifestations become evident in a predictable fashion. The earliest change noted is a fall in serum vitamin level, followed by an increase in the MCV, and release of hypersegmented neutrophils, and finally progressive anemia.

Following treatment, the earliest change noted is reversion of the bone marrow megaloblastosis to normoblastic cytology, which may begin as early as six to eight hours and is complete within four to six days. The maximal reticulocyte response is noted after five to seven days of treatment.

THE HEMOLYTIC ANEMIAS

Upon senescence, red cells are removed from circulation by the reticulo-endothelial system. Numerous changes occur in the aging red cells including loss of red cell enzyme activity, lipid peroxidation and progressive loss of cell membrane, increasing cell rigidity, and accumulation of oxidized heme breakdown products in the cytoplasm. How these changes trigger removal of the red cells from circulation is not entirely understood. Of probable importance is the observation that with aging, previously hidden red cell antigens become uncovered and bind autoantibodies directed against these determinants.

Hemolytic anemias result when the rate of peripheral destruction of red cells exceeds the rate of effective marrow production. Significant hemolysis may occur without anemia since erythroid production may be increased six- to eight-fold. Hemolysis may result from either extracellular or intracellular factors.

Although the direct quantification of red cell life span and destruction is best performed by direct measurement of red cell survival with ^{51}Cr, hemolysis is generally recognized by a reticulocyte index >3 and the laboratory tests characteristic of extravascular or intravascular red cell destruction.

The hemoglobin released during extravascular destruction is broken down into iron, which is reutilized; globin, which is split into amino acids destined to reenter the metabolic pool; and porphyrin ring, which is split at an α-methene bridge to release CO and biliverdin, which is quickly transformed to unconjugated bilirubin (Figure 61-23). The products of hemoglobin degregation can therefore be measured. The level of indirect acting (unconjugated) bilirubin reflects red cell destruction, but since it is rapidly eliminated within six to eight hours, a short episode of hemolysis will often be missed. In addition, it is not sensitive enough to be a reliable index of mildly shortened red cell life span. Urobilinogen excretion in the stool increases as bilirubin production and subsequent elimination into the bowel increases. These hemoglobin breakdown products and assays of their reference limits have been described in Chapter 11.

Cells may undergo intravascular destruction while still in the general circulation. In this case, the released hemoglobin is bound to the α_2 globulin, haptoglobin. This complex is absorbed and broken down by the reticulo-endothelial system. Usually the maximum hemoglobin binding capacity of the haptoglobin is 50 to 150 mg/dl, and as the complex is cleared, the haptoglobin tends to fall toward zero. When the binding capacity is exceeded, hemoglobin dimers pass through the glomerulus, where they are taken up in the tubular epithelial cells and intracellular hemosiderin formed. This can be detected in the sloughed cells of the urinary sediment. When the tubular resorption capacity is exceeded, hemoglobinuria occurs. If the released hemoglobin present in the circulation exceeds both the haptoglobin binding capacity and the glomerular filtration rate, the hemoglobin accumulates in the plasma and then undergoes oxidation to methemoglobin, which in turn loses free hematin that is either bound to β-glycoprotein, hemopexin, and cleared by the reticulo-endothelial system or bound to albumin to form methemalbumin, which circulates for several days prior to clearing by the reticuloendothelial system (Figure 61-24). Assays for plasma hemoglobin, methemalbumin and haptoglobin are discussed in Chapter 11.

In addition to the release of hemoglobin from hemolysed red cells, other intracellular constituents are released. Of diagnostic relevance is the release of red cell LDH, the serum level of which subsequently rises. Such LDH is comprised principally of LDH2 and, to a lesser degree, LDH1.

Anemias due to extracorpuscular hemolysis

Hemolysis due to extracorpuscular changes can have various causes: immunological (autoimmune and isoimmune); mechanical (malfunctioning heart valve prostheses, "march" hemoglobinuria, and microangiopathic hemolytic anemia);

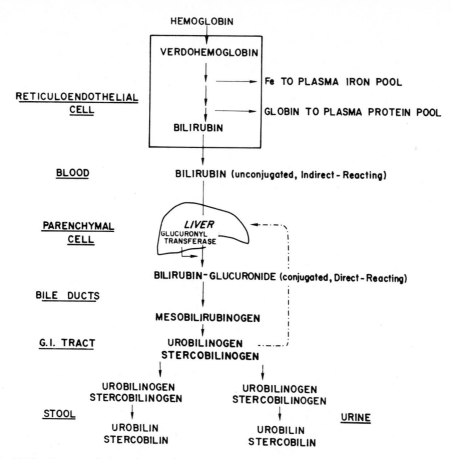

Fig. 61-23 Extravascular hemolysis and catabolic pathways of hemoglobin. *From Miale JB: Laboratory medicine: hematology, ed 6, St. Louis, 1982, Mosby–Year Book, Inc.*

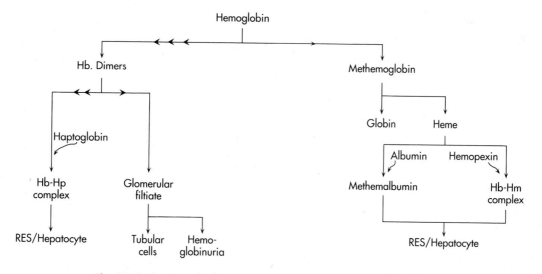

Fig. 61-24 Intravascular hemolysis and disposition of released hemoglobin.

infectious and toxic (*Clostridium* perfringens, *streptococcus*, malaria, *Babesia*, *bartonella*); chemical (heavy metals, drugs, metabolites); osmotic (water); and thermal, (Box 61-9). The anemia associated with hypersplenism is commonly considered one of the hemolytic anemias. However, it is doubtful that splenomegaly alone results in anemia. Although red cells are sequestered in the enlarged spleen, there is modest increased destruction of cells that are otherwise normal. Patients with anemia probably have either an intrinsic red cell defect or a decreased marrow production reserve.

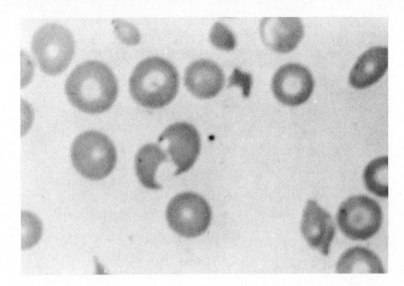

Fig. 61-25 Peripheral blood smear, shistocytes. (Wright's stain, ×1250.) *From Miale JB: Laboratory medicine: hematology, ed 6, St. Louis, 1982, Mosby–Year Book, Inc.*

Immune hemolytic anemia

Immune damage to red cells may be isoimmune (e.g., hemolytic transfusion reactions and hemolytic disease of the newborn); autoimmune (cold or warm antibodies); or drug induced. Elimination of these cells is by either intra- or extravascular lysis. This group will be discussed in Chapter 70.

Mechanical hemolytic anemias

Hemolysis of red cells may occur by mechanical trauma, which disrupts the integrity of the red cell, resulting in the production of shistocytes and helmet cells (Figure 61-25), the compensatory increased release of reticulocytes, and the discharge of free hemoglobin into the circulation. Hemolysis may be associated with cardiac valve dysfunction. Patients with malfunctioning valve prostheses often suffer angiopathic damage to red cells. Similar damage may be seen after prolonged and vigorous running or walking on hard surfaces, a condition known as march hemoglobinuria. Microangiopathic hemolytic anemia results from the passage of red cells through small vessels affected by significant endothelial damage, often containing small thrombi. It can therefore be seen in disseminated intravascular coagulation, thrombotic thrombocytopenic purpura, hemolytic-uremic syndrome, vasculitis, malignant hypertension, and diffuse carcinomatosis.

Hemolytic anemias due to infectious agents and toxins

Hemolysis of red cells during episodes of infectious diseases may occur as a result of the parasitization of red cells, which leads to their intravascular rupture or premature destruction by the reticulo-endothelial system (malaria, *Babesia*, *bartonella*). Destruction may also occur because of the production of toxins by bacteria that attack red cell membrane phospholipids (*Cl perfringens*, streptococci). Hemolytic snake venoms also contain such phospholipases and directly disrupt cell membrane integrity.

Discussed separately are hemolytic anemias resulting from immune damage to red cells occurring as a consequence of viral infections or in the course of disseminated intravascular coagulation complicating sepsis or rickettsial and parasitic diseases.

Anemias due to intracorpuscular hemolysis

Hemolysis due to intracorpuscular defects may be secondary to membrane defects including structural defects in the spectrin-actin cytoskeleton, abnormal permeability to ions, or unusual susceptibility to the action of complement; inherited red cell metabolic disorders (due to lack of normal activity of enzymes in the adult cell); or to abnormal hemoglobins that predispose the cells to shortened survival, (Box 61-9).

Hereditary spherocytosis and other membrane defects

The biconcave discoid shape and deformability of the red cell depends largely on the relationship of the surface area to its volume and the structure of the cell membrane. The quantity of membrane normally exceeds that required to enclose its volume by approximately 50%, thereby permitting the cell to relax within its redundant membrane and assume the form of a biconcave disc. A further increase in the surface area to volume ratio results in still more redundant membrane and the formation of a highly deformable target cell, while a reduction in the surface area to volume ratio of approximately one tends to result in the formation of a rigid spherocyte as the membrane is stretched tightly about the cellular contents (Figure 61-26).

The red cell membrane is a typical bilipid structure composed of phospholipid molecules arranged with their hydrophobic fatty acid tails facing internally, and their hydrophobic heads facing the external surface of the cell. Phosphatidyl choline and sphingomyelin make up the outer lipid layer, while phosphatidyl ethanolamine and phosphatidyl serine constitute the inner layer. The membrane also contains intercolated cholesterol molecules and several trans-

Box 61-9   Classification of hemolytic anemias

I. CAUSED BY EXTRACORPUSCULAR CONDITIONS

  A. Immune hemolysis
    1. Autoimmune hemolytic anemias
      a) Warm autoimmune hemolytic anemias
        Idiopathic
        Secondary
      b) Cold autoimmune hemolytic anemias
        Idiopathic
        Secondary
    2. Isoimmune hemolysis
      a) Hemolytic disease of the newborn
      b) Hemolytic transfusion reactions
    3. Drug-related hemolytic anemias
  B. Mechanical hemolysis
    1. Macrovascular hemolytic anemia
      a) Cardiac valve prosthesis dysfunction
      b) March hemoglobinuria
    2. Microangiopathic hemolytic anemias
      a) Disseminated intravascular coagulation
      b) Vasculitis
      c) Malignant hypertension
      d) Thrombotic thrombocytopenic purpura
      e) Hemolytic-uremic syndrome
  C. Hemolysis caused by other physical agents
    1. Burns
    2. Osmotic hemolysis
  D. Hemolytic agents caused by infectious agents and biologic toxins
    1. Malaria
    2. Bartonellosis
    3. Babesiosis
    4. Bacterial toxins (Cl, perfringens, streptococci)
    5. Venoms
  E. Hemolysis caused by direct action of drugs
    1. Heavy metal intoxications
    2. Others

II. CAUSED BY INTRACORPUSCULAR DEFECTS

  A. Membrane defects
    1. Abnormalities of the spectrin-actin cytoskeleton
      a) Hereditary spherocytosis
      b) Hereditary eliptocytosis
    2. Abnormalities in the membrane phospholipid content
      a) Abetalipoproteinemia
      b) Obstructive jaundice
      c) Others
    3. Abnormalities in cell permiability
      a) Hereditary stomatocytosis
      b) Hereditary xerocytosis
    4. Paroxysmal nocturnal hemoglobinuria
  B. Metabolic defects
    1. Defects of the E-B pathway
      a) Hexokinase deficiency
      b) Pyruvate kinase deficiency
      c) Others
    2. Defects of the hexose monophosphase shunt
      a) Glucose 6-phosphate dehydrogenase deficiency
      b) Glutathione reductase deficiency
      c) Others
    3. Defects of other enzymes
      a) Pyrimidine 5- nucleotidase deficiency
      b) Others
  C. Hemoglobinopathies
    1. Poorly soluble hemoglobins
      a) Sickle cell anemia
      b) S-C disease
      c) Sickle-thal disease
      d) Others
    2. Unstable hemoglobins

---

membranous proteins. Externally, sugar molecules are associated with either the phospholipids (glycolipids) or selected transmembranous proteins (glycoproteins). Below this membrane is a protein cytoskeleton, which is periodically linked to transmembrane proteins. The membrane and cytoskeletal proteins can be separated on polyacrylamide gels by electrophoresis following detergent solubilization (SDS-PAGE). Those stained with Coomasie Blue are designated by band number, while those heavily glycosylated are only stained with a PAS stain and are termed "glycophorins" (Figure 61-27).

The membrane lipids are freely mobile within the membrane, while the cholesterol is in free exchange with that in the plasma. The quantity of membrane lipids may increase when red cells are incubated in serum with markedly increased fatty acids and cholesterol. The glycolipid and glycoprotein moieties are associated with many red cell antigen systems.

Among the transmembrane proteins described, the following are of note: 1) band 3 protein functions as an anion transporter, is associated wtih the Ii antigen system, binds various enzymes (e.g., glyceraldehyde phosphate dehydro-

genase) and hemoglobin, and anchors the cytoskeleton; 2) the glycophorins are negatively charged due to their associated sialic acid moieties, possess blood group antigen determinants (glycophorin A is associated with MN antigens and glycophorin B is associated with Ss antigens), and anchor proteins of the cytoskeleton; 3) other proteins function as Na+ K+ pump ATPases, Ca++Mg++ATPases, and glucose transporters. In general these membrane proteins, as well as the cytoskeletal proteins, are essential for membrane integrity.

The submembranous cytoskeleton structure and its attachment to the membrane is highly complex (Figure 61-28). It is comprised largely of dimers of α and β spectrin (bands 1 and 2), which are linked together about actin and protein 4.1 moieties (band 5) to form tetramers or as oligomers complexed to tropomyosin (band 7) and protein 4.1. These fibers are, in turn, linked to band 3 protein via ankyrin (band 2.1) or to glycophorin A via protein 4.1, as shown. Both quantitative and qualitative abnormalities of spectrin and the other skeletal proteins or their associations with each other have been described. Such abnormalities may lead to abnormalities in membrane structure, stability, and

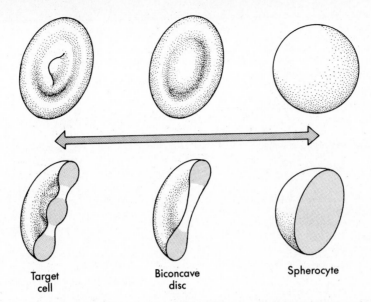

Fig. 61-26 Membrane surface-volume relationship to cell shape. The normal red cell possesses a greater membrane surface than necessary to contain the enclosed hemoglobin content. In such cells the hemoglobin pools on the periphery give rise to the usual biconcave disc appearance. With a reduced surface-volume relationship the cell is completely distended with hemoglobin, giving rise to a spherocyte. With an abnormally increased surface-volume relationship, redundant membrane bulges from the central region of the cell and contains hemoglobin, giving rise to a "target cell."

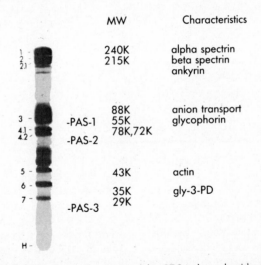

	MW	Characteristics
1	240K	alpha spectrin
2	215K	beta spectrin
2.1		ankyrin
3	88K	anion transport
-PAS-1	55K	glycophorin
4.1	78K,72K	
4.2 -PAS-2		
5	43K	actin
6	35K	gly-3-PD
7	29K	
-PAS-3		
H		

Fig. 61-27 Red cell membrane proteins separated by SDS-polyacrylamide gel electrophoresis after staining with Coomasie Blue. Each band is indicated by a number in order of decreasing molecular weight. The functional protein associated with the different bands is indicated. Not shown are glycoprotein bands, which would stain with PAS. *From Miller DR and Baehner RL: Blood diseases of infancy and childhood, ed 6, St. Louis, 1990, Mosby–Year Book, Inc.*

function of varying degrees including the types of hemolytic anemia listed previously.

Hereditary spherocytosis. This is the most common of the hereditary membrane defects and is often associated with significant hemolysis. It affects one in 5000 individuals and is generally transmitted as an autosomal dominant trait. The homozygous state is considered incompatible with life. Approximately 20% of cases occur in the absence of a family history and may represent *de novo* mutations. Rare cases are transmitted as recessive traits. These patients demonstrate a variety of defects that manifest as HS and are most commonly disturbances in the binding of spectrin to other cytoskeletal proteins. However, occasionally an absolute decrease in the amount of spectrin may be present (Table 61-3). The total surface-volume ratio is decreased either because of an inherent decrease in the amount of skeletal protein or an instability in the skeletal organization, which is thought to result in subsequent loss of membrane. This loss of membrane leads to rigid microspherocytes.

These spherocytes are not only less deformable than nor-

Table 61-3 Selected hereditary membrane protein abnormalities

Manifestation	Designation	Molecular defect	Transmission
Spherocytosis	HS (Sp⁺)	Decrease in Spectrin	Dominant, Recessive
	HS (Sp-4.1)	Decrease in Spectrin-4.1 binding	Dominant
	—	Increased binding of Spectrin to 4.1	?
Elliptocytosis	HE (4.1⁺)	Decrease of 4.1	Dominant Heterozygote
	HE (4.1⁰)	Absence of 4.1	Dominant Homozygote
	HE (SpDα-SpD) or HE (SpDβ-SpD)	Spectrin α or β A.A. chain substitutions leading to abnormal Spectrin Dimer Formation	Dominant
	HE (Sp-2.1)	Decrease in Spectrin-Ankyrin Binding	Recessive
	HE (2.1-3)	Defective Ankyrin-Band 3 Binding	Dominant
Pyropoikilocytosis	HPP (SpDα-SpD)	Spectrin α Chain A.A. Substitutions leading to Defective Dimer Formation with Reduced Spectrin Quantity	Double Heterozygote for Abnormal Spectrin α Chains

From: Palek J and Lux S: Red cell membrane skeletal defects in hereditary and acquired hemolytic anemias, Semin Hematol 20:189-244, 1980.

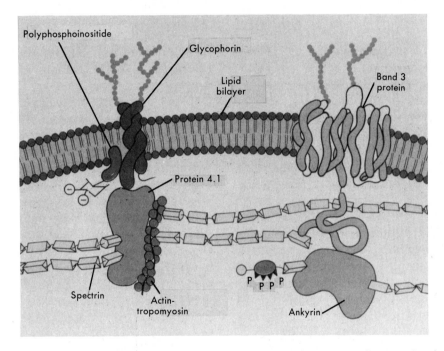

Fig. 61-28 Model of the erythrocyte membrane structural protein skeleton. *From Miller DR and Baehner RL: Blood diseases of infancy and childhood, ed 6, St. Louis, 1990, Mosby–Year Book, Inc.*

mal but are also abnormally permeable to Na+, requiring increased ATP consumption to maintain structural integrity. When these rigid spheres are caught in the splenic cords, hypoglycemia and acidosis decreases ATP synthesis and predisposes them to increased membrane loss and further rigidity. After repeated passages, these cells are no longer able to escape from the cords and are destroyed by the reticulo-endothelial system.

The clinical picture is variable. Severe forms are manifested by anemia, intermittent jaundice, splenomegaly (up to two- to eightfold) due to reticuloendothelial hyperplasia and congestion of the cords, bilirubin gallstones, and rarely, leg ulcers. Intermittently, hemolysis may markedly increase during episodes of infection (hemolytic crisis), or temporary red cell aplasia (aplastic crisis) may occur as previously discussed.

The anemia may be normochromic and normocytic, but more commonly the MCV tends to be low and the MCHC increased. The peripheral smear shows anisocytosis with microspherocytes and polychromasia (Figure 61-29). There is a reticulocytosis, which is roughly proportional to the severity of the anemia unless secondary folate deficiency or aplasia intervenes.

The cells show increased autohemolysis on incubation at 37°C for 48 hours. Autohemolysis is largely prevented by addition of glucose to the whole blood. The osmotic fragility test (Figure 61-30) shows that the cells have an increased susceptibility to osmotic stress. This test is performed by incubating venous blood diluted to a .5% concentration in saline solutions of varying strengths (.85% to .30% sodium chloride). When performed at room temperature and when

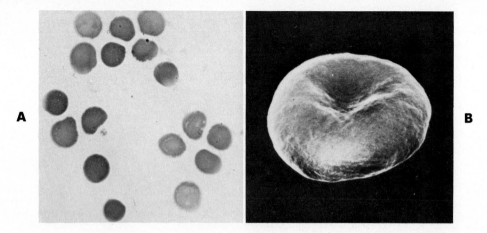

Fig. 61-29 The microspherocyte. **A,** Blood smear from patient with hereditary spherocytosis (Wright's stain). **B,** Scanning electron microscope photograph. (Courtesy Dr. M. Bessis.) *From Miale JB: Laboratory medicine: hematology, ed 6, St. Louis, 1982, Mosby—Year Book, Inc.*

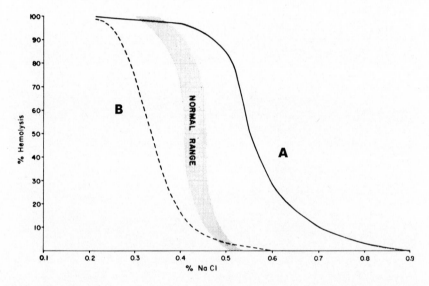

Fig. 61-30 Normal and abnormal osmotic and fragility curves. **A,** Increased osmotic fragility. **B,** Decreased osmotic fragility. *From Miale JB: Laboratory medicine: hematology, ed 6, St. Louis, 1982, Mosby—Year Book, Inc.*

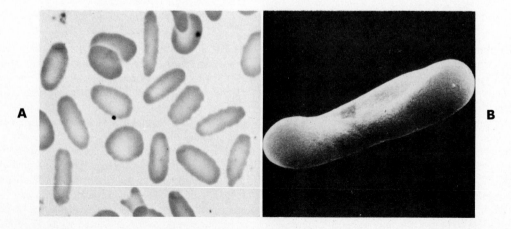

Fig. 61-31 The elliptocyte. **A,** Blood smear, hereditary elliptocytosis (Wright's stain). **B,** Scanning electron microscope photograph. (Courtesy Dr. M. Bessis.) *From Miale JB: Laboratory medicine: hematology, ed 6, St. Louis, 1982, Mosby—Year Book, Inc.*

incubation is carried out for 20 minutes, normal cells are resistant to hemolysis in saline solutions of greater than .45% to .50% strength.

Hereditary elliptocytosis. This is a very common membrane defect (Figure 61-31). Its exact incidence has been estimated at approximately one in every 2000 to 5000 individuals. The incidences cited are greater than in previous years because the previously held opinion that some normal individuals may possess up to 15% elliptocytes has been revised. It is now believed that healthy individuals possess less than 1% elliptocytes. Elliptocytosis is associated with a wide variety of molecular defects (Table 61-3). Although generally mild, some patients experience more severe hemolysis.

In some patients HE is associated with the presence of spherocytes *(Spherocytic HE)*. Spherocytes seem to be present when molecular defects involve the linkage of the cytoskeleton to the membrane. Such patients have mild ongoing hemolysis, which is usually compensated. A few patients who are double heterozygotes for defects involving spectrin heterodimer formation develop a severe hemolytic anemia, characterized by large numbers of poikilocytes, few elliptocytes, and a marked propensity of cells to fragment when exposed to mild increases in temperature (i.e., 45°C). (The term *hereditary pyropoikilocytosis* has been assigned to this condition.) Some patients are homozygous for more common HE gene products and tend to have poikilocytosis in the peripheral smear in addition to numerous elliptocytes.

Hereditary stomatocytosis. Hereditary stomatocytosis is one of a group of rare hemolytic anemias resulting from abnormal cation permeability. In this condition the membrane is abnormally permeable to Na+, which, in spite of increased Na+ pump activity, accumulates in the cell. A resultant influx of water into the cell leads to overhydrated cells (hydrocytes), cells with a decreased MCHC that have lost their biconcave disc shape to assume the form of a cup. Such cells, when seen on fixed peripheral smear, appear to have a central or peripheral mouth-like slit from which the term "stomatocyte" is derived (Figure 61-32). A still rarer familial abnormality associated with hemolysis is when cells are abnormally permeable to K+ diffusion out the cell, leading to progressive dehydration and appearance of small spiculated cells with an increased MCHC. This condition is termed *hereditary xerocytosis* (Figure 61-33).

Acanthocytosis and spur cell anemia. Alterations in the lipid composition of the red cell membrane also lead to structural abnormalities, which, when marked, lead to hemolysis. Such alterations in lipid composition occur as cells age in a variety of clinical conditions. Patients with congenital abetalipoproteinemia experience a progressive increase in the red cell sphingomyelin:lecithin ratio. Such an increase is associated with transformation of erythrocytes into cells possessing one or more irregular spiculations, termed "acanthocytes" (Figure 61-34). These cells have a shortened survival. Similarly, patients with obstructive liver disease and cirrhosis may develop a deficiency in plasma lecithin-cholesterol acyl transferase (LCAT) resulting in increased membrane cholesterol. The increased membrane mass, if moderate, results in the formation of target cells with a normal red cell life span (Figure 61-35). However, continued accumulation of cholesterol results in the formation of acanthocytes. Acanthocytes with multiple-pro-

jecting spiculations are also known as "spur" cells. The hemolytic anemia associated with severe obstructive liver disease is also known as spur cell anemia. In addition, children with vitamin E deficiency or the McLeod syndrome have numerous acanthocytes in their peripheral blood smears.

Paroxysmal nocturnal hemoglobinuria. Paroxysmal Nocturnal Hemoglobinuria (PNH) is an acquired stem cell defect. Twenty-five percent of cases arise in patients with aplastic anemia. Occasionally, patients with myeloproliferative diseases and leukemia also develop PNH, which occurs in both sexes equally. Approximately 50% of cases occur between the ages of 20 and 40. In this disorder, a population of red cells is unusually susceptible to the action of complement fixed on the cell membrane via the alternate pathway.

The abnormal cell population coexists with a population of apparently normal cells (PNH type I cells). Although the underlying membrane defect is poorly understood, a major contributing factor is the absence of glycophorin-associated decay accelerating factor (DAF), an inhibitor of the C3 convertase complexes fixed to the membrane by either the classical or alternate pathways. These cells are heavily laden with clusters of C3b molecules, and thus are likely to initiate the formation of membrane attack complexes. Although complement-sensitive cells from different patients all demonstrate a lack of DAF, they vary in their propensity to form attack complexes. The PNH cells of most patients tend to form large numbers of complexes and are extremely liable to undergo hemolysis (PNH type III cells), while the cells of other patients tend to form fewer complexes and are less predisposed to hemolysis (PNH type II cells). Although the significance of the finding is unknown, Type II and Type III cells demonstrate a lack of membrane-associated acetylcholinesterase activity, while Type I cells have normal amounts of activity.

In these patients, ongoing intravascular hemolysis may increase during sleep for unknown reasons and is periodically further accentuated during episodes of infection or allergic reactions when fluid phase complement activation may occur. Patients usually have a hematocrit below 30%. The reticulocyte index is high unless the patient has developed iron deficiency secondary to the intravascular hemolysis. The peripheral smear varies according to whether or not iron deficiency is present. Among the usual laboratory findings of intravascular hemolysis, hemosiderinuria is a constant and usually dramatic finding.

In addition to the anemia, about 50% of patients are neutropenic and thrombocytopenic. The leukocyte alkaline phosphatase is low. It is believed that neutrophils and platelets are extremely sensitive to complement activation as well. Fixation of C3 on the neutrophil surface may induce a defect in chemotactic and phagocytic functions, while attachment to platelets induces the release reaction. This latter phenomenon may be responsible for the high incidence of life-threatening venous thromboses seen in these patients. The median survival is thought to be from five to 10 years. Infection and thrombotic episodes account for most deaths. Some patients develop acute leukemia.

The susceptibility of the cell to complement can be detected by provoking cell lysis following exposure of cells to a mild fall in pH (acidified serum lysis or Ham test), or

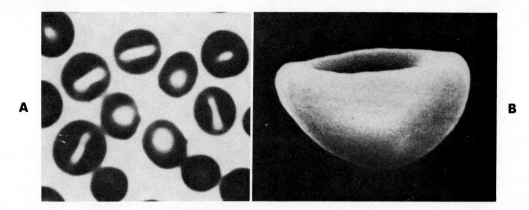

Fig. 61-32 The stomatocyte. **A,** Blood smear (Wright's stain). **B,** Scanning electron microscope photograph. (Courtesy Dr. M. Bessis.) *From Miale JB: Laboratory medicine: hematology, ed 6, St. Louis, 1982, Mosby–Year Book, Inc.*

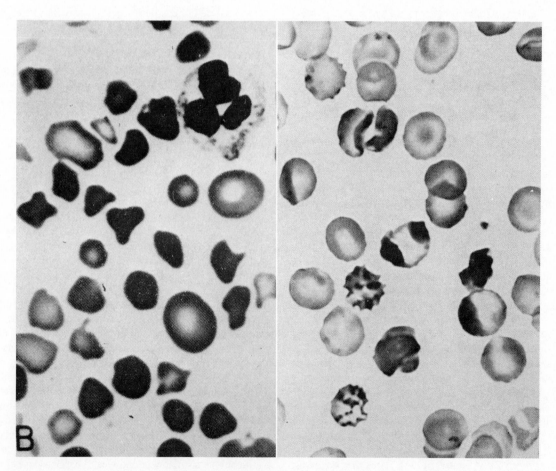

Fig. 61-33 Xerocytes. *From Glader BE, et al: N Engl J Med 291:492, 1974.*

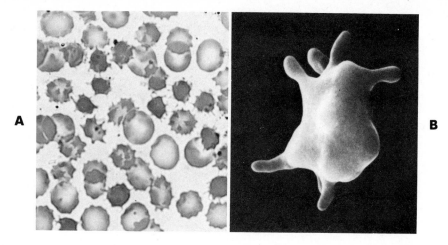

Fig. 61-34   The acanthocyte. **A,** Blood smear (Wright's stain). **B,** Scanning electron microscope photograph. (**A** courtesy Dr. K. Singer; **B** courtesy Dr. M. Bessis.) *From Miale JB: Laboratory medicine: hematology, ed 6, St. Louis, 1982, Mosby—Year Book, Inc.*

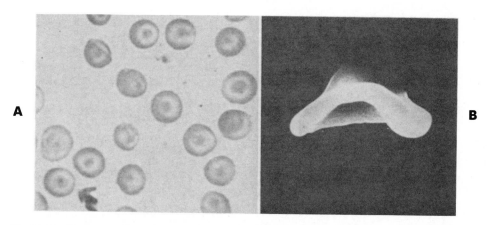

Fig. 61-35   The target cell. **A,** Blood smear (Wright's stain). **B,** Scanning electron microscope photograph. (Courtesy Dr. M. Bessis.) *From Miale JB: Laboratory medicine: hematology, ed 6, St. Louis, 1982, Mosby—Year Book, Inc.*

by fixing complement after membrane absorption of aggregated serum globulins when the cells are exposed to low ionic strength sucrose solution (sucrose hemolysis test).

The acidified serum lysis test is performed by incubating the patient's red cells, obtained from defibrinated blood, at 37°C with both fresh autologous and ABO compatible homologous sera adjusted to pH 6.5 with dilute hydrochloric acid. The amount of hemolysis observed is quantified photometrically at 450 nm as cyanmethemoglobin following addition of Drabkin's solution, and then compared to a completely hemolysed autologous standard. A positive test is when 10% to 80% hemolysis of the cells is observed. This test, although less sensitive than the sucrose hemolysis test, is highly specific if performed with the proper controls (e.g., the use of non-acidified serum and heating serum to 56°C). In addition, HEMPAS cells from patients with type II congenital dyserythropoietic anemia will also demonstrate

hemolysis following incubation with some homologous acidified sera but not with autologous serum. As previously explained, such cells are lysed via the classical pathway following sensitization of the cells with antibodies contained in the sera.

The sucrose-hemolysis test is performed by incubating citrated red cells from the patient with a sucrose solution and a small amount of ABO compatible serum, and then calculating the percentage of cells hemolysed, as in the acidified serum lysis test. Lysis in PNH varies from 10% to 80%. HEMPAS cells give a negative test.

Glucose 6-phosphate dehydrogenase deficiency and other red cell enzymopathies

Immature red cells (normoblasts) possess full complements of the structural and enzymatic machinery necessary for aerobic and anaerobic glucose metabolism, protein synthesis, and fat metabolism.

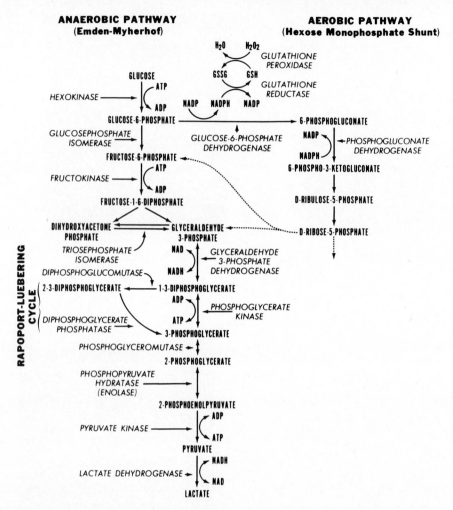

ANAEROBIC PATHWAY
(Emden-Myherhof)

AEROBIC PATHWAY
(Hexose Monophosphate Shunt)

Fig. 61-36 Major pathways of glucose metabolism in the red blood cell. *From Miale JB: Laboratory medicine: hematology, ed 6, St. Louis, 1982, Mosby—Year Book, Inc.*

With loss of the mitochrondria and microsomal units from the reticulocyte, the mature red cell is only able to metabolize glucose through two pathways (Figure 61-36): the anaerobic Embden-Meyerhoff pathway (90% to 95%) and the hexose-monophosphate shunt (5% to 10%). The E-B pathway generates two moles of ATP per mole of glucose consumed. One of the principal functions of ATP is to maintain the integrity of the Na^+ and Ca^{++} pumps. This pathway is also the principal source of NADH required as a cofactor in the reduction of methemoglobin by methemoglobin diaphorase. Lastly, 2,3 DPG is formed from 1,3 DPG in the Rapaport-Luebring shunt and binds reversibly with hemoglobin to regulate O_2 release to the tissue. The HMP shunt is the major source of NADPH in the red cells and therefore the major pathway through which glutathione is maintained in the reduced state. Peroxide-generating reactions oxidize GSH to GSSG through glutathione peroxidase and thereby increase shunt activity. GSH is therefore essential in protecting both enzymes and hemoglobin against oxidation and membrane against lipid peroxidation.

In addition, all capability for the synthesis of protein, lipid, heme, and nucleotides is lost with the maturation of the reticulocyte to a mature red cell. Preserved, however, is the capacity for purine nucleotide salvage, requiring a phosphoribosyl transferase, as well as purine metabolism, requiring adenosine deaminase and other enzymes.

Inherited red cell metabolic defects may be manifested as congenital non-spherocytic hemolytic anemias and result from a decreased activity of enzymes present in the adult cell, which are essential to glycolysis or HMP shunt activity. These disorders are usually the result of amino acid substitutions producing molecules with deficient kinetic activity or with a shortened half-life because of sulfhydryl oxidation or molecular instability.

Glucose 6-phosphate dehydrogenase deficiency. HMP shunt defects result in decreased regeneration of intracellular GSH with increased oxidation of the cell constituents including lipid peroxidation of the membrane, denaturation of hemoglobin (Heinz bodies), and oxidation of enzymes predisposing the cells to hemolysis. The oxidant stress may be drugs (Box 61-10) or infection (macrophages

Box 61-10   Drugs causing hemolysis in G-6PD deficiency

CLINICALLY SIGNIFICANT HEMOLYSIS	NO SIGNIFICANT HEMOLYSIS UNDER NORMAL CONDITIONS
Antimalarials	Chloroquine
Pamaquine	Quinacrine
Pentaquine	Quinine*
Primaquine	Acetaminophen
Quinocide	Acetophenetidin
	p-Acetylsalicylic acid
Antipyretics and analgesics	Aminopyrine*
Acetanilide	Antipyrine*
	Sulfadiazine
Sulfonamides and sulfones	Sulfamerazine
N-acetylsulfanilimide	Sulfisoxazole
Nitrofurantoin	Sulfathiazole
Sulfacetamide	Sulfoxone
Sulfamethoxazole	p-Aminobenzoic acid
Diaminodiphenylsulfone	p-Aminophenol
Thiazosulfone	Aniline
	Antazolene
Others	Chloramphenicol
Adriamycin	Dimercaprol
BCNU	Diphenhydramine
Fava beans*	L-Dopa
Methylene blue	Isoniazid
Nalidixic acid	Menadione
Naphthalene	Phenylbutazone
Neoarsphenamine	Phenytoin
Phenylhydrazine	Probenecid
	Procainamide
	Pyrimethamine
	Streptomycin
	Trimethoprim
	Tripelennamine

From Valentine WN, et al: Ann Intern Med 103:245, 1985.
*Hemolysis in Caucasians only.

produce superoxide anion and hydrogen peroxide). These disorders vary in their clinical severity depending on the enzyme affected and the activity and stability of the mutation involved. Among those with severe hemolysis, red cells are constantly removed through ongoing extravascular splenic phagocytosis and fulminant intravascular hemolysis occurs if the oxidant stress is added. Patients with milder forms only undergo intermittent intravascular hemolysis with severe oxidant stress. Glucose 6-phosphate dehydrogenase deficiency is the prototype disorder and is the most common enzymopathy described. The next most common HMP disorders, glutathione reductase and pyruvate kinase deficiencies, occur with an incidence of perhaps only one thousandth the frequency of G6PD deficiency.

Numerous variants of G6PD are known. On the basis of electrophoretic migration, most commonly encountered variants can be designated as A or B. A variants migrate ahead of B variants on cellulose acetate at an alkaline pH (Figure 61-37). Whether or not the enzyme variant has a normal kinetic activity and T ½ and is therefore capable of maintaining normal activity in older red cells is designated

by + or −. The synthesis of G6PD and its variants is determined by the Gd gene or its variant alleles found on the X chromosomes. Type B is found in whites and 70% of black males. Type A is found exclusively in blacks. A-variants are associated with hemolysis only after oxidant stress. These enzymes have a half-life of 25 days (as opposed to the 60-day half-life of the normal A+ and B+ types), so that only the younger red cells have normal activity. Other types of body cells are not affected. Ten percent of the black male population carries the A-gene on the X chromosome, thus the trait is transmitted as a sex-linked "recessive." Rarely, female carriers with extreme Lyonization may show hemolysis as well. The B-variant enzyme in whites (Gd Mediterranean) and fast-moving variants in Orientals (e.g., Gd Canton) or North Africans (e.g., Gd Debrousse) have much shorter T ½ (often <10 days), so that most red cells are deficient in activity. Some patients with Gd Mediterranean exhibit marked hemolysis after ingestion of fava beans (favism). In these variants, other types of cells may also be deficient (e.g., granulocytes, hepatocytes, etc.).

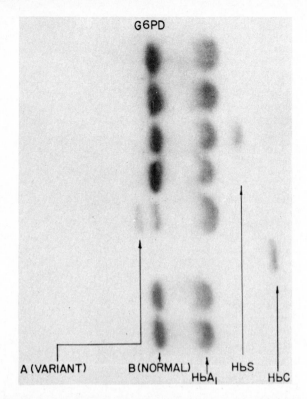

Fig. 61-37 Separation of G-6-PD (normal and variant) and simultaneous hemoglobin screening. (Courtesy Helena Laboratories, Beaumont, Tex.) *From Miale JB: Laboratory medicine: hematology, ed 6, St. Louis, 1982, Mosby–Year Book, Inc.*

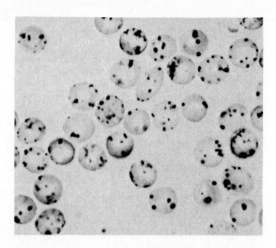

Fig. 61-38 Heinz body formation in drug-sensitive erythrocytes. Note multiple small bodies throughout cytoplasm. *From Beutler E, Dein RJ, and Alving AS: J Lab Clin Med 45:40, 1955.*

Patients with deficiency of G-6PD or other enzymes of the HMP shunt exhibit an increased sensitivity to oxidation of hemoglobin, so that incubation of cells with acetyl phenylhydralazine (an oxidant) results in oxidation and denaturation of hemoglobin, which stains with a supravital stain (Heinz body), (Figure 61-38). Other screening tests have been used to detect male hemizygous and female homozygous patients with severe G-6PD deficiency. None are capable of detecting the moderately depressed levels seen in female carriers. Among these tests are methemoglobin reduction, methylene blue reduction, and ascorbic cyanide tests. The most commonly employed screen is a fluorescent spot test, which is more specific than the others. The fluorescent spot test is based on the generation of fluorescent NADPH from substrate NADP$^+$ as follows:

EQ 61-5

$$\text{G6P} + \text{NADP}^+ \xrightarrow{\text{G-6PD}} \text{6PG} + \text{NADPH}$$
$$\text{(nonfluorescent)} \qquad \text{(fluorescent)}$$

In the test, which is marketed commercially, the sensitivity is augmented by the addition of glutathione to the reagent mixture of NADP and G6P. Following the addition of either patient or normal control blood, aliquots of the reaction mixture are placed on filter paper at five-minute intervals. The aliquots are then dried and placed under long-wave UV light. Patients with severe deficiency fail to show fluorescence of any spot samples. Not only does this technique display inadequate sensitivity to detect female carriers, but patients who have a high reticulocyte count incident to an episode of increased hemolysis may have a falsely negative test, because young cells have relatively increased quantities of G6PD activity. To adequately test such individuals, the assay should be repeated two to three months after the hemolytic episode or performed on a subpopulation of older cells separated by differential centrifugation or on a density gradient.

The quantitative determination of G6PD activity of red cells is also based on the conversion of NADP$^+$ to NADPH, which is measured spectrophotometrically at 340 nm. The quantity of enzyme present in a hemolysate prepared from an EDTA anticoagulated sample is therefore proportional to the rate of change in absorbance at 340 nm when the reaction is conducted at 37°C and is measured as IU/gm Hb. Although the World Health Organization accepts this determination as clinically useful and cites the reference range as approximately 10 to 18 IU/gm Hb, many workers recognize the fact that a fraction of this activity is due to the activity of red cell phosphogluconate dehydrogenase (PGD) in the hemolysate, since any 6-PG formed from G6P can be subsequently transformed to ribulose 5-P, a reaction which further generates NADPH from NADP$^+$. By repeating the assay after substituting 6-PG for G-6P in the reaction mixture, the activity of PGD can be determined and subtracted from the gross G-6PD value to give a corrected value, cited to be 6 to 12 IU/gm Hb b.

Pyruvate kinase (PK) deficiency. Enzymopathies of the E-B pathway are rare. The most common, PK deficiency, is perhaps a thousand times less frequent than G6PD deficiency and also less frequent than glutathione reductase (GR) deficiency. Most identified deficiencies in the E-B pathway cause cellular damage by failure to synthesize ATP. Those involving proximal enzymes in the pathway also result in decreased 2,3 DPG and NADH synthesis. Extravascular hemolysis probably results from failure of the Ca^{++} cation pumps of the cell membrane, which are ATPase dependent and result in the formation of rigid dehydrated cells that are trapped in the splenic cords.

PK Deficiency is transmitted as an autosomal recessive trait and is usually seen in northern Europeans. Most commonly, patients are double heterozygotes for different mutant genes. They are usually not markedly anemic, although the severely involved may have constant jaundice and most have splenomegaly. The patients tend to tolerate the anemia well because of the increased intracellular levels of 2,3 DPG characteristic of this enzymopathy. Some patients demonstrate positive autohemolysis tests. Heinz body preparations are negative.

The screening test commonly used is a fluorescent spot test, the principle of which is similar to that discussed previously. In this test, leukocyte depleted red cells, rather than whole blood, must be used because of the large quantity of PK present in leukocytes. The presence of normal levels of red cell PK is demonstrated by the ability of the red cell hemolysate to initiate a chain of reactions when added to a mixture of phospho(enol) pyruvate, ADP, LDH, and NADH, which culminate in the generation of nonfluorescent NAD$^+$ from NADH. The series of reactions involved are as follows:

EQ 61-6

$$PEP + ADP \xrightarrow{PK} ATP + Pyruvate$$

$$\underset{\text{(fluorescent)}}{Pyruvate + NADH + H^+} \xrightarrow{LDH} \underset{\text{(nonfluorescent)}}{Lactate + NAD^+}$$

The quantification of red cell PK is performed by a procedure similar to G-6PD determinations. However, the formed NAD$^+$ is detected by a decrease in optical density measured at 340 nm.

Sickle cell anemia and other hemoglobinopathies

Defects in the structure of the globin chains result from the transmission of mutant structural genes causing amino acid substitutions, additions, or deletions. These changes may cause alterations in charge of the molecules, which allows their detection in electrophoretic systems. Many of these abnormal hemoglobins do not cause alterations in function, but others cause striking abnormalities (hemoglobinopathies). Usually these dysfunctions can be directly related to changes in certain regions of the chain.

Substitutions in the A helical region often result in

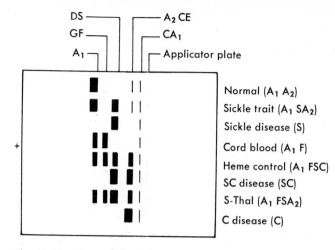

Fig. 61-39 Diagram of cellulose acetate electrophoretic patterns of normal and abnormal hemoglobins at pH 8.6. CA = carbonic anhydrase; + = anode. Heme Control is manufactured by Helena Laboratories, Beaumont, Tex. *From Sonnenwirth AC and Jarett L: Gradwohl's clinical laboratory methods and diagnosis, vol 1, ed 8, St. Louis, 1980, Mosby–Year Book, Inc.*

changes of solubility with formation of tactoids or puddling of hemoglobin (HbS, HbC, etc.).

Substitutions in the heme pocket or the $\alpha_1\beta_2$ contact region, along with deletions of amino acids or interruption of a helical chain by proline, may result in an unstable hemoglobin. These unstable hemoglobins tend to undergo oxidation and precipitate in the red cells.

Substitutions in the $\alpha_1\beta_2$ contact region or the C terminus of the β chain may alter the O$_2$ affinity of the hemoglobin, either increasing the affinity with resultant erythrocytosis or decreasing the affinity with "anemia."

Substitutions involving the proximal or distal histidine of the heme pocket may cause the production of methemoglobin (Hemoglobins M).

The primary screening method for the detection of an abnormal hemoglobin is hemoglobin electrophoresis. Most laboratories screen for hemoglobin variants by electrophoresis of hemolysates on cellulose acetate strips in an alkaline buffer (e.g., barbital or tris-EDTA-borate at pH 8.4). In this system, hemoglobin A (HbA) is the most negatively charged of the normal hemoglobins and migrates more rapidly toward the anode. The normal hemoglobins which migrate slower are HbA$_2$ and HbF. The principal slower variants are HbS and HbC. HbC migrates with HbA$_2$. Other variants that migrate like HbS include HbG and HbD, while HbE and HbO migrate together with HbA$_2$ and HbC. Hemoglobins that migrate ahead of HbA are termed "fast-moving" hemoglobins. They include HbH, HbBarts, and many of the unstable variants. Other hemoglobins migrate like HbA and these include HbM (Figure 61-39).

Numerous commercial systems are available and perform well, as long as precautions are taken to ensure good hemoglobin separation and to avoid protein trailing. The preparation of the hemolysate from packed red cells rather than whole blood and the packing of stroma into a discrete layer by the utilization of toluene together with distilled water in the hemolysing solution decreases protein trailing. Good

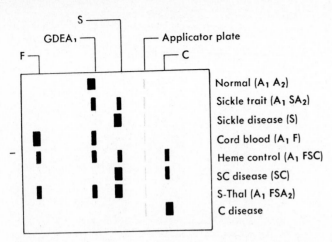

Fig. 61-40   Diagram of citrate agar, pH 6.2. electrophoretic patterns of normal and abnormal hemoglobins. Note separation of Hb D and Hb S and Hb E and Hb C; − = cathode. Heme Control is manufactured by Helena Laboratories, Beaumont, Tex. *From Sonnenwirth AC and Jarett L: Gradwohl's clinical laboratory methods and diagnosis, vol 1, ed 8, St. Louis, 1980, Mosby−Year Book, Inc.*

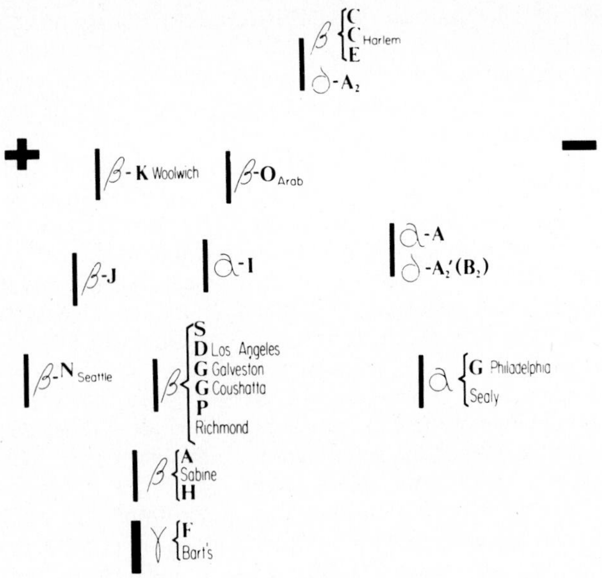

Fig. 61-41   Relative mobilities of globin chains, cellulose acetate, ureabarbital buffer, pH 8.7. *From Schmidt RM and Brosius EM: Basic laboratory methods of hemoglobinopathy detection, Atlanta, DHEW Publication No. (CDC) 76-8266.*

hemolysates can also be prepared from microsamples by using saponin as the hemolysing agent. Increased separation of the bands is achieved with a low ionic strength buffer (i.e., 0.05) and is favored by decreasing the voltage so as to minimize buffer evaporation due to generated heat. A voltage of 450 applied for 15 minutes usually results in good separation. Once separated, the hemoglobin bands can be stained with a protein stain (e.g., 0.5% Ponceau S). The identification of unknown bands is determined by comparing their migration positions with known control hemoglobins. The quantification of each band is usually performed by densitometry of the cleared electrophoretic strips or by eluting each separated band into buffer and then determining the OD of each band by spectrophotometry. As previously mentioned, the quantification of hemoglobins A_2 and F cannot be performed accurately by simple densitometry.

In the presence of very high levels of HbF, inadequate separation of hemoglobins is achieved by electrophoresis in order to accurately identify and quantify HbS and HbA by densitometry. Such a condition is noted in cord blood, and in this case, quantification is best performed by microcolumn chromatography using a cation-exchange resin (e.g., CM-Sephadex) and tris-maleate buffers at pH 6.8 and 7.4. When a hemolysate is applied over such a column and equilibrated with the pH 6.8 buffer, HbF passes to the bottom of the column, HbA settles in the middle of the column, and both HbS and HbC remain at the top. Subsequent passage of the pH 7.4 buffer through the column elutes HbA and HbS sequentially from the column. If desired, the eluted fractions can be collected and the hemoglobins quantified spectrophotometrically. As previously discussed, the accurate chromatographic quantification of HbA_2 is possible by using commercially available DEAE-Sephadex or cellulose micro-columns.

Hemoglobins can be further distinguished by their electrophoretic mobility in other media and pH (e.g., citrate agar at pH 6.1) (Figure 61-40); the electrophoretic mobility

of their constituent globin chains (Figure 61-41); or by their other properties (e.g., solubility, stability, or oxygen affinity). The separation of hemoglobins by citrate agar electrophoresis is now simplified by the availability of prepared plates and citrate buffers of the appropriate pH. Some have found that electrophoresis at 4° to 10°C reduces evaporation and permits neater separation of the hemoglobin bands, which are then stained with o-tolidene or another hemoglobin stain. This technique is of special help in distinguishing Hbs D and G from HbS and Hbs O and E from HbC. Some hemoglobins that have similar migration characteristics and cannot be separated by their other special properties are products of mutations in different chains (e.g., the α-chain variant, HbI, and the β-chain variant, HbN). Such variants can be readily distinguished if their globin chains are separated by a urea-2 mercaptoethanol buffer, and then electrophoresed on cellulose acetate strips. Other identification methods, such as isoelectric focusing and peptide fingerprinting, remain primarily research techniques.

Sickle cell anemia and trait.   HbS results from the substitution of #6 glutamic acid of the β chain with valine ($\alpha_2\beta_2^{6glu \rightarrow val}$). The gene is present in about 8% of black Americans. The presence of HbS predisposes the hemoglobin in a red cell to gelation. During gelation, HbS tetramers in the deoxy state tend to aggregate and polymerize into helical fibers, which then align themselves in parallel fashion to form intracellular precipitates termed "tactoids" (Figure 61-42). It has been proposed that gelation is initiated by molecules of deoxy Hb, which bind the N terminus of HbS β chains. All HbS molecules are able to participate in this polymerization. Heterozygotes tend to undergo sickling of the cells at much lower O_2 tensions than homozygotes, since HbA does not participate in the polymerization process. HbF likewise does not participate and high levels of

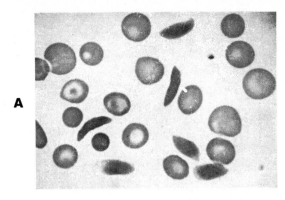

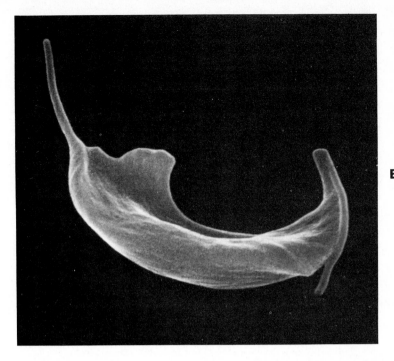

B

Fig. 61-42 Sickle cell anemia. **A,** peripheral smear. Note sickle cells, target cells, and polychromatophilic macrocytes. **B,** Sickle cell as seen with scanning electron microscope (× 5000). *From Weed RI: Clin Haematol 4:3, 1975. From Sonnenwirth AC and Jarett L: Gradwohl's clinical laboratory methods and diagnosis, vol 1, ed 8, St. Louis, 1980, Mosby–Year Book, Inc.*

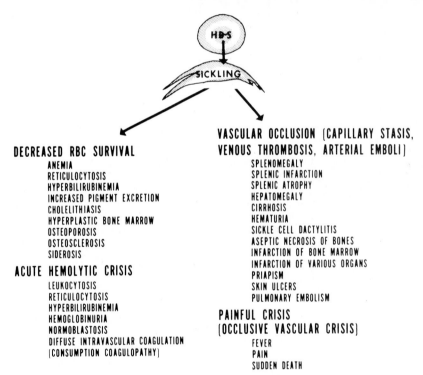

Fig. 61-43 Pathogenesis of the principle manifestations of sickle cell anemia. *From Miale JB: Laboratory medicine: hematology, ed 6, St. Louis, 1982, Mosby–Year Book, Inc.*

HbF are protective against HbS gelation. In addition to the concentrations of HbS and HbF in the cell and the O_2 tension to which the cell is exposed, the state of hydration is an important determinant of the propensity of the cell to sickle.

The formation of large numbers of sickle cells not only causes anemia by the extravascular hemolysis of these cells but also causes vascular occlusion with subsequent tissue ischemia and infarction resulting in organ dysfunction (kidneys, lung, bone, spleen, eye, CNS) (Figure 61-43).

Patients homozygous for HbS (sickle cell disease) show retarded growth, chronic anemia, and shortened life span. About 1/500-1/1000 black Americans have this disease. The degree of anemia is related to the survival of the in-

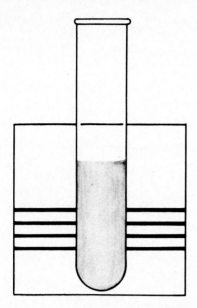

Fig. 61-44 Dithionite solubility tube test for sickling hemoglobins. Reduced HbS and other sickling hemoglobins tend to cause turbidity of the solution and obscure black lines behind the tube. *From Bauer JD: Clinical laboratory methods, ed 9, St. Louis, 1982, Mosby–Year Book, Inc.*

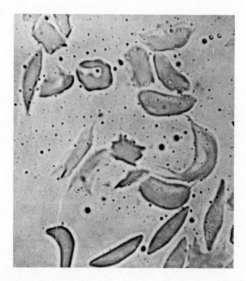

Fig. 61-45 Metabisulfite "sickle cell" preparation showing sickled cells. *From Miale JB: Laboratory medicine: hematology, ed 6, St. Louis, 1982, Mosby–Year Book, Inc.*

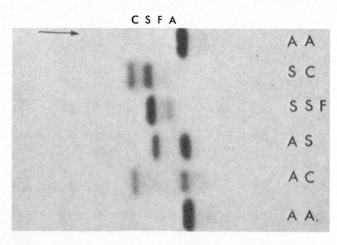

Fig. 61-46 Separation of various hemoglobins by electrophoresis on cellulose acetate, pH 8.6. *From Miale JB: Laboratory medicine: hematology, ed 6, St. Louis, 1982, Mosby–Year Book, Inc.*

hydration, stress, or infection. Chief among the manifestations due to vaso-occlusion are the intermittent painful crises that may arise in the trunk or extremities.

Early in life, splenomegaly is present, but after recurrent splenic infarcts it becomes a fibrous nodule. Microscopically, the spleen shows congestion of the cords and small veins with sickled cells as well as small areas of infarction during childhood. Later, areas of massive scarring contain calcific and ferruginized fibers ("Gamna-Gandy" bodies). As a result of autosplenectomy, the splenic pitting and culling function is lost and the number of Howell-Jolly bodies and siderocytes increases in the periphery. More importantly, there is a decreased clearance of blood-borne bacteria with a resultant increase in pneumococcal sepsis. This predisposition is further increased by a lack of oposonic activity in the blood of these patients. Microinfarctions of the renal medulla result in tubular dysfunction and isothenuria in almost all patients. Many patients have papillary infarction. Infarction of the bone leads to aseptic necrosis of the femoral heads as well as to foci which develop salmonella osteomyelitis. Cerebral infarcts are also common, as are retinal infarcts and detachment. In addition, expansion of the marrow results from the erythroid hyperplasia. Other changes related to hemolytic anemias are also seen, including cardiac dilatation, congestive heart failure, jaundice and gallstones.

The laboratory diagnosis is suggested by the presence of a large number of target cells and the findings of a hemolytic anemia in a black individual with hematocrit usually in the range of 18% to 25% vol. The indices are usually normochromic and normocytic. Howell-Jolly bodies are seen in asplenic patients. Occasionally, irreversibly sickled cells are seen in the peripheral smear. Blood smears taken from patients experiencing vaso-occlusive crises show increasing poikocytosis and numerous cells demonstrating varying degrees of sickling. With augmented hemolysis, the reticulocyte count may rise dramatically and nucleated red cells appear in the peripheral blood.

HbS can be demonstrated by its decreased solubility in

dividual cells. Because the level of HbF varies from cell to cell, those with the highest levels of HbF are largely protected, while those with the lowest levels tend to become irreversibly sickled and are taken out of circulation. Episodes of accelerated hemolysis occur with hypoxemia or during episodes of dehydration. Intermittently, the anemia is worsened by aplastic crises due to infection or to folate deficiency. In infancy, sudden worsening of the anemia may occur with sequestration of red cells in the spleen. Most other symptoms and signs result from the ischemic changes due to vaso-occlusion provoked by anoxic episodes, de-

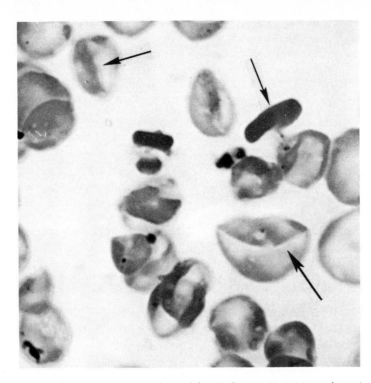

Fig. 61-47   Peripheral smear, homozygous hemoglobin C disease. Note intraerythrocytic and extra-erythrocytic hemoglobin C crystals and folding of red cell. *From Sonnenwirth AC and Jarett L: Gradwohl's clinical laboratory methods and diagnosis, vol 1, ed 8, St. Louis, 1980, Mosby—Year Book, Inc.*

high ionic strength reducing solutions such as sodium hydrosulfate, (dithionite tube test). In this test, the hemolysate that forms when a dithionite solution is added becomes opaque if HbS is present (Figure 61-44). The development of sickled cells in a preparation formed by mixing the blood sample with a reducing substance agent such as metabisulfite (sickle cell prep.) is also diagnostic of HbS, (Figure 61-45). Hemoglobin electrophoresis run on cellulose acetate at 8.4 (Figure 61-46) shows an absence of HbA and from 85% to 95% HbS, together with a variable elevation in HbF (1% to 15%), as well as the usual amount of HbA_2 (<3.5%). This pattern may be also seen in patients with hemoglobin S-β^0 thal disease, in which family or other special studies are required to make the diagnosis.

In patients heterozygous for HbS (sickle cell trait), the rate of HbA production is greater than HbS. They are usually asymptomatic and develop rare sickling crises only when the carrier is hypoxic. Rarely, splenic infarction occurs as does renal medullary infarction. The laboratory diagnosis rests upon cellulose acetate electrophoresis, which shows 60% to 65% HbA and 35% to 40% HbS (AS pattern) and a positive solubility test or sickle cell prep, (Figure 61-46). These findings must be distinguished from those found in patients with HbS-β^+ thal disease, in whom the electrophoretic pattern shows more HbS than HbA.

The neonatal diagnosis of sickle cell anemia or trait is possible by the detection of HbS and/or HbA in cord blood using column chromatographic techniques. Antenatal diagnosis is now based on the use of restriction enzyme fragment analysis of amniotic cell DNA. This approach has replaced the study of hemoglobin obtained from fetal blood aspirated during fetoscopy.

Hemoglobin C, hemoglobin D, and hemoglobin E diseases and traits. Hemoglobin C ($\alpha_2\beta_2^{6glu\rightarrow lys}$) is present in 2% to 3% of black Americans. It is less soluble than HbA and characerically puddles in the center of red cells. Peripheral smears therefore show numerous target cells. A mild hemolytic process is associated with splenomegaly in the homozygous state (CC). The slow drying of smears from CC patients may reveal rod-shaped crystals in the cells (Figure 61-47). The heterozygous state (AC) is not symptomatic. HbC cannot be diagnosed by simply examining the electrophoretic pattern obtained on cellulose acetate at pH 8.4; it needs to be confirmed on citrate agar at pH 6.2, since HbO and HbE variants migrate with HbC at an alkaline pH. Some patients with electrophoretic patterns consistent with the presence of hemoglobin C who do not possess hemoglobin S have a positive dithionite solubility test. Such patients have HbC Harlem.

HbE ($\alpha_2\beta_2^{26g/a\rightarrow lys}$), is the second most common variant worldwide. The gene's frequency is greater than 10% in some areas of the Far East. Heterozygotes have no anemia, but are microcytic, while homozygotes have mild anemia, microcytosis, and numerous target cells.

HbD variants, especially HbD Los Angeles, are encountered with some frequency in the United States. Homozygous patients are very rare and have a very mild anemia and numerous target cells in their peripheral smears.

SC and SD disease. The double-heterozygote SC patient has a mild to moderate anemia with splenomegaly, hematuria, and aseptic necrosis of the femoral head. Spontaneous abortions are frequent as well. The peripheral smear shows variable poikilocytosis, numerous target cells, and occasional sickled cells. The dithionite solubility test is positive, and the diagnosis is made by examining the electrophoretic patterns obtained with both cellulose acetate and citrate agar techniques.

Patients with SD disease usually present with a mild hemolytic anemia. Preliminary laboratory findings suggest SS disease, since the solubility test is positive and the cellulose acetate electrophoresis reveals only a hemoglobin S band. Further investigation with citrate agar electrophoresis reveals that in addition to hemoglobin S, hemoglobin D is present.

Unstable hemoglobin traits. While numerous unstable hemoglobins are described, only some result in clinically significant hemolysis. Many demonstrate increased or decreased oxygen affinity. These hemoglobins are only present in life in the heterozygous state and become clinically apparent at birth if they are an α-chain mutant, or later if they are a β-chain mutant. They tend to dissociate into dimers or spontaneously auto-oxidize to methemoglobin. The denatured hemoglobin precipitates against the cell membrane. These inclusions may be pitted from the red cell or the entire cell may be destroyed.

While some hemoglobins can be identified as slow- or fast-moving variants on electrophoresis (cellulose acetate pH 8.4), many of them migrate with HbA. Diagnosis of an unstable hemoglobin responsible for a congenital non-spherocytic hemolytic anemia often is initiated with the Heinz body preparation. In this test, heparinized blood is incubated with an acetyl-phenyl hydrazine solution and then a wet preparation consisting of a drop of the above mixture, and a drop of crystal violet solution is examined microscopically. The denatured hemoglobin is evident as numerous small intracellular Heinz bodies. As previously discussed, Heinz bodies are also noted in patients with thalassemia and G6PD deficiency. The presence of an unstable hemoglobin is further suggested by its rapid precipitation after the addition of the patient's hemolysate to a 17% isopropanol solution. In this test, stable hemoglobins precipitate slowly (>40 minutes). Similarly, unstable hemoglobins will precipitate out when the patient's phosphate buffered hemolysate is heated to 50°C for one hour. This heat instability test can quantify the amount of unstable hemoglobin in the hemolysate by measuring its optical density before and after heat treatment.

Hemoglobin M variants and methemoglobinemia. Hemoglobin can be oxygenated only when the iron is in the +2 state; if the iron is oxidized to the +3 state, the resultant methemoglobin cannot bind oxygen. Small amounts are continuously produced, but are then reduced through a NADH diaphorase enzyme system. Patients with a deficient NADH diaphorase system, or with an abnormal hemoglobin M, have congenital methemoglobinemia. The production of methemoglobin is increased in patients exposed to oxidant drugs or toxins.

The production of a hemoglobin M results in cyanosis, which appears at birth if the variant is an α-chain mutant or later if a β-chain mutant. As with other heterozygotic hemoglobinopathies, the quantity of hemoglobin M produced is usually approximately 40%. The homozygotic state is incompatible with life.

Methemoglobins are detected by spectrophoretic methods. Oxidized hemoglobin A (Methemoglobin A) demonstrates an absorption peak at 630 nm, while hemoglobin M shows a low peak at 600 nm without any peak at 630 nm. Following conversion of hemoglobin to cyanmethemoglobin, Hemoglobin M can be separated from HbA electrophoretically at pH 7.

Hemoglobins with altered oxygen affinity. The hemoglobins with either increased or decreased oxygen affinity are characterized clinically by the induction of a state of erythrocytosis or anemia respectively. Many cannot be isolated by their electrophoretic mobility and must be identified primarily by the study of the oxygen-dissociation curve. The finding of a shift to either the left or right, respectively, in the presence of normal 2.3 DPG levels confirms the diagnosis of such a hemoglobinopathy.

ERYTHROCYTOSIS

Erythrocytosis (polycythemia) denotes a condition in which the hematocrit exceeds 55 vol%, the red cell count exceeds 6 million/mm, or the hemoglobin concentration exceeds 18 gm/dl. It may follow either a decrease in plasma volume (spurious or relative erythrocytosis) or an increase in red cell mass (true polycythemia) (Box 61-11).

Spurious polycythemia may result either from an acute loss of plasma volume (e.g., burns, dehydration, etc.) or by a chronic decreased plasma volume ("Stress" erythrocytosis, or Gaisbock's syndrome). The latter occurs in middle-aged, tense men who are heavy smokers, frequently

---

Box 61-11 Classification of polycythemias

I. INCREASED RED CELL MASS

A. Primary polycythemia (polycythemia vera)

B. Secondary polycythemia
1. Hypoxic
   a. Chronic obstructive lung disease
   b. Cyanotic congenital heart disease
   c. Renal ischemia
   d. Hemoglobinopathies with high oxygen affinity
   e. Congenital decreased 2,3 DPG
2. Autonomous erythropoetin production
   a. Post-renal transplantation
   b. Renal cysts and hydronephrosis
   c. Renal adenomas
   d. Cerebellar hemangioblastomas
   e. Hepatocellular carcinoma
   f. Lyomyomata of the uterus
3. Benign familial polycythemia

II. NORMAL RED CELL MASS (RELATIVE ERYTHROCYTOSIS)

A. Acute hemoconcentration
1. Burns
2. Dehydration

B. Chronic decreased plasma volume
(Gaisbacks syndrome or "stress" erythrocytosis)

From: Bauer JD: Clinical laboratory methods, ed 9, St. Louis, 1982, Mosby–Year Book, Inc.

Table 61-4 Laboratory tests in the differential diagnosis of polycythemias in order of suggested protocol

Laboratory test	Polycythemia vera	Secondary polycythemia	Relative polycythemia
Hemoglobin	Increased	Increased	Increased
Hematocrit	Increased 60%-80%	Increased 60%-80%	Increased up to 60%
No. of WBCs	Normal or slightly increased	Normal	Normal
Immature RBCs	Occasional	None	None
No. of platelets	Increased	Normal	Normal
Bone marrow	Hyperplasia of all hematopoietic elements	Erythroid hyperplasia	Normal
LAP	Increased	Normal	Normal
Sedimentation rate	Decreased, 1 mm	Normal	Normal
Red cell volume	Increased	Increased	Normal
Plasma volume	Normal or decreased	Normal	Decreased
Arterial O_2 saturation	Normal	Decreased	Normal
Serum iron	Decreased	Increased	Normal
Plasma iron clearance and turnover	Accelerated	Normal	Normal
Uric acid	Increased	May be increased	Normal
Erythropoietin	Normal or decreased	Increased	Normal
Blood histamine	Increased	Normal	Normal
Unsaturated vitamin B_{12}-binding capacity	Increased	Normal	Normal
Serum vitamin B_{12}	Increased	Normal	Normal
Basophil count	Increased	Normal	Normal
Absolute reticulocyte count	Slightly increased	Increased	Normal

From Bauer JD: Clinical laboratory methods, ed 9, St. Louis, 1982, Mosby—Year Book, Inc.

obese, and have hypercholesterolemia and mild hyperuricemia.

True (absolute) polycythemia with an increased red cell mass and increased total blood volume is either secondary to increased erythropoietin drive or due to an autonomous proliferation of red cell precursors (polycythemia vera). Secondary erythrocytosis may then result from tissue anoxia with increased erythropoietin secretion from the kidney (hemoglobinopathies with increased O_2 affinity, depressed O_2 loading due to cardiopulmonary disease, or local vascular alterations leading to local renal hypoxia). It may also result from autonomous erythropoietin production of renal origin (hydronephrosis, renal cysts, and post-renal transplant) or extrarenal origin (cerebellar hemangioblastoma, hepatic carcinoma, uterine "fibroids" or androgen administration, and Cushing syndrome). Polycythemia vera is due to autonomous proliferation of red cell precursors. It is a stem cell defect of the myeloid tissue and is one of the myeloproliferative syndromes.

The laboratory evaluation of the patient with erythrocytosis usually begins with the calculation of the red cell mass utilizing ^{51}Cr, as previously described (Chapter 59). In the presence of a normal red cell mass, the diagnosis of relative erythrocytosis may be confirmed by the calculation of the patient's plasma volume.

The differential diagnosis of erythrocytosis is largely based on the medical history, arterial blood gas determinations and radiologic and imaging studies. When necessary, the patient's oxygen dissociation curve and 2.5 DPG levels can be calculated. The determination of erythropoietin levels is performed when the cause of the erythrocytosis remains obscure and the diagnosis of polycythemia vera is

being entertained, and in cases of neoplasias in which the level of erythropoietin can be used as a tumor marker in the management of the patient (Table 61-4).

Erythropoietin levels may be measured by either biologic or immunologic assays utilizing either plasma or 24-hour urine samples. The bioassays are performed in hypertransfused or hypoxic mice and measure the amount of active molecule circulating in the plasma or excreted in the urine. The immunologic assays are easier to perform but may measure nonfunctional molecules. Among such tests, the radioimmune assay is the most widely used. The normal upper level of erythropoietin is 10mU/ml. of plasma.

SUGGESTED READING

Bottomley SS: Sideroblastic anemias, Clin Haematol 11:389, 1982.

Chanarin I, Deacon R, Lumb M, et al: Cobalamine-folate interrelations: a critical review, Blood 66:479, 1985.

Cook JD: Clinical evaluation of iron deficiency, Semin Hematol 19:6, 1982.

Finch CA and Huebers H: Perspectives in iron metabolism, N Eng J Med 306:1520, 1982.

Ibrahim NG, Friedland ML, and Levere RD: Heme metabolism in erythroid and hepatic cells, Prog Hematol 13:75, 1983.

Karlson S and Nienhuis AW: Developmental regulation of human globin genes, Ann Rev Biochem 54:1071, 1985.

Kazazian HH and Boetim CD: Molecular basis and prenatal diagnosis of thalassemia, Blood 72:1107, 1988.

Kim HC: Laboratory identification of inherited hemoglobinpathies in children, Clin Pediatr 20:161, 1981.

Lindenbaum J: Status of laboratory testing in the diagnosis of megaloblastic anemia, Blood 61:624, 1983.

Schrier SL, ed: The red cell membrane, Clin Hematol 14:1, 1985.

Valentine WN, Tanaka, KR and Paglia DE: Hemolytic anemias and erythrocyte enzymopathies, Ann Int Med 103:245, 1985.

62

Laboratory diagnosis of granulocyte disorders

Robert F. Reiss

The differentiation and maturation of granulocyte precursors, their normal kinetics, and their regulation by various growth factors was described in Chapter 57. Similiarly, the cytologic characteristics of normal and abnormal white cell populations was extensively discussed in Chapter 58. The total leukocyte and differential cell counts vary with age, sex (Table 62-1), and race.

BENIGN KINETIC ABNORMALITIES

The developing granulocytic elements in the marrow are assigned to the stem cell, differentiation, and maturation compartments. Late band forms and mature granulocytes in the bone marrow constitute the storage compartment, while those present in the peripheral blood constitute the circulating cell compartment. The kinetic pattern of release and circulation of neutrophils is the best-studied granulocytic element and probably can be used as a model for the others. A part of the storage compartment is known as the marrow granulocyte reserve (MGR), which can be released under stress.

The cells in the differentiation, maturation, and storage compartments routinely are studied by examining marrow cellularity, M:E ratio, and differential cell count. The mitotic index of the granulocytic precursors in the differentiation compartment can also be determined. Release of cells from the MGR can be evaluated after the intramuscular injection of etiocholanolone. In research settings, the ability of bone marrow cells to form colonies in soft agar cultures and assays of growth factors, as well as their inhibitors, has helped in the understanding of abnormal neutrophil kinetics.

Cells in the circulating compartment are termed the total blood granulocyte pool (TBGP). Half of these cells do not actually circulate in the blood but are marginated along the vessel wall and are known as the marginal granulocyte pool (MGP). The half that does circulate in the blood is called the circulating granulocyte pool (CGP). The cells leave the marginal pool and migrate into the tissues after a mean transit time of six to eight hours. In the peripheral blood, mature granulocytes make up about 55% of the total white cells, while bands constitute about 5%. The total blood pool is studied most simply by the white cell and differential counts.

Neutropenia

Leukopenia is a decrease in the total white count to levels below 4000/mm³. "Leukopenia" should not be used interchangeably with "granulocytopenia" or "neutropenia." Similarly, granulocytopenia and agranulocytosis should be differentiated from true neutropenia.

Neutropenia results when the number of neutrophils falls below 1500/mm³ in whites or below 1300 mm³ in blacks. Neutrophils under 1000/mm³ may mean an increased incidence of infection, which becomes severe under 500/mm³. Numerous mechanisms can result in neutropenia:

Decreased neutrophil production due to a) reduced marrow pools (e.g., radiation and drug-induced granulocytic hypoplasia, aplastic anemia, myelophthsic neutropenia, chronic familial neutropenia, and cyclic neutropenia); b) increased ineffective granulopoesis, (folate and vitamin B_{12} deficiency); or c) decreased storage pool outflow with an enlargement of the storage pool (familial benign neutropenia).

Decreased survival of circulating neutrophils due to a) peripheral destruction with an inadequately increased diffentiation pool (e.g., immune neutropenia, early infection); or b) increased splenic trapping (hypersplenism).

"Pseudoneutropenia" due to an increased shift from the CGP to the MGP (e.g., hypersensitivity reactions, viremia).

Hereditary neutropenias

Infantile genetic agranulocytosis of Kostmann is a rare autosomal recessive trait characterized by severe isolated neutropenia and a maturation block of the neutrophil precursors at the promyelocyte or myelocyte level. It appears in early infancy.

Familial benign neutropenia is an autosomal-dominant condition characterized by mild to moderate granulocytopenia and a benign clinical course. The granulocytopenia results from a decreased release of mature cells from the marrow storage pool.

Cyclic neutropenia is an autosomal-dominant condition characterized by severe neutropenia occuring approximately every three weeks. Cyclic neutropenia results from cyclic decreases in committed progenitor cells.

Neutropenia associated with other abnormalities.

Table 62-1   Reference values (2.5 to 97.5 percentiles) for leukocyte differential counts, comparing 200-cell manual differentials with 10,000-cell Hemalog-D differentials*

	200-cell differential		Hemalog-D differential	
	Percentage counts	Absolute counts	Percentage counts	Absolute counts
ADULTS				
Neutrophils	43.5-79.5	2266-7676	47.5-76.8	2000-7150
Lymphocytes	13.0-43.0	832-3140	16.2-43.0	1100-3000
Monocytes	2.0-11.0	123-804	1.0-10.3	60-750
Eosinophils	0-7.5	0-492	0.4-5.9	25-380
Basophils	0-2.0	0-156	0.2-1.3	10-100
MALE CHILDREN (AGE 5-16 YR)				
Neutrophils	32.5-70.0	1420-5200	38.5-71.5	1700-5200
Lymphocytes	21.0-55.0	1200-3600	19.4-51.4	875-3300
Monocytes	2.5-12.5	120-886	1.1-11.6	28-825
Eosinophils	2.0-12.0	39-686	0.9-8.1	41-460
Basophils	0.0-2.5	20-118	0.2-1.3	16-80
FEMALE CHILDREN (AGE 5-16 YR)				
Neutrophils	36.0-73.5	1550-6500	41.9-76.5	1700-7500
Lymphocytes	18.0-53.0	1290-3600	16.3-46.7	1078-3000
Monocytes	2.0-13.0	112-850	0.9-9.9	45-750
Eosinophils	2.0-11.5	29-750	0.8-8.3	40-650
Basophils	0.0-3.0	20-130	0.3-1.4	7-140
CHILDREN (AGE 0-4 YR)				
Neutrophils	16.0-60.0	1000-12000	Total leukocyte count 3800 to 10,900/	
Lymphocytes	20.0-70.0	1500-8500	mm³ for adults, and 4000 to 9000 for	
Monocytes	0-7.0	0-450	children ages 5-16 years	
Eosinophils	0-8.0	0-600		
Basophils	0-1.0	0-400		

From van Assendelft OW, et al. In Koepke JA, ed: Differential leukocyte counting, Skokie, Ill, 1979, College of American Pathologists.

Among these conditions are X-linked agammaglobulinemia, reticular dysgenesis, Schwachman's syndrome, and dyskeratosis congenita.

Drug-induced neutropenias

Drugs may induce isolated neutropenia or generalized marrow hypoplasia by dose-related cytotoxicity or by a non dose-related idiosyncratic reaction. Dose-related damage tends to induce neutropenia earlier than thrombocytopenia because of the short peripheral survival of neutrophils and the relative greater sensitivity of their precursors as compared to megakaryocytes. In addition, some drugs may induce immune-mediated neutropenia.

Immune neutropenias

Antibody-mediated neutropenias are uncommon disorders that result from the action of cytotoxic allo- or auto-antibodies on circulating neutrophils.

Neutropenic syndromes due to alloantibodies include rare cases of neonatal alloimmune neutropenia, which results from the transplacental transmission of IgG antibodies directed against neutrophil-specific antigens on a newborn's cells (Table 62-2). Occasional cases of post-transfusion neutropenia may occur after platelet concentrates or other leukocyte containing blood components are transfused to HLA-sensitized patients, whose antibodies are leukoagglutinins.

Table 62-2   Neutrophil-specific antigens and given frequency*

Antigen	Frequency
NA1	0.377
NA2	0.633
NB1	0.83
NC1	?
9A	0.345
ND1	0.88
NE1	?

From Baehner RL: Disorders of granulopoiesis. In Miller DR and Baehner RL, eds: Blood diseases of infancy and childhood, ed 6, St. Louis, 1990, Mosby–Year Book, Inc.
*The antigens are found on myelocytes, metamyelocytes, bands, and polymorphonuclear neutrophils.

The neutropenia may occur in conjunction with neutrophil margination, resulting in non-cardiogenic pulmonary edema.

Drug-related immune neutropenia usually results from the sensitization of neutrophils by circulating drug-antidrug immune complexes and the subsequent fixation of complement on the cell surface. These complement-coated cells are removed from the circulation by macrophages of the RE system.

Autoimmune neutropenia may arise as an isolated disorder in conjunction with Felty's syndrome or as a manifestation of systemic lupus erythematosus. Both IgG and IgM antibodies are described. Many are directed against well-defined, neutrophil-specific antigens, while others do not possess specificity for any antigens which have been identified.

Some patients with chronic, isolated neutropenia have suppressor T-cell lymphocytosis. It is believed that in such patients the release of necessary growth factors for neutrophil progenitor cells is inhibited.

Neutrophilia

Leukocytosis describes an increase in the total white count to over 10,000/mm³. "Leukocytosis" should not be used interchangeably with the terms "granulocytosis" or "neutrophilia." Similarly, granulocytosis should be differentiated from true neutrophilia.

Neutrophilia results when neutrophils increase above 6500/mm³. Excessive neutrophilia with the presence of immature forms is termed "neutrophilic leukemoid reaction" and must be differentiated from chronic granulocytic leukemia. Marked neutrophilia without immature forms is termed "neutrophilic hyperleukocytosis." Numerous mechanisms can give rise to neutrophilia:

Increased neutrophil production due to a) a sustained increased proliferation and differentiation of neutrophil precursors (e.g., established infection, tissue necrosis, carcinomatosis, Hodgkin's disease) or b) an acute release of storage pool cells into the circulation (e.g., etiocholanolone or endotoxin).

Decreased neutrophil outflow from the circulating pool (e.g., corticosteroids, which also cause accelerated release from the storage pool).

"Pseudoneutrophilia" due to mobilization of cells from the MGP to the CGP (e.g., acute response to stress, exercise, or the administration of epinephrine).

Neutrophilia resulting from the increased proliferation and differentiation of precursor cells, which is seen in infection and tissue necrosis, results from the release of IL-1 and tissue necrosis factor (TNF) from monocytes and tissue macrophages and the subsequent augmented production of specific growth factors (e.g., GM-CSF and G-CSF) by lymphocytes, fibroblasts, and endothelial cells. The acute neutrophilia, which results when cells are released from the storage compartment, appears to be mediated by IL-1 and activated complement (C3a).

Abnormal kinetics of other myeloid elements

Eosinophilia

Eosinophilia is characterized by an eosinophil count in excess of 500/mm³. It may be found in allergic disorders, parasitic infestations, Hodgkin's disease, and the myeloproliferative disorders. Striking eosinophilia may be evident in primary eosinophilic syndromes.

The mechanisms by which eosinophilia occur are still obscure. In patients with asthma and atopic allergies, eosinophilia may appear in response to the release of specific chemotactic agents from degranulating mast cells and basophils, which have fixed IgE to their surfaces. In patients with parasitic infestations, the highest levels of eosinophilia

are noted in those which involve deep tissue infiltration (e.g., trichinosis) and in those complicated by pulmonary hypersensitivity reactions (Loeffler's syndrome).

Basophilia

Basophilia in excess of 200/mm³ may be seen in myeloproliferative syndromes.

Monocytosis

Monocytosis in excess of 1000/mm³ may be seen during recovery from marrow aplasia and isolated neutropenia; subacute bacterial endocarditis; chronic infections (e.g., tuberculosis, brucellosis, and listeria infections); and myeloproliferative disorders.

NEUTROPHIL ULTRASTRUCTURE

The neutrophil bilipid plasma membrane is associated with an external coat rich in glycoproteins, which function as receptors critically important to cell-cell and cell-surface interactions and to signal transmission from the cell surface to the cytoplasm.

One important group of such receptors is designated as the CD11/CD18 cluster group. Glycoproteins of this group are composed of specific alpha (CD11) and shared beta (CD18) subunits. Among those now defined by specific monoclonal antibodies against the alpha chains are a CR-3 receptor (CD11b/CD18 or Mol) involved in binding to C3bi-coated particles and surfaces; the LFA-1 receptor (CD11a/CD18) involved in binding to T cells, NK cells, and tumor cells; and the P150,95 receptor (CD11c/CD18) which binds to a variety of lipopolysaccharides, (Table 62-3).

Another critical receptor group associated with the external coat is the receptor for various chemotactic peptides, most notably the important class of N-formyl methionyl peptides, (NFMP), produced by bacteria. Activation of this receptor group is essential for signal transmission from the cell surface to the cytosol and therefore critical to the phagocytic function of the cell.

Other receptors have been identified for the fc fragment of IgG1 and IgG3, C3b (CR1 receptor), leukotrienes, histamine, and fibronectin.

The membrane itself also contains numerous enzyme systems (e.g., phospholipase, methyl transferase, adenyl cyclase, superoxide dismutase, protein kinase C, and NADPH oxidase) essential to normal cell function. The membrane also contains the proteins necessary to the structural integrity and deformability of the cell (e.g., actin binding protein).

The peripheral gel region of the cytoplasm contains a 10:1 ratio of actin and myosin as well as proteins that regulate actin polymerization (profillin and gelsolin). The central cytosol is rich in organelles, including remnants of the Golgi apparatus and rough endoplasmic reticulum, rare mitochondria, and the primary and secondary granules. The light microscopic characteristics of these granules and their contents have been previously discussed, (Chapter 58). Of note, NADPH oxidase activity is associated with the granule membrane. Additional NFMP and C3bi receptors have also been identified on secondary granule membranes. These serve to increase the number of such receptors expressed on the phagocytic cell surface during degranulation.

Table 62-3 The CD11/CD18 glycoprotein family

Glycoprotein (CD)	Cellular distribution	Functional capacity
LFA-1 (CD11a/ CD18)	All human leukocytes	Adhesion-promoting molecule facilitating lymphocyte blastogenesis; cellular cytotoxicity (CTL, NK, and K); lymphocyte-endothelial cell adhesion.
Mol (CD11b/ CD18)	Monocytes, neutrophils, NK cells	Receptor for C3bi (CR3); adhesion-promoting molecule facilitating PMN aggregation, PMN/Mo adhesion to substrates, PMN/Mo chemotaxis.
p150,95 (CD11c/ CD18)	Monocytes, neutrophils	Not well defined. May promote adhesion of PMN and Mo to substrates; may bind C3bi.

From Todd RF and Freyer DR: Hematol Oncol Clinics N America 2:13, 1988.
CTL = cytotoxic T lymphocyte; K = ADCC effector cells; Mo = monocyte;
NK = natural killing; PMN = polymorphonuclear neutrophil

ABNORMAL NEUTROPHIL MORPHOLOGY

Abnormalities in the cytoplasm, granules, or nucleus may be hereditary or acquired. Some may be associated with functional abnormalities, while others are simply morphologic aberrations. Toxic granules are larger, more prominent neutrophil granules associated with infections or other severe stress and appear to possess a mildly decreased bacteriocidal capability, (Figure 62-1). Giant granules are present in the neutrophils and other leukocytes in the Chediak-Higashi syndrome. This disorder is transmitted as an autosomal recessive trait and is associated with increased infections, ocular, and skin hypopigmentation, (Figure 62-2). In the Alder-Reilly anomaly, a failure of secondary granule formation and persistence of the azurophilic granules is associated with disordered mucopolysaccharide metabolism in gargoylism (Figure 62-3).

Döhle bodies are grayish-blue cytoplasmic inclusions representing ribosomal remnants. They are seen most often in severe infections. In the May-Hegglin anomaly, an autosomal dominant trait, Dohle bodies are associated with a decreased number of platelets and giant platelets (Figure 62-4).

The Pelger-Huet anomaly is characterized by defective segmentation of the neutrophil nucleus. In the typical heterozygous state, most cells have bilobed nuclei, while homozygotes have unsegmented round nuclei (Figure 62-5). Macropolycytes (hypersegmented neutrophils) have five or more lobes and are typical of the megaloblastic anemias.

NORMAL NEUTROPHIL FUNCTION

Microvascular margination, adhesion, emigration, chemotaxis, phagocytosis, and intracellular digestion are the essential granulocyte functions required for the killing of microbial agents.

Margination, adhesion, and emigration

These processes involve the ongoing displacement of circulating neutrophils from the central flow of circulating blood to the wall of the venules and capillaries, the adhesion of these marginated neutrophils to the endothelium in response to the expression of the cell's adhesion receptors of the CD11/CD18 group, and finally the diapedesis of these cells between interendothelial junctions and their passage through the basement membrane into the surrounding tissue.

Chemotaxis

Chemotaxis involves the unidirectional movement of phagocytes (granulocytes and then monocytes) toward microbes or other particulate matter they recognize as a target for phagocytosis or killing. Such directed movement is differentiated from random cellular movement, termed chemokinesis. Among the principal mediators of chemotaxis are the complement fragment C5a, the complex C567, leukotriene B_4, and NFMP and other bacterial products (Box 62-1). Neutrophils that reach the target particles may release other factors aside from leukotriene B_4, which are chemotactic for monocytes.

The binding of chemotactic agents to their specific receptors on the lead end of the cell initiates the following sequence of events:

1. activation of guanine nucleotide binding proteins (G proteins)
2. activation of membrane-associated phospholipase C
3. hydrolysis of phosphotidyl choline to generate inositol triphosphate (IP3) and diacylglycerol (DAG)
4. IP3-mediated release of intracellular calcium ion stores
5. further activation of membrane-bound protein kinase C by DAG and elevated calcium ion levels.

The generation of activated protein kinase C and the subsequent phosphorylation of membrane proteins contributes to the remodeling of the plasma membrane and establishment of cellular polarity, by which the lead end of the phagocyte assumes a positive charge relative to the rest of the cell. Other serial events that lead to further polarization are

1. the liberation of free arachadonic acid from the plasma membrane and the resultant augmented synthesis of leukotriene B_4;
2. further calcium ion flux following binding of this metabolite to membrane receptors;
3. reinforced activation of protein kinase C leading to still greater cell polarization; and
4. increased expression of the CD11/CD18 membrane receptors.

All of these cellular changes are preparatory to the actual movement of the neutrophil along the chemotactic agent concentration gradient. Such movement may be initiated by a falling concentration of calcium ion in the cell ectoplasm as these ions are shifted to the internal cytosol. Decreased calcium ion levels reduce the binding of actin to the regulatory proteins profilin and gelsolin. Actin polymerization is thereby permitted to occur and membrane-bound actin-binding protein is able to cross-link the formed actin filaments with myosin. In addition to favoring the formation of this contractile protein complex, the lowered calcium ion level also favors microtubule formation by tubulin and other essential proteins. The sequential formation and dissolution of these protein complexes is required not only for directed movement but for phagocytosis as well.

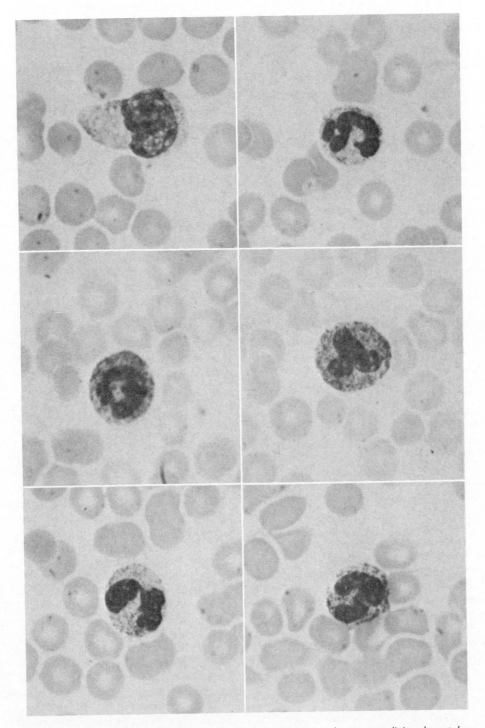

Fig. 62-1 Neutrophil containing toxic granulation. *From Miale JB: Laboratory medicine: hematology, ed 6, St. Louis, 1982, Mosby—Year Book, Inc.*

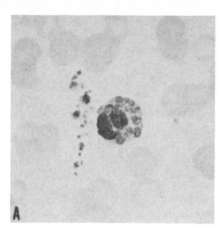

Fig. 62-2   Neutrophil in the Chediak-Higashi syndrome. *From Miale JB: Laboratory medicine: hematology, ed 6, St. Louis, 1982, Mosby—Year Book, Inc.*

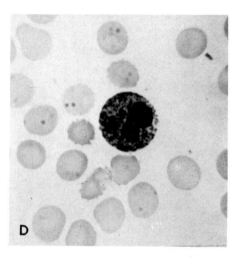

Fig. 62-3   Neutrophil in the Alder-Reilly anomaly. *From Miale JB: Laboratory medicine: hematology, ed 6, St. Louis, 1982, Mosby—Year Book, Inc.*

Box 62-1   Chemotactic agents for human neutrophils

ENDOGENOUS FACTORS

   Humoral
      C5a
      C567
      C3bB
      Factor Ba
      Fibrinopeptide B
   Cell-derived
      Arachidonate derivatives
         12-L-hydroxy-5,8,10,14-eicosatetraenoic acid (HETEs)
         12-L-hydroxy-5,8,10-heptadecatrienoic acid (HHT)
      Leukotriene B_4
      Lymphokine
   Neutrophil release products
      Urate crystal-induced glycoprotein
      Released on aggregated immunoglobulin G-coated surface
      Released from cells engaged in phagocytosis
   Release products of other cell types
      Macrophages
      Fibroblasts
      Damaged red cells
   Amphipathic or denatured proteins
      Casein
      α,1 and β-caseins
      Denatured serum albumin
      Denatured hemoglobin
      Collagen breakdown products
      Enzymatically altered immunoglobulin

EXOGENOUS FACTORS

   Formyl-methionyl peptides
   Bacterial signal peptides
   Undefined bacterial peptides with blocked N-termini
   Undefined bacterial lipids
   Other undefined bacterial factors
   Succinyl-melittin
   Products of specific immune reactions
   Migration of Ab-bearing cells to specific antigen
   Migration of neutrophils to antineutrophil-antibody

From Allen RA, et al: Hematol Oncol Clinics N America 2:33, 1988.

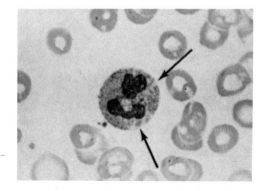

Fig. 62-4   Neutrophil containing a Dohle body. *From Bauer JD: Clinical laboratory methods, ed 9, St. Louis, 1982, Mosby–Year Book, Inc.*

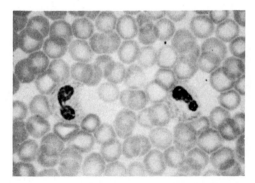

Fig. 62-5   Nuetrophil with the Pelger-Huet anomaly. *From Bauer JD: Clinical laboratory methods, ed 9, St. Louis, 1982, Mosby–Year Book, Inc.*

Phagocytosis

Upon adhesion to the target particle, neutrophil recognition and binding occurs. These activities depend on the interaction of membrane receptors with specific and nonspecific humoral opsonins coating the particle.

Specific opsonins are IgG1 and IgG3 antibodies directed against microbial surface antigens, which bind to fc receptors on the neutrophil. C3b and C3bi may also be found on target bacteria either following fixation by antigen-antibody complexes or by alternate pathway activation by the lipoprotein surface of non-capsulated microorganisms. These complement fragments bind to CR1 and CR3 receptors on the neutrophil membrane surface, respectively. In addition to the above opsonins, lipoprotein itself may be recognized by a CD11/CD18 group receptor, P150,95. Adherence may be further reinforced by fibronectin binding between the target particle and the neutrophil surface.

As a result of neutrophil binding, phagocytosis is initiated. This process is characterized by the evagination of pseudopods about the target particle and then its internatization following pseudopod fusion (Figure 62-6). The internalized particle is thus found within a vacule, the inner wall of which is formed by the pinched-off outer lipid layer of the neutrophil membrane. This vacule is termed a phagosome.

The molecular processes that permit the formation of pseudopods begin at the point of target binding, where a decreased calcium ion level develops in the neutrophil ectoplasm. As previously discussed, this lowered calcium ion concentration permits the formation of actin filaments, their crosslinkage with myosin, and their anchorage to membrane-bound actin binding protein. Subsequent contraction of bound actin filaments toward the membrane concentrates these filaments into a gel at the contact point and creates a relative sol state of either side, which permits the cytoplasm to bulge out into pseudopods.

As the pseudopods form, successive points of contact are made about the target particle, each of which creates it's own calcium ion flux and resultant ectoplasmic gelation. Simultaneously, calcium ions are also displaced back into gelation sites. The raised calcium ion level activates gelsolin, breaks down actin filament polymers and membrane linkages, and permits the cytoplasm to return to a sol state, which flows into the developing pseudopod as it encircles the target particle. In addition, as the actin filaments break down, neutrophil granules are able to migrate close to the developing phagosome.

Degranulation

Granules attach to and fuse with the developing phagosome, thereby forming the phagolysosome. Subsequently, the granules empty their contents into the vacule. The first granules to attach and degranulate are the secondary granules. Attachment often occurs while the phagosome is just forming and has not yet been internalized, so that up to 80% to 90% of the granule contents may be split from the cell. Attachment and degranulation of the primary granules occurs after most phagosomes are internalized, so that less than 10% of their contents are lost from the cell. During degranulation of the secondary granules, the availability of membrane-associated FMLP and C3bi receptors on the cell

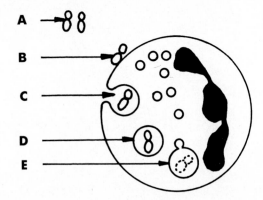

Fig. 62-6 Steps in the process of phagocytosis by a neutrophil. **A,** Bacteria. **B,** Recognition and binding. **C,** Ingestion. **D,** Phagosome formation. **E,** Phagolysosome. *From Bauer JD: Leukocyte function tests. In Sonnenwirth AC and Jarett L, eds: Gradwohl's clinical laboratory methods and diagnosis, vol 1, ed 8, St. Louis, 1980, Mosby–Year Book, Inc.*

surface is augmented and chemotaxis is consequently increased still further.

The movement of the phagosome into the cytoplasm and degranulation of the granules is in part due to contractile microtubules that form about them. How fusion of granule and phagosome membranes occurs is not known, but it may involve peroxidation of membrane lipoproteins following the activation of a membrane-bound NADPH oxidase system.

Following target recognition and the initiation of phagocytosis, the neutrophil exhibits a complex metabolic "burst," characterized not only by an increased rate of glycolysis but by a two- to threefold increase in oxygen consumption and a tenfold increase in HMP shunt activity. This metabolic activity furnishes energy for phagocytosis by ATP synthesis and activated oxygen products and hydrogen peroxide for the lipid peroxidation essential to membrane fusion and oxygen-dependent bacteriocidal activity.

Intracellular digestion

Before and after granule contents are discharged into the phagocytic vacule, digestion of the microbe proceeds in an environment isolated from the phagocyte's cytoplasm.

Before degranulation, active oxidizing radicals are generated by membrane-bound events, which depend on an intact membrane associated NADPH oxidase system. This oxidase system is a complex that includes flavin and cytochrome b molecules of the electron transport system essential to oxygen reduction.

$$2O_2 + NADPH \xrightarrow{\text{NADPH OXIDASE}} NADP^+ + H^+ + 2O_2^-$$
$$2O_2^- + 2H^+ \rightarrow {}^1O_2 \cdot + H_2O_2$$
$$2O_2^- + 2H^+ \xrightarrow{O_2^- \text{ Dismutase}} O_2 + H_2O_2$$

The superoxide radical (O_2^-) is not only a mild oxidant itself, causing lipid peroxidation of microbial membranes, but is also converted to singlet oxygen $({}^1O_2 \cdot)$, which oxidizes protein double bonds to form ketones and aldehydes. By the further action of superoxide dismutase, hydrogen peroxide is formed. Hydrogen peroxide accumulates in the phagosome and becomes available to participate in further oxidation reactions that follow degranulation. Among the granule contents critical to further bacteriocidal activity are lactoferrin and myeloperoxidase.

$$O_2 + H_2O_2 + H^+ \xrightarrow{Fe^{++} \text{ lactoferrin}} \cdot OH + H_2O + O_2$$
$$X^-(\text{halide}) + H_2O_2 \xrightarrow{\text{myeloperoxidase}} OX^- + H_2O$$
$$OX^- + H_2O_2 \rightarrow {}^1O_2 \cdot + X^- + H_2O$$

Hydrogen peroxide may form free hydroxyl radicals ($\cdot OH$) in the presence of oxygen, ferrous ion, and hydrogen after release of lactoferrin from secondary granules. These radicals are able to oxidize free carboxyl groups of amino acids to form ketones and aldehydes. The myeloperoxidase released from primary granules converts halide ions (especially chloride) to hypohalite ions (OX^-) in the presence of hydrogen peroxide. Hypohalite ions not only cause lipid peroxidation, but may be further converted to the previously mentioned, highly toxic singlet oxygen radicals. The metabolic pathways necessary for the production of hydrogen peroxide, as well as the pathways necessary to prevent its excessive accumulation, are shown in Figure 62-7. In addition to the activity of the HMP shunt in controlling hydrogen peroxide buildup, cytoplasmic catalase is able to directly inactivate this metabolic product.

Non oxygen-dependent bacterial killing and digestion is largely due to the bacteriostatic and bacteriocidal effects of the constituents of the primary and secondary granules (Table 62-4) and the accumulated lactate in the phagolysomes. Lysozymes digest peptidoglycans and therefore exert

Table 62-4 Neutrophil granule constituents

Constituent	Azurophilic granules	Specific granules
Microbicidal enzymes	Myeloperoxidase	Lysozyme
	Lysozyme	
Neutral serine proteases	Elastase	
	Cathepsin G	
Metalloproteinases	Proteinases	Collagenase
Acid hydrolase		
Acid hydrolases	N-Acetyl-glucuronidase	
	Cathepsin B	
	Cathepsin D	
	β-Glucuronidase	
	β-Glycerophosphatase	
	α-Mannosidase	
Others	Defensins	Lactoferrin
	Antibacterial cationic proteins	Vitamin B_{12} Binding Proteins
	Kinin-generating enzyme	Cytochrome *b*
	C5a-Inactivating factor	Histaminase
		Complement activator
		Monocyte-chemoat-tractant
		Plasminogen activator
		Protein kinase C inhibitor
		FMLP receptors
		C3bi receptors

From Boxer LA and Smoles JE: Hematol Oncol Clinics N America 2:101, 1988.

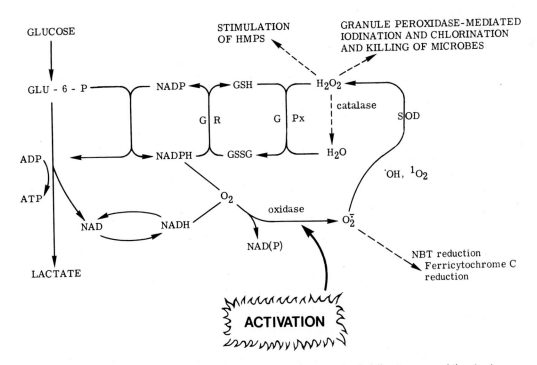

Fig. 62-7 Oxidative burst and the generation of active oxygen radicals following neutrophil activation. *From Wolach B, Baehner RL, and Boxer LA: Review: clinical and laboratory approach to the management of nuetrophil dysfunction, Isr J Med Sci 18:897, 1982.*

limited cidal effect against some bacteria and fungi. Cationic proteins, (e.g., permeability increasing factor and defensin), adhere to bacterial surfaces altering membrane permeability and interfering with membrane-associated respiratory function of the microbe. Apolactoferrin binds ferrous ion, which is essential to normal bacterial metabolism. As previously mentioned, this protein is also pivotal in oxygen-dependent killing. The decreased pH that develops with the accumulation of lactate in the phagolysosome is not only bacteriostatic for streptococci, but is also essential for the action of acid hydrolases, which are largely responsible for the digestion of dead bacteria.

TESTS OF NEUTROPHIL FUNCTION

The available laboratory tests of neutrophil function include assays of the humoral mediators of the different neutrophil functions, direct examination of the neutrophil's structural components, and physiological and biochemical tests of function.

Assays of humoral mediators

These assays include the quantitation of immunoglobulins, complement components, and fibronectin. In addition to the detection of decreased levels of IgG, IgM, or IgA, which may explain abnormal neutrophil function, the finding of a markedly elevated IgE level is diagnostically significant because it suggests Job's syndrome. Evaluation of complement activity is initiated by the determination of total complement activity (CH_{50}). Quantitation of the serum levels of the individual complement components is undertaken in patients who demonstrate decreased CH_{50}. Methods to determine the serum levels of immunoglobulins and complement components are discussed in Chapter 33.

Evaluation of neutrophil structure

Evaluation of neutrophil morphology and of the integrity of their structural components are essential steps in patients with suspected dysfunction. Direct examination of the peripheral smear permits detection of giant granules in Chediak-Higashi syndrome and a decrease in granularity in patients with secondary granule deficiency and some individuals with myeloproliferative syndromes. Further elucidation of morphologic abnormalities may require examination by electron microscopy. The enzymatic content of the granules themselves can be studied with cytochemical staining techniques (e.g., peroxidase activity in primary granules and leukocyte phosphatase activity in secondary granules). Similarly, the lactoferrin content of secondary granules may be determined by immunochemical staining. Recently, assay of the CD11/CD18 group of membrane glycoproteins has become relatively simple with fluorescent immunochemical staining techniques utilizing monoclonal antibodies and flow cytometry. The antibody most commonly used for this purpose is one with specificity for the alpha subunit of the CD11b/CD18 glycoprotein (Leu 15 or Mol).

Physiological and biochemical tests of function

Tests of varying specificity and sensitivity have been designed to evaluate the integrity of each aspect of neutrophil function, including adherence, chemokinesis and chemotaxis, phagocytosis, metabolic burst, degranulation, and bacterial killing

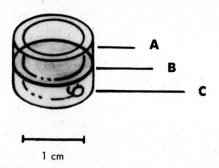

Fig. 62-8   Schematic diagram of the Boyden chamber. **A,** Upper compartment. **B,** Micropore membrane. **C,** Lower compartment and side opening. (From Mark-it Engineering Corp. Chicago.) *From Bauer JD: Leukocyte function tests. In Sonnenwirth AC and Jarett L, eds: Gradwohl's clinical laboratory methods and diagnosis, vol 1, ed 8, St. Louis, 1980, Mosby—Year Book, Inc.*

1. An in vivo skin test, the Rebuck Skin Window, can detect gross deficiencies in the first two of these functions. The test is performed by abrading the skin, sequentially tapping glass slides over the abrasion for variable periods of time, and then examining the Wright-stained slides to enumerate the number of neutrophils and other inflammatory cells that migrate and adhere to the slide. In general, large numbers of neutrophils adhere to the slide within three to six hours followed by monocytes in 12 hours. This test is usually a primary screening test along with a complete blood count and differential, examination of neutrophil morphology, and determination of serum immunoglobulin and complement levels in individuals suffering from recurrent bacterial infections.

2. In general, in vitro tests to measure neutrophil adherence are poorly standardized and are not often used. One of these tests measures C5a-dependent retention of neutrophils as blood is passed through a nylon wool column. In addition, neutrophil aggregation following exposure to C5a is also considered an index of adhesive ability.

3. In vitro assessment of neutrophil chemokinesis and chemotaxis is most commonly performed in a Boyden chamber, (Figure 62-8). This apparatus consists of a double chamber separated by a 100 micron-wide millipore filter, (pore size 3 to 8 microns). A standardized number of neutrophils are placed in one chamber, and after a period of incubation at 37°C, the number that migrate through the filter is determined and taken as a measurement of chemokinesis. Chemotaxis is assessed by repeating the experiment after the addition of a chemotactic substance to the other chamber. A positive chemotactic response is indicated by an increased neutrophil migration through the filter following addition of the agent.

   By modifying the conditions under which tests with the Boyden chamber are performed, the following facets of chemotactic function can be assessed:
   a. the response of the patient's cells to different chemotactic agents, (e.g., f-met-leu-phe [FMLP], soluble immune complexes, and mixtures of complement components), in order to detect intrinsic cellular dysfunction;
   b. the response of normal cells to the patient's serum in

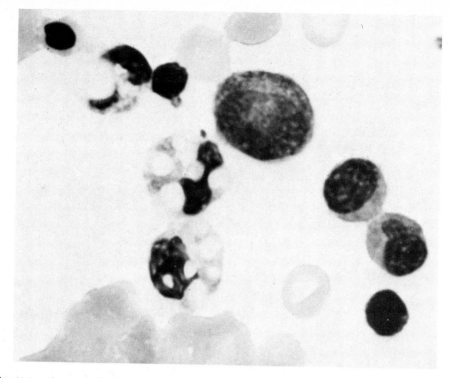

Fig. 62-9 Phagocytosis of opsonized oil droplets by bone marrow neutrophils. *From Altman AJ and Stossel TP: Br J Haematol 27:241, 1974.*

order to evaluate the chemotactic properties of the serum;

c. the response of normal cells to a mixture of normal serum and the patient's serum in order to detect the presence of a chemotactic inhibitor; and

d. the response of normal cells to normal serum and various drugs to assess the effects of drugs on chemotactic function.

The results of Boyden chamber tests are usually reported in an endpoint fashion as the percent of patient's cells that migrate through the filter after an incubation period of three hours, subsequent staining of the filter, and finally direct counting of the migrated cells appearing on the opposite side of the filter. This result is reported with the result of a control test performed with normal neutrophils. Alternatively, it may be more accurate to perform a kinetic assay. Such an assay can be performed by focusing up and down on the filter and then plotting the percentage of cells that have migrated through various depths of the filter after defined periods of incubation. The results are expressed as a curve, which is formed when the cumulative percent of migrating cells are plotted against the depth of migration. This curve can then be compared to that obtained with control neutrophils.

In some laboratories chemotactic assays are performed by direct vision of chemotaxis under agarose gels. In such tests, two wells—one containing the patient's neutrophils and one containing normal neutrophils—are spaced equidistant from a third well, which contains a chemotactic agent. The observer can periodically measure the orientation and movement of the cells toward the agent used. More detailed study can be performed by combining such a technique with time-lapse cinematography.

4. Neutrophil phagocytic activity can be assessed by visually examining stained smears for the mean number of opsononized bacteria or other reagent particles ingested per cell after a period of controlled incubation. Such tests are difficult to perform because particles adhering to the neutrophils are not easily distinguished from truly ingested particles. Extensive washing of the cells before counting tends to minimize this problem.

Tests that use opsononized bacteria (e.g., *S. aureus*) or *candida* can identify phagocytosed microbes by direct microscopic examination. Those tests can also quantify phagocytosed microbes by scintillation counting if they have been incubated with a radioactive tag before the test.

Other reagent particles used include oil droplets coated with lipopolysaccharide and complement and then stained with oil red O. These particles may be readily identified as stained bodies in phagosomes under direct microscopic examination (Figure 62-9), or the number phagocytosed can be quantitated by the spectrophotometric examination of the post incubation cell lysate.

These tests can be appropriately modified to test patient cells with reagent particles incubated in normal serum in order to examine the intrinsic phagocytic function of the cells or to assay the opsoninic potential of the patient's serum in which the target particles are incubated in the serum and then tested with normal neutrophils.

5. Numerous techniques have been introduced to examine the various biochemical aspects of the respiratory burst, including the measurement of oxygen consumption and superoxide generation, both at rest and following phagocytosis; detection of hydrogen peroxide synthesis and

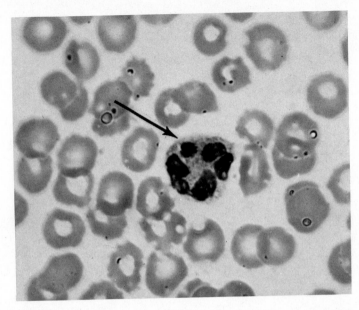

Fig. 62-10 NBT screening test. Neutrophil containing a formazan deposit (arrow). *From Bauer JD: Leukocyte function tests. In Sonnenwirth AC and Jarett L, eds: Gradwohl's clinical laboratory methods and diagnosis, vol 1, ed 8, St. Louis, 1980, Mosby–Year Book, Inc.*

singlet oxygen production; and quantitation of the different components of NADPH oxidase activity.

While the direct measurement of oxygen consumption and superoxide generation are performed in specialized laboratories, the detection of hydrogen peroxide and singlet oxygen production are becoming more common. Tests for hydrogen peroxide generation are based on hydrogen peroxide's ability to quench scopeletin fluorescence in the presence of horseradish peroxidase. Tests for singlet oxygen are based on the detection of chemiluminescence caused by photon emission during the oxidation of phagocytosed zymogen particles by singlet oxygen.

A screening test for the activity of the NADPH oxidase system is the nitroblue tetrazolium reduction (NBT) test. In this cytochemical test, colorless NBT is reduced to deep blue formazan by the transfer of hydrogen to the dye in the presence of normal oxidase system activity mediating the transformation of oxygen to superoxide. The test can be used as either a cytochemical screening test or a quantitative assay of oxidase activity.

The NBT screening test is performed by adding the NBT solution to heparinized whole blood. Following incubation of the mixture, a blood smear is made and examined. The percent of neutrophils containing blue formazan deposits is then determined (Figure 62-10). Reference values in most laboratories using a common commercial kit method is 2% to 30%. This test can be repeated after the addition of a membrane activator. The number of cells containing deposits should increase two to four times. Spontaneous increased NBT reduction is seen in the cells of normal individuals during the course of bacterial infections. For this reason this test is also used to differentiate bacterial from nonbacterial infections.

The quantitative NBT reduction test is performed by in-

cubating the patient's neutrophils with the NBT reagent and latex beads. After incubation, the neutrophils are isolated, washed, and lysed. Finally, the optical density of a pyridine extract of the supernatant solution is measured at 515 nm with a spectrophotometer.

Quantitating the various individual components of NADPH oxidase system is currently only performed in highly specialized laboratories. Such assays are indicated in cases of suspected chronic granulomatous disease of childhood in order that the precise defect can be identified. Cytochrome b activity can be quantified in extracts of intact neutrophils. In addition, identification of the cytochrome subunits can be carried out by Western blot analysis. The portion of the total cellular cytochrome b activity that is membrane associated can be determined on disrupted neutrophil fractions. Finally, maximal NADPH oxidase activity can be determined following the disruption of cells previously stimulated with opsonized zymosan.

6. Assays of degranulation depend on the detection of beta glucuronidase and lactoferrin released from the primary and secondary granules respectively into the suspending medium.

7. Finally, microbial killing can be directly assessed by the incubation of viable opsonized bacteria (e.g., *S. aureus*) with neutrophils, and following ingestion and further incubation, the lysing of the cells and subsequent culture of the lysate. A large number of viable bacteria indicate impaired killing. Alternatively, following ingestion of the target bacteria, the cells may be incubated with tritiated thymidine and its subsequent incorporation into the DNA of residual viable bacteria detected by radioautography. Some laboratories use candida instead of bacteria, and the viability of the ingested candida is assessed by their ability to exclude trypan blue dye.

NEUTROPHIL DYSFUNCTION

Defects in neutrophil function may be congenital or acquired and are due either to extracellular or intracellular defects. In the past, these disorders were classified according to the predominant function found (Box 62-2). In many of these abnormalities, however, more than one function is defective or the defect is poorly defined.

CD11/CD18 deficiency

This disorder, which is characterized by decreased adhesiveness of neutrophils, results from deficient expression of the CD11/CD18 glycoprotein group on the cell surface. It varies in severity depending on whether the alpha or beta subgroup is deficient. In the more severe variants, the beta subunit is deficient, and consequently the synthesis of all the glycoproteins is also deficient. Deficient synthesis of only one of the alpha subunits results in a milder disorder because two of the three glycoproteins are synthesized in normal amounts. The most common alpha variant results in the decreased expression of CD11b/CD18 (mol). Most cases are transmitted as an autosomal recessive trait, while occasional cases are sex-linked recessive.

The clinical manifestations include recurrent infections of the skin and subcutaneous tissues and otitis media, gengivitis, and pharyngitis; a history of delayed umbilical cord separation; and impaired wound healing.

Laboratory findings include persistent neutropenia, marked decrease in neutrophil migration into a Rebuck skin window, and decreased neutrophil adhesion. As would be expected of cells lacking adhesive ability, assays of chemokinesis and chemotaxis are abnormal. Because of the absence of CR3 receptors, patients with severe disease fail to form rosettes with C3bi-coated red cells. The diagnosis is confirmed by finding a decrease in CD11/CD18 glycoproteins in tests using fluorescent flow cytometry and monoclonal antibodies.

Chemotactic defects due to extrinsic causes

Patients with decreased levels of C3 and C5 show lowered ability to generate chemotactic factors, (e.g., systemic lupus and acute glomerulonephritis). In addition, a few patients with malignancies have serum inhibitors to chemotaxis (e.g., Hodgkin's disease, melanoma, carcinoma of the breast).

Hyperimmunoglobulin E syndrome (Job's syndrome)

This is a congenital disorder, characterized by the presence of an inhibitor to chemotaxis and extremely high levels of IgE in the serum. The nature of the inhibitor has not been defined, but it may be produced by the patient's mononuclear cells.

Patients suffer from recurrent pyogenic skin and respiratory tract infections after the age of six months. Associated are a chronic papular dermatitis and progressive osteoporosis related to the production of an osteoclast activating factor. Patients often have an associated cellular immune defect. The disorder is transmitted as an autosomal dominant trait with variable penetrance.

Laboratory findings include eosinphilia, extremely high serum IgE levels, elevated levels of IgE antibodies directed

---

Box 62-2 Granulocyte dysfunction

I. DEFECTS OF CELLULAR ADHESION

CD11/CD18 glycoprotein deficiency
Alcoholism

II. DEFECTS IN CHEMOTAXIS

A. Intrinsic defects
Neonates
Chediak-Higashi syndrome
Kartenger's syndrome
Increased microtubule assembly
Lazy leukocyte syndrome
Wiskott-Aldrich syndrome
Localized juvenile periodontitis
Congenital specific granule deficiency
B. Extrinsic defects
Hypogammaglobulinemia
C3 and C5 deficiency
Sickle cell anemia
Hyper IgE syndrome (Job's syndrome)
7q- syndrome
Acquired chemotactic inhibitors
(Rheumatoid Arthritis, Neoplasms)

III. DEFECTS IN PHAGOCYTIC ACTIVITY

A. Intrinsic defects
Actin anchoring deficiency
Actin dysfunction
B. Extrinsic defects
Hypogammaglobulinemia
C3 deficiency
Post-splenectomy with tuftin deficiency

IV. DEFECTS IN DEGRANULATION

Chediak-Higashi syndrome
Congenital secondary granule deficiency
Sepsis

V. DEFECTS IN BACTERICIDAL ACTIVITY

Chronic granulomatous disease of childhood
Glucose 6-phosphate dehydrogenase deficiency
Congenital myeloperoxidase deficiency
Glutathione regeneration pathway deficiencies
Acquired primary granule deficiency

---

against S. aureus, and circulating serum IgG-IgE immune complexes. Tests of neutrophil chemotaxis stimulated with endotoxin or FMLP are abnormal in most patients. Other neutrophil function tests are normal. Quantitation of T cell subsets often reveals decreased numbers of CD8 bearing cells. Although the patient's lymphocytes demonstrate normal responses to most mitogens, they may show decreased reactivity to candida.

Chediak-Higashi syndrome

As previously discussed, this syndrome is characterized morphologically by the presence of giant granules in the cytoplasm of neutrophils and other leukocytes. These giant granules result from the fusion of lysosomes. The neutrophils usually demonstrate abnormal structure of their microtubules, which may be due to alterations in tubulin alpha

Table 62-5 Classification of chronic granulomatous disease*

Type	Inheritance	Cytochrome *b* spectrum	NBT-positive cells	Intact cell O₂		NADPH Oxidase		Cell-free system		Relative frequency (%) cases)
				PMA	Zymosan	K_m* (mM)	V_{max}	Membrane oxidase	Cytosol factor	
I	X	0	0	0	0	—	0	0	Normal	~65%
IA	X	0	60-90% (weak)	1-10%	~3%	0.8-8.4	7-70%	0†	Normal†	5 cases
II	AR	100% (Normal)	0	0-0.7%	0-1%	—	0	Normal	0.2-2%	~30%
IIA	AR	100% (Normal)	85% (weak)	1.5%	4%	.17	85%	Normal	6%	1 case
III	AR	0-4%	0-4% (weak)	0	0	—	0	0	Normal	8 cases
IV	X	100% (Normal)	0	0.4%	0	NT	NT	0.6%†	Normal†	2 cases
IVA	X	8-100% (Normal)	80-100% (weak)	1-4%	16%	NT	NT	NT	NT	4 cases

Modified from Curnutte JT: Hematol Oncol Clinics N America 2:241, 1988.
*All data are presented as % normal except the K_m data, which are presented as NADPH concentration (mM). The normal K_m for NADPH is 0.04 mM. In the case of cytochrome *b* spectra, "Normal" refers to the appearance of the cytochrome spectrum, whereas the numbers refer to its quantitative level as a percentage of normal.
†One case studied (unpublished results from this laboratory).
X = X-linked; AR = autosomal recessive; NT = not tested; PMA = phorbol-12-myristate acetate; NBT = nitroblue tetrazolium.

chain structure or defective regulation of tubulin synthesis. Similar abnormalities are seen in the cytoplasmic granules of other cells including melanocytes, CNS Schwann cells, and platelets. These patients demonstrate defective degranulation and phagolysosome formation with resultant deficient bactericidal function. In addition, because of the defective degranulation, they also demonstrate a decrease of granule derived chemotactic receptors leading to abnormal chemotaxis.

Patients present with recurrent pyogenic skin infections, gingivitis, and periodontitis. *S. aureus* is most commonly responsible. With progression, approximately 50% develop a lymphoproliferative disorder, and many develop progressive cranial neuropathies. In addition, they have associated ocular-cutaneous hypopigmentation, mental retardation, photophobia, and a mild platelet dysfunction. The disorder is transmitted as an autosomal recessive trait.

Laboratory findings include neutropenia and the presence of the characteristic giant granules in the neutrophils (Figure 62-2). Patients demonstrate abnormal neutrophil migration into a Rebuck skin window and in vitro chemotaxis. Some also have a mild adhesion defect. Bactericidal killing is sluggish. Occasional patients also have a prolonged bleeding time and demonstrate a release defect during aggregation studies.

Phagocytic defects due to extrinsic causes

Most severe extrinsic defects are related to the absence of complement or IgG1 and IgG3 (e.g., sickle cell anemia, systemic lupus erythematosus, agammaglobulinemia). The neutrophils of splenectomized individuals also have deficient activity. It has been postulated that a small polypeptide, "tuftin," which is secreted by the spleen, increases the phagocytic activity of neutrophils. This polypeptide is lacking in splenectomized patients.

Chronic granulomatous disease

This disorder is actually a heterogenous group of related defects in the activity of the NADPH oxidase system, which results in the decreased ability of the neutrophils to synthesize normal amounts of superoxide. As a consequence, hydrogen peroxide and singlet oxygen generation is reduced or absent. The severity of this disorder varies according to the exact nature of the oxidase system defect.

These patients suffer recurrent infections during the first few years of life with catalase producing bacteria and fungi, which destroy the endogenous hydrogen peroxide produced by the microbe, (e.g., *S. aureus*, Gram negative-bacteria, *C. albicans*). These infections result in granulomatous lymphadenitis, hepatic abscesses, eczematoid dermatitis, and pneumonitis. Phagocytosed catalase negative microorganisms do not cause infections because the small amount of hydrogen peroxide they produce is sufficient to generate activated oxygen radicals and participate in myeloperoxidase mediated hypohalite synthesis.

Variants of chronic granulomatous disease can be classified according to the precise defect in the oxidase system, mode of inheritance, and clinical severity (Table 62-5). Type I CGD is the most common form, (65% of cases). It is due to a total lack of the cytochrome b constituent of the system and is transmitted as a sex-linked recessive trait. Neutrophils from these patients lack the ability to reduce NBT, and a totally negative NBT reduction test is highly suggestive of this diagnosis. Female carriers may show a mixed population of formazan positive and negative cells in the NBT test. Assays for cytochrome b in extracts of the patient's neutrophils reveal a total deficiency. As would be expected, superoxide production in response to various particulate and soluble stimuli is completely absent.

Cytochrome b positive variants tend to be milder in their clinical manifestations. In these forms, the NBT reduction test is not diagnostic since many neutrophils may contain small amounts of formazan, a finding which may be seen in other disorders that affect the respiratory burst. Differentiation from these other entities is made possible by measuring superoxide generation following stimulation, since variant CGD cells can generate only less than 10% of normal, while the cells from patients with other disorders generate significantly more.

Other enzymatic defects

Myeloperoxidase deficiency is a relatively common neutrophil enzymopathy. Although these patients are unable to generate bactericidal hypohalite ions, they generally do not suffer from recurrent severe infections, unless they are otherwise predisposed (e.g., diabetes mellitus). It appears that because they produce normal amounts of superoxide, other active oxygen species are able to kill phagocytosed bacteria.

Rare patients with severe glucose 6-phosphate dehydrogenase deficiency or deficiencies in the glutathione regeneration pathway may also suffer bactericidal defects resulting in recurrent infections because of their inability to resynthesize the NADPH required as a substrate for oxidase mediated synthesis of superoxide.

MYELOLEUKEMIC, MYELOPROLIFERATIVE AND MYELODYSPLASTIC DISORDERS

Leukemias are neoplastic disorders of hematopoietic cells that arise in the bone marrow and are associated with the replacement and loss of normal marrow elements. Leukemia is usually characterized by the presence of the abnormal cells in the peripheral blood. In a small number of patients, they are not found (aleukemic leukemia). Leukemias involving the proliferation and accumulation of immature cells (i.e., blasts and other very early cells) have a rapid course lasting two to four months without treatment, and usually affect younger age groups. These disorders are known as acute leukemia. Leukemias involving maturing elements have a protracted course and usually do not affect children. These are termed chronic leukemia. The cell line involved may be either lymphocytic or the cells of the various myeloid cell lines (granulocytic, monocytic, myelomonocytic, erythrocytic, or megakaryocytic). The proportion of newly diagnosed cases belonging to each principle category is 1. acute lymphocytic leukemia—25%; 2. acute myelogenous ("non-lymphocytic") leukemia—35%; 3. chronic lymphocytic leukemia—25%; 4. and chronic myelogenous leukemia—15%.

Although the prognosis of each category varies, they all tend to cause clinical manifestations in the same way. As they progress they cause anemia, thrombocytopenia, and with the exception of chronic myelogenous leukemia, neutropenia, due to replacement of normal marrow elements. Finally, in advanced cases, the leukemic cells infiltrate the parenchyma of other organs. Organs particularly predisposed to such infiltration vary according to the cell line giving rise to the leukemia. Lymphocytic leukemias tend to be characterized by lymphadenopathy and splenomegaly, while the myeloid leukemias tend to lack lymphadenopathy. In addition, the degree of infiltration, and therefore the degree of organomegaly, is more pronounced in the chronic forms. The lymphocytic leukemias will be discussed in Chapter 63.

The term myeloproliferative disorder was originally conceived to identify a group of chronic clonal disorders characterized by the purposeless proliferation of morphologically normally maturing marrow cells. They were grouped together because one marrow cell line is usually not singly affected, they are often difficult to distinguish from one another, and they all may develop into acute leukemia. Some investigators have included various idiopathic refractory anemias in the myeloproliferative group. They are more correctly referred to as myelodysplasic or dysmyelopoietic syndromes. They are characterized by abnormal cell division and maturation, thereby causing defective production of erythrocytes, granulocytes, and platelets. Some of these disorders are associated with a high propensity to evolve into acute leukemia ("preleukemic syndromes").

Etiopathogenesis of leukemia

Numerous etiologic factors have been implicated as contributing to the emergence of a neoplastic clone of hematopoietic cells which results in leukemia. It is generally true that more than one factor is operative and that they result in chromosomal alterations, which permit the expression of oncogenes and the emergence of a mutant that gives rise to the neoplastic clone. Among these factors are the following:

1. Hereditary predisposition: There is an increased incidence of acute leukemia among family members. In cases of ALL with an onset prior to one year of age, almost half of identical twins will also develop ALL. The incidence among twins decreases progressively with increasing age of onset. Patients with Down's syndrome and Bloom's syndrome have a much increased incidence of both AML and ALL. Those with Fanconi's anemia are predisposed to AML, while patients with various primary immunodeficiency syndromes (especially ataxia telangiectasia and Wiskott-Aldrich syndrome) are predisposed to ALL.
2. Radiation: Following radiation exposure there is a dose-related increasing incidence of both AML and CML. Onset usually occurs after a latent period of seven to 10 years. At high doses radiation may act as a direct leukemogen, (initiator), while at lower doses it may simply act as a predisposing agent for other tumorigenic factors. Its action is due to direct mutagenic effects (e.g., chromosomal breakage, etc.).
3. Chemical exposure: Benzene and alkylating drugs (e.g., chlorambucil, nitrosureas, cyclophosphamide) not only cause marrow hypoplasia, but are also mutagenic and leukemogenic. The occurrence of acute myelogenous leukemia following treatment of another malignancy (i.e., secondary leukemia) is a recognized complication of chemotherapy.
4. Viral infection: There is now conclusive evidence that RNA viruses (retroviruses) are able to cause leukemia in man. The human T cell lymphotrophic virus, type I, is the cause of adult T cell leukemia/lymphoma. Among the evidence implicating the virus as the cause of this disease is the demonstration of reverse transcriptase activity in leukemic cells, the demonstration of homology between the DNA of leukemic cells and the RNA of the virus, and epidemiological evidence that leukemia occurs with horizontal transmission of viral infection. In addition, infection with a DNA virus (cytomegalovirus) is now known to cause Burkitt's lymphoma in man.

The first three groups of etiologic factors listed above probably predispose to leukemic transformation by inducing chromosomal changes that permit the activation of normal cellular proto-oncogenes (c-oncs). Among these changes, translocations most often appear to be associated with leukemic transformation. They may juxtapose an oncogene next to a transcription promotor region, thereby inducing augmented production of the normal oncogene product responsible for growth activity. Alternatively, the translocation may induce the formation of a fusion gene between the translocated oncogene and another gene located at the breakpoint of the other chromosome, which codes for an abnormal new growth protein. More rarely, point mutations in an oncogene region may activate the gene, or deletions may release an oncogene from normal controls. The product of these activated oncogenes may include peptides with growth-promoting activity, protein products with homology to normal cell receptors for growth factors, or other proteins associated with nuclear chromatin that may participate in the control of DNA replication. Recently it has been proposed that some oncogene products may also prolong cell longevity. Specific examples of translocations, deletions, trisomies, and other alterations recognized to be associated with specific forms of leukemia and myelodysplastic syndromes will be discussed later in this chapter.

The mechanism by which retroviruses cause leukemia are still incompletely understood. The DNA transcripts of acute transforming viruses may express viral oncogenes (v-oncs), which become integrated into the host chromatin and are then activated. On the other hand, the DNA transcripts of retroviruses with long latency may either contain promoter and enhancer sequences inserted near a host c-onc or cause mutations in host regulatory genes leading to derepression of a c-onc or in the c-onc itself leading to its activation.

Acute non-lymphocytic leukemias

Acute non-lymphocytic leukemias (ANLL) or acute myelogenous leukemias (AML) are the most common types of leukemia in adults and also occur occasionally in children. They have a peak incidence in the third to fifth decade of life and have an overall incidence of approximately three per 100,000 individuals. Males have a slightly increased incidence of ANLL.

In these disorders, blasts accumulate because of the defective differentiation, prolonged cycle time, and an increased proportion of cells in Go. These blasts replace the normal population of maturing granulocytes, erythroid precursors, and megakaryocytes.

Common clinical and laboratory features

The various entities which belong to this group of disorders share many clinical characteristics and laboratory findings but can be distinguished by other clinical manifestations, morphologic differences, and both cytochemical and surface immune markers.

Clinically, the major manifestations of these disorders are progressive anemia, a hemorrhagic diathesis related to thrombocytopenia, infections due to neutropenia, and occasionally urate nephropathy secondary to increased serum urate levels. In addition to marrow replacement, subperiosteal collections of neoplastic cells may be associated with local pain. Nodular infiltrates (chloromas) may be found in the skin and about the orbits and spinal cord. Meningeal involvement is seen in less than 10% of cases. Intralobular

hepatic infiltration may result in hepatomegaly. Lymphadenopathy and splenomegaly are significant in only 10% of patients. The most common cause of death is infection, while hemorrhage can usually be controlled before becoming life threatening. Survival is only three to six months without treatment.

The peripheral white cell count is usually elevated and in 20% of cases is greater than 100,000/μl, a level often associated with the manifestations of leukostasis. In 25% of patients the count is less than 5,000/μl, which consist partially or wholly of blasts. Rarely, no immature myeloid cells are seen in the peripheral blood (aleukemic leukemia). The absolute number of mature granulocytes is decreased. A normochromic normocytic anemia is present in most patients. The hemoglobin concentration is below 7 gm/dl at the time of diagnosis in about 20% of cases. The reticulocyte index is reduced. Thrombocytopenia is almost universally present. Approximately 25% of cases have platelet counts below 20,000/μl at the time of diagnosis.

The bone marrow is hypercellular due to the leukemic infiltrate, which replaces normal cellular elements. The M:E ratio is markedly increased. The myeloid cells are immature, and their morphology varies according to the type of leukemia present. Megakaryocytes are markedly reduced in number. It is generally agreed that ANLL is only diagnosed when the immature elements constitute more than 30% of the total marrow cellularity. In addition, approximately 50% of cases have certain chromosomal abnormalities, the most frequent of which are trisomy 8 and monosomy 7.

Patients with ANLL tend to have 1) an elevated serum LDH level, the magnitude of which reflects the total body tumor burden; 2) a decreased serum potassium concentration, the cause of which is poorly understood; and 3) an increased serum uric acid level which results from the breakdown of leukemic cells. Rapid lysis of cells following the initiation of chemotherapy is associated with a further elevation of serum uric acid levels, hyperkalemia, hyperphosphatemia, and hypocalcemia.

Of special concern are the cases of ANLL that occur after treatment with radiotherapy or chemotherapy of another malignancy. These cases of secondary leukemia, which are often preceded by myelodysplasia, are usually accompanied by characteristic partial deletions of chromosomes 5 or 7, are refractory to treatment, and have an especially poor prognosis.

The French-American-British (FAB) classification of ANLL

This group of acute leukemias has been separated into different types based on morphologic criteria according to the French-American-British (FAB) Classification. Some types are also associated with specific cytochemical, immunophenotypic, and cytogenetic characteristics. Also, the clinical manifestations and course of these different types vary to some degree. They are classified as follows:

M1: acute myeloblastic leukemia without differentiation. This category is characterized by the proliferation of myeloblasts, which accumulate without undergoing further differentiation. Together with the M2 variant, it represents approximately half of all cases. These myeloblasts are usually large (20-25 μ) with large, round or bean-shaped nuclei

Table 62-6   French-American-British (FAB) classification of acute leukemias

FAB type	Characteristics of bone marrow
ACUTE NONLYMPHOBLASTIC (ANLL)	
M1: Myeloblastic, without maturation (AML)	<3% of blasts myeloperoxidase positive
M2: Myeloblastic, with maturation (AML)	Maturation to or beyond the promyelocyte stage, <20% monocytes
M3: Promyelocytic (APL)	Majority of cells are abnormal, hypergranular, promyelocytes
M4: Myelomonocytic (AMML)	Like M@, but with >20% monocytes (confirm with fluoride-inhibited esterase reaction)
M5: Monoblastic (AMoL)	Majority of cells monocytic, <20% granulocytic
M6: Erythroleukemia (EL)	>50% erythroblasts, or >30% if erythropoiesis is bizarre, must also have >30% myeloblasts and promyelocytes
M7: Megakaryoblastic (AMegL)	Blasts positive for platelet peroxidase reaction (by electron microscopy) or antibodies against platelet glycoprotein Ib, IIb/IIIa, IIIa or factor VIII, fibrosis

From Griffith RC and Janney CG: Hematopoietic system: bone marrow and blood, spleen, and lymph nodes. In Kissane JM, ed: Anderson's pathology, vol 2, ed 9, St. Louis, 1990, Mosby–Year Book, Inc.

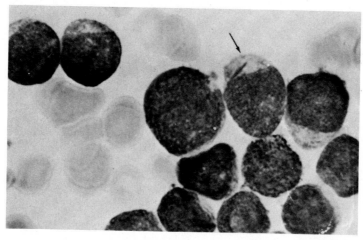

Fig. 62-11   Acute non-lymphocytic leukemia, bone marrow aspirate. FAB category M1. Auer rod in myeloblast (arrow). *From Bauer JD: Clinical laboratory methods, ed 9, St. Louis, 1982, Mosby–Year Book, Inc.*

containing 2 to 3 nucleoli, (Figure 62-11). A micromyeloblastic variant (<20 μ) is occasionally seen. M1 myeloblasts are particularly difficult to differentiate from lymphoblasts, which are smaller than most myeloblasts, have scantier cytoplasm, and possess nuclei containing only one or two nucleoli. Granules are not visible in the cytoplasm of these myeloblasts if stained with Wright's stain. However, the cells may contain large rod-like bodies that are intensely eosinophilic (Auer rods). Auer rods are thought to represent abnormal primary granules and are diagnostic of myeloid derived leukemic cells. Unless such rods are seen, the diagnosis of acute myeloblastic leukemia needs to be confirmed by cytochemical and/or immunophenotypic markers. Furthermore, the use of such markers assists in the differentiation of M1 leukemias from other types of ANLL.

Myeloblasts are usually peroxidase positive, and are differentiated from lymphoblasts by this finding. Myeloblasts, which are very primitive, may have insufficient enzyme activity to give a positive reaction. In these cases, the cells will be found to stain with Sudan black. Monoblasts may occasionally also stain with both peroxidase and Sudan black. Their differentiation from myeloblasts is made with either specific (chloroacetate) esterase or nonspecific (alpha-napthyl acetate) esterase following treatment with sodium fluoride, both of which only stain myeloblasts. Finally, myeloblasts do not stain or only stain slightly with PAS, while lymphoblasts show coarse PAS positive granularity in their cytoplasm.

Using the immunophenotyping techniques discussed in Chapter 60, M1 leukemias, which give inconclusive cytochemical staining results, can be shown to be myeloblastic in nature. More than 70% of such cells react with anti-CD13 (Leu M3 or MY7) and anti-CD33 (Leu M9 or MY9). Those cases which also react with anti-CD15 (LeuM1 or MY1) tend to respond well to therapy. It is important to recall that all these antibodies also react with receptors on early monocytic cells, which are differentiated because only they react with anti CD14 (MY4 or Mo2).

Approximately 50% of cases will have various chromosomal abnormalities. Together with the other variants, M1 types often demonstrate trisomy 8 and various deletions. Patients with these defects tend to have a worse prognosis.

M2: acute myelocytic leukemia with differentiation. This type is characterized by the accumulation of myeloblasts accompanied by some promyelocytes and myelocytes (Figure 62-12). The diagnosis is usually suspected from the cellular mileau in which the blasts are found. Cells with Auer rods may be present. Confirmation of the diagnosis is

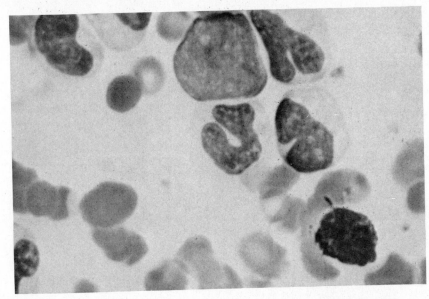

Fig. 62-12   Acute non-lymphocytic leukemia, peripheral smear. FAB category M2. *From Bauer JD: Clinical laboratory methods, ed 9, St. Louis, 1982, Mosby–Year Book, Inc.*

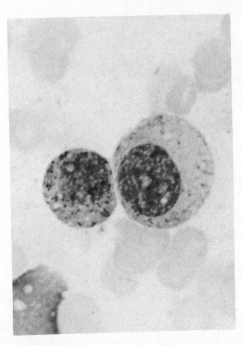

Fig. 62-13   Acute non-lymphocytic leukemia, bone marrow aspirate, FAB category M3. *From Miale JB: Laboratory medicine: hematology, ed 6, St. Louis, 1982, Mosby–Year Book, Inc.*

made with a peroxidase or Sudan black stain so that extensive cytochemical testing and immunophenotyping is not essential. Many patients with M2 leukemia have a unique chromosomal abnormality t(8:21). Taken alone, this finding does not appear to indicate a worse prognosis. Other chromosomal abnormalities common to all types of ANLL are seen as well.

M3: acute hypergranular promyelocytic leukemia. This unusual variant represents approximately 5% of all

cases of ANLL and is characterized by a predominant proliferation of promyelocytes with large primary granules and often numerous Auer rods (Figure 62-13). This entity is often complicated by disseminated intravascular coagulation due to the release of procoagulants from the granules. A characteristic cytogenetic finding in a large number of cases is t(15:17).

M4: acute myelomonocytic leukemia, (Naegeli type). This is a relatively common type of ANLL, accounting for approximately 30% of all cases. Morphologically, the blasts vary between myeloblastic and promonocytic in appearance (Figure 62-14). Many cells contain small peroxidase granules. However, the strength of reaction with peroxidase and Sudan black differs greatly from case to case as do the reactions with specific and nonspecific esterases. Occasionally, Auer rods are seen. Immunophenotyping may not be able to reliably distinguish this group from M1 and M2 variants. Cytogenetic studies have revealed t(9:11) and t(4:11) transpositions in many cases. Some patients release increased amounts of lysozyme from their leukemic cells resulting in high serum and urinary muramidase (lysozyme) levels. Overall, patients with M4 leukemia tend to have a somewhat worse prognosis than patients who show no monocytoid differentiation.

M5: acute monocytic leukemia, (Schilling variant). This unusual variant constitutes 10% of ANLL cases. Morphologically, the blasts are large, the nucleus is bean shaped, the cytoplasm contains few granules and may contain vacules, and on occasion, the cells appear to have stubby pseudopods bulging from their surface (Figure 62-15). The cells in most cases do not stain with peroxidase. However, in cells that do, staining with esterases and immunophenotyping with anti-CD14 help to confirm the diagnosis. Many cases also are characterized by the presence of t(9:11) transpositions. Patients with this variant also have high serum and urinary muramidase levels. The rather unique clinical findings of lymphadenopathy, splenomegaly, and gingival

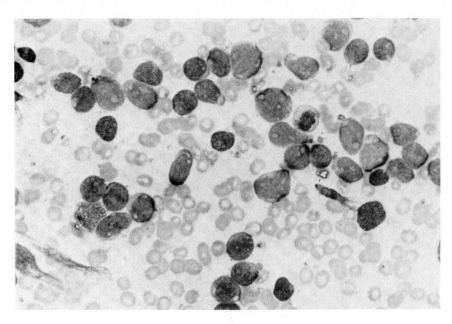

Fig. 62-14   Acute non-lymphocytic leukemia, peripheral smear. FAB category M4. *From Bauer JD: Clinical laboratory methods, ed 9, St. Louis, 1982, Mosby–Year Book, Inc.*

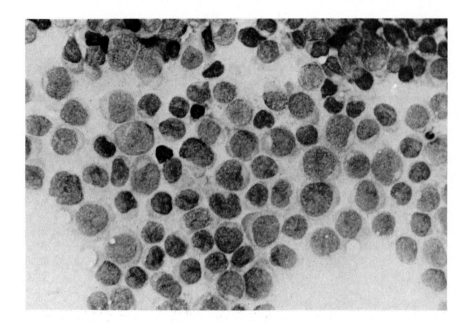

Fig. 62-15   Acute non-lymphocytic leukemia, bone marrow aspirate. FAB category M5. *From Bauer JD: Clinical laboratory methods, ed 9, St. Louis, 1982, Mosby–Year Book, Inc.*

"hypertrophy" due to leukemic cell infiltration are also frequently observed in these cases. As in the case of M4 leukemia, these patients have a poorer prognosis than those with the M1, M2, and M3 variants.

M6: acute erythroleukemia (acute erythroid myelosis or acute DiGuglielmo's syndrome). This rare variant constitutes about 5% of cases of ANLL. It is characterized by the striking erythroblastic proliferation of the marrow. The erythroblasts and other early erythroid precursors are usually megaloblastic. Many binucleate and multinucleate forms are often seen (Figure 62-16). These cells contain intracytoplasmic PAS positive deposits. Nests of myeloblasts are also seen. With a Prussian blue stain, ringed sideroblasts are often noted. The peripheral blood smear is characterized by numerous poikilocytes and nucleated red cells with megaloblastic features. With time, these cases tend to transform into more typical acute myeloblastic leukemia.

M7: acute megakaryocytic leukemia. This extremely

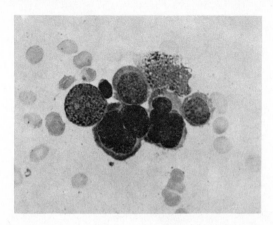

Fig. 62-16 Acute non-lymphocytic leukemia, bone marrow aspirate. FAB category M6. Note multinucleated normoblasts. *From Bauer JD: Clinical laboratory methods, ed 9, St. Louis, 1982, Mosby—Year Book, Inc.*

rare variant is characterized by the proliferation of immature atypical megakaryocytes, which is often accompanied by progressive fibrosis (acute myelofibrosis) and subsequently evolves into acute myeloblastic leukemia.

M0: acute undifferentiated leukemia. This category consists of acute leukemia, which possesses no cytochemical or immunophenotypic markers characteristic of acute lymphocytic or myelogenous leukemia.

Myeloproliferative disorders, (MPD)

The disorders belonging to this group are believed to originate from pluripotential stem cells which have preferentially, but not exclusively, differentiated into some myeloid cell line. In some, evidence of clonal nature is obtained by determining the G6PD type of cells in female patients known to be double heterozygotes. In others, distinctive chromosomal abnormalities are found in affected cells. The conditions classically included in this group include: Chronic myelogenous leukemia, in which the principal proliferating cells are granulocytes; Polycythemia vera, which principally involves erythroid precursors; Essential thrombocytopenia, in which megakaryocytes are the principal cells affected; and Myeloid metaplasia with myelofibrosis, in which all myeloid hematopoietic cells proliferate in extra-medullary sites and which is often associated with progressive fibrosis of the bone marrow.

Chronic myelogenous leukemia, (CML)

CML is a relatively common disorder that occurs with an incidence of 1 to 1.5 per 100,000 population. It most commonly affects individuals in middle age and demonstrates a slight male predisposition. Although some cases arise following exposure to radiation or benzene, most arise de novo. It is believed to arise from an early pluripotential stem cell. Approximately 90% of cases possess a characteristic chromosomal abnormality, the Ph_1 (Philadelphia) chromosome which results from the reciprocal translocation t(9:22) (Figure 62-17). In conjunction with this translocation, a proto-oncogene (c-abl) present on chromosome 9 forms a fusion gene with the break-point region gene (bcr)

of chromosome 22. The transcription product of this fusion gene is a protein with tyrosine-specific kinase activity found on the cell membrane, which is believed to have a growth promoting function. Using techniques of Southern blotting and more recently, polymerase chain reaction, approximately 50% of cases which appear to lack the Ph_1 chromosome can be shown to possess the c-abl bcr rearrangement and therefore are considered to be Ph_1 positive CML. Cases lacking evidence for this rearrangement are referred to as Ph_1 Negative CML, a group which some do not consider true CML and which has a worse prognosis. This chromosomal abnormality is not only in granulocytes, but also in erythroid and megakaryocytic precursors. Of particular note is the finding of the Ph_1 chromosome in B cells as well. Cytokinetically, CML is characterized by increased proliferative capacity of granulocytic precursors and often megakaryocytes, as well as a prolongation in the intravascular lifespan of the granulocytes.

Clinically, patients usually present with splenomegaly, which may be massive, and hepatomegaly, due to parenchymal infiltration of the splenic cords and hepatic lobules with proliferating CML cells. Later in the course of the disease, patients become symptomatic from progressive anemia. In patients whose counts are markedly elevated, thrombotic and hemorrhagic complications are common. A special neurological syndrome due to "leukostasis" in the small cerebral vessels is occasionally encountered with extreme elevations of the white cell count.

Examining the peripheral blood usually reveals a moderate normocytic normochromic anemia with reticulocytopenia and mild poikilocytosis. The white blood cell count is usually markedly elevated (50,000 to 400,000/µl). Granulocytic precursors of all degrees of differentiation and maturation as well as mature polymorphonuclear leukocytes are present in the peripheral blood smear. These polys often appear to have hypogranular cytoplasm. The number of blasts is less than 10%. Increased numbers of eosinophils and basophils are usually observed. Marked thrombocytosis is present in approximately 30% of cases (Figure 62-18).

The bone marrow shows marked hypercellularity, with myeloid hyperplasia which results in an increased M:E ratio. Basophils and eosinophils are usually increased. Megakaryocytes are numerous. Focal myelofibrosis is also commonly noted. Occasional Gaucher type macrophages are present in approximately 20% of cases and result from ingestion of debris from degenerating myeloid cells (Figure 62-19).

Among other laboratory findings, the leukocyte alkaline phosphatase (LAP) score is of special diagnostic importance because it permits the differentiation of CML from a leukemoid reaction. The neutrophils in CML are deficient in LAP, and therefore have a score of essentially zero, while those in leukemoid reactions give rise to an increased score. In addition, serum B_{12} levels are increased due to the production of transcobalamine I by the proliferating granulocytes. As would be anticipated given the increased cell turnover in this disease, serum uric acid levels are also increased. Lastly, as previously stated, routine cytogenetic studies reveal the presence of the Ph_1 chromosome in 90% of cases.

Normally the course of the disease is two to four years.

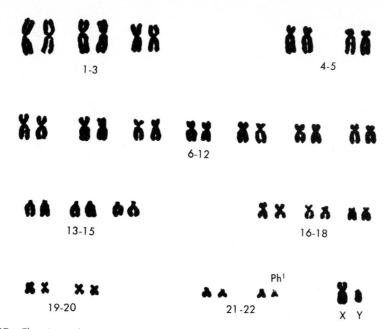

Fig. 62-17 Chronic myelogenous leukemia. Ph1 positive karyotype. *From Bauer JD: Clinical laboratory methods, ed 9, St. Louis, 1982, Mosby—Year Book, Inc.*

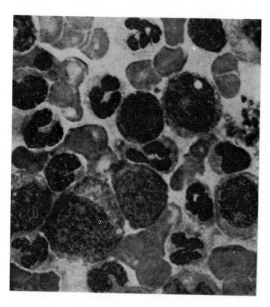

Fig. 62-18 Chronic myelogenous leukemia. Peripheral smear. *From Bauer JD: Clinical laboratory methods, ed 9, St. Louis, 1982, Mosby—Year Book, Inc.*

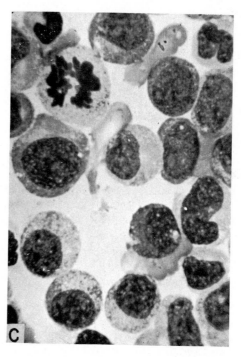

Fig. 62-19 Chronic myelogenous leukemia. Bone marrow aspirate. *From Miale JB: Laboratory medicine: hematology, ed 6, St. Louis, 1982, Mosby—Year Book, Inc.*

The disease eventually evolves into an accelerated phase, which is characterized by increasing splenomegaly, increasing anemia, difficulty controlling the white cell count with commonly used chemotherapeutic agents, an increasing LAP score, increasing basophilia, and a falling or rising platelet count. The bone marrow may show increasing fibrosis and nests of blasts. Cytogenetic studies reveal additional chromosomal abnormalities, including duplication of

the Ph_1 chromosome, trisomy 8, and an isochrome 17. Finally, the disease enters the phase known as "blast crisis," with the proliferation and accumulation of blasts that totally replace other marrow elements. The picture is that of an acute leukemia. Most cases transform into one of the forms of ANLL, including rare cases of M6 and M7 leukemia. In 20% of cases, the blasts have cytochemical characteristics of lymphoblasts (e.g., high concentration of terminal deoxy-

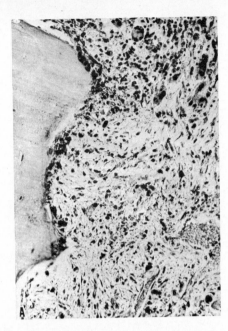

Fig. 62-20 Myeloid metaplasia with myeloid fibrosis. Bone marrow biopsy showing advanced myelofibrosis. *From Miale JB: Laboratory medicine: hematology, ed 6, St. Louis, 1982, Mosby–Year Book, Inc.*

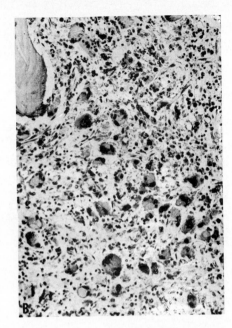

Fig. 62-21 Essential Thrombocythemia. Bone marrow biopsy showing striking megakaryocytic hyperplasia and mild to moderate fibrosis. *From Miale JB: Laboratory medicine: hematology, ed 6, St. Louis, 1982, Mosby–Year Book, Inc.*

nucleotidyl transferase) and appear to arise from a B cell line. The patients who undergo this transformation earliest appear to be truly Ph₁ negative (i.e., they show no evidence of a c-abl bcr gene rearrangement). In these patients, the typical course of CML is approximately one year.

Myeloid metaplasia with myelofibrosis (MMM)

This disease affects middle-aged and elderly individuals of both sexes. It is characterized by the clonal proliferation of all myeloid cell lines with the progressive accumulation of granulocytic, erythroid, and megakaryocytic precursors in the spleen, liver, and marrow. In most cases, however, this marrow proliferation is associated with myelofibrosis which may be related, in part, to the release of platelet-derived growth factor and other growth factors from platelets. With advancing disease, massive splenomegaly and marked hepatomegaly develops.

Patients usually have a normochromic, normocytic anemia and reticulocytopenia due to both myelofibrosis and hypersplenism. There is usually a mild neutrophilia associated with a variable platelet count. The peripheral smear reveals anisopoikilocytosis with numerous teardrop-shaped cells, which are characteristic of marrow replacement. The "leuko-erythroblastic picture" is completed by finding immature granulocytes and nucleated erythroid cells in the peripheral smear. See Chapter 61 (Figure 61-3).

Bone marrow aspiration commonly results in a "dry tap." The biopsy is characterized by the presence of myelofibrosis together with residual marrow tissue, which may appear hypercellular. Megakaryocytes are often large and bizarre (Figure 62-20). The fibrosis must be distinguished from secondary myelofibrosis due to carcinomatosis, lymphoproliferative disorders, or other myeloproliferative disorders.

The LAP score is increased. Measurement of serum LDH

and uric acid shows them to be elevated. Cytogenetic studies have shown a variety of chromosomal abnormalities. However, Ph₁ is not observed.

The course of the disease is markedly variable and the median survival is approximately five years. The cause of death is usually thrombosis, hemorrhage, or infection. About 20% of cases terminate in a blastic phase, similar to that previously discussed.

Essential thrombocythemia (ET)

This clonal disorder results in a striking proliferation of megakaryocytes together with a lesser increased proliferation of granulocytic precursors. It affects both sexes about equally, with a median onset age of 50 years.

Patients are usually asymptomatic until they develop thrombotic or hemorrhagic complications related to the extreme increase in platelet count or dysfunction. Most patients develop moderate splenomegaly.

Laboratory examination shows that patients have a mild to moderate normochromic, normocytic anemia with a reduced reticulocyte index. An absolute neutrophilia is usually present with a white count between 10 to 30,000/μl. The platelet count usually exceeds 1,000,000/μl and may reach 5,000,000/μl. Examining the peripheral smear shows mild poikilocytosis and polychromasia. Occasional nucleated red cells may be seen. Platelets are greatly increased with many megathrombocytes and megakaryocyte fragments present. Rarely, early myeloid precursors may be present as well.

The bone marrow aspirate is hypercellular and usually shows a somewhat increased M:E ratio. The most striking finding is the marked increase in megakaryocytes, many of which are large, have increased nuclear lobulation, and are surrounded by large numbers of budding platelets (Figure 62-21). Early in the disease, bone marrow biopsies reveal only a slight increase in reticulin. With progression, however, myelofibrosis becomes evident.

The LAP score is normal or increased. The serum potassium and acid phosphatase level may be increased when the platelet count is elevated to a degree that is characteristic of this disorder. Cytogenetic studies usually show a variety of abnormalities which appear to frequently involve chromosome #1.

The course of this disorder is prolonged. Patients may die from either thrombotic or hemorrhagic complications or from blastic transformation.

Polycythemia vera (PV)

PV is a clonal proliferative disorder of red cell precursors and, to a lesser degree, the other myeloid elements leading to erythrocytosis and often thrombocytosis and/or leukocytosis. It was this disorder in which the clonal nature of myeloproliferative syndromes was first demonstrated using G6PD markers, as previously described. PV is distinguished from other causes of true erythrocytosis related to increased erythropoietin production (Chapter 61). The disease is slightly more prevalent among males. The median age at the time of diagnosis is approximately 50.

The diagnosis is suggested by the finding of a hematocrit in excess of 47% in women or 54% in men in the absence of any signs or symptoms of cardiopulmonary disease. Splenomegaly is found in over 80% of patients, resulting from both extramedullary hematopoiesis and hypersplenism. Hepatomegaly is seen in approximately 50% of cases. With an increase in the hematocrit to above 60%, the viscosity of the blood increases dramatically, and tissue perfusion decreases. The increased red cell mass and thrombocytosis, which may exceed $1,000,000/\mu l$ may result in thrombotic tendency, as well as a paradoxical hemorrhagic diathesis. This hemorrhagic tendency is due to platelet dysfunction, the increased blood volume that distends venules and capillaries, and defective clot formation because of the masses of red cells entrapped in the clot.

In addition to the increased hematocrit, laboratory findings characteristic of PV include an increased red cell mass, the demonstration of normal arterial blood oxygen saturation, a normal P_{50} or oxygen dissociation curve, and a decreased erythropoietin level. Other findings include an increased LAP score, an increase in serum B_{12} levels, and hyperuricemia. Cytogenetic studies reveal chromosomal abnormalities in most cases. However, no constant and diagnostic changes have been found in this disorder.

The bone marrow shows marked hypercellularity with erythroid hyperplasia, which is accompanied by increased granulocytic and megakaryocytic elements and frequently focal fibrosis (Figure 62-22). The marrow contains depleted iron stores due to the marked increase in erythropoiesis and treatment by phlebotomy.

PV tends to evolve, over a period of five to 20 years, into a myelofibrotic stage. Among patients treated with alkylating agents, approximately 15% to 20% develop ANLL. Among those treated by phlebotomy alone, only about 1% develop this complication.

Myelodysplastic syndromes (MDS)

This group of disorders is comprised of idiopathic refractory anemias characterized by abnormal myeloid cell prolifera-

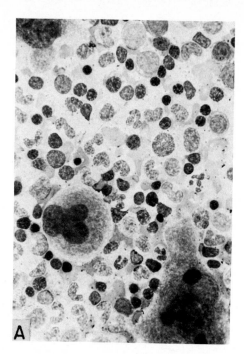

Fig. 62-22 Polycythemia Vera. Bone marrow aspirate showing hyperplasia of all precursor cells. *From Miale JB: Laboratory medicine: hematology, ed 6, St. Louis, 1982, Mosby—Year Book, Inc.*

tion and maturation. They affect patients over the age of 50. Although some have included those marked by a hypocellular marrow, (e.g., aplastic anemia and paroxysmal nocturnal hemoglobinuria without hypercellularity), the term is usually restricted to those characterized by marked hypercellularity and ineffective hematopoiesis. They have been classified by the FAB group, as outlined in Table 62-7. As previously stated, some of these disorders show a propensity for evolution into ANLL, are termed "pre-leukemic" syndromes, and may occur *de novo* or following chemotherapy of another malignancy. In these cases, chromosomal abnormalities, particularly 5q- and 7q-, are often observed.

Refractory anemia (RA)

Patients wth this variant of MDS present with a normochromic, normocytic anemia, and reticulocytopenia. Many patients have thrombocytopenia and granulocytopenia as well. Examining the bone marrow shows erythroid hyperplasia and mild to moderate nuclear cytoplasmic asynchrony of the erythroid precursors. The granulocytic and megakaryocytic cell lines appear normal in most patients. Blasts account for less than 5% of the cell population. Iron stores are increased. This form of MDS only rarely progresses into leukemia.

Refractory anemia with ringed sideroblasts (RARS) or idiopathic acquired sideroblastic anemia (IASA)

This disorder's presentation and laboratory findings are similar to RA. However, the bone marrow aspirate is remarkable, in that in excess of 15% of nucleated cells are ringed sideroblasts. This is the other form of MDS, which tends to behave in a benign manner.

Table 62-7 French-American-British (FAB) classification of myelodysplastic syndromes

Type	Blood findings	Marrow findings
Refractory anemia (RA)	Anemia, reticulocytopenia <1% blasts	<5% blasts, prominent erythroid hyperplasia with dyserythropoiesis
Refractory anemia with ringed sidero-blasts (RARS)	Anemia, reticulocytopenia <1% blasts	>15% ringed sideroblasts, <5% blasts
Refractory anemia with excess of blasts (RAEB)	<5% blasts	Hypercellular, trilineage dyspoiesis, 5% to 20% blasts
Chronic myelomonocytic leukemia (CMML)	Monocytosis (>1 × 10⁹/L) <5% blasts	<20% blasts, increased promonocytes
Refractory anemia with excess blasts in transformation (RAEBIT)	>5% blasts or Auer rods present	20% to 30% blasts or Auer rods present

From Griffith RC and Janney CG: Hematopoietic system: bone marrow and blood, spleen, and lymph nodes. In Kissane JM, ed: Anderson's pathology, vol 2, ed 9, St. Louis, 1990, Mosby—Year Book, Inc.

Refractory anemia with excess blasts (RAEB)

This type of MDS is characterized by pancytopenia, which tends to be somewhat more severe than the preceding two forms. Examination of the peripheral smear may show hypogranular polys, pseudo Pelger-Huet anomaly, or other signs of abnormal myeloid maturation. Occasional blasts may be seen as well, but they never account for more than 5% of the leukocytes seen. The marrow shows a definite increase in blasts, which ranges from 5% to 20% of the nucleated cells. RAEB often shows the cytogenetic abnormalities mentioned previously, and after a variable period, develops into ANLL.

Chronic myelomonocytic leukemia (CMML)

CMML presents with a similar clinical and laboratory picture as RAEB, except that the absolute monocyte count in the peripheral blood is in excess of 1000/mm³. The bone marrow shows a variable number of blasts, which never constitute more than 20% of the nucleated cells, together with monocytosis.

Refractory anemia with excess blasts in transformation

With this designation, disorders that resemble either RAEB or CMML are identified, but they have either an excess of 5% blasts in the peripheral smear, or between 20% and 30% blasts in the marrow. As a rule, the development of frank ANNL is imminent and would be diagnosed when the marrow contains in excess of 30% blasts.

SUGGESTED READING

Arnaout MA: Structure and function of the leukocyte adhesion molecule CD11/CD18, Blood 75:1037-1050, 1990.

Bennett JM, Catovsky D, Daniel MT, et al: Proposals for the classification of myelodysplastic syndromes, Br J Haematol 51:189-199, 1982.

Bennett JM, Catovsky D, Daniel MT, et al: Proposed revised criteria for the classification of acute myeloid leukemia, a report of the French-American-British cooperative group, Ann Int Med 103:620-625, 1985.

Chaganti RSK: Significance of chromosomal changes in hematopoetic neoplasms, Blood 62:515-524, 1983.

Curnutte JT, ed: Phagocytic defects, Hematol Oncol Clinics N America 2:1-334, 1988.

Deuel TF and Huang JS: Role of growth factor activities in oncogenesis, Blood 64:951-958, 1984.

Hyun BH: Bone marrow examination, Hematol Oncol Clinics N America 2:495-756, 1988.

McCullough EA: Stem cells in normal and leukemic hematopoesis, Blood 62:1-13, 1983.

Silver RT: Chronic myeloid leukemia: a perspective of the clinical and biological issues of the chronic phase, Hematol Oncol Clinics N America 4:319-335, 1990.

63

Laboratory diagnosis of lymphoid disorders

Robert F. Reiss

As previously discussed in Chapters 57 and 58, lymphoid cells develop from lymphoblasts through prolymphocyte and lymphocyte stages and evolve into B and T cells, which occupy distinct anatomic regions in the lymphoid organs. In the lymph node, B cells occupy follicles, the subcapsular region, and the medullary cords in which many of the B lymphocytes have evolved into plasma cells. T cells occupy deep cortical (paracortical) regions. In the spleen, B lymphocytes are found in the follicular regions of the peripheral white pulp, white T cells are concentrated about the periarteriolar sheath.

In the peripheral blood, the absolute and relative number of lymphocytes varies according to age and sex (Table 62-1). Lymphocytes vary in size, apparent cellular maturity as a reaction to immunological stimulation ("blast" transformation), and life span. The B cells tend to be short-lived and make up about 30% to 40% of the lymphocytes in the peripheral blood, while the T cells tend to be long-lived and make up 60% to 70% of the peripheral lymphocytes.

B cells were classically identified by their ability to form rosettes about complement-coated erythrocytes (EAC rosettes) and their lack of ability to rosette about sheep erythrocytes. Currently, mature resting B cells are recognized by the presence of both surface and cytoplasmic immunoglobulin (SIg and CIg) and by their reaction with monoclonal antibodies CD19 (Leu 12), 20, and 22. Plasma cells lose SIg but maintain high levels of CIg.

T cells, however, were once recognized by their ability to rosette with sheep erythrocytes (E rosettes). Resting T cells are now identified by their reactivity with the monoclonal antibodies CD5 (Leu 1) and CD7 (Leu 9). T cells are further defined as either CD4 reactive (helper-cytotoxic cells, which constitute 60% to 70% of the peripheral blood) or CD8 reactive (suppressor-inducer cells, which constitute 30% to 60% of the peripheral blood T cells).

BENIGN KINETIC ABNORMALITIES

Contrary to the case of myeloid cell precursors, the normal kinetics of lymphoid precursors and the subpopulations of mature lymphocytes is still poorly understood. Abnormalities of production, release, and peripheral survival may give rise to either increased or decreased numbers of lymphocytes in the peripheral blood or in lymphoid structures.

Although some clinicians include these benign kinetic abnormalities among the lymphoproliferative disorders, this discussion will reserve that term to describe chronic, malignant clonal proliferations of lymphoid elements.

Lymphocytopenia

Absolute lymphocytopenia is defined as less than $1500/\mu l$ lymphocytes in adults and less than $3000/\mu l$ in children. The various forms of lymphocytopenia are categorized according to the mechanisms responsible:

1. *Decreased lymphocyte production* is observed in individuals with a variety of congenital immune defects, aplastic anemia, and advanced malignancies.
2. *Increased lymphocyte destruction or loss* may occur in a variety of clinical circumstances. Infection with HIV-1 selectively destroys helper T cells. Treatment with high doses of alkylating agents and irradiation may be directly cytolytic, as are corticosteroids. Immune destruction of lymphocytes may occur in patients treated with antilymphocyte globulin or in patients who have formed lymphocytoxic autoantibodies. Finally, patients may lose lymphocytes when they develop intestinal lymphectasia, intestinal lymphatic obstruction, or severe right-sided heart failure.

Lymphocytosis

Relative lymphocytosis is a state in which neutropenia results in an increased proportion of lymphocytes in the peripheral blood but with a normal absolute lymphocyte count ($>45\%$ or $>70\%$ of white cells in adults and children, respectively). True (absolute) lymphocytosis ($>4000/\mu l$ in adults or $>7000/\mu l$ in children) may be seen in lymphoproliferative disorders, during viral infections, rare bacterial infections (e.g., pertussis), and immune disorders. The lymphocytosis associated with lymphoproliferative disorders is considered later. Reactive lymphocytosis is classically associated with infectious mononucleosis, infectious lymphocytosis, cytomegalovirus infection, and other viral infections.

Infectious mononucleosis

Infectious mononucleosis is a benign and generally self-limiting disorder due to viral infection of B cells with the

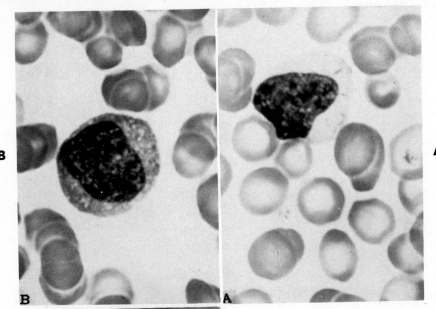

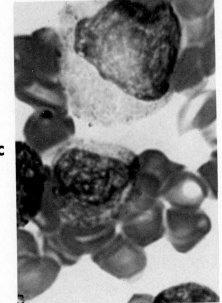

Fig. 63-1 Infectious mononucleosis, atypical lymphocytes in the peripheral smear. *Left to right:* Downey types 1, 2, and 3 cells. (Wright's stain; ×1450.) *From Miale JB: Laboratory medicine: hematology, ed 6, St. Louis, 1982, Mosby–Year Book.*

After an initial granulocytosis, the typical hematologic picture is one of lymphocytosis with total white cell counts in the 10,000 to 30,000/µl range. The peripheral smear shows numerous atypical lymphocytes (T cells), called "virocytes," which are immunologically responsive to the infection. These cells are of varying morphology and are classified by Downey into three categories (Figure 63-1):

1. *Downey type I* cells are relatively small (8 to 15 µ in diameter) and have either a peripheral notched or smooth nucleus and moderately basophilic cytoplasm, the latter cells appearing as plasmacytoid lymphocytes (Türk cells). In some cases, the cytoplasm may be vaculated.
2. *Downey type II* cells are the most prevalent. They are larger, with thin delicate cytoplasm, which is indented by the surrounding red cells. The nucleus is round or oval and possesses dark, smudged chromatin.
3. *Downey type III* cells are large, with an immunoblastic appearance (the cytoplasm appearing basophilic) and a nucleus containing visible nucleoli. These cells are the least common in smears.

Aside from the lymphocytosis, many patients have a mild normochromic, normocytic anemia. Reticulocytosis is noted in individuals with associated cold auto-immune hemolysis. Finally, mild to moderate thrombocytopenia is present as well.

Numerous serologic abnormalities are found in these patients including hypergammaglobulinemia, largely due to increased IgM levels; production of anti-IgG rheumatoid factor; cold agglutinins with anti-i specificity; and, in rare cases, the Wasserman antibody against cardiolypin. Distinctive serologic findings include production of IgM heterophile antibodies. Heterophile antibodies in humans against sheep cells occur in low levels of many *normal individuals* (Forssman type), in *serum sickness*, and in *infectious mononucleosis*, where they appear in the second week and persist about eight to 12 weeks. These three can be distinguished by the Paul-Bunnel-Davidsohn (PBD) dif-

Epstein-Barr (EB) virus. It is associated with a pronounced cytotoxic T cell reaction to the infected B cells. Infectious mononucleosis is an infectious disease of adolescents and young adults and affects both sexes equally. It is transmitted by the oral exchange of saliva. Infection is followed by an incubation period of four to six weeks. The first manifestations of the disease are pharyngitis followed by a reactive hyperplasia of the lymphoid organs, including pharyngeal lymphoid tissue, lymphadenopathy, and splenomegaly. The lymph node involvement is histologically a paracortical hyperplasia of large immunoblastic T lymphocytes. Hepatic involvement is also common, as reflected by an increased ALT, but leads to jaundice in only 10% of cases. A fine, macular skin rash is also seen in 10% of cases.

Table 63-1 Absorption patterns of various heterophil antibodies*

Condition	Absorbed by	
	Forssman antigen†	Beef erythrocytes
Normal	Yes	No or partial
Infectious mononucleosis	No or slight	Yes
Serum sickness or sensitization	Yes	Yes

From Miale JB: Laboratory medicine: hematology, ed 6, St. Louis, 1982, Mosby–Year Book, Inc.
*If absorption is "yes," there will be no agglutination, and if it is "no" there will be agglutination when the absorbed serum is added to sheep erythrocytes.
†Guinea pig or horse kidney.

ferential absorbtion test with guinea pig or horse kidney and beef red cells (Table 63-1). A recent discovery showed that the heterophile antibodies in these patients also react with horse red cells. Differential absorption tests using horse red cells as the indicator cell have now replaced the classical PBD test because of the threefold greater sensitivity of horse cells over sheep cells to infectious mononucleosis associated heterophile antibodies. The titer of the antibody response is not related to the severity of clinical disease. Rarely, patients may continue to produce sufficient heterophil antibody to give a positive test many months after resolution of the clinical infection. Serologic confirmation of infection in individuals giving false negative PBD tests is possible in most patients by the detection of IgM and IgG EB viral capsid antigen specific antibodies.

Although, as stated, the disease is normally self-limiting and resolves in four to six weeks, rare immunodeficient individuals are unable to mount a T cell response to the infection. Some of these patients have developed a progressive fatal B cell polyclonal immunoblastic disorder, which on occasion has evolved into a true monoclonal lymphoma.

Other lymphocytoses associated with infections

Seronegative infectious mononucleosis-like pictures are seen in patients infected with cytomegalovirus, *Toxoplasma*, rubella, and adenovirus. In these patients, the exact diagnosis can only be made with serologic techniques.

In addition, children with infectious lymphocytosis and pertussis also present with a fairly marked absolute lymphocytosis. As opposed to patients with infectious mononucleosis-like syndromes, the lymphocytes present in the peripheral blood appear morphologically as small to moderate mature cells rather than atypical lymphocytes.

Reactive lymphoid hyperplasia

Hyperplasia of lymphoid tissue may occur in response to a large variety of immunologic or particulate stimuli. A full discussion of these disorders is inappropriate for this chapter and the reader is referred to anatomic pathology texts. Briefly, B cell proliferation in nodes results in follicular hyperplasia and may also result in medullary plasmacytosis. As mentioned above, T cell proliferation results in paracortical hyperplasia. Lastly, nodal macrophages may also

undergo hyperplasia and initially present as sinus histiocytosis. Such changes can be seen in lymph nodes draining tumors and in dermatopathic lymphadenitis. In addition, a striking widespread histiocytosis is seen in patients with lipid and glycogen storage diseases.

As a rule, these hyperplastic reactions are nonprogressive. It has already been pointed out that immune incompetent patients may respond to an EB viral infection with an aggressive and progressive polyclonal B cell proliferative disorder.

Angioimmunoblastic lymphadenopathy is an unusual lymphoid reactive disorder with a benign, mixed cell histology. It presents with fever, rash, generalized lymphadenopathy, hepatosplenomegaly, polyclonal hypergammaglobulinemia, and often a hemolytic anemia. Histologically, the infiltrate is characterized by numerous immunoblasts, plasma cells, and small and large lymphocytes; a striking proliferation of small blood vessels; and varying amounts of homogenous, eosinophilic PAS positive material in interstitial spaces. These changes typically efface the nodal architecture, and in especially aggressive cases, the predominant feature is the proliferation of atypical immunoblasts. In many instances there is a preceding history of drug ingestion, but its relationship to the disorder is obscure. In most cases the course is progressive with survival usually under two years.

ACUTE LYMPHOCYTIC LEUKEMIAS (ALL)

ALL is a heterogeneous group of disorders characterized by the proliferation and accumulation of lymphoblasts. These disorders vary in age of onset, cell of origin, morphological characteristics, and clinical course. Overall, ALL occurs with an incidence of approximately two per 100,000 individuals. It is the most frequent malignancy of childhood and usually occurs between three and 10 years of age. ALL occurring in infants under 12 months has a poor prognosis. Adult ALL constitutes approximately 20% of cases. In all age groups, males are affected slightly more frequently than females.

Common clinical and laboratory features

As expected from the lymphoblastic infiltration of the bone marrow, the major manifestations of these disorders include progressive anemia, a hemorrhagic diathesis related to thrombocytopenia, and infections due to neutropenia. Urate nephropathy may occur secondary to the elevated serum urate levels present in these patients. Subperiosteal infiltrations of leukemic cells are common. The frequency of extramedullary infiltration with leukemic cells varies according to the form of ALL, but overall, adenopathy due to diffuse nodal infiltration is seen in 80% of cases. Infiltration in the splenic follicles and hepatic portal spaces is found in 70%. A distinctive feature of ALL is the infiltration of the meninges, noted in up to 70% of cases. As will be discussed, ALL of T cell origin tends to be associated with mediastinal masses and skin involvement.

The peripheral white count is elevated in most cases and an absolute lymphocytosis is present in 60% of patients. The degree of lymphocytosis varies according to the type of ALL. Examination of the peripheral smear reveals lymphoblastosis in over 90% of cases. Patients with markedly elevated lymphoblast counts have a poor prognosis. The morphologic characteristics of the lymphoblasts vary and form the basis for the FAB classification of ALL, discussed in the next section. The absolute number of granulocytes is decreased. Occasional patients have eosinophilia, which in rare cases may be so marked as to be associated with a hypereosinophilic syndrome. A normochromic, normocytic anemia is present in most patients at the time of diagnosis. The reticulocyte index is reduced. Thrombocytopenia is almost always present.

The bone marrow is hypercellular due to the leukemic infiltrate, which replaces normal cellular elements. The lymphoblasts vary in morphology according to the type of disease. Occasionally, the cells in the marrow develop a uropod projection and are termed "hand-mirror" variant cells. This morphologic alteration has no prognostic significance. ALL cells do not stain with Sudan black or myeloperoxidase stains, but are generally PAS positive. Furthermore, cells commonly possess nuclear terminal deoxytidal transferase (TdT), which can be detected by immunofluorescence. Further differentiation of these cells from myeloblasts and from other lymphoblasts can be made with immunophenotypic markers.

Patients tend to have elevated serum LDH levels, the magnitude of which reflects the total body tumor burden, and an increased serum uric acid level, which results from the breakdown of leukemic cells. Patients with ALL of T cell origin are often found to have hypercalcemia as well. Most patients also have chromosomal abnormalities, some of which tend to show relative specificity for an ALL type.

The French-American-British (FAB) classification of ALL

ALL has been separated into different types based on morphologic criteria according to the French-American-British (FAB) classification (Figure 63-2). These types tend to correlate with the different cells of origin as determined by immunophenotypic surface markers, the clinical presentation of disease, and the prognosis of the patient.

L1 ALL: This disorder is the most common type, accounting for about 70% of cases and is characterized by a predominant population of smaller lymphoid cells with a diameter of 8 to 10 μ, possessing scanty cytoplasm and large, regularly shaped nuclei. The nuclear chromatin of these cells is finely dispersed and their nucleoli are not visible. The cells usually stain with PAS and immunofluorescent stains for TdT. Overall, most cases of childhood ALL are the L1 morphologic type, and these patients have the best prognosis with treatment.

L2 ALL: L2 variants make up about 25% of all cases. The cytologic picture is dominated by large lymphoblasts with a variable amount of cytoplasm and large indented or folded nuclei possessing fine chromatin and prominent nucleoli. The staining properties of the cells are generally

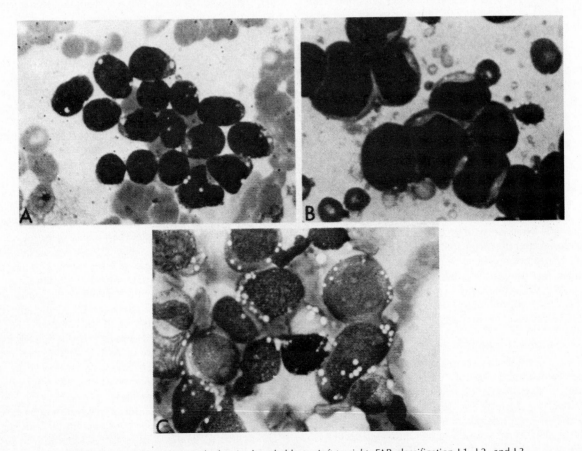

Fig. 63-2 Acute lymphocytic leukemia, lymphoblasts. *Left to right:* FAB classification L1, L2, and L3. *From Miller DR: Pediatr Clin North Am 27:269, 1980.*

similar to L1 lymphoblasts. However, some also stain focally for acid phosphatase. Cells that contain acid phosphatase activity are generally believed to be T cells. The L2 variant is more common in adults. These patients have a higher relapse ratio following therapy-induced remissions.

L3 ALL: This disorder is a rare form of ALL in which large lymphoblasts possess round nuclei with prominent, multiple nucleoli and numerous vacules in the cytoplasm. These vacules stain with Oil red 0, which shows that they contain lipid-like material. They usually stain negatively with PAS and TdT stains. As will be described, these variants are B cell malignancies. They are most commonly seen in late childhood and during adolescence. The prognosis is poor and most cases relapse within 12 months of treatment.

Immunologic classification of ALL

With the recognition of surface markers, which were able to differentiate T cells from B cells, investigators began to classify ALL by the cell of origin.

ALL of T cell origin was characterized by cells that formed E rosettes with sheep red cells. B cell ALL was a rare disease characterized by the presence of monoclonal surface immunoglobulin (SIg) on their cells. Other cases of ALL were found to possess isolated μ chains in the cytoplasm (CIg) and were termed Pre-B cell ALL. The remainder of cases were referred to as "null" or "non T, non B cell ALL." It was subsequently found that most cases of null cell ALL possessed a common surface antigen that reacted with antibodies prepared against ALL cells. This antigen, CALLA (common acute lymphoblastic leukemia antigen), was subsequently identified as an endopeptidase and has been assigned the cluster designation CD10. These null cell ALL were thus divided into CALLA positive and CALLA negative cases.

With the development of the current library of monoclonal antibodies, the separation of ALL according to the cell of origin has undergone further refinement. Many cases that were not known to be of defined B cell or T cell lineage have now been appropriately identified (Box 63-1).

T cell ALL

Cells of T cell ALL not only possess the E-rosette receptor, now designated CD2 (Leu 5), but also possess CD7 (Leu 9), and CD5 (Leu 1). Among these, reaction with anti-CD7 is probably the most sensitive T cell marker, while a reaction with anti CD5 is the most specific. (Anti-CD7 and CD2 may react with some cases of AML). In addition, a minority of cases react with anti-CD10. Notably, a few patients with T cell ALL are E rosette negative. Most cases possess an L2 morphology, while fewer can be classified as L1. Many patients are found to have a t(11:14) chromosomal translocation. T cell ALL accounts for approximately 15% of all cases in childhood but a larger proportion in adults. T cell ALL possesses several special clinical features, including frequent mediastinal masses, skin infiltration, hypercalcemia, and a relatively poor prognosis.

B cell ALL

Although investigators previously thought ALL of B cell lineage was a rare disorder, the use of monoclonal antibodies has shown that, in fact, most cases of ALL are of B cell

---

> **Box 63-1** Acute lymphocyte leukemias
>
> **IMMUNOPHENOTYPIC CLASSIFICATION**
> T cell ALL
> B cell ALL
>   B cell ALL—Burkitt's type
>   Pre-B cell ALL
>   ALL of early B cell origin—CALLA positive
>   ALL of early B cell origin—CALLA negative

---

origin. The presence or absence of other markers assists in the recognition of subtypes of prognostic importance. The most sensitive surface markers for B cell origin are HLA-DR and CD19 (Leu 12) antigens. While the former is nonspecific, the latter is highly specific. In addition, CD22 and CD20 are highly specific but less sensitive markers.

SIg and CIg are still commonly used to define cases of Burkitt's type B cell ALL and Pre-B cell ALL, respectively. B Cell ALL—Burkitt's Type invariably shows an L3 morphology, a unique chromosome translocation t(8:14), and is associated with a poor prognosis; Pre-B cell ALL usually shows an L2 morphology, is often associated with a t(1:19) translocation, and has a worse prognosis than those without CIg termed "ALL Of Early B Cell Origin." Ninety percent of remaining cases of early B cell origin are termed "CALLA (CD10) positive ALL," most of which have L1 morphology. Patients with CALLA negative ALL had been considered to have a somewhat poorer prognosis. This view has been questioned since most CALLA negative ALL occurs in infants under one year who are recognized to have a poor prognosis.

LYMPHOPROLIFERATIVE DISORDERS

Lymphoproliferative disorders are a loosely connected group of disorders characterized by the proliferation of the various cellular elements of the lymphoreticular system. Histopathologically, one disease merges with others and morphologic transitions may appear with time. However, this grouping may be less rational than the myeloproliferative disorders since most of the entities do not arise from such primitive multi-potential stem cells, but rather from precursor cells committed to one or another lymphoid cell line. Furthermore, although of myeloid origin, some investigators have included solid tumors of macrophage elements in this grouping. Lastly, development of acute leukemia in the course of chronic lymphoproliferative disorders is unusual.

Classification of lymphoproliferative disorders

This group includes 1) disorders that primarily originate in the bone marrow and show a tendency to involve the peripheral blood as a leukemia and 2) disorders that primarily involve the lymphoid organs and other sites as solid tumor-like collections termed "lymphomas."

Some lymphoproliferative disorders may involve cells with morphologic characteristics similar to mature normal cells. They often show a prolonged course. Leukemias of this type are termed "chronic." Others show varying degrees of blastic transformation which, rather than simply indi-

Table 63-2 Malignant lymphoproliferative disorders

T cell disorders	Acute lymphocytic leukemia (some)
	Chronic lymphocytic leukemia (some)
	Diffuse lymphoma (some)
	"Lymphoblastic" lymphoma
	Sezary syndrome
	Mycosis fungoides
	Leukemic reticuloendotheliosis (rare)
B cell disorders	Acute lymphocytic lymphoma (most)
	Chronic lymphocytic leukemia (most)
	Leukemic reticuloendotheliosis (most)
	Nodular lymphoma (all)
	Diffuse lymphoma (some)
	Waldenstrom's macroglobulinemia
	Multiple myeloma
	Plasmacytoma
	Heavy chain disease
M cell disorders	Malignant histiocytosis
Questionable origin	Hodgkin's disease

cating a reversion to a less differentiated progeny, may represent correlates of immunoblastic transformation. These types of disorders usually have a more accelerated course. The leukemic forms of this type are termed "acute."

From the point of view of lymphoreticular ontogeny, these disorders can be differentiated by T and B cell origin. According to this differentiation, the appended functional classification of malignant lymphoproliferative disorders is useful and is based on the identification of functional and immunophenotypic surface markers of the cells (Table 63-2).

Dysproteinemia and lymphoproliferative disorders

Some chronic B cell lymphoproliferative disorders are characterized by the secretion of large quantities of immunoglobulins leading to hypergammaglobulinemia and/or dysproteinemia. In most reactive disorders, multiple clones of cells—polyclonal disorders—are involved. In these cases, large amounts of different immunoglobulins may be secreted, leading to hypergammaglobulinemia of a polyclonal type, which on serum protein electrophoresis (SPEP) causes a broad-based β-γ hump whose area is greater than normal. On the other hand, the lymphoproliferative disorders result from the neoplastic emergence of one clone of cells. The more differentiated of the B cell malignancies may be characterized by a monoclonal immunoglobinopathy (dysproteinemia). Monoclonal gammopathy is characterized by production of a single class/subclass (IgG, IgM, IgA, etc.) and type/subtype (λ or κ) of immunoglobulin or fragment of heavy chain or free light chain (Bence-Jones protein). If produced in sufficient amount, it causes a narrow based globulin "M" spike in the α_2-γ region on SPEP (Figure 3). It is usually accompanied by a decrease in the amount of normal immunoglobulins produced. The class and type of these proteins cannot be identified by SPEP and requires immunoelectrophoresis (IEP) or immunofixation techniques. With IEP, these abnormal immunoglobulins (paraproteins) appear as a hump, having partial identity with the precipitin line formed between a known immunoglobulin

heavy or light chain and the appropriate anti-chain antibody (Figure 63-3).

Paraproteins may occasionally have identifiable antibody specificity; may precipitate or gel at low temperature (cryoglobulin); may, when present in large amounts, increase serum viscosity (IgM and to a lesser degree IgA and IgG_3); and are able to coat platelets and interfere with fibrin monomer polymerization. Monoclonal gammopathies are not only seen in patients with well-defined "plasma cell dyscrasias," but also in patients with chronic B cell lymphocytic leukemia and elderly patients with other malignancies, chronic infections, and rarely, no evidence of disease (benign monoclonal gammopathy).

Chronic lymphocytic leukemia (CLL)

CLL is a neoplastic medullary proliferation of mature-appearing immunoincompetent lymphocytes, which appear in the peripheral blood. It occurs predominantly in males 60 to 70 years of age, with an annual incidence of approximately two per 100,000 individuals. As a group, CLL tends to run a prolonged course and for a variable period of time, patients only show infiltration of the bone marrow and lymphocytosis. In more than 95% of cases, the neoplastic cells are B cells, while in less than 5%, the cells possess T cell markers. This latter form of CLL has a more aggressive clinical course. T cell CLL is now differentiated from adult T cell leukemia/lymphoma due to HTLV-1 infection, which will be discussed later.

The peripheral absolute lymphocyte count must be above 5000/μl for a diagnosis of CLL. However, the count is usually in excess of 20,000/μl. As stated above, CLL lymphocytes have the appearance of mature cells. B cell CLL is characterized by cells with round or oval nuclei, while T cell CLL is characterized by cells possessing notched or convoluted nuclei. Smudge cells, which are denuded, crushed lymphocyte nuclei, are common in the peripheral smear. The bone marrow aspirate reveals that more than 20% of the cells are lymphocytes. On biopsy, their distribution may be either focal or diffuse (Figure 63-4). Patients with a diffuse infiltration tend to have a more aggressive clinical course. With advanced infiltration of the marrow, a normochromic, normocytic anemia, thrombocytopenia and granulocytopenia develop. In 5% to 10% of cases an autoimmune hemolytic anemia also occurs.

B cell CLL is recognized by the presence of SIg (IgM, often with IgD) and reaction with anti-CD19, CD20, and CD21. Unlike normal B cells, they do not react with anti-CD22. T cell CLL is usually recognized as being derived from helper T cells and is CD2+, CD3+, CD4+, CD5+ and CD7+. Unusually, the T cells also are CD8+, or are recognized as suppressor CD4−CD8+ cells. A monoclonal gammopathy is demonstrated with serum protein electrophoresis in 5% to 10% of cases of B cell CLL. In more of these patients however, a monoclonal paraprotein in the serum can be demonstrated with more sensitive methods (e.g., immunofixation). Cytogenetic studies reveal trisomy 12 in over 50% of cases of B cell CLL. Patients with T cell leukemia may have trisomy 7 or 14q+.

Infiltration of other lymphoid organs occurs with progression. Lymphadenopathy is eventually present in 90% of individuals. The infiltration completely effaces normal nodal architecture and gives a picture of well-differentiated lymphocytic lymphoma. Infiltrative splenomegaly occurs in 70% of patients and is due to primary replacement of the follicles and later, non-follicular regions, while hepatomegaly occurs eventually in 65% of patients and is due to periportal infiltration. Patients with T cell CLL may also show extensive dermal infiltration, a situation known as "leukemia cutis," and hypercalcemia. Late stages are characterized by systemic symptoms such as weight loss and fever.

Investigators have attempted to define prognostically significant clinical stages at the time of diagnosis. In the United States, the Staging Classification of Rai, et al gained widespread acceptance (Table 63-3). This staging system was subsequently modified, as it was recognized that those with stage 0 disease (Low Risk), had the best prognosis, with a median survival of more than 10 years. Those with stages III and IV (High Risk) had a poor prognosis with a median survival of approximately two years. Patients with stages I

Table 63-3   Clinical staging system

Stage 0	Lymphocytosis only
Stage I	Lymphocytosis plus lymphadenopathy
Stage II	Lymphocytosis with splenomegaly or hepatomegaly (± lymphadenopathy)
Stage III	Lymphocytosis with hemoglobin <11gm/dl. (± lymphadenopathy or organomegaly)
Stage IV	Lymphocytosis with platelet count <100,000/mm^3 (± lymphadenopathy or organomegaly)

From Rai KR, Sawitsky A, Cronkite EP, et al: Clinical staging of chronic lymphocytic leukemia, Blood 42:219, 1975.

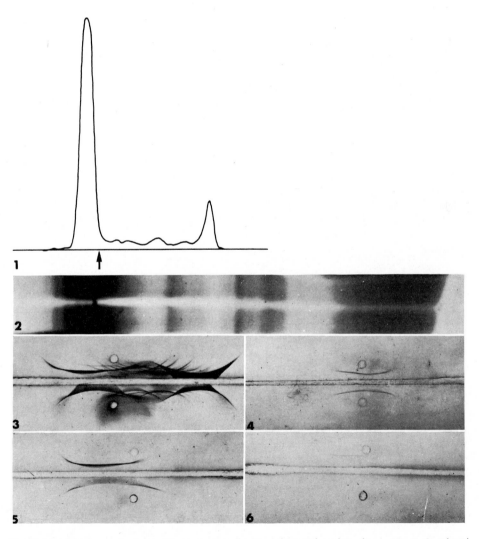

Fig. 63-3   Multiple myeloma. **1,** Electrophoresis showing abnormal peak in the γ area. **2,** Starch gel electrophoresis showing abnormal γ bands. **3-6,** Immunoelectrophoresis, normal control at top, patient at bottom: **3,** polyvalent antiserum; **4,** anti-IgA serum; **5,** anti-IgG serum showing abnormal γ component; **6,** anti-IgM serum showing decrease of IgM. *From Miale JB: Laboratory medicine: hematology, ed 6, St. Louis, 1982, Mosby–Year Book.*

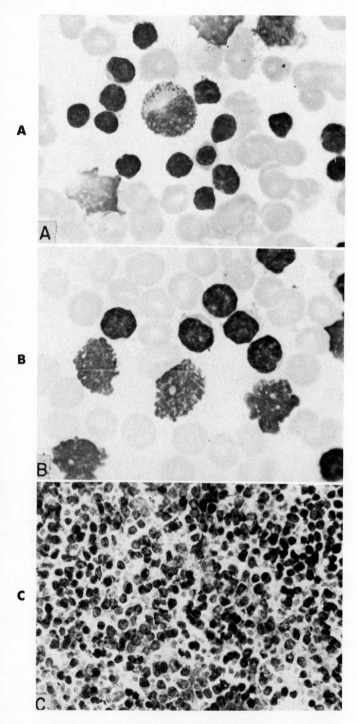

Fig. 63-4 Chronic lymphocytic leukemia. **A,** Bone marrow smear. (Wright's stain; ×950.) **B,** Peripheral blood smear. Note "smudge" cells. (Wright's stain; ×950.) **C,** Paraffin section of marrow. (Hematoxylin-eosin stain ×450.) *From Miale JB: Laboratory medicine: hematology, ed 6, St. Louis, 1982, Mosby–Year Book.*

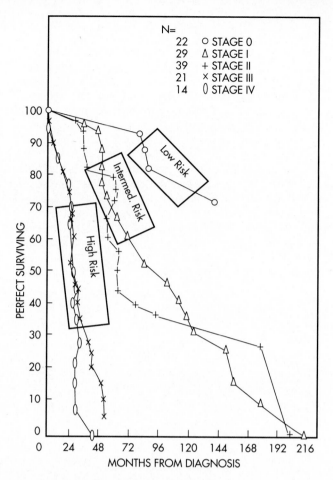

Fig. 63-5 Chronic lymphocytic leukemia. Survival curves of five stages demonstrating that according to prognosis they can be grouped into low risk, intermediate risk, and high risk. *From Rai RK and Han T: Clin Hematol/Oncol 4:450, 1990.*

and II (Intermediate Risk) had a median survival of six to seven years (Figure 63-5).

Complications of the disease include bleeding, infections due to granulocytopenia, diminished cellular immune response (rare), hypogammaglobulinemia (50% in late stages), and obstructive syndromes due to compression by large lymphoid masses. These leukemias do not terminate in blast crises. Some patients develop diffuse large cell lymphomas (Richter's syndrome).

A variant of CLL is characterized by the presence in the peripheral blood of atypical-appearing lymphocytes with more abundant bluish cytoplasm, oval or notched nuclei, and presence of occasional nucleoli (Figure 63-6). Cells of this type are often seen in patients with previously diagnosed lymphoma, which develop into leukemic phase. This variant is known as prolymphocytic leukemia. It usually arises de novo but may evolve from classical CLL. The clinical presentation differs from CLL because of prolymphocytic leukemia's very high peripheral white cell count (often >100,000/μl) and prominent splenomegaly. Both T and B cell variants of prolymphocytic leukemia are encountered. Cytogenetic abnormalities include t(6:12) and 14q+. Median survival is usually less than three years.

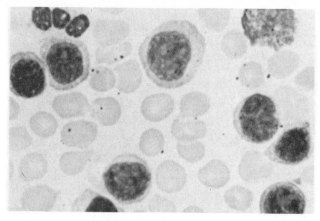

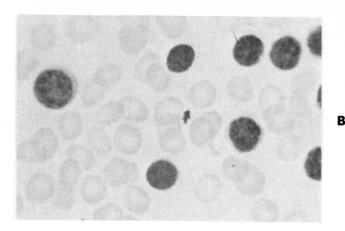

A   B

Fig. 63-6   Chronic lymphocytic leukemia with prolymphocytes. *Left,* Bone marrow smear. *Right,* Peripheral smear. (Wright's stain; ×950.) *From Miale JB: Laboratory medicine: hematology, ed 6, St. Louis, 1982, Mosby—Year Book.*

Adult T cell leukemia/lymphoma (ATL)

This neoplastic proliferation of T cells results from infection with HTLV-1, as previously described. Generally the cells that are infected, transformed, and then proliferate are CD4+ helper cells, although rare cases of CD8+ suppressor cell ATL are described. Patients with ATL generally present with lymphoadenopathy, hepatosplenomegaly, and extensive skin infiltrates and lytic bone lesions. Severe hypercalcemia occurs in 30% to 40% of patients.

This disease is endemic in southern Japan and the Caribbean and is seen among IV drug users in the United States. In endemic areas, most cases occur between the ages of 40 and 60 years. Males and females are affected equally. Only approximately 2% of individuals infected with the retrovirus develop ATL after a latency of up to 10 to 20 years.

Patients with ATL usually have elevated white blood cell counts and an absolute lymphocytosis. The leukemic lymphocytes have prominently lobulated or convoluted nuclei. Eosinophilia is common. As stated, these cells are most commonly CD4 positive T cells. Cytogenetic studies reveal that most cases demonstrate trisomy 7 and some 14q+. The diagnosis is further confirmed by the finding of elevated titers of HTLV-1 antibody in the serum, the specificity of which is confirmed by a Western blot technique.

The prognosis of ATL is very poor. Most patients die within one year of diagnosis.

Leukemic reticuloendotheliosis ("Hairy Cell Leukemia"—HCL)

This rare disorder involves the proliferation of large lymphocytic cells, with cytoplasmic projections (hairy cells) and nuclei with ropy chromatin in the bone marrow and spleen that subsequently appear in the peripheral blood (Figure 63-7). It affects men more commonly than women and occurs most commonly between the ages of 40 and 60. The disease tends to cause massive splenomegaly, while lymphopathy is less impressive. Bone marrow infiltration is usually diffuse and predominately involves the area next to the bone spicule. Marrow fibrosis is common.

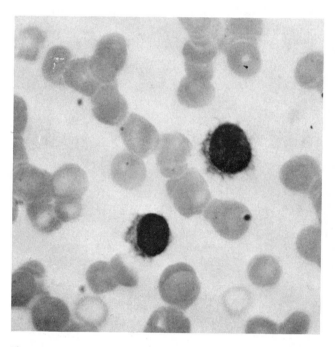

Fig. 63-7   Hairy cell leukemia. Peripheral smear. *From Bauer JD: Clinical laboratory methods, ed 9, St. Louis, 1982, Mosby—Year Book.*

The white count is usually normal or even decreased. Anemia and thrombocytopenia tend to develop slowly. Pancytopenia is seen in advanced cases and results from both marrow replacement and hypersplenism. The morphology of the hairy cell in the peripheral smear is best seen with phase contrast microscopy. Cytochemically, the LAP is increased and the abnormal cells stain positive for tartarate resistant acid phosphatase.

Cell marker studies show that most cases are of B cell origin, although cases of T cell HCL have been recently described. Some cytologic and functional features of monocytes have been noted in these cells, including phagocytosis.

Most patients have a chronic course with a median survival of more than five years. Patients develop infections from neutropenia, monocytopenia, T cell loss, and granulocyte dysfunction. In addition, patients may develop a wide variety of autoimmune disorders and bleeding due to thrombocytopenia and platelet dysfunction.

Chronic T gamma lymphocytosis syndrome (TGLS)

This chronic proliferation of large granular lymphocytes usually follows a benign clinical course and arises in late middle age. Men and women are affected equally. Although not conclusive, the bulk of currently available data derived from analysis of T cell receptor genes indicate that this proliferation is monoclonal. On the other hand, its increased incidence in individuals with autoimmune disorders (especially rheumatoid arthritis) and its associated polyclonal hypergammaglobulinemia are considered suggestive of a polyclonal reactive T lymphocyte proliferation. These cells have a suppressor/cytotoxic phenotype and probably represent abnormal NK cells. In addition to the proliferation of this lymphocytic subset, many patients are also neutropenic and have red cell aplasia. While the pathogenesis of the former manifestation is obscure, the latter is associated with suppression of CFU-E and BFU-E progenitors. Patients usually present with recurrent infections. Infiltrative splenomegaly occurs in 50% to 70% of patients. Hepatomegaly or lymphadenopathy is unusual. About a third of patients have a history of rheumatoid arthritis.

These patients usually have an elevated white cell count with absolute lymphocytosis and neutropenia. Most cells present in the peripheral blood are large granular lymphocytes. Patients with red cell aplasia have a normochromic, normocytic anemia and a reduced reticulocyte index. Thrombocytopenia is rare. The bone marrow is heavily infiltrated with lymphocytes.

The cells almost always express the expected markers of suppressor T cells, including CD2, CD3, and CD8. Rarely the cells express CD4, together with CD8 or alone. Surprisingly, they lack CD5. In addition, they possess fc receptors for IgG.

In addition to polyclonal hypergamma-globulinemia, patients may have rheumatoid factor and antinuclear antibodies in their serum. Antineutrophil and platelet antibodies may be found as well.

Multiple myeloma

Myeloma is a B cell disorder characterized by the medullary proliferation of malignant plasma cells. These cells may later be associated with myelomatous infiltration of parenchymal organs or spread into the peripheral blood (plasma cell leukemia).

Differentiated malignant plasma cells usually tend to produce both complete immunoglobulin and some excess light chains. Less-differentiated cells tend to produce isolated light chains, while the least-differentiated cells produce no detectable secretion product. According to the product, multiple myeloma can therefore be classified (Table 63-4). The light chain is κ twice as often as λ.

This disorder occurs with an annual incidence of three per 100,000 individuals. Both sexes are affected equally, and most cases occur in the 50- to 70-year age group.

Table 63-4 Incidence of myelomas according to secretory product

IgG myeloma	56%
IgA myeloma	25%
IgD myeloma	2%
IgE myeloma	<.01%
"Light-chain disease"	15%
"Non-secretory" myeloma	1%
IgM myeloma	rare cases

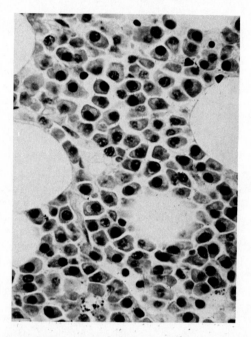

Fig. 63-8 Multiple myeloma. Paraffin section of marrow. (Hematoxylin and eosin ×450.) *From Miale JB: Laboratory medicine: hematology, ed 6, St. Louis, 1982, Mosby–Year Book.*

The primary manifestation of the marrow infiltration by myeloma is represented by osteolytic punched out lesions of axial skeletal bones or generalized osteoporosis. This change is due directly to marrow infiltration and is also related to an increased osteoclastic activity stimulated by the plasma cells. Pathologic fractures of vertebrae and long bones are a common complication. Hypercalcemia occurs in 10% to 30% of patients due to bony decalcification. The bone marrow infiltrates replace normal marrow elements and lead to progressive anemia, granulocytopenia, and thrombocytopenia.

A hyperviscosity syndrome may occur when the quantity of immunoglobulin is markedly elevated and is able to form multimers. It is manifested by sluggish passage of blood through small vessels and is associated with cerebral symptoms, retinal vein engorgement, epistaxis, and heart failure. It is more rarely seen in myeloma than in Waldenstrom's macroglobulinemia and is limited to patients with IgG_3 and IgA disease. Similarly, manifestations due to cryoglobulinemia and interference with coagulation are rarer than in

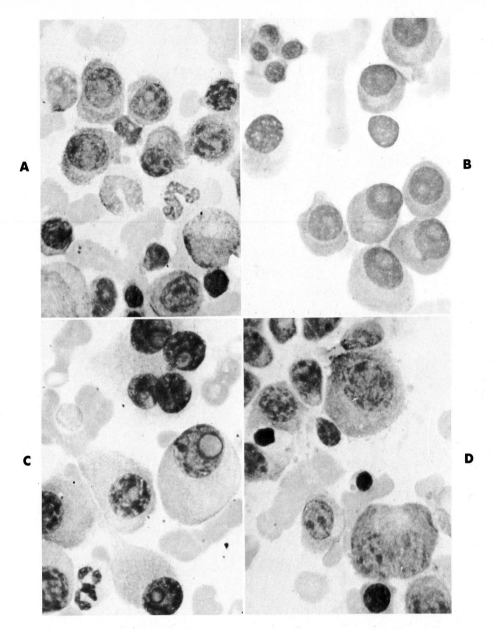

Fig. 63-9   Different degrees of maturity of plasma cells in multiple myeloma, bone marrow smears. **A,** Most mature. **D,** Least mature. (Wright's stain; ×950.) *From Miale JB: Laboratory medicine: hematology, ed 6, St. Louis, 1982, Mosby—Year Book.*

Waldenstrom's macroglobulinemia. Amyloidosis is seen in patients with long-standing myeloma. The excess light chains (Bence-Jones proteins) secreted are able to cross the glomerular basement membrane and tend to precipitate in the tubules. Precipitation in the tubules leads to a condition known as "myeloma kidney." The kidney is usually slightly shrunken and microscopically shows occlusion of the tubules with proteineceous casts of precipitated light chains, degeneration of the tubular epithelial cells and a profuse peritubular mononuclear cell inflammatory infiltrate often containing foreign body type giant cells. This condition is more common if the light chain is λ. Aside from myeloma kidney, other causes of renal failure in these patients include amyloidosis, renal calcinosis, and pyelonephritis.

Examination of the bone marrow reveals replacement by sheets of cells showing varying degrees of differentiation from atypical plasmablasts to mature appearing plasmacytes (Figures 63-8 and 63-9). In myeloma producing elevated amounts of paraprotein, some plasma cells may contain intracytoplasmic aggregates of immunoglobulin called Russell bodies (Figure 63-10). IgA myeloma may be characterized by the presence of plasma cells with a distinct eosinophilic coloration to the Golgi zone of the cytoplasm. Such cells are called "flame cells" or "thesaurocytes." With progressive infiltration of the marrow, patients develop a normochromic, normocytic anemia with a decreased reticulocyte index. Severe leukopenia and thrombocytopenia are unusual. When the marrow is heavily infiltrated, the blood

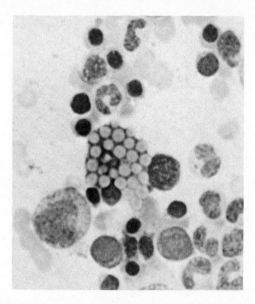

Fig. 63-10 Plasma cell containing Russell bodies. *From Bauer JD: Clinical laboratory methods, ed 9, St. Louis, 1982, Mosby—Year Book.*

smear may display a leukoerythroblastic reaction. Plasma cell leukemia is defined by an absolute plasma cell count of 2000/µl and may arise *de novo* or as a late manifestation in the course of 1% to 2% of myeloma patients. The rare IgE myeloma often presents as plasma cell leukemia. Rouleaux formation may be seen when the plasma immunoglobulin level is markedly increased, as the protein coats the cells and leads to increased cell-cell interaction.

As previously discussed, the monoclonal immunoglobulin produced is commonly detected by SPEP (Figure 63-3), is characterized by IEP (Figure 63-3) or immunofixation techniques, and is quantified by immunodiffusion or nephelometry. In the urine, Bence-Jones proteins were classically detected by their thermal characteristics (they precipitate on heating of the urine to 50° to 60°C and redissolve as the temperature is further raised to the boiling point). Because of the poor sensitivity of this screening method, detection of light-chain excretion is now made by urine IEP.

In cases of IgG_3 and IgA myelomas, the production of large amounts of paraprotein may be associated with increased serum viscosity. Viscosity is most commonly measured with an Ostwald viscometer. This instrument measures the rate of passage of serum heated to 37°C through a slender tube, as an index of viscosity. The result is reported as a ratio of the time obtained with serum compared with that obtained with distilled water. A normal serum viscosity is 1.4 to 1.8. Viscosity ratios greater than 4.0 to 5.0 may be associated with hyperviscosity syndromes, the incidence of which rises progressively with an increase in the ratio.

Table 63-5 Myeloma staging system

Criteria	Measured myeloma cell mass (cells × 10^{12}/m²)[a]
Stage I	
All of the following:	
1. Haemoglobin value >10 g/100 ml	
2. Serum calcium value normal (≤12 mg/100 ml)	
3. On x-ray, normal bone structure (scale 0) or solitary bone plasmocytoma only	<0.6 (low)
4. Low M-component production rates	
(a) IgG value <5 g/100 ml	
(b) IgA value <3 g/100 ml	
(c) urine light chain M-component on electrophoresis <4 g/24 h	
Stage II	0.6-1.20 (intermediate)
Fitting neither Stage I nor Stage III	
Stage III	
One or more of the following:	
1. Haemoglobin value <8.5g/100 ml	
2. Serum calcium value >12 mg/100 ml	
3. Advanced lytic bone lesions (scale 3)	
4. High M-component production rates	>1.20 (high)
(a) IgG value > 7 g/100 ml	
(b) IgA value > 5 g/100 ml	
(c) urine light chain M-component on electrophoresis > 12 g/24 h	
Subclassification	
A = relatively normal renal function (serum creatinine value <2.0 mg/100 ml)	
B = abnormal renal function (serum creatinine value ≥2.0 mg/100 ml)	
Examples:	
Stage 1A = low cell mass with normal renal function	
Stage IIIB = high cell mass with abnormal renal function	

From Durie BG and Salmon SE: Cancer 36:842, 1975.
[a]10^{12} cells = approximately 1 kg; m² = square meter of body surface area.

The overall prognosis of patients with multiple myeloma is poor, with median survival of three to four years, and is related to the calculated tumor mass, whch forms the basis of a commonly used staging system (Table 63-5). In addition, a poorer prognosis is associated with the presence of significant cytopenia at time of diagnosis; azotemia or hypercalcemia; the type of myeloma, IgA, and light-chain disease having a poorer prognosis than IgG; and the production of λ Bence Jones proteins. Finally, the prognosis of patients with *de novo* plasma cell leukemia is especially dismal, since most patients die within 12 months of diagnosis. The cause of death in most patients is either infection or renal failure as the disease becomes refractory to chemotherapy. Up to 7% of patients develop secondary acute non lymphocytic leukemia.

A special form of this plasma cell dyscrasia is the extrammedullary soft tissue plasmacytoma, which occurs about 1/20 as frequently as multiple myeloma. It may be associated with "M" spike and is only rarely associated with the development of myeloma. Solitary bony plasmacytomas, on the other hand, are prone to develop into generalized multiple myeloma.

Waldenstrom's macroglobulinemia

This disease of B cells is characterized by the proliferation of so-called plasmacytoid lymphocytes in the bone marrow and the lymphoid tissues causing lymphadenopathy and hepatosplenomegaly with a histologic picture of lymphocytic lymphoma. It is associated with anemia in most patients but does not cause osteolytic lesions of the bone. The lymphocytes produce large amounts of IgM, which markedly increase serum viscosity. Hyperviscosity syndromes are common. A bleeding diathesis may also ensue because this paraprotein coats platelets and interferes with fibrin polymerization. Raynaud's phenomenon may be seen if the paraprotein is also a cryoglobulin. (Such cryoglobulins are IgM or, rarely, mixed IgM-IgG complexes resulting from IgM antibodies directed against circulating IgG). Rare cases

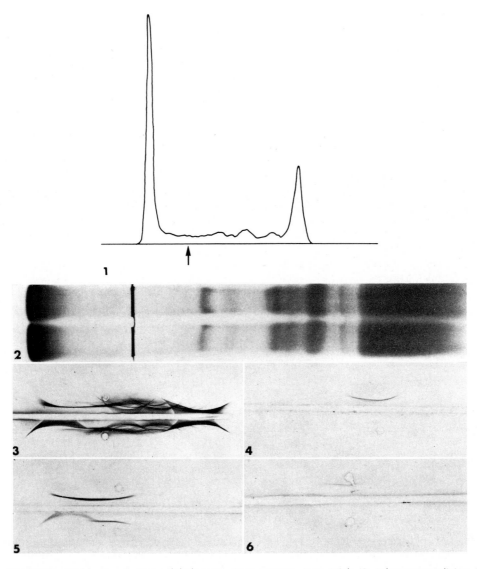

Fig. 63-11   Waldenstrom's Macroglobulinemia. Bone marrow. *From Miale JB: Laboratory medicine: hematology, ed 6, St. Louis, 1982, Mosby—Year Book.*

of cold autoimmune hemolytic anemia are also seen when the paraprotein has antibody specificity against the I antigen of the red cell. Bence-Jones proteinuria is unusual, occurring in only 10% of patients.

In most patients, a normochromic, normocytic anemia ensues. A decreased reticulocyte index is noted, except among patients with autoimmune hemolytic anemia in whom the index is usually increased and the direct Coombs test found to be positive. Examination of the peripheral smear shows the presence of distinctive large plasmacytoid lymphocytes with eccentric nuclei and prominent Golgi regions (Figure 63-11). The bone marrow aspirate shows an increase in lymphoid cells, which vary in appearance from small lymphocytes to plasmacytoid cells. Basophils and mast cells are often increased as well.

The paraprotein is usually readily detected by SPEP and confirmed by IEP. The monoclonal IgM usually exceeds 1 gm/dl. in the serum. As previously noted, free light chains are found in the urine in only about 10% of patients. Serum viscosity is almost always elevated and may cause a hyperviscosity syndrome at somewhat lower viscosity ratios than seen in myeloma.

With control of hyperviscosity and other manifestations of the high levels of paraprotein, the prognosis is relatively good, with a course similar to chronic lymphocytic leukemia.

Heavy chain diseases

These are rare disorders characterized by the proliferation of lymphocytic cells in both lymph nodes and soft tissue. Histologically, this infiltration is similar to a lymphoma. It is associated with the production of isolated γ, α, or μ heavy chains in the serum.

Gamma heavy chain disease presents as a lymphoma with lymphadenopathy and hepatosplenomegaly. Patients are usually anemic and have frequent infections. SPEP shows broad elevation in the β-γ region, which is shown to be isolated γ chains without light chains on IEP. Free γ chains are often found in the urine. Hypogammaglobulinemia is usually noted. Plasmacytoid lymphocytes are frequently noted in the peripheral blood, while the marrow is infiltrated with increased numbers of lymphocytes and plasma cells.

Alpha heavy chain disease is the most common heavy chain disease and tends to affect young adults from the Mediterranean basin. It presents as an intestinal lymphoma that results in a malabsorbtion syndrome. Free α chains are produced in only modest amounts so that SPEP is usually unremarkable; the paraprotein is detected by IEP of the serum and urine.

Mu heavy chain disease is a very rare disorder, occurring in patients with CLL or lymphoma. The free μ heavy chain is only found in the serum and not in the urine.

Benign monoclonal gammopathy

Elderly patients with other tumors or inflammatory conditions may respond with stimulation of one clone of immunocompetent cells and the production of a monoclonal immunoglobulin. In occasional cases, elderly individuals may produce such a monoclonal immunoglobulin without any identifiable primary cause. This finding is seen in up to 2% to 3% of healthy individuals over the age of 50. Benign monoclonal gammopathy is considered the appropriate di-

agnosis if the total M protein is less than 2 to 3 gms/dl, and no underlying plasma cell dyscrasia emerges after several years of observation.

MALIGNANT LYMPHOMAS AND RELATED DISORDERS

Malignant lymphomas present as localized tumors. Nodes infiltrated with lymphoma are enlarged, rubbery, and fish-flesh in color. They are replaced by a uniform cellular infiltrate that obliterates the normal nodal architecture. This includes loss of the normal follicular structure, invasion of the marginal sinuses, and extension of infiltrate beyond the capsule. Extension into the lumina of small vessels implies dissemination of disease. These infiltrations must be distinguished from various reactive lymphoid hyperplasias, which may involve the follicles, paracortical areas, or sinuses.

Lymphomas are currently divided into Hodgkin's and non-Hodgkin's types, not only because of differences in morphology, but also because of differences in biological behavior and possibly in ontogeny.

Hodgkin's disease

This disorder is characterized by a mixed infiltrate of lymphocytes, plasma cells, eosinophils, and large (15 to 45 μ in diameter), atypical reticular type cells, often containing multi-lobed or multiple nuclei with thick nuclear membranes and prominent eosinophilic nucleoli, termed "Reed-Sternberg" cells (Figure 63-12). These R-S cells, when found in the proper cellular milieu, are diagnostic of Hodgkin's disease but alone are insufficient to make the diagnosis. They are thought to be the neoplastic cells, with the other cells being reactive. Variant cells containing single nuclei are termed "Hodgkin" cells. The origin of these neoplastic reticular cells continues to be the subject of intense debate. Lymphocyte, macrophage, follicular dendritic cell, and even myeloid precursors have been proposed as the cell line of origin. In spite of the uncertainty of their origin, they are beginning to be characterized by their surface markers. Among these markers are HLA-DR antigens, fc receptors, IL-2 receptors, and receptors reacting with anti-CD15 and CD30. It is now considered very possible that different cell lines may give rise to different types of Hodgkin's disease. Overall, it is a disease of young adults that shows a slight male preponderance. The possibility of an infectious etiology has been suggested because of the clustering of cases reported.

Histological classification

Currently, four histologic categories with prognostic significance are defined according to the Rye modification of the Lukes-Butler classification. In general, the more lymphocytes present, the more favorable the prognosis. The classification and incidence of each type are listed in Table 63-6. These types are not immutably fixed in morphology with time. Thus, patients presenting as the lymphocyte-predominant type will, with time, often evolve into the lymphocyte-depleted type. Evolution is in the direction of poorer prognosis. The nodular sclerosis type, however, tends to remain the same throughout the course of the disease.

Lymphocyte predominant. This form consists of numerous mature lymphocytes with only a few atypical retic-

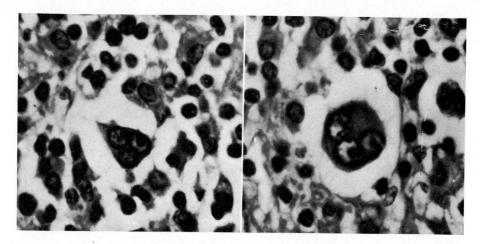

Fig. 63-12   Hodgkin's disease. Reed-Sternberg cells. *From Miale JB: Laboratory medicine: hematology, ed 6, St. Louis, 1982, Mosby–Year Book.*

Table 63-6   Histologic classification of Hodgkin's disease (rye conference)

Type	Reed-Sternberg cells	Lymphocytes	Collagen bands	Diffuse fibrosis	Eosinophils	Plasma cells	Frequency (% of total HD)	5 year survival (% of patients)
1. Lymphocyte predominance	+	+ + + + +	0	0	0	0	5	90
2. Nodular sclerosis	+ +	+ / + + +	+ / + + +	+	+	+	50	70
3. Mixed cellularity	+ +	+	0	+ +	+ +	+	40	70
4. Lymphocyte depletion							5	35
a. Diffuse fibrosis	+ +	0	0	+ + + + +	+	+		
b. Reticular	+ + + + +	+	0	+	+ +	+		

From Rosenthal DS: The malignant lymphomas. In Beck WS: Hematology, ed 2, Cambridge, 1977, MIT Press.

ular cells and rare R-S cells in a pattern of diffuse infiltration (Figure 63-13). Recently, a nodular type of lymphocyte-predominant Hodgkin's disease has been defined. This type of lymphoma is characterized by a relapsing, chronic, and nonprogressive behavior. It is believed that this variant is not truly Hodgkin's disease but represents a follicular B cell tumor. The R-S-like cells in this variant do not express CD15 and may not express CD30 either (Figure 63-14).

Nodular sclerosis. This is the most common type. Nodular sclerosis alone shows a slight female preponderance. It is characterized by the formation of distinct nodules of infiltrate, separated by thick bands of birefringent collagen (Figure 63-15). The infiltrate contains varying amounts of lymphocytes, plasma cells, eosinophils, and distinctive, variant types of mononuclear R-S cells called "lacunar" cells. These latter cells have single or lobulated nuclei with prominent nucleoli. They are surrounded by distinct pericellular halos, artifacts that depend on the tissue fixation.

Mixed cellularity. The infiltrate contains numerous reticular cells and R-S cells with many lymphocytes, eosinophils, and plasma cells in a pattern of diffuse infiltration (Figure 63-16). Focal necrosis and focal fibrosis are often present.

Lymphocyte depleted. The pattern may be cellular (the reticular variant) with large, bizarre, R-S like cells (Figure 63-17) or hypocellular (the diffuse fibrosis variant) with disorderly fibrosis.

Lymphocyte-predominant and nodular sclerosis types often present as localized disease, especially in the mediastinal and cervical nodes. Prior to the advent of modern chemotherapy, they had a much better prognosis than the mixed cellularity and lymphocyte depleted forms, even when the latter presented as localized diseases (Figure 63-18).

Spread of the disease and "staging"

It is now generally accepted that Hodgkin's Disease tends to spread in an orderly and predictable sequence to contiguous lymph nodes and eventually to spleen, liver, bone marrow, lungs, etc. Therefore, evaluating the extent of the spread of disease by clinical and surgical means has a high degree of prognostic usefulness and guides therapy. This determination of spread is known as "staging." Clinical staging incorporates a detailed physical examination and history, clinical laboratory determinations, chest X-ray, lymphangiograms, CAT scans, and bone marrow biopsy. Exploratory laparotomy may be necessary to rule out disseminated disease in persons who, following clinical staging, appear to have localized disease. At the time of laparotomy, splenectomy and multiple liver biopsies are per-

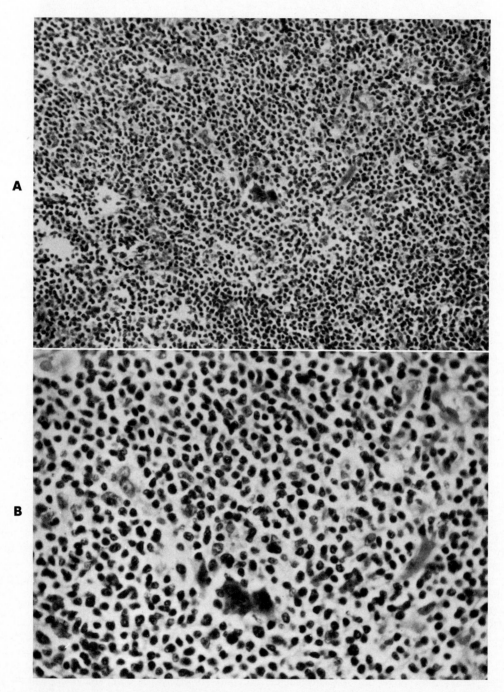

Fig. 63-13 Hodgkin's disease, lymphocytic predominance. Note the polyploid Reed-Sternberg cell, characteristic of this type. (Hematoxylin-eosin stain; **A,** ×350; **B,** ×850.) *From Maile JB: Laboratory medicine: hematology, ed 6, St. Louis, 1982, Mosby—Year Book.*

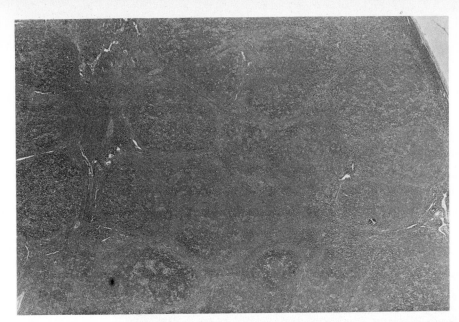

Fig. 63-14 Hodgkin's disease. Nodular lymphocytic predominant variant. *From Anastasi J: Hematology/Oncology Clin North Am 3:187, 1989.*

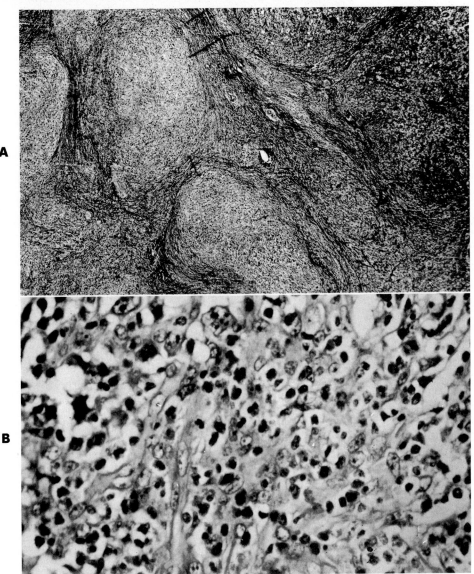

Fig. 63-15 Hodgkin's disease, sclerosing, nodular. (Hematoxylin-eosin stain; **A,** ×90; **B,** ×850.) *From Miale JB: Laboratory medicine: hematology, ed 6, St. Louis, 1982, Mosby–Year Book.*

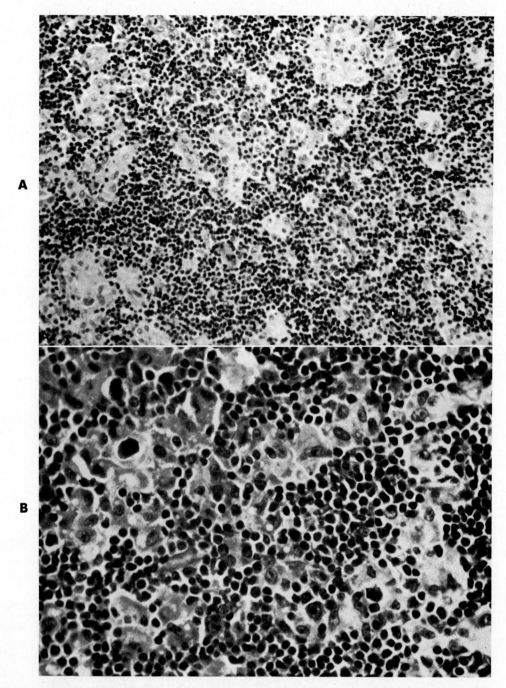

Fig. 63-16 Hodgkin's disease, mixed cellularity type. (Hematoxylin-eosin stain; **A,** ×350; **B,** ×850.)
From Miale JB: Laboratory medicine: hematology, ed 6, St. Louis, 1982, Mosby–Year Book.

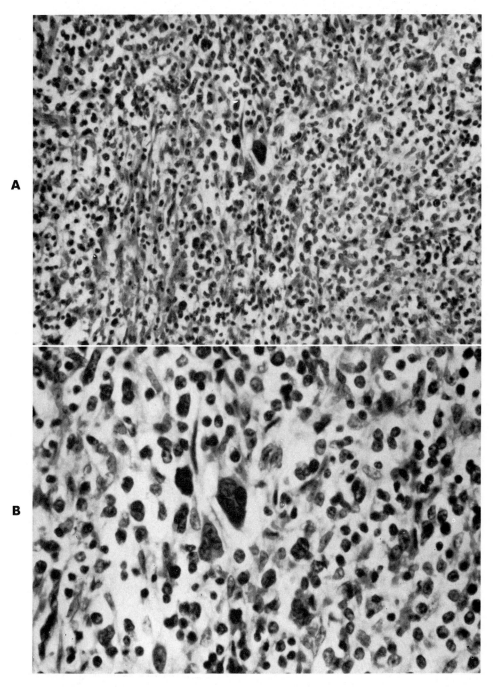

Fig. 63-17   Hodgkin's disease, lymphocytic depletion type (Hodgkin's sarcoma), with pleomorphic Reed-Sternberg cells. (Hematoxylin-eosin stain; **A,** ×350; **B,** ×850.) *From Miale JB: Laboratory medicine: hematology, ed 6, St. Louis, 1982, Mosby–Year Book.*

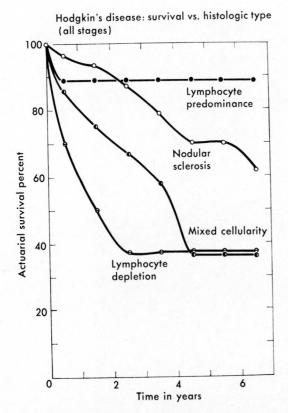

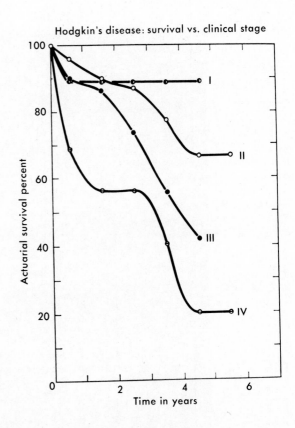

Fig. 63-18 Hodgkin's disease. Actuarial survival according to histologic type. *From Keller AR, et al: Cancer 22:487, 1968.*

Fig. 63-19 Hodgkin's disease. Actuarial survival according to stage. *From Keller AR, et al: Cancer 22:487, 1968.*

Table 63-7 Ann Arbor staging classification of Hodgkin's disease

Stage I:	Involvement of a single lymph node region (I) or of a single extralymphatic organ or site (IE).
Stage II:	Involvement of two or more lymph node regions on the same side of the diaphragm (II) or localized involvement of an extralymphatic organ or site and of one or more lymph node regions on the same side of the diaphragm (IIE).
Stage III:	Involvement of lymph node regions on both sides of the diaphragm (III), which may also be accompanied by localized involvement of an extralymphatic organ or site (IIIE) or by involvement of the spleen (IIIS), or both (IIISE).
Stage IV:	Diffuse or disseminated involvement of one or more extralymphatic organs or tissues with or without associated lymph node enlargement.
Each stage is subdivided into A and B categories:	
A:	No systemic symptoms.
B:	Unexplained weight loss greater than 10% of the body weight in the previous 6 months and/or
	Unexplained fever with temperatures above 38°C and/or
	Night sweats.

From Moormeier JA, et al: Hematol Oncol Clin N America 3:237, 1989.
Pathologically confirmed extralymphatic disease is further defined by subscripts: H, liver; S, spleen; L, lung; P, pleura; M, marrow; O, bone; D, skin.

formed together with excision of intra-abdominal and paraaortic lymph nodes. When laparotomy is used, the staging is termed "pathological" or "surgical" staging. The currently accepted staging classification can be seen in Table 63-7. In general, the prognosis of patients with limited disease is better than a prognosis of widespread disease. Prior to modern therapy, these differences were striking (Figure 63-19). With progressive spread, there is an increasing incidence of "B" type systemic symptoms (weight loss, fever, and sweats). Furthermore, there is an increased incidence of viral and fungal infections due to a defect in cell-mediated immunity.

Non-Hodgkin's lymphomas

While the classification of Hodgkin's Disease is well established and generally accepted, the classification of the non-Hodgkin's lymphomas continues to undergo major evolutionary changes due to increasingly sophisticated immunocytology techniques and growing knowledge of the natural history of this group of diseases. A host of classifications have evolved, and those that have gained widespread usage with successive generations of hematopathologists in the United States will be briefly described. In the oldest classification, "lymphosarcoma" and "reticulum cell sarcoma" were the main types described. The term "giant follicular lymphoma" was used when the microscopic pattern was markedly nodular, and it implied an origin from the lymphoid follicles. Subsequently, the *Rappaport classification* found acceptance among oncologists, since its classes showed correspondence with prognosis and response to treatment. This classification was based on the histologic pattern as seen under the light microscope (nodular and diffuse) as well as on the cytologic characteristics of the cells (well-differentiated lymphocyte, poorly differentiated lymphocyte, and "histiocyte"). Nodular (or follicular) lymphomas tended to have a better prognosis than most diffuse lymphomas and with progression of disease tended to evolve into a diffuse histology. Diffuse lymphomas not only evolved from nodular lymphomas but also arose de novo. No reference was made to immunological lineage of cells. By using immunologic methods, *Lukes and Collins* showed that most of the histiocytic types classified by Rappaport were in fact derived from lymphocytes. They defined a classification based on the immunologic cell of origin (T cell, B cell, and true histiocyte) and on the histological pattern. It was proposed that nodular (follicular) lymphomas actually take origin from the follicles and as such are derived from B cells, while the diffuse lymphomas either represent evolution from nodular lymphomas or arise de novo from B or T cells in non-follicular regions of the nodes or tissue. Features of the classification and an understanding of the prognostic significance of defined cytologic and histologic features have been incorporated in the currently utilized *Working Formulation Classification For Clinical Usage*.

The Rappaport system

The original Rappaport classification was modified after it was realized that some cytologic types never presented in a nodular pattern (Box 63-2). The figures that illustrate the various types of lymphomas are identified by both the Rappaport and Working Formulation Classifications.

Box 63-2 Modified Rappaport classification of non-Hodgkin's lymphomas

I. Nodular lymphomas
  A. Lymphocytic, poorly differentiated
  B. Mixed cell, lymphocytic and histiocytic
  C. Histiocytic
II. Diffuse lymphomas
  A. Lymphocytic, well diffferentiated
  B. Lymphocytic, poorly differentiated
  C. Mixed cell, lymphocytic and histiocytic
  D. Histiocytic
  E. Lymphoblastic
  F. Undifferentiated, Burkitt type
  G. Undifferentiated, non-Burkitt type

Well-differentiated lymphocytic lymphoma. The cells of this tumor are small, with hyperchromatic, round nuclei resembling mature lymphocytes. These cells have the surface characteristics of B cells and probably originate from perifollicular or medullary cord lymphocytes. The histologic pattern is always diffuse (Figure 63-20). An identical morphologic pattern is seen in chronic lymphocytic leukemia involving lymph nodes and in Waldenstrom's macroglobulinemia, in which the cells are plasmacytoid.

Poorly differentiated lymphocytic lymphoma. The cells of this tumor are larger, more polymorphic, and have prominent "cleaved" or indented nuclei. Their cytoplasm is scanty and small nucleoli may be present (Figure 63-21). These tumors occur in nodular or diffuse forms, with the nodular form more common. Most cases are of B cell origin.

Lymphoblastic lymphoma. This distinct clinico-pathological picture occurs primarily in children and adolescents, with a strong male preponderance. It arises as a mediastinal mass, probably originating from the thymus. It has a characteristic clinical history of rapid progression, with involvement of the bone marrow and peripheral blood, to simulate a picture of acute lymphocytic leukemia. The tumor is composed of large lymphocytes with strikingly irregular, deep nuclear convolutions, which present with a diffuse histology (Figure 63-22). These lymphomas are of T cell origin.

"Histiocytic" lymphoma. Rappaport used this category to include lymphomas composed of cells larger than poorly differentiated lymphocytes, both nodular and diffuse. Nodular lymphomas in this group are composed of large cells with varying amounts of basophilic cytoplasm and round nuclei with prominent nucleoli and distinct nuclear membranes and have been shown to be of B cell origin. Diffuse lymphomas in this category are composed of still larger cells with pleomorphic nuclei and eosinophilic cytoplasm and apparently represent either B or T cells (Figure 63-23). These were termed "reticulum cell sarcoma" in older terminology. T cell lymphomas arise with a diffuse histology, while B cell lymphomas may have arisen de novo in a diffuse pattern or evolved from a nodular pattern.

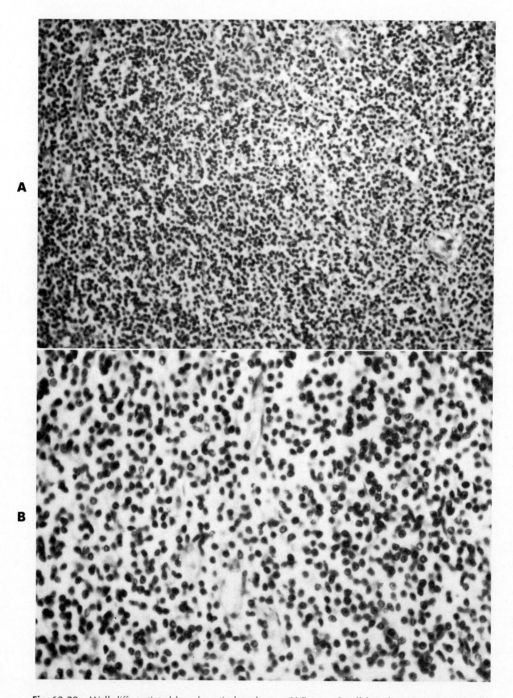

Fig. 63-20 Well-differentiated lymphocytic lymphoma. (WF type: Small lymphocytic.) (Hematoxylin-eosin stain; **A,** ×350; **B,** ×850.) *From Miale JB: Laboratory medicine: hematology, ed 6, St. Louis, 1982, Mosby–Year Book.*

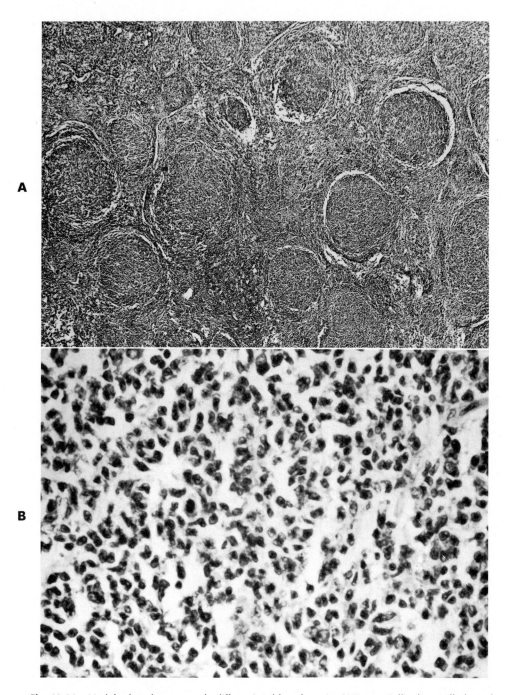

Fig. 63-21   Nodular lymphoma, poorly differentiated lymphocytic. (WF type: Follicular small cleaved cell.) (Hematoxylin-eosin stain; **A,** ×100; **B,** ×850.) *From Miale JB: Laboratory medicine: hematology, ed 6, St. Louis, 1982, Mosby–Year Book.*

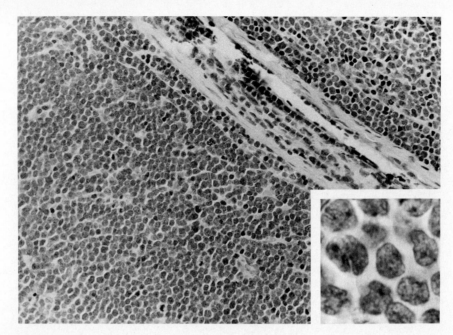

Fig. 63-22   Lymphoblastic lymphoma. (WF type: lymphoblastic.) *From Griffith RC and Janney CG: Hematopoietic system: bone marrow and blood, spleen, and lymph nodes. In Kissane JM: Anderson's pathology, ed 9, St. Louis, 1990, Mosby—Year Book.*

"Mixed" lymphoma. Rappaport originally described this lesion as a (virtually always) nodular tumor composed of lymphocytes and "histiocytes" in various proportions (Figure 63-24). Now it is recognized that this represents two populations of B cell lymphocytes.

Undifferentiated lymphoma. Two variants present as a diffuse lymphoma. The Burkitt's lymphoma consists of uniform cells smaller than those typical of histiocytic lymphomas, with nuclei containing visible nucleoli and moderate amounts of cytoplasm. A striking finding is the classical "starry sky" pattern due to the presence of large phagocytic cells containing ingested materials released from necrotic cells, which reflects the elevated cell turnover of these rapidly progressive tumors (Figure 63-25). There are two forms: Burkitt's lymphoma in Africa has been associated with the Epstein-Barr virus, affects children, and involves the mandibular-maxillary region. In the Western world, the tumor is not associated with EB viral infection and involves the abdominal organs and retroperitoneal space.

The rare pleomorphic undifferentiated non-Burkitt's lymphoma is composed of cells that are variable in size with prominent nucleoli and mitotic figures.

Lukes and Collins classification

The Lukes and Collins classification of lymphomas not only required separation of the various cells based on their immunologic characteristics but also identification of certain cytologic features, which appear to correlate with morphologic changes seen in antigenically stimulated transformed B lymphocytes within and without the follicular germinal centers and stimulated T cells.

Briefly described, the morphologic changes that accompany antigenic stimulation of B and T cells are as follows:

Mature small B lymphocytes are present outside the germinal center. With antigenic stimulation follicular center cells progressively transform through the stages: small cleaved (nuclei) follicular center cell (SCFCC); large cleaved (nuclei) follicular center cell (LCFCC); small noncleaved (nuclei) follicular center cells (SNCFCC); and large noncleaved (nuclei) follicular center cells (LNCFCC) with prominent nucleoli. The latter cells leave the follicular center appearing first as immunoblasts (IBS-B) and finally as plasma cells. The small T cells in the T cell regions of the node respond to stimuli by first forming cells with small nucleoli termed "epitheloid lymphocytes," then convoluted (nuclei) cells, which may become markedly convoluted Mycosis/Sezary cells and then finally appear as immunoblasts (IBS-T).

The correlation between these cell types and the cell types defined by Rappaport can be seen (Figure 63-26). Each cell type might give rise to a different lymphoma with a distinctive morphology. According to Lukes and Collins, rare true histiocytic lymphomas may exist but are not to be confused with the histiocytic denomination of Rappaport. The Lukes and Collins classification incorporates these concepts of cellular detail (Box 63-3).

The working formulation of NHL for clinical use

The Working Formulation is a consensus classification devised by an international group of experts who wished to correlate the morphological characteristics of lymphomas with prognosis. These experts also wished to avoid erroneous inferences regarding the ontogeny of these tumors. The Working Formulation integrated features of the Rappaport and other classifications (Table 63-8). Although it has been criticized because it does not clearly define the

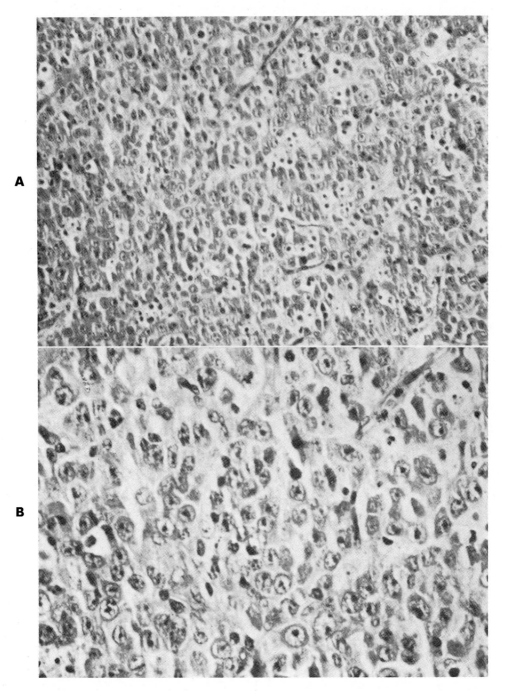

Fig. 63-23   Diffuse lymphoma, histiocytic. (WF type: Diffuse, large cell.) (Hematoxylin-eosin stain; **A,** x350; **B,** ×850.) *From Miale JB: Laboratory medicine: hematology, ed 4, St. Louis, 1972, Mosby–Year Book.*

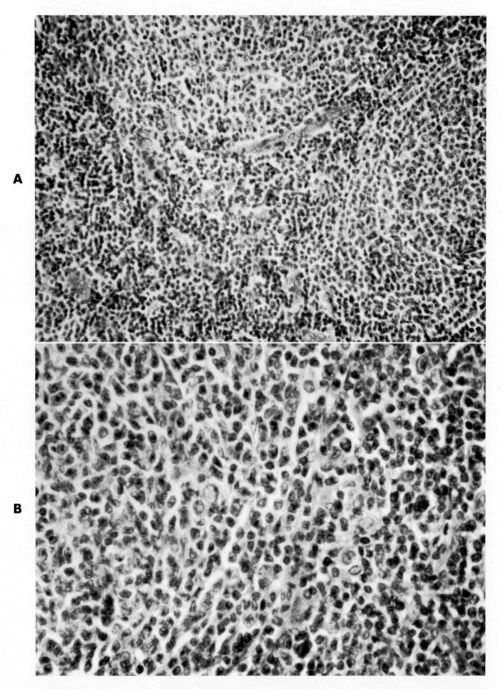

Fig. 63-24 Nodular lymphoma, mixed cell. (WF type: Follicular, mixed, small cleaved, and large cell.) (Hematoxylin-eosin stain; **A,** ×350; **B,** ×850.) *From Miale JB: Laboratory medicine: hematology, ed 6, St. Louis, 1982, Mosby–Year Book.*

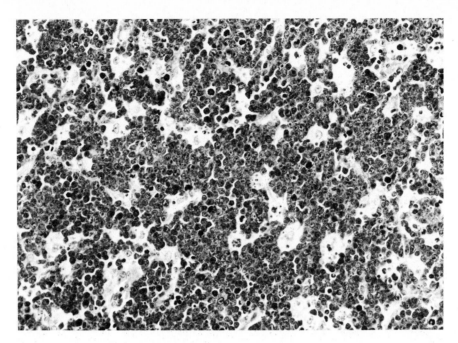

Fig. 63-25   Undifferentiated lymphoma, Burkitt's type in the ilium. (WF type: Small non-cleaved cell.) Note large benign phagocytic histiocytes dispersed throughout the infiltrate ("starry sky" appearance). *From Griffith RC and Janney CG: Hematopoietic system: bone marrow and blood, spleen, and lymph nodes. In Kissane JM: Anderson's pathology, ed 9, St. Louis, 1990, Mosby—Year Book.*

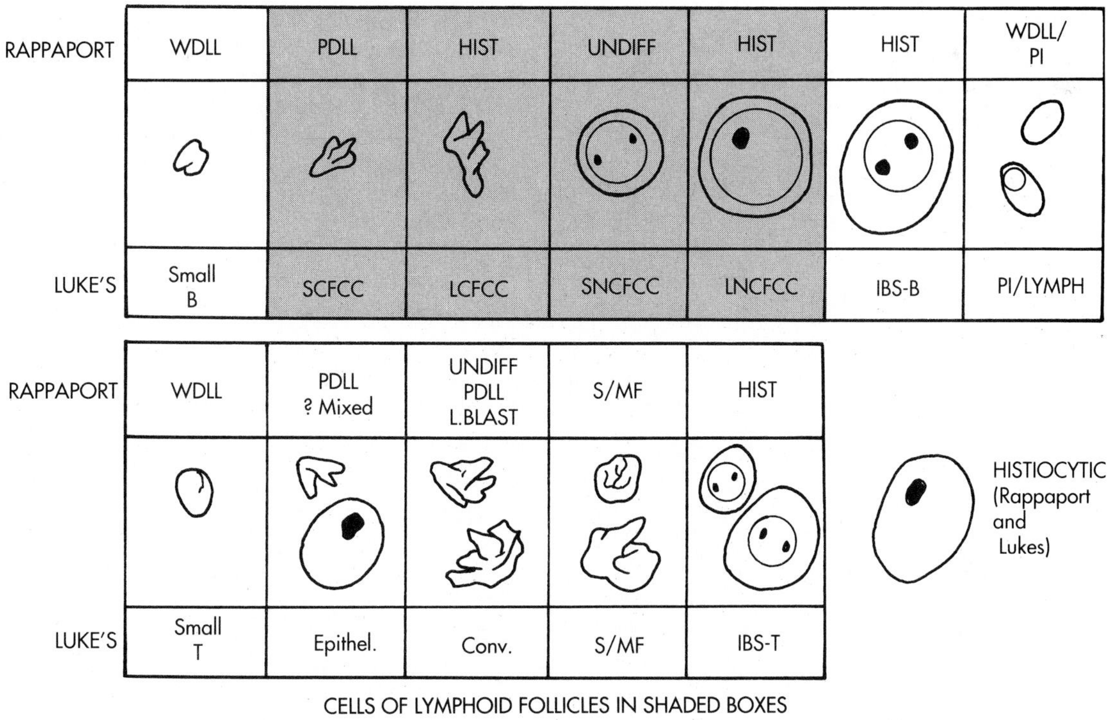

RAPPAPORT	WDLL	PDLL	HIST	UNDIFF	HIST	HIST	WDLL/PI
LUKE'S	Small B	SCFCC	LCFCC	SNCFCC	LNCFCC	IBS-B	PI/LYMPH

RAPPAPORT	WDLL	PDLL ? Mixed	UNDIFF PDLL L.BLAST	S/MF	HIST
LUKE'S	Small T	Epithel.	Conv.	S/MF	IBS-T

HISTIOCYTIC
(Rappaport
and
Lukes)

CELLS OF LYMPHOID FOLLICLES IN SHADED BOXES

Fig. 63-26   Morphologic alterations of B and T cells with immune stimulation. Correlation of lymphomas comprised of these cell types and classified according to Lukes with lymphomas classified according to Rappaport. *Redrawn from Tindle B: Revised classification of malignant lymphomas based on modern immunology. In Bryne GE, Chandor SB, Hurtubise P, Sheehan WW, and Tindle B: A unifying concept of lymphoma-morphology and immunology, Chicago, 1979, American Society of Clinical Pathology.*

ontogeny of lymphomas, this classification is gradually gaining preeminence and has been incorporated into many experimental chemotherapeutic protocols.

In this classification the various morphologic categories are grouped according to prognosis as low-grade, intermediate-grade, and high-grade lymphomas. Low-grade lymphomas have a better prognosis than the others; high-grade lymphomas have the worst prognosis.

Etiopathogenesis of non-Hodgkins lymphomas

The underlying etiologic agents of most non-Hodgkins lymphomas are unknown. However, it is presumed that, alone or in concert with other factors, these agents ultimately may lead to chromosomal changes that permit the emergence of a neoplastic clone, as has been previously described with leukemias. Underlying factors that have been identified include viral infection, chronic intense immunologic stimulation, and immune suppression.

Box 63-3 Lukes and Collins Classification of lymphomas

U cell types (undefined)
T cell types
    Small lymphocyte
    Convoluted lymphocyte
    Immunoblastic sarcoma
    Mycosis fungoides and Sezary syndrome
B cell types
    Small lymphocyte/plasmacytoid
    Follicular center cell
        Small cleaved cell
        Large cleaved cell
        Small non-cleaved cell
        Large non-cleaved cell
    Immunoblastic sarcoma
Histiocytic type

Viral agents are implicated as either direct or indirect causes of these neoplasms. As previously discussed, the retrovirus HTLV-1 is the causative agent of adult T cell leukemia/lymphoma.

Preceding infection with the Epstein-Barr virus is associated with the development of the African type of Burkitt diffuse small non-cleaved cell lymphomas. These tumors are characterized by the presence of EBV genomes in their cells, a finding now also encountered in cells from North American tumors. It is recognized, however, that infection alone is insufficient to cause the emergence of a malignant clone. Current opinion favors the theory that ongoing intense immunologic stimulation of children infected with EBV with a succession of infections and infestations, particularly falciparum malaria, induces B cell hyperplasia and thus increases the probability of mutation. The characteristic mutation of both the African and American varieties of Burkitts lymphoma is a t(8:14). This translocation juxtaposes the c-myc protooncogene, located on chromosome 8, band q24 to the immunoglobulin heavy chain gene located on chromosome 14, band q32. Interestingly, the precise breakpoint on chromosome 8, band q24 in the African disease is different from that in the American variant. Other less frequent translocations have also been observed in Burkitts lymphoma, including t(2:8) and t(8:22), which juxtapose the c-myc oncogene next to the kappa or lambda light chain locus respectively. The precise role of these transpositions in the emergence of a malignant clone is still unclear. EB viral infection may also be an important cofactor in the pathogenesis of lymphomas occurring in immunosuppressed patients.

Immune suppression is associated with a marked propensity toward the development of lymphomas. Primary immune deficiency syndromes, HIV-induced acquired immune deficiency syndrome (AIDS), iatrogenic post-transplant, and chemotherapeutic immune suppression have all been implicated. Common to all is a decrease in T cell control of B cell proliferation. Most of these neoplasms are

---

Table 63-8 Non-Hodgkin's lymphomas: correlation of classifications in use

Working formulation classification	Modified Rappaport classification	Lukes-Collins classification
Small lymphocyte (L.G.)	Lymphocytic, well diff.	B cell, small lymphocyte/plasmacytoid lymph.
Follicular, small cleaved cell, (L.G.)	Nodular, lymphocytic, poorly diff.	Follicular center cell small cleaved, follicular
Follicular, mixed, small cleaved and large cell (L.G.)	Nodular, mixed lymphocytic and histiocytic	Follicular center cell, mixed small cleaved and large cleaved, follicular
Follicular, large cell (I.G.)	Nodular, histiocytic	Follicular center cell, large cleaved or large non-cleaved, follicular
Diffuse, small cleaved cell (I.G.)	Diffuse, lymphocytic, poorly differentiated	Follicular center cell, small cleaved, diffuse
Diffuse, mixed small and large cell (I.G.)	Diffuse, mixed lymphocytic and histiocytic	Follicular center cell, mixed small cleaved and large cleaved or noncleaved, diffuse
Diffuse, large cell (I.G.)	Diffuse, histiocytic	Follicular center cell, large cleaved or non-cleaved, diffuse
Large cell, immunoblastic (H.G.)	Diffuse, histiocytic	Immunoblastic sarcoma, B or T cell
Lymphoblastic (H.G.)	Lymphoblastic	Convoluted T cell
Small, non-cleaved cell (H.G.)	Undifferentiated, Burkitt's and non-Burkitt's types	Follicular center cell, small non-cleaved, diffuse
L.G. = low grade	I.G. = intermediate grade	H.G. = high grade

B cell tumors, particularly large cell and immunoblastic lymphomas. Many are preceded by progressive polyclonal B cell proliferative syndromes. These tumors tend to be extranodal, and many are primary CNS lymphomas.

Among the primary immunodeficiency states, the Wiskott-Aldrich syndrome, Ataxia Telangectasia, common variable immunodeficiency disease, subacute combined immunodeficiency disease, and X-linked lymphoproliferative syndrome all are associated with a high incidence of B cell lymphomas.

Among patients with AIDS, non-Hodgkins lymphomas are the second most common malignancy after Kaposi's sarcoma. EB viral infection may be a significant cofactor in the causation of these tumors—it is believed that these patients are unable to mount an adequate T cell response to the EB virus and permit the persistence of high numbers of infected B cells that may give rise to lymphomas.

Lymphomas occurring during the post-transplant period appear soon after transplantation. In addition to the occurrence of CNS lymphomas, these tumors tend to involve the allograph. The frequency and rapidity with which lymphomas develop is greatest in patients treated with high-dose cyclosporin. Cyclosporin inhibits the development of cytotoxic T cells and permits the expression of suppressor T cells that may permit tolerance not only to the allograph but to a malignant B cell clone as well.

Non-Hodgkins lymphomas occur as a second malignancy in patients with other hematologic neoplasms. Large-cell lymphomas occurring in the course of chronic lymphocytic leukemia is known as Richter's syndrome. Together with acute non-lymphocytic leukemia, non-Hodgkins lymphomas are the second most common treatment-related malignancies in patients with Hodgkin's disease, usually following combined radiation and chemotherapy.

Clinical staging and prognosis of non-Hodgkin's lymphomas

Staging is much less useful than in Hodgkin's disease because these lymphomas, which arise multifocally and do not disseminate in a regularly predictable manner, tend to skip contiguous nodal groups and spread erratically. They are more often widely disseminated at the time of clinical presentation. For these reasons, patients usually undergo clinical staging, but aside from a bone marrow biopsy, the use of invasive procedures is reserved for special diagnostic situations.

Only 15% of patients present with stage 1 disease. Prior to the currently used chemotherapeutic protocols, prognosis correlated well with histologic types. Early studies using the Rappaport classification revealed that lymphocytic types had a better prognosis than histiocytic types, and that the nodular pattern showed a distinctly more favorable prognosis than the diffuse pattern (Figure 63-27). Later data revealed marked differences in prognosis between the low-, intermediate-, and high-grade histologic types when lymphomas were classified according to the Working Formulation (Figure 63-28).

Extranodal lymphoma

Many lymphomas originate in extranodal lymphoid tissue. The region usually affected is the gastrointestinal tract. About 5% of Hodgkin's disease presents extranodally. This presentation does not seem to have the same serious prognosis as secondary spread of Hodgkin's disease to extranodal sites. Alpha chain disease typically presents with intestinal lymphoma or, rarely, isolated respiratory tract involvement. As previously stated, non-Hodgkins lymphomas in childhood, and particularly the Burkitt's lymphoma, are primarily extranodal lymphomas. In addition, large B cell lym-

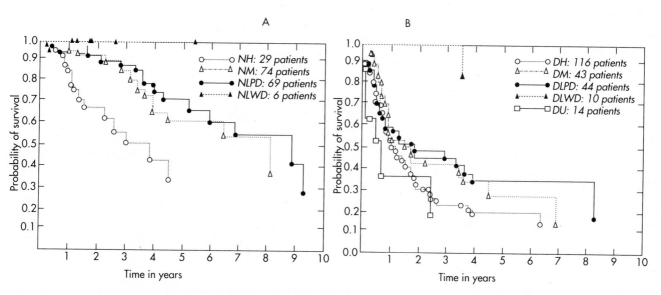

Fig. 63-27   Actuarial survival of patients with all types of nodular (left) and diffuse (right) non-Hodgkin's lymphomas, which were classified according to the Rappaport scheme. (See text.) *From Jones SE, Fuhs Z, Bull M, Kadin ME, Dorfman RF, et al: Non-hodgkin's lymphomas, clinicopathologic correlation in 405 cases, Cancer 31: 806, 1973.*

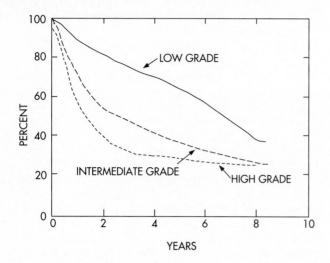

Fig. 63-28   Actuarial survival of patients with non-Hodgkin's lymphomas, which were classified according to the Working Formulation classification and then grouped prognostically as described in Table 11. *From: Rosenberg SA and the Non-Hodgkin's Lymphoma Pathologic Classification Project: National Cancer Institute Study of Classification of Non-Hodgkin's Lymphomas: Summary and description of a working formulation for clinical usage, Cancer 49:2122, 1982.*

phomas arising in immunosuppressed patients are also usually extranodal. A special type of histiocytic lymphoma that presents in the long bones is called "Reticulum cell sarcoma of bone."

Mycosis fungoides and Sezary syndrome

Mycosis fungoides is a T cell lymphoma (CD4 positive helper cells) that arises in the upper dermis and later infiltrates into the lower epidermis. The early lesions appear as macular-desquamative patches (premycotic phase). This lesion evolves into firm, raised purple-red placques (infiltrative phase). Lastly, large tumor masses develop and ulcerate (fungoide tumefation). In about 50% of cases, a secondary involvement of visceral organs eventually occurs. In the skin and visceral lesions, these lymphomas cells may be called "mycosis cells."

Sezary's syndrome is probably a variant of mycosis fungoides in which the skin involvement consists of a diffuse dermal infiltrate, causing a confluent macular rash (erythroderma) and invasion of the blood stream with tumor cells called "Sezary cells" (Figure 63-29).

Histiocytoses

This group of histiocytic proliferative disorders is divided into the frankly Malignant Histiocytoses, involving the clonal proliferation of histiocytes; those called Progressive Histiocytoses, involving the non-neoplastic proliferation of differentiated histiocytes; and the Reactive Systemic Histiocytoses, including those due to lipid and glycogen storage diseases.

Malignant histiocytoses

Among the malignant histiocytoses are cases of rare histiocytic leukemia and a disorder marked by the malignant proliferation of histiocytes within the red pulp of the spleen and in the subcapsular spaces and sinuses of lymph nodes known as Histiocytic Medullary Reticulosis. Histologically, these disorders show progressive proliferation of true histiocytes throughout various tissues of the body. A striking cytological finding is the abundant erythrophagocytosis of the proliferating histiocytes. Malignant histiocytoses are disorders of adults. They all progress rapidly to a fatal conclusion.

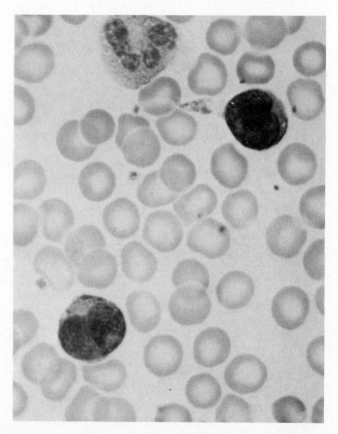

Fig. 63-29   Sezary cells in peripheral blood. *From Bauer JD: Clinical laboratory methods, ed 9, St. Louis, 1982, Mosby–Year Book.*

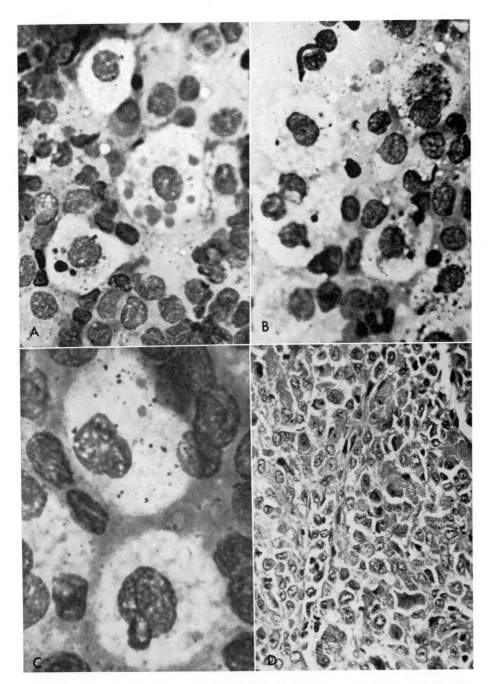

Fig. 63-30   Letterer-Siwe disease. **A-C,** Smear of lymph node aspiration. (Wright's stain; **A** and **B,** ×400; **C,** ×950.) **D,** Paraffin section, lymph node. (Hematoxylin-eosin stain; ×400.) *From Miale JB: Laboratory medicine: hematology, ed 6, St. Louis, 1982, Mosby–Year Book.*

Progressive histiocytoses

Among these disorders are those characterized by the aggressive, differentiated proliferation of functional histiocytes that are responsible for marked erythrophagocytoses, and others that involve the proliferation of cells indistinguishable from the normal Langerhans cells found in the epidermis and to a lesser degree in the reticuloendothelial system throughout the body. These latter histiocytic proliferations were originally grouped together as Histiocytosis X because of their similar pathologic features. With the further characterization of the proliferating cell, the term "Langerhans Cell Histiocytosis" is preferred.

The progressive erythrophagocytic histiocytoses include a nonreversible Familial Erythrophagocytic Histiocytosis, which has an unrelenting fatal course and is transmitted as an autosomal recessive trait, and a reversible Viral-associated Erythrophagocytic Histiocytosis, the pathogenesis of which is unclear.

The etiopathogenesis of the Langerhans cell histiocytosis (LCH) is unknown. However, an immune abnormality is suspected because of the natural role of Langerhans cells in antigen presentation to T cells and the loss of suppressor T cells in this disorder. An inherent abnormality of these histiocytic elements or an infectious etiology has not been entirely ruled out.

The clinical presentation and course of LCH has led to their usual separation into three separate diseases, which may show transition from one to another. The acute disseminated form, Letterer-Siwe disease, affects infants and children under the age of three years with infiltration of the skin, lymph nodes, liver, spleen and bone marrow by rapidly proliferating histiocytes (Figure 63-30). Flooding of the bone marrow leads to severe pancytopenia, with a rapidly fatal course. In the chronic disseminated form, Hand-Schuller Christian disease, bone involvement may be prominent, due to multifocal destructive lesions. Infiltrations are composed of foamy histiocytes (phagocytosis of lipid debris) mixed with eosinophils, lymphocytes, plasma cells, and neutrophils (Figure 63-31). A classical picture of diabetes insipidus, exophthalmos (due to lesions in the sella turcica and the orbit), and radiolucent defects on skull X-ray has often been described. This usually affects children and may become disseminated to extraosseous sites. Isolated unifocal bone lesions without the accompanying skin or visceral involvement are found in older children and adults. These behave in a very benign fashion and are called Eosinophilic Granuloma of Bone.

Although the presumptive diagnosis of LCH can usually be made on the basis of clinical presentation and histopathology, definitive diagnosis rests on the detection of surface HLA-DR antigens and receptors for anti-CD1a (an antigen shared with thymocytes), peanut lectin, and anti S-100 protein. Alternatively, the diagnosis can be confirmed by electron microscopy if the proliferating cells contain intracytoplasmic Birbeck granules, which are characteristic of Langerhans cells.

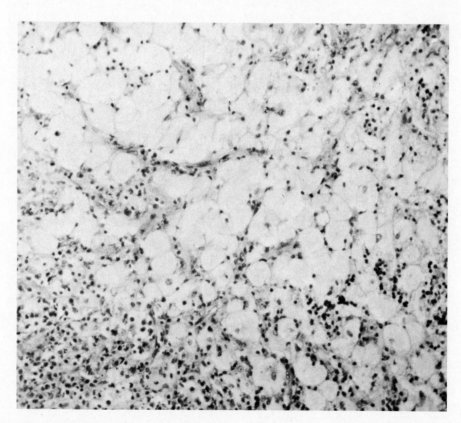

Fig. 63-31 Spleen, Hand-Schuüller-Christian disease. (Hematoxylin-eosin stain; ×250.) *From Miale JB: Laboratory medicine: hematology, ed 6, St. Louis, 1982, Mosby–Year Book.*

Reactive systemic histiocytoses

The reactive-systemic histiocytoses are associated with lysosomal disorders of sphingolipid, mucopolysaccharide, glycogen, or glycoprotein metabolism giving rise to histiocytic storage of metabolites and secondary cellular proliferation. The reticuloendothelial system shows preeminent involvement in Gaucher's disease, Niemann-Pick disease and Ceroid histiocytosis (Sea-blue histiocyte syndrome). For this reason, the resultant hypersplenism and marrow replacement tend to give rise to pancytopenia in these conditions.

Gaucher's disease results from a hereditary deficiency of glucocerebrosidase, which is transmitted as an autosomal recessive trait. Reticuloendothelial storage of cerebrosides is most pronounced in the chronic adult form (Type I). The macrophages become distended with the secondary lysosomes filled with this metabolite. These Gaucher cells are large and possess small, dense nuclei and abundant characteristic cytoplasm, classically described as "wrinkled tissue paper" (Figure 63-32). The cytoplasm stains positively with PAS stain, but not with Oil red 0 (Table 63-9). As stated, patients become progressively pancytopenic as their bone marrow is replaced with the infiltrate (Figure 63-33).

Niemann-Pick disease results from a hereditary deficiency of sphingomyelinase, which is transmitted as an autosomal recessive trait. In this disorder, the macrophages accumulate sphingomyelin and appear as distended cells with foamy cytoplasm (Figure 63-34), which stain with fat stains but may not stain with PAS stain (Table 63-9). In this disorder, marrow replacement is not as marked as in Gaucher's disease and the resultant anemia and thrombocytopenia tend to be mild.

The sea-blue histiocyte syndrome is a rare storage disorder of unclear pathogenesis that may be transmitted as an autosomal-recessive trait. It is characterized by the collection of large amounts of oxidized unsaturated lipids, termed "ceroid," in macrophages of the spleen, liver, and bone marrow. Examination of the bone marrow reveals diffuse infiltration with macrophages characterized by blue or blue-green cytoplasm (Figure 63-35), which stains with both PAS and fat stains (Table 63-9).

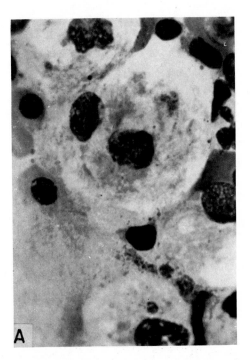

Fig. 63-32 Gaucher's disease. Bone marrow smear. (Wright's stain; ×950.) *From Miale JB: Laboratory medicine: hematology, ed 6, St. Louis, 1982, Mosby—Year Book.*

Table 63-9 Cytochemical reactions of some storage cells in fresh smears or frozen sections*

Stain	Gaucher's	Niemann-Pick	Ceroid storage†
Hematoxylin-eosin	Colorless	Greenish-yellow	Brownish-yellow
Wright-Giemsa	Colorless	Blue-green‡	Blue-green
PAS	Positive	Variable	Positive
Oil red O	Negative to slight	Positive‡	Positive
Sudan black B	Slight	Positive‡	Positive
Baker's acid hematin	Negative	Positive	Positive
Luxol fast blue	Negative	Positive	Doubtful
Acid-fast	Negative	Positive	Positive
Autofluorescence	Positive (diffuse)	Positive (nodular)	Positive (nodular)
Acid phosphatase	Positive	Negative	Negative

From Miale JB: Laboratory medicine: hematology, ed 6, St. Louis, 1982, Mosby—Year Book, Inc.
*Formalin fixation and paraffin embedding removes phospholipid from Niemann-Pick cells, voiding the positive reaction for phospholipid with Baker's acid hematin and Luxol fast blue.
†Primarily the sea-blue histiocyte syndrome, but applies to other accumulations of ceroid-like material.
‡Varies from cell to cell.

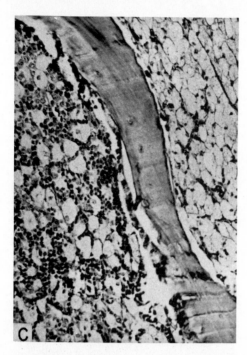

Fig. 63-33   Gaucher's disease. Bone marrow massively infiltrated with Gaucher's cells. (Hematoxylin-eosin stain; ×100.) *From Miale JB: Laboratory medicine: hematology, ed 6, St. Louis, 1982, Mosby— Year Book.*

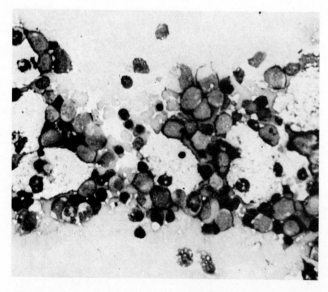

Fig. 63-34   Nieman-Pick disease. Bone marrow smear. *From Ladisch S and Miller DR: The spleen and disorders involving the monocyte-macrophage system. In Miller DR and Baehner RL: Blood diseases of infancy and childhood, ed 6, St. Louis, 1989, Mosby—Year Book.*

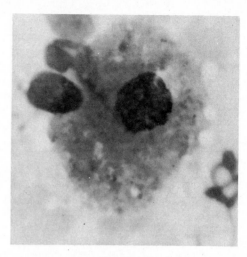

Fig. 63-35   Sea-blue histiocyte syndrome. Spleen imprint. (Wright's stain; ×950.) *From Miale JB: Laboratory medicine: hematology, ed 6, St. Louis, 1982, Mosby—Year Book.*

Of note is the frequent observation that rather typical Gaucher's cells or sea-blue histiocytes may be found in the bone marrow aspirates of patients with myeloproliferative disorders. The formation of these cells is not related to an intrinsic enzyme defect in the marrow macrophages but rather to an overload of lipid breakdown products from the proliferating myeloid elements in these disorders.

SUGGESTED READING

Anastasi J, Bitter MA, Vardiman JW: The histopathologic diagnosis and subclassification of Hodgkin's disease, Hematol Oncol Clinics, N America 3:187-204, 1990.

Behm J: Morphologic and cytochemical characteristics of childhood lymphoblastic leukemia, Hematol Oncol Clinics, N America 4:715-741, 1990.

Biemer JJ: Malignant lymphomas associated with immunodeficiency states, Ann Clin Lab Sci 20:175-191, 1990.

Borowitz MJ: Immunologic markers in childhood acute lymphoblastic leukemia, Hematol Oncol Clinics, N America 4:743-765, 1990.

Heerema NA: Cytogenetic abnormalities and molecular markers of acute lymphoblastic leukemia, Hematol Oncol Clinics, N America 4:745-820, 1990.

Leikin SL: Immunobiology of histiocytosis X, Hematol Oncol Clinics, N America 1:49-61, 1987.

McKenna RW: Infectious mononucleosis: part 1: morphologic aspects, Lab Med 10:135-139, 1979.

Ophoren J: Infectious mononucleosis, Part 2: serologic aspects, Lab Med 10:203-206, 1979.

Rai KR and Han T: Prognostic factors and clinical staging in chronic lymphocytic leukemia, Hematol Oncol Clinics, N America 4:447-456, 1990.

Rosenberg SA and the Non-Hodgkin's Lymphoma Pathologic Classification Project: National Cancer Institute sponsored study of classifications on non-Hodgkin's lymphoma, summary and description of a working formulation for clinical usage, Cancer 49:2112-2135, 1982.

Slivnick DJ, Nawrocki JF, Fisher RI: Immunology and cellular biology of Hodgkin's disease, Hematol Oncol Clinics, N America 3:205-220, 1990.

PART TEN

HEMOSTASIS

64 Normal hemostasis

Robert F. Reiss

The term "hemostasis" denotes the totality processes concerned with the control of bleeding. It includes vascular factors, the formation of a clot through the interaction of platelets and plasma coagulation factors with the damaged vessel, and the action of various control factors that limit the extension of the clotting phenomenon.

Vascular contraction is usually the initial response to arterial vascular damage. Platelet plug formation is the major mechanism of hemostasis in the microvasculature and the initial step in the definitive control of hemorrhage from larger vessels. Platelet plug formation is often referred to as primary hemostasis. Coagulation results in the formation of fibrin strands that further reinforce the platelet plug and thereby form a clot in larger vessels. The coagulation process is often referred to as secondary hemostasis. Numerous mechanisms control the extent of platelet clumping and coagulation. These control mechanisms are sometimes called tertiary hemostasis.

Following its formation, a clot's further evolution is related to its dissolution and eventual reconstitution of an intact vessel wall. Clot dissolution begins within a few hours of formation. The clot's platelets disintegrate and then lysis occurs by plasmin activated in the clot and proteolytic enzymes released by leukocytes incorporated into the clot. Proliferation of smooth muscle cells and fibroblasts in the vascular defect follows and repair of the damaged wall is completed by growth of endothelial cells over the defect. The proliferation of smooth muscle and endothelial cells is stimulated by the release of various mitogens including platelet-derived growth factor.

Failure to achieve an adequate balance between the factors promoting and regulating normal hemostasis may result in a hemorrhagic tendency on the one hand or the development of intravascular clotting (thrombosis) on the other.

PLATELETS AND FORMATION OF THE PLATELET PLUG

Platelets are disc-shaped anucleate cell fragments formed by fragmentation of megakaryocytes in the bone marrow and lung. The number of platelets in the circulating blood varies according to the method of measurement (see Chapter 58). By most methods the normal values in adults range from 140,000 to 400,000/μl of blood. Preteen children reportedly have higher counts than adults (Table 64-1).

Table 64-1 Platelet counts in normal children (per μL)

Age group	Median count	5th Percentile	95th Percentile
1-12 mo	425,000	300,000	750,000
1-3 yr	375,000	250,000	600,000
3-7 yr	325,000	250,000	550,000
7-12 yr	325,000	200,000	450,000

From: Nowak Rn, Tschantz JA, and Krill CE: Normal platelet and mean platelet volumes in pediatric patients, Lab Med 18:613-614, 1987.

Thrombopoiesis and platelet kinetics

The fragmentation of megakaryocyte cytoplasm occurs after maturation of the megakaryocyte to an average ploidy number of 16N to 32N. The differentiation and maturation of megakaryocytes, as well as the release of platelets into the blood, is stimulated by the hormonal-like substance termed thrombopoietin. The thrombopoietin activity in plasma appears to relate inversely with the circulating platelet mass. Experimentally, the injection of plasma from a thrombocytopenic animal can cause increased incorporation of intravenously injected 75 Se-selenomethionine into developing megakaryocytes and newly released platelets while transfusion of platelets causes decreased platelet incorporation. Chemical characterization of thrombopoietin or identification of its production site has yet to be achieved. However, it is known that other growth factors including IL-3 also stimulate the proliferation and differentiation of megakaryocytic precursors (see Chapter 57). The young platelets are believed to be the larger platelets identified as megathrombocytes. Their number is usually inversely related to the total circulating platelet mass and directly related to the number of marrow megakaryocytes. It appears that these megakaryocytes are more active hemostatically. There is evidence that, upon release from the marrow, young platelets are sequestered in the spleen for two to three days and then released into the circulation. Two thirds of the platelets circulate, while the other third are sequestered in the spleen. The platelets in each of these two pools are freely interchangeable. Platelets have a life span of nine to 10 days (Figure 64-1). Their removal from the circulation is primarily according to age, but some random loss also occurs. Removal may be triggered by increased binding of IgG to senescent platelets.

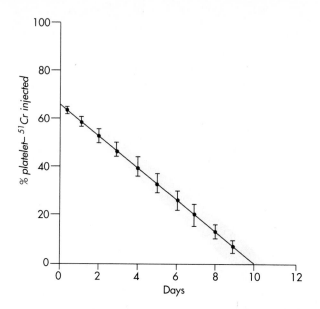

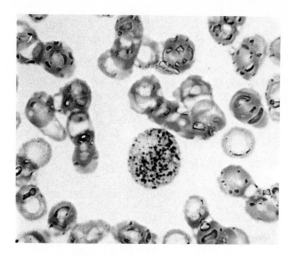

Fig. 64-2   Megathrombocyte (×1250). *From Bauer JD: Clinical laboratory methods, ed 9, St. Louis, 1982, Mosby–Year Book, Inc.*

Fig. 64-1   Normal platelet survival curve using Cr⁵¹ labelled platelets. The mean recovery ± (1 S.D.) is shown. The mean recovery immediately after infusion is 60% to 65%, the life span is 8.5 to 10.5 days, and the T 1/2 is four to five days. *From Harker LA and Finch CA: Thrombokinetics in man, J Clin Invest 48:963-974, 1969.*

Platelet structure

The morphology of megakaryocytes is reviewed in Chapter 58. In peripheral smears prepared from EDTA-anticoagulated blood and stained with Romanowsky stains, platelets are bluish-gray in color, possess a granular cytoplasm, and measure approximately 1.0 to 2.5 μ in diameter (see Chapter 58). Platelets have a volume of 2 to 13 μ^3 (mean 7 to 10 μ^3) when blood is anticoagulated with EDTA. Ten percent of platelets (megathrombocytes) have a diameter greater than 2.5 μ and about 5% to 10% have a volume greater than 13.5 μ^3 (Figure 64-2).

Electron microscopy shows that platelets are complex structures (Figure 64-3). Surrounded by a cell membrane rich in phospholipid, platelets contain various structural proteins and enzymes. The membrane invaginates into the cytoplasm, forming an extensive, open canalicular system. An exterior coat, rich in glycoproteins, separates the membrane from the surrounding plasma. The glycoproteins are identified by separating membrane proteins on polyacrylamide gel electrophoresis following SDS solubilization of the membranes (SDS-PAGE).

The cytoplasm is divided into peripheral and central zones. The peripheral zone is characterized by a circumferential microtubular system rich in tubulin and the calcium-dependent contractile protein, platelet actomyosin (thrombasthenin). The peripheral zone also contains numerous actin microfilaments and filaments anchored to the platelet membrane by a structural protein termed actin-binding protein. The protein terminus of one of the external-coat glycoproteins (glycoprotein IIIa), termed α-actinin, may be anchored to the actin-binding protein and reinforces the binding of actin to the membrane.

The central zone contains various organelles including mitochondria, peroxisomes, lysosomes, electron dense bodies, and lighter-staining alpha granules. The dense bodies contain quantities of ADP, ATP, serotonin, and calcium ion. The alpha granules contain various substances whose function is still being elucidated, including β-thromboglobulin, platelet factor 4 (antiheparin factor), thrombospondin ("thrombin-sensitive protein"), fibronectin, platelet-derived growth factor, and platelet-derived coagulation factors (fibrinogen, factor V, von Willebrand factor). Finally, channels that appear to be connected to the peripheral microtubular system, termed the dense tubular system, are found in the cytoplasm. This appears to be derived from rough endoplasmic reticulum and contains high concentrations of calcium ion and some of the enzymes involved in prostaglandin synthesis.

Platelet function
Platelet adhesion

Under normal circumstances, platelets do not adhere to the walls of the larger blood vessels. Damage to the endothelial lining of the vessels exposes sub-endothelial basement membrane and collagen, to which circulating platelets first adhere (contact adhesion) and then spread (spreading adhesion).

At high shear rates, as in small blood vessels, contact adhesion to collagen fibrils and elastin-associated non-collagenous microfibrils require the presence of a glycoprotein Ib and IX complex in the membrane exterior coat and high molecular weight multimers of von Willebrand protein. For contact adherence to occur, first von Willebrand factor must bind to the subendothelial fibrils, and subsequently platelets adhere to the bound vWF by means of the glycoprotein Ib-IX vW receptor. At low shear rates, as in large blood vessels, contact adhesion does not require von Willebrand factor, but involves collagen receptors on platelets. These collagen receptors may be associated with glycoprotein Ia or a IIb-IIIa complex.

Platelet release reactions

Following contact adhesion, platelets release their granule contents. Although adhesion to collagen may result in

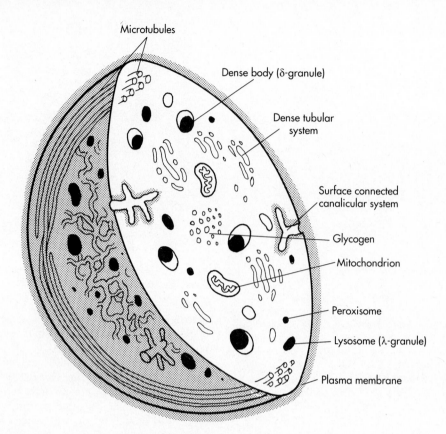

Fig. 64-3   Diagrammatic representation of platelet ultrastructure as identified by electron microscopy and cytochemistry. *Redrawn from Bentfield-Barker ME and Bainton DF: Identification of primary lysosomes in human megakaryocytes and platelets, Blood 59:479, 1982.*

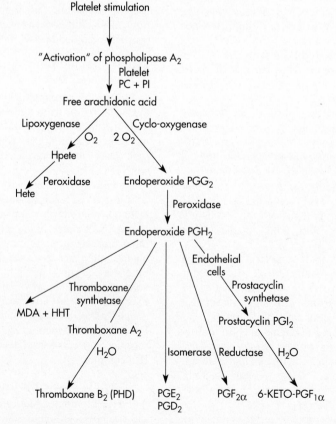

Fig. 64-4   Prostaglandin synthesis following platelet stimulation. *From Marcus AJ: The role of lipids in platelet function, J. Lipid Res 19:793-826, 1978.*

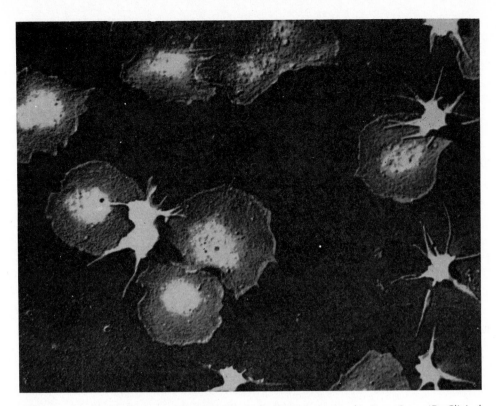

Fig. 64-5   Pseudopod formation by normal platelets (electron micrograph). *From Bauer JD: Clinical laboratory methods, ed 9, St. Louis, 1982, Mosby—Year Book, Inc.*

some direct release, most depends on the generation of prostaglandins. After binding to collagen, a phospholipase A associated with the cell membrane is activated and releases arachidonic acid from platelet membrane phospholipid. Arachidonic acid is then converted into intermediate prostaglandins and a derivative, Thromboxane A_2 (TxA_2) (Figure 64-4). Elevated levels of TxA_2 result in decreased adenyl cyclase and increased phosphodiesterase activity, which decrease levels of cyclic AMP. This decreased level of cyclic AMP and increased level of TxA_2 in turn cause increased mobilization of calcium from the dense tubular system into the cytoplasm. These changes stimulate the cells to undergo a shape alteration, becoming swollen, spiny spheres with long pseudopods containing newly formed actin filaments (Figure 64-5). They also cause the peripheral microtubular system to detach from its membrane anchor, partially disassemble, and constrict about the organelles in the central portion of the cytoplasm. The increased cytoplasmic calcium, in part complexed to a calcium-binding protein, calmodulin, may be responsible for these contractile processes by permitting ATP-dependent phosphorylation of both myosin, necessary for actin-myosin contraction, and actin-binding protein, necessary for the production of actin filaments involved in pseudopod formation. A portion of the contents of the dense granules are then released through the open canalicular system to the outside (Release Reaction I). The ADP released from platelets, damaged tissue, and red cells attaches to the ADP receptors on the surface of platelets. Binding of ADP to the membrane is accompanied by an alteration in surface charge and increased formation and exposure of the glycoprotein IIb-IIIa complex.

As a glycoprotein IIb-IIIa complex forms, it functions as a receptor for several "adhesive" proteins, including fibrinogen, fibronectin, and von Willebrand factor. The pseudopods of the adherent platelets then spread over the subendothelial collagen fibrils. Spreading adhesion is mediated by these adhesive proteins. At low shear there may be additional mechanisms to mediate platelet spreading. These additional mechanisms are not dependent on the glycoprotein IIb-IIIa complex.

Platelet aggregation

The ADP released from adherent platelets also binds to platelets circulating nearby. Membrane-bound ADP may directly cause mobilization of calcium and activation of prostaglandin synthesis, thereby causing the newly attracted platelets to undergo the previously described shape changes. These altered platelets are then attracted to those already adherent to the damaged site and cause the formation of large tangled clumps of sticky platelets with long pseudopods. This process is known as aggregation and these clumps are known as primary hemostatic plugs. Aggregation of platelets is largely due to calcium-dependent fibrinogen binding between GP IIb-IIIa complexes of their external coats. Aggregation is therefore dependent not only on ADP release, but on availability of fibrinogen.

In addition to exposure to collagen and ADP, thrombospondin released from alpha granules and phospholipid material released from both leukocytes and platelets ("platelet-activating factor") can also cause the release reaction and aggregation by mechanisms not fully elucidated. Through the positive feedback mechanism of ADP release and binding to newly aggregated platelets, further release of dense and alpha granule contents occurs from all platelets (Release Reaction II). At this point the contraction of the microtubular system is such that the central portion of the platelets are only masses of contractile gel.

Platelet factor 3 availability

During the release reaction and throughout the process of aggregation, the platelet membrane undergoes poorly described conformational changes, which make phospholipid receptors available to bind factor X and factor II on the membrane surface, thus localizing coagulation to the hemostatic plug (Platelet factor 3 availability). Concurrently, the coagulation process is initiated and is favored by the release of platelet coagulant proteins, including fibrinogen, factor V, factor VIII, factor XI, high molecular weight kininogen, and platelet factor 4. The small amount of thrombin generated initially is bound to thrombin receptors (possibly Glycoprotein Ib) on the platelet's external coat and induces further irreversible platelet aggregation, which terminates in fusion of platelets with loss of their individual structural integrity to form the definitive hemostatic plug.

Clot retraction

Fibrin strands generated by the coagulation pathway strengthen the plug, thereby forming a clot, which then retracts and expresses serum. This retraction results in a more compact clot resistant to dissolution. Retraction is thought to be due to the contraction of thrombasthenin.

Control of platelet plug formation

The growth of the platelet plug is limited to the site of injury by 1) the dilution of ADP and other aggregation mediators by blood flow and 2) the antagonistic effects of other substances produced during hemostasis. Prostacyclin, produced by endothelial cells in response to thrombin binding, inhibits aggregation by raising intracellular levels of platelet cyclic AMP. Plasmin released during hemostasis also inhibits aggregation by a noncyclic, AMP-dependent mechanism. Finally, adenosine produced by the enzymatic digestion of ADP by endothelial cells inhibits aggregation.

THE COAGULATION CASCADE

Coagulation involves the formation of cross-linked fibrin strands produced from the soluble protein, fibrinogen, by the enzymatic action of thrombin. This transformation is the final step of a cascade of enzymatic reactions mediated by the serial formation of enzymes (activated clotting factors) acting in concert with other non-enzymatic cofactors. The initial steps of coagulation may proceed either from the interaction of certain clotting factors with subendothelial collagen fibrils (intrinsic pathway) or by the release of a lipoprotein "tissue factor" (extrinsic pathway). Both pathways culminate in the activation of factor X, which has been localized on platelet surfaces in the developing clot and which then participates in the final steps of fibrin strand formation (common pathway).

The plasma coagulation factors

The coagulation factors involved in this process are identified by Roman numerals, according to an internationally adopted nomenclature. Many of these factors have proper names as well. These factors, their half-lives, and their normal concentrations in plasma are listed in Table 64-2. Except for fibrinogen, the concentration is measured in terms of coagulant activity rather than actual protein concentration. One unit of factor activity is defined as the amount of coagulant activity present in one ml of pooled normal plasmas. The concentration of these factors varies markedly in normal individuals and depends on the method of measurement (see Chapter 65).

Many of the coagulation factors are zymogens, which, upon activation, act as serine proteases. These include factors XII, XI, X, IX, VII, II (Prothrombin), and Prekallikrein (Fletcher factor). These activated factors (denoted by subscript a) are proteases that contain a serine residue at their active site. They act upon specific peptide bonds containing argenine. Factor XIII is also a zymogen which, upon activation, becomes an enzyme capable of forming an amide bond between a carboxyl group of glutamine and an amino group of lysine. Fibrinogen (factor I) is the soluble protein substrate which, after thrombin (II_a) mediated proteolysis, forms fibrin monomer. Factors V and VIII are co-factors which non-enzymatically accelerate the activation of prothrombin to thrombin by factor X_a, and factor X to X_a by IX_a respectively. Their cofactor activity is markedly increased if they have undergone limited proteolysis by trace amounts of thrombin. These altered factor V and VIII cofactor molecules are variously denoted as modified (subscript m) or activated (subscript a). Lastly, high molecular

Table 64-2 Nomenclature of well-described clotting factors. Except as noted, the concentration of functional coagulation factors is given in terms of percent of activity, (i.e., the number of units per deciliter of plasma).

International nomenclature	Common name	Normal range	Mean half-life
Factor I	Fibrinogen	150-400 mg/dl	4 days
Factor II	Prothrombin	70%-130%	60 hr.
Factor V	Proaccelerin	50%-150%	15 hr.
Factor VII	Proconvertin	70%-150%	5 hr.
Factor VIII C	Antihemophiliac Factor	50%-200%	12 hr.
Factor IX	Plasma Thromboplastin Component	70%-130%	25 hr.
Factor X	Stuart-Power Factor	70%-130%	40 hr.
Factor XI	Plasma Thromboplastin Antecedent	70%-130%	48 hr.
Factor XII	Hogeman Factor	40%-150%	48 hr.
Factor XIII	Fibrin-Stabilizing	15-45 µg/ml	8 days
Prekallekein	Fletcher Factor	35-50 µg/ml	36 hr.
HMWK	Fitzgerald or Williams Factor	70-90 µg/ml	6 days

Table 64-3 Factor content of various blood fractions and products

	I	II	V	VII	VIII	IX	X	XI
Fresh normal plasma	Yes	Yes	Yes	Yes	Yes	Yes	Yes	Yes
Aged normal plasma	Yes*	Yes	No	Yes	No	Yes	Yes	Yes
Serum	No	Yes†	No	Yes	No	Yes	Yes	Yes
Al(OH)₃-adsorbed citrated plasma	Yes‡	No	Yes	No	Yes	No	No	Yes (reduced)
BaSO₄-adsorbed oxalated plasma	Yes‡	No	Yes	No	Yes	No	No	Yes (reduced)
Seitz-filtered plasma	Yes	No	Yes	No	Yes	No	No	Yes (reduced)
Plasma from intensive bishydroxycoumarin-treated patient	Yes	Reduced	Yes	Reduced	Yes	Reduced	Reduced	Yes

From Maile JB: Laboratory Medicine: hematology, ed 6, St Louis, 1982, Mosby–Year Book.
*But reduced and of dimished reactivity on prolonged storage.
†Significant amounts remain just after clotting, gradually diminishing as serum ages.
‡Prolonged or intensive adsorption removes significant amounts of fibrinogen and other factors.

weight Kininogen (HMWK) and a poorly described factor, Passavoy factor, appear to be non-enzymatic co-factors that participate in the initial steps of the intrinsic pathway (contact phase).

The plasma coagulation factors, with the exception of factor VIII, are synthesized solely in the liver. Factors II, VII, IX, and X are known as the prothrombin complex and depend on vitamin K for their synthesis. Vitamin K is necessary for the gamma-carboxylation of the glutamic acid (gla) residues near the N terminus of these factors. Such carboxylation is required for the calcium-mediated bonding of the vitamin K-dependent factors to platelet phospholipid or tissue lipoprotein surfaces that localize their coagulant activity. They are absorbed from citrated plasma by Al(OH)₃ and from oxalated plasma by BaSO₄ (Table 64-3).

Factors XII, XI, prekallekrein and HMWK are involved in the "contact" phase of the intrinsic pathway of the coagulation cascade and are therefore called contact factors.

Factors I, V, VIII, and XIII are known as consumable factors because they are enzymatically destroyed by plasmin (all) and by activated protein C (V, VIII) during clotting and are therefore absent from serum (Table 64-3). Factors I and VIII increase in concentration during periods of stress, pregnancy, and administration of oral contraceptives.

Fibrinogen is a protein made up of pairs of three polypeptide chains termed Aα, Bβ, and γ (Figure 64-6). The N terminals of the three chains are closely bound into a central (E) domain by disulfide bridges, while the carboxy terminals of the Aα and γ chains form terminal (D) domains. The most central portion of the E domain is known as the disulfide knot (N-DSK). Thrombin acts on the molecule by splitting off fibrinopeptides A and B from the N terminus portions of the A and B chains, and the resultant fibrin monomers polymerize by side-to-side bonding between E and D domains and lengthwise bonding between D domains.

Factor VIII procoagulant (VIII C, formerly termed VIII:AHF) is a small protein that circulates in the plasma bound by non-covalent bonds to multimers of the von Willebrand protein, having an average molecular weight in excess of 10⁶ (VIII C/vWF) (Figure 64-7). Factor VIII C

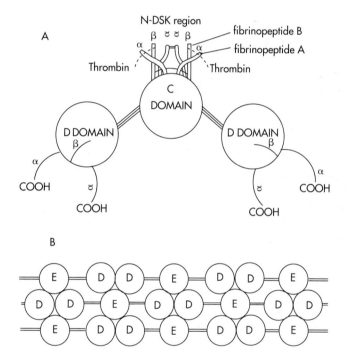

Fig. 64-6 Representation of the structure of fibrinogen showing the central E domain near the N terminus and the terminal D domains at the C terminus **(A)**; the polymerization of fibrin monomers **(B)**. *From Rosenberg RD. In Beck WS, ed: Hematology, ed 3, Cambridge, Mass, 1981, MIT Press.*

molecules are also antigens (VIII C:Ag) neutralized by human antibodies. The synthesis of these molecules is regulated by an X-linked gene. VIII C is synthesized in the liver and other unidentified tissues. The size of the multimeric complex of von Willebrand's protein (previously termed VIII:vWF, VIII R:RC, or Ristocetin Cofactor) depends on the number of protein monomers (M.W. 2×10^5). The largest of these multimers (M.W. up to 10^7) supports the normal adhesion of platelets to endothelium and the various in vitro tests of platelet function including bleeding time,

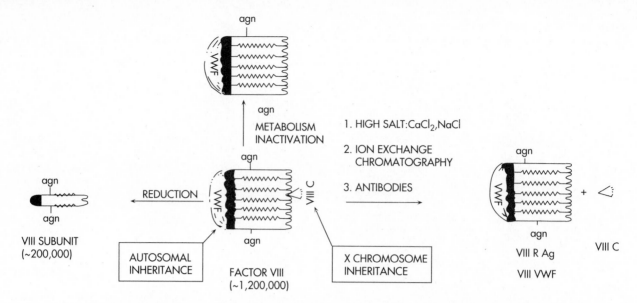

Fig. 64-7   Representation of the factor VIII C/VWF complex. von Willebrand factor (VWF) was formerly identified as VIII:VWF or VIII:RRC (factor VIII related ristocetin cofactor). The antigenic properties of VWF were denoted by VIII R:Ag. *From Hoyer LW: von Willebrands disease, Prog Hemostasis Thromb 3:321, 1976.*

retention in glass bead columns, and ristocetin-induced platelet agglutination. This protein is produced by endothelial cells throughout the body and in megakaryocytes. Its production is regulated by an autosomal-dominant gene. It possesses antigenic properties detected by precipitating antibodies produced in rabbits (formerly termed vWF:Ag VIII R:Ag or VIII:AGN).

Factor I, factor VIII, vWF, and factor XIII are precipitable in the cold. Together with these factors, a high molecular weight glycoprotein called fibronectin (cold insoluble globulin) is found in these cryoprecipitates. Fibronectin is produced by many cell types in the body, including endothelial cells and platelets, and is found in plasma. Its functions may include mediation of cell-cell adhesion, attachment of cells to substrates and regulation of cell locomotion. Its role in hemostasis is still being delineated. Fibronectin assists in platelet adhesion to collagen. In addition, fibrin attachment to collagen and retraction of the fibrin clot by fibroblast may also be mediated by fibronectin.

Tissue factor

Tissue factor is a lipoprotein produced by monocytes, endothelial cells, smooth muscle cells, and fibroblasts. Certain tissues appear especially rich in tissue factor (e.g., brain, lung, placenta). The tissue factor apoprotein has now been purified. It is complexed to liposomes composed of the zwitterionic phospholipids, phosphatidylethanolamine, and phosphatidylcholine. Tissue factor lacks proteolytic activity and functions as a cofactor for VII and VII$_a$ in the activation of X.

Coagulation pathways

The intrinsic pathway

The intrinsic pathway is initiated by the activation of factor XII and progresses through the activation of factor X (Figure 64-8). This activation was thought to involve the non-enzymatic conformational change of factor XII following its binding to negatively charged surfaces. Although surface contact activation of factor XII by collagen and a variety of other substances, such as glass, celite, or kaolin, has been demonstrated in vitro, it has never been conclusively shown that in vivo collagen induced surface activation of factor XII occurs. It is now felt that after binding to such surfaces, trace amounts of kallekrein or other serine proteases causes activation. Once the intrinsic cascade is initiated, more factor XII is activated enzymatically, in the presence of high molecular weight kininogen (Williams, Fitzgerald, or Flaujeac factor), by kallikrein, factor XII$_a$, and, to a lesser extent, by factor XI$_a$ and plasmin.

The factor XII$_a$ formed activates factor XI to factor XI$_a$, prekallikrein (Fletcher factor) to kallikrein (which in turn transforms kininogen to bradykinin), and plasminogen proactivator to plasmin activator (which in turn transforms plasminogen to plasmin). These reactions are accelerated by the presence of high molecular weight kininogen, which participates in the binding of these zymogens to charged surfaces. Another poorly described factor, Passavoy factor, may also be involved in accelerating the activation of the contact factors. Finally, platelets appear to promote proteolytic activation of "contact" factors that bind to platelets. It has therefore been hypothesized that platelets may be able to support activation of factor XI in the absence of factor XII.

Factor XI$_a$ activates Factor IX in the presence of calcium ions. It is thought that this reaction may occur on the platelet membrane. Factor IX$_a$ binds to this phospholipid surface (platelet factor 3) along with factor VIII$_a$ and factor X in the presence of calcium ions. There is some evidence that factor V produced by platelets may need to participate in the binding of factor X. In the presence of the complex formed by activated factor VIII, factor IX$_a$, and Ca, factor X is enzymatically activated to factor X$_a$, which remains bound to the phospholipid surface.

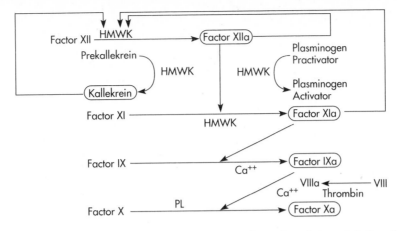

Fig. 64-8 Cascade concept of coagulation. The intrinsic pathway through the activitation of factor X. The activated factors are circled.

The extrinsic pathway

The extrinsic pathway involves the initial activation of bound factor VII to factor VII$_a$ by an unidentified protease and the subsequent activation of factor X by VII$_a$ (Figure 64-9). It is known that factors XII$_a$ and X$_a$ may also cause VII activation. VII$_a$ complexes to tissue factor and Ca, and this complex in turn activates bound factor X. There is some evidence that native factor VII in the presence of tissue factor may also slowly activate X. This latter reaction may be key to initiation of the extrinsic pathway, while further factor VII activation occurs enzymatically by a positive feedback system through the action of factor X$_a$. As opposed to the intrinsic system, the extrinsic system is faster and is generated within a matter of seconds. In addition to the activation of factor X, the tissue factor VII$_a$ complex may also activate factor IX. Such an indirect pathway through factor IX accounts for about 30% of all factor X activation.

Recent evidence shows that factor X may also be localized on perturbed endothelial cells and that these cells may then produce tissue factor resulting in the activation of factors X by VII$_a$.

The common pathway

The common pathway involves the activation of prothrombin (II) to thrombin and the subsequent formation of fibrin from fibrinogen (Figure 64-10). Prothrombin is bound on a platelet phospholipid surface in the presence of calcium ion and then activated to thrombin by the proteolytic action of a prothrombinase complex formed by factor X$_a$ and cofactor V$_a$. Thrombin represents the carboxy terminal half of the prothrombin molecule freed from the bound amino terminus. Activation of prothrombin may also proceed on the surface of perturbed endothelial cells that have previously bound factor X$_a$.

Thrombin acts on fibrinogen to form fibrin monomer by the splitting off of small fibrinopeptides A and B from the amino terminals of Aα and Bβ chains of the fibrinogen molecule. These monomers undergo side-to-side polymerization by peptide bonding between the carboxy terminals of the γ chains (D domain) and the remaining portions of the N terminals of the central portion of the Aα chains (E

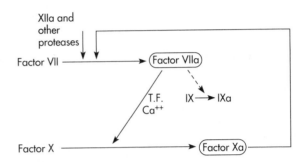

Fig. 64-9 Cascade concept of coagulation. The extrinsic pathway through the activation of factor X. The activated factors are circled.

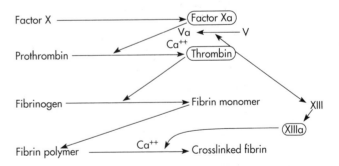

Fig. 64-10 Cascade concept of coagulation. The common pathway through the formation of cross-linked fibrin. The activated factors are circled.

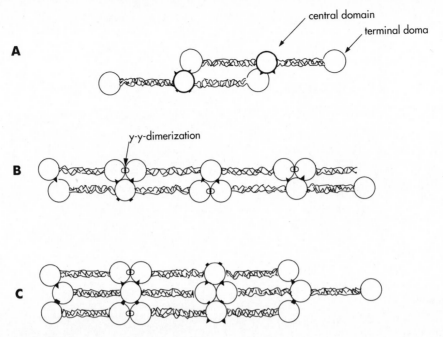

Fig. 64-11 Representation of fibrin monomer polymerization. **A,** Overlapping of fibrin monomers and bonding between central and terminal domains. **B,** End-to-end bonding of successive fibrin monomers and polymers. **C,** Side-to-side thickening of the fibrin fiber. *From Doolittle RF. In Bloom AL and Thomas DP: Haemostasis and thrombosis, Edinburgh, 1981, Churchill Livingstone.*

domain). This polymerization is reinforced by hydrophobic and electrostatic bonding. These polymers are lengthened and stabilized by end to end cross linking transamidation bonds between the carboxy terminals of γ chains (D domains) of initiated fibrin polymers. This reaction is catalyzed by factor XIII activated by thrombin. Thickening of these fibrin polymer chains occurs by successive lateral central-terminal domain binding and end to end γ-γ cross linking (Figure 64-11). Excess fibrin monomers complex with fibrinogen to form soluble fibrin monomer complexes (SFMC).

REGULATION OF HEMOSTASIS

Once activated, the hemostatic process would appear to be self-perpetuating and to proceed until all the procoagulant substances are exhausted. Obviously, limiting mechanisms must be concurrently operative to avoid progressive clotting of the intravascular circulation and limit the clot to the immediate area of damage. The mechanisms limiting the formation of the platelet plug have been previously discussed. Numerous control systems limit the extent of coagulation. Among them are the following:

1. the inherent instability of activated factors, which tend to rapidly lose biologic activity;
2. the rapid dilution of the local high concentration of activated factors by blood flow;
3. the rapid clearance of activated factors and soluble fibrin monomer-fibrinogen-complexes by the reticuloendothelial system;
4. the presence of certain globulins in the plasma that inhibit or inactivate the serine protease clotting factors;

5. the inactivation and subsequent clearance of the cofactors V and VIII by activated protein C and plasmin; and
6. the activation of the fibrinolytic pathway during coagulation and the release of a protease from leukocytes within the clot, which cause clot digestion.

These last three mechanisms are discussed in greater depth.

Inhibitors of activated coagulation factors

Several globulins function as enzyme inhibitors or inactivators of serine proteases. In general, they bind in a one-to-one molar ratio with activated coagulation factors. The bond involves the active serine site of the protease and an arginine site of the inactivator. The principle globulins that function in this manner to regulate coagulation are antithrombin III, heparin cofactor II, and α2 macroglobulin. In addition, C1 inhibitor and α1 antitrypsin may inhibit the activity of the serine proteases involved in coagulation to a lesser extent.

Anti-thrombin III (AT III) slowly binds and inactivates thrombin and factors X_a, IX_a, XI_a, and XII_a. This activity is almost instantaneous in the presence of heparin (Figure 64-12). It is thought that under physiologic conditions, vascular tissues catalyze AT III activity by the production of mucopolysaccharides possessing heparin-like activity. Absence of AT III not only makes an individual refractory to anticoagulation with heparin but also predisposes the individual to thrombosis. Other substances that interfere with the conversion of fibrinogen to fibrin had also been loosely termed "anti-thrombins." Such agents included fibrin itself (antithrombin I), which tends to absorb thrombin and the

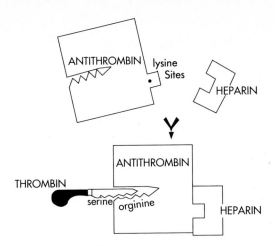

Fig. 64-12 Heparin facilitates and markedly accelerates the binding and inactivation of thrombin and other activated serine protease clotting factors by antithrombin III. *From Rosenberg RD: Protein Inhibitors of Blood Coagulation. In Human hemostasis, Washington DC, 1975, American Association of Blood Banks.*

fibrinogen/fibrin degregation products (antithrombin VI), which interfere with fibrin monomer polymerization.

Heparin cofactor II is a second heparin activated inhibitor that selectively inactives thrombin. Although its in vitro activity may require higher levels of heparin than does AT III, it may be the principle anti-thrombin protein in vivo under physiologic conditions.

α2-macroglobulin (α_2 M) is thought to bind to thrombin and kallikrein and partially inhibit their activity. These complexes are cleared from the circulation by the reticuloendothelial system. α_2 M, however, binds most avidly to plasmin. It has been proposed that such complexes may serve as circulating reserves of proteolytic activity.

Inhibitors of activated cofactors

Protein C (PC) is a zymogen that depends on vitamin K for its synthesis. This zymogen is activated to a serine protease by thrombin complexed to thrombomodulin, a protein produced by endothelial cells. Activated protein C (APC) enzymatically inactivates factors V and VIII. The rate of activation of PC is further positively modulated by the quantity of factor V_a bound at the site of clot formation, the presence of negatively charged phospholipid or platelet surfaces, and the action of a vitamin-K-dependent cofactor designated protein S. Factors V and VIII previously activated by thrombin are more susceptible to the action of APC. The activity of APC is neutralized by a distinct serine protease inhibitor (Activated Protein C Inhibitor).

Fibrinolytic mediators

The fibrinolytic mechanism operative in modulating the progression of the clotting process is due to the formation of the serine protease, plasmin, from its zymogen, plasminogen, by various activators. Plasminogen is a β globulin that circulates in two forms, one has an N-terminal glutamic acid group, the other an N-terminal lysine. The former has a plasma half-life of approximately two days, while the latter's half-life is one day.

Although small amounts of plasmin may be continuously generated by minute quantities of tissue-type plasminogen activator (t-PA) released by endothelial cells, under normal circumstances plasminogen is incorporated into the clot and activation in this site leads to local fibrinolytic activity. Fibrinolysis is localized in the clot because of plasminogen binding to platelet proteins (e.g., thrombospondin) and phospholipids and because of plasmin binding to fibrin.

Release of tissue plasminogen activator is increased by fibrin formation and various physiologic stimuli, such as stress and exercise, as well as by pathologic stimuli, such as shock. However, the major regulator of total plasminogen activation is not the level of t-PA, but rather the level of its inhibitor, which is also produced by endothelial cells.

Factor XII_a or kallekrein generated during coagulation enzymatically transforms circulating plasminogen proactivator to plasminogen activator, which then converts plasminogen to plasmin.

Lastly, urokinase in the urine is capable of rapidly transforming plasminogen to plasmin. A urokinase-related plasminogen activator has been isolated from leukocytes.

Plasmin causes the enzymatic proteolysis of the fibrin structure by cleavage of the molecule into progressively smaller fragments called fibrin split or fibrin degradation products (fdp). The abnormal accumulation of plasmin in the plasma can lead to progressive proteolysis of fibrinogen and factors V and VIII. These fibrinogen split or degradation products (FDP) are similar to fdp, but have not undergone early thrombin proteolysis and therefore the larger fragments still possess the fibrinopeptide A segments of the Aα chains. The largest fibrinogen degradation fragment is called X, which is in turn broken into a Y and D fragment. The Y fragment subsequently breaks into a D and E fragment (Figure 64-13). Fragments X and Y are the earliest products of plasmin digestion, while D and E fragments are later digestion products. Continued digestion leads to the formation of small fragments, which have been poorly characterized. Fragment X is slowly clottable by thrombin. However, the resultant polymer is unable to undergo transamidation cross-linking. The later fragments are soluble and actually interfere with fibrin formation from fibrinogen, either because of direct inhibition of thrombin activity or disruption in fibrin monomer polymerization, since they form the soluble fibrin monomer complexes previously described. In addition, these degradation products, when present in high concentrations, have been shown to inhibit platelet aggregation. Fibrin degradation products from digestion of non cross-linked fibrin (fdp) have been designated X^0, Y^0, D^0, and E^0. These fragments have anticoagulant properties similar to fibrinogen degradation products. Increased levels of circulating soluble fibrin monomer complexes, produced by these fdp, are reduced by their uptake and degregation in the reticuloendothelial system. Digestion of cross-linked fibrin leads to the formation of dimers of D fragments, and complexes of D and E fragments rather than the series of distinct fragments described previously.

Activity of the fibrinolytic system in the circulation and in the clot is depressed by activity of inhibitors that complex with plasmin. Foremost among them are α2 antiplasmin, and plasminogen activator inhibitor, while α2 macroglobulin exerts lesser protease inhibitor activity against plasmin.

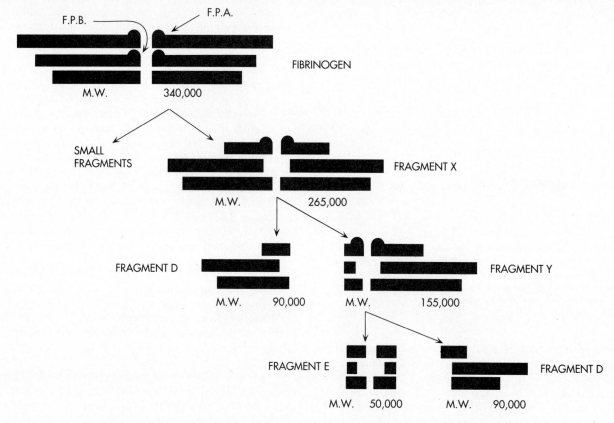

Fig. 64-13 Sequential degredation of fibrinogen or fibrin monomer by plasmin into fibrinogen split (or degredation) products.

SUGGESTED READING

Andrew M, Paes B, Milner R, Johnston M, Mitchell L, Tollejsen DM, Castle V, and Powers P: Development of the human coagulation system in the healthy premature infant, Blood 72:1651-1657, 1988.

Chesterman CN and Berndt MC: Platelet and vessel wall interaction and the genesis of atherosclerosis, Clin Haematol 15:323-353, 1986.

Colman RW: Surface mediated defense reactions: the plasma contact activation system, J Clin Invest 73:1249-1253, 1984.

Erickson LA, Schleef RR, Ny T, and Loskintoff DJ: The fibrinolytic system of the vascular wall, Clin Haematol 14:513-530, 1985.

Hessel LW and Kluft C: Advances in clinical fibrinolysis, Clin Haematol 15:443-463, 1986.

Kane WH and Davie EW: Blood coagulation factors V and VIII: Structural and functional similarities and their relationship to hemorrhagic and thrombotic disorders, Blood 71:539-555, 1988.

Kaplan AP and Silverberg M: The coagulation-kinin pathway of human plasma, Blood 70:1-15, 1987.

Lammle B and Griffin JH: Formation of the fibrin clot: the balance of procoagulant and inhibitory factors, Clin Haematol 14:281-342, 1985.

Montgomery RR, Marlar RA, and Gill JC: Newborn haemostasis, Clin Haematol 14:443-460, 1985.

Mosesson M and Amrani DL: The structure and biologic activities of plasma fibronectin, Blood 56:145-158, 1980.

Naworth P, Kisiel W, and Stern D: The role of endothelium in the haemostatic balance of haemostasis, Clin Haematol 14:531-546, 1985.

Nemerson Y: Tissue factor and hemostasis, Blood 71:1-8, 1988.

Phillips DR, Charo IF, Parise LV, and Fitzgerald LA: The platelet membrane glycoprotein IIb-IIIa complex, Blood 71:831-843, 1988.

Salem HH: The natural anticoagulants, Clin Haematol 15:371-391, 1986.

Thompson AR: Structure, function and molecular defects of factor IX, Blood 67:565-572, 1986.

Thompson CB and Jakubowski JA: The pathophysiology and clinical relevance of platelet heterogeneity, Blood 72:1-8, 1988.

Zimmerman TS and Fulcher CA: Factor VIII procoagulant protein, Clin Haematol 14:343-358, 1985.

Laboratory evaluation of hemostasis

Robert F. Reiss

Evaluation of the integrity of the hemostatic system in the patient with a bleeding diathesis involves first the review of medical history and the assessment of the type and degree of bleeding. The subsequent ordering of appropriate laboratory tests is, in part, dependent on this prior clinical evaluation. The laboratory approach to the bleeding patient will be discussed later. Laboratory tests have been devised to study the various components of primary hemostasis, coagulation, and fibrinolysis.

LABORATORY EVALUATION OF PRIMARY HEMOSTASIS

Since primary hemostasis is dependent on adequate numbers of normally functioning platelets, evaluation first entails the performance of a platelet count. The finding of decreased numbers of platelets (thrombocytopenia) requires subsequent laboratory investigations to elucidate the mechanism by which thrombocytopenia developed. Further investigation of primary hemostasis in the presence of a normal number of platelets, or occasionally in patients with thrombocytopenia, involves the assessment of platelet function.

Quantitative evaluation of primary hemostasis

As previously described (Chapter 59), the platelet count may be estimated from the peripheral blood smear, counted manually in a chamber with light or phase-contrast microscopy, or electronically in an impedance particle counter or an optical light scattering measurement device. The reference values for platelet counts vary not only with age, but also according to the method used.

Although thrombocytopenia associated with increased peripheral destruction is often characterized by increased numbers of megathrombocytes in the peripheral smear, such a finding is not specific for, or adequate to assure that, thrombopoesis is increased and effective. Direct assessment of thrombopoesis by bone marrow examination is essential. Both the number and morphology of megakaryocytes require evaluation (see Chapter 58).

Peripheral sequestration and or destruction of platelets is best evaluated in the laboratory by platelet survival and sequestration studies with chromium-51 or Indium-111 tagging (see Chapter 59). With these methods, it can be shown in normal individuals that 50% to 60% of injected platelets circulate, that they have a life span of 10 days, and that

they are removed in a slightly curvilinear fashion, with a half-life of approximately 4.5 days.

Platelet function tests

Overall platelet function is best performed in vivo by means of the bleeding time test. Laboratory tests that attempt to measure each individual parameter of platelet function have also been devised, including those that evaluate adhesion, release reactions, aggregation, platelet factor 3 availability, and clot retraction. The clinical utility of these tests varies considerably and not all have found a place in routine practice.

Bleeding time tests

These tests attempt to quantify the efficacy of hemostasis in the superficial capillary bed of the dermis. Since coagulation does not play a role in the control of microvascular bleeding, these tests measure the number and function of platelets, as well as structural integrity of the microvasculature. All measure the blood loss from superficial incisions as a function of time.

Duke's bleeding time test was performed by making small incisions in the earlobe. Standardization was difficult and the procedure has been generally abandoned. Most of the currently used tests are based on Ivy's bleeding time test. The original Ivy procedure entailed making duplicate incisions on the volar surface of the forearm with a blood pressure cuff applied and inflated to 40 mm Hg; the subsequent blotting of blood every 30 seconds with filter paper while avoiding contact with the incised skin; and the recording of the time required for cessation of bleeding (Fig. 65-1). Not only was it found that the incision length and depth are difficult to standardize, but also that other factors influence bleeding time. Of particular note is the influence of the direction of incision, the presence of superficial small veins in the path of the incision, and the age of the patient. In order to standardize the length and depth of the incisions, two modifications to the Ivy technique are now in routine use, the template method of Mielke and the Simplate method.

The template method utilizes a disposable polystyrene template with a 9-mm long central slit and a blade that fits through the slit, extending 1 mm beyond the template surface. Application of the template to the skin and incision

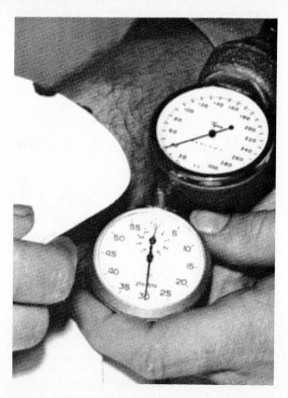

Fig. 65-1 Ivy bleeding time. Horizontal incision made in volar aspect of forearm, with blood pressure cuff inflated to 40 mm Hg and the resultant blood drops blotted at 30-second intervals. *From Mielke CH and Rodvien R: Bleeding time procedures. In Schmidt RM (editor): CRC handbook series in clinical laboratory science, vol I: Hematology, Baton Rouge, La, 1972, CRC Press.*

Table 65-1 Bleeding times: reported reference range

Method	Time (min)
Duke's	1.0-3.5
Original Ivy	1.0-5.0
Template (horizontal)	5.1 ± 1.4*
Template (vertical)	4.2 ± 1.0*
Simplate	4.0 ± 2.2*
Hemalet	3.7 ± 2.1*

*$\bar{x}$ = ±1 SD.

Box 65-1 Common drugs reported to affect platelet function

ANTI-INFLAMMATORY DRUGS

Corticosteroids*
Aspirin†
Ibuprofin†
Indomethacin†
Phenylbutazone†
Colchicine§
Sulfinpyrazone†

VASODILATOR DRUGS

Dipyridamole‡
Aminophylline‡
Theophylline‡
Papaverine‖

ANTIBIOTICS

Penicillin§
Carbenicillin§
Gentamicin§
Ticarcillin§

OTHER COMMON DRUGS

General anesthetics§
Diphenhydramine§
Dextran‖
Ethanol‖
Propranolol‖
Clofibrate‖
Furosemide‖
Glyceryl guaiacolate‖
Psychotropic drugs
Phenothiazines§
Tricyclic antidepressants§

*Inhibit phospholipase.
†Inhibit cyclooxygenase.
‡Inhibit phosphodiesterase.
§Stabilize biologic membranes.
‖Other or unknown action.

along the slit permits standardization. The Simplate method creates standardized incisions 5 mm in length and 1 mm in depth by use of a spring-loaded disposable blade. More recently, another device, the Hemalet, which combines features of the template and spring-loaded blade devices, has been introduced. It makes uniform incisions, 5 mm in length and 1.5 mm in depth. With all the devices, two incisions are made and the bleeding times are averaged. If the two times differ by more than 20% of the longer time, a third time should be determined. Reference limits for bleeding time tests vary according to the method used (Table 65-1). Performance of the bleeding time along a horizontal plane, parallel to the antecubital crease, tends to give a time that is about 1 minute longer than when performed vertically to the antecubital crease.

Prior to the performance of the bleeding time and all other platelet function tests, the history of possible ingestion of drugs that can affect function (Box 65-1) should be reviewed. In particular, the ingestion of aspirin during the 7 days before test performance needs to be ruled out. Such ingestion tends to prolong the bleeding time by several minutes. Pronounced prolongation with 600 mg of aspirin taken 2 hours prior to the test is seen in patients with hemophilia and von Willebrand's disease (aspirin stress test).

Prolongation of the bleeding time is due to either thrombocytopenia, platelet dysfunction, or connective tissue ab-

normalities, which lead to vascular fragility. The platelet count below which the bleeding time becomes prolonged has been cited to be 100,000/μl (Fig. 65-2). A constant relationship between the degree of thrombocytopenia and the prolongation has been represented by the formula:

$$\text{Bleeding time} = 30 - \frac{\text{Platelet count/}\mu l}{4000}$$

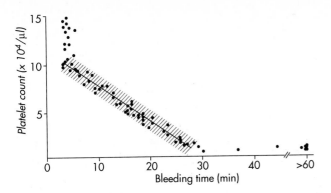

Fig. 65-2 Linear inverse relationships between the platelet count and Ivy bleeding time. *From Harker LA and Slichter S: The bleeding time as a screening test for evaluation of platelet function, New Engl J Med 287:155, 159, 1972.*

Many investigators have not found such a predictable relationship between the platelet count and bleeding time, and have also observed normal test times with counts of 80,000/μl or lower.

At counts of 100,000/μl and above, prolonged bleeding times indicate platelet dysfunction. Patients with marked thrombocytopenia characterized by increased platelet turnover may have normal or shorter than predicted bleeding times. This finding may correlate with the increased numbers of megathrombocytes that are present in such conditions.

The performance of a bleeding time test carries with it the complication of scarring. It has been suggested that incisions made perpendicular to the antecubital crease are less likely to scar than those made parallel to the crease. Similarly, it has been stated that the Simplate technique is more likely to cause scarring. The risk for scarring, or even for keloid formation, is greatest in black patients.

Platelet adhesion tests

These tests are better referred to as retention tests because rather than simply measuring adhesion, they are tests of global platelet function. The various glass bead platelet retention tests, patterned after the method of Hellem, measure the in vitro retention of platelets from native or anticoagulated whole blood as it passes through a column of glass beads. This test not only measures adhesion of platelets to these beads, but also measures subsequent aggregation of platelets to each other. The reference value for this test, as modifed by Bowie, is the retention of >65% of platelets passing through the column, measured as the difference between the platelet count of the subject and the platelet count of the blood after it has passed through the column. Decreased retention is due to either an intrinsic abnormality of platelet function or a decrease in functional von Willebrand's factor concentration in the plasma. Because of the difficulty in standardizing the test and the lack of information obtained that is not available from other function tests, these determinations are no longer widely performed.

The Borchgrevink retention test measures the in vivo retention of platelets in the incision made as part of Ivy's bleeding time determination. Retention is represented as the difference in platelet count between blood taken from the incision at the start of the test and that taken just prior to the cessation of bleeding. Reference values are reported to be between 56% and 95% of the initial count. Adhesion, and then subsequent aggregation, can be directly visualized by the Baumgartner procedure. This test, used primarily in research laboratories, entails the observation of platelet interaction with de-endothelialized aortic strips under varying experimental conditions.

Demonstration of platelet release reactions

Platelet release is usually examined in vitro as an intrinsic part of aggregation testing. It may also be directly examined by measuring the release of adenosine triphosphate (ATP) and vasoactive amines from dense granules and secretory proteins from alpha granules. The release of ATP is discussed later in this chapter. The release of carbon-14 serotonin, which had been previously absorbed by platelets during a period of incubation, can be measured following stimulation with adrenalin, adenosine diphosphate (ADP), or collagen. Similarly, β-thromboglobulin or platelet factor 4, released after platelet stimulation, can be measured. More commonly, the concentration of these secretory proteins in the plasma is measured as an index of in vivo platelet activation.

Tests of platelet aggregation

Laboratory tests to demonstrate the aggregation response of platelets to various mediators (agonists) that have bound to receptors on their external coat are based on detection of a change in either turbidity or electrical resistance (impedance). Among the agonists used are collagen, ADP, epinephrine, and occasionally, thrombin. Although ristocetin is commonly included in this list, it is not an agonist in the usual sense since, at the recommended concentration, it does not provoke true calcium-dependent aggregation, but simply mediates electrostatic agglutination of platelets to each other.

At appropriate concentrations, agonists other than collagen cause de novo aggregation (primary wave). Following this initial aggregation, the platelets are activated and, after a lag period, undergo the release reaction. As a consequence of endogenous ADP release, further aggregation occurs (secondary wave). Lesser than optimum concentrations of agonists permit disaggregation of the formed aggregates, whereas elevated concentrations of agonists cause irreversible aggregation de novo and masks evidence of the platelet release reaction. Exposure to collagen does not provoke a biphasic curve, but simply results in a monophasic response following a latent period during which endogenous ADP is released.

The most commonly performed tests are conducted in aggregometers, which detect changes in turbidity of citrated platelet-rich plasma (PRP) following addition of the appropriate agonist. An initial decrease in light transmission may be seen after addition of the agonist due to the change in shape, from disk or sphere, of the suspended platelets. Sub-

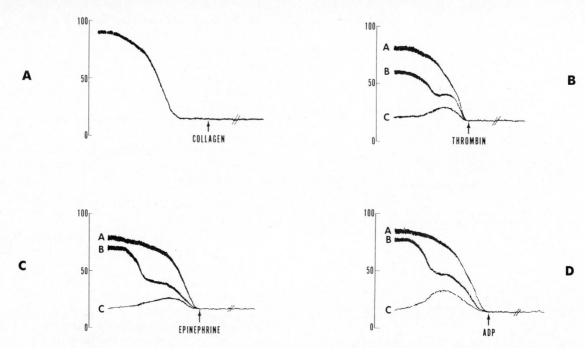

Fig. 65-3 Normal platelet aggregation patterns obtained by addition of commonly used agonists to platelet-rich plasma; collagen (**a**); thrombin (**b**); epinephrine (**c**); and ADP (**d**). *From Miale JB: Laboratory medicine: hematology, ed 6, St Louis, 1982, Mosby–Year Book.*

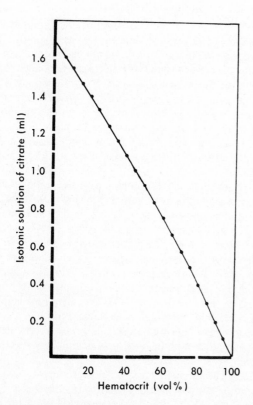

Fig. 65-4 Nomogram relating hematocrit to the amount of 3.8% citrate anticoagulant required to maintain a constant 0.64% citrate concentration in plasma. *From Hellem AJ, Scand J: Clin Lab Invest [Suppl] 51:1, 1960.*

sequently, as aggregation occurs in the plasma, there is a decrease in turbidity and an increase in light transmission through the suspension (Fig. 65-3).

Various aggregometers that measure turbidity are commercially available. All require careful standardization of technique. Among the variables that must be optimized are (1) Concentration of citrate in the prepared PRP. At normal hematocrits, optimum concentration is reached with whole blood: 3.8% sodium citrate ratio of 9:1. An adjustment to this ratio can be made for different hematocrits (Fig. 65-4). (2) Adjustment of the platelet count of the PRP to 200 to 300,000/μl with platelet-poor plasma. Performance of aggregation tests on plasma with lower platelet counts requires the preparation of a control PRP of a similar count to be run concurrently. (3) Storage of PRP in capped plastic syringes or containers for 30 to 120 minutes at 22° C prior to use. Capping prevents loss of CO_2 and maintains pH at an optimum, whereas storage prior to use for moderate periods of time increases the sensitivity of platelets to agonists. (4) Optimum concentration of agonists to elicit biphasic aggregation (usually found to be approximately 2μM ADP, 2μM epinephrine, 0.2 μ/ml thrombin) and soluble collagen (approximately 0.8 μg/ml). Of note is the fact that the exact final concentration of the agonist necessary to acheive optimum results may vary from specimen to specimen, and will require some empiric experimentation with each test. (5) Reaction temperature is set at 37°C. Extreme lipemia or hemoglobinemia and demonstrably icteric plasma interferes with the performance of accurate aggregometry because of their intrinsic optical density.

Up to 30% to 40% of normal individuals will not show a biphasic response with epinephrine in optimal concentrations. Occasionally, individuals will also not show a biphasic response to ADP. Spontaneous aggregation may be seen in some individuals. It has been claimed that these persons may be "hypercoagulable" and predisposed to thrombotic disease.

More recently, aggregometers capable of measuring aggregation as a function of impedance to electrical current have been developed. Their main advantages stem from the possibility of measuring aggregation in small volumes of whole blood as well as platelet-rich plasma. With such instruments, it is now easier to study infants and make measurements in hemolyzed, icteric, and lipemic blood. In addition, it has been proposed that studies carried out in whole blood may more closely reflect the physiologic situation than do those that are carried out in platelet-rich plasma.

Such devices measure the increase in resistance to the passage of an electrical current (impedance) through blood or platelet-rich plasma, as platelets aggregate on the electrodes placed in the blood or plasma. Following addition of an agonist, initial aggregation occurs. This is followed, in turn, by release of endogenous ADP and further aggregation. Distinct biphasic patterns may not be seen with these instruments.

Adenosine triphosphate release following aggregation induced by agonists (an index of the release reaction) may also be directly measured in some aggregometers. Its release provokes the development of luminescence by a firefly luciferin-lucerifase mixture and is detected in a photomultiplier tube.

Individuals who do not show platelet aggregation at all with any concentration of agonist either lack platelet receptors for fibrinogen or are afibrinogenemic. Those who do demonstrate a primary wave of aggregation but not a secondary wave either are unable to release endogenous ADP from dense granules, lack ADP in the dense granules, or have decreased numbers of dense granules. Further evaluation of such individuals with either "release" defects or "storage pool" disorders may require the performance of those specialized release reaction tests referred to previously and special assays of platelet enzyme activities, as well as an estimation of storage pool nucleotides and electron microscopy. The estimation of the adequacy of the storage pool of nucleotides can be performed by determining the ratio of total platelet ATP to ADP. An increased ratio would indicate decreased granule content of nucleotides, since the ATP:ADP ratio in the granules is normally less than in the cytoplasma metabolic pool. Election microscopy permits the direct estimation of granule number in platelets.

Ristocetin-Induced agglutination

Agglutination of platelets after the addition of a 1.5 mg/ml ristocetin solution occurs in the presence of high molecular weight multimers of von Willebrand's factor and glycoprotein Ib-IX on the external coat of the platelet. In the aggregometer, this concentration of ristocetin causes a single wave of agglutination (Fig. 65-5). At lower concentrations it is possible to obtain a biphasic curve due to the induction of a platelet release reaction and subsequent true aggregation.

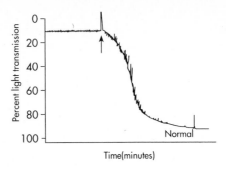

Fig. 65-5 Platelet agglutination obtained with the addition of ristocetin to platelet-rich plasma. *From Hoyer LW: von Willebrands Disease, Prog in Hemostasis and Thrombosis 3:231, 1976.*

This test may be modified so as to quantify high molecular weight von Willebrand multimers present in the plasma, rather than measuring platelet function. In this modification, the degree of ristocetin-induced agglutination of formalin-fixed reagent platelets suspended in the patient's plasma is compared to the degree of agglutination observed with the same reagent platelets when they are suspended in serial dilutions of normal pooled plasma. The concentration of von Willebrand's factor in a patient's plasma is reported as the percentage of activity indicated on a standard curve constructed by plotting the observed degree of agglutination seen with each reagent platelet against the normal plasma dilution specimen (Fig. 65-6). Alternatively, the amount of von Willebrand's factor in the plasma can be determined immunologically by the Laurell technique (Fig. 65-7) and the distribution of multimer sizes can be estimated by crossed immunoelectrophoresis (Fig. 65-8).

Platelet factor 3 availability

Tests to demonstrate platelet factor 3 (PF3) availability are coagulation tests that compare the relative abilities of platelet-rich plasma and platelet-poor plasma to either accelerate coagulation or become deplete of consumable coagulation factors. The former tests are modified assays of the intrinsic system (e.g., activated clotting times) or the common pathway (e.g., Stypven time). The latter tests are modifications of the prothrombin consumption test. They will be discussed in limited detail later in this chapter. These tests are no longer commonly performed since abnormalities in platelet factor 3 availability only rarely exist as isolated defects. Generally, these defects will accompany abnormalities in the release reaction identified by aggregometry.

Clot retraction

Measurement of the retraction of a formed whole blood clot may be performed in conjunction with a whole blood clotting time and a whole blood clot lysis time. Following complete formation of the clot and incubation for 1 hour, the clot is removed and the amount of expressed serum is measured. Normal clot retraction is indicated if the expressed serum is 40% of the volume of the whole blood that had clotted. Abnormal clot retraction may be seen in patients with thrombocytopenia <50,000 or with Glanzmann's thrombasthenia. This poorly standardized test may

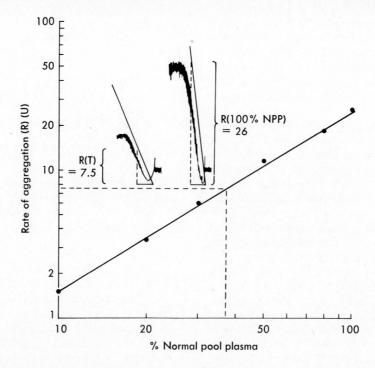

Fig. 65-6   Normal pooled plasma (NPP) dilution curve for quantitation of von Willebrand's factor activity. Each dilution of NPP is plotted against its ristocetin cofactor activity (reflected as the slope of the aggregation wave resulting from ristocetin-induced agglutination of reagent platelet suspended in the dilutions of NPP). Activity of undiluted test plasma (T) is calculated by plotting its agglutination slope against the reference curve. *From Sonnenwirth AC and Jarett L: Gradwohl's clinical laboratory methods and diagnosis, vol 1, ed 8, St Louis, 1980, Mosby–Year Book.*

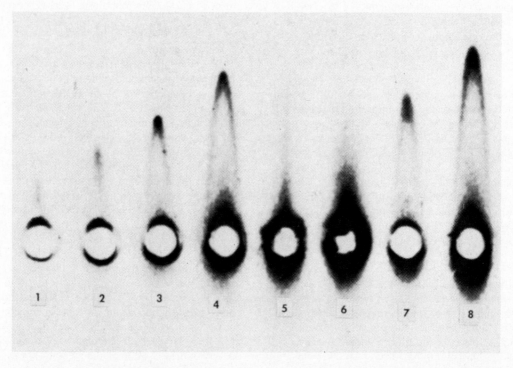

Fig. 65-7   Electroimmunodiffusion quantitation of von Willebrand's protein. Serial dilutions of pooled normal plasma *(wells 1-4);* von Willebrand's plasma *(wells 5-6);* and hemophilia A plasma *(wells 7-8). From Heimburger N and Karges HE: Med Lab 5:1, 1978.*

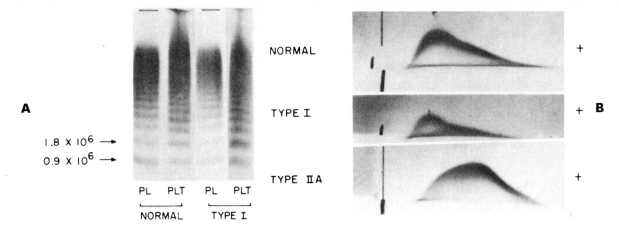

Fig. 65-8 von Willebrand's protein multimers in normal plasma. Separation of multimers by SDS-polyacrylamide gel electrophoresis (a) and distribution of multimers by crossed immunoelectrophoresis (b). The heaviest multimers remain near the origin (cathode) at the top and left of the electrophoretic patterns respectively. *Modified from Weiss H and others: Heterogenous abnormalities in the multimeric structure, antigenic properties, and plasma-platelet content of factor VIII/von Willebrand factor in subtypes of classic (type 1) and variant (type IIA) von Willebrand's disease, J Lab Clin Med 101:413, 1983.*

also be abnormal in patients with hypofibrinogenemia, increased fibrinolysis, polycythemia, or hemophilia. It is now rarely performed, having been largely replaced by aggregometry and tests of global hemostatic function, including thromboelastography and related tests.

Some laboratories still utilize a modification of this test to demonstrate antidrug antibodies in cases of drug-associated immune thrombocytopenia. This test is based upon the demonstration that platelet interaction with antibody leads to cellular damage the interferes with platelet functions, including clot retraction. In this case, the preincubation of a whole blood in the presence of serum containing a drug-dependent antibody and the drug leads to inhibition of clot retraction. In addition, this test has been utilized for the detection of platelet-specific antibodies associated with posttransfusion purpura. In general, however, tests measuring the inhibition of clot retraction have been replaced by more sensitive and specific immunologic assays performed in specialized laboratories.

LABORATORY EVALUATION OF COAGULATION

Screening tests of coagulation separately evaluate the integrity of the extrinsic and intrinsic pathways and the final conversion of fibrinogen to fibrin. All of these tests measure the time required for platelet-poor plasma to clot after exposure to laboratory reagents that reproduce the in vivo actions of tissue factor, platelet phospholipid, or thrombin, respectively. These tests are termed the prothrombin time, partial thromboplastin time, and thrombin time. Prolonged clotting times indicate either decreased levels of one or more coagulation factors, the presence of inactive factors, or the presence of inhibitors, including heparin, which can be detected by specialized assay systems.

Screening tests

The screening tests may be performed manually by tilt tube techniques or in semiautomated and automated timer devices that detect clot formation by changes in either electrical impedance or optical density.

In general, clotting times obtained with manual tests are longer and less reproducible than those obtained with semi-automated or automated instrumentation, and therefore have been largely abandoned. Photoelectric clot timers tend to record shorter times than impedance clot sensors when similar reagents are used.

Although it is generally recommended that tests be performed in duplicate, that agreement between the two results be within a set percentage of the shorter value for the various tests, and that the average time be reported, it has been proposed that the reproducibility of the tests performed with automated instruments is so great that replicate testing may be unnecessary.

Performance of coagulation tests in any of the aforementioned systems require careful standardization of technique. A description of the variables that must be optimized follow. (1) Phlebotomy should be performed in such a way to avoid contamination of the sample with tissue factor or hemolysis of the sample. Reference laboratories recommend the performance of a two-plastic syringe technique or, if using the Vacutainer system, a two-tube technique with submission of the second sample. (2) An appropriate concentration of citrate in the platelet-poor plasma should be regulated. At normal hematocrits, optimum concentration is reached with a whole blood: 3.8% sodium citrate ratio of 9:1. An adjustment to this ratio can be made for elevated or decreased hematocrits (See Fig. 65-4). (3) Stoppered centrifuged whole blood samples collected in Vacutainer tubes should be stored at either room temperature or 4° C,

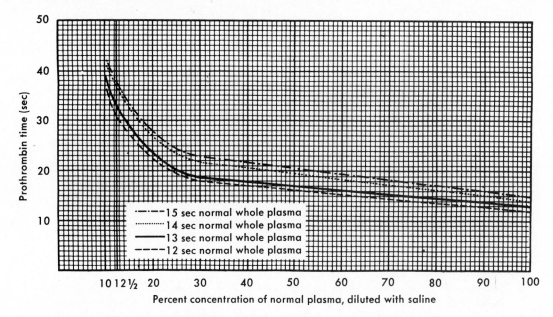

Fig. 65-9 Prothrombin activity curves with representative normal plasmas. *From Bauer JD: Clinical laboratory methods, ed 9, St Louis, 1982, Mosby–Year Book.*

or syringe-drawn samples should be stored in stoppered plastic or siliconized glass tubes at 4°C (melting ice bath) for up to 6 hours. Such storage prevents loss of CO_2 and changes in plasma pH from an optimum of 7.2 to 7.4. (4) Incubation and reaction temperatures should be set at 37°C. (5) Incubation times of reagent and plasma mixtures should be carefully followed to comply with manufacturers' specifications. (6) Reagents should be standardized, and lot-to-lot variation should be controlled, as will be discussed.

It is usual practice in many laboratories to report the patient's clotting times together with control times obtained by testing lyophilized, normal, citrated reagent plasma. Although these control plasmas were designed to be used together with abnormal citrated plasma reagents as quality control checks on the instrument and reagents in use, they have been erroneously thought to always represent a normal standard against which the patient's clotting time should be measured. In utilizing such a control reagent as a normal standard, it is assumed that the plasma pool utilized has been assayed to document 100% activity of all relevant coagulation factors. This is not the case with many commercially available controls. In addition, such a comparison fails to take into account the expected range of values found in normal individuals. For this reason, laboratories should determine their own reference limits for each clotting time test and report results together with these reference values. They should also determine whether the clotting time of the control reagent corresponds to the mean clotting time obtained with normal individuals.

These facts not withstanding, it is common practice to utilize normal level reference plasmas to help interpret the significance of observed clotting times of patient plasmas in the following special situations: the determination of the ratio of patient clotting times to normal times in the regulation of anticoagulant therapy (see Chapter 67), and the construction of dilution curves with $Al(OH)_3$ or $BaSO_4$ absorbed plasma, single factor deficient plasma, or saline (Fig.

65-9). Such curves may be used to regulate anticoagulation with coumarin-type drugs, estimate degrees of factor depletion or dilution in patient plasmas, or as a step in lot-to-lot quality control of laboratory reagents, respectively.

The day-to-day quality control of screening tests utilizing the same lots of reagents consists in the replicate testing of standardized, pooled, reference plasmas with clotting times known to be within the normal (level I), moderately abnormal (level II), and severely abnormal (level III) ranges. The times obtained at each level should fall within 2 SD of the cumulative mean of the preceding day's data. Values found to be out of control or that constitute a continuing drift away from the prior mean should result in reevalution of procedures and reagents prior to the commencement of routine testing.

The change in lots of reagents used for these screening tests requires the determination of whether or not they behave differently than the lots previously in use at varying levels of procoagulant activity. Dilution curves may be constructed for each combination of reagent lots in use, and the characteristics of these curves compared for lot-to-lot variation. In addition, replicate testing of the new lots of levels I, II, and III reagent-pooled plasmas should be carried out and these means compared to those obtained with the prior lots. If the characteristics of the dilution curves are found to be different, or if there is greater than a 2 SD difference between current and prior control times, new reference limits for each screening test should be determined from normal individuals.

Prothrombin time and allied tests

Prothrombin time (PT) examines the integrity of the extrinsic and common pathways by measuring the clotting time of platelet-poor plasma after addition of a prepared "complete thromboplastin" (a substitute equivalent to tissue factor) and Ca^{2+}. Different locally produced and commercial thromboplastins are in use. Most are saline or acetone extracts of either human brain or rabbit lung and brain. Saline extracts of human brain are the thromboplastins in common use in Europe. Many are standardized against reference thromboplastins in an attempt to minimize laboratory-to-laboratory variation (e.g., the British Comparative Thromboplastin and International Reference Preparation). In the United States, commercially available thromboplastins are acetone extracts of rabbit lung and brain. Prothrombin times performed with these reagents are less sensitive to decreases in the concentration of factors VII and the other vitamin K-dependent factors, and therefore tend to give shorter clotting times than those performed with human brain thromboplastin. The reference limits for the clotting times obtained with the former reagents are usually between 10 and 12 seconds, whereas those obtained with the latter thromboplastins are usually between 13 and 15 seconds. Recently, a thromboplastin derived from human placenta has been introduced into use in the United States. This reagent has been standardized against reference thromboplastin and gives similar reference limits.

Using automated techniques, the coefficient of variation for replicate test times within the normal reference limits is reported to be within 1%. Repeat testing of a given sample with prothrombin times in this range should give values within approximately 0.5 seconds of the shorter time.

The prothrombin times in newborn infants between the second and fifth days of life are longer than those found in adults because of decreased levels of factors VII, X, and II, resulting from physiologic vitamin K deficiency. The prothrombin time is the screening test that shows the greatest sensitivity to treatment with coumarin-type anticoagulants (see Chapter 67). In pathologic states, prolongation of the prothrombin time results from a decrease in the procoagulant activity of one or more of the following factors or cofactors: VII, X, V, II, and fibrinogen, or inhibitors to one of these factors or thromboplastin. In addition, inhibitors to the final conversion of fibrinogen to fibrin may cause prolongation of the prothrombin time. As will be discussed (see Chapter 67), the prothrombin time is less sensitive to heparin than is the partial thromboplastin time, which is in turn much less sensitive than the thrombin time.

The sensitivity of the prothrombin time to a decrease in a single factor activity can be determined by the use of dilution curves resulting from plotting the results of prothrombin times performed on serial dilutions of normal pooled plasma made with factor deficient plasmas. Tests using brain thromboplastin usually become abnormal with factor VII levels <40% to 50%, whereas those tests utilizing rabbit thromboplastin may become abnormal only with factor VII levels <30%. The sensitivity of the prothrombin time to decreases in vitamin K-dependent factors can be determined by the use of similar dilution curves resulting from serial dilution with $Al(OH)_3$ or $BaSO_4$ adsorbed plasma (see Chapter 67), whereas the sensitivity of this screening test to multiple factor decreases (e.g., hemodilution) can be estimated by serial dilutions in saline.

The Stypven time also measures the conversion of X to Xa as well as the rest of the common pathway after the addition of Russell's viper venom to plasma. The test is performed to distinguish factor VII deficiency from other causes of prolongation of the prothrombin time. Factor VII and tissue factor are not required for this conversion, since

this snake venom is capable of directly activating X. The test is therefore normal when simple VII deficiency is present, but is generally abnormal if procoagulants required in the common pathway are decreased. Rare variants of factor X deficiency may also be associated with a normal Stypven time. This test is very sensitive to the presence of platelet phospholipid and therefore has also been used as a test for platelet factor 3 activity.

Partial thromboplastin time and allied tests

Partial thromboplastin time (PTT) examines the integrity of the intrinsic system and, to a lesser degree, the common pathway by measuring the clotting time of platelet-poor plasma after addition of a partial thromboplastin (a phospholipid emulsion equivalent to platelet phospholipid) and Ca^{++}.

Numerous different partial thromboplastins are in use. They include: chloroform or ether extracts of acetone-dried bovine or human brian, soybean asolectin, and various other commercial preparations. They have different sensitivities to the factors involved in the intrinsic and common coagulation paths. Most laboratories currently perform the activated partial thromboplastin time (APTT). In these modified tests finely particulate materials are added, with which the contact factors may interact and accelerate the clotting times. Kaolin, celite, silica, and ellagic acid are the materials added to commercially available partial thromboplastins. These substances demonstrate different degrees of clotting activation and sensitivity to the various contact factors. Depending on the partial thromboplastin and activator combination selected, the reference range is usually found to be between 25 and 45 seconds. As with prothrombin time, partial thromboplastin time is prolonged in newborn infants.

Using semiautomated and automated techniques, the coefficient of variation for replicate-activated partial thromboplastin times within the normal reference limits is reported to be within 1.5% to 4%. Repeat testing of a given sample with partial thromboplastin times in this range should give values within 1.5 seconds of the shorter time.

Because of its greater sensitivity to the integrity of the intrinsic pathway, prolongation in the partial thromboplastin time results from a moderate decrease in the procoagulant activity (below 20% to 50% normal activity) of one or more of the following factors or cofactors: XII, prekallikrein, HMWK, XI, IX, and VIII; a more severe decrease in activity of X, V, II (below 10% to 20% activity) and fibrinogen (below 80 to 100 mg/dl); or inhibitors to one of these factors or the partial thromboplastin (lupus-type inhibitor). In addition, inhibitors to the final conversion of fibrinogen to fibrin cause prolongation of the partial thromboplastin time (e.g., fibrin split products and heparin). The fact that heparin causes a gradual prolongation of the partial thromboplastin time in a dose-dependent fashion makes this test that which has found the greatest usefulness in monitoring heparin therapy (see Chapter 67).

The sensitivity of the partial thromboplastin time to a decrease in a single factor activity can be determined by the use of dilution curves resulting from plotting the results of partial thromboplastin times performed on serial dilutions of normal pooled plasma made with factor-deficient plasmas. Laboratories performing tests in facilities that treat large numbers of hemophiliac patients should examine dilution curves made with factor VIII- and factor IX-deficient plasmas to understand the sensitivity of their test systems to these factors.

Generally, the clotting times of these tests become abnormal with factor VIII and IX levels under 25% to 50%. The sensitivity of the partial thromboplastin times to multiple factor decreases (e.g., hemodilution) can be estimated by serial dilutions in saline. Finally, the sensitivity of the different activated partial thromboplastin time tests to varying concentrations of heparin differ, and can be estimated by testing normal pooled plasma mixed with serial dilutions of heparin (see Chapter 67).

The whole blood clotting time was the prototype screening test for demonstrating abnormalities of the intrinsic pathway. It is a manual test that measures the time required to clot nonanticoagulated whole blood in a glass tube, without the addition of extrinsic phospholipid, calcium^{++}, or surface-activating material. Depending on the technique used, normal clotting times are between 5 and 15 minutes. As previously mentioned, the test can be performed in conjunction with subsequent observation of clot retraction and lysis. Because of its insensitivity to all but severe decreases in the clotting factors involved in the intrinsic pathways, it had been largely abandoned as a screening test. A modification of this test (the Lee-White clotting time) is still utilized to measure the adequacy of heparinization (see Chapter 67). Its use in the control of heparin treatment has now been abandoned by most laboratories in favor of either the activated whole blood clotting time (see text that follows) or the partial thromboplastin time.

The recalcification time permits the performance of either whole blood or more commonly, platelet-rich plasma clotting times on blood anticoagulated with sodium citrate. In these tests, calcium is added to the anticoagulated blood or plasma and then the clotting time is recorded. Tests with whole blood are performed manually and give shorter times than those performed with platelet-rich plasma, which can be performed with semiautomated or automated instruments and give longer clotting times (90 to 150 seconds). As with the whole blood clotting time, these tests' relative insensitivity to all but severe decreases in the factors involved in the intrinsic pathway accounts for their decreased use in routine practice. The plasma recalcification time performed simultaneously on platelet-poor and platelet-rich plasma from a patient yields a rough indication to the adequacy of factor 3 availability.

The activated clotting time, as is usually performed, measures the clotting time of nonanticoagulated whole blood that is drawn into tubes containing celite and incubated at 37°C. Although it is more sensitive to decreases in the activities of factors involved in the intrinsic pathway than the whole blood clotting time, its principle use is not found in screening for the integrity of the intrinsic pathway, but in monitoring the adequacy of heparinization. Reference limits for this test are from 1 to 2 ½ minutes. The availability of prepared Vacutainer tubes containing celite and a simple incubator-clot timer device (Hemochron System, International Technidyne Co, Edison, NJ) has made the activated clotting time a frequently used system for intraoperative management of heparin therapy during open heart surgery (see Chapter 67).

Thrombin time and allied tests

Thrombin time (TT) examines the final step in the common pathway leading to the formation of noncross-linked fibrin from fibrinogen. In this test, performed by manual, semiautomated, or automated techniques, thrombin is added in a low enough concentration to result in the clotting of normal citrated plasma in a time range of approximately 15 to 20 seconds. The control time obtained is then compared to the clotting time of patient test plasma. Times greater than 1.3 times the control plasma are considered abnormal. Prolonged thrombin times result from severe hypofibrinogenemia (under 80 to 90 mg/dl), dysfibrinogenemia, inhibitors to fibrin polymerization (e.g., fibrin split products and paraproteins), and heparin. This test is exquisitely sensitive to the presence of even trace amounts of heparin, which may contaminate specimens drawn from arterial lines previously used to obtain samples of blood for blood gas analysis. Because of this sensitivity, which results in the extreme prolongation of the thrombin time with very small amounts of heparin, this test cannot be used to monitor heparin therapy.

In order to eliminate the possibility that prolonged thrombin times are due to heparin contamination, the plasma may be incubated with a solution of protamine sulfate and then the test should be repeated. Protamine sulfate will neutralize any heparin present, but will not alter prolonged thrombin times due to the other causes listed. More conveniently, the reptilase time may be performed to rule out or identify heparin as the cause of a prolonged thrombin time. In this test, the clotting time is determined by substituting a solution of a snake venom from *Bothrops atrox* for thrombin. This snake venom splits fibrinopeptide A from fibrinogen molecules and permits loose, noncross-linked polymerization of the resulting monomers. The reptilase time is prolonged more than 1.3 times the control value in the presence of severe hypofibrinogenemia, dysfibrinogenemia, high levels of fibrin split products, or paraproteins. The reptilase time is normal if the thrombin time prolongation was due to heparin.

Factor assays

Factor assays may be performed by measuring the quantity of active factor in plasma as reflected in the clotting time obtained with appropriately modified screening tests of coagulation, or by measuring the total amount of protein present in the plasma by either immunological or chemical techniques. In addition, more recently, the procoagulant activity of some coagulation factors, as well as the activities of various inhibitors of coagulation, have been measured by the use of chromogenic and fluorogenic substrate techniques.

Prior to the widespread availability of the reagents required to directly assay individual factor activities, laboratories first performed differential prothrombin and partial thromboplastin time tests in order to make presumptive qualitative diagnoses of suspected single factor deficiencies. Thereafter, and when possible, quantification of activity was carried out.

The differential prothrombin time measures the relative ability of normal aged serum (deficient in factors II and V) and normal Al(OH)$_3$-adsorbed citrated plasma or normal BaSO$_4$-adsorbed oxalated plasma (deficient in factors II,

Table 65-2 Combined use of activated partial thromboplastin time (aPTT) and prothrombin time (PT) differential studies*

| Results of original tests | | Correction studies | | | | Probable factor deficiency |
| | | aPTT | | PT | | |
aPTT	PT	Adsorbed plasma	Serum	Adsorbed plasma	Serum	
P	N	C	NC	—	—	VIII
	N	C	C	—	—	XI, XII†
P	N	NC	C	—	—	IX
P	P	C	NC	C	NC	V
P	P	NC	C	NC	C	X‡
P	P	NC	NC	NC	NC	II
N	P	—	—	NC	C	VII

From Bauer JD: Clinical laboratory methods, ed 9, St Louis, 1982, Mosby–Year Book.
*P, prolonged; C, clotting time corrected; —, does not apply; NC, clotting time not corrected.
†Suggested additional test is differential aPTT with celite-adsorbed plasma.

VII, and X) to correct a prolonged prothrombin time when added in a ratio of 1:9 to patient plasma. Similarly, the differential partial thromboplastin time measures the relative ability of these reagent preparations and celite-adsorbed plasma (deficient in factor XI) to correct a prolonged partial thromboplastin time when added in a ratio of 1:9 or 1:5 to patient plasma (Table 65-2).

Fibrinogen assays

Fibrinogen may be measured either as functional fibrinogen in a clotting time test system, as total clottable protein, or as an antigen in an immunologic assay.

Tests that measure functional fibrinogen based on the rate of conversion to fibrin by utilizing a modified thrombin time are the procedures that are most widely utilized. In these tests, all based on the original Clauss method, excess thrombin is added to overcome the presence of inhibitors to the conversion of fibrinogen to fibrin, so that the clotting time obtained usually depends solely on the amount of functional fibrinogen present. Only levels of fibrin degradation products (FDP) >100 μg/ml or very high concentrations of heparin influence this test. Quantification is obtained by comparing the test clotting time with a reference curve constructed from clotting times of standard dilutions of a normal plasma with a known fibrinogen concentration that had been plotted on a log-log paper (Fig. 65-10). With these methods, the fibrinogen concentration reference values are usually found to be between 160 and 400 mg/dl.

The measurement of total clottable fibrinogen can be determined by either chemical or turbidimetric techniques. In the chemical methods based on the original method of Ware and Seegars, the fibrinogen in plasma is clotted by addition of thrombin and then the total protein or tyrosine content of the resultant clot is determined by the biuret reaction or by the addition of the Folin-Ciocalteu reagent, respectively. The results are compared to those obtained using plasma of standardized fibrinogen concentration. These accurate methods are laborious and time-consuming. In the turbidimetric procedure of Ellis and Stransky, the total change in turbidity of plasma following the addition of thrombin and subsequent standardized incubation is an

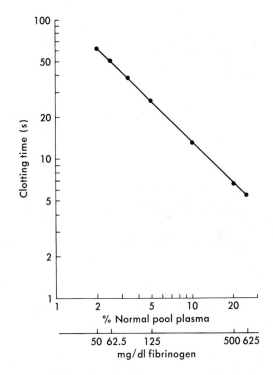

Fig. 65-10   Reference curve for fibrinogen assay (Clauss). *From Sonnenwirth AC and Jarett L: Gradwohl's clinical laboratory methods and diagnosis, vol 1, ed 8, St Louis, 1980, Mosby–Year Book.*

index of the amount of clottable fibrinogen that had been converted to fibrin. Reference values for methods that measure total clottable fibrinogen tend to be higher (200 to 400 mg/dl) than those clotting time assays that measure the rate of fibrin formation. These tests are also less sensitive to the presence of inhibitors than the clotting time tests. A marked discrepancy between the fibrinogen concentration obtained by measuring total clottable protein and that obtained by measuring the clotting time is highly suggestive of dysfibrinogenemia.

Immunologic methods including radial immunodiffusion,

electroimmunodiffusion, or radioimmunoassays, may be unreliable because nonclottable fibrin monomers and dimers, as well as fibrinogen and fibrin degradation products are all measured. The principle utilization of these assays is for the determination of the levels of degradation products in serum.

Factor XIII assays

Screening tests for severe (<2%) factor XIII are dependent on the dissolution of noncross-linked fibrin clots in either a 5 M urea or 2% monochloroacetic acid solution. In these tests, the patient's plasma is first clotted by recalcification; the resultant clot is then suspended in either of these two solutions and finally incubated at 37°C for up to 24 hours. Clots formed from plasma containing less than 2% activity of factor XIII show dissolution of the clot. Mild to moderate factor XIII deficiency is not detected by this method. Quantitative assays for factor XIII concentration in plasma is most easily performed by immunologic assays, particularly electroimmunodiffusion.

Assays of procoagulant activity of other factors

The procoagulant activity of the other clotting factors may be measured as percent activity (i.e., IU/dl of plasma) by comparing the activity of the test plasma to the ability of a pool of citrated normal plasmas (i.e., containing 100% activity or 100 IU/dl) to correct the clotting time of factor-deficient plasma. The clotting tests most commonly used are one-stage assays that are modifications of either the prothrombin time (factors X, VII, V, II) or activated partial thromboplastin time (factors VIII, IX, XI, XII, prekallikrein, HMWK). The reference ranges for each of the factors vary widely, as previously cited (see Chapter 64). Patients with disseminated intravascular coagulation, whose plasma often contain free thrombin and activated X factor, may tend to give falsely elevated factor levels in one-stage tests.

A prototype procedure for single-stage assays is illustrated by the factor VIII procoagulant assay. In this test, the clotting time of a mixture of equal portions of factor VIII-deficient plasma, known to be free of inhibitors, and the patient's diluted plasma (1:5 or 1:10) is compared to a standard curve. The standard curve is obtained by determining and plotting on log-log paper, the clotting times of serial dilutions (1:5 or 1:10 to 1:320) of citrated normal plasma (100% VIII activity), mixed with an equal volume of factor VIII-deficient plasma (Fig. 65-11).

Chromogenic and fluorogenic assays

The proteolytic activity of serine proteases, including activated coagulation factors, can be measured by detecting the release of chromophores or flurophores from synthetic substrates by hydrolysis. The specificity and sensitivity of these enzymatic reactions is determined by the primary, secondary, and tertiary structure of the peptide to which the indicator substance is linked. These peptides are manufactured to closely match the peptide structure of the enzyme's natural substrate.

The chromophore most commonly utilized is para-nitro-analine, which has been bound to the C terminus of the substrate by an acylamide bond. The serine protease hydrolyzes the bond, releasing this chromophore which is then measured spectrophotometrically at 405 nm (Fig. 65-12). The enzyme activity is proportional to the absorbance intensity and is measured as either an end point or a kinetic determination. More recently, fluorophores such as 7-amino, 4-methyl coumarin have been attached to peptide substrates and the intensity of fluorescence released by the enzyme was measured.

Among the manufactured peptide substrates, the best standardized substrates are those for thrombin, Xa, plasmin, kallikrein. In addition, substrates for XIIa, XIa, IXa, and tissue plasminogen activator are becoming available. By appropriate modifications of these assays, the substrates may also be used to assay for their respective zymogens, other factors in multistep indirect assays, and inhibitors of these enzymes. The applications of chromogenic and fluorogenic procedures to assay elements of the fibrinolytic pathway and inhibitors will be referred to later in this section.

The concentration of enzymatic activity measured with these assays can be represented either as percent activity, when the proteolytic activity of the test plasma is compared to that of a known standard, or in nanokatals (one nanokatal equals the activity that converts one nanomole of substrate/second).

The potential advantages of chromogenic and fluorogenic assays include: (1) their potential for standardization, (2) the greater sensitivity and precision of these tests as compared to clotting assays, (3) the requirement for small quantities of plasma, (4) the decreased need for factor-deficient plasma in the laboratory, (5) their great potential for automation. Aside from use with classical spectrophotometric and fluorometric equipment, these assays have been incorporated into several of the automated clot timer devices now available.

The major disadvantages of these tests remain the great cost of some substrates and the lack of available substrates for the direct assay of many coagulation factors.

Immunologic assays of clotting factors

Immunological measurements (e.g., electroimmunodiffusion and radial immunodiffusion) of factors other than fibrinogen are available. These tests are unable to differentiate functional from nonfunctional, but immunologically related molecules. Discrepancy between the results obtained with these assays and those that measure factor procoagulant or proteolytic activity suggests the synthesis of a dysfunctional factor.

Assays for acquired coagulation inhibitors

The presence of acquired inhibitors results in the prolongation of clotting times when various screening tests are performed. Such inhibitors include antibodies directed against coagulation factors or platelet phospholipid, paraproteins, fibrin(ogen) degradation products, and heparin. Assays for the presence of these latter inhibitors, as well as the natural inhibitors of coagulation (serine protease inhibitors and protein C) are dealt with later in this section, while assays for antibodies are discussed shortly.

Screening tests for inhibitor antibodies

The presence of an antibody to one or another coagulation factor is suspected when a patient's prolonged clotting time

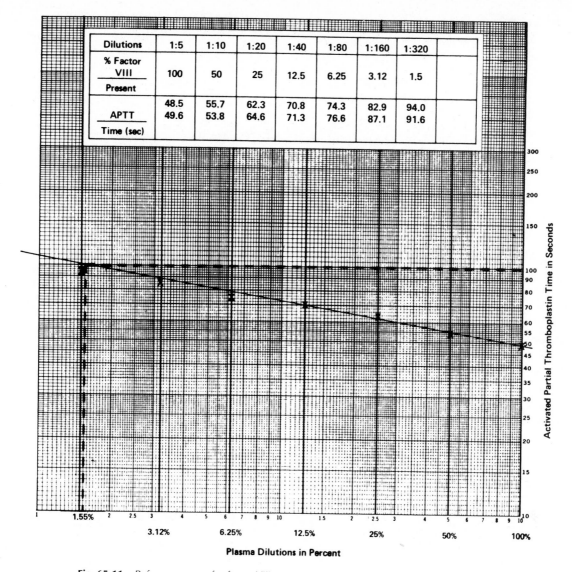

Dilutions	1:5	1:10	1:20	1:40	1:80	1:160	1:320	
% Factor VIII Present	100	50	25	12.5	6.25	3.12	1.5	
APTT Time (sec)	48.5 49.6	55.7 53.8	62.3 64.6	70.8 71.3	74.3 76.6	82.9 87.1	94.0 91.6	

Fig. 65-11   Reference curve for factor VIII assay. *American Hospital Supply Corporation.*

Peptide —— NH— ⬡ —NO₂ $\xrightarrow{\text{ENZ}}$ Peptide——OH + NH₂— ⬡ —NO₂

Fig. 65-12   Chromogenic assays for proteolytic activity. Hydrolytic release of chromophore (para-nitro-analine) from substrate.

is not corrected by the addition of pooled normal plasma. The test is performed by determining clotting times (prothrombin time or activated partial thromboplastin time, as appropriate) on samples of normal pooled plasma, on patients' plasma, and on an equal volume-to-volume mixture of patients' plasma and normal pooled plasma immediately after preparation of the test samples and following an incubation period of 20 to 60 minutes at 37°C. Failure to correct the prothrombin time or activated partial thromboplastin time by the addition of normal plasma to within 2 to 3 or 5 to 6 seconds, respectively, of the times obtained with the normal plasma alone is presumptive evidence of

such an inhibitor. The incubation of the mixture prior to performance of the test is often essential for the detection of slow-acting VIIIC inhibitors.

Weak or low-level inhibitors may fail to be detected with 1:1 test mixtures and their detection may depend on comparing the behavior of varying mixtures of test plasma and normal pooled plasma with similiar mixtures of test plasma and factor-deficient plasma.

Quantitation of factor VIII inhibitors

Acquired inhibitors to factor VIIIC are IgG antibodies that not only develop in 5% to 10% of severe hemophiliacs, but also develop rarely in elderly individuals, postpartum women, and patients with lupus or other autoimmune disorders. Quantitation of these inhibitors is determined by the degree that the factor VIII activity of pooled normal plasma is inhibited by an equal volume of patient plasma in an activated partial thromboplastin time system after 2 hours of incubation at 37°C. The strength of the inhibitor is expressed in Bethesda units/ml of plasma. One Bethesda unit/ml is the concentration of inhibitor in undiluted plasma that is capable of reducing the residual postincubation factor VIII activity of pooled normal plasma to one-half of its starting activity.

Low concentrations of inhibitor (<2 Bethesda units/ml) may be quantified by comparing the residual factor VIII level of the post-incubation plasma mixture with the post-incubation activity of pooled normal plasma (Fig. 65-13).

At a level of greater than 2 to 3 Bethesda units/ml, the accuracy of quantitation is improved by measuring the degree that serial dilutions of patient plasma inhibit the activity of pooled normal plasma and then correcting the calculated inhibitor level for the appropriate dilution factor.

Assays for the lupus inhibitor

These inhibitors are usually IgG antibodies directed against platelet phospholipids that are not infrequently encountered in a wide variety of patients. Their clinical importance and laboratory diagnosis will be discussed later (see Chapter 67).

LABORATORY EVALUATION OF FIBRINOLYSIS

Screening tests for increased fibrinolysis were recognized to be relatively insensitive, but remained in widespread use until convenient assays for the quantitation of fibrin(ogen) degradation products and, more recently, the various components of the fibrinolytic pathway were developed.

Screening tests of fibrinolysis

These tests quantify the time required for formed clots or fibrin plates to undergo lysis. The prototype clot lysis test is the whole blood clot lysis time, which may be performed in conjunction with the whole blood clotting time and clot retraction tests. If normal whole blood is allowed to clot in a glass tube and subsequently incubated at 37°C, no evidence of clot lysis is seen at the end of 48 hours. In the presence of markedly increased fibrinolytic activity, the clot may lyse in as little as a few minutes and is seen as the progressive clot fragmentation and fallout of released red cells (Fig. 65-14). The plasma clot lysis time is a modification of the aforementioned test in which citrated plasma is clotted with thrombin and then the time to clot lysis is measured. The direct observation of whole blood clot lysis is intrinsic to the performance of in vitro global assays of hemostasis (i.e., thromboelastograph and related tests), which will be discussed later in this chapter.

The euglobulin lysis time is not a true screening test of overall fibrinolytic activity. It is a modification of the plasma clot lysis time test, which is a relatively rapid procedure for the detection of increased plasminogen activation and subsequent fibrinolysis, but does not detect decreased fibrinolytic inhibition. In this test, the euglobulin fraction of diluted citrated plasma is precipitated in the cold by acetic acid. This fraction contains fibrinogen, plasminogen, and plasminogen activators, but does not contain fibrinolytic inhibitors. After redissolving this precipitate, the euglobulin solution is clotted with thrombin. The clotted sample is in-

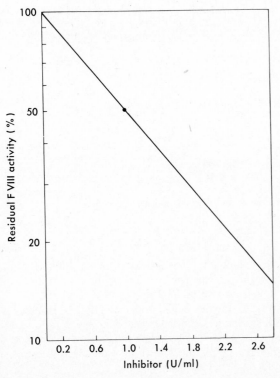

Fig. 65-13 Reference curve for the quantitation of factor VIII inhibitors (Bethesda units). *From Sonnenwirth AC and Jarett L: Gradwohl's clinical laboratory methods and diagnosis, vol 1, ed 8, St Louis, 1980, Mosby–Year Book.*

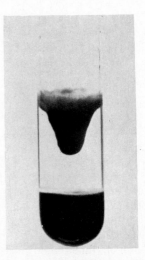

Fig. 65-14 Increased fibrinolysis; incubation of whole blood clot at 37°C. *From Miale JB: Laboratory medicine: hematology, ed 6, St Louis, 1982, Mosby–Year Book.*

cubated at 37°C, and observed at 10 minute intervals until the clot lyses. A euglobulin lysis time of less than 2 hours indicates increased plasminogen activation. Sources of error in the performance of tests include the presence of low levels of fibrinogen, causing the clot to be so small as to make interpretation difficult, and factors that cause local release of tissue plasminogen activator at the venipuncture site, such as vigorous rubbing of the area or maintenance of tourniquet pressure for an extended period to time.

Lysis of fibrin plates by a test plasma is also not truly a global screening test for increased fibrinolysis, but is instead a semiquantitative test to assess the net activity of plasminogen activators, plasmin, and plasmin inhibitors in a test plasma. This activity is proportional to the radius of fibrin lysis about the site of plasma inoculation, when the test is carried out at 37°C incubation for 16 hours (Fig. 65-15). If the test is carried out on plates that have been previously heated to 80°C for 60 minutes, and thus have had their contained plasminogen inactivated, the test only measures

the plasmin and antiplasmin present in the sample. This procedure has been largely abandoned because of the ready availability of assays for the individual components of the fibrinolytic system and the quantification of fibrin(ogen) degradation products.

Specific assays of the fibrinolytic system components

Assays for the various components of the fibrinolytic system include both immunologic tests, which quantitate the amount of antigenically recognizable factor, and functional assays. Among these latter tests, those that are currently most commonly utilized are the chromogenic and fluorogenic assays.

Assays of plasminogen and plasmin

Plasminogen can be measured immunologically by radial immunodiffusion and radioimmunoassay techniques. The finding of normal or elevated levels of immunologically

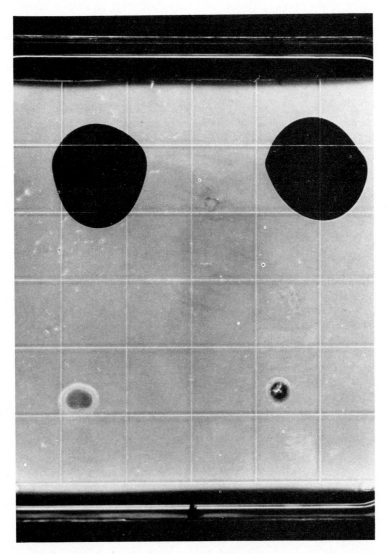

Fig. 65-15 Fibrin plate lysis test. Varying activity shown by different patient samples. *From Sonnenwirth AC and Jarett L: Gradwohl's clinical laboratory methods and diagnosis, vol 1, ed 8, St Louis, 1980, Mosby–Year Book.*

detectable plasminogen with decreased levels of functional plasminogen, as determined in the assays that follow, indicate the presence of dysfunctional plasminogen.

The standard reference methods for assaying the level of functional plasminogen and preformed plasmin rely on the conversion of all plasminogen in the test sample to plasmin by the sequential addition of hydrochloric acid to inactivate antiplasmin and then streptokinase. Following the conversion of plasminogen to plasmin, casein is added to the mixture. The degree of casein digestion is measured in either an ultraviolet spectrophotometer at 275 nm, or in a standard spectrophotometer at 750 nm. The preferred method is that which utilizes the ultraviolet spectrophotometer and is the reference method of the Committee on Thrombolytic Agents (CTA). Plasminogen activity is represented as CTA units/ ml of plasma. The reference range is usually found to be approximately 2.5 to 4.5 μm/ml. Because of the tediousness of these caseinolytic procedures, plasminogen, as well as free plasmin, is now usually measured by chromogenic and fluorogenic assays.

Plasminogen is measured in these assays after conversion to plasmin by streptokinase, whereas free plasmin can be measured by assaying plasma activity without addition of streptokinase. Decreased levels of plasminogen are found in hyperfibrinolytic states, whereas elevated levels may be associated with pregnancy and inflammatory conditions.

Assays of plasminogen activators

Measurement of plasminogen activators is difficult to perform and standardize. A rough assessment can be made by the concurrent observation of fibrin plate lysis and performance of the euglobulin lysis time in conjunction with direct measurement of plasminogen and plasmin levels. Direct measurement is dependent on performance of chromogenic and fluorometric assays, utilizing a recently developed substrate for plasminogen activator. Decreased levels have been proposed as a predisposing factor for thrombosis.

Assay of α₂-antiplasmin

Radial immunodiffusion and electroimmunodiffusion plates are available for measurement of total α₂-antiplasmin as well as measurement of α₂-macroglobulin and other serine protease inhibitors with antiplasmin activity.

Quantitation of total antiplasmin activity is performed by methods that test the ability of plasma to inhibit reagent plasmin. Residual plasmin activity is then measured by caseinolytic, fibrin plate lysis, chromogenic or fluorogenic assays.

Decreased α₂-antiplasmin levels are seen in cases of liver disease, disseminated intravascular coagulation, thrombolytic therapy, and as a congenital disorder (Miyasato disease), whereas increased levels may be associated with a thrombotic tendency.

Assays for fibrin(ogen) degradation products and allied tests

Fibrin and fibrinogen degradation products have been assayed by both nonimmunologic and immunologic tests, the latter constituting the usual methods in use today. The tests vary in their sensitivity to the different early and late products of plasmin digestion.

Nonimmunologic assays for degradation products

The presence of high levels of these products in serum may be suspected by finding a prolongation of the thrombin time if the fibrinogen concentration and its activity is normal and heparin is absent. The staphylococcal clumping test is a sensitive assay for the early degradation products, but also adequately detects the presence of later fragments in either the free form or complexed to fibrin monomer. The test is based on the ability of fibrinogen to clump certain strains of coagulase-negative *Staphylococcus aureus*. It consists of determining the highest dilution of patient serum capable of causing clumping of suspension of bacteria and then calculating the concentration of degradation products from fibrinogen standards run concurrently. The reference limits for this test are usually found to be 0.5 to 2.0 μg/ml. With the development of simple immunologic assays, this test has been largely abandoned by most laboratories.

Immunologic assays for degradation products

The original reference method for the quantitation of degradation products is the tanned red cell hemagglutination assay. In this test, the patient blood is clotted in the presence of a pharmacological inhibitor of fibrinolysis (e.g., ε–aminocaproic acid); the resultant serum is then incubated with serial dilutions of antihuman fibrinogen antiserum and the residual activity of these absorbed antisera to agglutinate a suspension of fibrinogen-coated, tanned red cells is determined in microtiter plates. Inhibition of the activity of the fibrinogen antiserum indicates the presence of fibrin(ogen) degradation products in the patient's serum. The amount of these degradation products is inversely proportional to the dilutional titer of the antiserum still able to agglutinate the coated red cells. Quantitation is determined by comparing this dilutional titer to serial dilutions of a normal plasma of known fibrinogen concentration. Laboratory reference ranges will usually be found to be less than 4 μg/ml. As with the staphylococcal clumping test, the tedious nature of this test has led to its abandonment by many laboratories in favor of the semiquantitative assays discussed shortly.

Simple latex bead agglutination tests are quick, yield semiquantitative results that are clinically useful, and are commercially available in kit form. In one of these kits, the latex beads are coated with antibody fibrinogen, whereas the other beads are coated with antibody to fragments D and E. Although the use of different antibodies would be expected to cause these kits to have different specificities and sensitivities, clinically significant differences have not been found in routine practice. With these tests, levels of degradation products are determined by sample dilution and reported as <10 μg/ml (no diagnostic significance), 10 to 20 μg/dl, 20 to 40 μg/ml, and >40 μg/dl. Both these kits may also detect nonclottable fibrin monomer and fibrinogen (e.g., cryofibrinogen) and thereby falsely indicate the presence of elevated levels of degradation products. As stated, these tests do not discriminate between fibrinogen and fibrin degradation products.

In order to differentiate between positive reactions due to dysfibrinogens, fibrin monomer, and the different degradation products, paracoagulation tests for fibrin monomer, and more recently, the D-D dimer agglutination test, have

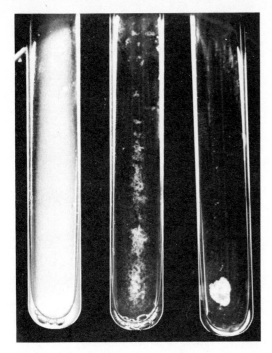

Fig. 65-16   Protamine sulphate paracoagulation test. Serial dilutions of test sample containing fibrin monomers and fibrin degradation products, and showing amorphous precipitation, fibrin strands, and gelation (left to right). *From Niewiarowski S and Gurewich V: J Lab Clin Med 77:665, 1971.*

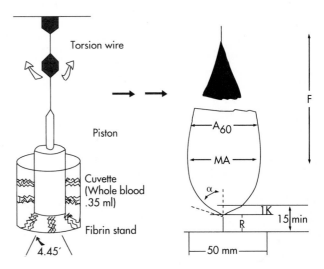

Fig. 65-17   Thromboelastogram. Principle of instrument operation *(left)* and normal tracing *(right)*. See text for details. *From Truman KJ and others: Effects of progressive blood loss on coagulation as measured by thromboelastography, Anesth Analg 66:856, 1987.*

been found to be useful. The paracoagulation tests specifically detect the presence of large fibrin degradation products (X°) and fibrin monomers. In these tests, agents that cause paracoagulation (1% protamine sulfate or 50% ethanol) are able to split fibrin monomers from circulating soluble fibrin monomer-degradation product and fibrin monomer-fibrinogen complexes, and permit monomers and X° fragments to polymerize. A visible gel is formed, which then precipitates. A positive test implies that thrombin was generated and clotting occurred (Fig. 65-16), and thereby differentiates fibrin monomer and fibrin degradation products from fibrinogen degradation products. The recently introduced D-D dimer test is a modification of the classic latex agglutination tests in which latex beads are coated with a monoclonal D-D dimer antibody. This test, although lacking the high sensitivity of other latex agglutination tests, has a high specificity for fibrin degradation products.

IN VITRO TESTS OF GLOBAL HEMOSTATIC FUNCTION

As previously described, the whole blood clotting time and the subsequent observation of the formed clot can be a rough measure of multiple facets of in vitro hemostasis including: adequacy of platelet count, platelet function, the intrinsic pathways of coagulation, and fibrinolysis. The usefulness of whole blood clotting time is greatly limited by the time required to complete the study through clot incubation and its poor sensitivity to changes in the extrinsic pathway of coagulation, mild impairments in platelet function, and moderate increases in fibrinolytic activity. It therefore can-

not be considered a clinically useful measure of global hemostatic function.

Subsequent modifications of the aforementioned procedure, in which the viscoelastic properties of blood are measured during clot formation, and its subsequent evolution, have found their way into clinical practice. Although the sensitivity and time requirements for test performance have been greatly improved by the use of these procedures, they still do not qualify as optimum tests of global hemostatic function. They are predominantly used to monitor the hemostatic integrity of surgical patients undergoing massive transfusion, or procedures known to be associated with significant hemostatic perturbations (e.g., cardiopulmonary bypass and liver transplantation).

The thromboelastographic instruments available detect changes in the viscoelastic properties of the blood during and after clotting by measuring shear elasticity (Fig. 65-17). In this procedure, a cuvette containing the patient's whole blood is rotated. During clotting, fibrin strands form between the wall of the cuvette and a central piston. Shear develops on the central piston as the cuvette rotates. As the fibrin strands develop, the central piston is placed in motion. The movements of the central piston are recorded, and the various parameters shown in Fig. 65-17 are measured over time.

The initial reaction time (R) is dependent on levels of procoagulant and the presence of anticoagulants, whereas the subsequent time measurement of initial clot buildup (K) is primarily a reflection of procoagulant levels and factor XIII activity. The R value corresponds to the other clotting

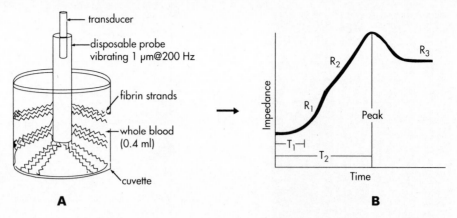

Fig. 65-18   Sonoclot. **A,** Principle of instrument operation. **B,** normal tracing. See text for details. *From Anesthesiol News July, p 34, 1988.*

assays of the intrinsic pathway. The rate of clot development (K) and the maximal clot development (MA) are dependent on the fibrinogen level, platelet count, and platelet function. An index of clot lysis can be derived by measuring amplitude of the clot at 1 hour and dividing by the maximal clot amplitude (A60/MA). The whole blood clot lysis time may be measured as well (F).

A more recently introduced technology (Sonoclot, Sienco Inc, Morrison, Colo) measures the viscoelastic properties of blood during clotting by changes in impedance to vibration (Fig. 65-18). In this procedure, the patient's blood is placed in a stationary cuvette and clotting is detected as fibrin strands form between the cuvette wall and a vibrating probe. The subsequent changes in impedance are then recorded. The onset time (T) is related to the level of procoagulants and the presence of anticoagulants, whereas the primary rate of clot formation (R1) is related principally to the levels of procoagulant. The secondary rate of clot formation (R2) is principally related to fibrinogen concentration, platelet count, and platelet function. The rate of clot retraction (R3) is an index of platelet function. Fibrinolysis is reflected in the degree that the formed clot tracing after retraction tends to return toward the baseline.

SUGGESTED READING

Coller BS: Platelet aggregation by ADP, collogen and ristocetin: a critical review of methodology and anaylsis. In Schmidt RM (editor): CRC handbook series in clinical laboratory science. Section I: hematology. Boca Raton, Fla, 1972, CRC Press.

Day HJ: Laboratory tests in platelet function. In Schmidt RM (editor): CRC handbook series in clinical laboratory science. Section I: hematology. Boca Raton, Fla, 1972, CRC Press.

Giddings JC and Peake IR: Laboratory support in the diagnosis of coagulation disorders, Clin Haematol 14:571, 1985.

Italian CISMEL Study Group: Multicentre comparison of nine coagulometers and manual tilt-tube methods for prothrombin time performance, Clin Lab Haematol 5:177, 1983.

Mielke CH and Rodvien R: Bleeding time procedures. In Schmidt RM (editor): CRC handbook series in clinical laboratory science. Section I: hematology. Boca Raton, Fla, 1972, CRC Press.

Triplett DA: Synthetic substrates: a revolution in the diagnostic coagulation laboratory. In Triplett DA (editor): Recent advances in hemostasis and thrombosis, Chicago, 1982, American Society of Clinical Pathologists.

66 Laboratory diagnosis of hemorrhagic disorders

Robert F. Reiss

Hemorrhage may be due to either the primary physical disruption of the vascular continuity or to a defect in the normal hemostatic mechanism because of failure of primary hemostasis (formation of a platelet plug), secondary hemostasis (clot formation), or fibrinolytic inhibition (increased fibrinolysis).

DISORDERS OF PRIMARY HEMOSTASIS
Hemorrhagic manifestations of primary defects

Regardless of whether or not the cause is due to decreased numbers of platelets (thrombocytopenia), platelet dysfunction, or primary vascular abnormality (Box 66-1), hemorrhagic diathesis results from a failure of normal capillary integrity. The spontaneous bleeding seen is therefore largely from small blood vessels. In the skin, this is seen as petechiae and ecchymosis. Hemorrhage most frequently arises from the mucous membranes (e.g., gastrointestinal tract, urinary tract, and respiratory tree). The severity of bleeding is related to the degree of the thrombocytopenia or type of dysfunction. With severe defects in primary hemostasis, intracerebral bleeding occurs.

Thrombocytopenia

Platelet counts below 100,000/μl are associated with a progressive increase in bleeding time. Spontaneous bleeding is rare at counts above 30,000/μl and surgical hemostasis is usually normal with counts above 50,000/μl. As the count falls below 30,000/μl, the risk of hemorrhage had been considered to increase significantly. At counts under 10,000/μl, there is concern that patients are at a significant risk of intracranial hemorrhage (Fig. 66-1). In situations characterized by numerous megathrombocytes with thrombocytopenia and increased platelet turnover (e.g., autoimmune thrombocytopenia), the hemorrhagic risk is often less than would have been predicted on the basis of a platelet count corresponding to the relatively short bleeding time seen in these instances (Fig. 66-2). Recently, it has been shown that spontaneous blood loss from the bowel does not increase until the platelet count falls below 5000/μl if the function of the platelets is normal (Fig. 66-3).

The diagnosis of thrombocytopenia based upon results obtained by a particular counter should be confirmed by examination of the peripheral smear in order to rule out pseudothrombocytopenia. This is a condition in which platelets may be agglutinated together or about leukocytes (plate-

let satellitism) by autoantibodies, which are often ethylenediamine tetracetic acid (EDTA)-dependent (Fig. 66-4). The agglutinated platelets are therefore not counted by the particle counter.

Thrombocytopenia can result from simple underproduction, ineffective thrombopoesis with intramedullary destruction, disorders of distribution (i.e., splenomegaly), increased destruction due to immune destruction, or increased consumption. The various etiologies of thrombocytopenia are described in Box 66-2.

Hypoproliferative thrombocytopenias

Thrombocytopenias associated with congenital or acquired marrow hypoplasia, isolated megakaryocytopenia, or marrow replacement result in the decreased production of platelets that have a normal or modestly decreased peripheral survival. The bone marrow contains decreased numbers of megakaryocytes, which in many conditions tend to be larger than usual with increased ploidy due to a continued thrombopoietic stimulus.

Congenital thrombocytopenias may be inherited and associated with Fanconi's anemia or an isolated defect in congenital thrombocytopenia with absent radii (TAR syndrome); may follow intrauterine infections; or may be subsequent to the ingestion of drugs during pregnancy. Acquired megakaryocytic hypoplasia may occur in aplastic anemia or as an isolated defect following marrow irradiation, during or after infections (e.g., sepsis, hepatitis), and after drug ingestion. Hypoplastic thrombocytopenia associated with marrow replacement is characterized by the presence of megathrombocytes and a leukoerythroblastic reaction in the peripheral blood.

Ineffective thrombopoiesis also results in hypoproliferative thrombocytopenias. These conditions are characterized by increased numbers of megakaryocytes that are smaller than usual with decreased ploidy. The platelets produced have relatively normal peripheral survival. Congenital syndromes are generally inherited and include isolated thrombocytopenias transmitted as autosomal-dominant traits, as well as several complex syndromes. In the May-Hegglin anomaly, which is transmitted as an autosomal-dominant trait, moderate thrombocytopenia is associated with megathrombocytes and the presence of Döhle's bodies in neutrophils. Thrombocytopenia with megathrombocytes may be seen in Alport's syndrome, which is associated with ne-

1025

Box 66-1 Vascular purpura

Hereditary hemorrhagic telangiectasia
Osteogenesis imperfecta
Marfan syndrome
Ehlers-Danlos syndrome
Pseudoxanthoma elasticum
Senile purpura
Stasis purpura
Schönlein-Henoch syndrome
Autoerythrocyte sensitivity
Scurvy
Dysproteinemias

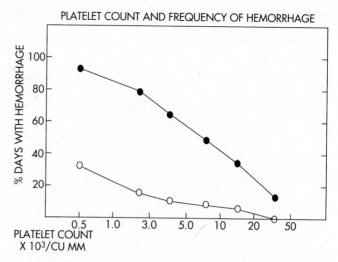

PLATELET COUNT AND FREQUENCY OF HEMORRHAGE

Fig. 66-1 The frequency of hemorrhage as it relates to platelet count. The frequency of all episodes of hemorrhage rises as the platelet count falls under 30,000/mm³ *(closed circles)* and the frequency of severe hemorrhage rises significantly as the count falls under 10,000/mm³ *(open circles). Redrawn from Gaydos and others: N Engl J Med 266:906, 1966.*

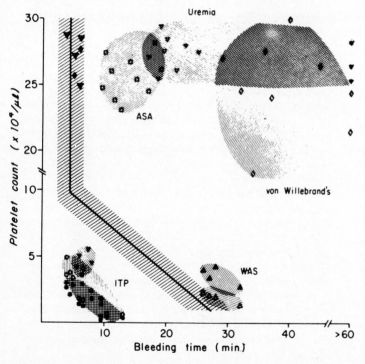

Fig. 66-2 Unexpectedly short bleeding times found in patients with thrombocytopenia and increased platelet turnover. Such patients include those with autoimmune thrombocytopenia *(circles)* and some in whom marrow function is returning after chemotherapy related myelosuppression *(inverted solid triangles). From N Engl J Med 287:155, 1972.*

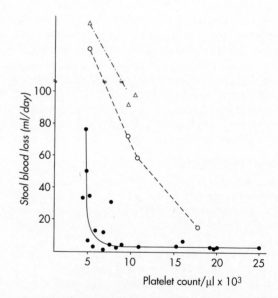

Fig. 66-3 Fecal blood loss in aplastic thrombocytopenic patients increases as the platelet count falls below 5000 to 10,000/mm³(•), unless the patient is treated with systemic corticosteroids (20 to 60/mg prednisone, 0) or semisynthetic penicillin (Δ). *From Slichter SJ and Harker LA: Clin Haematol 7:3, 531, 1978.*

phritis and nerve deafness. The Bernard-Soulier syndrome is an autosomal-recessive disorder characterized by mild thrombocytopenia, megathrombocytes in the peripheral smear, and abnormal platelet adhesion. This syndrome is described more fully later in this chapter. The Wiskott-Aldrich syndrome is an X-linked disorder of male children in which thrombocytopenia, microthrombocytes, and ab-

normal platelet aggregation are associated with decreased IgM levels, eczema, and an increased incidence of infections. Patients who survive early infancy have a predisposition for the development of lymphoid malignancies. Acquired ineffective thrombopoiesis is most commonly seen in patients with folate or vitamin B_{12} deficiency, or rarely, as an idiopathic disorder in patients with myelodysplastic syndromes.

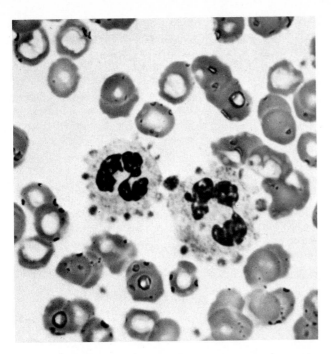

Fig. 66-4   Platelet satellitism about neutrophils. *From Bauer JD: Clinical laboratory methods, ed 9, St Louis, 1982, Mosby—Year Book.*

Box 66-2   Etiopathogenesis of thrombocytopenia

HYPOPROLIFERATION

Marrow hypoplasia (drugs, chemicals, radiation, infection, congenital)

Marrow replacement (leukemia, lymphoma, carcinoma, fibrosis)

Ineffective thrombopoiesis (vitamin B_{12} and folate deficiency, familial)

DISORDERS OF DISTRIBUTION (SPLENOMEGALY)
(congestive, myeloid metaplasia, tumor, parasite)

INCREASED CONSUMPTION
Nonimmune consumption

Altered vascular surface (vasculitis, TTP, prosthetic device)
Sepsis
Disseminated intravascular coagulation

Immune consumption

Autoantibodies and immune complexes (ITP, SLE, lymphomas, viral)
Alloantibodies (neonatal, post-transfusion)
Drug-related antibodies

DILUTIONAL THROMBOCYTOPENIA (massive transfusion)

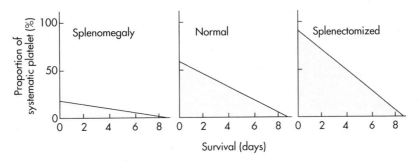

Fig. 66-5   Platelet survival studies with Cr-51—labeled platelets, comparing the decreased recovery found in patients with splenomegaly with the 50% to 60% recovery seen in normal individuals and near 90% recovery seen in splenectomized patients. Note the normal survival of recovered platelets. *From Thompson AR and Harker LA: Manual of hemostasis and thrombosis, ed 3, Philadelphia, 1983, FA Davis.*

Hypersplenism

Patients with hypersplenism have thrombocytopenia due to increased sequestration of platelets in the spleen. Most characteristically, this is accompanied by anemia, as previously described (Chapter 64). The platelet count rarely falls below 50,000/μl, regardless of the degree of splenomegaly, because of the compensatory increase of platelet production. Postinfusion recovery and survival studies show decreased recovery of the infused platelets, but a normal survival of those that circulate (Fig. 66-5).

Consumptive thrombocytopenias

Consumptive thrombocytopenias result from a significantly shortened peripheral life span of platelets which is not compensated by an increased platelet production in the bone marrow. The bone marrow aspirate contains increased numbers of megakaryocytes and the peripheral blood may contain an increased proportion of megathrombocytes. These thrombocytopenias may be classified into those caused by increased nonimmune consumption and those caused by immune destruction.

Nonimmune consumption. Platelets may be consumed on large, de-endotheliazed surfaces (e.g., extensive surgical dissections), in diffuse vasculitis, on prosthetic devices, or on the surfaces of extracorporeal oxygenators during open heart surgery, as will be discussed. Patients with sepsis are often severely thrombocytopenic. Not only do those patients have suppressed megakaryocytic proliferation, but the circulating platelets tend to become sequestered in foci of infection. Platelets are consumed rapidly in patients with disseminated intravascular coagulation, as will be discussed later in this chapter.

Thrombotic thrombocytopenic purpura (TTP). This is also known as Moschcowitz's syndrome, and is characterized by progressive thrombocytopenia; the formation of widespread hyaline thrombi in small blood vessels leading to cerebral, hepatic, and renal insufficiency; and a microangiopathic hemolytic anemia. Its cause is unknown; however, its temporal clustering and frequent antecedent history of a viral infection is suggestive of an infectious or postinfectious immune etiopathogenesis. Histopathologic evidence appears to implicate a primary vascular abnormality characterized by subendothelial hyaline change. This thesis is supported by the observation that endothelial cells from patients with TTP synthesize reduced quantities of prostacylin. Other data implicate humoral factors as the major mediators of this disorder. Although a platelet aggregating factor has been isolated from the plasma of some patients that is inhibited by normal plasma, it is believed that aggregation may not be a primary event. Indeed, it is likely that the agglutination phenomenon observed may not be true aggregation, since the release of granule contents (e.g., β-thromboglobulin) has not been observed. More recently, it has been found that patients with TTP possess increased levels of von Willebrand's factor (vWF) and unusually large vWF multimers of the protein. It has been postulated that during periods of disease activity, these superlarge multimers bind to platelets and are capable of causing platelet agglutination. It is thought that normal plasma contains a depolymerase that regulates the size of vWF multimers. These observations form the basis for treatment of TTP with plasma infusions and/or exchange.

The origin of these ultralarge monomers is unknown, but it is suggested that they may be released from damaged endothelial cells. The clinical presentation of this disorder varies from an acute, rapidly progressive form to a more insidious, slowly developing syndrome. Most patients with TTP present with neurologic changes and fever. In addition, some patients also present with progressive renal failure and hematuria. Patients with a clinical picture predominated by renal disease may be considered to have hemolytic-uremic syndrome.

Laboratory studies reveal a microangiopathic hemolytic anemia with a falling hematocrit, the presence of schistocytes in the peripheral smear, reticulocytosis, reduced haptoglobin, increased indirect bilirubin and elevated red cell lactate dehydrogenase (LDH) serum levels, as well as thrombocytopenia. Resolution of the disease is heralded by a rising platelet count and reduction in LDH to normal levels. The disappearance of schistocytes from the peripheral smear may be delayed for weeks after resolution of the disease. Some patients may undergo dramatic permanent remission, whereas others may experience a chronic relapsing form.

Immune thrombocytopenias. Immune-mediated destruction of platelets may be caused by autoantibodies or alloantibodies directed against antigens located in the platelet glycocalyx, circulating immune complexes, or drugs. Techniques to demonstrate increased levels of platelet-associated IgG (PAIgG), other immunoglobulins, or complement were developed in an attempt to devise sensitive and specific tests for the diagnosis of immune thrombocytopenias, which are analogous to the direct Coombs' test. The types of tests developed to quantify PAIgG are based upon either the demonstration of subsequent complement binding, direct reaction with the platelet surface, or reaction of an antiglobulin serum or staphylococcal protein A with eluted antibody or solubilized membranes.

The degree of complement binding to PAIgG is proportional to the quantity of IgG on the platelet membrane, and is quantified by the degree that preincubation with the test platelets inhibits complement-mediated lysis of sensitized red cells. This complement lysis inhibition assay (CLI) was one of the first tests produced to detect PAIgG. The test not only detects platelet-bound IgG_1 and IgG_3 antibodies, but also detects immune complexes. Although sensitive and accurate, it is tedious to perform and difficult to standardize.

The various types of direct antiglobulin tests are more sensitive to the presence of IgG antibodies on the platelet surface than to the presence of immune complexes. Many of the older tests discussed shortly are sensitive and accurate, but are also tedious and difficult to standardize. The original method utilized was the Fab-anti-Fab technique, in which PAIgG on test platelets proportionally binds reagent anti-Fab and decreases the amount of anti-Fab that is available to combine with iodine[125] labelled Fab fragments, and subsequently precipitates as a quantifiable immune complex. A related test is the quantitative antiglobulin consumption test (ACT). In this test, preincubation of anti-IgG with platelets bearing PAIgG inhibits the subsequent reaction of an antiglobulin reagent with IgG on sensitized red cells in the presence of complement, thereby inhibiting the lysis of these red cells.

Newer developed direct antiglobulin tests are somewhat simpler and more easily standardized. The radioimmune antiglobulin test (RIAT) measures the direct binding of iodine[125] labelled anti-IgG to the surface of test platelets and then compares the bound radioactivity with that observed when platelets from normal controls are incubated with the antiglobulin reagent. The platelet suspension immunofluorescence test (PSIFT) measures the strength of immunofluorescence acquired by paraformaldehyde-fixed test platelets after incubation with fluorescent-labeled anti-IgG and direct examination by fluorescent microscopy. Quantitative measurement is possible by cytofluorometry. In this widely used test, positive results due to fixation of immune complexes are weaker. Also in these cases, eluates prepared from nonformalinized platelets are found to be nonreactive with fixed reagent platelets. Enzyme-linked immunosorbent assays (ELISA) have been developed. Those utilizing microdilution plate technology entail the fixation of patient platelets to the wells of the plate, incubation with perioxidase-conjugated anti-IgG, and detection of antiglobulin fixation by the addition of a suitable substrate. Quantification of IgG sensitization is determined photometrically in an ELISA reader. More recently, the quantification of bound PAIgG has been performed with iodine[125] labelled staphylococcal protein A binding assay (SPA). In this assay, the platelets under study are lysed by freeze-thawing, and serial dilutions of an initial standardized suspension are incubated in microtiter plate wells to allow platelet protein adherence. Following this step, anti-IgG is added to each well and the amount of immune complex formed is quantitated by subsequently measuring the amount of iodine[125] labelled staphylococcal protein A bound. This test is sensitive to the presence of

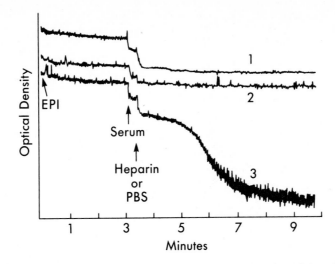

Fig. 66-6   Platelets in platelet-rich plasma from a patient with heparin-associated thrombocytopenia, to which had been added a subaggregatory dose of epinephrine, undergo aggregation with the sequential addition of the patient's serum and heparin (3), whereas no aggregation is seen if phosphate-buffered saline is substituted for heparin (2) or nonimmune plasma is substituted for the patient's plasma (1). *From McMillan RE (editor): The immune cytopenias, New York, 1983, Churchill Livingstone.*

all IgG subclasses except IgG_3.

In addition to the aforementioned tests, simple immunoassays have been developed to directly measure the amount of associated IgG present on solubilized platelets. These assays measure the formation of immune complexes in standard immunodiffusion (ID), electroimmunoassay (rocket technique, EIA), or nephelometric tests. Although simple to perform, accurate testing is dependent on the preparation of purified platelet suspensions and careful standardization.

Techniques to demonstrate antiplatelet antibodies include tests that measure the effect of these antibodies on normal platelet function and tests that measure the formation of PAIgG on normal platelets (indirect PAIgG assays). Among the former type of tests, the simplest technique is the clot retraction inhibition test. In this test, the presence of antibody in patient serum inhibits the retraction of a clot formed in normal blood. This test has been found to be insensitive and is rarely performed. It's only currently used in some laboratories to demonstrate some antidrug antibodies responsible for immune complex-mediated thrombocytopenia (e.g., quinidine). In this test, addition of the drug to the test system is essential to inhibit clot retraction. Platelet factor 3 release and serotonin release methods have also been developed to demonstrate allo- and autoantibodies. These techniques are also no longer widely utilized except to demonstrate antidrug antibodies, including those responsible for heparin-associated thrombocytopenia. Induction of platelet aggregation by serum antibodies is a technique that has found its greatest utility in the demonstration of antiheparin antibodies. In this test, platelets sensitized with subaggregation doses of epinephrine undergo aggregation following subsequent addition of patient serum and heparin to the test system (Fig. 66-6).

Most allo- and autoantibodies are detected best by immunological assays. All of the PAIgG-antiglobulin assays previously described have been adapted as indirect tests.

Among those most commonly utilized are the ELISA and PSIFT tests. In addition, the Chromium[51] release procedure has found wide application for the demonstration of allo- and autoantibodies. In this test, the presence of complement-fixing antibodies is elucidated by demonstrating cytolysis of Chromium[51] labeled reagent platelets that have been pretreated with either bromelin or papain. This test has also found extensive application in the demonstration of drug-dependent antibodies.

Idiopathic thrombocytopenia purpura (ITP). This term describes a group of disorders characterized by immune-mediated destruction of platelets in the reticuloendothelial system, which are not secondary to other immune disorders, caused by alloantibodies or associated with drug therapy. Included in this group are those disorders that may be caused by either circulating immune complexes or autoantibodies.

Acute ITP is usually a disorder of childhood. Both sexes are equally affected. In over 80% of the cases, the disease appears 1 to 6 weeks after the onset of a viral infection. Most commonly, these infections are nonspecific respiratory illnesses. It is thought that immune complexes formed by viruses and antiviral antibodies attach to the fc receptors on the platelet glycocalyx. Recent evidence has also implicated the formation of antibodies directed against glycocalyx constituents in some cases. These platelets are then cleared from the circulation by the RES. The period of thrombocytopenia lasts from 4 to 6 weeks, and in more than 80% of the cases, the patients undergo permanent remission. Overall mortality is about 1% and is due to intracerebral bleeding. The pathogenesis of thrombocytopenia associated with human immunodeficiency virus (HIV) infection is unclear, but may in part also be mediated by removal of immune complex-coated platelets. The HIV-associated thrombocytopenia will be discussed separately.

Thrombocytopenia is usually severe. Megathrombocytes are seen on the peripheral smear. Examination of the bone marrow reveals increased numbers of megakaryocytes,

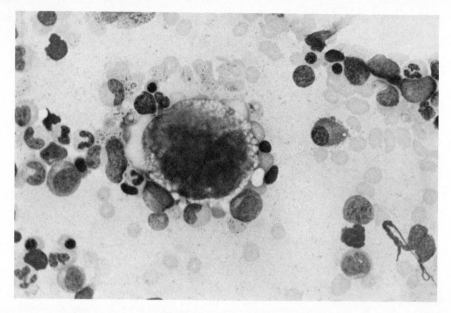

Fig. 66-7 Megakaryocyte with vacuolated cytoplasm and reduced numbers of budding platelets in ITP. *From Bauer JD: Clinical laboratory methods, ed 9, St Louis, 1982, Mosby–Year Book.*

which may appear vacuolated and have reduced numbers of budding platelets at their margins (Fig. 66-7). The survival of transfused platelets is markedly shortened, with half-lives measured in hours rather than days. As stated, the bleeding time is usually found to be shorter than would have been anticipated from the platelet count (Fig. 66-2).

Although increased PAIgG is found on the surface of platelets of many patients, the diagnostic specificity of this finding is poor except in laboratories with carefully determined reference value ranges for normal subjects and patients with other immune and nonimmune thrombocytopenias, as will be described. Tests of the patients' serum to detect specific antibodies directed against platelet surface antigens are most often negative.

Chronic ITP is most commonly a disease of young and middle-aged adults. Women are affected three times as frequently as men. It generally appears insidiously and is associated with the HLA-DR2 antigen. Chronic ITP is believed to be due to the formation of autoantibodies directed against specific glycoproteins of the platelet glycocalyx. Fewer than 10% of patients with chronic ITP undergo spontaneous remission.

The thrombocytopenia is generally not as severe as that seen in acute ITP and usually ranges from 30,000 to 80,000/μl. The bone marrow findings and platelet survival studies are similar to acute ITP. Although some patients have shorter than anticipated bleeding times, in others, they may be markedly prolonged. It is believed that the autoantibodies may block expression of the functional activities of the surface glycoproteins.

Most of the various methodologies described are able to detect increased PAIgG in 85% to 95% of patients (Table 66-1). In addition, increased bound IgM and C3 is found in 50% to 60% of patients. Although the diagnostic specificity of increased PAIgG is limited, there appears to be a direct relationship between the severity of the reduction in platelet count and the quantity of PAIgG. Many believe that the routine determination of PAIgG and other platelet-associated immunoglobulins or complement add little essential information to the diagnosis of ITP and that these techniques should remain research tools.

Antiplatelet antibodies are found in 30% to 90% of cases depending on the technique utilized. They are usually IgG$_1$ antibodies and most commonly have specificity for the GPIIbIIIa complex, and more rarely for GPIb. Patients who respond to corticosteroids, splenectomy, or other immunosuppressive therapy will have decreased levels of PAIgG and reduced titers of antiplatelet antibody in their sera after treatment.

Since the antibody causing ITP is usually an IgG molecule, it crosses the placenta. For that reason, about 50% of babies born to women with ITP are thrombocytopenic. Since some believed that severely thrombocytopenic (<50,000 μl) babies should not be exposed to the trauma of vaginal delivery, it is a common procedure to determine the platelet count of a baby prior to birth by either scalp skin sampling under direct vision or umbilical vein sampling with ultrasound guidance.

Table 66-1 PAIgG in chronic ITP

Method	No. patients	Percent elevated (%)
C L inhibition	367	87
Fab-Anti-Fab	31	94
I-125 Antiglobulin	131	84
Staphylococcal protein A	70	89
ELISA	20	90
PSIFT	70	89

Modified from Morse BS and Giuliani D: Measurement of platelet-associated antibody with immunodiffusion and nephelometry. In McMillan R (editor): *Immune cytopenias*, New York, 1983, Churchill Livingston.

An ITP-like syndrome may be associated with a wide variety of other immune disorders, including patients with lupus erythematosus, malignant lymphoma, chronic lymphatic leukemia and, HIV infection. Up to 2% of patients with ITP subsequently develop lupus erythematosus, whereas not unusually, patients with lupus develop immune-mediated thrombocytopenia. Although in some cases anti-platelet antibodies have been demonstrated, most cases are due to immune complex deposition on the patient's platelets. A lupus-like syndrome with thrombocytopenia can be seen in patients treated with procainamide.

The thrombocytopenia associated with HIV infection is complex and may be related to multiple mechanisms acting together. Aside from inhibition of hematopoiesis, a moderate to severe ITP-like syndrome is seen in many patients with HIV infections, acquired immunodeficiency syndrome (AIDS), or AIDS-related complex (ARC). Laboratory tests reveal increased levels of PAIgG and circulating immune complexes.

Alloimmune thrombocytopenias. These disorders are due to the interaction of alloantibodies with antigens belonging to one of the platelet-specific antigen systems (Table 66-2). Among these various antibodies, the antibody against the PL^A1 antigen is that which is most commonly responsible for the two syndromes seen in clinical practice.

Alloimmune (isoimmune) neonatal thrombocytopenia is caused by the transplacental passage of an IgG antibody against a platelet-specific antigen and is a consequence of sensitization of an antigen-negative woman through pregnancy or transfusion. An antigen-positive fetus experiences severe thrombocytopenia ($<50,000/\mu l$) that persists for 2 to 3 weeks. The disease may affect the firstborn. Laboratory examination shows the mother to be PL^A1 negative in about 50% of cases, and in 80% to 90% of these cases, she is shown to possess anti-PL^A1 antibody in her serum, which is best detected by PSIFT and Chromium[51] release assays. The newborn's platelets possess increased PAIgG. The performance of platelet counts on predelivery umbilical cord or fetal scalp vein sampling can assist in deciding whether or not delivery by vaginal or caesarean section is preferable (as was previously discussed). Treatment is based on the transfusion of platelets from volunteer donors known to be PL^A1-negative or washed platelets from the mother obtained by plateletpheresis.

Posttransfusion purpura is a rare syndrome characterized by the sudden onset of severe thrombocytopenia 1 to 2 weeks after transfusion of red cell or platelet concentrates in an individual possessing an alloantibody against one of the platelet-specific antigens, most commonly PL^A1 (70% to 80%). Its pathogenesis is poorly understood, since no adequate explanation has been offered for the destruction of the patient's own antigen-negative cells during the reaction between the alloantibody and transfused antigen-positive platelets. A suggestion has been made that the PL^A1 antigen may elute off the transfused platelets and bind to the patient's own platelets, thereby exposing them to the action of antibody. Patients are almost always multiparous women who became sensitized during previous pregnancies. The thrombocytopenia can last for several weeks before spontaneously resolving itself. The antibody can be demonstrated in over 90% of cases occurring in PL^A1-negative patients. The PSIFT and Chromium[51] release assays appear to be the most sensitive for detecting antibody in this condition. In many cases the presence of the PL^A1 antibody is accompanied by anti-HLA antibodies.

Drug-associated immune thrombocytopenias. A wide variety of drugs have been associated with the immune destruction of platelets (Box 66-3). The most frequent mechanism accounting for thrombocytopenia is the formation of drug–anti-drug immune complexes attaching to the fc receptors present on the platelet surface. Although quinidine has been the drug most commonly associated with this mechanism, such thrombocytopenia is reported with numerous other medications, including gold, cimetidine, and trimethoprim-sulfamethoxazole. In virtually all cases of immune complex drug-associated thrombocytopenia, PAIgG is elevated. Following suspension of the offending drug, the platelet count rises as the PAIgG falls. Numerous techniques have been utilized to demonstrate the drug-related antibodies implicated in the causation of disease. They vary in sensitivity from the low sensitivity of simple clot retraction inhibition tests to the 80% to 90% seen with PSIFT and Chromium[51] release methods.

The occurrence of severe thrombocytopenia during treatment with heparin has been widely reported and investigated. To date, the mechanism responsible for the immune destruction of platelets has not been satisfactorily elucidated. Although immune complexes and increased PAIgG

Table 66-2   Platelet-specific antigen systems

System name	Alternate designation	Glycoprotein association	Alleles described	Phenotypic frequency (%)
Pl^A	Zw	IIIa	Pl^A1 (Zw^a)	98
			Pl^A2 (Zw^b)	26
Ko	Sib	Ib	Ko^a	14
			Ko^b	99
Pl^E	—	Ib	Pl^E1	99
			Pl^E2	5
Bak	Lek	IIb	Bak^a	95
			Bak^b	65
Pen	Yuk	IIIa	Yuk^a	2
			Pen (Yuk^b)	>99
Duzo	—	?	Duzo	18

Box 66-3   Drugs associated with immune thrombocytopenia

ANALGESICS

Salicylates*
Acetaminophen
Phenylbutazone*
Antipyrine

ANTIBIOTICS

Cephalosporine
Penicillin
Streptomycin
Para-amino salicylic acid (PAS)
Rifampin
Novobiocin
Various sulfa drugs*

CINCHONA ALKALOIDS

Quinidine*
Quinine*

HYPNOTICS

Phenobarbital
Meprobamate*
Sedormid*
Dilantin
Chlorpromazine

ORAL HYPOGLYCEMICS

Chlorpropamide*
Tolbutamide

HEAVY METALS

Gold
Mercury
Bismuth
Organic arsenicals*

DIURETICS

Acetazolamide
Chlorothiazide*
Mercurial diuretics

OTHERS

Digitoxin*
Ergot
Methyldopa
Propylthiouracil
Disulfiram (Antabuse)
Chloroquine*
Stibophen (Fuadin)
Heparin

Modified from Triplett D: Hematology. In Seligson D (editor): Handbook of clinical laboratory science, vol I, Boca Raton, Fla, 1982, CRC Press.
*Drugs most frequently associated with immunologic thrombocytopenia.

have been demonstrated in many cases, it is unclear whether they are the principle causes of thrombocytopenia. Onset of the thrombocytopenia occurs about 1 to 2 weeks following initiation of treatment in those who had not previously been treated with heparin, and earlier in those previously exposed. In some patients the thrombocytopenia is associated with arterial thrombosis, which is frequently fatal. The clinical aspects of this disorder are discussed at greater length, together with its laboratory diagnosis, in Chapter 67.

Thrombocytosis

Thrombocytosis is defined by a platelet count $>400,000/\mu l$. This condition may result as a reactive manifestation of a variety of inflammatory and neoplastic conditions associated with certain hypoproliferative anemias, and following splenectomy (Box 66-4). Reactive thrombocytosis is associated with an increase in thrombopoietic-stimulating factors and resultant moderate megakaryocytic hyperplasia. In general, the platelet counts usually remain under $1,000,000/\mu l$. Thrombocytosis following splenomegaly is often greater than $1,000,000/\mu l$. Reactive thrombocytoses are only rarely associated with thrombotic or hemorrhagic manifestations.

Primary thrombocytosis (essential thrombocythemia) is classified as one of the myeloproliferative disorders characterized by the autonomous proliferation of megakaryocytes and a resultant isolated increase in platelet count, which commonly exceeds $1,000,000/\mu l$. Severe thrombocytosis is also often a feature of polycythemia vera, chronic myelogenous leukemia, and myeloid metaplasia. These types of thrombocytosis are commonly accompanied by thrombosis or hemorrhage. They are discussed in detail elsewhere (Part IX).

Box 66-4   Classification of secondary thrombocytosis

SECONDARY TO INFLAMMATORY REACTIONS

Rheumatoid arthritis
Ulcerative colitis
Regional enteritis
Tuberculosis
Osteomyelitis

ASSOCIATED WITH ANEMIAS

Acute hemorrhage
Iron deficiency anemia
Hemolytic anemias

ASSOCIATED WITH MALIGNANCY

Carcinomas
Hodgkin's disease
Non-Hodgkin's lymphomas

OTHER REACTIVE THROMBOCYTOSES

Postchemotherapy rebound
Postoperative
Postsplenectomy

Platelet function defects

Disorders are described in which any one or several of the facets of platelet function are defective, including adhesion, aggregation, platelet factor 3 availability, and clot retraction. These disorders may be either congenital or acquired. The congenital disorders are hereditary and are generally characterized by single function abnormalities, whereas acquired disorders most commonly are characterized by defects in multiple functions (Box 66-5). Platelet dysfunction is diagnosed by the finding of a prolonged bleeding time in the presence of a normal platelet count (Fig. 66-2).

Hereditary platelet dysfunction

Disorders of platelet adhesion. These disorders include those that are intrinsic defects of the platelets and those that are due to the absence of adequate levels of high molecular weight von Willebrand (vWF) multimers in the plasma. As previously described in this chapter, the Bernard-Soulier syndrome is an autosomal-recessive disorder characterized by mild thrombocytopenia, megathrombocytes in the peripheral smear (Fig. 66-8), and abnormal platelet adhesion due to absent glycoproteins Ib and IX. In addition to a prolonged bleeding time, the platelets from these patients demonstrate absent agglutination with ristocetin when suspended in normal plasma (Fig. 66-9), but normal aggregation with other agonists. Von Willebrand's disease is a designation applied to a heterogenous group of disorders, all of which are characterized by platelet adhesion defects due to reduced plasma levels of high molecular weight vWF multimers and associated ristocetin cofactor activity and variable descreases of VIIIC activity. This group of disorders will be discussed later in this chapter.

Box 66-5   Congenital and acquired defects of platelet function

CONGENITAL DEFECTS

Disorders of adhesion

Bernard-Soulier syndrome
von Willebrand's disease

Disorders of primary platelet aggregation

Glanzmann's thrombasthenia
Afibrinogenemia

Disorders of platelet release reaction

Phospholipase deficiency
Cyclooxygenase deficiency
Thromboxane synthetase deficiency

Storage pool deficiencies

Dense granule deficiencies (e.g., Hermansky-Pudlak syndrome and Wiskott-Aldrich syndrome)
Alpha granule deficiency (grey platelet syndrome)

Platelet factor 3 deficiency

Rare isolated defect

ACQUIRED DEFECTS

Uremia
Cardiopulmonary bypass
Autoimmune disorders
Myeloproliferative disorders
Hyperfibrinolysis
Dysproteinemias
Drugs

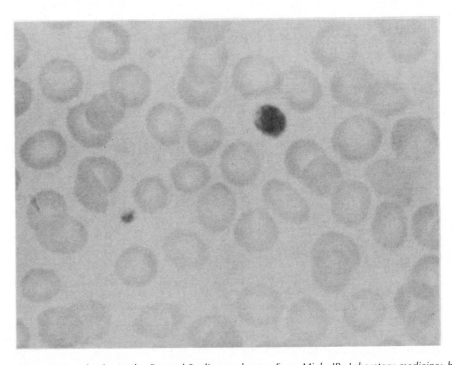

Fig. 66-8   Giant platelet in the Bernard-Soulier syndrome. *From Miale JB: Laboratory medicine: hematology, ed 6, St Louis, 1982, Mosby-Year Book.*

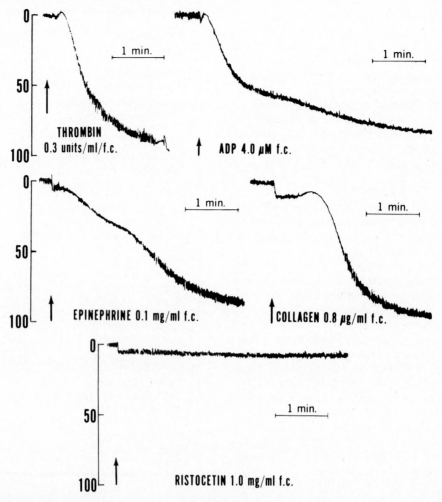

Fig. 66-9 Bernard-Soulier syndrome and von Willebrand's disease. Autologous platelets suspended in autologous plasma. Normal aggregation patterns are seen following stimulation with collagen, ADP, thrombin, and epinephrine. Absent agglutination is seen following the addition of ristocetin. *From Miale JB: Laboratory medicine: hematology, ed 6, St Louis, 1982, Mosby–Year Book.*

Defective primary aggregation. This group also includes an intrinsic disorder of primary aggregation of affected platelets and a defect due to an absence of adequate levels of fibrinogen in the plasma. Glanzmann's thrombasthenia is a rare hereditary defect, transmitted as an autosomal recessive trait and characterized by deficient fibrinogen mediated primary aggregation due to absent glycoprotein IIb-IIIa complex. In this disorder, the bleeding time is usually greatly prolonged. Examination of a peripheral smear made from nonanticoagulated capillary blood obtained by finger stick shows that the platelets are not grouped into aggregates, as is normally seen. Observation of clot retraction reveals a striking decrease in expected clot retraction. The most sensitive and specific test for thrombasthenia remains aggregometry. Platelets from these patients demonstrate absent primary aggregation to even elevated levels of commonly used agonists (Fig. 66-10). Patients with severe afibrinogenemia not only have a severe coagulopathy, but also demonstrate a prolonged bleeding time and absent respon-

siveness of the patient's platelets suspended in autologous plasma to all usual agonists. This disorder will be discussed later in this chapter.

Defective release reaction. Rare congenital disorders are characterized by deficient release of dense granule contents following platelet stimulation with thrombin or interaction with collagen. All of these disorders result from the congenital deficiency activity of one of the enzymes involved in the synthesis of thromboxane A_2. Deficiencies of phospholipase, cyclooxygenase, and thromboxane synthetase have been described. These disorders are characterized by a mild prolongation of the bleeding time. Aggregation studies show complete aggregation with high doses of adenosine disphophate (ADP), but show absent primary aggregation with collagen and absent secondary aggregation with low-dose ADP and other agonists (Fig. 66-11). Similar aggregation study results are obtained with the storage pool disorders, which must be differentiated from these release reaction dysfunctions.

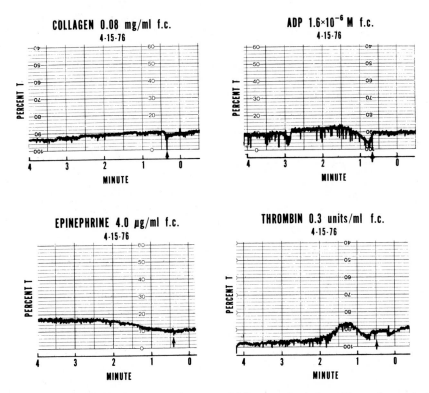

Fig. 66-10 Thrombasthenia. No aggregation is noted following stimulation with usual agonists. *From Miale JB: Laboratory medicine: hematology, ed 6, St Louis, 1982, Mosby–Year Book.*

Storage pool disorders. This group of disorders is characterized by either a decrease or virtual absence of dense and/or alpha granules, or a decrease in the dense granule content of ADP, serotonin, and calcium ion. The grey platelet syndrome is characterized by a marked decrease in the number of alpha granules. Bleeding times are slightly prolonged and a marked decrease in release of β-thromboglobulin and platelet factor 4 is noted after platelet stimulation. A mild bleeding diathesis may be related to the lack of reinforcement of fibrinogen-modified aggregation by adhesive proteins contained in the alpha granules (e.g., thrombospondin, fibronectin). Decreases in dense granules are usually associated with other congenital abnormalities. In the Hermansky-Pudlak syndrome dense granule deficiency is associated with oculocutaneous albinism, whereas in the Wiskott-Aldrich syndrome it is associated with thrombocytopenia, microthrombocytes, decreased levels of IgM, and recurrent infections and eczema. This syndrome affects male children and is transmitted as an X-linked disorder. In general, this group of disorders is characterized by a moderate to pronounced prolongation of the bleeding time, aggregation studies similar to those described with release reaction defects, decreased release of dense granule contents, and characteristic electron microscopic structure in those syndromes due to a decrease in granule number.

Platelet factor 3 deficiency. Poorly described defects in reduced platelet factor 3 (PF3) activity related to an abnormal phospholipid composition of the platelet membrane have been found to be associated with other functional abnormalities. One case of isolated procoagulant deficiency resulting in a significant bleeding disorder has been reported. In this case, the bleeding time was normal, but PF3 activity was abnormal.

Acquired platelet dysfunction (acquired thrombocytopathies)

A wide variety of dysfunctions may become evident in the course of other illnesses or during treatment with a large number of drugs. As previously stated, many of these abnormalities are complex and affect more than one function.

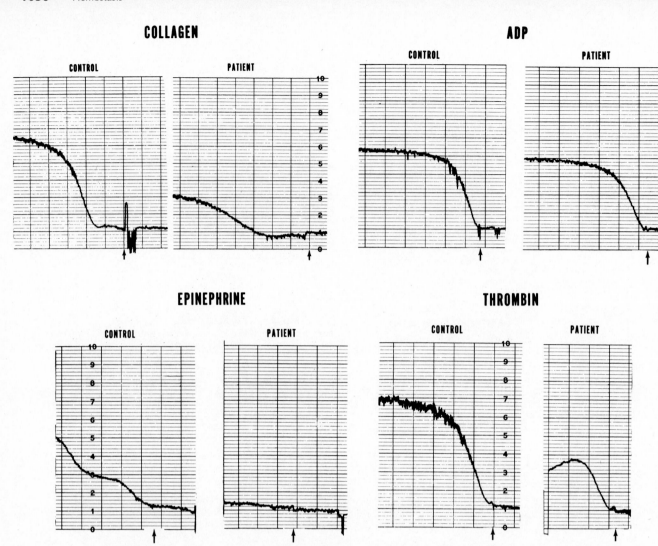

Fig. 66-11 Thrombocytopathy. Absent secondary aggregation in patient with defective release reaction. Study is atypical in that pronounced primary aggregation is obtained with low-dose ADP and disaggregation is only evident when thrombin is used as an agonist. *From Miale JB: Laboratory medicine: hematology, ed 6, St Louis, 1982, Mosby–Year Book.*

Furthermore, some are accompanied by coagulopathies and give rise to complicated hemostatic defects.

Uremia. Patients with renal insufficiency have a markedly prolonged bleeding time and a mild to moderate hemorrhagic diathesis. The bleeding time is not predictably correlated with the patient's blood urea nitrogen (BUN) or creatinine levels. In vitro testing most commonly shows secondary aggregation with the usual agonists and impaired PF3 availability. The secondary aggregation defect can be reproduced experimentally by adding metabolites that accumulate in the sera of uremic patients, such as guanidinosuccinic acid, to the test system. The mechanism that causes this defect is unclear.

Cardiopulmonary bypass. In addition to the dilutional thrombocytopenia and various acquired coagulopathies to be discussed later in this chapter, patients undergoing open heart surgery have a significantly prolonged bleeding time and may have an associated hemorrhagic diathesis. This prolongation is most pronounced while the patient is hypothermic and partially corrects itself when the patient's core temperature returns to normal. In vitro testing has shown a variety of defects, most commonly, defective aggregation with epinephrine. The primary cause of such abnormalities may be related to the progressive release of alpha-granule contents during bypass and subsequent loss of the platelet-associated adhesive protein (e.g., thrombospondin). Dense granule release does not usually occur.

Autoimmune disorders. Patients with acquired antibodies to vWF have been described who manifest a prolonged bleeding time, defective platelet adhesion, and absent agglutination with ristocetin (acquired von Willebrand's disease). In addition, patients with idiopathic thrombocytopenic purpura, autoimmune hemolytic anemia, and lupus erythematosus are found to have prolonged bleeding times and abnormal aggregation with the usual agonists. These abnormalities may be due to fixation of immune complexes or antibodies directed against surface glycoproteins, which result in dense granule discharge or interference with expression of receptors for aggregatory agonists.

Myeloproliferative disorders. As previously described, patients with myeloproliferative disorders associated with thrombocytosis may suffer a paradoxical bleeding tendency manifested by a prolonged bleeding time and abnormal aggregation following stimulation with epinephrine.

Other hematologic disorders. Patients with severe fibrino- and fibrinogenolysis; and elevated levels of degradation production may have poorly described platelet dysfunction, apparently related to interference with in vivo aggregation. Individuals with lymphoproliferative disorders and dysproteinemia may also have hemostatic defects associated with prolonged bleeding time and abnormal aggregation studies.

Drugs causing platelet dysfunction. A wide variety of drugs interfere with platelet function by diverse mechanisms (Box 66-6). Patients treated with aspirin develop a mildly prolonged bleeding time and a defective release reaction during aggregation tests due to acetylation of platelet cyclooxygenase and failure to synthesize thromboxane A_2. This defect is nonreversible during the life of the platelet and the bleeding time is corrected as new platelets are released. Other nonsteroidal anti-inflammatory agents also inhibit endoperoxide synthesis. The resultant dysfunction is, however, quickly reversible upon suspension of the offending drug. Administration of high doses of penicillin and

---

Box 66-6 Drugs causing platelet dysfunction

INHIBITORS OF PHOSPHOLIPASE A_2

Corticosteroids

INHIBITORS OF CYCLOOXYGENASE

Aspirin
Indomethacin
Butazolidin
Ibuprofin
Sulfinpyrazone
Furosemide

ACTIVATORS OF ADENYL CYCLASE

Prostaglandins (e.g., PGE_1)
Isoprenaline

INHIBITORS OF PHOSPHODIESTERASE

Dipyramidole
Aminophylline
Caffeine

STABILIZERS OF MEMBRANES

Xylocaine and other local anesthetics
Antihistamines (e.g., diphenhydramine)
Tricyclic antidepressants (e.g., imipramine)
Beta blockers (e.g., propranolol)
Penicillin and cephalosporins

OTHER

Alcohol, dextran, clofibrate, glycerol guaiacolate

Modified from Rao AK and Walsh PN: Acquired qualitative platelet disorders: Clin Haematol 12:201, 1988.

---

cephalosporin-type antibiotics commonly result in a prolongation of the bleeding time and an increased hemorrhagic tendency in septic thrombocytopenic patients. Dextran administration also results in prolongation of the bleeding time, a decrease in platelet adhesion, and defective PF3 availability. It is believed that this highly charged molecule may coat surface glycoprotein receptors, thereby interfering with function. Finally, the chronic ingestion of alcohol induces a mild platelet dysfunction with a prolonged bleeding time, defective secondary aggregation, and decreased PF3 availability. The mechanism by which alcohol induces these abnormalities is unclear.

DISORDERS OF COAGULATION AND FIBRINOLYSIS

Patients with abnormalities in coagulation and fibrinolysis suffer increased bleeding following minimal trauma or during surgery. Bleeeding is localized in the traumatized area, with resultant intramuscular hematomas, retroperitoneal hemorrhages, or hemarthroses. Severe coagulopathies may be associated with intracerebral bleeding. The most severe hemostatic disorders result when these abnormalities develop together with primary defects. Decreased factor levels may be due to deficient synthesis, synthesis of inactive molecules, the presence of inhibitors, excessive factor consumption, or dilution by infusion of intravenous fluids.

Congenital disorders

Congenital disorders of coagulation and fibrinolysis are usually characterized by the decreased synthesis of a single soluble plasma factor or synthesis of an abnormal molecule that manifests decreased procoagulant activity. Single factor deficiencies of the intrinsic pathway are most commonly encountered.

Factor VIII deficiency (hemophilia A)

Hemophilia A is a hereditary deficiency of factor VIIIC activity, which is transmitted as a sex-linked recessive trait (Fig. 66-12) and is caused by one of a number of point mutations or deletions of the VIIIC gene. Approximately 20% to 30% of the cases arise as a spontaneous mutation without a family history of a bleeding disorder. Over all, one in 8,000 to 10,000 males are affected.

The severity of the disease is related to the level of factor VIIIC activity (Table 66-3). Over 50% of patients have severe hemophilia with levels of <1% and a severe hem-

Table 66-3 Hemophilia A and B: severity and factor activity

Severity	Activity (%)	Manifestations
Severe	<1	Multiple bleeding episodes since infancy; frequent severe hemarthroses
Moderate	1-5	Increased bleeding episodes; occasional hemarthroses
Mild	>5	Bleeding with surgical procedures; no hemarthroses
Carrier	20-50 (usual)	Usually asymptomatic

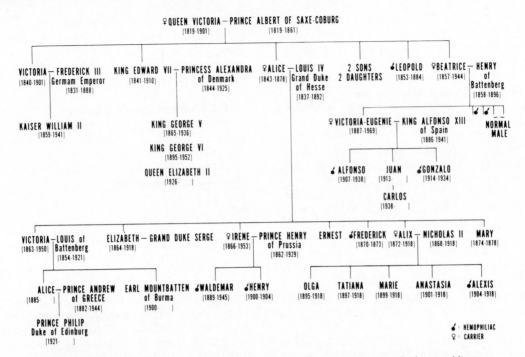

Fig. 66-12 Sex-linked transmission of hemophilia in the Royal House of Stuart and other royal lineages. *From Miale JB: Laboratory medicine: hematology, ed 6, St Louis, 1982, Mosby—Year Book.*

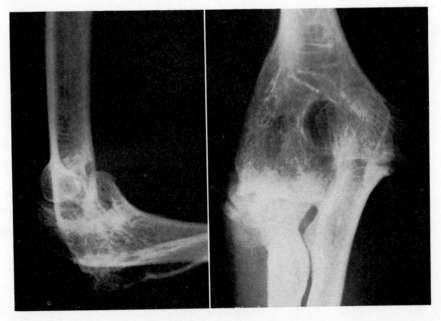

Fig. 66-13 Hemophiliac arthropathy of elbow, resulting from recurrent hemarthrosis. *From Miale JB: Laboratory medicine: hematology, ed 6, St Louis, 1982, Mosby—Year Book.*

orrhagic diathesis with spontaneous hemarthroses (Fig. 66-13). The moderate form is characterized by a factor VIIIC activity of 2% to 5% and occasional hemarthrosis. Mild hemophilia is characterized by levels of factor VIIIC of 6% to 30% and increased bleeding with trauma and surgery. Neutralizing antibodies to factor VIIIC, usually IgG₄, develop in 5% to 10% of severe hemophilias following variable periods of replacement treatment. They may be low titer antibodies that do not increase following transfusion, or high titer antibodies that rapidly increase after infusion of plasma containing blood components.

Laboratory findings include a normal prothrombin time (PT) and thrombin time (TT), a prolonged partial thromboplastin time (PTT), decreased factor VIIIC activity, and normal to increased vWF(VIIIRAg) (Fig. 66-14). In patients who are not immunized to factor VIIIC, correction

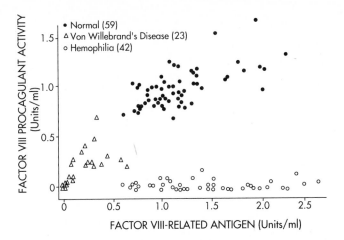

Fig. 66-14   Relationship of factor VIIIC to factor VIII RAg in normal individuals, hemophiliacs, and patients with von Willebrand's disease. *From Hoyer LW: J Lab Clin Med 80:822, 1972.*

of the PTT is seen with the addition of normal plasma. The detection and quantifications of factor VIIIC inhibitors has been previously discussed (Chapter 65).

Although some female carriers may be detected by finding reduced levels of factor VIIIC activity (<50%), sole dependence on such a finding is an insensitive method for carrier detection. This lack of sensitivity is due to the broad reference range of factor VIIIC activity (50% to 200%) and the fact that extreme lyonization in the carrier could result in the total inactivation of the affected X chromosome with resultant normal factor VIIIC levels. Increased detection of carriers is achieved by comparing the relative levels of factors VIIIC and VIIIRAg or VIIICAg. Normal women will have VIIIC:VIIIRAg or VIIICAg ratios that approximate 1.0, while carriers will have ratios of about 0.5. However, in the presence of extreme lyonization, some carriers will have normal ratios and will therefore not be detected. Markedly improved sensitivity of carrier detection is possible by Southern blot analysis of restriction fragments obtained by endonuclease digestion of deoxyribonucleic acid (DNA) derived from patient leukocytes. Application of polymerase chain reaction techniques promises to further simplify and improve carrier detection.

Antenatal diagnosis has been performed on blood obtained by umbilical vein sampling by determining factor VIII:C:VIII:CAg ratios. Techniques are being developed to utilize direct DNA analysis technique on chorionic villus samples or amniocytes obtained during amniocentesis.

von Willebrand's disease

Von Willebrand's disease is the term used to designate a heterogenous group of disorders, all of which are characterized by decreased plasma levels of high molecular weight multimers of vWF and variable decreases of factor VIIIC. Numerous variants are described that vary according to clinical severity, molecular defect, and mode of transmission.

Classical von Willebrand's disease (type I) is a variably mild to moderately severe disease transmitted as an autosomal-dominant trait with variable penetrance that is characterized by concordant decreases in factor VIIIRAg, as-

sociated factor VIIIRCoF activity, and factor VIIIC procoagulant activity (Fig. 66-14). The incidence of this disease is approximately 1 per 1000. These forms of the disease present primarily as a defect in primary hemostasis, but those patients with significantly depressed factor VIIIC levels may also have a tendency to develop increased deep tissue bleeding following trauma. Laboratory diagnosis is suggested by a prolonged bleeding time that is generally associated with a prolonged PTT. The mildest forms may be characterized by a borderline normal bleeding time and a normal PTT. In such cases, administration of aspirin (aspirin stress test) prior to performance of the bleeding time results in a prolonged bleeding time. Platelet function tests reveal decreased adhesion of platelets suspended in autologous plasma to glass beads or de-endothelized aortic strips and decreased platelet agglutination with ristocetin. Aggregation tests with other agonists are normal. Factor VIIIC activity is decreased in proportion to the reduction in factor VIIIRAg. Analysis of multimer distribution of this protein by crossed immunoelectrophoresis or SDS digestion, gel electrophoresis, and immunofixation reveals a normal pattern.

Type II von Willebrand's disease is the term given to those forms in which the total amount of plasma VIIIRAg is only slightly reduced or normal, but the plasma VIIIRCoF is decreased because of the absence of large multimers that support normal platelet adhesion. Bleeding times are prolonged. Factor VIIIC levels are usually normal. About 20% of all cases of von Willebrand's disease are type II. Patients with the type II A variant not only possess decreased or absent large multimers in the plasma, but also lack these multimers in their platelets. Patients with the type II B variant have an isolated defect characterized by decreased levels of large plasma multimers, whereas the platelet level is normal. Platelets from these patients demonstrate normal or heightened agglutination responses to ristocetin, even when suspended in autologous plasma. It is hypothesized that this form results from increased degradation of the large multimers to smaller molecules. Both types II A and II B variants are transmitted as autosomal-dominant traits.

Type III von Willebrand's disease is a severe defect characterized by extremely low levels of factors VIIIRAg, VIIIRCoF, and VIIIC. It presents a clinical picture similar to hemophilia A and is transmitted as an autosomal-recessive trait. It is a very rare disorder with an incidence of approximately 1:1,000,000.

Numerous other variants have been and continue to be reported. Final classification of von Willebrand's disease variants awaits further elucidation of the molecular basis of these disorders.

Factor IX deficiency (hemophilia B: Christmas disease)

Hemophilia B is a hereditary deficiency of factor IX procoagulant activity, which is transmitted as a sex-linked recessive trait, and is caused by one of a number of point mutations or deletions of the factor IX gene. This disorder occurs less frequently than hemophilia A, with 1 in 100,000 males affected.

As with hemophilia A, the severity of disease is related to the level of factor IX activity (Table 66-3). About 3% of the patients develop IgG inhibitor antibodies.

Laboratory findings are identical to hemophilia A except that the factor VIIIC levels are normal and the factor IX level is decreased. Unusual variants of factor IX interfere with factor VII-ox brain tissue factor interaction and thereby cause a unique prolongation of the prothrombin time performed with this reagent thromboplastin. Affected individuals are said to have hemophilia Bm. Approaches to the detection of the carrier state and antenatal diagnoses are identical to those described for hemophilia A.

Factor XI deficiency (hemophilia C: Rosenthal's disease)

Hemophilia C is a fairly rare hereditary deficiency of factor XI procoagulant activity and is transmitted as an autosomal-recessive trait. These patients demonstrate an absolute decrease in the amount of factor XI synthesized. Homozygous patients have less than 20% activity, but have a relatively mild bleeding disorder.

Laboratory screening tests are similar to hemophilia A and B, with decreased levels of demonstrable factor IX activity.

Afibrinogenemia and dysfibrinogenemia

Congenital afibrinogenemia is a rare hereditary abnormality characterized by a marked reduction in the synthesis of fibrinogen. It is transmitted as an autosomal-recessive trait. Most homozygous patients are found to have fibrinogen levels below that detectable with routine laboratory methods. These patients have a severe bleeding disorder, often evident at birth with prolonged umbilical bleeding, hematomas, and gastrointestinal hemorrhage. This bleeding diathesis is due to both a coagulopathy resulting from deficient fibrin formation and a defect in primary hemostasis resulting from depressed platelet aggregation.

Coagulation screening tests performed on homozygous patients reveal prolonged prothrombin, partial thromboplastin, and thrombin times. Assays for fibrinogen by modified thrombin time methods and tests for total clottable protein both show comparable reductions in fibrinogen concentration. Trace amounts of fibrinogen may be detected by immunologic means. In addition these patients may demonstrate a marked prolongation in bleeding time and clot retraction times. Aggregation tests performed with a patient's platelets suspended in autologous plasma demonstrate reduced responsiveness to stimulation with the usual agonists. Heterozygous patients are usually asymptomatic and are found to have fibrinogen levels over 75 mg/dl. Tests of primary hemostasis are normal.

Dysfibrinogenemias are a heterogenous group of disorders, all of which are characterized by the synthesis of abnormal fibrinogen molecules responsible for a wide spectrum of clinical pictures that range from asymptomatic states to severe coagulopathies. A few of these abnormal fibrinogens have been associated with thrombosis. These various abnormal fibrinogens are identified according to the city in which they were first described (e.g., Paris I, Bethesda I). Most of these traits are inherited as autosomal-dominant characteristics. The structural defects most commonly involve amino acid substitutions of the Aα chain, although some are due to amino acid deletions or chain elongations. These defects may be responsible for abnormalities in fi-

brinopeptide cleavage, fibrin monomer polymerization, or fibrin polymer cross-linkage.

The laboratory diagnosis is based upon the finding of prolonged screening clotting time tests and disproportionately decreased levels of fibrinogen as measured by modified thrombin time assays. Total clottable protein and immunologic tests usually reveal normal fibrinogen levels, although some dysfibrinogenemias are associated with mild hypofibrinogenemia.

Factor XIII deficiency

Factor XIII deficiency is an unusual congenital disorder characterized by either the decreased synthesis of a normal factor XIII protein or the production of a nonfunctional molecule that results in the formation of an unstable fibrin clot. The disorder is usually transmitted as an autosomal-recessive trait, however, rare cases may be sex-linked. They are characterized by delayed bleeding from wounds and easy bruising in homozygous patients. The coagulopathy is often first detected at birth with umbilical bleeding. Heterozygous patients are asymptomatic, since only 2% to 3% activity is required to achieve normal hemostasis.

Routine laboratory tests are normal. The defect is diagnosed by the finding that formed plasma clots are readily lysed by a 5 M urea solution, whereas clots formed from normal plasma are stable in these solutions for more than 24 hours.

Other congenital deficiencies

Congenital deficiencies of other coagulation factors and inhibitors of fibrinolysis are rare. Among them, isolated deficiency of factor VII is most common. It presents with an isolated prolongation of the prothrombin time in the presence of a normal partial thromboplastin time. Isolated deficiencies of factors V, X, or II present with prolongation of both screening tests. Patients with factor V deficiency tend to have a disproportionate prolongation of the prothrombin time. Deficiencies of the content factors XII, prekallikrein, and high molecular weight kininogen deficiencies all present with an isolated prolongation of the partial thromboplastin time, which is usually discovered incidentally as these deficiencies are not associated with bleeding diathesis. Decreased levels of hemolytic inhibitors, especially α_2-antiplasmin, are rare causes of a hemorrhagic diathesis. Deficiencies of such inhibitors may be characterized by an accelerated whole blood or clot lysis time and a decreased plasma level of the inhibitor involved.

Acquired coagulopathies

Acquired coagulopathies are usually multifactorial and result in the prolongation of both the PT and PTT. Exceptions to this general rule include the acquired inhibitors of specific clotting factors.

Vitamin K deficiency

Deficiency in the availability of vitamin K results in the formation of noncarboxylated inactive molecules of factors II, VII, IX, X, and (PIVKA), as well as decreased synthesis of active protein C. Deficiency results in the early prolongation of the prothrombin time, reflecting the short half-life of factor VII and the subsequent prolongation of the partial thromboplastin time. These abnormalities are reversed within 6 to 24 hours of the parenteral administration of vitamin K, if liver function is normal. Vitamin K deficiency is a contributing cause of hemorrhagic disease of the newborn and occurs in older individuals as a consequence of prolonged treatment with antibiotics and parenteral nutrition, biliary obstruction, malabsorption, and treatment with coumarin-type anticoagulants.

Hemorrhagic disease of the newborn is a complex syndrome resulting from both vitamin K deficiency and functional immaturity of the liver. It is most severe in premature infants who are unable to adequately respond to vitamin K administration. Patients unable to eat and who are treated with parenteral nutrition may become depleted of vitamin K, which is usually supplied in foodstuffs, especially green leafy vegetables and dairy products. Such depletion occurs most commonly when such dietary deficiency occurs in patients being treated with oral antibiotics, in whom the normal vitamin K-producing intestinal flora has been eliminated. Biliary obstruction prevents the secretion of bile salts essential for absorption of this fat-soluble vitamin. Both this condition and malnutrition syndromes result in the decreased absorption of vitamin K and resultant deficiency. The action of coumarin anticoagulants is extensively discussed in the next section.

Amyloidosis

Occasionally, patients with generalized amyloidosis may develop a deficiency of factor X. It is believed that factor X is taken up by the amyloid.

Circulating anticoagulants

As previously discussed, 5% to 10% of patients with severe factor VIII deficiency, and rare patients with factor IX deficiency may develop antibodies with resultant refractoriness to usual replacement therapy. The spontaneous appearance of factor VIIIC autoantibodies occurs in patients with lupus erythematosus and rheumatoid arthritis, occasional postpartum women, and individuals experiencing an allergic reaction to penicillin. These antibodies may disappear spontaneously or with immunosuppressive therapy. Rare patients have developed antibodies to vWF, fibrinogen, and factors V, IX, X, XI, and XIII. The most common inhibitor encountered in practice is the so-called lupus anticoagulant, which is described in depth in the next section.

Liver dysfunction

Patients with hepatocellular dysfunction develop a coagulopathy, the severity of which is related to the severity of liver disease. Those with relatively mild dysfunction present with decreased synthesis of the vitamin K-dependent factors, which results in prolongation of the prothrombin time (PT) and a somewhat lesser prolongation of the activated partial thromboplastin time (aPTT). With progressive dysfunction, the levels of factor V and fibrinogen also fall progressively, resulting in increasingly prolonged PT and aPTT clotting tests. Factor VIIIC activity remains normal. As the level of functional fibrinogen falls to below 80 to 100 mg/dl, the thrombin time becomes prolonged as well. In addition, the synthesis of abnormal fibrinogen molecules (dysfibrinogenemia), the accumulation of fibrinogen deg-

radation products due to their decreased clearance, and the decreased synthesis of plasmin inhibitors may cause further prolongation of the thrombin time. Elevated levels of immunologically detected serum fibrinogen/fibrin split products are often present, but tests for thrombin generation, including fibrin monomers and D-D dimers, are negative. In addition to coagulation defects, patients with portal hypertension may also develop moderate thrombocytopenia secondary to hypersplenism.

Disseminated intravascular coagulation

Disseminated intravascular coagulation (DIC) is an intermediary mechanism of disease, characterized by diffuse vascular thromboses and a secondary hemorrhagic diathesis due to both fibrinolysis and consumption of platelets and procoagulant materials. In acute severe forms, bleeding may predominate when secondary fibrinolysis is prominent, whereas clotting phenomena may predominate in the more chronic low-grade forms.

The most characteristic pathologic finding of DIC is the presence of small vessel thrombi in both arterioles and venules (Fig. 66-15). If fibrinolysis is prominent, these thrombi may not be demonstrable on histological examination. These thrombi are most evident in the intestinal submucosa, preglomerular arterioles, adrenal medulla, liver, brain, and pituitary gland. They may be associated with infarction of end-organ tissues (hemorrhagic enterocolitis, renal cortical necrosis, etc.). When the thrombotic component is very pronounced, thrombosis of the large veins may occur (e.g., femoral, iliac, renal, and adrenal). Pulmonary embolism may also occur. Bleeding in these patients is most pronounced from the mucosal surfaces. Rare patients with fulminant DIC may develop extensive ecchymosis with subepithelial necrosis and sloughing (purpura fulminans). With very low levels of platelets, intrapulmonary and intracranial hemorrhage may result.

Initiation of clotting in this syndrome is due to factors that may cause diffuse damage to vascular endothelium, vascular stasis, and circulation of activated procoagulants (Box 66-7). As clotting progresses, platelets are incorporated into the clots, and some coagulation factors are consumed. Secondary plasmin activation occurs and leads to fibrin and fibrinogenolysis, and digestion of factors V, VIII, and XIII. The resultant bleeding diathesis is due to thrombocytopenia, decreased levels of consumed clotting factors, destruction of fibrin clots by secondary fibrinolysis, and the anticoagulant effect of fibrin and fibrinogen degradation products.

Thrombocytopenia is present with megathrombocytosis. In the acute severe case, the screening tests will show prolonged PT, PTT, and TT. Factor assays show decreasing levels of factors I, V, and VIII. The euglobulin lysis time may be somewhat shortened and there will be increased amounts of fibrin degradation products (FDP) in the serum. Increased fibrin monomers may be demonstrable (Table 66-4). In more chronic cases and in those cases in which the thrombotic component is more accentuated, the PTT may be normal or even shortened, factors I and VIII not as decreased, and the test for fibrin monomers markedly positive. A characteristic morphological change in the appearance of red cells may be noted in these cases and consists

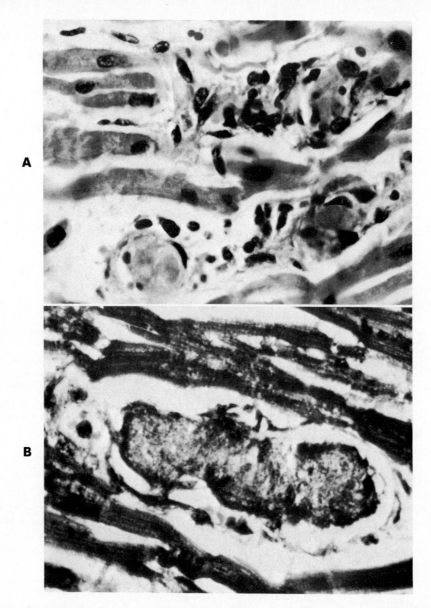

Fig. 66-15 Fibrin thrombi occluding microvasculature in the myocardium of 2 1/2-week-old infant who died of gram-negative sepsis and disseminated intravascular coagulation. *From Miale JB: Laboratory medicine: hematology, ed 6, St Louis, 1982, Mosby–Year Book.*

in the finding of fragmented red cells (schistocytes) in the peripheral blood. This change results from physical trauma to the cells as they pass over and about blood clots in the circulation.

Primary fibrinogenolysis

In some cases of urinary tract trauma, or in cases of widespread malignancy, large quantities of plasminogen activators may be released into the blood. Large amounts of plasmin may then be generated, and a very rare condition known as primary fibrinogenolysis may ensue. As stated elsewhere, a similar condition may occur in patients with liver disease who cannot synthesize plasmin inactivators, and during cardiopulmonary bypass. A bleeding diathesis develops that mimics, to a great degree, the consumption coagulopathy seen with DIC. As opposed to this, however,

the platelet count is usually normal, the peripheral smear is normal, fibrin monomers and dimers are not detectable, the euglobulin lysis time is markedly shortened, and fibrinogen split products are markedly elevated (Table 66-4).

Dilutional coagulopathy

The coagulopathy associated with massive blood loss and replacement with nonplasma volume expanders when not associated with other phenomena occurs after the loss of approximately 50% of the plasma volume, at which time the prothrombin time becomes prolonged. Continued dilution then causes prolongation of the partial thromboplastin time and progressive prolongation of the prothrombin time at a rate that tends to follow the theoretical dilution curve observed in vitro as plasma is diluted with saline. Severe dilution is associated with prolongation of the thrombin

Box 66-7   Pathologic processes associated with disseminated intravascular coagulation

IN INFECTIOUS DISEASE

Sepsis (various organisms)
Gram-negative shock
Viral or rickettsial infections
 Varicella (hemorrhagic, purpura fulminans)
 Generalized vaccinia
 Smallpox
 Rubella (hemorrhagic)
 Rubeola (hemorrhagic black measles)
 Generalized varicilla zoster
 Hemorrhagic fevers (Thailand, Bolivian, Argentinian, Philippine, Kyasanur Forest disease)
 Rocky Mountain spotted fever
 Scrub typhus
 Viral hepatitis

IN OBSTETRIC COMPLICATIONS

Premature separation of placenta
Retained dead fetus or placental tissue
Septic abortion
Amniotic fluid embolism
Hydatidiform mole
Placenta previa
Placenta accreta
Eclampsia
Ruptured uterus
Cesarean section

IN INTRAVASCULAR HEMOLYSIS

Hemolytic transfusion reaction
Acute hemolytic anemias (except PNH)
Venomous snake bite
Hypotonic hemolysis (intravenous hypotonic solution, transurethral prostatectomy)

IN NEOPLASMS

Acute leukemia (acute progranulocytic)
Lymphomas
Carcinoma (pancreas, prostate, ovary, breast, bladder, stomach)

Neuroblastoma, metastatic
Rhabdomyosarcoma, metastatic
Kasabach-Merritt syndrome
Hemangiomatous transformation of the spleen or liver

IN AUTOIMMUNE DISEASE AND HYPERSENSITIVITY REACTIONS

Drug reactions
Lupus erythematosus
Acute glomerulonephritis
Renal homograft rejection
Other autoimmune reactions

POSTOPERATIVE

Pulmonary surgery
Shock

IN BENIGN TUMOR (giant cavernous hemangioma of liver)

Kasabach-Merritt syndrome

MISCELLANEOUS

Heat stroke
Extensive burns
Cyanotic congenital heart disease
Sarcoidosis
Hyaline membrane disease
Asphyxia (newborn)
Combat casualties
Hypobaric erythrocytosis (experimental)
Fat embolism
Dissecting aneurism of aorta
Amyloidosis

Modified from Miale JB: Laboratory medicine: hematology, ed 6, St Louis, 1982, Mosby–Year Book.

Table 66-4   Differentiation of acute disseminated intravascular coagulation (DIC) from primary fibrinogenolysis

Test	DIC	Fibrinogenolysis
Prothrombin time	Prolonged	Prolonged
Partial thromboplastin time	Prolonged	Prolonged
Thrombin time	Prolonged	Prolonged
Fibrinogen	Low	Low
Factor V	Low	Low
Factor VIII	Decreased	Normal to decreased
Fibrinogen split products	Increased	Increased
Euglobulin lysis time	Normal or shortened	Shortened
Paracoagulation tests	Positive	Negative
D-D Dimer	Positive	Negative
Platelet count	Decreased	Normal
Erythrocyte morphology	Schistocytes	Normal

time, as the fibrinogen level falls to below 80 to 100 mg/dl. Factor VIII level tends to be maintained in spite of continued dilution as a consequence of the accelerated synthesis associated with stress. Dilutional coagulopathy is associated with the dilutional thrombocytopenia previously discussed. The bleeding diathesis resulting from simple dilution is more likely related to the thrombocytopenia until dilution is severe.

Previously healthy young men bleeding from trauma have been found to develop excess bleeding when more than one and a half to two blood volumes have been replaced with red cells and nonplasma volume expanders. In many patients, however, the dilutional hemostatic defect is associated with other preexisting or concurrent hemostatic abnormalities that may give rise to a severe bleeding diathesis with blood losses that would be otherwise considered modest. Patients undergoing open heart surgery not only have a predictable dilutional coagulopathy, but are routinely noted to have a disporportionate fall in factor V, without other evidence of disseminated intravascular coagulation, and the acquired storage pool disease characterized by alpha granule depletion previously discussed. Furthermore, such patients may have preexisting liver disease associated with chronic passive congestion, bleeding associated with inadequate heparin neutralization, and evidence of disseminated intravascular coagulation or primary fibrinogenolysis. Patients undergoing liver transplantation may develop severe hemodilution associated with dramatic blood loss unless replacement therapy is aggressively pursued. In these patients, not only does severe thrombocytopenia develop, but the coagulation defect often complicates preexisting hepatocellular insufficiency. Some patients may develop significant fibrinogenolysis during the anhepatic phase of the surgical procedure.

SUGGESTED READING

Coleman RW and Rao AK (editors): Platelets in health and disease, Hematol Oncol Clin N Amer 4:1, 1990.

Hoyer LW: Molecular pathology and immunology of factor VIII, Hum Pathol 18:153, 1987.

King DJ and Kelton JG: Heparin-associated thrombocytopenias, Ann Int Med 100:535, 1984.

McMillan RE (editor): The immune cytopenias, New York, 1983, Churchill Livingstone.

Ruggeri ZM and Zimmerman TS: Von Willebrand factor and Von Willebrand disease, Blood 70:895, 1987.

Schafer AI: Bleeding and thrombosis in the myeloproliferative disorders, Blood 64:1, 1984.

Thompson AR: Structure, function and molecular defects of factor IX, Blood 67:565, 1986.

White JC and Shoemaker CB: Factor VIII gene and hemophilia A, Blood 73:1, 1989.

67

Laboratory diagnosis and management of thrombotic disorders

David Ciavarella

The clinical laboratory's role in the diagnosis and management of thrombotic disorders has grown increasingly important over the past decade. Compared to the critical role of the laboratory in the diagnosis, prognosis, and on-going clinical management of bleeding disorders, thrombotic disorders remained for many years in the domain of the anatomic pathologist. The intrinsic properties of the blood are of primary, even overwhelming, importance in the pathogenesis of bleeding disorders, whereas abnormalities of the blood vessels and rheologic abnormalities are of equal or greater importance in thrombotic disorders.

The great importance of thrombotic disease, which still accounts for more deaths in the Western world than any other disease entity, has led to intense study of all three elements that predispose to thrombosis. Advances in rheology, protein and lipid chemistry, endothelial cell and platelet biochemistry and physiology, and molecular biology, and the accumulated evidence of many multicenter trials testing antithrombotic therapies have led to wide availability and greater understanding of diagnostic laboratory tests for thrombotic disorders. Unfortunately, the prognostic value of tests for thrombotic disorders is very limited. This is perhaps understandable and inevitable, since hemodynamic alterations and blood vessel pathophysiology are poorly studied ex vivo. With few exceptions, pathologic thrombosis results from simultaneous derangements in at least two of the three classic predisposing factors, whereas most bleeding disorders are manifest by altered physiology of the blood alone. For example, deep-venous thrombosis and myocardial infarction are both complex disorders in which vessel alterations and blood flow patterns are of greater consequence than properties of the blood. In common, hemorrhagic disorders, such as hemophilia A or severe thrombocytopenia, "spontaneous" bleeding (i.e., without apparent inciting cause) is a frequent occurrence. Parallels exist in a few, well-defined thrombotic disorders, such as hereditary antithrombin III deficiency. However, at our present state of knowledge, these types of disorders are uncommon compared to acquired, multifactorial disorders.

Another dissimilarity between thrombotic and bleeding disorders, or perhaps an explanation for the aforementioned phenomenon, is that severe (homozygous) hereditary thrombotic disorders are rare, probably because they are incompatible with life. Severe hereditary bleeding disorders are neither rare nor incompatible with life, even without precise replacement therapy, as any study of the history of hemophilia will reveal. For the most part, then, the clinical laboratory's role in thrombosis testing involves ruling out those well-defined disorders for which accurate laboratory tests are available and in careful laboratory monitoring of antithrombotic therapy, perhaps the laboratory's most critical role.

In this chapter, an overview of conditions that place patients at increased risk of thrombosis will be discussed. The prethrombotic or hypercoagulable states vary greatly in their definition, pathophysiology, and, most importantly, our understanding of their pathogenesis. Clinically useful tests, and the disorders in which they are used, will be emphasized, and an attempt made to place these tests in their appropriate clinical context. Finally, antithrombotic therapy will be discussed primarily from a laboratory monitoring perspective.

THE PRETHROMBOTIC OR HYPERCOAGULABLE STATE

The definition of the prethrombotic or hypercoagulable state varies from author to author. One might practically define the hypercoagulable state as any condition in which a system perturbation that is controlled in a normocoagulable person leads to thrombosis in the hypercoagulable person. Further, this definition lends itself to a separation of perturbations into those that primarily cause thrombosis and those that support or facilitate thrombosis. In general, abnormalities of blood flow facilitate thrombosis, whereas endothelial damage or deficiency of blood substances critical to normal blood patency (e.g., antithrombin III) are direct causes of thrombosis. Of course, one may argue for a clinical approach, in other words, a hypercoagulable state is any condition in which there is a well-documented increased risk of thrombosis. This definition is useful in the design of epidemiologic and antithrombotic research trials, but is not overly helpful to our understanding of pathogenesis or approach to the individual patient.

From a laboratory point of view, tests for the hypercoagulable state should predict degree of risk in an individual, have clear therapeutic implications, and permit on-going monitoring of the degree of risk and response to therapy. Only a few tests meet these criteria. These include assays for antithrombin III and protein C deficiencies and some abnormalities of fibrinogen and plasminogen. Remaining tests, such as platelet count or products of platelet activation, serve either to place the patient in a broad category of patients at increased thrombotic risk or are useful in research settings, where they are used to explore pathogenesis and have not yet (or never will) become available and useful clinical laboratory tests.

CLASSIFICATION OF THROMBOTIC DISORDERS

A number of classifications of thrombotic disorders have been proposed. Primary disorders are those with a presumed clear-cut pathogenesis, often inherited rather than acquired. These are relatively few, and together, affect only a minority of patients with clinical thrombotic disease. Secondary thrombotic disorders are typically complex, less completely understood disorders, such as the myeloproliferative disorders and atherosclerosis.

In this chapter, an attempt is made to classify disorders by their pathophysiology. Accordingly, disorders of blood rheology and blood vessels will be discussed first, followed by disorders of platelet number and function, coagulation factors, fibrinolysis, and coagulation factor inhibitors. Clearly, much overlap is inevitable in this schema, since more than one mechanism operates in the great majority of thromboses. These interrelationships will be emphasized when possible, and therefore, the classification should not be rigidly interpreted (Table 67-1). Disorders with a complex or multifactorial etiology are listed in more than one category. Parentheses are used to indicated an etiology of secondary importance.

Disorders of blood rheology

In general, low flow or abnormal flow situations are additive to other stimuli in causing thrombosis. Normal blood flow occurs in a laminar pattern, which can be visualized as a series of parallel sheets of varying composition flowing past one another at varying speeds. Blood flow is most rapid in the central laminae, which are enriched with cells, and approaches zero at the vessel wall. The blood viscosity, defined as shear stress divided by shear rate, depends primarily upon the aggregation of red blood cells with fibrinogen and other large and asymmetric plasma proteins.

Situations of low blood flow due to increased blood viscosity can predispose to thrombosis by disrupting several of the natural rheologic control mechanisms. These include the transport of activated clotting factors to the liver or other organs, where they are removed from circulation; the breakup of small platelet aggregates on the endothelium; the dilution of activated platelets or clotting factors and their activators, which require an appropriate surface and concentration to proceed to full thrombosis formation; and the approximation by mixing of activated factors with endothelial-based and circulating inhibitors. Besides changes in blood viscosity, changes in the laminar flow pattern also predispose to thrombosis. Flow separation is the term used to describe flow that is circular and separated from the main flow volume. This occurs at sites of changes in flow volume, such as at bifurcations. Concentration of activated platelets, vasoactive substances of platelet release or metabolism, and activated clotting factors can occur, with depletion of inhibitory proteins. Damage to the endothelium occurs via hypoxia or directly by vasoactive substances. Thus, prolonged immobilization, heart failure, and structural abnor-

Table 67-1 Classification of thrombotic disorders*

DISORDERS OF BLOOD RHEOLOGY	DISORDERS OF BLOOD VESSELS	DISORDERS OF PLATELET NUMBER AND FUNCTION
Hyperviscosity syndrome	Atherosclerosis and other occlusive disorders	Thrombocytosis/Myeloproliferative syndrome
Polycythemia	Homocystinuria	Heparin-induced thrombocytopenia
Congestive heart failure and other low flow states	Vasculitis syndromes	(Hyperaggregable states)
Sickle-cell anemia	Postphlebitic damage	(Diabetes mellitus)
Hyperleukocytosis syndrome	Artificial surfaces	(Hyperlipidemia)
Immobilization/Stasis	Lupus anticoagulant/Antiphospholipid antibodies	(Sickle-cell anemia)
(Structural abnormalities of blood vessels)	Thrombotic thrombocytopenic purpura/ Hemolytic-Uremic syndrome	
(Pregnancy/Oral contraceptive use)	Tobacco-associated injury	**DISORDERS OF COAGULATION INHIBITORS**
(Thrombocytosis)	Nephrotic syndrome	Antithrombin III deficiency
	(Sepsis)	Heparin cofactor II deficiency
DISORDERS OF COAGULATION	(Leukoagglutination)	Protein C deficiency
Increased levels of clotting factors	Tissue injury/Trauma	Protein S deficiency
Malignancy		
Dysfibrinogenemias	**DISORDERS OF FIBRINOLYSIS**	
Infusion of activated clotting factors	Deficiency/Abnormalities of plasminogen	
Pregnancy/Oral contraceptive use	Defects in plasminogen activator	
Paroxysmal nocturnal hemoglobinuria	Increases in plasminogen activator inhibitor	
Sepsis	(Pregnancy/Oral contraceptive use)	
(Tissue injury/Trauma)	(Vasculitis syndromes)	
(Sickle-cell anemia)		

*Disorders with complex or multifactoral etiology are listed in more than one category. Parentheses indicate etiology of secondary importance.

malities of blood vessels are often preludes to development of thrombosis, particularly when a stimulus to clotting, such as tissue injury, is superimposed.

In the hyperviscosity syndrome, seen with elevated levels of IgM and rarely IgG or IgA, low flow occurs particularly in small vessels, where resultant hypoxia damages endothelium. Vasodilation and a bleeding disorder occur more frequently than overt thrombosis, but cerebral ischemia is common. Classical polycythemia vera is associated with hypervolemia and hyperviscosity, and overt arterial and venous thrombosis are common. As with other myeloproliferative disorders, thrombocytosis can add to the thrombotic risk. It is believed that mechanical disruption of flow, with vessel hypoxia, is the etiology of thrombosis in the hyperleukocytosis syndrome. Typically, this syndrome occurs with very high (>100,000/µl) peripheral blood levels of large, immature myeloblasts, or rarely, lymphoblasts. Cerebral and pulmonary ischemia is common.

In sickle-cell anemia, the complete pathogenesis of vaso-occlusion has not been elucidated. The inciting event may be adhesion of sickle cells to endothelium, but is probably multifactional. Areas of stasis are prone to sickling, and once sickling occurs, hypoxia, acidosis, and further decreased flow exacerbate the process with resultant ischemia and infarction. Careful studies have revealed evidence of platelet and coagulation factor activation in sickle crisis; however, the true role of the hemostatic system in producing or promoting the clinical features of sickle-cell anemia is not clear. Finally, although the pathogenesis of the thrombotic diathesis seen in the puerperium and in users of oral contraceptives is not well understood, disturbances in coagulation, fibrinolytic, and hemodynamic mechanisms have been documented. Marked vasodilation with stasis occurs in pregnancy and with use of oral contraceptives.

Disorders of blood vessels

Disorders of blood vessels, including atherosclerosis, are clearly the most frequent cause of thrombotic disease. Decades of intense research in endothelial and subendothelial structure, chemistry, and physiology have revealed much useful information about the pathogenesis of vascular disease. Endothelial cells have multiple functions, including control of fluid dynamics across the vessel wall; production of hemostatic inhibitory factors or complexes; synthesis and release of von Willebrand factor (vWF) and tissue plasminogen activator (t-PA), and the provision of a cell surface active in the coagulation mechanism. These disparate and indeed conflicting functions point out the major regulatory role served by endothelial cells. As described in previous chapters, exposure of the blood to subendothelial structures leads to platelet adhesion, aggregation, and granule release. Thrombin formation is stimulated and a stable clot is subsequently formed. The control of this process is believed to be dependent upon normal endothelium nearby the site of thrombus formation. Membrane phospholipids contain arachidonic acid, which can be converted by the endothelial cell to prostacyclin (PGI_2), a vasodilating agent that elevates platelet cyclic AMP (cAMP) and thus inhibits platelet aggregation. The endothelial surface contains heparin, heparan, and other glycosaminoglycans, antithrombin III (AT-III) and thrombomodulin, which bind thrombin and either inactivate its procoagulant activity (AT-III–heparin) or activate the anticoagulant serine protease protein C (thrombomodulin-thrombin). Thus, normal endothelium can dampen a thrombotic stimulus, and, via release of t-PA, mediate thrombolysis. Endothelial damage, either acute or chronic, thereby presents an enormous stimulus to thrombus formation, and the site (i.e., microvessels, arteries, veins), extent, and nature of the damage are important variables in the production of thrombotic disease.

Most of the disorders classified as disorders of blood vessels are complex, with incompletely understood pathophysiology. Abnormalities of any of the endothelial cell functions can be found in these disorders, for example, PGI_2 deficiency has been reported in thrombotic thrombocytopenic purpura and disturbances of t-PA release have been described in a number of vasculitis syndromes. Diagnostic or prognostic tests of endothelial or hemostatic function are not available, however, for most of these disorders.

Both arterial and venous thrombosis may occur in childhood in the genetic disorders that result in homocystinemia and homocystinuria. Multiple organ systems are involved in homocystinuria, whose most frequent cause is cystathione β-synthetase deficiency. Endothelial damage by elevated plasma levels of homocystine are thought responsible for the thrombotic diathesis. Definitive diagnosis requires detection of homocystinuria.

Atherosclerosis, the vasculitis syndromes, and the interaction of blood with artificial surfaces are complex disorders beyond the scope of this chapter. The uncommon disorder, thrombotic thrombocytopenia purpura (TTP), and the related syndrome, the hemolytic-uremic syndrome (HUS), are syndromes of unclear etiology, manifested by microvascular thromboses, and subsequent microangiopathic anemia and thrombocytopenia. Primary endothelial damage is suggested by the findings of endothelial cell proliferation and subendothelial hyaline deposits. Antiendothelial cells antibodies have been described in a few patients, but confirmation in a larger group is lacking. In addition to endothelial cell damage, plasma abnormalities have been proposed as the primary etiology. A circulating platelet aggregating factor has been described in TTP plasma that can be inhibited by normal plasma. However, such factors have been described in other thrombocytopenic disorders.

In 1982, Moake and colleagues described unusually large complexes of vWF in the plasma of four patients with recurrent TTP. The highest molecular weight complexes disappeared from plasma during relapses, leading the authors to speculate that an interaction between vWF and platelets was important in the clinical manifestations. However, infections or inflammatory diseases of many varieties produce similar high molecular weight complexes of vWF, and a specific or unique nature of these complexes in TTP has not been shown. Laboratory monitoring of TTP is generally accomplished by following the platelet count or serum levels of lactate dehydrogenase (LDH), which is a sensitive indicator of hemolysis. More sensitive measures of platelet function or damage, such as plasma levels of alpha granule contents, have not been systematically studied in TTP.

A marked increase in glomerular capillary permeability to plasma proteins results in the nephrotic syndrome. Massive proteinuria as well as hypoalbuminemia and hyperlipidemia are laboratory hallmarks. Venous thromboembolism is seen frequently in this disorder. The exact cause of the thrombotic diathesis is unclear, although a host of abnormalities in the concentrations of coagulation and inhibitory proteins have been described. Elevated levels of factors VIII and fibrinogen can be seen as well as diminished levels of AT-III, antiplasmin, factor IX, and the contact factors, presumably secondary to urinary losses. The hyperlipidemia has been associated with platelet hyperreactivity; however, several groups have implicated hypoalbuminemia as an important factor in the inability of nephrotic plasma to nullify production of thromboxane A_2. Theoretically, this could lead to platelet activation; however, whether this mechanism operates in vivo is speculative.

The effects of tobacco smoke inhalation on endothelial cells have been studied *ex vivo* and in animal models. Endothelial injury by nicotine or other elements of tobacco smoke in vitro has been shown in a number of investigations, and PGI_2 production has been reported diminished in animals and humans exposed chronically to tobacco smoke. The association of tobacco smoke and vascular injury (especially atherosclerosis) is well established.

Both tissue injury and sepsis are associated with formation of a number of substances that directly or indirectly damage endothelium and/or activate the clotting mechanism. Endotoxin, damaged or necrotic tissue, and other inflammatory stimulants lead to widespread activation of the complement, coagulation, kinin, and arachidonic acid-related prostaglandin systems and to the release of toxic cytokines, such as interleukin-1 and tumor necrosis factor. Leucocyte procoagulant activity, shown to be primarily monocyte-macrophage–associated tissue thromboplastin, can be generated by a number of stimuli, including endotoxin, immune complexes, complement fragments, and viruses. In addition, complement fragments can lead to neutrophil agglutination and margination, with generation of toxic oxygen compounds and release of proteases that can cause endothelial desquamation. Platelets may be activated by leukocytes, probably via oxygen radicals, and platelets and platelet activation products (such as prostaglandins) can augment monocyte tissue thromboplastin activity. Thus, tissue injury and sepsis are broad prothrombotic stimuli and some of the biochemical reactions already noted are likely responsible for the increased risk of thrombosis seen with surgery, trauma, infection, and inflammation.

Lupus anticoagulant/antiphospholipid antibodies

The association of autoimmune dysfunction and a circulating plasma factor with anticoagulant properties was recognized nearly 50 years ago. Since patients with systemic lupus erythematosus (SLE) had the highest incidence of this inhibitory factor, it was given the name lupus anticoagulant (LA) in 1972 by Feinstein and Rapaport.

The LA is one of several antibodies with specificity toward negatively charged phospholipids. Other antiphospholipid antibodies (APL) include antibody to cardiolipin (ACL). The LA and other APL are nonspecific inhibitors of coagulation in that they are not directed toward a specific clotting factor. Instead, their antiphospholipid action inhibits the binding of clotting factors and/or Ca^{2+} to the phospholipid added to the reagent mixture in routine coagulation screening tests. The LA has been identified in about 50% of patients with SLE (idiopathic or drug-induced) and in variable but smaller percentages of patients with other autoimmune disorders. It can also be seen in patients with infectious diseases, where it is usually a transient phenomenon, and most importantly, after ingestion of certain medications, especially phenothiazines, phenytoin, quinidine, and procainamide.

A bleeding diathesis with LA is distinctly unusual, and seen only when accompanied by severe thrombocytopenia and/or prothrombin deficiency. Instead, both LA and ACL are predominantly associated with thrombotic disorders, including deep-venous thrombosis (DVT), cerebral and peripheral artery thrombosis, and thrombosis of renal, retinal, and placental veins, the latter giving rise to a syndrome of recurrent abortions. It is estimated that some 2% of patients with pathologic venous thrombosis have LA. About one third of patients with LA have pathologic thrombosis, of which two thirds is DVT, one quarter is cerebral arterial, and one tenth is peripheral arterial thrombosis.

Classically, LA have not been associated with an increased incidence of coronary thrombosis, but recent studies have associated ACL with an increased risk of graft occlusion after bypass surgery. Although LA are most common in females, thrombosis is more common in male patients with LA. Patients under 10 years with LA and patients with transient LA associated with infectious diseases appear not to have an increased risk of thrombosis. Unfortunately, most LA patients at especially high risk of thrombosis cannot be identified by accompanying clinical or laboratory features. Neither the presence of ACL, a false-positive VDRL, moderate thrombocytopenia (which is common in patients with LA), nor the strength of the LA or titer of ACL or other APL are predictive of the patients at highest risk for thrombosis.

The *in vivo* mechanism by which APL predispose to thrombosis is unclear. Platelet activation, with subsequent thrombin formation, has been suggested by the phospholipid specificity of the antibodies and the frequent finding of thrombocytopenia. Alternatively, endothelial damage is suggested by reports of diminished production of PGI_2 in cultured endothelial cells exposed to the LA and a report of LA inhibition of soluble and endothelial-based thrombomodulin, with resultant diminished protein C activation. The membrane damage mechanism was furthered by reports suggesting that the phospholipid specificity of the LA is directed against a pathologically altered structural array of lipids. Lastly, the heterogeneity of LA and the inability of any given APL assay or configuration of assays to accurately predict which APL patients are at highest risk of thrombosis may indicate that these antibodies are epiphenomena, and the thrombotic diathesis is a manifestation of a yet to be discovered abnormality.

Laboratory features

Typically, tests of intrinsic coagulation are prolonged in the presence of LA, whereas the prothrombin time (PT) is usually normal. An abnormal PT in the setting of an LA should always prompt a specific assay for prothrombin, since prothrombin deficiency (<40%) can accompany an LA and is an important prognostic factor for abnormal bleeding. Interestingly, the prothrombin deficiency is caused by

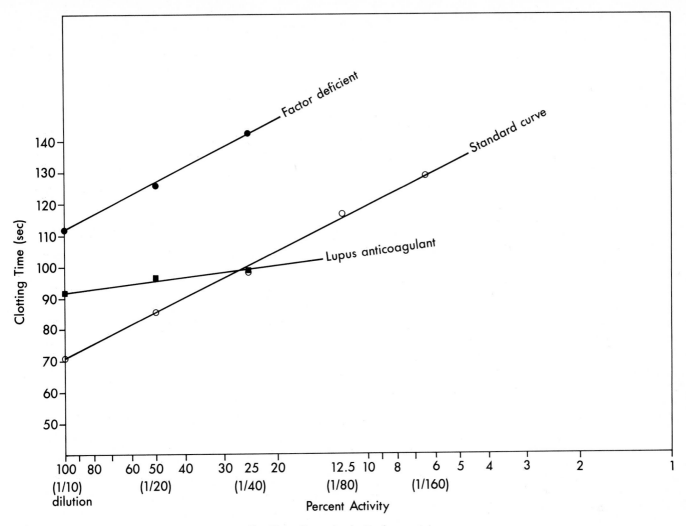

Fig. 67-1   Curves in clotting factor assays.

antibodies that do not neutralize the procoagulant activity of prothrombin, but are thought to mediate its rapid removal from circulation. Prolongations of the thrombin time (TT) are unusual as well, and usually signify an antibody of another specificity that interferes with fibrin polymerization.

The standard activated partial thromboplastin time (aPTT) detects most cases of LA, although sensitivity varies with the manufacturer. As is characteristic of inhibitors of coagulation, repeating the aPTT using a 1:1 mix of test and normal plasma will not shorten it. In fact, mixing studies often result in a further prolongation of the aPTT. Lupus anticoagulant can be distinguished from specific inhibitors of clotting factors by the lack of progressive inhibition with time, in other words, the inhibition does not increase with incubation at 37° C for 1 to 2 hours. Specific factor assays are normal in LA plasma (with the rare exception of true prothrombin deficiency), although one-stage assays based on the aPTT will be low if judged at low dilution points. At higher dilutions, the LA activity is diluted out, and the correct factor level is obtained. This results in a test curve that is nonparallel to the standard curve (Fig. 67-1).

Tests that do not utilize added phospholipid, or that use diluted phospholipid, are the most sensitive to the LA. Tests

without added lipid include the whole blood clotting time, the platelet-rich or platelet-poor recalcification time, and the activated clotting time (ACT). Assays that have used diluted phospholipid to detect LA include the diluted Russell's viper venom time (dRVVT) and the tissue thromboplastin inhibition test (TTI). In the dRVVT, Russell's viper venom (RVV) is diluted to give a normal RVV-phospholipid time of 20 to 25 seconds. The phospholipid is then diluted 1:8 or greater with buffered saline and both test and normal plasmas are run. A prolongation of test plasma above normal plasma of 5 seconds (about 3.5 to 4 SD) is considered positive. In the TTI, tissue thromboplastin is diluted 1:100 or 1:1000, and PTs are obtained on both test and normal plasma. A ratio of PT (test) to PT (normal) of >1.3 is considered positive. Several comparison studies of the TTI, dRVVT, and aPTT have shown that each can sensitively detect the lupus anticoagulant.

It is important to understand other conditions that can give a positive result in these tests. All tests, of course, are abnormal in factor deficiencies. The aPTT is also prolonged by factor VIII inhibitors and therapeutic levels of heparin. The dRVVT is somewhat less sensitive than the aPTT to heparin, and because Russell's viper venom acts on factor

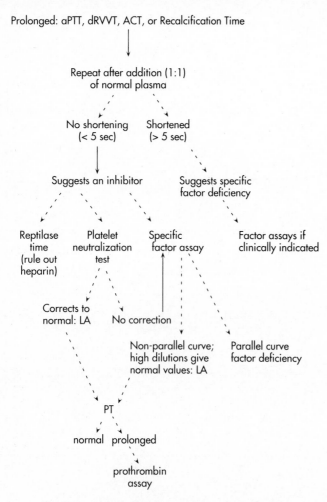

Prolonged: aPTT, dRVVT, ACT, or Recalcification Time

Repeat after addition (1:1)
of normal plasma

No shortening (< 5 sec)   Shortened (> 5 sec)

Suggests an inhibitor   Suggests specific factor deficiency

Reptilase time (rule out heparin)   Platelet neutralization test   Specific factor assay   Factor assays if clinically indicated

Corrects to normal: LA   No correction

Non-parallel curve; high dilutions give normal values: LA   Parallel curve factor deficiency

PT

normal   prolonged

prothrombin assay

Fig. 67-2   Suggested work-up of a lupus anticoagulant.

X, factor VIII inhibitors do not prolong the dRVVT. The dRVVT, the aPTT, and the TTI would be prolonged by a factor V inhibitor (a rare occurrence). The TTI is also abnormal in the presence of heparin and, surprisingly, in the presence of factor VIII inhibitors. This finding indicates that, at dilute tissue thromboplastin concentrations, amplification of factor X activation by factor VIIa-mediated factor IX activation is discernible using the PT system. The specificity of the aPTT and dRVVT in detecting the LA can be enhanced by substituting freeze-thawed or ionophore-activated platelets for phospholipid. Phospholipid in the platelet membrane neutralizes the LA (the platelet neutralization test), and thus significant shortening of these tests is seen with platelet substitution in LA plasma. Specific inhibitors are not neutralized, and no shortening of the aPTT or dRVVT occurs in these patients.

A simplified approach to the detection of LA, based on these studies, can be constructed (Fig. 67-2). If an LA is suspected due to the finding of a prolonged aPTT that does not correct itself by addition of normal plasma, a specific factor inhibitor can be ruled out by a platelet neutralization test and/or specific factor assays. If an LA is the presumptive diagnosis, a concurrent prolonged PT should prompt a

prothrombin assay. If a request to rule out LA is received, several sensitive tests can be utilized to detect the inhibitor. If these screening tests of intrinsic coagulation are normal, LA is very unlikely. However, a PT and TT may be performed to detect the presence of less common LA-like inhibitors that have activity against tissue thromboplastin-dependent complexes or that inhibit fibrin polymerization. If clinical thrombosis is present and the LA is absent, a test for ACL or APL should then be obtained. These tests are performed in specialized laboratories using an enzyme-linked immunoassay method. At the present time, testing for ACL or APL in plasma with a known LA is redundant, since no further diagnostic or prognostic information will be obtained.

Disorders of platelet number and function

The demonstration of thrombocytosis is a simple task in most laboratories, but some clinical correlation is often required before a definite thrombotic diathesis can be diagnosed. Transient or secondary thrombocytosis, such as postsplenectomy in hematologically normal patients, or caused by iron deficiency or inflammation, is generally not believed to represent a prethrombotic state. However, there is a well-recognized increased incidence of venous and microvascular thromboses in patients with thrombocytosis secondary to a myeloproliferative disorder. The mechanism of this thrombotic risk, which generally increases as the platelet count increases above $1 \times 10^6/\mu l$, is unclear. Hyperreactive platelets have been noted in patients with thromboses, but this simple concept is clouded by (1) a lack of understanding of the cause of the hyperreactivity when demonstrated; (2) the more frequent demonstration of hyporeactive platelets in the myeloproliferative disorders, including alterations in ultrastructure, granule content, membrane receptor activity, and prostaglandin metabolism; and (3) the finding of a bleeding diathesis in thrombocytosis, which occurs as frequently as thrombotic complications. Unfortunately, no laboratory test alone predicts clinical bleeding or thrombosis in an individual patient, although the finding of hyperreactive platelets in a patient with thrombosis is often seen as an indication for antiplatelet therapy.

Platelet hyperreactivity is a general term that encompasses several different laboratory definitions. Platelet survival and platelet turnover have been studied in patients suffering from or at risk of thrombotic disorders. Presumably, increased platelet turnover or diminished survival would indicate ongoing platelet activation by a foreign surface or a damaged vessel, or, perhaps, incorporation into a thrombus. Platelet survival and turnover are generally measured using platelets tagged with radioisotopes, either chromium-51 or indium-111. Platelet consumption is increased in arterial thrombotic disorders without significant concurrent activation of the coagulation system, as measured by fibrinogen consumption. Thus, in patients with atherosclerotic disease, prosthetic valves, arterial grafts, and homocystinuria, platelet turnover may be increased and survival shortened. Both platelet and fibrinogen consumption are accelerated in thrombotic disorders of the venous system, a finding consistent with morphologic differences between venous and arterial thrombi. Unfortunately, platelet survival and turnover studies are of relatively little use as clinical predictors of thrombosis in individual patients, nor are these studies valuable diagnostically. At present, they are used primarily in research settings.

Enhanced platelet aggregability to adenosine diphosphate (ADP), epinephrine, and other agonists has been described in patients with atherosclerosis, diabetes mellitus, and hyperlipidemia, where increased membrane lipid can be demonstrated and is likely responsible for in vitro abnormalities. Spontaneous in vitro platelet aggregation, in other words, without addition of an agonist, has been reported in myeloproliferative disorders with thrombocytosis. Similarly, increases in the in vitro expression of platelet procoagulant activity (formerly referred to as platelet factor 3 activity) have been noted in association with arterial and venous thrombotic disorders. As with the demonstration of increased platelet turnover, however, all these tests have no predictive or diagnostic utility in the setting of thrombotic disease.

An attempt to improve predictability of platelet function tests in this regard led to the description of a test for circulating (in vivo) platelet aggregates in the mid-1970s. In this test, venous blood is drawn into two syringes, one with formalin-EDTA (ethylenediamine tetraacetic acid) solution and the other with EDTA alone. Platelet counts are performed on platelet-rich plasma (PRP) from each sample and a ratio is derived—platelet count in formalin-EDTA:platelet count in EDTA only. The normal value ranges from 0.77 to 1.00. Presumably, the PRP of patients with circulating aggregates has a lower platelet count due to centrifugation of the higher density aggregates during preparation of PRP. Abnormalities in patients with chronic or acute arterial and venous thrombosis have been described, but the test has not found widespread applicability as a clinical or research tool.

Many studies have reported association of elevated plasma levels of the platelet alpha-granule proteins, β-thromboglobulin (βTG), and platelet factor 4 (PF4), with other abnormalities of platelet function or with established thrombotic disease. These proteins are measured by radioimmunoassay, and are thus not readily available in most clinical laboratories. Furthermore, extreme care is necessary in collection of blood samples for testing, since platelet alpha granule release in vitro is easily stimulated. Some investigators have therefore utilized urinary levels of βTG, which vary consistently with plasma levels, or by using the ratio of βTG to PF4, taking advantage of the very rapid plasma clearance of PF4 compared to βTG. Despite several reports of predictive value of βTG in cerebrovascular disease, further study in this and other thrombotic disorders has produced results that are conflicting and difficult to interpret. Elevated levels of these proteins are associated with vascular disorders, but at present, their utility is limited to the research setting.

Heparin-induced thrombocytopenia

Heparin-induced thrombocytopenia is a relatively frequent complication of heparin therapy, at both low and full doses. The most recent studies put the estimated frequency of this effect at 3% to 10%, depending upon the source of the heparin (bovine > porcine) and the ability of study authors to carefully eliminate nonheparin-related causes of thrombocytopenia.

Heparin has a wide variety of effects on the hemostatic system, reflecting the heterogeneous nature of the preparations and its highly negative charge. In addition to its well-described interaction with AT-III, it has variable effects on platelet function, having been reported to cause platelet hyper- or hyporeactivity. Increased in vitro aggregation and granule release have been reported, as have decreased platelet aggregation and prolongation of the template bleeding time. These findings vary greatly among individuals, as well as among heparin preparations, where high molecular weight fractions tend to interact with platelets more than low molecular weight fractions. During heparin therapy, mild thrombocytopenia (defined as platelet count above 50,000/μl or a drop of 40% or less below the pretreatment count), occurs most frequently (3% to 10% of heparin-treated patients), but is without significant clinical sequelae. In fact, mild thrombocytopenia may resolve very shortly after or even during heparin treatment and is not associated with serious bleeding or thrombotic problems. Severe thrombocytopenia (defined as platelet count less than 50,000/μl or >40% diminution compared to pretreatment count) however, is associated with serious clinical thrombotic sequelae, mostly arterial, including myocardial, cerebral, and acute limb infarction, resulting in amputation. Death occurs in some one quarter to one third of patients with heparin-induced thrombocytopenia and arterial thrombosis, and it appears to occur more frequently with bovine as opposed to porcine preparations. Fortunately, arterial thrombosis is only a rare complication of severe heparin-induced thrombocytopenia. Nevertheless, discontinuation of heparin therapy is recommended when severe thrombocytopenia develops.

The cause of heparin-induced thrombocytopenia with or without arterial thrombosis remains a mystery. Most investigators favor an immunologic mechanism, namely IgG heparin-dependent antiplatelet antibodies. In the laboratory, most attempts at diagnostic tests have focused on the demonstration of the aggregation of normal platelets in the presence of patient plasma or serum and heparin. Controls for this test would include mixtures without heparin and with normal plasma or serum instead of patient plasma or serum. Kelton and colleagues reported that heparin-dependent dense granule release (measured as serotonin release) achieved a 90% specificity in their study. Thus, a positive test is useful when obtained. With a reported sensitivity of under 40%, however, a negative test cannot rule out the syndrome. Platelet-associated IgG was not discriminatory and heparin-dependent aggregation was not as predictive as serotonin release in their experience.

In summary, heparin-induced thrombocytopenia remains primarily a clinical diagnosis, awaiting a better understanding of its pathophysiology. Demonstration in vitro of heparin-dependent platelet aggregation or dense granule release appears to be a useful confirmation of the diagnosis, but negative test results cannot rule out the syndrome.

Disorders of coagulation

Ultimately, the coagulation system is involved in all pathologic thrombi, and thus the classification of specific disorders as coagulation disorders is somewhat arbitrary. The question of whether increased concentrations of normal clotting factors alone could predispose to thrombosis is unan-

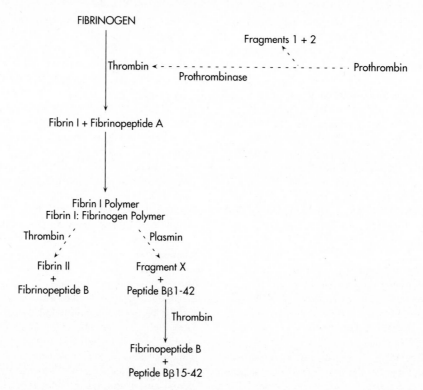

Fig. 67-3 *Generation of prothrombin and fibrinogen peptide fragments. Redrawn from Kaplan KL: Coagulation proteins in thrombosis. In Colman RW and others (editors): Hemostasis and thrombosis, ed 2, Philadelphia, 1987, JB Lippincott.*

swered. An increased level of factor VIII will shorten the aPTT, and other global tests of coagulation may reveal more rapid thrombin generation when clotting factor levels are elevated. In addition, epidemiologic studies have shown an increased risk of coronary and cerebral artery thrombosis when elevated levels of fibrinogen or factor VIII are present. Nevertheless, large studies have not shown that the aPTT, fibrinogen level, or factor VIII level can reliably predict the development of thrombosis in any patient group.

Standard tests of coagulation (PT, aPTT, fibrinogen level, TT, fibrin degradation products) are not useful in predicting risk for an individual. Theoretically, a shortened PT or aPTT may be evidence of factor Xa or thrombin generation in vivo; however, pretest variables, such as the conditions of blood collection and the inherent variability in the test itself, make these tests too nonspecific for this purpose.

Major advances in elucidation of the biochemistry and physiology of fibrinogen and its reactions have led to a number of very sensitive and specific tests for thrombin (and plasmin) action (Fig. 67-3). Radioimmunoassays and/or enzyme-linked immunosorbent assays (ELISA) for prothrombin fragments 1 and 2, fibrinopeptides A (FpA) and B (FpB), and fibrinogen peptide fragments Bβ1-42 and 15-42 have been developed. A radioimmunoassay for thrombin–AT-III complexes has been developed and specific assays for fibrinogen degradation products, such as fragment X and fragment E, are also available. The greatest clinical experience has been acquired with FpA and, secondarily, Bβ1-42.

Elevated levels of FpA are found in venous thrombosis,

pulmonary embolism, after tissue injury, in infectious states, in SLE, and indeed in disseminated intravascular coagulation (DIC) of any cause. Thus, an elevated FpA level is the closest thing to a true marker for hypercoagulability. In venous thrombosis, FpA levels promptly fall upon heparin anticoagulation, and subsequent increases are associated with recurrence or clot extension. If tissue injury is present however, such as in pulmonary infarction, FpA levels may remain elevated, signaling either ongoing thrombin generation or extravascular clot formation. A better measure than FpA alone is the FpA/Bβ1-42 ratio, which reflects the balance in circulation of thrombin vs. plasmin action. However, despite some predictive ability, the FpA/Bβ1-42 ratio was not found to be specific in the detection of asymptomatic thrombosis.

Overall, the use of these ultrasensitive tests of thrombin generation and action is limited to research settings. Great care must be taken in sample collection and processing to ensure reliable results.

Specific disorders

A small number of the 100+ dysfibrinogens that have been described are associated with an increased thrombotic risk. As with dysfibrinogens of all types, a prolonged TT and/or reptilase time is the rule, and the fibrinogen level is somewhat reduced when assayed with a functional method (e.g., Clauss). A number of biochemical mechanisms for the disorder have been described, including resistance to plasmin action or decreased plasminogen binding.

Infusion of activated clotting factors, especially those

designed to bypass factor VIII inhibitor activity, can lead to pathologic thrombosis. Patients with liver disease, who are unable to clear from circulation these activated factors, are at particular risk.

Malignant disorders of many types are associated with an increased risk of thrombosis, both localized and widespread. Venous thrombosis is common in cancer patients, afflicting perhaps 10% of patients. An associated syndrome of recurrent venous thrombophlebitis, occurring in superficial and deep veins in unusual sites, so-called migratory thrombophlebitis, was described in 1865 by Trousseau. Sensitive tests of thrombin activation reveal subclinical activation of clotting in many cancer patients, due both to release of thromboplastin-like materials from the tumor and to widespread vascular damage, with subsequent activation of intrinsic and extrinsic pathways. In addition, platelet turnover is often increased in cancer and hyperaggregable platelets have been demonstrated in some patients. Both standard and nonstandard measures of coagulation are not specific for cancer, but may be best utilized to follow the course of an individual patient. Tumor burden is roughly correlated with activation of coagulation.

Hemostatic abnormalities that have been associated with pregnancy or oral contraceptive use include diminished vascular tone, increased platelet adhesion, elevation of coagulation proteins (fibrinogen, factors II, VII, IX, X, and XII), and an increase in plasminogen levels associated with progressive increase in the euglobulin lysis time, which may indicate a diminished fibrinolytic capability. Antithrombin III levels have been reported as diminished or not changed. The relative roles of these factors in producing the clear hypercoagulable state associated with oral contraceptive use and the peripartum period are undefined. Sensitive tests of thrombin generation often reveal subclinical activation of clotting, however, and the rapidity with which DIC can develop with obstetrical disorders implies that an abnormal coagulation system is an important predisposing factor to thrombosis in these patients. The etiology of the activated coagulation systems is unclear.

Paroxysmal nocturnal hemoglobinuria is a malignant stem cell disorder associated with an increased risk of thrombosis. Complement-induced hemolysis of abnormal red blood cells is the likely trigger event, although platelet lysis and activation may be important in pathogenesis as well. Although the exact mechanism leading to clot formation is not known, it is presumed that the acute hemolysis leads to red blood cell membrane-related activation of clotting, as with other hemolytic disorders.

Sepsis and tissue injury both lead to a variety of systemic and local reactions that can culminate in thrombin formation. Endotoxin can damage endothelium and induce the appearance of tissue factor activity (TFA) on the surface of leukocytes, especially in the macrophage-monocyte line. Leukocyte TFA can also be stimulated by immune complexes, complement fragments, and other plasma constituents. In conjunction with factor VII, this TFA has clearly been shown to activate coagulation and is most likely responsible for the hypercoagulable or subclinical consumptive state, which sometimes develops into overt DIC, in sepsis. Tissue injury leads to activation of coagulation, complement, kinin, and other systems involved in inflammation.

Endothelial damage and tissue injury are the proximate causes, and tissue injury/trauma should be considered a hypercoagulable state. Platelet and fibrinogen turnover are increased in even controlled injuries (i.e., elective surgery) and the magnitude of the increase is proportional to the extent of injury.

Finally, using sensitive tests of thrombin generation, coagulation system activation has been documented in sickle-cell crisis, presumably due to the distorted red blood cell membranes of sickled cells. Whether or not this is of primary importance or secondary to and synergistic with the stasis and ischemic vascular damage caused by vessel occlusion in sickle-cell disease has not been determined.

Disorders of fibrinolysis

Fibrinolytic disorders leading to thrombosis include dysplasminogenemia, plasminogen activator defects, and increases in plasminogen activator inhibitor. Historically, the techniques and experience necessary to demonstrate these fibrinolytic defects were limited to research centers. Although simple functional and immunoassays are now commercially available for some of these proteins, their specificity is often poor, and fibrinolytic defects are rarely diagnosed without specialized laboratory assistance.

Dysplasminogenemia

Functional plasminogen deficiency has been reported as both a classic type I defect (true deficiency of protein) and as a type II defect (normal amount of a dysfunctional protein). Dysplasminogenemia is suspected by the finding of a prolonged euglobulin lysis time. Both chromogenic and fluorogenic assays for functional plasminogen (as plasmin) are available, as are standard immunoassays, such as radial immunodiffusion. They have been previously described in Chapter 65.

Defects in plasminogen activator and plasminogen activator inhibitor

Several groups have reported large families with adolescent onset of recurrent venous thromboembolic disease associated with a decreased plasminogen activator (PA) activity, or an increased plasminogen activator inhibitor (PAI) activity. Inheritance appears to be autosomal-dominant, and long-term warfarin therapy is indicated in these patients. Although the previously described assays for PA are available, they are not highly specific and this lack of specificity has led to a need for confirmatory studies to document the true role of defects in PA or PAI as a cause of thrombotic disease.

Disorders of inhibitors of coagulation

The physiologic importance of plasma protease inhibitors is illustrated by the well-described disorders associated with their deficiencies. Deficiency of the plasmin inhibitor, α-2-antiplasmin, is associated with a hemorrhagic disorder, whereas thrombotic disorders result from deficiencies of the thrombin inhibitors, antithrombin III (AT-III) and heparin cofactor II (HC-II). In addition to these classic inhibitory proteins, the anticoagulant protease, protein C, and its cofactor, factor S, have critical physiologic roles, since deficiencies of these proteins can also result in a thrombotic disorder.

Antithrombin III

Antithrombin III is the most important inhibitor of procoagulant serine proteases including thrombin, Xa, and IXa. Antithrombin III is a glycoprotein of molecular weight of 58,000 and has markedly increased antiprotease activity when bound to heparin, either in solution or on the endothelial cell surface.

The incidence in the general population of congenital AT-III deficiency is on the order of 1 per 2000 to 5000, and both deficiency states and abnormal protein have been described. Antithrombin III abnormalities are inherited in an autosomal-dominant fashion, and heterozygotes with levels of less than 50% of normal are affected. Recurrent thromboses of primarily the venous system may occur early in adolescence, often in conjunction with pregnancy, surgery, or trauma.

Acquired deficiency of AT-III has been reported in heparin therapy, liver disease (the site of synthesis), DIC, nephrotic syndrome, and in patients taking oral contraceptives. Whether these conditions of acquired deficiency represent a true thrombotic risk is difficult to acertain, although many investigators believe it to be the major thrombotic predisposing factor in nephrotic syndrome and with oral contraceptive use.

Antithrombin III levels may be measured immunologically by radial immunodiffusion or by the Laurell rocket method. Functional activity is usually measured by the ability of plasma to inhibit thrombin or factor Xa in the presence of heparin (heparin cofactor activity). In practice, heparin is mixed with normal plasma of varying dilutions and thrombin or factor Xa is added. The residual thrombin or factor Xa is measured using a chromogenic substrate. Patient plasma is compared to the normal plasma standard to calculate percent activity. Normal functional values vary between 75% to 120% of normal, with the normal protein levels varying between 18 to 30 mg/dl.

Antithrombin III deficiency has been classified into three types: type I, in which concurrent and parallel deficiencies of functional activity and immunoreactive protein are found; type II, in which protein levels are normal but functional activity is decreased; and type III (a variant of type II), in which functional defects are noted only in the presence of heparin. Types II and III therefore most likely represent different protein abnormalities. Thus, both immunologic and functional assays must be performed to rule out AT-III deficiency.

Lyophilized AT-III concentrates are now available for replacement therapy, and they may be given with heparin (at 20 to 40 μ/kg) to treat acute thrombotic episodes. Long-term therapy is successfully achieved with warfarin anticoagulation. It has been reported that warfarin therapy may increase AT-III levels, but the mechanism remains obscure.

Heparin cofactor II

Heparin cofactor II is a recently described, heparin-dependent thrombin inhibitor. It differs from AT-III in at least two respects: it has no activity against other serine proteases and its antithrombin activity is accelerated by glycosaminoglycans other than heparin, such as dermatan and heparan sulfates.

Like AT-III, heparin cofactor II (HC-II) is synthesized in the liver, and acquired deficiencies in liver disease and DIC have been reported. The congenital deficiency state is inherited in an autosomal-dominant fashion. Compared to AT-III, the prevalence of HC-II deficiency is low and it is believed to represent only a weak risk factor for thrombosis.

Heparin cofactor II can be measured by immunoassay and by functional assay. Normal values range from 75% to 180%. Two different techniques are used to measure functional HC-II activity. In the first, AT-III is either depleted by immunoadsorption onto sepharose or neutralized by addition of specific AT-III antibodies. Heparin cofactor activity can then be measured by a thrombin or factor Xa substrate assay. The second technique utilizes dermatan sulfate as a cofactor, thus eliminating the problem of AT-III interference when using the heparin cofactor activity.

Protein C

Protein C is a vitamin K-dependent protein that functions as a protease anticoagulant. Protein C is converted to its proteolytic form, activated protein C (APC), by an endothelial-based complex of thrombin and thrombomodulin, a protein whose molecular weight is 74,000 and which is synthesized by endothelial cells. Interestingly, thrombin is rendered incapable of clotting fibrinogen or of activating platelets while bound to thrombomodulin.

Activated protein C degrades factors V and VIII, as well as the factor X receptor on platelets (the receptor thought responsible for platelet procoagulant activity). Activated protein C also increases plasminogen activator activity, perhaps by degradation of plasminogen activator inhibitor. Like AT-III, an hereditary deficiency of protein C (levels less than 50% of normal) is associated with an increased risk of premature venous thrombosis. This disorder is inherited in an autosomal-dominant manner, and the incidence of heterozygotic deficiency is only about a third as frequent as AT-III deficiency. An unusual manifestation of protein C deficiency is neonatal purpura fulminans, a severe thrombotic disorder of infancy thought to be a manifestation of homozygous protein C deficiency. Like AT-III, protein C is synthesized in the liver, and acquired deficiencies can be found in liver disease as well as DIC, and during warfarin anticoagulation.

Immunoassays for protein C antigen are available, both by rocket electroimmunoassay and by ELISA. A number of functional assays have been described. These assays are available primarily in research laboratories and are based on either isolation of protein C by barium sulfate or aluminum hydroxide, followed by thrombin activation, and measurement using either a chromogenic substrate or the aPTT, or the addition of thrombomodulin and thrombin to form a complex to activate protein C. Several crossover assays that use both principles have been developed. The use of functional assays appears to be warranted to rule out protein C deficiency, since there have been reports of functional deficiency of clinical significance in the face of a normal immunoassay. At present, treatment of symptomatic protein C deficiency is long-term warfarin therapy.

Protein S

Protein S is a vitamin K-dependent protein that circulates partially (60%) bound to complement C4b-binding protein. Free protein S acts as a cofactor in the inactivation of factor

V by APC. Like AT-III and protein C deficiency, heterozygotic protein S deficiency is associated with early onset thromboembolic disease.

Measurement of protein S is problematic even with standard immunoassays due to the presence of bound protein S. Prolonged room temperature electrophoresis is required to dissociate the bound protein; alternatively, an immunoradiometric assay using high dilutions can be used. At present, functional assays are imprecise and are performed in only a few research centers.

ANTITHROMBOTIC THERAPY

Our understanding of the role and limitations of antithrombotic therapy has increased markedly in recent years. Although two drugs, heparin and warfarin, continue to be the most useful and widely prescribed agents, better use of antiplatelet drugs and thrombolytic therapy have added greatly to the prevention and management of thrombotic disorders.

The ideal antithrombotic agent would prevent pathologic thrombi in susceptible patients, prevent the propagation of established thrombi, preferably by effecting clot lysis, and do so promptly so that clinical sequelae of thrombi are obviated or minimized. Hemorrhagic and other side effects would be minimal, and laboratory tests to judge indications, efficacy, and risk-benefit ratio would be routinely available.

For many, but not all, clinical thrombotic states, available medications do meet these specifications. The indications, laboratory monitoring, and side effects of antiplatelet drugs, anticoagulant drugs, and thrombolytic agents will be discussed in this section.

Antiplatelet agents

A variety of drugs that inhibit platelet function have been utilized to prevent or modify thrombotic disorders, including aspirin and dipyridamole. Because of the well-known role of platelet activation and consumption in arterial thrombotic disorders, antiplatelet therapy plays a more important role in arterial rather than venous thrombosis, where both platelet and clotting factor consumption occur.

Unfortunately, in vitro correlates of in vivo efficacy of antiplatelet therapy do not exist. Therefore, both overall utility and appropriate dose regimens can only be judged by in vivo trials that measure clinical (pathologic) end points.

The most frequently used antiplatelet agent is aspirin, which inhibits the platelet release reaction by irreversibly inactivating platelet cyclooxygenase, an enzyme important in the generation of thromboxane A_2 from arachidonic acid. Thromboxane A_2 is a potent vasoconstrictor and platelet-activating agent. Its importance in clinical hemostasis is judged by the bleeding disorders seen after aspirin ingestion and due to congenital absence of enzymes, including cyclooxygenase, important in its generation. Aspirin has been successful in the prevention of initial and recurrent myocardial infarction in males, in the treatment of unstable angina, and in the prevention of graft occlusion after coronary artery bypass surgery. Aspirin has been shown to decrease the incidence of stroke and death in patients with transient ischemic attacks, but has not been shown efficacious in the prevention of recurrent strokes. In conjunction with dipyridamole, aspirin therapy has been shown to slow the progression of peripheral arterial disease. Less clear-cut indications for aspirin include prosthetic heart valves, where it has been used in conjunction with oral anticoagulants, thrombotic thrombocytopenia purpura, and in the prevention of venous thromboses in patients undergoing hip surgery. In symptomatic patients with thrombocytosis and platelet hyperreactivity, aspirin has been reported to both correct in vitro hyperreactivity and to prevent thrombotic complications.

As expected, all antiplatelet drugs pose a threat of hemorrhagic and other side effects. At present, laboratory monitoring of drug effects plays no role in clinical management. The decision to use antiplatelet therapy in any disorder is always made with full cognizance of its risks.

Anticoagulation therapy

Heparin

Heparin is a potent global anticoagulant that acts in concert with protein cofactors to inhibit a number of serine proteases important in blood coagulation. Heparin is a complex carbohydrate, consisting of a repetitive glycine-serine peptide backbone to which long (8 to 20 residues), highly sulfated mucopolysaccharides are bound to the serine residues. This highly negative-charged proteoglycan has multiple anticoagulant and nonanticoagulant effects. All heparin preparations are not alike, since the relative binding of heparin to its anticoagulant cofactors, activated clotting factors, or other molecules depends upon the residue length, degree of negative charge, and other factors. Low molecular weight heparin fractions, which appear to have potent anticoagulant effects with minimal antiplatelet or other side effects, are under clinical evaluation, and may be especially useful for patients with heparin-associated thrombocytopenia.

As stated in a previous section, heparin interacts with plasma and endothelial-based cofactors, especially AT-III and HC-II, to accelerate the antiprotease effect of these cofactors. Heparin can be safely administered either subcutaneously or intravenously, and is used prophylactically (i.e., to prevent thrombosis) or therapeutically (i.e., to prevent further growth of an established thrombus).

For prophylactic purposes, large doses of heparin are too often associated with bleeding to be useful. Therefore low-dose or "mini" heparin—subcutaneous administration of 5,000 to 10,000 units every 8 to 12 hours—has been tried and found useful in preventing thrombosis in general surgery patients and other patients at moderate risk of thrombosis. In patients at greater thrombotic risk, however, such as patients undergoing hip operations or with gynecologic malignancies, low-dose heparin is not an effective prophylaxis. It is likely in high-risk disorders that the rate of procoagulant formation is too high to allow low doses of heparin to fully neutralize procoagulant action. Full-dose heparin is generally given intravenously, and has a plasma half-life of about 1 hour. Half-lives are decreased with larger thrombi and with pulmonary emboli, and larger doses may be needed in these situations. A bolus injection of 5,000 to 10,000 units is generally followed by a constant infusion of 800 to 2000 units per hour. Full-dose heparin can be given subcutaneously, where every 12-hour injection can maintain therapeutic levels. After subcutaneous injection, peak levels are typically reached 4 to 5 hours after injection.

Unfortunately, the optimum dose in an individual patient—the smallest dose at which clot progression is just halted—cannot be determined. Instead, animal studies and clinical studies in humans have used pathologic end points to determine the dose at which thrombus growth can be prevented in the great majority of subjects. Heparin monitoring is typically performed by using the standard aPTT, since the PT is very insensitive to the presence of heparin and even small amounts of heparin will infinitely prolong the standard thrombin time (Fig. 67-4). Advantages of the aPTT include its widespread availability and the long experience that has been gained in its standardization and use in heparin monitoring. The earliest heparin-monitoring test was the whole blood (Lee-White) clotting time test. Whole blood was placed in three glass tubes (1 ml each) and the first tube was tilted every 30 seconds until a clot formed. The second and third tubes were similarly treated. The time to clot formation (an average of the three tubes) was taken as the clotting time. This test is both unreliable and too insensitive for heparin monitoring and it has been supplanted by the aPTT. In human and animal studies, enough heparin to prolong the aPTT to 1.5 to 2.0 times the value obtained using pooled normal plasma has been shown to prevent clot

propagation in a great majority of subjects. This corresponded to a heparin concentration of 0.2 to 0.5 u/ml in these studies, and aPTT and heparin levels were highly correlated. This aPTT end point (1.5 to 2.0 times normal plasma value) has become standard, although proper use of the aPTT requires an understanding of the variable sensitivities of different manufacturers' reagents to heparin. Reagents with poor sensitivity to heparin can lead to over-heparinization if the end point of 1.5 to 2.0 times normal plasma value is strictly adhered to (Fig. 67-5). Each laboratory should determine the range of aPTT for its reagent corresponding to a heparin concentration of 0.3 to 0.5 u/ml (Box 67-1). It should be noted that the type of equipment or technique used to detect clot formation is not an important variable in heparin monitoring by the aPTT.

Another disadvantage of the aPTT is the ability of elevated factor VIII levels to decrease its sensitivity to heparin, in other words, the aPTT may be shorter than expected for a given heparin concentration when the factor VIII level rises above 150%. In animals with experimental thrombi, infusion of additional factor VIII (via cryoprecipitate) shortened the aPTT to 1.0 to 1.5 times the normal plasma value,

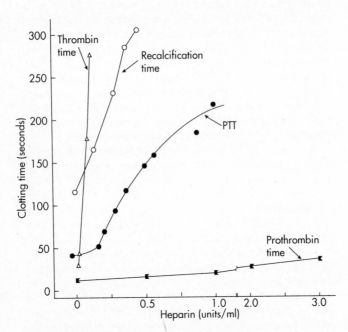

Fig. 67-4 Sensitivity of various coagulation screening tests to heparin. *Redrawn from Thompson AR and Harker LA: Manual of hemostasis and thrombosis, ed 3, Philadelphia, 1983, FA Davis.*

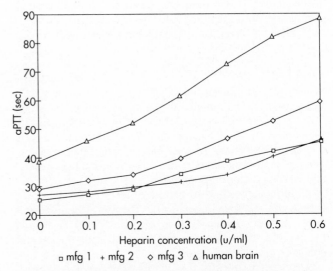

Fig. 67-5 Sensitivity of different aPTT reagents to heparin. Heparin was added to pooled normal plasma in varying concentrations and aPTT was obtained according to manufacturer's instructions.

Box 67-1 Correlation of heparin level with aPTT at the therapeutic range

aPTT TIMES NORMAL PLASMA VALUE AT THERAPEUTIC RANGE OF HEPARIN (0.3 to 0.5 u/ml)

	Mfg 1	Mfg 2	Mfg 3	Human brain
aPTT (times normal plasma level)	1.30-1.68	1.20-1.56	1.38-1.86	1.58-2.08

CORRESPONDING HEPARIN-LEVEL AT aPTT 1.5-2.0 TIMES NORMAL PLASMA VALUE

	Mfg 1	Mfg 2	Mfg 3	Human brain
Heparin level (u/ml)	0.40-0.65	0.46-0.75	0.35-0.57	0.27-0.46

despite heparin levels of 0.4 to 0.5 u/ml, which gave aPTTs of 2.2 to 2.4 times normal plasma value in noncryo-precipitate-treated animals. Nevertheless, fibrinogen accretion on the experimental thrombosis was impeded equally in treated and untreated animals. Therefore, in patients with a normal or marginally prolonged aPTT despite high doses of heparin (2000 u/hour), a heparin level in the blood should be measured directly. The finding of therapeutic levels (0.3 to 0.5 u/ml) indicates an appropriate heparin response and adequate anticoagulation. If heparin levels are low (heparin resistance), accelerated clearance may be occurring (as is seen with pulmonary emboli). Alternatively, AT-III deficiency is theoretically a possibility. However, in vitro studies by Hirsh and colleagues have indicated that AT-III deficiency blunts the aPTT response to heparin only when levels decrease to <25%. This low AT-III level is unusual, even in heterozygotic-deficient patients, since heparin therapy only modestly decreases AT-III levels. In the case of true heparin resistance, however, an AT-III assay is indicated.

A less widely used alternative to the aPTT in heparin monitoring is a modified thrombin time, sometimes called a thrombin clotting time (TCT). In the TCT, 0.2 ml of test or normal plasma is warmed to 37° C and 0.1 ml of a thrombin-calcium reagent (thrombin concentration 7 NIH u/ml; calcium concentration 0.8 to 1.0 M) is added. Excellent correlation with heparin levels over the range 0.1 to 0.6 u/ml can be demonstrated. The advantage of the TCT is that the effects of factor VIII and other clotting factors are eliminated. However, the test as described is prolonged by fibrinogen levels below 150 mg/dl. In addition, one might expect that the TCT would be less sensitive than the aPTT to moderate AT-III deficiency, since amounts of AT-III–heparin that inhibit factor Xa may not inhibit thrombin.

The activated clotting time (Chapter 65) can also be used to monitor heparin therapy, although it is primarily used in operating rooms during cardiopulmonary bypass procedures. In this setting, overheparinization is less worrisome than underheparinization, which can have disastrous consequences during operation of the extracorporeal circuit. The activated clotting time (ACT), often performed via automated devices, is simple and easily available in this setting. In most hands, heparin is given to maintain an ACT above 180 seconds.

Specific heparin assays are now readily available through the use of automated devices based upon chromogenic or fluorogenic methods. The techniques are variants of the reaction utilized to measure AT-III. Thrombin or factor Xa is added to dilutions of patient or normal plasma (containing a known amount of heparin). Surplus AT-III is added to avoid a limiting concentration of this inhibitor. Excess thrombin or factor Xa (remaining after neutralization by heparin–AT-III) is then measured using chromogenic or fluorogenic substrates.

Warfarin

Warfarin (3-[α-acetonyl-benzyl]-4-hydrocoumarin) is the most frequently used of the several available vitamin K antagonists. It has better solubility (and thus bioavailability) than its cousin dicumarol and is less toxic than the inanedione class of drugs. Warfarin is available as a racemic

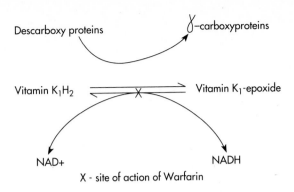

Fig. 67-6 Inhibition of vitamin K_1H_2 regeneration by warfarin.

mixture of its two enantiomorphs, levo- and dextrowarfarin, of which levowarfarin is the more active. The precise and complete mechanism of warfarin's anticoagulant effect is not yet determined, but it is known that warfarin antagonizes the action of vitamin K (Fig. 67-6), resulting in the production of non γ-carboxylated forms of factors II, VII, IX, X, and proteins C and S (Chapter 64).

Warfarin is well absorbed when taken orally, and although its half-life varies greatly among individuals, the half-life in any individual is consistent. The two enantiomorphs have different half-lives; a useful rule of thumb for the racemic mixture is a value of about a day and a half (32 to 46 hours). Warfarin is nearly completely complexed with albumin in circulation, although only uncomplexed drug is active as a vitamin K antagonist. This albumin-binding characteristic is extremely important clinically, since drugs such as nonsteroidal anti-inflammatory agents, which displace warfarin from its albumin-binding sites, can greatly increase free warfarin levels and lead to marked anticoagulation. A host of other drugs alter warfarin metabolism, some by increasing metabolism (barbiturates and rifampin), which leads to lessened warfarin effect, or by prolonging warfarin half-life (antabuse, trimethoprim-sulfamethoxazole), which increases its effect. In addition, conditions or drugs that lead to vitamin K deficiency (malabsorption, lipid-binding drugs, broad-spectrum antibiotics) also markedly increase the warfarin effect.

The PT is widely utilized to monitor the anticoagulant effect of warfarin in vivo since it is sensitive to three of the four vitamin K-dependent procoagulant factors: II, VII, and X. Plasma warfarin levels can be measured precisely with advanced chromatographic techniques, but this is rarely necessary.

Unlike heparin, where a therapeutic effect can be assumed at drug concentrations of 0.2 to 0.5 u/ml, drug levels of warfarin are highly variable among individuals. In an individual patient, there is consistent correlation between the PT and warfarin levels, but for routine monitoring purposes, warfarin levels offer no advantage over the PT. Warfarin levels are useful in detecting surreptitious drug ingestion or rare cases of true warfarin resistance, in which high plasma drug levels do not result in vitamin K antagonism.

Warfarin is best administered orally as small doses (5 to 10 mg) on successive days rather than in large, loading doses. The half-lives of the vitamin K-dependent procoagulant proteins vary greatly: factor VII, 4 to 6 hours; factor IX, 20 to 30 hours; factor X, 25 to 60 hours; and factor II, 50 to 80 hours. Thus, a large dose of warfarin will result in decreased factor VII levels in a day; the PT will be prolonged, but most investigators believe that the full anticoagulant effect does not occur until stable and diminished levels of all four factors have been achieved. This requires 3 days at minimum and probably 6 to 7 days for the full effect. Typically, therefore, warfarin therapy is begun concurrently with, or soon after, heparin therapy, so that at the time of heparin discontinuation at 7 to 10 days, a full and stable anticoagulant effect with warfarin has been achieved.

It is believed by many investigators that the differential effect of warfarin on plasma levels of the vitamin K-dependent proteins is responsible for the rare disorder, warfarin-induced skin necrosis. This disorder is marked by microvascular thromboses in subcutaneous tissue, with infarction and necrosis. It occurs suddenly after beginning warfarin therapy, particularly after a large loading dose, and may be related to a paradoxical prothrombotic effect of the drug. This effect is believed to be caused by relative protein C deficiency early on in warfarin therapy, since protein C has a short half-life (6 hours). Thus, relative protein C deficiency without a balancing anticoagulant effect may occur in patients with low normal protein C levels in the first 24 to 48 hours of therapy. For this reason as well, overlap between warfarin therapy and heparin anticoagulation is desired for several days before stopping heparin.

Several randomized studies and a long experience in the use of warfarin have documented its efficacy in both the prophylaxis and treatment of arterial and venous thromboembolic disorders. Warfarin is indicated as a primary prophylaxis, or after an episode of thrombosis, in congenital thrombotic disorders, such as AT-III, protein C, and plasminogen activator deficiency states. High-risk patients, including those with an established thrombosis or those about to undergo a surgical procedure with a high risk of postoperative thrombosis (e.g., hip surgery) also benefit from warfarin. Warfarin is also clearly indicated in patients with cardiac mural thrombi, in selected patients with atrial fibrillation, in patients with prosthetic or tissue heart valves, and in the prevention of recurrent myocardial infarction, particularly anterior wall infarctions.

Warfarin therapy is best monitored by the one-stage PT. Great progress has been made in an international effort to standardize the reporting of the PT for this purpose. Thromboplastin reagents vary considerably in their sensitivity to deficiencies of the pertinent factors, and therefore, interlaboratory differences made interpretation of studies about the optimal PT range for warfarin monitoring problematic. Standard methods of interpreting PTs for patients receiving warfarin therapy include the percent activity and the PT ratio. Patients are monitored to achieve a percent activity range of 10% to 25%. However, since markedly different end points can be reached depending upon whether saline or adsorbed plasma is used as the diluent to construct the activity curve, 25% activity in one laboratory may or may not correspond to 25% activity reported by another laboratory. The PT ratio is simply the number obtained by dividing the patient's PT by the PT of pooled normal plasma. This simple technique is available to all laboratories; how-

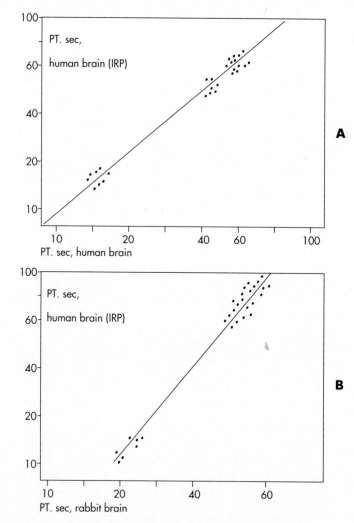

Fig. 67-7 Calibration of rabbit brain thromboplastin against the international reference thromboplastin preparation using a log/log plot. The International Sensitivity Index (ISI) denotes the slope of the calibration line in the log PT plot when the IRP is represented on the vertical axis. The International Normalized Ratio (INR) is calculated from the measured ratio and the slope according to the following equation: patient PT normal PT[151]. **A,** Log/log plot in seconds of human brain thromboplastin PT vs, the IRP; ISI = 1.0. **B,** Log/log plot in seconds of rabbit brain thromboplastin vs. the IRP; ISI = 1.6. *Redrawn from Gambino R: Lab Report for Physicians 8:45, 1986.*

ever, assayed, pooled, normal plasma rather than controls, which often contain nonphysiologic concentrations of factors, should be utilized. Early clinical studies recommended that warfarin-treated patients be treated to obtain a PT ratio of 2 to 2.5. At this level, the majority of thromboembolic phenomena were suppressed and bleeding side effects were judged acceptable. However, these studies utilized human brain thromboplastin. Rabbit brain thromboplastin, which is widely utilized in the United States, is less sensitive than human brain thromboplastin. Thus, patients in the United States with a PT ratio of 2.0 to 2.5 are overanticoagulated compared to patients in these early studies. Partly to ameliorate this problem, a new placenta-derived thromboplastin

Table 67-2   Recommendations on degree of warfarin anticoagulation using the PT in various disorders*

Disorder	Recommended INR	Recommended rabbit brain PT ratio
Patients with mechanical heart valves	3.0-4.5	1.5-2.0
Patients with systemic thromboembolism of cardiac origin	3.0-4.5	1.5-2.0
Patients with recurrent thromboemboli in lower dose warfarin therapy	3.0-4.5	1.5-2.0
Prophylaxis against venous thromboembolism in high-risk patients	2.0-3.0	1.2-1.5
Treatment (after heparin therapy) in patients with venous thromboembolism	2.0-2.0	1.2-1.5
Prevention of systemic embolism in patients with heart disease	2.0-3.0	1.2-1.5

*PT, prothrombin time; INR, international normalized ratio.

is now available in North America. This thromboplastin has a sensitivity similar to human brain thromboplastin. Recently, several studies have documented the efficacy of warfarin prophylaxis in high-risk patients, maintained by achieving a PT ratio of 1.3 to 1.5 using rabbit brain thromboplastin. These studies were also impressive in that this lower PT ratio was associated with fewer bleeding side effects than the 2.0 to 2.5 ratio.

The International Committee for Standardization in Haematology and the International Committee on Thrombosis and Haemostasis have issued recommendations for the standardization of thromboplastin reagents. Manufacturers of thromboplastins are encouraged to compare their reagent to the World Health Organization (WHO) International Reference Preparation (IRP), made from human brain. A log/log plot of PTs from patients on warfarin therapy, comparing the manufacturer's thromboplastin reagent to the IRP is constructed (Fig. 67-7). With the IRP reagent results plotted on the y-axis, the International Sensitivity Index (ISI) is calculated as the comparative slope of the log/log plot. The average commercial rabbit brain thromboplastin has an ISI of 2.4. The International Normalized Ratio (INR) is then calculated as: $INR = [patient\ PT \div normal\ plasma\ PT]^{ISI}$. Each manufacturer is encouraged to solve this equation over a wide range of PT values in warfarin-treated patients, and thus provide a table to translate the patient's PT ratio obtained using a commercial INR. Each batch of thromboplastin must be correlated in this fashion to the WHO IRP. Using this system, patients may be assured of consistent warfarin therapy monitoring from laboratory to laboratory. Recommendations using the INR have been made regarding the suggested level of anticoagulation in differing clinical circumstances (Table 67-2).

Other antithrombotic agents

Other antithrombotic drugs include dextran and defibrinogenating enzymes. Low molecular weight (less than 70,000 daltons) dextrans are utilized to expand plasma volume as well as antithrombotic agents. These branched polysaccharides are adsorbed to platelets and can interfere with fibrin polymerization as well. These properties make dextran a useful agent in microvascular procedures, in which it provides both anticoagulation and hemodilution, thereby improving microvascular blood flow. Dextran has proven effective as prophylaxis against deep vein thrombosis (DVT) and pulmonary embolism in high-risk surgical patients; its efficacy vis-à-vis mini heparin in lower risk patients has not been proven. Laboratory monitoring is not routinely performed for dextran therapy; instead, fixed dosage regimens are used (e.g., 500 ml of 10% dextran daily for 1 to 3 days) without regard to effects on laboratory tests. Dextran therapy is associated with bleeding complications, allergic reactions, and volume overload.

A number of defibrinogenating enzymes are available for use as antithrombotic agents. The enzymes are snake venoms extracted for clinical or laboratory use. Ancrod (from *Agkistrodon rhodostoma*) and batroxobin (from *Bothrops atrox moojeni*) are the best studied enzymes. They act by cleaving FpA, but not FpB, from fibrinogen, which results in an unstable fibrin polymer and ultimately, its rapid dissociation and dissolution by plasmin. Upon clinical administration, fibrinogen concentration falls markedly and rapidly, and the formed fibrin monomer induces release of t-PA. Fibrin degradation products rise as a result. Often, this profibrinolytic stimulus results in diminution of the circulating plasminogen level and serious in vivo thrombotic complications will result if the fibrinolytic inhibitor ε-aminocaproic acid is given concurrently. The cellular blood elements are not affected. The resultant fall in protein levels leads to a several-fold decrease in blood viscosity, which may add to the therapeutic effect.

Ancrod and batroxobin are given at 2 to 3 units/kg every 12 to 24 hours and the fibrinogen level is measured every 12 hours to ensure sufficient hypofibrinogenemia (less than 75 mg/dl). No further laboratory monitoring is necessary. Clinically, these agents are safe and efficacious in the prevention and treatment of DVT and pulmonary embolus.

Thrombolytic therapy

The advent of clinical agents that can effect fibrin clot lysis has been an important adjunct to the treatment of thrombotic disorders. Thrombolytic therapy is most precisely termed fibrinolytic therapy, since these agents generate plasmin (i.e., they are plasminogen activators), which degrades the fibrin portion of the clot, but which is comparatively ineffective at degrading cellular components of the thrombus.

The first generation of activators useful in thrombolytic therapy includes streptokinase and urokinase. Streptokinase is manufactured by purifying a filtrate of streptococcal bacteria, whereas urokinase is isolated from human urine or produced in culture from transformed renal cells or by recombinant DNA technology. Streptokinase must first combine with circulating plasminogen to form an active plasminogen activator complex, whereas urokinase is active as an uncomplexed agent. Both streptokinase and urokinase are capable of plasminogen proteolysis in the fluid or solid phase; as a consequence, these drugs produce not only fibrin lysis, but fibrinogen lysis as well.

A second generation of agents has been developed with an aim toward increasing the fibrin-specific (i.e., solid phase) activity of the activator, thus localizing to the greatest degree possible the generation of plasmin at the site of a thrombus. Second-generation activators include acylated plasminogen; streptokinase activator complex (APSAC); single-chain urokinase (scu-PA, or prourokinase), and tissue type-plasminogen activator produced by recombinant DNA technology (t-PA or rt-PA).

Although in vitro conditions can be defined in which these second-generation activators do not cause fibrinogenolysis in the fluid phase, in clinical use, all three activators show some evidence of free plasmin action. This is referred to as the *lytic* state. There are several laboratory indicators of free plasmin generation, including decreases in plasma fibrinogen, plasminogen, factor V, factor VIII, and antiplasmin levels, and increased levels of plasmin-antiplasmin complexes and fibrin(ogen) degradation products. Other laboratory hallmarks of the lytic state include a shortened euglobulin lysis time due to increased plasminogen activator levels; prolonged PT, PTT, TT, and reptilase time due to diminished factor V, factor VIII, and fibrinogen levels; and an increase in measurable free plasmin levels by the fibrin plate assay, by a chromogenic substrate assay, or by using other plasmin assay systems.

Despite the relative fibrin specificity of the second-generation activators, the doses used clinically result in some fibrinogenolysis, and therefore, any of these tests can be used to document a lytic state. Many studies, in a wide variety of clinical situations, have failed to reveal the superiority of one test or another in regard to establishing the presence of a lytic state. Furthermore, none of these laboratory tests are useful in predicting either the efficacy of response to therapy or which patients will develop hemorrhagic side effects. Although instinct would predict that patients rendered hypocoagulable by thrombolytic therapy, in other words, those in whom procoagulant levels are reduced below hemostatic levels, would be at greater risk for bleeding complications, this has not been shown in clinical trials. Thus, dosage regimens have been standardized for all agents, and laboratory monitoring is limited to documentation (by any means) of a lytic state.

Table 67-3 Laboratory tests in the diagnosis and treatment of thrombotic disorders*

READILY AVAILABLE TESTS

Clinically useful	Useful in research setting	Doubtful value
Blood viscosity	(Platelet factor 4)	Circulating platelet aggregates
Complete blood count	(β Thromboglobulin)	"Spontaneous" platelet aggregation
PT, PTT, TT, ACT	(Plasminogen activator)	Platelet procoagulant activity
Reptilase time	(Fibrinopeptide A)	Whole blood clotting time
Fibrinogen (F + I)	(Fibrinogen fragments Bβ1-42, Bβ15-42)	
Plasminogen (F + I)		
Protein C (I)		
Heparin-Induced platelet aggregation and release		
Heparin assay		
Sugar water test		
Tests for lupus anticogulant		
Fibrin(ogen) degradation products		
Euglobulin lysis time		
Antithrombin III (F + I)		

TESTS AVAILABLE IN SPECIALIZED LABORATORIES

Clinically useful	Useful in research setting	Uncertain value
Protein C (F + I)	Prothrombin fragments 1 + 2	Thrombin-Antithrombin III Complexes
Protein S (F + I)	Fibrinopeptides A and B	Thrombin-α_2 macroglobulin complexes
Antiphospholipid antibodies	Fibrinogen fragments Bβ1-42, Bβ15-42	
Heparin cofactor II (F + I)	Fragment E	
	Platelet factor 4	
	β Thromboglobulin	
	Plasminogen activator	
	Plasminogen activator inhibitor	
	Thromboxane A_2†	
	Prostacyclin (PGI$_2$)‡	
	Platelet survival and turnover	
	Fibrinogen survival and turnover	

*F, functional; I, immunological.
†As thromboxane B_2.
‡As 6-keto-PGFI$_\alpha$.

Summary of laboratory tests for thrombosis

A summary of laboratory tests for thrombosis (Table 67-3) reveals that few of the new, more specific tests are both readily available and clinically useful. Many of the tests listed in the research categories make use of techniques now familiar to most laboratorians, especially radioimmunoassay and/or ELISA. However, because their interpretation is not straightforward, and/or they add little to patient management decisions at present, they cannot be considered mainstream tests. In addition, these tests often require very careful and specialized collection techniques, suited less to a busy hospital laboratory than to a research setting. Therefore, most clinical laboratories will not perform these tests, and instead, will make use of reference or research laboratories when these tests are requested. In is axiomatic, though, that as our understanding of the thrombotic process increases, subcategories of patients for whom these specialized tests are of clinical importance will be identified. At that point, some of these research tests will make their way into the lexicon of the clinical laboratory.

SUGGESTED READING

Coleman RW and others (editors): Hemostasis and thrombosis: basic principles and clinical practice, ed 2, Philadelphia, 1987, JP Lippincott.

Corriveau DM and Fritsma GA (editors): Hemostasis and thrombosis in the clinical laboratory, Philadelphia, 1988, JP Lippincott.

Davies JA: The pre-thrombotic state, Clin Sci 69:641, 1985.

DeCamp MM and Demling RH: Posttraumatic multisystem organ failure, JAMA 260:530, 1988.

Hirsh J: Mechanism of action and monitoring of anticoagulants, Seminars in Thrombosis and Hemostasis 12:1, 1986.

Kelton JG: Heparin-induced thrombocytopenia, Haemostasis 16:173, 1986.

Kitchens CS: Concept of hypercoagulability: a review of its development, clinical application, and recent progress, Semin Thromb Hemost 11:293, 1985.

Kwaan HC and Samama MM (editors): Clinical thrombosis, Boca Raton, Fla, 1989, CRC Press.

Mannucci PM and Tripodi A: Laboratory screening of inherited thrombotic syndromes, Thromb Haemost 57:247, 1987.

Owen J and others: Thrombin and plasmin activity and platelet activation in the development of venous thrombosis, Blood 61:476, 1983.

Rodgers GM and Schuman MA: Congenital thrombotic disorders, Am J Hematol 21:419, 1986.

Salem HH, Mitchell CA, and Firkin BG: Current views on the pathophysiology and investigations of thrombotic disorders, Am J Hematol 25:463, 1987.

Schafer AL: The hypercoagulable states, Ann Int Med 102:814, 1985.

Triplett DA and others: Laboratory diagnosis of lupus inhibitors: a comparison of the tissue thromboplastin inhibition procedure with a new platelet neutralization procedure, Am J Clin Pathol 79:678, 1983.

Triplett DA and others: The relationship between lupus anticoagulants and antibodies to phospholipid, JAMA 259:550, 1988.

PART ELEVEN

IMMUNOHEMATOLOGY AND TRANSFUSION PRACTICE

68

Blood group antigens and antibodies

Carol L. Johnson

Blood groups are inherited antigenic structures expressed on the surface of the red blood cell. They belong to polymorphic systems and in some cases include multiple allelic forms. Because of their immunogenic properties, blood groups are of primary importance to the field of transfusion medicine. Compatibility testing in blood banks is designed to detect blood group antibodies in the sera of transfusion candidates and to identify compatible donor blood.

A number of red-cell phenotypes have also been associated with abnormal clinical conditions, and some antigens are known to act as receptors for pathogenic organisms. These observations have sparked research interests that promise significant insight into undiscovered aspects of cellular metabolism and genetic regulation.

BLOOD GROUP GENETICS
Patterns of inheritance

Blood group antigens are inherited as codominant traits. At a single locus, if different alleles occur on each chromosome, both antigens are expressed, and a heterozygous genotype can be inferred. Only in this case, however, can blood group genotype be assumed. If a phenotype should include only one of these antigens, several genetic explanations are possible. Most likely the individual is homozygous, with the same allele carried on both chromosomes. It is possible, however, that the person is heterozygous with a silent gene on one chromosome. This silent allele may code for an antigen that cannot be identified with available reagents or techniques; it may make no product at all; or it may represent a deletion of genetic material (Box 68-1).

Although a homozygous genotype can never be proven, its probability can be assessed by observing inheritance of the trait in a family pedigree. An antigen positive individual may be homozygous for the allele if, in a mating with an antigen negative individual, all offspring type positive. Alternatively, the person may be heterozygous and by the chance assortment of genes may have passed the allele for the expressed antigen to every child. However, as the number of antigen positive offspring increases without the birth of a child who lacks the antigen, homozygosity of the parent becomes more probable.

Most blood group genes are inherited as autosomal traits, but some blood group expression is controlled by the X chromosome. Males have only one X chromosome and are considered hemizygous for the X-linked genes they carry. Because fathers pass their Y chromosome to their sons, no male-to-male transmission of X-linked genes occurs. Daughters, however, must receive their fathers' X chromosomes and are therefore obligate carriers of all paternal X-linked genes. Since females have two X chromosomes, the frequency distribution of X-linked traits is higher among them than among males (Figure 68-1).

Null phenotypes

Occasional red cells express none of the antigens in a particular blood group. These null-phenotype cells result from the inheritance of two silent genes at the blood group locus. This phenotype occurs in approximately 25% of the offspring from a mating between two individuals who each carry one silent gene (Figure 68-2). Silent gene frequencies are low in the random population and the chance of inheriting a null phenotype is unusual. However, in families that carry a rare silent gene and in which consanguinity has occurred, the probability of carrier matings that produce null phenotypes is greatly increased.

Gene interaction

Although blood group inheritance is straightforward, antigen expression may be influenced by other circumstances (Box 68-2). Red-cell phenotypes are often—perhaps always—affected by the interaction of numerous genes. For example, the manner in which genes are physically arranged in relation to each other produces positional effects. Weakened expression of some alleles is the result of a *trans*-positional effect by others on the opposite chromosome. *Cis*-modifying alleles affect expression of other alleles on the same chromosome.

Another influence is the action of modifying genes, which are inherited independently of the blood group locus they affect. Normal synthesis of some red-cell antigens requires the action of both a blood group gene and a modifier, and a change at the modifying locus may produce aberrant phenotype.

Perhaps the best illustration of gene interaction is provided by carbohydrate-determined antigens. The primary products of the blood group genes responsible for these structures are transferase enzymes, which confer antigen specificity by adding terminal sugar residues to appropriate

Box 68-1 Hypothetical blood group system with known antigens Q and R

RED-CELL PHENOTYPE	POSSIBLE GENOTYPES
Q+R+	*QR*
Q+R−	*QQ*
	Qq
Q−R+	*RR*
	Rr

q, r = silent genes

Box 68-2 Gene interactions that influence expression of blood group antigens

—Positional effects
—Modifying genes
—Consecutive transferase action

Autosomal inheritance

X-linked inheritance

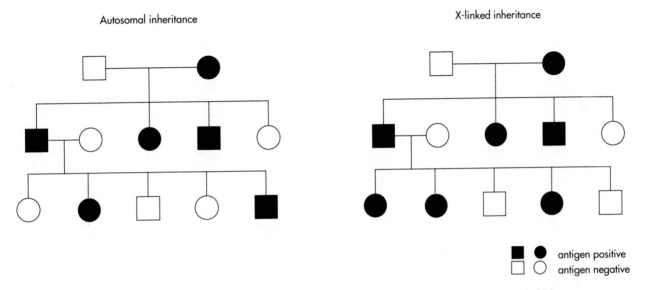

■ ● antigen positive
□ ○ antigen negative

Fig. 68-1 Autosomal traits are distributed equally among males and females. The frequency of X-linked traits is higher among females than males.

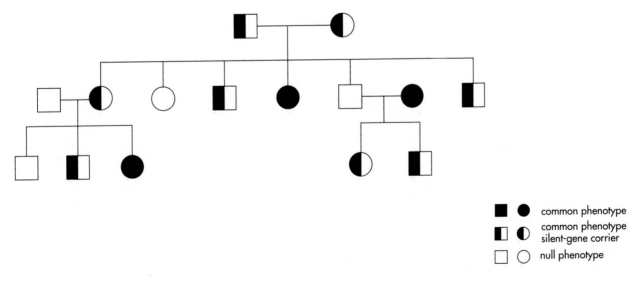

■ ● common phenotype
◧ ◑ common phenotype silent-gene corrier
□ ○ null phenotype

Fig. 68-2 Inheritance of a null phenotype.

oligosaccharide receptors. The work of more than one enzyme, and consequently more than one gene, is necessary for construction of these carbohydrate chains. They result from consecutive attachment of a number of sugar residues, each acting as a substrate for action of the next transferase enzyme in the series. Specific examples of all the above mechanisms will be given as this chapter proceeds.

The concept of one gene ordering production of one protein has become archaic in this era of molecular genetics. We now know that individual genes can be variably expressed by interaction with other genes and through a myriad of RNA-processing mechanisms. Our understanding of the leap between genotype and phenotype will widen as we inevitably learn more steps that occur between inheritance of a blood group gene and expression of its antigen on the red-cell surface.

Calculation of gene frequency

In a given population the gene frequency for alleles *a* and *b* in a two-antigen blood group system can be calculated by use of the Hardy-Weinberg formula. The sum of these frequencies equals 1.00, as in the equation

$$p + q = 1.00$$

where p and q represent the frequency value for each allele. The Hardy-Weinberg formula states

$$p^2 + 2pq + q^2 = 1.00$$

where

$$p^2 = aa \text{ genotype frequency}$$
$$q^2 = bb \text{ genotype frequency}$$
$$2pq = ab \text{ genotype frequency}$$

If, for example, 65% of the population type positive for antigen a, it has a phenotype frequency of 0.65, which includes the genotypes *aa* and *ab*. The gene frequency q can be calculated as follows:

$$(p^2 + 2pq) + q^2 = 1.00$$
$$0.65 + q^2 = 1.00$$
$$q^2 = 1.00 - 0.65$$
$$q^2 = 0.35$$
$$q = 0.59$$

Therefore,

$$p + (q) = 1.00$$
$$p + 0.59 = 1.00$$
$$p = 0.41$$

Phenotype frequency can be calculated for antigen b and will include genotypes *ab* and *bb*:

$$2(0.41 \times 0.59) + (0.59)^2 = 0.83$$

RED-CELL ANTIGENS AND MEMBRANE STRUCTURE

The bilipid membrane of the red cell is characterized by surface-attached carbohydrates that form glycosphingolipids and by transmembrane proteins attached to the cell's pe-

---

Box 68-3 Red-cell membrane structures with blood group activity

—Glycosphingolipids
—Transmembrane proteins
  Glycophorins
  Band 3
  Unique proteins

---

ripheral protein skeleton. Blood group activity is associated with the surface glycosphingolipids and several transmembrane proteins, including the glycophorins and band 3. (Box 68-3). The specific associations of defined blood groups with these various membrane structures will be examined in this chapter.

IMMUNE RESPONSE TO BLOOD GROUP ANTIGENS

Until Karl Landsteiner's observation in 1900 that mixing the red blood cells from one individual with serum from another often caused hemagglutination, all human red cells had been considered essentially the same. When he presented the ABO blood group classification, Landsteiner suggested these differences might explain the serious clinical consequences that frequently resulted from blood transfusion. Nearly a century later sophisticated techniques of biochemical analysis and molecular genetics are revealing intricacies of blood group structure never before imagined. However, no finding has had as profound consequences on the practice of transfusion therapy as Landsteiner's original discovery of blood group allogeneity among individuals and their ability to produce antibodies against non-self red-cell antigens.

The earliest blood group antibodies described were capable of causing direct agglutination when mixed on a slide with antigen positive red cells. These agglutinins were considered "naturally-occurring," since their presence appeared to require no provocation from red cells. Anti-A and anti-B appeared in the sera of all individuals whose red cells lacked these respective antigens. Animal studies subsequently led to the discovery of anti-P_1 and anti-M by Landsteiner and Levine in 1927, and other agglutinin specificities have since been defined.

Many non-agglutinating blood group antibodies were later found in individuals with previous exposure to homologous red cells either by transfusion or pregnancy, events presumed responsible for the resultant antibody production. In contrast to "naturally-occurring" antibodies, these were termed "immune." Accumulated evidence now indicates that human blood group antigens are not necessarily unique to the red cell. Analogues have been found elsewhere in nature, in plants, and in microbial life. Certain strains of *Escherichia coli,* for example, have been responsible for some examples of anti-A, anti-B, and anti-K1. All blood group antibodies are the result of an immune response, although the antigenic challenge need not come from red cells.

Exposure to non-self red-cell antigens does not always result in antibody production. An immune response is in fact uncommon; fewer than one percent of transfusion re-

PRIMARY RESPONSE:	SECONDARY RESPONSE:
—occurs over period of weeks	—occurs over period of days
—requires large antigen dose	—requires small antigen dose
—produces large amount of antibody	—produces small amount of antibody
—produces IgM antibody	—produces IgG antibody
—antibody titer drops shortly after reaching its peak	—antibody titer is sustained

cipients produce antibodies. Antibody production depends on a number of factors:

1. *Immunogenic potential of the antigen.* The most competent immunogen is the Rh antigen D. Other antigens in the Rh system are not especially potent.
2. *Dose of the antigen.* When first exposed to antigen, antibody production is more likely when a large dose is given. In one study, 80% of D negative individuals made antibody when transfused with 200 milliliters (ml) of D positive blood, but less than 50% formed antibody when the dose volume was less than one ml.
3. *Immunocompetence of the recipient.* Individuals vary by genetic makeup in their ability to respond to antigen. In the above study, most subjects who failed to produce Rh antibody after the 200 ml transfusion also remained free of antibody after repeated exposures to antigen. Some disease states may depress or amplify immune function, as in autoimmune conditions when the normal regulatory mechanism of suppressor T-cells is disturbed.

When immunization to red cells does occur, the primary response occupies a period of several weeks after initial encounter with antigen. During this time, the transfused red cells are removed from the circulation, antigen is processed, appropriate B cells are selected, clonal proliferation begins, and IgM antibody is produced. When first produced, the concentration of serum antibody is low, and the titer declines shortly after reaching its peak.

Upon next exposure to the same antigen, immune memory causes a more rapid and dramatic event. This secondary response typically occurs within a few days. It requires a much lower dose of provoking antigen and results in production of more antibody, which maintains its titer for a longer period of time and demonstrates higher affinity for its antigen. During the secondary response, the structure of immunoglobulin produced switches from IgM to IgG (Box 68-4).

Immunization to blood groups that is provoked by a source other than red cells is not subject to a secondary response. Despite repeated exposure to antigen, antibody production continues as IgM and does not increase in titer.

Blood group antibodies produced as part of some pathologic conditions may be monoclonal, but the usual immune response to polyclonal. Red-cell antigens are complex structures with numerous epitopes, each capable of initiating the clonal expansion of a different B cell. Although serologic testing may appear to indicate a single antibody specificity, most reactive sera contain a heterogeneous mixture of antibody molecules with subtle differences in specificity, affinity for antigen, and other characteristics.

HEMOLYTIC POTENTIAL OF BLOOD GROUP ANTIBODIES

Immune destruction of red blood cells may occur at two sites. Intravascular hemolysis takes place within the blood vessels. It is mediated by red cell bound antibody capable of activating the complement cascade to completion, resulting in cell lysis. The physiologic reaction is rapid, severe, and sometimes fatal.

Fortunately, most immune hemolysis occurs in the extravascular space of the reticulo-endothelial (RE) system, where the effect is less dramatic. Here tissue-bound macrophages clear antibody-coated red cells from the circulation by receptor recognition of the Fc portion of IgG and of the C3b component of complement. Extravascular hemolysis occurs slowly, and although it may produce significant clinical symptoms, it is rarely fatal.

The following variables act together to determine a blood group antibody's hemolytic potential:

1. *Antigen density.* A large number of antigen sites on the red-cell surface allows heavy immunoglobulin coating, increasing the possibility for immune destruction. In addition to number, the architecture of antigen sites is important. Sites close to each other facilitate complement activation when IgG antibody is bound by permitting the necessary juxtaposition of available Fc fragments, while the distance antigen sites project from the cell surface or their steric relationship to other membrane structures influences their accessibility to antibody molecules.

2. *Immunoglobulin class and subclass.* With rare exception blood group antibodies are either IgM or IgG. Both may cause intravascular hemolysis, but because macrophages recognize only IgG, IgM-coated cells that have not bound complement are not destroyed extravascularly. Among IgG molecules, subclasses IgG1 and IgG3 are recognized most readily by macrophages and are best able to mediate hemolysis. Occasional examples of IgG2 may also be recognized, but IgG4 generally is not.

Both IgM and IgG antibodies activate complement. When antibody binds with cellular antigen, it is believed to undergo a configurational change that exposes the complement activation site on its Fc portion. This receptor interacts with C1q, initiating the activation sequence. Two immunoglobulin monomers, however, must reside near each other on the membrane surface and provide two receptors to which C1q can bind. An IgM molecule, with its pentamer structure, does this easily, but two individual IgG molecules must attach to the cell in tandem before complement is activated. IgG1 and IgG3 activate complement efficiently. Some IgG2 antibodies may bind complement weakly, but IgG4 binds none.

If both C3b and IgG are bound to red cells, the potential for extravascular destruction is increased exponentially. However, when inactivators convert bound C3b to C3d, it is no longer recognized and enhanced clearance does not occur. Cells coated with C3b alone are not readily destroyed.

3. *Thermal amplitude and environmental conditions.* Agglutination of red cells by IgM antibodies in cold ex-

tremities is readily reversed as the blood circulates and is reheated to 37°C, but complement activation and fixation may occur at low temperatures (below 30°C), and this complement remains bound to the red cells as they circulate. Occasionally, sufficient complement is fixed to cause shortened red cell survival, but usually only those antibodies that react at physiologic temperature (above 30°C) will cause in vivo hemolysis.

4. *Availability of complement.* Ongoing complement activation during episodes of severe hemolysis may lead to depletion of C2 and the interruption of complement fixation.

5. *Concentration and avidity of antibody.* Blood-bank workers know empirically that high-titer serum antibodies cause more hemolysis than those with low titers. Flow cytometry studies have confirmed this with examples of IgG1 autoantibodies by showing that patients with the greatest number of antibody molecules (and no complement) coating their cells are the most likely to experience hemolysis. Antibodies that bind tightly to their antigens are better able to carry out hemolytic functions than those that dissociate easily.

6. *Amount of red blood cells.* In general, the degree of hemolysis increases as the number of antigen positive red cells exposed to the patient's antibody increases. With an excessive amount of incompatible cells, however, hemolysis may temporarily subside due to depletion of antibody and/or complement and an overwhelmed RE system.

7. *Soluble antigen.* When an immunized patient is exposed to antigen positive red cells suspended in plasma that contain a soluble form of this antigen, the soluble substance may neutralize the patient's antibody, reducing its capacity to cause hemolysis.

8. *Activity level of macrophages.* The vigor with which macrophages can destroy cells coated with immunoglobulin or complement varies in individuals. Macrophages from persons with autoimmune conditions, for example, are known to be more active than those from healthy individuals. On the other hand, blockade of macrophage function by corticosteroids and other drugs (e.g., Vinca alkaloids) or by splenectomy may permit continued circulation and survival of sensitized red cells.

Clinical experience has shown that one of the best indices of a blood group antibody's hemolytic potential is its specificity. Most examples of a given specificity react predictably in laboratory tests, and unless atypical serologic results present, broad transfusion recommendations on this basis alone can be made for the management of common alloantibodies.

Each antibody specificity will be discussed in detail, but some generalizations regarding the most common may be a helpful beginning. Antibodies of the Lewis, P, and MN systems are usually IgM and react best at temperatures below 30°C. They do not bind complement well enough to cause immune hemolysis, and antigen negative blood is not often supplied for patients with these antibodies. Those antibodies directed toward antigens of the Rh, Ss, Kell, Duffy, and Kidd blood groups are usually IgG. They react optimally at temperatures above 30°C. Their ability to bind complement varies. However, all have the potential to cause extravascular hemolysis. Of all common specificities, only ABO antibodies are capable of causing intravascular hemolysis, and the majority of fatal hemolytic transfusion reactions can be attributed to this incompatibility.

ABO BLOOD GROUP

ABO is the simplest red-cell antigen system to detect serologically, but its complex genetic background and biochemical structure grant it status among the most sophisticated blood groups. ABO structures result from interaction of a number of genes. Interruption of their synthesis may occur at many different stages, and an array of variant phenotypes are possible.

Genetics

Each ABO antigen is determined by a specific sugar residue placed in an immunodominant position on the appropriate precursor molecule by a glycosyl transferase enzyme. *A*- and *B*-specified transferases are the respective products of the *A* and *B* genes. These two allelic forms, plus the silent allele *O*, appear at the *ABO* gene locus on chromosome 9. Six genotypic configurations and four red-cell phenotypes are known (Table 68-1).

Another gene, *H*, which is inherited independently of *ABO*, acts as a modifier of ABO expression. Its product, the *H*-specified transferase, prepares substrate for ABO transferases by attaching a specific sugar residue to the precursor. A silent allele, *h*, may appear at the *H* locus. In an *hh* homozygous individual, no *H*-specified transferase is produced and consequently no acceptor substrate is available for production of ABO antigens. This rare blood type is named Bombay, for the city in which it was discovered (Table 68-2).

Table 68-1 ABO genotypes and frequency of resultant phenotypes

Genotype	Phenotype	Phenotype frequency (%) in US population	
		Whites	**Blacks**
AA			
AO	A	40	27
BB			
BO	B	11	20
AB	AB	4	4
OO	O	45	49

Table 68-2 Products of the *ABO* and *Hh* genes.

Genotype		Transferase	Phenotype
AA	*HH* or *Hh*	A, H	A
AO	*HH* or *Hh*	A, H	A
BB	*HH* or *Hh*	B, H	B
BO	*HH* or *Hh*	B, H	B
AB	*HH* or *Hh*	A, B, H	AB
OO	*HH* or *Hh*	H	O
AA	*hh*	A	Bombay (O$_h$)
AO	*hh*	A	Bombay (O$_h$)
BB	*hh*	B	Bombay (O$_h$)
BO	*hh*	B	Bombay (O$_h$)
AB	*hh*	A, B	Bombay (O$_h$)
OO	*hh*		Bombay (O$_h$)

Table 68-3 Phenotype products of *ABO*, *Hh*, and *Sese* genes.

Genotype			Red Cell Phenotype	Soluble Substance
AA or *AO*	*HH* or *Hh*	*SeSe* or *Sese*	A	A, H
BB or *BO*	*HH* or *Hh*	*SeSe* or *Sese*	B	B, H
AB	*HH* or *Hh*	*SeSe* or *Sese*	AB	A, B, H
OO	*HH* or *Hh*	*SeSe* or *Sese*	O	H
AA or *AO*	*HH* or *Hh*	*sese*	A	
BB or *BO*	*HH* or *Hh*	*sese*	B	
AB	*HH* or *Hh*	*sese*	AB	
OO	*HH* or *Hh*	*sese*	O	
AA or *AO*	*hh*	*SeSe*, *Sese* or *sese*	Bombay (O$_h$)	
BB or *BO*	*hh*	*SeSe*, *Sese* or *sese*	Bombay (O$_h$)	
AB	*hh*	*SeSe*, *Sese* or *sese*	Bombay (O$_h$)	
OO	*hh*	*SeSe*, *Sese* or *sese*	Bombay (O$_h$)	

ABO and *Hh* genes function independently of each other. Perhaps in this and in similar situations the phrase "gene product interaction," rather than "gene interaction," more accurately applies, since the *hh* genotype prevents *ABO* expression only at a phenotypic level. It has no direct impact on the *ABO* gene, as evidenced by the presence of *ABO*-specified transferases in the sera of Bombay individuals. Offspring of Bombay individuals exhibit normal ABO expression, providing they inherit an *H* gene from the other parent.

Routine red-cell typing tests with anti-A and anti-B reagents will not distinguish between group O and Bombay phenotypes. Only an anti-H reagent can define Bombay red cells. All other blood types will express H, although with varying reaction strength. Group A and group B red cells will react less strongly with anti-H than will group O cells due to the steric interference of their immunodominant sugars.

Another independent gene, *Se*, is also involved in *ABO* expression. Individuals with this gene carry soluble substances that have A, B, and H reactivity, as determined by individual genotype, in their secretions and other body fluids, including saliva, tears, milk, and urine. These persons, approximately 80% of the population, are known as secretors; non-secretors result from the genotype *sese*, in which two silent alleles are inherited (Table 68-3).

Biochemistry

The immunodominant sugars that determine A, B, and H antigen activity are N-acetyl-galactosamine (GalNAc), D-galactose (Gal), and L-fucose (Fuc), respectively. They are each linked to the terminal residue of a three-sugar oligosaccharide chain. The *H*-specified transferase adds Fuc directly to this short chain by specified linkage, creating H antigen and providing *A*- and *B*-specified transferases with available substrate for the attachment of their sugars (Figure 68-3).

Two types of oligosaccharide chains exist that differ only in their linkage between the N-acetyl-glucosamine (GlcNAc) and terminal Gal residues. Type 1 chains link Gal to the number 3 carbon of GlcNAc; type 2 chains link Gal to the number 4 carbon. ABO specificity may be conferred on either chain type.

Paragloboside is a glycosphingolipid, which is formed when a short sugar chain of either type is attached by way

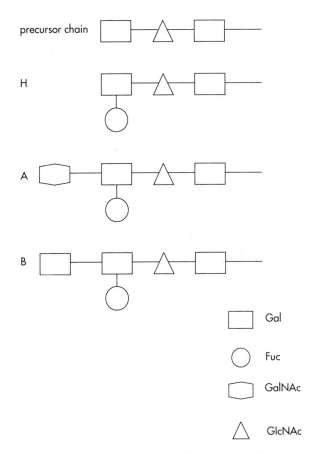

Fig. 68-3 Terminal sugar specificity of A, B, and H blood group antigens.

of a glucose residue to the lipid backbone ceramide. Glycosphingolipids carrying ABO antigen activity are found in both plasma and on the red cell, but not in other body secretions. In plasma they have both type 1 and type 2 chains, but only structures with type 2 chains are found on the red-cell membrane.

When a short sugar chain is joined by a GalNAc residue to a polypeptide backbone, a glycoprotein is formed. Glycoproteins carrying ABO activity may be found with both chain types in secretions and on the red-cell membrane.

ABO subgroups

Group A subdivides into phenotypes A_1, A_2, and a variety of weakly expressed subgroups that make up less than one percent of the total A population. Approximately 80% of A individuals are A_1, and about 20% are A_2. Although the same immunodominant sugar, GalNAc, determines specificity in both A_1 and in A_2 phenotypes, differences exist between the two *A* alleles and their transferase products. In A_1 individuals, transferase levels are higher, and the enzyme functions more efficiently than in A_2 individuals. The A_1-specified transferase acts on branched and on linear chains of H precursor. The A_2-specified transferase is limited to linear chains, leaving more exposed H receptor on the cell surface. In serologic tests, A_1 cells react more strongly with the lectin *Dolichos biflorus* than do A_2 cells.

Weak subgroups of A include A_3, A_m, A_{end}, A_x, and A_{el}. The variant genes responsible for these phenotypes produce transferases with varying levels of low efficiency. A antigen expression is often so weak that red cells will not agglutinate in typing tests with the anti-A reagents, although they are capable of absorbing antibody. Category assignments are based on red-cell reaction strength with anti-A and with anti-A,B, which is usually stronger, and on the results of tests for serum anti-A_1, secreted A- and H-active substance, and *A*-specified transferase. In a clinical setting, detection of A subgroups is important, especially in blood donors, who might otherwise be mistakenly typed as group O. However, specifying subgroup category is not critical.

Several subgroups of B have been defined, but these are rare. *B*-specified transferase appears to act with more consistency among different individuals than *A*-specified transferase.

Cis AB phenotype

In this unusual phenotype both *A* and *B* are inherited from the same chromosome. B-antigen expression is usually weaker than normal, and anti-B may appear in the serum. Both *A*- and *B*-specified transferase have been found in some of these individuals, suggesting that unequal crossing-over of chromosomal material during meiosis produced a recombinant gene. However, in other cases, a single variant enzyme is present, suggesting a mutation. It appears *cis* AB is a heterogeneous condition that may arise from more than one genetic event.

B(A) phenotype

Under appropriate experimental conditions, *A*-specified transferase is capable of transferring Gal to an H-active acceptor molecule, thereby producing B antigen, and conversely, *B*-specified transferase can transfer the A-active sugar, GalNAc, to form A antigen. This laboratory-manipulated phenomenon of overlapping specificities was assumed not to occur in vivo until the recent discovery of some group B individuals who exhibit weak, but reproducible reactivity with a monoclonal anti-A reagent. Extended studies of these B(A) phenotype individuals revealed they have enhanced *B*-specified transferase activity. This level of enzyme is believed to produce sufficient numbers of A-antigen determinants to be detectable by the highly sensitive monoclonal anti-A.

ABO antigens in disease

The red blood cells of Bombay individuals lack ABO and H antigens and yet they function normally and survive the expected length of time in vivo. ABH antigens are not essential structures to cell function or viability; however, they are coincidentally involved in some disease states.

Acquired B antigen

This phenotype is a transient expression of B antigen in individuals whose genetically-determined blood type is A. Its observed association with intestinal cancer or bowel infection suggested it was caused by action from a bacterial enzyme on the red-cell surface. Bacterial acetylase is believed to degrade the terminal A sugar, N-acetyl-galactosamine, to N-galactosamine, a structure similar to the B sugar D-galactose and capable of cross-reacting with anti-B. A is lost gradually as B is acquired, and both antigens are detected in serologic tests. This phenotype is difficult to distinguish from *cis* AB, unless the patient's clinical condition is known, follow-up serologic studies are performed, or a family study of ABO inheritance is possible.

Leukemia

Weakened expression of ABO antigens has been observed in some cases of myeloid leukemia and related disorders. Cells transfused to these individuals remain unchanged, indicating this condition is not acquired from the action of an extrinsic agent. No responsible chromosomal aberration has been found at the *ABO* locus. In some instances decreased transferase levels have been reported. Abnormalities in hemopoietic disorders may be a reflection of deficient cell-line differentiation and are potential markers for following disease progression.

Carcinomas

ABO antigens are normally expressed on epithelial tissue. In malignant tumors this activity is sometimes lost, and lack of these antigens has been associated with metastasis. Continued ABO expression on tumor cells is generally considered a favorable clinical indicator.

ABO-like antigens may appear as *de novo* structures in malignant cell lines, frequently in gastrointestinal tumors. Forssman or carcinoembryonic antigens, which are expressed in some neoplastic cells, are biochemically similar to the A blood group antigen and in some cases may account for A-like activity.

ABO antibodies

Individuals whose red cells lack A or B antigen exhibit the respective antibody in their sera. Immunization is provoked by a variety of environmental agents, and infants begin to produce these antibodies shortly after birth. Anti-A and anti-B serum levels peak between five and ten years of age; thereafter the titer gradually declines. Expected antibodies may be missing from newborns, elderly people, or patients with pathologic conditions that affect antibody production, such as lymphocytic leukemia or hypogammaglobulinemia.

ABO antibodies are the most clinically important of all blood group specificities. Their natural occurrence in nearly all patients and the serious consequences of this incompatibility make ABO the single most important consideration when developing pretransfusion testing policies and procedures. These antibodies are potent hemolysins, capable of causing intravascular hemolysis. They react well at physiologic temperature, bind complement with great efficiency, and usually exist at high titers. Both IgM and IgG components are produced.

More than one million copies of ABO antigen occur per red cell. This high-site density accounts for the ability of both IgG and IgM antibody molecules to bind complement. IgG antibody may, in fact, be more threatening than the IgM component, since IgM is more easily neutralized by the soluble antigen present in ABO incompatible plasma.

Group O persons produce a greater proportion of ABO antibody that is IgG than do individuals who are type A or B. In addition to anti-A and anti-B, they also produce a third antibody, anti-A,B, as a single component. These characteristics account for the especially dramatic hemolysis seen in group O people who encounter ABO-incompatible blood.

A_2B and A_2 individuals sometimes produce anti-A_1, but this antibody is weakly reactive and incapable of mediating hemolysis in vivo. A_1B and A_1 individuals, whose red cells carry the least amount of H antigen of all ABO blood groups, may produce an anti-H, which is also rarely of clinical significance. This antibody, however, contrasts sharply with the powerful anti-H made by all Bombay individuals, who must be transfused only with blood of their own phenotype.

During pregnancy, ABO IgG antibodies cross the placenta and may cause hemolytic disease of the newborn (HDN) in an antigen positive fetus. HDN due to ABO incompatibility, however, is rarely severe because of the neutralizing effect of the infant's soluble antigen and in part because of the incomplete development of ABO red-cell antigens in the neonate. A and B, like all transferase-dependent antigens, are not fully expressed until an infant's enzyme production is competent.

Because ABO antigens are present on tissues other than red cells, their antibodies have implications in the transplantation of highly vascularized organs. ABO incompatibility can cause rapid organ rejection. Passive transplantation of lymphocytes can also occur and result in production of incompatible donor antibody in the recipient. ABO antigens are not expressed on red-cell precursors; therefore, bone marrow transplant donors need not be ABO-matched with recipients. Bone marrow preparations should be treated, however, to remove incompatible mature red cells.

Rh BLOOD GROUP

First knowledge of the Rh blood group was presented in 1939 by Levine and Stetson in their legendary report of a fetal death due to HDN. The mother also suffered hemolysis after transfusion with her husband's blood. The authors postulated that an antibody found in the woman's serum was responsible for both hemolytic episodes. The following year Landsteiner and Wiener produced an antibody they called anti-Rh in guinea pigs and rabbits by immunizing them with Rhesus-monkey red cells. The antibody described by Levine and Stetson, as well as other examples of serum antibodies believed responsible for transfusion reactions,

demonstrated the same specificity as the animal anti-Rh. Later the animal antibody was found to be different, but by this time human anti-Rh had been widely reported, and the animal antibody was renamed anti-LW.

These early antibodies were directed toward the Rh antigen, now known as D. Many other Rh specificities have since been discovered; however, transfusion services rarely deal with more than the five most common antigens: D, C, c, E, and e. Rh is unrivalled among blood groups for its polymorphism, today boasting more than 40 antigens. In addition to these qualitative differences, variation in quantitative expression of individual antigens also contributes to the phenotypic diversity of the Rh blood group.

Genetic theories and nomenclature

Two genetic models for inheritance of Rh were proposed in the early 1940s. Fisher and Race designed the *CDE terminology*. On the basis of serological evidence, they suggested the Rh gene is composed of three subloci, which are so closely linked that crossing-over between them never occurs. The entire gene complex is inherited as a unit. According to their design, *D*, and its hypothetical allele *d*, for which no product has been detected, occupy one locus; *C* and *c* occupy another; and *E* and *e* occupy the third. Eight different gene complex combinations are possible (Table 68-4). Every individual inherits two complexes, one from each parent, making 36 Rh genotypes possible. Several genotypes may produce the same phenotype (Table 68-5). Less common alternative alleles may also appear at the *Rh* locus and some will be discussed later.

Wiener developed the *Rh-Hr terminology* based on a single-gene theory of Rh inheritance. He believed each gene produces an agglutinogen, which is composed of specific blood factors (Table 68-6). Although they were never imagined in 1943, this model can accommodate the many Rh alleles that have since been defined.

Everyday usage of Rh terminology is a hybrid language derived from both nomenclature systems. It evolved from selecting the easiest terms to say and not from any preferential support for either genetic theory. Although this usage is inconsistent, it can be justified by its expediency in a clinical setting. Individual antigens and their responsible genes are usually called by CDE names, but genotypes are referred to by the Wiener nomenclature.

A third nomenclature system was proposed in 1962 by Rosenfield and his colleagues. It is merely a numerical list-

Table 68-4 Frequency of *Rh* gene complexes.

Gene complex	Frequency (%) in US population	
	Whites	Blacks
CDe	42	17
cDE	14	11
CDE	rare	rare
cDe	4	44
cde	37	26
Cde	2	2
cdE	1	rare
CdE	rare	rare

Table 68-5   Phenotypic expression of selected Rh genotypes.

Rh genotype	Red-cell phenotype	Serologic reactions with anti-				
		D	*C*	*E*	*c*	*e*
CDe/CDe CDe/Cde	CDe	+	+	0	0	+
cDE/cDE cDE/cdE	cDE	+	0	+	+	0
CDe/cde CDe/cDe	CcDe	+	+	0	+	+
CDe/cDE CDE/cde	CcDEe	+	+	+	+	+
cDe/cde cDe/cDe	cDe	+	0	0	+	+
cde/cde	ce	0	0	0	+	+
Cde/cde	Cce	0	+	0	+	+
cdE/cde	cEe	0	0	+	+	+

Table 68-6   Comparison of Fisher-Race and Wiener Rh nomenclature.

Gene complex		Agglutinogen product	Selected genotypes		Antigen	Blood Factor
Fisher-Race	Wiener	Wiener	Fisher-Race	Wiener	Fisher-Race	Wiener
CDe	R^1	Rh_1	CDe/CDe	R^1R^1	D	Rh_o
cDE	R^2	Rh_2	cDE/cDE	R^2R^2	C	rh'
CDE	R^z	Rh_z	CDe/cDE	R^1R^2	E	rh''
cDe	R^o	Rh_o	cDe/cde	$R^o r$	c	hr'
cde	r	rh	cde/cde	rr	e	hr''
Cde	r'	rh'	Cde/cde	r'r		
cdE	r''	rh''				
CdE	r^y	rh^y				

ing of antigens and makes no presumptions regarding their genetic background. As the Rh blood group has become more complex, this nomenclature is used more commonly for newly defined antigens. It is probably the most appropriate means of referring to Rh antigens until their genetics are better understood.

D^u phenotype

Considerable variation in the strength of D antigen expression exists among Rh positive individuals. Those red cells that have an especially weak D belong to the D^u phenotype. As will be discussed, some of these do not agglutinate in direct tests with anti-D typing serum and require the addition of an antiglobulin reagent to promote a positive reaction.

Several genetic mechanisms account for this phenotype. Low-grade D^u's, those with the weakest expression, have inherited a unique Rh gene that codes for a weakly reactive antigen product. High-grade D^u's present less profound depression due to the *trans* position effect of *C*. Specifically, when a *C* allele is present on the chromosome opposite to the *D* allele, as in the genotype *cDe/Cde*, the red cells type as D^u. In the genotype *CDe/cde*, the cells are phenotypically the same, except that D is expressed normally. The definitive difference is that the gene responsible for low-grade D^u is a variant and will always produce a weak antigen *regardless*

of its position; the gene involved in high-grade D^u is capable of producing a robust D antigen and only produces a D^u red cell *because* of its position. A third situation may also be responsible for the D^u phenotype. The D antigen is believed to consist of a number of discrete epitopes and may not be complete in some individuals. Those who are missing a portion of D, a condition known as D^{mosaic}, may be immunized and produce an antibody that reacts with all random D positive cells, but not with their own cells. The antibody is presumably directed against only that portion of the antigen that they lack. Some D^{mosaic} cells react weakly in Rh typing tests with anti-D. D^{mosaic} types have been categorized based on results from cross-testing their red cells and sera. More definition of this classification is expected from the use of monoclonal anti-D reagents, which are undoubtedly specific for narrower components of the D antigen.

Although the D^u phenotype was once regarded as "D negative, D^u positive," this thinking is now obsolete. D^u red cells are D positive. When processing donor blood, all samples that do not react by direct agglutination with anti-D typing sera must be tested for D^u. D^u phenotype donors are labelled as Rh positive and transfused only to Rh positive patients. Most transfusion services now perform only direct anti-D typing on patient samples and transfuse those who are non-reactive with Rh negative blood. Others, however,

Table 68-7 Compound antigens of the Rh blood group by different nomenclature systems.

Fisher-Race	Wiener	Rosenfield	Other
ce	hr	Rh6	f
Ce	rh$_i$	Rh7	
CE	rh	Rh22	Jarvis
cE	rh$_{ii}$	Rh27	

prefer to conserve their use of Rh negative blood. These blood banks test for D^u on such patients and if positive, transfuse them with Rh positive blood. Immunization of D^u individuals against D is rare and can only occur in D^{mosaic} patients, since only they encounter a D antigen qualitatively different from their own.

Compound antigens

Two Rh antigens, such as C and e, may form an epitope that can produce a single antibody, namely anti-Ce. This antibody reacts only with red cells derived from a gene complex that includes both alleles, and not with red cells that are positive for both antigens, but result from a genotype in which they are part of different gene complexes. For example, red cells positive for the antigens C and e may be determined by the genotypes *CDe/CDe* and *CDE/cde*, among others. However, only the former produces the compound antigen Ce that will react with anti-Ce (Table 68-7).

Rh antibodies directed toward compound antigens are considered unusual, in part because they rarely appear in a serum by themselves, and other antibody components mask their activity. Anti-f(ce), for example, is often accompanied by separable components of anti-c or anti-e, and the serum will react with all c positive or e positive red cells, regardless of their genetic background. To date, all compound antigens involve the Cc and Ee antigen sets, suggesting that these products are positioned in tandem on the cell surface.

G antigen

All red cells positive for C or D also carry an antigen called G. Rare examples of C negative, D negative, but G positive cells have also been identified by their surprising reactivity with sera that was thought to be a mixture of anti-C and anti-D but was actually anti-G. The responsible gene complex, r^G, appears to direct weak e expression, no c antigen, and a C antigen that reacts with only some examples of anti-C.

Other variant phenotypes

Numerous other phenotypes have been reported as part of the Rh blood group. Many can be grouped into broad categories. Some antigens, such as C^X and C^W, or E^W and E^T, are the products of alleles that occur with low frequency at the *Cc* and *Ee* loci, respectively.

Another category includes the e variants that occur almost exclusively in Blacks. Similar to D, the e antigen appears to be a mosaic structure, and some Blacks lack either the hr^S or hr^B component. The antigens V and VS are seen with low frequency in Whites, but are not uncommon in Blacks, and they may also be related to e.

A third group includes the low-frequency antigens that serve as markers for rare complexes. Go^a, for example, always occurs with D^{mosaic} Category IV, and the Evans antigen always occurs with the ·D· gene complex.

Deleted phenotypes

In the rare red cells with deleted Rh phenotypes, no Ee antigens, and in some cases neither Ee nor Cc antigens, are detectable. The partially deleted gene complex noted as *cD*- produces elevated expression of D, weakened expression of c, and no Ee antigens. The -D- and ·D· complexes produce only D, and in both cases D activity is enhanced, but it is especially strong on -D- cells. The low-frequency antigen Evans is associated with the ·D· complex. It marks the presence of this genotype, which is masked in a heterozygous individual when the other *Rh* gene complex produces normal Cc and Ee activity.

Rh$_{null}$ and Rh$_{mod}$ phenotypes

Rh$_{null}$ individuals express no Rh antigens at all. Pedigree analysis of families in which this phenotype has been described show two different inheritance patterns. The least common, but perhaps purest form of Rh$_{null}$ results from inheritance of two silent genes at the *Rh* locus. This is known as the amorphic type. Most Rh$_{null}$ persons, however, are of the regulator type. In this case, Rh antigen synthesis is interrupted by the modifying gene, $X^o r$, which segregates independently of *Rh*. The gene that is usually present at this locus, $X^I r$, allows normal production of Rh antigens. The *Rh* gene in the regulator type of Rh$_{null}$ can be normally expressed in offspring, and the parents of these individuals may each possess two normal *Rh* genes (Figure 68-4).

Red cells of the Rh$_{mod}$ phenotype have detectable but weakly expressed Rh antigens. A third allele at the modifying gene locus, $X^o r$, may be responsible for this type. The inheritance pattern of Rh$_{mod}$ is identical to that of the regulator type of Rh$_{null}$, and the two phenotypes differ only in their degree of Rh suppression.

Rh$_{null}$ cells lack a number of antigens other than Rh, suggesting a structural relationship between Rh and other blood groups. Rh$_{null}$ cells are LW negative; they also lack Fy5, a Duffy blood group antigen present on all random cells except type Fy(a − b −). Interestingly, both the *Rh* and *Duffy* genes have been mapped to chromosome 1; however, their inheritance is not linked. Many Rh$_{null}$ cells are also weakly reactive for S, s, and U antigens.

LW blood group

Both Rh positive and Rh negative red cells carry LW antigen, but it is expressed most strongly on Rh positive cells. The preference of anti-LW for D antigen accounts for the early impression that human anti-D and the animal antibody provoked by Landsteiner and Wiener were identical. Despite their phenotypic relationship, Rh and LW have no common genetic background. The *Rh* gene resides on chromosome 1, and *LW* is inherited from chromosome 19. The LW negative phenotype occurs in the presence of normally expressed Rh antigens. All Rh$_{null}$ individuals, however, are LW negative, and it appears LW expression requires the production of Rh antigens.

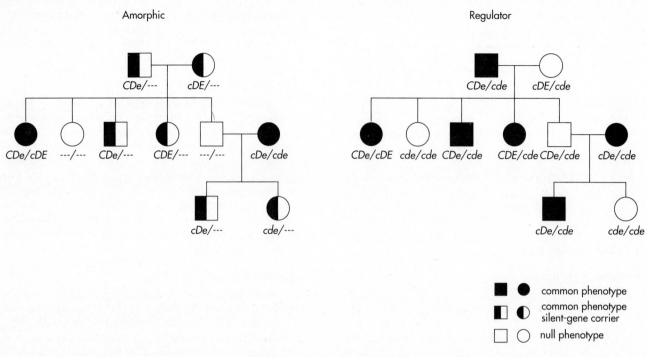

Fig. 68-4 Rh$_{null}$ inheritance patterns.

The LW blood group consists of two antithetical alleles, LW^a and LW^b. Most individuals considered LW negative lack the high-frequency antigen LW^a, but one example of LW(a−b−) has been reported. Because the LW negative phenotype is rare, few examples of LW alloantibodies have been seen. Autoanti-LW, however, has been reported in antigen positive individuals.

Biochemistry

D antigen resides on a transmembrane protein that has a molecular weight of approximately 30,000 daltons. It is associated with the membrane skeleton, perhaps through another protein rather than by direct connection. Rh protein carries no carbohydrate. Some studies have indicated that membrane lipids are essential for the D antigen to be immunoreactive.

Rh antigens and disease

Rh$_{null}$ persons, of both the amorphic and regulator types, have aberrant red-cell morphology and hemolytic anemia. On a peripheral smear these cells appear stomatocytic and spherocytic. The hemolytic anemia is usually mild and well compensated, but severity varies, and one individual required splenectomy. The osmotic fragility of Rh$_{null}$ cells is increased, and they have defective cation transport with both increased K$^+$ permeability and an increased number of pump sites.

Occasional cases of Rh antigen loss have been reported in association with myeloid cell line disorders. These patients exhibit a mosaic population of some red cells that carry Rh antigen and others, considered the products of an abnormal clone, that are missing those antigens. In one case the proportion of red cells without antigen matched the

proportion of nucleated cells that showed a specific cytogenetic change on the short arm of chromosome 1, allowing the position of the *Rh* gene to be localized.

Rh antibodies

The most immunogenic Rh antigen is D, followed by c and E. Because Rh negative transfusion recipients are generally matched with D negative donors, anti-D is not frequently found in these patients. Anti-E is the most commonly encountered Rh alloantibody.

Rh$_{null}$ individuals produce a "total" antibody, anti-Rh29, that will react with any Rh antigen. Surprisingly, these people are not readily immunized, and may make Rh antibodies with other specificities before producing anti-Rh29.

Rh alloantibodies are generally IgG1 or IgG3, although isolated examples of IgM, usually with anti-E specificity, have been reported. Even when an IgG3 component is present, Rh antibodies do not bind complement and therefore cannot mediate intravascular hemolysis. Nevertheless, they react well at physiologic temperature and have high titers, enabling them to cause severe extravascular hemolysis.

Only 10,000 to 30,000 copies of D antigen are estimated per red cell. This factor may contribute to the inability of Rh antibodies to bind complement, but it cannot be solely responsible. Duffy and Kidd blood group antigens occur with the same surface density, and yet their antibodies, especially Kidd antibodies, bind complement quite well.

The Rh blood group is perhaps most famous from a clinical perspective for its involvement in HDN. In addition, Rh is the most common specificity defined among IgG red-cell autoantibodies. These issues are discussed comprehensively later in this book (Chapter 70).

Table 68-8   Frequency distribution of common blood group phenotypes.

Blood group	Phenotype	Frequency (%) in US population	
		White	Blacks
Lewis	Le (a+b−)	22	23
	Le (a−b+)	72	55
	Le (a−b−)	6	22
P	P_1	79	94
	P_2	21	6
MNSs	M+N−	28	26
	M−N+	22	30
	M+N+	50	44
	S+s−	11	3
	S−s+	45	69
	S+s+	44	28
Lutheran	Lu (a+b+)	8	*
	Lu (a−b+)	92	*
Kell	K+k+	9	3
	K−k+	91	97
Duffy	Fy (a+b−)	17	9
	Fy (a−b+)	34	22
	Fy (a+b+)	49	1
	Fy (a−b−)	rare	68
Kidd	Jk (a+b−)	28	57
	Jk (a−b+)	23	9
	Jk (a+b+)	49	34
Xg^a	Xg (a+) male	66	*
	female	89	*
	Xg (a−) male	34	*
	female	11	*

* = insufficient data

OTHER BLOOD GROUPS

Aside from the ABO and Rh systems, hundreds of other antigens are detectable on the human red cell. Serologic studies and observation of inheritance patterns have separated some into distinct systems. Molecular technology is beginning to reveal information about their structure. The following describes blood groups that have been well defined and are most frequently encountered in clinical situations (Table 68-8).

Lewis blood group

A number of antigens have been placed in the Lewis blood group, but it is not a multi-allelic system. It has one productive allele, called *Le.* A silent gene, *le,* is believed to occupy the locus in its absence.

Lewis antigens, like A, B, and H, are carbohydrate-determined and constructed on the same precursor. *Le-* specified transferase, however, can only act on type 1 chains; therefore Lewis antigens can only be synthesized on plasma glycolipids and on glycoproteins in secretions. Red-cell Lewis antigens are not an intrinsic part of the membrane, but are adsorbed from plasma onto the cell surface.

In non-secretor individuals who have the *Le* gene, the *Le*-specified transferase adds a Fuc residue to the subterminal GlcNAc residue on type 1 chains, producing Le^a plasma antigen and red-cell phenotype Le(a+b−). When *Se* and *H* are also present, gene interaction comes into play. As described previously, the *Se* gene also directs action on

type 1 chains and produces soluble antigen by adding an Fuc residue to the terminal Gal. In Lewis positive secretors, two Fuc substitutions can be made on the same molecule, forming Le^b antigen and the red-cell phenotype Le(a−b+) (Figure 68-5). The observation that all Lewis positive Bombay individuals are type Le(a+b−) indicates that the *H, Se,* and *Le* genes are all necessary for production of Le^b. The *Le*-specified transferase can also act on type 1 chains that carry A or B activity and create the compound antigens ALe^b or BLe^b.

Le(a−b−) individuals have no *Le* gene, but they do produce antigens that are considered part of the Lewis system. The structure of these antigens is still speculative. Le^c is found in non-secretors and may represent type 1 chain precursor. Le^d occurs in secretors and appears to be type 1 chain to which a terminal Fuc has been added by action of the *Se* gene.

Le^a and Le^b are not well developed on cord red cells. Another Le antigen, Le^x, is expressed on all Le(a+b−) and Le(a−b+) adult cells and is strongly expressed on Lewis positive cord cells. Le^x is believed to represent early development of Le and to consist structurally of the Fuc-GlcNAc subterminal disaccharide common to both Le^a and Le^b antigens.

With rare exception, anti-Le^a and anti-Le^b are produced only by Le(a−b−) individuals. Both specificities commonly appear in the same serum. An occasional Le(a+b−) person makes anti-Le^b, but Le(a−b+) individuals never

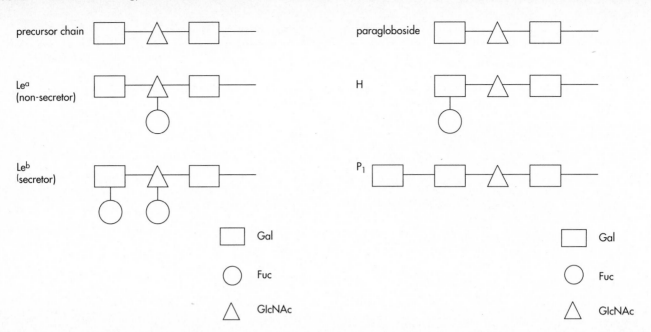

Fig. 68-5 Terminal sugar specificity of Lewis blood group antigen.

Fig. 68-6 Terminal sugar specificity of H and P_1 blood group antigens.

produce anti-Le^a. Le^b antibodies may be either anti-Le^{bH} or anti-Le^{bL}. Anti-Le^{bH} reacts more strongly with Le(b+) cells that are group O than with cells of other ABO types. Anti-Le^{bL} reacts equally well with Le(b+) cells of any ABO group.

Lewis antibodies are usually IgM and react best below physiologic temperature. Some examples of anti-Le^a bind complement well and can cause hemolysis, but in general, Lewis incompatible transfusions occur without event, because soluble Lewis antigen in transfused plasma neutralizes recipient antibody. By the time serum antibody is replenished, the transfused red cells have lost Lewis antigen by lipid exchange with the patient's Lewis negative plasma.

Pregnancy is often associated with reduced expression of Lewis antigens, and the mother may develop transient Lewis antibody. Lewis antibodies are usually IgM, and incapable of crossing the placenta. Even when IgG antibodies do enter fetal circulation, HDN does not occur, because Lewis antigens, like all blood groups that depend on transferase-generated synthesis, are not well-developed on fetal cells.

Ii blood group

I and i antigens are carbohydrate determinants that also share the same membrane structure with A, B, H, and Lewis antigens. Some compound antigens, such as IH, form among this blood group and the various epitopes of its neighbors. I and i also appear on glycoprotein molecules in secretions and are especially concentrated in milk.

Unlike the carbohydrate antigens of other blood groups, I and i both carry the same immunodominant sugars. Repetition of the terminal sequence Gal—GlcNAc of the sugar chain precursor, when repeated in linear structure forms i antigen, but when it is repeated as a branched structure, I antigen is formed.

I antigen is present on the red cells of all adults, but only a small amount appears on cord cells. Its antithetical antigen i shows the reverse pattern of weak expression on adult cells and strong expression on cord cells. During the first 18 months of life, transition from i to I as predominant antigen takes place. The i antigen also serves as a maturation marker during erythropoiesis, and enhanced i activity may be observed in adults if immature red cells have been released into the peripheral circulation.

A rare inherited I negative phenotype also exists. The red cells of these i_{adult} individuals remain strongly positive for i antigen throughout their lifetimes and display only a trace amount of I.

Individuals with the rare i_{adult} phenotype may produce an alloanti-I, but anti-I specificity is most commonly found among IgM autoantibodies that react optimally below physiologic temperature. Autoanti-I is found in the serum of many healthy individuals and is usually clinically benign. Increased titers (>1:64) may be seen in the course of mycoplasma and some viral infections. Anti-I is also the specificity responsible for hemolysis in most cases of cold hemagglutinin disease. Here it reacts over a broader thermal range, has a higher titer, and effectively binds complement.

Autoanti-i also occurs but is much less common. Often it is seen as a secondary effect of infectious mononucleosis.

P blood group

Antigens of the P system reside on two different red-cell glycolipids. The P_1 antigen is determined by the transferase-directed attachment of a Gal group to paragloboside, joining A, B, H, Lewis, and Ii antigens on the same precursor (Figure 68-6). Antigens P and P^k are produced on another molecule, lactosylceramide, a glycolipid that carries a two-sugar chain. The addition of Gal forms P^k, and subsequent addition of GalNAc creates globoside, which has P activity.

Both P-system glycolipid structures are produced independently, but their serologic behavior indicates an interaction between them that is not yet understood. A number of possible mechanisms have been proposed, but to date they remain largely speculative.

Common red cells carry both P and P^k activity, and may be either P_1 positive (P_1) or P_1 negative (P_2). Rare P negative individuals, who apparently lack the necessary transferase to produce P, carry P^k activity that is stronger than normal on the cell surface. These P^k cells may be P_1 positive (P_1^k), in which case the P_1 antigen is only weakly expressed, or they may be P_1 negative (P_2^k). The very rare null phenotype, p, also known as Tj(a−), displays no P_1, P, or P^k activity at all.

Glycolipid P and P^k activity is detected in plasma, and soluble glycoprotein P-system antigens are expressed in hydatid cyst fluid. The P antigen has been found on some tumor cells and is expressed on epithelial cells lining the urinary tract, where it is specifically recognized as an attachment site by organisms that cause pyelonephritis.

The most common P antibody specificity is anti-P_1, which is often produced by P_2 individuals. Most examples are IgM, have a low titer, and react best below physiologic temperature. This antibody is almost always incapable of causing hemolysis.

In contrast, a much stronger IgM antibody, anti-P, is present in the sera of all P^k individuals. Some examples of the biphasic autohemolysin associated with paroxysmal cold hemoglobinuria also have P specificity.

All individuals of the p type produce an especially potent hemolysin, anti-PP_1P^k. It is usually IgM, but several examples of IgG have been reported. This is one of the few blood group specificities—other than ABH—capable of causing intravascular hemolysis. Separable components of anti-P, anti-P_1, and anti-P^k have been recovered from some sera containing this antibody. Studies have indicated an association between the presence of anti-PP_1P^k and abortion in early pregnancy, but a direct cause-and-effect relationship between the two events has not been proven.

MNSs blood group

This blood group contains two sets of antithetical antigens, MN and Ss. Family studies have shown that the genes directing production of MN and Ss antigens are inherited together as a complex (Figure 68-7). Evidence of this linkage includes the observation that the antigen combination of N and s occurs with five times greater frequency than does N with S.

MN and Ss antigens reside on surface-exposed regions of the transmembrane proteins glycophorin A (GPA) and glycophorin B (GPB), respectively. Carbohydrate side chains, which include predominantly sialic acid, are attached near the terminal ends of these molecules and are responsible for the negative surface charge of the red cell. Although these sugar groups may be included in the binding sites for some MN antibodies, the specificity of MNSs antigens is determined in the protein moiety of the glycophorin molecule.

GPA is an abundant molecule that displays about 500,000 copies per red cell. The antigens M and N are determined by amino acid substitutions at positions 1 and 5. The MN

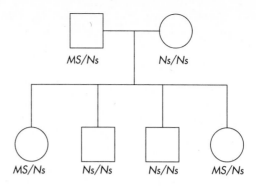

Fig. 68-7 Linkage of the *MN* and *Ss* genes. Each time the M antigen is inherited, the S antigen is also inherited.

null phenotype, En(a−), occurs in those rare individuals who lack the entire GPA molecule.

GPB is a smaller molecule and occupies fewer sites on the red-cell surface. Its first 25 amino acids maintain a sequence identical to those of GPA in an N positive individual, producing an N-like antigen referred to as 'N'. The difference between S and s antigens is determined by the amino acid at position 29. U negative is the rare Ss null phenotype found in Black Americans and is believed to result from either an altered form of GPB or absence of the entire molecule.

The extremely rare genotype M^kM^k results in no production of either GPA or GPB and consequently no MNSs blood group activity. Cells deficient in GPA and/or GPB maintain normal morphology and function, indicating these components are not essential to red-cell viability.

GPA and GPB also carry uncommon determinants referred to collectively as satellite antigens. Some of these, including M^g, M^c, and He, all variants inherited from the *MN* locus, result from differences in amino acid sequence. Others, such as M_1, Tm, and Can are variations in the carrier molecule's sugar moiety. A third group of antigens, which include Hil, St^a, and Dantu are markers on hybrid molecules that may form as the result of an unusual meiotic crossing-over event.

Anti-M antibodies are IgM or IgG, while most examples of anti-N are IgM. They react optimally below physiologic temperature and are clinically benign. Anti-M occurs more commonly than anti-N, and occasionally reacts above 30°C, in which case it should be regarded as potentially hemolytic.

An antibody with 'N' specificity has been described in some hemodialysis patients. These antibodies are the apparent result of N antigen alteration by the formaldehyde used to sterilize reusable dialysis membranes.

Most examples of S and s antibodies are IgG, although IgM anti-S does occur. These antibodies usually react best at physiologic temperature and are therefore capable of causing hemolysis.

Anti-En^a and anti-U, produced by null-phenotype individuals, are invariably potent antibodies that can cause significant hemolysis. These specificities have also been identified among autoantibodies.

Lutheran blood group

Lutheran antigens are probably glycoprotein in nature. The Lutheran blood group includes three sets of antithetical antigens: Lu^a and Lu^b, Lu9 and Lu6, Lu14 and Lu8. Informative family studies indicate these antigen pairs are the allelic products of three closely linked genes, probably subloci within the *Lutheran* complex. Lu^a is expressed on eight percent of random red cells, but Lu9 and Lu14 each are extremely rare. The alternative antigens Lu^b, Lu6, and Lu8 all occur with high frequency and only very rare cells lack any one of them. Other high-frequency antigens are absent from *Lutheran* null cells, which express no Lutheran antigens, and they are therefore phenotypically associated with this blood group, but no evidence has proven that they are inherited from the *Lutheran* gene complex (Table 68-9).

The Lutheran null phenotype, commonly referred to as Lu(a−b−), results from several genetic mechanisms. Inheritance in a few families indicates Lu(a−b−) can result from two silent genes at the *Lutheran* locus. This pattern is analogous to the amorphic type of Rh$_{null}$, but in the Lutheran system it is called the recessive Lu(a−b−) type.

Most Lu(a−b−) individuals, however, can transmit a functional *Lutheran* gene to their offspring, and their phenotype must result from an independent modifying gene. These Lu(a−b−) red cells, called the dominant type, may express a small amount of Lutheran antigen. In some cases they display a poikilocytic morphology, but the effect is variable, even within a given family. Initially, the Lutheran modifying gene was named *In(Lu);* however, it was subsequently shown to have a suppressive effect on several other blood group antigens, including P$_1$, i, Au^a and AnWj. A broader terminology, *SYN-1B,* has been proposed in consideration of the gene's impact on synthesis of more than one blood group.

Finally, an example of Lu(a−b−) phenotype was recently reported that demonstrates X-linked inheritance and is the apparent result of an X-borne modifying gene. Antigens other than Lutheran are suppressed by action of this gene, but they are different from those influenced by the autosomal modifier.

In 1951, linked inheritance between the *Lutheran* and *Sese* gene loci was reported. This was the first example of human autosomal linkage. Since then *Lutheran* has been assigned to chromosome 19 and linked with the gene responsible for myotonic dystrophy.

Reduced in vivo survival time has been cited in a few reports of Lutheran incompatible red-cell transfusions, but in general Lutheran antibodies are not clinically significant. They react at low titers and with poor avidity in serologic tests. They may be either IgM or IgG, and IgG4, a subclass unlikely to mediate hemolysis, is often a primary component. Lutheran antibodies have occasionally caused mild HDN, but severe disease is unlikely due to the poor development of *Lutheran* antigens on fetal cells.

Kell blood group

In 1945, development of a new antiglobulin technique allowed in vitro detection of non-agglutinating blood group antibodies. Anti-Kell, followed by anti-Cellano, were among the first antibodies discovered by this method. The antigens they detected, Kell (K or K1) and Cellano (k or K2), were the beginning of the Kell blood group, which today includes 24 members. The early Kell nomenclature has been supplemented by a numeric system, which is now used exclusively in naming new additions to the blood group.

The Kell blood group includes four sets of antithetical antigens: K1 and K2; K3, K21, and K4; K6 and K7; K17 and K11. As described above with the Lutheran blood group, each antigen set represents alternative products of a different sublocus within the *Kell* gene. Frequency data show an interesting distribution of these antigens that varies across racial lines (Table 68-10). Most of the remaining antigens in the Kell system occur with high frequency and

Table 68-9 Lutheran blood group antigens.

Antithetical pairs		Other antigens
Low frequency	**High frequency**	**High frequency**
Lu^a	Lu^b	Lu3
Lu^9	Lu6	Lu4
Lu14	Lu8	Lu5
		Lu7
		Lu11
		Lu12
		Lu13

Table 68-10 Frequency distribution of Kell blood group antigens.

Antigen notation		Frequency (%) in US population	
Original	**Numeric**	**Whites**	**Blacks**
K (Kell)	K1	9	3
k (Cellano)	K2	99.8	>99.9
Kp^a	K3	2	<0.1
Kp^c	K21	<0.1	*
Kp^b	K4	>99.9	100
Js^a	K6	<0.1	20
Js^b	K7	100	99
	K17	0.3	*
	K11	>99.9	*

* = insufficient data

were initially related to Kell by their absence from cells of the rare null phenotype, Ko. Ko cells express no Kell antigens and result from inheritance of two silent alleles at the *Kell* locus.

Two other Kell antigens, K10 and K23, occur with low frequency. Accumulated information from a number of family studies was required to demonstrate the K^{10} allele is inherited in linkage to *Kell*. In 1987, however, when K23 was discovered, biochemical techniques were available that allowed immediate proof the antigen is part of the *Kell* protein. Kell is a 93,000 dalton transmembrane glycoprotein and is linked to the red-cell skeleton. Nearly all antigens related to Kell by serologic activity have now been shown to reside on this protein, confirming they are all products of the *Kell* gene.

Weakened expression of Kell antigens is inherited in two situations. It occurs as a consequence of McLeod syndrome, an X-linked condition. It also results from a *cis*-positional effect of the K^3 allele in individuals with the K^3K^3 or K^3K^o genotype. Acquired and transient Kell antigen depression may also occur as a symptom of red-cell autoimmunity when the responsible antibody has Kell specificity. Some reported examples of depressed Kell activity have none of the above associations and are broadly categorized as K_{mod}.

The K1 antigen is surpassed only by D in its ability to induce antibody production, and anti-K1 is one of the most common antibody specificities seen in blood banks. Antibodies to other Kell antigens, however, are rarely found. Immunized Ko individuals produce anti-K5, which reacts with all red cells that express Kell antigens.

Kell antibodies are capable of mediating significant immune hemolysis. They have high titers, high affinity for their antigens, and react optimally at physiologic temperature. Only 17% of Kell antibodies, however, have been found to bind complement, perhaps due to the low density of Kell antigens, estimated at only 3000 to 7000 sites on the red-cell surface.

Most Kell antibodies are IgG, but some IgM examples, usually with K1 specificity, have been reported in patients with no previous pregnancy or transfusion histories. These antibodies are often transient and occur subsequent to a septic episode. One strain of *Escherichia coli* ($O_{125}B15$) is known to carry a K1-like antigen, and was the likely stimulus for IgM anti-K1 in one infected newborn.

Kell specificity is demonstrated in a small percentage (approximately 0.5%) of IgG red-cell autoantibodies, and about 10% of Kell autoantibodies produce hemolytic anemia. As mentioned previously, a transient weakening of all Kell antigen activity on the patient's red cells often accompanies this autoimmune condition and may provide protection against antibody-mediated hemolysis. The antigen weakening appears the result of an extrinsic influence, possibly action of a bacterial enzyme, since red cells transfused to these patients also lose their Kell reactivity. Cases of autoimmunity that involve blood groups other than Kell have been reported, where expression of the corresponding red-cell antigens is also weakened.

Kx antigen and McLeod syndrome

By its involvement with Kx antigen and McLeod syndrome, the Kell blood group provides a unique dimension of interest. McLeod syndrome was originally recognized as a red-cell phenotype, with X-linked inheritance from a locus named *Xk,* which was characterized by weakened expression of Kell antigens and absence of the otherwise ubiquitous antigen Kx. Follow-up of these patients revealed acanthocytic red-cell morphology, mild hemolytic anemia, and eventually a broad clinical syndrome involving multiple cell lines that usually presents during their middle years. McLeod patients demonstrate a mild to occasionally severe muscle atrophy with elevated serum creatine kinase levels. McLeod syndrome also shows high association with chronic granulomatous disease (CGD), an X-linked defect of phagocytic neutrophils.

Kell and Kx antigens clearly have a serological relationship. McLeod cells are Kx negative and express Kell antigens weakly. All other red-cell phenotypes are Kx positive, but the strength of Kx expression varies inversely with that of Kell antigens. Most cells express Kell antigens strongly and Kx weakly; however, Ko cells and other non-McLeod individuals with weak Kell phenotypes demonstrate an exalted quantity of Kx. It appears that Kx is necessary for Kell antigen synthesis, but the mechanism involved is unknown.

Biochemical studies show Kell and Kx mark different membrane proteins. The results of these studies are consistent with serologic reaction patterns (Table 68-11).

It is interesting that Kx, but not Kell, appears an important functional component of the red-cell membrane. Ko cells, which lack Kell antigens but are Kx positive, have a normal shape and survive in vivo the expected length of time. The specific biochemical defect in McLeod red cells remains a mystery. Most functional parameters are normal, but the cells do show increased phosphorylation of some membrane components, decreased water permeability, changes in ability to exchange lipids, and an aberration of the inner leaflet of the lipid bilayer.

Table 68-11 Comparison of serologic and biochemical activity of Kell and Kx.

Kell phenotype of red cells studied	Serologic tests		Biochemical tests	
	Kell antigens	Kx antigens	Kell protein	Kx protein
Common	present	weak	present	weak
K$_o$	none	present	none	present
McLeod	weak	none	weak	none

Table 68-12   Serologic specificity of Duffy blood group antibodies.

Red cell:	Anti-Fyᵃ	Anti-Fyᵇ	Anti-Fy3	Anti-Fy4*	Anti-Fy5**
Fy (a+b−)	+	O	+	+/O	+
Fy (a−b+)	O	+	+	+/O	+
Fy (a+b+)	+	+	+	O	+
Fy (a−b−)					
Black	O	O	O	O	O
White	O	O	O	O	+

*non-reactive with all red cells from whites
**non-reactive with Rh$_{null}$ cells

Duffy blood group

Duffy was the first blood group to receive assignment to a human autosome. The Duffy gene is located on chromosome 1, syntenic to *Rh,* but the two genes are not linked and segregate independently.

The primary Duffy antigens, Fyᵃ and Fyᵇ, are the allelic products of a single locus. The Fy(a−b−) phenotype is common among Blacks, with a frequency of 68%, but it occurs in less than one percent of other individuals. The antibody produced by Fy(a−b−) individuals, anti-Fy3, reacts with all Fy(a+) and/or Fy(b+) red cells. Only a few examples of this antibody have been reported and of these, about half have occurred in non-Black individuals. Initially, Fy(a−b−) was assumed to result from two silent *Fy* alleles, but the realization that few Blacks produce anti-Fy3, even though the majority are Fy(a−b−), suggested that this phenotype might not have the same genetic background in all population groups.

Another antibody specificity was then described that supported this idea. Anti-Fy4, as it was called, reacted preferentially with all Fy(a−b−) cells from Blacks, with some Fy(a+b−) and Fy(a−b+) cells from Blacks, and was nonreactive with Fy(a+b+) cells from Blacks and with all red cells from Whites regardless of Duffy phenotype (Table 68-12). It appeared that a silent gene, *Fy,* in double dose, was responsible for the Fy(a−b−) phenotype in Whites and that another allele, named *Fy⁴,* was present at the *Duffy* locus in Fy(a−b−) Blacks.

One genetic model proposes that *Fyᵃ, Fyᵇ,* and *Fy* are all alleles at one locus, and that *Fy³* and *Fy⁴* occupy another locus within the *Duffy* gene. Other explanations are also possible. For example, Fy3 may not be the direct product of a single *Fy³* allele, but rather the result of interaction among several genes. It cannot, however, be a fourth allele at the proposed *FyᵃFyᵇFy* locus, because Fy(a+b+) individuals are also Fy3 positive.

Several other antigens have been placed in the Duffy system. Fy5 is serologically similar to Fy3 except that it is missing from Rh$_{null}$ cells and is present on Fy(a−b−) cells from Whites. Fy5 may be an interaction product of the *Duffy* and *Rh* genes. Fyˣ is a weak variant of Fyᵇ. It appears qualitatively identical to Fyᵇ, but is expressed in less quantity. Fy6 is defined by a murine monoclonal antibody that reacts like Anti-Fy3. Fy6 differs, however, in its sensitivity to in vitro treatment with various protease enzymes. Studies in nonhuman primates suggest Fy6 is involved in red-cell invasion by malarial parasites. Fs antigen demonstrates a possible relationship to Duffy by its presence on a significantly higher percentage of Fy(a−b−) cells than cells of other blood group phenotypes. Biochemical studies of Duffy indicate it resides on a protein of approximately 40,000 dalton molecular weight.

Duffy antigens are not strongly immunogenic. One study estimates Kell antigens are nine times more potent in their capacity to initiate antibody production. Anti-Fyᵃ, however, is fairly common, and can cause significant hemolysis. It is IgG, reacts optimally at physiologic temperature, and may activate complement. Although patients with this antibody should always be transfused with Fy(a−) blood, on a relative scale it cannot be considered as clinically important as Rh or Kell antibodies. Many infants with HDN caused by anti-Fyᵃ, for example, are not severely affected.

Anti-Fyᵇ occurs less frequently and is generally less capable of initiating hemolysis than anti-Fyᵃ. Anti-Fy3 and anti-Fy5 have been implicated in hemolytic events, but anti-Fy4 has not. However, only a few examples of these specificities have been reported and generalizations about their clinical significance should not be made.

The possibility that blood groups can play functional roles was clearly realized with the dramatic discovery that Duffy antigens serve as receptors for red-cell invasion by the malarial parasite *Plasmodium vivax.* It had been known since the mid-1950s that most Blacks are resistant to *P. vivax* malaria. However, association between malarial resistance and the Fy(a−b−) phenotype was not recognized for another two decades. Expanded work with the monoclonal anti-Fy6 and red cells from nonhuman primates now suggest that Fy6—not Fyᵃ or Fyᵇ—is the actual receptor. *Plasmodium falciparum,* which causes a more malignant disease than *P. vivax,* is not dependent on Duffy antigens for red-cell invasion. This organism appears to recognize sialic acid, since invasion of cells deficient in glycophorin molecules is reduced.

Kidd blood group

Kidd is a small blood group, consisting of only one pair of alleles, *Jkᵃ* and *Jkᵇ,* and a silent gene, *Jk,* which produces the Jk(a−b−) null phenotype when inherited in double dose. Recent studies of two Japanese families indicate the Jk(a−b−) phenotype may also result from action of an independent modifying gene.

Kidd antigens are not strongly immunogenic, but when

antibody is produced, it is usually IgG and optimally reactive at physiologic temperature. Anti-Jk3, the specificity produced by Jk(a − b −) individuals, reacts with all red cells positive for Jk^a and/or Jk^b antigens. Autoantibodies with Kidd specificity, usually anti-Jk^a, have also been reported.

Kidd antibodies are very important clinically, because they bind complement well and are therefore capable of causing intravascular, as well as extravascular hemolysis. They are of particular concern because many examples react weakly in vitro, and immunized persons do not generally maintain high levels of antibody. Kidd antibodies can easily go undetected in pretransfusion tests, and if antigen positive blood is given, it will stimulate a secondary immune response, during which the transfused cells are destroyed. Kidd antibodies are commonly implicated in these delayed transfusion reactions, but perhaps due to their low titration scores, Kidd antibodies are not often associated with HDN.

Xg^a blood group antigen

The Xg^a antigen is inherited from the X chromosome and therefore occurs with greater frequency in females than in males. *Xg^a* has been linked with some genetic traits, and early calculations suggested that it might be measured close enough to *Xk* that it would be a useful marker for genetic counselling of families that carry the *McLeod* gene. Further work indicated, however, that it is not located within meaningful distance to this site.

Anti-Xg^a is an uncommon blood group antibody. It is usually IgG and reacts optimally at physiologic temperature, but it has not been implicated in transfusion reactions or HDN.

Other antigens of high and low frequency

Many other red-cell antigens exist that are unrelated to any of the previously discussed blood groups. Some are inherited together as allelic products of the same gene; others are genetically independent. Most occur with very high (>99.9%) or with very low (<0.1%) frequency. Discussion of each individual specificity is beyond the scope of this chapter; however, some selected comments about this category are appropriate.

As with all blood groups, these antigens may occur with varying frequency in different population groups. For example, the rare Diego antigen Di^a demonstrates highest prevalence among South American Indians. Some phenotypes that lack high-frequency antigens, such as At(a −), Cr(a −), Jo(a −), and Hy − predominate in Blacks. Screening efforts to identify these rare individuals are most efficient if they can be confined to the populations in which they occur most commonly.

Antibodies to low-frequency antigens are usually encountered when the reactive serum happens by chance to be tested with a cell positive for the rare corresponding antigen. It is an interesting but unexplained observation that several antibodies to different low-frequency antigens often appear in the same serum, commonly from patients with autoimmune hemolytic anemia.

In contrast, antibodies to high-frequency antigens are reactive with all random donors. These antibodies are usually IgG and vary in their clinical importance. One specificity, anti-Vel, should always be considered clinically sig-

nificant. Many examples of anti-Vel are IgM; it invariably binds complement well and may cause intravascular hemolysis of Vel positive red cells. Another specificity, anti-Yt^a, directed toward an antigen in the Cartwright system, has a less predictable hemolytic potential. Some examples can mediate significant hemolysis, while others appear to be harmless.

Antibodies to high-frequency antigens are unusual and therefore clinical experience with many of them is limited. Considering the difficulty in finding compatible blood for patients who have them, in vivo survival studies are often warranted to determine if the antibody's hemolytic ability justifies an exhaustive search for antigen negative blood. Whenever antigen negative blood is indicated, compatible donors are most likely to be found among the patient's family members, especially siblings.

Sd^a antigen

One unique high-frequency red-cell antigen, Sid (Sd^a), is also expressed in soluble form in body fluids. Sd^a has been characterized as an epitope on the Tamm and Horsfall glycoprotein in human urine and is strongly expressed in the urine of Sd(a +) humans and in that of guinea pigs. Anti-Sd^a is found quite commonly in human serum but does not cause destruction of transfused Sd(a +) red cells.

HTLA antibodies

A number of high-frequency antigens have been defined by antibodies categorized as high-titer low-avidity (HTLA). These antibodies characteristically react very weakly and with poor reproducibility. However, their reactivity persists through multiple serial dilutions. They are commonly encountered antibodies but are rarely associated with significant in vivo hemolysis of antigen positive cells.

Cost-Stirling(Cs^a)/York(Yk^a) and Knops-Helgeson (Kn^a)/McCoy (McC^a) are two of the best delineated systems within the HTLA category. The frequency distribution of various phenotypes within these two systems varies considerably between Blacks and Whites.

The antigens of another blood group within this category, Chido (Ch^a)/Rodgers (Rg^a), are markers on the C4 molecule of human complement. They are not synthesized by the red cell but are detected on the surface of complement-coated cells.

Red-cell antigens shared with other tissues

Bg^a, Bg^b, and Bg^c are three related determinants weakly expressed on the red cell but proven to be red-cell analogues of human leukocyte antigens (HLA), which are expressed predominantly on leukocytes and other body tissues. The red-cell antigens Ii, U, Jk3, Kx, and Gerbich (Ge) have been detected on granulocytes; A and B antigens are found on platelets.

Polyagglutination

Human red cells carry hidden determinants, known as cryptantigens, that are not normally detected on the membrane surface. Due to some extrinsic action on the red-cell membrane, such as that of a bacterial enzyme, these antigens are sometimes exposed. Affected red cells react in the presence of all human serum, which normally contains agglutinating antibodies directed against these antigens.

The two most common polyagglutination specificities are T and Tn, carried by tetrasaccharide side chains attached to GPA and GPB. Cleavage of sialic acid by a bacterial neuraminidase exposes Gal, the immunodominant sugar of the T antigen.

Tn, unlike other polyagglutination specificities, is not acquired but results from a somatic mutation that prevents production of the *T*-specified transferase. Carbohydrate synthesis of the tetrasaccharide is interrupted, leaving GalNAc, which is normally a subterminal sugar, exposed as the immunodominant determinant that forms Tn antigen. White cells and platelets may also be affected. Some patients with Tn polyagglutination develop hemolytic anemia, leukopenia, and thrombocytopenia.

PARENTAGE TESTING

To be considered in cases of disputed paternity, genetic markers must exhibit a clear pattern of inheritance, they must be polymorphic, and their various phenotypes must be clearly distinguishable by tests that provide reproducible results. Blood groups satisfy these criteria, and in the mid-1930s, the American legal system began to admit red-cell typing results as evidence in paternity cases.

Power of exclusion

Every blood group system carries a power of exclusion (PE) rate, which is determined by the number of alleles it contains and the frequency with which they each occur. When several systems are included in a paternity testing protocol, the power increases and can be calculated as a cumulative power of exclusion (CPE). This figure represents the percentage of falsely accused men who will be excluded from paternity on the basis of that particular protocol. The red-cell typings available today allow a CPE of approximately 70%—a limited improvement over the CPE of 50% in the 1930s.

Two types of exclusion may occur. A direct exclusion occurs when the alleged father does not express an antigen that the mother's cells also lack, but which is expressed by the child. For example, a direct exclusion is provided when an alleged father is group O, the mother is also group O, but the child is group A. In this case the biological father is obligated to contribute the *A* gene.

Indirect exclusions occur when the alleged father expresses a marker that the child does not express. These situations are less conclusive, because the trait does not have to be inherited unless the alleged father is homozygous for the responsible gene. The child may in fact have inherited a silent gene from the alternative gene locus. For example, an indirect exclusion appears when the alleged father's red cells type Jk(a+) and both mother and child are Jk(a−). The alleged father's genotype may be *Jk^aJk^a*, in which case he is excluded. Alternatively, his genotype may be *Jk^aJk*, in which case inheritance of the *Jk* allele could account for the child's negative phenotype.

In the late 1960s the legal system began to rule in favor of more financial support for illegitimate children. Several US Supreme Court decisions as well as a 1975 amendment to the Social Security Act (PL 93-647) recognized the needs of this increasingly large population of children and mandated legal obligation for biological fathers, as well as for public funds, to contribute to their support. Consequently, more paternity actions were brought to the courts. As the caseload increased, so did the demand for more definitive evidence. Joint guidelines published by the American Medical Association (AMA) and the American Bar Association (ABA) recommended that evidence introduced should have a CPE of at least 90%. Tests of other genetic systems were then included in paternity study protocols to supplement the exclusion rate achieved by blood group antigens. These included serum proteins, red-cell enzymes, and HLA.

The four subloci of the HLA genome each have a large number of possible alleles, and are so closely linked that the rate of recombination among them is less than one percent. The resultant haplotypes are inherited as a unit, providing a high degree of polymorphism and allowing the HLA system by itself a CPE of more than 90%. Many laboratories include HLA typing, along with tests for red-cell antigens to achieve an acceptable paternity testing protocol, and only perform the biochemistry assays for serum proteins and red-cell enzymes if that is within their particular expertise.

As paternity testing included more systems, the courts began to place increasing value on genetic evidence. Exclusionary evidence now carries strong credibility and rarely requires substantiation by expert testimony.

Probability of inclusion

When an alleged father is not excluded, the probability that he is the biological father may be high. This value is indicated by the paternity index (PI). The PI compares the probability (X) that the alleged father could provide the obligatory genes required to satisfy the paternal contribution to the child, with the probability (Y) that they could be provided by a random man in the same population. The comparison is expressed as PI = X/Y. When multiple genetic systems are used, a combined paternity index (CPI) is obtained by calculating the products of the individual X and Y values. When the PI is expressed as a percentage, it is referred to as the relative chance of paternity (RCP). In 1979 the Uniform Parentage Act allowed these statistical estimates to become admissible in paternity cases.

DNA probe technology

The introduction of DNA probes into paternity testing now adds even more weight to inclusionary evidence. This testing presents PI values that move close to actual proof of paternity. The new technology detects previously undisclosed genetic markers in the blood referred to as restriction fragment length polymorphisms (RFLPs). Testing consists of DNA digestion with restriction enzymes that cleave at specific sequence sites. This creates DNA fragments of varying lengths, depending on the individual's genotype. The fragments are separated by electrophoresis and then challenged with DNA probes of known specificity in a Southern Blot technique. Banding patterns of the mother and child are then compared with that of the alleged father. Nearly 100 systems have proven useful in paternity testing. Most two-allele systems alone have a PE of about 0.80; using two systems yields a CPE of 0.96, and three systems raises it to 0.99.

Other legal considerations

Genetic results must fulfill several evidentiary requirements to be admissible in paternity cases. A chain of sample custody must be established to substantiate sample identification. Assurance must be provided that all tests are performed properly using reliable reagents and that the results are interpreted by a qualified individual.

Since these cases are civil rather than criminal proceedings, paternity need not be established "beyond reasonable doubt." Only a "preponderance of evidence" is required. It is sometimes disconcerting for scientists to realize that no matter how convincing for or against paternity genetic tests results may be, they remain only one piece of evidence. Prior evidence, including reports of cohabitation or reduced fertility, and allegations or denial of sexual activity, among other events, are all considered in the court's decision.

SUGGESTED READING

Allen RW, Wallhermfechtal M, and Miller WV: The application of restriction fragment length polymorphism mapping to parentage testing, Transfusion 30:552, 1990.

Beattie KM: A review: The Duffy blood group system, Immunohematology 5:45, 1989.

Bryant NJ: Paternity testing: Current status and review, Transf Med Rev 2:29, 1988.

Freedman J: The significance of complement on the red cell surface, Trans Med Rev 1:58, 1987.

Garratty G: The significance of IgG on the red cell surface, Transf Med Rev 1:47, 1987.

Issitt PD: The Rh blood group system, 1988: Eight new antigens in nine years and some observations on the biochemistry and genetics of the system, Transf Med Rev 3:1, 1989.

Levene C, Levene NA, Buskila D, and Manny N: Red cell polyagglutination, Transf Med Rev 2:176, 1988.

Marsh WL and Redman CM: Recent developments in the Kell blood group system, Transf Med Rev 1:4, 1987.

Marsh WL and Redman CM: The Kell blood group system: a review, Transfusion 30:158, 1990.

Mougey R: A review: the Kidd system, Immunohematology 6:1, 1990.

Pierce SR and Macpherson CR, eds: Blood group systems: Duffy, Kidd, and Lutheran, Arlington, Va, 1988, American Association of Blood Banks.

Reid ME and Bird GWG: Associations between human red cell blood group antigens and disease, Transf Med Rev 4:47, 1990.

Rolih SD: High-titer, low-avidity (HTLA) antibodies and antigens: a review, Transf Med Rev 3:128, 1989.

Tippett P: Regular genes affecting red cell antigens, Transf Med Rev 4:56, 1990.

Unger PJ and Laird-Fryer B, eds: Blood group systems: MN and Gerbich, Arlington, Va, 1989, American Association of Blood Banks.

Vengelen-Tyler V and Pierce SR, eds: Blood group systems: Rh, Arlington, Va, 1987, American Association of Blood Banks.

Walker RH: DNA probe technology in parentage testing, Immunohematology 5:31, 1989.

Wallace ME and Gibbs FL, eds: Blood group systems: ABH and Lewis, Arlington, Va, 1986, American Association of Blood Banks.

69

Laboratory techniques in immunohematology

Arlene S. Gingras

The 1980s was an era of redefinition and streamlining in serologic methodology. Because of cost, only test procedures that enhanced detection of clinically significant antibodies were required and encouraged. Changes in traditional methods (e.g., eliminating the room temperature phase of the antibody screen and the minor crossmatch procedure) have resulted in a more efficient approach to compatibility testing. There is still controversy over which antigens need to be absent from donor red cells for transfusion to a patient possessing the corresponding antibody. Recent applications of flow cytometry in analyzing RBC antibody sensitized in vitro are now being used to evaluate cell survival in vivo. Widespread application of this method may result in redefining the clinical significance of many antibodies as related to transfusion practice.

The blood banker is challenged to choose donor, prenatal, and pretransfusion tests that meet high performance standards. At the same time, the blood banker must respect increasing cost constraints. The purpose of this chapter is to present an overview of in vitro antigen-antibody reactions and a systematic approach to problem solving when unexpected test results occur.

FACTORS AFFECTING ANTIGEN-ANTIBODY DETECTION

In routine blood bank methods, the observed endpoint is either agglutination or hemolysis of RBCs triggered by the formation of antigen-antibody complexes. To achieve optimum sensitivity, the serologist must control the conditions under which the events leading to hemolysis or hemagglutination occur.

Before the discovery of anti-human globulin sera (Coombs' sera), only antibodies capable of causing direct agglutination of red cells suspended in saline (complete antibodies) could be recognized. With the addition of the anti-globulin phase to antibody detection tests, antibodies not capable of causing such direct agglutination (incomplete antibodies) could also be demonstrated by observing hemagglutination resulting from the reaction of added anti-IgG and/or anti-complement with sensitized RBCs. Hemolysis, the recognizable end point of an antigen-antibody reaction

activating the entire complement cascade, is also interpreted as a positive result.

It is hypothesized that the agglutination of red blood cells by an antigen-antibody reaction occurs in two stages that may proceed simultaneously. The first stage involves the binding of antigen and antibody (sensitization), the second stage involves the actual lattice formation of the red cells to which antibody has bound (hemagglutination).

First stage: sensitization

The rate and strength of this reaction is determined by the kinetics of the formation of antigen-antibody complexes (association) and breakdown of the complexes to free antigen and antibody (dissociation). The greater the strength of the bonding between antigen and antibody (avidity), the more stable the end point (association).

$$[Ag] + [Ab] \underset{k2}{\overset{k1}{\rightleftarrows}} [AgAb] \text{ or } \frac{[AgAb]}{[Ag] + [Ab]} = \frac{k1}{k2} = K$$

This equilibrium constant (K) is affected by: the concentration of antigen and antibody, pH, temperature, and ionic strength.

Antigen-antibody concentration

As the relative concentration of antibody to antigen is increased, the avidity of the reaction is augmented. This state is reached by increasing the serum-cell ratio in the test suspension. In addition to affecting the avidity of the sensitization reaction, the efficiency of hemagglutination may be increased, as will be discussed.

pH

The majority of blood group antibodies demonstrate optimal activity between a pH of 6.5 and 7.5. Some examples of anti-M reportedly are enhanced by decreasing the suspending medium's pH.

Temperature

For most blood group antibodies, changing the temperature of the reaction has little effect on the amount of antigen-antibody complex formed. However, the rate at which the complexes are formed may be remarkably altered by changing the temperature. In blood banks where speed and avidity are critical, optimum temperature conditions for antibody detection is closely observed. The incubation temperature for enhancing cold agglutinins is room temperature or below; for warm agglutinins, 37°C.

Ionic strength

Decreasing the ionic strength of the medium results in an increase in the rate at which antigen-antibody complexes are formed. When the ionic strength of the medium is decreased (e.g., decreasing the concentration of $Na+$ ions), the negative charge of the cell surface is no longer neutralized by clustered cations. This results in an increased attraction between the negatively charged red cells and the slightly positively charged antibody molecules.

Suspending red cells in Low Ionic Strength Solution (LISS) increases the speed of reactivity with both IgG and IgM antibodies. However, false positive antiglobulin phase reactions may result from complement activation by aggregated serum immunoglobulins. Thus, the addition of monospecific IgG antisera rather than polyspecific or broad spectrum (IgG and anti-complement) antisera at the antihuman globulin phase is recommended when using LISS.

Second stage: hemagglutination

The second stage, agglutination of sensitized red cells, is influenced by several elements: zeta potential of the red cells, characteristics of the antibody molecules, characteristics of the test medium, location and density of antigen determinants, and the concentration of antigen and antibody.

Zeta potential

The negative electrical charge of red cells results from the N-acetyl neuraminic acid (NANA) residues (sialic acid) on the red cell surface. This charge is responsible for the normal repulsion of RBC's from one another.

The negatively charged red cell membrane in an ionic solution attracts a cloud of positively charged ($Na+$) cations. The edge of this ionic cloud of uniformly suspended $Na+$ ions travels with the cell and is called the boundary of shear (Figure 69-1). The zeta potential, measured in millivolts, is the difference in energy between the cell surface and the boundary of shear. A decrease in the zeta potential permits red cells to come closer together. $Na+$ ions and other cations are attracted to the negative red cell surface charge and thereby result in a decrease in the zeta potential.

Antibody characteristics

The difference in physical properties of IgG and IgM antibodies has a bearing on lattice formation between sensitized red cells. IgG molecules are thought to be Y or T shaped. IgG molecules have two combining sites about 140 A° apart when their Fab sites are maximally extended from each other. IgM molecules are circular and have 10 potential Fab combining sites. The maximum distance between Fab sites is 300 A°. Because of their size and number of potential binding sites, IgM antibodies can agglutinate red cells in a

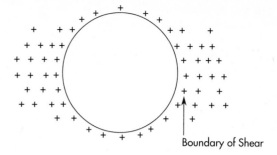

Fig. 69-1 Layer of sodium ions at the boundary of shear, which move with the red cell in an electrolyte solution. *Redrawn from Bovine Albumin, Raritan, NJ, 1980, Ortho Diagnostics.*

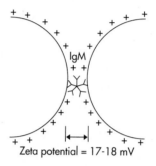

Fig. 69-2 Agglutination of red cells suspended in 0.9% NaCl by IgM antibodies. *Redrawn from Bovine Albumin, Raritan, NJ, 1980, Ortho Diagnostics.*

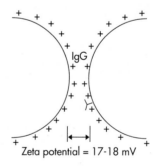

Fig. 69-3 Inability of IgG antibodies to agglutinate red cells suspended in 0.9% NaCl. *Redrawn from Bovine Albumin, Raritan, NJ, 1980, Ortho Diagnostics.*

saline medium (complete antibodies), whereas the majority of IgG molecules (incomplete antibodies) fail to do so because the zeta potential precludes the formation of antibody bridges by these smaller molecules (Figures 69-2 and 69-3).

Characteristics of the test system

The suspending medium or the reacting red cell surface can be altered to lower the zeta potential and promote the detection of IgG antibodies in direct agglutination tests. Colloids such as gelatin, PVP, dextran, and bovine albumin can decrease the zeta potential more effectively than saline. Bovine albumin, for example, dissipates electrical charge, since it is a dipolar molecule, which upon orientation in the test medium attracts both the positively charged Na ion and the negatively charged RBC surface (Figure 69-4). Some antibodies—notably Rh—that fail to agglutinate red cells suspended in saline may demonstrate agglutination of red cells in albumin (Figure 69-5).

Treating red cells with proteases (ficin, papain, bromelin,

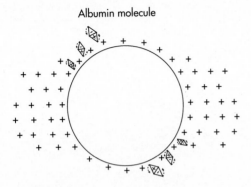

Fig. 69-4   Reduction in zeta potential from orientation of dipolar albumin molecules in an electric field. *Redrawn from Bovine Albumin, Raritan, NJ, 1980, Ortho Diagnostics.*

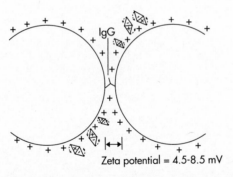

Zeta potential = 4.5-8.5 mV

Fig. 69-5   Hemagglutination by some IgG antibodies suspended in albumin additive. *Redrawn from Bovine Albumin, Raritan, NJ, 1980, Ortho Diagnostics.*

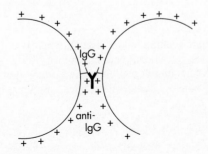

Fig. 69-6   Agglutination of IgG-sensitized red cells by anti-IgG molecules. *Redrawn from Bovine Albumin, Raritan, NJ, 1980, Ortho Diagnostics.*

or trypsin) results in the liberation of sialic acid and thereby reduces the zeta potential. In addition, the destruction of some antigens that are structurally part of NANA (M, N, S, Fy^a, Fy^b) may make other blood group antigens (notably Rh) more accessible to the activity of the antibodies. Therefore the reactions of certain antibodies will be enhanced with enzyme treatment of the test cells while others will be depressed.

Some antibodies, such as examples of Kidd, are not detected in systems that simply lower the zeta potential of test cells. In order to detect prior sensitization with IgG or complement, it is necessary to test the sensitized red cells with an anti-IgG and/or anti-C3b (or C3d) antiserum. These antisera are added after cells are extensively washed. Hemagglutination will then result from the bridging between cells by antiglobulin (Figure 69-6).

Antigen structure

The more antigen sites on the red cells (density), the better the opportunity for antibody binding to occur. In addition, the location of the antigens on the red cell determines their relative accessibility to the corresponding antibody. The A and B antigens, for example, are glycolipids protruding from the RBC membrane surface and are readily exposed for antibody uptake. This may explain, in part, why some IgG antibodies, such as anti-A, may directly agglutinate red cells. Other blood group antigens, such as Rh, are protein and are part of the membrane structure itself; thus they are less available for antibody attachment.

Antigen-antibody concentration

The relative proportions of antigen and antibody will affect RBC lattice formation and consequently RBC agglutination (Figure 69-7).

If the relative concentration of antigens is greatly decreased (e.g., by making the red cell suspension weaker or increasing the ratio of antibody to antigen), too many antibody molecules compete for too few antigen sites on the red cell, and a prozone effect may occur. If the relative antigen concentration is greatly increased, few bridges between red cells occur. Prozone and excess antigen in the test system both affect the second stage of antibody detection by decreasing RBC lattice formation.

In the usual blood bank setting, in which a 2% to 5% red suspension is used, the consequences of excess antibody are only encountered in situations with very high cold agglutinin titers. More often, weak antibody concentrations are undetected by routine test procedures. In practice, increasing the serum-to-cell ratio (i.e., three or four drops of serum from the usual two drops added to one drop of a 2% to 5% suspension of cells) usually increases the sensitivity of antibody detection.

In vitro hemolysis

Activating complement by IgM and, rarely IgG (IgG_3 and IgG_1 subclasses), may result in in vitro hemolysis. A single IgM molecule, which provides two adjacent Fc regions for such activation, is more effective at binding C1q than IgG molecules, which are usually bound randomly over the RBC surface and less likely to align. Such IgM antibodies, when present in high titer and characterized by a high thermal

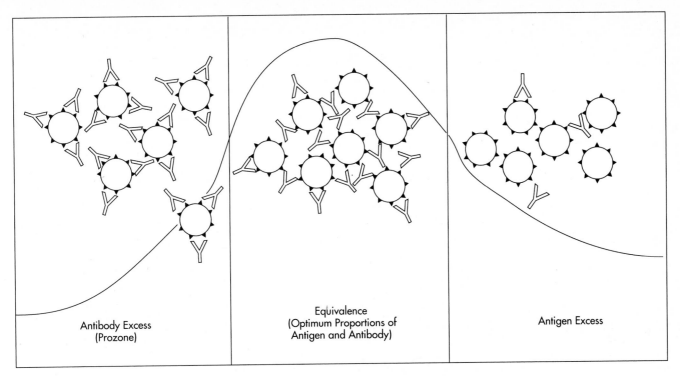

Fig. 69-7 Schematic representation of the effects of varying concentrations of antigen and antibody on lattice formation. *Redrawn from Pittiglio DH: Modern blood banking and transfusion practices, Philadelphia, 1983, FA Davis Co.*

Table 69-1 Grading and scoring of hemagglutination reactions

Grade	Score	Appearance
4+	12	complete agglutination—no nonagglutinated red cells
3+s	11	intermediate between 3+ and 4+
3+	10	strong reaction—a few detached masses of agglutinated red cells
2+s	9	intermediate between 2+ and 3+
2+	8	moderate reaction—large agglutinates in a sea of smaller agglutinates.
1+s	6	intermediate between 1+ and 2+
1+	5	weak reaction—many agglutinates of up to 20 red cells, with some smaller agglutinates and nonagglutinated red cells.
±	3	weak granularity of red cell suspension—scattered agglutinates of six to eight red cells with many nonagglutinated red cells.
w	2	a few small agglutinates of three or four red cells, but with a majority of nonagglutinated red cells.
0	0	no agglutination

From March WL: Scoring of hemagglutination reactions, Transfusion 12:352, 1972.

amplitude, may not only fix the early components of the complement cascade but also may activate the system through formation of a lytic complex.

GRADING AND SCORING SYSTEMS

No matter which grading system is used, test results should be performed consistently and recorded accurately. Whether using slide or modified tube test methods, reading after each step should be observed against a white or lighted background for RBC agglutination or lysis. Antiglobulin tests accomplished by the tube method are read both macroscopically and microscopically with low magnification. Agglutination reactions are interpreted with the tube method

by attempting to re-suspend the button of cells formed by centrifugation or by settling. Re-suspension is performed by swirling the suspending medium and intermittently tilting the test tube. Violent shaking or tapping of the tubes may disrupt fragile agglutinates, thus causing false negative reading. The supernatant should be carefully observed for the presence of hemolysis. Two methods for evaluating agglutination reactions—one a grading system and one a scoring system—are used in the clinical setting (Table 69-1).

The grading system of 0-4+, ranging from no agglutination (0) to the formation of one solid aggregate of RBC's (4+) is most widely used in cell typing and in the direct and indirect antiglobulin tests.

The Marsh scoring system is used more frequently in semi-quantitating antibody titers. When scoring titers for prenatal studies, a numerical value is assigned to each tube and then totaled. A change in score by 10 on the present serum sample from a previous one may be judged clinically significant and less biased than a system evaluating a twofold change in titer level.

Ordinarily, readings above 5 or 1+ are considered macroscopic observations, readings below are viewed microscopically.

False positive readings due to pseudoagglutination must be distinguished from true antigen-antibody reactions. Rouleaux formation is discerned microscopically and gives a characteristic "penny-stacking" appearance. Use of saline-washed RBC suspensions rather than whole blood can prevent rouleaux during cell or front typing. The saline replacement technique, in which saline replaces serum, is used to disperse rouleaux during serum or back-typing and antibody detection. The cell washing steps prior to the addition of the antiglobulin reagent eliminates the effects of rouleaux in the antiglobulin tests.

THE BLOOD SAMPLE

A clotted specimen is used for most routine type and cross-match procedures and prenatal studies. Serum separated from a clotted sample is preferable to plasma for antibody detection testing. The presence of fibrin clots in plasma samples may interfere in the interpretation of hemagglutination results. In addition, the anticoagulant in plasma samples chelates calcium ions, and thereby precludes the binding of complement that had been considered necessary for detecting some antibodies such as Kidd and Lewis.

An anticoagulated sample (EDTA tube) is ideal for ABO typing and evaluating a direct antiglobulin test because it is easier to prepare an RBC suspension, since one avoids having to break up the clot. EDTA samples may be necessary for slide testing or testing with automated blood grouping instruments. Furthermore, EDTA anticoagulated blood specimens prevent the occurrence of false positive direct antiglobulin tests due to complement activation in vitro by the cold autoagglutinins naturally found in the serum.

Some antigens, such as P, deteriorate upon sample storage as do levels of complement and antibody activity. Complement stability deteriorates more rapidly at room temperature. Therefore, testing should be performed on fresh blood specimens or on samples stored in the refrigerator after serum has been separated from the clot if complement binding is thought to be essential to antibody detection. Antibodies of the Kidd blood group system are notorious for demonstrating weakened expression upon storage. In general, samples should not be stored for more than seven days. Furthermore, it is considered good practice to use samples drawn from patients who have been pregnant or transfused within the prior three months for a period of only 48 to 72 hours. This prevents formation of new antibodies by the patient between the time the specimen is drawn and the time it is used.

BLOOD GROUPING

The correct determination of the ABO blood group and Rh type of a donor, prenatal patient, or transfusion candidate is very important. Much attention is therefore devoted to properly interpreting test results and to choosing suitable reagents.

ABO grouping

Most laboratories performing ABO typing use commercially prepared anti-A, anti-B, and anti-A,B to test whole blood or a 2% to 5% RBC saline suspension for front or cell typing, depending on whether slide or tube testing is performed. Serum or plasma is added to and mixed with a 2% to 5% RBC suspension of commercially prepared A_1 and B cells in reverse or serum typing.

Human anti-A,B is required to detect individuals who are subgroups of A and might otherwise be mistaken for type "O" or "B." Anti-A,B can be omitted in testing pre-transfusion candidates for mistaken identity in a weak-subgroup of A will not have adverse consequences since "O" RBCs would be used for transfusion to an A sub-group individual and "B" RBCs for transfusion to A sub B individuals. A_2 cells are not routinely used in serum typing of donors or recipients unless investigation of serum and cell discrepancies from room temperature reacting antibodies is warranted. Traditionally, human anti-sera (polyclonal) has been used in both the slide and rapid tube methods for ABO typing. The commercial availability of monoclonal anti-A sera has negated the need for human anti-A,B to detect weak expressions of the A antigen. Unfortunately, this monoclonal antibody has been found to be responsible for fragile agglutination of B cells if the technologist used gentle agitation of the test tube. Moderate agitation will negate this weak agglutination. If unclear results continue, a polyclonal antisera or another manufacturer's reagent must be used.

ABO typing discrepancies

Discrepancies between the front typing and back typing can occur under the following circumstances:

1. *Rouleaux formation* resulting in erroneous front typing is seen in hypergammaglobinemia or contamination of cord blood samples with Wharton's jelly when the cells are inadequately washed. Similarly, back typing errors may be caused by rouleaux in hypergammaglobinemia. (Table 69-2)
   Resolution: Wash cells four to six times before front typing; perform a saline replacement test in the back typing by substituting the serum with saline after initial reaction, and observing for dissipation of rouleaux.

2. *Strong cold agglutinins.* Strong autoagglutinins coat autologous RBCs in vitro at room temperature (RT). In addition, sera containing potent cold-reacting auto- and alloantibodies, such as anti-I,-M,-N,-P or Le, can agglutinate back typing cells with the corresponding antigen. (Table 69-3)
   Resolution: In order to dissociate adherent autoagglutinins from autologous cells, wash the RBCs with warm (37°C) saline several times. These cells can then be typed with appropriate antisera. If that fails, pretreatment of the cells with 2-mercaptoethenal (2-ME) or dithrothreital (DDT) will destroy the adherent cold-reacting IgM antibody. Pre-warming the back typing cells and the patient's serum or plasma will avoid agglutination by cold antibodies present in the serum.

Table 69-2 Rouleaux formation causing discrepant backtyping

		Reagent antisera					Reagent RBCs			
		anti-A	anti-B	anti-A, B	Cell type		A_1 RBCs	B RBCs	Serum type
Example:	Patient or donor RBCs					Patient or donor plasma/serum			
		+	+	+	AB		$+^w$	$+^w$	O
	Probable type: AB								

Agglutination Key   + = positive $+^w$ = weaker than expected
                          0 = negative $+^{mf}$ = mixed field appearance

Table 69-3 Cold agglutinins causing agglutination of both patient and reagent red cells

		Reagent antisera					Reagent RBCs			
		anti-A	anti-B	anti-A, B	Cell type		A_1 RBCs	B RBCs	Serum type
Example:	Patient or donor RBCs					Patient or donor plasma/serum			
		+	$+^w$	+	AB		$+^w$	+	O
	Probable type: A								

Table 69-4 Hypogammaglobulinemia causing absent expected back-typing results

		Reagent antisera					Reagent RBCs			
		anti-A	anti-B	anti-A, B	Cell type		A_1 RBCs	B RBCs	Serum type
Example:	Patient or donor RBCs					Patient or donor plasma/serum			
		0	0	0	O		0	0	AB
	Probable type: O								

Table 69-5 Weakened ABO antigens causing diminished front-typing results

		Reagent antisera					Reagent RBCs			
		anti-A	anti-B	anti-A, B	Cell type		A_1 RBCs	B RBCs	Serum type
Example:	Patient or donor RBCs					Patient or donor plasma/serum			
		0	$+^w$	$+^w$	B^w		+	0	B

3. *Hypogammaglobinemia* seen in newborns, the elderly, and immune deficiency states may cause negative reactions of a patient serum when tested against A_1 and B cells. (Table 69-4)
Resolution: Incubate the back typing cells at room temperature for 15 to 30 minutes to enhance detection of isohemagglutinins. If still negative, place the test tubes at 4°C and include an auto control. Note that the auto control must be negative, since cold autoagglutinins reacting at that temperature may interfere with the interpretation of test results.

4. *Weakened antigens* due to the decreased production of glycosyltransferases in patients with leukemia and myeloproliferative disorders must be differentiated from weak subgroups or gene suppression. (Table 69-5)
Resolution: Identify the diagnosis of the patient. Demonstrate weakened expression of blood group antigens other than ABH. Absorption of anti-A or anti-B onto the alleged cells with the subsequent recovery of the corresponding antibody or antibodies in the eluate confirms a specific blood group typing.

5. *Subgroups of A* may account for discrepancies between front and back typing as previously described. Approximately 2% of A_2 and 25% of A_2B people demonstrate anti-A_1. (Table 69-6)
Resolution: Include human anti-A,B or monoclonal sera in the test system and observe microscopically. The use of plant lectins *Dolichos biflorus* (anti-A_1) and *Ulex europeus* (anti-H) are inexpensive cell typing reagents for identifying subgroups of A. Secretor studies of individuals and family members can be useful in determining the specific blood type of the patient/donor.

6. *Polyagglutination* is a condition in which RBC's are agglutinated by a high proportion of blood-group compatible, normal adult sera. (Table 69-7)
Resolution: Polyagglutinable cells cause weak typing and, unlike IgG-coated cells, the autocontrol will probably be negative. Proteases destroy the T and Tn receptors. Therefore enzyme-treated cells can be retyped in cases of such polyagglutination.

7. *Acquired B-like antigen.* As previously described,

Table 69-6   Subgroups of A may cause apparent typing discrepancies

		Reagent antisera					Reagent RBCs		
Example:	Patient or donor RBCs	anti-A	anti-B	anti-A, B	Cell type	Patient or donor plasma/serum	A₁ RBCs	B RBCs	Serum type
		$+^w$	0	+	A^w		$+^w$	+	O
	Probable type: A₂ with anti-A₁								

Table 69-7   Polyagglutination causing cells to type as group AB

		Reagent antisera					Reagent RBCs		
Example:	Patient or donor RBCs	anti-A	anti-B	anti-A, B	Cell type	Patient or donor plasma/serum	A₁ RBCs	B RBCs	Serum type
		$+^w$	$+^w$	$+^w$	AB^w		+	+	O
	Probable type: O								

Table 69-8   Acquired B-like antigen cause apparent typing discrepancies

		Reagent antisera					Reagent RBCs		
Example:	Patient or donor RBCs	anti-A	anti-B	anti-A, B	Cell type	Patient or donor plasma/serum	A₁ RBCs	B RBCs	Serum type
		+	$+^w$	+	AB		0	$+^w$	A
	Probable type: A with acquired B-like antigen								

Table 69-9   Chimerism causes typing discrepancies

		Reagent antisera					Reagent RBCs		
Example:	Patient or donor RBCs	anti-A	anti-B	anti-A, B	Cell type	Patient or donor plasma/serum	A₁ RBCs	B RBCs	Serum type
		$+^{mf}$	0	$+^{mf}$	A^{mf}		0	+	A
	Probable type: A/O								

certain strains of *E. coli* have the capacity to deacetylate N-acetyl-D-galactosamine into galactosamine, which is similar in structure to D-galactose. (Table 69-8)

Resolution: If B typing is weak and patient is septic, the acquired B-like antigen—and not a subgroup of B—should be suspected.

8. *Chimerism* is a rare cause of such discrepancy. It is seen in twins in whom an exchange of hemopoietic tissue has occurred during fetal development or following transplantation. (Table 69-9)

Resolution: Inquire if individual is a twin or has undergone an ABO unidentical allogeneic bone marrow transplant. Following cell separation techniques, perform typing studies on family members, including the twin or the bone marrow donor.

Rh system

Reagents used in Rh typing have been modified repeatedly since being introduced in the 1940s. The original Rh reagent was a saline-agglutinating human IgM anti-D. It could not be used in the antiglobulin D^u test. IgG anti-D reagents were subsequently introduced. In order for these antisera to agglutinate saline suspended cells, bovine albumin (22% to 30%) and other potentiators were added to the medium. With the widespread use of this high-protein anti-D (HP-D) came reports of spontaneous agglutination of Rh negative RBCs coated with immunoglobulin. This prompted manufacturers to include a parallel patient control—the diluent of the anti-Rh sera (HP-C). Antisera or control diluent are mixed with 2% to 5% RBC suspension in the modified tube technique or mixed with whole blood for slide testing. If the immediate spin phase (IS, the first centrifugation step at room temperature) is negative, the test is carried to the antiglobulin phase (AHG, serial washing of the test red cells and addition of anti-IgG). Still routinely used, results with HP-D on immediate spin are interpreted as correct in the presence of a negative Rh control. The positive D^u test cannot be interpreted as valid if the direct antiglobulin test is positive, since the final step of the procedure is the addition of anti-globulin reagent to the cells.

The introduction of chemically modified anti-D (CM-D)

in the 1970s revolutionized Rh typing. In the manufacture of these antisera, the disulfide bonds that maintain the rigidity of the hinge region of the IgG molecule are broken, allowing the antibody to stretch a greater distance and agglutinate RBCs in a low protein medium (6% to 8% albumin). Since spontaneous agglutination of IgG-sensitized cells in the immediate spin phase of testing with HP-D is not usually experienced with these reagents, the testing of an Rh control tube in parallel with the anti-sera tube is not required by regulatory agencies provided a control system is run concurrently with typing. ABO typing serves as a control.

Individuals other than group AB whose cells do not react with both anti-A and Anti-B can be considered to have typed appropriately with CM-D as Rh positive. Apparent group AB positive individuals will require the use of a separate Rh control (e.g., 6% to 8% albumin).

Monoclonal IgM anti-D blended with polyclonal anti-D was introduced in the 1980s. This reagent not only demonstrated more avid reactions, but did not require a second diluent control tube. Manufacturers of monoclonal anti-Rh sera also claim that these reagents can detect weak expressions of the D antigen on direct saline agglutination.

OTHER BLOOD GROUP ANTIGEN TYPING

Although transfusion candidates are routinely typed for ABO and Rh only, it may be necessary to type them for other blood group antigens in order to confirm the identity of antibodies detected in their sera. Donor RBCs are typed to ensure lack of antigens corresponding to clinically significant antibodies detected in the recipient prior to or concurrent with compatibility testing. Occasionally, it may be desirable to determine a patient's phenotype of the most common antigens to which clinically significant antibodies are produced prior to initiating long-term transfusion therapy or if the recipient is already deemed a "responder."

Some methods employ immediate centrifugation spin (IS) at room temperature with IgM antisera (e.g., anti-Le, -P1, -M), while others using IgG antisera employ a 37°C incubation followed by addition of an antiglobulin reagent (e.g., anti-Kell, -Duffy, -Kidd, -SsU).

ANTIBODY SCREENING AND COMPATIBILITY TESTING

Protocols governing pre-transfusion testing vary from one institution to another. Until recently, it was common practice for hospital laboratories to perform a complete blood type, antibody screen, and a direct antiglobulin test or autocontrol on all pre-transfusion candidates, prenatal patients, and whole blood donors. A major and minor crossmatch that included room temperature testing, 37°C incubation, and antiglobulin phases was also part of compatibility testing. Most transfusion services have now dropped the minor crossmatch, since antibody screenings are routinely performed on donor units. Many facilities have further reduced procedures for routine antibody detection and compatibility testing by eliminating the room temperature phase of the antibody screen, the direct antiglobulin test, and the serum autocontrol. Recently, licensing and accreditation organizations have relaxed their criteria for compatibility testing by permitting an optional Coombs' crossmatch, provided

that the routine testing ensures major ABO compatibility between donor RBC's and recipient serum, and that the antibody screen run prior to or concurrently with the crossmatch is negative for clinically significant alloantibodies reactive at 37°C and at the antiglobulin phase.

The antibody screen

Before commercially prepared screening cells were available, compatibility testing was based solely on the results of the crossmatch between donor and recipient. Currently, laboratories performing pre-compatibility tests rely heavily on the premise that detecting irregular antibodies in the serum of the recipient can predict results of the crossmatch. Such detection is accomplished by observing the reactions of the individual's serum against a battery of at least two "O" reagent donor cells with known major blood group phenotypes. Briefly, the antibody screening is performed by mixing serum with a 2% to 5% suspension of reagent RBCS, incubating at 37°C, and carrying to the antiglobulin phase. Whether this screening test is accomplished prior to or concurrently with the crossmatch, this phase of compatibility testing, together with the ABO and Rh determination, represents a critical in vitro manuever to forecast survival of transfused RBCs.

The screening cells

As stated, hospital transfusion services and free-standing blood banks are required to use at least two separate reagent RBC's for pre-transfusion testing. The test system must detect antibodies that are reactive at 37°C and capable of causing destruction of donor RBC's carrying the corresponding antigen, or of causing hemolytic disease of the newborn. Some weak antibodies may escape detection if serum is tested against reagent or donor cells with heterozygous expression of the corresponding antigen. Therefore, in order to demonstrate antibodies influenced by "dosage effect," reagent RBCs should be homozygous for such commonly analyzed antigens such as C, c, E, e, (i.e., genotypes R_1R_1 and R_2R_2); Fy(a) and Fy(b); and Jk(a) and Jk(b) (Table 69-10). Such conditions are not always met in the two-cell set; therefore, some blood banks utilize a three-cell screening which usually includes an rr donor cell. Some manufacturers also provide screening cell packages negative for most RBC cross-reactive HLA antigens, so that Bg antibodies, which are clinically unimportant and commonly seen in the multiparous and multiply-transfused patients, will be undetected.

Enhancement and antiglobulin reagents

The selection of reagents and test conditions will determine which antibodies are detected. Enhancement solutions, such as albumin and LISS added at the 37°C incubation phase, are not required by licensing agencies as part of the testing procedure. However, these additives can influence the speed at which antigen-antibody complexes are formed. In addition, some additives are able to potentiate the detection of certain antibodies. Most clinically significant antibodies can be demonstrated by a saline system incorporating a one-half to one-hour 37°C incubation phase. The addition of albumin can reduce incubation time to 15 to 30 minutes, enzymes to 10 minutes, and LISS to 5 to 10 minutes.

Table 69-10   Example of a two-cell antibody screening set

CELL	GENO-TYPE Donor	Rh-Hr								Kell						Duffy		Kidd		Lewis		P	MN				Lutheran	
		D	C	c	E	e	f	V	Cw	K	k	Kpa	Kpb	Jsa	Jsb	Fya	Fyb	Jka	Jkb	Lea	Leb	P1	M	N	S	s	Lua	Lub
I	R1R1	+	+	0	0	+	0	0	0	+	+	0	+	0	+	+	0	+	0	0	0	+	+	0	+	0	+	0 +
II	R2R2	+	0	+	+	0	0	0	0	0	+	0	+	0	+	0	+	+	+	+	0	+	+	0	+	0	+	0 +

Table 69-11   A reagent red cell panel for alloantibody identification

Sample #	Rh genotype	Rhesus						Kell	Duffy		Kidd		P	Lewis		MN			
		C	Cw	c	D	E	e	K	Fya	Fyb	Jka	Jkb	P1	Lea	Leb	M	N	S	s
1	r'r	+	0	+	0	0	+	0	+	0	+	+	+	0	+	+	+	0	+
2	R1wR1	+	+	0	+	0	+	+	+	+	0	+	+	+	0	+	+	0	+
3	R1R1	+	0	0	+	0	+	0	+	+	+	+	0	0	+	+	0	+	+
4	R2R2	0	0	+	+	+	0	0	0	+	0	+	+	+	0	0	+	0	0
5	r"r	0	0	+	0	+	+	0	+	+	0	+	0	0	+	+	+	+	0
6	rr	0	0	+	0	0	+	0	0	+	+	0	+	0	0	+	+	0	+
7	rr	0	0	+	0	0	+	+	0	+	+	0	+	0	+	+	0	+	0
8	rr	0	0	+	0	0	+	0	+	0	0	+	+	+	0	0	+	0	+
9	rr	0	0	+	0	0	+	0	0	+	+	0	0	0	+	0	+	+	0
10	R0r	0	0	+	+	0	+	0	0	0	+	+	+	0	0	+	+	+	+

From Walker RH, ed: AABB Technical Manual, ed 10, Arlington, Va, 1990, AABB.

Room temperature incubation is not only unnecessary but undesirable when using these reagents because nonsignificant cold auto- and alloantibodies may react. Effects of cold agglutinins that react at higher temperatures can be minimized if monospecific anti-IgG is used in the antiglobulin phase rather than broad spectrum (anti-IgG and anti-C3d) Coombs' serum. Since some IgM antibodies readily activate complement components, polyspecific antisera in the antiglobulin phase will detect this complement fraction from activity carried over from IS testing. The possibility of missing complement-activating IgG antibodies such as anti-Jk^a, must be taken into consideration, although most Kidd antibodies can be detected with anti-IgG alone.

Limitations of the antibody screening procedure

Some of the most commonly occurring technical errors that result in a false negative test result and consequently lead one to conclude that the serum is absent of clinically significant alloantibodies include:

Omission of the patient's serum in the test system. There is no reagent indicator that can infallibly determine whether the serum has been added to the test tube. By routinely placing the serum in the test tube first, one can minimize this problem, because its absence might be noticed when the cell suspension is added.

Inadequate washing of RBCs or interruption in washing prior to the addition of Coombs' sera. The amount of residual immunoglobulin from the patient's serum defines the number of full-tube washings required to prevent neutralization of the anti-human globulin reagent. Whether using manual or automatic washing devices, each fill and decant process should allow no residual saline to remain between washes. The procedure should be rapid and uninterrupted, allowing minimum time before adding antiglobulin sera, so as to preclude elution of adherent antibody into the saline wash.

Omission of the anti-human globulin reagent. IgG-coated RBC's, added after apparent negative reactions, monitor the reactivity of anti-IgG and polyspecific antisera. Absence of agglutination invalidates the test results. This may occur from inadequate washing, which results in neutralization of the antisera, or from failing to add the reagent at that phase of testing. Manufacturers have dyed polyspecific and monospecific antisera green in order to prevent omission.

Antibody identification

If the antibody screen in positive, the serum can be further tested in similar fashion with a panel of eight or more reagent RBCs of known phenotypes. The panel should allow for a high level of confidence in assessing the identity of clinically significant antibodies. Each RBC is typed for antigens of the Rh, Kell, Duffy, Kidd, Lewis, MNS, and P blood group systems, which are represented horizontally on the panel sheet as indicated in Table 69-11. Antigen specificity is represented by a unique vertical pattern. Antibodies in the serum can then be selectively identified, with some degree of certainty, according to their unique pattern by an elimination process, if the following considerations in selection and testing of the panel cells are taken into account:

1. The exclusion process should only be done by eliminating those antigens present on reagent cells giving

Table 69-12   The serologic characteristics of some commonly encountered alloantibodies

System	Specificity	Reaction phase					Complement binding	In vitro hemolysis	Dosage
		4 C	RT	37 C	IAT	Enzymes			
Duffy	Fy^a/Fy^b				*	X	(*)	X	(*)
Kell	all		(*)	(*)	*	*(W)	(*)	X	(*)
Kidd	all				*	*e	*	(*)	(*)
Lewis	all	*	*	(*)	(*)	(*)e	(*)	(*)	X
Lutheran	all		(*)		*	*	X	X	(*)
MN	M/N	*	*	(*)	(*)	X	X	X	(*)
	S		(*)	(*)	*	X	(*)	X	(*)
	s				*	*	(*)	X	(*)
P	P_1	*	*	(*)	(*)	(*)e	(*)	(*)	X
Rhesus	D			(*)	*	*e	X	X	X
	all other			(*)	*	*e	X	X	(*)
Xg	Xg^a		(*)	(*)	*	X	(*)	X	X

From A handbook of serologic techniques for use in investigative immunohematology, 1975, BCA, Organon-Teknica.
* = invariably; X = rarely or not at all; ( ) = some examples; e = enhanced; w = weakened; RT = room temperature; IAT = indirect antiglobulin test

a negative result in all phases of testing of the patient or donor sera. This will ensure that additional antibodies will not be inadvertently eliminated.

2. Attention must be paid to the zygosity of the reagent cells prior to omitting a particular antibody known to show dosage effect. Therefore the elimination process should be done only after a negative serum reaction to donor cells homozygous (i.e., MM), rather than heterozygous (i.e., MN), for the antigen being observed. Special considerations therefore must be taken into account when excluding antibodies to the Rh, Duffy, Kidd, and MNS antigens.

3. The reactivity of some antibodies are known to be influenced by various test conditions, including temperature, enhancement medium, and type of antiglobulin reagent. As previously discussed, IgM antibodies generally react optimally at room temperature and colder temperatures, whereas IgG antibodies react better at 37°C and at the anti-human globulin phase. Some Kell antibodies react less optimally with LISS and therefore are better demonstrated with a saline medium or albumin additive system. Antigens of the Duffy and MNS Blood Group Systems are depressed with enzyme-treatment of the RBCs, whereas weak expressions of Rh, Kidd, P, and Lewis antibodies are often enhanced with this media. Some reactions of the Kidd antibodies appear stronger with the use of polyspecific anti-globulin sera. Many users of the LISS additive system prefer to use anti-IgG routinely in the antiglobulin phase in order to avoid enhancing clinically insignificant cold agglutinins. Some serologists believe that enzymes should not be used routinely, since these reagents enhance the detection of most cold-reacting antibodies. Furthermore, interpretation of reactions at the Coombs phase should depend on macroscopic observations only when using enzyme-treated reagent RBCs. Some antibodies, such as Lewis, I, Vel, and Tj^a, demonstrate hemolysis at 37°C, particularly with enzyme-treated RBC's. The characteristics of these various antibodies are summarized in Table 69-12.

Table 69-13   Probability of antibody identification

# RBC samples tested	# RBC(s) reactive	# RBC(s) nonreactive	Probability (p)
6	1	5	1/6
6	2	4	1/15
6	3	3	1/20
6	4	2	1/15
8	5	3	1/56
10	6	4	1/210

From Dixon MR: American association of blood banks' technical workshop on complex serological problems, Arlington, Virginia, 1988.

4. Grading variations in the test phases of each donor cell must be carefully documented. The strength of agglutination can vary when there is more than one antibody in the serum, if dosage effect is an influencing factor, or if the specific antigen is known to have a different degree of expression from donor to donor. The latter is known to occur particularly with the P antigen. Antigens not completely developed at birth, including the I and Lewis antigens, are weaker on cord cells. Some manufacturers include a cord cell or incorporate an I negative adult donor cell into their panel system.

5. The finding of a positive autocontrol may indicate the presence of alloantibodies to antigens on recently transfused donor RBC's or the presence of sensitization of the patient's autologous cells, which would be revealed by the direct Coombs' test.

6. To prove the existence of a particular antibody(ies) in the serum requires testing the antibody(ies) against a sufficient number of donor cells that lack and carry the corresponding antigen. This minimizes chance as responsible for a diagnostic reactivity pattern. Usually, testing three positive cells and three negative cells gives a probablity (p) value of 1/20 (0.05), the minimum value at which the deciding factor is statistically valid (Table 69-13). Some commercially or

Table 69-14   A reagent red cell panel demonstrating the presence of anti-E

Sample #	Rh genotype	Rhesus						Kell	Duffy		Kidd		P	Lewis		MN				Serum		
		C	C^w	c	D	E	e	K	Fy^a	Fy^b	Jk^a	Jk^b	P$_1$	Le^a	Le^b	M	N	S	s	IS	37°	AHG
1	r'r	+	0	+	0	0	+	0	+	0	+	+	+	0	+	+	+	0	+	0	0	0
2	R$_1^w$R$_1$	+	+	0	+	0	+	+	+	+	0	+	+	+	0	+	+	0	+	0	0	0
3	R$_1$R$_1$	+	0	0	+	0	+	0	+	+	+	+	0	0	+	+	0	+	0	0	0	0
4	R$_2$R$_2$	0	0	+	+	+	0	0	0	+	0	+	+	+	0	0	+	0	+	0	0	+
5	r"r	0	0	+	0	+	+	0	+	+	0	+	0	0	+	+	+	+	0	0	0	+
6	rr	0	0	+	0	0	+	0	0	+	+	0	+	0	+	+	0	+	0	0	0	0
7	rr	0	0	+	0	0	+	+	0	+	+	0	+	0	+	+	0	+	0	0	0	0
8	rr	0	0	+	0	0	+	0	+	0	0	+	+	+	0	0	+	0	+	0	0	0
9	R$_2$r	0	0	+	+	+	+	0	0	+	+	0	0	0	+	0	+	+	0	0	0	+
10	R$_0$r	0	0	+	+	0	+	0	0	0	+	+	+	0	0	+	+	+	+	0	0	0

Patient RBC's   0   0   0

in-house produced reagent panels are unable to provide such statistically valid results for some antigens. In such cases, additional selected donor cells may be sought from other panels for definitive identification.

The panel in Table 69-14 depicts the resolution of an antibody identification problem in which a single antibody, anti-E, is identified. Utilizing the systematic approach of "crossing-out antigens," all other possible antibodies are excluded.

The direct antiglobulin test (DAT)

To perform the DAT, a suspension of washed RBC's is mixed with broad spectrum or polyspecific antihuman globulin sera, centrifuged, and observed for the presence of hemagglutination. The presence of IgG and/or complement components may be found not only on the red cells of patients with hemolytic anemia, but also on the red cells of non-hemolyzing patients and otherwise healthy donors.

After detecting a positive DAT on a routine clotted sample, further evaluation is performed with an EDTA anticoagulated blood sample in order to more easily wash cells, prepare an eluate, or eliminate the possibility of complement coating after drawing the blood sample. Once the test is found positive, monospecific antisera to IgG or complement is used to determine specificity. Both polyspecific and monospecific test results should be observed microscopically in order to detect not only weak agglutination, but the presence of mixed-field reactivity. This discovery may be the first clue to the presence of a mixture of autologous RBC's with antibody-sensitized, transfused RBC's.

Most reagent manufacturers try to purify their antisera by removing most of the C4 reactivity, since detection of this component alone is usually clinically insignificant. Some manufacturers have prepared a blend of rabbit IgG and murine (mouse) C3b/C3d polyspecific antisera and respective monospecific counterparts, which they believe cause few false positive results.

The test system must include a control of IgG-coated RBC's and/or complement-coated RBC's to verify negative test results. Absence of agglutination after adding these "check" cells may be attributed to unacceptable reagents or inadequate removal of extraneous protein from the RBC suspension, thereby neutralizing the Coombs' sera. Dilution of the antisera with residual saline can also negate a weak antiglobulin reaction. This can be avoided by leaving a "dry" button of cells in the test tube after washing. Furthermore, direct agglutination of RBC's can occur before the addition of anti-globulin sera from strong cold agglutinins. Therefore, careful observation of an RBC suspension in saline alone, acting as the control tube, should be compared to the antiglobulin test tube. Presence of RBC agglutination in the saline control invalidates the test results.

Elution procedures

If IgG is present on the cells, and if the patient has been recently transfused, is hemolyzing, or has atypical antibodies, most serologists proceed to further identify the immunoglobulin coating the RBC's. Excepting IgG anti-A and anti-B which can be identified in eluates with a negative antiglobulin test, most laboratories attempt elutions only in the presence of detectable IgG on the red cells.

The objective of any elution technique is to break the binding forces between antigen and sensitizing antibody molecules without destroying antibody activity. This can be accomplished by various treatments that usually rupture the RBC membrane with subsequent release of the antibody molecule into the suspending medium. Methods using organic solvents, freeze-thawing, heat and sonication, or alteration of pH or salt concentration are employed.

The technologist may be restricted by local safety regulations in the use of highly flammable (ether and xylene) or carcinogenic (chloroform and xylene) organic solvents. Consequently, many facilities opt for commercially prepared reagents in kit form (i.e., cold glycine acid, digitonin) or simple, physical techniques (i.e., heat [56°C], thaw-freeze). The heat and freeze-thaw methods are best reserved for the investigation of suspected ABO hemolytic disease of the newborn, or when ABO antibodies are thought to be responsible for the observed positive direct Coombs test (i.e., ABO minor incompatibility due to ABO mismatched plasma products). Warm-reactive allo-or autoantibodies are best recovered with methods like the cold glycine acid removal.

Whichever method is employed, it is critical that the antibody captured in the eluate consist solely of the IgG coating the RBCs. Therefore, it is essential to wash the cells four to six times to remove serum antibodies from the cell suspension before elution technique is begun. This is particularly critical when the patient also possesses alloantibodies in the serum.

Testing the eluate

The eluate is usually tested against "O" screening cells. If positive, the eluate is then tested against a full panel of reagent RBC's. The detection and subsequent identification of IgG antibody eluted from the RBC's relies on proper incubation at 37°C followed by rapid washing of the RBC's and addition of anti-IgG reagent. Some serologists recommend that the washing process be done only once with low ionic strength solution (LISS), since the eluate, unlike sera, is essentially free of extraneous protein. It is advisable to test the last wash in parallel with the eluate to ensure adequate removal of plasma antibody. The last wash should test negative. It may be important to concentrate the amount of antibody in the supernatant, particularly if the DAT is very weak. Alternatively, the strength of agglutination may be enhanced by increasing the eluate-to-cell ratio.

The reactive eluate—auto or alloantibody. When the antibody in the eluate appears to have specificity for blood group antigens, the patient can then be typed for the presence or lack of corresponding antigens. If the patient has not been recently transfused, the presence of the antigen confirms that the antibody is autoantibody, which may often demonstrate broad Rh specificity.

The non-reactive eluate. If the eluate does not react when tested against a panel of "O" reagent RBC's, it is important not to dismiss this as a negative finding until concentration techniques have been attempted. If the patient has been recently transfused with plasma-containing components (e.g., platelet concentrates or fresh frozen plasma) that are not ABO compatible with the recipient's RBC's, the incorporation of A and B reagent RBC's into the test system can detect the presence of isoagglutinins passively acquired from incompatible donor plasma. A nonreactive eluate may indicate insufficient antibody in the supernatant for detection by routine procedures, or that the recovered immunoglobulin is not directed against a specific RBC antigen (e.g., directed against a drug).

Testing the eluate with drug-coated RBC's. Negative reactions of eluates with routine reagent RBC's are seen with anti-drug antibodies (e.g., penicillins and cephalosporins), which have coated the patient's red cells. In these cases, group O reagent RBC's can be treated with the suspected drug and the reactivity of the eluate against such treated cells measured.

When testing the eluate against drug-coated cells, a negative control known to lack antibodies against the suspected drug and, if available, a positive control consisting of serum or eluate containing those anti-drug antibodies should be run in parallel. In addition, a suspension of the same group "O" RBC's used in the preparation of the drug-coated cells should remain untreated and also tested in parallel.

QUALITY CONTROL OF ROUTINE SEROLOGIC PROCEDURES

An adequate and comprehensive immunohematology quality control (QC) program includes a check of all reagents employed on the day of use. This not only ensures that the reagents are functioning properly, but also serves as a verification of proper technique. The reactivity of certain antigens may diminish as the reagent ages or is exposed to temperature variations. For this reason, the reagent RBC's acceptable level of activity is monitored against a known standard antisera. Similarly, a good quality control program includes a check of blood grouping and anti-human globulin sera against a known standard RBC control to ensure that acceptable levels of specific antibodies are present in each vial.

Overt discrepancies between the results obtained and those expected must be promptly resolved. Usually, subtle discrepancies are the result of variation in technologists' grading. If, however, repeat testing continues to manifest the same discrepancy, investigation is mandatory.

Possible explanations for false negative test results and their resolution include:

1. Cells not properly washed causing the Coombs' antisera to be neutralized by residual serum globulin. Check manual washing technique or automated cell washer function. Use IgG and/or C3-sensitized reagent cells to ensure serologic activity at the antiglobulin phase.
2. Antibody has eluted from the cells during incubation or washing. Ensure that proper incubation times were used and that the cell-washing procedure was uninterrupted. Check temperature of waterbaths and incubators and monitor cell washer function.
3. RBC's and antiseras have lost expected reactivity. Recheck for proper storage of reagents and expiration dates.
4. Reagents or sera have been inadvertently omitted. Repeat procedure to ensure addition of appropriate reagents or patient sera.
5. Tests are inadequately centrifuged. Recheck that the centrifugation speed and time designated for the specific phase of testing was employed. Check instrument for functional calibration.
6. Weak agglutination is missed. Check resuspension technique for too vigorous shaking.

Factors that may cause false positive reactions include:

1. Reagent screening or panel cells are unexpectedly demonstrating positive reactions. Check the direct antiglobulin test of reagent RBC's. Observe vials for discoloration, turbidity, or hemolysis due to microbial contamination or improper storage.
2. Tests are overcentrifuged or undershook. Check that proper centrifugation (speed and time) was carried out according to procedure.
3. Fibrin from a clotted sample. Check by observing the suspension microscopically.

AUTOMATED METHODS IN BLOOD BANKING

In the last 20 years, breakthroughs in automation and computerization have brought about a wide variety of instruments that test and interpret routine laboratory procedures which were otherwise performed manually. Utilization of bar code specimen labels have dramatically reduced clerical errors in sample identification. Furthermore, computerized sensing devices can interpret and record results objectively.

Although many thought these technological advances would have widespread appeal in the hospital blood bank, automated testing instruments developed to date are mainly used in the donor testing areas of large blood centers with high volume, batched-testing capabilities.

Instruments such as the continuous flow Autoanalyzer (Technicon, Tarrytown, NY) allow hemagglutination to occur without the need for the centrifugation steps. The agglutinated RBC's in a positive reaction settle to the bottom of the reaction tubing and are blotted onto a moving filter after a decant process. The unagglutinated cells in a negative test are hemolyzed and read spectrophotometrically. Although such an instrument, the Autogrouper 16C (Technicon), has been adapted to perform ABO grouping and Rh typing, this type of equipment is not suitable for antibody detection or crossmatching.

Robotization of the manual hemagglutination testing steps, including a centrifugation step, is the technologic concept used in the Groupamatic Models 360 and G2000 Mark II (Kontron Instruments, Everett, Ma). Agglutination and interpretation of the blood type is determined electronically by comparative optical density readings.

The use of a terraced microplate is the principal feature of the Olympus PK7100 (Olympus Lake Success, NY). When agglutination occurs due to an antigen-antibody reaction, RBC lattice formation causes a settling pattern, producing an even coating of the terraced wall in the wells of the microplate. When agglutination lacks antigen-antibody reaction, the individual RBC's settle into a button on the bottom of the well.

Some manufacturers, aware of the need for cost-effective, non-batch testing for smaller blood banks, are now marketing smaller versions of automated instruments. Instruments such as the Micro Groupamatic (Kontron), Micro Bank (Dynatech), and Pro-Group (Olympus/Cetus), are intended for small donor centers and busy hospital transfusion services. Still, the cost of this equipment and the inability of many hospitals to accept the concept of batch testing in a non-scheduled transfusion setting has limited their use to blood collection facilities performing high volume ABO and Rh typings.

Two instruments developed by Gamma Biologicals (Houston, Tx.), the STS-M for ABO/Rh typing and the STS-A for antibody screening, crossmatching, DAT, antigen typing, and antibody identification are semiautomated systems. Although they utilize costly disposables and equipment, they offer the benefits of decreased technologist time, and smaller reagent and sample volumes. Results are read by an optical system that scans the distribution of cells in the dome of a Microtear™ well. Nonagglutinated cells stream down the front of the well, whereas agglutinated cells remain as tight buttons in the dome of the well.

Other methods of streamlining antibody screening are employing the concepts of solid-phase antiglobulin testing. Based on the principles of a solid-phase RBC adherence test, a commercially prepared system Capture R™ (Immucor Inc, Norcross, Ga.) was developed to immobilize either the RBC or antibody to the surface of a microtiter well. The presence of bound antibody to antigen is detected by centrifugation of the plates after addition of anti-IgG sensitized indicator RBC's. If positive, the bound antibody will cause layering of the indicator cells in the well; if negative, the indicator cells will form a central pellet after centifugation. The major advantage of a solid-phase system for type and antibody screening is the clear stable endpoints of the reaction, which can be observed manually or electronically. This system can be adaptable to the average transfusion service or hospital-based blood bank.

COMPLEX ANTIBODY PROBLEMS
The panagglutinin with a negative autocontrol

One may encounter a situation in which most or all of the panel cells react with the patient's serum in the antiglobulin phase. This serological presentation restricts the routine process of exclusion for antibody problem solving, and is attributed to the presence of multiple antibodies or an antibody

Table 69-15 Apparent panagglutinin demonstrated by testing the patient's RBC's against a panel of untreated reagent cells. Enzyme treatment abolishes reactivity of anti-Fy$_b$ with Fy$_b$ positive cells. Anti-c is thus evident at 37°C. Anti-K may also be present, since the serum reacts with cell #3 possessing the Kell antigen. Anti-E cannot be excluded since the serum is reactive with R$_2$R$_2$ RBC's bearing both the E and c antigens

Sample #	Rh geno-type	C	C^w	c	D	E	e	K	Fy^a	Fy^b	Jk^a	Jk^b	P$_1$	Le^a	Le^b	M	N	S	s	IS	37°	AHG	IS	37°	AHG
		Rhesus						**Kell**	**Duffy**		**Kidd**		**P**	**Lewis**		**MN**				**Untreated RBCs** Serum			**Enzyme treated RBCs** Serum		
1	r'r	+	0	+	0	0	+	0	+	0	+	+	+	0	+	+	+	0	+	0	0	+	0	+	++
2	R$_1^w$R$_1$	+	+	0	+	0	+	+	+	+	0	+	+	+	0	+	+	+	+	0	0	+	0	0	+
3	R$_1$R$_1$	+	0	0	+	0	+	0	+	+	+	+	0	0	+	+	0	+	0	0	0	+	0	0	0
4	R$_2$R$_2$	0	0	+	+	+	0	0	0	+	0	+	+	+	0	0	+	0	+	0	0	+	0	+	++
5	r''r	0	0	+	0	+	+	0	+	+	0	+	0	0	+	+	+	+	0	0	0	+	0	+	++
6	rr	0	0	+	0	0	+	0	0	+	+	0	+	0	+	+	0	+	0	0	0	+	0	+	++
7	rr	0	0	+	0	0	+	+	0	+	+	0	+	0	+	+	0	0	+	0	0	+	0	+	++
8	rr	0	0	+	0	0	+	0	+	0	0	+	+	+	0	0	+	0	+	0	0	+	0	+	++
9	rr	0	0	+	0	0	+	0	0	+	+	0	0	0	+	0	+	0	+	0	0	+	0	+	++
10	R$_0$r	0	0	+	+	0	+	0	0	0	+	+	+	0	+	+	+	+	+	0	0	+	0	+	++
Patient RBC's		+	0	0	+	0	+	0	0	+	+	+	+	+	0	+	+	+	+	0	0	0	0	0	0

to a high frequency antigen. The technologist must carefully document the presence of different reaction strengths and be alerted to patterns demonstrated at the various phases of testing.

Multiple antibodies

In order to differentiate the presence of multiple antibodies from a single antibody to a high frequency antigen, one or more of the following techniques may be of assistance.

Enzymese. It is recommended that an enzyme-treated RBC panel be part of the protocol for resolving complex antibody problems. Information gained from this testing may be very beneficial if the mixture contains an antibody or antibodies affected by enzymes. If all panel cells react similarly, there may be either multiple antibodies which are not altered by enzymes (i.e., anti-K, -s), or are depressed by enzymes (i.e., anti-Fy^a, -Fy^b, -M, -S), or there is only one alloantibody in the serum directed against a high frequency antigen (i.e., anti-k, not altered by enzymes, or anti-Vel, depressed by enzymes). If some of the panel cells show enhanced and others depressed reactions, the technologist should be aware of the possible existence of more than one antibody. For example, an anti-c masked by anti-Fy^b could be unveiled and even enhanced by use of an enzyme-treated RBC panel. (Table 69-16).

Phenotyping donor/patient. If the patient blood sample does not contain circulating donor RBC's from a recent transfusion, phenotyping the autologous RBC's for blood group antigens can be successfully accomplished with a minimum of difficulty. Most technologists begin their typing with the Rh system, since antibodies to members of this blood group system are often encountered in a mixture.

Further investigation may include extensive antigen typings of the Kell, MNS, Duffy, and Kidd systems. If the patient tests positive for the antigen, corresponding antibodies can then be eliminated, thus limiting the possible choices in the antibody identification process. Note that the patient is negative for the E antigen in Table 69-15. Therefore anti-E cannot be eliminated. Antibodies to the Kidd system can be excluded since the patient types Jk(a+b+).

Mixed field agglutination can be encountered when phenotyping the recently transfused or newly-engrafted allogeneic bone marrow transplant patient as previously described. Methods employing cell separation techniques in order to isolate the patient's cells are based on the principle that transfused older cells are denser than autologous cells newly released from the bone marrow. Recipient RBC's can be separated from circulating donor RBC's by centrifugation through solutions of phthalate esters with varying specific gravities in microhematocrit tubes. The lighter autologous RBC's are then harvested from the area above the ester layers. Some serologists have demonstrated acceptable results without the use of phthalate esters by centrifuging microhematocrit tubes filled with packed RBC's and gathering the top 5 mm layer. Another method that can separate the patient's own cells from transfused cells in cases of Hgb SS or SC disease is based on the premise that RBC's containing Hgb S resist hemolysis in a hypotonic saline solution (0.45% NaCl); transfused RBC's with hemoglobin A can then be hemolyzed in this solution permitting autologous cells to remain intact for further phenotyping.

Selected cell panel. One can choose selected donor cells from additional panel sets to construct a "selected cell panel." For example, if one desires to disclose the existence of possible antibodies in addition to the anti-c and anti-Fy^b (Table 69-15), one could formulate a panel with cells negative for the c and Fy^b antigens, but one positive for K, another for E, etc. Considerations to zygosity when selecting reagent donor cells must be taken into account in preparing a suitable panel. It may be difficult to find reagent RBC's representative of the antigen combination needed to meet the above criteria. Therefore, adsorption of a known antibody to a high percentage of antigens on reagent cells, and then testing that adsorbed serum on a variety of selected cells, may be of some benefit in solving complex combinations of antibodies. A more detailed instruction on adsorption techniques will be presented on managing autoantibodies in the serum.

Altering test conditions. IgM antibodies such as anti-Le^a and Le^b, although occasionally detected at the 37°C and AHG phases, are optimally demonstrated at room temperature. Instead of utilizing anti-IgG in the Coombs phase, the incorporation of polyspecific antisera may enhance the expression of complement-binding antibodies such as anti-Lewis and anti-Kidd. By lowering the pH of the test media to 6.0 with a weak solution of HCl, weakly-reactive examples of anti-M can be enhanced in vitro. Some examples of anti-K react weakly with cells suspended in LISS, while albumin additives may augment reactivity.

Inhibition studies. Neutralization techniques are based on the premise that some natural substances demonstrate specificity to RBC antigens (Box 69-1). The activity of one of the antibodies in the mixture may be suppressed with

---

Box 69-1 Neutralizing substances

1. Lewis substances. Le^a and Le^b substances are present in the saliva of persons of the appropriate Lewis phenotype. Le^a substance is present in the saliva of Le(a+b−) individuals, and both Le^a and Le^b substances are present in the saliva of Le(a−b+) individuals. Commercially prepared Lewis substance is available.

2. P_1 substance. Soluble P_1 substance is present in hydatid cyst fluid. A reagent preparation derived from pigeons is commercially available.

3. Sd^a (Sid) substance. Sd^a blood group substance is present in soluble form in various body fluids. The most abundant source is urine. If anti-Sd^a is suspected, urine from a known Sd(a+) individual can be used to inhibit the antibody. A pool of 8 to 10 random urines is also suitable since 91% will contain Sd^a substance.

4. Chido and Rodgers substances. Characteristically, these antibodies produce fragile agglutinates, and the reaction scores are low. Anti-Ch^a and anti-Rg^a, unlike other HTLA antibodies can be inhibited by plasma from Ch(a+), Rg(a+) individuals. A pool of 8 to 10 AB plasmas is suitable for inhibition procedures since 95% will be Ch(a+) Rg(a+).

From Walker RH, ed: American Association of Blood Banks Technical Manual, ed 10, Arlington, Va, 1990, AABB.

such a substance and thereby indirectly prove its presence. After neutralization, additional underlying antibodies may be unmasked. As with any modification in serum concentration, there is a risk that a lower titer antibody may become undetectable due to the dilutional effect of the reagent. A control system, run in parallel with the serum diluted by the neutralizing substance, must show reactivity with similar dilutions in saline in order to validate the test results. Suppressed reactivity with the neutralized serum on donor cells positive for the corresponding antigen is a positive result. The absence of agglutination indirectly proves the existence of the suspected antibody. An unchanged reactivity with the substance and serum constitutes a negative test result, thereby disproving the presence of the alleged antibody.

Antibodies to a high frequency antigen

The search for antibody identity may lead to the conclusion that an antibody in the serum is directed against a high-incidence RBC antigen in the population. This deduction is proven when further testing leads to nonreaction with a reagent cell negative for a high incidence antigen [e.g., anti-K, -U, -I, -Vel, -Tjª].

The apparent finding of an antibody against a high-frequency antigen may be confused with rare antibodies directed against preservatives in the suspension of reagent red cells. One can eliminate interference from or demonstrate the formation of antibodies to non-RBC antigens or proteins by washing the panel cells free of the preservative and resuspending the reagent cells in saline. Such an antibody is suggested when crossmatching donor units is nonreactive, but screening against all panel cells is reactive.

Although the definitive determination of whether a high-frequency antibody is capable of causing shortened survival of transfused RBC's depends on the results of red cell survival studies determined by Cr⁵¹ tagged RBC's, some indication as to an antibody's clinical significance may be suggested by its serologic properties at 37°C. Unfortunately, some clinically insignificant antibodies (e.g., most high-titer, low-avidity antibodies (HTLA) and Sdª antibodies) may also react at 37°C. The HTLA group antibodies (Ch, Rg, Yk, Cs, Mc, Kn, JMH, Gy, Hy and Ytª) and anti-Sdª are generally reactive in the antiglobulin phase with most RBC's. HTLA antibodies typically give weak reactions that persist with sequential serum titration. If testing with enzyme-treated cells reveals markedly reduced reactivity, the antibody may be directed against Ch, Rg, JMH or Ytª. Some blood bankers also include a neutralization step, using pooled AB plasma, to investigate the possible presence of anti-Ch or Rg, or pooled dialyzed urine for anti-Sdª. The use of ZZAP, a reagent that contains 0.2M DDT and cysteine-activated papain in a PBS at pH 7.3, is capable of creating an HTLA "null" cell. If the serum is nonreactive with the treated cells, the antibody could belong to the HTLA group. Caution must be taken in arriving at this conclusion, since LW, and Kell antigens are also destroyed with this reagent.

Although they are not antibodies to high frequency antigens, Bg antibodies behave serologically similar. Due to cross-reactivity and inconsistencies with manufacturers' typing of cells for the Bg antigens, many blood bankers needlessly spend a great deal of time trying to solve unexplained reactions due to Bg antibodies. Two procedures use commercially prepared reagents that aid in avoiding their detection. One procedure involves adsorption with pooled platelet concentrates possessing a wide variety of HLA types. A negative antibody screen with the adsorbed serum suggests the presence of Bg antibodies. Another procedure uses chloroquine diphosphate-treated RBC's to create a Bg "null" cell. Nonreactivity of the serum tested with the chemically treated cells indirectly proves the presence of Bg antibodies.

The panagglutinin with a positive autocontrol

When an individual's serum reacts with all or most donor cells and with autologous cells, autoantibody is usually present. However, in the recently transfused patient this picture could represent the recent production of alloantibody directed against an antigen or antigens on circulating donor RBC's. These auto- or alloantibodies can be identified by determining whether the eluate of the DAT or autocontrol is positive, or by analyzing the serum testing results, as previously described. When allo- and auto-antibodies occur simultaneously in the serum, there is a risk that the clinically significant alloantibodies will be masked by the autoantibody reacting with all reagent panel and donor RBC's. It is therefore important to characterize and identify warm and cold-type autoantibodies (Box 69-2) and to have a clear understanding of how to handle the serologic problems resulting from such situations.

Cold autoantibodies. In order to identify and accurately titer cold-reacting autoantibodies for diagnostic and clinical purposes, serum should be separated from a blood sample, transported, and maintained at 37°C. This will reduce the degree of absorption of cold-reacting antibody onto the autologous cells, thereby maintaining an antibody concentration truly representative of its in vivo level. A titer of serially-diluted serum in saline incubated with "1" RBC's is usually determined by its reactivity at 4°C. Testing can also be accomplished at RT, 30°C and 37°C, if thermal amplitude is considered an indicator for assessing the clinical significance of the autoantibody.

The use of a prewarmed technique minimizes interference from cold antibodies in detecting clinically significant alloantibodies. The reactivity of some high-titer cold autoantibodies is not always eradicated, even in the antiglobulin phase under the strictest prewarming conditions. Treating serum with thiol agents, dithiothreitol (DTT) or 2-mercaptoethanol (2-ME), can eliminate the reactivity of IgM au-

---

Box 69-2   Serologic characteristics of cold & warm autoantibodies

COLD TYPE	WARM TYPE
IgM	IgG
Reacts optimally at <37°C	Reacts optimally at 37°C, AHG
Destroyed by DTT, 2ME	Not destroyed by DTT, 2ME
Absorbed at 4°C	Absorbed at 37°C

toantibodies. These reagents have two major drawbacks: both clinically significant and nonsignificant cold-reacting IgM antibodies are destroyed, and a weak antibody may be overlooked due to the dilution of serum with reagent. Some blood bankers prefer to adsorb strong cold-reacting antibodies onto rabbit erythrocyte stroma, which contains a large amount of I antigen; others employ a cold 4°C autologous adsorption technique in which autologous cells have been treated with enzymes to facilitate the uptake of anti-I. As with any adsorption process, the possibility of adsorbing significant antibodies on other antigens of the adsorbing medium always exists. When using commercially-prepared adsorbent surfaces, strict adherence to the manufacturer's directions must be followed and the limitations of interpretation must be clearly understood. In addition, most technologists avoid performing autoadsorptions for removing cold or warm autoantibodies if the individual has been transfused or pregnant in the last few months, because developing alloantibodies can be inadvertently adsorbed onto the corresponding antigen contained on transfused donor RBC's.

Warm autoantibodies. Methods that determine specificity of warm autoantibodies by eluate testing have been previously discussed. In addition to identifying the autoantibody, the technologist must accurately phenotype the patient and diminish autoantibody activity in the serum in order to reveal possible underlying alloantibodies.

Phenotyping the patient with IgG autoantibodies is complex because IgG antisera suspended in a high-protein diluent may result in false positive typings, as the RBC's are coated with IgG in vivo. For Rh phenotyping, methods that use saline antisera can be employed. When using other antiglobulin reactive reagents, the results of the antigen typing can be compared to the reactivity of the direct anti-human globulin test. Accuracy of such test results are questionable. Most serologists attempt to remove immunoglobulin from the cells prior to antigen typing. One simple method uses a mild 45°C heat elution. Drawbacks to this technique include some hemolysis of the RBC's and incomplete removal of the bound antibody. Another method uses a 20% chloroquine diphosphate solution to dissociate IgG from the RBC's. It is necessary to use an anti-IgG reagent rather than chemically modified antisera when typing with reagents by the indirect anti-globulin test. Since this treatment does not dissociate C3 components from RBC's, monospecific IgG sera is used.

Adsorption techniques are the most widely used methods for removing autoantibody from the serum prior to compatibility testing. If the patient has not been transfused for three months, autologous RBC's can be treated with enzymes or ZZAP reagent (dithiothreitol and cysteine-activated papain) for enhancement of autoantibody uptake. The treated cells are then washed and incubated with the serum at 37°C. The adsorbed serum is then examined for alloantibody activity after one to four adsorption processes, depending on autoantibody titer and binding affinity.

If the patient has been transfused or pregnant in the previous three months, autoadsorption techniques should proceed with utmost caution. In this situation, many blood bankers employ homologous adsorbing cells of various phenotypes, such as R_1R_1, R_2R_2, and rr with different Kell, Duffy, Kidd, and MNS antigen profiles.

The following points should be considered when performing homologous adsorptions:

1. If the Rh phenotype of the pre-transfusion candidate can be accurately determined, then use two or more homologous donor cells of the same Rh phenotype as the adsorbing cells. This is usually not an option and most blood bankers find it easier to use separate suspensions of R_1R_1, R_2R_2, and rr cells.

2. If the adsorbing cells are treated with enzymes, then RBC's with antigens known to be destroyed by that reagent [i.e., Fy(a) and Fy(b)] will not be capable of adsorbing the corresponding antibody. Consequently, that particular antibody, if present in the serum, will remain in the adsorbed serum and can be identified by further testing with a cell panel. The same holds true for treatment with ZZAP reagent, which alters not only the Duffy antigens, but all antigens of the Kell system.

3. If the autoantibody in the serum has no relative Rh specificity, then the autoantibody will be adsorbed equally well with any Rh phenotype.

4. If the autoantibody does exhibit relative Rh specificity, then the absorbing cells positive for that particular antigen, such as "e" (e.g., rr and R_1R_1), will be more effective in adsorbing the corresponding antibody than R_2R_2 cells.

THE MAJOR CROSSMATCH

Testing the patient's serum or plasma with a 2% to 5% suspension of donor RBC's constitutes the essential elements of the major crossmatch. The immediate spin phase of the crossmatch confirms ABO compatibility between donor and recipient. This one simple step constitutes the minimum standard requirement of most licensing and accrediting agencies for compatibility testing, as long as the patient has no detectable atypical antibodies active at 37°C. Some authorities dispute the degree of reliability of the immediate spin (IS) crossmatch for judging ABO compatibility, particularly when titers of the isoagglutinins are below detectable levels in the patient's serum. Therefore, accurate ABO typing of the patient and donor remains critically important.

Antigen typing of the donor units

Before crossmatching is performed for patients with clinically significant alloantibodies, antigen negative units should be selected, since units heterozygous for the antigen in question might give a negative crossmatch test result if the antibody exhibits weak reactions. The technologist determines the number of units to screen according to the probability of finding antigen negative units in the general population. For example, if the Kell antigen is known to be lacking on 91% of random donor RBC's, then approximately nine out of 10 units should be negative. When more than one antibody is detected, the percentage of donor cells negative for the antigens among random units is calculated by multiplying the frequency of antigens negative in the donor pool by each other.

If the probability of discovering antigen negative units is so low that more than the number of available units in the facility's blood bank are required to find sufficient units, or if there is less than a 10% chance of finding antigen negative units in the random donor population, it is appropriate to request the assistance of a blood center reference laboratory. Such a facility is equipped to handle rare blood requests because it possesses adequate blood resources and can perform automated antigen typings. An alternate source of RBC units for patients with clinically significant antibodies against high frequency antigens is the family of the propositus. Such individuals may be typed while the regional blood center attempts to locate compatible units in their rare donor files.

The Coombs' crossmatch

Limited blood resources and cost-containment issues have prompted serologists to evaluate the usefulness of the antiglobulin phase of the crossmatch. The classical Coombs' crossmatch requires extended incubation at 37°C, a washing step, and the addition of antiglobulin serum. Occasionally, the Coombs' crossmatch is found to be incompatible with a negative antibody screening. Such a serologic situation can be attributed to one of the following factors:

1. Basic clerical or technical routine tasks are performed erroneously: The ABO type of the patient has been incorrectly determined, the wrong type unit has been chosen from stock inventory, or the serum tube has been misidentified.
2. The DAT on the donor RBCs is positive: the antiglobulin phase of the crossmatch appears to be incompatible, since the cells of the donor are already coated with immunoglobulin.
3. Some antibodies may be missed because of antibody screen test limitations: There is an antibody in the serum of the patient to a private or low frequency antigen found on the donor cells and not on the reagent cells. A negative antibody screen missed a weak reaction now being discerned with stronger antigen expression of the donor cells (i.e., dosage effect).

For the above reasons, some transfusion services have decided to retain the antiglobulin phase of the crossmatch. Each facility must weigh the cost/benefit ratio of the Coombs' crossmatch as it applies to their own establishment by analyzing the incidence of delayed transfusion reactions, the technical ability of their staff, performance on proficiency testing, and the frequency with which incompatible units on apparent negative antibody screenings have occured.

Type & screen

Most blood bankers have observed that unnecessary crossmatching and reserving of units results in excessive inventories and increased outdating. This observation led to the promotion of the Type and Screen (T&S) policy, whereby only a complete ABO grouping and antibody screening is performed for patients undergoing particular surgical procedures less likely to require transfusion; they do not have units crossmatched and reserved in advance, unless they have atypical antibodies. In the event transfusion is warranted in the individual with a negative antibody screen, units of blood can be released upon the IS of the crossmatch with a great assurance of survival following transfusion.

The fate of the traditional Coombs' crossmatch is soon to be decided, for the T&S policy is already being adapted to the nonsurgical setting. Some facilities have opted to complete the antiglobulin phase of the crossmatch after release of the unit, while others have chosen to eliminate that portion of the crossmatch based on expected low risk to the patient without atypical antibodies and the benefits of reduced workload and expenses.

Whichever immunohematologic methods are employed, an efficient transfusion service is defined by its ability to provide compatible and safe blood components to the patient with minimum delay. Likewise, blood collection facilities, in their quest to streamline testing of donors for ABO type and atypical RBC antibodies, need to assure transfusion services that they have followed appropriate practices in order to provide quality components for transfusion.

SUGGESTED READING

Dixon MR and Ellison SS: Selection of methods and instruments for blood banks, Arlington, Va, 1984, American Association of Blood Banks.

Lauenstein KJ, Martin BG, and Winkelman JW: Modifications for expense reduction, part 1: blood bank, Laboratory Medicine, Vol 15, No 9: 609-613, 1984.

Oberman HA, Barnes BA, and Steiner EA: Role of the crossmatch in testing for serologic compatibility, Transfusion 22:12-16, 1982.

Plapp FV: New techniques for compatibility testing, Arch Pathol Lab Med. 113:262-269, 1989.

Polan CS: Automation in blood banking and hemotherapy. In Clinics in Laboratory Medicine, Vol 8, No 4: 675-687, 1988.

Rolih SD, ed: High-titer low-avidity antibodies and antigens: a review, Transf Med Rev 3:128-139, 1989.

Shulman IA and Nelson JM: When should antibody screening tests be done for recently transfused patients? Transfusion 30:39-41, 1990.

Smith DM and Judd JW: Blood banking in a changing environment, Arlington, Va, 1984, American Association of Blood Banks.

Treacy M and Bertsch JA, eds: Selecting policies and procedures for the transfusion service, Arlington, Va, 1982, American Association of Blood Banks.

Wallace ME and Green TS, eds: Selection of procedures for problem solving, Arlington, Va, 1983, American Association of Blood Banks.

70 Immune hemolysis

Robert F. Reiss

As previously discussed (Chapter 68), the in vivo effects of antigen-antibody interaction depend in part on: the number and distribution of antigen sites; the class and subclass of antibody; the availability of complement; the environmental conditions at the time of interaction; and the functional capacity of the reticulo-endothelial system.

INTRAVASCULAR AND EXTRAVASCULAR IMMUNE HEMOLYSIS

Although the reversible vasoocclusion of small blood vessels by red cell agglutinates may occur with IgM cold-reacting antibodies, the principle effects of in vivo antigen-antibody reactions are related to the intravascular or extravascular hemolysis of sensitized red cells. The diagnosis of immune hemolysis rests with the elucidation of laboratory findings characteristic of hemolysis, and with demonstration of antibody or complement on the cell surface (direct Coombs' test). The demonstration of the responsible antibody in the serum is also helpful in evaluating the mechanism of the anemia. The responsible antibody may be 1) an alloantibody as in the cases of hemolytic transfusion reaction and hemolytic disease of the newborn, 2) an autoantibody in the case of the various autoimmune hemolytic anemias, or 3) a drug related antibody.

Extravascular hemolysis

Most antibodies, especially those of the IgG type, are not hemolysins, but simply coat the red cells. These sensitized red cells then pass through the spleen, where the macrophages recognize the fc fragment of the attached antibody. This interaction is largely specific for subclasses IgG_1 and IgG_3. The action of the phagocyte with the red cell results in the formation of spherocytes, which subsequently undergo accelerated extravascular hemolysis.

Agglutinates of red cells coated with IgM tend to disperse as IgM elutes from the cell during circulation. If any agglutinates persist, they are rapidly cleared by the reticulo-endothelial system. Complement-fixing IgM antibodies do not usually fix all the components of the complement system, and activation ceases at the C3 stage. Cells coated with C3b are sequestered by the reticulo-endothelial cells in the liver, which possess receptor sites for C3c. These cells may

undergo erythrophagocytosis in the liver sinusoids, or, if such a process is delayed, the C3b coating the cells may be lysed into C3c and $C3d_g$ by C3b inactivator. If such an event occurs, C3c remains attached to the macrophage while $C3d_g$-coated cells are freed to circulate normally.

Intravascular hemolysis

The in vivo action of some antibodies on red cells bearing the appropriate antigen may be rapid complement fixation through formation of a lytic complex, and subsequent intravascular hemolysis. Free hemoglobin is liberated with consequent hemoglobinemia and hemoglobinuria. In some cases, shock, acute renal shutdown, and a severe bleeding diathesis ensue. The mechanism of some of these manifestations is poorly understood but may be related to the thromboplastinic properties of the red cell stroma released in the free circulation, which provokes disseminated intravascular coagulation and/or to the activation of complement with a subsequent liberation of vasoactive amines.

ALLOIMMUNE HEMOLYSIS
Hemolytic transfusion reactions

Infusing red cells into an individual possessing a preformed antibody may result in intravascular or extravascular hemolysis as will be discussed in Chapter 73.

Hemolytic disease of the newborn

Hemolytic anemia occurring in utero and continuing into the perinatal period due to passively acquired IgG antibodies from the mother defines hemolytic disease of the newborn. IgM antibodies do not cross the placenta and therefore do not cause this disease. It may be caused by acquired alloantibodies stimulated in the mother or by the transfer of IgG anti- A or anti- B from a group O mother. The more severe but less common form of hemolytic disease of the newborn is seen in cases caused by non-ABO antibodies. Over 97% of these cases were caused by anti-D prior to advent of Rh prophylaxis.

Rh hemolytic disease

This condition is caused by the passive transfer of IgG anti-D antibodies from the maternal circulation across the

Table 70-1 Classification of severity of Rh erythroblastosis

Mild	Only moderate jaundice, no anemia. No treatment required.	50%
Moderate	Jaundice severe (icterus gravis), anemia mild to moderate. Will develop kernicterus if not treated.	25%-30%
Severe	Hydrops fetalis will develop before 40 wk gestation if not treated.	20%-25%
	1. Hydropic after 32-33 wk 10%-15%	
	2. Hydropic before 32-33 wk 8%-10%	

From Bowman JM: Rh erythroblastosis fetalis, Semin Hematol 12:190, 1975.

placenta to a D positive fetus. Sensitization occurs either through transfusion of D positive blood to a D negative female or by sensitization through a D positive pregnancy. Such sensitization occurs because small amounts of fetal red cells leak into the maternal circulation. Such leakage may occur throughout pregnancy but is most severe at delivery. While most cases of sensitization occur following delivery, approximately 10% occur during pregnancy. Sensitization is much less than expected since most fetal-maternal hemorrhages are less than 1 ml, ABO incompatibility destroys the cells immediately so that sensitization to D does not occur, and approximately 20% to 30% of women appear to be non-responders to immunization with the D antigen. In women not previously sensitized by transfusion, the first D positive pregnancy is usually unaffected. Subsequent pregnancies may be involved.

Coating of the fetal cells with anti D results in extravascular hemolysis, and the resultant bilirubin is cleared through the mother. If intrauterine red cell production is insufficient to match cell destruction closely enough to prevent severe anemia, the fetus will develop heart failure and die. When death occurs near term, the stillborn will have massive edema *(hydrops fetalis)*. If the production can match the hemolysis, the anemia will be compatible with life and characterized by large numbers of circulating young red cells *(erythroblastosis fetalis)*. Hepatosplenomegaly is due to abundant extra-medullary hematopoiesis. Peripheral edema may develop if post-natal heart failure supervenes. After birth, the infant will develop jaundice within a few hours due to increasing levels of indirect bilirubin in the plasma *(icterus gravis)*. Continued accumulation of indirect bilirubin to high levels is associated with the development of basal ganglia degeneration *(kernicterus)*. The risk of this complication increases dramatically in term infants when the level of bilirubin exceeds 20 mg/dl. Premature infants and newborns suffering from acidosis, hypoxia, and hypoalbuminemia may experience kernicterus at significantly lower levels of bilirubin. Cases of Rh hemolytic disease can be classified according to severity (Table 70-1).

Laboratory tests indicate a severe hemolytic anemia with large numbers of circulating nucleated red cells and reticulocytes, decreased platelet count, and a strongly positive direct Coombs' test of the D positive cord red cells from

which anti-D can be eluted. A cord hemoglobin under 13 mg/dl is associated with severe disease. The bilirubin level may be only slightly elevated at birth, but in severe cases the level increases rapidly, since bilirubin cannot be conjugated by the immature liver. A cord bilirubin of greater than 5 mg/dl in a term infant or rapidly rising bilirubin indicates that without treatment by exchange transfusion, the critical level of 20 mg/dl may be reached. The risk that the bilirubin level will reach this critical level in the immediate postnatal period is also indicated by a serum bilirubin level (gm/dl) that exceeds the age of a term neonate in hours. Premature infants will experience a corresponding risk with levels 2 to 3 mg/dl less at any given age.

Since hemolysis continues throughout gestation and becomes more severe as term is approached, it is prognostically important to detect the sensitized mother and the involved fetus during pregnancy so that an optimal therapeutic approach is planned. Each pregnant woman should be screened early in gestation (i.e., 12th week of gestation) for irregular antibodies in the serum and in the case of Rh negative women, the Rh genotype of the husband determined.

If no antibody is found at 12 weeks, the antibody screen is repeated at 24 to 28 weeks. If an IgG antibody (e.g., anti D) is identified, it should be titered and the serum frozen for future comparative titration with samples obtained later in pregnancy. Repeat testing is carried out every month in cases where an antibody had been identified at 12 weeks. A significant rise in concentration of antibody is signaled by a twofold increase in titer when a current sample is run in parallel with the previously frozen serum. Alternatively, laboratories utilizing a scoring system judge the concentration to have increased significantly if the score increases by more than 10. Although there is only a modest correlation between the concentration of antibody and the severity of disease, a high concentration or rapidly increasing concentration of antibody indicates the presence of a fetus positive for the D or other responsible antigen.

In general if the maximum titer observed in the case of Rh sensitization is less than 1:16, the resultant disease is not severe. If there is a strong history of previously affected infants, the anti D titer is greater than 1:16-1:32, the titer is rapidly rising, or the fetus shows decreased activity, the bilirubin concentration of fetal blood from the umbilical vein may be determined, or amniocentesis may be performed to determine the content of bilirubin in the amniotic fluid, by spectrophotometry. This concentration as determined by a $\triangle$OD at 450 nm (Figure 70-1) is correlated to known normals for the age of gestation (Figure 70-2). Significant elevations (Zone III) indicate dangerous rates of hemolysis in the fetus. Prior to 32 weeks, this may require intrauterine transfusions into the fetal peritoneal cavity to partially correct anemia and the resultant high output failure. After 32 weeks, early delivery is planned before term depending on the severity of disease and estimation of lung maturity according to the level of glycerol phosphatidyl or the lecithin/sphingomyelin ratio in the amniotic fluid. Upon delivery, infants with evidence of severe disease should undergo exchange transfusion with 10 to 20 ml liquots of Rh negative red cells of the appropriate ABO group reconstituted with

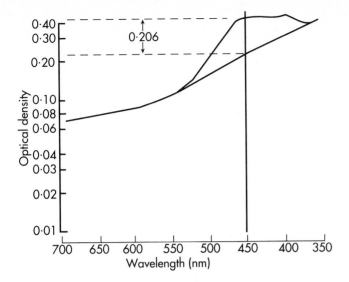

Fig. 70-1 The concentration of bilirubin in the amniotic fluid of a sensitized Rh positive pregnant woman. It is represented by the △ O.D. measured at 450 nm as the difference between the observed O.D. and the hypothetized base line O.D. In this case the △ O.D. is 0.206. *Redrawn from Mollison PL: Blood transfusion in clinical medicine, ed 8, Oxford, 1987, Blackwell Scientific Publications.*

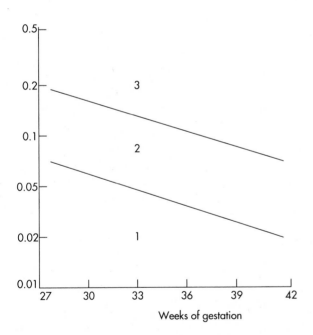

Fig. 70-2 Liley's chart plotting the measured △ O.D. against the age of pregnancy. The △ O.D. falls into one of three risk zones at any gestational age. Zone 1 (low risk of severely affected infant); Zone 3 (high risk of hydrops fetalis); and Zone 2 (intermediate). *Redrawn from Mollison PL: Blood transfusion in clinical medicine, ed 8, Oxford, 1987, Blackwell Scientific Publications.*

type specific plasma. The amount exchanged is usually twice the blood volume. The exchange transfusion is performed to: reduce the danger of kernicterus by removing bilirubin; correct anemia; remove coated red cells, the potential source of bilirubin; and remove unbound antibodies from the infant's plasma. Mild degrees of hyperbilirubinemia are treated with exposure to ultraviolet light, which photochemically converts bilirubin to excretable degradation products.

Sensitization of Rh negative mothers following pregnancy with an Rh positive fetus can be prevented by administering high titered Rh immune globulin to the mother within 72 hours of delivery or at the time of abortion. It is good practice to also administer Rh immune globulin at 28 weeks. This prevents the 10% of cases of sensitization that occur during pregnancy. This mode of prevention termed mediated immune suppression, has drastically reduced the incidence of Rh HDN. The mechanism of action is unclear but may be related to the partial coating of D antigen sites on the fetal red cells. The usual dose of 300 µgm will protect against all but unusually large fetal-maternal hemorrhages (i.e., >15 ml of red cells), which are seen in 1% to 2% of cases.

Several techniques can detect and quantitate large fetal-maternal hemorrhages, which require increased doses of Rh immune globulin. These techniques depend on the detection of D positive cells or cells containing large amounts of hemoglobin F in the maternal circulation. The simplest test is a D^u test on a post-delivery sample to demonstrate conversion of a previously negative D^u test to the finding of a positive mixed field reaction. Unfortunately the smallest hemorrhage detected with this technique is represented by greater than 2% to 3% of the total cell population (i.e., 30 to 45 ml red cell hemorrhage in a woman with a red cell mass of 1500 ml). The more sensitive Rosette screening test for circulating D positive fetal cells relies on formation of rosettes of fetal D positive cells about reagent R_2R_2 red cells after the addition of chemically modified anti D. The number of rosettes that indicate a hemorrhage of greater than 15 ml usually varies by test system. Positive results indicate a need to more precisely quantitate the fetal hemorrhage by examining a peripheral smear stained with the Acid Elution Stain (Kleinauer-Betke). The dose of Rh-immune globulin is determined by dividing the observed hemorrhage (ml of red cells) by 15 and multiplying the result by 300 µgm.

ABO hemolytic disease

In occasional pregnancies involving a group O mother with IgG anti A, anti B, or anti A,B and a group A or B fetus, sufficient antibody coats the fetal red cells to cause anemia. Upon birth, these babies will usually have mild hemolysis and hyperbilirubinemia, neither of which require therapy. Rarely, the hyperbilirubinemia is sufficient to necessitate exchange transfusion with group O red cells reconstituted with plasma compatible with the baby's own red cells. The cord red cells of infants with even relatively severe disease may demonstrate only a weak or negative Direct Coombs' Test, but anti A, anti B, or anti A,B antibody is able to be eluted from these cells (Table 70-2).

Table 70-2   Comparison of ABO and Rh hemolytic disease of the newborn

	Rh HDN	ABO HDN
Incidence	Uncommon since advent of RhIG	1-3%
Anemia	Moderate to severe	Absent to moderate
Hemoglobin concentration	Low	Normal to moderately low
Bilirubin	Increased at birth; may be severe	Increased after 24 hr; usually mild
Direct antiglobulin test	Strongly positive	Weakly positive or negative
Eluate of infant cells	Anti-Rh	Anti-A or anti-B
Nucleated red cells	Moderate to marked	Mild to moderate
Reticulocyte count	Moderate to marked increase	Mild to moderate increase
Spherocytes	Inconspicuous	Common
Pregnancy	After the first	First likely
Prenatal testing useful	Yes	No
Therapy required	Often	Rarely
Prevention by antibody	Yes	No

From Bauer JD: Clinical laboratory methods, ed 9, St. Louis, 1982, Mosby-Year Book, Inc.

AUTO-IMMUNE HEMOLYTIC ANEMIA

The development of autoantibodies directed against red cells may be idiopathic, secondary to disease, or associated with the administration of some medications. These autoantibodies may or may not be associated with hemolysis. The antibodies involved are usually IgG (warm) or IgM (cold). They cause hemolysis by different mechanisms and have different presentations, prognoses, and therapies.

Warm autoantibody hemolytic anemia

Eighty percent of autoimmune hemolytic anemias (AIHA) are caused by warm-acting IgG antibodies. Seventy percent of warm AIHA cases are secondary to other diseases (SLE, CLL, lymphoma, cirrhosis, ulcerative colitis and ovarian teratoma) or drugs (e.g., alpha-methyldopa). Occasionally the immunological reaction can also be directed against platelets, which leads to thrombocytopenia (Evans syndrome).

Pathologically, the important findings are limited to splenomegaly in 50% of cases due to reticuloendothelial proliferation and congestion, as well as hepatomegaly in about 25% to 30%. Peripheral smears show spherocytosis and polychromatophylic macrocytes (reticulocytes). The bone marrow shows erythroid normoblastic hyperplasia. If folate deficiency intervenes, the marrow maturation will become megaloblastic.

The direct Coombs' test in about 30% of cases reveal coating with only IgG, 55% with both IgG and C3, and 15% with only C3 (probably representing small amounts of IgG not detectable by routine methods that fixed complement). The serum usually shows lesser amounts of free unbound antibody. As a rule, 90% of patients with detectable amounts of IgG on their cells have shortened cell life spans, while 50% of those with only C3 have shortened life spans. In more than 90% of cases in which IgG is detected on the cell, no exact specificity can be determined for the coating antibody. However, it is usually directed against some determinant in the Rh complex, as shown by reactions against all cells except Rh null cells. Rare patients with warm AIHA have negative direct Coombs' tests. In some of these patients, the quantity of IgG antibody on the cell is below that detectable with usual techniques. In others, the antibody is IgA.

The serologic determination of the specificity of the antibody begins with the preparation of an eluate from the patient's sensitized red cells, as previously described. In these disorders, the preparation and evaluation of an eluate from cells bearing no detectable IgG, using a monospecific antiglobulin reagent is generally futile. The prepared eluate is then tested against a commercially available panel of phenotyped reagent red cells. Usually, no distinct specificity is observed and the eluted antibody reacts as a panagglutinin in the Coombs phase. When specificity is found, it is usually within the Rh system, generally anti-e. The determination that a panagglutinin has relative specificity for one or another Rh antigen or is directed against a high frequency antigen within the Rh system or in another system (e.g., Kell) follows testing of serial dilutions of the eluate against selected phenotypes (R_1R_1, R_2R_2, rr) (Table 70-3) and subsequently the neat eluate against partially Rh deleted (e.g., -D-) and Rh null red cells (Table 70-4). Determining specificity is of limited clinical utility, since patients are transfused with antigen negative units in only limited clinical circumstances, as will be discussed. In previously transfused patients, the finding of clear specificity in the eluate should alert the technologist of the possibility of a delayed hemolytic transfusion reaction, and lead to a reexamination of the direct Coombs' test to detect possible mixed field agglutination and to careful cell typing for the presence of a minor population of antigen positive red cells.

Of greater importance is carefully examining the serum to detect the presence of alloantibodies, which may be present along with any autoantibody. In the presence of a very weak reacting autoantibody, a striking variation in the strength of reaction between the patient's serum and various panel cells will often permit ready identification of the alloantibody. In cases where the autoantibody reacts strongly, the reaction may mask the presence of an alloantibody. Two methods are used to uncover its presence. First, some workers have proposed that the serum be diluted and then retested against the red cell panel, in the hope that the autoantibody would become relatively more diluted than the alloantibody, and that this latter antibody would then be readily detected. Generally, this technique is fraught with the obvious concern

Table 70-3 Serial titrations of eluate in WAIHA detecting anti-e relative specificity

	1	2	4	8	16	32	64	128
R_1R_1	+4	+4	+3	+3	+2	+1	+1	±
R_2R_2	+4	+3	+2	+1	±			
r r	+4	+4	+3	+3	+2	+1	+1	±

that the undetected alloantibody is weaker reacting than the autoantibody and would therefore be lost during dilution. In the preferred method, the serum undergoes autoabsorption and the absorbed serum is then reexamined for the presence of residual alloantibodies. In order to effectively absorb out the serum autoantibody, the patient's cells must be stripped of bound autoantibody with one of the elution techniques previously discussed. When employing this technique, it is important to remember that an absence of alloantibodies following autoabsorption of a serum from a recently transfused patient must be accepted with caution, since the transfused cells may have absorbed any alloantibodies present.

Although the mainstay of initial therapy is treatment with corticosteroids, some patients may require transfusion if the anemia is associated with manifestations of tissue hypoxia. Since most randomly selected red cell units will not undergo post-transfusion hemolysis at a rate exceeding the destruction of the patient's own cells by the antibody, the principle risk lies in the transfusion of red cells possessing an antigen against which the patient has formed an alloantibody. The transfusion of red cells to patients in whom the presence of an alloantibody cannot be eliminated should be carried out with caution. Some advocate the slow transfusion of 50 ml of red cells and then examining the patient's plasma for free hemoglobin prior to further infusion. Patients who experience accelerated hemolysis following transfusion or suffer frank hemolysis transfusion reactions should be examined for relative specificity of their autoantibody, and if feasible, antigen negative units should be selected. With continued transfusion, relative red cell specificity is often lost and the antibody reacts equally with all donor units.

Cold autoantibody hemolytic anemias
Cold agglutinin syndromes

As stated previously, most cold AIHA are caused by IgM antibodies, and these cases account for approximately 20% of AIHA cases.

Although almost everyone has cold autoantibodies in low titer and active only *in vitro* at 4°C, rare individuals possess these complement fixing antibodies potent enough to cause AIHA. These potent antibodies have a higher titer and a thermal amplitude that reaches higher temperatures (up to and above 30°C). The specificity of the responsible antibody is generally found within the Ii system, although rare antibodies are found to belong to the Pr (Sp) system. In these patients, they tend to bind to red cells in cold extremities and then fix complement. Usually this C3 coating causes extravascular hemolysis but occasionally the entire complement cascade may be activated, leading to intravascular

Table 70-4 Reaction patterns of anti-nl, anti-pdl and anti-dl and some alloantibodies that are similar

Phenotype of test red cells	Reactions of autoantibodies		
	Anti-nl	Anti-pdl	Anti-dl
Normal Rh phenotype (i.e. R_1R_1, R_1R_2, r'r", rr, etc.)	+	+	+
D-deletion (i.e. D——, Dc—, DC^w—)	0	+	+
Rh_{null}	0	0	+

Alloantibodies with similar reaction patterns		
Anti-Hr	Anti-Rh29	Anti-En^a
Anti-Hr_o	Anti-LW^a	Anti-Wr^b
Anti-Rh34	Anti-LW^{ab}	Anti-Kp^b
	Anti-U	Anti-K13

From Issitt PD: Applied blood group serology, ed 3, Miami, 1985, Montgomery Scientific Publications.

hemolysis. Polyclonal high titered auto-anti I of acute onset may be seen secondary to mycoplasma infections and in patients with CLL and lymphocytic lymphoma. Patients with infectious mononucleosis may develop an auto-anti i, which may be associated with hemolysis. A rare idiopathic form of chronic Cold Agglutinin Disease is also described in elderly men in whom the antibody is monoclonal. As opposed to the acute form, this disease is characterized by splenomegaly and often lymphadenopathy. Many consider Cold Agglutinin Disease to be a lymphoproliferative disorder in its own right.

Patients with cold auto immune anemia are found to have a normocytic normochromic anemia, with reticulocytosis. Spherocytes are not usually seen in large numbers, however, shistocytes may be present. In those patients experiencing intravascular hemolysis, hemoglobinemia, hemoglobinuria, hemosiderinuria, and absent serum haptoglobin may be present. The MCV calculated by automated cell counters may be elevated because of the increased reticulocytes and presence of adherent red cells (doublets) passing through the counting field.

The direct Coombs test is positive due to the presence of C3b and C3d on the circulating red cells. With rare exceptions, IgG is not found on the cells. The serum antibody appears as a cold agglutinin with reaction at room temperature in saline. Almost uniformly, the antibody is a

Table 70-5 Examples of Anti-I, Anti-i, and Anti-I^T in titration studies

Cell type and antibody	Serum dilutions												
	None	2	4	8	16	32	64	128	256	512	1024	2048	4096
ANTI-I													
Adult I	4+	4+	4+	4+	4+	4+	3+	3+	2+	2+	+	+	0
i cord	4+	4+	3+	2+	+	0	0	0	0	0	0	0	0
Adult i	4+	3+	2+	+	0	0	0	0	0	0	0	0	0
ANTI-i													
Adult I	4+	4+	3+	2+	+	0	0	0	0	0	0	0	0
i cord	4+	4+	4+	4+	4+	4+	3+	3+	2+	2+	+	0	0
Adult i	4+	4+	4+	4+	4+	4+	3+	3+	3+	2+	+	+	0
ANTI-I^T													
Adult I	4+	4+	3+	2+	+	+	0	0	0	0	0	0	0
i cord	4+	4+	4+	4+	3+	2+	2+	+	+	+	0	0	0
Adult i	4+	3+	+	+	0	0	0	0	0	0	0	0	

From Issitt PD: Applied blood group serology, ed 3, Miami, 1985, Montgomery Scientific Publications.

Table 70-6 Some differences between pathological and benign cold-reactive autoantibodies

	Pathological autoantibody in CHD	Benign autoantibody in hematologically normal persons
Highest temperature at which most autoantibodies act as agglutinins[*1]	30-32°C	Usually <25°C
Highest temperature at which most autoantibodies activate complement[*1]	30-37°C	Usually <25°C
Titer at 4C[*1]	Often >500	Usually <64
Titer at 22C[*1]	Often >128	Usually <16
Thermal range and titer increased in in vitro test systems in which bovine albumin is used	Usually yes	Usually no
Ability of autoantibody to hemolyze enzyme-treated red cells in an in vitro system using acidified serum	Almost 100%[*2]	Uncommon but not unknown
Nature of autoantibody	Monoclonal in idiopathic CHD, polyclonal in secondary hemolytic episodes	Polyclonal

From Issitt PD: Applied blood group serology, ed 3, Miami, 1985, Montgomery Scientific Publications.
*1 In test systems using saline suspended red cells and serum dilutions made in saline
*2 If the antigen defined is not denatured when red cells are treated with proteases

panagglutinin. In patients who are not group O, the autologous cells often react more weakly than the reagent screening or panel cells, because partial anti H specificity is demonstrated by the antibody. Antibodies directed against the Ii system are enhanced by pretreatment of the reagent cells with proteolytic enzymes, while those within the Pr (Sp) system are abolished by such treatment. Specificities within the Ii system can be differentiated by observing the strength of reactions of the serum against normal adult cells, cord cells, and adult i cells (Table 70-5). Anti I antibodies in patients who are not group O usually show IH specificity. Other complex specificities (e.g., iH, IP$_1$, ILe^b) are well described. An accurate determination of antibody titer depends on the proper collection of blood and separation of serum at 37°C to minimize the autoabsorption of the antibody, and the observation of agglutination strength of serial dilutions of serum, which is carried out at 4°C. As stated, low titered anti I active only at very low temperature is present in most normal individuals. An anti I titer less than

1:64 possesses little diagnostic significance and is generally not active at room temperature. It is usually found that with increasing titer, the thermal amplitude of the antibody increases and the propensity to fix complement also increases. A diagnostically significant cold agglutinin titer for mycoplasma infection is cited at 1:64. Most patients who demonstrate hemolysis are found to have antibodies with a titer greater than 1:512 or 1:1024. Patients with monoclonal cold agglutinin disease may have a titer greater than 1:10,000 (Table 70-6).

Patients with cold antibody AIHA do not usually respond to steroids or splenectomy. Transfusion in these patients is undertaken as little as possible, but is not fraught with the danger of increasing antibody titer as in warm antibody AIHA. Furthermore, the possible presence of clinically significant IgG antibodies may be easily detected following 4°C autoabsorption of the patient's serum with autologous anticoagulated red cells collected and separated at 37°C. Further cross-matching is carried out at 37°C.

Paroxysmal cold hemoglobinuria

An unusual form of cold antibody AIHA is due to an IgG complement fixing autoantibody known as the Donath-Landsteiner antibody. This antibody arises idiopathically or after viral infections and in patients with latent syphilis. Donath-Landsteiner antibody characteristically causes a low-grade, ongoing hemolysis, with intermittent marked intravascular hemolysis often during cold weather, giving rise to a condition known as Paroxysmal Cold Hemoglobinuria.

In this condition, aside from the laboratory findings associated with intravascular hemolysis, the direct Coombs' test is positive. The cells are found to be coated with C3b and C3d. Since the IgG antibody elutes off the cell at increased temperatures, IgG is not usually detected on the red cell surface. The responsible antibody is a biphasic hemolysin, which is detected with the "Donath-Landsteiner" test. In this test, incubation of reagent red cells with the patient's serum at 4°C for 30 minutes does not result in hemolysis but permits reaction with the IgG antibody and the subsequent fixation of complement followed by hemolysis as the reaction mixture is incubated as 37°C for up to 60 minutes. The specificity of this antibody is usually found to be against the P antigen, although rare IH and iH antibodies have been described.

Transfusion of antigen negative units is generally not possible, given the rarity of P negative red cells (less than 1 in 200,000). Most patients are able to be transfused with random blood units with satisfactory clinical responses. Some workers have advocated the infusion of washed red cells in order to eliminate the infusion additional complement. There is little evidence that this practice is able to slow the rate of hemolysis or increase the post-transfusion survival of donor red cells.

DRUG RELATED IMMUNE HEMOLYSIS.

The binding of immunoglobulin to the red cell and, in some cases, the subsequent destruction of these cells by the reticuloendothelial system may be related to the ingestion of drugs. Common to all of these situations, regardless of whether or not hemolysis ensues, is the demonstration of a positive, direct Coombs' test. The drugs implicated (Table 70-7) cause the coating of the red cells by different mechanisms. Four types of mechanisms are described.

Haptenic mechanism

The drug binds firmly to the red cell surface and then fixes preformed IgG antibodies specific for the drug (Figure 70-3). In these situations the direct Coombs' test is positive when performed with anti IgG and generally negative with anti C3b and anti C3d. Eluates prepared from these cells are non-reactive with reagent red cells but react with cells coated with the suspected drug. Penicillin and, rarely, the cephalosporins administered intravenously and in high dose act in this manner. Hemolysis occurs in some patients in whom the drug is continued after sensitization occurs. Hemolysis ceases with suspension of the drug.

Circulating immune complex mechanism

The circulating drug combines with anti-drug antibody. A circulating complex then attaches to the red cell membrane

Table 70-7 Drugs involved in immunohemolysis

Type	Drug
Antibiotics and anti-bacterial and anti-protozoal agents	Stibophen
	Para-aminosalicylic acid (PAS)
	Penicillin
	Sulfonamide
	Isoniazid (INH)
	Cephalosporins
	Streptomycin
Anti-inflammatory and analgesic agents	Phenacetin
	Mefenamic acid
	Phenylbutazone
	Indomethacin
Anti-convulsants and sedatives	Chlorpromazine
	Phenantoin (Mesantoin)
	Phenytoin (Dilantin)
Miscellaneous	Quinidine
	Quinine
	Methyldopa (Aldomet)
	Levodopa
	Sulfonylurea
	Chlorpropamide
	Melphalan
	Insecticides (chlorinated hydrocarbons)

From Bauer JD: Clinical laboratory methods, ed 9, St. Louis, 1982, Mosby-Year Book, Inc.

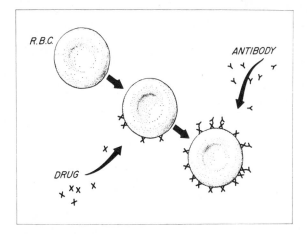

Fig. 70-3 Drug-related red cell sensitization: Haptenic mechanism. *From Garatty G: A seminar on problems encountered in pre-transfusion tests, Washington, DC, 1972, American Association of Blood Banks.*

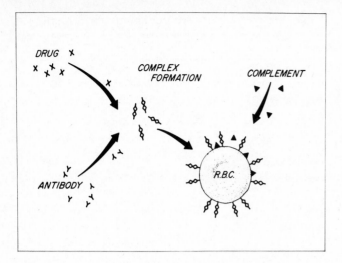

Fig. 70-4 Drug-related red cell sensitization: Immune complex mechanism. *From Garatty G: A seminar on problems encountered in pre-transfusion tests, Washington, DC, 1972, American Association of Blood Banks.*

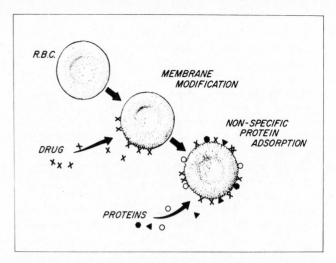

Fig. 70-5 Drug-related red cell sensitization: Non-immunologic surface adsorption. *From Garatty G: A seminar on problems encountered in pre-transfusion tests, Washington, DC, 1972, American Association of Blood Banks.*

(innocent bystander). Complement is subsequently fixed and often the immune complex thereafter dissociates, leaving only complement coating the cell (Figure 70-4). The direct Coombs' test is positive when performed with anti C3b and anti C3d but is generally negative when performed with anti IgG. The patient's serum is found to react with reagent red cells only when they are incubated together in the presence of the responsible drug. Quinidine and quinine are the drugs classically associated with hemolysis via this mechanism. However, many others cause a positive direct Coombs' test by this mechanism. Hemolysis due to this mechanism ceases within a few days of suspension of the offending drug.

Nonspecific protein absorption mechanism

The cephalosporins may also cause an alteration of the red cell membrane, such that normal serum proteins adhere to the cells. If this includes γ-globulin or complement, these will be detected by the antiglobulin reaction (Figure 70-5). Hemolysis does not result from this nonspecific protein absorption.

Red cell specific antibody mechanism

Some drugs, notably α-methyldopa, L-Dopa, mefenamic acid, and procainamide may alter the red cell membrane and/or the immune system thereby inducing the formation of true anti red cell antibodies. These antibodies are similar to those causing warm antibody AIHA in that they appear as autoantibodies that often have specificity within the Rh

group. The most common drug causing a direct Coombs' reaction by this mechanism is α-methyldopa (10%). However, only 1% of people taking the drug develop hemolysis. Because the immune reaction is a true autoimmune phenomenon rather than a simple reaction to the drug itself, the direct Coombs' test may remain positive for up to six months after suspension of the drug.

SUGGESTED READING

Bowman JM: Treatment options for the fetus with alloimmune hemolytic disease, Transf Med Rev 4:191-207, 1990.

Garratty G, ed: Hemolytic disease of the newborn, Arlington, Va, 1984, American Association of Blood Banks.

Gravenhorst JB: Management of serious alloimmunization in pregnancy, Vox Sang 55:1-8, 1988.

Giles CM: The role of complement in immunohematology, Transfusion 29:803-811, 1990.

Goldfinger D: Acute hemolytic transfusion reactions—a fresh look at pathogenesis and considerations regarding therapy, Transfusion 17:85-98, 1977.

Kelton JG: Platelet and red cell clearance is determined by the interaction of the IgG and complement on the cells and the activity of the reticuloendothelial system, Transf Med Rev 1:75-84, 1987.

Petz LD: Drug-induced hemolysis, N Eng J Med 313:510, 1985.

Plapp F and Beck M: Transfusion support in immune hemolytic disorders, Clin Haematol 13:167-183, 1984.

Schmidt PJ: The mortality from incompatible transfusion. In Sandler SG, et al, eds: Immunobiology of the erythrocyte, New York, 1980, Alan J Liss, Inc.

Tovey LAD: Hemolytic disease of the newborn—the changing scene, Brit J Obstct Gynecol 93:960, 1986.

71 Blood collection, processing, and storage

Joan Uehlinger

The collection, processing, and storage of blood and its components for transfusion has become increasingly complex. The safety of both the donor and the recipient, as well as the current legal and regulatory climate, demands scrupulous attention to procedures and their documentation. The continual addition of new tests performed on donor blood affects not only the safety of the blood supply, but also the integrity of the testing process.

Federal, state, and local agencies regulate blood processing. These regulations are meant to be only *minimum* required standards. This chapter will only address national or federal regulations as detailed in the references at the end of this chapter. State and local health codes may be more stringent than those given here; for any questions, contact the state or local Department of Health.

All regulations require detailed records of each step in blood collection, processing, and storage, from donor registration through transfusion to the recipient. These records must be retained for a minimum of 5 years in order to allow the subsequent trace of any unit of blood. The record of blood collection must include all donor-identifying information, an indication that all questions have been understood and answered, the results of the limited physical examination, and consents for the donation as well as the laboratory testing. Documentation must be made of the separation of any unit of blood into its components. Records of laboratory testing must include all results and follow-up and disposition of units with abnormal results. In order to facilitate any subsequent recall, records of release or distribution must be complete. Each facility must keep a detailed procedure manual, which is updated with modifications in either policy or technique. All past procedure manuals must be retained, with documentation of the dates that these were in force.

CRITERIA FOR DONOR SELECTION

Donor screening procedures have two aims: protection of the donor and protection of the recipient. The criteria for protection of the donor are generally concerned with prevention of iron depletion and assuring stable hemodynamics during the donation. These risks are always balanced with the expected medical benefit to the recipient of the product. The criteria for the protection of the recipient are generally concerned with preventing either infectious or immunologic complications of transfusion. A careful donor history is the crucial first safety check for any transfusion.

Homologous whole blood donors

The selection criteria for volunteer whole blood donors apply to all other donors, except as noted shortly. There is a minimum interval between donations of 8 weeks. There are no federal restrictions on donor age. The American Association of Blood Banks' *Standards* state that donors shall be at least 17 years old. An upper age limit may be set by local regulation. The lower age limit depends on local law regarding minors and their ability to give consent. Donors who weigh more than 110 lb may donate 450 ± 45 ml. The American Association of Blood Banks' *Standards* state that donors who weigh less may give a smaller volume, provided the amount of anticoagulant is proportionally reduced. The concern is that the anticoagulant solution, which is distributed in the plasma, should not be too concentrated. The necessity for a reduction in anticoagulant has been a subject of controversy.

Physical examination

The oral temperature must be less than 37.5° C (99.5° F). The pulse must be between 50 and 100 beats per minute, with no pathologic irregularity. The systolic blood pressure must be between 100 and 180 mm Hg, and the diastolic blood pressure less than 100 mm Hg. Donors with uncontrolled hypertension have more vasomotor instability with the hemodynamic challenge of phlebotomy. There must be, on inspection of both arms, no evidence of intravenous drug use or rash at the site of venipuncture.

Hemoglobin concentration in whole blood may be determined by a number of acceptable methods. The method used may be determined by each facility. Factors to be considered in the decision include: workflow, accuracy, cost, deferral rates, as well as the training required for each method. When finger puncture is used as the source, deferral rates are about 5% higher than when earlobe puncture is used. The donor hemoglobin standard has recently been the subject of some debate. The Code of Federal Regulations sets a minimum of 12.5 g/dl. The largest single cause of donor deferral, about 50% in most centers, is a low hemoglobin level. Of donors deferred for a low hemoglobin, 75% are women. Iron deficiency without anemia is common in menstruating women who are blood donors. This has caused concern about a lowered standard for women. However, there is little evidence that iron deficiency without anemia is harmful.

Medical history

Donors should be asked about their medical history in an open-ended fashion. Leading questions should be avoided. A number of preexisting medical conditions may increase the risk of donation. Donors must therefore be questioned about heart disease, cerebrovascular disease or stroke, seizures, fainting, pulmonary or renal disease, blood diseases or bleeding tendency, and recent surgery or pregnancy.

Donors must be questioned about exposure to infectious disease. If there has been exposure, the donor should be deferred for at least the length of the incubation period of the disease. Specific questions should be asked about hepatitis risk, including any history of hepatitis or possible exposure within the preceding 12 months. This would include contact with the body fluids of a person with hepatitis, acupuncture, tattoos, ear piercing, or transfusion. Some centers defer donors who have been exposed to dialysis patients or institutionalized patients. However, because of the widespread use of hepatitis B vaccination and isolation precautions in these situations, this deferral may no longer be necessary. Donors who have been exposed to hepatitis B and have received hepatitis B immune globulin should be deferred for 1 year, since this may prolong the incubation period of hepatitis B.

Unless they received live vaccine, recent immunization in an asymptomatic subject is not a contraindication to donation. Examples of live vaccines and their deferral periods are measles, mumps, yellow fever, or oral polio (2 weeks); rubella (4 weeks); rabies (1 year).

Donors with respiratory infections, colds, or sore throats should be deferred while they are symptomatic. Those with a history of travel to a malarious area should be deferred for 6 months. Immigrants from malaria endemic areas, or travelers who have taken antimalarial prophylaxis or treatment, should be deferred for 3 years. Donors with a history of dental procedures should be deferred for 3 days because of the possibility of transient bacteremia. Recipients of human pituitary growth hormone are deferred permanently because of reports of Creutzfeldt-Jakob disease in these patients.

Information must be provided to all donors about activities associated with a high risk of exposure to human immunodeficiency virus (HIV), and that they must not donate if any apply (Box 71-1). Questions about the symptoms of AIDS (unexplained fever, weight loss, night sweats, lymphadenopathy, oral thrush, purple skin lesions, persistent cough, or diarrhea) should be asked and the donor deferred if there is no explanation for the symptom.

Donors must be offered an additional opportunity to confidentially indicate that their blood should not be used for transfusion to another person. The reason for this confidential unit exclusion (CUE) is that high-risk individuals may be under social pressure to donate blood. By using CUE, they may maintain the appearance of donation, but ensure that the blood is discarded. Mechanisms that have been used

---

> **Box 71-1**   Persons who should not donate blood or blood components due to risk of HIV-1 or HIV-2 (Food and Drug Administration recommendations, December 5, 1990):
>
> - Persons with clinical or laboratory evidence of HIV infection
> - Men who have had sex with another man, even once, since 1977
> - Past or present intravenous drug users
> - Persons with hemophilia or related clotting disorders who have received clotting factor concentrates
> - Persons born in or emigrating from countries where heterosexual activity is thought to play a major role in transmission of HIV-1 or HIV-2 infection (i.e., Haiti, sub-Saharan Africa, and islands located near these areas of Africa). This exclusion is not necessary after implementation of HIV-2 testing.
> - Persons who have had sex with any person meeting the above description
> - Men and women who have engaged in sex for money or drugs since 1977 and persons who have engaged in sex with such people during the preceding 12 months
> - Persons who have had or been treated for syphilis or gonorrhea during the preceding 12 months.

---

include separate forms labeled with the number of the unit, barcode labels to be placed on the registration form, and special telephone numbers for donors to call after the donation.

Medication histories should be directed at the underlying disease and the risk it poses to the donor. There are few medications that might directly harm the recipient. Exceptions include potentially teratogenic drugs such as Accutane (isoretinoin), which requires deferral for at least 1 month after the completion of therapy. Permanent deferral is indicated following the use of Tegison (etretinate), since it is highly tissue-bound.

Blood from donors who have previously been permanently deferred because of infection risk must not be used for transfusion. Examples include those who have been implicated in posttransfusion hepatitis cases and those who have had laboratory results that result in permanent deferral (see text that follows). Each blood collection facility must have a mechanism to check previous donation histories and remove such units from inventory.

Directed whole blood donors

With increasing public awareness of the hazards of transfusion, patients may request that they select donors whose blood will be made available for them. There is no clear evidence that these directed donations are any safer than the community blood supply. In fact, studies of prevalence of infectious disease markers in this population suggest that they are higher than in the volunteer donor population.

There have been reports of fatal graft-versus-host disease in immunocompetent transfusion recipients whose donors were homozygous for one of the recipient's human leukocyte antigen (HLA) haplotypes. In this situation, donor lymphocytes are not recognized as foreign by the recipient, but are able to recognize the recipient as foreign. Most of these cases have received "fresh" blood, but the interval from donation to transfusion was not stated.

Directed blood donors must meet all the criteria for homologous donors, and must be tested by the same procedures used for homologous donors. A written policy must be developed detailing the circumstances, if any, under which such blood will be collected. Several issues might be addressed in such a policy. These include:

1. Restrictions on who may donate for a particular patient. For example, many centers will not allow donation for a woman of childbearing age from her spouse or sexual partner, because of the possibility of red cell alloimmunization.

2. Any special consents from either the donor or the recipient.

3. Whether blood typing will be performed on either donor or patient prior to the donation.

4. The minimum time required to make such units available for transfusion.

5. The circumstances under which the blood might subsequently be entered into the general inventory. This involves two issues: (1) whether or not directed donor blood should be used for other patients, and (2) if so, how long the blood bank is obligated to hold the blood for the intended recipient. The first issue is the question of the safety of these donations. Some blood bankers have been hesitant to use these donations for other patients because these donors may not give a totally honest health history, in their desire to help the recipient. Other blood bankers have argued that if this blood will be used, and therefore is presumably safe for the intended recipient, then it should be safe for any other recipient. Crossover of directed donations to the general inventory requires a policy decision by the facility. If the blood is held for the intended recipient too long, some will be outdated. If it is not held long enough for the needs of the recipient, the blood bank will be the subject of complaints from donors, patients, and physicians. The policy that is developed must take into account the inventory system in the blood bank and what data is easily accessible. Whatever decision is made, it must be clearly disclosed to all the interested parties.

Autologous whole blood donors

The criteria for acceptance of autologous predeposit donors need not be as strict as those for homologous donors. However, unless both the donor and the units meet the requirements for homologous use, the units must be labeled, "For Autologous Use Only." The statement, "Autologous Donor" must be permanently affixed in either case. Written guidelines should be established by each facility for the acceptance of donors who do not meet the usual criteria. The FDA has issued guidelines on the testing of autologous blood (March 15, 1989), stating that all required tests should be performed, and that blood confirmed to be anti-HIV-1 positive or HBsAg reactive should not be used.

The volume of blood collected at each donation should be proportional to the donor's/patient's weight. Preexisting cardiac or cerebrovascular disease need not be a cause for deferral, but may require medical review prior to the first donation. The patients at greatest risk are those with symptomatic coronary artery disease or aortic stenosis. Patients with coronary artery disease may have worsened ischemia with the decrease in venous return due to phlebotomy. Those with aortic stenosis may not be able to increase cardiac output in response to phlebotomy.

At least 72 hours should elapse between donations, and between the last donation and any surgical procedure. This interval is the minimum necessary to replace the volume lost by phlebotomy. The hemoglobin should be at least 11 g/dl. Some donor centers request that referring physicians prescribe iron supplements for the autologous donor/patient. Normal iron requirements are 2 mg/day for menstruating women and 1 mg/day for other adults. Each unit of blood contains approximately 250 mg of iron. For those donors with marginal iron stores, or for those who will donate multiple units in a short time, iron may become the limiting factor for further donation.

No autologous donation should be undertaken when the donor has, or is suspected to have, bacteremia. Because blood is an excellent culture medium, this could result in a unit that is heavily contaminated with organisms. Transfusion of such blood usually results in endotoxic shock, and is sometimes fatal. Collecting autologous blood from patients with cancer will not result in further cancer dissemination. If there are tumor cells in the blood at the time of collection, then hematogenous spread has already occurred.

In addition to autologous predeposit, intraoperative collection of autologous blood for transfusion during the procedure is also used to avoid or reduce exposure to homologous blood. In this procedure, blood is aspirated from the surgical site, filtered, washed, and then returned to the patient. It is not clear whether the washing step is necessary, but early reports of disseminated intravascular coagulation (DIC) in these recipients have resulted in its widespread use, especially when large volumes are to be reinfused.

Intraoperative autologous transfusion is most commonly used during cardiac, vascular, and orthopedic procedures. It has also significantly changed blood utilization for liver transplantation. It is generally not used for procedures in which there is fecal contamination because of concerns about bacterial contamination. Oncologic surgeons are also hesitant about intraoperative salvage of blood from the site of a local malignancy, since theoretically this could result in hematogenous dissemination.

Postoperative collection of shed blood is another means of autologous transfusion. This has been used most widely in cardiac surgery. Chest tubes are routinely placed at the end of these procedures, and the output monitored. With the addition of a closed system for collection, mediastinal-shed blood can be reinfused. The system must be changed every 4 hours, and any blood that is not reinfused at that point must be discarded. Some studies have shown a significant decrease in homologous blood requirements with the use of postoperative autotransfusion.

Special considerations for the apheresis donor

Donor apheresis procedures accomplish, by either automated or manual methods, the separation of specific components from a single donor. The same general criteria used for whole blood donors apply to apheresis donors. Each institution should have written protocols that include the minimal acceptable criteria for donors, the collection procedures in use, a procedure for management of donor reactions, and equipment maintenance procedures.

Platelets are usually collected by automated methods. Donors should be deferred who have taken aspirin in the preceding 3 days, especially in the preceding 36 hours. The minimum interval between plateletpheresis procedures is 48 hours, with no more than two procedures in a 7-day period or 24 procedures per year. If procedures are performed more frequently than permitted for whole blood, a platelet count must be performed. The results should be reviewed prior to the next procedure. Donors with platelet counts less than $150,000\mu l$ should be deferred until the count returns to normal. The accumulated laboratory data on the donor must be reviewed at least every 4 months by a physician. An informed consent must include all reasonable risks of the procedures in use.

Granulocytes are also collected by automated methods. In addition to the aforementioned remarks concerning platelet donation, three further considerations apply also to granulocyte donation. First, there is an unavoidable red cell loss during granulocyte donation, which should be limited to less than 25 ml per week. Second, because of the red cells contained in granulocyte products, donors should be selected who are known to be ABO-compatible with the recipient. Third, drugs may be given to facilitate leukapheresis. A sedimenting agent such as hydroxyethyl starch (HES) or pentastarch is used to improve separation of granulocytes. These are both also volume expanders. After infusion, 40% of HES and 90% of pentastarch is excreted within 24 hours. Since HES is slowly eliminated, there has been concern about the frequency of donor procedures with this agent. Pentastarch is eliminated more rapidly. Corticosteroids are given to raise the peripheral white count and thereby improve yields. Oral prednisone or oral dexamethasone both have their peak effect on the peripheral white count at 3 to 5 hours after ingestion. There is a second peak at about 12 hours. If a single oral dose is desired, either dexamethasone 4 to 6 mg/M^2 4 hours before the procedure or prednisone 30 mg 5 hours before the procedure may be used. An optimal effect may be achieved with two oral doses of dexamethasone 3 mg/M^2 at 12 and 3 hours prior to the procedure. However, two doses may be impractical for some centers. The informed consent obtained from the donor must additionally state any reasonable risks from these drugs, such as fluid retention from sedimenting agents and headache, mood changes, or insomnia from corticosteroids. Contraindications to the use of these agents include congestive heart failure, active peptic ulcer disease, or uncontrolled hypertension. Donors with these conditions should not undergo apheresis procedures whether or not these drugs are used.

Plasmapheresis is the procedure for obtaining plasma from a donor. It can be performed by either manual or automated methods. Detailed regulations regarding donor suitability, informed consent, laboratory and physical examinations, and medical supervision can be found in the Code of Federal Regulations. State or local regulations may be more strict.

DONATION PROCEDURES

All phlebotomy procedures should be performed by trained staff under the direction of a qualified physician. Before phlebotomy is begun, the donor record form, blood bags, and pilot tubes should be labeled and the numbers checked to assure corresponding identification of both the donor and the unit. The correct expiration date must be recorded on the bag. Materials used in phlebotomy must be sterile; disposable materials are preferred. Blood must be collected into sterile, pyrogen-free containers approved for this purpose by the FDA. There must be sufficient anticoagulant in the container for the volume of blood collected.

Preparation of the venipuncture site is a critical step in assuring a sterile unit. The skin should be free of lesions. Many acceptable procedures for skin preparation are available. Most involve a scrub with alcohol or an iodine-containing scrub solution, followed by application of iodine or iodophor. For donors who are sensitive to iodine, alternate preparations, such as green soap scrub followed by acetone-alcohol, can be used. If the venipuncture is not to be performed immediately after the preparation, the area should be covered with sterile gauze. The vein should not be palpated again after the preparation.

Whole blood donation

Prior to phlebotomy, the container should be inspected for defects. A mechanism is required both to monitor the amount of blood withdrawn and to mix the blood with the anticoagulant. Phlebotomists should wear gloves for their own protection while performing the venipuncture. The procedure for phlebotomy is as follows:

1. Apply a tourniquet or blood pressure cuff above the chosen site. The pressure applied should be less than the systolic blood pressure, but sufficient to make the vein prominent.
2. Perform a single, uninterrupted venipuncture, minimizing as much as possible trauma to the surrounding tissue.
3. Tape the tubing to the donor's arm below the site to prevent needle dislodgment. Place sterile gauze over the venipuncture site.
4. Instruct the donor to squeeze the fist intermittently.
5. When the collection is complete, the tubing should be clamped or knotted. Specimens should be collected for testing by any method that does not compromise the sterility of the unit. For example, some bags are equipped with in-line needles, tubes, or pouches for specimen collection. If there is a straight-tubing set, tubes may be filled either from the donor needle after it is withdrawn, or by clamping and cutting the tubing, filling tubes from the proximal (donor) end.
6. With the tubing clamped, release the tourniquet or deflate the blood pressure cuff. Withdraw the needle and apply pressure to the site for a few minutes with sterile gauze. Apply a bandage to the site.
7. Complete the documentation of the donation. Recheck donor identification and the numbers on the donor record form, the bags, and specimen tubes.

The needle must be cut off and discarded into a container designed to prevent accidental needlesticks. Blood remaining in the tubing between the clamp and the bag should be stripped into the primary bag. Segments may be made using a manual or dielectric sealer with care to preserve the segment identification number. If platelets are to be made from the unit, blood should be kept at room temperature. Otherwise, the blood should be kept at 1° C to 6° C.

Following completion of the procedure, donors should rest and be given postdonation instructions. Donors should never be left unattended during or after donation. Fluids and/or light refreshments may be offered when an upright position can be tolerated. The donation process should be made as pleasant as possible and all participants should be thanked.

Apheresis procedures

Specific blood components may be collected from a single donor by a variety of methods. The disadvantage of manual procedures is that blood must be removed from the donor, disconnected, separated, and then reinfused. The risk of misidentification of the original unit is present. Additionally, manual procedures are more time-consuming and less efficient than automated procedures. Except for plasmapheresis and some unusual circumstances, most donor apheresis procedures are therefore performed using automated techniques. Automated apheresis procedures can accomplish separation by centrifugation, filtration, or both. See Table 71-1 for examples of equipment.

Collection of cellular components using currently available equipment is by centrifugation, with either continuous or discontinuous flow centrifuges. During centrifugation, layering of components occurs according to size and weight. The desired component is separated by detection of the interface between layers and collection from that point. Con-

tinuous flow centrifugation requires two venipunctures; one line is used for blood withdrawal and the other for return. Blood is continuously collected, centrifuged, and returned. The configuration of the centrifuge varies depending on the manufacturer. These devices have the advantage of a small extracorporeal volume, generally about 100 cc. Continuous flow centrifugation is preferred for the collection of leukocytes because it results in optimal yields. For discontinuous flow procedures, a centrifuge bowl is filled with whole blood. After component collection, the blood is returned and this sequence is repeated in cycles. Discontinuous flow procedures can be performed with a single venipuncture, and are therefore preferred by some donors. Both continuous and discontinuous flow devices are available with FDA-approved closed system software to collect platelets with a 5-day expiration.

Membrane filtration may be used, either alone or combined with centrifugation, in some devices designed specifically for plasmapheresis. Filtration is accomplished with a microporous membrane, which separates components depending on the pore size. When membrane filtration alone is used, the extracorporeal volume can be quite low (50 to 100 cc). These procedures take about as much time as pure centrifugation procedures, and are limited to plasmapheresis. When membrane filtration is combined with centrifugation, the necessary extracorporeal volume is 250 to 500 cc. However, the time required is much shorter and it is possible to collect platelets simultaneously.

Management of donor reactions

All personnel caring for donors must be trained to recognize donor reactions and their initial management. Careful observation of the donor is necessary during any reaction. See Table 71-2 for a description of the most common donor reactions. There should be a written protocol on the treatment of donor reactions. General measures should be undertaken at the first symptoms. Donors should be given nothing by mouth until all symptoms subside. Medications are rarely needed in the treatment of donor reactions.

Vasodepressor or vasovagal reactions are the most common donor reactions. They may occur before, during, or after blood collection. There is vascular dilatation with a resultant fall in arterial blood pressure. The normal cardiac compensation for this does not occur, because of vagal stimulation. This autonomic activity results in a fall in cardiac output and bradycardia. When such a reaction occurs during or after donation, these effects are worsened due to the loss

Table 71-1 Examples of FDA-approved donor apheresis instruments

Manufacturer	Instrument	Method
Haemonetics	V-50	Discontinuous flow centrifugation
Haemonetics	PCS	Discontinuous flow centrifugation
Baxter	Fenwal CS-3000	Continuous flow centrifugation
Baxter	Autopheresis C	Filtration/Centrifugation
COBE/IBM	2997	Continuous flow centrifugation
COBE/IBM	Spectra	Continuous flow centrifugation

Table 71-2 Donor reactions and their management

Type	Symptoms/signs	Management
Vasovagal	Apprehension; pallor; sweating, dizziness; hypotension and/or bradycardia; loss of consciousness; rarely, seizures	Reassurance; place in recumbent position; stop blood collection; give fluids if necessary; assure airway; prevent injury by mild restraint
Hematoma	Swelling at venipuncture site	Remove needle, apply pressure
Hyperventilation	Deep or fast breathing, twitching or muscle spasm	Divert donor's attention, rebreathing into paper bag
Citrate toxicity	Perioral or peripheral paresthesias, anxiety, muscle spasms	Reassurance, decrease rate of blood return, oral calcium replacement

of blood volume by phlebotomy. The symptoms generally begin with light-headedness, pallor, diaphoresis, and restlessness. If cerebral blood flow is inadequate, these may progress to loss of consciousness (syncope), and further, to seizures. Diverting the donor's attention and simple reassurance are usually sufficient to control the psychological factors that contribute to mild vasovagal reactions. Once symptoms begin, the donor should be placed in the supine position with the legs elevated in order to maximize venous return. If symptoms are prolonged, severe, or if a significant volume of blood has been collected, intravenous hydration with normal saline may be required. This will help to more rapidly restore arterial pressure. The decision to begin intravenous hydration should be made by the responsible physician, either according to a written protocol or on an individual basis.

Hematomas are usually caused by extravasation of blood from the venipuncture site. If they are recognized at the time of donation, they can be limited by applying direct pressure at the site. If they cause pressure on a nerve, they may cause pain and/or loss of function, which may take weeks or months to resolve. Arterial punctures are rare; they are usually recognized because of the bright-red color of the blood. It may or may not appear to be pulsatile, depending on the equipment used for blood collection. When arterial puncture is suspected, the needle should be withdrawn and firm direct pressure applied to the venipuncture site for at least 10 minutes. The radial pulse should be assessed once bleeding has been controlled.

Extremely nervous donors may hyperventilate sufficiently to cause a respiratory alkalosis. This may cause a lowered ionized calcium, and therefore twitching or muscle spasm. Hyperventilation may be most effectively controlled by having the donor rebreathe into a paper bag.

Citrate is the anticoagulant most commonly used for donor apheresis procedures; it is added to whole blood as it is withdrawn. Citrate acts by binding calcium and may lower ionized calcium. Mild citrate-related symptoms such as paresthesias can be easily controlled by decreasing the rate of blood return to the donor. If necessary, oral calcium replacement may be used. Chills are sometimes seen in apheresis donors due to cooling of blood in the extracorporeal circuit. This can be corrected by warming the donor with blankets.

The nature of any reaction and any treatment given should be recorded on the donor record form. The written protocol should include a policy on acceptance of donors after reactions. It is advisable to permanently defer donors who have had loss of consciousness or seizures during a donation. If the severity of the reaction warrants deferral of the donor, this should be documented as well.

DONOR TESTING

Tests performed on donated blood are similar or identical to those used in diagnostic testing, and the interpretation of results for the purposes of donor notification are the same. The interpretation of results to determine the acceptability of units of blood for transfusion is made using different criteria. The major consideration is to maximize safety. In the following discussion, these differences will be noted.

All laboratory testing is performed on specimens taken at the time of donation. Reagents used for testing donor blood must be licensed by the FDA for this purpose.

All equipment used in testing should be checked on receipt or after repairs for proper functioning and then receive periodic maintenance. Operating temperatures of all temperature-regulated equipment (water baths, heat blocks) should be checked daily, and the results recorded. Serologic centrifuges should be calibrated to determine the optimal speed and time for different procedures. After initial calibration, the time of centrifugation and number of revolutions per minute should be checked every 3 to 4 months. Thermometers should be checked for both accuracy and consistency, against a thermometer certified by the National Bureau of Standards. When any of these findings are outside the acceptable range, corrective action should be taken and documented.

Serologic testing

ABO and Rh types must be determined on each unit of blood. Previous donor records are not sufficient for identification of units of blood, but may be used as a quality control check. Details of the methods used may be found in Chapter 69. ABO type is determined by testing the red blood cells with anti-A and anti-B sera and the serum or plasma for the expected antibodies with A_1 and B red blood cells. No unit may be issued unless these results are in agreement.

Rh testing must be performed with anti-D serum. If the results are negative, the sample must be tested using a method that can detect the D^u phenotype, as described in Chapter 69. If either D or D^u is positive, the unit is labeled "Rh Positive." If they are both negative, the unit is labeled "Rh Negative." This is in contrast to the testing necessary for blood recipients, for whom the test for D^u is not required. A D^u recipient who receives D-negative blood will not be harmed, but anti-D may be formed by a D-negative recipient who receives a D^u-positive unit.

Tests for unexpected antibodies are not required by the Code of Federal Regulations. However, the American Association of Blood Banks' Standards require tests for donors with a history of transfusions or pregnancy. Blood found to contain unexpected antibodies should be prepared into components that contain minimal amounts of plasma. If the plasma is used, it must be labeled with the specificity of the antibody.

Transmissible disease testing

In the years from 1985 to 1988, four tests were added to routine donor screening (anti-HIV, alanine aminotransferase [ALT], anti-HBc, and anti-HTLV I/II [human T-cell lymphotropic virus, types I and II]). It is probable that additional tests will be added as knowledge of transfusion-transmitted disease improves and technology becomes available. The FDA requires that all donated blood be tested for syphilis, hepatitis B surface antigen (HBsAg), and antibody to HIV. Decisions to perform other tests are based on recommendations made by blood banking professional organizations such as the Council of Community Blood Centers and the American Association of Blood Banks. The tests recom-

*HBsAg, hepatitis B surface antigen; ALT, alanine aminotransferase; HBc, hepatitis B core antigen; HIV, human immunodeficiency virus; HTLV-I/II, human T-cell lymphotropic virus type I and II; HCV, hepatitis C virus.

mended to be performed on donated blood as of mid-1990 are listed in Box 71-2. Details of the methods used can be found in previous chapters. Blood banking tests for exposure to infectious agents, in contrast to diagnostic testing, generally assess total immunoglobulin or IgG, rather than IgM. Discussion of the infectious complications of transfusion can be found in Chapter 73.

The safety of the recipient is directly related to the sensitivity of donor screening tests. Positive screening tests are repeated in duplicate. Decisions about the disposition of blood units are based on screening test results regardless of confirmatory test results. Donor deferral and counseling are based on the more specific confirmatory tests.

The need for syphilis screening is controversial. Theoretically, fresh blood components are more likely to transmit syphilis, since spirochetes are unlikely to survive refrigerated temperatures. Units of blood that are reactive on serologic tests are discarded. Fluorescent treponemal antibody (FTA) testing may be used for confirmation. Syphilis is a reportable disease in many states and notification of public health authorities may be required.

Hepatitis B surface antigen (HBsAg) screening is used to detect the viremic state of acute hepatitis B as well as the chronic carrier state. All donor blood must be tested by a method approved by the FDA, usually by enzyme-linked immunosorbent assay (ELISA) or by radioimmunoassay (RIA). All components must be destroyed if HBsAg is positive. Confirmation is performed using a neutralization test. Current prevalence of HBsAg in the donor population is 0.01% to 0.03%. Donors found to be positive are counseled and permanently deferred. Local law may necessitate reporting of HBsAg-positive donors.

Serum alanine aminotransferase (ALT) levels correlate with the transmission of non-A, non-B hepatitis to the recipient. This test was first added as a surrogate test. The use of this test requires that an arbitrary cutoff value be set. In 1981, two studies suggested either a fixed cutoff at 45 IU or a cutoff set at 2.25 SD above the mean log for normal subjects, which was to be defined locally. In 1987, the American Association of Blood Banks recommended that units with an ALT greater than 2 SD above the mean of the donor population be discarded, and that donors be deferred permanently after two such donations, or after one donation with an ALT greater than twice the cutoff. However, ALT has been shown to vary with sex, race, body mass index, and geographic location. Because of this, a national reference standard for ALT is being developed to normalize ALT cutoffs between centers. With the introduction of testing for antibody to hepatitis C (anti-HCV), this test was retained, since it may serve to identify some hepatitis C virus carriers who have not yet developed anti-HCV.

Another test originally introduced as a surrogate test for non-A, non-B hepatitis is antibody to hepatitis B core antigen (anti-HBc). The prevalence of anti-HBc in the donor population was about 4% prior to the institution of screening. Centers that defer these donors permanently now have a much lower prevalence. Anti-HBc screening was continued after the introduction of anti-HCV for the identification of HBsAg-seronegative carriers of hepatitis B (HBV) and HBV-delta virus carriers. This screening is generally performed using an ELISA method. Units found to be positive are discarded. Plasma from these units may be used for fractionation into plasma derivatives.

A new virus, named hepatitis C virus (HCV), is the major causative agent of non-A, non-B hepatitis. An ELISA test for antibody to HCV based on a single viral peptide has been developed, and was implemented for blood bank screening in May of 1990. This test is expected to reduce the risk of posttransfusion hepatitis to 0.5% to 2.5% per transfusion episode. Clinical trials indicate that 0.5% to 1.0% of volunteer donors will test repeatedly reactive by this test, and of these, 40% to 70% may show false-positive results. As of this writing, there is no licensed confirmatory test. Repeat reactive donors are permanently deferred. It is expected that improved tests using multiple viral antigens may be developed in the future.

Screening for antibody to human immunodeficiency virus (anti-HIV-1) is usually performed using an ELISA method. All components of units found repeat reactive in the ELISA are discarded. Donors who are repeat reactive on ELISA on one donation are placed in a deferral registry. Future donations by these donors must be discarded even if the test results are negative. Prior to donor notification, reactive ELISA results must be confirmed by a more specific method, usually Western blot. In the Western blot assay, proteins of an HIV-1 lysate are separated according to size by polyacrylamide gel electrophoresis. These are then transferred onto nitrocellulose and reacted with the test serum. Antihuman IgG conjugated with an enzyme substrate results in colored bands in the presence of HIV antibodies. Confirmed positive donors must be notified and counseled regarding disease transmission and told not to donate blood in the future. Current prevalence of confirmed positives is about 0.01% to 0.02%. Donors whose ELISA is repeat reactive but whose Western blot is negative may be removed from permanent deferral using an FDA-approved protocol if they have negative ELISA and Western blot results over a period of more than 6 months. Samples must be tested with ELISAs manufactured from virus grown in two different cell lines. The most recent sample must be tested with an FDA-licensed Western blot.

Screening for antibody to HTLV I/II is performed using an ELISA method. Units found repeat reactive on screening are discarded. Confirmatory testing is performed using Western blot and, when necessary, radio immunoprecipitation assay (RIPA). No Western blot or RIPA has yet been licensed by the FDA. Confirmed positive donors are counseled and permanently deferred. Current prevalence of confirmed positive donations is 0.02%. Donors whose ELISA is repeat reactive, but whose Western blot and/or RIPA are negative or indeterminate, are permanently deferred if the ELISA is repeat reactive on any subsequent donation. There is no re-entry protocol for anti-HTLV I/II, because there is no licensed confirmatory test.

Special considerations

For some recipients, specially tested components are necessary in specific clinical situations. Because these procedures are not routine, they are generally used according to the local guidelines of the transfusion facility.

Anti-CMV (cytomegalovirus) testing

The frequency of anti-CMV in the donor population varies depending on location; in the United States, from 20% to 80% of donors are seropositive for CMV. Obviously, donors cannot be routinely screened for CMV. Currently, the methods most commonly used to detect antibodies to CMV are ELISA or indirect latex agglutination for total anti-CMV.

Cytomegalovirus infection may be transmitted to immunocompromised hosts by transfusion of cellular blood components; granulocyte concentrates carry the greatest risk. Severely immunosuppressed patients who are CMV-seronegative are at greatest risk of CMV infection. These include premature infants whose mothers are CMV-seronegative and who weigh less than 1200 grams at birth, and recipients of bone marrow or solid organ transplants (when the donor is also CMV-seronegative). The risk can be reduced by providing CMV-seronegative blood or frozen deglycerolized red cells (if only red cells are required). Infants whose mothers are seropositive and who require transfusion support may be at higher risk of maternally acquired CMV if they receive only seronegative products, since they would not be passively immunized.

Screening for hemoglobin S

In selected clinical situations, it is optimal to provide red blood cells known to lack hemoglobin S. For instance, red cell exchange may be necessary in patients with sickle-cell disease in order to increase the percentage of circulating hemoglobin A. In this situation, screening for hemoglobin S is logical. Red cells from donors with sickle trait may sickle under conditions of low oxygen tension. Therefore, some transfusion services also provide red cells that lack hemoglobin S for intrauterine transfusion or for hypoxic neonates.

Screening for hemoglobin S may also be useful in testing red cells before freezing, depending on the frequency of sickle trait in the donor population. Deglycerolization of these cells by the usual methods results in hemolysis of the unit. When cells are known to have AS hemoglobin before deglycerolization, a modified method may be used to prevent hemolysis. See the discussion of frozen cells that follows for more details.

COMPONENT PREPARATION AND STORAGE

Procedures for the separation of blood components from whole blood must ensure the sterility of the final product. Blood that will be separated should be collected into bags that have attached satellite bags in order to maintain a closed system. A closed system can also be maintained using a commercial device that interconnects additional bags in a sterile manner. A closed system should be entered only using aseptic methods and sterile, pyrogen-free equipment and solutions. Once it is entered, a closed system becomes an open system, substantially reducing the shelf-life of the product: components stored between 1° C and 6° C must be transfused within 24 hours; those stored between 20° C and 24° C must be transfused within 4 hours; those stored frozen must be transfused within 6 hours.

Centrifuges used in preparation of blood components must be maintained and used properly. Cups and holders should be balanced and bags overwrapped to contain spills and aerosols. Conditions of speed and time to separate components should be determined by each laboratory with the equipment in use. After calibration, speed should be checked every 3 to 4 months. Suggested guidelines can be found in the references at the end of this chapter. Continuous recording thermometers and audible alarms are required for refrigerators and freezers in which blood is stored. These must be checked periodically to assure appropriate storage of the product. Temperature records must be retained for a minimum of 1 year.

Labeling

There are precise requirements for labeling of blood and its components. These can be found in both the Code of Federal Regulations and the American Association of Blood Banks' Standards. The time of labeling is the crucial point at which all necessary checks are performed before a unit of blood is said to be suitable for transfusion. Every component must be labeled with:

1. The name of the component.
2. Identification of the collecting facility.
3. Alphanumeric or numeric identification in order to be able to subsequently trace the unit. This information may also be machine-readable. The transfusing facility can add a local number for identification, but may not remove the original number of the collecting facility.
4. Identification of the donor as either volunteer, paid, or autologous. Blood collected from autologous donors that is not suitable for homologous use for whatever reason should be labeled "For Autologous Use Only."
5. Expiration date, including day, month, and year. If the dating period is 72 hours or less, the hour must be included.
6. Storage temperature.
7. The approximate volume of the component, for whole blood, platelets, low volume red blood cells, fresh-frozen plasma, plasma, liquid plasma, pooled components, and components made by hemapheresis.
8. Except for components prepared by hemapheresis, the name of the anticoagulant and the approximate amount of blood collected.

Table 71-3 Biochemical changes of blood stored in CPD and CPDA-1

		CPD		CPDA-1			
		Whole blood		Whole blood	Red blood cells	Whole blood	Red blood cells
Variable	Days of storage:	0	21	0	0	35	35
% viable cells (24-hour posttransfusion)		100.0	80.0	100.0	100.0	79.0	71.0
pH (measured at 37°C)		7.20	6.84	7.6	7.55	6.98	6.71
ATP (% of initial value)		100.0	86.0	100.0	100.0	56.0 (±16)	45.0 (±12)
2,3-DPG (% of initial value)		100.0	44.0	100.0	100.0	<10.0	<10.0
Plasma K$^+$ (mmol/L)		3.9	21.0	4.2	5.1	27.3	78.5*
Plasma Na$^+$ (mmol/L)		168.0	156.0	169.0	169.0	155.0	111.0
Plasma hemoglobin (mg/L)		17	191	82	78	461	6580*

From Walker RH, ed.: Technical manual, ed. 10, Arlington, Va, 1990, American Association of Blood Banks.
*Values for plasma hemoglobin and potassium concentrations may appear somewhat high in 35-day stored red blood cell units; the total plasma in these units is only about 70 mL.

Table 71-4 Biochemical changes of red blood cells stored in additive systems (AS)

Variable	AS-3*		AS-1**
Days of storage	42	49	49
% Viable cells (24 hours post-transfusion)	83 ± 10	72 ± 9	76 (64-85)
ATP (% of initial value)	58	45	64
2,3-DPG (% of initial value)	<10	<15	<5.0
Plasma K$^+$ (mmol/L)	NA	NA	6.5
pH	6.5	6.4	6.6
Glucose (mmol/L)	28	27	31
% hemolysis	0.8	0.9	0.5

From Walker RH, ed.: Technical manual, ed 10, Arlington, Va, 1990, American Association of Blood Banks.
*From Simon TL.[7]
**Based on manufacturer's submission to FDA (1983)

9. ABO and Rh type and the interpretation of unexpected antibody tests when positive. For cryoprecipitated antihemophilic factor (AHF), the Rh type may be omitted. The American Association of Blood Banks' Standards does not require Rh type for liquid plasma, plasma, or fresh-frozen plasma.

10. For components intended for transfusion, instructions to the transfusionist and the following statements:

    "See circular of information for the use of human blood and blood components"

    "Caution: Federal law prohibits dispensing without prescription"

    "Properly identify intended recipient"

Certain components have special labeling requirements. Pooled components must have a unique pool number. Identification of each unit in the pool must be part of the record. The number of units in the pool must be indicated, along with its final volume. The ABO and Rh types in the pool must be indicated; if there is more than one, the label must indicate the types contained in the mixture. The label for frozen, deglycerolized, or washed red blood cells need not indicate the anticoagulant used in the original unit or the interpretation of a positive unexpected antibody test.

Additional information is necessary for autologous whole blood or red blood cells. The name of the patient, the hospital, and the date of donation may be indicated either on the container or on a tie-tag. The FDA recommends that autologous components that test positive for anti-HIV-1 or HBsAg not be used for transfusion, but may be used after receipt of a written, signed, and dated request from the patient's physician. In this circumstance, the blood should be permanently labeled with a biohazard label.

Whole blood

Blood that has not been separated into components is called whole blood. It is stored at 1° C to 6° C. The expiration date of whole blood depends on the anticoagulant-preservative solution in which it was collected. Whole blood collected in citrate-phosphate-dextrose (CPD) or acid-citrate-dextrose (ACD) has an expiration date 21 days after phlebotomy. Whole blood collected in citrate-phosphate-dextrose-adenine (CPDA-1) has an expiration date 35 days after phlebotomy. Red blood cells collected in additive systems (AS) containing saline-adenine-dextrose have an expiration date 42 days after phlebotomy. During storage, some important biochemical changes occur that are dependent on the anticoagulant-preservative in which the blood was collected. See Tables 71-3 and 71-4 for details.

There is a progressive fall in red cell adenosine triphosphate (ATP) with storage, associated with a decreased posttransfusion viability of the stored cells. The levels of 2,3-diphosphoglyceric acid (2,3-DPG) also fall with storage as the pH of stored blood drops due to red cell metabolism. Transfused blood with low 2,3-DPG levels temporarily releases less oxygen to tissues, but the levels are restored in vivo. With storage, sodium-potassium transport across the red cell membrane is slowed, and equilibration occurs. There is a resulting increase in extracellular potassium and an increase in intracellular sodium. The anticoagulant-preservative solutions used to store blood were developed in order to minimize this storage lesion. Additionally, during storage, there is progressive formation of microaggregates from senescent leukocytes, platelets, and fibrin. The significance of these is unclear. Pilot samples, either in separate tubes or as integral bag segments, must accompany the unit of whole blood or red blood cells to its final destination, for use in confirmation of ABO and Rh types, crossmatching, and investigation of adverse reactions.

Red blood cells

After plasma has been removed by centrifugation or sedimentation from a unit of whole blood, the product is known as red blood cells and must be refrigerated at 1° C to 6° C. Its expiration date is the same as the unit of whole blood from which it was separated. A portion of the plasma must be left with the red cells to ensure cell viability. The hematocrit of red blood cells should not exceed 80%.

Red blood cells may be modified by certain additive solutions, which can restore ATP and 2,3-DPG concentrations. Systems that have a second preservative in the satellite bag intended for red cells (AS-1 and AS-2, as mentioned in Table 71-4) allow longer storage of red cells in the liquid state. Rejuvenation solutions containing pyruvate, inosine, phosphate, and adenine can improve oxygen-carrying capacity of older units. The rejuvenation solution must be washed out before the unit is used for transfusion. Such units may be glycerolized and frozen, or used as washed red blood cells.

Frozen, deglycerolized, and washed red blood cells

Cryoprotectants permit frozen storage of viable red cells for many years. In freezing red blood cells, ice forms first outside the cells. As extracellular water is taken up into ice crystals, osmolality increases and water is lost from the cells, resulting in dehydration. Cryoprotectants act as an antifreeze. The optimal temperature must be maintained throughout the storage period. Washing must be performed to remove the cryoprotectant prior to transfusion. The expiration date and required storage temperature depend on the method used. Three methods of red cell freezing are compared in Table 71-5. High glycerol is the method most commonly used.

Glycerol is the cryoprotectant generally used and the final product is called red blood cells, deglycerolized. Red blood cells should be frozen within 6 days of collection, or rejuvenated before freezing. Automated cell washers are used for deglycerolization or for preparation of washed cells. Thawed red cells are initially equilibrated with a hypertonic solution, then washed with progressively less hypertonic solutions until they are finally suspended in an isotonic solution. When sickle trait cells are deglycerolized, they are equilibrated as already mentioned, but the hypertonic wash is omitted. These cells also require more wash cycles than other units. Since washing necessitates entering the closed

Table 71-5 Comparison of the three basic methods of red blood cell freezing

Consideration	High glycerol	Agglomeration	Low glycerol
Final glycerol concentration (w/v)	Approx. 40%	Approx. 40%	Approx. 20%
Initial freezing temperature	−80°C	−80°C	−196°C
Freezing rate	Slow	Slow	Rapid
Freezing rate control	No	No	Yes
Type of freezer	Mechanical	Mechanical	Liquid nitrogen
Storage temperature (maximum)	−65°C	−65°C	−120°C
Change in storage temperature	Can be thawed and refrozen	Cannot be refrozen	Critical
Type of storage container	Polyvinyl chloride; polyolefin	Polyvinyl chloride	Polyolefin
Shipping	Dry ice	Dry ice	Liquid nitrogen
Special deglycerolizing equipment required	Yes	No	No
Deglycerolizing time (minutes)	20-40	35	30
Hematocrit (%)	0.55-0.70	0.85	0.50-0.70
WBC removed (%)	94-99	80-90	95

From Walker RH, ed.: Technical manual, ed 10, Arlington, Va, 1990, American Association of Blood Banks.

Table 71-6 Leukocyte depletion of red blood cells (RBC) by filtration

Filter	Vendor	Filter material	Initial processing	Prime/flush	Final leukocyte count	% RBC recovered
Imugard	Terumo	Cotton wool	RBC	Yes	1×10^8	85
IG500			Remove 30 ml BC	Yes	5×10^6	NG
Erypur	Organon Teknika	Cellulose acetate	RBC	Yes	6.5×10^7	97
			Remove BC	Yes	$2\text{-}5 \times 10^6$	90-99
Sepacell	Asahi Fenwal	Polyester	RBC	Yes	2.6×10^6	95
R-500			Remove 30 ml BC	Yes	$0.4\text{-}1.5 \times 10^6$	75
Cellselect	NPBI	Cellulose acetate	Remove 30 ml BC	Prime	$0\text{-}11 \times 10^6$	75
Miropore	Fenwal		Remove 30 ml BC	Yes	2×10^6	—
RC100	Pall		2 U/whole blood	No	$2\text{-}5 \times 10^6$	94
			2 U RBC, no BC	No	$<1 \times 10^6$	92

Modified from Meryman HT: Transfusion-induced alloimmunization and immunosuppression and the effects of leukocyte depletion, Trans Med Rev III:188, 1989.

system, deglycerolized or washed red blood cells stored at 1° C to 6° C have a 24-hour expiration time.

Leukocyte-poor red blood cells

Leukocyte-poor red blood cells are indicated for patients with repeated or severe febrile reactions to transfusion. Recent data also suggest that alloimmunization can be prevented by the use of blood products with less than 5×10^6 residual leukocytes per transfusion. They can be prepared by a variety of methods, including centrifugation, filtration, or washing of red cells. The American Association of Blood Banks' Standards requires that leukocyte-poor red blood cells have less than 5×10^8 leukocytes in the final component and retain at least 80% of the original red cells.

Centrifugation is inexpensive and can usually be accomplished without entering the system. Unfortunately, it is the least efficient method, with residual leukocyte counts on the order of 1 to 5×10^8. Very effective leukocyte depletion at reasonable cost can be accomplished by the use of filter technology. Current commercially available filters require entry of the system, shortening the expiration to 24 hours. See Table 71-6 for comparison of these filters. The spin/cool/filter method is appropriate when leukocyte-depleted products are being used because of febrile reactions. Some of these filters allow leukocyte depletion to less than 5×10^6 residual leukocytes. Washed or deglycerolized red blood cells are leukocyte-poor, with residual leukocyte counts on the order of 10^7. Leukocyte depletion of these products must be documented during standardization of procedures at each facility. This method is much more expensive than either filters or centrifugation. However, these products are also free of plasma, which may be helpful in selected clinical situations.

Plasma and plasma components

Plasma may be prepared from whole blood or by plasmapheresis. In order to be labeled fresh frozen plasma, plasma must be separated from the red blood cells and frozen solid at $-18°$ C or below, within 6 hours of collection from the donor. Plasma contains all coagulation factors, including factors V and VIII, which are not stable at refrigerated temperatures. Fresh-frozen plasma has an expiration date of 12 months after the blood is collected. If plasma has not been separated and frozen within 6 hours, if cryoprecipitate has been removed, or if fresh-frozen plasma has not been used after 1 year of storage, it is named plasma. When refrigerated at 1° C to 6° C, liquid plasma may be stored for no more than 5 days after the expiration of the original unit of whole blood. Plasma may be stored at $-18°$ C for up to 5 years after the date of phlebotomy.

Cryoprecipitated AHF (antihemophilic factor) is the part of plasma that is insoluble when fresh-frozen plasma is thawed at 1° C to 6° C. It is produced by partially thawing fresh-frozen plasma and removing the liquid supernatant. It contains factors VIII and XIII, von Willebrand's factor, and fibrinogen. The Code of Federal Regulations requires an average of 80 units of factor VIII per unit of cryoprecipitate. Testing for other factors is not required. Cryoprecipitate must be stored at $-18°$ C or lower for not more than 12 months. 1-Deamino-8-D-arginine vasopressin (DDAVP), given to donors by either the intravenous or intranasal route,

has been shown to increase factor VIII yields in the collected plasma or cryoprecipitate. This drug has not yet been approved for this purpose in the United States by the FDA.

Platelets

Platelets may be prepared from whole blood, or they may be prepared by plateletpheresis of a single donor. Platelets are prepared from whole blood by two centrifugation steps; first, a "light" spin to separate platelet-rich plasma from red cells, and then a "heavy" spin to separate platelets from platelet-poor plasma. They must contain at least 5.5×10^{10} platelets per unit in at least 75% of the units tested. Lactic acid, as a product of metabolism, is released into the plasma in which platelets are resuspended, thereby lowering the pH progressively with storage. Platelet concentrates, regardless of the method of preparation, must be resuspended in sufficient plasma so that they have a pH of not less than 6.0 at the end of the dating period. Platelets must be stored at 20° C to 24° C with continuous agitation. The type of rotator used for storage is selected according to the bag used. The dating period depends on the ability of the container to maintain platelet viability. Bags are available with either 3-day or 5-day expiration dates. Polyvinylchloride (PVC) plasticized with dihexylethyl phthalate (DEHP) has limited ability to allow gas exchange, and therefore aerobic metabolism. Polyolefin, a thinner plastic, or PVC plasticized with other materials, allows improved gas exchange and longer storage. Platelets prepared by apheresis must contain 3.0×10^{11} platelets in at least 75% of units tested. Storage is the same as for platelets prepared from whole blood. Either an open apheresis system (with a 24-hour expiration) or a closed system (with a 5-day expiration) may be used. If at any time during a closed system procedure there is a break in the integrity of the system (including a repeat venipuncture), the platelets have a 24-hour expiration time. Platelets are particularly prone to bacterial contamination and overgrowth, since they are stored at room temperature.

Granulocytes

Granulocyte concentrates are prepared by leukapheresis of a single donor. The preferred method of collection is by continuous flow centrifugation. There must be at least 1.0×10^{10} granulocytes in at least 75% of units tested. Although granulocytes may be stored for up to 24 hours, they rapidly lose viability and should be transfused as soon as possible following collection. They should be stored at 20° C to 24° C without agitation.

Irradiation of blood components

Severely immunosuppressed recipients can develop graft-versus-host disease (GVHD) after transfusion of viable, immunocompetent lymphocytes. These lymphocytes are able to engraft, since the recipient cannot prevent it, and recognize recipient tissues as foreign. Transfusion-associated GVHD typically begins within 1 to 2 weeks after transfusion. Clinically, the patient manifests a diffuse skin rash, which progresses to erythroderma, high fever, nausea, vomiting, and diarrhea. Liver enzymes are frequently elevated, as is bilirubin. There is almost always bone marrow aplasia or severe hypoplasia. In most recognized cases, this has led to a rapidly fatal outcome within days to weeks. Further discussion of transfusion-associated GVHD may be found in Chapter 73.

Patients at highest risk are those with congenital immunodeficiencies, transplant recipients, premature neonates, fetuses receiving intrauterine transfusion, and those with aggressively treated neoplastic disease, such as leukemia and lymphoma. The only products that are known not to carry a risk of GVHD are those that are frozen without a cryoprotectant (fresh-frozen plasma, cryoprecipitate). The most efficient means of prevention is irradiation of components prior to transfusion to these recipients. A dose of 500 rads may be sufficient to abolish the ability of lymphocytes to proliferate in the mixed lymphocyte culture assay. However, higher doses are required to reduce the mitogenic response of lymphocytes; 5000 rads results in a 98.5% reduction. The results of these in vitro lymphocyte functional assays must be extrapolated with caution to the in vivo phenomenon of GVHD. With prolonged storage of red cells after irradiation, there may be some hemolysis and therefore higher plasma potassium levels. However, this has not yet been studied over the entire storage period. Platelets are relatively radioresistant. Irradiation may adversely affect granulocyte function. A dose of 1500 to 3000 rads per unit is most commonly used in order to balance optimal lymphocyte inactivation with minimal damage to the blood product. Irradiators must be monitored to ensure accurate delivery of dose and to prevent leakage. Irradiated blood has unaltered therapeutic properties under most circumstances, and may therefore be given to patients who do not require irradiated blood.

SUGGESTED READING

Code of Federal Regulations, Title 21, Parts 600 to 799, Washington, DC, 1989, U.S. Government Printing Office.

Garratty G: Should donor hemoglobin standards be lowered?: Pro, Transfusion 29:261, 1989.

Goldfinger D: Directed blood donations: Pro, Transfusion 29:70, 1989.

Insalaco SJ and Menitove JE (editors): Transfusion-transmitted viruses: epidemiology and pathology, Arlington, Va, 1987, American Association of Blood Banks.

Keating LJ: Should donor hemoglobin standards be lowered?: Con, Transfusion 29:259, 1989.

Leitman SF and Holland PV: Irradiation of blood products: indications and guidelines, Transfusion 25:293, 1985.

Meryman HT: Frozen red cells, Trans Med Rev III:121, 1989.

Meryman HT: Transfusion-induced alloimmunization and immunosuppression and the effects of leukocyte depletion, Trans Med Rev III:180, 1989.

Page PL: Directed blood donations: Con, Transfusion 29:65, 1989.

Sohmer PR and Schiffer CA (editors): Blood storage and preservation, Arlington, Va, 1982, American Association of Blood Banks.

Standards for blood banks and transfusion services, ed 13, Arlington, Va, 1989, American Association of Blood Banks.

Tegtmeier GE: The use of cytomegalovirus-screened blood in neonates (editorial), Transfusion 28:201, 1988.

Walker RH (editor): Technical manual of the American Association of Blood Banks, ed 10, Arlington, Va, 1990, American Association of Blood Banks.

72

Transfusion of blood components and fractions

Robert F. Reiss

As previously described in Chapter 71, blood components are the cellular and liquid constituents separated from whole blood by differential sedimentation or centrifugation. Recently, attempts have been initiated to inactivate viral contaminants in cellular components by exposure to ultraviolet or visible light energy and by addition of photoactive chemicals such as psoralen and merocyanine. Plasma fractions are protein constituents that have been separated by physiochemical and/or immunological means. Cohn fractionation is the classical method for separating these proteins and is based on their differential solubility in varying concentrations of ethanol at different temperatures. Further disinfection and purification of plasma and its fractions results from other processing steps, including heating, treatment with solvents and detergents, and immunoabsorption. Most recently, methods are being developed to produce selected plasma proteins by recombinant deoxyribonucleic acid (DNA) technology. Finally, nonplasma-derived volume expanders and drugs that stimulate endogenous production of various blood constituents have been introduced into clinical practice. This chapter deals with the utilization of these components and fractions.

Transfusion is undertaken for well-defined criteria of need and with an understanding of the expected therapeutic benefit. In addition, the selection of the appropriate component or fraction assumes a thorough knowledge of the contents of each component or fraction, and in the case of components, an understanding of the alterations that occur during the storage period. Lastly, transfusion must be undertaken with full appreciation of the risks involved (Chapter 73).

The intravenous administration of blood components necessitates the use of an in-line filter. For most purposes, the common 170-micron pore filter integral to most blood infusion sets is satisfactory. Microaggregate and leukocyte depletion filters should be used for well-defined clinical indications, as will be described.

The rate of infusion should be such that the component would be transfused within 3 to 4 hours. Most adult patients can safely receive one unit in one to two hours. Patients with limited cardiac reserve should be transfused slowly. In such cases, it may be preferable to divide the unit in smaller aliquots that are issued sequentially from the laboratory. Monitoring the central venous or pulmonary wedge pressures during transfusion can minimize the risk of circulatory overload in such patients. In some patients receiving large volumes of refrigerated blood, as well as in patients with cold autoagglutinins, it is appropriate to transfuse blood that has been warmed. Such warming should occur in-line during transfusion, either by passage through coils placed in a monitored 37°C waterbath or through commercially available blood heaters.

TRANSFUSION OF RED BLOOD CELLS

Red blood cell transfusion is performed to correct inadequate oxygen transport because of decreased red blood cell mass or hemoglobin concentration. Other clinical considerations merely affect the type and age of the red cell preparation administered.

Acute blood loss is the most common, and often the most urgent indication for transfusion. Correction of chronic anemia with appropriate hematinics, or treatment of the underlying disorder implicated in the causation of the anemia is usually preferable to transfusion. Transfusion may have to be undertaken in patients who are so severely symptomatic as to not tolerate continuing anemia while diagnostic studies are performed and subsequent specific therapy instituted. In such cases, all samples required for diagnosis must be drawn prior to transfusion. In addition, transfusion may be indicated for those patients whose anemia cannot be otherwise treated. The decision to perform transfusions in such individuals should depend on the adequacy of their cardiovascular function and exercise tolerance; not solely on laboratory parameters. Little objective data have ever been offered to substantiate the thesis that patients with hemoglobin levels less than 7 gm/dl should receive transfusions; that patients undergoing surgery should have hematocrits greater than 30% (patients undergoing cardiac bypass surgery with hemodilution routinely tolerate hematocrits less than 30%); or that optimal wound healing requires a similar hematocrit. Finally, exchange transfusion is performed for the treatment of several disorders, (e.g., hemolytic disease of the newborn, severe coagulopathies in neonates and infants, and certain complications of sickle-cell anemia).

1121

Red blood cell concentrates

Packed red cells separated from plasma and stored in the residual 40 to 70 ml of citrate anticoagulant-preservative, or in the added 100 ml of saline-adenine-glucose (AS) preservative solution have storage times of 35 and 42 days, respectively, as was previously described (Chapter 71).

The progressive decrease of cellular adenosine triphosphate (ATP) and consequent loss of cell viability over the storage period has relatively little importance in transfusion therapy for most patients, but is a factor that must be taken into account when planning transfusions for neonates, who have a limited capability for handling the increased bilirubin load resulting from the transfusion of senescent cells, and for the chronically transfused (e.g., patients with thalassemia, hemoglobinopathies, and aplastic anemia), who are also at risk for transfusion-associated hemosiderosis and posttransfusion infections. These special patients should be infused with fresher cells (i.e., less than 3 to 5 days old), which in some cases, should also have had nonviable cells removed (e.g., frozen-thawed red cells).

Since low levels of 2,3-diphosphoglyceric acid (2,3-DPG) cause the O_2 dissociation curve to shift to the left, concern has been expressed that massive transfusion of stored blood could be associated with tissue hypoxia. Although direct evidence to support this view is extremely limited, and it is known that transfused red cells resynthesize DPG during the 24 hours following transfusion, some prefer to infuse blood less than 7 to 10 days old when performing massive transfusions on seriously ill patients or neonates.

The potassium load that accumulates during storage usually will not result in hyperkalemia in heavily transfused individuals with normal renal function. In fact, hypokalemia has been reported, and may be related to uptake of potassium by red cells in the posttransfusion period. In patients with compromised renal function, the potassium load may be avoided by the transfusion of citrated red cells less than 7 to 10 days old, freshly washed citrated red cells, or packed cells prepared at the time of transfusion from AS-preserved red cells or whole blood.

The concurrent transfusion of citrate in citrate-preserved red cells concentrates tends to attenuate the anticipated acidosis resulting from massive transfusion with stored blood in patients with normal hepatic function, because citrate is metabolized to bicarbonate in the liver. Such an effect is especially pronounced when large amounts of whole blood are transfused, in which case metabolic alkalosis may be induced. In patients with impaired hepatic function who receive frequent transfusions, the metabolism of citrate is impaired and a progressive fall in ionized calcium level may be seen. This effect is more pronounced with whole blood transfusions.

Infusion of microaggregates in transfused stored blood and their subsequent trapping in the pulmonary microcirculation has been of considerable hypothetical concern because it had been implicated as a possible cause of respiratory insufficiency in animals receiving transfusions. Studies in humans have not conclusively demonstrated that these microaggregates are a major cause of adult respiratory distress syndrome. These theoretical concerns, however, have prompted some transfusionists to recommend the use of special microaggregate filters when infusing large volumes of stored blood over a brief period of time (e.g., 4 units in 2 to 3 hours), or when transfusing blood to patients with chronic obstructive pulmonary disease or passive congestion of the lungs. Both 20-μ and 40-μ polyester screen filters and depth filters comprised of Dacron wool, cotton wool, or nylon fibers are in wide use. Since clinical efficacy is difficult to demonstrate given the lack of evidence to support the implication of microaggregates in the causation of respiratory distress syndrome, the increased in vitro effectiveness of some depth filters in removing these aggregates must be measured against the reduced cost of the screen filter.

The different characteristics of packed red cells and whole blood make the use of packed red cells preferable to the transfusion of whole blood for many patients. The reduced volume, sodium, and albumin in citrated packed red cells are advantages when transfusing blood to patients with limited cardiac reserve. Similar benefits accrue with transfusion of AS-preserved packed red cells after removal of the preservative medium. The reduced amount of citrate present in packed cell preparations is important when transfusing patients with hepatocellular disease who would be unable to efficiently metabolize citrate. Contrary to commonly held opinion, the transfusion of routinely available packed cell concentrates does not have the advantage of reducing the potassium, lactate, ammonia, and free hemoglobin load present in whole blood. As outlined previously, it is the removal of the plasma from whole blood or the preservative solution from AS-preserved red cells at the time of transfusion that results in a packed red cell preparation depleted of these substances. Finally, the use of packed red cells is mandatory when transfusing compatible but non-ABO–identical red cells since one can reduce the quantity of passively acquired isoagglutinins contained in the transfused blood.

Concerns about the use of packed cells in routine surgery were largely predicated upon the increased viscosity and the resultant slower infusion rate of such units. The infusion time of units preserved in citrated anticoagulants can be decreased to that of whole blood by the addition of 50 to 100 ml of saline to the unit (Fig. 72-1). Units preserved with AS solutions have flow rates similar to whole blood units. Other intravenous solutions or drugs should not be added to blood because they may result in hemolysis or clotting of the unit.

Table 72-1   Granulocyte transfusion studies at the National Cancer Institute: 1972-1977

		Survival*		
		Bone marrow recovery		
Patient group	No.	Yes	No	Total
PMN† transfusion	28	11/11	13/17	24/28
Control	33	9/10	1/23	10/33

From Herzig RH: Granulocyte transfusion therapy: results of clinical trials, Proceedings of The Haemonetics Research Seminar, Boston, Mass, 1978.
*No. survivors/Total no. patients in group.
†PMN, polymorphonuclear leukocyte.

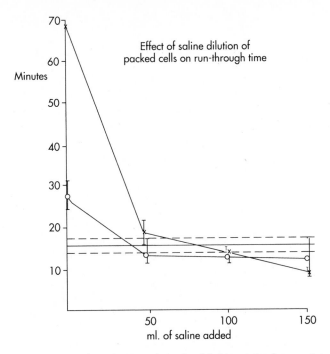

Fig. 72-1   Run-through times of platelet-rich *(x)* and platelet poor *(o)* packed red cells can be normalized by the addition of 50 ml of saline. *Redrawn from Reiss RF and Katz AJ: Microaggregate content and flow rates of packed red cells, Transfusion 17:484, 1977.*

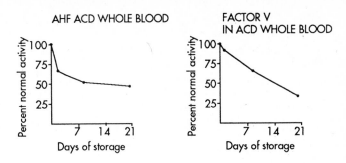

Fig. 72-2   Rates of decay of factors VIII C and V stored in ACD whole blood over 21 days of storage. *Redrawn from Huestis DW: Fresh blood: fact or fancy. In Seminar on current technical topics, American Association of Blood Banks, 117-128, 1974.*

Whole blood

Whole blood collected and stored in citrate anticoagulant-preservative solutions is the component of choice in only a few special clinical circumstances. Furthermore, prior to the selection of whole blood for transfusion, the transfusionist must consider the thesis that to make adequate amounts of other blood components available, the preferential use of packed red cells is essential. Aside from the increased volume of these preparations when compared to packed red cells due to the presence of approximately 200 to 250 ml of plasma and anticoagulant, these units contain large amounts of coagulation factors. The stable factors remain at essentially 100% of their initial activity throughout the storage period at 4°C, whereas the labile factors (V and VIII) decay at rates slower than commonly thought. Their levels remain at greater than 50% at the end of 1 week of storage (Fig. 72-2). The principle use for available whole blood is transfusion replacement of massive blood loss in order to maximize ease of transfusion and minimize the risk of dilutional coagulopathy.

Leukocyte-poor red blood cells

These concentrates had been defined as those that have been processed to contain less than 30% of the leukocytes present in the unit prior to leukodepletion while containing more than 70% of the red cells of the original unit. More recently, the American Association of Blood Banks has defined such units as those containing less than 5×10^8 leukocytes while containing more than 80% of the red cells in the original unit. A wide variety of preparations exist that meet the former criteria and several available products meet the latter criteria. Because the extent of depletion varies greatly, not

all products are equally useful for all clinical needs. Leukocyte-poor red cells were originally prepared to permit transfusion of blood to patients who suffer febrile reactions during red cell transfusion; however, their use has been expanded to the transfusion of blood to patients in whom one wishes to avoid alloimmunization to leukocyte antigens.

Among the most widespread methods in use for the production of leukocyte-poor red cells is the simple upright or inverted centrifugation of a whole blood unit with subsequent removal of both plasma and buffy coat. As previously described (Chapter 71), buffy coat depleted units contain more leukocytes (1 to 5×10^8) than units prepared by other methods; however, the degree of leukodepletion is sufficient to permit the uneventful transfusion of more than 50% of patients who previously suffered febrile reactions.

Washed red cells prepared by manual techniques have only slightly fewer leukocytes than those prepared as simple buffy coat depleted units, whereas those prepared by automated cell washers contain $<10^7$ cells. These units are considerably more expensive than simple buffy coat-depleted units. Their principle use should be as a transfusion product for patients who have had urticarial reactions resulting from the infusion of soluble allergens in the plasma of red cell units. Until recently, the reduced number of white cells in washed red cells prepared by automated techniques made such units an alternative component for those patients who continued to have febrile reactions when transfused with buffy coat-depleted red cells. The availability of less expensive and more efficient filtration methods have caused a marked reduction in the demand for washed units.

The filtration of older units of red cells through standard microaggregate filters following centrifugation to promote clumping of leukocytes and platelets has been found to be a simple way for the transfusion service laboratory to prepare a red cell unit sufficiently depleted of leukocytes to permit the transfusion of blood to most individuals with a prior history of febrile reactions without incident. As was previously described (Chapter 71), it was subsequently found that transfusion of red cells after filtration through one of the recently developed cotton wool, cellulose acetate, or polyester filters designed especially for leukofiltration in the laboratory is very effective in markedly reducing the number of leukocytes to the recipient.

With the latest in-line polyester filters, greater than 99.5% to 99.9% of the leukocytes are removed and only 1 to 5×10^6 leukocytes are found in the filtered red cells. This number of leukocytes is less than the 5 to 10×10^6 believed to be the minimum number necessary to cause alloimmunization to human leukocyte antigens (HLA) present on white cells. Clinical trials are underway to confirm the clinical effectiveness of such filtered units in preventing alloimmunization. The use of in-line filtered red cell units is also increasing in out-patient transfusion facilities in order to reduce the incidence of febrile reactions and the special management problems such reactions cause when they occur in an out-patient setting.

During the thawing and washing process required to deglycerolize frozen red cells prior to transfusion, plasma and almost all of the leukocytes, platelets, and cell debris are removed from the red cells. In addition to the use of cryo-preservation for the storage of rare red cell units, frozen, thawed red cells are the component of choice for the transfusion of blood to patients who suffer allergic reactions to ashed red cells or to sensitized IgA-deficient patients who are prone to suffer anaphylactic reactions when transfused with components containing even traces of plasma. Because of the marked depletion of leukocytes in these units, frozen red cells had been not only utilized for the transfusion of blood to patients who suffer febrile transfusion reactions with other leukocyte-poor red cell products, but had also become the preferred component for transfusion-dependent renal transplant candidates in an attempt to avoid sensitization to HLA antigens and thereby decrease the rate of allograft rejection of cadaver kidneys. The use of frozen blood for these patients declined markedly when it was observed that renal transplant recipients who had received frozen red cell transfusions had poorer allograft survivals than those who received other red cell products. Frozen red cells continue to be utilized for patients who are bone marrow transplant candidates in an attempt to prevent alloimmunization; however, with the demonstrated effectiveness of the leukocyte depletion filters and the considerable additional cost of frozen red cell units, their use to prevent alloimmunization should disappear.

Red blood cell substitutes

Recently, the introduction of recombinant human erythropoietin (rHuEPO) into clinical practice promises to reduce transfusion requirements of large numbers of patients with chronic hypoproliferative anemias and intact marrow potential. The routine use of rHuEPO in patients with chronic renal failure has had a marked impact on red cell usage by these patients. Current clinical trials are underway to evaluate the effectiveness of rHuEPO in correcting the anemia of chronic disease and other hypoproliferative anemias. In addition, its usefulness in permitting more autologous donations by patients participating in presurgical deposit plans has been proposed.

The development of oxygen-carrying volume expanders and their use as non-red cell resuscitation fluids has been an active field of research. Early promising results obtained with the experimental use of perfluorocarbons were not confirmed in clinical trials. Cross-linked purified hemoglobin solutions with prolonged intravascular half-lives and high P_{50} values show promise as clinically useful therapeutic products.

TRANSFUSION OF PLATELET CONCENTRATES

The transfusion of platelet concentrates is indicated therapy for bleeding associated with significant thrombocytopenia or platelet dysfunction, and may be indicated for the prophylactic treatment of profound thrombocytopenia without bleeding. Factors to be evaluated in deciding the need for platelet transfusion include the etiopathogenesis of the thrombocytopenia or platelet dysfunction, the degree of thrombocytopenia or dysfunction, the presence or absence of bleeding, the clinical history of the patient, and the degree of response demonstrated to previous transfusions.

In general, prophylactic platelet transfusions are utilized for patients who have hypoproliferative thrombocytopenia or platelet dysfunction due to an intrinsic cellular defect. It is anticipated that transfusion to patients with consumptive thrombocytopenia would have limited benefit because of the reduced post transfusion recovery and/or shortened circulating life span of the infused platelets. Similarly, patients with acquired extracellular causes for platelet dysfunction (e.g., renal failure, medications, paraproteinemia) will expose the transfused platelets to the same noxious environment and may render them dysfunctional.

Prophylactic transfusions are undertaken to reduce the serious risk of hemorrhage. Spontaneous hemorrhage in adults is rare with functional platelets and a count greater than $30,000/\mu l$. As previously described, with platelet counts less than $20,000/\mu l$, patients with hypoproliferative thrombocytopenia had been found to have an increased risk of bleeding that increased progressively with lowered counts (Chapter 66). At counts below $10,000/\mu l$, many hematologists have considered the risk of intracerebral bleeding to increase dramatically. For these reasons, some feel that it is imperative to transfuse platelets to patients with hypoproliferative thrombocytopenia with counts under $20,000/\mu l$, whereas most will transfuse platelets to patients with counts under $10,000/\mu l$. Recent work has shown, however, that spontaneous fecal blood loss does not increase until platelet counts under $5000/\mu l$ are reached if the patient is not infected or treated with drugs that affect platelet function. Patients with consumptive thrombocytopenia associated with increased platelet turnover (e.g., immune thrombocytopenic purpura), have a reduced relative risk of hemorrhage at very low platelet counts and should not normally be subjected to prophylactic transfusion. The degree of platelet dysfunction as reflected by in vitro testing has not been well correlated with the risk of bleeding; however, it is generally established that patients with bleeding times less than 15 minutes do not have increased risk for severe hemorrhage.

Patients who are bleeding and have significant thrombocytopenia should receive platelet transfusions. Most patients with platelet counts in excess of $50,000/\mu l$ and normal platelet function experience normal hemostasis in surgery. Bleeding in such patients will therefore usually not be halted by the infusion of platelets. Patients with consumptive thrombocytopenia should receive transfusions only in the presence of severe hemorrhage. Neonates are at a markedly increased risk for severe bleeding, including intracerebral hemorrhage, as compared to infants, older children, or adults. Patients who are septic tend to bleed at higher platelet counts than noninfected patients. Finally, patients with platelet dysfunction due to underlying disease (e.g., renal failure) or medications (e.g., aspirin, synthetic penicillins) tend to bleed at higher platelet counts than others. Individuals who have a lengthy history of thrombocytopenia without signs of bleeding may not require transfusion when equally low counts are encountered during the patients' clinical course. This is especially important when managing patients with aplastic anemia who may be bone marrow transplant candidates, and in whom alloimmunization to HLA antigens must be avoided in order to not jeopardize the engraftment of donor marrow.

Achievement of inadequate postinfusion recovery and survival of transfused platelets may indicate HLA alloimmunization of the patient if other causes for the poor response cannot be found. Once patients become alloimmunized and are refractory to transfusion of platelets from random donors, it is prudent to withhold future transfusions with incompatible platelets unless truly life-threatening bleeding occurs, as will be discussed.

The anticipated response from each of the single units of platelets separated from random units of whole blood, containing a mean of approximately 7×10^{10} platelets, is $10,000/\mu l/m^2$ BSA at 1 hour and $7500/\mu l/m^2$ BSA at 24 hours posttransfusion. Optimally, survival studies of transfused platelets would show a half-life of 4.0 to 4.5 days, a value similar to that found with autologous platelets. Good 1 hour posttransfusion recovery is deemed to be $>7500/\mu l/m2$ BSA whereas such corrected increments of $<4500/\mu l$ are considered unacceptable.

Although ABO compatible platelets may give somewhat higher postinfusion increments, the administration of ABO mismatched concentrates to most patients results in a satisfactory response. It is desirable to refrain from the transfusion of large numbers of platelet concentrates containing incompatible plasma, if possible.

Among possible reasons for inadequate postinfusion recovery and survival of transfused platelets that must be differentiated from alloimmunization are those relating to the transfusion itself and those relating to the clinical condition of the patient.

Inappropriate storage at 1°C to 6°C will markedly decrease postinfusion platelet recovery, whereas decreased numbers of platelets will be transfused if pooling or transfusion of concentrates is performed without gently agitating or rinsing the platelet bags. In addition, transfusion through some depth-type microaggregate filters will remove platelets, and their use would account for poor postinfusion recoveries.

Patients with splenomegaly will have postinfusion recoveries decreased below the expected 50% to 60%, but have normal survival of the circulating transfused platelets. Decreased survival and recovery of transfused platelets is noted in patients who are actively bleeding, febrile, or septic, or are experiencing consumptive coagulopathy.

Patients not affected by any of the aforementioned conditions, who have repeatedly inadequate 1-hour or 24-hour corrected increments, are termed refractory. According to this criterion, 30% to 70% of multiply transfused patients become refractory. It is generally assumed that they have developed antibodies directed against antigens present on the platelet surface. Although a minority of patients will be

---

Box 72-1 Donor-Recipient match categories for HLA-A and HLA-B antigens

A   Four-antigen match
B1   Three-antigen match, fourth donor antigen is unknown (B1U) or crossreactive (B1X)
B2   Two-antigen match, third and fourth donor antigens are unknown (B2U) or cross-reactive (B2X) or both (B2UX)
C   One donor antigen major mismatch
D   Two or more donor antigen major mismatch
R   Random

From Duqnesnoy RJ: Donor selection in platelet transfusion therapy of alloimmunized thrombocytopenic patients. In The blood platelet in transfusion therapy, New York, 1978, Alan R. Liss.

---

found to have inadequate increments because of ABO incompatibility, and rare patients will be sensitized to platelet-specific antigens, most refractory individuals are believed to have developed antibodies to HLA antibodies. Screening tests for cytotoxic HLA antibodies will not be found to be positive in all patients who are clinically refractory. Whenever possible, the presence of these antibodies should be demonstrated before concluding that the refractory patient has been sensitized to HLA antigens. Up to 20% to 30% of patients who receive chronic transfusions will develop such antibodies. The number of transfusions and the duration of transfusion therapy required to sensitize these patients varies greatly.

The management of refractory patients has been based upon the provision of platelets from HLA-matched donors obtained by plateletpheresis (Box 72-1). In order to be able to provide such platelet support to these myelosuppressed patients, it is important to obtain HLA typing on patients with aplastic anemia and acute leukemia at the time of diagnosis. Some also recommend that such typing also be obtained on patients with non-Hodgkin's lymphomas and selected solid tumors undergoing chemotherapy. HLA-matched donors may be sought among the patient's siblings or recruited from files of typed donors maintained by many regional blood centers. Of alloimmunized patients, 70% to 80% respond well to A or B matched platelet transfusions (Fig. 72-3). It has been proposed that matching for public HLA antigens might be more feasible and effective than classical HLA matching.

The required size of the volunteer donor pool may be less than that anticipated given the polymorphism of the HLA system, because of the nonimmunogenicity of antigens cross-reactive with those of the patient, and because HLA-C locus antigens are not present on platelets. Furthermore, HLA-A2 and many HLA-B antigens are weakly expressed on platelets and therefore the transfusion of platelets possessing these antigens may result in satisfactory increments. It is estimated that with a pool of 1500 donors, a mean of 89 (range, 1 to 334) potential satisfactory donors can be found for a given refractory patient.

Clinical studies are underway to determine if the selection of compatible platelets by cross-matching will result in rates of satisfactory posttransfusion increments comparable to

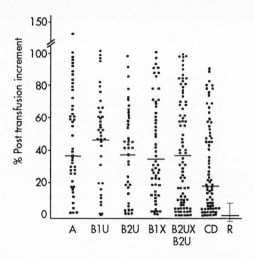

Fig. 72-3 Recoveries of platelets 24 hours after infusion into alloimmunized thrombocytopenic patients, according to degree of histocompatibility. *R* indicates response to random pooled platelets.*Redrawn from Duquesnoy RJ: Donor selection in platelet transfusion therapy of alloimmunized thrombocytopenic patients. In The blood platelet in transfusion therapy, New York, 1978, Alan R Liss.*

those seen with selecting donors on the basis of HLA type.

It has been determined that some refractory patients have improved responses if transfused with ABO-compatible platelets. Suggestions to the effect that improved recovery and survival can be seen in refractory patients if platelet concentrates depleted of leukocytes are transfused has not been substantiated.

Selected refractory patients without available HLA-compatible donors have been managed on a long-term basis with ε-amino-caproic acid, as such treatment has been suggested to prevent or reduce bleeding in severely thrombocytopenic patients. The mechanism of action is not understood. It has also been suggested that bleeding emergencies in these refractory patients will sometimes be successfully managed by the infusion of a large bolus of incompatible platelets administered following either a slow platelet infusion designed to absorb the circulating HLA antibodies, or reduction of antibody titer by plasmapheresis or immunoabsorbtion. In some research centers, patients with acute leukemia in remission are subjected to plateletpheresis, and their harvested platelets are stored frozen for future transfusion.

The prevention of alloimmunization to HLA antigens in patients undergoing long-term transfusion support is an area of continuing investigation. In general, the provision of HLA-matched patients to nonsensitized myelosuppressed patients is not logistically feasible. Some data have suggested that the provision of random single donor platelets obtained by apheresis techniques may delay the onset of the refractory state. Others have found that the provision of cellular transfusion products depleted of leukocytes, including the antigen-preventing cells that have been found to be critical to the immunization process, will prevent sensitization. Such leukodepletion is most easily achieved by filtration of red cells and pools of platelet concentrates with available leukodepletion filters. The residual numbers of leukocytes in these products can be reduced to the range of 1 to 5 $\times$ 10^6, which is below the level thought to be required for sensitization. Finally, it has been shown that ultraviolet irradiation of platelet concentrates may impair the immunogenicity of the contained leukocytes. Studies are underway to evaluate the efficacy of ultraviolet irradiation in preventing sensitization and to compare it to filtration methodologies.

TRANSFUSION OF GRANULOCYTES

The major cause of death in severely myelosuppressed patients is infection. The rate of infection increases dramatically as the granulocyte count falls under 500/μl. Patients with acute leukemia and documented infection, especially gram-negative sepsis, were found to have improved survival rates when they received transfusions of granulocyte concentrates in addition to appropriate antibiotics and supportive care (Table 72-1). Candidates for granulocyte transfusions should have documented or strongly suspected infections not responsive to treatment with appropriate antibodies for at least 48 to 72 hours and a granulocyte count <500/μl. Some refrain from transfusion of granulocytes until the granulocyte count falls below 100/μl or 200/μl. The minimum daily effective dose of granulocytes obtained from single donors by apheresis techniques is considered to be 1 $\times$ 10^{10}. Treatment is usually continued until 48 hours past the clinical resolution of the infection or recovery of the granulocyte count to greater than 500/μl. The effectiveness of therapy is determined exclusively by clinical response because a posttransfusion increment in circulating leukocytes is generally not seen. With the development of modern antibiotic treatment, the use of granulocyte transfusions for patients with aplastic anemia or with myelosuppression due to chemotherapy has all but disappeared in many major medical centers.

As opposed to the decreasing use of granulocytes for replacement therapy in septic granulocytopenic patients with aplastic anemia and postchemotherapy hypoplasia, the transfusion of granulocytes to septic neutropenic neonates has tended to become standard therapy. Sepsis in neonates carries with it an overall mortality rate of 20%, whereas premature infants with neutropenia have up to a 50% mortality rate. There is strong evidence that transfusion of 1 to 2 $\times$ 10^9 neutrophils/kg to these infants results in significantly reduced mortality.

TRANSFUSION OF PLASMA COMPONENTS

Once frozen, the procoagulant activities of all factors in fresh-frozen plasma (FFP) are maintained for up to 1 year. Since factors V and VIII both are labile with storage at refrigerated temperatures, liquid plasma and plasma frozen after liquid storage are products that cannot be utilized as sources of these two factors.

The infusion of plasma components should be undertaken for the treatment of clinically significant mixed coagulopathies with bleeding, or single factor deficiencies for which lyophilized pooled concentrates are not available (e.g., factor V or XI deficiencies). In addition, the infusion of fresh-frozen plasma is currently considered to be critical to the induction of remission in patients with thrombotic thrombocytopenia purpura. Finally, patients with protein C or antithrombin III deficiencies may be successfully treated with plasma. The infusion of plasma components for volume expansion is inappropriate, given the infectious and other risks involved and the availability of safer plasma fractions (i.e., albumin and plasma protein fraction) and synthetic expanders (e.g., hydroxyethyl starch).

Since the level of the various procoagulants in each unit of plasma varies from donor to donor, and the postinfusion recovery of the transfused factors vary, the methods of determining dosage are empirical. In general, approximately 10 ml/kg is administered, and the clinical response (e.g., cessation of bleeding) and the correction of coagulation screening tests is confirmed. The ability to administer adequate amounts of plasma to patients with severe coagulopathies is sometimes limited by the volume of plasma that can be safely administered in a brief period of time. The central venous or pulmonary wedge pressure is helpful in monitoring the volume of plasma infused. Patients with an extremely limited intravascular reserve may require partial exchange transfusion with the plasma in order to administer adequate volume.

The frequency of transfusion for the correction of coagulopathies should be determined by the in vivo half-lives of the various procoagulants. In this regard, it is useful to recall that the half-life of factor VII may be as short as 4 to 6 hours. This explains the futility of attempting to maintain a normal prothrombin time in cases of severe hepatocellular disease.

In general, plasma is over transfused. Prophylactic transfusion in most patients with mixed coagulopathies is not able to fully correct the abnormalities, and the correction seen is often very transitory. Because of the striking patient-to-patient variation in rates of procoagulant synthesis and relatively low levels of clotting factors required for hemostasis, the use of empiric formulas relating the need for plasma infusion to units of blood transfused to prevent dilutional coagulopathy are generally inappropriate.

TRANSFUSION OF CRYOPRECIPITATE

Cryoprecipitate is rich in factor VIII C (approximately 80 to 100 u/bag), von Willebrand's factor (vWF equivalent to the quantity of factor VIII C), fibrinogen (approximately 200 mg/bag), and large amounts of both factor XIII and fibronectin.

The principle clinical use of cryoprecipitate is the replacement therapy of patients with von Willebrand's disease, in which infusion not only corrects the ristocetin agglutination defect and shortens the bleeding time of these patients, but also may cause a sustained rise of procoagulant activity by the increased endogenous synthesis and stabilization of the VIII C molecule. The calculation of dosage for patients with moderate to severe von Willebrand's disease is 10 to 15 units of factor VIII/kg/day in divided doses every 12 hours. Larger doses may be required for major surgery and severe bleeding. The infusion of cryoprecipitate may often be avoided in patients with mild to moderate type I disease in whom administration of desmopressin acetate (DDAVP) induces the release of vWF and subsequent synthesis and stabilization of factor VIII C.

Cryoprecipitate has been also transfused to selected patients with moderate and severe hemophilia A, in whom no markers to indicate exposure to hepatitis have yet appeared. In such patients without inhibitors, cryoprecipitate raises the factor VIII C procoagulant level in a predictable manner. Following transfusion of the initial dose (Box 72-2), the factor VIII C activity decays with a half-life of 8 to 12 hours. Subsequent doses are calculated to maintain the desired level of factor VIII C activity, and are usually half the original dose administered every 8 hours. With the increasing safety of current factor VIII concentrates, the use of cryoprecipitate for hemophiliac patients will decline even further.

The transfusion of cryoprecipitate as a source of fibrinogen is restricted to rare patients with afibrinogenemia, dysfibrinogenemia, or mixed coagulopathies with disproportionate hypofibrinogenemia. In addition, cryoprecipitates have been used to manufacture fibrin glue for intraoperative use by the addition of bovine thrombin to the cryoprecipitate.

Cryoprecipitate has been used experimentally in other clinical situations. Because of the opsonizing properties of its contained fibronectin, cryoprecipitate had been used in the treatment of trauma patients with sepsis. Similarly, reports that cryoprecipitate infusions were able to reverse platelet dysfunction in uremic patients, and the suspicion that the contained large multimers, vWF, were responsible for this effect, eventually led to the use of DDAVP for this purpose.

COAGULATION FACTOR CONCENTRATES

Two major lyophilized procoagulant protein concentrates prepared from large pools of donor plasma are commercially available. Efforts continue to prepare these proteins by DNA recombinant technology. These two preparations are factor IX or prothrombin complex concentrates, containing the vitamin K-dependent factors II, VII, IX, and X, and factor VIII concentrates. Because of the incidence of posttransfusion infections and other complications associated with these fractions, various previously described procedures have been incorporated into the manufacturing process to reduce their incidence and severity.

Factor IX or prothrombin complex concentrates are principally utilized in the management of patients with hemophilia B; in the rare patients with factor II, VII, or X deficiency; and in selected patients with severe overdoses of coumarin-type drugs. These concentrates carried with them a high risk of posttransfusion hepatitis and human immu-

---

Box 72-2 Calculation of dosage: factor VIII C in cryoprecipitate

Patient data: 70-kg man with 10% factor VIII C activity
Treatment goal: Raise activity to 50%
Factor VIII C content in cryoprecipitate: 80 units/bag
Calculation of plasma volume: 70 kg $\times$ 40 ml/kg = 2800 ml
Calculation of dose:
  2800 ml $\times$ .40 = 1120 units
  1120 $\div$ 80 = 14 bags of cryoprecipitate

nodeficiency virus (HIV) infection. All currently marked products are heat-treated to reduce their infectivity. There is evidence that these heat-treated concentrates may not be infectious for the HIV-1 virus, but still are capable of transmitting hepatitis C (non-A, non-B hepatitis). In addition, some activated coagulation factors may be present in lots of these concentrates. They are thought to be a cause of the thrombogenicity noted with their infusion in some patients. Lots with larger amounts of these activated factors, which apparently bypass the requirement for factor VIII in the activation of factor X, have been utilized to induce hemostasis in hemophilia A patients with moderately high titer factor VIII inhibitors. More recently, the routinely prepared lots of factor IX concentrates have been found to contain bypassing activity as well.

Factor VIII concentrates have been used exclusively for the management of hemophilia A. Preparations prepared from cryoprecipitate and processed by most methods contain low levels of von Willebrand activity. Recently, it has been reported that pasteurized factor VIII concentrates do possess large amounts of high molecular weight vWF multimers and can be utilized in replacement therapy of patients with von Willebrand's disease.

Those concentrates that have been subjected to heat treatment after drying are reported to be capable of transmitting hepatitis C; however, those that have undergone disinfection with solvent-detergent methods, or purified by absorption with monoclonal antibody columns are reported to be free of viral contaminants.

Patients with low-level factor VIII inhibitors may be treated effectively with increased doses of factor VIII concentrate. Porcine factor VIII concentrates have been utilized in the management of patients with high titer inhibitors. As previously mentioned, lots of factor IX concentrates containing inhibitor bypassing activity are commonly utilized in the management of hemophilia A patients with moderately high titer antibodies. Finally, clinical trials continue on the induction of tolerance in patients with inhibitors by the long-term administration of large doses of factor VIII concentrates.

INFUSION OF ALBUMIN SOLUTIONS

Albumin solutions for infusions are available as a partially purified plasma protein fraction (PPF) and more purified albumin fractions.

Plasma protein fraction is prepared by the coprecipitation of fractions IV and V from pools of plasma subjected to Cohn fractionation. It consists of at least 83% albumin and less than 17% globulins, of which not more than 1% may be gamma globulin. Albumin solutions are prepared from fraction V and must be at least 96% albumin and less than 4% globulin. Both products undergo heat treatment for viral inactivation (60°C for 10 hours) after the addition of sodium caprylate and sodium acetyl tryptophanate for protein stabilization. These derivatives do not transmit hepatitis or other viral illnesses.

Five percent albumin in saline and PPF solutions are utilized for simple volume replacement in patients when use of colloids rather than crystalloids is desired. The use of albumin rather than PPF is preferred by many because of the occurrence of hypotensive episodes that have been reported to be related to the presence of bradykinin in the frac-

tion that was formed from kininogen during heat treatment.

Twenty-five percent albumin solutions are utilized for the correction of acute hypoalbuminemia in order to maintain an acceptable plasma oncotic pressure of 20 mmHg, and for the mobilization of extravascular edema fluid in selected cases of adult respiratory distress syndrome. Utilization for protein replacement in patients with undernutrition, chronic nephrotic syndromes, or cirrhosis is considered unjustified.

It has been reported that expenditures for albumin may constitute up to 20% of pharmacy budgets and that most of the albumin used has been infused inappropriately. Clearly, guidelines for usage should be established and compliance monitored closely.

ADMINISTRATION OF GAMMA GLOBULIN

Gamma globulin concentrates are prepared from Cohn fraction II, and are subsequently heated to 60°C. Concentrates for either intramuscular or intravenous administration are now available.

The administration of immune serum immunoglobulin (ISG) preparations have been utilized for replacement in hypogammaglobulinemia patients. Following an initial dose of 0.25 gm/kg, maintenance doses of 0.025 gm/kg/week are administered.

Recently, the intravenous infusion of large doses of IgG has been shown to be effective in rapidly raising the platelet count of patients with idiopathic thrombocytopenic purpura (ITP) who are bleeding or who must be prepared for surgery. Most commonly, infusions of 400 mg/kg/day for 5 days are administered. The effects are transitory, but permit hemostasis in the bleeding or surgical patient who has not responded to more conservative measures. It is unclear whether or not this effect is related to retriculoendothelial blockade or the infusion of anti-idiotype antibodies. The usefulness of infusion of large doses of IgG for other immune disorders (e.g., autoimmune hemolytic anemia) is undocumented.

Hyperimmune gamma globulin preparations are now available for the passive immunization of patients at risk who have been exposed to hepatitis B, measles, tetanus, herpes zoster, rabies, and cytomegalovirus. Immune serum globulin (ISG) is also effective in the prevention of hepatitis A. Its efficacy as prophylaxis for hepatitis C has not been proven. The utilization of Rh immune globulin for the prevention of maternal sensitization of Rh(D)-negative mothers by their Rh-(D) positive fetuses has been previously discussed.

Risks associated with the infusion of immunoglobulin preparations are minimal. Documented transmission of infectious agents with currently prepared products has not been reported. The passive transfer of antibodies present in immunoglobulin concentrates has resulted in occasional instances of positive direct Coombs' tests due to red cell antibodies, or in transitory positive tests for antibodies to various infectious diseases.

QUALITY ASSURANCE AND TRANSFUSION PRACTICE

With the increasing awareness of the significant risks associated with transfusion of blood components and fractions, and the limited supplies of these products, quality assurance programs to encourage that blood products are used for appropriate clinical indications, at minimum doses that offer patients optimal benefit, are a requirement placed on the institution by the Joint Commission on Accreditation of Health Organizations (JCAHO).

The director of the transfusion service, transfusion committee, and the quality assurance group, as well as the clinicians themselves are responsible for the implementation and conduct of a comprehensive program. Such a program has as its goals the elimination of transfusion for inappropriate clinical indications, the reduction of excess transfusions, the documentation of the clinical benefit from transfusion, the education of the patient as to the risks and benefits of transfusion, the assurance of provision of an adequate blood supply in a timely manner, the minimization of blood wastage, and the reduction of the risks associated with required transfusions. Critical facets of this program are described in the text that follows.

Constitution of an effective hospital transfusion committee

The transfusion committee is responsible to the medical board and is charged with the task of recommending policies for optimal transfusion practice, reviewing the quality of both transfusion practice and operation of the blood bank or transfusion service, and assisting the director, both in implementing programs and in obtaining required resources.

The size and composition of the committee is dependent on the size and characteristics of the hospital and the services it offers. As a minimum, the director of the blood bank or transfusion service, senior representatives of the major clinical services (surgery, medicine, obstetrics and gynecology, and pediatrics), and appropriate representatives of the hospital administration should comprise the committee's membership. Large centers offering subspeciality services that are heavy consumers of blood components and laboratory services (e.g., neonatology, cardiothoracic surgery, and oncology), should also represent these services. Finally, it may be appropriate to include the laboratory supervisor and a representative of the regional blood center as ex officio members. Acceptance of the policies and quality assurance decisions adopted by the committee is usually facilitated if the committee chairperson is not the director of the blood bank or transfusion service.

Among the specific tasks that the transfusion committee undertakes are: (1) creation of criteria for blood utilization and audit review; (2) performance of utilization audits; (3) review and approval of the maximum surgical blood order schedule; (4) review and interpretation of blood use, wastage, and laboratory workload statistics; (5) review of the timeliness and quality of laboratory and clinical services offered; (6) monitoring that proper transfusion procedures are followed, including patient identification and completion of transfusion documentation; and (7) review of severe transfusion reactions. In order to adequately fulfill these tasks, the committee must meet at least quarterly, and larger institutions should meet more often.

Indications for appropriate blood use and utilization audits

Indications for the appropriate usage of blood, components, and in many institutions, plasma fractions, are written and promulgated by the director of the transfusion service and

members of the transfusion committee together with user consultants. They should be reviewed by the chiefs of services, and then distributed to all attending physicians, house staff, and nursing units. Many institutions have found the National Institutes of Health Consensus Statements to be of great assistance in drafting a document outlining appropriate indications for component use. Included in this document must be instructions on the proper documentation of the rationale for transfusion and the results of the treatment.

Once written and disseminated, the transfusion committee must decide on the appropriate mechanism for auditing medical practice and utilization. In some institutions this responsibility may be shared with the quality assurance group, whereas in others, the transfusion committee assumes the entire responsibility.

It is currently required by certain review organizations that all transfusions be reviewed until it is demonstrated that the disseminated guidelines for blood product use are generally followed. Subsequently, a representative fraction of transfusions must be reviewed in order to demonstrate continued compliance. In small institutions, the physician members of the transfusion committee may be able to review all transfusions utilizing the guidelines as written. In most institutions, however, audit of transfusions is performed by nonphysician reviewers in the medical records, quality assurance, or laboratory departments. Only those transfusions that do not comply with established guidelines for the use of blood components are referred to the transfusion committee for peer review.

In order to enable nonphysician reviewers to expeditiously examine the medical records and carry out this retrospective audit, simple criteria must be established that enable the reviewer to easily interpret guidelines and identify essential data in the patient chart or laboratory records. Such audit criteria are usually organized into three sections: elements of the criteria, exceptions to the criteria, and instructions and definitions (Table 72-2). In some large centers, paraprofessional staff may do preliminary screening reviews. In these cases, further organization of easily researched audit criteria into a decision tree format may be useful.

The maximum surgical blood order schedule

In order to encourage thoughtful surgical transfusion practice, minimize the required blood inventory, and reduce the outdating and wastage of blood, the director of the transfusion service and the transfusion committee should review historical blood utilization for various surgical procedures and criteria for red cell utilization with representatives of surgical specialty sections, and then agree on the number of units of blood that can reasonably be expected to be transfused in procedures performed in that institution. From these consultations, an agreed upon maximum surgical blood order schedule should be written and utilized as a guide for ordering by surgeons. According to this schedule, only a type and screen procedure need be performed and no blood crossmatched for those surgeries that only infrequently require transfusion, if the patient has a negative antibody screen (Table 72-3). Acceptance of a type and screen procedure in lieu of crossmatching is dependent upon the provision of blood in a timely manner in case of sudden need. Timely provision may require release of blood without a full Coombs' crossmatch or entirely without any cross-

Table 72-2 Elements of audit: red blood cell transfusion in adults

Elements	Exceptions	Instructions and definitions

Justification for transfusion of red cells into adults
1. Hypovolemia due to surgery, trauma, gastrointestinal, or other blood loss documented by *one* of the following:
  a. fall in blood pressure >20%, *or*,
  b. fall in systolic blood pressure to <100 mmHg, *or*
  c. pulse >100 per minute, *or*,
  d. 750 ml or greater estimated blood loss, *or*,
  e. orthostatic change in blood pressure or pulse.
	None	1-3a. Progress notes, admissions notes, operative notes, anesthesia record, laboratory data, or graphic vital sign sheet must document one of the criteria. Subsequent notes or laboratory data *must* reflect clinical response (correction of abnormal parameter toward normal *and* document a follow-up hemoglobin or hematocrit value).

2. Symptomatic anemia, whatever the cause, if no other medicinal therapy (iron, folate, vitamin B$_{12}$, etc.) or surgical therapy (splenectomy, repair of site, etc.) has or is likely to correct the anemic state.	None	b. Admission note or progress notes *must* document indication for transfusion (i.e., symptoms of anemia other than in 1-3a above, tachypnea or angina pectoris or fatigue on minimal exertion or dyspnea at rest).
3. Anemia requiring correction prior to anesthesia (hematocrit less than 27% or hemoglobin less than 9 g per dl).	None	c. Record *must* reflect that transfusion is the preferred form of therapy as opposed to medicinal or surgical therapy or in addition to those therapies. Record *must* also document follow-up hemoglobin or hematocrit value *and* clinical response. d. A statement that no acute complications occurred *must* be in the record.

From Simpson M: Audit criteria for transfusion practices. In The hospital transfusion committee, Washington, DC, 1982, American Association of Blood Banks.

Table 72-3 Maximum surgical blood order schedule*

GENERAL SURGERY

Aneurysm resection	6
Breast biopsy	T/S
Colon resection	2
Exploratory laparotomy	4
Femoropopliteal bypass	T/S
Hernias	T/S
Mastectomy—radical	1
Pancreatectomy	4
Splenectomy	2
Thyroidectomy	T/S

GYNECOLOGY

AP repair	1
D & C	T/S
Hysterectomy—Abdominal	T/S
Radical	2

OBSTETRICS

C-Section—Hysterectomy	2
C-Section	T/S
L & D Admission	T/S

THORACIC-CARDIAC

Bypass procedures	
Adult	6
Children	4

VASCULAR

Aortic bypass	6
Endarterectomy	1
Renal artery repair	6

ORTHOPEDICS

Arthroscopy	T/S
Laminectomy	3
Spinal fusion	8
Total hip	5
Total knee	T/S

UROLOGY

Prostatectomy	
Perineal	2
Transurethral	T/S
Renal Transplant	2
TUR	T/S

From Sharpe MA: Inventory management. In *Selecting policies and procedures for the transfusion service*, Washington, DC, 1982, American Association of Blood Banks.
*AP, Anterior and posterior repair; D & C, dilation and curettage; C-section, cesarean section; L & D, labor and delivery; TUR, transurethral resection.

match. In such cases, the director of the transfusion service must be willing to assume responsibility for the provision of such blood. A requirement for the surgeon to sign a release for uncrossmatched blood may undermine compliance with the maximum surgical blood order (MSBO) schedule.

Documentation of transfusion practice

Written documentation is required of all steps in the ordering and transfusion of blood components. Such documentation must be sufficient to create a paper trail that identifies the patient; the physician who orders the product; the degree of urgency of the transfusion (emergent, stat, routine); the indication for transfusion; the consent of the patient to be transfused; the completion of appropriate pretransfusion tests on the component utilized and the patient; the source of the units released; the initiation of transfusion to the properly identified recipient; the documentation of completion of transfusion; and finally, the result of the transfusion and any complications of the transfusion encountered. Following transfusion, complete records must be kept of the evaluation of any reported transfusion reaction or transfusion-transmitted infection. These records are required to be held for a minimum of 5 years according to the recommendation of the American Association of Blood Banks and the Code of Federal Regulations. Local regulations may require more prolonged storage of such records. Increasingly, records are kept many years after transfusion for legal purposes and to trace the recipients of blood components donated by individuals who subsequently develop acquired immune deficiency syndrome (AIDS) or other infectious diseases.

Further documentation of both compliance with transfusion policy and protocol and adequacy of laboratory support can be obtained by maintaining the following statistical data: (1) number of inadequate samples and or incomplete order forms; (2) number of emergent or stat requests and the turnaround time for their supply; (3) number of units outdated in the laboratory or wasted by clinical staff after release for transfusion; (4) the crossmatch-to-transfusion ratio, which reflects compliance with ordering according to the agreed-upon MSBO schedule (it is generally agreed that such a ratio should be in the range of 1.5 to 2.5 and may vary according to the characteristics of individual transfusing facilities); (5) number of single red cell unit transfusions (although there may be legitimate clinical rationales for the transfusion of a single unit, some review organizations persist in requiring that this data be maintained); and (6) number of inappropriate blood transfusions, as determined by audit review. In larger institutions, such data are best maintained according to clinical division so that it may be more easily analyzed by both the transfusion committee and, when appropriate, by departmental chiefs.

In addition to the aforementioned records, the laboratory staff should maintain appropriate workload statistics that will enable them to both document ongoing personnel needs and plan for the distribution of work or staff.

SUGGESTED READING

Code of Federal Regulations: Additional standards for human blood and blood products, Part 640, Washington, DC, 1990, U.S. Government Printing Office.

Consensus Development Conference Statement: Fresh frozen plasma: indications and risks, Bethesda, Md, 1984, National Institutes of Health.

Consensus Development Conference Statement: Perioperative red cell transfusion, Bethesda, Md, 1988, National Institutes of Health.

Consensus Development Conference Statement: Platelet transfusion therapy, Bethesda, Md, 1986, National Institutes of Health.

Kahn RA, Allen RW, and Baldassare J: Alternate sources and substitutes for therapeutic blood components, Blood 66:1, 1985.

Kim HC: Red blood cell transfusion in the neonate, Perinatol 7:159, 1983.

Simpson M: Audit criteria for transfusion practices in the hospital transfusion committee, Arlington, Va, 1982, American Association of Blood Banks.

Slichter SJ: Prevention of platelet alloimmunization. In Transfusion medicine: recent technological advances, New York, 1986, Alan R. Liss.

Tullis JL: Albumin 1. Background and use, JAMA 237:355, 1977.

Tullis JL: Albumin 2. Guidelines for clinical use, JAMA 237:460, 1977.

73 Complications of blood transfusion

Harold S. Kaplan

Transfusion therapy, like any other therapy, incurs both risks and benefits. Although the risks are usually outweighed by the benefits of transfusion, they underscore the importance of rational transfusion decisions. This chapter reviews the major complications of transfusion therapy and their prevention and management.

Different estimates suggest that an adverse reaction is detectable in 0.5% to 4.0% of all transfusions (independent of transfusion-transmitted disease). Different criteria of reaction, such as degrees of fever, as well as the diligence of observation, reporting, and recording, are some of the factors contributing to this variability in occurrence. Regardless of the exact number, the majority of these adverse effects or reactions are benign and self-limited. The primary concern is to ascertain as quickly as possible whether or not a suspect reaction is potentially life-threatening.

IMMUNOLOGIC COMPLICATIONS

Immunologic complications include observable transfusion reactions to red cells and other components, alloimmunization to red cells and other antigens that may complicate future transfusion therapy, immune suppression of the recipient, and graft vs. host disease.

Hemolytic transfusion reactions

Acute hemolytic transfusion reactions

Hemolytic transfusion reactions (HTR) are the main concern in transfusions compromised by red cell incompatibility. The transfused components may contain incompatible red cells or, less commonly, incompatible plasma. The Mayo Clinic, during the period from 1978 to 1980, documented that immediate hemolytic reactions occurred at a rate of 1/17,000 transfusions. A fatal HTR occurs once in a million transfusions, as estimated on the basis of mandatory reporting of transfusion-related fatalities to the Food and Drug Administration (FDA). ABO mismatches caused by, or following, clerical errors are responsible for the majority of these fatal reactions.

Acute hemolytic reactions may involve predominantly intravascular or extravascular hemolysis. Antibodies that are hemolytic in vitro are most likely to cause HTR. Anti-A and anti-B antibodies are ubiquitous, potent, and lytic, and are the most frequent causes of acute intravascular HTR. Anti-Jk^a antibodies, although less impressive in vitro, may

also cause dramatic intravascular red cell destruction.

Some of the possible symptoms of an acute intravascular HTR present in an alert patient include complaints of dyspnea, a burning sensation in the vein used for transfusion, flank pain, back pain, headache, fever and chills, and apprehension. In an anesthetized surgical patient, these signals of HTR cannot be detected. Shock, hemoglobinuria, and/or unexplained bleeding may be the only clues to a hemolytic reaction in the surgical patient, although other causes may be responsible. Increased bleeding and hypotension may result in the further transfusion of incompatible blood.

The mechanisms by which antigen-antibody reactions initiate the endocrine, coagulation, and complement changes leading to shock and the other serious effects of HTR are not completely understood. However, activation of complement by lytic antibodies is thought to play an important role, along with activation of the coagulation cascade leading to disseminated intravascular coagulation and the release of vasoactive amines.

Even in the case of ABO incompatibility, the majority of red cell destruction may be extravascular rather than intravascular. In the case of most other antibodies, the red cell removal is extravascular, although hemoglobinemia may occur. More typically, this slower process, involving removal by the reticuloendothelial system (RES), results in bilirubinemia rather than hemoglobinemia, and is generally less dramatic and less threatening. Typically, red cells coated with IgG and/or C3b are removed by the RES. The spleen is the primary site of RES removal of the sensitized red cells. The liver is another major RES site of red cell removal, especially when the cells carry large amounts of bound antibody and complement.

A direct relationship exists between the volume of incompatible blood transfused and the severity of outcome in an HTR. Therefore, it is critical to interrupt each suspect transfusion and suspend further transfusion until any question of incompatibility is resolved.

Initial steps in the investigation of suspected transfusion reactions

1. After interrupting the transfusion, check for clerical error. The clerical check quickly establishes whether or not an obvious clerical error has occurred. Was a component of the correct blood type given to the intended recipient?

2. Next, check for hemolysis by visual inspection of a centrifuged sample. Although not all immediate transfusion reactions result in visible hemolysis, hemolysis in the bloodstream of as little as 5 ml of red cells will give a pink tinge to plasma. Visual inspection of plasma or serum is a sensitive means of detecting hemolysis. Hemoglobinemia can be reliably detected, all the way from the pink tinge of plasma with 20 mg/dl of hemoglobin, to the clearly red color of plasma with 100 mg/dl of hemoglobin.

3. Finally, test the red cells of this sample for serological incompatibility by direct antiglobulin testing. This will be found positive in cases of acute hemolytic reactions involving extravascular hemolysis.

These are the important initial steps. In addition, confirming the ABO group of the donor segment and the post-transfusion recipient sample should provide a reasonable level of confidence that red cell incompatibility is not the cause of the reaction.

Clinical circumstances may not allow for complete diagnostic satisfaction before initiating therapy. However, other indications and measures of hemolysis, including haptoglobin determinations, hemoglobinuria, hemosiderinuria, and bilirubin determinations may be of importance in individual cases.

Additional tests and evidence of hemolytic transfusion reaction

1. Haptoglobin levels. Hemoglobin released into the plasma is bound to the plasma protein, haptoglobin. Haptoglobin binds hemoglobin dimers in a one-to-one ratio. This hemoglobin-haptoglobin complex is cleared by the reticuloendothelial system and is not excreted by the kidneys. The resultant fall in haptoglobin may be a useful measure of hemolysis.

2. Hemoglobinuria. Saturation of haptoglobin occurs at about 100 to 150 mg/dl. When this binding capacity is exceeded, free hemoglobin appears in the plasma. If free hemoglobin reaches levels of 25 mg/dl in the plasma, it is excreted in the urine, resulting in hemoglobinuria. Visual examination of the urine is an easy and rapid way of detecting hemoglobinuria. It is not usually necessary to use dipsticks to detect hemoglobinuria, because their increased sensitivity, particularly in the presence of hematuria, may lead to spurious results. Confusion of hematuria with hemoglobinuria frequently causes investigation of a spurious HTR. Simply centrifuging the urine and demonstrating a button of red blood cells in the bottom of the tube along with a clear supernatant quickly differentiates the "red" urine of hematuria from hemoglobinuria. Hematuria is, of course, not a sign of hemolysis nor of an acute HTR.

3. Hemosiderinuria. Some of the hemoglobin reabsorbed by the renal tubules is stored as iron and hemosiderin in the tubule cells. At free plasma hemoglobin levels between 25 and 50 mg/dl, hemosiderinuria may appear in the urine several days following a hemolytic event. Its appearance may allow documentation of hemolysis in cases in which such verification was not done at the time of its occurrence.

4. Serum bilirubin determinations. Bilirubin, a product of hemoglobin catabolism, may appear in the plasma at a maximum level in about 3 to 6 hours following red cell destruction. Its presence may persist for several hours after the clearance of any hemoglobin released into the plasma. The slow rate of bilirubin's release into the plasma and its excretion are, in general, balanced. Plasma bilirubin levels do not rise as dramatically as the amount of red cell destruction might suggest.

Since the fatality associated with HTR is usually intractable hypotensive shock, aggressive treatment of the hypotension is vital. Vigorous efforts to maintain renal flow with diuretics and careful hydration to prevent irreversible renal tubular damage are also essential. Even though renal failure is not the usual cause of death in HTR, it is of major importance.

Delayed hemolytic transfusion reaction

Red cell incompatibility may cause a delayed hemolytic reaction following transfusion to a sensitized patient with antibody undetected by routine compatibility tests. Such delayed reactions have been referred to as "sleeping" incompatibilities. They may occur as often as 1/1500 units transfused. These reactions are more frequently observed in individuals who receive multiple transfusions and in women who have had multiple pregnancies. The detection of delayed reactions is closely related to the diligence with which they are sought. The majority go undetected. Transfused red cells provide the antigenic stimulus for an anamnestic reaction. The secondary antibody response may be very rapid and, in some cases, result in intravascular hemolysis with severe clinical results. More typically, these reactions are relatively benign and occur about a week or so following transfusion. Antibodies of the Rh and Kidd systems are often identified. The triad of fever, bilirubinemia, and unexplained fall in hemoglobin in a patient who received a transfusion the prior week, suggests this diagnosis. A positive direct antiglobulin test with a mixed field pattern, or the appearance of a previously undetected antibody reactive with samples of the transfused red cells confirms the diagnosis.

Febrile nonhemolytic reactions

Febrile nonhemolytic reactions (FNHR) are the most common of the immediate transfusion reactions, occurring in about 1% to 3% of all transfusions. They are generally benign but may infrequently be severe. Febrile nonhemolytic reactions are defined by a rise in temperature of at least 1°C (without other cause of fever) and may be accompanied by a shaking chill. Different authors define these reactions to occur during transfusion or within 8 hours, or up to as long as 24 hours following transfusion.

Multiparous women and patients who have received multiple transfusions are the most likely candidates for an FNHR. Human leukocyte antigen (HLA) antibodies and granulocyte-specific antibodies have each been proposed as the major cause of the reactions. Current evidence suggests that HLA antibodies and granulocyte-specific antibodies are equally likely to be the cause, and granulocytes the target cells, resulting in the severest reactions.

Although complement activation may cause some flushing of the face a few minutes after the start of transfusion, the rise in temperature is usually not apparent until an hour or two after transfusion.

Although the reaction is almost invariably self-limited, fever may be the first sign of a much more serious reaction. The transfusion must therefore be interrupted and investigation begun. The diagnosis of FNHR is made by exclusion. If the diagnosis is made for the first time in a patient without a history of prior transfusions or pregnancies, there is only a 1 in 8 chance of a repeat reaction with the next transfusion. Removal of at least 90% of the leukocytes from blood components will prevent subsequent reactions in a patient who has received multiple transfusions and who has a history of two episodes of FNHR. The fever responds to antipyretics. Because of aspirin's effect on platelet function, acetaminophen rather than aspirin is used in bleeding patients.

Acute noncardiogenic pulmonary edema

A striking acute noncardiogenic pulmonary edema may result when donor plasma contains a high titer of antileukocyte antibody. Antigen-antibody reaction accompanied by complement activation and its direct effect on smooth muscle, white cell damage with release of vasoactive amines from mast cells and lysomal enzymes from granulocytes, as well as platelet aggregation are the probable mechanisms responsible. The pulmonary edema is accompanied by X-ray changes, including pulmonary infiltrates and perihilar nodules without evidence of heart failure. There is no sign of cardiac enlargement or blood vessel distension. These reactions have been treated with intravenous steroids and the administration of oxygen. In almost all the published reports, the donors were multiparous women with leukoagglutinins (most likely granulocyte-specific antibodies) present in their plasma. The identification of such donors and their deferral from subsequent donation is an important preventive measure. It is not surprising that pulmonary symptoms may also occur when granulocytes are transfused into a recipient with a potent granulocyte-specific antibody.

Allergic reactions

Allergic reactions are the second most common of the immediate reactions. They range from the relatively ubiquitous, localized urticaria to the very rare anaphylactic reaction. They are unaccompanied by fever and occur after a small volume of blood has been transfused.

Urticaria

Urticaria, or hives, are areas of erythema and itching. They are often localized, with one or two raised wheals and no other symptoms. Such localized reactions may be treated by slowing the transfusion without stopping it, and administering an antihistamine. If the urticaria subsides, the transfusion may be slowly continued. This exception of not interrupting the transfusion appears reasonable because the benign nature of the localized urticaria only reaction is well established. The cause of these reactions is not known, although they are assumed to involve a soluble antigen in the donor plasma. Some patients have repeated episodes of localized urticaria, and prevention by administering antihistamine prior to transfusion is an effective prophylactic measure.

Anaphylaxis

Respiratory, vascular, and gastrointestinal symptoms may signal an anaphylactic reaction. Glottal edema with coughing, wheezing, difficult breathing, nausea and vomiting, hypotension, vascular collapse, and loss of consciousness may occur rapidly. A quickly progressing urticaria may herald these dramatic changes. This is clearly different from an isolated, localized urticaria, and it underscores the need to observe transfusion recipients carefully and to evaluate any untoward reaction.

The majority of anaphylactic reactions are due to anti-IgA antibody in an IgA-deficient individual who has received a transfusion or who has been pregnant in the past. The prior sensitizing event is not always known. Anaphylactic reactions are fortunately very rare, even though the frequency of IgA deficiency is 1/700 persons. IgA-deficient individuals may make both class- (heavy chain) specific and type- (light chain) specific antibody to IgA. Some IgA-normal individuals make type-specific antibodies, and some of these antibodies may be involved in limited urticarial reactions.

Unlike a localized urticarial reaction, anaphylaxis requires immediate interruption of transfusion. Maintenance of the intravenous line is important. Treatment of the symptoms with subcutaneous epinephrine and intravenous steroids is necessary and cannot await serological diagnosis. Subsequently, a presumptive diagnosis may be based on a lack of detectable IgA on immunoelectrophoresis. The use of IgA-free blood components is required to prevent further reactions. Repositories of IgA-deficient donor blood and files of IgA-deficient individuals willing to donate are maintained nationally by the American Red Cross and other blood centers. Extensively washed red cells may also be used in such circumstances, as may autologous donations.

Posttransfusion purpura

Immediate antigen-antibody reactions involving platelets are often seen as febrile reactions and/or a poor response to platelet transfusion. Posttransfusion purpura (PTP) is a delayed reaction in which a striking thrombocytopenia occurs about 1 week following transfusion of platelet-containing components. This syndrome occurs characteristically, but not exclusively, in women who have been sensitized by a previous pregnancy. Approximately 70% to 80% of these individuals typically lack Pl^{A1} antigen on their platelets and have anti-Pl^{A1} antibody in their plasma. The fall in platelets is usually at its nadir about 1 week after transfusion. The diagnosis of posttransfusion purpura is usually made at that time.

The thrombocytopenia is thought to be due to an "innocent bystander" attachment of the patient's own Pl^{A1}-negative platelets to immune complexes composed of the anti-PL^{A1} antibody and transfused Pl^{A1}-positive platelets. Persistence of the thrombocytopenia for more than a month, if untreated, suggests that some other mechanism, such as cross-reactivity with the alloantibody, may also be involved. Treatment with intravenous gamma globulin has had reported success. Plasmapheresis has also been effective. Steroids have been effective in only a few cases.

Alloimmunization

The formation of antibodies against one or more of the cellular and plasma antigens contained within a blood component is not an uncommon consequence of transfusion. The frequency and rate of alloimmunization is a subject of continuing interest, particularly as it may relate to future problems in compatibility. There is a great deal of variation in individual propensity to make antibody. In addition, the immunogenicity of the different blood groups, as well as their relative frequency of positive-donor, negative-recipient combinations affects the likelihood of alloimmunization. Despite the difficulty of prediction in any individual circumstance, several studies have shown that about 12% of transfusion recipients make antibody to red cell antigens, and about 4% make more than one new antibody. The incidence of antibody increases with the number of transfusions, anti-K and anti-E being found most frequently, given the fact that most Rh-negative individuals are transfused with D-negative red cells.

Graft-vs.-host disease

Acute graft-vs.-host disease (GVHD) has long been a serious concern in bone marrow transplantation recipients. It has been less appreciated as a problem in transfusion recipients in whom there is a lower incidence of GVHD but a higher mortality (exceeding 90%).

Transfusion-associated graft-vs.-host disease (TA-GVHD) develops when there is engraftment of donor T-lymphocytes that proliferate and react against recipient tissue. There is a wide range of findings, including diarrhea, gastrointestinal ulceration, dermatitis, hepatosplenomegaly, lymphadenopathy, and pancytopenia. One hypothesis suggests that the pathological symptoms of acute GVHD are caused by the alloreactive T suppressor (TS) cells of the donor.

The disease occurs most often in immunocompromised patients, especially those with a severe cellular immunologic defect, including hematological malignancy, chemotherapeutic aplasia, prematurity, and congenital immunodeficiency. A fatal progressive TA-GVHD may occur in such patients because they are unable to mount an effective immune response against transfused allogeneic lymphocytes. Irradiation of cellular blood components with at least 1500 rads has been used to eliminate the proliferative capacity of these lymphocytes, and in so doing, prevent TA-GVHD in such patients.

Until recently, TA-GVHD has been thought to be essentially limited to immunocompromised patients. Recent reports from Japan, Israel, and the United States have documented the occurrence of TA-GVHD in immunocompetent individuals. For a number of years the entity of postoperative erythroderma was recognized to occur particularly in patients who had undergone cardiopulmonary bypass. It was estimated that in Japan, the syndrome occurred following cardiovascular surgery in as many as 1/300 to 1/700 procedures, and was almost invariably fatal. A drug reaction was initially considered to be the cause, but typing of an affected patient's lymphocytes demonstrated that GVHD was the actual pathologic mechanism. Engraftment of donor lymphocytes has been documented in the majority of cases

in which HLA typing was performed. The engrafted lymphocytes have been demonstrated to be homozygous for one of the recipient's haplotypes. The host's immune competence is not a factor here. The transfused homozygous cells appear to the host as "self," and are not attacked. At the same time, the host's heterozygous cells appear to the mature engrafting cells as foreign and are destroyed.

In circumstances in which transfusion practices may shrink the size and genetic variability of the donor pool, such as in family member donation, the chances of GVHD may increase. Two cases reported from Israel suggest GVHD to be due to a haplotype that was homozygous in the offspring donor and shared as heterozygous in the parent recipient.

The current recommendations for irradiation of first-degree, family member (parent-child, sibling) directed donations seem prudent. Until further information is available, it is not known whether or not reduction of the number of lymphocytes by filtration will provide an equivalent degree of protection.

ALTERED IMMUNE RESPONSE: RECURRENT CARCINOMA

It has been found that renal transplant recipients who received pretransplant blood transfusions have enhanced allograft survival. Although in this instance an altered immune response caused by transfusion has been beneficial, concerns have been raised regarding a possible deleterious immunological effect of transfusion in other clinical circumstances, particularly postoperative infections and cancer recurrence. Experimental animal studies demonstrate that blood transfusions have a complex interaction with immune mechanisms. The question of whether or not transfusions could lead to a diminished protective response to malignancy was first raised in patients undergoing colorectal cancer surgery. This retrospective study indicated a shortened recurrence-free survival in patients who received transfusions compared with that of patients who did not receive transfusions. However, in the only prospective study also done on colorectal surgical patients, there was no evidence of an effect of blood transfusion on the tumor recurrence rate during more than 3 years of postsurgical follow-up. Other investigators, using both animal and clinical models with a variety of tumors and infectious agents, have shown divergent results. To date, the clinical studies showing deleterious effects have all been retrospective case reviews in which the usual methodological difficulties leave significant questions.

NONIMMUNOLOGIC COMPLICATIONS
Circulatory overload

Circulatory overload can be easily induced in some clinical situations unless there is a proactive approach to prevent its occurrence. Depending on the clinical circumstances, even relatively small volumes of transfusion may precipitate or worsen congestive heart failure. Patients with an already increased plasma volume due to chronic anemia, or with cardiac or pulmonary compromise, or small infants, are likely candidates. Careful attention must be paid to both the rate and volume of transfusion. Dyspnea, coughing, cyanosis, and other signs of congestive heart failure may occur.

These clinical problems usually respond to interruption of the transfusion, administration of oxygen, and placement of the patient in a more upright position. When planning transfusion for such patients, prior arrangements should be made to subdivide the unit of red cells under aseptic conditions and maintain aliquots in the blood bank refrigerator. This procedure allows sequential portions of the unit to be administered slowly (about 100 ml/hour) without undue concern about bacterial contamination.

Hypothermia

Very rapid infusions of large amounts of cold blood have caused cardiac arrest. In infants undergoing exchange transfusion, the large volumes of blood required are relatively easily reached. In adults, these circumstances are less readily achieved and usually require the massive transfusion associated with major surgical hemorrhage. The site of infusion is also of importance, since introduction of the blood directly into the region of the right heart significantly increases the hypothermic effect.

Prevention of this complication is achieved by anticipating it and providing a safe means for warming the blood. The proper selection, calibration, and maintenance of the commercially available blood warmers are important. Unless other specific arrangements are made, the transfusion service is considered responsible for this quality assurance. Provision for documenting test operating temperature and the correct function of the temperature alarm of each instrument is the minimum required. If care is not exercised, warming of the blood can result in its hemolysis.

Metabolic derangements

The metabolic derangements observed in selected infants undergoing exchange transfusion and in adults undergoing massive transfusion, which are related to the infusion of free lactate, potassium, and citrate loads, as well as microaggregates, were previously discussed (Chapter 72).

Hemosiderosis

The mechanisms for preserving the body's iron stores are very effective; less than 1 mg of iron is lost per day. A single unit of blood contains about 250 mg of iron. Unless an individual loses additional iron due to bleeding, transfusion of multiple units over time may lead to a significant increase in the deposit of iron in the tissues. In patients who receive chronic transfusions, this iron deposition or transfusion hemosiderosis is a major clinical problem.

Contaminated blood

Bacterial contamination, although rare, has potentially catastrophic consequences. Refrigerator temperatures, not generally optimal for bacterial growth, are quite satisfactory for growth of some psychrophilic bacteria. These are most often gram-negative, endotoxin-producing organisms. Transfusion of this endotoxin causes a disastrous "warm" septic shock. This is characterized by a dry, flushed (reddened) skin and a shaking fever accompanied by severe hypotension, vomiting, diarrhea, abdominal cramps, and pain in the extremities. This potentially fatal reaction must be treated immediately with antibiotic, antihypotensive drugs, and steroidal therapy.

Careful attention to aseptic technique in blood collection and in component preparation is critical for preventing such contamination. The thawing of fresh-frozen plasma and cryoprecipitates in 37°C water baths is another potential point of contamination. Examination of the thawed plasma unit for any leaks due to small breaks in the previously frozen plastic bag is a prudent routine. Inappropriate storage temperatures may accelerate growth and increase the quantity of endotoxin produced. Some of the gram-negative bacteria reported in such instances of growth in refrigerated blood are *Escherichia coli*, *Pseudomonas* spp., *Yersinia enterocolitica*, and *Citrobacter freundii*. Recent reports of *Y. enterocolitica*-contaminated units that resulted in fatal septic transfusion reactions suggested no break in collection techniques nor in component preparation. It is thought that low levels of organisms may circulate in the donor's bloodstream following gastrointestinal infection. Subsequent growth of the bacteria and production of endotoxin is thought to occur in the refrigerated unit. Although the presence of contamination may be undetected by the eye or even by Gram's stain examination, visual inspection is required. The gram-negative organisms may produce hemolysis, clots, or a purple color of the contaminated stored blood.

Nonimmune hemolysis of blood

Not infrequently, hemolysis associated with transfusion is due to something other than immunological incompatibility. Inappropriate storage of red cells in an unmonitored refrigerator may freeze and lyse red cells. Use of the same transfusion line for the infusion of hypotonic solution such as 5% dextrose in water may cause hemolysis.

Transfusion-associated infection

Some of the characteristics of infectious diseases most relevant to transfusion transmission are: an infectious blood-borne phase, prevalence, severity of the disease, length of incubation period, chronic asymptomatic disease or carrier state with no disease but the potential for transmission, and presence or absence of a reliable means of screening.

Hepatitis virus agents

Viral hepatitis is an inflammation of the liver that may be classified by etiologic agent into one of at least five distinct types, designated hepatitis A through E (Table 73-1). Transfusion-associated hepatitis (TAH) is the most common of the serious complications of transfusion. A decade ago, two prospective studies of more than 2000 transfusion recipients documented that close to 7% of these recipients developed TAH.

Hepatitis B virus. Hepatitis B virus (HBV) has long been an important complication of transfusion. It may result in acute and chronic disease, as well as in a carrier state. The incubation period is typically 6 to 26 weeks following transfusion. The incidence of transfusion-associated hepatitis B (TAHB) has been significantly reduced over the last 2 decades. At the present time, the proportion of patients with hepatitis B reporting transfusion as a risk factor is only 1%. This decrease followed the introduction of a screening test for hepatitis B surface antigen (HBsAg) and the use of volunteer rather than paid blood donors. The prevalence of HBsAg in the volunteer donor population is 0.01% to

Table 73-1 The five major types of viral hepatitis

Type	Designation	Blood-borne (BB) or oral-fecal (OF)	Carrier state	Screening test
Hepatitis A	HAV	OF	No	—
Hepatitis B	HBV	BB	Yes	HBsAg
Hepatitis C	HCV	BB	Yes	anti-HCV
Hepatitis D	Delta/HDV	BB*	Yes*	—
Hepatitis E	HEV	OF†	?	—

*The delta virus is an incomplete virus requiring the helper function of HBV for its infectivity. HDV multiplies only in liver cells already infected by HBV.
†Seen in epidemics associated with fecally contaminated water sources in underdeveloped countries.

0.03%. Current third-generation enzyme-linked immunosorbent assay (ELISA) test methods are able to detect levels of HBsAg in the range of 1 ng/ml of serum. In about 10% of patients with acute hepatitis, HBsAg may not be detectable in the serum, even with the most sensitive tests. The continued use of antihepatitis B core testing as a surrogate test for HCV infection may further reduce the approximately 10% of TAH due to HBV. Anti-HBc antibody screening would detect donors in the later phases of acute HBV infections when HBsAg falls and the anti-HBc antibody rises to detectable levels. This window period, in which anti-HBc antibody is the only serological marker of recent infection, may last for several weeks or more.

In 1982, the Transfusion Transmitted Virus (TTV) study reported that, of 1553 transfusion recipients, 15 (1%) had developed serologic evidence for HBV infection. Of these 15 patients, 1 developed clinically evident hepatitis and 1 developed chronic HB.

The chronic state is characterized by the persistence of elevated serum transaminase levels for more than 6 months and a persistent HBsAg with a concomitant lack of detectable anti-HBs. The rate of development of chronic hepatitis B in adults is in the range of 7% to 10%. In newborns and neonates the rate is approximately 70% to 80%.

This increased vulnerability in the very young is due to their immature immunological defenses. Along with age, immunosuppression and the male gender are also predisposing factors for chronic hepatitis. Why males are more prone to develop chronic hepatitis than females is not understood. Over time, varying from months to years, chronic hepatitis B shows a gradual decrease in the elevated transaminase levels. This may then progress to a carrier state with the presence of HBsAg, anti-HBc, and anti-HBe. Cirrhotic symptoms or hepatoma may result years later.

Hepatitis C virus. Hepatitis C virus (HCV), or non-A, non-B (NANB) hepatitis, the most frequent of the infectious complications of transfusion, is associated with both a carrier state and chronic disease. It accounts for 90% of the cases of TAH. First identified in 1975, it has been estimated that 3% to 7% of the population carry the virus. A patient requiring a 4.5- to 5-unit transfusion has about a 1% to 2% chance of becoming infected with HCV. Transfusion is a risk factor in only about 5% to 10% of the cases of hepatitis C in the population at large. Forty percent of the cases of HCV have no known risk history.

Seventy-five percent of recipients infected by transfusion have no clinical evidence of infection. However, prospective studies have shown significant and prolonged elevation of alanine aminotransferase (ALT) enzyme levels in as many as 50% of all infected individuals, whether symptomatic or not. There is a 20% risk of progression to cirrhosis and, in some instances, hepatic carcinoma.

The major, if not the only, agent of transfusion-associated NANB hepatitis, HCV, was discovered using the techniques of molecular biology. Viral nucleic acid was extracted from large volumes of infected chimpanzee plasma and was used in the cloning of viral DNA and synthesis of the corresponding protein. This nonstructural viral protein was used as an antigen in the current immunoassay to detect antibodies (anti-HCV) directed at its dominant epitope. This assay demonstrated the presence of anti-HCV antibody in more than 90% of the sera in the well-characterized NANB hepatitis cases of the National Institutes of Health (NIH) test panel.

Chronic cases are more likely to have demonstrable antibody than cases in which there is self-limited acute infection. The period between the time of infection and the appearance of detectable antibody may typically range from 2 to 4 months. An even more prolonged window period of up to 1 year has been documented.

The surrogate tests ALT and anti-HBc produce a small but significant overlap of positivity with anti-HCV. In donors with both surrogate tests positive, there is a 45% prevalence of anti-HCV. With either of the surrogate tests positive, there is a 5% prevalence of anti-HCV. The majority of donors who transmit HCV infection may be the chronic carriers detected by the test for anti-HCV. There cannot, however, be exclusive reliance on this test because of the prolonged window period. Continued use of surrogate tests has been recommended despite their nonspecificity. It is unlikely that a specific test for viral antigen will afford any help. The very low levels of circulating virus were a major reason for the lack of success of conventional approaches to its detection. New methods such as polymerase chain reaction (PCR) technology may be of eventual benefit, but, for the time being, surrogate tests are the best available help in detection of false-negative donors in the window period. The continued use of ALT and anti-HBc assays is also recommended because of the possibility of other causes of NANB hepatitis, and because TAHB still occurs.

The lack of a true confirmatory assay is another limitation of anti-HCV testing. Given a false-positive rate of approximately 40% in blood donors, identifying donors and recipients who may require follow-up and counseling is a serious public health challenge. Measurement of ALT levels in these donors is one important means of evaluating the significance of a screening test for anti-HCV positivity. In addition, positive samples may be frozen to allow their possible eventual reevaluation by a newly developed confirmatory procedure.

Retroviral agents

Retroviruses have only recently been recognized to cause human disease. They are discussed in more detail elsewhere in the text. The retrovirus virion is composed of an outer glycoprotein coat and a central core of protein and single-stranded ribonucleic acid (RNA). The term *retrovirus* comes from the reverse transcription or copying of single-stranded viral RNA into double-stranded deoxyribonucleic acid (DNA) by the virus through an enzyme, reverse transcriptase. Although the known retroviruses have a number of features in common, they vary significantly in their cellular effects and their likelihood of causing human disease (Table 73-2).

Human immunodeficiency virus. Acquired immunodeficiency syndrome (AIDS) is a complex of clinical manifestations resulting from a severe immune deficiency caused by infection with human immunodeficiency virus (HIV). As stated previously, HIV is a cytopathic retrovirus containing genomic RNA and reverse transcriptase in its core. The viral RNA is retrocopied into DNA by the reverse transcriptase, and the DNA is inserted into the genome of the infected host. The virus has a predilection for helper T lymphocytes.

The discovery that AIDS could be transmitted by blood was, in a very real sense, the "Three Mile Island" of transfusion medicine. This was a signal event, a term used by social scientists to denote an occurrence that, although localized, has a signal potential of perceived risk that is enormous. The fear of AIDS has led to an increased awareness in physicians and the public that blood transfusion decisions are important ones. An increase in transfusion utilization review, a decrease in unnecessary transfusion, and an increase in the use of autologous transfusion are some of the positive effects of this new awareness. Unfortunately, an unrealistic fear of transfusion has also caused dangerous delay in needed transfusion, sometimes in order to accommodate directed donation.

As in hepatitis prevention, donor exclusion by history of exposure risk was the first safety measure put in place. The initial exclusion included individuals in known risk groups: male homosexuals, intravenous drug users, Haitian immigrants, hemophiliacs, and the sexual partners of individuals in these groups. In addition to donor education for voluntary self-exclusion before donation, provisions were made for people to go through the donation process and to confidentially indicate that their donated units not be used for transfusion. A screening test for anti-HIV-1 was developed, and national testing of the blood supply was implemented in 1985. Chapter 71 discusses current donor screening practices.

The time between infection and detection of antibody by the current generation of anti-HIV-1 screening tests is about 6 to 8 weeks. This window period, before anti-HIV antibody is made or before it reaches a detectable level, accounts for false-negative screening tests. The potential usefulness of HIV viral antigen tests instead of antibody tests to "close this window" in volunteer blood donors has not been confirmed. Studies in over one million volunteer blood donors revealed no instance in which a positive antigen test result was not accompanied by a positive test for HIV antibody. Current estimates of the rate at which infective window period false-negative units may enter the blood supply is about 1 per 150,000, with a range of estimates from 1 per 40,000 to 1 per 250,000. The cumulative total of transfusion-associated AIDS cases reported through April 1990 is shown in Table 73-3.

Table 73-2   Retroviruses: terminology, target cell effects and human disease states*

Virus	Old/Alternate terminology	Cytopathic/Proliferative	Transformation	Human disease
HIV-1		+	−	AIDS
HIV-2		+	−	AIDS
HTLV-I		−	+	ATL
				TSP
HTLV-II		−	+	? Hairy cell leukemia
HTLV-IV (STLV-III Simian)		− ?	−	No known human disease

*HIV, human immunodeficiency virus; HTLV, human T-cell lymphotropic virus; AIDS, acquired immune deficiency syndrome; LAV, lymphadenopathy associated virus; ATL, adult T-cell leukemia; TSP, tropical spastic paraparesis; STLV, Simian T-cell lymphotropic virus.

Table 73-3   Transfusion-associated AIDS cases

Category	Risk factor	Cumulative total	(%)
Adult/adolescent	Transfusion/Tissue	3119*	2
	Hemophilia/Coagulation	1171	1
	All other causes	125962	97
Pediatric (<13 yrs old)	Transfusion/Tissue	226	10
	Hemophilia/Coagulation	114	5
	All other causes	1918	85

*Includes eight transfusion recipients who received HIV antibody-screened blood and one tissue recipient.

In instances in which blood donors have been confirmed to be infected by HIV, the national practice has been to "look back" over the donor's history of previous donations and to inform, test, and counsel recipients of these prior donations, the rationale being that the donor, even if test negative previously, may have been in a window period of infectivity. The public health aspects of preventing spread to sexual partners and to newborns were the main impetus to this effort, but the availability of potential treatments such as azidothymidine (AZT) further drive this look back effort. Some of the units were collected from currently positive donors before the availability of screening tests for anti-HIV antibody, and, as already indicated, some units that tested negative, may have been collected and tested when the donor was in the window period.

The recipients of these units have shown about a 50% HIV seroconversion rate. The chances of infection increase with proximity to the date of the detectable positive donation. In contrast to this figure is the rate of 95% seroconversion in recipients of known positive units.

A variant of HIV, designated HIV-2 and identified in some African locations, has been of concern because, despite a very high degree of cross-reactivity, it is not invariably detected by current tests for HIV-1. The prevalence of HIV-2 in the United States is extremely low. There is no evidence that HIV-2 has entered the U.S. blood supply. There is, however, general interest in the availability of a combined test for HIV-1 and HIV-2 in order to anticipate any eventual increase in its prevalence in blood donors.

Human T-cell lymphotropic virus types I and II (HTLV-I/HTLV-II). Human T-cell lymphotropic virus type I was the first retrovirus reported in association with human disease. It stimulates lymphocyte proliferation and brings about neoplastic transformation of T lymphocytes. The antigens of HTLV-I do not cross-react significantly with those of HIV.

Human T-cell lymphotopic virus type I infection is endemic primarily in southwestern Japan, the Caribbean, and some areas of Africa. In some parts of Japan, a reported prevalence of antibody runs as high as 15% in the general population and twice that rate in the older population. No systematic study of prevalence in the United States' general population has been made, but prevalence in blood donors has been estimated at 0.025%.

Human T-cell lymphotropic virus type I infection caused by transfusion of infected cellular components has been clearly documented in Japan. Seroconversion rates as high as 60% prior to screening blood donors for anti-HTLV-I fell sharply with the advent of screening. Transmission of infection has not been documented for plasma components.

Although infection has been well documented, there have been rare reports of direct evidence for disease transmission by transfusion. This may be the case in part because the diseases etiologically associated with HTLV-I infection — adult T-cell leukemia/lymphoma (ATL) and tropical spastic paraparesis/HTLV-I – associated myelopathy (TSP/HAM) — have prolonged latency periods. This is especially true for ATL, in which the lifetime risk of ATL is estimated to be about 2% in individuals infected with HTLV-I (Japanese studies) and 4% in individuals infected before 20 years of age (Jamaican studies). Tropical spastic paraparesis, al-

though perhaps more likely to occur than ATL, is nonetheless thought to be of very low lifetime risk.

The relationship of HTLV-II and disease is less clear. Although a few patients with the atypical T-cell variant of hairy-cell leukemia have been found to have recoverable virus, many patients show no evidence of infection with HTLV-II. In addition, most infected individuals show no evidence of disease.

Other viral agents

Cytomegalovirus. Cytomegalovirus (CMV) is one of the herpes viruses. These cell-associated DNA viruses may cause transfusion-associated primary infection, reinfection, or reactivation of a latent virus infection. Cytomegalovirus infection results in alterations of T-cell subsets, with an increase in the absolute number of suppressor cells and a decreased number of helper cells.

The presence of antibodies to CMV is evidence of prior exposure. However, these antibodies are not uniformly protective; infection may occur despite their presence. In fact, blood positive for antibodies to CMV may transmit infection, and the selection of seronegative donor blood is an effective way to prevent CMV. The infectious seropositive donor is not readily identifiable. There is, however, some evidence that IgM-specific anti-CMV–positive donors may be more likely to be infectious.

Cytomegalovirus seronegative immunocompetent patients do not require selection of CMV seronegative blood, since infection in such individuals is, for practical purposes, not clinically significant. In immunocompromised recipients, including low birthweight newborns and transplant recipients, however, CMV infection can have serious consequences. Such patients may require CMV-free blood components. Reducing the number of white blood cells by filtration or washing, as well as the use of CMV immune globulin, may also decrease the risks of infection in selected patients. Granulocyte concentrates have the highest risk of transmitting CMV infection.

In the newborn, the majority of transfusion-associated perinatal infections are subclinical and go unnoticed. However, there is a significantly increased risk of severe damage in infants with concurrent medical problems such as prematurity and respiratory distress syndrome. Pneumonitis, hepatosplenomegaly, and lymphadenopathy may result. Other more subtle long-term neurological effects may occur as well.

Low birth weight infants (<1250 g) of seronegative mothers are especially at risk. These infants receive seronegative blood in the usual transfusion circumstances. As a practical routine, all low birth weight infants may receive seronegative blood, because the mother's serological status is often undetermined. Some evidence suggests that in infants of seropositive mothers, perinatal acquired infection may result in clinical disease if the infant's passive immunity is diluted by transfusion with exclusively seronegative blood. If these initial observations are validated, then seropositive blood may be better suited for the low birth weight infant of the seropositive mother.

In the immune competent adult, transfusion-associated CMV infection is typically limited to asymptomatic seroconversion. Infrequent symptomatic infections were first described in cardiovascular surgical patients who had a mild self-limited mononucleosis-like syndrome. This heterophile-negative postperfusion syndrome is now known as posttransfusion mononucleosis.

In the immunocompromised adult there is a range of practice in regard to prevention of transfusion-transmitted CMV. In patients whose immunity is suppressed secondary to chemotherapy for solid tumors and hematological malignancies, the usefulness of CMV seronegative blood is not clear. In the immune suppression associated with bone marrow transplantation, however, there is a body of evidence in favor of the use of CMV-negative blood and anti-CMV IgG in preventing or ameliorating infection. This is because of the established potential for serious and even fatal complications of CMV infection, including interstitial pneumonitis.

Epstein-Barr virus. Epstein-Barr virus (EBV), the agent of infectious mononucleosis (IM), is a herpes virus and typically causes an asymptomatic infection with subsequent latent infection. Transfusion-associated EBV infection is very rare, and even this is most likely asymptomatic. The frequency of prior EBV exposure in the population (90% of blood donors) and the fact that neutralizing antibody persists longer in circulation than infected lymphocytes help make this a rare event. The primary setting in which transfusion-associated IM might occur is in an immunocompromised EBV-negative recipient transfused with a single, relatively fresh unit collected from a donor during incubation of EBV infection. In this circumstance, neutralizing antibodies would not be available.

Human parvovirus, B19 virus. Human parvovirus (HP), also known as B19 virus, is the agent of "fifth disease," or erythema infectiosum of children. Infection with B19 virus, which is usually minor or asymptomatic, may cause a mild febrile illness with the rash of erythema infectiosum, or an arthropathy in adults. However, the parvovirus has a specific cytotoxic effect on erythroblasts, and is probably the most frequent cause of aplastic crisis in chronic hemolytic anemia, altering the usual balance between shortened red cell survival and compensatory increased production. Despite a brief period of antigenemia, parvovirus has been transmitted by blood and plasma products.

Bacterial infections

Syphilis (Treponema pallidum). Syphilis is no longer considered a significant complication of transfusion. This is due in part to the fragility of *Treponema pallidum* under refrigeration and the frequent use of antibiotics in transfusion recipients. In addition, routine screening tests do not detect the spirochete phase. However, the test is still required, more perhaps for its possible contribution as a test of sexually transmitted disease and high risk behavior than for its original purpose. The majority of positive screening tests are false-positive results, the "biological false-positive." The rare case of transfusion-associated disease appears as the rash of secondary syphilis.

Lyme disease. Lyme disease (Lyme borreliosis) is due to the spirochete, *Borrelia burgdorferi*. It is transmitted by the bite of an infected tick, *Ixodes dammini*. Although it occurs predominantly in the northeast, it is known to occur in 43 states. Its initial manifestation is a slowly expanding circular rash originating at the site of the tick bite. If untreated, it can, in some cases, lead to serious arthritic, neurological, and cardiac complications. Experimental inoculation of the spirochete into human blood collected in citrate-phosphate-dextrose and stored at 4°C showed viability of the organism up to 60 days. To date there is no case report to support transmission of Lyme disease by blood transfusion. If a significant blood-borne phase occurs, it is thought that it occurs early in the disease when the infected individual would be symptomatic and not qualified to donate. In studies of patients with positive blood cultures, all had fever and muscle pains at the time of positive culture. However, because of its potential for chronic infection, a history of Lyme disease, even in a completely asymptomatic individual, should preclude donation, unless a course of antibiotic therapy has been completed.

Parasitic infections

Malaria. The increase in air travel and immigration in recent years has contributed to an increased risk of malarial transmission in nonmalarious areas. Although the increased risk in these areas remains relatively small, this increase, along with the fact that plasmodia may be found in an asymptomatic person's red cells years after infection (*Plasmodium falciparum,* although usually resolved by 1 year, may rarely take up to 2 to 3 years. *Plasmodium malariae* as long as 10 to 46 years), requires care in evaluation of the donor's history of travel, residence, and ingestion of antimalarials.

Small numbers of infected red cells may transmit malaria, and plasmodia survive for at least a week in stored blood. Transmission has occurred with red cell concentrates, whole blood, platelets, granulocytes, and even cryoprecipitate. Plasmodia may survive for years in frozen red cells.

Direct microscopic examination of blood smears, as well as serologic tests for malaria, may be beneficial in the diagnosis of transfusion-transmitted malaria (TTM). Serologic tests for malaria are generally positive within a week to 12 days following infection, often shortly after the onset of symptoms. If TTM is correctly recognized and treated without undue delay, it responds well without relapse. However, it may be severe or even fatal, because the diagnosis, particularly in nonendemic areas, is often delayed, if recognized at all. It may also be superimposed on a serious underlying medical problem in a transfusion recipient. Pregnant women and splenectomized or immune-suppressed patients are at special risk.

Chagas' disease (Trypanosoma cruzi). This is another parasitic disease that, because of immigration, may increase in importance in nonendemic areas. Only two cases of transfusion-transmitted Chagas' disease have been reported in the United States. However, the frequency of this infection in Latin America; the entry of large numbers of immigrants from these countries; the large numbers of asymptomatic, chronically infected individuals; the high percentage of parasitemia in the chronically infected (50%); the severe effects of chronic disease, including cardiomyopathy; and the relative untreatability of these complications have made it a matter of increased concern in regard to transfusion.

Because of its current rarity, there has not been a general policy of donor assessment beyond deferral of donors with a history of Chagas' disease. In addition, currently available screening tests are not yet of practical usefulness. Broad exclusion of donors from endemic areas has been considered in some instances. A more rational approach might be to focus on individuals from such areas who have been bitten by the reduviid (triatomid) bug, or who have lived in the thatched roof huts in which the insect vector seems to have its relatively restricted territory.

Babesiosis. Babesiosis is caused by the intraerythrocytic parasite, *Babesia microti.* The deer tick, *Ixodes dammini,* is the vector for the parasite. Babesiosis is endemic in areas within the northeastern United States and Europe, and its range appears to be increasing. Splenectomized patients, patients with altered immunocompetence, and the elderly have an increased vulnerability to the more severe consequences of this infection. These include hemolysis, renal failure, and death. Six cases of transfusion-associated infection have been reported over the last decade. Red cells, both liquid and frozen, and platelets have been implicated in transmission. Prevention currently relies on the exclusion of donors with a history of babesiosis.

SUGGESTED READING

Alter HJ and others: Detection of antibody to hepatitis C virus in prospectively followed transfusion recipients with acute and chronic non-A, non-B hepatitis, N Engl J Med 321(22):1494, 1989.

Baldwin S, Stagno S, and Whitley R: Transfusion-associated viral infections, Curr Probl Pediatr 17(7):391, 1987.

Berkman SA and Groopman JE: Transfusion associated AIDS, Transfusion Med Res 2:18, 1988.

Brunson ME and Alexander JW: Mechanisms of transfusion-induced immunosuppression, Transfusion 30(7):651, 1990.

de Rie MA and others: The serology of febrile transfusion reactions, Vox Sang 49(2):126, 1985.

Goodnough LT and Shuck JM: Reviews: risks, options, and informed consent for blood transfusion in elective surgery, Amer J Surg 159(6):602, 1990.

Hogman CF: Immunologic transfusion reactions, Acta Anaesthesiol Scand (Suppl) 89:4, 1988.

Holland PV: Prevention of transfusion-associated graft-vs-host disease, SO Arch Pathol Lab Med 113(3):285, 1989.

Leitman S and Holland P: Irradiation of blood products: indications and guidelines, Transfusion 25(4):293, 1985.

Marcus RR and Huehns ER: Transfusional iron overload, Clin Lab Haematol 7:195, 1985.

PART TWELVE

CYTOGENETICS

74 Cytogenetics

Peter A. Benn

In 1956, J.H. Tjio and A. Levan described a technique to obtain high-quality chromosome preparations from human fibroblast cultures and correctly interpreted the human chromosome number as 46. This milestone in genetics opened a new era in which specific disorders could be diagnosed from an analysis of chromosomes. In 1959, Lejeune and others reported the first chromosome aberration in humans; the presence of three copies of chromosome 21 in Down syndrome. The diagnosis of cytogenetic abnormality was simplified by Nowell, who pointed out that mitotic cells could be readily obtained from a peripheral blood sample. Following the introduction of chromosome banding techniques in the early 1970s, each chromosome could be individually recognized and the diagnostic value of cytogenetics was vastly expanded. The combination of molecular genetics and cytogenetics now promises to further enhance this burgeoning field.

THE HUMAN CHROMOSOMES
Description of metaphase chromosomes

The normal diploid 46-chromosome complement consists of 22 pairs of chromosomes that are identical in males and females (the autosomes) and a 23rd pair (the sex chromosomes) consisting of two X chromosomes in females, or an X and a Y chromosome in males.

Abnormality in the human chromosome complement may involve a numerical deviation (aneuploidy), which can include additional chromosomes (trisomy), loss of chromosomes (monosomy), or extra chromosome sets (triploidy, tetraploidy, or polyploidy). Other abnormalities include exchange between two chromosomes (translocation) and deletion or duplication of a particular chromosome segment.

Chromosomes viewed under the microscope show primary constrictions or centromeres that are the attachment sites for spindle fibers during mitosis. Chromosomes with the centromere in the middle are referred to as metacentrics (chromosomes 1,3,19, and 20) and chromosomes with a centromere near one end are acrocentrics (13,14,15,21, 22, and Y). The other chromosomes are submetacentrics. A broken chromosome without a centromere is referred to as an acentric fragment. The ends of chromosomes are the telomeres.

Nomenclature

For describing human chromosome complements, a standardized nomenclature has been established. According to this scheme, the number of chromosomes present is specified, followed by a listing of the sex chromosomes present. For example, a 47,XXY karyotype describes an individual with 47 chromosomes that includes two X chromosomes and a Y chromosome (Klinefelter syndrome).

Prior to the introduction of chromosome banding, the human chromosomes were divided into seven groups—A group consisting of large metacentrics or submetacentrics (1 to 3), B group containing large submetacentrics (4 to 5), C group containing medium-sized submetacentrics (6 to 12,X chromosome), D group containing medium-sized acrocentrics (13 to 15), E group containing short submetacentrics (16 to 18), F group containing small metacentrics (19 to 20), and G group containing small acrocentrics (21 to 22, with the Y chromosome usually included in this group).

With the introduction of chromosome banding, a more complete description was established. The short arm of each chromosome is designated p and the long arm is designated q. Chromosome arms are divided into regions, with bands within regions. Chromosome bands, which stain lightly or darkly, are numbered from the centromere. Thus 4p12 refers to chromosome 4, short arm, region 1, band 2. For high resolution studies additional numbers are added to designate the separation of further chromosome bands. Figures 74-1 and 74-2 show diagrammatic representations (idiograms) of the bands observed with the most widely used banding techniques.

Terminology exists for describing translocations, deletions, duplications, inversions, products of meiotic recombinations, and polymorphisms. Box 74-1 lists some of the most commonly used abbreviations.

Chromosome banding

Using appropriate chromosome banding techniques, each chromosome can be individually identified. The number of bands visualized may vary depending on the level of contraction of the chromosome. Routine chromosome analysis is generally carried out at the 550 band per haploid set level, whereas high-resolution studies (with 850 bands or more

Box 74-1 Common abbreviations in cytogenetics

ace	Acentric fragment	mat	Maternal origin
cen	Centromere	−	Loss of
chi	Chimera	mos	Mosaic
:	Break	p	Short arm of chromosome
: :	Break and reunion	pat	Paternal origin
cs	Chromosome	+	Gain of
ct	Chromatid	q	Long arm of chromosome
del	Deletion	r	Ring chromosome
der	Derivative chromosome	rcp	Reciprocal
dic	Dicentric	rec	Recombinant chromosome
dir	Direct	rob	Robertsonian translocation
dup	Duplication	sce	Sister chromatid exchange
fra	Fragile site	;	Separates chromosomes and chromosome regions in structural rearrangements involving more than one chromosome
g	Gap		
h	Secondary constriction		
ins	Insertion	/	Separates cell lines in describing mosaics or chimeras
inv	Inversion	t	Translocation
MI	First meiotic metaphase	ter	Terminal
MII	Second meiotic metaphase	var	Variable chromosome region
mar	Marker chromosome		

For additional information on correct usage, see: An international system for human cytogenetic nomenclature birth defects: original article series IXV, no. 8, New York, 1978, The National Foundation.

per haploid set) are carried out when a specific subtle abnormality is suspected.

The most widely used staining technique involves treatment of chromosomes with a protease such as trypsin followed by staining with Giemsa stain (G-banding). A number of variations exist in the procedure involved with obtaining G-banding, but each reveal the same characteristic pattern (Fig. 74-3). Light and dark staining regions are thought to reflect both structural and functional differences in chromatin, and the differential extraction of protein prior to staining is thought to be important in the mechanism of G-banding.

Another widely used technique involves staining with quinacrine dihydrochloride (Q-banding). The banding pattern obtained is similar to that obtained with G-banding with the exceptions of the centromeric regions of chromosomes 1,9, and 16 and the acrocentric satellite regions (Fig. 74-4). Q-banding is particularly useful for identifying polymorphic variation between chromosomes of different individuals and detecting Y chromosome abnormality. Quinacrine dihydrochloride binds to deoxyribonucleic acid (DNA) by intercalation and external ionic binding, with banding influenced by the protein composition of the various chromosome regions.

Constitutive heterochromatin located at the centromeres of chromosomes can be selectively stained darkly using C-banding techniques. This staining is useful for characterizing abnormality involving centromeric regions. Because individual variation in the size of C-bands can be substantial, it is sometimes necessary to band chromosomes by this technique to distinguish between unusual variants and structural abnormality (Fig. 74-5).

Bands that are darkly stained by G-banding stain light by reverse banding (R-banding). This banding can be ob-

tained by incubating slides in hot saline solution followed by Giemsa staining.

The chromosome regions containing actively transcribed genes for ribosomal ribonucleic acid (rRNA) can be selectively stained by staining with silver nitrate (NOR-staining). Proteins adjacent to the nucleolar organizer regions stain an intense black color. The short arms of the acrocentrics (chromosomes 13,14,15,21, and 22) are the locations of this staining and considerable individual variation exists in the extent of staining (Fig. 74-6).

Another specialty staining technique involves staining with two dyes, DAPI (4,6-diamino-2-phenyl-indole) and distamycin A to obtain a fluorescent banding pattern that highlights the centromeric regions of chromosomes 1,9,16, the short arm of chromosome 15, and the distal long arm of the Y chromosome (DAPI/DA staining) (Fig. 74-7).

Finally, methods exist to selectively stain early and late replicating regions. The incorporation of the thymidine analog, 5-bromodeoxyuridine (BrdU), into chromosomes will result in alteration in the subsequent staining of chromosomes. If incorporation is confined to early or late replicating segments, these regions can be selectively identified. The approach is particularly useful for distinguishing between early and late replicating X chromosomes and identifying the spread of X inactivation in X-autosome translocations. Incorporation of BrdU for two cell cycles allows differential identification of individual chromatids, and detection of exchanges between chromatids provides an important assay for mutagenesis studies.

Detailed descriptions of methods for chromosome banding and staining are reviewed elsewhere (Rooney and Czepulkowski, 1992). The mechanisms of chromosome banding have been reviewed by Sumner (1982).

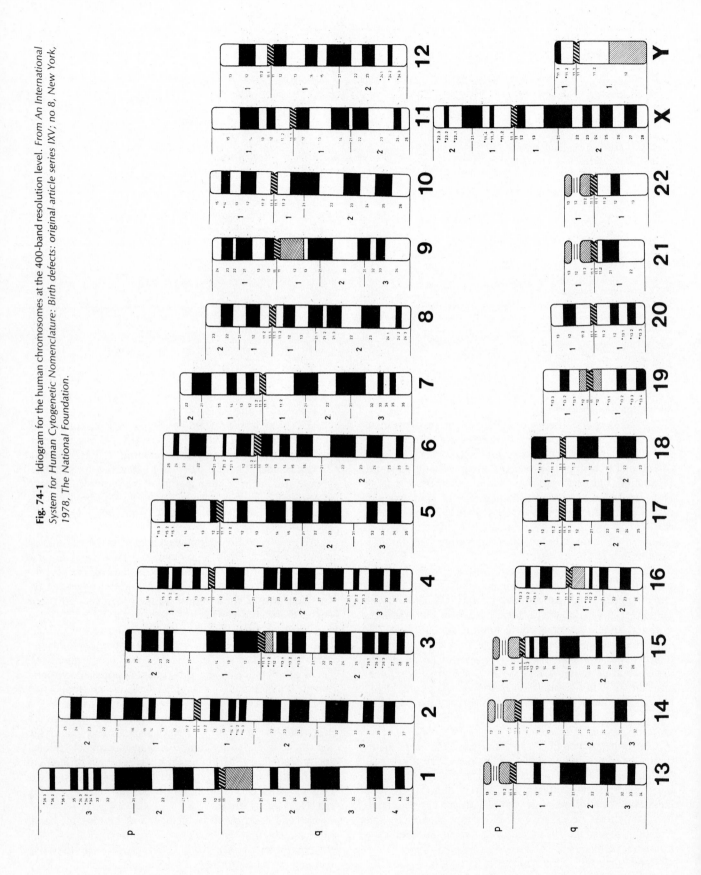

Fig. 74-1 Idiogram for the human chromosomes at the 400-band resolution level. *From An International System for Human Cytogenetic Nomenclature: Birth defects: original article series IXV; no 8, New York, 1978, The National Foundation.*

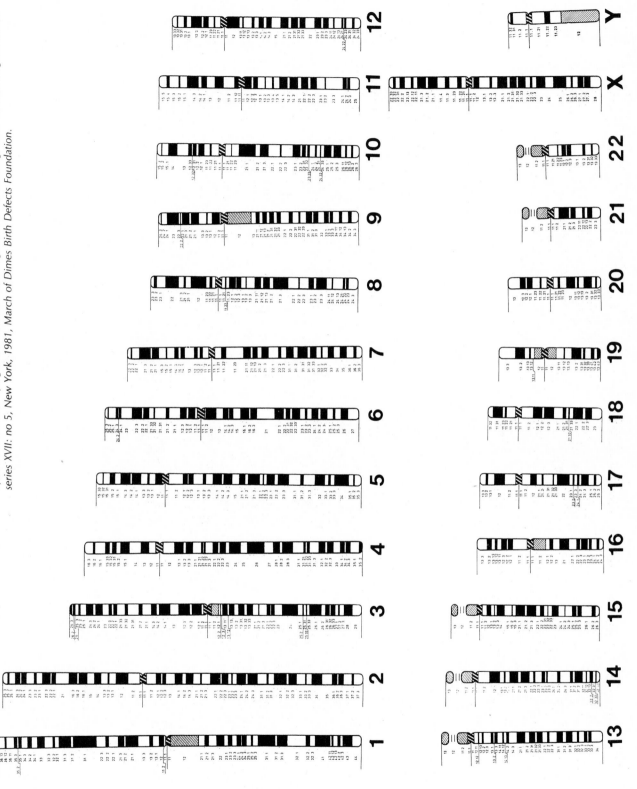

Fig. 74-2 Idiogram for the human chromosomes at the 850-band resolution level. *From An International System for Human Cytogenetic Nomenclature High-Resolution Banding: Birth defects: original article series XVII: no 5, New York, 1981, March of Dimes Birth Defects Foundation.*

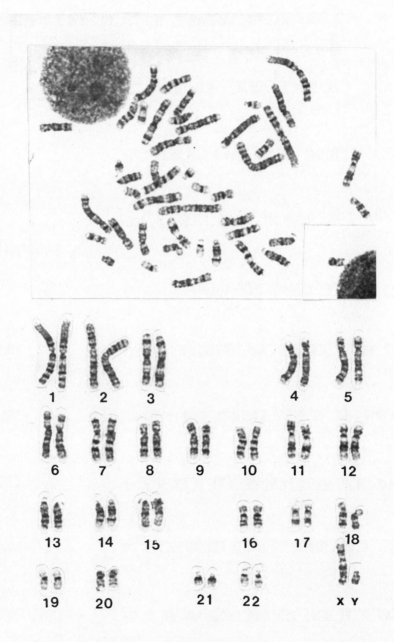

Fig. 74-3   A normal male 46,XY cell (G-banded) with karyotype shown below.

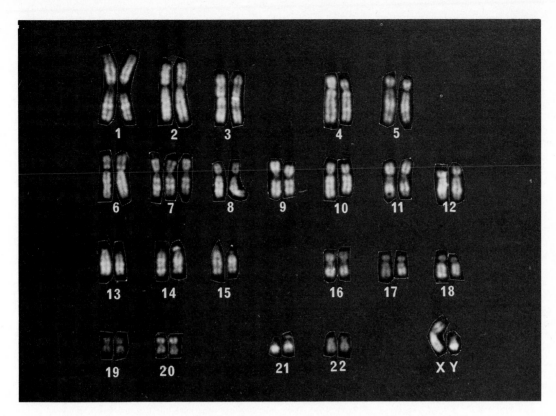

Fig. 74-4 Q-banded karyotype showing trisomy 7. The karyotype is described as 47,XY,+7.

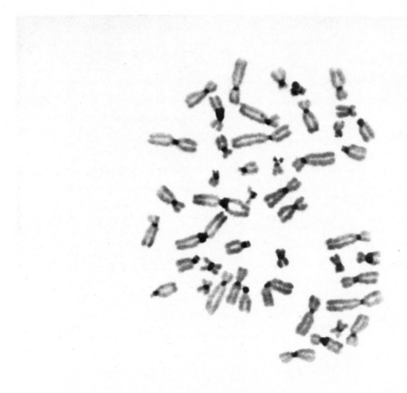

Fig. 74-5 A normal male C-banded cell.

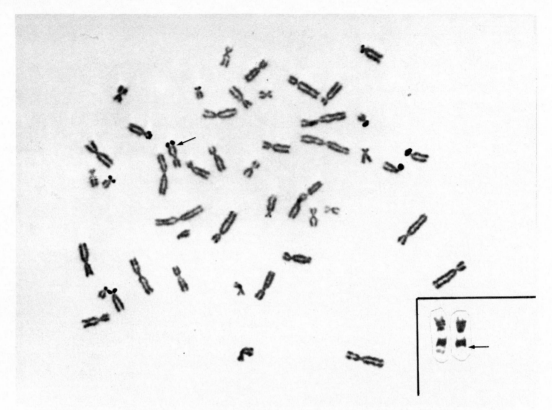

Fig. 74-6 A cell showing NOR-staining. The cell is from an individual with the karyotype 46,XY,der(11),t(11;13)(q23;p12)mat. The patient has an abnormal derivative chromosome 11 in which a satellited region from chromosome 13 is translocated to the distal long arm *(arrow)*. The normal and abnormal chromosome 11 is shown G-banded in the inset, lower right hand corner.

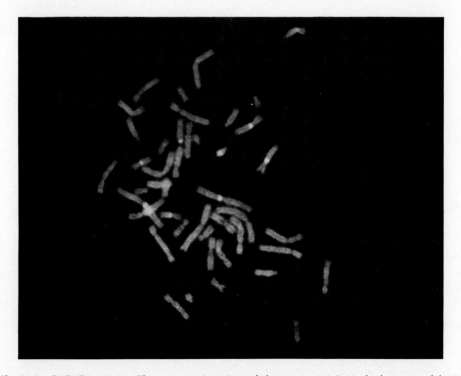

Fig. 74-7 DAPI/DA staining. The centromeric regions of chromosomes 1,9,16, the long arm of the Y, and the short arm of chromosome 15 stain brightly.

Incidence of chromosome abnormalities

It is estimated that at least 0.7% of all newborns have a chromosome abnormality. Box 74-2 summarizes the incidence of the more common abnormalities. This overall frequency of abnormality probably represents an underestimation since some of the newborn survey studies were conducted prior to the introduction of chromosome banding. In addition, many cases of mosaicism may have been missed since relatively few cells were analyzed in many of the studies.

The incidence of fetal chromosome abnormality is much higher. It is thought that about 15% of all recognized pregnancies spontaneously abort, mostly during the first trimester. The overall frequency of chromosome abnormalities among these abortuses is about 50% of which 24% have a 45,X chromosome constitution, 49% are trisomic, 15% are triploid, and 12% have unbalanced translocations or other abnormalities. This distribution of abnormalities differs substantially from the newborn situation reflecting the differential nonviability of genetic imbalances.

PRENATAL DIAGNOSIS
Indications for prenatal diagnosis

The indications for prenatal diagnosis are summarized in Box 74-3. The well-known association between the increased frequency of Down syndrome (trisomy 21) births with advanced maternal age in fact applies to most chromosome abnormalities. Amniocentesis has been widely offered to women over the age of 35, although it should be noted that risk increases gradually and that recognition of an increased risk at a particular age is somewhat arbitrary. The proportion of cases with a chromosome abnormality at the time of prenatal diagnosis exceeds the liveborn rate because of the significantly higher risk for spontaneous abortion of chromosomally abnormal fetuses throughout pregnancy (Table 74-1).

Because of the much larger number of births to women under the age of 35, most chromosomally abnormal births are in fact among younger women. The recognition that a low maternal serum alpha-fetoprotein level is weakly as-

---

Box 74-2   Incidence of chromosome aberrations in newborns

Type of abnormality	Approximate incidence
Sex chromosome abnormalities in males:	
XYY	1/1000
XXY	1/1000
Fragile X	1/1200
Other	1/1300
Sex chromosome abnormalities in females:	
45,X	1/10000
XXX	1/1000
Fragile LX	1/2000
Other	1/3000
Autosomal aberrations	
+13	1/20000
+18	1/8000
+21	1/800
Other trisomy	1/50000
Balanced rearrangement	1/500
Unbalanced rearrangement	1/2000
Total Chromosome Aberrations	1/130

Based, in part, on data from Hook EB and Porter I: Population cytogenetics: studies in humans, New York, 1977, Academic Press.

Box 74-3   Indications for prenatal diagnosis*

Advanced maternal age
Low serum AFP, high hCG, low uE
High serum AFP
Carrier of chromosome rearrangement
Previous child with chromosome abnormality
X-linked biochemical disorder
Exposure to known clastogenic agent
Extreme anxiety

*AFP, alpha-fetoprotein; hCG, human chorionic gonadotropin; uE, unconjugated estriol.

Table 74-1   The incidence of chromosome abnormality (%) with increasing maternal age

Maternal age (years)	From liveborn studies		From amniocentesis	
	47, +21	All chromosome abnormalities	47, +21	All chromosome abnormalities
33	0.16	0.29	0.24	0.48
34	0.20	0.36	0.30	0.66
35	0.26	0.49	0.40	0.76
36	0.33	0.60	0.52	0.95
37	0.44	0.77	0.67	1.20
38	0.57	0.97	0.87	1.54
39	0.73	1.23	1.12	1.89
40	0.94	1.59	1.45	2.50
41	1.23	2.00	1.89	3.23
42	1.56	2.56	2.44	4.00
43	2.00	3.33	3.23	5.26
44	2.63	4.17	4.00	6.67
45	3.33	5.26	5.26	8.33

sociated with increased risk for a chromosomally abnormal fetus has resulted in the widespread use of serum alpha-fetoprotein testing as a useful screening tool for identifying those younger women for whom prenatal cytogenetic diagnosis should be offered. Raised serum alpha-fetoprotein concentration is associated with an increased risk of a neural tube defect or of other fetal abnormalities. Recently, considerable attention has been paid to human chorionic gonadotropin levels as an additional screening test for chromosome abnormality and unconjugated estriol is also used as a further screening test for the same purpose. Results of these screening tests can be combined with maternal age to provide an individual patient-specific risk figure. Accurate gestational ages are needed for the interpretation of these screening tests and highly misleading risk figures can arise with incorrect dating.

A small, but important group of individuals at risk for chromosomally abnormal offspring are couples in whom one parent is a carrier of a translocation or other cytogenetic abnormality. The precise risk for abnormality will vary depending upon the specific rearrangement present, whether or not the original recognition of abnormality was through examination of a liveborn with an unbalanced karyotype (mode of ascertainment), and whether or not the father or the mother is the carrier of the translocation. An increased risk for chromosomally abnormal offspring also exists for pregnant women who have had a previous child with a noninherited chromosome aberration. Couples who have had a history of recurrent fetal loss or subfertility may themselves be carriers of a chromosome abnormality, and prenatal diagnosis may be an option for this group when parental chromosome studies have not already been carried out.

Chromosome analysis is sometimes carried out for sex determination for obligate carriers of an X-linked disease when a definitive biochemical test is not available. Prenatal diagnosis for fetal sex determination solely for social reasons has been widely discouraged.

Women undergoing prenatal diagnosis to detect a specific biochemical defect, neural tube defect, or other fetal anomaly, will also generally be offered chromosome analysis. Extreme parental anxiety is also a reason for some prenatal testing. Although an association between the incidence of chromosome abnormality and paternal age has been claimed, there is little evidence of any substantial effect.

Amniocentesis

Karyotyping amniotic fluid cells has been carried out since the mid-1960s. Because of the extensive experience and low risk associated with the amniocentesis procedure, it has become the most widely acceptable approach. Amniocentesis has generally been carried out at 15 to 19 weeks' gestational age, but in recent years it has been increasingly performed for earlier gestational ages. Sampling of amniotic fluid is carried out under ultrasonic guidance and the associated risk for fetal mortality is thought to be less than 0.5%.

The cells in amniotic fluid are grown in tissue culture for 7 to 10 days. Two strategies are widely used for cell culture. In the first approach, cells are grown in several flasks and cultures are trypsinized from each flask during the harvest procedure. Representative metaphases from the cell suspensions from at least two cultures are routinely analyzed. The second method involves growing the cells on coverslips or vessels, where the harvesting procedure does not disrupt individual colonies of cells. Multiple colonies are then analyzed from at least two cultures. This latter technique generally allows earlier harvest, can be advantageous in distinguishing between chromosome abnormality arising *in vivo* or *in vitro,* and may allow for a broader analysis.

Amniotic fluid samples can also be analyzed for the detection of open neural tube defects and other fetal anomalies associated with raised alpha-fetoprotein concentrations. The concentration of alpha-fetoprotein in normal pregnancies is dependent on the gestational age. Raised alpha-fetoprotein levels can be due to spina bifida, anencephaly, ventral wall defects, fetal distress or demise, polycystic kidneys, and other abnormalities. Elevation can also be due to contamination of samples by fetal blood. Acetylcholinesterase assay and tests to distinguish between fetal and adult hemoglobin are used to confirm abnormality.

Chorionic villi

In recent years considerable interest has been shown in the prenatal diagnosis of genetic disorders by analyzing chorionic villi samples (CVS). Sampling is carried out at 9 to 11 weeks, either transcervically or transabdominally under ultrasound guidance. Tissue is obtained from the chorion frondosum, which is the tissue that later forms the embryonic portion of the placenta. The risk of fetal loss for the transcervical procedure is estimated to be 0.8% greater than that for amniocentesis, after adjustment for gestational age differences. Although the chance to obtain a successful cytogenetic diagnosis is very high, it is often necessary to make more than one attempt at biopsy.

After a satisfactory sample is obtained, the specimen is divided into two portions, one of which is used for a direct chromosome preparation and the other for tissue culture. Direct analysis involves washing the specimen to remove any blood or debris present, incubating overnight in tissue culture media, and chromosome preparation using standard techniques. The cultured portion is carefully dissected to remove maternal cellular material, disaggregated with trypsin and collagenase, and cells cultured typically for 3 to 7 days as is performed for amniotic fluid cells. The number and quality of the mitoses in the preparations from the cultured material is generally highly superior to that obtained from the direct analysis.

It has been recommended that both direct and indirect analyses be carried out. The direct analysis involves the analysis of trophoblastic cells and the indirect approach reflects the mesenchymal cell population. Although the mesenchymal cell population more accurately reflects the status of the fetus, the analysis can still lead to ambiguous or even erroneous results due to mosaicism. The distribution of normal or abnormal cells in placental tissues may not necessarily be an accurate reflection of the fetus. Maternal cell contamination can also complicate interpretation, particularly for the cell culture results (see also the problems discussed in the prenatal diagnosis section).

Problem diagnoses can be resolved later in pregnancy by

amniocentesis. It should be noted that chorionic villi analysis provides no information on neural tube defects. Consequently, alpha-fetoprotein serum screening should still be considered at approximately 16 weeks' gestational age.

Fetal blood sampling

Fetal blood sampling by cordocentesis or percutaneous umbilical blood sampling (PUBS) is a procedure limited to testing in special high-risk situations. Although considered safer than fetoscopy, the procedure still carries a fetal mortality rate of 1% to 2%. The procedure is generally carried out after 18 weeks' gestation by inserting a needle in the umbilical cord under ultrasound guidance. The procedure requires considerable obstetric skill. Samples of the fetal peripheral blood obtained in the procedure can be used for cytogenetic studies or other diagnostic procedures and is sometimes an option to help resolve equivocal amniocentesis results.

Problems in prenatal diagnosis

The finding of cells with both a normal and an abnormal karyotype in a prenatal diagnosis specimen can be problematical because it is not always possible to distinguish between true *in vivo* abnormality (mosaicism) and artifacts arising in culture (pseudomosaicism). Although multiple independent cultures are generally analyzed, the number of cells growing in any one culture and subsequently analyzed may be relatively small. A diagnosis of true mosaicism is only made when two cell populations are seen in multiple independent cultures. Based on several collaborative surveys involving over 100,000 amniocenteses, the overall incidence of true mosaicism in amniotic fluid specimens is 0.2% and approximately 3.3% of cases have at least one cell that is karyotypically abnormal. The frequency of mosaicism in CVS has been reported to be 0.8% to 1.0%, with pseudomosaicism at frequencies comparable to amniocentesis data. Because of cell sampling, some cases of true mosaicism will be missed or dismissed as pseudomosaicism despite optimal laboratory procedures. Even when abnormal cells are found in more than one cell culture, the frequency of abnormal cells in the fetus may not be clinically significant or the abnormality may be confined to extrafetal tissues. Although large amounts of data have been collected on mosaicism and pseudomosaicism, complete long-term follow-up and confirmatory studies are infrequently carried out and information on a specific abnormality is often scant.

Maternal cell contamination is found in approximately 0.3% of amniotic fluid cell prenatal diagnoses and is probably largely due to maternal cells trapped in the needle during insertion. Usually, both maternal and fetal cells are present and consequently, misdiagnoses are rare. Survey data has indicated that 0.05% of cases have entirely maternal cells. Maternal cell contamination is rare in the direct analysis of CVS, but 1.9% of long-term cultures have been reported to contain maternal cells. The efficiency of separating maternal and fetal elements of CVS is clearly important.

The prenatal detection of structurally abnormal chromosomes generally requires cytogenetic studies on parents. Familial balanced translocations are generally considered to be of no adverse clinical consequence, but *de novo* trans-

locations pose significant counseling problems. The incidence of de novo translocations is higher among the mentally retarded, and limited amniocentesis data support the idea of a risk of approximately 7.5% for phenotypic abnormality. Common polymorphisms (1qh+, 9qh+, 16qh+, inv(9)) do not generally require family studies, but highly unusual chromosomes that subsequently turn out to be extreme examples of polymorphism are sometimes encountered.

Perhaps most problematical is the finding of a supernumerary chromosome. Supernumerary chromosomes are additional marker chromosomes that cannot be fully identified in terms of their chromosomal origin even after the application of multiple banding techniques. The frequency of cases with supernumerary markers is approximately 0.09% at amniocentesis. Some supernumerary chromosomes apparently have no adverse clinical consequences, whereas others clearly are associated with severe phenotypic abnormality. Mosaicism for cells with and without supernumerary markers is common and it is often necessary to analyze substantial numbers of parental cells because of the propensity for these accessory chromosomes to be lost. Even when identified as familial and mosaic in nature, there is a concern about tissue-specific variation in the distribution of cells with and without the additional chromosome.

Despite these problems, prenatal cytogenetic analysis is a powerful and accurate diagnostic tool. The extensive experience of amniocentesis allows interpretation of most unexpected findings. Currently, about 0.8% of CVS patients subsequently require amniocentesis because of ambiguity in diagnosis, but this number is likely to decline with experience. When problems do arise, genetic counseling is essential.

CYTOGENETIC ABNORMALITY IN NEWBORNS
Indications for analysis

The reasons for carrying out cytogenetic analysis are extremely varied and the cytogenetics laboratory receives referrals from pediatricians, endocrinologists, obstetricians, hematologists, oncologists, and others. Box 74-4 summarizes some of the diverse reasons for routine chromosome analysis.

Babies born with multiple congenital anomalies should be referred for chromosome analysis. Even when clinical evaluation reveals an obvious disorder such as Down syndrome, cytogenetic analysis should always be used for confirmation. Distinguishing between the usual trisomy 21 and an unbalanced translocation can have important recurrence implications. Although gross chromosome imbalances are

---

Box 74-4 Indications for routine peripheral blood chromosome analysis

Multiple congenital anomalies with mental retardation
Confirm known chromosome abnormality
Unexplained mental or growth retardation
Ambiguous genitalia in newborns
Infertility, amenorrhea, azoospermia, etc.
Multiple miscarriages

generally associated with severe abnormality, cytogenetic analysis is also sometimes indicated for milder unexplained mental or growth retardation.

Newborns with ambiguous genitalia require chromosome analysis to establish correct gender. Females who fail to develop secondary sexual characteristics or have primary amenorrhea, sterility, or short stature are often referred for cytogenetic analysis to rule out Turner syndrome. Similarly, males with hypogonadism, sterility, and tall stature are referred with suspected Klinefelter syndrome. Patients with milder gonadal dysfunction, such as azoospermic or oligozoospermic males and females with secondary amenorrhea, are also evaluated cytogenetically. Couples with a history of miscarriage often receive cytogenetic analysis to rule out the presence of a translocation or other chromosome structural anomaly.

Routine lymphocyte cell culture

Routine cytogenetic analysis can be readily carried out from a sample of peripheral blood collected in sodium heparin. Cells are cultured in the presence of tissue culture media, fetal bovine serum, and the mitogen phytohemagglutinin (PHA). Phytohemagglutinin is an extract of the red kidney bean *Phaseolus vulgaris*, which preferentially stimulates T lymphocytes (and some T-cell dependent B lymphocytes) into mitotic activity. Large numbers of mitotic cells are present in cultures at 48 to 96 hours, with maximum metaphases at approximately 64 to 68 hours. Other mitogens are known (pokeweed mitogen (PMW), concanavalin A (con A), lipopolysaccharide from *Escherichia coli* (LPS), 12-0-tetradecanolylylphorbol-13-acetate (TPA)), which stimulate different cell populations but are relatively ineffective.

Harvesting cells for chromsome preparations is preceded by the addition of colchicine (or more usually colcemid), which inhibits formation of the mitotic spindle. This inhibition lasts for 30 minutes to 2 hours. A longer time of incubation with colcemid results in larger numbers of mitoses, but the additional metaphase cells tend to have very short chromosomes.

At the end of the cell culture process, cells are exposed to a hypotonic solution that preferentially lyses erythrocytes and causes swelling of the leukocytes. Following several fixations with modified Carnoy's fixative (three parts methanol and one part glacial acetic acid), the cells are spread onto glass slides and chromosomes are stained (see chromosome banding).

High-resolution chromosome analysis

In rare situations very subtle cytogenetic abnormality is suspected. Chromosome analysis is then carried out in late prophase, prometaphase, or early metaphase, at which time the chromosomes are much longer and many more bands can be visualized (up to 1000 or more). Since relatively few of these cells are generally present in routine cultures, techniques exist to synchronize the cell population. The most commonly used approach involves culture in the presence of amethopterin (methotrexate), which blocks DNA replication and allows cells to accumulate in the G_1 phase, immediately prior to the S phase. The block is released by washing out the methotrexate and 4 to 6 hours later, chromosome preparations are made following essentially stan-

---

Box 74-5 Some indications for high-resolution chromosome analysis with chromosome band of interest

Disorder	*Band*
Prader-Willi syndrome	del(15)(q11-12)
Angelman syndrome	del(15)(q11-12)
Langer-Giedion syndrome	del(8)(q24.1)
Smith-Mageris syndrome	del(17)(p11.2)
Miller-Dieker syndrome	del(17)(p13.3)
DiGeorge syndrome	del(22)(pter-q11)
X-linked chondrodysplasia punctata	del(X)(p22.32)
Retinoblastoma	del(13)(q14)
Aniridia-Wilms' tumor	del(11)(p13)

---

dard techniques. Short colcemid times and good spreading of chromosomes are required to minimize problems of overlapping chromosomes (Fig. 74-8).

There are a number of disorders for which this analysis is appropriate (see Box 74-5). This analysis is also sometimes requested in situations where multiple congenital anomalies are present, highly suggestive of a cytogenetic defect, but where routine analysis has failed to identify any abnormality.

Fragile X chromosome analysis

The fragile X syndrome is an X-linked disorder associated in males with moderate to severe mental retardation, prominent jaw and forehead, and large ears. Macro-orchidism is a common characteristic in postpuberty males. Fragile X syndrome is also sometimes associated with autism and hyperactivity. The incidence of males with fragile X syndrome may be as high as 1 in 1000. Females carrying a fragile X chromosome may have normal or reduced intelligence, but appear to be otherwise generally phenotypically normal.

Cytogenetic detection of the fragile X chromosome involves culturing cells in conditions that directly inhibit thymidylate synthetase. Use of fluorodeoxyuridine (FUdR), L-methionine, diazepam, or trimethoprim and the use of folic acid free medias such as TC-199 with low serum concentration are commonly used for this purpose. For cells grown in such conditions, a proportion of cells from patients with a fragile X chromosome will display the characteristic nonstaining gap usually involving both chromatids at band Xq27.3 (Fig. 74-9). A number of other chromosome regions also show similar gaps, but these other regions do not appear to be associated with any clinical disorder. Of particular importance in correctly diagnosing fragile X syndrome are nonclinically significant fragile sites occurring at band Xq27.2 because these can easily be misinterpreted as being at band Xq27.3.

In a male with fragile X syndrome, the percentage of cells that express the cytogenetic abnormality may be quite variable, and generally, 100 cells or more may have to be scored to rule out the presence of a fragile X chromosome. Some obligate carrier males fail to express a fragile X chromosome and are clinically normal. Expression of the fragile X chromosome in females is even more problematical with

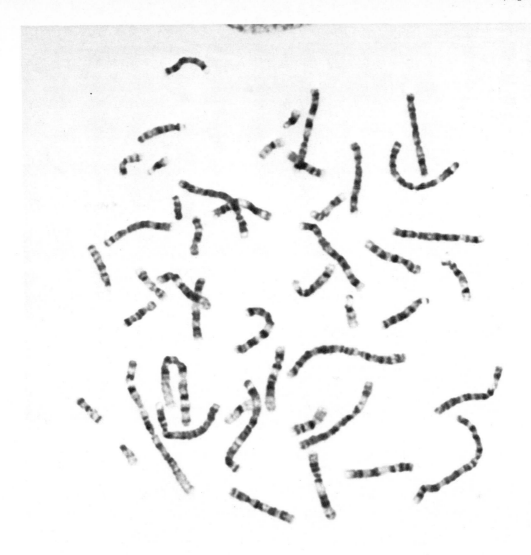

Fig. 74-8 Higher resolution chromosomes. The banding level for this particular cell is estimated to be approximately 750 to 800 bands.

the frequency of expression correlated with mental impairment. Failure to detect a fragile X chromosome in females by cytogenetic analysis does not exclude carrier status. Expression of a fragile X chromosome is difficult for tissues other than lymphocytes, although prenatal diagnosis is possible. Recombinant DNA technology can improve detection using closely linked restriction fragment length polymorphisms (RFLPs). Recent advances in the molecular characterization of the fragile X are likely to lead to substantially improved diagnostic testing. Patients with the fragile X syndrome show amplification of a specific CEG trinucleotide repeat sequence within a gene, FMR-1 that maps to the fragile site at Xq27.3. Detection of the amplified sequence should provide definative identification of the fragile X.

Fragile sites can also be seen on chromosomes when they are exposed to bromodeoxyuridine, 5-azacytidine, and other chemicals. Fragile sites are sometimes referred to as either common sites, which can be expressed in the cells of any individual, or as rare sites, which are limited to some individuals and which are inherited in a Mendelian dominant fashion.

Autosomal abnormality
Down syndrome

Trisomy 21 was the first chromosome abnormality described in humans. The clinical disorder is usually referred to as Down syndrome and the term *mongolism* is discouraged because of its racial implication. The syndrome is characterized by hypotonia, a round flat face, palpebral fissures slanted upward and outward, brushfield spots, small ears, and a flat nape. Cardiac abnormalities are present in approximately 40% of the cases. The extent of mental retardation is quite variable. Mean life expectancy at birth is 16.2 years, with a 30% mortality rate in the first year.

Nearly all cases of Down syndrome are attributable to the presence of an additional copy of chromosome 21, but a small proportion of individuals have unbalanced translocations with additional chromosome 21 material. Robertsonian translocations (fusion of two acrocentric chromosomes) account for most translocation cases, with fusion of chromosomes 14 and 21 the most common. Approximately 90% of trisomy 21 appears to be due to errors in maternal meiosis. Absence of pairing of chromosomes or reduced

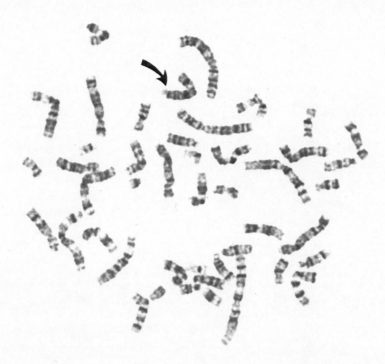

Fig. 74-9 Typical appearance of the fragile-X chromosome *(arrow).*

recombination appears to contribute to non-disjunction in a significant proportion of cases. A small proportion of cases (approximately 3%) are mosaic, with both normal and trisomy 21 cells present. Mosaic cases are associated with variable clinical findings.

Trisomy 18

Trisomy 18, or Edwards syndrome, is associated with severe malformations that include growth retardation, hypoplasia of skeletal muscles, micrognathia, occipital protuberance, fawnlike ears, overlapping fingers, narrow pelvis, rocker-bottom feet, and a high frequency of arches. Mean survival is approximately 6 months, with cardiac malformations the cause of most deaths. Free trisomy accounts for nearly all cases, with few translocations seen for this disorder. Mosaicism is present in about 10% of the cases.

Trisomy 13

Trisomy 13, occasionally referred to as Patau syndrome, is characterized by microcephaly, harelip, (usually bilateral and accompanied by a cleft palate), microphthalmia, hexadactyly, and other severe abnormalities. Mean life expectancy is 130 days, with nearly half of the newborns with trisomy 13 dying within the first month. Approximately 80% of cases show free trisomy, with rare cases showing mosaicism. Robertsonian translocations, particularly involving chromosomes 13 and 14, account for most of the remaining cases.

Trisomy 8

The most characteristic anomalies in trisomy 8 are facial dysmorphism (high protruding forehead with elongated face and eversion of the lower lip), spinal abnormalities (including additional vertebrae, hemivertebrae, butterfly vertebrae, spina bifida occulta), broad dorsal ribs, narrow hypoplastic iliac wings, absent or hypoplastic patellae, deep plantar furrows, osteoarticular anomalies, and moderate mental retardation. Most, if not all, newborns with trisomy 8 are, in fact, mosaic, although nonmosaic trisomy 8 is seen in first trimester spontaneous abortions. The proportion of trisomic cells may vary substantially in different tissues, and it has been reported that the percentage of trisomic metaphases decreases with age.

Trisomy 9

Trisomy 9 is a very rare disorder characterized by microcephaly; enophthalmy; microretrognathia; dislocation of hips, knees, or elbows; deformities of the spinal cord and ribs; and inner organ anomalies. Mosaicism is present in approximately 50% of the cases.

Other autosomal duplications

Other autosomal trisomies (either mosaic or nonmosaic) appear to be extremely rare in newborns. Trisomy for chromosomes 3,7,10,12,14,15,19,20, and 22 have been described with, in some instances, inconsistent clinical findings and sometimes with dubious cytogenetic documentation. Trisomy for nearly every chromosome (with the exception of trisomy 1) has, however, been found in spontaneous abortion tissues.

Partial trisomies (in which a particular chromosome segment is present in three copies) can arise as a result of unbalanced translocation. Predicting clinical consequences in such karyotypes can be problematical, especially when deletion of other chromosome segments may also be present. In general, the larger the duplication, the more severe the associated clinical anomalies.

Autosomal deletions

A number of syndromes have been described with deletion of specific chromosome segments. The most well known of these is 5p monosomy or cri du chat syndrome. This disorder is characterized clinically by microcephaly, distinctive mewing cry (that may disappear after a few months or years), moonlike face, hypertelorism, short fingers with clinodactyly of the little fingers, and muscular hypotomia. Most cases (80% to 90%) arise as a *de novo* deletion, the remainder being the segregation products of parental translocations. Most of the clinical features of this syndrome appear to be due to the deletion of a critical region at 5p15.1.

Wolf-Hirschhorn syndrome is another relatively frequent deletion syndrome involving the short arm of chromosome 4. Patients with this disorder have severe growth retardation, severe mental deficiency, microcephaly, and a highly characteristic facial dysmorphism that includes the "Greek warrior helmet" appearance. The specific segment of the short arm of chromosome 4 that appears to be associated with these features is band 4p16.

Other well-documented deletion syndromes include 9p2, 11q2, 18p, 18q monosomies, together with other numerous, less common deletions. In some instances the deleted segments may be very small and higher resolution studies are required. Box 74-5 lists some referral indications for high-resolution analysis and the chromosome regions that may be deleted. It is of interest to note that two disorders, Prader-Willi syndrome and Angelman syndrome, which are clinically quite distinct, appear to share a common deleted chromosome segment (15q11-15q13). Evidence would suggest that it is the parental origin of the deleted chromosome or genetic imprinting that determines which of these two syndromes will be present. For the diagnosis of extremely subtle deletions, the application of DNA probe technology is likely to ultimately replace high-resolution chromosome studies.

Sex chromosome abnormalities

Turner syndrome

Patients with Turner syndrome have short stature, primary amenorrhea, with streak gonads that are devoid of primordial follicles. Many patients also show lymphedema of the hands and feet at birth, a triangular face with hypoplasia of the mandible and retrognathia, a short webbed neck with a low posterior hairline, shortening of the fourth and fifth metacarpals, multiple pigmented nevi, space-form perceptional deficit, lack of emotional arousal, and many other features.

A 45,X karyotype is observed in approximately 55% of the cases. In the remaining cases, mosaicism with normal

male, normal female, or other abnormal karyotypes are seen. Some common karyotypes that may be seen, with or without additional normal or abnormal cell lines, are: 46,X i(Xq); 46,X i(Xp); 46,X del (Xp); 46,X del (Xq); 46,X,r(X); and 46,X,del(Yp) with variable degrees of expression of the Turner phenotype. Patients with Xp deletion usually have short stature but may show normal ovarian tissue function with a critical region for ovarian function possibly at Xp11. Patients with Xq deletion may also show short stature and ovarian dysfunction possibly determined by loci at Xq13-21 and Xq24-Xq26.

Klinefelter syndrome

Klinefelter syndrome is present in approximately 1 in 1000 male births. The disorder is undiagnosable on the basis of dysmorphism at birth, but is recognizable at puberty or later on the basis of gynecomastia, testicular atrophy, and sterility. Intelligence may be slightly lower than normal and problems with social relationships, gender role development, criminal behavior, and mental illness all appear to be more prevalent in patients with Klinefelter syndrome. In 80% of the cases, the karyotype is 47,XXY, whereas in the remaining cases, mosaicism and/or another karyotype may be seen. Alternate karyotypes include 48,XXY, 48,XXXY, and so on, with or without other cell lines present.

XXX and XYY

Females with a karyotype 47,XXX are relatively common (approaching 1 in 1000 females) and generally have a normal phenotype. Premature ovarian failure is sometimes found and average intelligence may be somewhat lower, with increased mental retardation risk and behavioral disturbances. With an increasing number of X chromosomes (48,XXXX; 48,XXXXX; etc.), abnormality becomes more apparent. In the latter disorders, a dysmorphology somewhat like Down syndrome is seen with mild to moderate mental retardation.

Males with a karyotype 47,XYY are also relatively common (approximately 1 in 1000 males) and have a generally normal phenotype. Such individuals are generally tall (due to long legs), usually fertile, but may have a slight deficit of intelligence, show excessive negative moods, impulsiveness, aggressiveness, and other mild behavioral problems that may lead to an increased chance for internment in an institution for mentally retarded delinquents. The presence of additional Y chromosomes (48,XYYY; 49,XYYYY; etc.) results in progressively more pronounced physical and mental abnormalities.

X-inactivation

In considering the consequences of abnormality of the X chromosome in females, consideration has to be given to lyonization. In normal females, one of the X chromosomes is inactivated at random early in embryogenesis; a phenomenon known as lyonization. However, female carriers of X-autosome translocations usually show nonrandom X-inactivation patterns, depending on the nature of the translocation. For balanced translocations, there is preferential inactivation of the normal X chromosome. In unbalanced translocations the abnormal X chromosome is frequently inactivated and the X-inactivation can spread into the autosomal segment of the rearranged chromosome. Thus, selection appears to favor cells with the minimum genetic balance and the phenotype of the individual may be less abnormal than might first be expected, based on the size of the imbalance alone. Individuals with more than two X chromosomes inactivate all but one X chromosome.

Other sex chromosome abnormalities

Pericentric inversions of the Y chromosome involving bands p11 and q11 appear to have no clinical significance and this inversion is seen in approximately 1 to 2 per 1000 males. Partial deletion of the distal, brightly fluorescent segment of the long arm of the Y chromosome (Yq12) or polymorphic variation of this band also seems to have no clinical significance. Deletion of the short arm, however, results in Turner syndrome stigmata, indicating that a male-determining factor is located on the short arm of the Y chromosome.

The location of a testes-determining factor (tdf) on the short arm of the Y chromosome helps explain rare individuals with sex reversal. Males with a 46,XX karyotype have been described who are sterile but have testicular tissue present; have no ovaries and no female internal genitalia. Similarly, there are examples of females with a 46,XY karyotype showing sterility, streak ovaries without follicles but no testicular tissue, and female internal genitalia. At least some males with a 46,XX karyotype can be explained by translocation of tdf, often to the X chromosome as a result of an aberrant meiotic crossover or by translocation to an autosome. Females with a 46,XY karyotype could arise by similar mechanisms with segregation of the reciprocal translocation products. Use of DNA probes has been highly informative in identifying such exchanges.

True hermaphroditism is defined by the presence of both male and female gonadal tissue. The karyotype may be 46,XX; 46,XY; 46,XX/46,XY; 46,XY/45,XO; or other mosaicism. In pseudohermaphroditism, there is ambiguity of genitalia but with the exclusive presence of either a male or female type. Female pseudohermaphroditism is due to secondary virilization of a female fetus (46,XX) by male hormone (as a result of congenital adrenal hyperplasia, hormonal therapy during pregnancy, or ovarian tumor). Male pseudohermaphroditism includes testicular feminization (caused by absence of testicular hormone receptors), true gonadal dysgenesis, and mixed gonadal dysgenesis. Male pseudohermaphrodites usually show a 46,XY karyotype, although 46,XY/45,X or other mosaicisms may be seen.

Noonan's syndrome is an autosomal-recessive disorder in which individuals with a normal karyotype show a Turner-like phenotype.

Other karyotype abnormalities and normal variation

Triploidy and polyploidy

Triploid chromosome complements (69,XXX; 69,XXY; or 69,XYY) are some of the most common cytogenetic abnormalities seen in first trimester spontaneous abortions and rare cases result in full-term newborns. Such infants show severe growth deficiency, with multiple congenital abnormalities usually resulting in death within hours or days. Less severe abnormalities are present in cases where there is mosaicism with a normal cell line. In such cases there is often cranial, body, or limb asymmetry.

Tetraploidy is also sometimes seen in spontaneous abortions and there have been isolated reports of newborns with tetraploidy and multiple congenital abnormalities. Mosaicism with normal cells is also found, but interpretation is often complicated by the fact that a variable percentage of tetraploid cells are often seen in the blood or cell cultures established from normal individuals.

Translocations and inversions

Robertsonian translocations are relatively common (0.09% of the newborn population have a Robertsonian translocation), most of which are familial. Other reciprocal translocations are seen at a comparable frequency (0.08%) and approximately one third appear to be *de novo*. Non-Robertsonian translocations seem to be largely unique to particular families, a notable exception being the t(11;22)(q23:q11), which has been widely reported in diverse populations.

Translocation carriers can give rise to unbalanced karyotypes in progeny depending upon the segregation of the rearranged chromosomes, which can include 3:1 segregations. Pericentric inversion with crossovers within the inversion loop at meiosis can result in unbalanced karyotypes in progeny. Paracentric inversion with crossover within the loop results in dicentric and fragment chromosomes that are unstable. Aneusomie de Recombinaison is a term used to describe the at least theoretical possibility that as a result of a translocation or inversion, crossover between a normal and abnormal chromosome can arise with displacement of a region, and this can lead to an unbalanced karyotype. For a full explanation of segregation and recombination of rearrangements see, for example, Therman, listed in the suggested reading at the end of this chapter.

Balanced translocation and inversion carriers are heterozygous for mutations at the breakpoint, which presumably could be occasionally of clinical significance. Many translocations that appear to be balanced at the cytogenetic level are in fact probably unbalanced at the molecular level, with extensive deletion or duplication possible. Position effects may also influence gene activity and these factors may explain the risk associated with *de novo* translocation (see problems in prenatal diagnosis).

Polymorphism and other normal variation

The human karyotype can show extensive variability from individual to individual and considerable caution is required before concluding that a particular karyotype is indeed abnormal. Some common regions that show variability in size are the heterochromatic regions of chromosomes 1,9,16, and Y, which can readily be identified by C-banding. Darkly staining C-band regions can show variation in rare instances for many, perhaps all, other chromosomes. The size of the short arms of acrocentric chromosomes also show considerable variation from individual to individual. This variation in part reflects variation in nucleolar organizer regions (NOR), the activity of which can be identified by silver staining. There is doubt that the presence of double NORs are associated with nondisjunction as was originally proposed. Pericentric inversion of chromosome 9 is extremely common (inv(9) (p11q12 or q13)) and is thought to have no clinical significance. Other rarer inversions that probably have little or no clinical significance include inv(2) (p11q13), inv(3) (p11q12), inv(19) (p11 or p13q13), and inv(Y) (p11q11). As previously pointed out (in problems in prenatal diagnosis), even the presence of an additional supernumerary chromosome may not necessarily indicate an abnormal phenotype.

In most chromosome analyses from normal individuals, a small proportion of abnormal cells is generally found. As well as random loss of chromosomes, a low level of chromosome rearrangements, broken chromosomes, and other lesions are seen. In lymphocyte cultures, an age-related hypodiploidy involving a loss of sex chromosomes and probably a gain of X chromosomes in females is seen. In early passage skin fibroblast cultures established from adults, clones of cytogenetically abnormal cells are common, but these are not seen in fetal skin fibroblasts cultured under identical conditions.

CHROMOSOMES IN NEOPLASIA

Since cancer is a heterogenous group of diseases, each of which can be considered as the consequence of multiple genetic alterations, it is to be expected that cytogenetics plays an important role in diagnosis. In this section, three aspects are considered. First the association between chromosome breakage and increased cancer incidence; second, constitutional cytogenetic abnormality associated with particular cancers; and third, cytogenetic abnormality in tumor cells.

Chromosome breakage and cancer
Ataxia-telangiectasia and Nijmegen breakage syndromes

Ataxia-telangiectasia is a rare autosomal-recessive disorder characterized by cerebellar degeneration, oculocutaneous telangiectasias, immunological dysfunction, cancer proneness, and increased radiation sensitivity. In addition to showing high levels of chromosome breakage when cells are X-irradiated or exposed to radiomimetic chemicals, a high frequency of spontaneous chromosome abnormalities is seen. Specific chromosome bands are involved in translocations and inversions, with the emergence of clones of lymphocytes in the peripheral blood carrying an identical abnormality. The chromosome bands that are most frequently involved in clones are 14q11, 7p14 and 7q35, and 14q32. The first three of these bands contain T-cell receptor genes (14q11 TCRA and TCRD, 7q35 TCRB and 7p14 TCRG) and 14q32 contains a putative oncogene *tcl*-1. The involvement of T-cell receptor gene loci appears to reflect aberrant V-D-J joining during the processes by which these genes rearrange to form antigen-specific receptors; there may also be a possible deregulation of the *tcl*-1 oncogene (see also the section on chromosome abnormality in tumor cells and lymphoid cell disorders).

Interestingly, an identical spectrum chromosome abnormality, sensitive to radiation and susceptible to cancer, is seen as an entirely different genetic disorder, the Nijmegen breakage syndrome. This latter disorder is characterized clinically by variable immune deficiency, microcephaly, and developmental delay. No cerebellar ataxia and no telangiectasias are seen. Precisely how the disorders may be related remains to be established.

Bloom syndrome

Bloom syndrome is an extremely rare autosomal-recessive disorder associated with a greatly increased risk for cancer. Patients with this disorder show low birth weight, stunted growth, sun-sensitive erythema, immunologic deficiencies, and characteristic facial appearance. The characteristic cytogenetic findings are a greatly increased rate of sister chromatid exchange, chromosome aberrations, and chromatid interchanges between homologous chromosomes. Chromatid interchanges between homologous chromosomes are seen in cytogenetic preparations as highly characteristic symmetrical, quadraradial configurations that are only rarely seen in preparations from normal individuals. Increased mutation rate, loss of tumor suppressor gene activity, or activation of specific oncogenes may account for the cancer predisposition.

Fanconi anemia

Fanconi anemia is an autosomal-recessive disorder in which a pancytopenia develops between the ages of 5 to 9 years. This anemia is sometimes associated with congenital abnormalities that include low birth weight, growth retardation, abnormal skin pigmentation, hypoplasia or aplasia of the radius and thumb, and kidney malformations. Cytogenetic analysis frequently reveals an increase in the frequency of spontaneous chromosome breakage. This is seen as chromosome gaps and breaks, chromatid gaps and breaks, rearrangements, fragments, and so on. Exposure of Fanconi anemia cells to agents such as diepoxybutane (DEB) greatly enhances the frequency of breakage as compared to that seen in normal cells exposed to DEB.

Other chromosome instabilities and acquired aberrations

Cytogenetic analysis of peripheral blood from patients with xeroderma pigmentosum show normal levels of chromosome damage. Although an ultraviolet radiation sensitivity exists for these cells, spontaneous levels of chromosome damage are normal. Patients with Werner syndrome (a premature aging disorder) may show an increased frequency of cytogenetically abnormal cells in fibroblast cultures.

Induced chromosome breakage can be seen in preparations from normal individuals following exposure to ionizing radiation and some other carcinogenic agents. Also, many but not all carcinogens induce an increased frequency of sister chromatid exchanges.

Constitutional cytogenetic abnormality and cancer

Although inheritance plays an important role in the risk of developing most types of cancer, in general cytogenetics currently has a minor role in evaluating individuals at risk for developing cancer. There are, however, some rare situations in which constitutional abnormalities are associated with extremely high relative risks for particular types of cancer, and these situations have been highly informative in understanding mechanisms in cancer development.

One such example is retinoblastoma. Retinoblastoma is a rare malignant eye tumor of children that may involve one eye (one third of the cases) or two eyes (two thirds of all cases). For bilateral retinoblastoma and some case of unilateral retinoblastoma, the mode of inheritance is autosomal-dominant with about 90% penetrance. There is also an additional increased risk for osteosarcoma. Approximately 2% to 3% of patients with retinoblastoma have a cytogenetically detectable deletion of chromosome 13, band q14. Other patients with the hereditary form have a submicroscopic deletion or mutation that inactivates the gene product of the so-called Rb locus. The tumor cells appear to have homozygous loss of the Rb gene product. This important example provided the first clear evidence to support the Knudson two-hit hypothesis to explain some types of cancer.

In patients with the hereditary form of Wilms' tumor that is frequently associated with aniridia, genitourinary anomalies, and mental retardation (WAGR), deletion of chromosome band 11p13 is sometimes seen. In Wilms' tumor, deletion of loci on 11p13 are common and the mechanism for tumor development thus appears to parallel that seen in retinoblastoma.

The deletions in retinoblastoma and Wilms' tumor are best identified using DNA probe technology rather than cytogenetics. The use of molecular genetics is resulting in the identification of numerous other situations where loss of specific loci (tumor-suppressing genes) are thought to be important in tumor evolution. Cytogenetics has, however, been extremely helpful in some rare families in whom striking familial patterns of cancer inheritance is paralleled by inheritance of a specific translocation.

It should also be noted that some common constitutional chromosome abnormalities are associated with increased cancer risk. For example, Down syndrome patients show an increased risk of leukemia and patients with 45,X/46,XY mosaicism can show a high propensity for the development of gonadal tumors.

Cytogenetic abnormality in tumor cells

The extent of the chromosome changes that may be present in a particular cancer may be enormous. In addition to aneuploidy, marker chromosomes representing the products of translocation are extremely common. In some cases specific abnormalities are highly diagnostic or have important prognostic value, whereas other changes appear to be entirely random. In general, there is an association between chromosome breakpoints and known oncogenes, and in some cases, the relationship between the observed cytogenetic abnormality and oncogene activation is becoming clear. Deletion can result in the loss of tumor-suppressor genes. Translocation can result in deregulation of gene(s) adjacent to breakpoints or can fuse two genes, resulting in chimeric protein products with aberrant functions. There also appears to be an association between chromosome breakpoints in cancer and fragile sites, although the significance of this is uncertain.

There are some types of chromosome abnormalities that appear to be almost exclusively confined to cancer cells. Double minutes (DMs) are small but variably sized, fragment-like chromosomes that are sometimes seen in some tumor cell preparations (Fig. 74-10). The number of double minutes may vary substantially from cell to cell. In tumors in which double minutes are present, so-called homogenously staining regions (HSRs) are also often seen. These are large regions of chromosomal material that fail to show a normal banding pattern, but show a uniform staining along the entire chromosomal segment (Fig. 74-11). Both DMs and HSRs are the cytogenetic presentation of amplification of chromosomal regions. Whereas gross amplification of a particular gene may confer an advantage to a particular tumor cell, the potential exists for DMs to arise and the integration of amplified chromosomal material into another chromosome can result in an HSR.

Chromosome analysis of tumor cells is often technically difficult. For leukemia, bone marrow or peripheral blood can be processed directly or cultured for 1 to 3 days in the absence of any mitogen and chromosome preparations made using the standard techniques. For solid tumors, tissue must be minced or digested with enzymes to obtain single-cell suspensions and then cultured. The yield of metaphase cells may be low, the quality of the chromosome preparation is often poor, and identification of marker chromosomes is sometimes complex. Nevertheless, more than 125 specific structural abnormalities have now been described in 39 different tumor types. A disproportionately large number relate to hematologic disorders because these have been easier to analyze. It is clear that the list of abnormalities will grow substantially in the coming years and the application of DNA probe technology will make detection easier as well as clarify the significance of many of the changes.

The following sections provide an overview of cytogenetic abnormalities of tumor cells. The Catalogue of Chromosome Aberrations in Cancer and Human Gene Mapping Reports are important resources for additional information.

Myeloid cell disorders

Box 74-6 summarizes some of the most common chromosome abnormalities in various myeloid leukemias, myeloproliferative disorders, and myelodysplastic syndromes.

The first chromosome abnormality to be described in a human cancer was the presence of the Philadelphia chromosome (Ph) in chronic myeloid leukemia (CML), which was subsequently shown to be a derivative of chromosome 22 arising from the translocation t(9;22)(q34;p11) (Fig. 74-12). Although variant or complex translocations (those that involve additional chromosomes other than 9 and 22) and Ph-negative CML have been widely described, molecular genetic data indicate that true CML is perhaps always characterized by the juxtaposition of chromosome 9 sequences (the c-*abl* oncogene) and chromosome 22 sequences (the so-called breakpoint cluster region gene BCR or *phl*). This may be present even when cytogenetic analysis fails to detect a Ph chromosome. As a result of the translocation, a fusion *phl-abl* gene is produced and the resulting chimeric protein is strongly implicated in the pathogenesis of CML. The breakpoints on chromosome 22 within the *phl* gene are confined to a small segment referred to as the breakpoint cluster region, *bcr,* and the rearrangements can be readily detected using DNA probes to the *bcr.*

Another highly consistent chromosome abnormality is the t(15;17)(q22;q11-q12) and variant translocations seen in 60% to 100% of individuals with acute promyelocytic leukemia, subtype M3. The leukemic cells in this disorder are characterized by coarse granules with strong myeloperoxidase activity. The translocation fuses the retinoic acid receptor alpha gene (*RAR*x) located on chromosome 17 with a chromosome 15 locus called *Myl* resulting in the synthesis of an *myl/RAR*x fusion messenger RNA.

The translocation t(6:9)(p23:q23) (found in approxi-

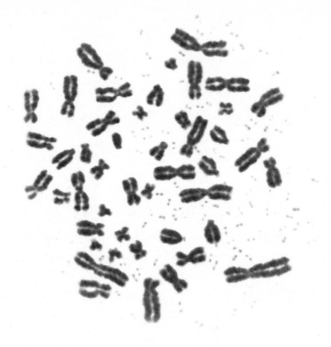

Fig. 74-10 Double minutes in a cell from a neuroblastoma line *(unbanded)*.

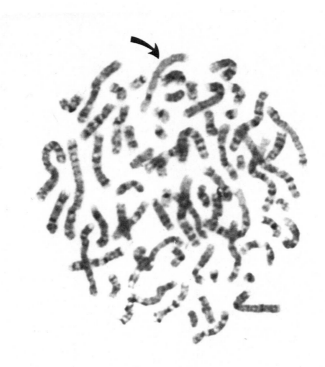

Fig. 74-11 An HSR on the short arm of chromosome 19 in a neuroblastoma cell line.

Box 74-6 Common cytogenetic abnormalities in myeloid leukemias; myeloproliferative disorder, and myelodysplasia*

Cytogenetic abnormality	Disease
t(9;22)(q34;q11) + variants	CML
t(9;22), +8, +19, +Ph, i(17q)	CML, blast crisis
t(8;21)(q22;q22)	AML-M2, AMMoL-M4
t(15;17)(q22;q11-12) + variants	APL-M3
inv(16)(p13q22) or t(16;16)(p13;q22)	AMMoL-M4Eo
t(11q22) or del(11)(q23)	AMMoL-M4
t(9;11)(p22;q23)	AMoL-M5
+8	ANLL, MDS, MPD
−7, 7q−	ANLL, MDS, MPD
−5, 5q−	ANLL, MDS, MPD, 5q− syndrome
t(6;9)(p23;q34)	ANLL
20q−	MDS, MPD
inv(3)(q21q26) or t(3;3)(q21;q26)	ANLL with high platelet count

*Disorders are organized in accordance with the French-American-British (FAB) classifications. CML, chronic myeloid leukemia; AML-M2, acute myeloblastic leukemia with maturation; AMMoL-M4, acute myelomonocytic leukemia; APL-M3, acute promyelocytic leukemia; AMMoL-M4Eo, acute myelomonocytic leukemia with abnormal eosinophils; AMoL-M5, acute monoblastic leukemia; ANNL, acute nonlymphocytic leukemia; MDS, myelodysplastic syndrome; MPD, myeloproliferative disorder.

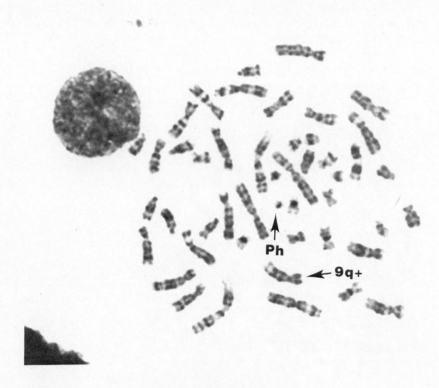

Fig. 74-12 The Philadelphia chromosome (Ph) in a cell line with the common t(9;22)(q34;q11) in CML.

mately 2% of acute myeloid leukemias) has also been characterized in detail at the molecular level. This translocation fuses a gene of unknown function (*DEK*) with a regulatory gene (*CAN*).

The involvement of chromosome 16 (inversion or translocation at bands p13 and q24) is highly specific for myelomonocytic leukemia with abnormal eosinophils (AM-

Mol-M4E). The precise significance of this translocation is, however, currently unclear.

The specific translocations listed in Box 74-6 not only have diagnostic value, but also provide important prognostic information. Patients with acute myelocytic leukemia and a t(8;21) have the longest survival rate, and those with inv(16), 11q deletion or translocation also have favorable

Box 74-7   Common cytogenetic abnormalities in lymphoid neoplasia*

t(1;19)(q23;p13)	ALL (pre-B)
t(9;22)(q34;q11)	ALL
t(8;14)(q24;q32)	BL, ALL-L3
t(2;8)(p12;q24)	BL, ALL-L3
t(8;22)(q24;q11)	BL, ALL-L3
t(14;18)(q32;q21)	ML
t(11;14)(q13;q32)	B-CLL, MM/PCL, B-PLL
t(2;14)(p13;q32)	B-CLL
+ 12	B-CLL
t(8;14)(q24;q11)	T-ALL
t(8;14)(p13;q11-13)	T-ALL
t(10;14)(q24;q11)	T-ALL
t(1;14)(q32;q11)	T-ALL
t(7;14)(q35-36;q11)	T-ALL
t((14;14)(q11-12;q32)	T-ALL, T-CLL
inv(14)(q11q32)	T-CLL, T-PLL, ATL
t(4;11)(q21;q23)	ALL
6q −	ML, ALL, CTCL, ATL, B-PLL

*ALL, acute lymphocytic leukemia; BL, Burkitt's lymphoma; ALL-13, Burkitt's leukemia; ML, malignant lymphoma; CLL, chronic lymphocytic leukemia; MM/PCL, multiple myeloma/plasma cell leukemia; PLL, prolymphocytic leukemia; ATL, adult T-cell leukemia; CTCL, cutaneous T-cell lymphoma. T- refers to T-cell neoplasia and B- refers to B-cell neoplasia.

prognoses. Loss or deletion of chromosomes 5 and 7, inv(3) (q21q26), or t(3;3)(q21;q26) are associated with a poor prognosis. The t(15;17) may also be unfavorable. Patients with all normal cells (NN) or some normal cells (AN) generally have a better prognosis than patients with only abnormal metaphases (AA). A highly complex cytogenetic abnormality is generally worse than the presence of a single abnormality such as a simple translocation or single additional chromosome. Patients with acute nonlymphocytic leukemia arising from treatment of another malignancy generally have a poor prognosis and these patients usually have the cytogenetic abnormalities that are associated with poor outcome.

Lymphoid cell disorders

Box 74-7 lists some characteristic chromosome abnormalities seen in various lymphocytic leukemias and non-Hodgkin's lymphomas. Many of the cytogenetic changes seen in this group of disorders involve immunoglobulin genes and T-cell receptor genes, and it has become clear that aberrant exchanges between these and other specific genes characterize many lymphoid neoplasias.

The immense diversity of immunoglobulins and T-cell receptors required for the rejection of invading foreign materials and cells from the body is achieved, at least in part, by the somatic rearrangement of the immunoglobulin heavy chain genes (IGH, located at 14q32), kappa light chain genes (IgG-κ, 2p11), lambda light chain genes (IgG-λ, 22q11), T-cell receptor beta chain genes (TCRB, 7q35-36), T-cell receptor alpha chain genes (TCRA, 14q11), T-cell receptor gamma chain genes (TCRG, 7p15), and T-cell receptor delta chain genes (TCRD, 14q11). These submicroscopic rearrangements occur within normal cell populations, giving rise to polyclonal B- and T-cell populations that mediate the immune response. Specific abnormal rearrangements sometimes arise in which immunoglobulin or T-cell receptor genes are juxtaposed with oncogenes, with uncontrolled pro-

liferation of the aberrant clone. This occurs, for example, in the B-cell disorder, Burkitt's lymphoma, where an immunoglobulin gene (usually IGH) is translocated adjacent to the c-*myc* oncogene. Cytogenetically, this is seen as a t(8;14)(q24;q32), or t(2;8)(p11;q24), or t(8;22)(q24;q11), depending on the immunoglobulin gene involved. These same translocations are seen in occasional cases of non-Hodgkin's lymphoma and acute lymphocytic leukemia (Fig. 74-13). Parallel types of aberrant exchange occur in T cells, in which the T-cell receptor genes are brought into close association with the putative oncogenes, *tcl*-1 (14q32), *tcl*-2 (11p13), and *tcl*-3 (10q24). A locus on chromosome 1, band p32 or p33, with a gene referred to as TCL5, SCL, or *tal*, appears to be involved with rearrangement; TCRD in rare T-cell leukemias and other specific loci have also been described that are involved in rearrangement with T-cell receptor genes.

The translocation t(14;18)(q32;q21) is seen in most follicular lymphomas, but also in some lymphomas with large cell or diffuse morphology. This translocation brings together IGH and a gene from chromosome 18, known as *bcl*-2. As a result of the translocation, the *bcl*-2 gene is deregulated and the presence of this protein appears to be at least a contributing factor to the malignant phenotype. Similarly, the translocation t(11;14)(q13;q32) is an aberrant positioning of IGH with a gene referred to as *bcl*-1. This translocation is found in some non-Hodgkin's lymphomas, CLL, and multiple myeloma.

The translocation t(9;22)(q34;q11) is seen in up to 20% of acute lymphocytic leukemias (ALL) and is cytogenetically indistinguishable from that seen in CML. In approximately 50% of Ph-positive ALL, the breakpoints are within the *bcr*, whereas in the remaining 50%, the breakpoints are located in a separate region of the *phl* gene. These variable breakpoint locations result in different *phl-abl* fusion products, which may have differing activities in terms of their transforming effects.

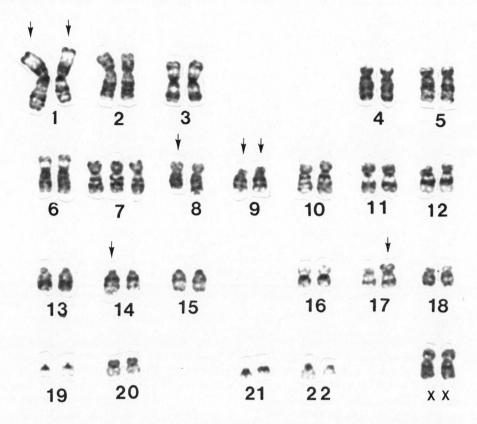

Fig. 74-13 A karyotype from a patient with ALL. As well as having a translocation t(8;14)(q24;q11), the patient also has abnormalities involving both chromosomes 1, both chromosomes 9, and one chromosome 17. An additional chromosome 7 is also present.

Box 74-8 Chromosome abnormalities seen in solid tumors

Bladder carcinoma	Abnormalities of chromosomes 1,5,11
Brain tumors	del(22)(q11-13)
Breast carcinoma	Abnormalities of chromosomes 1,3,7,11
Colon carcinoma	Abnormalities of chromosomes 1,7,17
Ewing sarcoma	t(1;16)(q11;q11), t(11;22)(q24;q12)
Extraskeletal mxyoid chondrosarcoma	t(9;22)(q22-31;q11-12)
Leiomyoma	t(12;14)(q13-15;q23-24), del(7)(q11-32)
Leiomyosarcoma	Abnormalities of lp
Lipoma	t(3;12)(q27-28;q13-14), t(12;?)(q13-14;?)
Liposarcoma	t(12;16)(p13;p11)
Lung carcinoma	del(3)(p14p23)
Malignant histiocytosis	t(2;5)(p21-23;q35)
Malignant melanoma	Abnormalities of chromosomes 1,6,7,10,11,19
Mesothelioma	Abnormalities of 3p
Neuroblastoma	del or t(1)(p32-36)
Ovarian carcinoma	del(3)(p13-21), del(6)(q15-q23), t(6;14)(q21;q24)
Pleomorphic adenomas	t(12;14)(q13-15;q23-24), t(9;12)(p13-22;q13-15), t(3;8)(p21;q12)
Prostate carcinoma	del(7)(q22), del(10)(q24)
Retinoblastoma	i(6p), del(13)(q13.3q14.3)
Renal cell carcinoma	del(3)(p21-p14)
Rhabdomyosarcoma	t(2;13)(q35-37;q14)
Synovial sarcoma	t(X;18)(p11;q11)
Testicular carcinoma (and other male germ cell tumors)	i(12p)
Uterus carcinoma	Abnormalities of chromosome 1, del 6(q21)
Wilms' tumor	Abnormalities of chromosome 1, del 11(p13)

A further example of the production of a chimeric protein arising as a result of translocation has also been described. The translocation t(1;19)(q23;p13), seen in pre–B-cell acute lymphoblastic leukemia, appears to involve the fusion of the E2A regulatory gene (chromosome 19) with a gene referred to as *prl* (chromosome 1).

The different cytogenetic abnormalities seen in lymphoid neoplasia have variable prognostic significance. In children with ALL, a hyperdiploid karyotype has a better prognosis than a normal or hypodiploid karyotype. Translocation t(4;11)(q21;q23), the presence of Ph, abnormality involving 8q24 or 14q+, are all associated with poor prognosis, but longer survival is seen in children with a 6q- cytogenetic abnormality. For adults with ALL, a karyotype provides less prognostic information. Detection of a t(14;18) (q32;q21) translocation is usually, but by no means invariably, associated with the relatively slowly progressing follicular lymphoma, whereas t(8;14)(q24;q32) is seen in more aggressive lymphomas.

Solid tumors

Substantial technical difficulties are associated with the cytogenetic analysis of solid tumors. Some tumor cells grow very poorly in tissue culture because non-tumor cell outgrowth is frequently a problem, often there are few mitotic cells, the complexity of the karyotypes make interpretation difficult, and there can be considerable variation from one cell to the next. Consequently, solid tumors are not usually referred for routine analysis. Nevertheless, in recent years, considerable progress has been made in identifying some highly specific cytogenetic changes and the combination of cytogenetic and molecular genetic approaches has provided some profound insights.

Box 74-8 lists some of the most consistent findings seen in solid tumors. Some cytogenetic changes appear to be present in widely different tumor cell types, whereas others are clearly specific for a particular tumor type. For both types of abnormalities, the observations point clearly to specific genetic lesions being important in the initiation and evolution of cancer. In the coming years the full significance of these genetic changes will be appreciated from the application of molecular genetic techniques. This will result in highly specific diagnostic tests, prognostic evaluations, and also the identification of subgroups of patients who will derive the most benefit from any particular type of treatment.

SUGGESTED READING
Bloomfield CD, Trent JM, and van Den Berghe H: Report of the committee on structural chromosome changes in neoplasia, Cytogenet Cell Genet 46:344, 1987.

Borgaonkar DS: Chromosomal variation in man: a catalog of chromosomal variants and anomalies, ed 4, New York, 1984, Alan R Liss.

Grouchy J de and Turleau C: Clinical atlas of human chromosomes, ed 2, New York, 1984. John Wiley.

Hsu LYF: Prenatal diagnosis of chromosome abnormalities. In Genetic disorders and the fetus, ed. Milunsky A, New York, 1986, Plenum.

Mitelman F: Catalogue of chromosome aberrations in cancer, ed 3, New York, 1988, Alan R. Liss.

Rooney DE and Czepulkowski BH: Human cytogenetics: a practical approach, ed. 2, Oxford, 1992, Oxford Press.

Sandberg AA: The chromosomes in human cancer and leukemia, New York, 1980, Elsevier Science.

Schinzel A: Catalogue of unbalanced chromosome aberrations in man, Berlin, 1983, W de Grugter.

Smith DW: Recognizable patterns of human malformation, ed 3, Philadelphia, 1982, WB Saunders.

Sumner AT: The nature and mechanisms of chromosome banding, Cancer Genet Cytogenet 6:59, 1982.

Therman E: Human chromosomes: structure, behavior, effects, ed 2, New York, 1985, Springer-Verlag.

Thompson JS and Thompson MV: Genetics in medicine, ed 4, Philadelphia, 1986, WB Saunders.

Trent JM, Kaneko Y, and Mitelman F: Report of the committee on structural changes in neoplasia, Cytogenet Cell Genet 49:236, 1988.

APPENDICES

A

Chemistry reference intervals

Analyte	Reference Interval	Chapter
Acetaminophen, serum	10-20 mcg/mL	27
Acid phosphatase, serum	0.5-1.9 IU/L* 37°C	14
Acid phosphatase, prostatic	<1.2 IU/L* 37°C	14
Adrenocorticotropic hormone	10-80 pg/mL	16
Alanine aminotransferase, serum (ALT, SGPT)	5-45 IU/L* 37°C	14
Albumin, serum		12
0-1yr	29-55 g/L	
1-31 yr	35-50 g/L	
after 40 yr	declines	
Alcohol, serum (Ethanol)	undetectable	27
Aldolase, serum		14
adult male	4-12 IU/L* 37°C	
adult female	1.5-7.9 IU/L* 37°C	
Aldosterone, serum	<10 ng/dL	16
secretion rate	40-200 mcg/day	16
Akaline phosphatase, serum	35-105 IU/L* 37°C	14
Alpha₁acid glycoprotein, serum	0.55-1.4 g/L	
Alpha₁antitrypsin, serum	0.78-2.0 g/L	12
neonates have much lower values		
Alpha₁fetoprotein, serum	1×10^{-5} g/L	
Alpha₂macroglobulin, serum	1.5-4.2 g/L	
Alpha lipoprotein, serum	2.5-3.9 g/L	
Alprazolam, serum	20-60 ng/mL	27
Aluminum, serum	0-10 mcg/L	25
on dialysis	>60 mcg/L	
chronic exposure	>100 mcg/L	
urine	0-30 mcg/24 hr	25
possible toxic?	>50 mcg/24 hr	
Amikacin, serum	5-10 mcg/mL	27
Aminoglycosides	Trough Values	27
Amikacin, serum	5-10 mcg/mL	
Gentamicin, serum	1-2 mcg/mL	
Kanamycin, serum	5-10 mcg/mL	
Netilmicin, serum	0.5-2 mcg/mL	
Streptomycin, serum	<5 mcg/mL	
Tobramycin, serum	1-2 mcg/mL	
Amitriptyline, serum (+nortriptyline)	125-300 ng/mL	27
Ammonia, plasma		13
child 1-5 yr	10-40 umol/L	
5-19 yr	11-35 umol/L	
adult male	11-35 umol/L	
adult female	11-35 umol/L	
Amobarbital, serum	1-10 mcg/mL	27
Amylase, serum	25-115 IU/L* 37°C	14
Anion gap, serum	5-14 mmol/L	7
Antidiuretic hormone, plasma	5-8 ng/mL	16

*Enzyme values are method dependent.

Analyte	Reference Interval	Chapter
Anticonvulsant drugs, serum		27
Carbamazepine, serum	4-12 mcg/mL	
Ethosuximide, serum	40-100 mcg/mL	
Phenobarbital, serum	15-40 mcg/mL	
Phenytoin, serum	10-20 mcg/mL	
Primidone, serum	5-12 mcg/mL	
Valproic acid, serum	50-120 mcg/mL	
Arsenic, whole blood	5-60 mcg/L	25
chronic exposure	100-500 mcg/L	
acute exposure	>600 mcg/L	
urine	0-100 mcg/L	
chronic exposure	100-200 mcg/L	
acute exposure	>200 mcg/L	
hair	0-65 mcg/100 g	
chronic exposure	>100 mcg/100 g	
nails	90-180 mcg/100 g	
chronic exposure	>200 mcg/100 g	
Ascorbic acid see Vitamin C		
Aspartate aminotransferase, serum (AST, SGOT)	15-45 IU/L* 37°C	14
Barbiturates, serum		27
Amobarbital	1-10 mcg/mL	
Butabarbital	1-10 mcg/mL	
Butalbital	1-10 mcg/mL	
Pentobarbital	1-6 mcg/mL	
Phenobarbital	15-40 mcg/mL	
Secobarbital	1-6 mcg/mL	
Thiopental	<4 mcg/mL	
Benzene, serum	none detected	27
Beta core human chorionic gonadotropin, serum	not established	21
Beta HCG see human chorionic gonadotropin		
Beta lipoprotein, serum (LDL)	2.5-4.4 g/L	12
Beta$_2$microglobulin, serum	1.0-2.6 mg/L	21
urine	30-370 mcg/24 hr	
Bilirubin, total, serum		13
0-1 month	1-12 mg/dL	
1 mo to adult	0-1.2 mg/dL	
Bilirubin, conjugated, serum (direct)	0-0.2 mg/dL	
Blood gases, whole blood		7
arterial pH	7.35-7.45	
pCO$_2$	35-45 mm Hg	
pO$_2$	80-100 mm Hg	
HCO$_3^-$	22-26 mmol/L	
total CO$_2$	23-27 mmol/L	
O$_2$ saturation	94-100%	
venous pH	7.33-7.43	
pCO$_2$	38-50 mm Hg	
pO$_2$	30-50 mm Hg	
HCO$_3^-$	23-27 mmol/L	
total CO$_2$	24-28 mmol/L	
O$_2$ saturation	60-85%	
Bromide, serum	500-1500 mcg/mL	27
BUN see urea nitrogen		
Butabarbital	1-10 mcg/mL	27
Butalbital	1-10 mcg/mL	27
CA 15-3, serum	<30 U/mL	21
CA 19-9, serum	<37 U/mL	21
CA 50, serum	<17 U/mL	21
CA 125, serum	<35 U/mL	21
CA 195, serum	not established	21
CA 549, serum	<11 KU/mL	21
Cadmium, whole blood	0.5-1.1 mcg/L	25
toxic	7-10 mcg/L	
urine	<1 mcg/L	
toxic	>10 mcg/L	

Continued.

Analyte	Reference Interval	Chapter
Caffeine, serum	<15 mcg/mL	27
Calcitonin, plasma males	<40 ng/L	21
females	<20 ng/L	
Calcium, ionized, plasma	1.14-1.29 mmol/L	10
Calcium, total, serum		10
children	2.2-2.7 mmol/L	
adults	2.1-2.55 mmol/L	
Carbamazepine, serum	4-12 mcg/mL	27
Carbon monoxide, whole blood, (carboxyhemoglobin)		27
nonsmoker	<2%	
smoker	<8%	
Carbon dioxide, serum	24-32 mmol/L	6
Carboxyhemoglobin see carbon monoxide		
Carcinoembryonic antigens, serum (CEA)		21
nonsmoker	<2.5 mcg/mL	
smoker	<5 mcg/mL	
Carotenes see Vitamin A		
Catecholamines see epinephrine and norepinephrine		
c-erbB-2, breast tissue	not established	21
CEA see carcinoembryonic antigens		
Ceruloplasmin, serum	0.15-0.6 g/L	12
Chloral hydrate, serum (Trichloroethanol)	<10 mcg/mL	27
Chloramphenicol, serum	<40 mcg/mL	27
Chlordiazepoxide, serum	<1 mcg/mL	27
Chloride, serum	101-111 mmol/L	6
urine	110-150 mmol/L	
sweat	<35 mmol/L	
Chlorpromazine, serum	<0.5 mcg/mL	27
Cholesterol, serum		9
desirable	<200 mg/dL	
borderline	200-239 mg/dL	
high	>=240 mg/dL	
Cholinesterase (pseudo), serum	1800-4800 mIU/mL	27
Chorionic gonadotropin see human chorionic gonadotropin		
Chromium, serum	0.2-0.5 mcg/L	25
whole blood	0.7-2.8 mcg/L	
urine	<1.0 mcg/24 hr	
hair	0.1-3.6 mcg/g	
CK see creatine kinase		
Cobalt, serum	0.2-2.0 mcg/L	25
whole blood	2.0-2.8 mcg/L	
urine	0.7-10 mcg/24 hr	
hair	0.2-1.0 mcg/g	
Copper, serum		25
males	700-1400 mcg/L	
females	800-1550 mcg/L	
Complement, C_3, serum	0.55-1.8 g/L	12
Complement, C_4, serum	0.8-1.4 g/L	12
Cortisol, plasma am	50-230 mcg/L	16
urine free (extracted)	4.9-35.3 mcg/24 hr	
urine (unextracted)	46-131 mcg/24 hr	
Creatine kinase, serum (CK)	25-250 IU/L* 37°C	14
Creatine kinase isoenzymes, serum		
CK (MM)	>95%	
CK (MB)	<5%	
CK (BB)	about 0%	
Creatinine, plasma		13
infant 0-1 yr	2-10 mg/L	
child 1-5 yr	2-10 mg/L	
5-19 yr	4-13 mg/L	
adult male	5-12 mg/L	
adult female	4-10 mg/L	
Creatinine, urine		6
male	1.0-2.0 gm/24 hr	
female	0.8-1.8 gm/24 hr	

Analyte	Reference Interval	Chapter
Creatinine clearance		6
(surface adj) male	97-137 mL/min	
(surface adj) female	88-128 mL/min	
Cyclosporine, whole blood	Abbott TDx Monoclonal	27
Therapeutic ranges depend on assays used and organ transplanted		
Kidney & kidney/pancrease		
<6 months	250-375 ng/mL	
>6 months	100-250 ng/mL	
Liver		
<=1 month	350-450 ng/mL	
2-6 months	250-350 ng/mL	
>6 months	170-240 ng/mL	
Cardiac		
<6 weeks	300-420 ng/mL	
6-12 weeks	180-300 ng/mL	
>12 weeks	120-180 ng/mL	
Desipramine, serum (+imipramine)	150-300 ng/mL	27
Dehydroepiandrosterone sulfate, serum		19
cord blood	72-200 mcg/mL	
serum, 0-1 month	15-265 mcg/mL	
1-6 months	0-29 mcg/mL	
6 mo-7 years	0-12 mcg/mL	
8-15 years	5-200 mcg/mL #	
# during puberty, DHEA-S values rise to adult values		
male 15-40 years	150-550 mcg/mL	
41-50 years	100-400 mcg/mL	
51-60 years	60-300 mcg/mL	
61-127 years	30-200 mcg/mL	
female 15-30 years	100-500 mcg/mL	
31-40 years	60-350 mcg/mL	
41-50 years	40-250 mcg/mL	
51-127 years	20-150 mcg/mL	
Diazepam, serum	0.2-2.0 mcg/mL	27
Digoxin, serum	0.5-2.2 ng/mL	27
Digitoxin, serum	<35 ng/mL	27
Disopyramide, serum	2-4 mcg/mL	27
Dopamine, plasma	10-130 pg/mL	16
Doxepin, serum (+desmethyldoxepin)	75-200 mcg/mL	27
Dopamine, urine	60-400 mcg/24 hr	16
Epidermal growth factor receptor, serum		21
(EGF-R)	not established	
Epinephrine, plasma	25-50 pg/mL	16
Epinephrine, free, urine	0.5-25 mcg/24 hr	16
Estriol, serum	varies with gestational age	18
urine	varies with gestational age	
Estrogen receptor, breast tissue	>10 fmol/mg	21
Ethanol see alcohol		
Ethchlorvynol, serum	<10 mcg/mL	27
Ethosuximide, serum	40-100 mcg/mL	27
Ethylene glycol, serum	none detected	27
Ferritin, serum	20-200 ng/mL	11
Fluoride, blood	<0.5 mcg/mL	27
Fluoride, urine	<1 mcg/mL	27
Fluoxetine, serum	<1200 ng/mL	27
Flurazepam, serum	<20 ng/mL	27
Folate, serum	<3.0 mcg/L	20
RBC	<140 mcg/L	
Follicular stimulating hormone, serum (FSH)		16
Prepubertal, male & female	<9 mIU/mL	
adult, male	<20 mIU/mL	
adult, female		
follicular	<17 mIU/mL	
mid-cycle	20-30 mIU/mL	
post menopausal	30-150 mIU/mL	

Continued.

Analyte	Reference Interval	Chapter
Follicular stimulating hormone, urine (FSH)		16
male to age 8 yr	<5 mIU/mL	
male greater 8 yr	<22 mIU/mL	
female to age 8 yr	<5 mIU/mL	
female age 9 to 15 yr	<22 mIU/mL	
female greater 15 yr	<30 mIU/mL	
FTI Free thyroxine index	1.2-3.2	17
Gamma glutamyltransferase, serum	15-70 IU/L* 37°C	14
Gastric acid, gastric juice		32
basal acid output		
male	0-10 mmol/hr	
female	0-6 mmol/hr	
maximal acid output		
male	7-48 mmol/hr	
female	5-30 mmol/hr	
Gastrin, serum	30-100 pg/mL	15
Gentamicin	1-2 mcg/mL	27
Glucose, serum	70-110 mg/dL	8
Gluthethimide, serum	<10 mcg/mL	27
Glycohemoglobin, whole blood	6-8%	11
Growth hormone, plasma, males	0-5 ng/mL	16
females	0-10 ng/mL	16
Haloperidol, serum	<15 ng/mL	27
Haptoglobulin, serum	0.4-1.8 g/L	12
HDL see Alpha lipoprotein		
HDL-Cholesterol, serum		9
desirable	>65 mg/dL	
borderline	35-65 mg/dL	
at risk	<35 mg/dL	
Hemoglobin, blood		11
males	>130 g/L	
females	>120 g/L	
Hemoplexin, serum	0.5-1.0 g/L	12
HIAA-5, urine	<15 mg/24 hr	15
Homovanillic acid, urine	<13 mg/24 hr	16
Human chorionic gonadotropin, serum		21
(beta-hCG) males and nonpregnant		
premenopausal females	<5 IU/L	
postmenopausal females	<7 IU/L	
pregnant females	> 20 IU/L	
rising to in first trimester	>100,000 IU/L	
IgA, serum	0.7-3.2 g/L	12
IgD, serum	0.015-0.2 g/L	12
IgE, serum	6×10^{-4} g/L	12
IgG, serum	8.0-12 g/L	12
IgM, serum	0.5-2.8 g/L	12
Interleukin-2 receptor, T cells	not established	21
Insulin, serum	<1042 pg/mL	15
Imipramine, serum (+desimipramine)	150-300 mcg/mL	27
Iron, serum		11
males	500-1600 mcg/L	
females	400-1500 mcg/L	
Iron, urine	10-250 mcg/mL	27
Iron binding capacity, total		11
serum	2500-4000 mcg/L	
Iron saturation, serum	20-55%	
Isopropanol, serum	none detected	27
Kanamycin	5-10 mcg/mL	27
17-Ketosteroids, urine	5-15 mg/24 hr	18
Lactic dehydrogenase, serum (P->L)	90-320 IU/L* 37°C	14
Lactic dehydrogenase isoenzymes		14
LD 1	18-33%	
LD 2	28-40%	
LD 3	18-30%	
LD 4	6-16%	
LD 5	2-13%	

Analyte	Reference Interval	Chapter
Lead, whole blood	0-200 mcg/L	25
chronic exposure	200-700 mcg/L	
acute exposure	>700 mcg/L	
urine	0-80 mcg/24 hr	25
possible exposure	80-120 mcg/24 hr	
toxicity associated	>120 mcg/24 hr	
Lecithin-sphingomyelin (LS) ratio, amnionic fluid	>2 is mature	19
LDL see Beta lipoprotein		
LDL-Cholesterol, serum		9
desirable	<130 mg/dL	
borderline	130-159 mg/dL	
high	>=160 mg/dL	
Lidocaine, serum	1.2-5 mcg/mL	27
Lipase, serum	4-24 U/dL	14
Lipid associated sialic acid, plasma		21
(LASA-P)	<20 mg/dL	
Lithium, serum	0.5-1.3 mcg/mL	27
Luteinizing hormone, serum		16
Prepubertal, male & female	<15 mIU/mL	
adult, male	<26 mIU/mL	
adult, female		
follicular	<33 mIU/mL	
mid-cycle	30-200 mIU/mL	
post menopausal	30-130 mIU/mL	
Luteinizing hormone, urine		16
Prepubertial	<7 mIU/mL	
Childhood	<40 mIU/mL	
Adult	<45 mIU/mL	
Magnesium, plasma	0.6-1.1 mmol/L	10
Manganese, whole blood	<10 mcg/L	25
serum	1-3 mcg/L	
urine	<1mcg/24 hr	
hair	0.1-2.1 mcg/g	
Maprotilene, serum	120-300 ng/mL	27
Meperidine, serum	<1 mcg/mL	27
Mephenytoin, serum	5-16 mcg/mL	27
Meprobamate, serum	<20 mcg/mL	27
Mercury, whole blood	0-5 mcg/L	25
toxic	20-30 mcg/L	
urine	0-20 mcg/24 hr	25
exposure to organic form	>100 mcg/24 hr	
exposure to inorganic form	>200 mcg/24 hr	
WBC/plasma ratio		
organic	5-20	
inorganic	1.0	
Methanephrine, urine	0.2-1.3 mg/24 hr	16
Methanol, serum	none detected	27
Methaqualone, serum	<5 mcg/mL	27
Methotrexate, serum at 24 hr post	<4.5 mg/L	26
Methylmalonic acid, urine	2.7-8.6 mg/L	
Molybdenum, whole blood	1-15 mcg/L	25
serum	0.1-6 mcg/L	
urine	10-16 mcg/L	
hair	0.06-0.2 mcg/L	
N-acetylprocainamide, serum (see also procainamide)	9-19 mcg/mL	27
Netilmicin	0.5-2 mcg/mL	27
Niacin, urine ratio pyridone/methyl nicotinamide	>=1.0	20
Nickel, whole blood	0-1.05 mcg/L	25
urine	0-7 mcg/24 hr	
toxic values	>20 mcg/24 hr	
serum	0.05-1.1 mcg/L	
Norepinephrine, plasma	100-400 pg/mL	16
Norepinephrine, free, urine	10-70 mcg/24 hr	16
Nortriptyline, serum	50-150 ng/mL	27
5' Nucleotidase, serum	3-15 U/L* 37°C	14
Oxazepam, serum	<500 ng/mL	27
Oxytocin, serum	1-2 mcU/mL	16

Continued.

Analyte	Reference Interval	Chapter
Osmolality, serum	282-300 mOsm/kg	6
Osmolality, urine	50-1200 mOsm/kg	6
Parathyroid hormone, plasma	0-97 pg/mL	10
Pentobarbital, serum	1-6 mcg/mL	27
Phenobarbital, serum	15-40 mcg/mL	27
Phenytoin, serum	10-20 mcg/mL	27
Philadelphia chromosome, bone marrow cells		21
(Ph[1])	present/absent	
Phosphatidyl glycerol, amnionic fluid	present when lungs mature	19
Phosphorus, serum	1.45-2.76 meq/L	10
Porphyrin, blood	500-600 mcg/L	11
urine	<200 mcg/L	
feces	<60 mg/dry gram stool	
Potassium, serum	3.6-5.0 mmol/L	6
Potassium, urine	2.5-125 mmol/24 hr	6
Pre-albumin, serum varies with age	0.2-0.4 g/L	12
Pre-beta lipoprotein, serum (VLDL)	1.5-2.3 g/L	12
Primidone, serum	5-12 mcg/mL	27
Procainamide, serum	4-10 mcg/mL	27
N-acetylprocainamide+procainamide	5-30 mcg/mL	
Progesterone, serum		19
male prepubertal	0.11-0.26 ng/mL	
male adult	0-0.4 ng/mL	
female prepubertal	0.10-0.34 ng/mL	
female adult follicular	0.10-1.5 ng/mL	
luteal	2.5-28 ng/mL	
pregnant	9-255 ng/mL	
postmenopausal	0.03-0.3 ng/mL	
ectopic pregnancy	<13-13.5 ng/mL	
normal pregnancy	>15-20 ng/mL	
Progesterone receptor, breast tissue	>10 fmol/mg	21
Prolactin, serum, males	6-15 ng/mL	16
females	8-25 ng/mL	16
Properidin factor B, serum	0.12-8.0 g/L	12
Propoxyphene, serum	<0.5 mcg/mL	27
Propranolol, serum	<100 ng/mL	27
Prostate specific antigen, serum (PSA)	<4 mcg/mL	21
Protein, total, serum	6.6-6.8 g/dL	6
urine	40-150 mg/dL	
cerebrospinal fluid	15-45 mg/dL	
Protoporphyrin, RBC free erythrocyte	150-800 mcg/L cells	11
PSA see prostate specific antigens		
Pyruvate, serum	<8.8 mg/L	8
Pyridoxal phosphate see Vitamin B_6		
Quinidine, serum	2-5 mcg/mL	27
Ras oncogenes, tissue	not established	21
Retinoblastoma gene prod, tissue	not established	21
Riboflavin see Vitamin B_2		
Salicylate, serum	<300 mcg/mL	27
Secobarbital, serum	1-6 mcg/mL	27
Selenium, serum	78-320 mcg/L	25
whole blood	100-340 mcg/L	
urine	15-100 mcg/L	
hair	0.6-2.6 mcg/g	
Seminal fluid analysis		31
volume	2.0 or more	
pH	7.2-7.8	
sperm concentration	20×10^6 sperm/mL or more	
total sperm	40×10^6 spermatozoa	
motility	50% with forward progression	
morphology	50% with normal morphology	
viability	50% or more live	
WBC	$<1 \times 10^6$/mL	
Zinc	2.4 mcmol or more/ejaculate	

Analyte	Reference Interval	Chapter
Citrate	52 mcmol or more/ejaculate	
Fructose	13 mcmol or more/ejaculate	
MAR	Fewer than 10% spermatozoa with adherent particles	
Immunobead test	Fewer than 10% spermatozoa with adherent beads	
Sodium, serum	135-145 mmol/L	6
urine	40-220 mmol/L	6
SGOT see Aspartate aminotransferase (AST)		
SGPT see Alanine aminotransferase (ALT)		
Squamous cell carcinoma antigen, serum		21
(SCC)	<2.5 mcg/mL	
Streptomycin	<5 mcg/mL	27
Sulfa, serum	<250 mcg/mL	27
T3-Uptake, serum	25-35%	17
T4 see thyroxine		
TAG-72 see Tumor associated antigen-72		
Testosterone, total, serum		18
males	270-1070 ng/dL	
females	6-86 ng/dL	
urine		
males	25-125 ng/dL	
females	5-35 ng/dL	
Testosterone, free, serum		
males	absolute % of total	
20-39 yr	1.7-4.1 ng/dL, 0.32-0.76%	
40-59 yr	1.4-3.4 ng/dL, 0.26-0.63%	
60-79 yr	0.9-2.8 ng/dL, 0.17-0.52%	
females 20-39 yr	0.08-0.32 ng/dL, 0.17-0.68%	
40-59 yr	0.04-0.27 ng/dL, 0.08-0.57%	
60-99 yr	0.02-0.22 ng/dL, 0.04-0.47%	
Theophylline, serum adult	10-20 mcg/ml	27
serum neonate (Apnea)	5-15 mcg/mL	
Thiamin see Vitamin B_1		
Thiopental, serum	<4 mcg/mL	27
Thyroid stimulating hormone, serum	2 mcU/mL (mean)	17
Thyroxine, free, serum	2.2 ng/dL (mean)	17
Thyroxine, total, serum (T4)	8 mcg/dL (mean)	17
cord blood	6.6-18.1 mcg/dL	
2-5 days	8.5-22.0 mcg/dL	
3-12 months	7.6-16.0 mcg/dL	
1-5 yr	7.3-15.0 mcg/dL	
6-10 yr	6.4-13.3 mcg/dL	
11-16 yr	5.6-11.7 mcg/dL	
>16 yr	4.5-11.5 mcg/dL	
TIBC see Iron binding capacity, total		
Tissue plasminogen activator, serum		
(TPA, a genetically engineered drug)	not established	
Tissue polypeptide antigen, serum (TPA)	not established	21
Tobramycin, serum	1-2 mcg/mL	27
Toluene, serum	none detected	27
TPA see Tissue poylpeptide antigen and Tissue plasminogen activator		
Transferrin, serum	2.52-4.29 g/L	11
Transforming growth factor-alpha, serum (TGF-alpha)	<2 mcg/mL	21
Trazodone, serum	<1600 ng/mL	27
Trichloroethanol see Chloral hydrate		
Triglycerides, serum		9
1-29 yr	<140 mg/dL	
30-39 yr	<150 mg/dL	
40-49 yr	<160 mg/dL	
50-59 yr	<170 mg/dL	
>60 yr	<200 mg/dL	
Triiodothyronine, free, serum (T3)	0.4 ng/dL (mean)	17
Triiodothyronine, reverse, serum (rT3)	25 ng/dL (mean)	17

Continued.

Analyte	Reference Interval	Chapter
Triiodothyronine, total, serum (T3)	130 ng/dL (mean)	17
cord blood	24-77 ng/dL	
2-5 days	99-227 ng/dL	
3-12 months	96-219 ng/dL	
1-5 yr	92-215 ng/dL	
6-10 yr	84-194 ng/dL	
11-16 yr	75-172 ng/dL	
>16 yr	94-168 ng/dL	
Tumor associated antigen-72, serum	not established	21
Urea-nitrogen, serum		13
infant, 0-1 yr	60-450 mg/L	
child, 1-5 yr	50-170 mg/L	
5-19 yr	80-200 mg/L	
adult male	100-210 mg/L	
adult female	100-210 mg/L	
Urea-nitrogen, urine	7-16 g/24 hr	6
Uric acid, serum		13
infant, 0-1 yr	10-76 mg/L	
child, 1-5 yr	18-50 mg/L	
5-19 yr	30-60 mg/L	
adult male	40-90 mg/L	
adult female	30-60 mg/L	
Urinalysis		29
Chemical findings		
specific gravity	1.003-1.040	
pH	4.8-7.5 (mean 6.0)	
protein	neg to trace	
glucose	negative	
ketones	negative	
urobilinogen	<1 mg/dL	
bilirubin	negative	
occult blood	negative	
WBC esterase	negative	
nitrite	negative	
Microscopic findings		
RBC	0-3/HPF	
WBC	0-5/HPF	
bacteria	few/HPF	
epithelial cells		
renal tubular	0-1/HPF	
transitional	0-2/HPF	
squamous	varys/HPF	
mucus	<1+	
crystals		
calcium oxalate	few	
amophorous urates	few	
amophorous phosphates	few	
casts		
hyaline	0-2/LPF	
granular	0-1/LPF	
spermatozoa, in male	may be present	
spermatozoa, in female	may be present	
Yeast	negative	
Trichomonas	negative	
Urine protein, total	40-150 mg/24 hr	12
Urinary gonadotropin peptide, urine (UGP)	<8 nmol/L	21
Valproic acid	50-120 mcg/mL	27
Vanillylmandelic acid, urine (VMA)	2-7 mg/24 hr	16
VLDL see Pre-beta lipoprotein		
Vitamin A, plasma deficiency	<0.1 mg/L	20
Vitamin B$_1$, RBC deficiency (Thiamin)	ETR index >1.25	20
Vitamin B$_2$, RBC deficiency (Riboflavin)	ETR index >1.4	20
Vitamin B$_6$, plasma (Pyridoxal phosphate)	<15 nmol	20

Analyte	Reference Interval	Chapter
Vitamin B$_{12}$, true-serum	<100 ng/L	20
Vitamin C, serum deficency	<2.4 mg/L	20
Vitamin D, plasma	20-76 ng/L	10
plasma deficiency	<20 ng/L	20
Vitamin E, plasma deficiency	<5.0 mg/L	20
Vitamin K, plasma deficiency	<0.5 mcg/L	20
Zinc, serum	700-1500 mcg/L	25
urine	0.15-1.0 mg/24 hr	
hair	100-280 mcg/g	
d-Xylose, serum	at 2 hr 30-50 mg/dL	9
urine	4-8.2 g/5 hr	

g = gram, mg = milligram, mcg = microgram, ng = nanogram, pg = picogram, mol = mole, mmol = millimole, mcmol = micromole, nmol = nanomole, fmol = fentomole, meq = milliequivalent, mm = millimeter, mOsm = milliosmole, U = unit, IU = International Unit, mIU = milli-International Unit, mcU = micro unit, LPF = low power field, HPF = high power field

Appendix B

Periodic Table of the Elements

KEY:

1	Atomic number
H	Symbol of element
1.008	Atomic weight

Transition elements

Period	IA	IIA	IIIB	IVB	VB	VIB	VIIB	VIIIB			IB	IIB	IIIA	IVA	VA	VIA	VIIA	0 (Inert gases)
1	1 **H** 1.00794																1 **H** 1.00794	2 **He** 4.00260
2	3 **Li** 6.941*	4 **Be** 9.01218											5 **B** 10.81	6 **C** 12.011	7 **N** 14.0067	8 **O** 15.9994*	9 **F** 18.998403	10 **Ne** 20.179
3	11 **Na** 22.98977	12 **Mg** 24.305											13 **Al** 26.98154	14 **Si** 28.0855*	15 **P** 30.97376	16 **S** 32.06	17 **Cl** 35.453	18 **Ar** 39.948
4	19 **K** 39.0983	20 **Ca** 40.08	21 **Sc** 44.9559	22 **Ti** 47.88*	23 **V** 50.9415	24 **Cr** 51.996	25 **Mn** 54.9380	26 **Fe** 55.847*	27 **Co** 58.9332	28 **Ni** 58.69	29 **Cu** 63.546*	30 **Zn** 65.38	31 **Ga** 69.72	32 **Ge** 72.59*	33 **As** 74.9216	34 **Se** 78.96*	35 **Br** 79.904	36 **Kr** 83.80
5	37 **Rb** 85.4678*	38 **Sr** 87.62	39 **Y** 88.9059	40 **Zr** 91.22	41 **Nb** 92.9064	42 **Mo** 95.94	43 **Tc** 97 (98)	44 **Ru** 101.07*	45 **Rh** 102.9055	46 **Pd** 106.42	47 **Ag** 107.8682*	48 **Cd** 112.41	49 **In** 114.82	50 **Sn** 118.69*	51 **Sb** 121.75*	52 **Te** 127.60*	53 **I** 126.9045	54 **Xe** 131.29*
6	55 **Cs** 132.9054	56 **Ba** 137.33	57-71 **La-Lu** Rare earths	72 **Hf** 178.40*	73 **Ta** 180.9479	74 **W** 183.85*	75 **Re** 186.207	76 **Os** 190.2	77 **Ir** 192.22*	78 **Pt** 195.08*	79 **Au** 196.9665	80 **Hg** 200.59*	81 **Tl** 204.383	82 **Pb** 207.2	83 **Bi** 208.9804	84 **Po** (209)	85 **At** (210)	86 **Rn** (222)
7	87 **Fr** (223)	88 **Ra** 226.0254	89-103 **Ac-Lw** Actinides	104 **†** (261)	105 **†** (262)	106 **†** (263)												

Shell electrons:
He: 2;
Ne: 2, 8;
Ar: 2, 8, 8;
Kr: 2, 8, 18, 8;
Xe: 2, 8, 18, 18, 8;
Rn: 2, 8, 18, 32, 18, 8;
Lu: 2, 8, 18, 32, 9, 2;
Lr: 2, 8, 18, 32, 18, 9, 2

Rare earths (Lanthanides)

57 **La** 138.9055*	58 **Ce** 140.12	59 **Pr** 140.9077*	60 **Nd** 144.24*	61 **Pm** (145)	62 **Sm** 150.36	63 **Eu** 151.96	64 **Gd** 157.25*	65 **Tb** 158.9254	66 **Dy** 162.50*	67 **Ho** 164.9304	68 **Er** 167.26*	69 **Tm** 168.9342	70 **Yb** 173.04*	71 **Lu** 174.967

Actinides

89 **Ac** 227.0278	90 **Th** 232.0381	91 **Pa** 231.0359	92 **U** 238.0289	93 **Np** 237.0482	94 **Pu** (244)	95 **Am** (243)	96 **Cm** (247)	97 **Bk** (247)	98 **Cf** (251)	99 **Es** (252)	100 **Fm** (257)	101 **Md** (258)	102 **No** (259)	103 **Lr** (260)

(From Kaplan LA, Pesce AJ: Clinical chemistry: theory, analysis, and correlation, ed. 2, St. Louis, 1989, Mosby-Year Book, Inc.) Chart modified from Toporek, M.: Basic chemistry of life, St. Louis, 1981, Mosby-Year Book, Inc., and from Fisher Scientific 1983 Catalog, Pittsburgh, Pa, 1983, Fisher Scientific Co. Data in this chart have been checked by the National Bureau of Standards' Office of Standard Reference Data. Atomic weights corrected to conform to the most recent values of the Commission on Atomic Weights.

*These weights are considered reliable to ±3 in the last place. Other weights are reliable to ±1 in the last place, except for the weight of hydrogen, which is reliable to ±7 in the last place.

†The International Union for Pure and Applied Chemistry has not adopted official names or symbols for these elements. Because of scientific and political controversy, for 104, neither rutherfordium (Rf) nor kurchatovium (Ku) is satisfactory; for 105 hahnium (Ha) has not been accepted yet; for 104 to 106 the IUPAC has declined to use the old cumbersome forms unnilquadium (Unq), unnilpentium (Unp), and unnilhexium (Unh), which etymologically mean 'one zero four' etc.

Index